Liver Disease in Children

Third Edition

Liver Disease in Children

Third Edition

EDITED BY

Frederick J. Suchy, M.D.

Professor and Chair, Department of Pediatrics
Mount Sinai School of Medicine of New York University
Pediatrician-in-Chief, Mount Sinai Hospital
New York, New York

Ronald J. Sokol, M.D.

Professor and Vice Chair, Department of Pediatrics
Chief, Section of Pediatric Gastroenterology, Hepatology, and Nutrition
University of Colorado School of Medicine and The Childern's Hospital
Denver, Colorado

William F. Balistreri, M.D.

Dorothy M. M. Kersten Professor, Department of Pediatrics
University of Cincinnati College of Medicine
Director, Pediatric Liver Care Center
Cincinnati Children's Hospital Medical Center
Cincinnati, Ohio

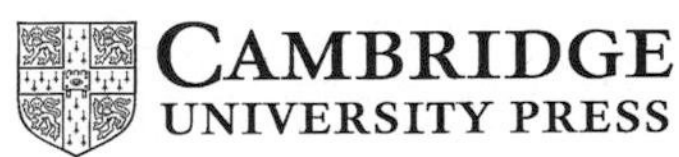

CAMBRIDGE UNIVERSITY PRESS
Cambridge, New York, Melbourne, Madrid, Cape Town, Singapore, São Paulo

Cambridge University Press
32 Avenue of the Americas, New York, NY 10013-2473, USA

www.cambridge.org
Information on this title: www.cambridge.org/9780521856577

Third edition 2007

Printed in the United States of America

A catalog record for this publication is available from the British Library.

Library of Congress Cataloging-in-Publication Data

Liver disease in children / edited by Frederick J. Suchy, Ronald J. Sokol, William F. Balistreri. – 3rd ed.
p. ; cm.
Includes bibliographical references and index.
ISBN: 978-0-521-85657-7 (hardback)
1. Liver–Diseases. 2. Pediatric gastroenterology. I. Suchy, Frederick J. II. Sokol, Ronald J.
III. Balistreri, William F.
[DNLM: 1. Liver Diseases–diagnosis. 2. Adolescent. 3. Child. 4. Infant.
5. Liver Diseases–physiopathology. 6. Liver Diseases–therapy.
WS 310 L784 2007] I. Title.
RJ456.L5L575 2007
618.92′362–dc22 2006035202

ISBN: 978-0-521-85657-7 hardback

To my wife, Patty, and children, Kristin, Fred, Michael, and Peter, for their love, understanding, and support; to my parents for their love and support; and to Dr. William K. Schubert for his guidance, example as a leader in academic pediatrics, and for rousing my interest in the clinical and research aspects of pediatric hepatology. – FJS

To my wife, Lori, and children, Skylar and Jared, for their love, patience, encouragement, and understanding; to my parents, brothers, and sister for their love and support; and to my mentor, Dr. Arnold Silverman, for his encouragement to pursue investigative pediatric gastroenterology and for his guidance and friendship. – RJS

To Becky and our children, Tony, Jenny, and Billy, for their love and support. – WFB

Contents

SECTION V: OTHER CONDITIONS AND ISSUES IN PEDIATRIC HEPATOLOGY

Color plates appear after page 366

Contributing Authors

Estella M. Alonso, M.D. Professor, Department of Pediatrics, Northwestern University, Chicago, Illinois; Director of Hepatology, Department of Gastroenterology, Hepatology, and Nutrition, Children's Memorial Hospital, Chicago, Illinois

Maria H. Alonso, M.D. Assistant Professor, Department of Surgery, University of Cincinnati College of Medicine, Cincinnati, Ohio; Associate Surgical Director, Liver Transplant Program, Department of Pediatric and Thoracic Surgery, Cincinnati Children's Hospital Medical Center, Cincinnati, Ohio

Fernando Alvarez, M.D. Professor of Pediatrics, Department of Pediatric Gastroenterology, CHU Sainte-Justine and Université de Montréal, Montréal, Québec, Canada

Karl E. Anderson, M.D. Professor of Medicine, Department of Preventive Medicine and Community Health, University of Texas Medical Branch, Galveston, Texas

Jerry Angdisen, B.S. Graduate Student, Department of Molecular Medicine, Wake Forest University School of Medicine, Winston-Salem, North Carolina; Research Technician, Department of Gastroenterology, University of Missouri–Columbia, Columbia, Missouri

Kenneth H. Astrin, Ph.D. Associate Professor, Department of Genetics and Genomic Sciences, Mount Sinai School of Medicine of New York University, New York, New York

William F. Balistreri, M.D. Dorothy M. M. Kersten Professor, Department of Pediatrics, University of Cincinnati College of Medicine, Cincinnati, Ohio; Director, Pediatric Liver Care Center, Department of Pediatric Gastroenterolgy, Hepatology, and Nutrition, Cincinnati Children's Hospital Medical Center, Cincinnati, Ohio

Jorge A. Bezerra, M.D. Professor, Department of Pediatrics, University of Cincinnati College of Medicine, Cincinnati, Ohio; Division of Pediatric Gastroenterology, Hepatology, and Nutrition and the Pediatric Liver Care Center, Cincinnati Children's Hospital Medical Center, Cincinnati, Ohio

Kevin E. Bove, M.D. Professor of Pathology and Pediatrics, Department of Pediatrics, University of Cincinnati College of Medicine, Cincinnati, Ohio; Pediatric Pathologist, Division of Pathology and Laboratory Medicine, Cincinnati Children's Hospital Medical Center, Cincinnati, Ohio

John C. Bucuvalas, M.D. Professor, Department of Pediatrics, University of Cincinnati College of Medicine, Cincinnati, Ohio; Clinical Director, Medical Director of Liver Transplantation, Department of Gastroenterology, Hepatology, and Nutrition, Cincinnati Children's Hospital Medical Center, Cincinnati, Ohio

T. Andrew Burrow, M.D. Resident, Department of Pediatrics, University of Cincinnati College of Medicine, Cincinnati, Ohio; Resident, Division of Human Genetics, Cincinnati Children's Hospital Medical Center, Cincinnati, Ohio

Majed Dasouki, M.D. Associate Professor, Department of Pediatrics and Internal Medicine, University of Kansas Medical Center, Kansas City, Kansas

Valeer J. Desmet, M.D., Ph.D. Professor, Department of Pathology, Katholieke Universiteit Leuven, Leuven, Belgium

Robert J. Desnick, M.D., Ph.D. Professor and Chairman, Departments of Genetics and Genomic Science and Pediatrics, Mount Sinai School of Medicine of New York University, New York, New York; Attending Physician, Department of Pediatrics, Mount Sinai Hospital, New York, New York

Josée Dubois, M.D., F.R.C.P. Professor of Radiology, Department of Radiology, CHU Sainte-Justine and Université de Montréal, Montréal, Québec, Canada

Nissa I. Erickson, M.D. Assistant Professor, Department of Pediatrics, University of Wisconsin, Madison, Wisconsin; Medical Director, Pediatric Liver Program, Division of Pediatric Gastroenterology, Hepatology, and Nutrition, University of Wisconsin Children's Hospital, Madison, Wisconsin

MICHAEL K. FARRELL, M.D. Professor, Department of Pediatrics, University of Cincinnati College of Medicine, Cincinnati, Ohio; Division of Pediatric Gastroenterology and Nutrition, Cincinnati Children's Hospital Medical Center, Cincinnati, Ohio

ANDREW P. FERANCHAK, M.D. Assistant Professor, Department of Pediatrics, University of Texas Southwestern Medical Center, Dallas, Texas; Department of Pediatric Gastroenterology and Hepatology, Children's Medical Center of Dallas, Dallas, Texas

MILTON J. FINEGOLD, M.D. Professor, Department of Pathology and Pediatrics, Baylor College of Medicine, Houston, Texas; Head of Pathology Department, Texas Children's Hospital, Houston, Texas

FAYEZ K. GHISHAN, M.D. Professor and Head, Department of Pediatrics, University of Arizona Health Sciences Center, Tucson, Arizona

GLENN R. GOURLEY, M.D. Professor, Department of Pediatrics, and Research Director, Division of Pediatric Gastroenterology, University of Minnesota, Minneapolis, Minnesota

GREGORY A. GRABOWSKI, M.D. Professor, Department of Pediatrics, University of Cincinnati College of Medicine, Cincinnati, Ohio; Director, Division of Human Genetics, Cincinnati Children's Hospital Medical Center, Cincinnati, Ohio

NEDIM HADŽIĆ, M.D. Senior Lecturer, Institute for Liver Studies, King's College London School of Medicine at King's College Hospital, London, England; Consultant in Paediatric Hepatology, Department of Children's Health, King's College Hospital, London, England

STEPHEN HARDY, M.D. Instructor, Department of Pediatrics, Harvard Medical School, Boston, Massachusetts; Attending Physician, Department of Pediatric Gastroenterology, Massachusetts General Hospital, Boston, Massachusetts

JAMES E. HEUBI, M.D. Professor and Associate Chair for Clinical Investigation, Department of Pediatrics, University of Cincinnati College of Medicine, Cincinnati, Ohio; Program Director, General Clinical Research Center, Cincinnati Children's Hospital Medical Center, Cincinnati, Ohio

JAY A. HOCHMAN, M.D. Clinical Associate Professor, Division of Pediatric Gastroenterology, Emory University School of Medicine, Atlanta, Georgia; Attending Physician, Children's Center for Digestive Health Care, LLC, and Children's Healthcare of Atlanta, Atlanta, Georgia

JAMAL A. IBDAH, M.D., PH.D. Professor and Chief, Division of Gastroenterology and Hepatology, University of Missouri–Columbia, Columbia, Missouri; Director, Digestive Health Center, University of Missouri Hospital and Clinic, Columbia, Missouri

MAUREEN M. JONAS, M.D. Associate Professor, Department of Pediatrics, Harvard Medical School, Boston, Massachusetts; Associate in Gastroenterology, Department of Medicine, Division of Gastroenterology, Children's Hospital Boston, Boston, Massachusetts

BINITA M. KAMATH, M.B. B.CHIR. Assistant Professor of Pediatrics, University of Pennsylvania School of Medicine, Philadelphia, Pennsylvania; Attending Physician, Division of Gastroenterology, Hepatology, and Nutrition, Department of Pediatrics, Children's Hospital of Philadelphia, Philadelphia, Pennsylvania

SAUL J. KARPEN, M.D., PH.D. Associate Professor of Pediatrics and Molecular and Cellular Biology, Faculty, Transitional Biology and Molecular Medicine Program, Department of Pediatrics, Baylor College of Medicine, Houston, Texas; Director, Texas Children's Liver Center, Department of Pediatric Gastroenterology, Hepatology, and Nutrition, Texas Children's Hospital, Houston, Texas

RONALD E. KLEINMAN, M.D. Professor, Department of Pediatrics, Harvard Medical School, Boston, Massachusetts; Acting Physician-in-Chief, Department of Pediatrics, Massachusetts General Hospital, Boston, Massachusetts

ALEX S. KNISELY, M.D. Professor of Pathology, Institute of Liver Studies, King's College Hospital, London, England

RICHARD L. KRADIN, M.D. Associate Professor, Department of Pathology, Harvard Medical School, Boston, Massachusetts; Associate Pathologist and Physician, Departments of Pathology and Medicine, Massachusetts General Hospital, Boston, Massachusetts

GREGORY Y. LAUWERS, M.D. Associate Professor of Pathology, Department of Pathology, Harvard Medical School, Boston, Massachusetts; Director of Gastrointestinal Pathology, Department of Pathology, Massachusetts General Hospital, Boston, Massachusetts

DOLORES LÓPEZ-TERRADA, M.D., PH.D. Assistant Professor, Department of Pathology, Baylor College of Medicine, Houston, Texas; Pathologist, Department of Pathology, Texas Children's Hospital, Houston, Texas

GIORGINA MIELI-VERGANI, M.D., PH.D. Alex Mowat Professor of Paediatric Hepatology, Department of Liver Studies and Transplantation, King's College London School of Medicine at King's College Hospital, London, England; Director of the Paediatric Liver Centre, Department of Children's Health, King's College Hospital, London, England

GRANT MITCHELL, M.D. Professor, Department of Pediatrics, CHU Sainte-Justine and Université de Montréal, Montréal, Québec, Canada

Michael R. Narkewicz, M.D. Professor of Pediatrics, Section of Pediatric Gastroenterology, Hepatology, and Nutrition, University of Colorado School of Medicine, Denver, Colorado; Medical Director, Pediatric Liver Center, Children's Hospital, Denver, Colorado

Vicky Lee Ng, M.D., F.R.C.P.C. Assistant Professor, Department of Paediatrics, University of Toronto, Toronto, Ontario, Canada; Medical Director, Liver Transplant Program, Staff Physician, Division of Pediatric Gastroenterology, Hepatology, and Nutrition, The Hospital for Sick Children, Toronto, Ontario, Canada

Donald A. Novak, M.D. Professor of Pediatric Gastroenterology, Hepatology, and Nutrition, Department of Pediatrics, University of Florida College of Medicine, Shands AGH Children's Hospital, Gainesville, Florida

Nancy C. O'Connell, M.S., C.C.R.C., C.C.R.A. Research Scientist, Clinical Mass Spectrometry Laboratory, Cincinnati Children's Hospital Medical Center, Cincinnati, Ohio

Judith A. O'Connor, M.D. Pediatric Gastroenterology, Sacred Heart Children's Hospital, Spokane, Washington

Devin Oglesbee, Ph.D. Fellow in Molecular Genetics, Mayo Clinic, Rochester, Minnesota

Antonio R. Perez-Atayde, M.D. Associate Professor of Pathology, Department of Pathology, Children's Hospital Boston, Boston, Massachusetts

David H. Perlmutter, M.D. Vira I. Heinz Professor and Chair, Department of Pediatrics, Professor of Cell Biology and Physiology, University of Pittsburgh School of Medicine, Pittsburgh, Pennsylvania; Physician-in-Chief and Scientific Director, Children's Hospital of Pittsburgh, Pittsburgh, Pennsylvania

David A. Piccoli, M.D. Biesecker Professor of Pediatrics, University of Pennsylvania School of Medicine, Philadelphia, Pennsylvania; Chief, Division of Gastroenterology, Hepatology, and Nutrition, Department of Pediatrics, Children's Hospital of Philadelphia, Philadelphia, Pennsylvania

Piero Rinaldo, M.D., Ph.D. Professor of Pathology and Pediatrics, Department of Laboratory Medicine and Pathology, Mayo Clinic, Rochester, Minnesota

Eve A. Roberts, M.D., F.R.C.P.C. Professor, Department of Paediatrics, Medicine, and Pharmacology, University of Toronto, Toronto, Ontario, Canada; Staff Physician, Division of Gastroenterology, Hepatology, and Nutrition, The Hospital for Sick Children, Toronto, Ontario, Canada

Philip Rosenthal, M.D. Professor of Pediatrics and Surgery, Department of Pediatrics, University of California–San Francisco, San Francisco, California; Medical Director, Pediatric Liver Transplant Program, Department of Pediatrics, University of California–San Francisco Children's Hospital, San Francisco, California

Tania A. D. Roskams, M.D., Ph.D. Full Professor, Head of Liver Research Unit, Department of Morphology and Molecular Pathology, Katholieke Universiteit Leuven, Leuven, Belgium; Head of Clinics, Department of Pathology, University Hospital Leuven, Leuven, Belgium

Pierre A. Russo, M.D. Professor of Pathology and Pediatrics, Department of Pathology and Laboratory Medicine, Children's Hospital of Philadelphia, Philadelphia, Pennsylvania

Frederick C. Ryckman, M.D. Professor, Department of Surgery, University of Cincinnati College of Medicine, Cincinnati, Ohio; Surgical Director, Liver Transplant Program, Department of Pediatric and Thoracic Surgery, Cincinnati Children's Hospital Medical Center, Cincinnati, Ohio

Kathleen B. Schwarz, M.D. Professor, Department of Pediatrics, Johns Hopkins University School of Medicine, Baltimore, Maryland; Director, Pediatric Liver Center, Department of Pediatrics, Johns Hopkins Children's Center, Baltimore, Maryland

Jeffrey B. Schwimmer, M.D. Associate Professor of Pediatrics, Division of Gastroenterology, Hepatology, and Nutrition/Pediatrics, University of California–San Diego, San Diego, California; Director, Fatty Liver Clinic, Department of Pediatrics, Rady Children's Hospital, San Diego, California

Kenneth D. R. Setchell, Ph.D. Professor, Department of Pathology and Laboratory Medicine, Cincinnati Children's Hospital Medical Center, Department of Pediatrics, University of Cincinnati College of Medicine, Cincinnati, Ohio

Benjamin L. Shneider, M.D. Visiting Professor, Department of Pediatrics, University of Pittsburgh, Pittsburgh, Pennsylvania; Director of Pediatric Hepatology, Department of Pediatrics/Gastroenterology, Children's Hospital of Pittsburgh, Pittsburgh, Pennsylvania

Ronald J. Sokol, M.D. Professor and Vice Chair, Department of Pediatrics, Chief of Pediatric Gastroenterology, Hepatology, and Nutrition, University of Colorado School of Medicine, Denver, Colorado; Chair, Department of Pediatric Gastroenterology and Hepatology, Children's Hospital, Denver, Colorado

Nancy B. Spinner, Ph.D. Professor of Human Genetics in Pediatrics, Department of Pediatrics, University of Pennsylvania School of Medicine, Philadelphia, Pennsylvania; Director, Cytogenetics Laboratory, Department of Pathology and Clinical Laboratories, Children's Hospital of Philadelphia, Philadelphia, Pennsylvania

Robert H. Squires, M.D. Professor of Pediatrics, Divison of Pediatric Gastroenterology and Hepatology, Children's Hospital of Pittsburgh, Pittsburgh, Pennsylvania

Frederick J. Suchy, M.D. Professor and Chair, Department of Pediatrics, Mount Sinai School of Medicine of New York University, New York, New York; Pediatrician-in-Chief, Department of Pediatrics, Mount Sinai Hospital, New York, New York

Marshall L. Summar, M.D. Associate Professor, Department of Pediatrics and Molecular Physiology and Biophysics, Vanderbilt University Medical Center, Nashville, Tennessee

Greg Tiao, M.D. Assistant Professor, Department of Surgery, University of Cincinnati College of Medicine, Cincinnati, Ohio; Attending Surgeon, Department of Pediatric and Thoracic Surgery, Cincinnati Children's Hospital Medical Center, Cincinnati, Ohio

Diego Vergani, M.D., Ph.D. Professor of Liver Immunopathology, Department of Liver Studies and Transplantation, King's College London School of Medicine at King's College Hospital, London, England

Paul A. Watkins, M.D., Ph.D. Professor, Department of Neurology, Johns Hopkins University School of Medicine, Kennedy Krieger Institute, Baltimore, Maryland

Peter F. Whitington, M.D. Sally Burnett Searle Professor, Department of Pediatrics, Northwestern University, Chicago, Illinois; Division Head, Department of Gastroenterology, Hepatology, and Nutrition, Children's Memorial Hospital, Chicago, Illinois

Torsten Wuestefeld, Ph.D. Postdoctoral Fellow, Cell and Developmental Biology Program, Fox Chase Cancer Center, Philadelphia, Pennsylvania

Kenneth S. Zaret, Ph.D. Senior Member and Program Leader, Cell and Developmental Biology Program, Fox Chase Cancer Center, Philadelphia, Pennsylvania

Mona Zawaideh, M.D. Assistant Professor, Department of Pediatrics, University of Arizona Health Sciences Center, Tucson, Arizona

Preface to the Third Edition

Liver Disease in Children has become the premier reference on pediatric liver disease. This third edition provides authoritative coverage of every aspect of liver disease affecting infants, children, and adolescents. This edition has been thoroughly revised and updated. In addition, it features new contributions on liver development, cholestatic and autoimmune disorders, fatty liver disease, and inborn errors of metabolism. The book offers an integrated approach to the science and clinical practice of pediatric hepatology and charts the substantial progress in understanding and treating these diseases. Chapters are written by international experts and address the unique pathophysiology, manifestations, and management of these disorders in the pediatric population.

In the six years since the publication of the second edition of *Liver Disease in Children*, pediatric hepatology has continued to evolve as a discipline. Our knowledge of the structural and functional development of the liver continues to grow, aided by sophisticated approaches in molecular biology. For example, the genetic basis of inherited cholestatic disorders has been further elucidated, and the clinician is now provided with useful information about the natural history, spectrum, and options for therapy. Investigators can couple this information with emerging science in their own laboratories. Several canalicular membrane transport proteins were actually discovered based upon their role in inherited disorders of cholestasis. These advances have allowed detailed studies regarding the behavior of these transporters in acquired cholestasis. New information has also come from microarray (gene chip) studies about the coordinate expression of regulatory genes that may differentiate the embryonic and perinatal forms of biliary atresia. These insights have led to a better animal model of the disorder that is helping to define further the immunopathogenesis of biliary atresia and develop targets for therapy. The spectrum of mitochondrial and fatty acid oxidation disorders has also expanded as a result of the continuing advances in molecular biology and molecular genetics.

The third edition of *Liver Disease in Children* also reflects the unexpected change in the incidence and spectrum of pediatric liver disease. For example, when the first edition was published in 1995, Reye's syndrome was occasionally seen and still warranted detailed coverage in a separate chapter. This disorder has all but disappeared. Nonalcoholic fatty liver disease (NAFLD) associated with obesity was briefly covered but now is the most common cause of chronic liver disease in children and thus warrants a separate chapter in which the disorder is extensively reviewed. Fewer infants are now classified as having "idiopathic" neonatal hepatitis owing to improved imaging, advances in virology and immunology, and the application of sophisticated biochemical and molecular methods to the diagnosis of inherited disease. The entities that were dissected out of this "default" category are dealt with in discrete chapters.

We are proud of the efforts of all contributing authors and we thank them for their efforts. We believe that *Liver Disease in Children*, third edition, will be an essential reference for all physicians involved in the care of children with liver disease.

Frederick J. Suchy, M.D.
Ronald J. Sokol, M.D.
William F. Balistreri, M.D.

Preface to the First Edition

The last decade has seen an explosion of activity in the clinical and research aspects of pediatric hepatology. The discipline has grown from a cataloging of the many unique disorders that can occur during infancy and childhood to a more profound understanding of the genetic, biochemical, and virologic basis for many pediatric liver diseases. The increasing availability of orthotopic liver transplantation in pediatric patients has contributed significantly to this renaissance in interest. More than ever before, the practitioner can offer therapies that can be curative, or at least improve the growth and development of children until transplantation is required. During the past 2 years, as this book was being planned and completed, many important advances have been made. For example, studies have demonstrated the potential beneficial effects of interferon treatment of chronic viral hepatitis in children. Novel therapies have also been developed for the treatment of children with hereditary tyrosinemia, several of the glycogenoses, some of the lysosomal storage disorders, and defects in bile acid metabolism. We are also at the dawn of efforts to selectively correct inborn errors of metabolism by somatic gene transfer into hepatocytes or the biliary tree. Increasingly, advances in the basic sciences are being incorporated directly into clinical practice of hepatology. As a result, clinicians must now view liver disease in ways not possible or even imagined by their predecessors.

The goal of this first edition of *Liver Disease in Children* is to both provide a framework to understand the pathophysiology of the various hepatobiliary disorders and offer authoritative analyses of the clinical and laboratory manifestations of specific diseases and the strategies for managing them. A number of superb texts exist in internal medicine that deal effectively with the mechanisms and manifestations of liver disease. In this text, there has been no attempt to duplicate the material that is available in these scholarly works. Rather those aspects of the structure and function of the developing liver are covered that are required to understand pathophysiology unique to children. It should be recognized that a diverse group of physicians is now involved in the care of children with acute and chronic liver diseases, including pediatric gastroenterologists, pediatricians with a particular interest in liver disease, pediatric surgeons, transplant surgeons, and transplant physicians who have a background primarily in internal medicine. Therefore, there is a need for a text that provides comprehensive coverage of the pathophysiology, diagnosis, and treatment of hepatobiliary disease in pediatric patients.

This book offers an integrated approach to the science, technology, and clinical practice of pediatric hepatology. Each chapter is written by an authority or authorities who are often actively engaged in advancing the field of knowledge in the subject matter. Each has been asked to deal with the topic comprehensively and to highlight areas of uncertainty and controversy in the field. Overall, it is hoped that this text will be a valuable resource to clinicians at various stages of their training and those in the multiple disciplines that now contribute to the diagnosis and treatment of hepatobiliary disease in children.

Frederick J. Suchy, M.D.

Section I: Pathophysiology of Pediatric Liver Disease

1

LIVER DEVELOPMENT: FROM ENDODERM TO HEPATOCYTE

Torsten Wuestefeld, Ph.D., and Kenneth S. Zaret, Ph.D.

The liver is derived from the endoderm, one of the three germ layers formed during gastrulation. The initial endodermal epithelium consists of approximately 500 cells in the mouse [1], from which cells will be apportioned to the thyroid, lung, stomach, liver, pancreas, esophagus, and intestines. How is the endoderm patterned to generate such diverse tissues? Once the hepatic primordium is formed, how are the different hepatic cell types generated? How do they generate a proper liver architecture? And how do the principles of liver development apply to liver regeneration and the possibility of generating hepatocytes from stem cells? This chapter focuses on all of these questions.

A BRIEF OVERVIEW OF EMBRYONIC LIVER DEVELOPMENT

By late gastrulation in the mouse (embryonic day of gestation 7.5 [E7.5]) the anteroposterior pattern of the endoderm is already established [2], so that during E8.5–9.5 (mouse) the anterior-ventral domain develops the organ buds for the liver, lung, thyroid, and the ventral rudiment of the pancreas [3]. This corresponds to about 2–3 weeks' gestation in humans. The specification of liver progenitors occurs through a combination of positive inductive signals from the cardiogenic mesoderm and septum transversum mesenchyme and repressive signals from the trunk mesoderm [4–6]. This occurs at about 8.5 days gestation in the mouse, when the embryo contains six to seven pairs of somites, which are clusters of skeletal and muscle progenitors. The cells adopting the hepatic fate are characterized by the expression of two of the liver-specific markers, albumin and α-fetoprotein (AFP). Although albumin was initially considered to be an adult liver marker, it is now well established that it is among the earliest liver-specific markers to be expressed in development, along with AFP. The nascent hepatic epithelium, consisting of hepatoblasts, then invades a stromal cell field containing angioblasts, which are precursors to the blood vessels, and the septum transversum mesenchyme. Under the influence of the stromal cells, the hepatoblasts proliferate to form the liver bud, and then differentiate to form the fetal liver.

At E10–11 in the mouse, hematopoietic stem cells originating from the yolk sac and aorta-gonad-mesonephros regions colonize the fetal liver and expand their mass and lineage diversity. Therefore, the fetal liver in mammals is a primary site of hematopoiesis. At the same time, the resident hematopoietic cells secrete growth signals that promote maturation of the liver [7–10]. Around birth, hematopoietic cells migrate out of the liver and a functional switch from a hematopoietic microenvironment to a metabolic organ occurs.

DISTINCT HEPATIC PROGENITOR DOMAINS IN THE MAMMALIAN EMBRYO

A recent study investigated in detail which populations of undifferentiated endoderm cells generate the embryonic liver bud [11]. The authors isolated mouse embryos at E8.0, which is prior to hepatic specification, and used vital dyes to label different clusters of endoderm cells in different isolated embryos. They then cultured the embryos whole, into the organogenic phase, and then determined which tissues inherited the labeled cells. By comparing the descendant cell populations arising from different labeled endoderm cell domains in different embryos, they were able to develop a "fate map." The fate map (Figure 1.1) indicates the location of progenitor domains in the undifferentiated endoderm that will give rise to the embryonic liver bud. Interestingly, the authors found that two distinct types of endoderm-progenitor cells, lateral and medial, arising from three spatially separated embryonic domains, generate the epithelial cells of the liver bud (see Figure 1.1). The movement of these cells and the morphologic changes in the embryo during this period position the distinct progenitor domains close to the hepatic-inducing tissues. Although both lateral and medial liver bud descendants express early hepatoblast genes in common, it remains to be determined if the different progenitor domains give rise to functionally different cell populations in the adult liver.

LIVER-INDUCTIVE ROLE OF CARDIAC MESODERM

To be induced to a liver fate, the ventral endoderm has to interact with other tissues. An early finding was that the ventral

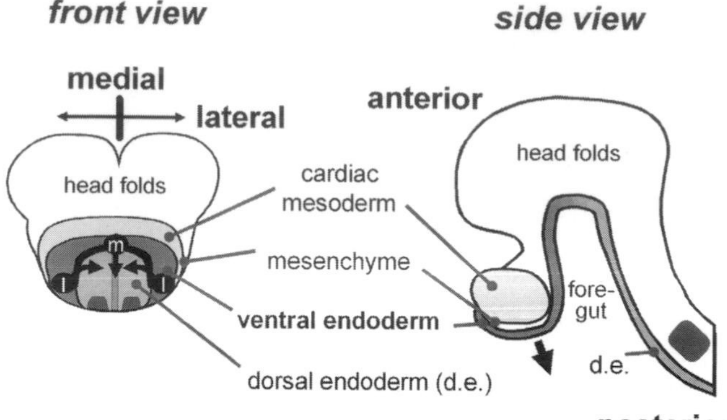

Figure 1.1. Fate map of liver progenitors in the ventral foregut endoderm. The ventral foregut endoderm is denoted by the dark-shaded area and surrounds the anterior intestinal portal of the foregut. Anterior halves of embryos are shown, corresponding to about day 8.0 of mouse gestation (~2.5 weeks of human gestation). The dark spots designated *m* (for medial) and *l* (for lateral) indicate progenitor domains of undifferentiated endoderm cells that will contribute to the liver bud [11]. The arrows indicate tissue movement. Also shown are the location of the cardiac mesoderm and prospective septum transversum mesenchyme cells ("mesenchyme"), both of which signal to the endoderm during this period to promote hepatic induction.

endoderm has to be in close contact with cardiac mesoderm (Figure 1.1), as first shown by transplant experiments with chick embryos [4,6,12]. This is consistent with the morphologic changes that occur during this time of embryo development. At the five- and seven-somite stages, the future hepatic part is brought in close proximity to the cardiac mesoderm through invagination of the foregut. Although the cardiac mesoderm is necessary for the induction of the hepatic fate, it is not sufficient. Further studies showed that the endoderm needs a second stimulus from the septum transversum mesenchyme [13–15] (Figure 1.1). Results in the chicken were confirmed in the mouse [5,16], suggesting a general mechanism of liver development in higher vertebrates. Although these pure morphologic studies showed clearly the importance of both cardiac mesoderm and septum transversum mesenchyme for liver development, they left open the question of what signals are produced by these tissues to facilitate hepatic lineage commitment.

Gualdi et al. [5] developed an in vitro assay to analyze hepatic specification, and showed that the signal from the cardiac mesoderm requires close proximity to the endoderm. Using this explant system, it was then found that fibroblast growth factor 1 (FGF1) and FGF2 could substitute for cardiac mesoderm to induce the hepatic fate (Figure 1.2) [17]. This is in agreement with the ability of FGFs to act locally, as secreted FGFs stay in close contact with the extracellular matrix. As the FGFs are secreted from the cardiac mesoderm, Jung et al. [17] found that the endodermal cells express FGF receptor 1 (FGFR1) and FGFR4, receptors specific for these FGF molecules. Although the group found weak liver gene inductive potential for FGF8, they showed that this factor has a positive effect on the outgrowth of hepatic cells, after the initial specification.

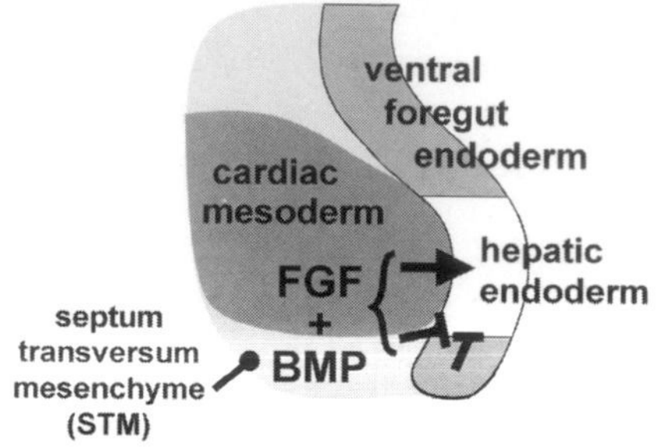

Figure 1.2. Signaling that induces hepatic genes in the endoderm in the mouse. See text for details.

Interestingly, in the absence of the FGF signaling from the cardiac mesoderm, the domain of the ventral foregut endoderm that normally becomes the liver rapidly defaults to a pancreatic fate [18]. Recent work by Serls et al. [19] showed that the FGF signals do not work as on/off switches for the liver program; rather, there are different thresholds of FGF concentrations that pattern the ventral foregut. This group cultured ventral endoderm explants in medium with different concentrations of FGF2. In the absence of FGF, the explants expressed pancreatic genes. At low concentrations of FGF, they expressed hepatic genes, and at high concentrations, lung marker genes were expressed.

Although it is clear that FGF1 and 2 can induce liver development and both factors are expressed by the cardiac mesoderm, it is important to keep in mind that no liver defects have been described in FGF1 and FGF2 double-knockout mice [20]. Because there are 22 known members of the FGF protein family, it is likely that other members can compensate for the loss of FGF1 and 2 or that other FGFs are involved in the induction of hepatic fate. For example, Cai et al. [21] showed in a study investigating heart development that FGF8 and 10 are expressed in the cardiac mesoderm. Therefore, there may be considerable redundancy of FGF signaling here, as in many other developmental contexts.

Further evidence for the importance of cardiac mesoderm as an inductive tissue for liver development comes from experiments with embryonic stem cells. Co-culture experiments of mouse embryonic stem cells with cardiac mesoderm found that under these conditions, the embryonic stem cells differentiate into hepatocyte-like cells [22]. The cells activate the crucial endodermal transcription factors, such as SOX17α, FOXA2, and GATA4, and express albumin and AFP. These results emphasize the predictive value of information from developmental biology on the productive differentiation of stem cells.

LIVER-INDUCTIVE ROLE OF SEPTUM TRANSVERSUM MESENCHYME

The septum transversum mesenchyme, the second most important tissue for liver fate decision, originates from the lateral plate mesoderm and gives rise to the epicardium of the heart and the diaphragm. Rossi et al. [23] used the in vitro hepatic induction assay and included the bone morphogenetic protein (BMP) inhibitor Xnoggin. When they cultured cardiac mesoderm, septum transversum mesenchyme, and ventral endoderm together with the inhibitor, albumin gene induction was not observed. Addition of BMPs could rescue this phenotype, but not the addition of FGFs. This shows that in addition to FGFs, BMPs play a role in the hepatic fate decision (Figure 1.2). This group then used knock-in mouse embryos containing an LacZ reporter transgene controlled by BMP4 transcriptional regulatory elements. They found high expression of BMP4^{LacZ} at the eight-somite stage within the septum transversum mesenchyme. In situ hybridization experiments for BMP2 and 4 also showed the expression of these genes in the septum transversum mesenchyme [24], supporting the role of the septum transversum mesenchyme as the source of BMP signaling for liver development (Figure 1.2). In addition to the cell fate decision, the secretion of BMPs seems to be important for the outgrowth of the budding hepatoblasts [23].

Summarizing our knowledge, the model suggests that FGF and BMP signals act cooperatively on the endoderm to induce hepatic cell fate and the outgrowth of the hepatoblasts. Interestingly, there is another example of cooperation of these two pathways in development in that the factors together induce cardiogenesis during chick development [25,26].

TRANSCRIPTION FACTORS IMPORTANT FOR THE HEPATIC FATE DECISION

Foxa transcription factors are important for liver-specific gene expression. Lee et al. [27] used in vitro transcription assays to show that Foxa1 can relieve the transcriptional repression of the *Afp* gene in chromatin-assembled DNA templates. Furthermore, FoxA1 and FoxA2 are expressed within the ventral endoderm prior to the induction of the hepatic fate [28–30]. Foxa1-null mice have no defect in early embryonic development [31,32] but this might result from compensation through Foxa2 (see below). In contrast, FoxaA2-null embryos show major developmental defects in the formation of the node, the notochord, the floor plate of the neural tube, and the morphogenesis of the foregut endoderm [33–35]. The early endoderm defect prevented an assessment of the role of Foxa2 on liver specification. To address this question, conditional gene inactivation approaches were used.

First, Sund et al. [36] made an AlbCre-FoxA2$^{loxp/loxp}$ mouse. These mice have loxp recombination sites flanking the *Foxa2* gene, so that in liver cells, where the AlbCre construct is expressed, the Cre recombinase will delete the *Foxa2* gene and the phenotype can be assessed. However, these mice developed a normal liver morphology. Because in this context the Cre recombinase is expressed late in development, the conclusion is that Foxa2 is not required for maintaining the hepatic fate. With FoxA3Cre-FoxA2$^{loxp/loxp}$ mice, in which the *Foxa2* gene is inactivated in the endoderm prior to liver induction, Lee et al. [37] also found normal hepatic induction and growth. However, this might be still through compensation by Foxa1. Lee et al. [37] pursued this further with an impressive set of genetic experiments to simultaneously knock out both the *Foxa1* and *Foxa2* genes in the undifferentiated endoderm. These embryos completely lacked the formation of the liver bud, and no liver-specific genes were activated. Thus, both *Foxa* genes cooperate in the establishment of the hepatic primordium and thus promote the hepatic competence of the foregut endoderm.

Narita et al. [38] found that the transcription factor Gata4 is intrinsically required for ventral foregut endoderm development. In addition, it was shown that this factor is necessary for early liver gene expression [39]. Gata4 and its family member Gata6 are expressed in the endoderm before the hepatic fate is induced [40,41]. The expression of Gata4 in the lateral mesoderm is downstream of BMP4 [42]. Corresponding with this, Gata4 mRNA could be detected within the hepatic endoderm in explant studies of ventral endoderm in co-culture with cardiac mesoderm and septum transversum mesenchyme. Adding the BMP inhibitor Xnoggin to the explants abolished Gata4 expression [39], and explants from BMP4$^{-/-}$ mice also exhibited a strong down-regulation of Gata4 [23]. Gata4 expression is activated by binding of forkhead and Gata transcription factors to a distal enhancer element [42]. The activity of this enhancer element is initially broad but eventually becomes restricted to the mesenchyme surrounding the liver. This activity of the enhancer is attenuated by the BMP antagonist Noggin, and the enhancer is not activated in BMP4-null embryos. This suggests a direct requirement of BMP signaling for the enhancer activity and that Gata4 is a downstream effector of BMP signaling in lateral mesoderm. Gata4$^{-/-}$ embryos show defects in foregut development similar to Foxa2 knockout embryos [40], again indicating that Foxa2 and Gata4 are acting on the same developmental process. Additional studies in *Drosophila* and *Caenorhabditis elegans* suggest that cooperation between Foxa2 and Gata transcription factors is crucial for the endoderm specification [43].

These factors also cooperated at a transcriptional enhancer sequence for the albumin gene, which binds both Foxa and Gata factors in the gut endoderm prior to albumin gene activation [5,39,44,45]. This suggests that these factors are mediators of competence in the foregut endoderm. Interestingly, Foxa and Gata4 can bind to their specific binding sites in compacted chromatin [46], which is usually inaccessible to transcription factors. Foxa and Gata4 were found to locally open the chromatin structure, allowing other transcription factors to enter and bind their specific nearby sites. From these results, it was proposed that Foxa and Gata4 represent "pioneer" transcription factors that could mark genes as competent, through opening of the local chromatin structure. These genes are finally expressed if they receive the correct inductive signals via the expression of other transcription factors. Supporting this idea is the fact that Foxa was found to relieve the p53-mediated transcriptional repression of the *Afp* gene in chromatin-assembled DNA templates [27,47,48].

Gata factors also exhibit genetic redundancy [36,49,50] and have roles in the early embryo, prior to liver induction [34,40,41,51–53]. To circumvent a requirement for Gata6 in yolk sac development [52,53], tetraploid embryo chimeras were used to give Gata6$^{-/-}$ embryos a wild-type extra-embryonic endoderm [54]. Zhao et al. [54] could show that the Gata6 tetraploid chimeric embryos still induced the hepatic fate decision of the ventral endoderm, but exhibited a failure in the outgrowth of the liver bud beyond day 9.5 of gestation. As Gata4 is still expressed in the ventral endoderm of Gata6 knockout embryos, Gata4 may compensate for Gata6 loss. Gata4 is expressed only transiently in the prehepatic endoderm during hepatic specification and then the expression is normally lost during outgrowth of the liver bud.

Consistent with this finding in the mouse, zebrafish need Gata6 for liver bud growth. Experiments in the fish depleting both Gata4 and Gata6 found an earlier block in liver development and a complete lack of the liver bud [55]. Summarizing these results, it is now clear that both Gata factors have both redundant and specific functions during liver development.

Wandzioch et al. [56] showed another role for the septum transversum mesenchyme. The LIM homeobox gene *Lhx2* is expressed in hepatic stellate cells in the adult liver. In addition, liver development in Lhx2$^{-/-}$ mice is disrupted. In the embryo, *Lhx2* expression can be found in cells from the septum transversum mesenchyme, E9 onward. These cells build a subpopulation of mesenchymal cells in the liver and become hepatic stellate cells. The Lhx2 knockout mice show a disrupted cellular organization and altered gene expression pattern in intrahepatic endoderm cells. An increased deposition of extracellular matrix proteins precedes these abnormalities. Therefore, the septum transversum mesenchyme is not only an inductive tissue for the early liver; it also contributes to nonparenchymal cells.

STIMULATION OF HEPATOBLAST GROWTH

The second important step after the induction of the hepatic fate in endoderm cells and the differentiation into hepatoblasts is the proliferation of these cells. The mesenchymal component of the liver, derived from the septum transversum mesenchyme, is essential for proliferation of hepatoblasts [6,14,16].

There are other essential interactions for liver bud growth. Experiments with flk$^{-/-}$ mice [57], which lack endothelial cells [58], show a failure of hepatic endoderm morphogenesis and mesenchyme invasion, after the primary specification of hepatic endoderm. The requirement for endothelial cells for hepatic endoderm growth could be recapitulated with embryo tissue explants, showing that the effect is independent of oxygen and factors in the bloodstream. The important interactions between endothelial and liver cells appear to persist in the adult liver [59].

A signaling pathway that controls the proliferation of the fetal liver cells involves hepatocyte growth factor (HGF). Genetic studies in mouse embryos showed that the proliferation and outgrowth of the liver bud cells require the interaction of HGF with its receptor, c-met. Either knockout of HGF (expressed in the hepatic mesenchyme) or c-met (HGF-receptor expressed in hepatoblasts) showed similar phenotypes, a hypoplastic liver at E14.5 [60–62]. This again shows a clear interaction between the mesenchyme and the hepatoblasts. Interestingly, during regeneration of the adult liver, this pathway is important for the proliferation of the hepatocytes, since conditional c-met knockout mice show an inhibition in the proliferation after partial hepatectomy [63]. This is a good example in which pathways for the development of an organism function in a similar way in the adult.

The transcription factors Xbp1 and Foxm1b are also required for the liver bud cell proliferation [64]. Foxm1b knockout mice die in utero by E18.5. The fetal liver shows a 75% reduction in the number of hepatoblasts. This diminished proliferation of the hepatoblasts contributes to abnormal liver development. In addition, these animals do not develop intrahepatic bile ducts. Therefore, this factor seems to be critical for the hepatoblast precursor cells to differentiate toward the biliary epithelial cell lineage. The Xbp1 knockout mice also show hypoplastic livers [65]. These animals die from anemia caused by reduced hematopoiesis, with a reduced growth rate and increased apoptosis of hepatocytes. This again shows a link between hematopoiesis and liver development. Xbp1 is also highly expressed in hepatocellular carcinomas [65].

Using ex vivo cultured fetal mouse liver, Monga et al. [66] found a function of the Wnt pathway for fetal liver cell proliferation. Blocking the expression of β-catenin, a key component of the Wnt signaling pathway, leads to reduced cell proliferation. Consistent with these findings are studies in chicken embryos, in which an inhibition of Wnt signaling results in reduced liver size. In contrast, the overexpression of β-catenin increases the liver size [66,67].

Hlx is a homeodomain transcription factor whose expression is restricted to the hepatic mesenchyme. In studies by Hentsch et al. [68] and Lints et al. [69], deletion of this factor led to severe hepatic hypoplasia; the liver failed to expand and reached only 3% of its normal size. This was not associated with an increase in apoptotic cells. The animals also had severe anemia because the small liver provided insufficient support for fetal hematopoiesis.

The expression of the homeobox factor Hex is restricted to the ventral endoderm at the ten-somite stage. During further development, the expression is even more restricted to two areas, the future liver and thyroid [70,71]. Studies in Hex knockout mice established the importance of this factor for liver development [70,71]. More detailed investigations showed that at E9.0, the presumptive hepatic bud is formed but no albumin or Afp expression could be detected. Further analysis using reverse-transcriptase polymerase chain reaction of earlier stage embryos could detect the expression of Alb, Ttr, and Prox1 in the ventral endoderm [72]. This shows that Hex seems not to be necessary for the establishment of the hepatic fate but for the outgrowth of the hepatoblasts. It was further established that Hex promotes the hepatic endoderm to transition to a pseudostratified epithelium, which in turn allows hepatoblasts to emerge into the stromal environment and continue differentiating [73]. The function of Hex seems to be conserved in higher vertebrates, as in Hex$^{-/-}$ zebrafish no liver develops [74]. Zhang et al. [75] showed in the chicken that the expression of

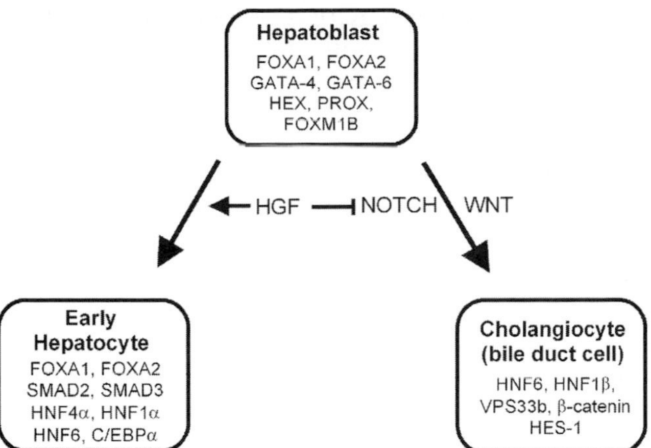

Figure 1.3. Transcription factors and signals promoting hepatoblast growth and differentiation into hepatocytes and cholangiocytes (bile duct cells). See text for details.

Hex in the ventral endoderm requires both FGF and BMP signaling. This is in agreement with a BMP-responsive element in the promoter of the *Hex* gene [76]. Other promoter studies show the binding of Foxa2 and Gata4 to the Hex promoter [77]. Both transcription factors are important for the promoter activity and contribute to liver-enriched expression of Hex (Figure 1.3).

Burke and Oliver [78] showed that the expression of homeobox transcription factor Prox1 is restricted to regions developing into mammalian pancreas and liver in the early endoderm. The liver of Prox1 knockout mice embryos at E14.5 is significantly smaller compared with control animals [79]. Still, these animals formed distinct liver lobes, but the hepatocytes were restricted to the central rudiment. At E10.0–E12.5, hepatoblasts were absent from the developing liver lobes. The proliferation of the hepatoblasts was strongly reduced in the knockout embryos. Further, it was shown that the $Prox^{-/-}$ cells failed to delaminate from the liver diverticulum. As these cells express Alb and Afp, Prox1 seems not to be necessary for the induction of the hepatic fate but for the expansion of the hepatoblasts (Figure 1.3). A newer study presented data that the early expression in hepatoblasts is evolutionarily conserved, as the same expression profile was found in chicken, mouse, rat, and human embryos [80–83]. Interestingly, this group showed that adult hepatocytes still express Prox1 and that the expression is strongly up-regulated in hepatoma cell lines. This might provide a link between a developmental factor and cancer.

FETAL HEMATOPOIESIS DURING LIVER DEVELOPMENT

As mentioned previously, after the liver bud emerges from the gut tube, hematopoietic cells migrate there and proliferate. The hematopoietic cells secrete oncostatin M (OSM), a growth factor belonging to the interleukin-6 (IL-6) family, and the surrounding liver cells express the gp130 receptor subunit OSMR. Supporting the importance of this interaction in fetal hepatocyte cultures, OSM stimulates the expression of hepatic differentiation markers and induces morphologic changes and multiple liver-specific functions as ammonia clearance, lipid synthesis, glycogen synthesis, detoxification, and cell adhesion [81–83].

Oncostatin M not only induces hepatic differentiation but also suppresses fetal liver hematopoiesis. For these experiments, Kinoshita et al. [8] used fetal hepatic cells from different developmental stages in co-culture with hematopoietic stem cells. Hepatic cells from E8.5 support the expansion of hematopoietic stem cells and give rise to myeloid, lymphoid, and erythroid lineages. The addition of OSM and glucocorticoid strongly suppresses this. In contrast, hepatic cells from E14.5 no longer support hematopoiesis in co-cultures. However, the hematopoietic cells induce further differentiation of hepatoblasts, and in consequence, the liver stops supporting local hematopoiesis and induces the hematopoietic stem cell switch to the bone marrow.

During liver development, the expression of the cyclins D1, D2, and D3 are down-regulated [83]. These cyclins are important for the initiation of the cell cycle and therefore for cell proliferation. In primary cultures of fetal hepatocytes, OSM can induce the down-regulation of the cyclins D1 and D2 [83]. This down-regulation is mediated by Stat3, which is activated through OSM and OSM receptor complex interaction.

SPECIFYING THE HEPATOCYTE AND BILIARY LINEAGE

Other studies showed that mice lacking either hepatocyte nuclear factor (HNF)6 or HNF1β in the liver show defects in the development of the biliary cell lineage, but little effects were found on the hepatocyte lineage [84,85]. Weinstein et al. [86] investigated the liver development in $Smad2^{+/-}$ and $Smad3^{+/-}$ mice; Smads are the downstream effectors of transforming growth factor-β (TGF-β). They found that the livers of these mice at E14.5 were dramatically hypoplastic, with a strong reduction of hepatocyte proliferation (Figure 1.3). In addition, there was more apoptotic cell death and the liver architecture was disrupted. These abnormalities were likely related to a defect in cell–cell adhesion, as β1-integrin was very strongly down-regulated. Interestingly, this phenotype could be rescued through the addition of HGF. Therefore, it seems that the TGF-β and HGF pathways cooperate on this aspect of liver development.

It is well known that hepatocytes and bile duct cells originate from a common precursor, the hepatoblast [87]. Notch signaling promotes hepatoblast differentiation into the biliary epithelial lineage, and HGF antagonizes this [88,89]. The expression of the Notch intracellular domain in hepatoblasts inhibits their differentiation into hepatocytes. In contrast, if Notch signaling was down-regulated by application of an siRNA against Notch2 mRNA, hepatic differentiation occurred. Therefore, HGF-based antagonism of Notch signaling would promote the commitment to the hepatocyte lineage (Figure 1.3).

Supporting the idea of HGF as a promoter for the hepatic fate decision is a study from Suzuki et al. [90]. They found that HGF induces the expression of C/EBPα in albumin-negative fetal liver cells. When C/EBPα activity is blocked through expression of a dominant negative form of C/EBPα, there is no transition of alb− to the alb+ stage (Figure 1.3).

The importance of the Notch signaling for biliary development is evolutionarily conserved. In humans, a haploinsufficiency of Jagged1 (a Notch ligand) leads to the Alagille syndrome. This disease is characterized by a reduction in intrahepatic bile ducts [91,92]. Notch signaling is also required for the biliary development in zebrafish [93], where disruption of signaling leads to a phenotype similar to humans with the Alagille syndrome. In mice, the Notch pathway controls the expression of the helix-loop-helix protein Hes1 [94,95]. Mice deficient in this factor show an absence of the gallbladder and severe hypoplasia of extrahepatic bile ducts, and the tubular formation of intrahepatic bile ducts is completely absent. In addition, the biliary epithelium of Hes1$^{-/-}$ mice ectopically expresses the proendocrine gene *Neuro3*, and pancreatic differentiation programs are activated. Thus, biliary epithelium has the potential for pancreatic differentiation, and Hes1 seems to determine biliary organogenesis by blocking the pancreatic cell fate (Figure 1.3).

Wnt signaling might be involved in regulating biliary epithelial cell fate. Ex vivo fetal liver culture experiments show that the addition of Wnt3A supports the biliary epithelial cell differentiation. In agreement with this finding, the inhibition of β-catenin prevents hepatoblasts from expressing biliary markers [66,96]. One important factor for activating this differentiation program is HNF6. HNF6 is expressed in hepatoblasts, in the gallbladder primordium, and in biliary epithelial cells of the developing intrahepatic bile ducts. HNF6 knockout mice developed no gallbladder, and the development of the intrahepatic and extrahepatic bile ducts was abnormal. The intrahepatic bile ducts had a similar phenotype in conditional HNF1β knockout mice. HNF1β was down-regulated in HNF6$^{-/-}$ mice, and HNF6 could activate the HNF1β promoter [84,85]. These results suggest that the effect of HNF1β is downstream of HNF6 (Figure 1.3). Supporting this relationship between HNF6 and HNF1β are results from zebrafish, which showed a biliary phenotype in HNF6-deficient animals and that this phenotype can be rescued by overexpressing HNF1β [97].

Another study in zebrafish found an additional gene involved in this cascade. The vps33b ortholog of a mammalian vacuolar sorting protein is expressed in the developing liver and intestine. A knockdown study showed similar biliary defects as in the HNF6 knockdown. The expression of vps33b is reduced in HNF6-deficient and vhnf1 mutated zebrafish embryos. This implies that vps33b is a downstream target gene of HNF6/vhnf1 [98]. It is important to realize that many of these pathways work together. HNF6 synergizes with Foxa2 to potentiate Foxa2 transcriptional activity by recruiting the p300/C/EBP coactivator proteins [99]. For a full understanding of liver development, it will be important to discern the feedback and regulatory loops between all pathways involved. For this, the use of bioinformatics will be crucial.

REGULATION OF LIVER-SPECIFIC GENE ACTIVITY AND DIFFERENTIATION

Odom et al. [100] have demonstrated the importance of HNF4α for gene regulation in hepatocytes. Microarray data suggest that HNF1α binds to 222 target genes in human hepatocytes corresponding to 1.6% of the genes assayed. HNF6 bound to 227 (1.7%), and HNF4α bound to 1575 (12%) of the genes, which means that HNF4α bound to nearly half of the active genes in the liver that were tested. In addition, most of the genes bound by HNF1α or HNF6 were also bound by HNF4α, but only a few genes were bound by both HNF1α and HNF6.

HNF4α knockout embryos have a severe defect in visceral endoderm formation, which prevents gastrulation and causes a stop in development at E6.5 [101]. This is consistent with the expression pattern of HNF4α, which is in the primary and extraembryonic visceral endoderm before gastrulation and in epithelial cells at the beginning of liver, pancreas, and intestine formation [102]. To circumvent this early mortality in HNF4α knockout mice, Duncan et al. [103] performed tetraploid rescue experiments. Applying this technology, the HNF4$\alpha^{-/-}$ embryos developed through gastrulation and developed a fetal liver. Analysis of the liver in rescued E12.5 embryos showed a critical function of HNF4α in the regulation of pregnane X receptor (PXR) and cross-regulation with HNF1α [104]. In addition, the expression of several liver genes, such as albumin, AFP, and transferrin was reduced. Using another strategy, Parviz et al. [105] made a conditional HNF4α knockout mouse specific for the fetal liver. At E18.5, the liver of these animals failed to store glycogen. Consistent with this, genes important for glucose homeostasis were down-regulated and the liver architecture was abnormal, including a decreased expression of cell adhesion and cell junction molecules in hepatocytes. Both these studies and others [106] together show clearly that HNF4α is broadly involved in diverse aspects of hepatocyte differentiation (Figure 1.3). As Gata4 is important for hepatic fate decision and HNF4α seems to be a downstream target, this again links the early steps of liver development with the later ones. To summarize, HNF4α is important for the regulation of many genes involved in the physiologic function of the liver, but this factor seems to be dispensable for the initial hepatic fate decision.

THE PHENOMENON OF TRANSDIFFERENTIATION

Transdifferentiation is the name used to describe the conversion of one differentiated cell type to another [107,108]. There is some evidence for a transdifferentiation of pancreas cells into hepatocyte-like cells. The first experiment to show this was performed by Scarpelli and Rao [109]. They used a methionine-deficient protocol to induce the regeneration of pancreas in the hamster. Analyzing the tissue, this group found hepatocytes in the regenerating pancreas. The authors suggested that the conversion of pancreas cells into hepatocytes was triggered by a single dose of the carcinogen N-nitrosobis (2-oxopropyl) amine, given during the S-phase in the regenerating pancreatic cells. Since then, there have been different protocols in different animal systems that induce hepatocytes in the pancreas (e.g., rat [110–112], mice [113]). In addition to these experimental conditions, Paner et al. [114] found hepatocytes naturally in human pancreatic tumors.

In this context, the establishment of the pancreatic cell line AR42J was helpful. AR42J cells were originally isolated from a pancreatic carcinoma of an azaserine-treated rat [115,116]. These cells have an amphicrine character, meaning they possess both exocrine and neuroendocrine properties. A subclone of the parent cell line named AR42J-B13 was isolated later by Mashima et al. [117]. Shen et al. [118] showed that treatment with dexamethasone and OSM induces the formation of hepatocyte-like cells from AR42J-B13 or AR42J. These hepatocyte-like cells express liver markers such as albumin, glucose-6-phosphatase, transferrin, and transthyretin. The group found that the cells are induced to express the liver transcription factor C/EBPβ and that the ectopic expression of C/EBPβ alone induces the differentiation of AR42J cells into hepatocytes. Expression of liver inhibitory protein (LIP), a dominant negative form of C/EBPβ, blocks the transdifferentiation. In the same paper, the authors describe the use of isolated pancreatic buds from E11.5 mouse embryos. Cultures of the pancreatic bud exposed to dexamethasone and OSM leads to the transdifferentiation from an exocrine phenotype to a hepatic phenotype. These experiments suggest that C/EBPβ is an important switch for inducing transdifferentiation, and the experimental results support the idea that pancreatic exocrine cells have the potential to differentiate into hepatocyte-like cells. Still, it remains to be shown if these cells can completely function as hepatocytes in vivo.

Our knowledge of liver-to-pancreas cell transdifferentiation is more limited. Pancreatic-type exocrine tissue has been found in livers of rats treated with polychlorinated biphenyls [111], in fish liver tumors induced by chemical carcinogens [119], and in the liver of a human patient with hepatic cirrhosis [120]. But until now, there has been no clear evidence of transdifferentiation from hepatocytes to pancreatic cells. The pancreatic cells in the liver could come from oval cells or another kind of progenitor.

These reactions might be better understood in a developmental context. As mentioned before, the endoderm reacts to FGF signaling in a dose-dependent manner, and without FGF signaling, the endoderm takes the default pancreas fate. Therefore, both organs are strongly linked developmentally, and adult cells of these organs might retain the ability to activate the other determination program. For the future, it might be interesting to see if the ability for transdifferentiation is dependent on specific competence factors, such as Foxa and Gatas.

STEM CELLS AND THE LIVER

Recent studies suggest that bone marrow cells can differentiate into hepatocytes and cholangiocytes in the liver. Petersen et al. [121] performed bone marrow transplantation in mice, and then they induced liver damage and compensatory regeneration. Rare bone marrow donor cells migrated to the liver and differentiated into hepatocytes and bile duct cells. Theise et al. [122] showed later that this differentiation does not require liver damage or regeneration. Investigations in human patients who underwent bone marrow transplantation found hepatocytes derived from bone marrow cells [123,124]. Lagasse et al. [125] determined which bone marrow cell subpopulation possesses this ability. Only highly purified hematopoietic stem cells, but not other bone marrow cells, were able to restore liver function in mice. Interestingly, Ishikawa et al. [126] showed recently that bone marrow cells differentiate into hepatocytes via hepatoblast intermediates. They used green fluorescent protein–marked bone marrow cells for bone marrow transplantation experiments in carbon tetrachloride–treated mice (induces liver damage and consequently regeneration). In this model, FGF is an important growth factor for the differentiation process of bone marrow cells to hepatocytes. Treatment of these mice with recombinant FGF2 increased the repopulation by bone marrow cells and increased the expression of hepatoblast marker genes. In addition, these animals showed a higher survival rate. This links the phenomenon of bone marrow cell differentiation into hepatocytes to the events occurring during liver development.

A different perspective on these studies was gained from work on restoring liver function in fumarylacetoacetate hydrolase (FAH)-deficient mice, in which the application of myelomonocytic cells was sufficient [127,128]. Notably, it was shown that cell fusion is the source of apparent bone marrow–derived hepatocytes. That is, rare bone marrow–derived cells fuse with resident hepatocytes and activate the *Fah* gene on a bone marrow cell chromosome, thereby complementing the host cell Fah1 defect. A recent study using monkey embryonic stem cells also showed cell fusion events [129]. Monkey embryonic stem cells were cultured to form embryoid bodies. In these embryoid bodies, hepatocyte-like cells were found and transplanted into immunodeficient, urokinase-type plasminogen-activator transgenic mice. When these mice developed liver failure, hepatocytes expressing monkey albumin were identified. A more detailed analysis of the cells, however, showed that they originated from cell fusion. Interestingly, if undifferentiated embryonic stem cells were applied, cell fusion and liver repopulation did not occur. Therefore, cell fusion might occur more with partially differentiated cells and might be another mechanism distinct from stem cell differentiation.

Schwartz et al. [130] isolated multipotent adult progenitor cells (MAPCs) from postnatal bone marrow from human, mouse, and rat. Culturing these cells on Matrigel with FGF4 and HGF caused the cells to differentiate into hepatocyte-like cells. The cells expressed the typical liver genes *Foxa2*, *Gata4*, cytokeratin 19, transthyretin, *Afp*, and albumin. But more importantly, these cells showed functional characteristics of hepatocytes, such as the secretion of urea and albumin, expression of phenobarbital-inducible cytochrome P450, taking up of low-density lipoprotein, and storage of glycogen. These results are more supportive of the idea of a stem cell differentiating into hepatocytes, as in the cell culture system, no cell fusion with hepatocytes should be possible.

Recent studies have shown that embryonic stem cells can efficiently be differentiated into definitive endoderm [131,132]. The differentiated cells could be purified to near homogeneity. Kubo et al. [133] described a protocol for the induction of differentiation into definitive endoderm from embryonic stem cells. After the embryonic stem cells differentiated into embryoid bodies, the cells were cultured in the presence of activin A under serum-free conditions. This induced the development of endoderm from a brachyury-positive population that also displays mesoderm potential. Activin belongs to the TGF-β family and, as discussed previously, members of this family are important for endoderm formation during normal development. Interestingly, it was previously shown that hepatic differentiation could be induced in embryonic stem cells by co-culturing them with cardiac mesoderm [22]. This, again, is a link to a process during development, in which the cardiac mesoderm is essential for hepatic fate decision. Additional studies have identified growth factors that allow direct hepatic fate specification from embryonic stem cells in cell culture [134]. A combination of FGF1, FGF4, and HGF can induce the hepatic fate, and the later addition of OSM to the cell culture induced an even more differentiated hepatocyte-like cell. Again, this in part is a recapitulation of the events during development. This study also showed that the transplantation of the differentiated cells into mice with cirrhosis had a significant therapeutic effect. This is a very important control to confirm that hepatocyte-like cells can function as hepatocytes in vivo. Using microarray analysis, the same group later showed that the gene expression profile of the appropriately differentiated embryonic stem cells is highly similar to that of adult mouse liver [135]. In addition, they used siRNA against Foxa2 and identified this transcription factor as having an essential role in hepatic differentiation from embryonic stem cells. This agrees with the findings during normal liver development.

For the future, studies of embryonic stem cells to endoderm or hepatocyte differentiation can increase our understanding of the molecular basis of liver development, as this technique overcomes the limitations of the small amount of tissue during normal development. The exact understanding of these developmental processes that lead to a specific cell fate might help us to recapitulate the events in vitro and engineer artificial liver cells and tissue to combat pediatric liver diseases.

REFERENCES

1. Wells JM, Melton DA. Early mouse endoderm is patterned by soluble factors from adjacent germ layers. Development 2000;127:1563–72.
2. Lawson KA, Meneses JJ, Pedersen RA. Cell fate and cell lineage in the endoderm of the presomite mouse embryo, studied with an intracellular tracer. Dev Biol 1986;115:325–39.
3. Wells JM, Melton DA. Vertebrate endoderm development. Annu Rev Cell Dev Biol 1999;15:393–410.
4. Fukuda-Taira S. Hepatic induction in the avian embryo: specificity of reactive endoderm and inductive mesoderm. J Embryol Exp Morph 1981;63:111–25.
5. Gualdi R, Bossard P, Zheng M, et al. Hepatic specification of the gut endoderm in vitro: cell signaling and transcriptional control. Genes Dev 1996;10:1670–82.
6. Le Douarin NM. An experimental analysis of liver development. Med Biol 1975;53:427–55.
7. Kinoshita T, Miyajima A. Cytokine regulation of liver development. Biochim Biophys Acta 2002;1592:303–12.
8. Kinoshita T, Sekiguchi T, Xu MJ, et al. Hepatic differentiation induced by oncostatin M attenuates fetal liver hematopoiesis. Proc Natl Acad Sci U S A 1999;96:7265–70.
9. Kamiya A, Kinoshita T, Miyajima A. Oncostatin M and hepatocyte growth factor induce hepatic maturation via distinct signaling pathways. FEBS Lett 2001;492:90–4.
10. Kamiya A, Gonzalez FJ. TNF-alpha regulates mouse fetal hepatic maturation induced by oncostatin M and extracellular matrices. Hepatology 2004;40:527–36.
11. Tremblay KD, Zaret KS. Distinct populations of endoderm cells converge to generate the embryonic liver bud and ventral foregut tissues. Dev Biol 2005;280:87–99.
12. Fukuda S. The development of hepatogenic potency in the endoderm of quail embryos. J Embryol Exp Morph 1979;52:49–62.
13. Le Douarin N. Etude expérimentale de l'organogenèse du tube digestif et du foie chez l'embryon de poulet. Bull Biol Fr Belg 1964;98:543–676.
14. Le Douarin N. Synthese du glycogene dans les hepatocytes en voie de differentiation: role des mesenchymes homologue et heterologues. Dev Biol 1968;17:101–14.
15. Le Douarin NM, Jotereau FV. (1975). Tracing of cells of the avian thymus through embryonic life in interspecific chimeras. J Exp Med 1975;142:17–40.
16. Houssaint E. Differentiation of the mouse hepatic primordium. I. An analysis of tissue interactions in hepatocyte differentiation. Cell Differ 1980;9:269–79.
17. Jung J, Zheng M, Goldfarb M, Zaret KS. Initiation of mammalian liver development from endoderm by fibroblast growth factors. Science 1999;284:1998–2003.
18. Deutsch G, Jung J, Zheng M, et al. A bipotential precursor population for pancreas and liver within the embryonic endoderm. Development 2001;128:871–81.
19. Serls AE, Doherty S, Parvatiyar P, et al. Different thresholds of fibroblast growth factors pattern the ventral foregut into liver and lung. Development 2005;132:35–47.
20. Miller DL, Ortega S, Bashayan O, et al. Compensation by fibroblast growth factor 1 (FGF1) does not account for the mild phenotypic defects observed in FGF2 null mice. Mol Cell Biol 2000;20:2260–8.
21. Cai CL, Liang X, Shi Y, et al. Isl1 identifies a cardiac progenitor population that proliferates prior to differentiation and contributes a majority of cells to the heart. Dev Cell 2003;5:877–89.
22. Fair JH, Cairns BA, Lapaglia M, et al. Induction of hepatic differentiation in embryonic stem cells by co-culture with embryonic cardiac mesoderm. Surgery 2003;134:189–96.
23. Rossi JM, Dunn NR, Hogan BLM, Zaret KS. Distinct mesodermal signals, including BMPs from the septum transversum mesenchyme, are required in combination for hepatogenesis from the endoderm. Genes Dev 2001;15:1998–2009.
24. Furuta Y, Piston DW, Hogan BL. Bone morphogenetic proteins (BMPs) as regulators of dorsal forebrain development. Development 1997;124:2203–12.
25. Barron M, Gao M, Lough J. Requirement for BMP and FGF signaling during cardiogenic induction in non-precardiac

mesoderm is specific, transient, and cooperative. Dev Dyn 2000;218:383–93.

26. Lough J, Barron M, Brogley M, et al. Combined BMP-2 and FGF-4, but neither factor alone, induces cardiogenesis in non-precardiac embryonic mesoderm. Dev Biol 1996;178:198–202.
27. Lee KC, Crowe AJ, Barton MC. p53-mediated repression of alpha-fetoprotein gene expression by specific DNA binding. Mol Cell Biol 1999;19:1279–88.
28. Ang SL, Wierda A, Wong D, et al. The formation and maintenance of the definitive endoderm lineage in the mouse: involvement of HNF3/forkhead proteins. Development 1993; 119:1301–15.
29. Monaghan AP, Kaestner KH, Grau E, Schutz G. Postimplantation expression patterns indicate a role for the mouse forkhead/HNF-3 alpha, beta, and gamma genes in determination of the definitive endoderm, chordamesoderm and neuroectoderm. Development 1993;119:567–78.
30. Sasaki H, Hogan BLM. Differential expression of multiple fork head related genes during gastrulation and pattern formation in the mouse embryo. Development 1993;118:47–59.
31. Kaestner KH, Katz J, Liu Y, et al. (1999). Inactivation of the winged helix transcription factor HNF3alpha affects glucose homeostasis and islet glucagon gene expression in vivo. Genes Dev 1999;13:495–504.
32. Shih DQ, Navas MA, Kuwajima S, et al. Impaired glucose homeostasis and neonatal mortality in hepatocyte nuclear factor 3alpha-deficient mice. Proc Natl Acad Sci U S A 1999;96: 10152–7.
33. Ang S-L, Rossant J. *HNF-3b* is essential for node and notochord formation in mouse development. Cell 1994;78:561–74.
34. Dufort D, Schwartz L, Harpal K, Rossant J. The transcription factor HNF3b is required in visceral endoderm for normal primitive streak morphogenesis. Development 1998;125:3015–25.
35. Weinstein DC, Ruizi Altaba A, Chen WS, et al. The winged-helix transcription factor *HNF-3b* is required for notochord development in the mouse embryo. Cell 1994;78:575–88.
36. Sund NJ, Ang SL, Sackett SD, et al. Hepatocyte nuclear factor 3beta (Foxa2) is dispensable for maintaining the differentiated state of the adult hepatocyte. Mol Cell Biol 2000;20:5175–83.
37. Lee CS, Friedman JR, Fulmer JT, Kaestner KH. The initiation of liver development is dependent on Foxa transcription factors. Nature 2005;435:944–7.
38. Narita N, Bielinska M, Wilson DB. Cardiomyocyte differentiation by GATA-4 deficient embryonic stem cells. Development 1997;122:3755–64.
39. Bossard P, Zaret KS. GATA transcription factors as potentiators of gut endoderm differentiation. Development 1998;125:4909–17.
40. Kuo CT, Morrisey EE, Anandappa R, et al. GATA4 transcription factor is required for ventral morphogenesis and heart tube formation. Genes Dev 1997;11:1048–1060.
41. Molkentin JD, Lin Q, Duncan SA, Olson EN. Requirement of the transcription factor GATA4 for heart tube formation and ventral morphogenesis. Genes Dev 1997;11:1061–72.
42. Rojas A, De Val S, Heidt AB, et al. Gata4 expression in lateral mesoderm is downstream of BMP4 and is activated directly by Forkhead and GATA transcription factors through a distal enhancer element. Development 2005;132:3405–17.
43. Zaret K. Identifying specific protein-DNA interactions within living cells, or in "in vivo footprinting." Methods 1997;11:149–50.
44. Cirillo LA, McPherson CE, Bossard P, et al. Binding of the winged-helix transcription factor HNF3 to a linker histone site on the nucleosome. EMBO J 1998;17:244–54.
45. Chaya D, Hayamizu T, Bustin M, Zaret KS. Transcription factor FoxA (HNF3) on a nucleosome at an enhancer complex in liver chromatin. J Biol Chem 2001;276:44385–9.
46. Cirillo L, Lin FR, Cuesta I, et al. Opening of compacted chromatin by early developmental transcription factors HNF3 (FOXA) and GATA-4. Mol Cell 2002;9:279–89.
47. Ogden SK, Lee KC, Wernke-Dollries K, et al. p53 targets chromatin structure alteration to repress alpha-fetoprotein gene expression. J Biol Chem 2001;276:42057–62.
48. Wilkinson DS, Ogden SK, Stratton SA, et al. A direct intersection between p53 and transforming growth factor beta pathways targets chromatin modification and transcription repression of the alpha-fetoprotein gene. Mol Cell Biol 2005;25:1200–12.
49. Hiemisch H, Schutz G, Kaestner KH. Transcriptional regulation in endoderm development: characterization of an enhancer controlling Hnf3g expression by transgenesis and targeted mutagenesis. EMBO J 1997;16:3995–4006.
50. Kaestner KH, Hiemisch H, Schütz G. Targeted disruption of the gene encoding hepatocyte nuclear factor 3g results in reduced transcription of hepatocyte-specific genes. Mol Cell Biol 1998;18:4251.
51. Duncan SA, Navas MA, Dufort D, et al. Regulation of a transcription factor network required for differentiation and metabolism. Science 1998;281:692–5.
52. Morrisey EE, Tang Z, Sigrist K, et al. GATA6 regulates HNF4 and is required for differentiation of visceral endoderm in the mouse embryo. Genes Dev 1998;12:3579–90.
53. Koutsourakis M, Langeveld A, Patient R, et al. The transcription factor GATA6 is essential for early extraembryonic development. Development 1999;126:723–32.
54. Zhao R, Watt AJ, Li J, et al. GATA6 is essential for embryonic development of the liver but dispensable for early heart formation. Mol Cell Biol 2005;25:2622–31.
55. Holtzinger A, Evans T. Gata4 regulates the formation of multiple organs. Development 2005;132:4005–14.
56. Wandzioch E, Kolterud A, Jacobsson M, et al. Lhx2-/- mice develop liver fibrosis. Proc Natl Acad Sci U S A 2004;101: 16549–54.
57. Matsumoto K, Yoshitomi H, Rossant J, Zaret KS. Liver organogenesis promoted by endothelial cells prior to vascular function. Science 2001;294:559–63.
58. Shalaby F, Rossant J, Yamaguchi TP, et al. Failure of blood-island formation and vasculogenesis in Flk-1-deficient mice. Nature 1995;376:62–6.
59. LeCouter J, Moritz DR, Li B, et al. Angiogenesis-independent endothelial protection of liver: role of VEGFR-1. Science 2003;299:890–3.
60. Sonnenberg E, Meyer D, Weidner KM, Birchmeier C. Scatter factor/hepatocyte growth factor and its receptor, the c-met tyrosine kinase, can mediate a signal exchange between mesenchyme and epithelia during mouse development. J Cell Biol 1993;123:223–35.
61. Schmidt C, Bladt F, Goedecke S, et al. Scatter factor/hepatocyte growth factor is essential for liver development. Nature 1995;373:699–702.
62. Uehara Y, Minowa O, Mori C, et al. Placental defect and embryonic lethality in mice lacking hepatocyte growth factor/scatter factor. Nature 1995;373:702.

63. Borowiak M, Garratt AN, Wustefeld T, et al. Met provides essential signals for liver regeneration. Proc Natl Acad Sci U S A 2004;101:10608–13.
64. Krupczak-Hollis K, Wang X, Kalinichenko VV, et al. The mouse Forkhead Box m1 transcription factor is essential for hepatoblast mitosis and development of intrahepatic bile ducts and vessels during liver morphogenesis. Dev Biol 2004;276: 74–88.
65. Reimold AM, Etkin A, Clauss I, et al. An essential role in liver development for transcription factor XBP-1. Genes Dev 2000;14:152–7.
66. Monga SP, Monga HK, Tan X, et al. Beta-catenin antisense studies in embryonic liver cultures: role in proliferation, apoptosis, and lineage specification. Gastroenterology 2003;124: 202–16.
67. Suksaweang S, Lin CM, Jiang TX, et al. Morphogenesis of chicken liver: identification of localized growth zones and the role of beta-catenin/Wnt in size regulation. Dev Biol 2004; 266:109–22.
68. Hentsch B, Lyons I, Ruili L, et al. *Hlx* homeo box gene is essential for an inductive tissue interaction that drives expansion of embryonic liver and gut. Genes Dev 1996;10:70–9.
69. Lints TJ, Hartley L, Parsons LM, Harvey RP. Mesoderm-specific expression of the divergent homeobox gene Hlx during murine embryogenesis. Dev Dyn 1996;205:457–70.
70. Keng VW, Yagi H, Ikawa M, et al. Homeobox gene Hex is essential for onset of mouse embryonic liver development and differentiation of the monocyte lineage. Biochem Biophys Res Commun 2000;276:1155–61.
71. Martinez-Barbera JP, Clements M, Thomas P, et al. The homeobox gene *hex* is required in definitive endodermal tissues for normal forebrain, liver and thyroid formation. Development 2000;127:2433–45.
72. Bort R, Martinez-Barbera JP, Beddington RS, Zaret KS. *Hex* homeobox gene-dependent tissue positioning is required for organogenesis of the ventral pancreas. Development 2004;131: 797–806.
73. Bort R, Signore M, Tremblay K, et al. Hex homeobox gene controls the transition of the endoderm to a pseudostratified, cell emergent epithelium for liver bud development. Dev Biol 2006;290:44–56.
74. Wallace KN, Pack M. Unique and conserved aspects of gut development in zebrafish. Dev Biol 2003;255:12–29.
75. Zhang W, Yatskievych TA, Baker RK, Antin PB. Regulation of Hex gene expression and initial stages of avian hepatogenesis by Bmp and Fgf signaling. Dev Biol 2004;268:312–26.
76. Zhang W, Yatskievych TA, Cao X, Antin PB. Regulation of Hex gene expression by a Smads-dependent signaling pathway. J Biol Chem 2002;277:45435–41.
77. Denson LA, McClure MH, Bogue CW, et al. HNF3b and GATA-4 transactivate the liver-enriched homeobox gene, *Hex*. Gene 2000;246:311–20.
78. Burke Z, Oliver G. Prox1 is an early specific marker for the developing liver and pancreas in the mammalian foregut endoderm. Mech Dev 2002;118:147–55.
79. Sosa-Pineda B, Wigle JT, Oliver G. Hepatocyte migration during liver development requires Prox1. Nat Genet 2000;25:254–5.
80. Dudas J, Papoutsi M, Hecht M, et al. The homeobox transcription factor Prox1 is highly conserved in embryonic hepatoblasts and in adult and transformed hepatocytes, but is absent from bile duct epithelium. Anat Embryol (Berl) 2004;208:359–66.
81. Kamiya A, Kinoshita T, Ito Y, et al. Fetal liver development requires a paracrine action of oncostatin M through the gp130 signal transducer. EMBO J 1999;18:2127–36.
82. Kojima N, Kinoshita T, Kamiya A, et al. Cell density-dependent regulation of hepatic development by a gp130-independent pathway. Biochem Biophys Res Commun 2000;277:152–8.
83. Matsui T, Kinoshita T, Hirano T, et al. STAT3 down-regulates the expression of cyclin D during liver development. J Biol Chem 2002;277:36167–73.
84. Clotman F, Lannoy VJ, Reber M, et al. The onecut transcription factor HNF6 is required for normal development of the biliary tract. Development 2002;129:1819–28.
85. Coffinier C, Gresh L, Fiette L, et al. Bile system morphogenesis defects and liver dysfunction upon targeted deletion of HNF1beta. Development 2002;129:1829–38.
86. Weinstein M, Monga SP, Liu Y, et al. Smad proteins and hepatocyte growth factor control parallel regulatory pathways that converge on beta1-integrin to promote normal liver development. Mol Cell Biol 2001;21:5122–31.
87. Shiojiri N. The origin of intrahepatic bile duct cells in the mouse. J Embryol Exp Morphol 1984;79:25–39.
88. McCright B, Lozier J, Gridley T. A mouse model of Alagille syndrome: Notch2 as a genetic modifier of Jag1 haploinsufficiency. Development 2002;129:1075–82.
89. Tanimizu N, Miyajima A. Notch signaling controls hepatoblast differentiation by altering the expression of liver-enriched transcription factors. J Cell Sci 2004;117:3165–74.
90. Suzuki A, Iwama A, Miyashita H, et al. Role for growth factors and extracellular matrix in controlling differentiation of prospectively isolated hepatic stem cells. Development 2003;130:2513–24.
91. Oda T, Elkahloun AG, Pike BL, et al. Mutations in the human Jagged1 gene are responsible for Alagille syndrome. Nat Genet 1997;16:235–42.
92. Li L, Krantz ID, Deng Y, et al. Alagille syndrome is caused by mutations in human Jagged1, which encodes a ligand for Notch1. Nat Genet 1997;16:243–51.
93. Lorent K, Yeo SY, Oda T, et al. Inhibition of Jagged-mediated Notch signaling disrupts zebrafish biliary development and generates multi-organ defects compatible with an Alagille syndrome phenocopy. Development 2004;131:5753–66.
94. Kodama Y, Hijikata M, Kageyama R, et al. The role of notch signaling in the development of intrahepatic bile ducts. Gastroenterology 2004;127:1775–86.
95. Sumazaki R, Shiojiri N, Isoyama S, et al. Conversion of biliary system to pancreatic tissue in Hes1-deficient mice. Nat Genet 2004;36:83–7.
96. Hussain SZ, Sneddon T, Tan X, et al. Wnt impacts growth and differentiation in ex vivo liver development. Exp Cell Res 2004;292:157–69.
97. Matthews RP, Lorent K, Russo P, Pack M. The zebrafish onecut gene hnf-6 functions in an evolutionarily conserved genetic pathway that regulates vertebrate biliary development. Dev Biol 2004;274:245–59.
98. Matthews RP, Plumb-Rudewiez N, Lorent K, et al. Zebrafish vps33b, an ortholog of the gene responsible for human arthrogryposis-renal dysfunction-cholestasis syndrome, regulates biliary development downstream of the onecut transcription factor hnf6. Development 2005;132:5295–306.
99. Rausa FM, Tan Y, Costa RH. Association between hepatocyte nuclear factor 6 (HNF-6) and FoxA2 DNA binding domains

stimulates FoxA2 transcriptional activity but inhibits HNF-6 DNA binding. Mol Cell Biol 2003;23:437–49.
100. Odom DT, Zizlsperger N, Gordon DB, et al. Control of pancreas and liver gene expression by HNF transcription factors. Science 2004;303:1378–81.
101. Chen WS, Manova K, Weinstein DC, et al. Disruption of the HNF-4 gene, expressed in visceral endoderm, leads to cell death in embryonic ectoderm and impaired gastrulation of mouse embryos. Genes Dev 1994;8:2466–77.
102. Duncan SA, Manova K, Chen WS, et al. Expression of transcription factor HNF-4 in the extraembryonic endoderm, gut, and nephrogenic tissue of the developing mouse embryo: HNF-4 is a marker for primary endoderm in the implanting blastocyst. Proc Natl Acad Sci U S A 1994;91:7598–602.
103. Duncan SA, Nagy A, Chan W. Murine gastrulation requires HNF-4 regulated gene expression in the visceral endoderm: tetraploid rescue of Hnf-4(-/-) embryos. Development 1997;124:279–87.
104. Li J, Ning G, Duncan SA. Mammalian hepatocyte differentiation requires the transcription factor HNF-4alpha. Genes Dev 2000;14:464–74.
105. Parviz F, Matullo C, Garrison WD, et al. Hepatocyte nuclear factor 4alpha controls the development of a hepatic epithelium and liver morphogenesis. Nat Genet 2003;34:292–6.
106. Hayhurst GP, Lee YH, Lambert G, et al. Hepatocyte nuclear factor 4alpha (nuclear receptor 2A1) is essential for maintenance of hepatic gene expression and lipid homeostasis. Mol Cell Biol 2001;21:1393–403.
107. Slack JM, Tosh D. Transdifferentiation and metaplasia – switching cell types. Curr Opin Genet Dev 2001;11:581–6.
108. Tosh D, Slack JM. How cells change their phenotype. Nat Rev Mol Cell Biol 2002;3:187–94.
109. Scarpelli DG, Rao MS. Differentiation of regenerating pancreatic cells into hepatocyte like cells. Proc Natl Acad Sci U S A 1981;78:2577–81.
110. Reddy JK, Rao MS, Qureshi SA, et al. Induction and origin of hepatocytes in rat pancreas. J Cell Biol 1984;98:2082–90.
111. Rao MS, Subbarao V, Reddy JK. Induction of hepatocytes in the pancreas of copper-depleted rats following copper repletion. Cell Differ 1986;18:109–17.
112. Rao MS, Dwivedi RS, Subbarao V, et al. Almost total conversion of pancreas to liver in the adult rat: a reliable model to study transdifferentiation. Biochem Biophys Res Commun 1988;156:131–6.
113. Krakowski ML, Kritzik MR, Jones EM, et al. Pancreatic expression of keratinocyte growth factor leads to differentiation of islet hepatocytes and proliferation of duct cells. Am J Pathol 1999;154:683–91.
114. Paner GP, Thompson KS, Reyes CV. Hepatoid carcinoma of the pancreas. Cancer 2000;88:1582–9.
115. Longnecker DS, Lilja HS, French J, et al. Transplantation of azaserine-induced carcinomas of pancreas in rats. Cancer Lett 1979;7:197–202.
116. Christophe J. Pancreatic tumoral cell line AR42J: an amphicrine model. Am J Physiol 1994;266:G963–71.
117. Mashima H, Shibata H, Mine T, Kojima I. Formation of insulin-producing cells from pancreatic acinar AR42J cells by hepatocyte growth factor. Endocrinology 1996;137:3969–76.
118. Shen CN, Slack JM, Tosh D. Molecular basis of transdifferentiation of pancreas to liver. Nat Cell Biol 2000;2:879–87.
119. Lee BC, Hendricks JD, Bailey GS. Metaplastic pancreatic cells in liver tumors induced by diethylnitrosamine. Exp Mol Pathol 1989;50:104–13.
120. Wolf HK, Burchette JL Jr, Garcia JA, Michalopoulos G. Exocrine pancreatic tissue in human liver: a metaplastic process? Am J Surg Pathol 1990;14:590–5.
121. Petersen BE, Bowen WC, Patrene KD, et al. Bone marrow as a potential source of hepatic oval cells. Science 1999;284:1168–70.
122. Theise ND, Nimmakayalu M, Gardner R, et al. Liver from bone marrow in humans. Hepatology 2000;32:11–16.
123. Alison MR, Poulsom R, Jeffery R, et al. Hepatocytes from non-hepatic adult stem cells. Nature 2000;406:257.
124. Theise ND, Badve S, Saxena R, et al. Derivation of hepatocytes from bone marrow cells in mice after radiation-induced myeloablation. Hepatology 2000;31:235–40.
125. Lagasse E, Connors H, Al-Dhalimy M, et al. Purified hematopoietic stem cells can differentiate into hepatocytes in vivo. Nat Med 2000;6:1229–34.
126. Ishikawa T, Terai S, Urata Y, et al. Fibroblast growth factor 2 facilitates the differentiation of transplanted bone marrow cells into hepatocytes. Cell Tissue Res 2006;323:221–31.
127. Willenbring H, Bailey AS, Foster M, et al. Myelomonocytic cells are sufficient for therapeutic cell fusion in liver. Nat Med 2004;10:744–8.
128. Wang X, Willenbring H, Akkari Y, et al. Cell fusion is the principal source of bone-marrow-derived hepatocytes. Nature 2003;422:897–901.
129. Okamura K, Asahina K, Fujimori H, et al. Generation of hybrid hepatocytes by cell fusion from monkey embryoid body cells in the injured mouse liver. Histochem Cell Biol 2006;125:247 57.
130. Schwartz RE, Reyes M, Koodie L, et al. Multipotent adult progenitor cells from bone marrow differentiate into functional hepatocyte-like cells. J Clin Invest 2002;109:1291–302.
131. Yasunaga M, Tada S, Torikai-Nishikawa S, et al. Induction and monitoring of definitive and visceral endoderm differentiation of mouse ES cells. Nat Biotechnol 2005;23:1542–50.
132. D'Amour KA, Agulnick AD, Eliazer S, et al. Efficient differentiation of human embryonic stem cells to definitive endoderm. Nat Biotechnol 2005;23:1534–41.
133. Kubo A, Shinozaki K, Shannon JM, et al. Development of definitive endoderm from embryonic stem cells in culture. Development 2004;131:1651–62.
134. Teratani T, Yamamoto H, Aoyagi K, et al. Direct hepatic fate specification from mouse embryonic stem cells. Hepatology 2005;41:836–46.
135. Yamamoto Y, Teratani T, Yamamoto H, et al. Recapitulation of in vivo gene expression during hepatic differentiation from murine embryonic stem cells. Hepatology 2005;42:558–67.

2

Functional Development of the Liver

Frederick J. Suchy, M.D.

The liver attains its highest relative size at about 10% of fetal weight at the ninth week of gestation. Early in gestation the liver is the primary site for hematopoiesis. At 7 weeks of gestation, hematopoietic cells outnumber hepatocytes. Primitive hepatocytes are smaller than mature cells and are deficient in glycogen. As the fetus nears term, hepatocytes predominate and enlarge with expansion of the endoplasmic reticulum and accumulation of glycogen. Hepatic blood flow, plasma protein binding, and intrinsic clearance by the liver (reflected in the maximal enzymatic and transport capacity of the liver) also undergo significant postnatal maturation [1]. These changes correlate with an increased capacity for hepatic metabolism and detoxification. At birth the liver constitutes about 4% of body weight compared with 2% in the adult. Liver weight doubles by 12 months of age and increases threefold by 3 years of age.

The functional development of the liver that occurs in concert with growth requires a complicated orchestration of changes in hepatic enzymes and metabolic pathways that result in the mature capacity of the liver to undertake metabolism, biotransformation, and vectorial transport. Greengard [2] has established a paradigm for hepatic development based on a group of several hepatic enzymes studied in the rat and, less extensively, in humans. In one pattern of hepatic development, enzymatic activity is high in a fetus and falls during postnatal development. Examples would include thymidine kinase and ornithine decarboxylase [3]. The activities of other enzymes are expressed initially during early fetal development and continue to increase progressively after birth [2]. Examples include glutamate, dehydrogenase, fructose-1,6-diphosphatase, and aspartate aminotransferase [4]. Another group of enzymes is expressed perinatally and continues to increase progressively after birth. These enzymes include phosphoenolpyruvate carboxykinase and uridine 5′-diphosphate glucuronyl transferase (UGT). A final pattern of development occurs with enzymes that are expressed significantly after birth and peak at weaning, including alanine aminotransferase and alcohol dehydrogenase.

The stepwise appearance of new groups of enzymes during development may be related causally to sequential changes in the level of circulating hormones [4]. For example, total serum thyroxine and triiodothyronine levels of the human fetus undergo a sudden increase between the ninth and tenth weeks of gestation. Similarly, fetal plasma concentrations of cortisol and cortisone are as high by the third month of gestation as at term. There is also a sudden increase in plasma glucagon at birth, which may influence the expression of the neonatal cluster of enzymes in rat liver. The final steps of biochemical differentiation, including the synthesis of enzymes necessary to process a solid diet, occur just before weaning in the rat. A natural surge in cortisone and thyroxine at this time may be important in mediating this change.

With advances in cellular and molecular biology, mechanisms underlying these developmental changes have been found to be extremely complicated and regulated at transcriptional, translational, and posttranslational levels. A complete discussion of this topic is beyond the scope of this review. Only selected examples of developmental changes in the functional capacity of the liver are discussed, particularly those with relevance to understanding susceptibility to liver disease.

HEPATIC ENERGY METABOLISM IN THE FETUS AND NEONATE

Carbohydrate Metabolism

The fetus is completely dependent upon the mother for the continuous transfer of glucose across the placenta [5]. At birth the neonate must rapidly transition to independent control of glucose homeostasis. The tenuous nature of perinatal-neonatal glucose metabolism is exemplified by the multiplicity of disorders associated with neonatal hypoglycemia, including many liver diseases [6].

Glycogen synthesis begins in the fetus at about the ninth week of gestation, with glycogen stores rapidly accumulating near term, at which time the fetal liver contains an amount of glycogen two to three times higher than that in the adult liver (40–60 mg/g liver) [7]. These large stores of hepatic glycogen are important for maintenance of blood glucose levels during the perinatal period, before other energy sources are available and before the onset of hepatic gluconeogenesis. Because

Table 2.1: Metabolic Changes During Liver Development

Accumulation of glycogen in fetal liver (to levels two- to threefold higher than in the adult by term)
Low rates of gluconeogenesis by fetal liver
Low rates of glucose use by fetal liver
Amino acids an important energy source for fetal liver (extensive transamination and oxidative degradation)
High capacity of fetal liver for fatty acid synthesis
Rapid induction of ability to oxidize fatty acids during first days of life
Fatty acid oxidation critical to support of hepatic gluconeogenesis
Rapid increase in hepatic ketogenesis after birth

efficient regulation of the synthesis, storage, and degradation of glycogen develops only near the end of a full-term gestation, there is propensity to hypoglycemia in preterm infants (Table 2.1) [8]. Other sources of carbohydrates, particularly galactose, are converted to glucose, but there is substantial dependence on glucogenesis for supplies of glucose early in life, especially if glycogen stores are low. There is significant reaccumulation of glycogen around the second postnatal week, so that stores reach adult levels at about 3 weeks in normal full-term infants [8]. The blood glucose concentration in the neonate can be maintained for about a 10- to 12-hour fast by glycogenolysis until hepatic glycogen is reduced to less than 12 mg/g liver. The mechanisms underlying the initiation of hepatic glycogenolysis postnatally are not defined completely. The initiation of glycogenolysis may be stimulated by the concomitant rise in plasma glucagon and fall in plasma insulin that occur after birth [7].

After birth and before the onset of suckling there is a time lapse in which the newborn undergoes a unique kind of starvation. During this period glucose is scarce and ketone bodies are not available, because of the delay in ketogenesis. Under these circumstances, the newborn is supplied with another metabolic fuel, lactate, which is utilized as a source of energy and carbon skeletons [9]. Neonatal rat lung, heart, liver, and brain utilize lactate for energy production and lipogenesis. Recent studies using stable isotopes have shown that gluconeogenesis from lactate and pyruvate is established by 4–6 hours after birth [10]. Gluconeogenesis from pyruvate contributes as much as 30% to total glucose production in healthy term babies between 5 and 6 hours after a feed. Both glycogenolysis and gluconeogenesis are stimulated by the surges of serum catecholamines and glucagon associated with birth.

Gluconeogenesis, the synthesis of glucose from lactate, amino acids, and other small molecules, does not occur at significant rates in the fetal liver [7]. Fetuses are hyperinsulinemic, and insulin is known to behave as an inhibitor of the gluconeogenic gene expression program [11]. In animal studies, fetal glucose utilization has been shown to be approximately equal to umbilical glucose uptake over a wide variety of maternal glucose concentrations. The enzymes necessary for hepatic gluconeogenesis are present in the near-term fetus. However, the level of activity of the rate-limiting enzyme of gluconeogenesis, phosphoenolpyruvate carboxykinase (PEPCK), is extremely low in the late-gestation fetus and increases rapidly after birth [8].

Changes in several other hepatic enzymes underlie differences in carbohydrate metabolism between the fetus and neonate [8,9]. For example, there is a deficiency of hepatic glucokinase, a high K_m glucose phosphorylating enzyme, until the time of weaning. In contrast, the amount of activity of hexokinase I, a low K_m glucose phosphorylating enzyme, is high in fetal liver and declines at the end of gestation. Hepatic glucose uptake may be limited by the ability to phosphorylate glucose in the fetal and neonatal liver. The activity of hepatic galactokinase, the enzyme that phosphorylates galactose, the other major hexose in the neonatal diet, rapidly increases near term, probably to assimilate the large intake of galactose in the newborn diet. Glucose may be taken up by the fetal liver, but this process is inhibited by lactate, amino acids, and fatty acids and is not stimulated by insulin as it is postnatally. Glucose utilization by the fetal liver is low, owing to the use of alternative fuels such as amino acids and lactate. A mechanism possibly available to increase hepatic glucose uptake is an increase in glycolytic flux resulting from a decrease in the hepatic concentration of glucose-6-phosphate. The levels of activity of several key enzymes that can decrease glucose-6-phosphate, including glucokinase and pyruvate kinase, are low in fetal liver, impairing the ability of the fetal liver to increase glucose uptake by decreasing the hepatic concentration of glucose-6-phosphate [8]. There appears to be little hepatic glucose uptake in the neonate. Animal studies have shown preferential hepatic uptake of galactose and lactate after a meal, with incorporation of galactose into glycogen or its conversion to glucose. Glucose appears to be delivered for use by peripheral tissues; galactose is used preferentially by the liver for carbohydrate synthesis.

Another important feature of fetal hepatic carbohydrate metabolism is a deficiency of glucose-6-phosphatase activity [6,7]. This enzyme, which is present in liver and kidney, is a microsomal enzyme that is involved in the last step of hepatic glucose synthesis. Gluconeogenic flux is directed into hexose and pentose phosphate pools and to glycogen formation with minimal fetal glucose production in the liver. The level of glucose-6-phosphatase increases to near adult levels at term and rises further after birth.

After birth and initiation of suckling, glucagon- and glucocorticoid-mediated pathways regulating gluconeogenesis are rapidly activated, and insulinemia declines. The molecular mechanisms underlying this dramatic change have not been completely elucidated. PEPCK catalyzes the initial step in hepatic gluconeogenesis and is tightly regulated by glucagon, glucocorticoids, thyroid hormone, insulin, and glucose. A number of transcription factors that bind to the PEPCK gene promoter appear be important in the process, including the glucocorticoid receptor (GR), the retinoic acid receptor, the retinoid X receptor, forkhead box family members, C/EBPα, CREB, COIP-TFI, and hepatocyte nuclear factor (HNF)4α [11]. The peroxisome proliferator-activated receptor-coactivator 1α (PGC1α) is a transcriptional coactivator thought to be a master regulator of liver energy metabolism through its capacity to activate genes involved in gluconeogenesis including HNF4α and GR [12]. FOXO1 is another transcription factor shown to be required for the gluconeogenic action of PGC1α. However, PGC1α is expressed at much higher levels in rat fetal than in adult liver [11]. After birth PGC1α is not induced further unless the animals are fasted even as gluconeogenesis is markedly induced. It is unknown why PGC1α seems to be partially dis-associated from regulation of gluconeogenesis in the fetus and newborn. These data give some sense of the complexity of the changes that occur in gene expression that allow maintenance of blood glucose concentrations after birth.

Amino Acid Metabolism

Amino acids are an important source of energy for the fetus [8]. Amino acids as a metabolic fuel provide an amount of energy for the fetus equivalent to that provided by glucose. Even essential amino acids are oxidized for energy in the fetus. In animal studies, amino acids account for approximately one third of fetal carbon uptake and over 40% of fetal energy requirements. In rodent studies, the uptake of glutamine, alanine, and lysine by the liver is much greater than their incorporation into protein. The large uptake of amino acids by the liver and the increase in hepatic concentrations of free amino acids during gestation, which decline after birth, likely contribute to the synthesis of other substrates, such as glycogen and glucose. Interorgan cycling between the fetal liver and placenta has been proposed for nonessential amino acids like glycine and serine [13].

The use of amino acids by the fetal liver may differ significantly from that by the adult [9]. For example, there is preferential use of the β-carbon of serine for DNA synthesis by fetal liver and for RNA synthesis by adult liver. The high concentration of free amino acids in fetal liver may have a key role in regulation of hepatic growth. For example, high concentrations of free amino acids suppress intralysosomal proteolysis.

The capacity for urea synthesis by the fetal liver is well established by mid-gestation, and the liver serves as the major site for ammonia clearance in the fetus [8]. There is significant endogenous fetal ammonia production by peripheral tissues, with hepatic clearance. Owing to a mature complement of urea cycle enzymes by mid- to late gestation, there is a capacity to increase urea production with increased ammonia and nitrogen uptake.

Many amino acids are transported actively by the placenta through specific carrier mechanisms [14,15]. Net flux of amino acids from placenta to fetus has been demonstrated for all essential amino acids and most nonessential amino acids except for aspartate, glutamate, and serine [9]. Most amino acids also are taken up avidly by the fetal liver [16]. There is evidence for net production of serine, glutamate, and aspartate by the fetal liver, with no umbilical uptake. Studies in the pregnant sheep model indicate that maternal serine is not transferred to the fetus, but is metabolized, in large part to glycine, which is transferred to the fetus and taken up by the fetal liver [17]. Fetal serine requirements are largely met by production in the liver via the action of serine hydroxymethyltransferase and the glycine cleavage system [13]. The uptake of some neutral and basic amino acids by the placenta is in considerable excess of the estimated growth requirements, providing further evidence that some amino acids undergo extensive transamination and oxidative degradation in the fetus [9].

The fetal hepatic uptake of glutamine appears to be greater than that of any other amino acid [18]. The placenta is a major source of the glutamine that enters the fetal circulation [19]. Net flux of glutamine from the maternal circulation, large in comparison to the net fluxes of other amino acids, occurs into the placenta and is augmented by placental glutamine synthesis. After transport into the fetal circulation, the fetal liver is the primary site for fetal glutamine uptake and glutamate production, and, as such, determines the glutamate supply to the placenta [20]. Glutamine is converted to glutamine and NH_2 by glutaminase. The placenta can also produce glutamate by branched-chain amino acid transamination. Although glutamine is a gluconeogenic amino acid, its uptake by the fetal liver is not coupled with a significant amount of fetal hepatic gluconeogenesis. The fetal liver releases glutamate, which is taken up by the placenta and for the most part rapidly oxidized. A significant proportion of the remaining glutamine that is not metabolized to glutamate in the liver and transported to the placenta is used by the fetal tissues for growth.

Most of the enzymes required for regulation of amino acid metabolism are expressed at birth [9]. However, there may be delayed appearance of the activity of *P*-hydroxy phenyl pyruvate oxidase, a key enzyme in the degradation of tyrosine. A relative deficiency of this enzyme is thought to cause transient neonatal tyrosinemia.

The transulfuration pathway is an aspect of amino acid metabolism that has been well studied and has important implications for nutrition of the infant [21]. A low level of cystathionase activity impairs the transulfuration pathway by which dietary methionine is converted to cysteine [22]. Thus, cysteine may be an essential amino acid for the fetus and neonate. After birth there is a rapid increase in cystathionase activity in the human liver. The level of cysteine is 50% higher than that of methionine in human milk, supporting the notion that this amino acid may be essential to the neonate. Similar dietary requirements may exist for other sulfur-containing amino acids, such as taurine.

The distribution and zonation of enzymes involved in glutamine metabolism during development have been evaluated extensively [8]. Glutamine synthetase catalyzes the reaction of glutamate and α-ketoglutarate with the production of glutamine. This ammonia-scavenging pathway has been studied in developing rodent liver. In adult liver, glutamine synthetase protein and mRNA are localized exclusively to the hepatocytes immediately adjacent to central veins [1]. This restricted localization correlates with hepatic uptake of metabolic precursors used by glutamate synthetase, such as glutamate and α-ketoglutarate. Ornithine aminotransferase also is colocalized to this area. In contrast, in fetal liver glutamine synthetase, mRNA is expressed in all fetal hepatocytes at mid-gestation and at term. In the rodent liver, the shift to the adult pattern of glutamine synthetase localization in the perivenous hepatocytes occurs postnatally. This mature pattern of perivenous expression of glutamate synthetase is a permanent feature of the adult liver. There is no regression to the fetal pattern with liver injury or with regeneration.

Lipid Metabolism

Fatty acid oxidation provides a major energy source, augmenting glycogenolysis and gluconeogenesis [23]. The fetus obtains fatty acids through de novo synthesis, passive diffusion of nonesterified fatty acids across the placenta, and selective maternofetal placental transport for certain fatty acids, particularly physiologically important long-chain, polyunsaturated fatty acids [24,25]. The modest amounts of free fatty acids transferred across the placenta are stored in the liver and adipose tissue and are not used by peripheral tissues. The capacity for fatty acid synthesis by the fetal liver is high, peaking in mid-gestation [17]. In rodent models, the level of acetyl CoA carboxylase, the rate-limiting enzyme for fatty acid synthesis in adult liver, is low, suggesting an alternative mechanism for provision of CoA derivatives [23]. Maternally derived ketones and glucose may be precursors for fatty acid synthesis by the fetal liver.

Although some fatty acids can passively diffuse across the placenta, much less is known about transport of other lipids. Recent studies have found that apolipoprotein B (apo B) and microsomal triglyceride transfer protein (MTP) mRNAs are expressed in the human placenta [26]. Term placental tissue was found to produce and secrete apo B-100 particles in vitro. The apo B–containing lipoproteins carry cholesterol and triglyceride as well as fat soluble vitamins and glycoproteins. The term placenta weighs approximately four times more than the fetal liver so is likely to make a significant contribution to the fetal plasma pool of apo B–containing lipoproteins.

Fat that accumulates in the fetal liver is mobilized soon after birth, not for export of free fatty acids but for local utilization [27]. The oxidation of fat results in significant generation of adenosine triphosphate (ATP) for energy and ketone body formation for use by peripheral tissue [17]. Similar to adult liver, a lysosomal acid lipase mediates the breakdown of triacylglycerols. There is rapid maturation of the ability of the liver to oxidize fatty acids during the first days of life. The liver is the main source for synthesis of ketone bodies used by other tissues. The concentrations of ketone bodies, including acetoacetate, 3-hydroxybutyrate, and acetone, increase in the blood during the first 24 hours after birth. In the liver, the postnatal development of long-chain fatty acid oxidation and ketogenesis is regulated by pancreatic hormones, the levels of which change markedly at birth, with a fall in insulin and a rise in glucagon levels [28].

The postnatal increase in hepatic fatty acid oxidation is critically important in supporting hepatic gluconeogenesis [17]. Milk feedings provide the major source for calories postnatally; this high-fat, low-carbohydrate diet supports active gluconeogenesis to maintain levels of blood glucose [29]. Both long- and medium-chain fatty acids from the diet stimulate gluconeogenesis by increasing the hepatic supply of gluconeogenic precursors and activating hepatic gluconeogenesis. In rodent models, the rate of hepatic lipogenesis decreases just prior to birth, as a result of a reduction in the activity of lipogenic enzymes. The large amounts of nonesterified free fatty acids present during the suckling period may underlie the inhibition of acetyl CoA carboxylase activity. At weaning, the lipogenic capacity of the liver increases in response to a high-carbohydrate diet. The specific activity and amount of mRNA for fatty acid synthase and acetyl CoA carboxylase increase significantly in the liver [8].

There is a marked increase in plasma free fatty acid concentrations after birth in infants [29]. Fatty acids varying in their chain length and degree of saturation have very specific roles in metabolism. Short-chain fatty acids may act as local growth factors in the intestine; medium- and saturated long-chain fatty acids are important sources of energy; polysaturated long-chain fatty acids are involved in metabolic regulation; and very long–chain fatty acids are important structural components of membranes [29]. Free fatty acids may supply approximately 42 kJ/kg/d of energy for the newborn [8]. Fat stores complementing gluconeogenesis in a newborn may be particularly important for the infant who is small for gestational age. The induction of fatty acid oxidation that occurs at birth is part of a coordinate increase in hepatic gluconeogenesis that occurs after birth in an effort to adapt to an alteration in energy supply.

Biotransformation

The liver is the main site for metabolism of drugs and xenobiotics and therefore is unusually susceptible to structural and functional injury following exposure to drugs and toxins. Infants and children may be more or less vulnerable to toxic liver injury than adults. Immaturity of pathways for biotransformation may prevent efficient degradation and elimination of a toxic compound; in other circumstances the same immaturity may limit the formation of a reactive metabolite.

Many variables influence drug metabolism, including liver size, liver blood flow, plasma protein binding, and intrinsic clearance (a product of the enzymatic and transport capacity of the liver) [30]. Infants and young children actually have a greater liver-to–body mass ratio than adults, but many of the functions of the hepatocyte involving detoxification, energy metabolism, and excretion of wastes require significant pre- and postnatal maturation to attain the capacity of the adult. The underlying pharmacogenetics may also influence either the affinity or the capacity of an enzyme responsible for biotransformation of a drug or toxin [31]. The development of the array of mechanisms involved in the process for the most part is not completely defined.

Three general stages of drug metabolism occur in the liver: phase I reactions (oxidations–reductions and hydrolyses), phase II reactions (synthetic conjugations with sulfate,

Table 2.2: Developmental Changes in Biotransformation

Decreased capacity of the neonatal liver to metabolize, detoxify, and excrete many drugs
Deficiency of many enzymes required for oxidative, reductive, hydrolytic, and conjugation reactions
Early expression of many cytochrome P450 enzymes in the embryo and fetus, such as CYP3A7, which is involved in steroid metabolism
Delayed expression of other cytochrome P450 enzymes, such as CYP1A2, important in drug metabolism
Reduced activity of many phase II enzymes, including uridine diphosphate glucuronyl transferases in fetus and neonate

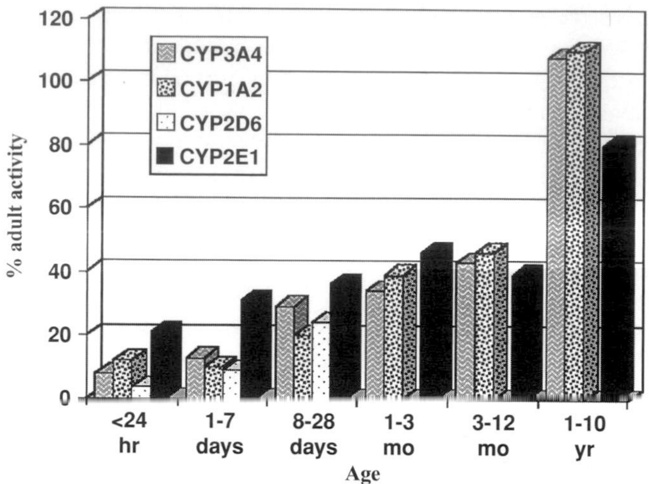

Figure 2.1. Development of cytochrome P450 enzymes. (Data compiled from references [30,34,41,42]).

acetate, glucuronic acid, glycine, and glutathione), and phase III processes (export out of the liver via transporters on the sinusoidal and canalicular membranes) [32,33]. Many phase I and phase II enzymes that are critically important for drug metabolism are polymorphically expressed, developmentally regulated, and subject to considerable inducibility because of exposure to drugs, xenobiotics, and environmental factors (Table 2.2) [34].

There have been many recent advances in understanding of the mechanisms that regulate the expression of genes encoding the enzymes and transporters involved in drug metabolism. The xenobiotic nuclear receptors (NRs), the pregnane X receptor (PXR, also known as the steroid and xenobiotic receptor, or SXR), the constitutive androstane receptor (CAR), and the aryl hydrocarbon receptor (AhR) coordinately induce genes involved in the three phases of xenobiotic metabolism, including oxidative metabolism, conjugation, and transport [35,36]. Many xenobiotics are ligands for the orphan NRs, CAR and PXR, that both heterodimerize with the retinoid X receptor (RXR) and transcriptionally activate the promoters of many genes involved in drug metabolism [33,37]. Similarly, the AhR, which dimerizes with the AhR nuclear translocator (Arnt), in response to many polycyclic aromatic hydrocarbons (PAHs) regulate cytochrome P450 genes. There is little known about the development of these NRs in humans and animals. A recent survey of NR development in the rat showed minimal expression of PXR mRNA and protein in the fetus, but there was a gradual increase to adult levels after weaning [38]. Miki and associates [39] found very low expression of PXR mRNA and protein (also known as SXR) in human fetal and neonatal liver compared with young adults. In another report, expression of CAR mRNA and protein was very low but not absent in neonatal human and mouse livers [40].

Cytochrome (CYP) P450 enzymes perform the majority of phase I reactions. In humans, 57 CYP enzymes have been identified and are classified into families according to sequence homology [33]. Overall expression is highest in the liver, but significant and even exclusive expression can be found for some CYPs in other tissues [33]. Developmental expression of CYP enzymes is one of the key factors determining the pharmacokinetic status pre- and postnatally [41]. Drug-metabolizing cytochrome P450 enzymes, the major phase I enzymes, are active in human liver at very early stages of intrauterine development, albeit at much lower concentrations than in the adult. The liver of the human fetus and even the embryo possesses relatively well-developed metabolism of xenobiotics. There is experimental evidence for the presence of CYP1A1, CYP1B1, CYP2C8, CYP2D6, CYP2E1, CYP3A4, CYP3A5, and CYP3A7 in the fetal liver after the embryonic phase (approximately 8 to 9 weeks of gestation) [42]. Significant xenobiotic metabolism also occurs during organogenesis (before 8 weeks of gestation). The major increase in both activity and number of different enzymes takes place after birth, probably during the first year of life. Information concerning these developmental changes in the human is incomplete [34]. Figure 2.1 shows the postnatal development of several of the more important CYP450 enzymes.

The CYP3A subfamily is the most abundant of the CYP enzymes, involved in the metabolism of approximately 50% of commonly used medications [43,44]. CYP3A7, the major fetal hepatic cytochrome (30–50% of total liver P450), is uniquely present during organogenesis, and it is involved in steroid metabolism [45]. Expression declines after the first postnatal week and is nondetectable in most livers by 1 year of age. Variably detectable in the fetus, CYP3A5 is expressed at significant levels in about half of all children [46]. CYP3A4 is the major functional member of the CYP3A subfamily expressed postnatally and metabolizes over 75 drugs [42]. CYP3A4 expression is low in the fetus and newborn, but reaches 50% of adult values between 6 and 12 months of age [44]. CYP3A4 is induced by many drugs, including phenytoin and rifampin, and can be inhibited by erythromycin, cimetidine, and many other commonly used agents.

CYP1A1 is also present during organogenesis, and metabolizes exogenous toxins, some of which are procarcinogens [43]. CYP1A1 expression declines with age and is not detectable in adult liver. CYP1A2, important in its metabolism of caffeine and theophylline, is not expressed significantly in fetal liver, exists at a very low level in the neonate, but reaches adult levels by the fourth or fifth postnatal month [46].

The CYP2C subfamily metabolizes many clinically important drugs. CYP2C8 and CYP2C9 are minimally expressed in fetal liver [43]. CYP2C9, which metabolizes phenytoin, achieves the level of adult activity by 1–6 months postnatally and exceeds adult activity by 3–10 years of age. Eleven polymorphisms of CYP2C9 have been detected and add a further layer of complexity in considering the therapeutic efficacy or potential for toxicity of drugs such as ibuprofen and indomethacin, which are used in the neonate and are substrates for this enzyme.

CYP2E1 may be present in some second-trimester fetuses and is involved in metabolism of organic solvents including alcohol and is the primary enzyme involved in the generation of N-acetyl-P-benzoquinone-imine (NAPQI), the hepatotoxic metabolite of acetaminophen. CYP2E1 activity is low in the fetus, reaches 30–40% of adult levels by 1 year, and is fully expressed by age 10 years [43].

After birth, hepatic CYP2D6 becomes active. CYP2D6 has many genetic polymorphisms leading to differing capacities to metabolize exogenous drugs, including psychotropic drugs and antihypertensives [42].

The flavin-containing monooxygenases (FMOs), encoded by six genes, mediate the NADPH-dependent oxidative metabolism of a wide variety of drugs, such as chlorpromazine and promethazine, as well as environmental toxins [42]. FMO isoform switching occurs in the human from FMO1 in fetal liver to FMO3 in the adult [47]. FMO1 is most highly expressed at 8–15 weeks of gestation, declines through the rest of gestation, and is completely suppressed within 3 days after birth. FMO3 expression occurs by 1–2 years of age. A further increase in FMO3 expression is observed from 10–18 years of age.

The development of phase II enzymes, including glucuronosyl transferases, sulfotransferases, glutathione S-transferases (GSTs), *N*-acetyltransferases, and methyl transferases, has been studied less well than that of the cytochrome P450 system [42]. Sufficient information is available to indicate that important differences in the activities of these enzymes exist between children and adults and that each phase II enzyme in which these data are known follows a distinct pattern of development.

An important group of conjugation reactions are catalyzed by the uridine diphosphate UGP-glucuronosyltransferases (UGTs) [42]. The UGTs, with more than ten known isoforms, are involved not only in the glucuronidation of many hydrophobic drugs such as morphine and acetaminophen but also the biotransformation of important endogenous substrates, including bilirubin and ethinylestradiol. However, isoform specificity for these substrates has not been fully characterized. Serious adverse events associated with inadequate glucuronidation of chloramphenicol in the neonate have highlighted the importance of developmental changes in UGT activity. There are significant isoform-specific differences, which preclude a generalization of a simple developmental pattern for UGT activity. UGT2B7 is the only UGT isoform that has been characterized during ontogeny both in vitro and in vivo, using morphine as the probe drug [48]. Glucuronidation of morphine in 15–27-week fetuses is only 10–20% that of the adult. Morphine metabolism usually reaches adult capacity between 2 and 6 months, but may not fully mature in some individuals until 30 months of age. Genetic polymorphisms have been identified for the UGT family, for not only the *UGT1A* gene, which glucuronidates bilirubin, but also three other UGT isoforms. Mutations of the *UGT1A* gene lead to Crigler–Najjar and Gilbert's syndromes, inherited forms of hyperbilirubinemia. The impact of these genetic differences on drug metabolism remains to be established because of overlapping isoform specificity of the drugs studied as well as a lack of specific probe substrates to test the activity of individual UGT isoforms in relation to these gene mutations [48].

GSTs are a group of dimeric enzymes that conjugate glutathione to a wide variety of electrophilic compounds [49]. Thirteen GST subunits have been assigned to eight different families that demonstrate considerable overlap in substrate specificity [42]. The developmental expression of these enzymes is not well defined. Hepatic GSTA1 and GSTA2 have been detected at 10 weeks of gestation and attain adult levels by 1–2 years of age [50]. GSTM is minimally expressed in the fetus but dramatically increases to adult levels after birth. In contrast, GSTP1 is highly expressed in the first trimester and decreases progressively through gestation. Enzyme activity is still detectable in the neonate but is absent from adult liver. The functional significance of these ontogenic changes remains unknown.

The development of *N*-acetyltransferase 2 (NAT2) has been studied in human fetal liver. Genetic variation in the *NAT2* locus accounts for the rapid or slow acetylator status of individuals important in metabolism of isoniazid [51]. Acetylation activity by this enzyme was absent during the first 14 weeks of gestation, with some activity detected by 16 weeks gestation [42]. All infants between 0 and 55 days of age were phenotypically slow acetylators. Fifty percent of infants 122–224 days of age and 62% of those 225–342 days of age were found to be fast acetylators. NAT2 activity seemed to be fully expressed by 3 years of age, with 50% expressing the slow acetylation phenotypes, similar to the adult population [52].

Sulfotransferases (SULTs) catalyze the transfer of a sulfuryl group to a plethora of drugs, endogenous substrates, and xenobiotics [42]. There are at least 11 isoforms with overlapping substrate specificity. The pattern and extent of expression of the various SULT isoforms during development are not well defined [53]. Several isoforms have been studied in detail. Hepatic SULT2A1, important for steroid metabolism, is expressed at low levels at 25 weeks' gestation and increases to near adult levels in the neonate. Hepatic SULT1A3 is involved in catecholamine metabolism and is highly expressed in early gestation and progressively declines through the late fetal and neonatal periods. The enzyme cannot be detected in adult liver. Overall, fetal and neonatal livers have significant capacity for sulfation at a time when other phase II enzymes critical for detoxification, particularly UGTs, are poorly developed.

Epoxide hydroxylase is an enzyme critical to the hydrolysis of epoxide metabolites produced by phase I reactions

[54]. Microsomal (EPHX1) and cytosolic (EPHX2) forms exist. Substrates for microsomal epoxide hydroxolase include arene oxide intermediates of several aromatic anticonvulsants, such as phenytoin and carbamazepine. In human fetal liver, microsomal epoxide hydroxylase activity has been found to be correlated with both increasing gestational age and protein concentration. After 22 weeks of gestation, fetal activity is approximately 50% of that observed in adult liver [55]. There is less known about the ontogeny of EPHX2. Enzyme activity can be detected in fetal liver at 14 weeks of gestation and by 27 weeks, is about 20% of activity in adult liver [49].

There is limited information about the development of membrane transport proteins that participate in phase III of drug metabolism. The multidrug resistance gene 1 (*MDR1*) encodes a critical efflux pump, P-glycoprotein, located on the canalicular membrane of hepatocytes [32]. MDR1 mRNA was very low in human fetal and neonatal livers in comparison with young adults [39]. The multidrug resistance–related protein 2 (*MRP2, ABCC2*) is an ATP-dependent transport protein mediating the excretion of multivalent anionic molecules including glutathione conjugates and glucuronidated compounds. MRP2 mRNA has recently been studied in human fetal livers at gestational age 14–20 weeks and was present at 50% of the amount found in adult livers. Moreover, MRP2 showed mainly canalicular localization, which was indistinct compared with adult liver [56].

HEPATOBILIARY FUNCTION DURING DEVELOPMENT

Knowledge of the capacity for hepatic bile formation and excretory function during human development is incomplete and is derived largely from indirect evidence (Table 2.3) [57,58]. For example, biliary bile acid concentrations are low during fetal and neonatal development and increase progressively in response to maturation of pathways for bile acid biosynthesis and with increasing capacity for transport within the intestinal and hepatic limbs of the enterohepatic circulation [59]. Colombo et al. [60] found that total bile acid concentrations were extremely low (<0.05 mmol/L) in human fetal bile before 17 weeks of gestation but increased 20-fold between 16 and 20 weeks, reflecting a surge in bile acid synthesis. Even at birth in the full-term infant, however, biliary bile acid concentrations remain relatively low in comparison with those in the older child and adult [59]. The ability of the fetal and neonatal gallbladder to concentrate bile acids also appears to be less developed than that of the adult. The concentration of bile acids measured in collections of duodenal bile after stimulation with either a milk feeding or magnesium sulfate is reduced in comparison with the older child [61]. In several studies involving human neonates, intraluminal bile acid concentrations of 1–2 mmol/L have been found after meal stimulation and exhibit little variation throughout the day [57]. In term neonates, cholic acid pool size measured by isotopic dilution methods was smaller (290 ± 236 mg/m^2) than that of adults (605 ± 122 mg/m^2) [62].

Table 2.3: Ontogeny of Hepatic Excretory Function

Synthesis of unusual bile acids in the fetus and neonate
Decreased bile acid pool size
Low intraluminal bile acid concentrations in the intestine and gallbladder
Inefficient ileal bile acid readsorption
Low rate of bile acid clearance from portal blood
Elevated serum bile acid concentrations in the neonate

Total pool size was even smaller in premature infants and correlated directly with extremely low intraluminal bile acid concentrations measured in the duodenum postprandially [63]. Bile secretion and bile acid output appear to function near a maximum during early life and cannot be stimulated further by the hormonal milieu of the postprandial period. Bile acid synthesis, bile acid pool size, intraluminal bile acid concentrations, and presumably bile secretion increase gradually during the first year of life in the human [57,64]. The factors that control the development of the enterohepatic circulation of bile acids remain largely unexplored. It has been demonstrated that infants whose mothers were treated with dexamethasone before birth to induce lung maturation in the fetus also exhibited a significant increase in intraluminal bile acid concentrations during meals, which averaged 5.3 mmol/L in infants of treated mothers compared with 1.8 mmol/L in infants of untreated mothers [63]. This marked increase in intraluminal bile acid concentrations was associated with a fourfold increment in bile acid pool size. Thus, corticosteroids probably have a role in influencing the development of bile acid synthesis.

Bile acid synthesis and metabolism in the liver of human fetuses and neonates are significantly different from that occurring in the liver of adults [65,66]. The presence of relatively high proportions of hyocholic acid (often greater than cholic acid) and several 1β-hydroxycholanoic acid isomers indicates that C-1, C-4, and C-6 hydroxylation are important pathways in bile acid synthesis during development [67]. Relatively large amounts of unusual bile acids are detected during infancy, especially during the period up to 1 month of age. At that time, $1\beta,3\alpha,7\alpha,12\alpha$-tetrahydroxy-$5\beta$-cholan-24-oic, $7\alpha,12\alpha$-dihydroxy-3-oxo-5β-chol-1-en-24-oic, and $7\alpha,12\alpha$-dihydroxy-3-oxo-4-cholen-24-oic acids are predominant among the unusual urinary bile acids present [66]. These bile acids are unlikely to be good substrates for transport by basolateral and canalicular transporters and may not be ligands for the NR farnesoid X receptor (FXR), which is critical for regulation of bile acid homeostasis.

The development of hepatic excretory function in the infant has been followed using serum bile acid concentrations as a measure of the efficiency of hepatic transport [68]. Uptake of bile acids by the adult liver is extremely efficient, with a high first-pass extraction rate. The fractional extraction varies considerably according to bile acid structure but may exceed 90% for conjugates of cholic acid. The serum level of bile acids for

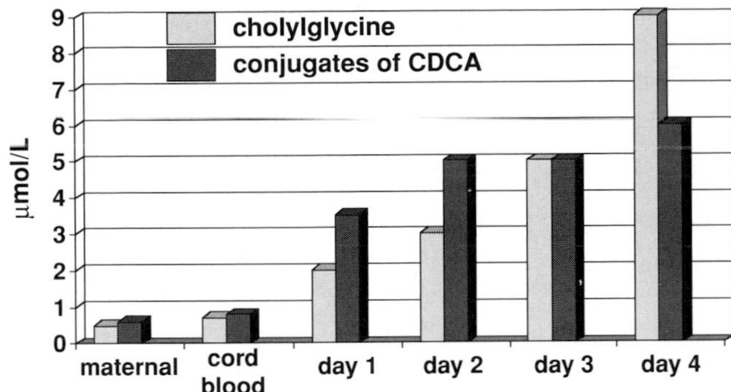

Figure 2.2. Serum concentrations of conjugates of cholic acid and chenodeoxycholic acid in normal newborns. (Redrawn from Suchy et al. [68], with permission).

a healthy human fetus is determined by spillover reaching the liver from the intestine. In the human fetus, it has been shown that the bile acid concentrations are lower in serum from the umbilical artery than from the umbilical vein, indicating that fetal serum bile acid concentrations are maintained at a relatively low level by net transport across the placenta to the mother [69]. Specific transport mechanisms of brush border and basal membranes of the human placental syncytiotrophoblast mediate the bidirectional transfer of bile acids, between the fetal and maternal circulations [70]. After birth, the conjugates of the primary bile acids cholate and chenodeoxycholate increase progressively in serum to reach concentrations during the first week of life that are significantly higher than in normal older children and adults and similar to patients with cholestatic liver disease (Figure 2.2) [68]. Unlike the transient physiologic hyperbilirubinemia of the newborn, serum bile acids levels remain elevated to a degree similar to that in infants 6–8 weeks of age. A gradual decline to adult level occurs only after 6 months of life [68]. It is important to recognize that serum bile acids are an enterohepatic "entity" with levels being determined not only by hepatic uptake but also by intestinal absorption. The rate of intestinal absorption of bile acids is determined by the load, by the intrahepatic concentrations, and by the kinetics of passive and active absorption from the intestine. The high levels observed in the serum of infants are remarkable because of the lower bile acid pool size and the immature mechanisms for intestinal reabsorption that also have been documented during this time of life [57]. The elevation of serum bile acid concentrations during the first year of life has been referred to in the literature as *physiologic cholestasis* or *physiologic hypercholanemia* of infancy [68].

Hepatocellular transport of a number of other organic anions, including the xenobiotics digoxin, eosin, indocyanine green, and bromosulfophthalein, has been studied during mammalian development [71]. The hepatic uptake of these compounds is decreased in developing compared with mature animals. Bromosulfophthalein, a substrate for the same plasma membrane carrier used by bilirubin, has been examined in several studies to evaluate the hepatic excretory function in normal human infants [72]. Tested at birth, full-term and premature infants demonstrated delayed clearance of bromosulfophthalein from serum compared with adults if given a dose comparable on the basis of body weight. Decreased uptake of bromosulfophthalein, as well as an altered volume of distribution, has been noted in the neonatal period. The ability to remove bromosulfophthalein from the circulation improved during the first month of life. The clearance of indocyanine green also was decreased in a group of normal full-term neonates [73]. The low rate of indocyanine green elimination and the low affinity constant compared with older children and adults were attributed to a possible altered hepatic blood flow or a decreased intrinsic capacity of the liver to extract this anion from the portal circulation.

Bile secretion starts at the beginning of the fourth month of gestation in the human, and thereafter the biliary system constantly contains bile, which is secreted into the gut and colors its contents (meconium) a dark green [65]. There is little additional information about the maturation of the process of bile formation in the human fetus and neonate. Owing to technical difficulties in performing physiologic studies in the fetus, there also is limited information about the process in animal models. Available studies indicate that the process is immature in the near-term fetus in comparison with the adult. For example, Little et al. [74] have demonstrated in the term fetal rhesus monkey that the sum of radiolabeled taurocholate recovered in fetal gallbladder plus intestinal contents averaged only 34% of a dose infused intravenously [74]. A substantial proportion (18–40%) was excreted across the placenta and was recovered in maternal bile. Immaturity of hepatic organic anion transport was demonstrated further by the failure of the fetal monkey liver to excrete unconjugated or conjugated (^{14}C) bilirubin into bile [75]. Spontaneous bile flow also was found to be significantly lower in near-term fetal sheep and dogs in comparison with that observed in adult animals, even though these species are thought to be precocious with respect to the maturation of hepatic excretory function [76,77].

Studies in neonatal and, to a lesser extent, fetal animals indicate that rates of bile secretion, bile acid excretion, and bile acid excretion in response to an exogenous infusion of bile acids are decreased in comparison with the adult [78,79]. Bile flow is lowest in the most immature animals and increases progressively with postnatal age. There are significant differences among species as to how much of this developmental change is related to bile flow stimulated by bile acids or the so-called bile acid–dependent fraction of bile flow. In both the rabbit and dog models, there was an increased biliary clearance of inulin in infant animals, suggesting increased entry at the level of the canalicular membrane or through the paracellular pathway [78,79]. It is possible that an increase in biliary permeability in the immature animal may allow greater excretion of water and electrolytes to maintain low rates of bile flow despite reduced bile salt secretion and a low rate of bile salt–independent flow. In keeping with the concept of a period of physiologic cholestasis in a neonate, the increase in biliary tract permeability frequently is observed in experimental models of cholestasis.

In the rat there is evidence that a developmentally related increase in bile flow rate was principally a result of the increase in bile acid–independent flow. Hepatic glutathione was low in the fetus but increased to approximate adult levels by 7 days postnatally. In contrast, significant efflux of glutathione and its constituent amino acids into bile did not occur until weaning (21 days of age). During weaning, there was a fivefold increase in the biliary glutathione and a twofold increase in bile flow rate. Biliary bile acid concentration remained constant throughout this period of development, with only a 30–50% increase in its secretion rate [80].

Factors such as hormones and second messenger systems regulate bile flow but have not been studied extensively during development [81,82]. In dogs studied during the first 3 days of life, the administration of secretin or glucagon failed to stimulate bile flow or produced only a minimal choleretic effect [81]. In these animals, biliary bicarbonate excretion in response to secretin increased with age and in parallel with the stimulation of bile flow. High plasma levels of these secretagogues have been detected in the young of other species. One interpretation of these findings is that spontaneous bile secretion in neonatal animals such as the dog is stimulated maximally by these hormones, so that exogenous administration no longer produces a choleretic effect. The age-related choleresis may indicate maturation of receptors for these hormones on the surface membrane of hepatocytes or biliary epithelial cells or of the postreceptor response to agonist binding.

Bile flow into the duodenum depends on bile acid secretion determined by hepatic secretory function and also on active contraction of the main biliary storage organ, the gallbladder. Recent studies have examined the volume and contractility of the gallbladder in neonates [59]. In term infants, it is not surprising that fasting gallbladder volume was larger than in premature infants [83]. Term neonates more readily showed significant gallbladder contraction. In preterm infants, significant contraction was observed after conceptual age of 31 weeks or with body weight greater than 1300 g [84]. In enterally fed term neonates, a 50% reduction in gallbladder volume was observed 15 minutes after starting the feeding, with return to a baseline volume by 90 minutes. In other studies, preterm infants of more than 33 weeks' gestation showed a gallbladder response to feeding with a contraction index of at least 50%. Very preterm infants (gestational age of 27–32 weeks) showed no postprandial gallbladder contraction, or the contraction index was under 50% [84,85]. In a follow-up study of nine very preterm infants, the contraction index exceeded 50% at a postconceptual age of 29–32 weeks [85]. The contraction index in these preterm infants was dependent on gestational age at birth and on the bolus volume of feeding.

The mechanical performance of the gallbladder in its ability to attain adequate intraluminal pressures has been examined in newborn piglets [86]. The intraluminal pressure was found to be lower at similar gallbladder volumes, and the increase in pressure subsequent to stimulation by cholecystokinin (CCK) was less in neonatal than in adult gallbladders. In situ, neonatal gallbladders were found to be three- to 12-fold less compliant than in the adult. Additional studies indicated that the neonatal gallbladder smooth muscle was responsive to both histamine and CCK; however, sufficient smooth muscle mass may not be present to lead to an appreciable change in gallbladder compliance. These data suggest that adequate intraluminal pressures probably are not generated in this neonatal model to overcome the resistances offered by the common bile duct and sphincter of Oddi.

CELLULAR MECHANISMS OF BILE FORMATION DURING DEVELOPMENT

Similar to the process in mature animals, bile formation during development is critically dependent on the functional capacity of the basolateral sodium pump as well as on the ontogenesis of specific carriers for bile acids and other ions on the plasma membrane [58]. Almost all of the information about the cellular mechanisms of hepatic transport are derived from studies using isolated hepatocytes and domain-specific plasma membrane vesicles in experimental animals.

The ontogenesis of Na^+-K^+ adenosine triphosphatase (ATPase) activity, which provides the driving force for many membrane transport processes involved in ion uptake and excretion, has been studied in rodent liver and differs somewhat from other tissues, such as intestine and kidney. Enzyme activity was significantly lower in basolateral membranes from late fetal (day 21 or 22 of gestation) and neonatal (day 1) rat liver compared with membranes from the adult [87]. Kinetic analysis of Na^+-K^+ ATPase activity at various concentrations of ATPase revealed that the maximum velocity (V_{max}) of the enzyme reaction was 70% and 90% of adult activity in the fetus and neonate, respectively. These differences in enzyme activity were statistically significant, but it is not known whether these differences in enzyme activity are of biologic importance because of the large reserve capacity of this transporter for ion pumping. Measurements of enzyme activity and protein content in membrane fractions in vitro may not correlate directly with the capacity of intact hepatocytes for cation pumping. In keeping with this concept, another study demonstrated greater ouabain-inhibitable uptake of Rb^+ (a substrate for the sodium-potassium pump) by hepatocytes isolated from neonatal compared with mature rats [88]. Available studies indicate that the activity of Na^+-K^+ ATPase is unlikely to be rate limiting during development in providing the driving forces for the transport system involved in bile formation.

Bile acid transport across the basolateral plasma membrane of the hepatocyte occurs largely through an Na^+-dependent cotransport mechanism [89]. Studies in hepatocytes and basolateral plasma membrane vesicles isolated from fetal and neonatal rats indicate that this process is developmentally regulated [87,90]. Transport activity is absent through much of gestation but is expressed just prior to birth. There is a progressive increase in transport activity during postnatal development. Adult rates of bile acid uptake are attained just after the time of weaning. Analysis of transport kinetics reveals no change in K_m, a possible reflection of carrier affinity for bile acids, but a fourfold increase in V_{max} between 7 and 56 days of life [91].

The mechanisms for the intracellular transport of bile acids and other organic anions from sinusoidal to the canalicular domain remain poorly understood in developing and mature liver. Possible age-related changes in intracellular compartmentalization have been demonstrated in isolated hepatocytes loaded with labeled taurocholate. In these studies, after preloading with radiolabeled plus cold bile acid (5–100 μmol/L), total taurocholate efflux, estimated by the decrease in cell taurocholate content, was unexpectedly greater from suckling compared with adult rat hepatocytes [92]. Insight into why intracellular sequestration of bile acids is less effective in the developing animal in comparison with the adult has been evaluated further by assessing the activity of a cytosolic bile acid–binding peptide. The activity of the bile acid–binding protein was found to be decreased markedly in fetal and neonatal rat liver in comparison to older age groups [93]. The concentration of the protein did not approach adult levels until 14 days postnatally. mRNA for the hepatic 3α-hydroxysteroid dehydrogenase, the major bile binder in rat liver, was detectable on fetal day 20 and increased progressively after birth [93]. Development of the capacity to bind bile acids within the cell seems to parallel the maturation of mechanisms for bile acid uptake, synthesis, and canalicular excretion.

Preliminary studies also have been done to define developmental changes in bile acid transport across the canalicular plasma membrane. An ATP-dependent process with properties virtually identical to that described in the adult also was present in 7 day–old rat liver canalicular membrane vesicles (F. J. Suchy and M. Ananthanarayanan; unpublished observations). V_{max} for ATP-dependent transport was approximately 60% of that determined in adult liver; K_m was similar at both ages. An ATP-dependent system is functional in neonatal liver and may be sufficient for biliary secretion of bile acids at a time when other components of the enterohepatic circulation of bile acids (including synthesis, pool size, ileal absorption, basolateral transport, and potential dependent canalicular excretion) are immature.

The molecular bases of developmental changes in anion transporters are being elucidated. Detailed studies on the basolateral sodium taurocholate cotransporting polypeptide (Ntcp) have shown that Ntcp mRNA is absent throughout much of rat gestation and first detected at day 20 of fetal life, reaching adult levels at day 7 after birth [94]. In addition, Ntcp protein is detected shortly after birth in a partially glycosylated form that persists up to 4 weeks of age. The level of transcription of the *Ntcp* gene, as assessed by nuclear run-on studies, is relatively low up to day 21 of gestation, with an abrupt increase at day 1 and reaching adult levels by 1 week of life. It is unknown how critical transcription factors, including HNF1 and the NRs RXR/retinoic acid receptor-α (RARα), which regulate transcription of *Ntcp*, are involved in the developmental expression of this transporter [95,96]. Transcriptional and posttranscriptional mechanisms seem to be involved in the developmental regulation of Ntcp expression.

Tomer et al. [97] have studied the development of the rat bile salt export pump (Bsep, ABCB11) at the level of transcription and by quantitation of Bsep mRNA and protein in fetal and neonatal rats [97]. Bsep mRNA was expressed minimally in the near-term fetus and increased abruptly to 50% of adult levels on postnatal day 1 and further to 90% of adult values by 1 week of life [97]. There was minimal expression of Bsep protein before birth, with an increase to 40% of the adult on the first day of life. Bsep protein levels increased to 90% of the adult by 1 week of life and further increased to adult values by 4 weeks of life. The patterns of mRNA and protein expression are quite similar prenatally and postnatally in two other studies [98,99]. There was minimal transcription of the *Bsep* gene assessed by nuclear run-on assays at the fetal age, with an abrupt increase in transcription on the first day of life. Transcription rates in adult nuclei were not significantly different from nuclei from 1-week old rat livers [97].

Zinchuk et al. [98] have localized Bsep in developing rat liver using immunofluorescence microscopy. Similar to the Western blotting results, Bsep immunofluorescence was not detected in fetal liver. In the newborn animals, the staining of bile canaliculi was indistinct, whereas in adults it was very compact and sharply defined. In livers of 1 week–old but not adult rats, fluorescence was frequently seen in subapical areas of hepatocytes possibly belonging to the so-called subapical vesicular compartment.

The development of BSEP has recently been studied in human fetal liver samples at gestational age of 14–20 weeks [56]. The mean expression levels of BSEP mRNA were 30% of adult values. The immunohistochemical localization of BSEP in fetal liver differed from the adult liver. In the adult liver, there was sharp-linear staining of bile canaliculi for BSEP. However, in fetal liver, BSEP showed a partially intracellular and partially canalicular pattern. These findings suggested decreased expression of BSEP and inefficient targeting of BSEP to the canalicular membrane in the fetus [56].

Mrp2 transports conjugated bilirubin and glutathione conjugates. Mrp2 mRNA levels were low through most of rat gestation, increased to about 30% of adult levels just after birth and reached adult levels by 1 week of age [99]. Nuclear run-on assays confirmed low transcription of *Mrp2* in the fetus and adult rates by 1 week of age [97]. There was minimal Mrp2 protein expression at the fetal stages (at fetal days 20 and 21), with an abrupt increase at postnatal day 1. At 1 week of life, Mrp2 protein expression reached 35% of the adult, and by 4 weeks of age, it was up to 70% of the adult level.

MRP2 expression was recently assessed in human fetal livers at 14–20 weeks of gestation [56]. MRP2 mRNA was present at approximately 50% of the adult concentration in these livers. MRP2 showed mainly canalicular localization on immunofluorescence microscopy, but the pattern of staining was indistinct compared to adults.

Bile salts can regulate the expression of transport systems through the action of critical NRs that are transcription factors that bind bile acids as ligands [100]. FXR, the most important of these receptors, is a member of the NR1 family of NRs and binds to an inverted repeat motif as a heterodimer with the retinoid X receptor alpha (RXRα). Bile salt transporter genes that are directly or indirectly regulated by FXR include *BSEP*, *MRP2*, rat *Ntcp*, *OATP-C*, and *OATP8* in hepatocytes, and *I-BABP* and *ASBT* (apical sodium-dependent transporter) in the intestine. Activation of the bile salt efflux pumps BSEP and MRP2 by bile acids is an important adaptive mechanism by which hydrophobic bile acids can promote their own excretion into bile [101]. Repression of bile salt transporter genes by FXR occurs indirectly. Rat *Ntcp*, human *OATP-C*, and mouse *ASBT* are transcriptionally repressed by bile salts through FXR-mediated induction of the small heterodimer partner (SHP). SHP is an NR (NR0B2) that does not bind ligands but interacts with other NRs to inhibit their effects on gene expression [100].

Because of the central role of several NRs in regulating bile acid homeostasis and other transport systems that contribute to bile formation, development of the most important NRs has recently been studied [102]. For the purposes of this review, only the data related to FXR and SHP are discussed.

Real-time polymerase chain reaction analysis of hepatic NR expression from fetal day 17 through adult revealed that steady-state mRNA levels for all NRs were low during the embryonic period [102]. FXR mRNA was barely detected at 1.5–5.9% of adult levels between embryonic days 17 and 21. However, on postnatal day 1, mRNA rose to 13.6%, and on day 7 there was a further rise to 101% of adult values. The level remained between 104% and 117% for the next 14 days but increased to 144% by day 21 of life. In contrast to FXR, the RXRα mRNA level remained relatively low, between 4.4% and 35%, between embryonic day 17 and postnatal day 7 and reached 69.9% of adult level during postnatal week 4. These data suggest that different mechanisms of transcriptional regulation are operative for FXR and RXRα.

SHP is a non–DNA binding protein of the NR family that acts as a strong repressor of many genes, including *cyp7a1* and *Ntcp*. The expression of SHP mRNA is low throughout the embryonic period (days 17–20), remaining at 0.25–0.35% of the adult. On embryonic day 21, SHP mRNA was 8.3% of the adult but increased and was maintained at 60% of adult values between postnatal days 1 and 14. The amount of mRNA reached adult levels by day 21.

The amount of FXR protein was at 16.8% of adult values on embryonic days 20 and postnatal day 7. However, because FXR mRNA was at 100% of adult level on postnatal day 7, posttranscriptional regulatory mechanisms are likely involved in determining FXR expression in the postnatal period. At 4 weeks of age, protein levels rose to 75.2% of the adult.

There was also significant disparity between mRNA and protein levels with regard to RXRα in the developing liver. Whereas the mRNA levels remained at 32.8–69.9% at postnatal days 7–28, protein levels were at 113.6% and 96.5% at days 7 and 28, respectively. Because RXRα heterodimerizes with all of the type II NRs, its availability, possibly enhanced by a long half-life, may not be limiting the activity of these receptors in the postnatal period.

Despite the extremely low levels of SHP mRNA during embryonic days 17–20 (0.25–0.35% of adult), SHP protein was 8.4% of the adult level at embryonic day 20. However, during the postnatal period, there was good correlation between the mRNA and protein levels for this potent repressor of cyp7a1 and Ntcp. On the basis of these data, it is likely that the repressive effect of SHP on transporter gene expression is significant only during the postnatal period.

The functional expression of FXR/RXRα was also assessed by electromobility shift assays (EMSAs). The complex formed by binding of FXR to its inverted repeat (IR-1) element was 32% of the adult amount on embryonic day 20 and reached adult levels by postnatal day 28. Comparison of the degree of FXR binding in the EMSA to the amount of its mRNA demonstrates more activity than can be accounted for by the level of mRNA, implying additional levels of posttranscriptional control. However, in the postnatal period, the temporal pattern of the EMSA compares well with mRNA levels (full activity at day 28), indicating transcriptional regulation as the major mechanism of control.

The clinical implications of immature hepatic excretory function are well known to pediatricians. Liver dysfunction in the neonate, regardless of the cause, commonly is associated with a failure of bile secretion and cholestatic jaundice. It is not uncommon to observe cholestasis in association with gram-negative infections, during a parenteral nutrition, and during the initial presentation of a variety of inborn errors of metabolism. Increasing numbers of reports of biliary sludge formation and gallstones in critically ill infants may be a reflection of immature hepatic excretory function, particularly in regard to the excretion of bile acids. It is likely that additional forms of inherited cholestasis will be proven eventually to represent exaggeration or persistence of a developmental deficit in hepatic ion transport or bile acid metabolism. Profound cholestasis and progressive liver failure can occur in infants with several inherited defects in the pathway for the biosynthesis of bile acids. In these disorders, the lack of primary bile acids critical for generating canalicular bile flow and the toxicity of abnormal bile acid precursors lead to cholestasis and progressive liver injury [103].

REFERENCES

1. Alcorn J, McNamara PJ. Pharmacokinetics in the newborn. Adv Drug Deliv Rev 2003;55:667–86.
2. Greengard O. Regulation of enzyme amounts in developing liver. Biochem J 1972;130:48P–49P.
3. Greengard O. Enzymic differentiation in mammalian liver injection of fetal rats with hormones causes the premature formation of liver enzymes. Science 1969;163:891–5.
4. Greengard O. Effects of hormones on development of fetal enzymes. Clin Pharmacol Ther 1973;14:721–6.
5. Cowett RM, Farrag HM. Selected principles of perinatal-neonatal glucose metabolism. Semin Neonatol 2004;9:37–47.
6. Hume R, Burchell A, Williams FL, Koh DK. Glucose homeostasis in the newborn. Early Hum Dev 2005;81:95–101.

7. Kalhan S, Parimi, P. Gluconeogenesis in the fetus and neonate. Semin Perinatol 2000;24:94–106.
8. Narkewicz MR. Hepatic energy metabolism in the fetus and neonate. In: Suchy FJ, ed. Liver disease in children. Philadelphia: Mosby–Year Book, 1994:39–56.
9. Battaglia FC, Meschia G. Principal substrates of fetal metabolism. Physiol Rev 1978;58:499–527.
10. Kalhan SC, Parimi P, Van Beek R, et al. Estimation of gluconeogenesis in newborn infants. Am J Physiol Endocrinol Metab 2001;281:E991–7.
11. Yubero P, Hondares E, Carmona MC, et al. The developmental regulation of peroxisome proliferator-activated receptor-γ coactivator-1α expression in the liver is partially dissociated from the control of gluconeogenesis and lipid catabolism. Endocrinology 2004;145:4268–77.
12. Herzog B, Hall RK, Wang XL, et al. Peroxisome proliferator-activated receptor gamma coactivator-1alpha, as a transcription amplifier, is not essential for basal and hormone-induced phosphoenolpyruvate carboxykinase gene expression. Mol Endocrinol 2004;18:807–19.
13. Cetin I. Amino acid interconversions in the fetal-placental unit: the animal model and human studies in vivo. Pediatr Res 2001;49:148–54.
14. Regnault TR, de Vrijer B, Battaglia FC. Transport and metabolism of amino acids in placenta. Endocrine 2002;19:23–41.
15. Jozwik M, Teng C, Wilkening RB, et al. Reciprocal inhibition of umbilical uptake within groups of amino acids. Am J Physiol Endocrinol Metab 2004;286:E376–83.
16. Teng C, Battaglia FC, Meschia G, et al. Fetal hepatic and umbilical uptakes of glucogenic substrates during a glucagon-somatostatin infusion. Am J Physiol Endocrinol Metab 2002; 282:E542–50.
17. McClellan R, Novak D. Fetal nutrition: how we become what we are. J Pediatr Gastroenterol Nutr 2001;33:233–44.
18. Neu J, Auestad N, DeMarco VG. Glutamine metabolism in the fetus and critically ill low birth weight neonate. Adv Pediatr 2002;49:203–26.
19. Battaglia FC. In vivo characteristics of placental amino acid transport and metabolism in ovine pregnancy—a review. Placenta 2002;23(Suppl A):S3–8.
20. Vaughn PR, Lobo C, Battaglia FC, et al. Glutamine-glutamate exchange between placenta and fetal liver. Am J Physiol 1995;268(4 Pt 1):E705–11.
21. Sturman J. Developmental aspects of amino acids metabolism with reference to sulfur amino acids. In: Blackburn GL, Grant JP, Young VR, eds. Amino acids: metabolism and medical applications. Boston: John Wright, 1983:29–36.
22. Zlotkin S, Anderson GH. The development of cystathionase activity during the first year of life. Pediatr Res 1982;16:65–8.
23. Herrera E, Amusquivar E. Lipid metabolism in the fetus and the newborn. Diabetes Metab Res Rev 2000;16:202–10.
24. Herrera E. Lipid metabolism in pregnancy and its consequences in the fetus and newborn. Endocrine 2002;19:43–55.
25. Haggarty P. Effect of placental function on fatty acid requirements during pregnancy. Eur J Clin Nutr 2004;58:1559–70.
26. Madsen EM, Lindegaard ML, Andersen CB, et al. Human placenta secretes apolipoprotein B-100-containing lipoproteins. J Biol Chem 2004;279:55271–6.
27. Bougneres P, Karl IE, Hillman LS, et al. Lipid transport in the human newborn: palmitate and glycerol turnover and the contribution of glycerol to neonatal hepatic glucose output. J Clin Invest 1982;70:262–70.
28. Pegorier JP, Prip-Buus C, Duee PH, Girard J. Hormonal control of fatty acid oxidation during the neonatal period. Diabetes Metab 1992;18:156–60.
29. Uauy R, Treen M, Hoffman DR. Essential fatty acid metabolism and requirements during development. Semin Perinatol 1989; 13:118–30.
30. Alcorn J, McNamara PJ. Ontogeny of hepatic and renal systemic clearance pathways in infants: part II. Clin Pharmacokinet 2002;41:1077–94.
31. Becquemont L. Clinical relevance of pharmacogenetics. Drug Metab Rev 2003;35:277–85.
32. Hoffmann U, Kroemer HK. The ABC transporters MDR1 and MRP2: multiple functions in disposition of xenobiotics and drug resistance. Drug Metab Rev 2004;36:669–701.
33. Wilkinson GR. Drug metabolism and variability among patients in drug response. N Engl J Med 2005;352:2211–21.
34. Choudhary D, Jansson I, Sarfarazi M, Schenkman JB. Xenobiotic-metabolizing cytochromes P450 in ontogeny: evolving perspective. Drug Metab Rev 2004;36:549–68.
35. Xu C, Li CY, Kong AN. Induction of phase I, II and III drug metabolism/transport by xenobiotics. Arch Pharm Res 2005; 28:249–68.
36. Tirona RG, Kim RB. Nuclear receptors and drug disposition gene regulation. J Pharm Sci 2005;94:1169–86.
37. Goodwin B, Moore JT. CAR: detailing new models. Trends Pharmacol Sci 2004;25:437–41.
38. Balasubramaniyan N, Shahid M, Suchy FJ, Ananthanarayanan M. Multiple mechanisms of ontogenic regulation of nuclear receptors during rat liver development. Am J Physiol Gastrointest Liver Physiol 2005;288:G251–60.
39. Miki Y, Suzuki T, Tazawa C, et al. Steroid and xenobiotic receptor (SXR), cytochrome P450 3A4 and multidrug resistance gene 1 in human adult and fetal tissues. Mol Cell Endocrinol 2005;231:75–85.
40. Huang W, Zhang J, Chua SS, et al. Induction of bilirubin clearance by the constitutive androstane receptor (CAR). Proc Natl Acad Sci U S A 2003;100:4156–61.
41. Kearns GL, Abdel-Rahman SM, Alander SW, et al. Developmental pharmacology—drug disposition, action, and therapy in infants and children. N Engl J Med 2003;349:1157–67.
42. Blake MJ, Castro L, Leeder JS, Kearns GL. Ontogeny of drug metabolizing enzymes in the neonate. Semin Fetal Neonatal Med 2005;10:123–38.
43. Hines RN, McCarver DG. The ontogeny of human drug-metabolizing enzymes: phase I oxidative enzymes. J Pharmacol Exp Ther 2002;300:355–60.
44. de Wildt SN, Kearns GL, Leeder JS, van den Anker JN. Cytochrome P450 3A: ontogeny and drug disposition. Clin Pharmacokinet 1999;37:485–505.
45. Hakkola J, Tanaka E, Pelkonen O. Developmental expression of cytochrome P450 enzymes in human liver. Pharmacol Toxicol 1998;82:209–17.
46. Hakkola J, Raunio H, Purkunen R, et al. Cytochrome P450 3A expression in the human fetal liver: evidence that CYP3A5 is expressed in only a limited number of fetal livers. Biol Neonate 2001;80:193–201.
47. Koukouritaki SB, Simpson P, Yeung CK, et al. Human hepatic flavin-containing monooxygenases 1 (FMO1) and 3 (FMO3) developmental expression. Pediatr Res 2002;51:236–43.

48. de Wildt SN, Kearns GL, Leeder JS, van den Anker JN. Glucuronidation in humans. Pharmacogenetic and developmental aspects. Clin Pharmacokinet 1999;36:439–52.
49. McCarver DG, Hines RN. The ontogeny of human drug-metabolizing enzymes: phase II conjugation enzymes and regulatory mechanisms. J Pharmacol Exp Ther 2002;300:361–6.
50. Strange RC, Howie AF, Hume R, et al. The development expression of alpha-, mu- and pi-class glutathione S-transferases in human liver. Biochim Biophys Acta 1989;993:186–90.
51. Pariente-Khayat A, Rey E, Gendrel D, et al. Isoniazid acetylation metabolic ratio during maturation in children. Clin Pharmacol Ther 1997;62:377–83.
52. Zielinska E, Bodalski J, Niewiarowski W, et al. Comparison of acetylation phenotype with genotype coding for N-acetyltransferase (NAT2) in children. Pediatr Res 1999;45: 403–8.
53. Coughtrie MW, Sharp S, Maxwell K, Innes NP. Biology and function of the reversible sulfation pathway catalysed by human sulfotransferases and sulfatases. Chem Biol Interact 1998;109: 3–27.
54. Omiecinski CJ, Hassett C, Hosagrahara V. Epoxide hydrolase—polymorphism and role in toxicology. Toxicol Lett 2000;112–113:365–70.
55. Omiecinski CJ, Aicher L, Swenson L. Developmental expression of human microsomal epoxide hydrolase. J Pharmacol Exp Ther 1994;269:417–23.
56. Chen HL, Chen HL, Liu YJ, et al. Developmental expression of canalicular transporter genes in human liver. J Hepatol 2005;43:472–7.
57. Balistreri W, Heubi JE, Suchy FJ. Immaturity of the enterohepatic circulation in early life: factors predisposing to "physiologic" maldigestion and cholestasis. J Pediatr Gastroenterol Nutr 1983;2:346–54.
58. Arrese M, Ananthananarayanan M, Suchy FJ. Hepatobiliary transport: molecular mechanisms of development and cholestasis. Pediatr Res 1998;44:141–7.
59. Halpern Z, Vinograd Z, Laufer H, et al. Characteristics of gallbladder bile of infants and children. J Pediatr Gastroenterol Nutr 1996;23:147–150.
60. Colombo C, Zuliani G, Ronchi M, et al. Biliary bile acid composition of the human fetus in early gestation. Pediatr Res 1987;21:197–200.
61. Ricour C, Rey J. Study of the hydrolysis and micellar solubilization of fats during intestinal perfusion: I. Results in the normal child. Rev Eur Etud Clin Biol 172;17:172–8.
62. Watkins J, Ingall D, Szczepanik P, et al. Bile-salt metabolism in the newborn: measurement of pool size and synthesis by stable isotope technic. N Engl J Med 1973;288:431–4.
63. Watkins J, Szczepanik P, Gould JB, et al. Bile salt metabolism in the human premature infant: preliminary observations of pool size and synthesis rate following prenatal administration of dexamethasone and phenobarbital. Gastroenterology 1975;69: 706–13.
64. Heubi JE, Balistreri WF, Suchy FJ. Bile salt metabolism in the first year of life. J Lab Clin Med 1982;100:127–36.
65. Suchy F, Bucuvalas JC, Novak DA. Determinants of bile formation during development: ontogeny of hepatic bile acid metabolism and transport. Semin Liver Dis 1987;7:77–84.
66. Balistreri W. Fetal and neonatal bile acid synthesis and metabolism—clinical implications. J Inherit Metab Dis 1991;14: 459–77.
67. Setchell KD, Dumaswala R, Colombo C, Ronchi M. Hepatic bile acid metabolism during early development revealed from the analysis of human fetal gallbladder bile. J Biol Chem 1988;263:16637–44.
68. Suchy FJ, Balistreri WF, Heubi JE, et al. Physiologic cholestasis: elevation of the primary serum bile acid concentrations in normal infants. Gastroenterology 1981;80(5 Pt 1):1037–41.
69. Itoh S, Onishi S, Isobe K, et al. Foetomaternal relationships of serum bile acid pattern estimated by high-pressure liquid chromatography. Biochem J 1982;204:141–5.
70. Dumaswala R, Setchell KD, Moyer MS, et al. An anion exchanger mediates bile acid transport across the placental microvillous membrane. Am J Physiol Gastrointest Liver Physiol 1993;264:G1016–23.
71. Klinger W. Biotransformation of drugs and other xenobiotics during postnatal development. Pharmacol Ther 1982;16:377–429.
72. Yudkin S, Gellis SS. Liver function in newborn infants with special reference to bromosulfophthalein. Arch Dis Child 1949; 24:12–14.
73. Helman G, Roth B, Gladke E. [Indocyanin green kinetics in neonates with transient hyperbilirubinemia.] Klin Wochenschr 1977;55:451–6.
74. Little J, Smallwood RA, Lester R, et al. Bile-salt metabolism in the primate fetus. Gastroenterology 1975;69:1315–20.
75. Bernstein R, Novy MJ, Piasecki GJ, et al. Bilirubin metabolism in the fetus. J Clin Invest 1969;48:1678–88.
76. Sewell R, Hardy KJ, Smallwood RA, et al. The hepatic transport of sodium [14C]taurocholate in foetal sheep. Clin Exp Pharmacol Physiol 1979;6:117–20.
77. Smallwood R, Lester R, Plasecki GJ, et al. Fetal bile salt metabolism: II. Hepatic excretion of endogenous bile salt and of a taurocholate load. J Clin Invest 1972;51:1388–97.
78. Shaffer E, Zahavi I, Gall DG. Postnatal development of hepatic bile formation in the rabbit. Dig Dis Sci 1985;30:558–63.
79. Tavoloni N, Jones MJ, Berk PD. Postnatal development of bile secretory physiology in the dog. J Pediatr Gastroenterol Nutr 1985;4:256–67.
80. Mohan P, Ling SC, Watkins JB. Ontogeny of hepatobiliary secretion: role of glutathione. Hepatology 1994;19:1504–12.
81. Tavoloni N. Bile secretion and its control in the newborn puppy. Pediatr Res 1986;20:203–8.
82. Harada E, Kiriyama H, Kobayashi E. Postnatal development of biliary and pancreatic exocrine secretion in piglets. Comp Biochem Physiol 1990;91A:43–51.
83. Ho M, Chen JY, Ling UP, et al. Gallbladder volume and contractility in term and preterm neonates: normal values and clinical applications in ultrasonography. Acta Paediatr 1998;87: 799–804.
84. Lehtonen L, Svedstrom E, Kero P, et al. Gall bladder contractility in preterm infants. Arch Dis Child 1993;68[1 spec no]:43–5.
85. Jawaheer G, Pierro A, Lloyd DA, et al. Gall bladder contractility in neonates: effects of parenteral and enteral feeding [published erratum appears in Arch Dis Child Fetal Neonatal Ed 1995;73:F198]. Arch Dis Child Fetal Neonatal Ed 1995;72: F200–2.
86. Kaplan G, Bhutani VK, Shaffer TH, et al. Gallbladder mechanics in newborn piglets. Pediatr Res 1984;18:1181–4.
87. Suchy FJ, Bucuvalas JC, Goodrich AL, et al. Taurocholate transport and Na^+-K^+-ATPase activity in fetal and neonatal rat liver

plasma membrane vesicles. Am J Physiol 1986;251(5 Pt 1): G665–73.

88. Bellemann P. Amino acid transport and rubidium-ion uptake in monolayer cultures of hepatocytes from neonatal rats. Biochem J 1981;198:475–83.
89. Trauner M, Boyer JL. Bile salt transporters: molecular characterization, function, and regulation. Physiol Rev 2003;83:633–71.
90. Suchy FJ, Courchene SM, Blitzer BL. Taurocholate transport by basolateral plasma membrane vesicles isolated from developing rat liver. Am J Physiol 1985;248(6 Pt 1):G648–54.
91. Suchy FJ, Balistreri WF. Uptake of taurocholate by hepatocytes isolated from developing rats. Pediatr Res 1982;16(4 Pt 1): 282–5.
92. Belknap WM, Zimmer-Nechemias L, Suchy FJ, Balistreri WF. Bile acid efflux from suckling rat hepatocytes. Pediatr Res 1988;23:364–7.
93. Stolz A, Sugiyama Y, Kuhlenkamp J, et al. Cytosolic bile acid binding protein in rat liver: radioimmunoassay, molecular forms, developmental characteristics and organ distribution. Hepatology 1986;6:433–9.
94. Hardikar W, Ananthanarayanan M, Suchy FJ. Differential ontogenic regulation of basolateral and canalicular bile acid transport proteins in rat liver. J Biol Chem 1995;270:20841–6.
95. Karpen SJ, Sun AQ, Kudish B, et al. Multiple factors regulate the rat liver basolateral sodium-dependent bile acid cotransporter gene promoter. J Biol Chem 1996;271:15211–21.
96. Denson LA, Sturm E, Echevarria W, et al. The orphan nuclear receptor, shp, mediates bile acid-induced inhibition of the rat bile acid transporter, ntcp. Gastroenterology 2001;121: 140–7.
97. Tomer G, Ananthanarayanan M, Weymann A, et al. Differential developmental regulation of rat liver canalicular membrane transporters Bsep and Mrp2. Pediatr Res 2003;53:288–94.
98. Zinchuk VS, Okada T, Akimaru K, Seguchi H. Asynchronous expression and colocalization of Bsep and Mrp2 during development of rat liver. Am J Physiol Gastrointest Liver Physiol 2002;282:G540–8.
99. Gao B, St Pierre MV, Stieger B, Meier PJ. Differential expression of bile salt and organic anion transporters in developing rat liver. J Hepatol 2004;41:201–8.
100. Kullak-Ublick GA, Stieger B, Meier PJ. Enterohepatic bile salt transporters in normal physiology and liver disease. Gastroenterology 2004;126:322–42.
101. Karpen SJ. Nuclear receptor regulation of hepatic function. J Hepatol 2002;36:832–50.
102. Balasubramaniyan N, Shahid M, Suchy FJ, Ananthanarayanan M. Multiple mechanisms of ontogenic regulation of nuclear receptors during rat liver development. Am J Physiol Gastrointest Liver Physiol 2005;288:G251–60.
103. Bove KE, Heubi JE, Balistreri WF, Setchell KD. Bile acid synthetic defects and liver disease: a comprehensive review. Pediatr Dev Pathol 2004;7:315–34.

3

Mechanisms of Bile Formation and Cholestasis

Saul J. Karpen, M.D., Ph.D.

With the recent findings of genetic causes of cholestasis (see Chapter 14), many of the previously ascribed "indeterminate" forms of cholestasis have been assigned molecular forms of causality because of specific impairments in critical genes involved in the formation of bile. In a similar vein, exploration of the effects of various endogenous and exogenous factors on the expression and function of these same essential bile formation genes has led to a greater molecular understanding of acquired forms of cholestasis. Thus, within the past 5–10 years, it has become possible to tease apart not only the means by which the liver is damaged by rare single-gene defects in critical hepatobiliary genes, but also how these gene products are engaged in the response and adaptation to cholestasis, and intriguingly, why these processes may not be fully adequate to protect the liver. In particular, see Chapter 14 and recent references [1–6] for our increasing knowledge of the expression, structure, and regulation of these genes and gene products in the underlying processes that lead to cholestasis. Among the more relevant findings has been that the processes of bile formation, cholestasis, and adaptation are inherently intertwined with structural, developmental, biochemical, intercellular communication, subcellular organization, cell signaling pathways, and physiologic components of the liver and liver function. In this chapter, attention focuses upon the basic mechanisms of bile formation as well as the *genetic* and *acquired* pathways that lead to cholestasis.

SUMMARY OF THE PHYSIOLOGY OF BILE FORMATION

Bile is formed mainly via secretion of solutes and water from both hepatocytes and cholangiocytes [7–9]. Among the many functions of bile and the maintenance of its flow is fulfilling the role of the liver as an excretory organ, with the end point of delivery to the intestinal lumen, or ultimately, fecal elimination. In general, toxic substances, drugs, endobiotics, and xenobiotics that are modified and detoxified by hepatocytes are efficiently excreted into bile to provide an overall survival benefit for the organism. Moreover, the role of intestinal luminal bile acids as a principal aid for the absorption of long-chain fats and fat-soluble vitamins links bile acid flow across the hepatocyte with nutrition. This has particular relevance for the growth impairments seen in children with many different forms of neonatal cholestasis.

The main driving force for bile flow is the secretion and recirculation of bile acids. Bile acids are efficiently taken up from the portal circulation via several resident transporter proteins, primarily the Na^+-dependent bile acid importer Ntcp (Slc10a1), and various organic anion transporters (members of the organic anion transporter family) [10]. Bile acids are rapidly transported across the cytoplasm of hepatocytes, mainly via unknown mechanisms, and efficiently secreted into the canalicular lumen via an adenosine triphosphate (ATP) cassette transporter known as the bile salt export pump (BSEP, ABCB11). It is the secretion of bile acids against a steep concentration gradient that is the ultimate rate-limiting step of bile secretion (see Figure 3.1). As expected, when this transporter is mutated, bile acid flow is reduced and bile acids are retained within hepatocytes, leading to the liver disease known as progressive familial intrahepatic cholestasis 2 (PFIC2).

The other main solutes in bile, phospholipids, cholesterol, and bilirubin conjugates are also secreted into bile via substrate-specific ATP-binding cassette (ABC) transporters. Phospholipids are secreted via a "flippase," the multidrug resistance protein 3 (MDR3; ABCB4) gene product, which, when mutated, leads to the disease PFIC3 [5]. Cholesterol is secreted via two combined half-transporters, ABCG5/G8, which, if either half-transporter gene is mutated, leads to the disease sitosterolemia and perhaps liver disease [11,12]. Finally, conjugated bilirubin appears to be excreted into bile primarily via the multidrug resistance–related protein 2 (MRP2) multispecific transporter (ABCC2), which, when mutated, leads to Dubin–Johnson syndrome [13]. These discoveries and assignments of specific genes to specific biliary transport functions has led to an exciting and expanding understanding of the molecular determinants of bile formation, but have also led to a greater understanding of how these physiologic processes can be suppressed with either mutations or alterations in gene expression and protein activity. For a detailed discussion of roles for familial intrahepatic

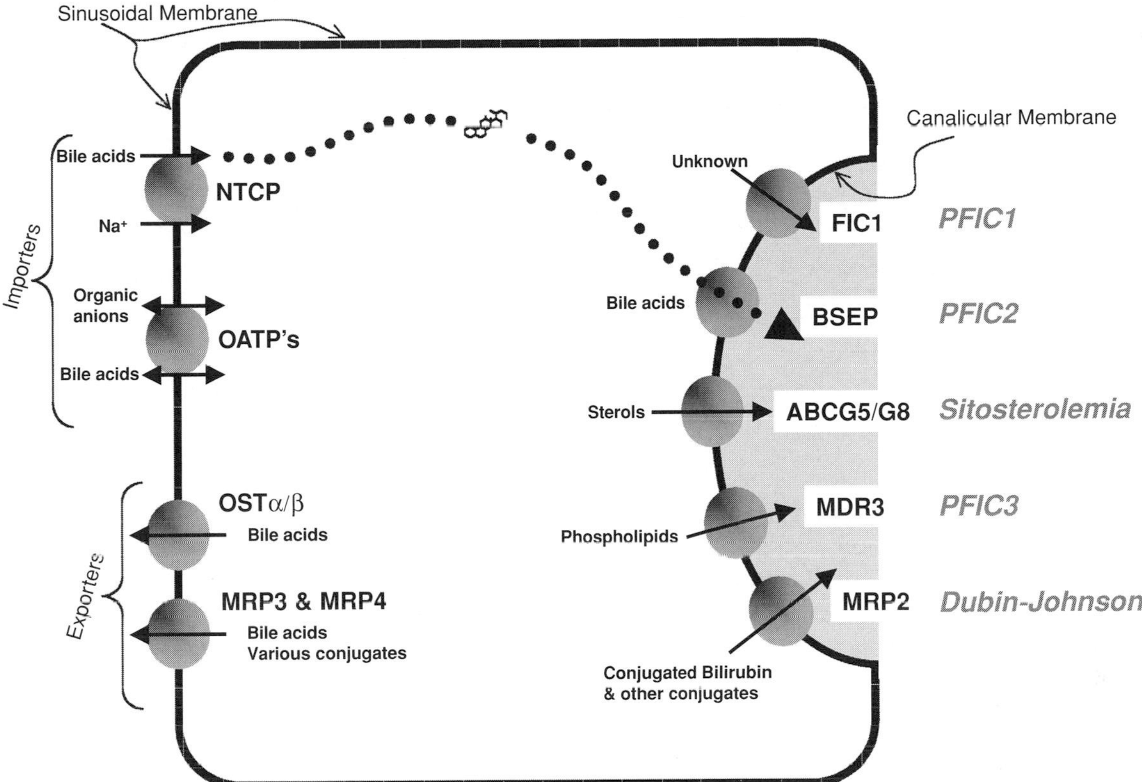

Figure 3.1. Roles for critical hepatic transporters in the formation of bile and adaptation to cholestasis. On the left is a representation of the sinusoidal surface and on the right, a canalicular surface. Diseases associated with defects in specific canalicular transporter genes are noted in *italics*. Note that bile acids have several means of transport across the sinusoidal membrane, both import and export, whereas there is one canalicular bile acid transporter, BSEP. These transporters allow for fine-tuning of intracellular bile acid concentrations as a means to adapt to a variety of cholestatic conditions. The principal means for bile acid flux across the hepatocyte is noted with the dotted line. NTCP, Na^+/taurocholate cotransporting polypeptide; OATP, organic acid transporting polypeptide; OST, organic solute transporter; MRP, multidrug resistance–related protein; FIC1, familial intrahepatic cholestasis 1; BSEP, bile salt export pump; MDR, multidrug resistance protein. Official gene designations: *FIC1* (*ATP8B1*), *BSEP* (*ABCB11*), *MDR3* (*ABCB4*), and *MRP2* (*ABCC2*).

cholestasis 1 (FIC1), BSEP, and MDR3 gene functions, and the diseases caused by their mutation, see Chapter 14.

Of clinical interest is the molecular distinction between bile acid flux across the hepatocyte and the export of conjugated bilirubin, although clinically the two are generally considered linked events during cholestasis. But because the two substances are transported by distinct transporters with different substrate affinities and regulation, there are certainly situations in which an individual can be cholestatic and have normal conjugated bilirubin flux, and times when elevated conjugated bilirubin levels are a marker for impaired MRP2 expression (e.g., Dubin–Johnson syndrome) while bile flow is normal. This is just one indication of the evolving nature of information about bile formation over the past few years, with an expectation that these discoveries will continue to improve our understanding of the molecular nature of bile formation.

In addition to flux of these solutes, bile formation is dependent upon ion flux in both hepatocytes and cholangiocytes. In humans, up to 40% of bile formation is derived from bile ducts [14], and a main determinant of bile flow is the secretion of chloride, which is primarily determined by the apical positioning of the CFTR gene product in cholangiocytes [8]. In diseases in which bile duct development is impaired, as in Alagille syndrome (see Chapter 15), cholestasis is a common clinical feature.

GENERAL PRINCIPLES OF CHOLESTASIS AND HEPATIC ADAPTATION

The definition of cholestasis as a blockage or severe impairment in the flow of bile is true in a few disease states that affect the overall "plumbing" of the liver (e.g., biliary atresia, common bile duct obstruction); however, with more sophisticated and recent genetic understanding of bile formation, it is clear that cholestasis can occur without frank ductal obstruction and can occur as an impairment in the functioning of proteins necessary for the formation of bile. Bile is composed of numerous substances, but the main solutes (salts, bile acids, phospholipids, cholesterol, bilirubin) each have a particular molecular means to become part of bile, mainly via substrate-specific canalicular transporters [5]. The main components of bile are bile acids, and it is the flux/recirculation of bile acids that is the main driving force in bile formation. The liver, and in particular the polarized hepatocyte, is the primary tissue that is responsible for the synthesis and transport of bile acids and thus is most likely to be damaged by bile acid retention when bile flow is reduced. Bile acid concentrations in peripheral circulation are generally less than 10 μmol/L, whereas in portal blood they vary from a low of 10–20 μmol/L between meals to upward of 100 μmol/L postprandially, when there is a significant gradient of concentrations in bile up to 3–30 mmol/L [15–17]. Thus, the highest concentration of bile acids is in the canalicular lumen, and it is the intracellular retention of bile acids that appears to be the most important disease-producing consequence of cholestasis and is the focus of adaptation. If bile flow is obstructed either downstream (e.g., Alagille syndrome–associated bile duct paucity or biliary atresia) or right at the canalicular membrane (e.g., PFIC2), bile acid concentrations will rise within hepatocytes. Bile acids are both detergents and signaling molecules, which, when retained within hepatocytes, lead to altered membrane composition and function, derangements of subcellular organelles, and broad changes in cell signaling pathways and gene expression [18]. Some of these changes lead to attempts at adaptation by reducing either the toxicity or concentration of retained bile acids by cytochrome P450–based mechanisms or sinusoidal export, respectively [19,20]. Prolonged retention of bile acids within the liver leads to activation of Kupffer cells, stellate cells, and myofibroblasts, with consequent increased expression of cytokines and progression of fibrosis. Thus, the overall effects of cholestasis, perhaps even long term, can in a broad way be ascribed to the effects of retained bile acids. Finally, little is known about the actual molecular causes of the enhanced susceptibility of the infant liver to cholestatic insults, although an immaturity of bile acid flux is present [21,22].

Over the past few years, much has been understood about how the hepatocyte responds and adapts to retained bile acids. Less is known about cholangiocytes. The hepatocyte is poised to respond to retained bile acids with a coordinated approach that treats retained bile acids as if they were a dangerous, foreign compound – that is, high levels of retained bile acids as xenotoxic endobiotics. Multiple processes, both transcriptional (mainly nuclear receptor [NR] mediated) and posttranscriptional, are engaged in the hepatocyte (see reviews [1,5,20, 23,24]), with the overall concept being to reduce concentration by suppressing bile acid import and synthesis, to reduce toxicity with hydroxylation and conjugation, and to increase export by sinusoidal – and to a lesser extent, canalicular – efflux. At the transcriptional level, bile acids are activators of at least three members of the NR superfamily, farnesoid X receptor (FXR), constitutive androstane receptor (CAR), and pregnane X receptor (PXR), and these three gene regulators are the primary means for effecting the transcriptional reprogramming of the hepatocyte in cholestasis. Genetically modified mice with mutations in any of these genes are essentially normal, except when exposed to cholestatic conditions. In cholestasis, mice without any one or more of these three genes rapidly develop hepatocyte apoptosis and necrosis, all apparently by an inability to adapt to retained bile acids. Conversely, in genetically normal mice, these NR-regulated adaptive mechanisms can be enhanced with small molecules that bind to the NR, lending an exciting prospect for future treatment paradigms (see the next section).

GENETIC MECHANISMS OF CHOLESTASIS AND DEVELOPMENT OF BILE FORMATION

There are multiple genetic mechanisms that lead to cholestasis, most involving mutations in critical hepatobiliary transporter genes or formation/structure of bile ducts (see Chapters 14 and 15 on Alagille syndrome and PFIC). An impaired ability to transport essential biliary substances across the canalicular membrane of the hepatocyte leads to obligate retention of that substance within hepatocytes (e.g., PFIC2, bile acids) or a deficiency of a substance in the biliary lumen (e.g., PFIC3, phospholipids), leading to bile acid–induced damage in hepatocytes or cholangiocytes, respectively [5]. However, why mutations in select gene products lead to disease is not always clear.

ACQUIRED MECHANISMS OF CHOLESTASIS

In addition to the single-gene defects that can lead to cholestasis, it is generally more prevalent that multifactorial, or structural, mechanisms are the main participants. Of these, drug-induced, total parenteral nutrition (TPN), or sepsis/inflammation-induced mechanisms are now being recognized to have molecular underpinnings.

Sepsis-Associated Cholestasis

Osler [25] was among the first to describe the association of nonhepatitic infections leading to a functional impairment in bile flow – "toxæmic jaundice." It has been well known, but poorly understood, that such cholestasis is not caused by damage or destruction of hepatocytes but is a functional impairment from either bacterial products (e.g., endotoxin) or inflammation-induced cytokines. Infants, in particular, are more susceptible to the effects of sepsis on bile flow, perhaps because of immaturity of bile formation or adaptive mechanisms [26–28]. Sepsis-associated cholestasis is a principal cause of cholestasis in adults as well, although it is not usually at the top of the list of differential diagnoses. Administration of endotoxin (bacterial lipopolysaccharides from gram-negative bacteria) to nearly all animal models leads to a rapid and sustained impairment in bile flow [1,29–32]. These effects appear to be caused by the release of endotoxin-induced cytokines from resident hepatic macrophages, Kupffer cells, which in turn act upon receptors in the sinusoidal membrane of neighboring hepatocytes to induce cell signaling changes that lead to reduced bile formation. It is also likely the endotoxin may act directly upon hepatocytes and cholangiocytes, since these cells have cell surface receptors for endotoxin and other microbial products [33]. In addition, the liver is a central player in the hepatic response to infection and injury – the acute phase response (APR), in which one may reasonably include sepsis-associated cholestasis as a component. The hepatic APR is a coordinated transcriptional reprogramming and prioritization of liver function as a means to restore homeostasis and help with injury repair and infection throughout the body. When activated by mediators of inflammation like endotoxin, the liver changes gene expression to increase secretion of many substances and enzymes to restore homeostasis (e.g., protease inhibitors), fight infection (e.g., complement, C-reactive peptide), and direct amino acids and lipids to the periphery, all coordinated intracellularly via complex and overlapping cell signaling pathways initiated by endotoxin and cytokines such as tumor necrosis factor (TNF)-α, interleukin (IL)-1β, and IL-6 [34–37]. The same cytokines that activate the expression of secretory substances from the liver during the APR are also involved in the suppression of function and expression of critical hepatobiliary transporters.

When exposed to lipopolysaccharides (LPS), bile flow is rapidly and profoundly reduced via a combination of molecular targeting of cell signaling pathways at existing membrane transporter proteins, as well as in the nucleus, at the control of transporter gene transcription [38]. Within 15–60 minutes after exposure to LPS, membrane localization of both BSEP and MRP2 proteins are significantly reduced, apparently because of both degradation and trafficking from canalicular membranes into submembrane vesicles [36,39–42]. Variable effects on FIC1, and MDR3 proteins have been seen in several experimental and human models. In the medium to long term, LPS and LPS-induced cytokines, primarily by activating members of the mitogen-activated protein kinase (MAPK) family, leads to marked alterations in the activity of several gene regulators of a broad number of transporters, namely those that are activated by members of the NR gene family.

Drug-Induced Cholestasis

It is well known that many drugs can lead to damage of liver parenchymal cells (e.g., acetaminophen), whereas some interfere with the basic mechanisms of the formation of bile (for an excellent review, see Navarro and Senior [43]). Cholestasis as a component of drug-related hepatotoxicity can involve a variety of mechanisms, including direct cholangiocyte toxicity and necrosis, impairments in bile acid transport, and thickening of biliary secretions [18]. An example of the latter includes supersaturating concentrations of select agents within bile, especially those with high biliary penetrance, such as cephalosporins, which can themselves lead to sludge/stone formation and obstructive cholestasis, (e.g., ceftriaxone) [44].

Infants and young children have reduced detoxification pathways compared to older children and adults, suggesting that there is an enhanced susceptibility to cholestatic effects of certain drugs [45]. This enhanced susceptibility is not fully understood but appears to involve developmentally regulated expression of detoxification and transport genes, immature protective measures against apoptosis/necrosis, and a role for altered inflammatory responses to damaged tissues.

TPN-Associated Cholestasis

Among the more prevalent associations of the rapid progression to end-stage liver disease is the setting of neonates with intestinal failure, who are dependent upon TPN, leading to a condition known as TPN-associated cholestasis (TPNAC). This entity was seen soon after the introduction of TPN in neonates, yet the underlying cause, or more likely causes, are unknown [46]. The typical clinical situation is a premature infant who has a damaged or resected small intestine with an inability to advance feeds. TPNAC can develop as soon as 2 weeks with hepatomegaly and conjugated hyperbilirubinemia, whereas cirrhosis has been reported in as little as 2 months [47]. Moreover, the cholestasis and injury can resolve if patients are weaned off TPN, attesting to the timeliness and confluence of these damaging factors in early infancy. Thus, there is an inherent susceptibility in this clinical setting, which is not readily replicated in older children or adults with TPN dependence.

There appear to be four main contributors to TPNAC – immaturity, infection, inadequate gut function, and a toxic/missing component in the TPN [48]. Despite TPN being administered for nearly 40 years, we still have little evidence as to which one of these four contributors is most relevant. Support for all four components has been addressed, yet the molecular, or cellular, etiologies remain elusive. The inherent immaturity of bile formation and flow, that is, "physiologic cholestasis of the newborn," [22] and drug metabolism pathways [45] support the concept that premature infant livers may be more susceptible to any cholestatic insult, although neither function has been adequately quantified in these babies. The scenario of infection and inflammation contributing to cholestasis in these infants is seen quite often, whereby bouts of infection are often heralded by elevations in serum levels of conjugated bilirubin [26,27]. Inadequate oral intake reduces the nutritional and hormonal input from the gut-to-liver function and bile flow, with evidence of an immaturity and impairment of certain gut hormones in intestinal failure and TPN dependence [49]. Finally, many components of the TPN solution have been implicated as cholestatic (minerals, amino acids, sterols, fatty acids, to name a few) or absent, but to date none has been definitively associated with causing cholestasis [48]. In one of the few epidemiologic studies to date, adults on TPN had lower hepatic complications on lower lipid infusions than higher, suggesting that there may be a component in the lipids that is cholestatic [50,51].

ADAPTATION TO CHOLESTASIS

The hepatocyte adapts to cholestasis by engaging broadly acting protective measures at the membrane, in the cytoplasm, and by a reprogramming of transcription in the nucleus. In

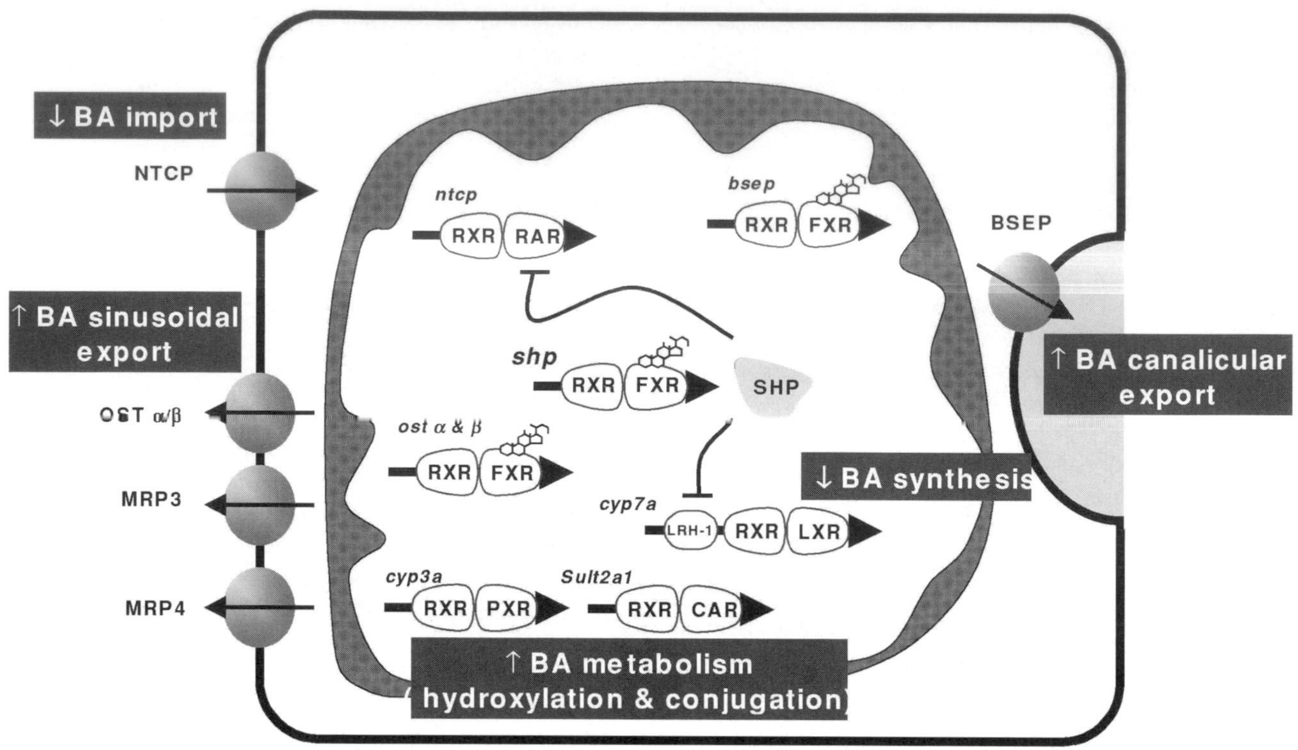

Figure 3.2. General overview of the nuclear adaptive response of the hepatocyte to bile acid retention. The hepatocyte engages multiple processes in order to reduce retention of intracellular bile acids. In addition to that shown here, there are direct effects on resident metabolic pathways and transporter and proteins. The overall process functionally involves reduction of sinusoidal import and synthesis, engagement of cytochrome P450–mediated hydroxylation and conjugation pathways for detoxification, and increased canalicular export. Shown are a few key target genes and members of the NR superfamily whose activation by ligands (e.g., bile acids for FXR) leads to these adaptive changes in gene expression. Relevant regulatory promoter regions are shown, although the list of target genes and transcriptional regulators is much more extensive [4,19,20,24,38]. Abbreviations of NR family members: RXR, retinoid X receptor; RAR, retinoic acid receptor; FXR, farnesoid X receptor; CAR, constitutive androstane receptor; PXR, pregnane X receptor; LXR, liver X receptor; SHP, small heterodimer partner.

addition to changes within hepatocytes, cell-to-cell communication, balancing immunologic responses to infected or damaged cells, with the endogenous capacity of the liver to regenerate, is an additional component to the liver's response to cholestasis. Over the past few years, it has become apparent that this coordination of response to cholestatic injury is multilayered, integrative, and quite complex but on a practical front, may be amenable to therapeutic intervention.

In general, the primary location of effecting a response to cholestasis resides within hepatocytes, likely because of this cell's role in handling bile acids, which can abruptly and profoundly rise in intracellular concentrations with all forms of cholestasis. Reducing the inherent toxicity of retained bile acids within hepatocytes is a major goal of the hepatocyte's response to cholestasis [20,24]. When bile acid concentrations rise within cells, there are profound effects on cell signaling and integrity of membranes and subcellular structures. As detergents, bile acids affect membrane fluidity and protein structure, while as cell signaling molecules, bile acids affect kinase pathways, initiate apoptosis, and alter gene expression, among many other critical cellular functions [6,10,52]. Over the past few years, the essential components of the hepatocyte's response to retained bile acids is coordinated to reduce sinusoidal import and synthesis, increase canalicular export, and engage cytochrome P450–based xenobiotic metabolism pathways (hydroxylation and conjugation) as a means to reduce intracellular concentrations and toxicity [6]. In addition, recent evidence suggests that at least two sinusoidal transporters are activated to export retained bile acids across the sinusoidal membrane (see Figure 3.1). These responses to bile acid overload are, in general, related to bile acids acting as gene regulators – as ligands for several NR family members (mainly CAR, FXR, and PXR), which then act as transcriptional activators for target genes whose proteins function to effect the changes noted previously (Figure 3.2). This is an evolving avenue of research that indicates that overall the hepatocyte has adaptive responses in place to handle cholestasis and that these pathways may be amenable to pharmacologic therapies [24].

FUTURE EXPECTATIONS

Although we have seen new identifications of genes associated with genetic forms of cholestasis (e.g., PFICs), it is still evident to practitioners that much remains to be discovered. On a diagnostic front, it is anticipated that we will be able to explore diagnostics as well as genotype–phenotype correlations as more and more of these disease-causing genes become available for commercial testing (see www.genetests.org for current lists) or are discovered as part of ongoing multicenter trials. Nutritional and supplemental means of enhancing the response of the liver to cholestasis as well as discoveries into the roles of immaturity, inflammation, and diet-derived substances that may, in fact, exacerbate ongoing cholestasis are expected to be revealed. Finally, with the discovery of the roles for inflammation and NR-mediated means of adaptation to cholestasis, anticholestatic therapeutic agents are expected to be available for testing, given the frank paucity of available agents at present [20,24].

REFERENCES

1. Wagner M, Trauner M. Transcriptional regulation of hepatobiliary transport systems in health and disease: implications for a rationale approach to the treatment of intrahepatic cholestasis. Ann Hepatol 2005;4:77–99.
2. Trauner M, Boyer JL. Bile salt transporters: molecular characterization, function, and regulation. Physiol Rev 2003;83:633–71.
3. Balistreri WF, Bezerra JA, Jansen P, et al. Intrahepatic cholestasis: summary of an American Association for the Study of Liver Diseases single-topic conference. Hepatology 2005;42:222–35.
4. Karpen SJ. Nuclear receptor regulation of hepatic function. J Hepatol 2002;36:832–50.
5. Oude Elferink RP, Paulusma CC, Groen AK. Hepatocanalicular transport defects: pathophysiologic mechanisms of rare diseases. Gastroenterology 2006;130:908–25.
6. Eloranta JJ, Meier PJ, Kullak-Ublick GA. Coordinate transcriptional regulation of transport and metabolism. Methods Enzymol 2005;400:511–30.
7. Hofmann AF. The continuing importance of bile acids in liver and intestinal disease. Arch Intern Med 1999;159:2647–58.
8. Feranchak AP, Sokol RJ. Cholangiocyte biology and cystic fibrosis liver disease. Semin Liver Dis 2001;21:471–88.
9. Scharschmidt BF, Lake JR. Hepatocellular bile acid transport and ursodeoxycholic acid hypercholeresis. Dig Dis Sci 1989;34(Suppl 12):5S–15S.
10. Kullak-Ublick GA, Stieger B, Meier PJ. Enterohepatic bile salt transporters in normal physiology and liver disease. Gastroenterology 2004;126:322–42.
11. Miettinen TA, Klett EL, Gylling H, et al. Liver transplantation in a patient with sitosterolemia and cirrhosis. Gastroenterology 2006;130:542–7.
12. Salen G, Patel S, Batta AK. Sitosterolemia. Cardiovasc Drug Rev 2002;20:255–70.
13. Keitel V, Nies AT, Brom M, et al. A common Dubin-Johnson syndrome mutation impairs protein maturation and transport activity of MRP2 (ABCC2). Am J Physiol Gastrointest Liver Physiol 2003;284:G165–74.
14. Nathanson MH, Boyer JL. Mechanisms and regulation of bile secretion. Hepatology 1991;14:551–66.
15. Hofmann AF. The enterohepatic circulation of bile acids in man. Clin Gastroenterol 1977;6:3–24.
16. Northfield TC, Hofmann AF. Biliary lipid output during three meals and an overnight fast. I. Relationship to bile acid pool size and cholesterol saturation of bile in gallstone and control subjects. Gut 1975;16:1–11.
17. Angelin B, Bjorkhem I, Einarsson K, Ewerth S. Hepatic uptake of bile acids in man. Fasting and postprandial concentrations of individual bile acids in portal venous and systemic blood serum. J Clin Invest 1982;70:724–31.
18. Jaeschke H, Gores GJ, Cederbaum AI, et al. Mechanisms of hepatotoxicity. Toxicol Sci 2002;65:166–76.
19. Eloranta JJ, Kullak-Ublick GA. Coordinate transcriptional regulation of bile acid homeostasis and drug metabolism. Arch Biochem Biophys 2005;433:397–412.
20. Karpen SJ. Exercising the nuclear option to treat cholestasis: CAR and PXR ligands. Hepatology 2005;42:266–9.
21. Watkins JB, Szczepanik P, Gould JB, et al. Bile salt metabolism in the human premature infant. Preliminary observations of pool size and synthesis rate following prenatal administration of dexamethasone and phenobarbital. Gastroenterology 1975;69:706–13.
22. Suchy FJ, Balistreri WF, Heubi JE, et al. Physiologic cholestasis: elevation of the primary serum bile acid concentrations in normal infants. Gastroenterology 1981;80(5 Pt 1):1037–41.
23. Rutherford AE, Pratt DS. Cholestasis and cholestatic syndromes. Curr Opin Gastroenterol 2006;22:209–14.
24. Boyer JL. Nuclear receptor ligands: rational and effective therapy for chronic cholestatic liver disease? Gastroenterology 2005;129:735–40.
25. Osler WH. Principles and practice of medicine. 4th ed. New York: Appleton, 1901.
26. Dunham EC. Septicemia in the newborn. Am J Dis Child 1933;45:229–53.
27. Rooney JC, Hill DJ, Danks DM. Jaundice associated with bacterial infection in the newborn. Am J Dis Child 1971;122:39–41.
28. Zimmerman HJ, Fang M, Utili R, et al. Jaundice due to bacterial infection. Gastroenterology 1979;77:362–74.
29. Green RM, Whiting JF, Rosenbluth AB, et al. Interleukin-6 inhibits hepatocyte taurocholate uptake and sodium-potassium-adenosinetriphosphatase activity. Am J Physiol 1994;267(6 Pt 1):G1094–100.
30. Bolder U, Tonnu HT, Schteingart CD, et al. Hepatocyte transport of bile acids and organic anions in endotoxemic rats—impaired uptake and secretion. Gastroenterology 1997;112:214–25.
31. Moseley RH. Sepsis-associated cholestasis. Gastroenterology 1997;112:302–6.
32. Moseley RH. Sepsis and cholestasis. Clin Liver Dis 2004;8:83–94.
33. Schwabe RF, Seki E, Brenner DA. Toll-like receptor signaling in the liver. Gastroenterology 2006;130:1886–900.
34. Baumann H, Gauldie J. The acute phase response. Immunol Today 1994;15:74–80.
35. Baumann H, Held WA, Berger FG. The acute phase response of mouse liver. Genetic analysis of the major acute phase reactants. J Biol Chem 1984;259:566–73.
36. Siewert E, Dietrich CG, Lammert F, et al. Interleukin-6 regulates hepatic transporters during acute-phase response. Biochem Biophys Res Commun 2004;322:232–8.
37. Moshage H. Cytokines and the hepatic acute phase response. J Pathol 1997;181:257–66.
38. Trauner M, Wagner M, Fickert P, Zollner G. Molecular regulation of hepatobiliary transport systems: clinical implications

for understanding and treating cholestasis. J Clin Gastroenterol 2005;39(4 Suppl 2):S111–24.

39. Bolder U, Jeschke MG, Landmann L, et al. Heat stress enhances recovery of hepatocyte bile acid and organic anion transporters in endotoxemic rats by multiple mechanisms. Cell Stress Chaperones 2006;11:89–100.
40. Elferink MGL, Olinga P, Draaisma AL, et al. LPS-induced down-regulation of MRP2 and BSEP in human liver is due to a post-transcriptional process. Am J Physiol Gastrointest Liver Physiol 2004;287:G1008–16.
41. Warskulat U, Kubitz R, Wettstein M, et al. Regulation of bile salt export pump mRNA levels by dexamethasone and osmolarity in cultured rat hepatocytes. Biol Chem 1999;380:1273–9.
42. Kubitz R, Wettstein M, Warskulat U, Haussinger D. Regulation of the multidrug resistance protein 2 in the rat liver by lipopolysaccharide and dexamethasone. Gastroenterology 1999;116:401–10.
43. Navarro VJ, Senior JR. Drug-related hepatotoxicity. N Engl J Med 2006;354:731–9.
44. Bonioli E, Bellini C, Toma P. Pseudolithiasis and intractable hiccups in a boy receiving ceftriaxone. N Engl J Med 1994;331: 1532.
45. Kearns GL, Abdel-Rahman SM, Alander SW, et al. Developmental pharmacology—drug disposition, action, and therapy in infants and children. N Engl J Med 2003;349:1157–67.
46. Abernathy CO, Utili R, Zimmerman HJ. Immaturity of the biliary excretory system predisposes neonates to intrahepatic cholestasis. Med Hypotheses 1979;5:641–7.
47. Sondheimer JM, Asturias E, Cadnapaphornchai M. Infection and cholestasis in neonates with intestinal resection and long-term parenteral nutrition. J Pediatr Gastroenterol Nutr 1998;27: 131–7.
48. Buchman AL, Iyer K, Fryer J. Parenteral nutrition-associated liver disease and the role for isolated intestine and intestine/liver transplantation. Hepatology 2006;43:9–19.
49. Teitelbaum DH, Han-Markey T, Drongowski RA, et al. Use of cholecystokinin to prevent the development of parenteral nutrition-associated cholestasis. JPEN J Parenter Enteral Nutr 1997;21:100–3.
50. Colomb V, Jobert-Giraud A, Lacaille F, et al. Role of lipid emulsions in cholestasis associated with long-term parenteral nutrition in children. JPEN J Parenter Enteral Nutr 2000;24: 345–50.
51. Cavicchi M, Beau P, Crenn P, et al. Prevalence of liver disease and contributing factors in patients receiving home parenteral nutrition for permanent intestinal failure. Ann Intern Med 2000;132:525–32.
52. Houten SM, Watanabe M, Auwerx J. Endocrine functions of bile acids. EMBO J 2006;25:1419–25.

4

THE CHOLANGIOPATHIES

Valeer J. Desmet, M.D., Ph.D., and Tania A. D. Roskams, M.D., Ph.D.

EMBRYOLOGY OF EXTRA- AND INTRAHEPATIC BILE DUCTS, DUCTAL PLATE, AND DUCTAL PLATE MALFORMATION

Development of Extrahepatic Bile Ducts

In the human embryo, the first anlage of the bile ducts and the liver is the hepatic diverticulum or liver bud. It starts as a thickening of the endoblastic epithelium in the ventral wall of the cephalad portion of the foregut (the future duodenum), near the origin of the yolk sac; this area is termed the *anterior intestinal portal.* This occurs around the 7-somite (2.5-mm) stage on the 18th day. In the 19-somite (3-mm, 22nd-day) embryo the diverticulum is formed. In the 22-somite embryo, the hepatic diverticulum is a well-defined hollow structure. From the ventral and lateral surfaces of the diverticulum, on which the endoderm is in contact with the bulk of the mesoderm of the septum transversum (between the pericardial and peritoneal cavities), short sprouts of endodermal cells extend into the septum transversum to form the earliest anlage of the liver [1].

In the embryo about 5 mm in length, the diverticulum also shows a protruding bud in its distal part. Some investigators accordingly distinguish in the hepatic diverticulum a cranial part (pars hepatica) and a caudal part (pars cystica) [2].

The caudal bud or pars cystica grows in length and represents the anlage of the gallbladder, the cystic duct, and common bile duct (ductus choledochus). For up to 8 weeks of gestation, the extrahepatic biliary tree further develops through lengthening of the caudal part of the hepatic diverticulum. This structure is patent from the beginning and remains patent and in continuity with the developing liver at all stages. These observations disprove the long-held concept that there is a "solid stage" of entodermal occlusion of the common bile duct lumen and hence refute the concept that extrahepatic bile duct atresia (EHBDA) may be caused by failure of recanalization of the common bile duct [3].

The gallbladder anlage is visible at 29 days after fertilization as a right anterolateral dilatation along the distal half of the hepatic diverticulum, with a cystic duct present at 34 days. At that stage, the gallbladder and cystic duct are provided with a lumen [3]. Outpockings appear in the gallbladder wall in the 42-mm embryo; folds develop on the interior surface of the bladder at the 78-mm stage [4]. The outer layers of the gallbladder and cystic duct develop from condensing mesenchyme around the original epithelial mass. Myoblasts develop around the 30-mm stage, resulting in the establishment of all three layers of the wall of the future gallbladder: the mucosa, the muscular layer, and the serosa. From 11 weeks of gestation onward, the gallbladder epithelium reacts with a monoclonal antibody directed against a 40-kDa epithelial autoantigen in ulcerative colitis, which simultaneously also appears in the gut and the skin [5].

The mRNA of the Onecut transcription factor hepatocyte nuclear factor 6 (HNF6) is expressed in mouse liver from the onset of its development, and is detected not only in hepatoblasts (see further) but also in the extrahepatic bile ducts and the gallbladder primordium [6,7].

In the mouse, development of the gallbladder further requires normal functioning of the forkhead box f1 gene (*foxf1* gene). Haploinsufficiency of the Foxf1 transcription factor results in gallbladder malformation, with inadequate external smooth muscle layer, insufficient mesenchymal cell number, and in some cases absence of a discernable cholangiocytic mucosal lining [8].

The caudal pars cystica of the hepatic diverticulum is associated closely with the ventral pancreatic bud. The portion of the hepatic diverticulum between the cystic duct and the gut (the choledochus) increases in length and a localized outgrowth develops from its dorsal wall: the ventral pancreas [1].

The pars cystica of the hepatic diverticulum begins initially from the anterior side of the future duodenum. About the fifth week, the duodenum rotates to the right, so that the attachment of the developing common bile duct becomes displaced to its definitive position on the dorsal side of the duodenum [4].

The hepatic duct (ductus hepaticus) develops from the cranial part (pars hepatica) of the hepatic diverticulum.

For a long time, the development of the proximal branches of the hepatic duct was not well understood [9]. The detailed investigations by Tan et al. [10,11] have documented this part of development.

In the 34-day embryo, the common hepatic duct is a broad, funnel-like structure in direct contact with the developing liver, without a recognizable left or right hepatic duct. During the fifth week, a rapid entodermal proliferation takes place in the dilated funnel-shaped structure above the junction of the common bile duct and cystic duct; this proliferation gives rise to several folds, resulting in several channels at the porta hepatis [10,11]. It is speculated that this remodeling at least partially explains the existence of the several normal variants in the configuration of the right and left hepatic ducts. The "normal" Y-shaped junction of right and left hepatic ducts with the common bile duct is found in only 57% of adults [10]. The distal portions of the right and left hepatic ducts develop from the extrahepatic ducts and are clearly defined tubular structures by 12 weeks of gestation. The proximal portions of the main hilar ducts derive from the first intrahepatic ductal plates [11]. The extrahepatic bile ducts and the developing intrahepatic biliary tree maintain luminal continuity from the very start of organogenesis throughout further development [11], contradicting a previous study in the mouse suggesting that the extrahepatic bile duct system develops independently from the intrahepatic biliary tree and that the systems are initially discontinuous but join up later [12].

Hes 1, the protein product of the *Hes1* gene is expressed in the epithelium of the extrahepatic bile ducts throughout their development. In vivo loss of Hes 1 (a transcription factor directly regulated by the Notch signaling pathway) results in agenesis of the gallbladder and hypoplasia of the extrahepatic bile ducts [13].

Development of Intrahepatic Bile Ducts

During the first 7 weeks of embryonic life, there is no intrahepatic bile duct system in the developing liver [14,15]. Different investigators have given varying reports of the precise moment of its first appearance. Its formation sets in at about the 18-mm [9,15,16] to 22-mm [14] stage or between the fifth and ninth gestational weeks [4]. A recent study mentions the seventh week as the timepoint for the first appearance of the intrahepatic bile duct system and describes a junction between the extrahepatic bile ducts and the earliest intrahepatic bile duct structure at the time of its first appearance in the liver hilum [17,18].

Several theories exist about the development of the intrahepatic bile ducts. One theory maintains that the intrahepatic biliary tree is derived from ingrowth of the epithelium of the extrahepatic ducts [19]. Another postulates that the entire intrahepatic bile-draining system develops from hepatocyte precursor cells (hepatoblasts) (reviewed in Desmet [20]). A third theory combines elements of both of the first two. Most investigators favor the second hypothesis. This concept was based on routine light microscopic and ultrastructural investigations.

The hepatoblastic origin of the intrahepatic bile duct system received additional support from several studies that reinvestigated the embryologic development of the intrahepatic bile ducts with immunohistochemical techniques [10,11, 15–28]. These studies made use of immunohistochemical stains for cytokeratins, tissue polypeptide antigen, carcinoembryonic antigen, epithelial membrane antigen, and other markers for parenchymal and bile duct cell phenotypes. However, lineage studies that firmly establish the hepatoblastic origin of the bile duct lining cells have not yet been performed. Newer techniques, like targeted somatic gene rearrangements using the Cre recombinase in transgenic mice might solve the problem [29].

Immunostaining for cytokeratins has been particularly useful for revealing changes in cellular phenotype. Cytokeratins are the intermediate filaments of the cytoskeleton characteristic for epithelial cells. Different cytokeratins have been identified and catalogued [28]. Normal adult human liver parenchymal cells express only the cytokeratins 8 and 18, intrahepatic bile duct cells express in addition the cytokeratins 7 and 19 [27] and 20 [26].

In its earliest developmental stages, the human embryonic liver is composed of epithelial liver cell precursors (hepatoblasts) that express the cytokeratins 8, 18, and 19 [24,25], and in addition cytokeratin 14 from 10–14 weeks of gestation [23].

The development of the intrahepatic bile ducts is determined by the development and branching pattern of the portal vein, starting at the hilum of the liver.

Around the eighth week of gestation, the primitive hepatoblasts adjacent to the mesenchyme around the largest hilar portal vein branches become more strongly immunoreactive for their cytokeratins 8, 18, and 19. This layer of cells, surrounding the portal vein branches like a cylindric sleeve, is termed the ductal plate [22], in analogy to the terminology of Hammar [19] (Figure 4.1). Recent studies unraveled that biliary cell differentiation is induced in the fetal liver by a periportal gradient of activin/transforming growth factor (TGF)-β signaling, the

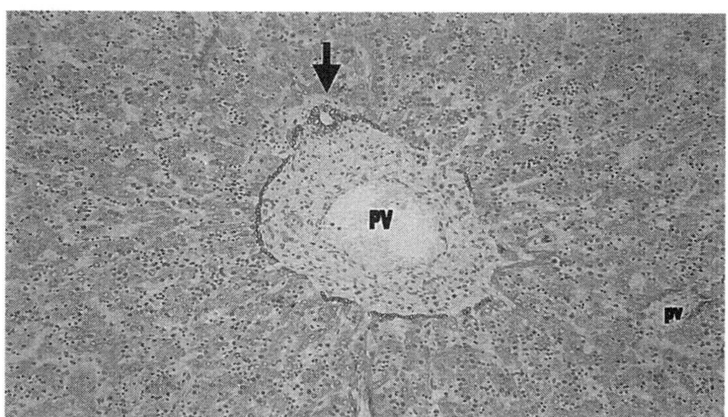

Figure 4.1. Autopsy liver specimen from an 18-week-old fetus. The picture shows a primitive portal tract containing a branch of the portal vein and its surrounding mesenchyme. Immediately surrounding the mesenchyme lies a layer of smaller cells with stronger immunoreactivity for cytokeratins. This layer is double over some segments. An early stage of remodeling of this ductal plate is seen at 12 o'clock, with development of a "tubular" lumen, lined by taller cells. (Monoclonal anticytokeratin antibody KL-1 immunostain [Immunotech, Marseille, France], hematoxylin counterstain, 312× magnification.) (Specimen courtesy of Dr. Philippe Moerman, Catholic University of Leuven, Leuven, Belgium.) For color reproduction, see Color Plate 4.1.

extent of which is controlled by the inhibitory influence of HNF6 and the Onecut factor OC-2. The Notch pathway may act in parallel or downstream of the activin/TGF-β signaling to further support the biliary differentiation or to repress the hepatocytic differentiation program in these cells [30]. The results of a study in murine liver indeed suggest an inhibitory role of *Notch1* on hepatocellular proliferation [31].

In mice, the forkhead box m1 transcription factor (Foxm1b) is also essential for normal intrahepatic bile duct cell differentiation, besides development of vessels and sinusoids [32].

The ductal plates adjacent to the mesenchyme (the portal ductal plate layer) become duplicated by a second layer of more keratin-rich cells over variably long segments of their perimeter (the second or lobular ductal plate layer) [17]. During the following weeks, ductal plates also appear around the smaller portal vein branches at a distance from the hilum. In the meantime, the hepatoblasts not involved in ductal plate formation gradually lose cytokeratin 19, and by 14 weeks of gestation the future parenchymal cells are immunoreactive only for cytokeratins 8 and 18, the cytokeratin pair normally expressed in adult liver parenchymal cells.

From about 12 weeks of gestation onward, a progressive "remodeling" of the ductal plates takes place, starting again in the earliest ductal plates around the larger portal vein branches near the hilum.

Over short segments of the perimeter of the double-layered ductal plates, a "tubular" dilatation occurs in the slit-like lumen, lined now by taller keratin-rich cells (Figure 4.2). These cells acquire epithelial membrane antigen and lose their biliary glycoprotein I [17]. The "tubular" parts of the ductal plate become incorporated into the mesenchyme surrounding the portal vein (the future portal tract) by ingrowth of mesenchyme between the lobular ductal plate layer and the hepatoblasts. The tubules incorporated into the portal mesenchyme are the future portal ducts; they remain connected, however, to the ductal plate and its adjacent parenchyma by thin epithelial channels, assuring continuity between the portal ducts and the already developed canalicular network located between the primitive hepatocyte precursor cells. Most of the excess epithelial components of the ductal plate that are not involved in tubule formation gradually disappear [20]. The ramification of the biliary tree continues throughout fetal life toward the liver periphery, but with a "slow-down period" of the progressive ramifications between the 20th and 32nd weeks of gestation, when the intraportal granulopoiesis of the liver is active [33].

By 20 weeks of gestation, weak immunoreactivity for cytokeratin 7 appears in the cells of the developing ducts, again appearing first in the older ducts near the hilum [22]. The immunoreactivity for cytokeratin 7 gradually increases and extends into more peripheral ducts, to reach the level of immunoreactivity observed in ducts of the adult liver at about 1 month after birth [22]. Other phenotypic markers appearing in the ducts include epithelial membrane antigens and carcinoembryonic antigens [17].

At the time of birth, the most peripheral branches of the intrahepatic biliary tree are still immature: The finest portal vein radicles still are surrounded by ductal plates, which require an additional 4 weeks after birth to develop into small portal ducts [17].

This indicates some degree of immaturity and incompleteness of the intrahepatic bile duct system in the neonate and may explain the lower ratio of the total number of bile ducts to the total number of portal tracts in premature infants [34].

The factors determining the developmental fate of the bipotential hepatoblasts remain incompletely known. There is evidence that components of the portal mesenchyme are crucial for inducing the phenotypic shift into bile duct–type cells in the layers of the ductal plate [35].

Several components, including laminin, fibronectin, collagen types I and IV, expression of corresponding cellular integrins, catenin, and neural cell adhesion molecule (N-CAM), have all been shown to be involved (for review, see Lemaigre [29]).

The process of intrahepatic bile duct development comprises schematically the following components: (a) a gradual phenotypic change of the hepatoblasts toward bile duct–type cells; (b) a remarkable remodeling of the tridimensional structure of the ductal plate; and (3) an ongoing further maturation of the remodeled, tubular ducts (reviewed in references [20,36–40]).

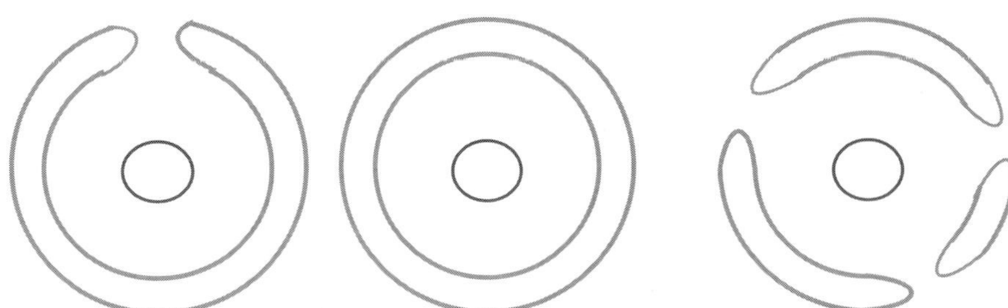

Figure 4.2. Schematic drawing of the appearance of the ductal plate malformation in cross sections, either in microscopic sections or in pictures of hepatic imaging. Lack of remodeling of the ductal plate results in persistence of the cylindric ductal plate (*center*). Moderate remodeling results in the appearance of a curved bile duct lumen in circular arrangement (*left*). Minimal remodeling creates the appearance of a "polypoid projection" in the lumen of a dilated bile duct (*right*). Inner circles represent portal vein; outer circles and structures represent ductal plate elements.

The phenotypic change from hepatoblast to cholangiocyte consists of a complex series of expressions of new molecules, including the de novo expression not only of cytokeratin 7 but also other molecules like carcinoembryonic antigens and epithelial membrane antigens, successively changing expression of surface glycoproteins and of glutathione S-transferase π, switching expression of integrins (loss of $\alpha 1$, induction of $\alpha 6$, and de novo expression of $\beta 4$, $\alpha 2$, and $\alpha 3$ chains) [41] and varying expression of the Ca^{2+}-dependent cell adhesion molecule epithelial cadherin and the linked cytosolic components α- and β-catenin [42]. The homeobox transcription factor Prox1 remains highly conserved in embryonic hepatoblasts but is absent in bile duct epithelium [43].The C/EBPα (CCAAT/enhancer-binding protein-α), which is expressed in hepatoblasts from the early stage of hepatic specification, is not observed in cholangiocytes of extra- and intrahepatic bile ducts [44].

The remodeling of the ductal plate involves epithelial changes – construction of new epithelial structures (by proliferation) and the simultaneous deletion of other parts (by apoptosis); mesenchymal influence; and determination by the portal vein.

Autocrine stimulation of ductal plate cell proliferation is suggested by the immunohistochemical positivity for TGF-α, hepatocyte growth factor, and parathyroid hormone–related peptide. Apoptosis in the remodeling ductal plate is indicated by positive histochemical terminal deoxynucleotidyl transferase–mediated bio-deoxy UTP nick end labeling (TUNEL) staining and expression of Fas, C-myc, and Lewis^y.

The importance of the periepithelial mesenchyme is indicated by the topographic expression of laminin and collagen type IV, and the matrix glycoprotein tenascin for the larger intrahepatic bile ducts; the expression of matrix metalloproteinases (MMP1) and their inhibitors (tissue inhibitor of MMP 1 [TIMP1] and TIMP2) [45]; patchy expression of N-CAM in duplicated ductal plates and incorporating ducts; and denser cellularity and nerve fibers close to incorporating ducts [46].

The determinating influence of the portal vein is evident from the exclusive development of intrahepatic bile duct structures around the branches of this afferent vessel [47]. The further maturation of the remodeled tubular ducts comprises, among others, a switch from apomucin MUC1 to MUC3, the further development of the peribiliary capillary plexus, and – for the larger intrahepatic bile ducts – the development of their peribiliary glands [39].

There is a close interaction of the developing intrahepatic bile ducts not only with the portal mesenchyme, but with the developing hepatic artery as well (arterial–ductal interaction). The sequence of events indicates that the ductal plates precede and determine the development of the intrahepatic branches of the hepatic artery. The appearance of α-smooth muscle actin-positive myofibroblasts and their organization into a vascular wall (vasculogenesis) follows the development of ductal plates [48]. The developing arterial branches in turn precede and presumably induce, during the remodeling process, the incorporation of the peripheral biliary cell tubules, which are accompanied by a denser myofibroblastic cell population that gives rise in turn to the peribiliary vascular plexus [49]. The dependence of arterial development on normal progression of bile duct development entails an involvement of the transcription factors HNF6 and HNF1β for both structures [50–52]. The arterial–ductal interaction is also reflected in the involvement of the same signaling pathways (Jagged1/Notch) in the development and in the maintenance of both the hepatic arterial system [53,54] and of the intrahepatic biliary tree [55–59]. Differences in the human and murine expression patterns for Jagged and Notch preclude at present a detailed mechanistic insight into the precise role of this pathway in bile duct development [29].

It thus appears that, in the embryologic development of the liver, it is the portal vein that determines the three-dimensional structure of the ramifying portal tracts and their essential tubular components (portal vein, bile duct, and hepatic artery) that constitute the basic angioarchitecture of the liver and its lobular organization.

Postnatal Development of the Intrahepatic Bile Ducts

The intrahepatic biliary system is not mature at the time of birth. During human fetal development, the major canalicular transporter genes are expressed at mid-gestational age, but differ in expression level and targeting pattern, indicating differential regulation and maturation [60]. Bile canaliculi between hepatocytes only acquire a mature appearance at the perinatal and early postnatal periods [61,62].

The remodeling of the intrahepatic bile ducts is not complete at the time of birth; it requires about six additional weeks for the ductal plates in the most peripheral (smallest) portal tracts to remodel [22]. This has implications for defining the "normal" bile duct–to–portal tract (BD/PT) ratio that is used to estimate the degree of ductopenia in the liver. A BD/PT ratio lower than 0.9 may be normal in the premature infant [22,33,34].

The expression of parathyroid hormone–related peptide (PTHrP) by cholangiocytes remains positive until the age of 4 years [63]. The end-stage maturity of the hilar peribiliary glands [64] and of the peribiliary capillary plexus [49] is only reached at the age of 15 years. Liver mass increases from 125 g at birth to 255 g at 1 year of age, 430 g at 2 years, and 530 g at 5 years. The adult liver weighs approximately 1400 g, more than ten times the weight of the newborn liver [65,66]. There is only scant information on the structural and lobular development of the human liver from birth to adulthood, possibly related to the unending search for the identity of the structural and functional unit of the liver: the classical lobule [67], the portal lobule [68], the acinus [69], the metabolic lobulus [70], the primary and composite lobule [71,72], its modular variant [73], and the smallest unit, termed *choleohepaton* [74]. An old investigation indicated that in the pig, the liver mass increases through increase in size and in number of the liver lobules, which themselves increase in size through increase in size and number of their constituting hepatocytes [75].

Consequently, the intrahepatic biliary tree is also growing after birth. Landing and Wells [76] propose, on the basis of observation and assumptions, that postnatal human liver growth occurs by an increase in number of peripheral lobules associated with branching and elongation of the accompanying portal tracts.

In the adult liver, the complete sequence of intrahepatic bile ducts from the hepatic ducts to the smallest ductules, as demonstrable on cholangiographic documents, comprises 11–12 orders of branching [77], but cholangiography fails to visualize an unknown number of finer ramifications. It is estimated that in the adult liver the biliary tree requires between 18 and 20 orders of branches in order to realize the ± 500,000 terminal bile ducts necessary to assure biliary drainage of the estimated 440,000 microarchitectural units (defined as lobules or otherwise) [65]. Because bile duct branching occurs in a three-dimensional treelike fashion, small ("peripheral") branches in small ("peripheral") portal tracts are formed not only in the hepatic periphery but also within the liver, just as terminal twigs and leaves are also found inside the crown mass of a tree [76].

Since shortly after birth ductal plates composed of immature cholangiocyte precursor cells have disappeared, and new bile ducts apparently arise from preexisting mature, tubular ducts by branching and elongation. This has been compared with blood vessel development: Formation from immature cells is referred to as *vasculogenesis*, whereas growth of preexisting vessels by sprouting is termed *angiogenesis*. In a similar way, it is suggested that *ductogenesis* and *cholangiogenesis* could be used as respective Latin- and Greek-derived terms to refer to bile duct formation before and after birth, respectively [48].

In human liver, Jagged1 is expressed in bile duct cells, hepatocytes, and vasculature, with, however, some variation between different reports [55,58].

The immunohistochemical localization of Notch1 and Notch2 in mature bile duct cells of pediatric normal liver suggests that Notch signaling continues to play a role in bile duct growth and remodeling in postnatal life, albeit that the precise tuning of the signaling may differ from what happens during development, because in the fetal liver the ductal plate cells express Jagged1, and Notch3 protein is found in the closely adjacent mesenchymal cells [59]. The results of a study in mice on inducible inactivation of *Notch1* point to a critical role of *Notch2*, and not of *Notch1*, for the maintenance of bile duct integrity [31].One has to keep in mind that the modalities of Notch signaling are not a linear picture; each step is subject to additional elements and features that modulate the activity and efficacy of the transmitted signals, and is further influenced by the developmental context [78,79].

The terminology of the adult intrahepatic bile duct system has recently been standardized by a consensus effort [80].

Ductal Plate Malformation

The normal development of intrahepatic bile ducts apparently requires finely timed and precisely tuned epithelial–mesenchymal interactions, which proceed from the hilum of the liver toward its periphery along the branches of the developing portal vein. Lack of remodeling of the ductal plate results in the persistence of an excess of embryonic bile duct structures remaining in their primitive ductal plate configuration. This abnormality has been termed the *ductal plate malformation* (DPM) [9].

Hnf6$^{-/-}$ and Hnf1$\beta^{-/-}$ mouse embryos show abnormal intrahepatic bile ducts corresponding to DPM, revealing the importance of the HNF6-HNF1β cascade in normal development of the intrahepatic bile ducts [50,52], as mentioned previously (see Development of Intrahepatic Bile Ducts).

Ductal plate malformation originally referred to a microscopic lesion [9]. Modern imaging techniques of the liver, however, such as ultrasonography and computed tomography, which produce the equivalent of sections through the liver, allow visualizion of the abnormalities of DPM also in the larger branches of the intrahepatic biliary tree [81–86].

Lack of remodeling of the ductal plate (or DPM) appears to be associated often with abnormalities in the branching pattern of the portal vein. Instead of giving rise to a regular, treelike branching pattern, resulting in individual portal tracts separated by intervening parenchyma, as occurs in the normal liver, the involved portal vein branch gives rise to multiple sprouts with diameters too small and spaced too closely together, resembling the branches of a "pollard willow" [87,88] (Figure 4.3).

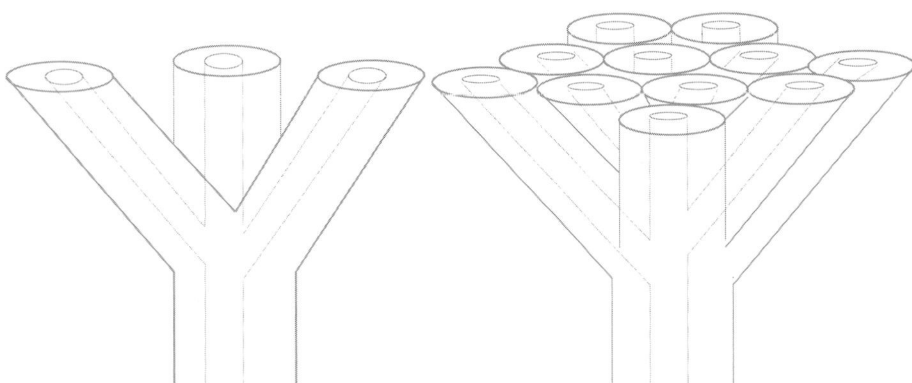

Figure 4.3. Schematic drawing, representing the normal branching pattern of the portal vein (*left*), and a "pollard willow" pattern (*right*). The circles around the cross-sectioned portal vein branches can be viewed both as portal tracts and as possible profiles of biliary ductal plates.

A transverse section through such a pollard willow appears as an enlarged portal area, which corresponds to the fusion of several smaller portal tracts, each containing a ductal plate (or incompletely remodeled parts thereof) surrounding a hypoplastic or even obliterated branch of the portal vein [87,88].

Ductal plate malformation is observed in several congenital diseases of the intrahepatic bile ducts [33,89]. The most frequent ones are discussed below together with other cholangiopathies.

CHOLANGIOPATHIES OF INTRAHEPATIC BILE DUCTS

Atretic Cholangiopathies

Extrahepatic Bile Duct Atresia, Biliary Atresia

Despite the older terminology of *extrahepatic bile duct atresia*, the disease is not restricted to the extrahepatic segments of the biliary tree; it also affects the intrahepatic bile ducts and thus represents a panbiliary disease [20,90,91]. For that reason, the term *biliary atresia* (BA) has become the preferred terminology for the disease.

Atresia of the extrahepatic bile ducts has been defined as absence of a lumen in part or all of the extrahepatic biliary tract, causing complete obstruction of bile flow.

A new era in the study and therapy of BA was inaugurated by the introduction of hepatic portoenterostomy as surgical treatment for this disease by Kasai et al. [92]. With the "Kasai operation," two important concepts entered into the pathology of BA [93]. First, it became evident that a variable number of bile-draining intrahepatic ducts are patent at the porta hepatis in nearly all patients during the first 2 or 3 months after birth. Interlobular bile ducts appeared to be destroyed rapidly and to decrease progressively in number after 2 months of age. Second, the radical approach of portoenterostomy with resection of the obliterated extrahepatic ducts provided unique specimens not previously available, allowing histopathologic study of the bile ducts before the terminal stage of the disease [93].

Histopathologic study of these "fibrous remnants" confirmed the concept that BA represents a necroinflammatory destructive cholangitis, resulting in progressive destruction and obliterating fibrosis of the ducts [94–96]. It was established further that the intrahepatic bile ducts participate in this dynamic inflammatory process and are equally subject to progressive destruction [97].

PATHOLOGY OF EXTRAHEPATIC BILE DUCTS IN BILIARY ATRESIA

Numerous anatomic types of BA can be distinguished and categorized as correctable and noncorrectable forms, according to the extent and the localization of the obliterated bile duct segments [90,98].

Several studies have been devoted to the histopathology of fibrous remnants of the resected extrahepatic biliary tree (summarized in Desmet and Callea [90]). These studies have focused on the topography and the nature of the lesions observed in the extrahepatic ductal remnants and on the correlation between the numbers and sizes of identifiable ducts at the porta hepatis and the success of postoperative bile flow after hepatic portoenterostomy.

The histologic appearances of the fibrous remnants of the resected extrahepatic biliary tree can be divided into three types. One histologic picture, termed *Gautier type 1* [99], corresponds to absence of any lumen lined by biliary epithelium: The bile duct segment is reduced to a fibrous cord. A second type of appearance (Gautier type 2) [99] corresponds to scattered or clustered lumina lined by epithelium, usually surrounded by inflammatory cells and often characterized by signs of necrosis and sloughing of the epithelial cells. A third pattern (Gautier type 3) [99] is characterized by a central structure that corresponds to an altered bile duct; in most specimens, part of the epithelial lining is still present but the rest of the perimeter appears eroded. The lumen may be filled with biliary concrement, cellular debris, and macrophages containing bile, and the degree of surrounding inflammation and fibrosis is variable.

All investigators agree that the variable histologic appearances reflect successive stages in a dynamic process of progressive inflammatory destruction of the extrahepatic ducts. The early stage corresponds to periductal inflammation with necrosis and sloughing of the epithelial lining, followed by progressive periductal fibrosis and narrowing of the lumen. The final stage is a complete fibrous scar of a destroyed epithelium-lined tube that remains identifiable as a fibrous cord [90].

The fibrous obliteration of the extrahepatic ducts increases with the age of the patient, in parallel with increasing fibrosis in the liver [100].

The search for a correlation between the number and size of the ducts observed at the porta hepatis and the success of hepatic portoenterostomy has yielded controversial results (summarized in Desmet and Callea [90]). Some investigators concluded that the size of the ducts at the porta hepatis has little influence on the postoperative course [101]; others insisted that the total diameter of all the prehilar bile duct structures is an important prognostic finding, with a total diameter of more than 400 μm indicating a favorable prognostic subtype [102]. A later study showed no correlation between duration of patient survival and the size of bile ducts at the resection margins [103]. At present, the need for frozen section examination of the liver at the site chosen for the portoenterostomy is no longer demanded [104].

PATHOLOGY OF THE LIVER AND OF INTRAHEPATIC BILE DUCTS IN BILIARY ATRESIA

CLASSIC BILIARY ATRESIA

The classic features of BA include histologic alterations that change during the course of the disease, allowing some chronologic staging in successive periods [105], although the timing of the stages is only approximate. The histologic alterations can be grouped in two categories: changes secondary to bile duct obstruction and lesions caused by primary bile duct disease. Obstructive features include bilirubinostasis, ductular reaction, and progressive fibrosis [106].

During the first 4 weeks or so, the liver is characterized by nonspecific features of bilirubinostasis, with bilirubin granules in hepatocytes and intercellular bile plugs. Parenchymal giant cells may be seen but usually in small numbers and without hydropic swelling. Kupffer cell bilirubinostasis increases with the duration of cholestasis. Foci of extramedullary hematopoiesis may persist to variable extent. The histopathology in this early period does not allow a firm diagnosis of BA because it virtually corresponds to that of so-called neonatal hepatitis [106].

Gradually, portal edema and ductular proliferation set in, associated with lymphocytic infiltration in the center of the portal tracts and polymorphs between the ductules.

The ductular reaction results from real multiplication of preexisting ductules and – with time – from ductular metaplasia of acinar zone 1 hepatocytes [107]. The increase in ductules is associated with progressive periductular fibrosis and soon is characterized by the appearance of bilirubin concrements in the ductular lumina (ductular bilirubinostasis) [106].

The ductular reaction is considered the most reliable, although not pathognomonic, criterion in diagnosing extrahepatic obstruction in liver tissue specimens [90,91,108]. Immunostaining for bile duct–type cytokeratins is valuable in highlighting this diagnostically helpful feature [109–111]. In rare instances, ductular proliferation may appear only late, between 9 and 12 weeks of age; therefore, sequential liver biopsies appear indicated in infants with unexplained conjugated hyperbilirubinemia and acholic stools until clinical improvement occurs or until BA can be excluded from the differential diagnosis [112]. Attention has been drawn to accompanying anomalies of the arterial system, consisting of hyperplastic and hypertrophic changes of the hepatic artery branches [113,114].

With ongoing cholestasis, portal and periportal fibrosis develops, associated with periportal extension of the ductular reaction and leading to development of portal–portal connections: the stage of biliary fibrosis. As in any type of longstanding cholestasis, the periportal and periseptal hepatocytes display changes corresponding to cholate stasis: swelling, coarse clumping of the cytoplasm, and accumulation of copper and copper binding protein [106]. The liver lesions at this time are advanced beyond the optimal stage for hepatic portoenterostomy.

A series of histopathologic changes, including syncytial giant cells, lobular inflammation, focal and bridging necrosis, and cholangitis, has been claimed to be predictive of portoenterostomy failure [115].

If the bile duct obstruction is not relieved, the lesions progress to the stage of secondary biliary cirrhosis, characterized by nodular regeneration of the parenchyma and perinodular septal fibrosis (at around 3 months) [105].

Besides ductular reaction, ductular bilirubinostasis, and progressive periportal fibrosis, the interlobular bile ducts show degenerative changes, which are part of the basic disease process of the biliary tree [51]. The appearance of the ductal lesions varies with the progression of the cholangiopathy. Interlobular ducts in an early stage of damage are characterized by irregularity of their lining epithelium, which shows vacuolization, nuclear pyknosis, atrophy, and infiltration by inflammatory cells (Figure 4.4). A gradual thickening of the basement membrane occurs, often linked with periductal fibrosis and associated with progressing atrophy and disappearance of the biliary epithelium. Finally, the duct disappears altogether. With increasing age of the patient, there is an increasing degree of ductopenia in BA [106]. The degree of damage and disappearance of interlobular bile ducts are important prognostic parameters predicting the success of hepatic portoenterostomy [102].

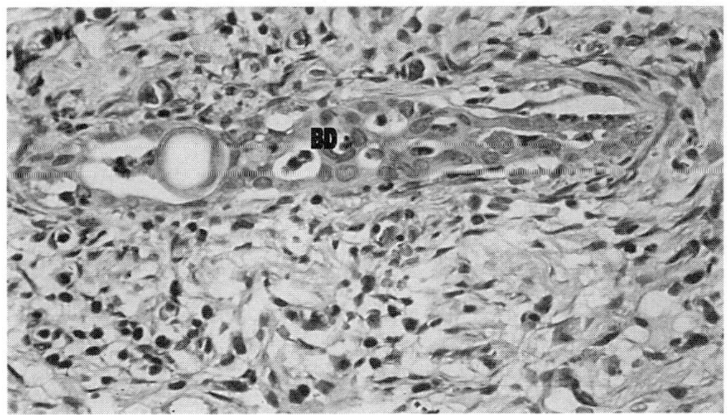

Figure 4.4. Small interlobular bile duct (BD) in liver biopsy from a 60-day-old baby with biliary atresia. Note the irregularity of the bile duct–lining cells, permeation by inflammatory cells, and presence of bile concrement. (Hematoxylin and eosin [H&E] stain, 500× magnification.)

Absence of interlobular bile ducts in later stages of BA probably results from several causes: damage resulting from bile retention caused by distal extrahepatic obstruction, strangulation by progressive fibrosis, ischemia resulting from compression of the peribiliary capillary plexus by periductal fibrosis, and – perhaps most importantly – the relentless progression of the primary process of sclerosing cholangitis that affects the bile ducts in BA [90]. Obliteration of the intrahepatic bile ducts is seen in radiographic investigation, which shows hypoplasia of the intrahepatic biliary tree [116,117].

The ductular reaction, which shows a rapid increase peaking around 200 days, is followed by regression of the ductules; the initially rapid loss of ductules slows down after 400 days [118]. The excess ductular structures disappear by apoptosis [119].

"EARLY SEVERE" BILIARY ATRESIA

In some patients with BA, the damaged intrahepatic bile ducts in the liver biopsy appear as unusually shaped duct structures in excessive numbers, corresponding to a more or less marked degree of DPM. The incidence of this lesion varies in different studies, between about 20% [120] and over 60%. In such patients, histology reveals an already advanced degree of fibrosis even at a very young age (4 weeks). These patients can be considered to suffer from an "early, severe" form of BA (Figure 4.5), which has been confirmed to carry a worse prognosis [121].

In several instances, the portal blood vessels have been surrounded by two or even more concentric rings of ductal plate

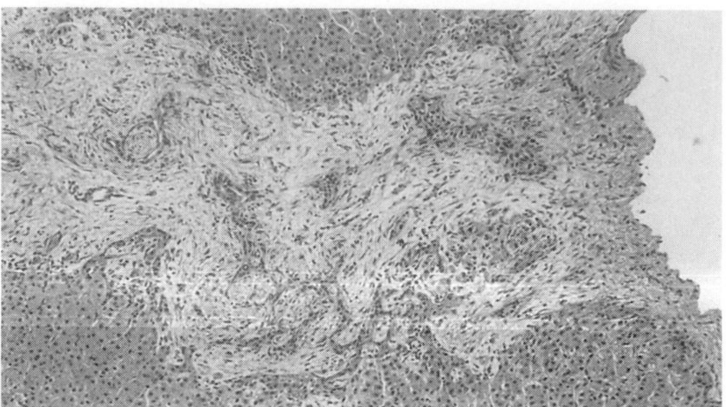

Figure 4.5. Liver biopsy specimen from a 30-day-old baby with biliary atresia. The picture shows an enlarged portal tract, corresponding to fusion of several portal areas (pollard willow pattern). Several profiles of incompletely remodeled ductal plates can be recognized (early severe type of biliary atresia). Some segments of the irregularly shaped ducts show epithelial damage. Note the extreme hypoplasia of the portal vein branches. (H&E stain, 125× magnification.) (Specimen courtesy of Dr. Francesco Callea, Rome, Italy.)

remnants. This observation suggests that repetitive formation of ductal plates has occurred in successive waves during the first few weeks of life. Concentric ductal plates may represent an embryonic or fetal type of ductular reaction [90]. Several enlarged portal areas seem to correspond to fused bundles of smaller portal tracts, because multiple aggregates of complex ductal plates surrounding arterial sprouts may be observed in the same large mesenchymal area. This fusion of portal areas corresponds to the pollard willow anomaly in the branching pattern of the portal vein that accompanies the DPM. The branches of the portal vein appear hypoplastic or may be missing altogether. In contrast, the hepatic artery branches are characterized by an increase in number resembling the arterial anomaly in mice with targeted deletion of HNF6 or HNF1β and DPM of the portal bile ducts [51]. The arterial wall often appears hypertrophic, indicating a remodeling of the arterial wall in association with the disappearance of the epithelial bile duct structures [113,114]. The occurrence of bile ducts in the ductal plate configuration in BA suggests an early antenatal start of the disease, at a time at which the interlobular bile ducts are still in their primitive, embryonic shape.

Apparently, the destructive cholangitis of BA involves an arrest in remodeling of the early embryonic plates and leads to progressive necroinflammatory destruction of the ducts in their immature shape of ductal plates [122].

LIVER LESIONS AFTER HEPATIC PORTOENTEROSTOMY

Some patients with BA are cured by hepatic portoenterostomy. Real cure appears, however, to be limited to a minority of patients. Most reports on long-term follow-up mention some abnormalities in liver enzyme and serum bile salt levels, hepatomegaly, splenomegaly, and often portal hypertension, occasionally with severe bleeding from esophageal varices. Most patients subsequently need liver transplantation [123–125].

In surgical reports, the complications of fibrosis, cirrhosis, and portal hypertension usually are ascribed to the occurrence of repetitive episodes of cholangitis, a dreaded complication of portoenterostomy. There is evidence, however, that the more serious long-term hepatic complications after portoenterostomy reflect the slow but relentless progression of the intrahepatic component of the "basic disease process" (sclerosing cholangiopathy) of BA [82,126,127].

Hepatic portoenterostomy exerts a beneficial effect on account of its relieving the extrahepatic obstructive component of the disease but does not influence per se the basic sclerosing cholangiopathy of BA.

The intrahepatic sclerosing cholangiopathy of BA continues after portoenterostomy but has a variable course in different patients. In some, it is highly active and progressive, in others, low-grade and smoldering, and occasionally it burns out after a variable period of time. The variability in activity, speed, and duration of the destructive cholangiopathy of BA may explain the differences in time span before the appearance of symptoms of complications. It explains the diversity of histologic lesions observed in follow-up liver biopsy specimens from children who have undergone successful portoenterostomy with a favorable postoperative course.

The hepatic lesions observed in follow-up biopsy specimens taken 4 to 5 years after portoenterostomy in "clinically cured" cases vary from mild periportal fibrosis, to advanced biliary fibrosis with ductopenia, to biliary cirrhosis [82,128].

In children who display ductal plate configuration of the interlobular bile ducts at the time of portoenterostomy, follow-up liver biopsies after four to five nearly symptom-free years reveal a histopathologic picture closely resembling that of congenital hepatic fibrosis (CHF) [128] (Figure 4.6). The lesion is interpreted as a "fetal" type of biliary fibrosis [90]. This remarkable observation indicates that interlobular bile ducts in

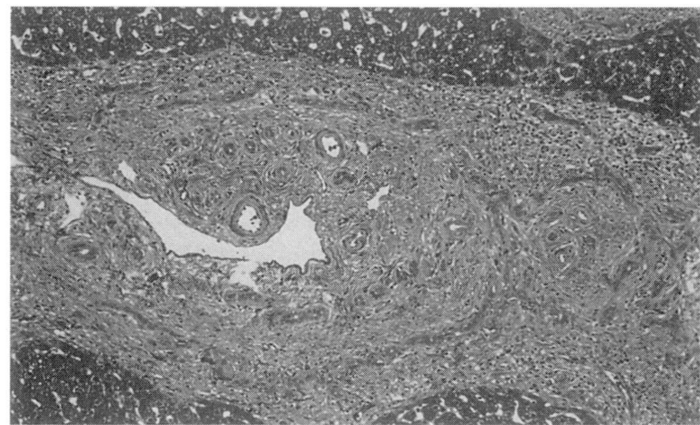

Figure 4.6. Follow-up liver biopsy specimen from a child who has undergone hepatic portoenterostomy for early severe biliary atresia, after 4 years of a favorable postoperative course. The liver shows a congenital hepatic fibrosis-like pattern, with perilobular fibrous bands carrying numerous irregular bile duct structures in ductal plate configuration. (Masson trichrome stain, 125× magnification.) (Specimen courtesy of Dr. Francesco Callea, Rome, Italy.) For color reproduction, see Color Plate 4.6.

DPM configuration, which are subject to a slowly progressive, sclerosing cholangiopathy, may give rise to a histopathologic lesion that is indistinguishable from CHF, provided that the patient is given the chance to survive long enough by hepatic portoenterostomy. This raises the suspicion that the disease known as CHF might be the result of an arrested or mild form of some sort of sclerosing cholangiopathy in children with immature interlobular bile ducts in DPM configuration at the time of birth.

ETIOLOGY AND PATHOGENESIS OF BILIARY ATRESIA

The etiology and pathogenesis of BA remain enigmatic. In spite of recent advances in developmental and cell biology, genetics, and genomics, no definite etiology has as yet unequivocally been proven and no pathogenetic pathway is firmly established. The present-day concept considers BA as the phenotypic expression of a variety of disparate disorders [129]. Any proposed pathogenetic disease mechanism has to account for the major clinical features that are exclusive to BA: the neonatal onset of the disease, the restriction of injury to the biliary system, and the lack of recurrence of typical BA lesions following liver transplantation [130]. Genetic predisposition, presumed environmental challenges, and aspects of susceptibility in the developing bile duct system are all parts of older and newer hypotheses, based on published observations that are still in need of further exploration.

Two major forms of BA can be distinguished: an embryonic or fetal form in a minority (20%) of cases and a perinatal or acquired form in the majority (80%) of patients [131]. Hypotheses concerning etiology and pathogenesis of BA have been the subject of extensive recent reviews [129,130,132,133]. These will be considered shortly, with some more detail on the embryonic form.

EMBRYONIC OR FETAL FORM OF BILIARY ATRESIA

A prenatal onset of the disease is suggested by the presence of nonhepatic malformations in a subgroup of patients with BA. The main associated malformations are poly- or asplenia, cardiovascular defects, abdominal situs inversus, intestinal malrotation, and anomalies of the portal vein and hepatic artery, pointing to potential defects in embryogenesis and asymmetric left–right determination of visceral organs [134]. A transgenic mouse model with a recessive mutation of the inversin gene shows similarities but not identity with the lesions in human BA [135], whereas mutational analyses in children with laterality defects and BA failed to identify mutations in the inversin gene [136].

Several other proteins are involved in establishment of left–right patterning; one is the CRYPTIC protein, encoded by the *CFC1* gene. Heterozygous *CFC1* mutations may predispose to BA but require an additional factor to produce the disease phenotype [137]. A mutation in *ZIC3* (encoding a transcription factor that influences left–right axis determination) is found in occasional cases of BA and heterotaxia [138]. A recent study on hepatic transcriptomes of patients with BA revealed that embryonic and perinatal forms are distinguished by gene expression profiling. In the embryonic form no differences were found in mRNA expression of a panel of laterality genes. However, the profile uncovered a coordinated expression of regulatory genes, comprising a unique pattern of genes involved in chromatin integrity/function, and the uniform overexpression of five imprinted gene programs, providing evidence for a transcriptional basis for the pathogenesis of the embryonic form of BA.The authors propose the novel hypothesis that epigenetic factors modulate the phenotypic manifestations of the embryonic or fetal form of the disease [139].

Sequence analysis of the *JAG1* gene in a group of children with BA and poor outcome revealed a high frequency of single nucleotide polymorphisms [140]. These data suggest that factors governing the morphogenesis of the biliary system may be involved in BA.

The above described "early severe" forms of BA, characterized by DPM at the time of diagnosis, also support the notion of an antenatal origin of the disease. Polymorphisms in *HNF6*, *HNF1B*, *JAG1*, or other genes involved in remodeling of the ductal plate may act as susceptibility factors or modifier genes necessary, but not sufficient, for the development of BA [132].

The intrahepatic bile duct system in these infants is characterized not only by an immaturity at the architectural level but also by signs of immaturity or inappropriate differentiation at the cellular level.The intermediate filament cytoskeleton of the cholangiocytes has an abnormal, immature cytokeratin composition [141], which is what may render the cells more susceptible to stress [142]. The cholangiocytes are characterized by an ectopic intracellular localization of TGF-β [143]; by inadequate regulation of their expression of E-cadherin and α- and β-catenin [144]; by disturbance in the regulation of apoptosis and the cell cycle, resulting in disorganized cell turnover [145]; and by persistent expression of N-CAM at the cell surface [46]. Collectively, these cellular characteristics point to a lack of adequate differentiation into a full biliary or cholangiocytic phenotype. Inappropriate differentiation of the cellular lining of tubes destined to drain a fluid with detergent properties, such as bile, may result in cell damage, apoptosis or necrosis, or both, in denudation of the underlying mesenchyme and initiation of chronic inflammation with ensuing scarring fibrosis. Such a pathogenetic mechanism might explain why the hilar and extrahepatic ducts show the most severe lesions at the time of diagnosis, because these structures are formed earlier than the progressively later-developing intrahepatic ducts, and hence are already longer exposed to the influence of bile and bile acids, the secretion of which starts around the 16th week of intrauterine life [146]. The formation of a hilar ductal network [147] would under such circumstances amplify the mass of periductal fibrosis, explaining the "fibrous cone" at the porta hepatis that is often observed in portoenterostomy resection specimens.

In this view, the bile (be it of normal composition or containing abnormal bile salts [148,149]), which flows through the intra- and extrahepatic bile ducts, would function as a damaging agent for the inappropriately prepared epithelial lining, thus realizing literally a "descending cholangitis" as proposed more than 100 years ago [150].

An alternative hypothesis to explain the constant involvement of the porta hepatis proposes a vulnerable stage in intrahepatic bile duct development between 11 and 13 weeks postfertilization, in which failure of ductal plate remodeling could lead to insufficient development of the mesenchymal cuff that normally surrounds the developing hilar ducts, resulting in ductal rupture, bile leakage, subsequent mesenchymal inflammation, fibrosis, and obstruction [3].

The finding that the development and maintenance of both hepatic artery branches and portal bile ducts appear to be assured by a common mechanism of Notch signaling (see Postnatal Development of the Intrahepatic Bile Ducts) together with the occurrence of arterial abnormalities (hypertrophy and hyperplasia) accompanying the ductal lesions also in EHBDA patients without DPM [113,114,151] suggests that in perinatal forms of EHBDA also, a genetic predisposition caused by abnormal final differentiation of the bile duct lining cells may play a role. If this is the case, the problem remains whether the triggering agent is an endogeneous or an exogeneous (environmental) factor.

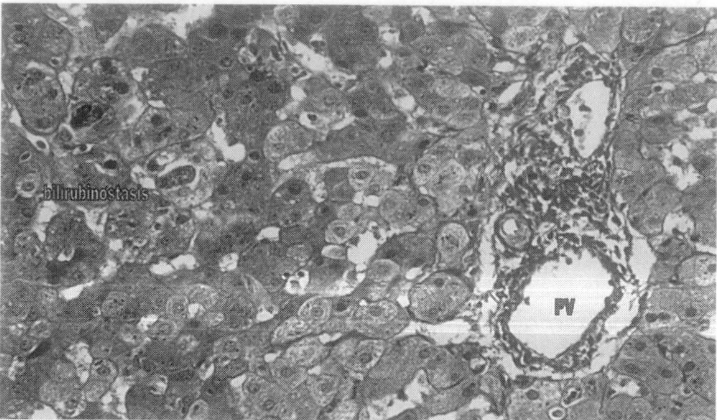

Figure 4.7. Detail from a liver biopsy specimen from a 5-year-old child with nonsyndromic paucity of interlobular bile ducts. The portal tract (*right*) is devoid of an interlobular bile duct. Note the bilirubinostasis in the lobular parenchyma at left. PV, portal vein. (Masson trichrome stain, 500× magnification.) For color reproduction, see Color Plate 4.7.

PERINATAL OR ACQUIRED FORM OF BILIARY ATRESIA

The theories for this form of BA consider environmental insults like toxins and infectious agents as well as disturbances in immune regulation. Several viruses have been considered. Hepatitis viruses A, B, and C have been studied and ruled out. Still under consideration, although awaiting futher consolidating evidence, are reovirus type 3, group C rotavirus, and cytomegalovirus (reviewed in Mack and Sokol [132]). Toxins have been suspected in unusual outbreaks of cholestatic hepatobiliary disease resembling human BA in lambs and calves in New South Wales, Australia, in 1964 and 1988, but causative phytotoxins or mycotoxins have not been found [152]. The search for a role of dysregulation of the immune system in disease pathogenesis through immune-mediated destruction of intrahepatic bile ducts in BA has focused on human leukocyte antigens, antigen-presenting cells, lymphocyte subsets, macrophages, cytokines, adhesion molecules, and chemokines, while attention has also been paid to autoantibodies in search of evidence for autoimmune mechanisms (reviewed in Mack and Sokol [132]).

Considering the present evidence that lesions of BA do not recur after liver transplantation, and with regard to the types of disease that produce posttransplant recurrence in adults, the theories of infectious etiology and autoimmune pathogenesis appear less plausible.

Paucity of Interlobular Bile Ducts

So-called atresia of the intrahepatic bile ducts usually is not complete but involves a reduced ratio of the number of interlobular ducts to the number of portal tracts. This explains the various synonyms: *atresia*, *hypoplasia* or *paucity of interlobular* (or *intrahepatic*) ducts, *ductular hypoplasia*, *ductular paucity*, and *ductopenia* (Figure 4.7).

A sound morphologic diagnosis of paucity of interlobular bile ducts (PILBD) requires a sufficiently large liver biopsy specimen and morphometric evaluation of bile ducts. Although originally a surgical wedge biopsy of the liver was recommended [153], it is felt that a simple percutaneous needle biopsy may suffice, provided the sample contains at least five portal tracts. Immunostains for cytokeratins or tissue polypeptide antigen are helpful for better visualization of interlobular ducts [154].

Paucity of interlobular bile ducts has been defined as a ratio of the number of interlobular ducts to the number of portal tracts of less than 0.5. In normal children this ratio lies between 0.9 and 1.8 [153].

It appears that this definition should not be used too strictly. It was a valid definition at the time of its formulation [153], but since 1975 evidence has accumulated that PILBD, like BA, is not a static condition resulting from agenesis or nonformation of the bile ducts but mostly (with the apparent exception of Alagille syndrome) corresponds to a progressive, necroinflammatory, destructive, and sclerosing cholangiopathy of unknown origin [90]. It follows that a reduced bile duct–to–portal tract ratio higher than 0.5 (i.e., a less pronounced degree of PILBD) can be considered "ductopenia," especially if besides a few portal tracts with missing ducts, ducts with degenerative changes also are observed [155].

Another word of caution concerns the size of the portal tracts and bile ducts. Instances occur in which there is a marked loss of the smallest terminal branches of interlobular ducts (bile duct–to–portal tract ratios of 0.3 or 0.2), but the larger, preterminal portal tracts virtually all retain their interlobular duct. Nondiscriminative counting of ducts and portal tracts of all sizes may lead to underestimation of the degree of disconnection between parenchyma and biliary tree in such instances.

A further complication is that the development and maturation of the biliary tree is not complete at the time of birth; full development of the finest ramifications of the intrahepatic biliary system takes an additional 4 weeks [22]. This explains why a ratio of bile ducts to portal tracts of less than 0.9 may be normal in premature infants [34].

The portal tracts devoid of bile ducts appear hypoplastic, and the total number of portal tracts per unit of tissue section is reduced compared with normal control subjects [156]. PILBD may be an isolated defect or associated with other extrahepatic anomalies. This allows patients with PILBD to be grouped into two categories: those with syndromic and those with nonsyndromic PILBD.

SYNDROMIC PILBD (ALAGILLE SYNDROME; ARTERIOHEPATIC DYSPLASIA; ALAGILLE-WATSON SYNDROME)

The preferred terminology has become *Alagille syndrome* (AGS). A description of the clinical fearures and associated extrahepatic malformations is given in Chapter 15. AGS is transmitted in an autosomal dominant way, with 94% penetrance and variable expressivity [157].

The histopathology of AGS has been described in detail in classic reviews [158,159]. DPM of interlobular bile ducts has not been reported in AGS.

Early changes (before 3 months of age) include prominent parenchymal giant cell transformation, marked hepatocellular and canalicular bilirubinostasis, and moderate copper accumulation in periportal hepatocytes. The number of interlobular bile ducts is not reduced or only a little reduced. The ducts often are surrounded by a mononuclear inflammatory infiltrate and show features of biliary epithelial degeneration and some degree of periductal fibrosis. Ductular reaction is not present [158,159].

Later changes (beyond 3 months of age) are characterized by moderate to severe parenchymal bilirubinostasis, less giant cell transformation, and a variable degree of periportal fibrosis. Duct paucity of variable degree, up to a complete lack of ducts, may be observed. However, occasional reports indicate that progression to paucity is not an absolute feature of the disease. The paucity of interlobular bile ducts is associated with a concomitant reduction in the number of portal tracts, indicating a deficiency in the branching of portal tracts during postnatal development [156,159]. As a result, the "real" paucity of interlobular ducts is not adequately reflected in the bile duct/portal tract ratio. Further changes include increased copper in periportal hepatocytes, cholestasis, and sinusoidal fibrosis. Ductular proliferation is occasionally seen. The histopathologic changes in the early stages of the disease do not allow prediction of the future development of fibrosis [158,159].

A narrowing of the extrahepatic biliary tree has been observed at autopsy or by operative cholangiography in patients with AGS [158].

Recently, the cause of the disease has been elucidated, but the pathogenesis remains unclear. AGS appears to be caused by the alteration of the gene *JAG1* [160] at chromosomal location 20p12 [99,100]. *JAG1* is the human homologue of rat Jagged1, which encodes a ligand for the Notch receptor, itself also a cellular transmembrane protein, of which four homologues have been identified in humans: Notch1, Notch2, Notch3, and Notch4. Both ligand and receptor are important participants in cell-to-cell signaling during morphogenesis [78,161] (see Postnatal Development of the Intrahepatic Bile Ducts).

At the molecular level, haploinsufficiency of *JAG1* (decreased gene dosage) seems to be the mechanism of clinically relevant mutations [162]. Mice doubly heterozygous for the Jag1 null allele and a *Notch2* hypomorphic allele exhibit developmental anomalies resembling AGS (but also impaired differentiation of intrahepatic bile ducts at birth, which is less characteristic for AGS), also suggesting haploinsufficiency as a disease mechanism [56]. A zebrafish animal model of AGS points to the importance of the dosage of the Notch signal for biliary development, supporting the notion that gene dosage best accounts for altered biliary development in compound *jagged/notch* morphants [163]. A recent study of Jagged1 mutant alleles in AGS patients leads to the suggestion of a dominant negative effect of some mutant protein as another possible molecular mechanism [164].

During normal embryonic and fetal liver development, bile duct epithelial cells express *NOTCH3*, whereas *JAG1* is expressed in mesenchymal cells (see Embryology of Intrahepatic Bile Ducts). In the neonate with AGS, the intrahepatic bile ducts are normally present at birth, indicating normal remodeling of the ductal plates and normal fetal development, in spite of *JAG1* mutation. This observation together with the strikingly variable clinical expression of the syndrome point to the importance of modulating factors, of which the Notch partners in the JAG/Notch signaling pathway are obvious candidates.

In livers of patients with AGS, two types of patterns of Jagged–Notch could be observed. In liver specimens characterized by marked ductular reaction, Jagged1 was expressed on ductular reactive cells, along with marked Notch2 and Notch3 staining. In contrast, in specimens with paucity, Notch2 and Notch3 were not expressed on remaining biliary epithelial cells (whereas in other cholestatic conditions (BA and α_1-antitrypsin deficiency) Notch expression was not observed on ductular reactive cells, but Notch2 and Notch3 were positive in stromal cells [59].

Evidence from several studies indicates a role for Notch2 in development and maintenance of bile duct epithelial cells [31,56,57,165] (see Postnatal Development of the Intrahepatic Bile Ducts). This correlates with the finding of absent Notch2 expression in liver specimens of AGS without ductular reaction. However, this dual observation in liver biopsies in AGS poses the problems of why ductular proliferation is only occasionally seen, whether this is a case of disproportionate sampling [166], and – if so – why.

An answer to this enigma may lie in the fact that apparently JAG1/Notch signaling is differently tuned during postnatal development than during fetal life, resulting in a lack of further development and maintenance of biliary epithelial cells. Such a scenario of absent postnatal bile duct development has been suggested in the past [154,167].

A recent report provides additional support for this hypothesis [168]. It concerns a detailed investigation of the explant liver of a 17-year-old male AGS patient at the time of transplantation. In this hepatectomy specimen, a central area, measuring

8.5 × 7 × 5 cm, showed a normal brown color and was sharply delineated from the pale-appearing peripheral part of the organ. Histologically, in the central area nearly all portal tracts (except a few ductless terminal ones) contained the normal triad of portal vein, hepatic artery, and interlobular duct and were free of periportal fibrosis. Some ducts showed mild damage with intramural infiltration by inflammatory cells, whereas immunostaining for cytokeratin 7 revealed some ductular reaction around the corresponding portal tracts. In contrast, the specimens sampled in the liver periphery showed prominent periportal fibrosis and some septa, and none of the portal tracts contained an interlobular bile duct. Cytokeratin 7 immunostaining revealed marked parenchymal positivity consistent with chronic cholestasis in the absence of any ductular reaction. The wall of the portal hepatic artery branches was characterized by hypertrophy of the muscular layer. A missense mutation in the *JAG1* gene was found in both parts of this liver.

In their interpretation of these findings, the authors propose that the central part corresponds to the "neonatal liver" of the patient, whereas the peripheral part represents the postnatally developed mass of the organ. The central area has the size of a liver at birth, and may explain the findings reported in liver imaging studies in several AGS patients. Scintigraphic imaging using hepatobiliary contrast agents early in life shows poor but diffuse biliary excretion of the tracer from the liver into the gallbladder and intestine. In contrast, imaging in older AGS patients shows clearance of the central hilar portion of the liver (measuring about 8 × 9 cm, corresponding to the maximal liver size during the first postnatal months) with simultaneous tracer retainment in the periphery of the liver [169–171]. Some reports mention the presence of bile ducts in the biopsied central area and their absence in the liver periphery [169–171]. The findings support the thesis that bile duct branching and elongation fail to occur in AGS [168] and further demonstrate the occurrence of intrahepatic arterial lesions as part of the more generalized vascular involvement in AGS [172].

Several questions remain in the pathogenesis of AGS [173]. The details of JAG1/Notch signaling involvement are not elucidated. What is the disease mechanism in the patients in whom no *JAG1* mutations have been identified? What is the reason for a reduced number of portal ramifications? What are the facors involved in the marked variability of clinical expression? What determines that some patients (15–20%) do not develop paucity of bile ducts? Why does the central "neonatal liver" show cholestatic features of (mild) bile duct lesions and ductular proliferation, in spite of clearance of tracers? What happens to the liver in those patients in whom cholestasis resolves in spite of ductopenia – is there a mechanism comparable to the "atresia" during metamorphosis of the sea lamprey *Petromyzon marinus L.* (a primitive vertebrate) [174]?

The prognosis for AGS usually has been considered favorable, characterized by resolution of jaundice and xanthomas and amelioration of pruritus in most patients. Cirrhosis develops in beween 10% and 50% of patients [167]. This latter investigation predicts a 20-year life expectancy for 75% of all patients, for 80% of those not requiring liver transplantation, and for 60% of those who did require liver transplantation [167]. One study, however, casts a shadow on this outlook by calculating only a 50% probability of survival until 19 years of age without liver transplantation [175].

Hepatocellular carcinoma has been reported as a rare complication in a total of about 15 patients [176], but may occur at a very young age [177].

NONSYNDROMIC PILBD

Nonsyndromic PILBD may be an isolated hepatic abnormality or one component of a more complex systemic process with or without a specific cause. Unlike syndromic PILBD, however, which is characterized by a set of well defined extra hepatic anomalies, nonsyndromic PILBD lacks these extrahepatic congenital anomalies or accompanies a variable number of other congenital anomalies. Nonsyndromic PILBD constitutes the most frequent diagnosis in patients with conjugated hyperbilirubinemia in the first month of life and occurs more frequently than BA [158]. It represents, however, a heterogeneous group of rare infectious and metabolic conditions, with unrelated pathogenesis and correspondingly diverse outcome [157]. Cases of nonsyndromic PILBD correspond to infections (cytomegalovirus, rubella, hepatitis B, syphilis), α_1-antitrypsin deficiency, endocrine disorders (hypopituitarism), chromosomal anomalies (trisomy 21, Turner's syndrome), Norwegian cholestasis, mucoviscidosis [178], and other miscellaneous disorders. Bile duct damage is part of the liver histopathology in progressive familial intrahepatic cholestasis (PFIC) type 3, caused by a mutation in the transporter *MDR3* gene [179]. Some cases are idiopathic [158]. Cholestatic diseases caused by defects in bile acid synthesis are not associated with bile duct damage or ductopenia [180].

The nonsyndromic variants of duct paucity represent a progressive cholangiopathy.

The hepatic pathology changes with advancing age of the patient. Up to 3 months, one finds parenchymal giant cell transformation, hepatocellular and canalicular bilirubinostasis, extramedullary hematopoiesis, perisinusoidal fibrosis, and mild periportal hepatocellular copper accumulation. Ductopenia in small and intermediate-sized portal tracts (bile duct–to–portal tract ratio lower than 0.6) may be noted; ductopenia with a ratio as low as 0.2 has been recorded as early as 1 week of age [158]. The remaining ducts show evidence of necroinflammatory destruction. After 3 months, lobular changes become less prominent. Ductopenia remains, and periportal fibrosis develops.

COMBINED BILIARY ATRESIA AND PILBD

Some investigators doubt whether AGS may coexist with BA in the same patient [92]. Intriguingly, sequence analysis of the *JAG1* gene in a group of children with BA and poor outcome revealed a high frequency of single-nucleotide polymorphisms [140]. Patients with AGS, however, may have hypoplasia of a segment of the extrahepatic bile ducts [158].

In the few patients in whom the hypoplastic ducts were examined histologically, the lesions in bile ducts in the porta hepatis were indistinguishable from those seen in BA [181]. This finding raises the question of whether so-called hypoplasia of an extrahepatic bile duct segment may represent an incomplete or arrested "atresia" of the duct [90,182]. This hypothesis is supported by the observation that hypoplasia of extrahepatic bile ducts may progress to total obliteration [183].

Nonsyndromic PILBD may coexist with BA in the same patient [158], and BA by itself results in intrahepatic ductopenia. These observations make one wonder about the factors that determine whether the "destructive cholangitis" preferentially hits the intrahepatic branches of the biliary tree (nonsyndromic PILBD), the larger extrahepatic segments (BA), or both, as mentioned in a study on "transitional types" between BA and nonsyndromic PILBD [184]. Furthermore, a sclerosing cholangitis with neonatal onset has been described that bears similarities to both BA and nonsyndromic PILBD [185].

Fibrocystic Cholangiopathies

Several liver diseases are characterized by some degree of dilatation of segments of the intrahepatic bile ducts associated with fibrosis (fibrocystic diseases); they constitute a merging spectrum of alterations, usually associated with renal abnormalities that also represent a continuous spectrum of lesions [186].

The older literature on these associated congenital liver and kidney lesions is confusing because of changes in classification, especially of cystic renal lesions. For instance, Caroli [187] described the pathologic condition that carries his name (Caroli's disease) as being associated with medullary sponge kidney or Cacchi–Ricci disease. What now is called *Cacchi–Ricci disease* or *medullary sponge kidney*, however, is basically different from the renal disease that usually accompanies Caroli's disease [188].

The basic lesion in all variants of fibrocystic liver diseases is DPM (Figure 4.8). DPM may affect all levels of the intrahepatic biliary tree: segmental ducts, septal ducts, interlobular ducts, and the smaller ducts of the more terminal portal tract ramifications. The immaturity of the intrahepatic bile ducts (DPM) at these different levels of the biliary tree determines the different anatomic–clinical entities known as *Caroli's disease*, *infantile polycystic disease*, and *adult polycystic disease*. DPM involving all segments of the entire intrahepatic biliary tree causes the combination of these various anatomic–clinical entities, which has been described in several case reports [189,190].

In some of these disorders, DPM seems to be associated with a progressive destruction of the immature intrahepatic bile ducts by a nonspecific necroinflammatory process, giving rise to the anatomic–clinical entities known as CHF and *Caroli's syndrome* [88].

The hepatic lesions are associated with renal abnormalities, which also may affect some or all levels of the nephron and may be accompanied by a slow destruction of the involved tubular segments in a nonspecific necroinflammatory process.

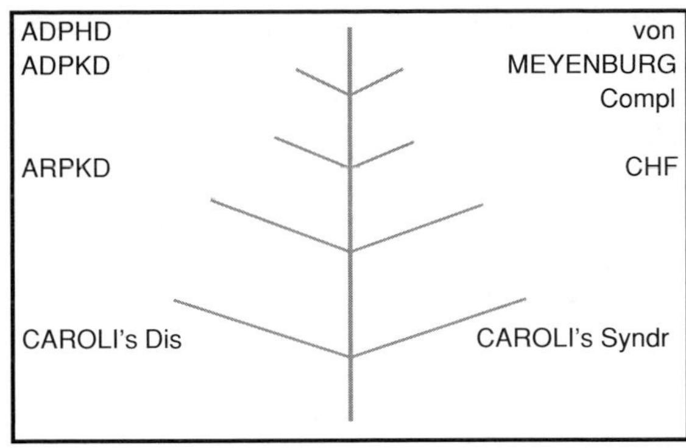

Figure 4.8. Schematic representation of the biliary tree and fibrocystic diseases discussed in this chapter. The placing of diseases at different levels of the tree indicates the approximate size of the bile ducts affected by ductal plate malformation in that particular disorder. The disorders mentioned on the left side are characterized by mild or marked dilatation of the bile duct structures; the entities listed on the right develop by a variable degree of involution ("destructive cholangitis") of the ductal plate remnants, associated with fibrosis. Although too schematic, this overview emphasizes a theme discussed in this chapter: that ductal plate malformation is a basic feature of all congenital bile duct disorders mentioned. ADPDK, autosomal dominant polycystic kidney disease; ADPHD, autosomal dominant polycystic hepatic disease; ARPKD, autosomal recessive polycystic kidney desease; CHF, congenital hepatic fibrosis. (Modified after Desmet [87].)

Autosomal Recessive Polycystic Kidney Disease (Formerly Infantile Polycystic Disease)

Because the "infantile" type of polycystic disease of liver and kidney may be observed in adults, the term has been replaced by the more accurate designation *autosomal recessive polycystic kidney disease* (ARPKD) [157,188,191]. ARPKD is a rare disease, with an incidence between 1 in 20,000 and 1 in 40,000 births [191,192]. It is inherited in an autosomal recessive pattern. The gene responsible for ARPKD has been localized on chromosome 6p21-p12 [192]. The gene is termed polycystic kidney and hepatic disease 1 (*PKHD1*) and encodes a receptor-like protein termed fibrocystin/polyductin [193] that is located in the primary cilium of renal tubular cells [194] and of cholangiocytes lining the intrahepatic bile ducts [195].

Although ARPKD may present on a broad spectrum of clinical and histopathologic phenotypes, two characteristics appear to be present constantly: bile duct abnormalities of the DPM type and fusiform dilatation of renal collecting tubules [196]. An extensive study into the long-term clinical consequences of *PKHD1* mutations in 164 patients with ARPKD suggested that the renal morbidities are positively related to hepatobiliary morbidities rather than organ-specific progression of ARPKD [197]. Animal models for ARPKD comprise the cpk mouse (a spontaneous mutation of the C57 BL/6J mouse) [198,199]. The *cpk* gene is expressed primarily in the kidney and liver and encodes a hydrophilic protein, termed cystin [200]. In the cpk model, expression of the biliary lesion is modulated by genetic background, and the specific biliary phenotype is determined by whether loss of function of the *cpk* gene occurs as a germline or a somatic event [199]. Further models include the Oak Ridge polycystic kidney disease (*orpk, Tg737^{orpk}*) mutant, a transgenic mouse line with a single transgene insertion that causes a recessively inherited kidney and biliary disease reminiscent of human ARPKD, with the protein polaris as disrupted gene product [201]; the Inv mouse [135]; and a recent mouse model generated by a targeted mutation of *Pkhd1,* the Pkhd1ex40 mouse [202]. Recently, a new rat model, the PCK rat, was described and the hepatic lesions were shown to correspond to DPM [203] with abnormal cilia in biliary cystic cells [204].

The different clinical phenotypes of ARPKD have been described according to age at presentation: perinatal, neonatal, infantile, and juvenile [205]. For a long time it remained uncertain whether the lethal neonatal form represented a genetic entity that is different from that which affects children who survive until later in infancy [191].

Linkage analysis in ARPKD families has indicated that ARPKD is genetically homogeneous [186]; however, the mutation detection rate is high in severely affected patients, lower in those with moderate ARPKD, and low – but significant – in adults with congenital hepatic fibrosis and Caroli's disease [206], which are mentioned below.

The hepatic lesions in ARPKD are fairly uniform; they seldom give rise to macroscopically visible cysts. Microscopically, the liver is characterized by portal tracts that may appear enlarged by connective tissue and that contain numerous somewhat dilated bile duct profiles, corresponding to (more or less) incompletely remodeled ductal plates (DPM) (Figure 4.9). Normal interlobular ducts in the center of the portal tract are often lacking. The number of abnormal bile duct sections varies, reflecting the variably insufficient degree of remodeling of the original embryologic ductal plate. These bile duct structures are in continuity with the rest of the biliary system (so-called communicating cystic disease) [207]. Similar lesions of larger bile ducts (Caroli's disease) may be associated [208]. The renal lesions correspond to bilateral enlarged kidneys, characterized by a fusiform dilatation of the collecting ducts; the affected part of the nephron corresponds to the division products of the ureteral bud and not the later developed products derived from the nephrogenic blastema: polycystic kidney of the type Potter I [209].

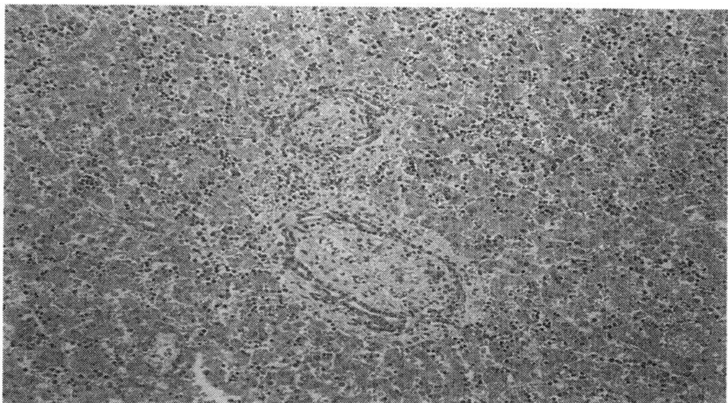

Figure 4.9. Ductal plate malformation. Detail from an autopsy liver specimen from a female baby who died a few minutes after birth from lung hypoplasia. Liver and kidneys showed lesions of autosomal recessive polycystic kidney disease. The picture shows two portal tracts with bile duct structures in ductal plate configuration. (H&E stain, 312× magnification.) (Specimen courtesy of Dr. Philippe Moerman, Catholic University of Leuven, Leuven, Belgium.)

Neonates with the perinatal form of ARPKD die in the first few hours of life from pulmonary insufficiency. Babies with the neonatal and infantile forms of ARPKD, characterized by a lower percentage of affected collecting ducts, may survive for months or even years [157,191]. In surviving children, a progression of the hepatic and renal lesions has been observed associated with increasing amounts of fibrosis [192,210,211]. With progressing age of the patient, often there is a decrease in the number of ductular profiles and an increase in fibrosis of the portal tracts; the renal cysts seem to become less numerous and more spherical, associated with increasing interstitial fibrosis [212], approaching the appearance of medullary sponge kidney [187] or even resembling that of adult polycystic disease [186,213].

From these observations comes the hypothesis that ARPKD corresponds to a defect in epithelial–mesenchymal inductive interactions, resulting in abnormalities of the renal collecting ducts and a more or less complete arrest of remodeling of the ductal plates during the development of the interlobular bile ducts. The latter would explain the sometimes reported absence of a mature bile duct in the center of the portal tract, and the variable number of ductal profiles in its periphery [88]. The association of ARPKD with Caroli's disease indicates an arrest of remodeling of the ductal plate not only during formation of the interlobular ducts but also during an earlier stage in which the larger segmental ducts are formed.

The variants of ARPKD in which patients survive for longer periods (neonatal, infantile, and juvenile forms) seem to be characterized by a slow but progressive involution of renal and biliary epithelial tubes, followed by fibrous scarring. This mysterious process of necroinflammatory involution of immature bile ducts and abnormal renal collecting ducts creates the link with the next fibrocystic congenital liver disease to be considered here: CHF [88].

The mechanisms involved in development of cystic dilatation of renal tubules and hepatic ducts in ARPKD are mentioned under the heading Cystogenesis.

CHF

CHF IN ARPKD

Congenital hepatic fibrosis [214] is an autosomal recessive disease, usually associated with renal abnormalities of ARPKD [215]. In a study on the long-term outcome of ARPKD patients, sequelae of CHF and portal hypertension were found to be developing in 44% of patients and were related with age [197].

Besides ARPKD, the liver abnormalities of CHF are also observed in a number of syndromes in autosomal dominant polycystic kidney disease [216–220] and in the recessive fibrocystic conditions termed Meckel–Gruber syndrome, Ivemark syndrome, Jeune syndrome, nephronophthisis, Bardet–Biedl syndrome, and Joubert syndrome [89]. Five patients have been reported in whom CHF was associated with phosphomannose isomerase deficiency or the type 1b carbohydrate-deficient glycoprotein syndromes [221,222]. Cases of CHF have also been described with other liver malformations, such as Caroli's disease, von Meyenburg complexes, and choledochal cyst [117,118].

From the point of view of clinical symptoms, different types of CHF are recognized: portal hypertensive, cholangitic, and latent forms [223]. The most common manifestations relate to portal hypertension (splenomegaly, cytopenias due to hypersplenism) [224]. Symptoms may appear early or late [225].

In view of the variable clinical expression, several researchers have emphasized that CHF does not constitute a single clinical entity but rather represents a broad spectrum of hepatic and renal lesions [213,226,227].

In the pure form of CHF (not associated with Caroli's disease – see further), the liver is of normal size without macroscopically visible cysts. It appears speckled, with irregular whitish areas regularly distributed over the liver surface or on cut sections [228].

The histopathologic picture is not uniform [228,229]. In some patients, CHF is characterized by fibrous enlargement of the portal tracts, which contain variable numbers of abnormally shaped bile ducts (Figure 4.10); in others, the liver shows bands of connective tissue of variable width linking adjacent portal tracts. Cases are on record with only partial involvement of the liver, for example, of one lobe [230] or of heterotopic liver tissue within the adrenal gland [231]. The fibrous areas contain increased numbers of bile duct profiles, which have been shown to be in continuity with the rest of the biliary system [228].

The portal vein branches are often hypoplastic [214,228], in contrast to the hepatic arterial branches, which may appear supernumerous [228]. Some investigators noted the existence of discrete signs of involution or epithelial degeneration of

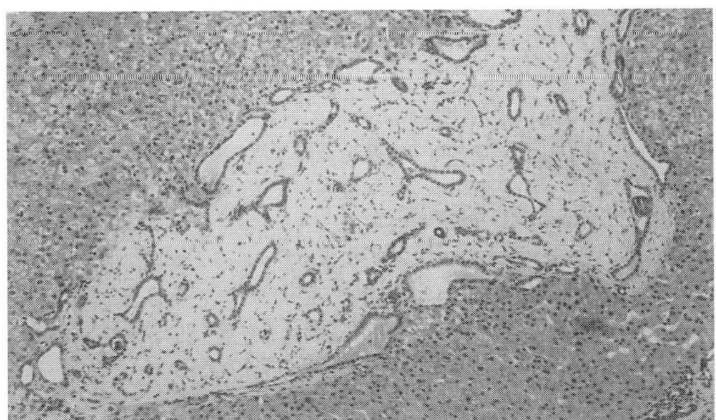

Figure 4.10. Liver biopsy specimen from a 6-year-old girl with congenital hepatic fibrosis. The picture shows an enlarged portal tract with numerous bile duct structures. The whole fibrous area can be interpreted as a fusion of several portal tracts containing incompletely remodeled ductal plates (pollard willow pattern). Note the extreme hypoplasia or virtual absence of portal vein branches. The lower right corner displays a more normal-appearing small portal tract. (H&E, 125× magnification.) For color reproduction, see Color Plate 4.10.

the aberrant bile ducts [9,232], mild features of parenchymal cholestasis [232,233], foci of ductular proliferation at the fibrous–parenchymal interface, and accumulation of copper and copper-binding protein (orcein-positive granules) in periportal hepatocytes. Usually, the latter features have been considered to result from bouts of cholangitis caused by the associated existence of Caroli's disease.

The liver lesions of CHF may progress with time [213,234] – in some patients, they remain relatively unchanged; in others, the fibrosis may increase – and the lesions may be modulated by superimposed bouts of cholangitis [211].

The abnormal bile duct structures in CHF were recognized as corresponding to (more or less) incompletely remodeled ductal plates of interlobular bile ducts by Jorgensen [9].

Sometimes duplications of ductal plates are seen, resulting in curved bile duct profiles arranged in concentric circles [235,236]. Such duplication of ductal plates has been interpreted as a fetal type of "ductular reaction" [90].

The observations of the multiple morphologic appearances of CHF, the evolution with time of the liver lesions in ARPKD [211], and the CHF-like appearance of the liver after successful portoenterostomy in early severe forms of BA have led to the following hypothesis on the morphogenesis of CHF [88]: The initial lesion of CHF corresponds to the liver lesion in ARPKD, that is, DPM of the interlobular bile ducts. The immature bile duct structures are subject to a slowly progressive destructive cholangiopathy, resulting in a gradual disappearance of bile duct profiles associated with increasing periportal fibrosis. The speed and the duration of the destructive cholangitis are variable in individual patients (akin to the variations in the basic disease process of BA after hepatic portoenterostomy): In some patients it is rapidly progressive, in others, slow and torpid. In still others it burns out spontaneously [88]. In this view, CHF can be considered a fetal type of biliary fibrosis, which may be more or less advanced and progressive or arrested. Occasional case reports have documented the possible progressive nature of a presumed destructive cholangiopathy in CHF [233,237].

This hypothesis on the pathogenesis of CHF explains a great number of diverse observations: the variability in the time of appearance of clinical symptoms, the possible progression of the fibrous component of the lesion, the variability in the number of bile duct profiles observed, the reported hypoplasia of the portal vein, the sometimes reported features of ductal degeneration and involution, the small foci of ductular reaction, the possible signs of parenchymal cholestasis, the elevated levels of alkaline phosphatase in the serum, and the association of CHF with renal lesions of ARPKD [88]. This hypothesis draws a parallel between the epithelial destruction of the abnormal bile ducts and the epithelial involution of the abnormal renal tubules that is part of the progression of the renal lesion [88,238].

CHF IN OTHER HEPATORENAL SYNDROMES

CHF WITH MATURITY-ONSET DIABETES MELLITUS OF THE YOUNG, TYPE 5 (MODY5)

Mutations of the human *HNF1β* gene (TCF2) are responsible for the autosomal dominant disorder MODY5. Patients present with early-onset type 2 diabetes mellitus caused by an impairment in insulin secretion. In addition, several patients have congenital abnormalities of the kidney and genitourinary tract, including polycystic kidneys and cystic dysplasia [239].

Autosomal recessive polycystic kidney disease is characterized by renal cysts and biliary dysgenesis and is caused by mutations in *PKHD1* (see above). HNF1β and the structurally related HNF1α bind specifically to the PKHD1 promoter and regulate its activity directly [240]. In mice, mutation of HNF1β inhibits *Pkhd1* expression and produces renal cysts [241]. The latter study represents a mouse model of the congenital renal abnormalities in MODY5 and predicts that humans with MODY5 will also have decreased expression of *PKHD1* in the biliary tract, because this is another site where the expression of HNF1β and *PKHD1* overlap. Liver-specific inactivation of HNF1β in transgenic mice produces DPM and biliary dysgenesis that resemble the lesions observed in the liver of ARPKD patients [52] (see Development of Intrahepatic Bile Ducts), and abnormalities in liver function and fibrosis have been observed in some patients with HNF1β mutations, although liver biopsies confirming an eventual biliary abnormality have not yet been performed [242]. These observations suggest that HNF1β may also be required for the expression of PKHD1 in the developing biliary tract and that mutations of HNF1β may produce biliary tract abnormalities through downregulation of PKHD1 [241]. Thus two renal cystic diseases, MODY5 and ARPKD, are linked in a common transcriptional pathway, and the mechanism of cyst formation in humans with mutations of HNF1β involves down-regulation of PKHD1 [240].

CHF WITH NEPHRONOPHTHISIS–MEDULLARY CYSTIC KIDNEY DISEASE

A group of renal cystic diseases has been summarized under the term *nephronophthisis–medullary cystic kidney disease* (NPH-MCKD) because they share similar clinical symptoms, macroscopic pathology, and renal histopathology. There are also three distinguishing features: mode of inheritance, age at onset of end-stage renal disease (ESRD), and type of extrarenal organ involvement. For the recessive forms of NPH-MCKD complex the term *nephronophthisis* (NPH) is used, whereas the designation *medullary cystic kidney disease* (MCKD) denotes the dominant variants of the complex [243,244]. A second distinction pertains to the age at onset for ESRD. For MCKD, terminal renal failure develops in adult life, comprising two variants, MCKD1 and MCKD2, with a median onset of ESRD at 62 years and 32 years, respectively. The gene mutated in MCKD2 is *UMOD* coding for the Tamm-Horsfall glycoprotein (also referred to as uromodulin), whereas the search for the gene of MCKD1 is getting closer to the aim [245]. In NPH, chronic renal failure occurs within the first three decades of life. The third distinguishing feature among variants of NPH-MCKD is the degree to which extrarenal associations occur; the latter have only been observed in recessive forms (NPH) and are seen virtually exclusively in juvenile NPH, with involvement of eyes, cerebellum, liver, and bones [243].

There is extensive gene locus heterogeneity with at least four different loci for NPH. Two loci are associated with juvenile NPH: *NPHP1* coding for nephronocystin on chromosome 2q13 and *NPHP4* coding for nephrocystin 4 (or nephroretinin) on chromosome 1p36 [246]. *NPHP2* on chromosome 9q22 codes for inversin (formerly termed nephrocystin 2) [247], involved in infantile NPH; and *NPHP3* on chromosome 3q22 codes for nephrocystin 3, involved in adolescent NPH [248]. The renal histopathology of NPHP4 shows the same characteristic features as those known for NPHP1 and NPHP3.

Nephronophthisis has been described in association with CHF [249]; in association with retinitis pigmentosa (Senior–Loken syndrome) [248,250]; in association with both CHF and retinitis pigmentosa [251]; in association with COACH (cerebellar vermis hypoplasia, oligophrenia, congenital ataxia, and hepatic fibrosis) with liver histopathology suggestive of CHF [252–257]; and in association with Joubert syndrome (cerebellar vermian hypoplasia, oligophrenia, congenital ataxia, coloboma, and hepatic fibrosis syndrome) [258,259].

The mechanism of cyst development is discussed under the heading Cystogenesis.

Caroli's Disease, Caroli's Syndrome

Caroli's disease corresponds to a congenital dilatation of the larger (segmental) intrahepatic bile ducts. Caroli described two varieties [260]: a pure form (Caroli's disease), characterized by ectasias of the intrahepatic bile ducts without further histologic abnormalities, and a combined form (Caroli's syndrome) in which Caroli's disease is associated with periportal fibrosis, the latter corresponding to CHF [261]. The mode of inheritance of Caroli's disease is controversial. According to some authors [227,262], Caroli's disease (unassociated with CHF) is not hereditary; in contrast, some rare observations of familial cases suggest a hereditary nature of the disease [263], and a recent report of 21 years of observation of a Japanese family suggests an autosomal dominant inheritance [264].

In Caroli's disease, the abnormalities of the bile ducts may be diffuse throughout the liver or more localized, and the disease is not associated with renal lesions of ARPKD (typically accompanying CHF). It may be associated, however, with choledochal cysts. The incidence of Caroli's disease is much lower than that of Caroli's syndrome [196], about 1 in 100,000 births [262].

In contrast, Caroli's syndrome (with associated CHF lesions) is transmitted as an autosomal recessive trait and is associated (like CHF) with the kidney lesions of ARPKD [265].

Similar to CHF, some cases of Caroli's syndrome have been reported that were associated with the adult type of polycystic disease (see further) or with a choledochal cyst [266].

Variations in anatomic patterns have been described – diffuse forms and localized forms [267] – as well as variations in clinical presentation: symptoms in the neonate, symptoms appearing later, and latent forms. Alertness is required for diagnosing the condition in children [268].

In Caroli's disease, the abnormality consists of moniliform or saccular dilatations of the larger intrahepatic bile ducts (left

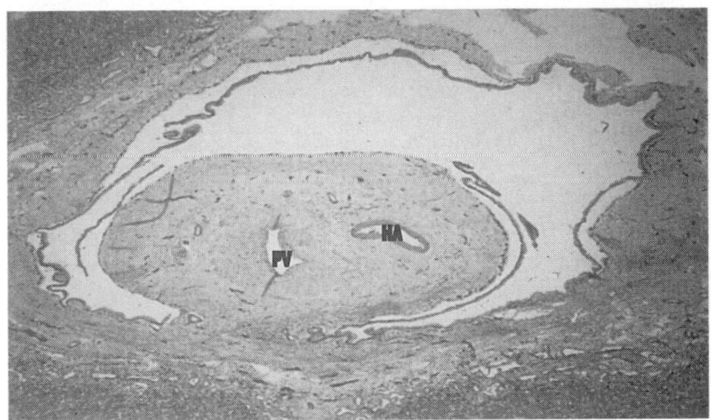

Figure 4.11. Low magnification of a cross-section through a dilated hilar bile duct from the liver of a patient with Caroli's disease. Ductal plate malformation with minimal degree of remodeling, appearing as a polypoid projection in the bile duct lumen. PV, portal vein; HA, hepatic artery. (H&E, 1× magnification.) (Specimen courtesy of Dr. Philippe Moerman, Catholic University of Leuven, Leuven, Belgium.) For color reproduction, see Color Plate 4.11.

and right hepatic ducts, segmental ducts, and some of their afferent branches), with predominant involvement of the segmental ducts [187]. The dilated parts are in continuity with the rest of the biliary system and hence contain bile (communicating type of cystic disease). Polypoid projections or cross-bridges have been noted in the dilated lumina [81,82,208] (Figure 4.11). The saccular dilatations of the ducts lead to stagnation of bile and in this way predispose to biliary sludge formation and intraductal lithiasis, often complicated by superinfection.

In Caroli's syndrome, the abnormalities of the larger ducts are associated with the lesions of CHF mentioned before. The duct anomalies of Caroli's disease predispose to repeated attacks of cholangitis, often complicated by biliary abcedation, septicemia, and pyemia. Further complications include amyloidosis [269] and cholangiocarcinoma [270]. The incidence of biliary carcinoma is up to 100 times higher than in the average population [271].

In patients with Caroli's syndrome, the clinical symptoms may be a combination of the classic symptoms of both Caroli's disease and CHF: cholangitis and portal hypertension.

The pathogenesis of Caroli's disease seems to involve a total or partial arrest of remodeling of the ductal plate of the larger intrahepatic bile ducts. The macroscopic appearance of the dilated ducts [208], as well as their visualization by modern imaging techniques [81,84–86,272–277], is most consistent with a DPM pattern. Caroli's syndrome has been diagnosed prenatally with ultrasound findings of a cystic liver mass and echogenic kidneys [265].

In Caroli's syndrome, the hereditary factors causing the partial or complete arrest in remodeling of the ductal plates appears to exert their influence not only during the early period of bile duct embryogenesis, in which larger ducts are formed, but also later on, during the development of more peripheral biliary ramifications (the interlobular bile ducts). This results in the development of the lesions of CHF in the more peripheral levels of the biliary tree.

This hypothesis, already proposed by Caroli himself [187], may explain the autosomal recessive transmission of the disease as well as its association with ARPKD. This pathogenetic mechanism implies the same basic defect in the two conditions that are combined in Caroli's syndrome: DPM in different levels of the biliary tree, developing in successive periods during the embryologic development of the intrahepatic bile ducts (Caroli's disease and CHF).

Ductal plate malformation of intrahepatic ducts often seems to be associated with some form of involution or destruction of the immature ducts. It is of interest in this respect that lesions of Caroli type (DPM of larger intrahepatic bile ducts) seem to explain the occurrence of biliary cysts observed in some infants with BA treated by portoenterostomy [278,279]. Caroli's disease may be associated with choledochal cyst, the pathogenesis of which remains unknown but may be related to bile duct atresia [280,281]. Furthermore, the choledochal cyst types IV A and V described by Todani et al. [282] correspond to Caroli's disease [277].

The PCK rat has been described as an animal model for Caroli's syndrome [203].

In short, the basic lesion of Caroli's disease corresponds to DPM of the larger intrahepatic bile ducts, which may be associated with DPM of the more proximal as well as of the more distal segments of the biliary system [87].

von Meyenburg Complexes

von Meyenburg complexes (VMCs) usually are described as bile duct microhamartomas, typically 0.1–0.3 cm in diameter [283]. These small, often multiple lesions are mostly asymptomatic incidental findings. Their incidence was originally reported in around 0.7% of surgical and autopsy liver specimens, but apparently more accurate figures, based on a study of 2843 consecutive autopsies, are 5.6% in adults and 0.9% in children. Among adults with autosomal dominant polycystc kidney disease (ADPKD), VMCs were found in 97% and hepatic cysts in 88%. ADPKD was found in 11% of adults with at least one VMC and in 40% of those with four or more VMCs.

A VMC is composed of a variable number of more or less dilated bile ducts embedded in a fibrous stroma. The lumen may contain inspissated bile concrements. Some of the duct structures may show polypoid projections in the lumen; others show in sections a central island of connective tissue covered with the same type of epithelium as that lining the wall of the dilated duct. The latter appearance is similar to the basic configuration of DPM (Figure 4.12). The complexes are localized in or close to portal tracts. In some complexes, the bile duct profiles are involutive and disappear in a hyalinized, scarring stroma.

von Meyenburg complexes remain stationary in most patients; only rarely are they the site of origin of cholangiocarcinoma [284], of which about 14 cases were reported until 2004 [285]. However, VMCs appear to be at the origin of the development of liver cysts in ADPKD (see further), as a result of progressive dilatation and fluid filling of the original clusters of bile duct structures [286,287].

According to some authors, the patient with multiple VMC lesions may be considered as having a very mild form of ADPKD,

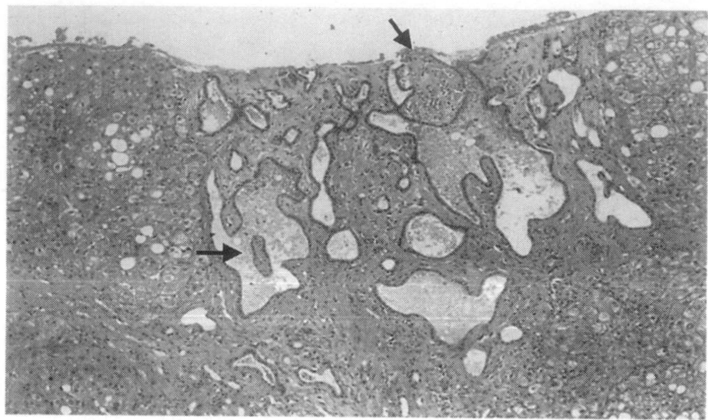

Figure 4.12. Detail from a liver biopsy specimen from a 74-year-old male patient with alcoholic liver disease. The von Meyenburg complex was an incidental finding. Note the pattern resembling ductal plate malformation, recognizable in a couple of the dilated ducts by the occurrence of a central fibrous axis covered with bile duct epithelium (*arrows*). (H&E, 125× magnification.)

with minimal progressive cystic dilatation of the lesions [288] (Figure 4.13). Another viewpoint reasons that because ADPKD accounts for only a minority (11%) of patients with VMCs, the lesions of VMC in the absence of ADPKD are manifestations of a different disease [289]. This interpretation especially applies to cases with smaller numbers of VMCs, to be considered as "local accidents" occurring in some of the developing peripheral branches of the portal vein and biliary tree, and is compatible with the still unsolved morphogenesis of individual VMC lesions.

The histologic appearance of VMCs has inspired the hypothesis that the lesions represent partially fibrosing (and on occasion, slowly involutive) remnants of DPM of the smaller, more peripheral branches of the intrahepatic biliary tree. This hypothesis invokes a factor arresting or perturbing the remodeling of ductal plates in the later phases of development of the intrahepatic biliary tree [87].

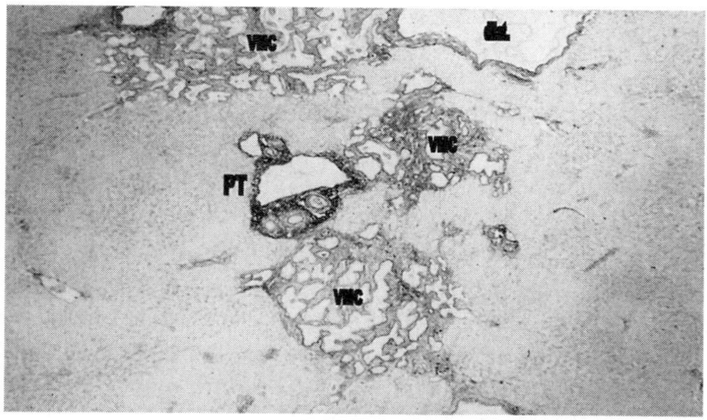

Figure 4.13. Liver specimen from a patient with autosomal dominant polycystic kidney disease. The picture shows a portal tract (PT) and three von Meyenburg complexes (VMC). Note the paraportal location of the complexes, and the contrast of their connective tissue matrix with that of the portal tract. One component bile duct structure (dilat.) is dilated. (Orcein stain, 25× magnification.) For color reproduction, see Color Plate 4.13.

A VMC may contain a large number of duct profiles, occasionally appearing like a conglomerate of approximated ductal plate remnants; one therefore has to suspect an abnormality in the arborization pattern of the peripheral branches of the portal vein: a "pollard willow" pattern of ramification, causing a close apposition and even fusion of the corresponding portal tracts [87] (see "Early, Severe" Biliary Atresia).

The paraportal localization of some VMCs, fused to normal-appearing portal tracts, suggests that one of the branches of the pollard willow may give rise to a normal portal tract with normal duct development, whereas the rest of the tuft evolves in hypoplastic vein branches with fusion of adjacent portal tracts and clustering of their ductal plates.

At first sight, this hypothesis may not be easily reconciled with the notion that part of the intrahepatic biliary system develops after birth in accordance with postnatal liver growth and lobule development. However, as mentioned previously, the present knowledge of human liver growth and related lobule formation after birth is rudimentary; furthermore, lobular development may be deviated from normal because the associated abnormal branching pattern of the portal vein suggests a derangement in normal growth and lobulation pattern. For that reason, the hypothesis of a DPM-like development of VMC is maintained until sound evidence provides a final alternative.

The classic theory states that the dilated ducts of the VMCs do not communicate with the rest of the biliary tree, as is the case in adult-type polycystic liver disease (the noncommunicating type of cystic disease) [207]. This hardly would be compatible with the DPM appearance of the lesions. However, investigations on a human complex [290] and studies in the *cpk* mouse and in infantile as well as adult types of human polycystic disease [291,292], and further, the presence of bilirubin-stained material in some lesional elements and the demonstration by radionuclide tracers of functional bile excretion in VMCs indicate the communicating nature of these bile duct abnormalities. Admittedly, some of the small cystic structures may have become secondarily pinched off by developing fibrosis in several of the VMCs.

Magnetic resonance imaging cholangiography appears very useful for the diagnosis of VMCs and their differentiation from hepatic metastases and other single or multiple focal lesions [293–295].

ADPKD (Formerly Adult Type Polycystic Disease)

The adult type of polycystic liver and kidney disease also may manifest itself in early childhood [296]. Consequently, the older nomenclature has been changed into autosomal dominant polycystic kidney disease (ADPKD) [297].

Autosomal dominant polycystic kidney disease is one of the most common hereditary disorders in humans, with an estimated prevalence of 1 in 1000 [157]. In the United States, 8–10% of cases of end-stage renal disease are due to ADPKD [298]. The clinical presentation of this disease is usually related to renal symptoms and abnormalities, but ADPKD is also a systemic disease with extrarenal manifestations involving several organs [296]. Besides renal and hepatic cysts, ADPKD may be associated with other malformations, such as pancreatic cysts, colon diverticula, heart valve abnormalities, berry aneurysms, aneurysms of the thoracic aorta, and inguinal hernias [299]. ADPKD may also be associated with Caroli's syndrome [266,300] and with CHF [219,220,301,302]. The most important noncystic extrarenal mainifestations of ADPKD are cardiovascular abnormalities [303].

At least two genetic loci are involved in ADPKD: *PKD1* and *PKD2* [304]. A third locus has been suggested (*PKD3*), but not yet been mapped [305]. *PKD1* has been localized to chromosome 16p13.3 [306,307] and accounts for 85% of cases. The *PKD1* gene has been cloned. It codes for a protein called polycystin-1 [196,197,308]. Polycystin-1 is a 462-kDa integral membrane protein with a large amino-terminal extracellular domain. Respective portions of the extracellular domain can engage in high-affinity homophilic interactions, recognize extracellular matrix proteins, and play a role as G-protein–coupled receptor.

Immunohistochemical studies and electron microscopy have localized polycystin-1 to the basolateral plasma membrane of epithelial cells of renal tubules, intrahepatic bile ducts, and pancreatic ducts, all sites of cystic change in ADPKD [309,310]. Polycystin-1 is more strongly expressed in the epithelial cells lining the renal cysts in ADPKD and in fetal kidneys than in normal adult renal tubules [311]. Polycystin-1 colocalizes with desmoplakin at newly assembled desmosomes and was found to be associated with the E-cadherin and catenin components of adherens junctions. Trafficking of polycystin-1 to the lateral membrane is dependent on tuberin (a multifunctional protein that is the product of the tuberous sclerosis gene *TSC2*) [312].

The *PKD2* gene is localized on the long arm of chromosome 4 (4q13-q23) [313–316]. Loss of somatic expression of *PKD2* is both necessary and sufficient for cyst development in ADPKD, suggesting that the disease type *PKD2* is caused by a recessive cellular mechanism [317].

The gene product of *PKD2* is an integral membrane protein termed polycystin-2 [318]. Polycystin-2 has been localized in lateral cell membranes at sites of renal tubular cell adhesion junctions and cell–matrix contacts (focal adhesions). It was also found in the endoplasmic reticulum and in the plasma membrane in close proximity to polycystin-1 [319]. This twofold localization has been reconciled by studies suggesting that the subcellular localization and function of polycystin-2 are directed by two adaptor proteins and phosphorylation/dephosphorylation reactions to either the plasma membrane or the endoplasmic reticulum and Golgi complex [312].

Both proteins, polycystin-1 and polycystin-2 are colocalized in the primary cilium of renal tubular cells, together with "cystoproteins" of animal models of renal polycystic disease (cystin and polaris) [320].

Polycystin-2 is the founding member of a growing family of transient receptor potential (TRP) channels, now also known as TRPP2. It functions as a Ca^{2+}-permeable, nonselective cation channel. Polycystin-1 and TRPP2 form a heterodimeric protein complex, suggesting that polycystin-1 acts as a novel type of receptor that regulates the channel activity of TRPP2 [312,321], one of the most versatile of all signaling molecules [322].

A striking feature of ADPKD is its phenotypic variability. PKD1-associated disease is more severe than in PKD2-associated families; bilineal inheritance of *PKD1* and *PKD2* mutations causes earlier and more severe disease manifestation; genomic deletion of *PKD1* and *TSC2* (a tuberous sclerosis contiguous gene) is unfavorable. Progression in ADPKD is modified by gender, genetics, and environmental and stochastic factors independent of the germline PKD mutations [323,324].

In ADPKD, not only renal cysts but also hepatic cysts are found in the majority of patients, with increasing prevalence as age increases [196,198]. Besides genetic factors, the development of liver cysts in ADPKD is modulated further by nongenetic factors including age, pregnancy, female gender, and severity of the renal lesions [297]. The size of the liver is variable; it may remain unchanged for many years, only to increase afterward. Macroscopically, the liver contains multiple cysts of variable diameter, disseminated throughout the organ or, more rarely, restricted to one lobe. The cysts are located either in or very close to portal tracts. The cavities are lined by a cuboidal, biliary type of epithelium [325] and surrounded by a fibrous capsule. The cysts frequently are associated with VMCs (see preceding section, von Meyenburg Complexes) or with zones of fibrosis of the CHF type [302] (Figure 4.14). Classically, the cysts are said to be of the noncommunicating type [302,326,327].

The cysts contain a clear fluid with a composition close to that of the bile salt–independent fraction of bile [328]. The fluid is secreted by the lining epithelial cells [329]. The hepatic cysts in ADPKD are considered to result from progressive further extension of the dilated ducts in VMCs [286–288]. Cysts may become infected and then are filled with pus.

A noncommunicating nature of the liver cysts in ADPKD, as reported in several textbooks, is difficult to reconcile with a DPM configuration. It is conceivable, however, that the ductal structures of a VMC originally communicate with the biliary

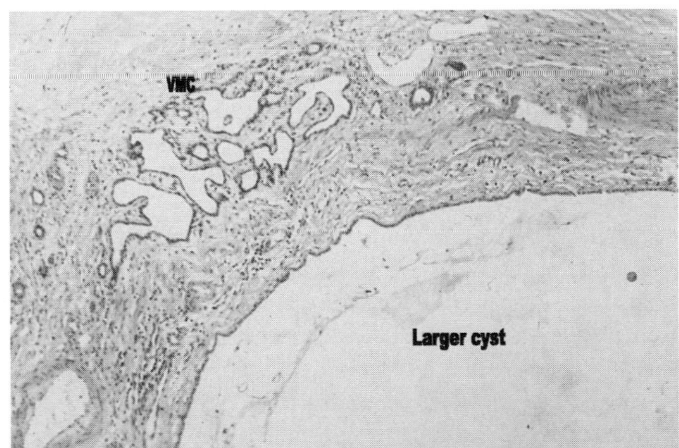

Figure 4.14. Liver cyst in autosomal dominant polycystic disease in a male patient 75 years of age. The picture shows a small cyst, lined by bile duct epithelium. The cyst can be viewed as a more dilated component in a cluster of less dilated, smaller bile duct structures of a von Meyenburg complex (*left upper portion*). (H&E, 125× magnification.) For color reproduction, see Color Plate 4.14.

tree but become separated and noncommunicating as a result of their progressive dilatation and strictures by the strangulating hyaline fibrosis that surrounds them. Some studies contradict the noncommunicating nature of the cysts in ADPKD [291,292]. Japanese studies have shown that peribiliary glands around the larger intrahepatic bile ducts also may contribute to hepatic cyst formation in ADPKD [330,331].

The association of ADPKD with CHF [219,220,302] and with Caroli's syndrome [266,300] suggests a lack of adequate remodeling of ductal plates at all levels of the biliary tree, invoking the influence of a causative agent throughout the whole period of embryogenesis of the intrahepatic biliary tree [87,90,332]. Similar associations have been described in a single kindred [216].

The different mode of inheritance in ADPKD compared with that in ARPKD (CHF, Caroli's disease) leads to the conclusion of a combination of at least two genetic factors in such cases [219] or of modulating factors capable of radically influencing the phenotype [333].

The mechanism of cyst development is discussed under the heading Cystogenesis.

Isolated Polycystic Liver Disease or Isolated Autosomal Dominant Polycystic Liver Disease or Autosomal Dominant Polycystic Hepatic Disease

The occurrence of isolated polycystic liver disease (PCLD) without associated renal cysts has been recognized for many years [287]. Evidence for a novel inherited disease came from family studies in which PCLD was described without linkage to PKD1 or PKD2 [334,335].

One gene for PCLD is *PRKCSH*, located on chromosome 19p13.2-13.1, which codes for "the β subunit of glucosidase II" or "protein kinase substrate 80K-H" (PRKCSH) or hepatocystin [336,337]. PCLD is genetically heterogeneous, as *PRKCSH* mutations cannot be demonstrated in all cases [337,338].

A second gene associated with PCLD is *SEC63*, which encodes an integral membrane protein of the endoplasmic reticulum that is part of the multicomponent translocon; the latter comprises the translocation machinery for integral membrane and secreted proteins. Mutations in *PRKCSH* and in *SEC63* together accounted for less than one third of cases in a studied cohort, indicating that there is at least one more locus associated with the disease [339].

The clinical manifestations and the management of PCLD are similar to those of ADPKD. Female patients have a significantly higher mean cyst score than do male patients [340]. The gross appearance of resected livers is indistinguishable from that of livers resected in ADPKD patients. Histologically, besides larger cysts, all specimens contain variable numbers of VMCs, and – as in ADPKD – cysts are considered to derive from dilatation of VMCs [340] and also from cystic enlargement of peribiliary glands accompanying the larger intrahepatic bile ducts [331]. Other lesions less consistently observed in PCLD consist of dilatation of intra- and extrahepatic bile ducts and focal biliary fibroadenomatosis [330,331,336].

For pathogenesis of cyst formation, see Cystogenesis.

Cystogenesis (Cell Biological Aspects of Renal and Hepatic Cystogenesis)

The mechanism(s) of cyst development in hereditary polycystic disease has (have) mainly been studied in the kidney. Although tissue-specific differences in cystogenesis certainly occur, there are strong suggestions and even evidence that a number of pathways are common to the conversion of tubes into cysts in general, be it in the kidney tubules, the hepatic bile ducts, or the pancreatic ducts. For this reason, a summary is given below of the present concepts of renal cystogenesis, followed by some remarks on tissue-specific aspects of cyst development in the liver.

RENAL TUBULAR CYSTOGENESIS

PRIMARY CILIA

Solitary cilia at the apical surface of tubular and ductal epithelia were first described in 1898 [341]. Their function remained unknown, and they were even considered as vestigial organelles. However, ciliary expression is widespread in multiple cell lineages (except hepatocytes, myeloid and lymphoid cells, and possibly endothelia) [342]. Investigations on polycystic kidney disease during the last years have moved this forgotten detail of cell biology into the focus of interest.

Cilia arise from centrioles. They form a fingerlike extension of the cytoplasm covered with the cell membrane and contain in their axis a system of nine pairs of longitudinal microtubules in circular arrangement (the axoneme). In contrast to motile cilia (e.g., in ciliated respiratory epithelium) that also contain a set of two centrally located microtubules (9 + 2 pattern), the single, immotile cilium lacks the centrally located doublet (9 + 0 pattern).

Assembly and maintenance of cilia is assured – as in flagella – by intraflagellar transport (IFT), which is a motility process taking place between the membrane and the outer doublet microtubules of all motile and immotile cilia and flagella. IFT moves axonemal precursors to the assembly site at the tip. The IFT particles, occurring in chains called "rafts," are moved antegrade to the tip by a heterotrimeric kinesin II, and retrograde to the base by cytoplasmic dynein 1B. Apparently, IFT is further involved in the ciliary sensory processes in that the IFT particles and their associated peptides are changed in the cilium and carry a message back to the cell body [343].

Primary cilia are not retained during cell division but are rapidly regenerated in early interphase. Solitary cilia are well developed in renal tubular cells (except for intercalated cells) and in epithelia lining the bile and pancreatic ducts; they also constitute the outer segment of rod and cone photoreceptors in the retina.

The solitary cilium is at present considered to represent a sensory antenna, functioning through the polycystin complex as a mechanotransducer: PKD1 acts as a cell surface receptor that upon activation binds to and activates in turn heterotrimeric G-proteins, resulting in opening of the Ca^{2+}-permeant cation channel of PKD2 (TRPP2) and increased cellular Ca^{2+}. The polycystin complex thus represents a sensing nanomachine that is used to signal relevant intratubular information and to maintain normal tubular architecture [344]. Loss of function of the complex results in perturbation of normal intracellular Ca^{2+} concentration, which underlies a multitude of pathologic reactions [345], including severe alterations in structure and function of tubular lining cells resulting in cyst formation (see Pathophysiology of Cystic Epithelium) [346].

It should be mentioned that apparently the node is not the first generator of laterality. Several findings suggest that laterality is established before ciliogenesis.This alternative model proposes that the asymmetric expression of ion exchangers such as H^+/K^+-ATPase and K^+ channels generate a voltage and a pH gradient across the midline [347] that may result from asymmetric mRNA localization driven by cytoplasmic motor proteins such as dynein and kinesin [348].

CILIARY PATHWAY OF CYSTOGENESIS

A tantalizing finding of recent years has been that most "cystoproteins," the mutation of which causes polycystic disease, have been localized in the primary cilia or basal bodies of tubular epithelial cells and embryonic nodal cells [349]. Such ciliar proteins include those involved in human disease: not only polycystin-1 and polycystin-2 [320] but also fibrocystin [194,350], inversin (nephrocystin-2) [247,351], nephrocystin-3 [248], nephrocystin-4 (nephroretinin) [246], gene product BSS8 of Bardet–Biedl syndrome [352], and proteins studied in animal models including polaris (Tg737) [353] and cystin-1 [354], but not the cystoproteins of isolated PCLD: hepatocystin and SEC63 [339].

The mutational mechanism leading to cystogenesis has mainly been studied in ADPKD.

An intriguing feature of ADPKD is the focal and sporadic nature of individual cyst formation in an age-dependent manner. It has been shown that cyst formation represents clonal growth aberration of single epithelial cells. Somatic inactivating mutations of *PKD1* and *PKD2* were documented in cell pools isolated from individual cyst linings in type 1 and 2 ADPKD, respectively. The somatic mutations in cells from different cysts were unique within the same patient and were consistently found to affect the copy of the *PKD* gene inherited from the unaffected parent (wild-type allele). The findings of monoclonality and somatic *PKD1/PKD2* mutations in human cystic epithelia provide the basis for the "two-hit" model of cystogenesis in ADPKD: Inactivation of both copies of PKD1 or PKD2 through germline and somatic mutations within an individual epithelial cell confers growth advantages for it to expand into a cyst [323]. Thus, ADPKD is a recessive disease at the level of the individual cells. *Cellular recessive* is used in this context to describe the convergence of two nonfunctional alleles through a mechanism that differs from the classical recessive model (i.e., one allele is transmitted as a germline mutation [not in itself sufficient for disease, hence *recessive*]) and the other arises as a de novo mutation in an individual cell (hence *cellular*) [304].

For the sake of completeness, it should be mentioned that some questions remain as to whether the two-hit mechanism is the only means to generate a cyst and whether the somatic events may be later events that are more important for cyst expansion and progression than initiation [349].

Mutations in the "cystoproteins" of the primary cilium of the renal tubule result in disturbance of its function in the normal sensing of fluid flow and tubular lumen and shape, resulting in a distorted message sent through the PKD1-TRPP2 receptor–channel complex to the cell interior and propagated to the neighboring cells through gap junctions. This results in cyst formation by a number of phenotypic changes characterizing the epithelial cyst–lining cells.

Renal cyst development in ARPKD appears also to be caused by disturbance in ciliary function due to mutation and inactivation of fibrocystin. In three-dimensional cell cultures of mouse inner medullary collecting duct cells, inhibition of fibrocystin disrupted tubulomorphogenesis; Pkhd1-silenced cells developed abnormalities in cell–cell contact, actin cytoskeleton organization, cell–extracellular matrix interactions, cell proliferation, and apoptosis [355]. Of interest, however, are the observations in a mouse strain with targeted mutation of Pkhd1. Because of disruption of exon 40, these Pkhd1ex40 mice develop severe malformations of the intrahepatic bile ducts but retain morphologically and functionally normal kidneys. This indicates that the role of fibrocystin/polyductin may be functionally divergent in liver and kidney because protein domains essential for bile duct development do not affect nephrogenesis in this mouse model [202].

A fascinating finding is the recent discovery of a direct transcriptional hierarchy between HNF1β and at least four cystic disease genes: *Umod* (medullary cystic kidney disease type 2), *Pkhd1* (ARPKD), *Pkd2* (ADPKD), and *Tg737/Polaris* (mouse cpk model of ARPKD). Interestingly, all of these identified HNF1β target gene products (except uromodulin/Tamm-Horsfall protein) are known to colocalize in the primary cilium. Although a defect in any of these genes in humans is sufficient to elicit cyst formation, this study revealed a concomitant downregulation of this subgroup of cystic disease genes. The combined defects in the expression of these genes might explain the massive cyst formation observed in this mouse model. Although HNF1β was shown not to be necessary for normal ciliar structure, this study demonstrates that the genetic program driven by the homeodomain transcription factor HNF1β involves the expression of genes that play a crucial role in the function of the cilium and regulates the terminal differentiation of renal tubular cells [239] together with – as shown before – the morphogenesis of hepatic bile ducts [52].

Although the ciliary model is a most attractive one, it should be kept in mind that possibly a cilium-mediated pathway may represent only one of several parallel pathways that control essential cellular functions such as proliferation apoptosis, adhesion, and differentiation [356,357].

PATHOPHYSIOLOGY OF CYSTIC EPITHELIUM

The Ca^{2+} signals modulate the expression, activity, and localization of many proteins and enzymes, other messenger systems, cell–cell communication, and tubular transport, reported during the last decade in an impressive number of studies [321].

Evidence has been produced for an increased proliferation of epithelial cyst-lining cells in ADPKD, comprising formation of papillary projections, and overexpression of Ki-67 and PCNA (proliferating cell nuclear antigen). The degree of proliferation appears to correlate with the level of apoptosis [304].

The cyst-lining cells appear relatively flattened with loss of the microvillous apical border, suggesting some degree of dedifferentiation. However, this dedifferentiation must be rather subtle or specific, leading to modulation rather than complete disruption of the phenotypic program that determines the higher-order structure of tubules. Indeed, the cells display no increased malignant potential and do not proliferate in compact cellular masses [304].

The epithelial lining cells have lost their "planar polarity" or "tissue polarity" (the ability to sense their position and orientation relative to the overall orientation of the epithelial sheet), resulting in a cyst that has no distinct longitudinal or circumferential axes [304].

In the renal cysts of ADPKD, the lining cells have undergone a switch from an absorptive to a secretory cell type, resulting in fluid secretion that is responsible (together with epithelial proliferation) for further cyst expansion [304].

BILIARY CYSTOGENESIS

Studies on the mechanisms for cyst development have mainly been devoted to renal cysts in polycystic kidney disease, and much less to cystogenesis in the liver.

The studies on primary cilia in cholangiocytes [195,204] and the evidence produced in recent years for the importance of the primary cilium in development and maintenance of epithelial tubules suggest that – at least to some extent – the cystogenesis in biliary ducts and ductules may be close to the concepts emerging from renal investigations. Obviously, organ- and tissue-specific differences are also to be expected.

In ADPKD, PKD1 and PKD2 are colocalized in bile duct epithelial cells [358] and the two-hit model of germline plus somatic mutation of PKD1 in focal liver cyst development appears applicable, as in the kidney cysts [359]. As in the kidney, biliary cyst expansion occurs by secretion of the cyst-lining epithelial cells. Autocrine and paracrine factors secreted into the cystic lumen modulate the rate of errant hepatic cyst growth, including interleukin (IL)-8, epithelial neutrophil attractant 78, IL-6, and vascular endothelial growth factor [360].

In ARPKD, findings suggestive for similarity with renal cystogenesis include the localization of Pkhd1 in the cilia of cholangiocytes in the PCK rat [195], which is a model for Caroli's syndrome [203], and the finding that HNF1β (localized in bile duct epithelium) regulates expression of Pkhd1 [240,241], together with other "cystoproteins" that colocalize into the cilium [239].

Differences in cystogenetic pathways between liver and kidney in ARPKD are indicated in animal models of the disease. The mouse *cpk* mutation is the most extensively characterized murine model, closely resembling human ARPKD, with the exception that the B6-*cpk/cpk* homozygotes do not express the lesion of DPM. However, homozygous mutants from outcrosses to some other strains express the DPM. Genetic analysis supports a loss-of-function model (two-hit model) for biliary cysts developing in an age-dependent fashion. There is no correlation between the severity of the DPM and the renal cystic disease. Expression of the biliary lesion is modulated by genetic background, and the specific biliary phenotype (DPM predominant or cyst predominant) is determined by whether loss of function of the *cpk* gene occurs as a germline or a somatic event [186].

In the mouse model generated by targeted mutation of *Pkdh1* (Pkdh1ex40 mouse), the animals develop severe malformation of their intrahepatic bile ducts but develop morphologically and functionally normal kidneys [202]. The cholangiocytes remain in a proliferative and TGF-β1-immunoreactive state that continuously stimulates mesenchymal cells to synthesize and deposit extracellular matrix, resulting in fibrosis. The findings suggest that fibrocystin/polyductin, already expressed in the embryonic ductal plate stage [361], acts as a matrix sensor and signal receptor during intrahepatic bile duct development and that its mutation results in a CHF-like picture. Its role in the liver and kidney appears to be functionally divergent, because protein domains essential for bile duct development do not affect nephrogenesis in this model [202]. Fibrocystin may serve as a key molecule for creating and/or maintaining the lumen of tubules and ducts [355].

In isolated PCLD, the mechanisms for cyst development appear to be different from those operative in ADPKD and ARPKD. The gene *PRKCSH* encodes a protein varyingly termed *protein kinase C substrate 80K-H* or *β subunit of glucosidase II* (GII β) [336,337]. The protein is widely distributed in tissues and highly conserved; it is predicted to be an endoplasmic reticulum luminal protein that recycles from the Golgi. The mutations found in PCLD are all predicted to cause premature chain termination, rendering loss-of-function changes most likely. The two-hit hypothesis for cyst formation in ADPKD appears extensible to PCLD. GII β plays a major role in regulation of proper folding and maturation of glycoproteins. It is conceivable that alterations in these mechanisms result in the development of biliary cysts. Polycystin-1, polycystin-2, and fibrocystin/polyductin are all glycoproteins. Mutations could compromise the processing of the N-linked oligosaccharide chains of the newly synthesized glycoproteins [337]. Improper association and trafficking of the polycystins caused by defective glycosylation by mutant GII β may link PCLD into the ADPKD pathway. This would be consistent with the marked similarity in clinical liver disease in both conditions [336,340].

The second gene involved in PCLD, *SEC63*, encodes a protein that is part of the multicomponent translocon of the endoplasmic reticulum. Sec63 is required in both the posttranslational and the cotranslational (or signal recognition particle [SRP]-dependent) targeting pathway. In the latter pathway, the ribosome is directly complexed with the Sec translocon and extrudes the nascent peptide through it; this is the main pathway in mammalian cells, including lumen-forming epithelia such as in the bile ducts. Cotranslational events include signal peptide cleavage, transfer and trimming of N-linked glycans, disulfide bond formation, transmembrane domain integration, chaperone binding, and protein folding. The transfer and trimming of N-glycans notably involves the activity of GII, the β subunit of which, PRKCSH, is the first gene found to be associated with PCLD. This is the functional link between the two genes known to be associated with PCLD.

If PCLD, like ADPKD, occurs by a cellular recessive two-hit mechanism, the mutation in either *SEC63* or *PRKCSH* will result in loss of proper folding of integral membrane proteins in bile duct cells that have undergone somatic second hits in later life. The lack of an observed abnormal kidney phenotype in PCLD may be due to the existence of alternative pathways for maturation of client proteins in renal tubular tissue [339].

Mesenchymal Hamartoma of the Liver

Mesenchymal hamartoma of the liver (MHL) was first described in 1956 [362]. It is, next to hemangiomas, the most common benign hepatic tumor in childhood. Nevertheless, MHL is relatively rare, and large children's hospitals are unlikely to see more than one new case every 2 years [363].

Most MHLs are large multicystic masses that present in the first 2 years of life typically with abdominal distention and/or an upper abdominal mass [364]. Less frequently, MHL is detected prenatally, in a newborn, in older children, and even in adults. Biochemical liver tests are usually normal, or only minimally deranged. In some patients, α-fetoprotein is moderately elevated. Ultrasound, computed tomography, and magnetic resonance imaging demonstrate a multiloculated cystic tumor with a variable amount of solid tissue, located in 75% of the patients in the right liver lobe. In some cases, the cysts may be very small so that the tumor appears as a solid lesion.

Histologically, the predominant component of the tumor consists of loose, edematous connective tissue, dilated vessels and lymphatics, and multiple cytokeratin 7 and 19–positive bile ducts, often in their early embryonic shape (DPM). Islands of parenchymal cells are scattered in between (Figure 4.15). Epithelium-lined cysts correspond to dilated bile duct structures, whereas cysts without epithelial lining correspond to areas of stromal liquefaction and dilated lymphatics. Small satellite lesions of similar outlook are sometimes found at the margin of the tumor. A variant MHL with myoid differentiation of the stromal cells was recently reported [365].

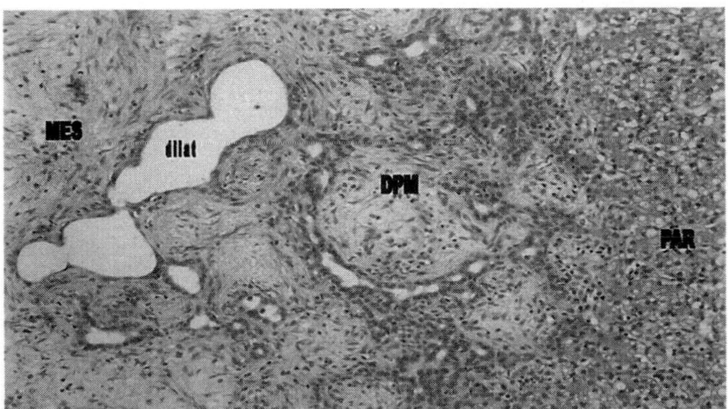

Figure 4.15. A mesenchymal hamartoma illustrating the basic components of the lesion: bile duct structures in ductal plate configuration (DPM), one dilated (dilat); loose myxoid type mesenchymal stroma (MES); and islands of liver parenchyma (PAR). (H&E, 125× magnification.)

The exact pathogenesis of mesenchymal hamartoma is unknown; the prevalent theory is that it represents aberrant development of primitive mesenchyme in portal tracts [366], apparently associated with disturbed remodeling of ductal plates. Another proposal favors the view of a regional ischemic lesion of a sequestered lobe [367].

Mesenchymal hamartoma of the liver was originally considered a benign hamartoma. However, several reports have highlighted an association between MHL and undifferentiated embryonal sarcoma (UES) [368]. Further evidence in favor of a relationship between MHL and UES are a similar cytogenetic abnormality involving the chromosome 19q13 region in both types of lesions and the occurrence of UES tumors that reveal areas with histology transitional between typical MHL and sarcomatous tissue of UES [364,369]. These data plead for a neoplasm rather than for a hamartoma.

The rapid enlargement of the tumor in young children is thought to be caused by cystic degeneration of the mesenchyme with secondary fluid accumulation within cysts, obstruction and dilatation of lymphatics, or both [363,370,371].

Treatment consists preferentially in total exeresis of the tumor. Recurrences have been noted, presumably caused by satellite lesions in the tumoral periphery. Although some rare cases progress to malignancy, the lesion behaves as a benign tumor in most cases, and even some spontaneous regressions are on record.

The literature on this puzzling lesion was systematically discussed in a recent review [364].

Solitary (Nonparasitic) Cyst

This lesion is not part of DPM. Solitary cysts of the liver are rare and are not associated with cysts in other viscera [326]. Because of the increased use of ultrasonographic examinations, nonparasitic cysts of the liver are more frequently encountered. They occur at all ages; they may be present at birth, but not all cases are clearly congenital. Solitary cysts involve more frequently the right lobe; the size is variable, but the vast majority are unilocular [326,372].

Microscopically, the outer layer of the cyst wall consists of loose connective tissue, the middle layer is more dense, and the inner layer is composed of less dense fibrous tissue and often shows an epithelial lining. The latter may be flat cuboidal or cylindrical; pseudostratified columnar epithelium and squamous epithelium also have been observed.

The expression and secretion of epithelial markers support the biliary origin of solitary, nonparasitic cysts [373]. The majority of solitary liver cysts are asymptomatic; however, there are possible complications that include infection, perforation, spontaneous hemorrhage, obstructive jaundice, and neoplastic degeneration [374]. Occasionally, a small solitary cyst present at birth may start expanding, even at high speed [375], indicating the usefulness of follow-up [376]. Treatment has included surgery and alcohol-induced sclerosis.

Ciliated Hepatic Foregut Cyst

Ciliated hepatic foregut cyst (CHFC) was first described in 1857 [377]. It is usually found in adults but occasionally in children as well [378].

Ciliated hepatic foregut cyst occurs preferentially in segment IV of the liver (medial segment of left lobe) underneath the anterior liver capsule [379]. It is typically a small lesion measuring 1–4 cm, containing viscous liquid. It is lined by respiratory epithelium, similar to that seen in bronchogenic and esophageal cysts. It is considered the result of maldevelopment, arising from remnants of the embryonic foregut; the latter forms the liver, the tracheobronchial tree, the esophagus, and other organs. Some reported cases were located in the gallbladder wall, usually without communication between the cyst and the gallbladder lumen, except one case that was documented with a patent connecting duct [380]. CHFC is mostly well defined with all imaging techniques [381] and is the only lesion with ciliated epithelium in the liver, enabling diagnosis by cytology. CHFC displays a benign behavior in most cases, but rare instances of invasive squamous carcinoma arising from a CHFC have been reported [382].

CHOLANGIOPATHIES OF EXTRAHEPATIC BILE DUCTS

Biliary Atresia

Biliary atresia has been discussed under the heading Cholangiopathies of Intrahepatic Bile Ducts, because the latter also are affected by this disease.

Anatomic Anomalies of Extrahepatic Bile Ducts

Anatomic variations and abnormalities of the extrahepatic bile ducts are of importance for radiologists and for biliary and transplant surgeons [82]. Variations are quite common; they can be demonstrated by radiographic techniques but are of no pathologic significance [383]. In contrast, abnormalities are pathologically significant deviations from the normal pattern. In a large series of operative cholangiograms, abnormalities were found in 18.4% of cases [383].

Agenesis of Extrahepatic Bile Ducts

Rare cases are on record of agenesis of the common bile duct: The common hepatic duct emptied into the gallbladder; bile was drained into the duodenum through a long cystic duct [384,385]. Schwartz et al. [386] reported four instances of agenesis of the proximal extrahepatic bile ducts and one case with total absence of the extrahepatic bile ducts and gallbladder, without fibrous remnant at the porta hepatis.

Aberrant and Accessory Bile Ducts

Accessory hepatic ducts have been reported that pass beyond the porta hepatis and terminate in other segments of the extrahepatic bile conduits [383]. The extra duct is usually the right hepatic duct [387]. The so-called aberrant hepatic duct corresponds to a dorsocaudal branch, which drains into the common hepatic duct or into the cystic duct [383].

Aberrant small biliary ducts in the gallbladder fossa were described by Luschka [388] and are termed ducts of Luschka or subvesicular or supravesicular ducts. These are often small bile ducts (<1 mm in diameter), running along the gallbladder fossa and the liver parenchyma. They branch from right hepatic or common hepatic ducts but are not accompanied by artery or vein and, having blind distal ends, do not drain any liver parenchyma and do not open into the gallbladder. Their importance lies in their common occurrence (30% of cases) and their possible injury or transsection during cholecystectomy, resulting in postoperative bile leak [389]. Ducts of Luschka show variations in localization, course, size, and termination [390].

Other variations include cystohepatic ducts (true bile ducts draining a portion of liver parenchyma and opening into the gallbladder or the cystic duct); vaginali ductuli (very small communications between two bile ducts or between a duct and the cystic duct); and duplication of the cystic duct or the gallbladder [389].

Bile Duct Duplication

Bile duct duplication is an exceedingly rare anomaly first described by Andreas Vesalius in 1543 [391], who reported a patient with two common bile ducts, one entering into the stomach antrum, the lower one entering into the duodenum.

The condition does not cause symptoms unless complications of obstruction or infection occur. Awareness about its existence is imperative for the biliary surgeon in order to avoid damage or section during operations [392]. The wide variations in the reported cases render any classification difficult; indeed, the dissimilarity among cases is such as to be in itself a characteristic of this anomaly [393,394]. Bile duct duplication may be associated with BA [395].

The embryologic development of the abnormality may be related to an incomplete division of the pars cystica and the pars hepatica of the hepatic diverticulum [396].

Congenital Bronchobiliary Fistula (Tracheocholedochal Tract; Biliotracheal Fistula with Trifurcation of the Bronchi; Carinal Trifurcation with Tracheobiliary Fistula)

A congenital fistula between the respiratory and biliary tract, first reported in 1952 [397], is very rare. About 24 cases had been reported in 2004 [398]. The clinical symptoms are cough, vomiting, and bronchopneumonia; some cases had associated malformations, such as diaphragmatic hernia, esophageal atresia, choledochal hypoplasia, and BA [399]. Fifty percent of the patients were less than 1 month at diagnosis, and the majority less than 6 months. Two thirds of the reported patients were female. The diagnosis has rested on clinical symptoms, bronchoscopy in former years, and different imaging techniques in later years [398]. Treatment consists of surgical resection of the fistula. The histopathology of the resected specimens generally shows bronchial tissue proximally with characteristics of esophagus or bile duct distally [400].

The embryologic morphogenesis is uncertain. An evagination from the pluripotential embryonic foregut located between the respiratory and hepatic diverticula, originally independent from both but with subsequent union to each embryonic organ, could conceivably be at the origin of the malformation [401,402].

Spontaneous Perforation of the Common Bile Duct

Spontaneous perforation of the common bile duct is a rare but specific entity, first described in 1932 [403], that occurs in the first 3 months of life. The cause is unknown; several factors have been suggested, including a congenital weakness of the bile duct wall at this site, mucous plugs, gallstones, and viral infection [90,372,387]. Radionuclide hepatobiliary scan is highly sensitive and specific for spontaneous perforation of the bile duct and is the preoperative test of choice when this diagnosis is suspected [404]. Treatment is surgical, with good prognosis.

Bile Duct Hypoplasia

Bile duct hypoplasia is a lesion characterized by an exceptionally small but grossly visible and radiographically patent extrahepatic biliary duct system [90]. It is thought not to correspond to a specific disease entity but to represent a manifestation of a variety of hepatobiliary disorders. It may be associated with atresia of extrahepatic ducts and with intrahepatic cholestasis of any cause [405].

Bile duct hypoplasia may represent an intermediate stage in the development of EHBDA [182]. A case was reported with the documented sequence of choledochal cyst, followed by biliary hypoplasia, followed by BA [183].

In patients with intrahepatic cholestasis (α_1-antitrypsin deficiency, syndromic PILBD), the hypoplasia of the extrahepatic bile ducts is thought to represent a form of disuse atrophy caused by decreased bile flow [406,407]. In the few patients with syndromic PILBD, however, in whom histologic study of the extrahepatic bile ducts was performed, inflammatory and epithelial degenerative lesions were found that were indistinguishable from those seen in BA [181]; this observation supports the concept that hypoplasia of extrahepatic bile ducts may represent a partial or arrested BA [90,182].

In patients with persistence of bile duct hypoplasia, liver cirrhosis is slowly progressive [408], comparable to the progressive biliary disease that develops in adults with narrowed extrahepatic ducts [409].

Anomalies of the Gallbladder and Cystic Duct

Anomalies of the gallbladder include absence of the gallbladder and double, bilobed, left-sided, folded, and intrahepatic gallbladder [410].

In 20% of subjects, the cystic duct does not join the common hepatic duct directly but instead runs parallel to it for some distance or occasionally makes a spiral turn around it. This variation is important for the biliary surgeon.

Congenital Bile Duct Cysts (Choledochal Cyst, Congenital Dilatation of the Common Bile Duct)

The incidence of this nonhereditary condition shows striking geographic differences: There is an unexplained higher frequency of choledochal cysts in Japan than in Western countries [326,411]. Females are affected more frequently than males. Advances in fetal imaging have allowed prenatal diagnosis in some cases [412,413].

The disorder occurs in multiple anatomic variants, which have been the subject of several classification systems [282,414–416]. The most used classification [282] takes into account that cysts need not be limited to the common bile duct but may occur in any segment of the extrahepatic biliary tree and may be associated with cystic dilatations of the intrahepatic bile ducts. This explains the term *congenital bile duct cysts.* This clinically relevant classification distinguishes five types. The types IV A and V combine cystic dilatations of the intra- and extrahepatic ducts. Type V corresponds to Caroli's disease [417,418].

The condition may cause symptoms at any age, with conjugated hyperbilirubinemia in infants and, more commonly, pain in patients older than 2 years [411]. The classic triad of pain, jaundice, and a palpable abdominal mass is seen in only about 25% of patients [419]. The patients who are not infants usually run a milder clinical course than those who are [411]. Spontaneous rupture in children is very rare, but possible [420].

The cause and pathogenesis of congenital bile duct cysts are unclear; neither is it known whether all variants share a common cause [326]. The proposed hypotheses include a "maldevelopment" resulting in an inherent abnormality of the ductal wall; acquired injury resulting from an anomalous arrangement of the distal pancreaticobiliary tree [421]; and an obliterative inflammatory process of the distal common bile duct analogous to BA [82]. Congenital bile duct cyst and BA may occur together [422].

The pathology of bile duct cysts is not very revealing of their etiology. The cysts vary greatly in size and have fibrous walls. An epithelial lining is often lacking, but islets of cylindric or columnar epithelium may be present. The wall may be thickened by inflammation and fibrosis and may be stained with bile. Occasional smooth muscle fibers are found in the wall [282,372].

Complications of congenital bile duct cysts occur in 16.5% of patients [419]. Stone formation is the most frequent and development of carcinoma the most dreaded long-term complications. Carcinoma develops in 4–8% of patients, usually beyond the age of 20 years [282,419]. Other complications include obstruction, cholangitis, and perforation [82,282, 419].

Treatment of choledochal cysts is surgical [281,282,419, 423], which should aim at complete removal of the cysts [424].

REFERENCES

1. Severn CB. A morphological study of the development of the human liver. II. Establishment of liver parenchyma, extrahepatic ducts and associated venous channels. Am J Anat 1972;133:85–107.
2. Dubois AM. The embryonic liver. In: Rouillen C, ed. The liver. New York: Academic Press, 1963:1–39.

3. Tan CEL, Moscoso GJ. The developing human biliary system at the porta hepatis level between 29 days and 8 weeks of gestation: a way to understanding biliary atresia. Part 1. Pathol Int 1994;44:587–99.
4. Dubois AM. The embryonic liver. In: Rouiller C, ed. The liver. New York: Academic Press, 1963:1–39.
5. Das KM, Squillante L, Chitayet D, et al. Simultaneous appearance of a unique common epitope in fetal colon, skin and biliary epithelial cells. A possible link for extracolonic manifestations in ulcerative colitis. J Clin Gastroenterol 1992;15:311–16.
6. Landry C, Clotman F, Hioki T, et al. HNF-6 is expressed in endoderm derivatives and nervous system of the mouse embryo and participates to the cross-regulatory network of liver-enriched transcription factors. Dev Biol 1997;192:247–57.
7. Rausa F, Samadani U, Ye H, et al. The cut homeodomain transcriptional activator HNF-6 is coexpressed with its target gene HNF-3 beta in the developing murine liver and pancreas. Dev Biol 1997;192:228–46.
8. Kalinichenko VV, Zhou Y, Bhattacharyya D, et al. Haploinsufficiency of the mouse Forkhead Box f1 gene causes defects in gall bladder development. J Biol Chem 2002;277:12369–74.
9. Jorgensen M. The ductal plate malformation: a study of the intrahepatic bile duct lesion in infantile polycystic disease and congenital hepatic fibrosis. Acta Pathol Microbiol Scand 1977;257(Suppl):1–88.
10. Tan CEL, Moscoso GJ. The developing human biliary system at the porta hepatis level between 11 and 25 weeks of gestation: a way to understanding biliary atresia. Part 2. Pathol Int 1994; 44:600–10.
11. Tan J, Hytiroglou P, Wieczorek R, et al. Immunohistochemical evidence for hepatic progenitor cells in liver diseases. Liver 2002;22:365–73.
12. Shiojiri N, Katayama H. Secondary joining of the bile ducts during the hepatogenesis of the mouse embryo. Anat Embryol 1987;177:153–63.
13. Mahlapuu M, Enerback S, Carlsson P. Haploinsufficiency of the forkhead gene Foxf1, a target for sonic hedgehog signaling, causes lung and foregut malformations. Development 2001;128:2397–406.
14. Bloom W. The embryogenesis of human bile capillaries and ducts. Am J Anat 1926;36:451–62.
15. Elias H, Sherrick JC. Morphology of the liver. New York: Academic Press, 1969.
16. Desmet VJ, Van Eyken P. Embryology, malformations and malpositions of the liver. In: Haubrich W, Schaffner F, Berk JE, eds. Bockus gastroenterology, 5th ed. Philadelphia, PA: Saunders, 1995:1849–57.
17. Blankenberg TA, Lund JK, Ruebner BH. Normal and abnormal development of human intrahepatic bile ducts. An immunohistochemical perspective. In: Abramowsky CR, Bernstein J, Rosenberg HS, eds. Perspectives in pediatric pathology. Transplantation pathology—hepatic morphogenesis. Vol. 14. Basel: Karger, 1991:143–67.
18. Ruebner BH, Blankenberg TA, Burrows DA, et al. Development and transformation of the ductal plate in the developing human liver. Pediatr Pathol 1990;10:55–68.
19. Hammar JA. Über die erste Entstehung der nicht kapillaren intrahepatischen Gallengänge beim Menschen. Z Mikrosk Anat Forsch 1926;5:59–89.
20. Desmet VJ. Embryology of the liver and intrahepatic biliary tract, and an overview of malformations of the bile duct. In: Bircher J, Benharnou JP, McIntyre N, et al., eds. The Oxford textbook of clinical hepatology. Oxford, UK: Oxford University Press, 1999:51–61.
21. Vijayan V, Tan CE. Developing human biliary system in three dimensions. Anat Rec 1997;249:389–98.
22. Van Eyken P, Sciot R, Callea F, et al. The development of the intrahepatic bile ducts in man: a keratin-immunohistochemical study. Hepatology 1988;8:1586–95.
23. Haruna Y, Thung S, Gerber M. Cell lineage specific markers during human liver organogenesis and regeneration. Hepatology 1994;20:210A.
24. Stosiek P, Kasper M, Karsten U. Expression of cytokeratin 19 during human liver organogenesis. Liver 1990;10:59–63.
25. Desmet VJ, Van Eyken P, Sciot R. Cytokeratins for probing cell lineage relationships in developing liver. Hepatology 1990, 12:1249–51.
26. Faa G, Van Eyken P, Roskams T, et al. Expression of cytokeratin 20 in developing rat liver and in experimental models of ductular and oval cell proliferation. J Hepatol 1998;29:628–33.
27. Van Eyken P, Sciot R, van Damme B, et al. Keratin immunohistochemistry in normal human liver. Cytokeratin pattern of hepatocytes, bile ducts and acinar gradient. Virchows Arch A Pathol Anat Histopathol 1987;412:63–72.
28. Moll R, Franke WW, Schiller DL, et al. The catalog of human cytokeratins: patterns of expression in normal epithelia, tumors and cultured cells. Cell 1982;31:11–24.
29. Lemaigre FP. Development of the biliary tract. Mech Dev 2003; 120:81–7.
30. Clotman F, Jacquemin P, Plumb-Rudewiez N, et al. Control of liver cell fate decision by a gradient of TGF beta signaling modulated by Onecut transcription factors. Genes Dev 2005;19:1849–54.
31. Croquelois A, Blindenbacher A, Terracciano L, et al. Inducible inactivation of Notch1 causes nodular regenerative hyperplasia in mice. Hepatology 2005;41:487–96.
32. Krupczak-Hollis K, Wang X, Kalinichenko VV, et al. The mouse Forkhead Box m1 transcription factor is essential for hepatoblast mitosis and development of intrahepatic bile ducts and vessels during liver morphogenesis. Dev Biol 2004;276:74–88.
33. Sergi C, Adam S, Kahl P, et al. The remodeling of the primitive human biliary system. Early Hum Dev 2000;58:167–78.
34. Kahn E, Markowitz J, Aiges H, et al. Human ontogeny of the bile duct to portal space ratio. Hepatology 1989;10:21–3.
35. Doljanski L, Roulet F. Ueber die gestaltende Wechselwirkung zwischen dem Epithel und dem Mesenchym, zugleich ein Beitrag zur Histogenese der sogenannten "Gallengangswucherungen." Virchows Arch [A] 1934;292:256–67.
36. Terada T, Kitamura Y, Nakanuma Y. Normal and abnormal development of the human intrahepatic biliary system: a review. Tohoku J Exp Med 1997;181:19–32.
37. Desmet VJ. Embryogenèse des voies biliaires. Med Ther 1995; 1:227–35.
38. Roskams T, van Eyken P, Desmet V. Human liver growth and development. In: Strain AJ, Diehl AM, eds. Liver growth and repair. London: Chapman and Hall, 1998:541–57.
39. Nakanuma Y, Hoso M, Sanzen T, et al. Microstructure and development of the normal and pathologic biliary tract in humans, including blood supply. Microsc Res Tech 1997;38: 552–70.

40. Balistreri W. Concluding remarks. 5th International Sendai Symposium on Biliary Atresia. In: Ohi R, ed. Biliary atresia. Tokyo: ICOM Associates, 1991:293–7.
41. Couvelard A, Bringuier AF, Dauge MC, et al. Expression of integrins during liver organogenesis in humans. Hepatology 1998;27:839–47.
42. Terada T, Ashida K, Kitamura Y, et al. Expression of epithelial-cadherin, alpha-catenin and beta-catenin during human intrahepatic bile duct development: a possible role in bile duct morphogenesis. J Hepatol 1998;28:263–9.
43. Dudas J, Papoutsi M, Hecht M, et al. The homeobox transcription factor Prox1 is highly conserved in embryonic hepatoblasts and in adult and transformed hepatocytes, but is absent from bile duct epithelium. Anat Embryol (Berl) 2004;208:359–66.
44. Shiojiri N, Takeshita K, Yamasaki H, et al. Suppression of C(EBP alpha expression in biliary cell differentiation from hepatoblasts during mouse liver development. J Hepatol 2004;41:790–8.
45. Quondamatteo F, Knittel T, Mehde M, et al. Matrix metalloproteinases in early human liver development. Histochem Cell Biol 1999;112:277–82.
46. Libbrecht L, Cassiman D, Desmet V, et al. Expression of neural cell adhesion molecule in human liver development and in congenital and acquired liver diseases. Histochem Cell Biol 2001;116:233–9.
47. Shiojiri N, Nagai Y. Preferential differentiation of the bile ducts along the portal vein in the development of mouse liver. Anat Embryol (Berl) 1992;185:17–24.
48. Libbrecht L, Cassiman D, Desmet V, et al. The correlation between portal myofibroblasts and development of intrahepatic bile ducts and arterial branches in human liver. Liver 2002;22:252–8.
49. Terada T, Nakanuma Y. Development of human peribiliary capillary plexus: a lectin-histochemical and immunohistochemical study. Hepatology 1993;18:529–36.
50. Clotman F, Lannoy VJ, Reber M, et al. The onecut transcription factor HNF6 is required for normal development of the biliary tract. Development 2002;129:1819–28.
51. Clotman F, Libbrecht L, Gresh L, et al. Hepatic artery malformations associated with a primary defect in intrahepatic bile duct development. J Hepatol 2003;39:686–92.
52. Coffinier C, Gresh L, Fiette L, et al. Bile system morphogenesis defects and liver dysfunction upon targeted deletion of HNF1beta. Development 2002;129:1829–38.
53. Xue Y, Gao X, Lindsell CE, et al. Embryonic lethality and vascular defects in mice lacking the Notch ligand Jagged1. Hum Mol Genet 1999;8:723–30.
54. Crosnier C, Attie-Bitach T, Encha-Razavi F, et al. JAGGED1 gene expression during human embryogenesis elucidates the wide phenotypic spectrum of Alagille syndrome. Hepatology 2000;32:574–81.
55. Louis AA, Van Eyken P, Haber BA, et al. Hepatic jagged1 expression studies. Hepatology 1999;30:1269–75.
56. McCright B, Lozier J, Gridley T. A mouse model of Alagille syndrome: Notch2 as a genetic modifier of Jag1 haploinsufficiency. Development 2002;129:1075–82.
57. Kodama Y, Hijikata M, Kageyama R, et al. The role of notch signaling in the development of intrahepatic bile ducts. Gastroenterology 2004;127:1775–86.
58. Nijjar SS, Wallace L, Crosby HA, et al. Altered Notch ligand expression in human liver disease: further evidence for a role of the Notch signaling pathway in hepatic neovascularization and biliary ductular defects. Am J Pathol 2002;160:1695–703.
59. Flynn DM, Nijjar S, Hubscher SG, et al. The role of Notch receptor expression in bile duct development and disease. J Pathol 2004;204:55–64.
60. Chen HL, Chen HL, Liu YJ, et al. Developmental expression of canalicular transporter genes in human liver. J Hepatol 2005;43:472–7.
61. De Wolf-Peeters C, De Vos R, Desmet V, et al. Electron microscopy and morphometry of canalicular differentiation in fetal and neonatal rat liver. Exp Mol Pathol 1974;21:339–50.
62. Kanamura S, Kanai K, Watanabe J. Fine structure and function of hepatocytes during development. J Electron Microsc Tech 1990;14:92–105.
63. Roskams T, Desmet VJ. Parathyroid hormone-related peptide and development of intrahepatic bile ducts in man. Int Hepatol Comm 1994;2:121–7.
64. Terada T, Nakanuma Y. Development of human intrahepatic peribiliary glands. Histological, keratin immunohistochemical, and mucus histochemical studies. Lab Invest 1993;68:261–9.
65. Crawford JM. Development of the intrahepatic biliary tree. Semin Liver Dis 2002;22:213–26.
66. Shankle WR, Landing BH, Gregg J. Normal organ weights of infants and children: graphs of values by age, with confidence intervals. Pediatr Pathol 1983;1:399–408.
67. Kiernan F. The anatomy and physiology of the liver. Philos Trans R Soc Lond 1833;123:711–70.
68. Mall FP. A study of the structural unit of the liver. Am J Anat 1906;5:227–308.
69. Rappaport AM. The microcirculatory hepatic unit. Microvasc Res 1973;6:212–228.
70. Lamers WH, Moorman AFM, Charles R. The metabolic lobulus, a key to the architecture of the liver. In: Gumucio JJ, ed. Revisiones sobre biologia cellular. Cell biology reviews. Vol. 19. Berlin: Springer International. 1989:5–26.
71. Matsumoto T, Komori R, Magara T, et al. A study on the normal structure of human liver, with special reference to its angioarchitecture. Jikeikai Med J 1979;26:1–40.
72. Matsumoto R, Kawakami M. The unit-concept of hepatic parenchyma – a re-examination based on angioarchitectural studies. Acta Pathol Jpn 1982;32:285–314.
73. Teutsch HF. The modular microarchitecture of human liver. Hepatology 2005;42:317–25.
74. Ekataksin W, Wake K. New concepts in biliary and vascular anatomy of the liver. In: Boyer JL, Ockner R, eds. Progress in liver disease. Philadelphia: WB Saunders Company, 1997:1–30.
75. Johnson F. The development of the lobule of the pig's liver. Am J Anat 1919;25:299–331.
76. Landing BH, Wells TR. Considerations of some architectural properties of the biliary tree and liver in childhood. In: Abramowsky CR, Bernstein J, Rosenberg HS, eds. Transplantation pathology – hepatic morphogenesis. Perspectives in pediatric pathology. Vol. 14. Basel: Karger, 1991:122–42.
77. Ludwig J, Ritman EL, LaRusso NF, et al. Anatomy of the human biliary system studied by quantitative computer-aided three-dimensional imaging techniques. Hepatology 1998;27:893–9.
78. Artavanis-Tsakonas S, Matsuno K, Fortini ME. Notch signaling. Science 1995;268:225–32.
79. Artavanis-Tsakonas S, Rand MD, Lake RJ. Notch signaling: cell fate control and signal integration in development. Science 1999;284:770–6.

80. Roskams TA, Theise ND, Balabaud C, et al. Nomenclature of the finer branches of the biliary tree: canals, ductules, and ductular reactions in human livers. Hepatology 2004;39:1739–45.
81. Marchal GJ, Desmet VJ, Proesmans WC, et al. Caroli disease: high frequency US and pathologic findings. Radiology 1986; 158:507–11.
82. Van Eyken P, Desmet VJ. Disordered embryogenesis of the hepatobiliary tract. In: Prieto J, Rodes JS, Shafritz DA, eds. Hepatobiliary diseases. Berlin: Springer, 1992:931–70.
83. Inui A, Fujisawa T, Suemitsu T, et al. A case of Caroli's disease with special reference to hepatic CT and US findings. J Pediatr Gastroenterol Nutr 1992;14:463–6.
84. Brancatelli G, Federle MP, Vilgrain V, et al. Fibropolycystic liver disease: CT and MR imaging findings. Radiographics 2005; 25:659–70.
85. Levy AD, Rohrmann CA Jr. Biliary cystic disease. Curr Probl Diagn Radiol 2003;32:233–63.
86. Zeitoun D, Brancatelli G, Colombat M, et al. Congenital hepatic fibrosis: CT findings in 18 adults. Radiology 2004;231:109–16.
87. Desmet VJ. Congenital diseases of intrahepatic bile ducts: variations on the theme "ductal plate malformation." Hepatology 1992;16:1069–83.
88. Desmet VJ. What is congenital hepatic fibrosis? Histopathology 1992;20:465–77.
89. Johnson CA, Gissen P, Sergi C. Molecular pathology and genetics of congenital hepatorenal fibrocystic syndromes. J Med Genet 2003;40:311–19.
90. Desmet VJ, Callea F. Cholestatic syndromes of infancy and childhood. In: Zakim D, Boyer TD, eds. Hepatology. A textbook of liver disease. Philadelphia: WB Saunders, 1996:1649–98.
91. Lefkowitch JH. Biliary atresia. Mayo Clin Proc 1998;73:90–5.
92. Kasai M, Kimuna S, Asakura S, et al. Surgical treatment of biliary atresia. J Pediatr Surg 1968;3:665–75.
93. Howard ER. Extrahepatic biliary atresia. A review of current management. Br J Surg 1983;70:193–7.
94. Ohya T, Fujimoto T, Shimomura H, et al. Degeneration of intrahepatic bile duct with lymphocyte infiltration into biliary epithelial cells in biliary atresia. J Pediatr Surg 1995;30:515–18.
95. Witzleben CL. The pathogenesis of biliary atresia. In: Javitt NB, ed. Neonatal hepatitis and biliary atresia. Washington, DC: US Department of Health, Education and Welfare, 1979:339–50.
96. Witzleben CL. Pathogenesis of bile duct paucity: observations in extrahepatic biliary atresia and arteriohepatic dysplasia. In: Waldschmidt J, Charissis G, Schier F, eds. Cholestasis in neonates. W Zuckschwerdt: München, 1988:53–61.
97. Haas JE. Bile duct and liver pathology in biliary atresia. World J Surg 1978;2:561–9.
98. Kasai M. Treatment of biliary atresia with special reference to hepatic porto-enterostomy and its modifications. In: Bill AH, Kasai M, eds. Progress of pediatric surgery. Baltimore: University Park Press, 1974:5–52.
99. Gautier M, Jehan P, Odièvre M. Histologic study of biliary fibrous remnants in 48 cases of extra-hepatic biliary atresia: correlation with postoperative bile flow restoration. J Pediatr 1976;89:704–9.
100. Miyano T, Surugo K, Tsuchiya H. A histopathological study of the remnant of extrahepatic bile duct in so-called uncorrectable biliary atresia. J Pediatr Surg 1977;12:19–25.
101. Suruga K, Miyano T, Arai T, et al. A study of patients with long-term bile flow after hepatic portoenterostomy for biliary atresia. J Pediatr Surg 1985;20:252–5.
102. Schweizer P. Extrahepatische Gallengangsatresie – Eine analytische Bewertung prognostischer Faktoren. Ein Beitrag zu einem rationelen Therapieansatz. Z Kinderchir 1990;45:365–70.
103. Tan CE, Davenport M, Driver M, et al. Does the morphology of the extrahepatic biliary remnants in biliary atresia influence survival? A review of 205 cases. J Pediatr Surg 1994;29:1459–64.
104. Dolgin SE. Answered and unanswered controversies in the surgical management of extra hepatic biliary atresia. Pediatr Transplant 2004;8:628–31.
105. Schweizer P, Muller G. Gallengangsatresie. Cholestase-Syndrome im Neugeborenen- und Suglingsalter. Stuttgart: Hippokrates Verlag, 1984.
106. Desmet VJ. Pathology of paediatric cholestasis. In: Lentze M, Reichen J, eds. Paediatric cholestasis. Novel approaches to treatment. Dordrecht: Kluwer Academic Publishers, 1992:55–73.
107. Cocjin J, Rosenthal P, Buslon V, et al. Bile ductule formation in fetal, neonatal, and infant livers compared with extrahepatic biliary atresia. Hepatology 1996;24:568–74.
108. Brough AJ, Bernstein J. Morphologic approach to the evaluation of infantile conjugated hyperbilirubinemia. In: Javitt NB, ed. Neonatal hepatitis and biliary atresia. DHEW publication no. (NIH) 79–1296. Washington, DC: US Department of Health, Education and Welfare, 1979;381–8.
109. Van Eyken P, Desmet VJ. Cytokeratins and the liver. Liver 1993; 13:113–22.
110. Roskams T, Desmet V. Ductular reaction and its diagnostic significance. Semin Diagn Pathol 1998;15:259–69.
111. Roskams T. The role of immunohistochemistry in diagnosis. Clin Liver Dis 2002;6:571–89, x.
112. Azar G, Beneck D, Lane B, et al. Atypical morphologic presentation of biliary atresia and value of serial liver biopsies. J Pediatr Gastroenterol Nutr 2002;34:212–15.
113. dos Santos JL, da Silveira TR, da Silva VD, et al. Medial thickening of hepatic artery branches in biliary atresia. A morphometric study. J Pediatr Surg 2005;40:637–42.
114. Ho CW, Shioda K, Shirasaki K, et al. The pathogenesis of biliary atresia: a morphological study of the hepatobiliary system and the hepatic artery. J Pediatr Gastroenterol Nutr 1993;16:53–60.
115. Azarow KS, Phillips MJ, Sandler AD, et al. Biliary atresia: should all patients undergo a portoenterostomy? J Pediatr Surg 1997;32:168–72; discussion 172–4.
116. Lilly JR, Alejandro M, Hernandez C, et al. Surgery of biliary atresia. In: Balistreri WF, Stocker JT, eds. Pediatric hepatology. New York: Hemisphere Publishing Corporation, 1990:19–27.
117. Lilly JR, Karrer FM. Contemporary surgery of biliary atresia. Pediatr Clin North Am 1985;32:1233–46.
118. Landing BH, Wells TR, Ramicone E. Time course of the intrahepatic lesion of extrahepatic biliary atresia. A morphometric study. Pediatr Pathol 1985;4:309–19.
119. Aronson DC, de Haan J, James J, et al. Quantitative aspects of the parenchyma-stroma relationship in experimentally induced cholestasis. Liver 1988;8:116–26.
120. Raweily EA, Gibson AAM, Burt AD. Abnormalities of intrahepatic bile ducts in extrahepatic biliary atresia. Histopathology 1990;17:521–7.
121. Low Y, Vijayan V, Tan CE. The prognostic value of ductal plate malformation and other histologic parameters in biliary atresia: an immunohistochemical study. J Pediatr 2001;139:320–2.
122. Desmet VJ. Cholangiopathies: past, present and future. Semin Liver Dis 1987;7:67–76.

123. Ryckman FC, Alonso MH, Bucuvalas JC, et al. Biliary atresia – surgical management and treatment options as they relate to outcome. Liver Transpl Surg 1998;4(5 suppl 1):S24–33.
124. Bates MD, Bucuvalas JC, Alonso MH, et al. Biliary atresia: pathogenesis and treatment. Semin Liver Dis 1998;18:281–93.
125. Laurent J, Gauthier F, Bernard O, et al. Long-term outcome after surgery for biliary atresia. Study of 40 patients surviving more than 10 years. Gastroenterology 1990;99:1793–7.
126. Fabbretti G, Gosseye S, Brisigutti M, et al. Liver transplantation after unsuccessful porto-enterostomy for extra-hepatic biliary atresia (EHBDA): morphologic study of 31 removed livers. In: Ohi R, ed. Biliary atresia. Tokyo: ICOM Associates, 1991: 70–4.
127. Petersen C. Surgery in biliary atresia – futile or futuristic? Eur J Pediatr Surg 2004;14:226–9.
128. Callea F, Facchetti F, Lucini L, et al. Liver morphology in anicteric patients at long-term follow-up after Kasai operation: a study of 16 cases. In: Ohi R, ed. Biliary atresia. Tokyo: ICOM Associates, 1991:304–10.
129. Perlmutter DH, Shepherd RW. Extrahepatic biliary atresia: a disease or a phenotype? Hepatology 2002;35:1297–304.
130. Bezerra JA. Potential etiologies of biliary atresia. Pediatr Transplant 2005;9:646–51.
131. Squires RH Jr. From whence does biliary atresia arise? Pediatr Transplant 2005;9:145 7.
132. Mack CL, Sokol RJ. Unraveling the pathogenesis and etiology of biliary atresia. Pediatr Res 2005;57(5 pt 2):87R–94R.
133. Sokol RJ, Mack C, Narkewicz MR, et al. Pathogenesis and outcome of biliary atresia: current concepts. J Pediatr Gastroenterol Nutr 2003;37:4–21.
134. Carmi R, Magee CA, Neill CA, et al. Extrahepatic biliary atresia and associated anomalies: etiologic heterogeneity suggested by distinctive patterns of associations. Am J Med Genet 1993;45:683–93.
135. Mazziotti MV, Willis LK, Heuckeroth RO, et al. Anomalous development of the hepatobiliary system in the Inv mouse. Hepatology 1999;30:372–8.
136. Schon P, Tsuchiya K, Lenoir D, et al. Identification, genomic organization, chromosomal mapping and mutation analysis of the human INV gene, the ortholog of a murine gene implicated in left-right axis development and biliary atresia. Hum Genet 2002;110:157–65.
137. Jacquemin E, Cresteil D, Raynaud N, et al. CFCI gene mutation and biliary atresia with polysplenia syndrome. J Pediatr Gastroenterol Nutr 2002;34:326–7.
138. Ware SM, Peng J, Zhu L, et al. Identification and functional analysis of ZIC3 mutations in heterotaxy and related congenital heart defects. Am J Hum Genet 2004;74:93–105.
139. Zhang DY, Sabla G, Shivakumar P, et al. Coordinate expression of regulatory genes differentiates embryonic and perinatal forms of biliary atresia. Hepatology 2004;39:954–62.
140. Kohsaka T, Yuan ZR, Guo SX, et al. The significance of human jagged 1 mutations detected in severe cases of extrahepatic biliary atresia. Hepatology 2002;36(4 pt 1):904–12.
141. Sasaki H, Nio M, Iwami D, et al. Cytokeratin subtypes in biliary atresia: immunohistochemical study. Pathol Int 2001;51: 511–18.
142. Omary MB, Ku NO, Toivola DM. Keratins: guardians of the liver. Hepatology 2002;35:251–7.
143. Tan CE, Chan VS, Yong RY, et al. Distortion in TGF beta 1 peptide immunolocalization in biliary atresia: comparison with the normal pattern in the developing human intrahepatic bile duct system. Pathol Int 1995;45:815–24.
144. Sasaki H, Nio M, Iwami D, et al. E-cadherin, alpha-catenin and beta-catenin in biliary atresia: correlation with apoptosis and cell cycle. Pathol Int 2001;51:923–32.
145. Funaki N, Sasano H, Shizawa S, et al. Apoptosis and cell proliferation in biliary atresia. J Pathol 1998;186:429–33.
146. Colombo C, Zuliani G, Ronchi M, et al. Biliary bile acid composition of the human fetus in early gestation. Pediatr Res 1987;21:197–200.
147. Yamamoto K, Fisher MM, Phillips MJ. Hilar biliary plexus in human liver. A comparative study of the intrahepatic bile ducts in man and animals. Lab Invest 1985;52:103–6.
148. Lester R, St Pyrek J, Little JM, Adcock EW. Nature of bile acids in the fetus and newborn infant. J Pediatr Gastroenterol Nutr 1983; 2(suppl 1):S197–206.
149. Hata Y, Sasaki F, Takahashi H, et al. Fetal bile acids in congenital biliary atresia. In: Ohi R, ed. Biliary atresia. Tokyo: ICOM Associates, 1991:182–6.
150. Rolleston H, Hayne L. A case of congenital hepatic cirrhosis with obliterative cholangitis (congenital obliteration of the bile ducts). BMJ 1901;1:758–60.
151. Uflacker R, Pariente DM. Angiographic findings in biliary atresia. Cardiovasc Intervent Radiol 2004;27:486–90.
152. Harper PAW, Plant JW, Unger DB. Congenital biliary atresia and jaundice in lambs and calves. Aust Vet J 1990;67:18–22.
153. Alagille D, Odievre M, Gautier M, et al. Hepatic ductular hypoplasia associated with characteristic facies, vertebral malformations, retarded physical, mental and sexual development and cardiac murmur. J Pediatr 1975;86:63–71.
154. Treem WR, Krzymowski GA, Cartun RW, et al. Cytokeratin immunohistochemical examination of liver biopsies in infants with Alagille syndrome and biliary atresia. J Pediatr Gastroenterol Nutr 1992; 15:73–80.
155. Faa G, Van Eyken P, Demelia L, et al. Idiopathic adulthood ductopenia presenting with chronic recurrent cholestasis. A case report. J Hepatol 1991;12:14–20.
156. Hadchouel M, Hugon RN, Gautier M. Reduced ratio of portal tracts to paucity of intrahepatic bile ducts. Arch Pathol Lab Med 1978;102:402–3.
157. Birnbaum A, Suchy FJ. The intrahepatic cholangiopathies. Semin Liver Dis 1998;18:263–9.
158. Kahn E. Paucity of interlobular bile ducts. Arteriohepatic dysplasia and nonsyndromic duct paucity. In: Abramowsky CR, Bernstein J, Rosenberg HS, eds. Perspectives in pediatric pathology. Transplantation pathology – hepatic morphogenesis, Vol. 14. Basel: Karger, 1991:168–215.
159. Hashida Y, Yunis EJ. Syndromatic paucity of interlobular bile ducts: hepatic histopathology of the early and endstage liver. Pediatr Pathol 1988;8:1–15.
160. Krantz ID, Piccoli DA, Spinner NB. Alagille syndrome. J Med Genet 1997;34:152–7.
161. Harper JA, Yuan JS, Tan JB, et al. Notch signaling in development and disease. Clin Genet 2003;64:461–72.
162. Balistreri WF, Bezerra JA, Jansen P, et al. Intrahepatic cholestasis: summary of an American Association for the Study of Liver Diseases single-topic conference. Hepatology 2005;42:222–35.
163. Lorent K, Yeo SY, Oda T, et al. Inhibition of Jagged-mediated Notch signaling disrupts zebrafish biliary development and generates multi-organ defects compatible with an Alagille syndrome phenocopy. Development 2004;131:5753–66.

164. Boyer J, Crosnier C, Driancourt C, et al. Expression of mutant JAGGED1 alleles in patients with Alagille syndrome. Hum Genet 2005;116:445–53.
165. Loomes KM, Taichman DB, Glover CL, et al. Characterization of Notch receptor expression in the developing mammalian heart and liver. Am J Med Genet 2002; 112:181–9.
166. Deutsch GH, Sokol RJ, Stathos TH, et al. Proliferation to paucity: evolution of bile duct abnormalities in a case of Alagille syndrome. Pediatr Dev Pathol 2001;4:559–63.
167. Emerick KM, Rand EB, Goldmuntz E, et al. Features of Alagille syndrome in 92 patients: frequency and relation to prognosis. Hepatology 1999;29:822–9.
168. Libbrecht L, Spinner NB, Moore EC, et al. Peripheral bile duct paucity and cholestasis in the liver of a patient with Alagille syndrome: further evidence supporting a lack of postnatal bile duct branching and elongation. Am J Surg Pathol 2005;29:820–6.
169. Aburano T, Yokoyama K, Takayama T, et al. Distinct hepatic retention of Tc-99m IDA in arteriohepatic dysplasia (Alagille syndrome). Clin Nucl Med 1989;14:874–6.
170. Torizuka T, Tamaki N, Fujita T, et al. Focal liver hyperplasia in Alagille syndrome: assessment with hepatoreceptor and hepatobiliary imaging. J Nucl Med, 1996;37:1365–7.
171. Jinguji M, Tsuchimochi S, Nakajo M, et al. Scintigraphic progress of the liver in a patient with Alagille syndrome (arteriohepatic dysplasia). Ann Nucl Med 2003;17:693–7.
172. Kamath BM, Spinner NB, Emerick KM, et al. Vascular anomalies in Alagille syndrome: a significant cause of morbidity and mortality. Circulation 2004;109:1354–8.
173. Spinner NB. Alagille syndrome and the notch signaling pathway: new insights into human development. Gastroenterology 1999;116:1257–60.
174. Makos BK, Youson JH. Serum levels of bilirubin and biliverdin in the sea lamprey, *Petromyzon marinus* L., before and after their biliary atresia. Comp Biochem Physiol 1987;87A:761–4.
175. Hoffenberg EJ, Narkewicz MR, Sondheimer JM, et al. Outcome of syndromic paucity of interlobular bile ducts (Alagille syndrome) with onset of cholestasis in infancy. J Pediatr 1995; 127:220–4.
176. Wegmann C, Munzenmaier R, Dormann AJ, et al. [Ticlopidine-induced acute cholestatic hepatitis]. Dtsch Med Wochenschr 1998;123:146–50.
177. Kim B, Park SH, Yang HR, et al. Hepatocellular carcinoma occurring in Alagille syndrome. Pathol Res Pract 2005;201:55–60.
178. Furuya KN, Roberts EA, Canny GJ, et al. Neonatal hepatitis syndrome with paucity of interlobular bile ducts in cystic fibrosis. J Pediatr Gastroenterol Nutr 1991;12:127–30.
179. Jansen PL, Sturm E. Genetic cholestasis, causes and consequences for hepatobiliary transport. Liver Int 2003;23:315–22.
180. Bove KE, Heubi JE, Balistreri WF, et al. Bile acid synthetic defects and liver disease: a comprehensive review. Pediatr Dev Pathol 2004;7:315–34.
181. Kahn EI, Daum F, Markowitz J, et al. Arteriohepatic dysplasia II. Hepatobiliary morphology. Hepatology 1983;3:77–84.
182. Gosseye S, Otte JB, De Meyer R, et al. A histological study of extrahepatic biliary atresia. Acta Paediatr Belg 1977;30:85–90.
183. Lilly JR. The surgery of biliary hypoplasia. J Pediatr Surg 1976; 11:815–21.
184. Yamagiwa I, Obata K, Hatanaka Y, et al. Clinico-pathological studies on a transitional type between extrahepatic biliary atresia and paucity of interlobular bile ducts. Jpn J Surg 1993; 23:307–14.
185. Amedee-Manesme O, Bernard O, Brunelle F, et al. Sclerosing cholangitis with neonatal onset. J Pediatr 1987;111:225–9.
186. Guay-Woodford LM, Galliani CA, Musulman-Mroczek E, et al. Diffuse renal cystic disease in children: morphologic and genetic correlations. Pediatr Nephrol 1998;12:173–82.
187. Caroli J, Corcos V. Maladies des voies biliaires intrah patiques segmentaires. Paris: Masson, 1964.
188. Welling LW, Grantham JJ. Cystic diseases of the kidney. In: Tisher CC, Brenner BM, eds. Renal pathology with clinical and functional correlations. Philadelphia: JB Lippincott, 1989:1233–75.
189. Henry X, Marrasse E, Stoppa R, et al. Association maladie de Caroli kyste du cholédoque fibrose hépatique congénitale polykystose rénale. Chirurgie 1987;113:834–43.
190. Buts JP, Otte JB, Claus D, et al. Kyste du cholédoque: un cas avec dilatation des voies biliaires intrahépatiques et fibrose hépatique congénitale. Helv Paediatr Acta 1980;35:289–95.
191. Cole BR. Autosomal recessive polycystic kidney disease. In: Gardner KD Jr, Bernstein J, eds. The cystic kidney. Dordrecht: Kluwer Academic Publishers, 1990:327–50.
192. Zerres K, Rudnik-Schöneborn S, Senderek J, et al. Autosomal recessive polycystic kidney disease (ARPKD). J Nephrol 2003; 16:453–8.
193. Onuchic LF, Furu L, Nagasawa Y, et al. PKHD1, the polycystic kidney and hepatic disease 1 gene, encodes a novel large protein containing multiple immunoglobulin-like plexin-transcription-factor domains and parallel beta-helix 1 repeats. Am J Hum Genet 2002; 70:1305–17.
194. Wang S, Luo Y, Wilson PD, et al. The autosomal recessive polycystic kidney disease protein is localized to primary cilia, with concentration in the basal body area. J Am Soc Nephrol 2004;15:592–602.
195. Masyuk TV, Huang BQ, Ward CJ, et al. Defects in cholangiocyte fibrocystin expression and ciliary structure in the PCK rat. Gastroenterology 2003;125:1303–10.
196. D'Agata ID, Jonas MM, Perez-Atayde AR, et al. Combined cystic disease of the liver and kidney. Semin Liver Dis 1994; 14:215–28.
197. Bergmann C, Senderek J, Windelen E, et al. Clinical consequences of PKHD1 mutations in 164 patients with autosomal-recessive polycystic kidney disease (ARPKD). Kidney Int 2005; 67:829–48.
198. Gattone VH 2nd, MacNaughton KA, Kraybill AL. Murine autosomal recessive polycystic kidney disease with multiorgan involvement induced by the cpk gene. Anat Rec 1996;245:488–99.
199. Guay-Woodford LM, Green WJ, Lindsey JR, et al. Germline and somatic loss of function of the mouse cpk gene causes biliary ductal pathology that is genetically modulated. Hum Mol Genet 2000;9:769–78.
200. Zou MH, Hou XY, Shi CM, et al. Modulation by peroxynitrite of Akt- and AMP-activated kinase-dependent Ser1179 phosphorylation of endothelial nitric oxide synthase. J Biol Chem 2002;277:32552–7.
201. Yoder BK, Tousson A, Millican L, et al. Polaris, a protein disrupted in orpk mutant mice, is required for assembly of renal cilium. Am J Physiol Renal Physiol 2002;282:F541–52.
202. Moser M, Matthiesen S, Kirfel J, et al. A mouse model for cystic biliary dysgenesis in autosomal recessive polycystic kidney disease (ARPKD). Hepatology 2005; 41:1113–21.

203. Sanzen T, Harada K, Yasoshima M, et al. Polycystic kidney rat is a novel animal model of Caroli's disease associated with congenital hepatic fibrosis. Am J Pathol 2001;158:1605–12.
204. Masyuk TV, Huang BQ, Masyuk AI, et al. Biliary dysgenesis in the PCK rat, an orthologous model of autosomal recessive polycystic kidney disease. Am J Pathol 2004;165:1719 30.
205. Blyth H, Ockenden BG. Polycystic disease of kidneys and liver presenting in childhood. J Med Genet 1971;8:257–84.
206. Rossetti S, Torra R, Coto E, et al. A complete mutation screen of PKHD1 in autosomal-recessive polycystic kidney disease (ARPKD) pedigrees. Kidney Int 2003;64:391–403.
207. Witzleben CL. Cystic diseases of the liver. In: Zakim D, Boyer TD, eds. Hepatology. A textbook of liver disease. 2nd ed. Vol. 2. Philadelphia: WB Saunders, 1990:1395–411.
208. Nakanuma Y, Terada T, Ohta G, et al. Caroli's disease in congenital hepatic fibrosis and infantile polycystic disease. Liver 1982;2:346–54.
209. Osathanondh V, Potter EL. Pathogenesis of polycystic kidneys. Arch Pathol 1964;77:466–73.
210. Lieberman E, Salinas-Madrigal L, Gwinn JL, et al. Infantile polycystic disease of the kidneys and liver. Clinical, pathological and radiological correlations and comparison with congenital hepatic fibrosis. Medicine 1971;50:277–318.
211. Bernstein J, Stickler GB, Neel IV. Congenital hepatic fibrosis: evolving morphology. APMIS Suppl 1988;4:17–26.
212. Premkumar A, Berdon WE, Levy J, et al. The emergence of hepatic fibrosis and portal hypertension in infants and children with autosomal recessive polycystic kidney disease: initial and follow-up sonographic and radiographic findings. Pediatr Radiol 1988;18:123–9.
213. Gang D, Herrin J. Infantile polycystic disease of the liver and kidneys. Clin Nephrol 1986;25:28–36.
214. Kerr DNS, Harrison CV, Sherlock S, et al. Congenital hepatic fibrosis. Q J Med 1961;30:91–117.
215. Alvarez F, Bernard O, Brunelle F, et al. Congenital hepatic fibrosis in children. J Pediatr 1981;99:370–5.
216. Matsuda O, Ideura T, Shinoda T, et al. Polycystic kidney of autosomal dominant inheritance, polycystic liver and congenital hepatic fibrosis in a single kindred. Am J Nephrol 1990;10:237–41.
217. Tazelaar HD, Payne JA, Patel S. Congenital hepatic fibrosis and asymptomatic familial adult-type polycystic disease in a 19-year old woman. Gastroenterology 1984;86:757–60.
218. Devos M, Barbier F, Cuvelier C. Congenital hepatic fibrosis. J Hepatol 1988;6:222–8.
219. Cobben JM, Breuning MH, Schoots C, et al. Congenital hepatic fibrosis in autosomal-dominant polycystic kidney disease. Kidney Int 1990;38:880–5.
220. Lipschitz B, Berdon WE, Defelice AR, et al. Association of congenital hepatic fibrosis with autosomal dominant polycystic kidney disease. Report of a family with review of literature. Pediatr Radiol 1993;23:131–3.
221. de Koning TJ, Nikkels PG, Dorland L, et al. Congenital hepatic fibrosis in 3 siblings with phosphomannose isomerase deficiency. Virchows Arch 2000;437:101–5.
222. Schwarzenberg SJ. Congenital hepatic fibrosis – is it really a matter of "a spoonful of sugar?" Hepatology 1999;30:582–3.
223. Clermont RJ, Maillard JN, Benhamou JP, et al. Fibrose hépatique congénitale. Can Med Assoc J 1967;97:1272–8.
224. Shneider BL, Magid MS. Liver disease in autosomal recessive polycystic kidney disease. Pediatr Transplant 2005;9:634–9.
225. Ghishan FK, Younoszai MK. Congenital hepatic fibrosis: a disease with diverse manifestations. Am J Gastroenterol 1981;75:317–20.
226. Murray-Lyon IM, Ockenden BG, Williams R. Congenital hepatic fibrosis – is it a single clinical entity? Gastroenterology 1973;64:653 6.
227. Summerfield JA, Nagafuchi Y, Sherlock S, et al. Hepatobiliary fibropolycystic disease: a clinical and histological review of 51 patients. J Hepatol 1986;2:141–56.
228. Potet F, Mulas Q, Feldmann G, et al. Problèmes anatomocliniques posés par la fibrose hépatique congénitale. Cah Med (Europa Medica) 1971;12:1015–30.
229. Nathan M, Batsakis JG. Congenital hepatic fibrosis. Surg Gynecol Obstet 1969;128:1033–41.
230. Hausner RJ, Alexander RW. Localized congenital hepatic fibrosis presenting as an abdominal mass. Hum Pathol 1978; 9:473–6.
231. Zlatkovic M, Duricic S, Plamenac P. Congenital hepatic fibrosis of heterotopic hepatic tissue. Pathol Res Pract 1998;194:523–6.
232. Phillips MJ, Poucell S, Patterson J, et al. The liver. An atlas and text of ultrastructural pathology. New York: Raven Press, 1987:524.
233. Bianchi L, Reichen J. A 20-year-old woman with portal hypertension and a cholestatic syndrome. Hepatology 1994;20:515–22.
234. de Ledinghen V, Le Bail B, Trillaud H, et al. Case report: secondary biliary cirrhosis possibly related to congenital hepatic fibrosis. Evidence for decreased number of portal branch veins and hypertrophic peribiliary vascular plexus. J Gastroenterol Hepatol 1998;13:720–4.
235. Parker RGF. Fibrosis of the liver as a congenital anomaly. J Pathol Bacteriol 1956;71:359–68.
236. Adams CM, Danks DM, Campbell PE. Comments upon the classification of infantile polycystic diseases of the liver and kidney, based upon three-dimensional reconstruction of the liver. J Med Genet 1974;11:234–43.
237. Takatori M, Iwabuchi S, Hayashi T, et al. Congenital hepatic fibrosis with fatal cholestatic liver damage. Intern Med 2000;39:930–5.
238. Bernstein J, Gardner KD Jr. Renal cystic disease and renal dysplasia. In: Walsh PC, Gitters RF, Perlmutter AD, Stamey TA, eds. Campbell's urology. 5th ed. Philadelphia: WB Saunders, 1986:1760–803.
239. Gresh L, Fischer E, Reimann A, et al. A transcriptional network in polycystic kidney disease. EMBO J 2004;23:1657–68.
240. Hiesberger T, Shao X, Gourley E, et al. Role of the hepatocyte nuclear factor-1beta (HNF-1beta) C-terminal domain in Pkhd1 (ARPKD) gene transcription and renal cystogenesis. J Biol Chem 2005;280:10578–86.
241. Hiesberger T, Bai Y, Shao X, et al. Mutation of hepatocyte nuclear factor-1beta inhibits Pkhd1 gene expression and produces renal cysts in mice. J Clin Invest 2004;113:814–25.
242. Montoli A, Colussi G, Massa O, et al. Renal cysts and diabetes syndrome linked to mutations of the hepatocyte nuclear factor-1 beta gene: description of a new family with associated liver involvement. Am J Kidney Dis 2002;40:397–402.
243. Hildebrandt F, Omram H. New insights: nephronophthisis-medullary cystic kidney disease. Pediatr Nephrol 2001;16:168–76.
244. Bissler JJ, Dixon BP. A mechanistic approach to inherited polycystic kidney disease. Pediatr Nephrol 2005;20:558–66.

245. Wolf MT, van Vlem B, Hennies HC, et al. Telomeric refinement of the MCKD1 locus on chromosome 1q21. Kidney Int 2004;66:580–5.
246. Mollet G, Salomon R, Gribouval O, et al. The gene mutated in juvenile nephronophthisis type 4 encodes a novel protein that interacts with nephrocystin. Nat Genet 2002;32:300–5.
247. Otto EA, Schermer B, Obara T, et al. Mutations in INVS encoding inversin cause nephronophthisis type 2, linking renal cystic disease to the function of primary cilia and left-right axis determination. Nat Genet 2003;34:413–20.
248. Olbrich H, Fliegauf M, Hoefele J, et al. Mutations in a novel gene, NPHP3, cause adolescent nephronophthisis, tapeto-retinal degeneration and hepatic fibrosis. Nat Genet 2003;34:455–9.
249. Boichis H, Passwell J, David R, et al. Congenital hepatic fibrosis and nephronophthisis. A family study. Q J Med 1973;42:221–33.
250. Fernandez-Rodriguez R, Morales JM, Martinez R, et al. Senior-Loken syndrome (nephronophthisis and pigmentary retinopathy) associated to liver fibrosis: a family study. Nephron 1990;55:74–7.
251. Proesmans W, Van Damme B, Macken J. Nephronophthisis and tapetoretinal degeneration associated with liver fibrosis. Clin Nephrol 1975;3:160–4.
252. Hunter AG, Rothman SJ, Hwang WS, et al. Hepatic fibrosis, polycystic kidney, colobomata and encephalopathy in siblings. Clin Genet 1974;6:82–9.
253. Gentile M, Di Carlo A, Susca F, et al. COACH syndrome: report of two brothers with congenital hepatic fibrosis, cerebellar vermis hypoplasia, oligophrenia, ataxia, and mental retardation. Am J Med Genet 1996;64:514–20.
254. Lewis SM, Roberts EA, Marcon MA, et al. Joubert syndrome with congenital hepatic fibrosis: an entity in the spectrum of oculo-encephalo-hepato-renal disorders. Am J Med Genet 1994;52:419–26.
255. Foell D, August C, Frosch M, et al. Early detection of severe cholestatic hepatopathy in COACH syndrome. Am J Med Genet 2002;111:429–34.
256. Kirchner GI, Wagner S, Flemming P, et al. COACH syndrome associated with multifocal liver tumors. Am J Gastroenterol 2002;97:2664–9.
257. Coppola G, Vajro P, De Virgiliis S, et al. Cerebellar vermis defect, oligophrenia, congenital ataxia, and hepatic fibrocirrhosis without coloboma and renal abnormalities: report of three cases. Neuropediatrics 2002;33:180–5.
258. Louie CM, Gleeson JG. Genetic basis of Joubert syndrome and related disorders of cerebellar development. Hum Mol Genet 2005;14(spec no. 2):R235–42.
259. Parisi MA, Bennett CL, Eckert ML, et al. The NPHP1 gene deletion associated with juvenile nephronophthisis is present in a subset of individuals with Joubert syndrome. Am J Hum Genet 2004;75:82–91.
260. Caroli J. Diseases of the intrahepatic biliary tree. Clin Gastroenterol 1973;2:147–61.
261. Mall JC, Chahremani GG, Boyer JL. Caroli's disease associated with congenital hepatic fibrosis and renal tubular ectasia. Gastroenterology 1974;66:1029–53.
262. Erlinger S. [Cystic dilatation of the biliary tract]. Rev Prat 2000; 50:2136–41.
263. Hoglund M, Muren C, Schmidt D. Caroli's disease in two sisters. Diagnosis by ultrasonography and computed tomography. Acta Radiol 1989;30:459–62.
264. Tsuchida Y, Sato T, Sanjo K, et al. Evaluation of long-term results of Caroli's disease: 21 years' observation of a family with autosomal "dominant" inheritance, and review of the literature. Hepatogastroenterology 1995;42:175–81.
265. Sgro M, Rossetti S, Barozzino T, et al. Caroli's disease: prenatal diagnosis, postnatal outcome and genetic analysis. Ultrasound Obstet Gynecol 2004;23:73–6.
266. Jordan D, Harpaz N, Thung SN. Caroli's disease and adult polycystic kidney disease: a rarely recognized association. Liver 1989;9:30–5.
267. Guntz PH, Coppo B, Lorimier G, et al. La maladie de Caroli unilobaire. J Chir (Paris) 1991;128:167–81.
268. Senyuz OF, Yesildag E, Kuruoglu S, et al. Caroli's disease in children: is it commonly misdiagnosed? Acta Paediatr 2005;94:117–20.
269. Fevery J, Tanghe W, Kerremans R, et al. Congenital dilatation of the intrahepatic bile ducts associated with the development of amyloidosis. Gut 1972;13:604–9.
270. Fozard JB, Wyatt JI, Hall RI. Epithelial dysplasia in Caroli's disease. Gut 1989;30:1150–3.
271. Etienne JC, Bouillot JL, Alexandre JH. Cholangiocarcinome développé sur maladie de Caroli. J Chir (Paris) 1987;124:161–4.
272. Choi BI, Yeon KM, Kim SH, et al. Caroli disease: central dot sign in CT. Radiology 1990;174:161–3.
273. Takehara Y, Takahashi M, Naito M, et al. Caroli's disease associated with polycystic kidney: its noninvasive diagnosis. Radiat Med 1989;7:13–15.
274. Hopper KD. The role of computed tomography in the evaluation of Caroli's disease. Clin Imaging 1989;13:68–73.
275. Hussman KL, Friedwald JP, Gollub MJ, et al. Caroli's disease associated with infantile polycystic kidney disease. J Ultrasound Med 1991;10:235–7.
276. Sood GK, Mahapatra JR, Khurana A, et al. Caroli disease: computed tomographic diagnosis. Gastrointest Radiol 1991;16:243–4.
277. Krause D, Cercueil JP, Dranssart M, et al. MRI for evaluating congenital bile duct abnormalities. J Comput Assist Tomogr 2002;26:541–52.
278. Fain JS, Lewin KJ. Intrahepatic biliary cysts in congenital biliary atresia. Arch Pathol Lab Med 1989;113:1383–6.
279. Takahashi A, Tsuchida Y, Hatakeyama S, et al. A peculiar form of multiple cystic dilatation of the intrahepatic biliary system found in a patient with biliary atresia. J Pediatr Surg 1997;32:1776–9.
280. Landing BH. Considerations on the pathogenesis of neonatal hepatitis, biliary atresia and choledochal cyst. The concept of infantile obstructive cholangiopathy. Prog Pediatr Surg 1974;6:113–39.
281. Ryckman F, Fisher R, Pedersen S, et al. Improved survival in biliary atresia patients in the present era of liver transplantation. J Pediatr Surg 1993;28:382–5; discussion 386.
282. Todani T, Watanabe Y, Narusue M, et al. Congential bile duct cysts. Classification, operative procedures and review of thirty-seven cases including cancer arising from choledochal cyst. Am J Surg 1977;134:263–9.
283. Burns C, Kuhns JG, Wieman TJ. Cholangiocarcinoma in association with multiple biliary microhamartomas. Arch Pathol Lab Med 1990;114:1287–9.
284. Jain D, Sarode VR, Abdul-Karim FW, et al. Evidence for the neoplastic transformation of Von-Meyenburg complexes. Am J Surg Pathol 2000;24:1131–9.

285. Eguchi S, Tajima Y, Yanaga K, et al. Hilar bile duct cancer associated with preoperatively undetectable von Meyenburg complex – report of a case. Hepatogastroenterology 2004;51:1301–3.
286. Melnick PJ. Polycystic liver. Analysis of seventy cases. Arch Pathol 1955;59:162–72.
287. Karhunen PJ. Adult polycystic liver disease and biliary microhamartomas (Von Meyenburg's complexes). Acta Pathol Microbiol Immunol Scand [A] 1986;94:397–400.
288. Tsui WM. How many types of biliary hamartomas and adenomas are there? Adv Anat Pathol 1998;5:16–20.
289. Redston MS, Wanless IR. The hepatic von Meyenburg complex: prevalence and association with hepatic and renal cysts among 2843 autopsies [corrected]. Mod Pathol 1996;9:233–7.
290. Ohta W, Ushio H. Histological reconstruction of von Meyenburg's complex on the liver surface. Endoscopy 1984;16:71–4.
291. Grimm PC, Crocker JF, Malatjalian DA, et al. The microanatomy of the intrahepatic bile duct in polycystic disease: comparison of the cpk mouse and human. J Exp Pathol 1990;71: 119–31.
292. Ramos A, Torres VE, Holley KE, et al. The liver in autosomal dominant polycystic kidney disease. Implications for pathogenesis. Arch Pathol Lab Med 1990; 114:180–4.
293. Lev-Toaff AS, Bach AM, Wechsler RJ, et al. The radiologic and pathologic spectrum of biliary hamartomas. AJR Am J Roentgenol 1995;165:309–13.
294. Mortele B, Mortele K, Seynaeve P, et al. Hepatic bile duct hamartomas (von Meyenburg complexes): MR and MR cholangiography findings. J Comput Assist Tomogr 2002;26:438–43.
295. Bruegel M, Rummeny EJ, Gaa J. Image of the month. Multiple biliary hamartomas as an incidental finding in a patient with neuroendocrine carcinoma of the pancreas. Gastroenterology 2005;128:259; answer 523.
296. Milutinovic J, Schabel SI, Ainsworth SK. Autosomal dominant polycystic kidney disease with liver and pancreatic involvement in early childhood. Am J Kidney Dis 1989;13:340–4.
297. Gabow PA. Autosomal dominant polycystic kidney disease. In: Gardner KD Jr, Bernstein J, eds. The cystic kidney. Dordrecht: Kluwer Academic Publishers, 1990:295–326.
298. Gabow PA. Autosomal dominant polycystic kidney disease. N Engl J Med 1993;329:332–42.
299. Gabow PA, Johnson AM, Kaehny WD, et al. Risk factors for the development of hepatic cysts in autosomal dominant polycystic kidney disease. Hepatology 1990;11:1033–7.
300. Mousson C, Rabec M, Cercueil JP, et al. Caroli's disease and autosomal dominant polycystic kidney disease: a rare association? Nephrol Dial Transplant 1997;12:1481–3.
301. Klinkert J, Koopman MG, Wolf H. Pregnancy in a patient with autosomal-dominant polycystic kidney disease and congenital hepatic fibrosis. Eur J Obstet Gynecol Reprod Biol 1998;76: 45–7.
302. Grunfeld JP, Albouze G, Junger P. Liver changes and complications in adult polycystic kidney disease. Adv Nephrol 1985;14:1.
303. Leier CV, Baker PB, Kilman JW, et al. Cardiovascular abnormalities associated with adult polycystic kidney disease. Ann Intern Med 1984;100:683–8.
304. Sutters M, Germino GG. Autosomal dominant polycystic kidney disease: molecular genetics and pathophysiology. J Lab Clin Med 2003;141:91–101.
305. Ariza M, Alvarez V, Marin R, et al. A family with a milder form of adult dominant polycystic kidney disease not linked to the PKD1 (16p) or PKD2 (4q) genes. J Med Genet 1997;34:587–9.
306. Consortium EPKD. The polycystic kidney disease 1 gene encodes a 14 kb transcript and lies within a duplicated region on chromosome 16. The European Polycystic Kidney Disease Consortium. Cell 1994;77:881–94.
307. Reeders ST. The genetics of renal cystic disease. In: Garder KD Jr, Bernstein J, eds. The cystic kidney. Dordrecht: Kluwer Academic Publishers, 1990;117–46.
308. Hughes J, Ward CJ, Peral B, et al. The polycystic kidney disease 1 (PKD1) gene encodes a novel protein with multiple cell recognition domains. Nat Genet 1995;10:151–60.
309. Geng L, Segal Y, Peissel B, et al. Identification and localization of polycystin, the PKD1 gene product. J Clin Invest 1996;98:2674–82.
310. Ibraghimov-Beskrovnaya O, Dackowski WR, Foggensteiner L, et al. Polycystin: in vitro synthesis, in vivo tissue expression, and subcellular localization identifies a large membrane-associated protein. Proc Natl Acad Sci U S A 1997;94:6397–402.
311. Ward CJ, Turley H, Ong AC, et al. Polycystin, the polycystic kidney disease 1 protein, is expressed by epithelial cells in fetal, adult, and polycystic kidney. Proc Natl Acad Sci USA 1996; 93:1524–8.
312. Kottgen M, Walz G. Subcellular localization and trafficking of polycystins. Pflugers Arch 2005;451:286–93.
313. Kimberling WJ, Kumar S, Gabow PA, et al. Autosomal dominant polycystic kidney disease: localization of the second gene to chromosome 4q13–q23. Genomics 1993;18:467–72.
314. Veldhuisen B, Saris JJ, de Haij S, et al. A spectrum of mutations in the second gene for autosomal dominant polycystic kidney disease (PKD2). Am J Hum Genet 1997;61:547–55.
315. Schneider MC, Rodriguez AM, Nomura H, et al. A gene similar to PKD1 maps to chromosome 4q22: a candidate gene for PKD2. Genomics 1996;38:1–4.
316. Peters DJ, Spruit L, Saris JJ, et al. Chromosome 4 localization of a second gene for autosomal dominant polycystic kidney disease. Nat Genet 1993;5:359–62.
317. Wu G, D'Agati V, Cai Y, et al. Somatic inactivation of Pkd2 results in polycystic kidney disease. Cell 1998;93:177–88.
318. Mochizuki T, Wu G, Hayashi T, et al. PKD2, a gene for polycystic kidney disease that encodes an integral membrane protein. Science 1996;272:1339–42.
319. Al-Bhalal L, Akhtar M. Molecular basis of autosomal dominant polycystic kidney disease. Adv Anat Pathol 2005;12:126–33.
320. Yoder BK, Hou X, Guay-Woodford LM. The polycystic kidney disease proteins, polycystin-1, polycystin-2, polaris, and cystin, are co-localized in renal cilia. J Am Soc Nephrol 2002;13:2508–16.
321. Nauli SM, Zhou J. Polycystins and mechanosensation in renal and nodal cilia. Bioessays 2004;26:844–56.
322. Berridge MJ, Bootman MD, Roderick HL. Calcium signalling: dynamics, homeostasis and remodelling. Nat Rev Mol Cell Biol 2003;4:517–29.
323. Pei Y. Nature and nurture on phenotypic variability of autosomal dominant polycystic kidney disease. Kidney Int 2005; 67:1630–1.
324. Fain PR, McFann KK, Taylor MR, et al. Modifier genes play a significant role in the phenotypic expression of PKD1. Kidney Int 2005;67:1256–67.
325. Perrone RD, Grubman SA, Rogers LC, et al. Continuous epithelial cell lines from ADPKD liver cysts exhibit characteristics of intrahepatic biliary epithelium. Am J Physiol 1995;269(3 pt 1): G335–45.

326. Witzleben C, Steigman C. Immunohistochemically defined duct element patterns in pediatric liver diseases. Lab Invest 1990;69:8P.
327. Piccoli DA, Witzleben CL. Disorders of the intrahepatic bile ducts. In: Walker WA, Durie RP, Hamilton JR, et al., eds. Pediatric gastrointestinal disease: pathophysiology, diagnosis, management Philadelphia: BC Decker, 1991:1124–40.
328. Patterson M, Gonzalez-Vitale JC, Fagan CJ. Polycystic liver disease. A study of cyst fluid constituents. Hepatology 1982;2: 475–8.
329. Everson GT, Emmett M, Brown WR, et al. Functional similarities of hepatic cystic and biliary epithelium: studies of fluid constituents and in vivo secretion in response to secretin. Hepatology 1990;11:557–65.
330. Itai Y, Ebihara R, Eguchi N, et al. Hepatobiliary cysts in patients with autosomal dominant polycystic kidney disease: prevalence and CT findings. AJR Am J Roentgenol 1995;164:339–42.
331. Kida T, Nakanuma Y, Terada T. Cystic dilatation of peribiliary glands in livers with adult polycystic disease and livers with solitary nonparasitic cysts: an autopsy study. Hepatology 1992; 16:334–40.
332. Desmet V. Pathogenesis of ductal plate abnormalities. Mayo Clinic Proc 1998;73:80–9.
333. Torra R, Badenas C, Darnell A et al. [Clinical, genetic and molecular studies on autosomal dominant polycystic kidney disease]. Med Clin (Barc) 1998;110:481–7.
334. Pirson Y, Lannoy N, Peters D, et al. Isolated polycystic liver disease as a distinct genetic disease, unlinked to polycystic kidney disease 1 and polycystic kidney disease 2. Hepatology 1996;23:249–52.
335. Iglesias DM, Palmitano JA, Arrizurieta E, et al. Isolated polycystic liver disease not linked to polycystic kidney disease 1 and 2. Dig Dis Sci 1999;44:385–8.
336. Li A, Davila S, Furu L, et al. Mutations in PRKCSH cause isolated autosomal dominant polycystic liver disease. Am J Hum Genet 2003;72:691–703.
337. Drenth JP, Tahvanainen E, te Morsche RH, et al. Abnormal hepatocystin caused by truncating PRKCSH mutations leads to autosomal dominant polycystic liver disease. Hepatology 2004;39:924–31.
338. Tahvanainen P, Tahvanainen E, Reijonen H, et al. Polycystic liver disease is genetically heterogeneous: clinical and linkage studies in eight Finnish families. J Hepatol 2003;38:39–43.
339. Davila S, Furu L, Gharavi AG, et al. Mutations in SEC63 cause autosomal dominant polycystic liver disease. Nat Genet 2004;36:575–7.
340. Qian Q, Li A, King BF, et al. Clinical profile of autosomal dominant polycystic liver disease. Hepatology 2003;37:164–71.
341. Zimmerman K. Bwitrage zur kenntnis einiger Drusen und epithelien. Arch Mikrosk Anat Entwicklungmech 1898;52:552–706.
342. Wheatley DN. Primary cilia in normal and pathological tissues. Pathobiology 1995;63:222–38.
343. Rosenbaum JL, Witman GB. Intraflagellar transport. Nat Rev Mol Cell Biol 2002;3:813–25.
344. Delmas P, Padilla F, Osorio N, et al. Polycystins, calcium signaling, and human diseases. Biochem Biophys Res Commun 2004; 322:1374–83.
345. Montell C. The latest waves in calcium signaling. Cell 2005; 122:157–63.
346. McGrath J, Somlo S, Makova S, et al. Two populations of node monocilia initiate left-right asymmetry in the mouse. Cell 2003;114:61–73.
347. Levin M. Motor protein control of ion flux is an early step in embryonic left-right asymmetry. Bioessays 2003;25:1002–10.
348. Tekotte H, Davis I. Intracellular mRNA localization: motors move messages. Trends Genet 2002;18:636–42.
349. Ong AC, Harris PC. Molecular pathogenesis of ADPKD: the polycystin complex gets complex. Kidney Int 2005;67:1234–47.
350. Ward CJ, Yuan D, Masyuk TV, et al. Cellular and subcellular localization of the ARPKD protein; fibrocystin is expressed on primary cilia. Hum Mol Genet 2003;12:2703–10.
351. Watanabe J, Asaka Y, Tanaka T, et al. Measurement of NADPH-cytochrome P-450 reductase content in rat liver sections by quantitative immunohistochemistry with a video image processor. J Histochem Cytochem 1994;42:1161–7.
352. Ansley SJ, Badano JL, Blacque OE, et al. Basal body dysfunction is a likely cause of pleiotropic Bardet-Biedl syndrome. Nature 2003;425:628–33.
353. Pazour GJ, Dickert BL, Vucica Y, et al. Chlamydomonas IFT88 and its mouse homologue, polycystic kidney disease gene tg737, are required for assembly of cilia and flagella. J Cell Biol 2000; 151:709–18.
354. Hou X, Mrug M, Yoder BK, et al. Cystin, a novel cilia-associated protein, is disrupted in the cpk mouse model of polycystic kidney disease. J Clin Invest 2002;109:533–40.
355. Mai W, Chen D, Ding T, et al. Inhibition of Pkhd1 impairs tubulomorphogenesis of cultured IMCD cells. Mol Biol Cell 2005;16:4398–409.
356. Watnick T, Germino G. From cilia to cyst. Nat Genet 2003; 34:355–6.
357. Ong AC, Wheatley DN. Polycystic kidney disease – the ciliary connection. Lancet 2003;361:774–6.
358. Ong AC, Ward CJ, Butler RJ, et al. Coordinate expression of the autosomal dominant polycystic kidney disease proteins, polycystin-2 and polycystin-1, in normal and cystic tissue. Am J Pathol 1999;154:1721–9.
359. Watnick TJ, Torres VE, Gandolph MA, et al. Somatic mutation in individual liver cysts supports a two-hit model of cystogenesis in autosomal dominant polycystic kidney disease. Mol Cell 1998;2:247–51.
360. Nichols MT, Gidey E, Matzakos T, et al. Secretion of cytokines and growth factors into autosomal dominant polycystic kidney disease liver cyst fluid. Hepatology 2004;40:836–46.
361. Nagasawa Y, Matthiesen S, Onuchic LF, et al. Identification and characterization of Pkhd1, the mouse orthologue of the human ARPKD gene. J Am Soc Nephrol 2002;13:2246–58.
362. Edmondson H. Differential diagnosis of tumors and tumor-like lesions of liver in infancy and childhood. AMA J Dis Child 1956;91:168–86.
363. DeMaioribus CA, Lally KP, Sim K, et al. Mesenchymal hamartoma of the liver. A 35-year review. Arch Surg 1990;125:598–600.
364. Stringer MD, Alizai NK. Mesenchymal hamartoma of the liver: a systematic review. J Pediatr Surg 2005;40:1681–90.
365. Gornicka B, Ziarkiewicz-Wroblewska B, Wroblewski T, et al. Myoid hamartoma of the liver – a novel variant of hamartoma developing in the hilar region and imitating a malignant liver tumor. Med Sci Monit 2004;10:CS23–6.
366. Dehner LP, Ewing SL, Summer HW. Infantile mesenchymal hamartoma of the liver. Histologic and ultrastructural observations. Arch Pathol 1975;99:379–81.

367. Lennington WJ, Gray GF Jr, Page DL. Mesenchymal hamartoma of liver. A regional ischemic lesion of a sequestered lobe. Am J Dis Child 1993;147:193–6.
368. O'Sullivan MJ, Swanson PE, Knoll J, et al. Undifferentiated embryonal sarcoma with unusual features arising within mesenchymal hamartoma of the liver: report of a case and review of the literature. Pediatr Dev Pathol 2001;4:482–9.
369. Lauwers GY, Grant LD, Donnelly WH, et al. Hepatic undifferentiated (embryonal) sarcoma arising in a mesenchymal hamartoma. Am J Surg Pathol 1997;21:1248–54.
370. Stocker JT, Ishak KG. Mesenchymal hamartoma of the liver: report of 30 cases and review of the literature. Pediatr Pathol 1983;1:245–67.
371. Cook JR, Pfeifer JD, Dehner LP. Mesenchymal hamartoma of the liver in the adult: association with distinct clinical features and histological changes. Hum Pathol 2002;33:893–8.
372. Ishak KG, Sharp HL. Developmental abnormality and liver disease in childhood. In: MacSween RNM, et al. Pathology of the liver. 3rd ed. Edinburgh: Churchill Livingstone, 1994:83–122.
373. Otani Y, Takayasu H, Ishimaru Y, et al. Secretion and expression of epithelial markers supports the biliary origin of solitary nonparasitic cyst of the liver in infancy. J Pediatr Surg 2005;40:e27–30.
374. Lin CC, Lin SC, Ko WC, et al. Adenocarcinoma and infection in a solitary hepatic cyst: a case report. World J Gastroenterol 2005;11:1881–3.
375. Raboei E, Luoma R. Definitive treatment of congenital liver cyst with alcohol. J Pediatr Surg 2000;35:1138–9.
376. Reichel S, Alzen G, Keller KM, et al. [Congenital, solitary hepatic cyst: observation of the development from birth upon the intervention in the 5th year of life]. Klin Padiatr 2002;214:332–3.
377. Friedrich N. Cyste mit flimmerepithel in der leber. Arch Pathol Anat 1857;11:466–9.
378. Kim S, White FV, McAlister W, et al. Ciliated hepatic foregut cyst in a young child. J Pediatr Surg 2005;40:e51–3.
379. Vick DJ, Goodman ZD, Deavers MT, et al. Ciliated hepatic foregut cyst: a study of six cases and review of the literature. Am J Surg Pathol 1999;23:671–7.
380. Koletsa T, Tzioufa V, Michalopoulos A, et al. Ciliated hepatic foregut cyst communicating with the gallbladder. Virchows Arch 2005;446:200–1.
381. Rodriguez E, Soler R, Fernandez P. MR imagings of ciliated hepatic foregut cyst: an unusual cause of fluid-fluid level within a focal hepatic lesion (2005.4b). Eur Radiol 2005;15:1499–501.
382. Furlanetto A, Dei Tos AP. Squamous cell carcinoma arising in a ciliated hepatic foregut cyst. Virchows Arch 2002;441:296–8.
383. Puente SG, Bannura GC. Radiological anatomy of the biliary tract. Variations and congenital abnormalities. World J Surg 1983;7:271–6.
384. Hashmonai M, Kam I, Schramek A. The etiology of "white bile" in the biliary tree. J Surg Res 1984;37:479–86.
385. Markle GB. Agenesis of the common bile duct. Arch Surg 1981;116:350–2.
386. Schwartz MZ, Hall RJ, Reubner B, et al. Agenesis of the extrahepatic bile ducts: report of five cases. J Pediatr Surg 1990;25:805–7.
387. Sherlock S. Diseases of the liver and biliary system. Oxford: Blackwell Scientific Publications, 1989.
388. Luschka H. Die Anatomie des Menschlichen Bauches Bd II. Tubingen: Laup und Siebeckle, 1863:248–55.
389. Sharif K, de Ville de Goyet J. Bile duct of Luschka leading to bile leak after cholecystectomy – revisiting the biliary anatomy. J Pediatr Surg 2003;38:E21–3.
390. Kitami M, Murakami G, Suzuki D, et al. Heterogeneity of subvesical ducts or the ducts of Luschka: a study using drip infusion cholangiography-computed tomography in patients and cadaver specimens. World J Surg 2005;29:217–23.
391. Boyden E. The problem of the double ductus choledochus (an interpretation of an accessory bile duct found attached to the pars superior of the duodenum). Anat Rec 1932;55:71–93.
392. Lamah M, Karanjia ND, Dickson GH. Anatomical variations of the extrahepatic biliary tree: review of the world literature. Clin Anat 2001;14:167–72.
393. Kodama T, Iseki J, Murata N, et al. Duplication of common bile duct – a case report. Jpn J Surg 1980;10:67–71.
394. Yamashita K, Oka Y, Urakami A, et al. Double common bile duct: a case report and a review of the Japanese literature. Surgery 2002;131:676–81.
395. Yamataka A, Yanai T, Hosoda Y, et al. A case of biliary atresia with duplication of the common bile duct. J Pediatr Surg 2001;36:506–7.
396. Casebolt BT. Duplication of the common bile duct. Case report. Mo Med 1973;70:171–4 passim.
397. Neuhauser EB, Elkin M, Landing B. Congenital direct communication between biliary system and respiratory tract. AMA Am J Dis Child 1952;83:654–9.
398. Hourigan JS, Carr MG, Burton EM, et al. Congenital bronchobiliary fistula: MRI appearance. Pediatr Radiol 2004;34:348–50.
399. Chan YT, Ng WD, Mak WP, et al. Congenital bronchobiliary fistula associated with biliary atresia. Br J Surg 1984;71:240–1.
400. DiFiore JW, Alexander F. Congenital bronchobiliary fistula in association with right-sided congenital diaphragmatic hernia. J Pediatr Surg 2002;37:1208–9.
401. Weitzman JJ, Cohen SR, Woods LO Jr, et al. Congenital bronchobiliary fistula. J Pediatr 1968;73:329–34.
402. Sane SM, Sieber WK, Girdany BR. Congenital bronchobiliary fistula. Surgery 1971;69:599–608.
403. Dijkstra C. Galuitstorting in de buikholte bij een zuigeling. Maandsch Kindergeneesk 1932;1:409–14.
404. Xanthakos SA, Yazigi NA, Ryckman FC, et al. Spontaneous perforation of the bile duct in infancy: a rare but important cause of irritability and abdominal distension. J Pediatr Gastroenterol Nutr 2003;36:287–91.
405. Alagille D. Cholestasis in the first three months of life. In: Popper H, Schaffner F, eds. Progress in liver disease. Vol. 1. New York: Grune and Stratton, 1979:471–85.
406. Gorelick FS, Dobbins JW, Burrell M, et al. Biliary tract abnormalities in patients with arteriohepatic dysplasia. Dig Dis Sci 1982;27:815–20.
407. Morelli A, Pelli MA, Vedovelli A, et al. Endoscopic retrograde cholangiopancreatography study in Alagille's syndrome: first report. Am J Gastroenterol 1983;78:241–4.
408. Krant SM, Swenson O. Biliary duct hypoplasia. J Pediatr Surg 1973;8:301–7.
409. Afroudakis A, Kaplovitz N. Liver histopathology in chronic common bile duct stenosis due to chronic alcoholic pancreatitis. Hepatology 1981;1:65–72.
410. Sherlock S. The liver in infancy and childhood. In: Sherlock S, ed. Diseases of the liver and biliary system. 8th ed. Oxford: Blackwell Scientific Publications, 1989:501–22.

411. Ryckman FC, Noseworthy J. Neonatal cholestatic conditions requiring surgical reconstruction. Semin Liver Dis 1987;7:134–54.
412. Okada T, Sasaki F, Ueki S, et al. Postnatal management for prenatally diagnosed choledochal cysts. J Pediatr Surg 2004;39:1055–8.
413. Wong AM, Cheung YC, Liu YH, et al. Prenatal diagnosis of choledochal cyst using magnetic resonance imaging: a case report. World J Gastroenterol 2005;11:5082–3.
414. Alonso Lej F, Rever WB, Pessagna DJ. Congenital choledochal cyst, with a report of two and an analysis of 94 cases. Surg Gynecol Obstet 1959;108:1–30.
415. Hadad AR, Westbrook KC, Campbell GS, et al. Congenital dilatation of the bile ducts. Am J Surg 1976;132:799–804.
416. Longmire WP, Mandiola SA, Gordon HE. Congenital cystic disease of the liver and biliary system. Ann Surg 1971;174:711–24.
417. Rizzo RJ, Szucs RA, Turner MA. Congenital abnormalities of the pancreas and biliary tree in adults. Radiographics 1995;15:49–68; quiz 147–8.
418. Tandon RK, Grewal H, Anand AC, et al. Caroli's syndrome: a heterogeneous entity. Am J Gastroenterol 1990;85:170–3.
419. Yamaguchi M. Congenital choledochal cyst. Analysis of 1.433 patients in the Japanese literature. Am J Surg 1980;140:653–7.
420. Chongsrisawat V, Roekwibunsi S, Mahayosnond A, et al. Spontaneous choledochal cyst rupture in a child. Pediatr Surg Int 2004;20:811–12.
421. Soreide K, Korner H, Havnen J, et al. Bile duct cysts in adults. Br J Surg 2004;91:1538–48.
422. Lam AH, Lam VK. Choledochal cyst with biliary atresia in an infant. Australas Radiol 1987;31:384–5.
423. Joseph VT. Surgical techniques and long-term results in the treatment of choledochal cyst. J Pediatr Surg 1990;25:782–7.
424. Jordan PH Jr, Goss JA Jr, Rosenberg WR, et al. Some considerations for management of choledochal cysts. Am J Surg 2004;187:434–9.

5

Acute Liver Failure in Children

Estella M. Alonso, M.D., Robert H. Squires, M.D., and Peter F. Whitington, M.D.

Acute liver failure (ALF) is a relatively rare but often fatal event in children. The frequency of ALF in all age groups in the United States is about 10 to 20,000 per year (about 17 cases per 100,000 population per year), but the frequency in the pediatric age group is unknown. ALF accounts for 10–15% of pediatric liver transplants performed in the United States annually. Even allowing for the probability that many children die without transplant, there may be as few as 50–100 cases per year in the United States.

Little is known about pediatric ALF; the rarity of the condition has precluded accumulation of a large experience. Several studies are under way to amass the experience of major transplant centers in an effort to learn more about the condition. Most cases of ALF in children have no identifiable cause, which has prevented a focus on the mechanism by which hepatocytes are killed. The mechanism of ALF remains elusive even if the cause is known. Orthotopic liver transplantation is a substantial advance in the therapy of ALF. Other therapies being studied in clinical trials include liver assist devices and hepatocyte transplantation. Medical therapy generally consists of supportive measures, with a focus on preventing or treating complications and early referral to a transplant center. Outcomes for children vary depending upon the etiology and degree of central nervous system (CNS) involvement.

DEFINITION

The broadest definition of ALF is the failure of the vital functions of the liver occurring within weeks or a few months of the onset of clinical liver disease. This definition implies that some agent or combination of agents has caused the sudden death of or severe injury to a large proportion of hepatocytes, leaving less parenchymal function than is needed to sustain life. Initial studies in ALF utilized a more narrow definition of ALF, which includes the onset of hepatic encephalopathy less than 8 weeks after the beginning of acute hepatic dysfunction and the absence of preexisting liver disease of any form [1]. The lack of preexisting liver disease is an important component of the definition because it implies that recovery is possible if the patient can be supported, the cause is eliminated, and the liver retains its capacity to regenerate. Some patients with acute hepatocellular disease develop encephalopathy more than 8 weeks into the course. Terms such as *subacute hepatic failure*, *subacute hepatic necrosis*, and *late-onset hepatic failure* have been used to describe cases in which encephalopathy develops 8–24 weeks after the onset of liver disease [2,3]. Experience suggests that the prognosis for spontaneous recovery is poorer for these cases than for ALF.

The group at King's College in London has defined ALF in children as "a multi-systemic disorder in which severe impairment of liver function, with or without encephalopathy, occurs in association with hepatocellular necrosis in a patient with no recognizable underlying chronic liver disease" [4]. This definition recognizes several problems in applying the narrow definition of ALF to children. First, it acknowledges markers of liver synthetic failure, such as an uncorrectable coagulopathy, as important indicators of liver failure. Second, it addresses the problems with detecting early stages of hepatic encephalopathy in children and infants. Finally, it attempts to distinguish the clinical presentation of patients who manifest signs and symptoms of ALF but in fact have an unsuspected chronic liver disease.

There remains a need for better definitions. A consensus of the members of the Pediatric Acute Liver Failure (PALF) Study Group [5], a multicenter and multinational consortium, developed a working definition for the clinical condition of ALF in children as the summation of clinical and biochemical parameters as follows:

1. The acute onset of liver disease with no known evidence of chronic liver disease.
2. Biochemical and/or clinical evidence of severe liver dysfunction: hepatic-based coagulopathy (prothrombin time [PT] ≥20 seconds or international normalized ratio [INR] ≥2.0) that is not corrected by parenteral vitamin K and/or hepatic encephalopathy (must be present if the PT is 15–19.9 seconds or the INR is 1.5–1.9, but not if the PT is ≥20 seconds or INR is ≥2.0).

Table 5.1: Causes of Fulminant Hepatic Failure in Children

	Disease	*Incidence*
	Neonates	
Infectious	Herpesviruses, echovirus, adenovirus, hepatitis B virus	Rare
Inborn errors of metabolism	Hereditary fructose intolerance, galactosemia, tyrosinemia	Rare
Immune mediated	Neonatal hemochromatosis	Rare
Ischemia and abnormal perfusion	Congenital heart disease, cardiac surgery, myocarditis, severe asphyxia	Rare
Other	Hemophagocytic syndrome	Rare
	Infants	
Infectious	Hepatitis A virus, hepatitis B virus, NANB hepatitis, herpesviruses	Moderately frequent
Drugs and toxins	Valproate, isoniazid, acetaminophen, *Amanita*	Moderately frequent
Inborn errors of metabolism	Hereditary fructose intolerance, others	Rare
Immune mediated	Autoimmune hepatitis, macrophage activation syndrome, hemophagocytic syndrome	Rare
Ischemia and abnormal perfusion	Congenital heart disease, cardiac surgery, myocarditis, severe asphyxia	Rare
Other	Malignancy	Rare
	2- to 10-year-olds	
Infectious	NANB hepatitis, others same as infants	Frequent
Drugs and toxins	Same as infants	Moderately frequent
Immune mediated	Autoimmune hepatitis, macrophage activation syndrome, hemophagocytic syndrome	Rare
Ischemia and abnormal perfusion	Budd–Chiari syndrome, others same as infants	Rare
Metabolic	Wilson's disease	Rare
Other	Malignancy, hyperthermia	Rare
	10- to 18-year-olds	
Infectious	Same as 2- to 10-year-olds	Frequent
Drugs and toxins	Acetaminophen overdose; same as 2- to 10-year-olds	Frequent
Immune mediated	Same as 2- to 10-year-olds	Moderately frequent
Ischemia and abnormal perfusion	Same as 2- to 10-year-olds	Rare
Metabolic	Wilson's disease, fatty liver of pregnancy	Rare
Other	Same as 2- to 10-year-olds	Rare

ETIOLOGY

ALF is a clinical syndrome that results from a variety of age-dependent etiologies (Table 5.1). Specific etiologies can be broadly categorized as infectious, autoimmune, metabolic, and toxin or drug related. A specific diagnosis is not established in over 50% of children with ALF – indeterminate ALF. Table 5.2 details the causes of ALF in children enrolled in the PALF study, representing the incidence of causation in 19 pediatric sites in the United States, Canada, and the United Kingdom [5]. A brief discussion of the various classes of disease that can cause ALF in children follows. The reader is referred to other chapters for more detailed discussion of each specific disease state.

Drug and Toxin-Related Hepatic Injury

Liver injury caused by drugs and toxins is a very common cause of fulminant hepatic failure (FHF) in children and adults [5–8].

Table 5.2: Final Diagnosis in Children with ALF in PALF Registry

	Age Category		
Diagnosis	*<3 Years (%)*	*>3 Years (%)*	*Total (%)*
Acetaminophen (N = 48)	2 (2)	46 (21)	48 (14)
Indeterminate (N = 169)	68 (54)	101 (46)	169 (49)
Autoimmune (N = 22)	6 (5)	16 (7)	22 (6)
Infectious (N = 20)	9 (7)	11 (5)	20 (6)
Adenovirus (N = 2)	1 (1)	1 (0)	2 (1)
Cytomegalovirus (N = 1)	1 (1)	0 (0)	1 (0)
Epstein–Barr virus (N = 6)	1 (1)	5 (2)	6 (2)
Enterovirus (N = 1)	1 (1)	0 (0)	1 (0)
Hepatitis A (N = 3)	0 (0)	3 (1)	3 (1)
Hepatitis C (N = 1)	0 (0)	1 (0)	1 (0)
Herpes simplex virus (N = 6)	5 (4)	1 (0)	6 (2)
Non-APAP drug induced liver disease (N = 17)	1 (1)	16 (7)	17 (5)
Mushroom (N = 2)	0 (0)	2 (1)	2 (1)
Anesthetic (N = 1)	0 (0)	1 (0)	1 (0)
Bactrim (N = 1)	0 (0)	1 (0)	1 (0)
Pemoline (N = 1)	0 (0)	1 (0)	1 (0)
Cyclophosphamide/phenytoin (N = 1)	0 (0)	1 (0)	1 (0)
Phenytoin (N − 1)	0 (0)	1 (0)	1 (0)
Isoniazid (N = 2)	0 (0)	2 (1)	2 (1)
Iron (N = 1)	0 (0)	1 (0)	1 (0)
Methotrexate (N = 1)	0 (0)	1 (0)	1 (0)
Minocycline (N = 1)	0 (0)	1 (0)	1 (0)
Pravastatin (N = 1)	0 (0)	1 (0)	1 (0)
Valproate (N = 3)	1 (1)	2 (1)	3 (1)
Metabolic (N = 36)	23 (18)	13 (6)	36 (10)
α_1-antitrypsin (N = 1)	1 (1)	0 (0)	1 (0)
Fatty acid oxidation defect (N = 4)	4 (3)	0 (0)	4 (1)
Galactosemia (N = 2)	2 (2)	0 (0)	2 (1)
Fructose intolerance (N = 1)	1 (1)	0 (0)	1 (0)
Mitochondrial disorder (N = 4)	2 (2)	2 (1)	4 (1)
Niemann–Pick type C (N = 1)	1 (1)	0 (0)	1 (0)
Respiratory chain defect (N = 7)	7 (6)	0 (0)	7 (2)
Reye's syndrome (N = 1)	0 (0)	1 (0)	1 (0)
Tyrosinemia (N = 4)	4 (3)	0 (0)	4 (1)
Urea cycle defect (N = 2)	1 (1)	1 (0)	2 (1)
Wilson's disease(N = 9)	0 (0)	9 (4)	9 (3)

(continued)

Table 5.2 (*continued*)

Diagnosis	*Age Category*		
	<3 Years (%)	*>3 Years (%)*	*Total (%)*
Other (N = 20)	11 (9)	9 (4)	20 (6)
Budd–Chiari (N = 2)	0 (0)	2 (1)	2 (1)
Hemophagocytic syndrome (N = 4)	2 (2)	2 (1)	4 (1)
Leukemia (N = 2)	1 (1)	1 (0)	2 (1)
Neonatal hemochromatosis (N = 6)	6 (5)	0 (0)	6 (2)
Veno-occlusive disease (N = 6)	2 (2)	4 (2)	6 (2)
Shock (N = 16)	7 (6)	9 (4)	16 (5)
Total	127 (36)	221 (64)	348 (100)

Drugs and toxins that result in severe liver injury can be broadly classified as *hepatotoxic* or having the potential for *idiosyncratic* injury [9]. Hepatotoxins predictably injure the liver dependant on dose and exposure. These agents include acetaminophen, solvents including carbon tetrachloride, and mushroom toxin, among many. The diagnosis of hepatotoxic liver injury is based upon the interval between drug ingestion and the onset of symptoms, the known hepatotoxicity of the offending agent, serum drug levels (if available), and liver biopsy findings. Many if not most prescription drugs have the potential for idiosyncratic drug reaction leading to severe liver injury. The diagnosis of idiosyncratic drug-related liver failure is based upon largely circumstantial evidence, so a degree of skepticism should be maintained regarding the role of drug exposure in causing the hepatic injury [10,11]. Exposure to drugs with a strong history of doing so – so-called black box drugs because of the warning for liver injury posted in Food and Drug Administration required drug information – should be considered strongly. These include isoniazid, propylthiouracil, and halothane, among many.

A careful history of exposure to hepatotoxins should be obtained from the family of any child presenting in ALF, including prescription and nonprescription drugs in the home that could have been ingested accidentally. In teenagers, a history of depression, illicit drug use (cocaine, ecstasy), or solvent sniffing should be sought. Any exposure to hepatotoxic drugs and chemicals should be considered possibly related to the liver injury. Mushroom ingestion has clearly been traced to ALF [12,13].

The evidence for idiosyncratic drug reaction as the cause of ALF is largely circumstantial [11,14]. Liver biopsy can assist in diagnosis. The pattern of injury observed histologically should be that expected from the drug to which the patient has been exposed. The patterns seen are hepatitis (hepatocellular necrosis), cholestasis, mixed cholestasis and hepatitis, and steatosis [9]. Drugs that cause hepatitis (isoniazid, propylthiouracil, and halothane) have the greatest potential for causing ALF. Drugs that cause steatosis (sodium valproate, amiodarone) may cause liver failure. Drugs that cause cholestasis (oxacillin) rarely produce liver failure, whereas drugs that cause mixed cholestasis and hepatitis (sulfa drugs) sometimes do. If the injury is not that expected from the drug in question, another cause should be sought. Exposure to a drug or toxin should not preclude a thorough search for other causes, particularly viral hepatitis.

Acetaminophen overdose is responsible for 21% of ALF cases in children over 3 years of age [5]. Diagnostic criteria for acute acetaminophen toxicity should include a toxic serum acetaminophen level as defined by the Rumack nomogram [15] or a history of an acute ingestion of 100–150 mg/kg of acetaminophen within a 24-hour period and exclusion of other common causes of acute hepatitis. Acetaminophen may also be responsible for some cases of ALF in which a cause is not readily identified. The role of fasting and alcohol consumption in potentiating acetaminophen toxicity in patients exposed to high doses (60–100 mg/kg) remains controversial [16,17]. New techniques to identify serum markers of acetaminophen hepatotoxicity in patients with ALF may help to unravel this question [18,19]. Patients with acetaminophen-related ALF have a higher rate of spontaneous recovery than do patients with viral hepatitis. Observation with supportive care should be maintained as long as possible before considering liver transplantation.

Neuroleptics are the most commonly prescribed medications associated with ALF. Valproic acid, phenytoin, carbamazepine, and felbamate are the most common offenders [20]. Valproic acid, when used to control seizures in children with the mitochondrial disease Alpers' syndrome, often precipitates ALF [21]. Antimicrobial agents such as isoniazid, ampicillin–clavulanic acid, roxithromycin, and nitrofurantoin as well as a number of antiviral agents used in the treatment of HIV have been reported to cause ALF [22]. Chemotherapeutic agents such as cyclophosphamide and dacarbazine are associated with hepatic vein injury resulting in veno-occlusive disease and ALF. Other potential medications that should be considered in the proper clinical setting include halothane (anesthetic), amiodarone (antiarrhythmic), propylthiouracil (hyperthyroidism), and trazodone (antidepressant) [9]. Ingestion of wild mushrooms, most notably *Amanita phalloides*, can result in ALF [12]. Recreational drug use, particularly cocaine and methylenedioxyamphetamine ("ecstasy"), is associated with ALF in teenagers and even younger children who live in environments where these compounds are accessible. Complementary or alternative medical therapies are utilized with increased frequency [23]. Examples of herbal remedies associated with ALF include pyrrolizidine alkaloids, germander, Chinese herbal medicine, ma huang, chaparral, black cohosh root, pennyroyal, and kava [24].

Infectious Diseases

A prodrome consisting of nonspecific complaints such as fever, nausea, vomiting, and abdominal discomfort will precede many cases of ALF in children. Therefore, it is not surprising that early accounts of ALF often attributed the cause to a virus or infection. As the ability to identify specific infectious agents through serology, culture, and polymerase chain reaction (PCR) technology has been applied, the common viruses have not often been found in ALF unless they were endemic to the region or in association with a community outbreak. Whereas an as yet unidentified infectious cause may account for some unexplained cases of ALF in children, efforts to identify rare infectious agents in adults have not been fruitful [25]. Therefore, a reasonable alternative is to classify as *indeterminate* any patient without an identifiable cause for the ALF until such time as a more specific diagnosis can be established.

Hepatitis Virus Infection

Acute hepatitis A virus (HAV) infection is a common cause of ALF in third-world and emerging countries but also has been recorded as a substantial cause in developed countries. HAV caused 31% of ALF in a series from London [26] and 26% of cases in a series from Paris [27]. In recent reports, HAV was identified in only 4.5% of ALF in adults [28] and 1% of children [5].

The reported risk of developing hepatic failure in patients with symptomatic HAV infection is very low (0.1–0.4%). However, HAV infection can complicate the course of other liver diseases to produce ALF. In a report from Italy, a large cohort of HAV-seronegative patients who had either chronic hepatitis B virus (HBV) or hepatitis C virus (HCV) infection were followed for 7 years to determine what happened if they became infected acutely with HAV [29]. Of 27 patients acquiring HAV, 7 of 17 with chronic HCV developed liver failure, all but one dying as a result. None of the 10 patients with coexistent chronic HBV developed failure. This experience supports the recommendation that hepatitis A vaccine should be administered to all children over 2 years of age with a chronic liver condition of any type.

Acute HBV infection resulting in ALF is uncommon in pediatric series from western Europe and North America, where HBV is not endemic. In the series from London, HBV infection could not be identified in any of the 31 children with FHF [26]. It plays a much greater role in endemic areas. In work from Taipei [30], HBV was identified in 11 of 16 children with virally caused FHF. Five of the patients' infections were transmitted from blood transfusions, whereas six were transmitted vertically. The prevalence of acute HBV infection in large series of adult patients with ALF ranges from 25–75% [2,31], making it a leading cause of ALF in adults.

The overall rate of FHF in acute HBV infection is estimated to be about 1%. In the large series of patients hospitalized with acute hepatitis in Melbourne [32], the case fatality rate of acute HBV was 0.84%. Fatality was substantially greater in patients older than 40 years of age (5.26%) and in individuals acquiring HBV infection as a result of blood transfusions (18.8%), and lower in patients 15–29 years old (0.23%) and in intravenous drug abusers (0.063%). Mutations in the HBV genome appear to be a risk factor in the development of ALF [33]. The risk seems to be relatively low in most pediatric patients – infants born to mothers who have chronic hepatitis B infection and are E antigen positive, and recipients of HBV-positive blood transfusions being the major exceptions [30].

Hepatitis C virus infection has rarely been identified as the cause for ALF [34], and ALF has not been observed in large studies of transfusion-acquired HCV infection [35]. In two studies, HCV RNA has not been detected in the serum of patients with sporadic fulminant hepatitis without defined cause [36,37] or in liver specimens from ALF victims using PCR techniques [38–40]. HCV RNA has been detected in the serum of 8 of 17 hepatitis B surface antigen (HBsAg)–positive patients with ALF, which suggests that coinfection or superinfection with HCV might play a role in producing severe hepatitis in patients with HBV infection [36].

Hepatitis D virus (HDV) infection can be acquired as a coinfection with HBV or as a superinfection in patients previously infected with HBV. In cases of acute hepatic failure, the prevalence of coinfection, rather than superinfection, varies from 50–75%. HDV coinfection has been found in about 30% of patients with acute HBV infection and ALF, so HDV appears to be an important determinant of the severity of acute HBV infection. Furthermore, superinfection with HDV can result in ALF in chronic carriers of HBV with or without chronic hepatitis. HDV infection probably plays little role in the etiology of ALF in children. In one study from Taiwan, anti-HDV was not detected in any child with ALF related to HBV infection [30].

Hepatitis E virus (HEV) infection is documented by association with epidemics of waterborne diseases not caused by HAV or by the presence of anti-HEV antibody in serum. Most experience with HEV comes from the Indian subcontinent. The case fatality rate from ALF among pregnant women in one study was 10.1%, with women in the third trimester particularly at risk. In a study involving 44 children with ALF in north India, 7 had isolated HEV infection and 16 had mixed HEV and HAV infection [41]. There are no reports of HEV involving children from western Europe or the United States, though HEV infection has been found in adults in England and Wales, possibly associated with swine as the viral carrier [42].

A few studies involving children have failed to demonstrate that hepatitis GB virus C/hepatitis G virus is a cause of either acute or chronic liver disease, and it has been specifically excluded in a small series of patients with ALF [43]. However, hepatitis G was recently reported in association with ALF in a pediatric patient [44]. Transfusion-transmitted virus, a recently described DNA virus about which little is known, has not been implicated in ALF.

Infection with Viruses Other than Hepatitis Viruses

The viruses in the herpes family are highly cytopathic and can cause severe hepatic necrosis often in the absence of significant inflammation. Herpes simplex virus, human herpesvirus 6 (HHV-6), varicella-zoster virus, cytomegalovirus, and Epstein–Barr virus have been reported to cause ALF in both immunocompromised and immunocompetent hosts. Epstein–Barr virus is most frequently implicated [45]. HHV-6 was detected in the explanted livers in 10 of 15 patients who underwent liver transplant for ALF of unknown cause [46]. However, HHV-6 is so prevalent as a latent infection in humans that causality may be difficult to prove in cases of ALF. Little is known about the incidence or case fatality rates among children with ALF secondary to herpesvirus infection. However, early detection utilizing newer diagnostic techniques, such as real-time PCR, and early institution of specific therapy may improve survival [47].

Acute liver failure in the neonate may result from infection with a wide variety of viruses that do not characteristically cause severe hepatitis in older individuals. The reasons for this susceptibility are poorly understood, but they probably include an immature immune system and perhaps overwhelming exposure, either transplacentally or by way of a gut with a poor immune barrier capability. Herpes simplex virus infections usually are associated with systemic features (skin rash, encephalitis). Cytomegalovirus hepatitis usually does not cause ALF in this age group, but rather a chronic or chronic progressive hepatitis, and usually is associated with systemic features (encephalitis, chorioretinitis, nephritis, bone marrow suppression). Epstein–Barr virus has been identified very rarely as the cause of ALF in neonates. Echovirus (principally type 11) and Coxsackie virus have been recorded as a cause of severe hepatitis in neonates and children.

Parvovirus B19 routinely infects children, causing one of the common childhood exanthemas. It rarely can cause severe bone marrow depression and has been associated with mild hepatitis. In one study involving six patients with ALF who developed aplastic anemia in the peritransplant period, viral DNA was identified in the liver of four, and all six had immunoglobulin G antibodies against the virus [48]. This virus has been sought and not found in other studies involving larger numbers of patients with ALF and aplastic anemia. The importance of parvovirus B19 in the syndrome is unclear at this point. It may exhibit latency, and its presence in liver tissue may only reflect prior infection, as would immunoglobulin G antibodies.

Another possible agent has been identified in London [49]. Toga virus–like particles were demonstrated by electron microscopy (EM) in hepatectomy specimens from 7 of 18 patients, including 3 children, undergoing orthotopic liver transplantation for the indication of ALF from apparent non-A, non-B (NANB) hepatitis. This group of patients experienced a high frequency of graft failure within a week of transplantation (5 of 7 patients) as a result of reinfection of the graft. No epidemiologic factors were identified that separated the group with infection from those with no identifiable viral agent.

Syncytial giant cell hepatitis with ALF was associated with paramyxovirus infection in a series from Toronto [50]. This infection is more likely to result in chronic progressive hepatitis or late-onset hepatic failure than ALF but should be considered in all three circumstances. Other viruses associated with ALF include adenovirus, dengue fever, and members of the enterovirus family that include echovirus (11 and 21) and Coxsackie A and B.

Nonviral Hepatitis

Infectious agents other than viruses only rarely have been recorded as producing ALF. Despite the rarity of occurrence, they should be considered carefully in every case because they are potentially treatable.

Systemic sepsis occasionally presents in a manner that is virtually indistinguishable from ALF. Reported infectious etiologies include *Neisseria meningitides* infection, septic shock and intra-abdominal abscesses, and portal sepsis with enteric organisms. Spirochetal infection can affect liver function and produce severe hepatitis, even hepatic failure. Congenital syphilis rarely has been determined to produce ALF but should be excluded carefully in any neonate with severe hepatitis. Leptospirosis very rarely causes hepatic failure. Finally, in endemic areas, brucellosis and *Coxiella burnetii* (Q fever), *Plasmodium falciparum*, and *Entamoeba histolytica* infections have presented as ALF.

Autoimmune Hepatitis

Autoimmune hepatitis (AIH) is recognized as an important and potentially treatable cause of ALF that occurs in all age groups. Presenting symptoms are not unique to AIH, and autoimmune markers may be not be present or specific, hypergammaglobulinemia may not be present, and liver biopsy may show confluent necrosis that hides the typical features of AIH, such as interface hepatitis (Figure 5.1). However, if autoantibodies are positive and other viral or drug-related causes are eliminated, the diagnosis of AIH should be strongly considered and treatment with corticosteroids initiated [51–53]. These findings are exemplified in a report of three children, 1–3 years of age, with severe acute hepatitis and hepatic failure caused by AIH [54]. Liver biopsy showed signs of chronic hepatitis (portal fibrosis and piecemeal necrosis) in addition to severe lobular hepatitis, and all had high titers of anti–liver-kidney-microsomal (LKM) antibodies in serum. The response to corticosteroid therapy was good. Cyclosporine also has been useful for this condition [55].

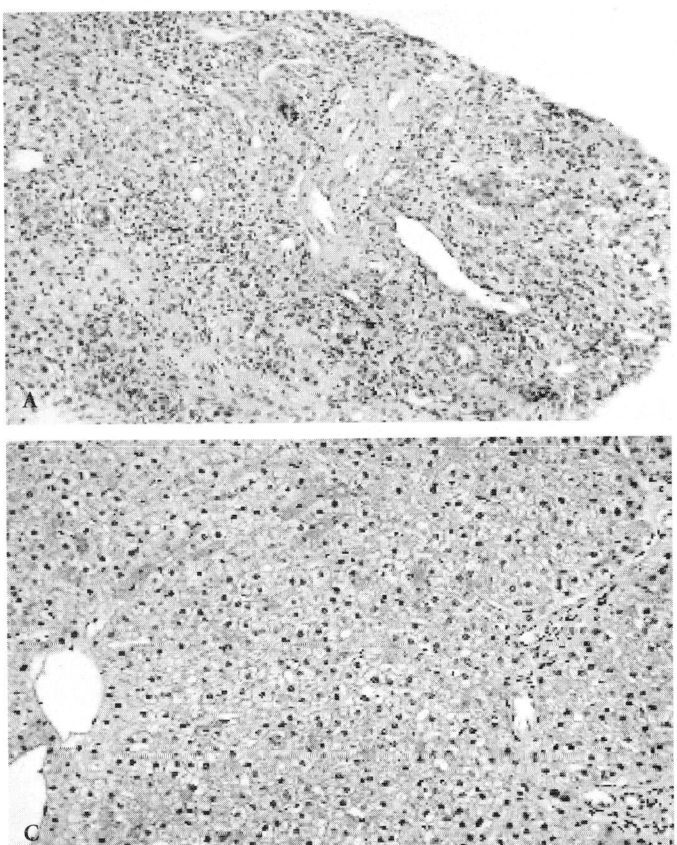

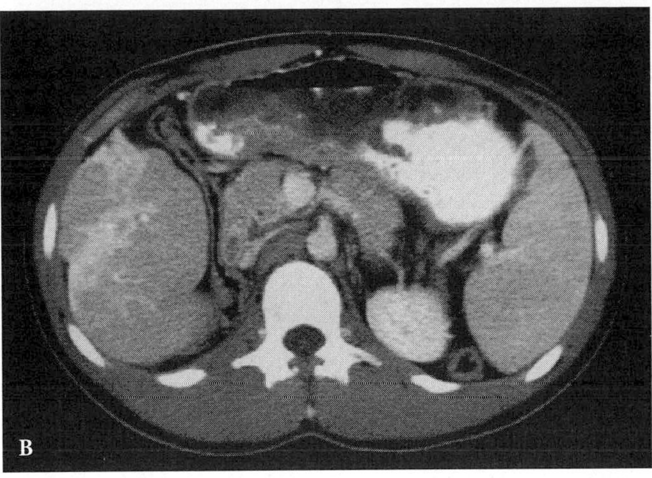

Figure 5.1. Findings in a teenage boy with anti-nuclear antibody positive type 1 autoimmune hepatitis and ALF. (**A**) Histopathology in a transjugular liver biopsy obtained at the time of presentation shows confluent necroinflammation. The diffuse inflammation prevented interface hepatitis to be clearly identified. Very few areas among several cores contained any viable hepatocytes (Hematoxylin and eosin [H&E], original magnification 100×). (**B**) Computed tomography of the liver with intravenous contrast performed at the time of presentation showed massive though heterogeneous necrosis. Only a small fraction of the liver in this plane was perfused with blood (lighter areas in liver profile). (**C**) Histopathology after clinical recovery with treatment with corticosteroids and azathioprine for 1 year shows normal hepatic architecture and no residual interface hepatitis. (H&E, original magnification 100×.)

Inherited and Metabolic Diseases

Consideration of the numerous inherited and metabolic diseases that severely affect hepatic function as causes of ALF is controversial, because all affected patients have preexisting liver disease by definition. These diseases are given only brief consideration here. The reader is referred to the full descriptions of these specific disorders elsewhere in this text.

Metabolic disorders that present in the neonatal period or infancy and can produce severe toxic hepatitis and even hepatic failure include galactosemia, hereditary fructose intolerance, and tyrosinemia type I. Neonatal hemochromatosis causes liver failure in the fetus and newborn, usually evident immediately post partum [56–58]. Inborn errors of bile acid synthesis can present as ALF in infancy [59]. α_1-Antitrypsin deficiency only rarely causes ALF. Two disorders that cause cerebral degeneration and disordered hepatic function, Zellweger syndrome [60] and Alpers' disease [21], have been recorded as causes of ALF, but confusion with primary hepatic failure seems unlikely because of the neurologic symptoms characteristic of these disorders. Disorders of fatty acid oxidation [61–63] and of oxidative phosphorylation [64] produce episodes of recurrent hepatic dysfunction and coma that can mimic ALF. Wilson's disease is the inherited disorder most likely to produce ALF in the older child [65,66].

Ischemia and Abnormal Perfusion

The liver is extremely resistant to hypoxic injury as evidenced by the fact that hepatic failure has been recorded rarely in near-drowning victims. Previous treatment with seizure medications, which induce cytochrome function and presumably the production of injurious free radicals during ischemia–reperfusion injury, can enhance hepatic injury during hypoxia [67]. Severe centrilobular necrosis is characteristic. Full recovery of hepatic function has been observed, but cerebral ischemic injury limits prognosis.

Abnormalities of hepatic perfusion occasionally cause ALF. The Budd–Chiari syndrome may present this way [68]. Severe congestive heart failure from congenital heart disease or acute myocarditis can result in acute congestive liver disease and hepatic failure. The cardiac findings usually predominate, and confusion with primary liver disease is unusual. Liver failure rarely complicates open heart surgery for correction of congenital defects [69].

Malignancy and Infiltrative Disorders

Primary hepatic malignancy (hepatoblastoma), metastatic malignancy (breast carcinoma, neuroblastoma), and massive blastic infiltration in leukemia and non-Hodgkin's lymphoma on occasion cause acute hepatic failure, as do X-linked lymphoproliferative syndrome and erythrophagocytic lymphohistiocytosis [70]. Therapy in all of these disorders involves treatment of the primary malignancy, and prognosis is poor.

Miscellaneous Diseases

Although rarely recorded in the pediatric age group, acute fatty liver of pregnancy can cause ALF in young adults [71,72]. Onset in the third trimester with symptoms usually including nausea, vomiting, malaise, and epigastric distress should lead to the consideration of this disorder. Rapid progression to coma occurs in about one half of affected patients, and the mortality rates are high in mothers and fetuses. Liver transplantation may be effective therapy for the mother. Heatstroke and malignant hyperthermia syndrome have been recorded as causing hepatic failure, usually in association with renal failure [73]. The prognosis is poor in both conditions. Celiac disease was recently reported to be associated with ALF [74]. Dietary intervention appeared to provide significant benefit.

Indeterminate Cause

An indeterminate cause for ALF is attributed to a patient if no specific etiology can be identified despite every effort to do so. The current feeling is that it might be a viral disease even though known viruses have been reasonably excluded as causing the syndrome. It has been described as *non-A-G hepatitis*, which is equivalent to NANB hepatitis as they relate to pediatric ALF [75].

One peculiar and puzzling characteristic of non-A-G hepatitis is its propensity to cause very severe hepatitis. It is clearly the most important cause of ALF in children in developed countries, comprising the vast majority of pediatric ALF cases in series from western Europe and the United States. In the King's College series, 26 of 31 children with ALF were felt to have NANB hepatitis [26].

An aspect of non-A-G hepatitis that provides compelling evidence of its viral cause is its association with aplastic anemia. In a series of 32 children and young adults receiving liver transplantation at four major centers for the indication of ALF secondary to NANB hepatitis, 9 developed aplastic anemia after successful transplantation [76]. This frequency (28%) contrasts with the absence of cases of aplastic anemia among 1463 other patients receiving liver transplantation in the same centers,

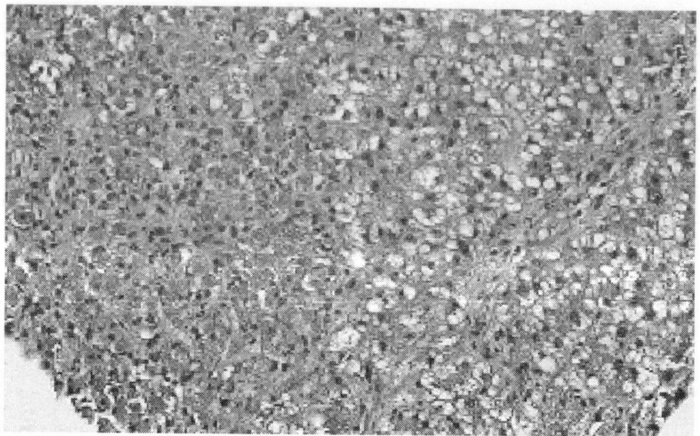

Figure 5.2. Liver histopathology of a transjugular biopsy from a 14-year-old white male with indeterminate acute liver failure with minimal hyperbilirubinemia (nonicteric ALF). Serum obtained on the second day of illness tested positive for acetaminophen protein adducts. Photomicrograph showing zonal distribution of the hepatic injury. A portion of a portal tract is present in the upper right corner of the image, with a centrilobular area in the lower left. Lobular zones 1 and 2 (*right aspect* of the image) show prominent hepatocellular vacuolation and steatosis, whereas centrilobular hepatocytes (zone 3, *left*) show extensive coagulative necrosis. (H&E stain, original magnification 100×.)

including 12 patients with ALF secondary to HAV or HBV infection and 18 patients with drug-induced ALF. Other centers have reported similar experiences [77–80]. It is apparent from these experiences that the non-A-G hepatitis virus infects bone marrow and that aplastic anemia is a second life-threatening event that confronts a significant proportion of children recovering from severe non-A-G hepatitis, with or without liver transplant.

Ten years ago, a series of children in Illinois and Colorado was reported with ALF of indeterminate cause and with minimal jaundice [81]. Other features distinguish these patients from those with typical non-A-G hepatitis. Histopathology is characterized by variable degrees of centrilobular necrosis (Figure 5.2), and the prognosis is better, with more than 50% of patients recovering. Exposure to acetaminophen in all patients in association with central necrosis, the lesion typically seen in acetaminophen overdose, suggested its possible role in the disease. Similar "epidemics" of nonicteric ALF have been recorded in Vancouver [82], Taiwan [83,84], and central California [85]. In the California cases, a potential hepatotoxin, pennyroyal oil, was ingested in the form of folk remedies, again suggesting an interaction of a viral agent with a toxin. It seems that this may be a separate and distinct form of non-A-G ALF. Among a group of children infected with influenza A serotype H3N2 during the influenza epidemic in Colorado in 2005 who had coincident ALF, only one had available liver histology: it, however, showed centrilobular necrosis reminiscent of the 1995 report [86].

A high case fatality rate (low rate of spontaneous recovery) appears to be characteristic of indeterminate ALF. The rate of spontaneous recovery in our own series was very low, only 1 (4%) of 26 patients [87]; in the London series, 8 (30%) of 26 children with NANB ALF survived [26]. In a series of 73 patients

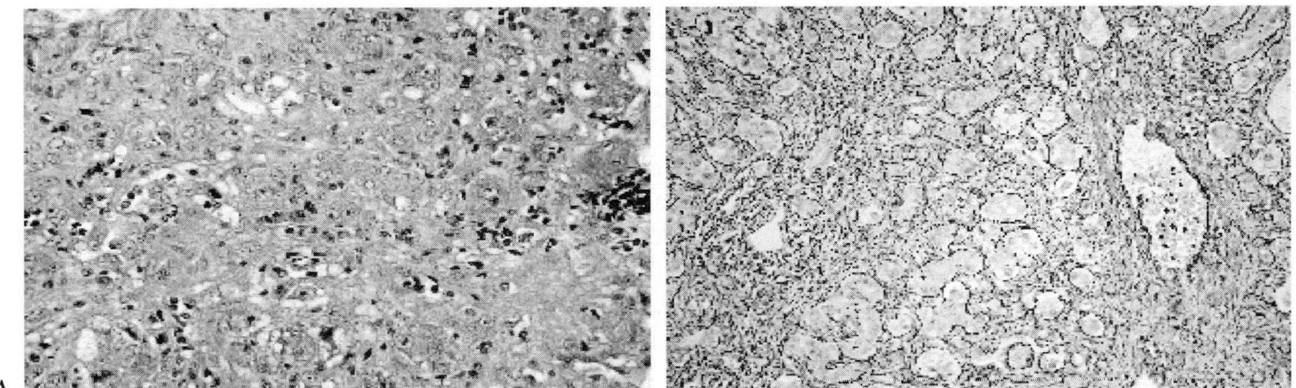

Figure 5.3. Liver histopathology from a patient with indeterminate ALF. (**A**) Transjugular biopsy at time of presentation shows confluent necrosis with little parenchymal inflammation. There were no viable hepatocytes evident in any of several cores. This section shows some tubular structures thought to represent attempted regeneration. (H&E, original magnification 200×.) (**B**) The reticulin stain shows focal collapse. The distance between the central vein on the right and portal area on the left is diminished, and the reticulin framework between is condensed. (Reticulin stain, original magnification 100×.)

of all ages with ALF in London, 44% had NANB hepatitis, only 1 with a significant exposure history [88]. The rate of spontaneous recovery was only 9.3%, in contrast to that with HAV infection (43.4%) and HBV infection (16.6%). In a series from Copenhagen, however, NANB infection in adults with ALF was not associated with a worse outcome than HAV or HBV infection [89]. In the prospective PALF study, the outcomes of 181 patients with indeterminate ALF at 3 weeks after entry into the study were 44% alive without a liver transplant, 11% dead without transplant, 40% alive with transplant, and 3% dead following liver transplantation [5]. Differences between this and previous studies are likely a reflection of dissimilar definitions of ALF, duration of follow-up, etiologic composition of the indeterminate group, and improvements in patient management that have occurred over the last 20 years. It is clear, however, that assessment of outcome in patients with indeterminate ALF remains challenging. As seen with the prior studies, virtually all the cases of "indeterminate" ALF were attributed to a yet-to-be-discovered viral agent. Such an assumption may narrow the diagnostic focus and thus cause other conditions, such as poor immune regulation, autoimmune disease, metabolic disease, and hepatotoxicity, to be overlooked.

PATHOLOGY AND BIOCHEMISTRY

Liver cell necrosis is characteristic of ALF resulting from viral infections, most toxic injury, ischemic injury, and some metabolic diseases. The degree of hepatocellular necrosis and its pattern vary by cause and by individual case. Establishing a pathologic diagnosis by liver biopsy has not been considered critical in patient management, largely because of the associated risks. The recent advent of the transvenous approach has so markedly reduced the risks of obtaining a liver biopsy that many more biopsies are being performed in the setting of ALF. As a consequence, much should be learned about the value of biopsy in this setting.

Most liver samples from children with ALF show massive confluent or multilobular necrosis (Figure 5.3). In many specimens, it is difficult to identify any remaining viable hepatocytes. The reticulin framework of the lobule is collapsed, and the mass of the liver is small. A moderate inflammatory infiltrate, usually consisting mainly of neutrophils, may be evident. In some patients, no evidence of regeneration can be found [90]; in others, there is proliferation of ductlike structures that probably results from attempts at regeneration. Occasionally, if orthotopic liver transplantation is performed early in the course of rapidly progressive ALF, the gross surgical and microscopic appearances of the liver are relatively normal. The lobular structure and framework may be intact, including a normal cord pattern, but the hepatocytes are necrotic. Inflammation is absent. This lesion suggests widespread, simultaneous lethal injury of hepatocytes. Much less commonly, the pathologic specimen demonstrates lesser degrees of necrosis. Diffuse hepatocellular necrosis, with patchy loss of hepatocytes throughout the lobule, may be seen in viral hepatitis. Nonicteric fulminant failure, some drug-induced liver disease (e.g., acetaminophen), and hypoxic–ischemic hepatitis are characterized by sublobular necrosis, with orientation of necrosis around central veins (Figure 5.4) [67,81].

The serum aminotransferase levels are characteristically elevated in ALF associated with necrosis. Peak levels are almost always above 1000 IU/L and may reach astronomically high values (e.g., 80,000 IU/L) in ischemic injury [67]. Peak values tend to be higher in patients who die, but aminotransferase values are not predictive of outcome [91]. Standard teaching suggests that rapidly falling aminotransferase values signify "exhaustion" of the hepatocyte mass and indicate imminent ALF. This is not necessarily the case; aminotransferase values fall equally fast in patients recovering from ALF if the inciting agent is eliminated [92]. For example, our observations in children with ischemic injury indicate that aminotransferase values fall with a serum half-life of 4–6 days in recovering patients (Figure 5.5) [67]. Rapidly falling aminotransferase values may indicate a good

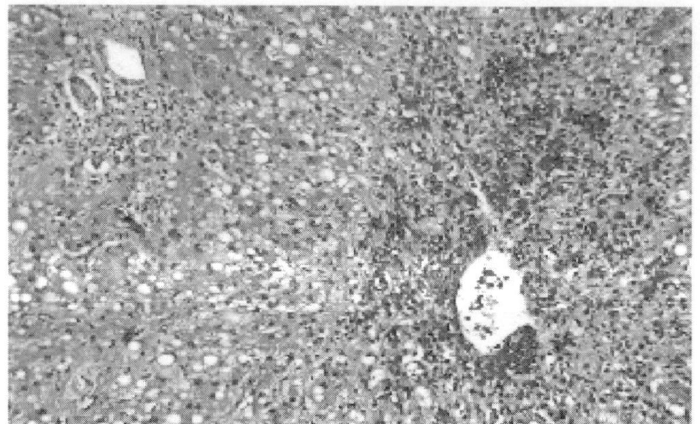

Figure 5.4. Hepatectomy specimen from a teenager who overdosed on acetaminophen. The specimen showed extensive sublobular necrosis throughout the liver. The central orientation of the necrosis is evident in this section because of the hemorrhage in and around the central vein on the right. The periportal zone is relatively spared, with a narrow rim of viable hepatocytes seen around the portal triad in the upper left. Between the frank necrosis and the rim of viable hepatocytes is a zone of hepatocyte injury notable by steatosis and ballooning of marginally viable hepatocytes. (H&E, original magnification 100×.)

prognosis if associated with evidence of functional recovery, such as improved coagulation and reduced encephalopathy. If seen in association with worsening function and rapid reduction of liver size, rapidly falling aminotransferase levels indicate a poor prognosis for recovery.

Marked jaundice often accompanies severe hepatic necrosis [93]. Serum bilirubin concentrations typically range from 10–60 mg/dL. The rate of increase in serum bilirubin often exceeds that expected with a normal rate of production and zero clearance. Increased production may result from catabolism of hepatic heme proteins or from hemolysis. Early in the course, the majority of serum bilirubin is in the conjugated form, indicating excretory dysfunction of viable hepatocytes. Later, the majority may be nonconjugated, indicating loss of conjugating ability. Because only about 1% of normal conjugation is necessary to maintain normal serum bilirubin concentration, inability to conjugate implies functional loss of essentially all hepatocytes and indicates a very poor prognosis. Occasionally, spontaneous recovery from ALF is associated with profound cholestatic jaundice, which may persist for a month or more after other functional recovery. The pathogenesis of this syndrome is poorly understood.

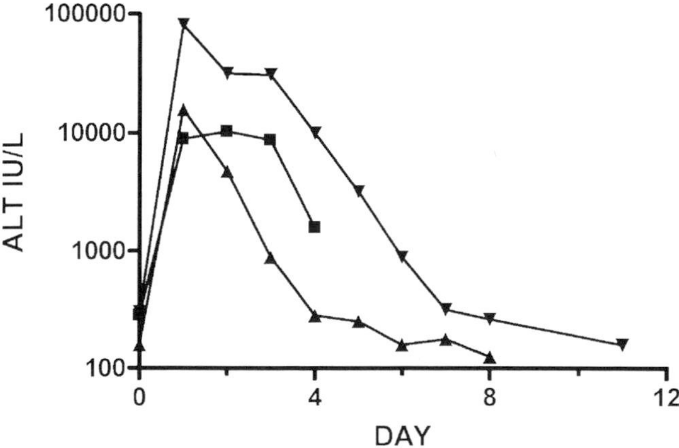

Figure 5.5. Pattern of aminotransferase change over time in three children with ischemic injury. Note the marked elevation of aspartate aminotransferase that can be seen with global hepatic ischemic injury from hypoxemia and the rapid recovery after the insult is eliminated. Two patients recovered normal liver function, whereas one patient (■) died of brain ischemia. (Replotted from data in Ussery et al. [67].)

Spontaneous recovery from ALF resulting from severe necrosis is uncommon. Functional recovery often is associated with complete histologic recovery, even if extensive necrosis is present [94,95]. Recovery from massive confluent necrosis is distinctly unusual and is associated with the development of postnecrotic cirrhosis [96].

Diffuse hepatic steatosis is observed rarely in ALF in children. This lesion is characterized by hepatocellular fat in a microvesicular pattern and is identical at a light-microscopic level to the hepatic lesion of Reye's syndrome. In adults, it is seen most often in fatty liver of pregnancy; in children, it is seen in association with toxic injury or inborn errors of metabolism (see Etiology). The absence of cell necrosis in association with failure of liver function implies organelle failure as the cause. Hepatomegaly is often evident. Serum aminotransferase levels usually are elevated, but only to a mild to moderate degree (usually <400 IU/L). Jaundice is minimal (serum bilirubin concentration usually <10 mg/dL), which suggests that certain organelle functions remain intact and also that bilirubin production probably is not increased. Full histologic recovery is the rule if the patient survives.

A third lesion characterized by diffuse swelling of hepatocytes with condensation of organelles and cytoplasmic elements (Figure 5.6) is seen in association with some inborn errors of metabolism. Hepatocyte necrosis is spotty and usually not prominent. Macrovesicular fat with displacement of nuclei is seen in a variable proportion of hepatocytes, sometimes a majority. This lesion suggests organelle injury that is severe enough to cause the death of some hepatocytes. Aminotransferase levels and serum bilirubin levels are elevated moderately. Full histologic recovery is the rule if the metabolic injury can be controlled.

PATHOGENESIS

Our understanding of the pathogenesis of ALF is limited. In most pediatric cases, the cause is not known, and even if a causative agent is known, how the agent produces injury to and death of hepatocytes is not. Several key steps or components involved in the overall pathogenesis of ALF can be identified.

Exposure

The initiating step in ALF is the exposure of a susceptible individual to an agent capable of causing widespread injury to

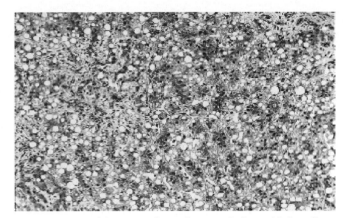

Figure 5.6. Liver biopsy specimen from an infant with hereditary fructose intolerance and hepatic failure. There is both diffuse hepatocyte necrosis and steatosis, mainly macrovesicular. Other findings include pseudotubule formation and condensation of organelles and cytoplasmic elements within hepatocytes. Interlobular bile ducts also are injured, with irregular shape of cholangiocytes and some vacuolization. The patient recovered normal liver function within 5 days of eliminating fructose from the diet. (H&E, original magnification 200×.)

hepatic parenchymal cells. The susceptibility of an individual to hepatic injury is determined by a variety of factors. There are strong age-related determinants, with newborns being more susceptible to herpes and other nonhepatitis viruses and elderly individuals more likely to develop ALF as a result of infection with HAV or HBV. The state of an individual's immunity is also important. Immaturity of immune function may be the key reason for susceptibility of newborns to herpesvirus infections, and immunodeficiency is related to susceptibility to severe viral infections in older individuals. In contrast, the severity of injury in HBV infection may be related to the vigor of the immune response. Individual biochemical polymorphisms may play a role in susceptibility to certain drug-induced injuries. Induction of drug-metabolizing enzymes that can lead to the formation of active intermediates can increase the susceptibility to certain drug-induced injuries and hypoxic injuries, as can depletion of protective mechanisms, such as glutathione.

The agent must be capable of producing severe hepatic injury or of inducing a response by the host that causes hepatic injury [97]. The interaction between the agent and the host apparently determines the prevalence of ALF, especially with regard to the hepatitis viruses. The proportion of individuals developing ALF after exposure to hepatitis viruses is small but varies among the hepatitis viruses. For example, epidemiologic data indicate that HAV infection has resulted in a fairly steady rate of ALF over several decades [98]. Whether this is related to the biology of the agent, how it is presented, or the susceptibility of the population is not clear. Viral mutations, such as HBV precore mutants, can result in an increased prevalence of ALF, which suggests that the biology of the infecting agent determines risk, at least to a certain degree [99]. Some agents, particularly hepatotoxins (*Amanita phalloides*, carbon tetrachloride), tend to produce severe injury in a large proportion of exposed individuals.

Hepatocyte Injury

The next important step involves the action of the offending agent to cause injury or death of hepatocytes. The mechanism varies according to the agent and in most patients is not known.

Hepatocyte necrosis is prominent in a large proportion of patients with ALF. The mechanism of cell necrosis is not known in most instances. Presumably, the virus either is directly cytopathic or induces an immune response that injures the cell (probably the exposed plasma membrane). Injury must be severe enough to result in loss of cell viability. The cascade of events leading to cell necrosis has not been determined in viral hepatitis, and why these events take place in some exposed individuals but not in a majority is unknown. The events leading to massive cell death after exposure to some hepatotoxins are better understood. For example, ingestion of the mushroom *Amanita phalloides* results in cell death because of the action of two hepatotoxins; phalloidin alters membranes of the hepatocyte and α amanitine inhibits hepatocellular RNA polymerase and inhibits protein synthesis [9,12].

In certain unusual instances, it appears that widespread functional impairment of hepatocytes without necrosis can cause liver failure. This is seen most often if the pathology reveals diffuse hepatosteatosis. In some circumstances, the mechanism of injury is known; for example, tetracycline can bind to transfer RNA in the hepatocyte, which can impair synthesis of proteins [9]. Failure to adequately package very-low-density lipoprotein results in accumulation of lipids within the cells. Fatty liver of pregnancy is assumed to have a similar pathogenesis, and disorders of fatty acid metabolism and oxidative phosphorylation and toxic injury from valproic acid may have similar mechanisms, at least in part [9,100,101]. General cellular dysfunction is also apparent in other metabolic disorders in which necrosis is insufficient to produce hepatic failure. For example, in the acute onset of hereditary fructose intolerance, functional hepatic failure may exist, but cell necrosis is rather limited. Also, there is usually no generalized accumulation of fat. Hepatocytes may be ballooned and demonstrate condensation of cytoplasmic elements, which suggest general impairment, but recover on elimination of fructose from the diet.

Potentiation

Events that take place after initial hepatocyte injury may amplify the injury and serve to accelerate what would be acute hepatitis into hepatic failure. Host differences in the response to injury, therefore, play a role in whether a particular injury leads to liver failure in any individual. Activation of Kupffer cells seems to play a key role in this process. Intrinsic activation seems to result from factors elaborated by injured hepatocytes; extrinsic activation seems to result from circulating endotoxin [102]. The source of endotoxin is probably the intestine. It can be detected in the serum of most individuals with FHF [103]. Increased gut permeability and decreased clearance both probably contribute to endotoxemia in these patients. Endotoxin can cause hepatocellular necrosis through activation of

Kupffer cells and neutrophils that in turn cause direct tissue damage and release cytokines, particularly tumor necrosis factor-α (TNF-α) and interleukin-6 [104,105]. These cytokines and endotoxin-mediated intravascular coagulation lead to circulatory changes and tissue ischemia. This leads to more injury, and a vicious cycle is created, leading to ALF [106]. Host idiosyncrasies play an important role in determining the fate of the individual. TNF-α phenotype has been shown to correlate with outcome in patients consuming overdoses of acetaminophen [107]. Circulating levels of TNF-α have been detected in patients with ALF, and levels correlate inversely with concentrations of interleukin-2 [108,109]. These data suggest that TNF may injure the host in a setting in which the host's immune response is impaired.

Regeneration

Liver cell necrosis leads to regeneration. Several growth factors are mediators of hepatic regeneration, including epidermal growth factor, transforming growth factor-α, and human hepatocyte growth factor/scatter factor [110–113]. Levels of circulating growth factors, particularly human hepatocyte growth factor, are influenced by the type and degree of hepatic injury [114]. The highest levels are seen in ALF, with lower levels observed after major hepatic resection. Levels are elevated minimally above normal in acute hepatitis and chronic liver disease. These growth factors have direct effects on hepatocyte renewal, and if the liver is able to respond, regeneration may keep pace with cell death.

In ALF, there also appears to be release of factors that inhibit cell replication [115,116]. These factors have low molecular weights and appear to emanate from necrotic hepatocytes. They inhibit DNA replication through an unknown molecular mechanism. Theoretically, excess circulating inhibitors may result in "hyporegenerative" hepatic necrosis.

The continued presence of the offending agent or an effect of the agent can injure or kill newly regenerated hepatocytes. This ongoing struggle between regeneration and hepatocyte death results in a balance being struck until one of several events terminates the course.

Termination

The events of ALF terminate under three circumstances. The first is terminal hepatic failure, if the liver is injured to such a degree that it cannot support life and regeneration has proved inadequate to effect its repair. In one study, all but 1 of 16 individuals with ALF who were thought to have died simply of inadequate liver function were found to have functional residual mass of less than 12% of normal [117]. The actual required functional hepatocyte mass to support life is unknown.

The second possible terminating event is spontaneous recovery. Elimination of the agent or the effect of the agent results in termination of hepatocyte injury. If the injury has not been too severe, hepatic regeneration can result in repair and ultimate recovery.

Finally, the overall process may become muted, slowed down by events taking place in the host, which may result in chronicity [94]. This appears to be the case in a small proportion of individuals with severe acute HBV infection [118]. A complication may intervene and terminate the patient's life, or liver transplantation may be performed before these events can play out.

CLINICAL MANIFESTATIONS AND COMPLICATIONS

Typical Clinical Presentation

The pediatric patient with ALF is most often a previously healthy, school-aged child, with no history of major medical problems and no history of blood transfusion or other exposure to hepatitis. Initially, the child has what appears to be "ordinary" hepatitis. Sometimes, the magnitude of aminotransferase elevations is alarming, but more often than not, nothing points to the potential for developing ALF. Over the next days to weeks, the child does not improve or has worsening symptoms. Parents may note increasing lethargy or occasionally hallucinations. Rarely a hemorrhagic diathesis or even more rarely systemic collapse brings to light the seriousness of the problem. When seen in the referral center, the child is desperately ill. The patient is typically deeply jaundiced. Fetor hepaticus is often evident but in the infant and young child it may not be. The patient is often somnolent, confused, combative, incontinent, responsive to only persistent or painful stimuli, or unresponsive. Other physical findings are limited. The liver size may be large, normal, or small. The patient may be bleeding from needle puncture sites, the nose, or the gastrointestinal tract. There is no difficulty recognizing the seriousness of the condition at this point. This is a characteristic presentation, by no means unusual. The promptness with which care providers respond can make the difference in survival: Immediate medical support in an intensive care unit (ICU) setting and rapid decision making regarding referral to a transplant center are imperative.

COMPLICATIONS

Encephalopathy

Brain dysfunction, an important component in the diagnosis of ALF, results from an effect of hepatocyte failure on the function of the brain [119–121]. The presence of impaired CNS function during acute liver disease is an indication for immediate hospitalization independent of any other clinical or biochemical findings because it indicates the failure of essential liver function. The neuropharmacologic events that result in hepatic encephalopathy are complex and not yet understood completely.

Clinically, acute hepatic encephalopathy can be defined as any brain dysfunction that occurs as a result of acute hepatic dysfunction. In ALF, the presumption is that hepatocyte

Table 5.3: Clinical Stages of Hepatic Encephalopathy

Stage	*Clinical Manifestations*	*Asterixis*	*Electroencephalographic Changes*
I (prodrome)	Slowness of mentation, mild, disturbed sleep–awake cycle	Slight	Minimal
II (impending coma)	Drowsiness, confusion, inappropriate behavior, disorientation, mood swings	Easily elicited	Usually generalized slowing of rhythm
III (stupor)	Very sleepy but arousable, unresponsive to verbal commands, markedly confused, delirious, hyperreflexia, positive Babinski sign	Present if patient cooperative	Grossly abnormal slowing
IV (coma)	Unconscious, decerebrate or decorticate, response to pain present (IV A) or absent (IV B)	Usually absent	Appearance of delta waves, decreased amplitudes

dysfunction has progressed to a point at which the liver fails to produce appropriate amounts of neuroregulatory substances or fails to eliminate neurotoxins (ammonia) or depressants (1,4-benzodiazepines), which results in brain dysfunction. Although the clinical manifestations and the progression through stages are highly variable, acute hepatic encephalopathy usually evolves over days through stages of personality changes and disturbances of mentation, to deepening difficulty with mentation and drowsiness, to hypersomnia and unresponsiveness, and finally to overt coma. A scale for grading clinical encephalopathy is presented in Table 5.3. This scale is useful for assessing encephalopathy in older patients, but it has little value in assessing neonates and infants, particularly in the early stages of encephalopathy. No study of the neuropsychiatric function of children with acute hepatic encephalopathy has been completed, and an age-dependent grading scale is badly needed.

The earliest abnormalities associated with hepatic encephalopathy may not be detectable by clinical assessment but are apparent to family members. Personality changes reflective of forebrain dysfunction include regression (childlike behavior in older patients and behaving as a younger child in children), irritability, apathy, and occasionally euphoria. The younger the child, the more likely irritability and apathy prevail as symptoms. The infant and young child may cry as if hungry but be apathetic about eating or suckle inattentively and ineffectively. The older child may assume infantile behavior, demanding attention and responding inappropriately when it is given. Sleep disturbances often are observed, including insomnia and sleep inversion. Intellectual deterioration may be observed in stage I hepatic encephalopathy but is usually not evident in acute encephalopathy as observed in ALF. Rather, children show inattentiveness to tasks. Constructional apraxia related to disturbed spatial recognition may be present. Simple, age-related tasks may be clinically useful tools for the day-to-day assessment of inattentiveness and apraxia. Subtraction of serial sevens, recall of events (such as recently viewed videos), writing, and figure drawing are appropriate tasks that older children can be asked to repeat daily in order to assess early encephalopathy. Younger children may be asked to color a figure in a simple coloring book while rounds are completed. On the physician's return to the patient's bedside, it may be found that the task is not completed (inattentiveness) or that the once excellent "colorer" has scribbled far outside the lines (constructional apraxia). Again, the age-appropriateness of the tools must be emphasized, and there are no useful tools for assessing early encephalopathy in young infants.

As the patient progresses more deeply into stage II hepatic encephalopathy, personality changes are more obvious and behavior can become very inappropriate, with outbursts of anger or crying. Drowsiness and lethargy are readily apparent. Mental deterioration is clearly evident – the tasks mentioned previously usually are not attempted by the patient. Gross motor impairment becomes evident, including ataxia, dysarthria, and apraxia. The older child may stumble about the room, appearing dazed or intoxicated. The infant more likely lays unmoving with widely open eyes. Infants, in our experience, also exhibit increasing irritability and often produce high-pitched, ear-piercing screams. They usually refuse to suckle or eat. Asterixis develops in stage II hepatic encephalopathy and is a useful sign. It cannot be elicited with regularity, however, in children younger than 8–10 years of age. Other neuromotor disturbances that can be detected at this stage include hyperreflexia, sustained clonus, rigidity, extensor posturing, and bizarre facial expressions. Electroencephalogram abnormalities are detectable at this stage.

Stage III hepatic encephalopathy is characterized by deepening somnolence and stupor. The patient is arousable by vigorous physical stimuli but often immediately returns to a sleep-like state. Children in this stage perform no tasks on command. If they attempt to speak, they sound intoxicated, with slurred speech. They are disoriented and often do not recognize family members. School-aged children and teenagers in deepening stage II and stage III coma often exhibit extreme agitation and rage. Biting may be a problem, and individuals caring for such children must be aware of the potential health risks involved. Seizures occur but are extremely rare. Neurologic findings are more profound.

Progression into stage IV hepatic encephalopathy is heralded by the onset of coma. The patient loses response to all stimuli. At first, the patient is flaccid and the coma resembles normal sleep. In deeper stage IV, the patient assumes decerebrate posturing. Brainstem reflexes are lost at this stage.

Hepatic encephalopathy may progress rapidly in ALF, with coma developing within hours of the earliest detectable signs. In clinical assessment of children with brain and liver dysfunction, however, it should be remembered that hepatic encephalopathy is secondary to liver failure and almost always has its onset well after other evidence of severe liver disease is apparent. Also, it is unlikely to be present with less than severe liver dysfunction unless other factors (such as the administration of benzodiazepine sedatives) are present. These considerations become important in establishing an appropriate diagnosis of systemic disorders that can affect both organ systems simultaneously (e.g., meningococcal sepsis, thrombotic thrombocytopenic purpura, and diffuse vasculitis).

Alterations in the electroencephalogram are nonspecific, but electroencephalography has been found to be of some use for monitoring hepatic encephalopathy [119]. Initially, there is a generalized slowing of the pattern and some suppression of the alpha rhythm. With progression, a high-voltage alpha rhythm appears with paroxysmal waves of five to seven cycles per second, beginning frontally. In deeper coma, there is a generalized slowing, and synchronous low-amplitude two- to three-cycle-per-second waves are recorded over the frontal lobes. Despite the fact that these changes parallel the progression of hepatic encephalopathy, it is unclear whether routine monitoring of the electroencephalogram provides any advantage over clinical assessment alone. Recorded evoked response potentials can provide some specificity for diagnosis but have found little clinical use [122].

The pathophysiologic mechanisms that lead to hepatic encephalopathy in ALF have not been defined fully. Hepatic encephalopathy in ALF is different in several ways from encephalopathy seen in chronic liver disease and in patients with portosystemic shunts. There are no neuropathologic abnormalities; acute hepatic encephalopathy is considered to be completely reversible after resolution of the hepatic dysfunction. Furthermore, hyperammonemia is observed more consistently in ALF-associated encephalopathy and may contribute more to its pathogenesis. This may be why seizures are more common in acute encephalopathy. Agitation is also more common, suggesting less dependence on neurodepressants.

Ammonia is clearly neurotoxic, and its accumulation in the systemic circulation is regarded widely as a contributor to acute hepatic encephalopathy. Ammonia is not solely responsible, however, and may not even be key to the pathogenesis of acute hepatic encephalopathy. The blood ammonia concentration does not correlate with the development or degree of hepatic encephalopathy in patients with acute liver disease. As a consequence, we do not rely on repeated measures of blood ammonia concentration to follow the course of encephalopathy in children with acute hepatitis. We do use blood ammonia concentrations to confirm the possible hepatic origin of encephalopathy, because all children with acute hepatic encephalopathy have elevated blood ammonia concentrations. Not all children with elevated ammonia levels, however, have encephalopathy; indeed, some children with three- to fivefold elevation may have no evidence of encephalopathy. Ammonia is mainly of gut origin, which makes it a target for treatment. Endogenous benzodiazepines also have an intestinal source. Much evidence suggests that increased concentration or availability of these compounds contributes to hepatic encephalopathy. The benzodiazepine receptor antagonist flumazenil has been shown to reverse the electrophysiologic abnormalities and neurologic findings in animals and humans with hepatic encephalopathy.

Despite the fact that the role that it plays is controversial, therapy to reduce ammonia production or accumulation is indicated in patients with hepatic encephalopathy. The essential components of therapy are diet, enteric antibiotics, enteral lactulose, and control of the complications of ALF that contribute to ammonia accumulation or its effects on the CNS.

Reduction of dietary protein intake is not usually an issue in children with ALF because they often have reduced oral intake or are being allowed nothing by mouth for medical reasons. Patients who are eating regularly should have the intake of protein limited to reduce ammonia production. To maintain ammonia production at a minimum, however, some protein (0.8–1.0 g/kg body weight) should be administered parenterally to reduce catabolism. The oral or rectal administration of nonabsorbable antibiotics (usually neomycin) is a time-honored approach to reducing ammonia production. Antibiotics reduce ammonia absorption by reducing bacterial urease and proteases responsible for ammonia production in the gut. No study of benefit and risk in children with ALF is available, but several studies of adults with acute and chronic hepatic insufficiency have shown that neomycin is effective in reducing blood ammonia levels. Lactulose, a nonabsorbable disaccharide, also can reduce ammonia absorption if administered orally or by enema. It acts principally as a cathartic, but also acidifies the colonic contents (trapping NH_{4+}) and qualitatively alters the bacterial flora. Lactulose is as effective as neomycin in reducing blood ammonia concentration. Although prolonged administration should be avoided because of potential toxic effects, neomycin administered orally (or by gavage) or by enema may be preferable to lactulose from a nursing standpoint, because of the diarrhea attendant to lactulose use. The two may be used together, and their effects may be additive. The dietary manipulations used to reduce ammonia accumulation as well as the use of antibiotics and lactulose also may reduce the accumulation of 1,4-benzodiazepines.

Many of the complications of ALF increase the potential for ammonia accumulation and its neurotoxicity. Gastrointestinal hemorrhage increases production. Measures should be used to prevent hemorrhage, and it should be controlled if it does occur. Dehydration and electrolyte and acid–base disturbances should be corrected, and blood glucose concentration should be maintained by administering 10–25% glucose solution.

Cerebral Edema

Brain death associated with cerebral edema is the most frequent cause of death in most series of ALF. It is also a major contributor to the reduced survival rate after orthotopic liver transplantation performed for this indication and is responsible for neurologic deficits in surviving patients. Every effort should be made to prevent this complication because the prognosis is poor once it occurs.

Cerebral edema develops in patients with deep coma (stage IV) usually after a prolonged time (2–3 days), although it may present within 24 hours of the onset of coma. It is heralded by changes in the neurologic examination: abnormally reacting or unequal pupils, muscular rigidity and decerebrate posturing, mild clonus or focal seizures, and loss of brainstem reflexes. Imaging of the brain by computed tomography or magnetic resonance imaging shows flattening of the gyri, reduction of the ventricular volume, and loss of the gray–white matter definition. At necropsy, the brain is heavy, the gyri are flattened, and there is evidence of herniation of the cerebral tonsils or the uncinate processes of the temporal lobes. The histologic pathology is normal except for a generalized cellular and interstitial edema and, in occasional patients, microscopic intravascular thrombi.

The pathophysiology of cerebral edema in ALF is poorly understood; several factors are thought to participate in the mechanism [121,123,124]. First, a change in the vascular integrity of the cerebral circulation might allow an increase in transfer of solute and water into the brain matter. This increased permeability might result from circulating endotoxin or toxic metabolites such as ammonia that accumulate during hepatocellular failure [125]. Next, there might be a failure of essential homeostatic mechanisms within brain cells that are responsible for maintaining the intracellular volume [126]. Finally, imbibement of water by the extracellular matrix by unknown mechanisms possibly related to astrocyte function could result in the pathologic findings observed in this condition [124]. Iatrogenic factors, including fluid overload, may contribute to cerebral edema. Cerebral edema in these patients usually is not associated with renal failure. Failure to maintain blood glucose concentrations can lead to anaerobic brain metabolism, which can result in fluid shifts. Likewise, failure to maintain systemic blood pressure can lead to cerebral ischemia and secondary edema. Most of the patients with cerebral edema are being ventilated artificially at its onset, although the contribution of ventilation to cerebral edema is not clear.

The treatment of cerebral edema in ALF is inadequate and ineffective, so every effort must be made to prevent it. There is some controversy about monitoring intracranial pressure in this setting [127]. It does not appear to improve overall outcome, although it appears to be helpful if liver transplantation is being considered as a therapeutic option. The intravenous infusion of mannitol may be helpful in controlling acute increases in intracranial pressure and in reversing acute neurologic changes associated with cerebral edema. Likewise, maintaining hypernatremia by infusions of hypertonic saline may be of benefit [128]. As this practice may be in conflict with the management of fluid and electrolyte balance in these patients, more data regarding benefits of therapy are needed before endorsing this therapy in general practice. Diligent effort should be made to maintain cerebral perfusion pressure (mean arterial pressure minus intercranial pressure). Controlled hypothermia also shows promise in preventing and perhaps treating cerebral edema in ALF [129–132].

Table 5.4: The Relationship Between Prothrombin Time and Factor VII Activity in Liver Disease

Mean Prothrombin Time, Sec	*Mean Factor VII Activity, % of Normal*
13	100
14	80
16	60
17	50
18	40
19	20
23	10

Data from Green G, Poller L, Thomson JM, et al. Factor VII as a marker of synthetic function in liver disease. J Clin Pathol 1976;29: 971–5.

Coagulopathy and Hemorrhage

Profound disturbances in hemostasis characteristic of ALF are contributed to by failure of hepatic synthesis of clotting factors and fibrinolytic factors, disturbances of platelet number and function, and intravascular coagulation [133]. The coagulopathy in ALF differs significantly from that seen in end-stage chronic liver disease in its severity and its pathogenesis, particularly the contribution of intravascular coagulation. Clinically significant hemorrhage frequently complicates ALF; coagulopathy certainly contributes to its severity, but factors that disrupt blood vessel integrity must be present for its initiation. The management of coagulopathy and hemorrhage constitutes a major part of the overall care of the child with ALF.

Severely depressed circulating levels of certain clotting factors reflect hepatocyte failure. The factors synthesized by hepatocytes include factors I (fibrinogen), II (prothrombin), V, VII, IX, and X. Failure to produce these in adequate amounts is the key contributor to the prolongation of the prothrombin time and partial thromboplastin time in ALF. The prothrombin time is the simplest clinical measure of failure of hepatic synthesis of clotting factors. Administering vitamin K parenterally assures the sufficiency of this essential cofactor but rarely affects the prothrombin time in ALF. The prothrombin time depends on the availability of factor VII (Table 5.4). Because of its shorter half-life, the plasma concentration of factor VII has been shown to decrease earlier and to a greater extent than other liver-derived clotting factors in ALF. As a result, the measurement of factor VII has been viewed as more sensitive for the detection of hepatic failure and recovery than the prothrombin time. Factor I concentrations are least depressed in ALF, and severe depression may indicate the presence of disseminated intravascular coagulation (DIC). The levels of factor VIII are not dependent on hepatocyte function because it is synthesized by vascular endothelium. Levels may be increased, possibly as an acute phase response or because of decreased utilization. Decreased levels of factor XIII may contribute to poor clot stabilization.

Up to half of patients with ALF have depressed platelet counts to less than 80,000 per microliter [133]. Profound thrombocytopenia, requiring platelet transfusion, is unusual in pediatric ALF and often indicates the presence of aplastic anemia. Other causes include hypersplenism and intravascular coagulation. The use of extracorporeal support devices also may contribute. Abnormal platelet structure and function also can be detected in patients with ALF and can contribute to prolonged bleeding times.

Intravascular coagulation can be detected in most patients with ALF. Abnormal concentrations of fibrin degradation products are measurable in almost all patients, albeit at low levels, indicating ongoing clot deposition and dissolution [133]. Also, the turnover of plasma fibrinogen has been shown to be increased. The major location for intravascular coagulation is probably the liver, as a consequence of tissue necrosis and the release of local cytokines [134]. Thrombosis in small vessels may be observed in liver specimens, but it is unclear whether local coagulation contributes to ongoing necrosis. Endotoxin-induced activation of factor XII also may contribute to intravascular coagulation within the liver [135]. DIC is not often significant. In the presence of secondary bacterial infection, however, DIC can contribute to organ damage. Also, the administration of clotting factors may precipitate disseminated coagulation [136].

Clinical bleeding occurs if vascular integrity is disrupted. Arterial puncture should be avoided except for the placement of an indwelling blood pressure monitor. Percutaneous liver biopsy is performed at high risk in these patients. Upper gastrointestinal tract bleeding is common, resulting from gastritis or the placement of nasogastric tubes. High-dose H_2-blockers or proton pump inhibitors should be administered to reduce the potential for upper gastrointestinal tract bleeding [137]. Intracranial bleeding also may occur. Petechiae reflect decreased platelet function, disturbed vascular integrity, or DIC.

The management of coagulopathy depends on the administration of fresh frozen plasma and platelets as needed [137]. It is impossible to maintain coagulation parameters (prothrombin time as expressed by INR) in the normal range, and no attempt should be made to do so. As a general approach, mild coagulopathy (INR <1.7) requires no therapy, and there is little to be gained by administering fresh frozen plasma. Moderate coagulopathy (INR 1.7–2.2) unaccompanied by hemorrhage also requires no therapy. In the event of significant bleeding, fresh frozen plasma should be administered at a rate to improve the prothrombin time (usually requiring about 10 mL/kg body weight every 6 hours). Marked coagulopathy (INR >2.2) should be corrected somewhat because of the risk of bleeding, particularly intracranial hemorrhage. Usually 10–15 mL/kg of fresh frozen plasma every 6 hours will bring the INR back into the 1.7–2.2 range, which is an adequate protective measure. If major bleeding occurs, additional attempts should be made to correct coagulation. The requirement for fresh frozen plasma may be as high as 20 mL/kg every 6 hours, or continuous infusions at a rate of 3 to 5 mL/kg/hr may be employed. Volume overload is a major problem under these conditions. Double-volume exchange transfusion with fresh blood may improve coagulation and control of hemorrhage temporarily. An alternative approach would be to use synthetic activated factor VII, which will nearly normalize the prothrombin time temporarily [138]. Such infusions do appear to reduce the risk of spontaneous and procedure-related hemorrhage. However, activated clotting factors may fuel intravascular coagulation and should not be used when significant levels of fibrin split products are detected. Platelet counts should be maintained above 50,000 per microliter by infusion of platelets. DIC is rarely severe enough to require heparin infusion, and exchange transfusion with fresh blood to rebalance coagulation may be more helpful in this event than is anticoagulation.

Aplastic Anemia

Bone marrow failure, a relatively common and usually ultimately fatal complication of ALF from sporadic NANB hepatitis (see Etiology) [76], probably results from hepatitis virus infection of bone marrow elements. It may not be evident before transplantation, but low blood counts should prompt examination of the bone marrow for this complication. The high mortality rate of patients who develop this complication provides a note of caution regarding management.

Hypoglycemia

Severe hypoglycemia (blood glucose concentration <40 mg/dL) is seen at some point in the majority of children with ALF. It may contribute to the severity of central nervous system impairment and other tissue or organ dysfunction. Frequent bedside monitoring of blood glucose concentrations (i.e., every 1–2 hours) should be performed to detect this complication. Factors contributing to hypoglycemia include failure of hepatic glucose synthesis and release, hyperinsulinemia (caused by failure of hepatic degradation), increased glucose utilization (resulting from anaerobic metabolism), and secondary bacterial infection. Glucose must be administered to compensate for reduced hepatic synthesis and release; inclusion of 10% glucose in intravenous fluids to provide an infusion rate of 6 mg/kg/min is usually adequate. Hyperinsulinemia can be a problem. Attempting to maintain a normal blood glucose concentration (i.e., >70 mg/dL) may be counterproductive. Increased glucose infusion can lead to increased insulin production, which leads to increased glucose need, a vicious cycle that can be avoided by permitting the blood glucose concentration to remain somewhat below normal (i.e., 40–60 mg/dL). Profound refractory hypoglycemia carries a grave prognostic implication.

Electrolyte and Acid–Base Disturbances

Disturbances in sodium homeostasis are observed in virtually all children with ALF; hyponatremia or hypernatremia may be observed. Hyponatremia is more common and occurs despite probable avid sodium retention by the kidney. It may result from decreased water excretion by the kidney and may be related to excess antidiuretic hormone. Disturbances in the sodium potassium pump, which are evident in peripheral leukocytes from patients with ALF, also may contribute [139]. Iatrogenic factors, particularly the excess administration of hypotonic saline, are clear contributors. Hypernatremia, which is less common, usually results from iatrogenic factors, particularly the administration of intravenous fluids or the vigorous use of lactulose.

Hypokalemia is often evident. The increased retention of sodium by the kidney as a result of a variety of mechanisms, including secondary hyperaldosteronism, plays a major role [140]. Decreased intake and vomiting also surely contribute. Iatrogenic factors that may result in hypokalemia include nasogastric suction and the vigorous use of diuretics. Occasionally hyperkalemia is observed in patients with massive hepatic necrosis or hemolysis.

Hypophosphatemia is a well-documented electrolyte disturbance in both children and adults with ALF [141,142]. Analysis of low serum phosphate in adults following major hepatic resection suggests that it may occur as a consequence of liver regeneration [143,144]. Severe hypophosphatemia may impair oxygen transport and leukocyte and platelet function and lead to generalized muscle weakness [145]. Thus, correction of serum phosphate levels is an important aspect of supportive care. It should also be noted that serum phosphate levels have been examined as a prognostic indicator in ALF with the assertion that low levels are a sign of significant liver regeneration [141,143,146,147]. However, as a single indicator, serum phosphate levels may not be as reliable as other accepted criteria. Hypocalcemia and hypomagnesemia frequently occur and should also be corrected.

A wide spectrum of acid–base disturbances is associated with ALF [148]. Respiratory alkalosis is observed in the spontaneously ventilating patient in the early stages of encephalopathy, as a result of central hyperventilation. Metabolic alkalosis is seen principally in the setting of hypokalemia and with the vigorous use of diuretics, particularly furosemide. Metabolic acidosis occurs as a result of metabolic failure with accumulation of a variety of organic acids, including lactate and free fatty acids. Ketosis is usually minimal. The vigorous administration of blood preserved with citrate can contribute to acidosis in the presence of failed liver metabolism. Failure to maintain arterial blood pressure and tissue perfusion may result in tissue hypoxia and anaerobic metabolism, with the production of lactate. Renal failure, if present, also can contribute to metabolic acidosis. Finally, respiratory failure occurs as coma deepens, which results in respiratory acidosis if the patient is not mechanically ventilated. Mechanical ventilation can contribute to metabolic acidosis.

Renal Dysfunction

Renal failure in ALF has poor prognostic significance. Renal function, however, returns quickly to normal after successful liver transplantation [149]. Oliguria is a particular problem because of the fluid volume required to provide other support for these patients. As a consequence, many patients require hemodialysis or hemofiltration support.

The spectrum of renal abnormalities seen in these patients is large. Azotemia and oliguria may result from failure to maintain adequate intravascular volume, and fluid challenge may be necessary for diagnosis, albeit with risk of volume overload. Monitoring central venous pressure may be helpful in preventing volume depletion. Azotemia may be contributed to by gastrointestinal tract bleeding with the absorption of nitrogenous substances. Failure of hepatic urea synthesis, however, can limit the degree of azotemia and confuse the diagnosis of renal insufficiency. A marked increase in blood creatinine concentration can be the result of decreased filtration or increased muscle breakdown. Functional renal failure (hepatorenal syndrome) is the most common cause of actual renal insufficiency in ALF, occurring in the majority of patients. Features include avid sodium retention (urinary sodium concentration <20 mEq/L), normal urinary sediment, and reduced urinary output (i.e., <1 mL/kg/hr). Acute tubular necrosis is seen in the minority of patients. Features include abnormal urinary sediment (i.e., granular and cellular casts), urinary sodium concentration greater than 20 mEq/L, failure of creatinine clearance (i.e., urine-to-plasma creatinine ratio <10), and usually profound oliguria. Although functional renal failure recovers quickly after orthotopic liver transplantation, acute tubular necrosis may complicate the postoperative management [149].

Ascites

The use of ultrasound in the pretransplant assessment of patients has provided evidence of excessive peritoneal fluid in all children with ALF. Clinically evident ascites occurs in about one half of patients and may be severe in a few. It probably results from acute portal hypertension from lobular collapse in addition to vasodilatation, poor vascular integrity, and reduced oncotic pressure. Ascites may be a site for secondary bacterial or fungal infection, a possibility that should be investigated using paracentesis in apparently infected patients. Therapy, except the correction of oncotic pressure and general fluid management, is not usually indicated or effective.

Pancreatitis

Pancreatic lesions consistent with acute pancreatitis have been found at autopsy in a significant proportion of adults with ALF. Clinically evident pancreatitis, however, is unusual. Children with hepatic steatosis and hepatic failure may have significant pancreatic lesions; this is particularly prominent in valproic acid toxicity. Significant pancreatitis, if present, may contribute to pain, hypotension, and disturbed calcium homeostasis.

Cardiovascular and Pulmonary Complications

Hemodynamics are deranged severely in patients with ALF. The majority of patients in grade IV hepatic coma have significant hypotension that is refractory to volume replacement and often to the administration of pressor agents. Independent causes of hypotension (hemorrhage, bacteremia) should be sought and managed appropriately, but in the majority of cases the cause of hypotension is not obvious. Patients frequently exhibit clinical evidence of reduced vascular resistance, such as warm extremities, facial flush, and erythema of palms and soles, despite profound hypotension ("warm shock"). Inappropriate bradycardia may be observed, suggesting a failure of central regulatory mechanisms, which may occur in the absence of clinically evident cerebral edema.

The consequences of peripheral vasodilatation relate to poor tissue perfusion and reduced usage of available oxygen [150]. In a study of adults with ALF and grade IV encephalopathy, patients who died were found to have more reduced tissue oxygen extraction and increased peripheral anaerobic metabolism than did survivors [151]. Similar studies have not been performed in children with ALF. The combination of hypotension, evidence of peripheral vasodilatation, and metabolic acidosis (or elevated blood lactate) is an indication of imminent death unless transplantation is performed.

The cause of reduced vascular resistance is not clear, and it may be the result of several factors. Substances released from a severely necrotic liver may contribute. Removal of the liver from an unstable patient in anticipation of transplantation has resulted in improved hemodynamic stability in a few cases, suggesting that substances released from necrotic hepatocytes may have an effect on vascular resistance. Gut-derived endotoxin also may contribute significantly.

Cardiac abnormalities are infrequent in children with ALF, although arrhythmias and other problems are observed in the majority of adults [152]. There have been no detailed studies reported of the electrocardiographic patterns or other cardiac abnormalities in children with ALF, but clinically significant arrhythmias or unexpected cardiac arrest is unusual. Abnormal electrocardiographic patterns including T wave and ST segment changes usually are related to electrolyte imbalance. In adults, significant arrhythmias tend to occur in patients with hypoxemia and metabolic acidosis. We have observed cardiac arrest refractory to all resuscitative measures only in children with multiorgan failure including cerebral edema. Necropsy findings usually include a dilated, flabby heart with pale myocardium and occasional focal hemorrhage of the endocardium. Small pericardial effusions are commonplace.

Defective ventilation and ventilatory response to chemical stimuli are virtually always present in patients with ALF [152]. Hyperventilation often accompanies stage III encephalopathy, and results in respiratory alkalosis. Patients in stage IV coma develop hypoventilation, hypoxia, and hypercapnia. Arterial blood gas analysis usually reveals a mixed respiratory–metabolic acidosis. Such patients may show an appropriate increase in ventilation to transient hypoxia but do not maintain increased minute ventilation if hypoxia is prolonged. Intubation and controlled mechanical ventilation guided by arterial blood gas analysis should be initiated at the first sign of ventilatory failure. Unfortunately, positive pressure ventilation, particularly if positive end-expiratory pressure is applied, can reduce hepatic perfusion and worsen lactic acidemia [153].

Poor oxygenation despite adequate ventilation can be the result of intrapulmonary shunting of blood, creating a secondary ventilation–perfusion mismatch [152]. The majority of children with grade IV encephalopathy on mechanical ventilation have large FIO_2 (fraction of inspired oxygen) requirements. This is apparently the result of microvascular dilatation similar to that seen in the peripheral circulation of these patients. Intrapulmonary shunting resolves promptly after orthotopic liver transplantation or spontaneous recovery.

About one third of adult patients with ALF demonstrate clinical or radiographic evidence of pulmonary edema [152]. This number is very much higher than in other situations of metabolic coma and higher than in children with ALF. In adults, renal failure, fluid overload, and hypoalbuminemia are not incriminated. Pulmonary edema is the likely consequence of vasodilatation and loss of vascular integrity. In children, mild pulmonary edema often is responsive to diuretics and correction of plasma oncotic pressure with albumin. Severe pulmonary edema with adult respiratory distress syndrome is unusual and carries a poor prognosis.

Pulmonary infection often complicates the courses of patients with ALF. The factors involved include pulmonary edema, intubation, mechanical ventilation, and general immune deficits. The organisms most often implicated include *Staphylococcus aureus*, gram-negative enterics, *Pseudomonas* species, and fungi. Prophylactic antibiotics should not be used, and patients with positive endotracheal tube cultures should not be treated unless there is clinical or radiographic evidence of pulmonary infection. In the event that the patient develops clinical or radiographic pneumonia, broad-spectrum antimicrobials should be administered, with therapy guided by endotracheal tube culture results.

Secondary Bacterial and Fungal Infections

The majority of adults and many children with ALF have their courses complicated by infection. Sepsis is the most frequent severe infection observed in both populations. The organisms most often implicated are gram-positive (*S. aureus*, *Staphylococcus epidermidis*, and streptococci), presumably of skin origin. Intensive care support contributes to the entry of skin bacteria, with a myriad of foreign bodies usually invading the integument. Occasionally gram-negative bacteria or fungal infection are observed. Urinary tract infections (complicating indwelling catheter use) and pulmonary infections are also common.

The frequency of infection in patients with ALF far exceeds that observed in similarly ill patients in intensive care settings, which has prompted an examination of the immune system. Both the cellular and humoral immune systems have significant impairment [154]. Neutropenia is observed commonly, sometimes in association with generalized aplastic anemia. Neutrophil function also is deranged, possibly as a consequence of the defective sodium pump. Defective opsonization results probably from low plasma levels of complement and fibronectin. Hepatic Kupffer cell function is not impaired grossly in most patients, as evidenced by hepatic scintigraphy, but there is much clinical evidence of impaired hepatic immune function. In summation, the immune defects, whether the result of the primary infection or toxin or secondary to failed hepatic function, result in a significant risk of secondary infection.

The approach to management includes daily surveillance cultures from all indwelling catheters. Positive cultures in the absence of clinical infection should result in removal or replacement of the infected catheter and a brief course of appropriate antimicrobials. Clinical infection should prompt aggressive antimicrobial therapy, with close attention to the possibility of additional, perhaps opportunistic infection.

MANAGEMENT

Management is directed at life support and prevention and treatment of complications to allow recovery to occur, if possible, or to provide a suitable candidate for liver transplantation.

General Measures

Management should be in an ICU setting. The evidence in favor of caring for children with ALF in an ICU is empiric and based on improved survival rates in adult patients with ALF in series in which intensive care was routinely applied [1,7,8]. It is logical to assume that improved life support, monitoring for the detection of complications, and the management of life-threatening complications in an intensive care setting improves the overall chance of survival.

All medical personnel should wear protective gowns, gloves, and masks if dealing with a child with ALF. Enteric isolation procedures must be enforced, and blood specimens should be labeled as potentially infectious. The older patient with aggressive delirium is a particular risk to care providers. Restraint and sedation may be necessary to protect staff. However, sedation usually is not needed, and the use of benzodiazepines should be avoided. Morphine or other opiates may be used in small doses to relieve pain associated with monitoring and catheter placement.

Venous access must be established immediately. A central venous catheter is useful for assessment of central venous pressure and volume status as is an indwelling arterial line for continuous measurement of blood pressure and to obtain blood for biochemical monitoring. A nasogastric tube is passed electively in the patient with altered mental status and a poor gag reflex. The tube is placed to gravity to avoid the gastric mucosal lesions associated with intermittent suction; it can also be used for regular gentle saline lavage to detect upper gastrointestinal hemorrhage. The urinary bladder is catheterized and strict output records maintained to help in the evaluation of fluid status and renal function. Ideally, the patient is placed on a bed that permits body weight to be recorded frequently.

Frequent evaluation of neurologic function is essential to follow the progress of hepatic encephalopathy. Conventional measures are taken to minimize the formation of nitrogenous substances by the intestine. Protein intake should be limited to 1.0 g/kg/d and should be administered parenterally. Infusion of dextrose is indicated to maintain blood glucose concentration. Laboratory monitoring, usually every 6–12 hours, should include complete blood count, plasma electrolyte measurement, and prothrombin time, with less frequent monitoring (daily) of plasma creatinine, aminotransferases, bilirubin, blood ammonia, cholesterol, and other biochemistries. Cultures should be obtained from all indwelling catheters daily. Chest radiography should be performed daily. If blood gas analysis demonstrates evidence of ventilatory failure, hypoxia, or hypercapnia, the patient should be intubated and placed on controlled mechanical ventilation.

Fluid balance is difficult to maintain with the competing forces of a large intake requirement and compromised renal function. Strictly maintained records of intake and output, frequently measured electrolyte concentrations, central venous pressure, and body weight guide fluid administration. Maintenance fluids usually consist of 10% dextrose in 0.25 normal saline. The rate of administration is guided by the other fluid requirements, and the total fluid intake should be maintained at near-normal maintenance requirements. A total sodium intake of 1.0 mEq/kg/d usually is adequate. Hyponatremia should not be corrected by the administration of additional sodium because total body sodium overload is the rule. As maintaining a state of hypernatremia may be of benefit in preventing cerebral edema [128], preventing hyponatremia by maintaining assiduous fluid restriction would seem prudent. Potassium requirements may be large, 3–6 mEq/kg/d, as guided by the serum concentration. Hypophosphatemia should likewise be corrected. Acid–base disturbances require appropriate action. Respiratory acidosis is treated by mechanical ventilation. Metabolic acidosis may require the administration of sodium bicarbonate, and alkalosis may require additional chloride. Anemia should be corrected, maintaining the hemoglobin concentration above 12 g/dL, to provide maximum oxygen delivery to tissue. Coagulopathy should be managed conservatively; the sometimes massive requirements for fresh frozen plasma may result in fluid overload and hypernatremia.

There are no data from controlled studies supporting the use of inotropes, but they seem to be effective and should be used as needed. Administering "renal doses" of dopamine may help to maintain renal perfusion. Should renal output diminish to below 1.0 mL/kg/hr, it is impossible to maintain fluid balance, and consideration should be given to therapy with hemofiltration or dialysis. The choice of therapy is determined by the presence of azotemia. As long as urine output is adequate, mannitol can be used to manage increased intracranial pressure. Hypotension should be treated promptly. Blood infusions are given to correct volume deficits from hemorrhage.

The management of increased intracranial pressure (ICP) depends on the administration of osmotic substances, usually mannitol. Mannitol is usually administered when changes in the neurologic examination or the onset of papilledema is detected. If intracranial pressure is being monitored, increases to more than 30 mm Hg should also be treated. The doses of mannitol required are usually in the range of 1.0 g/kg every 2–6 hours. Serum osmolarity should be monitored during mannitol therapy and should not exceed 320 mOsm/kg. Another potential option for treatment of increased ICP in the setting of ALF is mild hypothermia (32–35°C) [130,131]. Mild hypothermia may affect the course of cerebral edema by a number of mechanisms that include a reduction of ammonia crossing the blood–brain barrier, altering the pericellular osmotic gradient, decreasing cerebral blood flow, and decreasing cerebral metabolic rate [130,155]. Experimental work [129] and a multicenter adult study [132] suggest that mild hypothermia may provide a bridge to liver transplantation. Although the results are encouraging, the numbers of patients treated with mild hypothermia in the setting of ALF are small. More studies are needed to determine the proper duration of cooling, the rate of rewarming, and the potential effects upon liver transplantation. These early studies suggest an improvement in patients' survival, however, functional outcome of patients undergoing mild hypothermia is currently unknown.

Specific Therapies

A variety of experimental drugs has been used in treating ALF; however, none has proved effective. To date, there have been no multicenter treatment trials in children with ALF. As liver transplantation became the primary treatment for ALF, enthusiasm for multicenter medical treatment trials has diminished. However, with limited organ availability, efforts must continue to identify methods to improve hepatocyte function and patient survival. *N*-acetylcysteine (NAC) replenishes mitochondrial and cytosolic glutathione (GSH) stores, and has been shown in patients and in experimental animals to prevent or ameliorate the degree of injury and cell death [156–158]. Oral or intravenous NAC improves survival in patients with acetaminophen (APAP)-induced ALF, likely by replenishing hepatic GSH stores [159]. Evidence of patient benefit following the administration of NAC as late as 72 hours after acetaminophen overdose led to its use in non-APAP ALF cases [160]. A small uncontrolled study utilizing NAC in adult patients with ALF showed improvement in hemodynamics and oxygen transport in both APAP ($n = 12$) and non-APAP ($n = 8$) patients [161]. Mean arterial pressure, oxygen consumption, and oxygen delivery increased, as did the oxygen extraction ratio. As a result of these preliminary data, both the pediatric and adult ALF study groups are entering patients into a multicenter randomized, double-blinded, placebo-controlled trial to assess the safety and efficacy of NAC treatment for non-APAP ALF.

Attempts to develop an effective form of temporary hepatic support for patients with ALF continue. A variety of approaches have been used to assist the liver; these include double-volume exchange transfusion, plasmapheresis, extracorporal blood cleansing with activated charcoal and other binding resins, liver-assist devices containing cultured hepatocytes, and cross-circulation with animals. The goals of therapy are to provide support in order for the liver to repair and the patient to recover and to reduce or eliminate complications, particularly neurologic impairment.

The molecular adsorbent recirculating system has been used in adults with ALF with variable results [162–166]. This system allows the selective removal of albumin-bound substances that accumulate in liver failure by use of albumin-enriched dialysate. Continuous hemofiltration has been used in patients with and without renal failure to clear ammonia and other potential toxins, permit administration of large volumes of plasma to enhance coagulation, and improve fluid balance. Utilizing a single larger-bore vascular access site, plasma can be cleared against a charcoal filter designed to remove medium and small molecular weight solutes. This therapy usually requires controlled anticoagulation to prevent clotting of the filtration circuit. Many patients with ALF will require little or no anticoagulation. However, some patients with ALF may have a paradoxic coagulation status in which they appear "anticoagulated" based upon clotting times yet have a tendency to clot filtration circuits because of depressed levels of anticlotting factors and DIC. In this setting, use of citrate in the circuit can prevent this complication.

At present, liver transplantation holds the greatest lifesaving potential, but the decision process in the management of a child with acute hepatic failure is complex. The cause of the ALF is an important factor in determining whether transplant therapy should be used. Patients with drug-induced liver disease, such as that caused by acute acetaminophen intoxication, may have as good an outcome with intensive medical therapy as with transplantation. On the other hand, patients with ALF secondary to viral hepatitis have a very poor prognosis and should be offered transplantation. In children, the diagnoses of indeterminate (non-A-G hepatitis) ALF and fulminant Wilson's disease should lead to an immediate decision to transplant. If, while waiting for a donor, the patient experiences significant improvement, the decision can be reversed. Most of these patients, however, have rapidly deteriorating courses and require maximum medical therapy until a donor becomes available.

The shortage of donors affects the survival rate. Not only do children die without transplantation, but less than ideal donor organs often are accepted because of the urgency of the situation. Improved survival rates using living donors and split livers suggest that organ availability is a major factor in poor outcome. Postoperative infections seem to be more common than in other transplant patients, perhaps as a result of intrinsic immune deficits. The 1-year posttransplant survival rate approximates 60% in most series but has risen to 90% in the short term in recent experience [5,167]. Auxiliary liver transplants and hepatocyte transplantation have shown promise and may be useful as a support measure, with some patients recovering without the need for full liver replacement [13].

OUTCOMES AND PROGNOSIS

Causes of Death

Cerebral edema with brain death is the direct cause of death in most children with ALF. Overwhelming bacterial or fungal infection is implicated in a small proportion of patients, and pulmonary failure in very few. Hemorrhagic diathesis is a common cause of death in adult patients but is rare in children afforded effective management. Therapeutic intervention may be the cause of death of some patients. Experience with corticosteroid therapy indicates a risk of duodenal ulcer with perforation or hemorrhage. Extracorporal support devices are associated with technical failure (catheter dislodgment) and with numerous other complications that can lead to death.

There are no reliable criteria on which to base a determination of prognosis in a child with ALF. The absence of an obvious cause in a child with severe hepatitis with encephalopathy (indeterminate cause) is an indicator of poor outcome. It is desirable, however, to be able to predict the spontaneous recovery of a patient in order to avoid potentially life-threatening therapy, such as liver transplantation. Patients showing signs of stabilization (lack of progressive deterioration) or evidence of recovering function (improved coagulation parameters) while awaiting graft availability have an outlook for spontaneous recovery as good as that with liver transplantation [167]. Unfortunately, few affected children demonstrate these positive signs.

Many attempts have been made to correlate clinical variables and laboratory data with outcome, to little avail. Although some variables (such as etiology) correlate with survival rate, the accurate prediction of duration of survival in the individual patient with ALF is not possible. HAV infection generally is associated with higher survival rates than HBV and indeterminate etiology. Drug-induced liver disease, particularly acetaminophen overdose, has a better outcome than viral hepatitis. Among adults, age older than 40 years is associated with poorer prognosis. Among children with ALF, however, age is not a useful indicator [26,168]. The duration of illness before the onset of encephalopathy and the degree of encephalopathy at the time of presentation carry little prognostic significance.

Initial findings from the prospective PALF study has revealed that patient outcome was influenced by a number of factors, including age, diagnosis, the degree of hepatic encephalopathy, and severity of the coagulopathy [5]. The risk of death or liver transplantation in patients enrolled in the PALF study was highest among children less than 3 years of age. Although the numbers are relatively small, patients with grade IV encephalopathy at enrollment experienced a higher rate of spontaneous recovery than those who progressed to grade IV during the course of the study (50% vs. 20%). At the same time, 20% of children who never experienced clinical hepatic encephalopathy either died or received a liver transplant, suggesting that ALF associated with a poor outcome can develop in children without clinical signs of encephalopathy. Logistic regression analysis identified total bilirubin greater than 5 mg/dL, INR greater than 2.55, and hepatic encephalopathy to be risk factors to predict death or liver transplantation.

The onset of complications, particularly cerebral edema and renal failure, and multiorgan failure are associated with poor outcome. Physical evidence of a collapsing liver mass or a small liver is associated with a grave prognosis. Laboratory parameters correlate in some instances with the degree of necrosis and with outcome but provide little reliable predictive power. A prothrombin time longer than 50 seconds is a bad prognostic sign but does not necessarily predict a fatal outcome [169]. Other measures of disturbed synthesis of clotting factors provide little additional information beyond that provided by prothrombin time. The degrees of alteration in results of several clinical laboratory tests have failed to provide predictive power, including ammonia concentration, aminotransferase concentration, acidosis, blood ketone body ratio, lactic acid level, blood glucose concentration, and others. Quantitative liver function tests have not provided accurate predictive information. Hepatic histology correlates poorly with prognosis, and when liver biopsy is obtained, it is primarily for the purpose of excluding a treatable diagnosis. The availability of transjugular liver biopsy has significantly altered the risk–benefit ratio of liver biopsy in the setting of ALF, leading to a larger number of biopsies being obtained, especially in older patients. The mortality rate tends to be greater in patients with more extensive necrosis, but the degree of necrosis may not be unevenly distributed through the liver parenchyma, leading to sampling error. If a biopsy specimen is available, however, the extent of regeneration correlates with survival rate [95,170]. In one series, a fraction of viable hepatocytes of less than 35% of hepatic volume in premortem biopsy samples was associated with a 100% rate of death [170]. In another study, patients who died as a direct result of hepatic failure all had proportions of viable hepatocytes less than 12% of hepatic volume [117]. Complete absence of regenerative activity indicates very poor prognosis. Increased concentrations of serum α-fetoprotein (AFP) have been used as an index of regeneration and potential recovery. Elevated levels tend to occur late in the courses of patients who survive, although elevated AFP does not necessarily predict survival. Complete absence of regeneration is associated with low AFP levels, but some patients recover after never having developed increased levels.

Several attempts at multivariate analysis have provided tools with greater predictive power than is provided by any individual test [169,171,172]. A retrospective review of ALF cases at the University of Colorado was used to derive a risk score that estimated risk of mortality or liver transplantation as low, moderate, or high [93]. By using peak values for total bilirubin, INR, and ammonia, a model was developed with a C-index that was 90%, signifying high sensitivity and specificity. However, modeling that is based upon the combined outcome of death and/or liver transplantation may not be appropriate to determine individual patient decisions because it does not predict what would happen if liver transplantation were withheld or unavailable.

REFERENCES

1. Lee WM. Acute liver failure. N Engl J Med 1993;329:1862–72.
2. Bernuau J, Rueff B, Benhamou J-P. Fulminant and subfulminant liver failure: definitions and causes. Semin Liver Dis 1986; 6:97–106.
3. Gimson AES, O'Grady J, Ede RJ, et al. Late onset hepatic failure: clinical, serological and histological features. Hepatology 1986;6:288–94.
4. Bhaduri BR, Mieli-Vergani G. Fulminant hepatic failure: pediatric aspects. Semin Liver Dis 1996;16:349–55.
5. Squires RH Jr, Shneider BL, Bucuvalas J, et al. Acute liver failure in children: the first 348 patients in the pediatric acute liver failure study group. J Pediatr 2006;148(5):652–8.
6. Lee MG, Hanchard B, Williams NP. Drug-induced acute liver disease. Postgrad Med J 1989;65:367–70.
7. Lee WM. Acute liver failure in the United States. Semin Liver Dis 2003;23:217–26.
8. Schiodt FV, Atillasoy E, Shakil AO, et al. Etiology and outcome for 295 patients with acute liver failure in the United States. Liver Transpl Surg 1999;5:29–34.
9. Zimmerman HJ. Hepatotoxicity. The adverse effects of drugs and other chemicals on the liver. 2nd ed. Philadelphia: Lippincott Williams & Wilkins, 1999.
10. Lee WM. Drug-induced hepatotoxicity. N Engl J Med 2003;349: 474–85.
11. Navarro VJ, Senior JR. Drug-related hepatotoxicity. N Engl J Med 2006;354:731–9.
12. Mitchel DH. Amanita mushroom poisoning. Ann Rev Med 1980;31:51–7.
13. Rosenthal P. Auxiliary liver transplantation for toxic mushroom poisoning. J Pediatr 2001;138:449–50.
14. Larrey D. Epidemiology and individual susceptibility to adverse drug reactions affecting the liver. Semin Liver Dis 2002;22:145–55.
15. Rumack BH, Matthew H. Acetaminophen poisoning and toxicity. Pediatrics 1975;55:871–6.
16. Lee WM. Acetaminophen and the U.S. Acute Liver Failure Study Group: lowering the risks of hepatic failure. Hepatology 2004; 40:6–9.
17. Rumack BH. Acetaminophen misconceptions. Hepatology 2004; 40:10–15.
18. James LP, Farrar HC, Sullivan JE, et al. Measurement of acetaminophen-protein adducts in children and adolescents with acetaminophen overdoses. J Clin Pharmacol 2001;41:846–51.
19. Muldrew KL, James LP, Coop L, et al. Determination of acetaminophen-protein adducts in mouse liver and serum and human serum after hepatotoxic doses of acetaminophen using high-performance liquid chromatography with electrochemical detection. Drug Metab Dispos 2002;30:446–51.
20. Selim K, Kaplowitz N. Hepatotoxicity of psychotropic drugs. Hepatology 1999;29:1347–51.
21. Narkewicz MR, Sokol RJ, Beckwith B, et al. Liver involvement in Alpers disease. J Pediatr 1991;119:260–7.
22. Brown SJ, Desmond PV. Hepatotoxicity of antimicrobial agents. Semin Liver Dis 2002;22:157–67.
23. Stedman C. Herbal hepatotoxicity. Semin Liver Dis 2002;22: 195–206.
24. Stickel F, Patsenker E, Schuppan D. Herbal hepatotoxicity. J Hepatol 2005;43:901–10.
25. Umemura T, Tanaka E, Ostapowicz G, et al. Investigation of SEN virus infection in patients with cryptogenic acute liver failure, hepatitis-associated aplastic anemia, or acute and chronic non-A-E hepatitis. J Infect Dis 2003;188:1545–52.
26. Psacharopoulos HT, Mowat AP, Davies M, et al. Fulminant hepatic failure in childhood: an analysis of 31 cases. Arch Dis Child 1980;55:252–8.
27. Debray D, Cullufi P, Devictor D, et al. Liver failure in children with hepatitis A. Hepatology 1997;26:1018–22.
28. Schiodt FV, Davern TJ, Shakil AO, et al. Viral hepatitis-related acute liver failure. Am J Gastroenterol 2003;98:448–53.
29. Vento S, Garofano T, Renzini C, et al. Fulminant hepatitis associated with hepatitis A virus superinfection in patients with chronic hepatitis C. N Engl J Med 1998;338:286–90.
30. Chang MH, Lee C-Y, Chen D-S, et al. Fulminant hepatitis in children in Taiwan: the important role of hepatitis B virus. J Pediatr 1986;3:34–8.
31. Gimson AES, Tedder RS, White YS, et al. Serological markers in fulminant hepatitis B. Gut 1983;24:615–17.
32. McNeil M, Hoy JF, Richards MJ, et al. Etiology of fatal viral hepatitis in Melbourne. Med J Aust 1984;141:637–40.
33. Bartholomeusz A, Locarnini S. Hepatitis B virus mutants and fulminant hepatitis B: fitness plus phenotype. Hepatology 2001;34:432–5.
34. Farci P, Alter HJ, Shimoda A, et al. Hepatitis C virus-associated fulminant hepatic failure. N Engl J Med 1996;335:631–4.
35. Alter HJ, Purcell RH, Shih JW, et al. Detection of antibody to hepatitis C virus in prospectively followed transfusion recipients with acute and chronic non-A, non-B hepatitis. N Engl J Med 1989;321:1494–500.
36. Feray C, Gigou M, Samuel D, et al. Hepatitis C virus RNA and hepatitis B virus DNA in serum and liver of patients with fulminant hepatitis. Gastroenterology 1993;104:549–55.
37. Liang TJ, Jeffers L, Reddy RK, et al. Fulminant or subfulminant non-A, non-B viral hepatitis: the role of hepatitis C and E viruses. Gastroenterology 1993;104:556–62.
38. Fagan EA, Harrison TJ. Exclusion in liver by polymerase chain reaction of hepatitis B and C viruses in acute liver failure attributed to sporadic non-A, non-B hepatitis. J Hepatol 1994;21:587–91.
39. Hibbs JR, Frickhofen N, Rosenfeld SJ, et al. Aplastic anemia and viral hepatitis: non-A, non-B, non-C? JAMA 1992;267:2051–4.
40. Wright TL, Mamish D, Combs D, et al. Hepatitis B virus and apparent fulminant non-A, non-B hepatitis. Lancet 1992;339: 952–5.
41. Arora NK, Nanda SK, Gulati S, et al. Acute viral hepatitis types E, A, and B singly and in combination in acute liver failure in children in north India. J Med Virol 1996;48:215–21.
42. Ijaz S, Arnold E, Banks M, et al. Non-travel-associated hepatitis E in England and Wales: demographic, clinical, and molecular epidemiological characteristics. J Infect Dis 2005;192: 1166–72.
43. Perez RG, Zein NN, Freese DK, et al. No evidence of hepatitis G virus in fulminant hepatic failure in children. J Pediatr Gastroenterol Nutr 1999;28:400–3.

44. Anastassopoulou CG, Delladetsima JK, Anagnostopoulos G, et al. Fulminant hepatic failure in a pediatric patient with active GB virus C (GBV-C)/hepatitis G virus (HGV) infection. Hepatol Res 2002;23:85–9.
45. Feranchak AP, Tyson RW, Narkewicz MR, et al. Fulminant Epstein–Barr viral hepatitis: orthotopic liver transplantation and review of the literature. Liver Transpl Surg 1998;4:469–76.
46. Harma M, Hockerstedt K, Lautenschlager I. Human herpesvirus-6 and acute liver failure. Transplantation 2003;76: 536–9.
47. Ichai P, Roque Afonso AM, Sebagh M, et al. Herpes simplex virus-associated acute liver failure: a difficult diagnosis with a poor prognosis. Liver Transpl 2005;11:1550–5.
48. Langnas AN, Markin RS, Cattral MS, Naides SJ. Parvovirus B19 as a possible causative agent of fulminant liver failure and associated aplastic anemia. Hepatology 1995;22:1661–5.
49. Fagan EA, Ellis DS, Tovey GM, et al. Toga virus-like particles in acute liver failure attributed to sporadic non-A, non-B hepatitis and recurrence after liver transplantation. J Med Virol 1992;38:71–7.
50. Phillips MJ, Blendis LM, Poucell S, et al. Syncytial giant-cell hepatitis: sporadic hepatitis with distinctive pathological features, a severe clinical course, and paramyxoviral features. N Engl J Med 1991;324:455–60.
51. Gregorio GV, Portmann B, Reid F, et al. Autoimmune hepatitis in childhood: a 20-year experience. Hepatology 1997;25: 541–7.
52. Kessler WR, Cummings OW, Eckert G, et al. Fulminant hepatic failure as the initial presentation of acute autoimmune hepatitis. Clin Gastroenterol Hepatol 2004;2:625–31.
53. Squires RH Jr. Autoimmune hepatitis in children. Curr Gastroenterol Rep 2004;6:225–30.
54. Maggiore G, Porta G, Bernard O, et al. Autoimmune hepatitis with initial presentation as acute hepatic failure in young children. J Pediatr 1990;116:280 2.
55. Debray D, Maggiore G, Girardet JP, et al. Efficacy of cyclosporin A in children with type 2 autoimmune hepatitis. J Pediatr 1999;135:111–14.
56. Whitington PF, Kelly S, Ekong UD. Neonatal hemochromatosis: fetal liver disease leading to liver failure in the fetus and newborn. Pediatr Transplant 2005;9:640–5.
57. Whitington PF. Fetal and infantile hemochromatosis. Hepatology 2006;43:654–60.
58. Ekong UD, Kelly S, Whitington PF. Disparate clinical presentation of neonatal hemochromatosis in twins. Pediatrics 2005;116:e880–4.
59. Shneider BL, Setchell KD, Whitington PF, et al. Delta 4-3-oxosteroid 5 beta-reductase deficiency causing neonatal liver failure and hemochromatosis. J Pediatr 1994;124:234–8.
60. Danks DM, Tippett P, Adams C, Campbell P. Cerebro-hepato-renal syndrome of Zellweger. J Pediatr 1975;86:382–7.
61. Jackson S, Bartlett K, Land J, et al. Long-chain 3-hydroxyacyl-CoA dehydrogenase deficiency. Pediatr Res 1991;29:406–11.
62. Odaib AA, Shneider BL, Bennett MJ, et al. A defect in the transport of long-chain fatty acids associated with acute liver failure. N Engl J Med 1998;339:1752–7.
63. Alonso EM. Acute liver failure in children: the role of defects in fatty acid oxidation. Hepatology 2005;41:696–9.
64. Cormier V, Rustin P, Bonnefont J-P, et al. Hepatic failure in disorders of oxidative phosphorylation with neonatal onset. J Pediatr 1991;119:951–4.
65. Stremmel W, Meyerrose KW, Niederau C, et al. Wilson disease: clinical presentation, treatment, and survival. Ann Intern Med 1991;115:720–6.
66. Yarze JC, Martin P, Munoz SJ, Friedman LS. Wilson's disease: current status. Am J Med 1992;81:802–3.
67. Ussery XT, Henar EL, Black DD, et al. Acute liver injury after protracted seizures in children. J Pediatr Gastro Nutr 1989;9: 421–5.
68. Bourliere M, Le Treut YP, Arnoux D, et al. Acute Budd–Chiari syndrome with hepatic failure and obstruction of the inferior vena cava as presenting manifestations of hereditary protein C deficiency. Gut 1990;31:949–52.
69. Smith SD, Tagge EP, Hannakan C, Rowe MI. Characterization of neonatal multisystem organ failure in the surgical newborn. J Pediatr Surg 1991;26:494–9.
70. Dhawan A, Mieli-Vergani G. Acute liver failure in neonates. Early Hum Dev 2005;81:1005–10.
71. Hamid SS, Jafri SM, Khan H, et al. Fulminant hepatic failure in pregnant women: acute fatty liver or acute viral hepatitis? J Hepatol 1996;25:20–7.
72. Ockner SA, Brunt EM, Cohn SA, et al. Fulminant hepatic failure caused by acute fatty liver of pregnancy treated by orthotopic liver transplantation. Hepatology 1990;11:59–64.
73. Fidler S, Fagan E, Williams R, et al. Heatstroke and rhabdomyolysis presenting as fulminant hepatic failure. Postgrad Med J 1988;64:157–9.
74. Kaukinen K, Halme L, Collin P, et al. Celiac disease in patients with severe liver disease: gluten-free diet may reverse hepatic failure. Gastroenterology 2002;122:881–8.
75. Whitington PF, Alonso EM. Fulminant hepatitis in children: evidence for an unidentified hepatitis virus. J Pediatr Gastroenterol Nutr 2001;33:529–36.
76. Tzakis AG, Arditi M, Whitington PF, et al. Aplastic anemia complicating orthotopic liver transplantation for non-A, non-B hepatitis. N Engl J Med 1988;319:393–6.
77. Cattral MS, Langnas AN, Markin RS, et al. Aplastic anemia after liver transplantation for fulminant liver failure. Hepatology 1994;20:813–18.
78. Hagglund H, Winiarski J, Ringden O, et al. Successful allogeneic bone marrow transplantation in a 2.5-year-old boy with ongoing cytomegalovirus viremia and severe aplastic anemia after orthotopic liver transplantation for non-A, non-B, non-C hepatitis. Transplantation 1997;64:1207–8.
79. Kiem HP, Storb R, McDonald GB. Hepatitis-associated aplastic anemia. N Engl J Med 1997;337:424–5.
80. Roll C, Ballauff A, Lange R, Erhard J. Heterotopic auxiliary liver transplantation in a 3-year-old boy with acute liver failure and aplastic anemia. Transplantation 1997;64:658–60.
81. Alonso EM, Sokol RJ, Hart J, et al. Fulminant hepatitis associated with centrilobular necrosis in young children. J Pediatr 1995;127:888–94.
82. Gall DG, Cutz E, McClung HJ, Greenberg ML. Acute liver disease and encephalopathy mimicking Reye syndrome. A report of three cases. J Pediatr 1975;87:869–74.
83. Lii YP, Chi SC, Mak SC. Acute encephalopathy associated with centrilobular necrosis of liver mimicking Reye's syndrome–report of two cases [in Chinese]. Chung Hua I Hsueh Tsa Chih (Taipei) 1993;51:154–7.
84. Shibao K. Non-icteric fulminant hepatitis and Reye's syndrome: comparison of laboratory data. Acta Paediatr Jpn 1990;32:399–405.

85. Bakerink JA, Gospe SM Jr, Dimand RJ, Eldridge MW. Multiple organ failure after ingestion of pennyroyal oil from herbal tea in two infants. Pediatrics 1996;98:944–7.
86. Whitworth JR, Mack CL, O'Connor JA, et al. Acute hepatitis and liver failure associated with influenza A infection in children. J Pediatr Gastroenterol Nutr. In press.
87. Whitington PF, Soriano HE, Alonso EM. Fulminant hepatic failure in children. In: Suchy FJ, Sokol RJ, Balistreri WF, eds. Liver disease in children. 2nd ed. Philadelphia: Lippincott, Williams & Wilkins, 2001:63–88.
88. Gimson AES, White YS, Eddleston WF, Williams R. Clinical and prognostic differences in fulminant hepatitis type A, B and non-A, non-B. Gut 1983;24:1194–8.
89. Mathiesen LR, Skinoj P, Nielson JO, et al. Hepatitis type A, B, and non-A, non-B in fulminant hepatitis. Gut 1980;21:72–7.
90. Dupuy JM, Dulac O, Dupuy C, Alagille D. Severe hyporegenerative viral hepatitis in children. Proc R Soc Med 1977;70:228–32.
91. Davis MA, Peters RL, Redeker AG, Reynolds TB. Appraisal of the mortality in acute fulminant viral hepatitis. N Engl J Med 1968;278:1248–53.
92. Sawhey VK, Knauer CM, Gregory PB. Rapid reduction of transaminase levels in fulminant hepatitis. N Engl J Med 1980; 302:970.
93. Liu E, Mackenzie T, Dobyns EL, et al. Characterization of acute liver failure and development of a continuous risk of death staging system in children. J Hepatol 2006;44:134–41.
94. Horney JT, Galambos JT. The liver during and after fulminant hepatitis. Gastroenterology 1977;73:639–45.
95. Portmann B, Talbot IC, Day DW, et al. Histopathological changes in the liver following a paracetamol overdose: correlation with clinical and biochemical parameters. J Pathol 1975; 117:169–81.
96. Kalk H. Biopsy findings during and after hepatic coma and after acute necrosis of the liver. Gastroenterology 1959;36:870–7.
97. Popper H, Klepper D. Networks of interacting mechanisms of hepatocellular degeneration and death. Prog Liver Dis 1986;8: 209–35.
98. Willner IR, Uhl MD, Howard SC, et al. Serious hepatitis A: an analysis of patients hospitalized during an urban epidemic in the United States. Ann Intern Med 1998;128:111–14.
99. Liang TJ, Hasegawa K, Rimon N, et al. A hepatitis B virus mutant associated with an epidemic of fulminant hepatitis. N Engl J Med 1991;324:1705–9.
100. Schoeman MN, Batey RG, Wilcken B. Recurrent acute fatty liver of pregnancy associated with a fatty-acid oxidation defect in the offspring. Gastroenterology 1991;100:544–8.
101. Matern D, Hart P, Murtha AP, et al. Acute fatty liver of pregnancy associated with short-chain acyl-coenzyme A dehydrogenase deficiency. J Pediatr 2001;138:585–8.
102. Su GL, Gong KQ, Fan MH, et al. Lipopolysaccharide-binding protein modulates acetaminophen-induced liver injury in mice. Hepatology 2005;41:187–95.
103. Nolan JP. Endotoxin, reticuloendothelial function, and liver injury. Hepatology 1981;1:458–65.
104. Izeboud CA, Hoebe KH, Grootendorst AF, et al. Endotoxin-induced liver damage in rats is minimized by beta 2-adrenoceptor stimulation. Inflamm Res 2004;53(3):93–9.
105. Liu ZX, Han D, Gunawan B, Kaplowitz N. Neutrophil depletion protects against murine acetaminophen hepatotoxicity. Hepatology 2006;43:1220–30.
106. Jaeschke H, Ho YS, Fisher MA, et al. Glutathione peroxidase-deficient mice are more susceptible to neutrophil-mediated hepatic parenchymal cell injury during endotoxemia: importance of an intracellular oxidant stress. Hepatology 1999;29: 443–50.
107. Bernal W, Donaldson P, Underhill J, et al. Tumor necrosis factor genomic polymorphism and outcome of acetaminophen (paracetamol)-induced acute liver failure. J Hepatol 1998;29: 53–9.
108. Muto Y, Meager A, Eddleston ALWF, et al. Enchanced tumour necrosis factor and interleukin-1 in fulminant hepatic failure. Lancet 1988;2:72–4.
109. Sekiyama KD, Yoshiba M, Thomson AW. Circulating proinflammatory cytokines (IL-1 beta, TNF-alpha, and IL-6) and IL-1 receptor antagonist (IL-1Ra) in fulminant hepatic failure and acute hepatitis. Clin Exp Immunol 1994;98:71–7.
110. Borowiak M, Garratt AN, Wustefeld T, et al. Met provides essential signals for liver regeneration. Proc Natl Acad Sci USA 2004; 101:10608–13.
111. Huh CG, Factor VM, Sanchez A, et al. Hepatocyte growth factor/c-met signaling pathway is required for efficient liver regeneration and repair. Proc Natl Acad Sci USA 2004;101: 4477–82.
112. Pediaditakis P, Lopez-Talavera JC, Petersen B, et al. The processing and utilization of hepatocyte growth factor/scatter factor following partial hepatectomy in the rat. Hepatology 2001;34(4 Pt 1):688–93.
113. Phaneuf D, Moscioni AD, LeClair C, et al. Generation of a mouse expressing a conditional knockout of the hepatocyte growth factor gene: demonstration of impaired liver regeneration. DNA Cell Biol 2004;23:592–603.
114. Tomiya T, Nagoshi S, Fujiwara K. Significance of serum human hepatocyte growth factor levels in patients with hepatic failure. Hepatology 1992;15:1–4.
115. Gove CD, Hughes RD. Liver regeneration in relationship to acute liver failure. Gut 1991(suppl 2):S92–6.
116. Hughes RD, Yamada H, Gove CD, Williams R. Inhibitors of hepatic DNA synthesis in fulminant hepatic failure. Dig Dis Sci 1991;36:816–19.
117. Gazzard BG, Portmann B, Murray-Lyon IM, Williams R. Causes of death in fulminant hepatic failure and relationship to quantitative histological assessment of parenchymal damage. Q J Med 1975;44:615–26.
118. Karvountzis GG, Redeker AG, Peters RL. Long term follow-up studies of patients surviving fulminant viral hepatitis. Gastroenterology 1974;67:870–7.
119. Ferenci P, Lockwood A, Mullen K, et al. Hepatic encephalopathy – definition, nomenclature, diagnosis, and quantification: final report of the working party at the 11th World Congresses of Gastroenterology, Vienna, 1998. Hepatology 2002;35:716–21.
120. Blei AT, Cordoba J. Hepatic encephalopathy. Am J Gastroenterol 2001;96:1968–76.
121. Vaquero J, Chung C, Cahill ME, Blei AT. Pathogenesis of hepatic encephalopathy in acute liver failure. Semin Liver Dis 2003; 23:259–69.
122. Kugler CF, Taghavy A, Fleig WE, Hahn EG. Visual P300 in acute hepatic encephalopathy resulting from non-A, non-B fulminant hepatitis: analysis of the course before and after orthotopic liver transplantation. Z Elektroenzephalogr Elektromyogr Verwandt 1991;22:259–63.

123. Jalan R. Pathophysiological basis of therapy of raised intracranial pressure in acute liver failure. Neurochem Int 2005;47:78–83.
124. Blei AT. The pathophysiology of brain edema in acute liver failure. Neurochem Int 2005;47:71–7.
125. Clemmesen JO, Gerbes AL, Gulberg V, et al. Hepatic blood flow and splanchnic oxygen consumption in patients with liver failure. Effect of high-volume plasmapheresis. Hepatology 1999;29:347–55.
126. Bosman DK, Deutz NE, De Graaf AA, et al. Changes in brain metabolism during hyperammonemia and acute liver failure. Hepatology 1990;12:281–90.
127. Vaquero J, Fontana RJ, Larson AM, et al. Complications and use of intracranial pressure monitoring in patients with acute liver failure and severe encephalopathy. Liver Transpl 2005;11:1581–9.
128. Murphy N, Auzinger G, Bernel W, Wendon J. The effect of hypertonic sodium chloride on intracranial pressure in patients with acute liver failure. Hepatology 2004;39:464–70.
129. Belanger M, Desjardins P, Chatauret N, et al. Mild hypothermia prevents brain edema and attenuates up-regulation of the astrocytic benzodiazepine receptor in experimental acute liver failure. J Hepatol 2005;42:694–9.
130. Vaquero J, Rose C, Butterworth RF. Keeping cool in acute liver failure: rationale for the use of mild hypothermia. J Hepatol 2005;43:1067–77.
131. Jalan R, Olde Damink SW, Deutz NE, et al. Moderate hypothermia in patients with acute liver failure and uncontrolled intracranial hypertension. Gastroenterology 2004;127:1338–46.
132. Jalan R, Olde Damink SW, Deutz NE, et al. Moderate hypothermia prevents cerebral hyperemia and increase in intracranial pressure in patients undergoing liver transplantation for acute liver failure. Transplantation 2003;75:2034–9.
133. O'Grady JG, Langley PG, Isola LM, et al. Coagulopathy of fulminant hepatic failure. Semin Liver Dis 1986;6:159–63.
134. Andus T, Bauer J, Gerok W. Effects of cytokines on the liver. Hepatology 1991;13:364–75.
135. Chosay JG, Essani NA, Dunn CJ, Jaeschke H. Neutrophil margination and extravasation in sinusoids and venules of liver during endotoxin-induced injury. Am J Physiol 1997;272:G1195–200.
136. Tada K, Akamatsu K, Konno T, Ohta Y. Importance of measuring plasma thrombin-antithrombin III complex levels when using antithrombin III concentrate therapy in fulminant hepatic failure. Scand J Gastroenterol 1991;26:1188–92.
137. Pereira SP, Langley PG, Williams R. The management of abnormalities of hemostasis in acute liver failure. Semin Liver Dis 1996;16:403–14.
138. Brown JB, Emerick KM, Brown DL, et al. Recombinant factor VIIa improves coagulopathy caused by liver failure. J Pediatr Gastroenterol Nutr 2003;37:268–72.
139. Sewell RB, Hughes RD, Poston L, Williams R. Effects of serum from patients with fulminant hepatic failure on leucocyte sodium transport. Clin Sci 1982;63:237–42.
140. Panos MZ, Anderson AF, Payne N, et al. Human atrial natriuretic factor and renin–aldosterone in paracetamol induced fulminant hepatic failure. Gut 1991;32:85–9.
141. Quiros-Tejeira RE, Molina RA, Katzir L, et al. Resolution of hypophosphatemia is associated with recovery of hepatic function in children with fulminant hepatic failure. Transpl Int 2005;18:1061–6.
142. Chung PY, Sitrin MD, Te HS. Serum phosphorus levels predict clinical outcome in fulminant hepatic failure. Liver Transpl 2003;9:248–53.
143. George R, Shiu MH. Hypophosphatemia after major hepatic resection. Surgery 1992;111:281–6.
144. Pomposelli JJ, Pomfret EA, Burns DL, et al. Life-threatening hypophosphatemia after right hepatic lobectomy for live donor adult liver transplantation. Liver Transpl 2001;7:637–42.
145. Knochel JP. The clinical status of hypophosphatemia: an update. N Engl J Med 1985;313:447–9.
146. Schmidt LE, Dalhoff K. Serum phosphate is an early predictor of outcome in severe acetaminophen-induced hepatotoxicity. Hepatology 2002;36:659–65.
147. Baquerizo A, Anselmo D, Shackleton C, et al. Phosphorus ans an early predictive factor in patients with acute liver failure. Transplantation 2003;75:2007–14.
148. Record CO, Iles RA, Cohen RD, Williams R. Acid-base and metabolic disturbances in fulminant hepatic failure. Gut 1975;16:144–9.
149. Brown RS Jr, Lombardero M, Lake JR. Outcome of patients with renal insufficiency undergoing liver or liver-kidney transplantation. Transplantation 1996;62:1788–93.
150. Hanique G, Dugernier T, Laterre PF, et al. Significance of pathologic oxygen supply dependency in critically ill patients: comparison between measured and calculated methods. Intensive Care Med 1994;20:12–18.
151. Wendon JA, Harrison PM, Keays R, et al. Arterial-venous pH differences and tissue hypoxia in patients with fulminant hepatic failure. Crit Care Med 1991;19:1362–4.
152. Bihari DJ, Gimson AE, Williams R. Cardiovascular, pulmonary and renal complications of fulminant hepatic failure. Semin Liver Dis 1986;6:119–28.
153. Bonnet F, Richard C, Glaser P, et al. Changes in hepatic flow induced by continuous positive pressure ventilation in critically ill patients. Crit Care Med 1982;10:703–5.
154. Mackenjee MKR, Keipiela P, Cooper R, Coovadia HM. Clinically important immunological processes in acute and fulminant hepatitis, mainly due to hepatitis B virus. Arch Dis Child 1982;57:277–82.
155. Vaquero J, Blei AT. Cooling the patient with acute liver failure. Gastroenterology 2004;127:1626–9.
156. Ritter C, Reinke A, Andrades M, et al. Protective effect of N-acetylcysteine and deferoxamine on carbon tetrachloride-induced acute hepatic failure in rats. Crit Care Med 2004;32:2079–83.
157. Sheiner P, De-Majo W, Levy GA. Acetylcysteine and fulminant hepatic failure. Hepatology 1992;15:552–4.
158. Prescott LF, Illingworth RN, Critchley JA, et al. Intravenous N-acetylcystine: the treatment of choice for paracetamol poisoning. Br Med J 1979;2:1097–100.
159. Keays R, Harrison PM, Wendon JA, et al. Intravenous acetylcysteine in paracetamol induced fulminant hepatic failure: a prospective controlled trial. BMJ 1991;303:1026–9.
160. Harrison PM, Keays R, Bray GP, et al. Improved outcome of paracetamol-induced fulminant hepatic failure by late administration of acetylcysteine. Lancet 1990;335:1572–3.

161. Harrison PM, Wendon JA, Gimson AE, et al. Improvement by acetylcysteine of hemodynamics and oxygen transport in fulminant hepatic failure. N Engl J Med 1991;324:1852–7.
162. Krisper P, Haditsch B, Stauber R, et al. In vivo quantification of liver dialysis: comparison of albumin dialysis and fractionated plasma separation. J Hepatol 2005;43:451–7.
163. Lai WK, Haydon G, Mutimer D, Murphy N. The effect of molecular adsorbent recirculating system on pathophysiological parameters in patients with acute liver failure. Intensive Care Med 2005;31:1544–9.
164. Zhou XM, Miao JY, Yang Y, et al. Clinical experience with molecular adsorbent recirculating system (MARS) in patients with drug-induced liver failure. Artif Organs 2004;28:483–6.
165. Khuroo MS, Farahat KL. Molecular adsorbent recirculating system for acute and acute-on-chronic liver failure: a meta-analysis. Liver Transpl 2004;10:1099–106.
166. Sen S, Davies NA, Mookerjee RP, et al. Pathophysiological effects of albumin dialysis in acute-on-chronic liver failure: a randomized controlled study. Liver Transpl 2004;10:1109–19.
167. Emond JC, Aran PP, Whitington PF, et al. Liver transplantation in the management of fulminant hepatic failure. Gastroenterology 1989;96:1583–8.
168. O'Grady JG, Alexander GJM, Hayllar KM, Williams R. Early indicators of prognosis in fulminant hepatic failure. Gastroenterology 1989;97:439–45.
169. Tygstrup N, Ranek L. Assessment of prognosis in fulminant hepatic failure. Semin Liver Dis 1986;6:129–37.
170. Scotto J, Opolon P, Étévé J, et al. Liver biopsy and prognosis in acute liver failure. Gut 1973;14:927–33.
171. Bernuau J, Goudeau A, Poynard T, et al. Multivariate analysis of prognostic factors in fulminant hepatitis B. Hepatology 1986;6:648–51.
172. Christensen E, Bremmelgaard A, Bahnsen M, et al. Prediction of fatality in fulminant hepatic failure. Scand J Gastroenterol 1984;19:90–6.

6

CIRRHOSIS AND CHRONIC LIVER FAILURE

Stephen Hardy, M.D., and Ronald E. Kleinman, M.D.

DEFINITION

Cirrhosis is a form of chronic liver injury that represents an end stage of virtually any progressive liver disease. In fact, the process of cirrhosis may be superimposed on the primary liver disease and obscure the nature of the original insult. There is considerable overlap between the clinical features of the various forms of cirrhosis. In 1977, the World Health Organization defined cirrhosis as a diffuse liver process characterized by fibrosis and the conversion of normal liver architecture into structurally abnormal nodules [1]. Cirrhosis represents a dynamic state reflecting the competing processes of cell injury (necrosis), response to injury (fibrosis), and regeneration (nodule formation). Isolated hepatic fibrosis or nodule formation alone does not represent cirrhosis. As cirrhosis advances, it results in distortion of liver architecture and compression of hepatic vascular and biliary structures. These critical architectural changes lead to irregular delivery of nutrients, oxygen, and metabolites to various areas of the liver and may perpetuate the cirrhotic process even after the original insult has been brought under control or has ceased (Table 6.1).

CLASSIFICATION

Many schemes for categorizing cirrhosis have been proposed, including classification based on gross morphology, microscopic histology, etiology, and clinical presentation. Because cirrhosis is, in its later stages, a self-perpetuating process, the gross and microscopic appearances of the liver only occasionally reveal the nature of the original pathogenic process. The morphologic classification divides cirrhosis into micronodular, macronodular, and mixed types of cirrhosis. Micronodular cirrhosis (Figure 6.1) is characterized by thick fibrous septa separating small (<3 mm) hepatic nodules of almost uniform size [1]. The entire liver typically is involved. In its early stages, extrahepatic biliary atresia is micronodular. Cirrhosis associated with alcoholism is most commonly micronodular, although this is not always the case [2]. Macronodular cirrhosis (Figure 6.2) is characterized by nodules of varying sizes ranging from microscopic to 5 cm in diameter. These nodules are separated by irregular septa of varying width. Regenerative nodules larger than 2 cm in diameter are evidence that the cirrhotic process has persisted for at least several years. Macronodular cirrhosis is a feature of advanced Wilson's disease, α_1-antitrypsin deficiency, and chronic active hepatitis. This morphologic approach has not been proved to be a useful classification of cirrhosis because some patients have both micronodular and macronodular cirrhosis (characterized as "mixed" cirrhosis). In addition, micronodular cirrhosis can mature into either macronodular or mixed cirrhosis [3,4].

The histologic classification of cirrhosis emphasizes microscopic patterns of varying types of cirrhosis. Periportal (or biliary) cirrhosis is characterized by bile stasis, general reduction of bile ducts, and increased amounts of connective tissue within and extending from portal tracts (Figure 6.3). The lobular structure generally is preserved. This pattern often is ultimately seen in children with biliary atresia, cystic fibrosis, and progressive familial intrahepatic cholestasis I. In adults, it is seen in primary biliary cirrhosis, gallstone disease, and biliary and pancreatic neoplasms that result in biliary tree obstruction. Biliary cirrhosis presents clinically as severe cholestasis including jaundice, pruritus, dark urine, and light stools.

Postnecrotic cirrhosis, also known as *irregular* cirrhosis, is the result of chronic and recurrent liver cell destruction. It is usually not a result of a single necrotic injury [5] and is characterized by piecemeal necrosis that occurs at the interface between hepatocytes and portal tracts or fibrous septa. Bridging fibrosis, collapsed hepatic lobules, and regenerative nodules of varying sizes develop, usually producing micronodular cirrhosis (Figure 6.4). In children, postnecrotic cirrhosis may occur as a sequela of neonatal hepatitis. It is associated with chronic active hepatitis, caused by viral hepatitis B or C, or a result of autoimmune or idiopathic inflammation [6]. Drugs such as methyldopa or isoniazid, which may cause chronic active hepatitis, also can cause irregular or postnecrotic cirrhosis [7].

Cardiac cirrhosis develops as a result of centrilobular hemorrhagic necrosis. Increased right atrial pressure (resulting from congestive heart failure, congenital heart disease, or constrictive pericarditis) results in increased hepatic vein pressure and

Table 6.1: Diseases Resulting in Cirrhosis

Metabolic Disorders	*Biliary Malformations*
α_1-antitrypsin deficiency	Biliary atresia
Cystic fibrosis	Arteriohepatic dysplasia (Alagille syndrome)
Fructosemia	Intrahepatic biliary hypoplasia
Galactosemia	Choledochal cyst
Gaucher's disease	Congenital hepatic fibrosis
Glycogen storage disease, type III	Intrahepatic cystic biliary dilatation (Caroli's disease)
Glycogen storage disease, type IV	***Vascular lesions***
Hemochromatosis	Budd–Chiari syndrome
Indian childhood cirrhosis	Congestive heart failure
Histiocytosis X	Congestive pericarditis
Niemann–Pick disease, type D	Veno-occlusive liver disease
	Venacaval web
Tyrosinemia	***Toxic disorders***
Wilson's disease	Toxins found in nature (mushrooms)
Wolman's disease	
Infectious diseases	Organic solvents
Viral hepatitides	Hepatotoxic drugs
Cytomegalovirus	***Nutritional disorders***
Chronic hepatitis B +/− delta agent	Hypervitaminosis A
	Total parenteral alimentation
Chronic hepatitis C	Malnutrition
Herpes simplex virus	***Idiopathic diseases***
Rubella	Cerebrohepatorenal syndrome (Zellweger's)
Ascending cholangitis	
Neonatal sepsis	Familial intrahepatic cholestasis (Byler's disease)
Inflammatory diseases	
Autoimmune chronic active hepatitis	Neonatal hepatitis
Primary sclerosing cholangitis	

congestion of blood flow in centrilobular areas. Necrosis leads to formation of fibrous bridges between central veins. Vaso-occlusive disorders and the Budd–Chiari syndrome, which results from the congential or acquired obstruction of the hepatic veins, also result in cardiac cirrhosis.

Finally, various hepatic diseases that progress to cirrhosis have unique histologic patterns or findings. The cirrhosis of Wilson's disease and hemochromatosis is characterized by the presence of pigment (pigment cirrhosis) along with large regenerative nodules. The intracellular diastase-resistant inclusions of α_1-antitrypsin deficiency, seen with periodic acid–Schiff staining, and the gummas of hepatic syphilis identify these disorders even after fibrosis and cirrhosis are well established.

The histologic classification of cirrhosis is often unhelpful in clinical settings because so many cases of cirrhosis fail to fall distinctly into any specific pattern. Many forms of liver disease have specific histologic patterns early in disease, but as cirrhosis advances from early to late stages, these patterns merge, leaving these classifications confusing or unhelpful.

Grouping disorders that progress to cirrhosis by cause is helpful because it provides a framework for the diagnostic investigation of cirrhosis, provides a basis for prognosis, and forms a foundation for genetic counselling. Because several morphologic and histologic patterns often coexist in many disorders, this nosology may be the most clinically useful classification scheme (see Table 6.1).

The clinical classification of cirrhosis depends on the competing processes of liver destruction, fibrosis, and regeneration. If necrosis outpaces regeneration or repair, signs and symptoms of hepatocellular failure predominate. Failure of the liver to synthesize serum proteins and cofactors results in the appearance of ascites and coagulopathy. Inability of the liver to produce or secrete bile results in cholestasis, which is clinically evident as jaundice, pruritus, dark urine, and light stools. The accumulation of neurotoxic substances results in encephalopathy. Chronic active hepatitis and neonatal hepatitis are two examples of liver diseases often associated with primary hepatocellular failure. Primary biliary disease results in severe cholestasis, which may progress to biliary cirrhosis. This often is seen in infants with extrahepatic biliary atresia, or in older children with cystic fibrosis. If fibrosis and regeneration outpace necrosis, signs and symptoms of portal hypertension result. Hypersplenism may indicate the presence of portal hypertension, although life-threatening bleeding from esophageal varices may be the first presenting sign. Portal hypertension is described in detail in Chapter 7.

Often the cirrhotic process is silent or quiescent, in which case the term *compensated cirrhosis* is used. The patient is apparently healthy, and there are no signs or symptoms of liver disease. A detailed history provides no evidence of antecedent illness. There may be a large liver or palpable spleen, although this is not always the case. Biochemical tests may show mild increases in hepatic transaminase or alkaline phosphatase levels. Compensated cirrhosis is discovered in many patients during investigation of other often unrelated diseases, or as a result of family screening. Metabolic liver diseases such as α_1-antitrypsin deficiency or Wilson's disease often have a long compensated phase, during which liver disease is not suspected. Many cases of compensated cirrhosis, however, are cryptogenic.

As cirrhosis advances, eventually the clinical picture evolves to that of *decompensated cirrhosis*. Regardless of its cause, cirrhosis can result in failure to thrive, muscle weakness, fatigue, jaundice, edema, ascites, and steatorrhea. As with compensated cirrhosis, laboratory investigations may reveal elevated alkaline phosphatase, bilirubin, hepatic transaminase, and ammonia

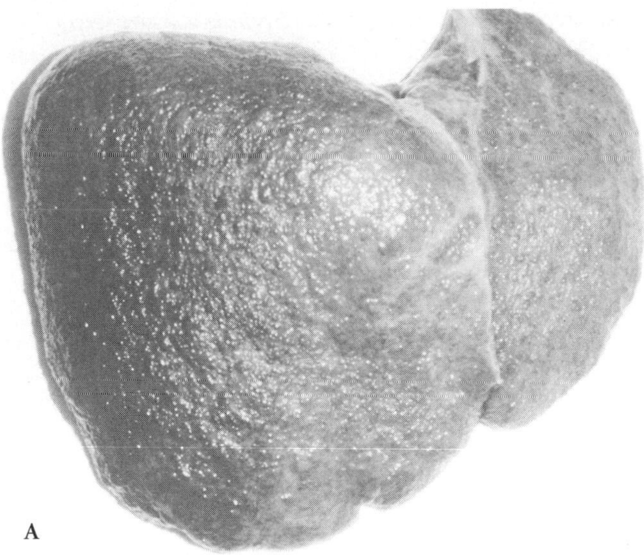

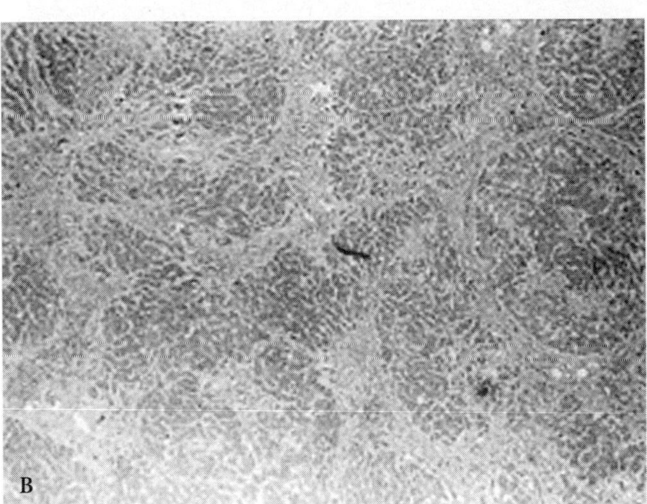

Figure 6.1. (**A**) Finely lobulated surface of the liver in micronodular cirrhosis. (**B**) Microscopic findings of micronodular cirrhosis include total destruction of hepatic architecture. Fibrous bands and regenerative nodules are prominent. (From Misiewicz JJ, Bartram CI, Cotton PB. Slide atlas of gastroenterology. London: Gower Medical Publishing, Ltd., 1987; with permission.)

levels. Hypersplenism also may be present. The distinction between compensated and decompensated cirrhosis often is based on the severity of clinical and laboratory findings and response to supportive medications.

PATHOPHYSIOLOGY

The response of the liver to injury is somewhat limited and stereotypic. Cell injury leads to cell death (necrosis), which is followed by scar formation (fibrosis) and, in some cases, nodule formation (regeneration). Cirrhosis is the result of these three processes.

Extracellular Matrix

The first step in the process that leads to cirrhosis is direct injury to the hepatocyte. This injury may occur as a result of almost any insult, including viral invasion, ischemia, and toxin exposure. After injury the parenchymal cells regenerate and replace the necrotic cell. This is associated with inflammation and deposition of additional extracellular matrix (ECM), including collagen. The cells responsible for intrahepatic fibrosis have not all been identified. The hepatic stellate cell is of high importance. Recently there has been interest in the identification of other, "nonresident" stem cells that might be involved in the process. It is unclear whether resident or extrahepatic stem cells become or differentiate into the nonparenchymal cells, such as

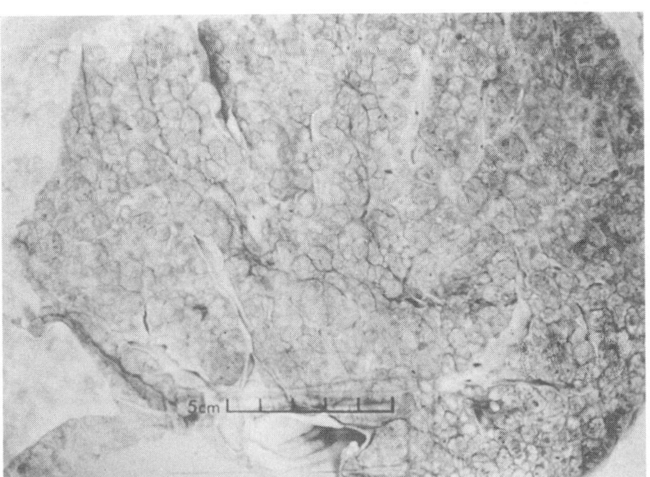

Figure 6.2. Large, irregular nodules typical of macronodular cirrhosis. (From Misiewicz JJ, Bartram CI, Cotton PB. Slide atlas of gastroenterology. London: Gower Medical Publishing, Ltd., 1987; with permission.)

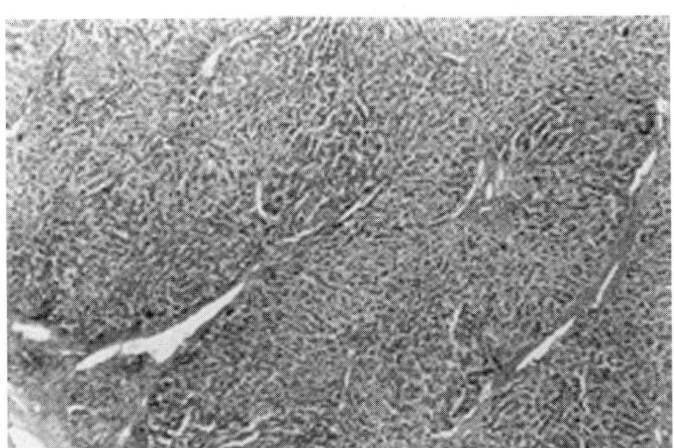

Figure 6.3. Periportal or biliary cirrhosis is characterized by fibrosis within and between portal tracts. Nodules are not present, and the general lobular structure is preserved. (Courtesy of Dr. Antonio Perez-Atayde.)

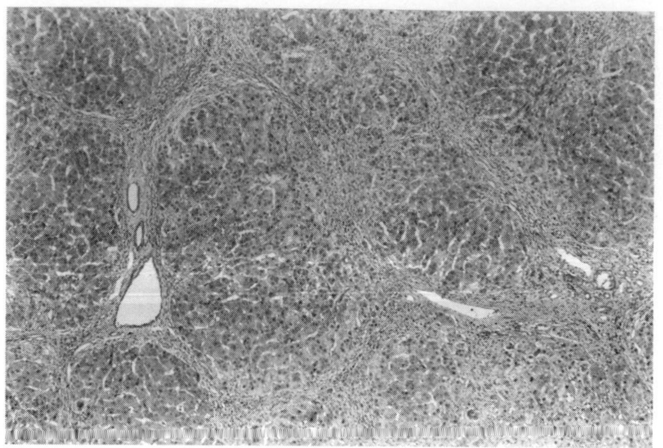

Figure 6.4. Postnecrotic or irregular cirrhosis is characterized by piecemeal necrosis and bridging fibrosis. Portal–portal and central-portal fibrotic bands and regenerative nodules of varying sizes are present. (Courtesy of Dr. Antonio Perez-Atayde.)

endothelial cells, hepatic stellate cells, and Kupffer cells, responsible for the fibrotic process. If stimulated by inflammatory cells or by various cytokines, hepatocytes and their supportive cells secrete an altered ECM. The ECM is vital to the survival and proper function of each cell; the ECM provides a stable environment within tissue compartments.

Extracellular matrix macromolecules can be divided into three distinct categories: collagens, proteoglycans, and glycoproteins [8]. Collagens are the most abundant protein in the ECM. Thirteen distinct types of collagens have been described. Types I, III, IV, V, and VI have been isolated from human liver tissue [9]. Proteoglycans are associated with basement membranes and appear to play a role in the regulation of cell permeability and cell proliferation [4,9]. Proteoglycans are composed of a protein linked covalently with at least one glycosaminoglycan [10]. In the liver, heparan sulfate is the most common glycosaminoglycan [11]. Glycoproteins serve to connect the ECM to the surrounding cells. Fibronectin and laminin are the most common glycoproteins in the liver. Both are complex multifunctional matrix proteins with multiple domains. Fibronectin (with at least ten different isoforms) mediates cellular adhesion to collagens [12], causes an increase in granulation tissue [13], and is a chemoattractant and growth factor for mesenchymal cells [14]. Laminin, a much-studied protein, also has several domains including receptors for collagen and epithelial cells [15,16]. Laminin acts on hepatocytes and regulates their growth and differentiation [17] and also plays a role in the organization of liver plates [18].

In cirrhosis, the ECM is altered qualitatively and quantitatively. In the normal liver, connective tissue proteins are seen along the basement membranes surrounding lymphatic and blood vessels, and around bile ducts. There is also scant collagen in the perisinusoidal space. The hepatocytes and greater part of the portal triads are virtually free of connective tissue. In cirrhosis, there are increased collagen types III and IV in the perisinusoidal space. The sinusoids are lined with a new basement membrane intimately associated with laminin and collagen type III [19]. In addition, collagen types IV, V, and VI increase eight- to tenfold; laminin increases threefold [10,18].

Extracellular matrix proteins that may control or contribute to fibrosis or regeneration continue to be described. Matrix metalloproteinase-2 is involved in ECM remodeling. It is expressed in myofibroblasts and may play a role in liver fibrosis. Recent studies have suggested that this enzyme may promote fibrogenesis. Active forms of matrix metalloproteinase-2 have been obtained from cultured myofibroblasts from the liver of patients with cirrhosis but are not found in specimens obtained from patients with no liver disease [20]. Investigators recently showed that alterations to the chemical composition or molecular structure of the liver ECM (in cell culture) are associated with specific changes in certain filament cytokeratins, demonstrating an intricate relationship between hepatocyte and ECM that can be disrupted in a pathologic state [21].

The altered proteins (mostly synthesized by hepatocyte stellate cells) are laid down at the space of Disse, and initially there is no effect on the function of the hepatocyte. As the collagen network becomes thicker, it becomes a barrier to the intimate interface between blood and hepatocytes and interferes with exchange of substances across the hepatocyte membranes. Laminin deposition increases along sinusoids and is related to the formation of a sinusoidal basement membrane [19,22]. This results in the so-called capillarization of sinusoids [23]. These altered sinusoids form conduits from portal to central veins, which shunt blood from the terminal portal veins and hepatic arteries to the central hepatic veins with little direct contact with hepatocytes. As the connective tissue network advances, connective tissue bands form, which run between portal triads or between portal triads and central veins. These septa may impede blood flow to entire hepatic lobules, resulting in further ischemic damage and cell dropout.

The reduction in the amount of viable, well-vascularized hepatic tissue leads to compensatory growth, or nodule formation. As hepatic nodules form, they increasingly impede blood flow to the lobules by direct compression of the hepatic arterial and venous blood flow. The cycle of necrosis, fibrosis, and nodule formation becomes self-sustaining and can persist independent of the initial insult.

Fibrogenesis

Although initially considered to be permanent, there is evidence suggesting that fibrosis is reversible, at least in some cases [24]. Experimentally induced fibrosis in rats has recently been shown to be reversible [25]. Some reversal of liver fibrosis has been seen in some liver diseases, such as chronic hepatitis C [24,26] and nonalcoholic steatohepatitis (NASH) [27]. Measuring the extent of liver fibrosis has been a vexing problem for clinicians treating patients with chronic liver disease.

Investigators have long sought to develop clinically relevant measures of hepatic fibrosis. The gold standard of these tests has been hepatic biopsy with its associated system for the scoring of hepatic fibrosis. These systems include the histology activity index (HAI: Knodell score) [28] with the Ishak modification [29], and the Metavir score [30]. The HAI system scores inflammatory activity from 0–18 by assessing periportal necrosis/inflammation, lobular necrosis and inflammation, and portal inflammation. Such biopsies, however, have considerable shortcomings. Liver biopsy, whether percutaneous or open, carries risks such as hemorrhage. Hepatic fibrosis is not a uniform process, and single biopsies may over- or underrepresent its extent. Furthermore, liver histology offers only a static picture of a dynamic process. For these reasons, liver histology may not correlate well with the prognosis of disease and liver function, and serial liver biopsies usually are not recommended as a means of following the progression of cirrhosis or fibrosis. Standard light microscopy might not sensitively identify early fibrosis. Immunohistochemical expression of matrix proteins such as laminin, fibronectin, and collagens III and IV may reveal early changes leading to cirrhosis, but even if such tests increase the sensitivity of biopsy interpretation greatly, percutaneous liver biopsy will remain overly invasive for frequent and routine analysis of ongoing liver disease.

Recently, biochemical assays for enzymes and metabolites associated with fibrogenesis have been developed. These may prove to be helpful in monitoring the progression of hepatic fibrosis, although their use in children has not yet been extensive. The aminoterminal extension peptide of type III procollagen (the serum procollagen III peptide [P3P]) is the most studied metabolite. As type III collagen is incorporated into the ECM, P3P is excised from procollagen III and can be recovered from the serum. P3P is found in higher than normal concentrations in acute liver disease, and it correlates with tests for hepatic necrosis such as alanine aminotransferase. Its level also is increased in patients with chronic liver disease and seems to correlate with fibrosis [31]. In one study, the level of P3P was increased in patients with active alcoholic liver disease. Significant correlations were seen between degree of P3P elevation and the extent of liver disease as measured by the Combined Clinical and Laboratory Index [32].

Serum laminin level also is elevated in patients with active fibrogenesis [33] and has been shown in some studies to correlate with the degree of portal hypertension [34,35]. More recent studies have not confirmed this association [36,37]. High levels of laminin correlate in a highly sensitive and specific way with the risk of severe complication in patients with cirrhosis and have been used to augment the Child criteria in cirrhosis [37]. Other macromolecules associated with fibrogenesis have been found in increased quantities in the serum of patients with fibrotic liver disease, including lysyl oxidase [38], prolyl-4-hydroxylase, hyaluronate, type IV collagen [33], and 7S collagen [31,39,40].

Although none of these tests has been applied to a pediatric population, they may prove to be valuable in the estimation of the activity of liver fibrogenesis in subjects of any age. P3P, for example, has been shown to have prognostic value in primary biliary cirrhosis [41]. A recent study found that a number of noninvasive tests might be helpful in correctly diagnosing cirrhosis. Of the 63 clinical, biochemical, radiographic, and endoscopic tests reviewed, serum hyaluronate and prothrombin index were the best overall predictors of cirrhosis [42].

Attempts are being made to treat liver fibrosis. The removal of the causative agent when possible is the first step in treating liver fibrosis and in some cases, may result in some reversal of the fibrotic process. In general, most treatments have not been widely applied or have not been tested in adults or children and thus are not used in children with progressive liver disease. Because inflammation is associated with the fibrotic process, anti-inflammatory medications such as corticosteroids have been used in patients with chronic liver disease. These drugs are especially effective in treating patients with autoimmune hepatitis [43]. Hepatic stellate cells (HSCs) are responsible for the excess production of ECM components, thus activation of HSC appears to be a key step toward the development of hepatic fibrosis. Inhibition of HSC activation has been of interest in reversing or preventing the development of hepatic fibrosis. Such treatments include the inhibition of transforming growth factor-β (TGF-β) [44], platelet-derived growth factor [44,45], and herbal extracts such as silymarin. Antioxidants such as vitamin E and silymarin protect hepatocytes from necrotic injury, inhibit hepatocyte stellate cell activation, and may result in decreased rates of fibrogenesis [46,47]. Antioxidants have been used with some success in patients with NASH [48]. Inhibition of the renin–angiotensin system has been shown to inhibit hepatocyte stellate cell activation and thus has been a target of antifibrotic therapy. Angiotensin II receptor antagonist therapy has been used with some success in the setting of NASH [49] and as a preventive measure after liver transplantation for hepatitis C [50]. Other experimental treatments include vasodilator therapy (prostaglandin-E$_2$ [PGE$_2$], used only in a rat model), the inhibition of collagen synthesis, and promotion of the degradation of collagen (urokinase-type plasminogen activators). Finally, it was demonstrated that extrahepatic bone marrow–derived stem cells reduced fibrosis in a rat model of induced liver injury [51]. The mechanism for improvement is not known, but such reports show the promise of potential new therapies in the future.

Regeneration

In the fully developed human liver, hepatocytes do not divide rapidly. Only 1 hepatocyte in 10,000–20,000 is dividing at any given time [52]. If stimulated, however, hepatocytes can proliferate rapidly. In response to insult by viral invasion, cirrhosis, ischemia, trauma, or partial hepatectomy, hepatocyte proliferation increases to replace lost cells. Hepatic regeneration is a complex process, highly regulated at the cellular level in an autocrine or paracrine manner by cytokines, some of which themselves are regulated by prostaglandins or by other cytokines. The highly regulated nature of hepatic regeneration is revealed by the observation in liver transplantation that the size of the donor organ may either expand or contract, according to the needs of the patient. Animal models of acute hepatocellular loss also show a prompt hepatocellular proliferation response [53]. Studies in the rat have shown that this proliferative response occurs if at least 10–20% of the hepatocytes are destroyed and that the response is proportional to the loss of viable hepatic mass [54]. The replacement of lost liver tissue is organized and synchronized, suggesting a high degree of regulation. Fausto and Mead [52] showed that proto-oncogenes are expressed in a sequential and regulated manner during liver regeneration. Regeneration requires not only the recruitment of new hepatocytes but also the restoration of the ECM.

Many hormones are known to influence the process of hepatic regeneration, including insulin, glucagon, growth hormone, adrenocorticotropic hormone (ACTH), vasopressin, cortisol, thyroxin, and estrogen. All of these can promote hepatic proliferation, but none appears to be the initiator of the process. The recent isolation and identification of specific cytokine hepatic growth factors has shed light on the initiation and control of hepatocyte proliferation as well as fibrogenesis.

Cytokines are glycoproteins, usually with a molecular mass of less than 80 kDa. Unlike the "classic" hormones, cytokines usually exert their effects in a paracrine or autocrine manner. Cytokines are produced in a variety of cells, including (but not limited to) lymphocytes, neutrophils, reticuloendothelial cells, fibroblasts, endothelial cells, and epithelial cells including hepatocytes. These peptide factors have become models for "contextual" peptide factors; that is, they have different effects on different cell types under various conditions. The liver is involved intimately with cytokines as a source, as a "target" organ, and as the site of cytokine clearance [55]. Interleukin-6 (IL-6), for example, is involved intimately with the hepatic acute phase response but also can play a role in hepatic regeneration. Epidermal growth factor (EGF), transforming growth factor-α (TGF-α) and TGF-β, hepatocyte growth factor (HGF), fibroblast growth factor (FGF), and IL-6 are the cytokines known to be important in the initiation and regulation of hepatic regeneration.

Epidermal growth factor is an important initiator of the hepatic regenerative response [56]. In association with insulin and glucagon, EGF promotes hepatocyte DNA synthesis [57]. Its action also is modulated by other hormones, including growth hormone, which enhances EGF expression, and estrogen, which inhibits EGF effect [58,59]. Intrahepatic EGF mRNA levels were increased 25-fold in one rat model of cirrhosis compared with noncirrhotic rats [60]. EGF has been shown to stimulate hepatic DNA synthesis in laboratory animals after partial hepatectomy, suggesting both the potential importance of this growth factor in regulating hepatic regeneration and its potentially therapeutic role in patients undergoing major hepatic resection [61].

Hepatocyte growth factor first was identified in 1985 as a serum substance (obtained from the serum of patients with fulminant hepatic failure [FHF]) that stimulates DNA synthesis in adult rat hepatocytes [62]. Its purification and analysis demonstrated that its identity was separate from other known growth factors [63–65]. Although not present in the serum of normal subjects, HGF is present in the serum of patients with acute and fulminant hepatitis. It is present in lower concentrations in the serum of patients with chronic hepatitis or cirrhosis and after partial hepatectomy. Furthermore, the serum level of HGF correlates with the level of hepatic coma [63] and, in the rat model, with the extent of hepatocellular necrosis [66]. These findings suggest that HGF is present in the blood in concentrations proportional to the loss of functional hepatic mass [67]. HGF also has been isolated from the ascitic fluid of cirrhotic patients [68]. Finally, interferon beta-2 has been shown to share immunologic identity with HGF and to compete with its receptor, regulating the hepatic response to HGF [69].

Transforming growth factor-α and TGF-β have been a focus of great interest. Although initially identified by its ability to transform cell lines in culture. TGF-α, a hepatocyte derived peptide, causes hepatocyte proliferation in vitro and is a physiologic regulator of hepatocyte regeneration [70]. TGF-α mRNA is associated with H3 histone mRNA, a marker of cell proliferative activity [71]. TGF-α and EGF bind to the same receptor, although TGF-α binds with much lower affinity. Nevertheless, TGF-α is more biologically active than EGF [72]. Serum TGF-α concentrations are elevated greatly in patients with cirrhosis, and these elevated levels correlate generally with the severity of disease as estimated by the Child–Pugh classification [73]. These findings suggest that TGF-α may play a role in the proliferative hepatic response.

Transforming growth factor-β is an inhibitor of epithelial cell lines (including hepatocytes) and a promoter of mesenchymal cell lines (such as fibroblasts and Ito cells). TGF-β is a negative regulator of hepatic regeneration [74]. It also is tied closely to fibrogenesis in liver disease, and it is thought to be a primary inducer of matrix protein synthesis in liver disease [75–77]. TGF-β mRNA is absent in normal livers; it is detectable in parenchymal and nonparenchymal cells in patients with liver disease [78]. TGF-β mRNA is associated with the appearance of serum P3P and procollagen I mRNA in hepatocytes and has been shown to stimulate collagen synthesis in human fibroblast cultures [71]. TGF-β is found in greatly increased levels in media obtained from activated human tonsillar T lymphocytes, which is known to stimulate collagen synthesis [79]. Inhibition of TGF-β synthesis prevents fibrosis in one experimental liver injury model [80]. Recent interest has been focused on the targets of TGF-β. Signals from TGF-β stimulate transmembrane receptor kinases to activate signaling intermediates called Smad proteins, which then modulate the transcription of target genes. The loss of the Smad3 receptor in mice is associated with a reduction in auto-induced TGF-β and a resistance to induced liver injury and fibrosis [81].

Fibroblast growth factor (endothelial cell derived) also is involved in hepatic embryogenesis as well as regeneration [82]. At high concentrations, paradoxically, it antagonizes the EGF-induced proliferative response and may act as a regulator of hepatic growth [83]. Intrahepatic levels of FGF mRNA have been found to be greatly elevated in rats with cirrhosis, suggesting that this growth factor may play an important part in the regenerative process [60].

Plasma IL-6 also plays a role in hepatocyte proliferation [69] as well as in the hepatic acute phase reaction, the maturation of hematopoietic stem cells, and the stimulation of B-cell immunoglobulin synthesis [84]. IL-6 also is found in elevated levels in patients with alcoholic hepatitis, suggesting that it may play a mediating role in the ongoing cell damage [85]. Kupffer cells, which make up 90% of the reticuloendothelial cells in the liver, are the source of IL-6. Kupffer cells are associated intimately with the hepatic regenerative response [86] and produce not only IL-6 but PGE_2, its regulator, as well [87].

The liver-derived insulin-like growth factors I and II also have been studied in patients with liver disease. Unlike HGF, their serum concentrations decrease with advancing liver disease, suggesting that serum levels of these proteins can reflect the residual capacity of liver function [88,89]. A recent study found that stimulation of insulin-like growth factor by injection of growth hormone correlated with severity of liver disease as estimated by the Child–Pugh score [90]. In patients with active alcoholic cirrhosis, insulin-like growth factor I levels correlate well with aminopyrine breath test values, but not with serum albumin or retinol binding protein levels [91]. Serum levels of insulin-like growth factor binding protein-3 also have been found to correlate with degree of liver dysfunction, especially hepatic synthetic capacity, in patients with cirrhosis [92]. Table 6.2 provides a summary of some cytokines known to be important in hepatic regeneration and fibrosis. Although the list of cytokines and chemokines that play a role in hepatocellular regeneration is expanding, there is currently no established consistent benefit from the use of these factors or their inhibitors in the treatment of progressive hepatic fibrosis in adults or children.

Table 6.2: Cytokines Associated with Hepatic Regeneration

Cytokine	*Source*	*Action*
Epidermal growth factor (EGF)	Salivary glands, Brunner's glands	Initiator of hepatic regenerative response. Stimulates hepatocyte DNA synthesis.
Hepatocyte growth factor (HGF)	Unknown	Stimulates hepatocyte DNA synthesis
Fibroblast growth factor (FGF)	Endothelial cells	Stimulates hepatocyte regeneration at low levels. High levels regulate epidermal growth factor EGF-induced proliferation.
Interleukin-6 (IL-6)	Kupffer cells	Promotes hepatocyte proliferation
Transforming growth factor-α (TGF-α)	Macrophage, hepatocyte	Promotes hepatic regeneration; also binds to EGF receptor
Transforming growth factor-β (TGF-β)	Hepatocytes	Inhibits epithelial cell proliferation, including hepatocytes; promotes mesenchymal cell proliferation. Primary inducer of matrix protein synthesis.

CLINICAL FEATURES OF CIRRHOSIS

The clinical presentation of cirrhosis depends on the cause of the primary liver disease as well as on the pace of progression of hepatocellular failure and fibrosis. Many children and adolescents present with findings discovered incidentally during routine physical examinations, or as a result of an investigation of an unrelated condition. In such patients, the cirrhosis is referred to as *latent* or *compensated.* In others, the discovery of chronic liver disease may be sudden and dramatic, such as with the onset of hematemesis, encephalopathy, ascites, or infection. If the signs and symptoms of cirrhosis are apparent and progressive, the term *decompensated* or *active* cirrhosis applies [93]. Finally some patients (usually adults) may never come to medical attention until cirrhosis is found at autopsy [94].

Cirrhosis is associated with a large number of specific findings, none of which, save growth failure, is unique to pediatric patients. It is rare to find all, or even a majority, of these signs in any particular patient, and some cirrhotic patients lack any obvious physical or laboratory evidence of their condition. Pediatric patients with cirrhosis or chronic liver disease also may present with signs of systemic illness such as failure to thrive, anorexia, easy fatigability, and muscle weakness. Nausea and vomiting may be present. Fever occasionally is present in decompensated cirrhosis. Jaundice may be present but is not always discernible by the patient or the patient's family.

Abdominal pain may be present and can be caused by peptic ulcer disease, gastritis, gastroesophageal reflux, gallstones, or, in acute hepatitis, the rapidly enlarging liver. Examination of the abdomen may reveal a large and tender liver, or one that is shrunken and nodular. The spleen may be enlarged, especially in the setting of portal hypertension. Ascites may be present and often is associated with hypoalbuminemia. Steatorrhea also may be present.

The encephalopathy of liver disease may be prominent, or it may present in subtle forms such as deterioration of school performance, depression, or emotional outbursts. A neurologic examination can reveal asterixis (rhythmic hand flapping on wrist extension), a prolonged relaxation phase of deep tendon reflexes, and a positive Babinski's sign. A history of epistaxis, hematemesis, and hematochezia may be related to the coagulopathy of liver disease or to portal hypertension with esophageal and rectal varices. Pallor may be present because of the anemia of chronic liver disease. Cyanosis and digital clubbing often are present and are related to chronic hypoxemia

Table 6.3: Physical Findings Associated with Chronic Liver Disease

Body Region	*Findings*
General	Poor growth, malnutrition, fever, muscle wasting
Skin and extremities	Jaundice, flushing or pallor, palmar erythema, spider angiomata, digital clubbing
Abdomen	Distention, caput medusa, ascites, larger tender liver or shrunken liver, large spleen, rectal varices
Central nervous system	Asterixis, positive Babinski's reflex, prolonged relaxation phase of deep tendon refluxes, mental status changes
Miscellaneous	Gynecomastia, testicular atrophy, feminization, delayed puberty

secondary to pulmonary–systemic collateral circulation and ventilation–perfusion mismatching. Skin and extremity changes include jaundice, cyanosis, and pallor. Skin flushing and spider angiomata also frequently are present in cirrhotic patients. Dupuytren's contracture is associated with longstanding cirrhosis but rarely is seen in childhood. Its pathophysiology may be related to the metabolism of hypoxanthine but is poorly understood [95]. Table 6.3 shows physical findings associated with chronic liver disease and cirrhosis.

Extrahepatic Manifestations of Cirrhosis and Chronic Liver Disease

Cirrhosis and chronic liver disease can affect virtually every organ system adversely. Data on the prevalence of extrahepatic manifestations of cirrhosis in children are limited. In the gastrointestinal tract, cirrhosis is associated with esophageal and gastric varices, which form as a consequence of portal hypertension. Hematemesis secondary to variceal bleeding may be the first clinical sign of cirrhosis. Bleeding from hemorrhoids, which arise from portosystemic shunting through the inferior mesenteric venous collateral system, is much less common. Chronic gastritis and peptic ulcer disease frequently are seen in patients with chronic liver disease. Excess gastric acid may be secreted in response to direct gastric stimulation by histidine, the decarboxylated form of histamine. In healthy people, histidine is cleared from the circulation by the liver; with hepatic disease, serum histidine levels are elevated [96]. Gastroesophageal reflux is seen in association with cirrhosis and probably is caused by increased intra-abdominal pressure secondary to ascites and hepatosplenomegaly. Diarrhea is a common manifestation of liver disease and may be a result of malabsorption, bile acid deficiency, or malnutrition.

Autopsy reports from adults show gallstones to be present in twice as many subjects (30%) with cirrhosis as those without cirrhosis or liver disease (13–16%) [97,98]. Unlike the general population, in whom cholesterol stones predominate, patients with cirrhosis develop pigment stones preferentially. The increased incidence of gallstones may be related to factors such as decreased bile acid pool, bile stasis, and estrogen-like feminization. The preponderance of pigment stones, however, suggests that hemolysis (secondary to hypersplenism) and abnormal bilirubin metabolism play a primary role in stone formation. Studies of biliary lipid secretion in patients with cirrhosis and gallstones show that the solubility of cholesterol in the bile of cirrhotic subjects is not less than that measured in normal subjects and that cirrhotics are not predisposed to the development of cholesterol stones [99].

The most important pulmonary manifestation of cirrhosis is the development of arteriovenous shunts, which lead to cyanosis and dyspnea. Hypoxemia is seen in up to 30% of children with cirrhosis and can be severe enough to cause cyanosis [100]. Digital clubbing often accompanies longstanding intrapulmonary shunting [101]. Attempts to locate discrete arteriovenous malformations have failed to show shunting of major or minor vessels. Rather, studies employing the use of radiolabeled, macroaggregated albumin show that the arteriovenous shunts are microscopic or at the level of pulmonary capillaries [100]. These shunts may result from increased vasodilation caused by vasoactive substances such as ferritin released from the diseased liver [101,102]. Other factors contributing to dyspnea include decreased pulmonary perfusion, portal–pulmonary collateral circulation, and decreases in lung vital capacity as a result of ascites or hepatosplenomegaly. Dyspnea related to cirrhosis can become disabling and may require hepatic transplantation. In some such patients, liver transplantation leads to reversal of the pulmonary disease.

Hematologic changes associated with cirrhosis include anemia and coagulopathy. The cause of the anemia of cirrhosis may be multifactorial and may include blood loss by way of the gastrointestinal tract, hemolysis secondary to hypersplenism, iron and folic acid deficiency secondary to malabsorption, malnutrition associated with malabsorption and anorexia, and dilution of red blood cell volume as a result of sodium and water retention [103]. The coagulopathy of cirrhosis also is multifactorial [104]. A decrease in the synthesis of liver-derived clotting proteins, including prothrombin and factors VII and IX, and increased consumption of clotting factors through increased fibrinolysis and disseminated intravascular coagulation (DIC) occur commonly in late, decompensated cirrhosis. Malnutrition, vitamin K deficiency, and thrombocytopenia as a result of hypersplenism may exacerbate the problem.

Cardiovascular manifestations of cirrhosis include a high cardiac output state related to changes in systemic vascular resistance, pulmonary vascular resistance, and hepatic blood flow (portal hypertension). The sustained increase in cardiac output results in the flushed appearance of patients with cirrhosis. Systemic hypertension is not common in cirrhosis.

Table 6.4: Stages of Encephalopathy

	Stage I	*Stage II*	*Stage III*	*Stage IV*
Mental status	Alert, oriented, irritable; sleep rhythm reversal	Lethargic, confused, combative	Stupor, marked confusion	Comatose; may respond to painful stimuli
Motor	Obeys commands; tremor, poor handwriting	Purposeful movement, grimacing, tremor	Local response to pain, intention tremor	Abnormal reflexes, no motor activity
Asterixis	Uncommon	Usually present	Present, if cooperative	Unable to elicit
Muscle tone	Normal	Increased	Increased	Increased or flaccid
Reflexes	Normal	Hyperreflexic	Hyperreflexic	Hyperreflexic/absent
Respiratory effort	Normal/ hyperventilation	Hyperventilation	Hyperventilation	Irregular
Eyes	Spontaneous opening	Open with verbal stimuli	Open with verbal stimuli	Sluggish or fixed; may open eyes with noxious stimuli
EEG	No gross abnormality	Grossly abnormal with slower rhythms	Theta activity and triphasic waves	Delta waves present

EEG, electroencephalogram.

Skin manifestations of chronic liver disease include spider angiomata and palmar erythema. Spider angiomata are easily recognizable as small, raised, dark lesions with radially distributed convoluted vascular branches. They arise because of vasoactive substances such as estradiol [105] in the circulation of patients with cirrhosis. Although it is not unusual to have several spider angiomata, the presence of more than five in the body region drained by the superior vena cava is abnormal and is suggestive of cirrhosis. Palmar erythema, a well-recognized sign of cirrhosis, is not specific to cirrhosis but is seen in other conditions associated with increased cardiac output or altered sex hormone metabolism [106]. Caput medusae may also be present. This refers to prominent abdominal wall veins seen in patients with portal venous hypertension. Nail changes characterized by horizontal white bands (Muehrcke's nails) may be seen in cirrhosis or in other conditions resulting in hypoalbuminemia [107].

Endocrine manifestations of cirrhosis result from failure of the liver to conjugate or metabolize hormones and include diabetes mellitus, which may present as subtle hyperinsulinemia without overt signs; syndrome of inappropriate secretion of antidiuretic hormone, presenting as hyponatremia; and feminization, including gynecomastia (benign proliferation of the glandular tissue of the male breast) and decreased axillary hair [108]. Gynecomastia may be caused by increased production of androstenedione and the increased conversion of estrone to estradiol [109]. Delayed puberty is common in children with chronic liver disease. In the mature adolescent, decreased libido, decreased facial hair, and impotence are caused by reduced testosterone synthesis in the liver [110].

The neurologic manifestations of chronic liver disease are grouped into stages as shown in Table 6.4. Changes in consciousness include hypersomnia, reversal of sleep pattern, apathy, slowed speech, decreased spontaneous movement, and eventually coma. Personality changes commonly seen in chronic liver disease include irritability, inability to cooperate, and childishness. These personality changes can be normal reactions to chronic disease in children, and their true cause may not be understood until frank encephalopathy is present. Intellectual deterioration with slight or gross confusion may be present. Focal defects in visual spatial skills also may appear, even if confusion is not present. Tests of constructional apraxia such as writing difficulty or the Reitan trail-making test may be difficult to administer if the child is at too early a developmental stage.

The most characteristic sign of central nervous system (CNS) dysfunction is asterixis, a flapping tremor that is demonstrated if the patient's arms are outstretched and wrists are hyperflexed. The tremor is absent at rest and present during voluntary movement. Asterixis also is seen in uremia, congestive heart failure, and respiratory failure. Deep tendon reflexes may be exaggerated in early encephalopathy, but in late stages the muscles become flaccid and the reflexes disappear. Hyperventilation suggests an extremely poor prognosis.

The deficits in immune function in patients with cirrhosis result in increased susceptibility to bacterial and mycobacterial infections, resulting in an increased rate of pneumonia [111] and spontaneous bacterial peritonitis (SBP). These deficits include abnormalities of reticuloendothelial phagocyte activity [112–114], opsonization [115], serum chemoattractant activity [116], serum complement levels including C2, C3, and C4 [117–119], and blood monocyte proliferative activity [120]. If portal hypertension is present, the patient is susceptible to prolonged and frequent bacteremia [121,122], which is important in the pathogenesis of SBP.

Renal and fluid complications often seen in cirrhosis include hypokalemia, which may be a result of potassium loss through vomiting, diarrhea, diuretic use, or secondary hypoaldosteronism.

Nutritional manifestations of cirrhosis include malnutrition, anorexia, malabsorption, steatorrhea, hypoalbuminemia, and fat-soluble vitamin deficiencies. Malnutrition is a common complication of liver disease, especially if the onset of liver disease is in infancy [123]. Standard weight and height values underestimate the extent of malnutrition in children; the triceps skinfold thickness is a more accurate assessment of a patient's nutritional status [124]. The poor nutritional status of children with chronic liver disease may result from poor caloric intake, which may be caused by anorexia or the general malaise that can accompany liver disease. Chin et al. [125] showed that in a group of 27 children awaiting orthotopic liver transplantation, mean protein-energy intake was only 70% of the recommended amount. In addition, patients with tense ascites or with hepatosplenomegaly may experience early satiety. Failure of linear growth often can be observed in children with advanced liver disease [126]. Malabsorption of ingested foods, especially fats, also is common in advanced liver disease. Deficiencies of fat-soluble vitamins can exacerbate other complications of cirrhosis, such as coagulopathy.

EVALUATION

Evaluation of a patient with liver dysfunction and suspected cirrhosis should focus on determining both the cause and the stage of liver disease. Table 6.5 lists the diagnostic tests that should be considered in evaluating a child with liver disease. Serologic testing for infectious diseases should include screens for hepatitis B and C. In appropriate clinical situations (fever in the setting of previous biliary tree surgery), bacterial cultures of blood and possibly liver tissue should be obtained.

Tests for metabolic liver disease should include quantitation of the serum α_1-antitrypsin level with determination of levels of protease inhibitor ("π-type"), fasting blood sugar (glycogen storage disease), urinary reducing substances (galactosemia), serum amino acids with urinary organic acids (tyrosinemia), serum iron, and iron binding capacity and ferritin (hemochromatosis), as well as the sweat chloride test (for cystic fibrosis). The initial evaluation for Wilson's disease should include serum copper, serum ceruloplasmin, a 24-hour urine collection for copper, and a slit-lamp ophthalmologic exam. Screens for autoimmune inflammatory disease include the erythrocyte sedimentation rate, anti–smooth muscle antibody, antimitochondrial antibody, anti–liver-kidney-microsomal antibody, and antinuclear antibody. Screening for ingested toxins such as acetaminophen should be done if appropriate.

An abdominal ultrasound examination aids in the evaluation of gallstones, choledochal cyst, and Caroli's disease (cystic dilation of the intrahepatic biliary tree). The anatomy and blood flow of the hepatic arterial and venous system also should be evaluated. In infants, in whom the consideration of extrahepatic biliary atresia is paramount, a biliary scintiscan should be done. In patients with suspected extrahepatic biliary tree obstruction, endoscopic retrograde cholangiopancreatography may be considered. The timing of liver biopsy in the investigation of suspected cirrhosis in children remains a matter of clinical judgment. A biopsy may be critical to confirm the presence of cirrhosis suspected on clinical grounds, or if the investigations outlined here fail to reveal the cause of the chronic liver disease.

Table 6.5: Diagnostic Tests in Chronic Liver Disease and Cirrhosis

Disorder	*Diagnostic Test*
Infections	
HBV	HBsAg, E antigen/antibody, HBV DNA
HCV	HCV antibody, HCV RNA
CMV	CMV serology, urine for CMV antigen
EBV	EBV serology, heterophile
Bacterial cholangitis	Blood and liver tissue culture
Autoimmune chronic active hepatitis	Sedimentation rate, ANA, anti–smooth muscle antibody, antimitochondrial antibody, anti–liver-kidney-microsomal antibody
α1-antitrypsin deficiency	Serum α1-antitrypsin level, Pi type
Glycogen storage disease	Lactic acid, fasting blood sugar, uric acid, liver and muscle tissue enzyme level
Galactosemia	Urinary non–glucose reducing sugar, red blood cell galactose-1-phosphate uridyl transferase level
Tyrosinemia	Serum amino acid levels, urine organic acids
Hemochromatosis	Serum iron TIBC, ferritin
Cystic fibrosis	Sweat chloride test, genotype analysis
Toxic ingestion	Toxic screen, serum acetaminophen level
Wilson's disease	Serum copper, serum ceruloplasmin, 24-hour urinary collection for copper, slit-lamp exam, liver copper concentration

ANA, antinuclear antibodies; CMV, cytomegalovirus; EBV, Epstein–Barr virus; HBsAg, hepatitis B surface antigen; HBV, hepatitis B virus; HCV, hepatitis C virus; TIBC, total iron-binding capacity.

Continuing Assessment and Prognosis in Cirrhosis

An accurate and informative test of liver function should indicate early in the patient's course whether irreversible and potentially fatal changes have occurred. In addition, it should pose no risk to the patient. The standard measurements of hepatic function involve a number of tests, few of which actually measure liver function. Most available tests have poor predictive value until almost complete liver failure has occurred, and none is specific for patients with cirrhosis. The advent of effective immunosuppression and improvements in surgical technique have made hepatic transplantation a widely used procedure for children with end-stage liver disease. With these advancements, liver function tests have taken on new importance. Patients with various complications, especially grade IV encephalopathy, have poor posttransplantation prognoses. Weight and age also are important factors for successful transplantation and should be monitored. Standard measurements of liver function (such as tests of hepatocellular injury, excretion of bilirubin, and measurement of hepatic synthetic function) do not provide helpful prognostic evaluation in most patients.

The hepatic transaminases, aspartate and alanine aminotransferase, are sensitive indicators of hepatocellular injury [127]. These proteins are intracellular enzymes normally present in low concentrations in the systemic circulation. They are released from the hepatocyte to the circulation with hepatocellular necrosis. High transaminase levels suggest acute hepatocellular disease, whereas moderate elevations suggest chronic liver disease [128]. In FHF, decreasing or low transaminase levels can herald complete destruction of the liver or demonstrate liver recovery. Elevation of the level of aspartate aminotransferase is not specific for liver disease. Cardiac disease (myocardial infarction, pericarditis, myocarditis), muscle disease (muscular dystrophy, myositis), and hemolysis (hemolytic anemia or red cell injury caused by traumatic phlebotomy) can cause elevations of serum aspartate aminotransferase levels. The alanine aminotransferase level, however, is more specific. The most serious shortcomings of measurement of serum transaminase levels are that it has no prognostic value and does not provide a true quantitative measure of liver function or synthetic capacity. As liver disease of any cause advances, transaminase levels may remain elevated or may be near normal until complete liver destruction has occurred.

Hyperbilirubinemia may be associated with hepatocellular dysfunction, with obstruction of bile flow, or with extrahepatic diseases such as hemolytic anemia. In obstructive biliary disease, serum alkaline phosphatase and 5′-nucleotidase usually are elevated along with bilirubin, because these enzymes are localized in the cellular membranes of canalicular cells [129]. In the hepatic disorders of childhood, these tests generally have poor prognostic value; that is, although greatly elevated levels may be associated with poor prognosis, mildly elevated levels provide no reassurance that there is not serious and progressive liver disease.

The liver metabolizes various substances by way of the hepatic microsomal systems. Tests using exogenous substrates have been developed to quantify microsomal function. Substrates used include bromsulphalein, aminopyrine, and caffeine. Bromsulphalein is taken up by, and conjugated in, the hepatocyte and then secreted into bile. The standard bromsulphalein test consists of a slow intravenous infusion followed by a blood sample drawn 45 minutes after infusion. This test may be useful in assessing liver dysfunction in the absence of jaundice. Because of the cost, inconvenience, and occasional severe adverse side effects, however, the bromsulphalein clearance test is no longer used [130]. The aminopyrine breath test employs aminopyrine labeled with radioactive carbon (^{14}C or ^{13}C) and measures $^{14}CO^2$ (carbon dioxide) or $^{13}CO^2$, respectively, as a result of hepatic demethylation of aminopyrine [131,132]. Studies in adults with alcoholic liver disease showed that decreases in labeled CO^2 production after the administration of aminopyrine were associated with increased mortality rates, although it was no more sensitive than serum levels of aspartate aminotransferase or albumin [133]. The aminopyrine breath test has not been used widely in children because the radioactive ^{14}C label is unsuitable for use in children and the ^{13}C label is expensive and cumbersome to measure. There is no consensus as to whether the results of the aminopyrine breath test are representative of generalized liver function or only reflect the hepatic microsomal mixed-function oxidase enzyme system.

Caffeine is metabolized almost exclusively by the P448 system of the liver [134]. There is high bioavailability after an oral dose, and saliva can be used as a test fluid for caffeine clearance [135], making the test relatively noninvasive. There is reduced caffeine clearance in cirrhotic patients in comparison with healthy controls. As in the aminopyrine breath test, it is unclear whether this test is a measure of hepatic microsomal activity alone or a broader test of liver function.

Investigations that reflect hepatic synthetic capacity are better predictors of survival. Hypoalbuminemia and clotting factor deficiencies have been associated with liver failure, and it has been suggested that decreased synthesis of these proteins by injured hepatocytes is responsible for these deficiencies. Post and Patek [136] showed that in patients with ascites, a serum albumin level of less than 2 g/dL was associated with a poor prognosis. Further studies have shown, however, that serum albumin concentrations alone are not reliable indicators of liver function or of prognosis [137]. This is because they reflect albumin distribution and degradation as well as liver-derived synthesis. Because albumin has a serum half-life of 21 days, serum levels often do not represent current albumin production. This is particularly true in the presence of ascites. Albumin is a component of ascitic fluid, and serum albumin slowly equilibrates with albumin in the ascitic fluid. The liver supplies essentially the entire intravascular pool of albumin and, with progressive ascites, an increasingly large extravascular albumin pool as well. Measures of albumin synthetic rates in patients with hypoalbuminemia and ascites have shown that such patients may have normal, decreased, or increased rates of albumin synthesis [138]. Liver disease often is associated with malabsorption, which can result in serious undernutrition; this alone may result in hypoalbuminemia [139].

Because of their short half-lives, serum clotting factors have been studied as indices of liver function, especially in acute settings. It generally is agreed that increased prothrombin time unresponsive to vitamin K implies poor hepatic synthetic capacity and decompensated hepatocellular disease. Because of its short half-life (6 hours), factor VII has been evaluated as a prognostic indicator in acute liver failure. Although some studies have shown that patients with extremely low factor VII levels have less chance of survival [140], other studies have failed to separate survivors from nonsurvivors based on factor VII levels alone [141]. As is often the case, single determinations of factor VII levels are not as helpful as serial determinations over time. Biland et al. [142] measured 20 coagulation parameters in 144 patients with various liver diseases and found that patients with low levels of factors V, VII, and XIII or plasminogen were likely to die in liver coma, although there were survivors in each of these groups. Studies of serum clotting factor activities are confounded by alterations in the degradation rates of the proteins being studied. The presence of DIC, for example, in some patients aggravates the clotting factor deficiency resulting from liver disease. Furthermore, all such studies have been done in subjects with advanced or fulminant liver disease. The prognostic value of clotting factor levels in early or milder forms of liver disease is not known. Isolated changes in the serum concentration of liver-derived proteins are nonspecific (changes may reflect extrahepatic disease) and insensitive (changes may lag behind changes in protein synthesis rates).

There have been few studies of prognostic factors in patients with chronic liver disease. One study analyzed, retrospectively, 162 clinical, laboratory, and histologic variables for prognostic value using log-rank analysis. A model was formed using eight variables with significant prognostic effect. These variables included age, gender, prothrombin time, acetylcholinesterase, and four histologic variables: the number of efferent veins in parenchymal nodules, the number of eosinophils in the liver parenchyma, the extent of focal liver cell necrosis, and the extent of an inflammatory response in the liver connective tissue [143]. A study such as this, conducted in an aged population, may not apply directly to a pediatric population. For example, some children undergo liver transplantation without undergoing a liver biopsy.

A similar attempt was made by Malatack et al. [144] to model prognosis for survival in children with liver disease. In this study, 216 children were evaluated for liver transplantation. Fifty-five percent of these received hepatic transplantation; another 25% died while awaiting an appropriate organ. Seventy variables obtained during transplantation evaluation were recorded. Of these, 23 were found to have prognostic significance. This number was reduced by eliminating those that gave redundant information, such as prothrombin time and partial thromboplastin time, and by eliminating those such as blood pH and serum calcium that are altered easily by therapeutic interventions. The four variables with the highest proportional risk – decreased serum cholesterol level, increased indirect bilirubin level, partial thromboplastin time prolonged by more than 20 seconds, and a positive history of ascites – were placed in a multiplicative exponential model, and this model was used to develop survival curves predictive of a patient's probability of survival over a given time [144]. A review of the model can be seen in Table 6.6. Prospective testing of this, or of any other proposed model, is necessary before it is employed in a regional organ allocation system.

Table 6.6: Prognostic Scores for Risk of Death from Chronic Liver Disease in Children*

Weighting Factor	*Variable*
+15	If cholesterol <100 mg/dL
+15	If positive history of ascites
+13	If indirect bilirubin >6 mg/dL
+11	If indirect bilirubin is 3–6 mg/dL
+10	If PTT is prolonged >29 seconds

PTT, partial thromboplastin time.

*Total score of 0–28 places patient in low-risk group (<25% risk of death within 6 months); score of 28–39 is associated with moderate-risk (25–75% risk of death within 6 months); score greater than 39 is associated with high risk (>75% of death within 6 months). From Malatack et al. [144].

MANAGEMENT OF THE CHRONIC COMPLICATIONS OF CIRRHOSIS

In many patients, the chronic complications of cirrhosis can be prevented, or at least ameliorated, by early detection. The physician must carefully and compulsively monitor patients with cirrhosis, even if it appears to be compensated. Ascites, bleeding, infection, and encephalopathy are serious and occasionally life threatening in patients with advancing liver disease.

Ascites

The development of ascites is one of the most common complications of cirrhosis. Although at first it may be subtle or undetectable, it eventually becomes incapacitating, limiting a patient's respiratory effort or mobility by sheer volume and mass. This accumulation of fluid represents a breakdown of intravascular volume homeostasis. Starling [145] proposed that fluid movement between blood and tissue is controlled by capillary hydrostatic pressure and plasma colloid osmotic pressure. Two important factors in ascites formation thus are portal venous pressure (which directly affects hydrostatic pressure in the liver) and plasma colloid oncotic pressure. Both are controlled by the integrated relationship of cardiac output, renal function, natriuresis, arterial vascular resistance, venous flow, albumin synthesis, and hepatic wedge pressure. Arginine vasopressin, the renin–aldosterone–angiotensin system, and sympathetic nervous system activity are the principle regulators of this integrated system that supports intravascular volume homeostasis. Portal hypertension is key to the development of ascites. Patients with liver disease but without portal hypertension do not develop ascites [146]. A portal pressure of greater than 12 mm Hg in adults is the threshold pressure above which ascites or edema might occur and below which it rarely arises [146,147].

Patients with cirrhosis and ascites have abnormal renal sodium retention. Total body sodium is dependent on the balance between sodium intake, sodium excreted in the urine, and the small and relatively fixed nonrenal sodium loss. That sodium plays an important role in the formation and maintenance of ascites is made clear by the observation that sodium restriction with or without natriuresis may result in improvements in sodium retention [148]. Sodium retention is an early change in renal function seen in patients with cirrhosis and can have prognostic importance [149]. Adult cirrhotics with a baseline urine sodium concentration of less than 10 mmol/d have a shorter median survival time than those with higher levels of urine sodium [150]. A subtle and variable vasoconstriction of the renal circulation also commonly is found in patients with cirrhosis and ascites [151].

Competing theories about the pathogenesis of ascites in patients with cirrhosis have attempted to incorporate normal and abnormal aspects of renal blood flow and sodium balance, as well as observed responses to stimuli such as fluid challenges. These theories are considered briefly here.

Underfilling Hypothesis

The primary abnormality in the "underfilling" hypothesis is increased hepatic sinusoidal pressure, which leads to a cascade of events resulting in fluid retention and ascites formation. Increased sinusoidal pressure results in elevated portal venous pressure and in increased splanchnic volume, which causes decreased systemic vascular resistance and decreased "effective" plasma volume. This is "sensed" by the plasma renin, aldosterone, norepinephrine, and arginine vasopressin feedback loops. Avid retention of sodium and water results, leading to the accumulation of ascites [152]. Increased sinusoidal pressure also leads to increased formation of hepatic lymph, which enters the abdominal cavity directly. If the observed increased serum levels of renin and aldosterone are a result of decreased effective plasma volume, repletion of the plasma volume should reverse ascites accumulation. In fact, rapid expansion of vascular volume by albumin infusion or by peritoneovenous shunting leads to suppression of serum renin, aldosterone, arginine vasopressin, and norepinephrine activities. In some patients with ascites, however, repletion of central volume and suppression of aldosterone activity do not lead to diuresis or to reversal of ascites accumulation. Furthermore, hepatic wedge pressure does not always decrease during diuresis [153,154]. It also has been observed that some patients with ascites have increased plasma volume, and inhibition of aldosterone secretion by aminoglutethimide does not always induce diuresis.

Overflow Hypothesis

The inadequacies of the underfill hypothesis prompted the speculation that inappropriate renal sodium and water retention is the primary abnormality in the pathogenesis of ascites: the "overflow" hypothesis of ascites formation. The triggering event for this primary abnormality is not known, although a hepatorenal reflex has been sought [155]. This postulated (but not proved) increased sodium and water retention would result in increased sinusoidal pressure "upstream." Experimental models support certain aspects of the overflow hypothesis. For example, in experimental animal models of cirrhosis, renal sodium and water retention preceded ascites formation [156]. The retention of renal sodium also preceded the development of hypoalbuminemia [157]. Sodium retention continued even after peritoneovenous shunts were created to avoid portal hypertension [158].

The failure to identify the agent or system primarily responsible for water and sodium retention mitigates support for the overflow hypothesis. Aldosterone usually is considered the salt-retaining hormone associated with ascites [159]. The metabolism of aldosterone is related directly to hepatic blood flow, which in portal hypertension and decompensated cirrhosis, is decreased. The aldosterone level, however, is not elevated consistently in patients with cirrhosis [160]. Intrahepatic baroreceptors [161] and atrial natriuretic factor also have been investigated as the primary abnormalities in ascites associated with cirrhosis. Patients with ascites and peritoneovenous shunts have an intact atrial natriuretic factor response to intravascular expansion, suggesting that this hormone does not have a primary role in ascites formation either [162]. In addition, the observation that the renin–angiotensin–aldosterone and α adrenergic sympathetic systems are activated in decompensated cirrhosis argues against the overflow hypothesis. These hormonal systems should be suppressed, not activated, with sodium retention and volume expansion [163,164].

Peripheral Arterial Vasodilation Hypothesis

Schrier et al. [165] have noted that patients with advanced cirrhosis and renal sodium and water accumulation have peripheral vasodilation with decreased arterial blood pressure as well as increased cardiac output, and they suggested that peripheral arterial vasodilation is the initiating event of ascites formation. The fact that patients with cirrhosis are prone to development of arteriovenous shunts implies the presence of vasoactive hormones not yet identified. It long has been known that patients with arteriovenous fistulas unassociated with cirrhosis have peripheral vasodilation and renal sodium retention [160]. The peripheral arterial vasodilation theory of ascites formation predicts that sodium and water retention in response to peripheral vasodilation increases plasma volume enough to cause ascites formation but not enough to totally refill the enlarged vascular compartment. Therefore the volume-control hormones such as arginine vasopressin, renin, aldosterone, and norepinephrine are not suppressed. Evidence supporting this theory includes the observation that the blockade of endogenous vasoconstrictor systems in patients with cirrhosis and ascites causes arterial hypotension, showing that these systems contribute to the maintenance of arterial pressure [166,167]. The administration of vasodilators to patients with cirrhosis without ascites can trigger sodium retention and ascites formation [168].

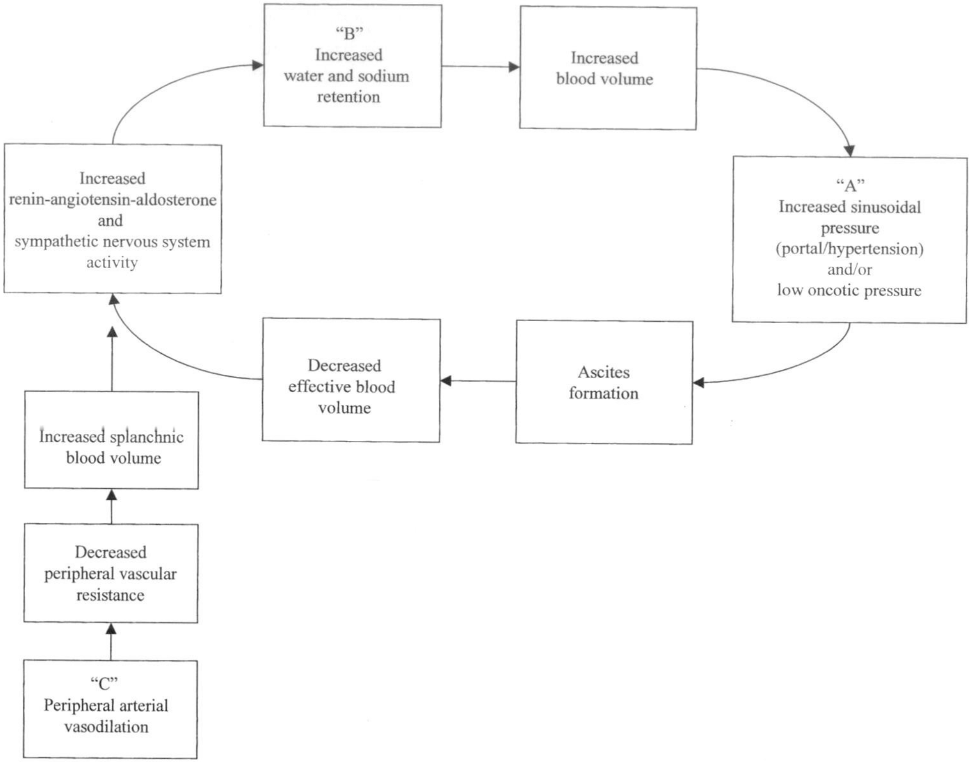

Figure 6.5. Pathophysiology of ascites formation. The "underfill" theory (**A**) states that ascites formation is primarily caused by increased hepatic sinusoidal pressure and low serum oncotic pressure, which leads directly to ascites formation and secondary water and sodium retention. The "overflow" theory (**B**) stresses the primary role of abnormal sodium and water retention, which leads to secondary ascites accumulation. The "peripheral vasodilation" theory (**C**) emphasizes the importance of peripheral arterial vasodilation, which results in decreased effective blood volume and increased sodium and water retention.

A number of factors have been implicated in the generation of vasodilation in patients with ascites. Portosystemic collaterals, which result in portocaval shunts, may help explain the lowered systemic vascular resistance [169,170]. However, circulating factors are likely to play a more substantial role in the altered vasodilation seen in cirrhotics. Glucagon, substance P, and prostaglandins have all been studied in patients with cirrhosis and ascites. Nitric oxide (NO), a potent vasodilator, has emerged as an important mediator of vasodilation in patients with cirrhosis. NO synthesis has been found to be higher in patients with cirrhosis than in controls [171]. In animal models, the inhibition of NO synthesis results in increased systemic vascular resistance [172,173]. Human data have shown that the increased levels of NO in cirrhotic patients appear to result from elevated levels of endotoxin that have been measured in their splanchnic circulation [174]. It appears that endotoxin is absorbed in the GI tract but is less efficiently cleared because of decreased reticuloendothelial cell function in cirrhosis [171,175].

Other secondary factors may play a role in ascites formation. Floras et al. [164] demonstrated that increased norepinephrine concentrations in patients with cirrhosis and ascites are caused by increased central sympathetic outflow. This may play a primary role in fluid retention in patients with cirrhosis. The roles of the catecholamines, atrial natriuretic factor, and antidiuretic hormone, however, have not been determined. Cirrhosis also is associated with diminished albumin synthesis. A low level of plasma albumin can result in low plasma oncotic pressure, which leads to changes in fluid exchange between plasma and extravascular fluid such that ascites formation is favored. These various models of ascites pathogenesis are not necessarily mutually exclusive. Early overflow secondary to renal sodium retention may initiate the process; in later phases, diminished effective plasma volume with its accompanying hormonal changes may predominate. Figure 6.5 combines the various hypotheses regarding the formation of ascites into one model.

The onset of ascites may be slow and insidious, or its appearance may be rapid. Sudden onset of ascites is associated with an acute insult to the liver such as hemorrhage, shock, infection, or occlusion of the portal vein. Slowly progressive liver failure is associated with the insidious onset of ascites.

The presentation of ascites in children may differ from that in adults. Accumulation of ascites is associated less frequently with peripheral edema in children than in adults. The first indication of ascites formation in children may be inappropriate weight gain. In early ascites, the only other abnormality might be dullness on percussion in the flanks. The area of dullness "shifts" if the patient changes position, indicating the presence of intra-abdominal fluid. A fluid wave can be present, although in children its presence may be difficult to determine. However, ascites may be difficult to detect. If abdominal ultrasonography is used as the reference standard, the physical examination has been found to have a sensitivity as low as 50%, and a specificity ranging from 30% to nearly 80% in adults [176]. The medical history can be helpful in separating ascites from obesity. Accumulation of ascitic fluid is often rapid and may be associated with shortness of breath or tachypnea.

As more fluid accumulates, the presence of ascites eventually might be notable by inspection alone. The abdomen is distended not only with fluid but also by intraintestinal air. If the patient is in a supine position, the fluid is first visible as bulging flanks. Later, the abdomen becomes grossly distended. Scrotal distention also may be obvious in males. Intra-abdominal organs may be ballotable as fluid accumulation continues, although in tense ascites the organs may not be palpable. Distended abdominal wall veins are indicative of portosystemic collaterals resulting from functional blockage of inferior vena cava return by tense ascitic fluid. Increased abdominal pressure also results in an everted umbilicus. Umbilical, femoral, inguinal, and incisional hernias also are associated with tense ascites, and abdominal striae may be present. The patient may have other signs of chronic liver disease, such as spider angiomata and muscle wasting. If ascites accumulates rapidly, the patient may become dehydrated as a result of relative depletion of intravascular fluid. Pleural effusions are associated with ascites, and the patient may present with dyspnea because of these effusions or increasing inferior pressure on the lungs. Edema often is seen in older children, especially if hypoproteinemia is present.

If ascites is suspected, abdominal ultrasonography can determine sensitively its presence. In a patient in the supine position, the ascites first collects in the pelvis. As the amount of fluid increases, it is detectable in the pericolic gutters (Morison's pouch) and around the liver and spleen. Echoes within the fluid suggest the presence of exudate, clotted blood, or malignancy [177] (Figure 6.6). Although not necessary for the diagnosis of ascites, the plain abdominal radiograph may show signs of ascites, including displacement of the colon from the properitoneal flank stripe, centrally located floating small bowel loops, separation of bowel loops, or fluid lateral to the liver or spleen [178,179]. The presence of fluid in the pelvis causes increased density above the bladder, producing the so-called dog-ears sign (Fig. 6.7). Computed tomography (CT) and magnetic resonance imaging (MRI) are not recommended for confirming the diagnosis of ascites, although they may help determine its cause in certain situations. Abdominal paracentesis is an efficient way to confirm a diagnosis of ascites. It can also function to document the presence of an infection of the ascitic fluid (see Spontaneous Bacterial Peritonitis). If ascitic fluid is obtained, it should be sent for cell count, culture, total protein, and albumin concentration. The cell count and culture will be useful in determining if the fluid is infected, whereas the albumin content can help determine whether portal hypertension is present. The albumin can be used to measure the serum-to-ascites albumin gradient, the difference between the serum albumin level and the ascites albumin level. A gradient of 1.1 g/dL or greater indicates that the patient has portal hypertension with great

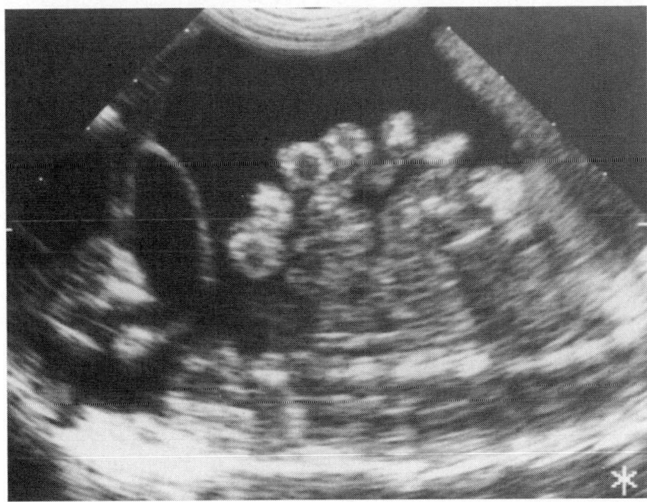

Figure 6.6. Abdominal sonogram showing a large accumulation of ascites. Loops of bowel are prominently outlined by surrounding ascites.

certainty, whereas a gradient of less than 1.1 g/dL indicates that the patient does not have portal hypertension [180]. Treating children and adolescents with ascites has challenges not encountered in treatment of adults. The goal of treatment is not only to reduce or eliminate ascites but also to encourage growth. Growth is in fact the more important consideration, especially in those patients in whom hepatic transplantation eventually will be necessary. Salt and fluid restriction result in a decrease

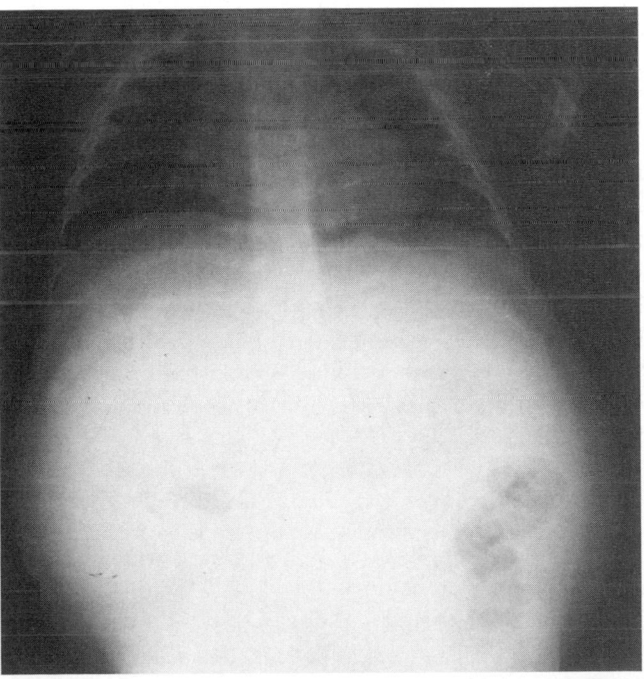

Figure 6.7. Abdominal radiograph of an infant with ascites showing several features of ascites, including bulging flanks, centrally located loops of "floating" bowel, and a hazy appearance of the abdomen in general.

in the rates of formation and absorption of ascites, but such restriction may not be optimal if the result is inadequate caloric intake. Dietary interventions should be offered in consultation with an experienced pediatric dietitian.

Patients with tense ascites or those with gross ascites resulting in dyspnea, abdominal pain, or limited movement, always should be treated. Small collections of fluid, discernible only sonographically, should be followed but not necessarily treated. Any patient with new or suddenly increased ascites should undergo diagnostic paracentesis. Paracentesis is also mandatory in the setting of unexplained fever. Sterile ascitic fluid appears clear, straw colored, or bile stained. The total protein content and leukocyte count should be measured, and a sample of the fluid should be stained for organisms (including acid-fast bacteria in appropriate settings). The fluid always should be cultured. Inoculating the culture media at the bedside increases the sensitivity of the culture [181]. The ascitic fluid may be sent for additional tests (amylase, cytology) as the clinical situation dictates. The protein concentration of ascitic fluid is usually less than 2.0 g/dL. A total protein content of less than 1.0 g/dL is associated with a low ascitic fluid complement content and poor opsonic activity and therefore suggests a high susceptibility to SBP [182]. Concentrations higher than 2.0 g/dL suggest infection, obstruction of the hepatic veins (Budd–Chiari syndrome), or pancreatic ascites. A leukocyte count of more than 250 neutrophils per high-power field suggests bacterial infection.

As treatment is started, several laboratory tests should be considered. Abdominal ultrasound confirms the presence of ascites and helps assess the possibility of an intra-abdominal abscess. Serum electrolytes (sodium, potassium, chloride, and bicarbonate), albumin, total protein, urea nitrogen, creatinine, hemoglobin, and white blood cell count should be measured. Measures of urinary sodium, potassium, creatinine, and urea may be helpful if compared with similar measures after diuretics are given. Sodium excretion in the urine can be especially helpful in determining the effectiveness of the treatment regimen for ascites. A 24-hour urine collection for sodium usually collects less then 10 mmol/d in afebrile cirrhotic patients, but this can increase to 1000 mmol/d with diuretic use. Measuring for urinary creatinine excretion (which should be in the range of 15–20 mg creatinine/kg/d) can reveal whether or not the urinary collection was complete. Because urinary sodium excretion is not uniform, "spot" urinary sodium specimens are not reliable.

In patients with tense or gross ascites, bed rest should be maintained and the patient should be hospitalized. The upright position may result in increased renin–aldosterone activity and increased retention of sodium and water. The patient's weight and abdominal girth should be measured at the same time each day, and fluid intake and output should be recorded carefully. These measurements serve to evaluate the effectiveness of the treatment regimen. Sodium and water restriction alone can result in substantial improvement in patients with mild ascites. Bed rest and salt restriction are the safest method for the treatment of ascites, allowing the patient to avoid drug-related side effects. Bed rest is associated with an increase in glomerular filtration rate. Adult or adolescent patients usually can tolerate a diet with daily sodium intake limited to 2000–3000 mg/d, and this often results in a negative sodium (and therefore water) balance. Younger children usually can be restricted successfully to 1000 mg/d, but only if their total caloric intakes remain adequate to sustain growth and if the concomitant use of sodium-wasting diuretics does not lead to hyponatremia. Fluid intake in children and adolescents may be limited to 1000–1500 mL/d, but this usually is unnecessary unless the serum sodium concentration is less than 120 mmol/L.

Diuretics

If bed rest and sodium restriction do not result in a decrease of ascites, diuretics should be used to promote sodium excretion. Because of the priority of maintaining growth in pediatric patients, diuretics may be the initial therapy for treatment of ascites. Loop diuretics (e.g., furosemide) and thiazide diuretics are strong natriuretic drugs that also promote potassium wasting. Aldosterone antagonists (e.g., spironolactone, triamterene, and amiloride) are more weakly natriuretic, but they spare potassium. Thiazides, aldosterone antagonists, and loop diuretics are the most commonly used diuretics in children. The goal of diuretic treatment is a negative fluid balance limited to 500–750 mL/d in adults and 10 mL/kg/d in children. If diuresis occurs at a rate faster than this, intravascular volume depletion may result and the glomerular filtration rate declines. There is evidence that diuresis rates more rapid than these can be achieved safely in patients in whom peripheral edema accompanies ascites [183]. If peripheral edema is not present (which is the more common scenario in children), diuretic-induced reduction of ascites should be done with caution.

Urinary sodium excretion determination can help assess the efficacy of any diuretic regimen. Insensible sodium losses equal approximately 10 mmol/d. If the patient is on a 2-g (88-mmol) sodium diet, weight loss is certain to occur if the 24-hour urinary sodium excretion exceeds 78 mmol/d [184].

Spironolactone is an aldosterone antagonist that spares renal potassium excretion. It takes up to 4 days to take effect after an initial dose or increase in dosage is given. The usual starting dosage in older children and adolescents is 100–200 mg/d in two divided doses. The dosage is increased 100 mg every 3 or 4 days up to a maximum dose of 600 mg, until satisfactory diuresis is reached or until the urinary concentration of sodium is higher than the urinary concentration of potassium. In such dosages, spironolactone alone causes a satisfactory diuresis in 50–90% of patients [185]. The initial response to spironolactone is so reliable that the renal function and plasma volume status of the patient should be investigated if diuresis is not achieved by a reasonable dose of spironolactone [186]. In infants and younger children, the starting dosage of spironolactone is 1 mg/kg/d, and the daily dose can be increased in increments of 1 mg/kg/d to a maximum dose of 6 mg/kg/d. All diuretics can produce various adverse side effects, including azotemia, hypokalemia, hyperkalemia, and volume contraction, and they can precipitate the hepatorenal syndrome (HRS) or hepatic encephalopathy, especially if used incautiously. Side effects specifically associated with spironolactone include hyperkalemia and skin rashes. Gynecomastia occurs in males after its long-term use.

Loop diuretics such as furosemide and bumetanide are often successful in patients who respond partially to spironolactone. They limit sodium reabsorption in the loop portion of the nephron and deliver it to the distal tubule. The distal tubule is unable to absorb the increased sodium so that sodium is excreted and, as always, water follows. The loop diuretics promote natriuresis more strongly and rapidly than spironolactone but also promote kaliuresis. Studies in adults reveal that up to 50% of patients with an initial satisfactory response to spironolactone eventually require the addition of a loop diuretic to maintain diuresis [187]. The starting dosage of furosemide is 40 mg/d divided into two doses. The dosage can be increased by up to 40 mg every other day to a maximum dose of 240 mg. Infants and young children should be started at 1–2 mg/kg/d, and this dosage may be increased by 1 mg/kg/d to a maximum dose of 6 mg/kg/d. Side effects associated with furosemide include ototoxicity (especially if used with aminoglycosides) and nephrocalcinosis (with long-term use, especially in neonates). Two newer loop diuretics, bumetanide and piretanide, have been used successfully as single drugs in the treatment of cirrhotic ascites in adults [188,189]. There is still limited experience with these drugs in children. Electrolyte disturbances and metabolic alkalosis are the most frequent complications of long term loop diuretic use. Hypokalemia is so common that routine replacement of potassium is recommended. If a combination of spironolactone and loop diuretic is used, potassium replacement may not be necessary. Serum electrolytes, creatinine, and blood urea nitrogen should be measured frequently at first and regularly for as long as diuretic or potassium supplementation continues.

Thiazide diuretics act at the cortical diluting site and proximal tubule to promote natriuresis. Thiazide diuretics often are used to maintain diuresis after initial successful diuresis with spironolactone with or without furosemide. The usual starting dosage of hydrochlorothiazide in adults is 50–100 mg/d divided into two doses. Pediatric dosages begin at 2–3 mg/kg/d. Side effects associated with thiazide diuretics include hypokalemia, hyperglycemia, hyperuricemia, and pancreatitis.

β-Blockers

There are reasons to believe that β-blockade may be helpful in the treatment of ascites. Propranolol lowers portal pressure [190] and inhibits renin secretion [191], and the combination of these effects may result in increased natriuresis. Propranolol, however, is known to increase sodium retention in congestive heart failure, and it reduces renal blood flow. Propranolol has not been shown to predictably alter baseline urine sodium excretion or aldosterone output [192]. In fact, it has been shown that propranolol substantially decreases sodium excretion and has no effect on weight loss in patients with ascites related to cirrhosis [193]. Although propranolol might be used in the treatment of portal hypertension, it is not indicated in the treatment of ascites associated with cirrhosis.

Paracentesis

Large-volume paracentesis has become a preferred intervention for patients with either tense ascites or ascites refractory to diet and diuretic therapy. Studies in adults have demonstrated that if combined with the intravenous infusion of albumin, 4–6 L of ascitic fluid can be removed safely at one time [194]. The fluid usually is removed through a large catheter placed in the median line below the umbilicus. Usually local anesthesia with lidocaine provides adequate pain control, even in children. One study showed no evidence of hypovolemia in nonedematous patients after removal of 5 L of ascitic fluid [195]. Another study, however, showed that patients receiving large-volume paracentesis without albumin infusions had decreased mean arterial blood pressure, decreased serum sodium concentration, increased serum potassium levels, and increased renin and aldosterone activities [196]. Total paracentesis also has been shown to be a safe treatment. In one study of 38 subjects, an average of 10.5 L of ascitic fluid was removed from each patient in one sitting. Albumin infusions were given during the paracentesis and 6 hours afterward. There was no impairment of glomerular filtration rate, free water clearance, plasma volume, or plasma renin activity in these patients [197]. Reinfusion of concentrated ascites has been performed in adults to provide plasma expansion with the patient's own proteins [198]. Almost half the patients in one study in adults developed fever after reinfusion, but more serious side effects were rare [199]. There are no published experiences with recycled protein reinfusions in children.

Because drug therapy is usually effective, large-volume or total paracentesis usually is not necessary in children with ascites. In subjects with respiratory compromise or ascites refractory to drug treatment, however, large-volume paracentesis may be considered as an initial therapy. Diuretics then may be used for maintenance therapy. Up to 100 mL/kg (up to 5 L) can be removed safely at a single sitting. Albumin is replaced at the rate of 6–8 g/L of ascitic fluid removed.

Transjugular Intrahepatic Portosystemic Shunts

Nonsurgical placement of an intrahepatic fistula between the hepatic veins and the portal venous system has been used in children for the relief of symptoms related to portal hypertension, including ascites. One early study of transjugular intrahepatic portosystemic shunts (TIPSs) for recurrent variceal bleeding reported resolution of ascites in most patients after the procedure [200]. A more recent study of 50 patients undergoing TIPS placement for the indication of refractory ascites reported resolution of ascites in nearly 75%. Complications resulting from TIPSs have included high-output cardiac failure, portal encephalopathy, rapidly progressive hepatic failure, and shunt stenosis or failure [201]. As in treatment for portal hypertension, a TIPS can result in short-term improvement of ascites. Long-term efficacy has not been proven for this treatment.

Surgical Peritoneovenous Shunts

LeVeen and Denver shunts permit unidirectional flow of ascitic fluid to the venous system. The insertion of such a shunt usually leads to prompt resolution of ascites. The use of these devices is controversial because recipients may be at increased risk for other complications of cirrhosis as well as the complications attributable to the shunt itself, such as coagulopathy, infection, cardiac failure, and renal failure. One large multicenter trial concluded that peritoneovenous shunts alleviated disabling ascites more rapidly than medical management but that the duration of survival was not prolonged. Survival was related instead to the severity of the illness at the time of entry into the trial [202].

HEPATIC ENCEPHALOPATHY

Hepatic encephalopathy refers to a variety of reversible neurologic abnormalities seen in patients with cirrhosis. Many neurologic functions may be involved in this syndrome, with effects including disturbed consciousness (including coma), personality changes, intellectual deterioration, and speech and motor dysfunction. The sudden onset and rapid reversibility of encephalopathy in liver disease suggest that it is of metabolic origin. The appearance of hepatic encephalopathy depends on three factors: portosystemic shunting, alterations in the blood–brain barrier, and the interactions of toxic metabolites with the CNS.

Portosystemic Shunting

Blood from the intestine can be shunted around the liver through collateral vessels or, in the setting of severe liver disease, through the liver as the blood passes by damaged or necrotic hepatocytes. Potentially neurotoxic nitrogenous intestinal metabolites, which usually are removed by the healthy liver, are found in the circulation in patients with liver dysfunction. Hepatic encephalopathy, therefore, is rare if liver function is good. Portosystemic shunting may result in encephalopathy, especially if the patient consumes a high-protein diet [203], although encephalopathy is rare in children with extrahepatic obstruction of the portal vein. If both shunting and hepatocyte dysfunction are present, the patient is most susceptible to the development of encephalopathy.

Changes in the Blood–Brain Barrier

The blood–brain barrier serves the important role of isolating the brain from various substances in the systemic circulation. The capillaries of the brain are lined by a specialized endothelium, which is impermeable to many substances. These endothelial cells do not have fenestrations otherwise seen in capillaries throughout the body. In acute liver failure, the blood–brain barrier undergoes changes in permeability so that marker substances such as inulin, horseradish peroxidase, and trypan blue pass to the brain more readily [204]. It has been shown in animal models that increased serum concentrations of ammonia and mercaptans cause increased blood–brain barrier permeability. Therefore, the neurotoxins may directly mediate the changes in blood–brain barrier permeability [205]. Although changes in the permeability of the blood–brain barrier are seen in the latter stages of encephalopathy, there is no evidence for changes that precede the onset of encephalopathy [206].

Toxic Metabolites

Many potentially toxic substances have been isolated from the blood, cerebrospinal fluid, or brain tissue of animals or humans with hepatic encephalopathy. None of these has been shown conclusively to be responsible for the mental changes that accompany chronic liver disease and cirrhosis. It is agreed, however, that hepatic encephalopathy can occur if toxic nitrogenous substances, ingested or formed in the intestine, reach the brain (through a "porous" blood–brain barrier) after incomplete hepatic removal, because of either impaired hepatocyte function or collateral circulation bypass of the liver [207]. The CNSs of patients with cirrhosis are hyperresponsive to these circulating toxins [208].

Ammonia Hypothesis

Altered ammonium metabolism has been implicated as the cause of hepatic encephalopathy for many years, and it still is considered an important factor in producing encephalopathy. Serum ammonia concentrations are increased in subjects with liver failure and chronic liver disease. Hyperammonemia also is seen in other encephalopathies, such as Reye's syndrome and organic acidemias. Serum ammonia is generated from both exogenous and endogenous sources. Ingested protein accounts for about half of the ammonia found in the blood. Amino acids from ingested proteins are metabolized by gut bacteria, with subsequent release of ammonia by bacteria-derived urease. Bacteria are not the sole source of serum ammonia derived from the intestine. In the absence of dietary protein, the gut continues to produce ammonia, using plasma amino acids (mostly glutamine) and urea as substrate [209]. Amino acid oxidases are the catalyst for this endogenous ammonia production, which accounts for the remainder of the serum ammonia [210]. In the healthy state, most of the serum ammonia is removed and detoxified by the liver. Up to 80% usually is removed from the portal vein blood in its "first pass" from the gut. The liver detoxifies ammonia through the urea cycle, or by way of the transamination of α-ketoglutarate to glutamate or glutamine. The remaining 20% is removed primarily by the kidneys, in which the ammonia is protonated and excreted as a means of maintaining systemic acid–base balance. Muscle tissue also can absorb and metabolize ammonia. During vigorous exercise, the relative importance of muscle detoxification of ammonia increases, and it can remove up to half the serum ammonia from the bloodstream [211]. The brain also can take up ammonia and detoxify it, mostly by production of glutamine, which then is metabolized to α-ketoglutarate.

In patients with liver disease, the liver is unable to metabolize ammonia, either because of shunting of portal blood around the liver or because of hepatocyte dysfunction. In either case, blood ammonia levels increase. Patients with advanced liver disease often have muscle wasting and are compromised further in their ability to metabolize ammonia that escapes the liver. The respiratory alkalosis associated with liver disease also causes the kidneys to retain ammonia. There is compelling evidence linking hepatic encephalopathy to increased serum ammonia. If patients with cirrhosis are given ammonium salts, large quantities of amino acids, or urea, they develop an encephalopathic state similar to that seen in hepatic encephalopathy. Measures taken to decrease serum ammonia result in decrease, or complete amelioration, of encephalopathy. Diets high in vegetable protein, which produce less ammonia than diets high in meat protein, produce less encephalopathy than diets emphasizing meat protein [212].

There is also evidence, however, that ammonia alone is not the main mediator of hepatic encephalopathy and that increased serum ammonia is only a marker for the encephalopathic process. There is poor correlation between blood ammonia levels and the stage of hepatic encephalopathy, especially in the early stages of encephalopathy. Patients do not often show increased serum ammonia levels in stages I and II of hepatic encephalopathy. There is better correlation between CNS concentrations of glutamine and α-ketoglutarate and the severity of encephalopathy. These products of brain ammonia metabolism may reflect high CNS ammonia levels. Further proof that ammonia alone cannot explain hepatic encephalopathy is that therapies sometimes effective in the treatment of encephalopathy, such as levodopa, do not affect blood ammonia level. There is also evidence that the encephalopathy induced by ingestion of ammonia is not the same as the encephalopathy of liver disease. Studies of visual-evoked responses in rabbits showed that abnormalities associated with hepatic encephalopathy were different from those induced by hyperammonemia [213]. Electroencephalogram abnormalities also differ between the two states [214]. Ammonia toxicity promotes excitation through reduced inhibition of the CNS, eventually resulting in seizure activity. Hepatic encephalopathy, on the other hand, is associated with CNS inhibition and only rarely is associated with seizures [215].

Synergistic Neurotoxin Hypothesis

Hepatic encephalopathy may result from the combined accumulation of several toxins, each of which itself would not produce encephalopathy. Interest in this hypothesis has centered on various toxins, including mercaptans and fatty acids, which are found in the blood in increased concentrations in patients with hepatic encephalopathy. Mercaptans are derived from intestinal bacterial metabolism of methionine [216]. Methylmercaptan and its metabolite, dimethyl sulfoxide, are the most common mercaptans. The presence of these compounds in the blood of patients with liver disease is responsible for fetor hepaticus [217]. Experimental infusions of these compounds have shown them to cause confusion, disorientation, and coma. Mercaptans have been shown to interfere with the urea cycle and thus with ammonia metabolism [218].

Short- and medium-chain fatty acids also are found in increased concentrations in subjects with hepatic encephalopathy. High levels are found in patients with coma; lower levels are associated with lesser degrees of encephalopathy [219]. As with ammonia and mercaptan compounds, these fatty acids are mainly derivatives of intestinal bacterial metabolism [220]. Feeding of medium-chain triglycerides to patients with cirrhosis increased their plasma and cerebrospinal levels [221]. Like mercaptans, fatty acids may interfere with urea cycle enzymes. Furthermore, high levels of fatty acids may displace other toxins from albumin, increasing their potential neurotoxicity. Much smaller doses of ammonia, mercaptans, and fatty acids are needed to produce encephalopathy if these toxins are given together than if each toxin is given individually. Smaller doses still are needed if hypoxemia or hypoglycemia is present [218,222].

False Neurotransmitter Hypothesis

Hepatic encephalopathy also may be caused by the accumulation of inhibitory neurotransmitters in the brain. These inhibitory neurotransmitters may be "false," or not ordinarily present in the systemic circulation or brain [223]. Octopamine, for example, is a weakly inhibitory neurotransmitter produced by the metabolism of tyrosine by gut bacteria. It usually is removed from the portal circulation by the liver. The inhibitory neurotransmitters may also be present in healthy people but occur in high concentrations in encephalopathic patients. Serotonin is derived from serum tryptophan. Both octopamine and tryptophan (as well as other aromatic amino acids) are found in high serum concentrations in the setting of acute liver failure. Furthermore, in hepatic encephalopathy, there is a decrease in excitatory neurotransmitters such as dopamine and norepinephrine [223,224].

Several findings argue against this hypothesis, however. Octopamine is not found in increased concentrations in the brain in subjects with cirrhosis [225], and coma cannot be induced in experimental animals by the introduction of octopamine to the CNS. Tryptophan has caused various neurologic symptoms in patients with cirrhosis, including dizziness and headache, but hepatic encephalopathy has not occurred [226]. Finally, hepatic encephalopathy is not reversed consistently by the administration of the excitatory neurotransmitter dopamine [223].

γ-Aminobutyric Acid–ergic Inhibitory Neurotransmitter Hypothesis

The amino acid γ-aminobutyric acid (GABA) is an inhibitory neurotransmitter found throughout the brain [227]. It is produced in the brain by the decarboxylation of glutamic acid. There has been considerable interest in GABA (and its receptor) as a major mediator of hepatic encephalopathy because of its important role in CNS inhibition. The GABA receptor is activated not only by GABA but also by barbiturates and benzodiazepines. Studies of visual-evoked potentials in rabbits with induced hepatic failure and hepatic encephalopathy showed abnormalities similar to those induced by barbiturates and benzodiazepines and different from those caused by other types of encephalopathy, such as ether-induced coma [228]. Although no specific compounds have been isolated, there is evidence that intestinal bacteria produce GABA-like agents and that these substances can reach the brain in the setting of liver failure. Portal vein blood has been shown to carry more GABA ergic activity than does blood from the aorta [228,229]. Ordinarily, this intestinal GABA would be inactivated by hepatic GABA transaminase, but in a rabbit model of liver failure, hepatic uptake of GABA was reduced [230].

Evidence in favor of this hypothesis includes the finding of increased GABA activity in plasma of patients with acute and chronic liver failure after gastrointestinal hemorrhage, a known precipitant of hepatic encephalopathy [231]. There also are increased GABA receptors in the brains of rabbits with induced liver failure compared with rabbits without liver disease [232]. It has further been shown in animal models that the direct introduction of GABA to the brain results in coma similar to that seen in hepatic encephalopathy [233,234].

Although the rabbit model of liver failure has provided promising evidence in favor of the GABA-ergic origin of hepatic encephalopathy, work in other animal models, including the guinea pig [75] and dog [206], has not been as promising. In humans with hepatic encephalopathy, there is no increase in plasma GABA activity [235], although plasma activity may not reflect CNS activity reliably and brain GABA receptors are normal in number and affinity [236]. The GABA-ergic hypothesis has been modified to include alteration of GABA activity by a benzodiazepine agonist [237]. Benzodiazepine and GABA receptors are associated closely in the brain, and benzodiazepine-binding sites are increased in the setting of acute liver failure [238].

Benzodiazepine-like substances have been isolated from the cerebrospinal fluid and plasma of patients with hepatic encephalopathy, although such substances may be metabolites of benzodiazepine drugs [239]. The reversal in some patients of hepatic encephalopathy after the administration of a benzodiazepine antagonist also supports the benzodiazepine hypothesis [240], although this effect is not consistent [241]. Although the GABA-ergic hypothesis of the pathogenesis of hepatic encephalopathy and the ammonia hypotheses appear to be unrelated, it has been shown that modest elevations in serum ammonia may contribute to encephalopathy by enhancing GABA-eric inhibitory neurotransmission [242,243].

In most patients, hepatic encephalopathy is initiated by a precipitating event. Common precipitants include gastrointestinal hemorrhage, infections (including SBP), administration of sedatives, and dehydration, often after aggressive diuresis with concomitant azotemia and hypokalemic alkalosis. In some patients, the identification and reversal of the precipitant may reverse the encephalopathic process. In many, however, the encephalopathy persists and requires separate treatment. After the onset of frank encephalopathy, it may become clear that mild encephalopathy was present before the precipitating event. The clinical course of hepatic encephalopathy usually fluctuates. Subjects may change neurologic status quickly, so repeated and frequent evaluations must be done.

The neurologic manifestations of chronic liver disease range from impairment of orientation to coma and are grouped into stages as shown in Table 6.4. Disturbance of sleep patterns, such as insomnia or hypersomnia, is common. The detection of subtle or "subclinical" changes in cerebral function is important in order to prevent the deterioration to frank encephalopathy. Although generalized neurologic deficits are more common, focal neurologic abnormalities, including hemiplegia, have been described as well [244].

Diagnostic models based on quantitative neuropsychological examinations have been developed to aid in the detection of early encephalopathy, but these models have not been adapted to children [245]. Electroencephalography may aid in the diagnosis of hepatic encephalopathy. In general, there is a slowing from the normal alpha-range frequency to the delta range. Stimuli such as opening the eyes fail to reduce the abnormal background activity. These abnormalities may precede biochemical changes as well as behavioral changes. Proton magnetic resonance spectroscopy shows characteristic abnormalities, but so far these changes have not proved to be an aid in the diagnosis of subclinical hepatic encephalopathy [246]. When considering the diagnosis of hepatic encephalopathy, every effort should be made to consider alternative explanations for the observed neurologic changes. A CT or MRI scan of the brain may indicate head trauma, subdural hematoma, and/or the presence of cerebral edema.

The first step in the treatment of hepatic encephalopathy is to identify and treat directly any precipitating factors. In general, the prognosis is better if a clear precipitant is present. Because of the fluctuating course of hepatic encephalopathy, the patient should be observed closely and repeatedly. For most, initial admission to an intensive care unit is advisable. Supportive measures should be provided as needed, including respiratory support, with airway protection. Sedatives should be avoided because these can precipitate or exacerbate hepatic encephalopathy. If a sedative is necessary, a benzodiazepine or opiate should not be used.

All dietary and intravenous protein intake should cease during the acute onset and treatment of encephalopathy. Protein may be reintroduced as the encephalopathy subsides. Standard therapy for chronic hepatic encephalopathy in adults includes restriction of protein to 40 g/d. In children, protein restriction may result in growth failure and should be undertaken only with specific attention to the overall nutritional state and needs of the patient. Cleansing enemas may reduce further the amount of exogenous ammonia from the intestine, particularly if hepatic encephalopathy follows a gastrointestinal

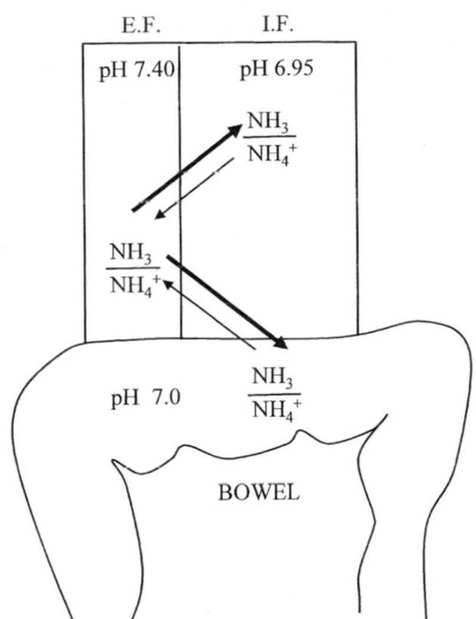

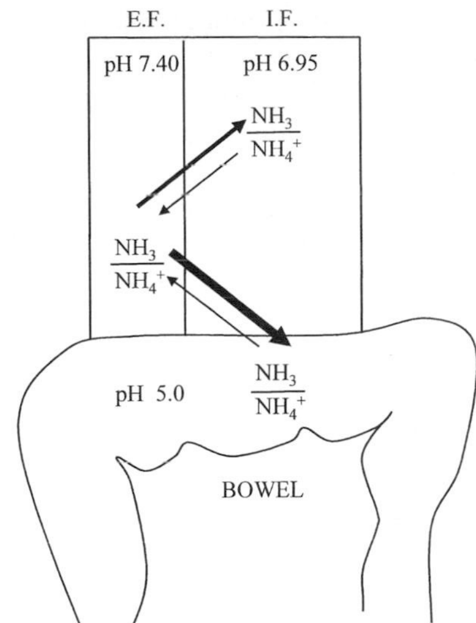

Figure 6.8. Mechanism of action of lactulose. In normal situations (*left*), the pH or extracellular fluid (EF) is more alkaline than the pH of the intracellular fluid (IF) and more alkaline than the pH of the bowel lumen. This favors the diffusion of ammonia from the EF to the bowel. In subjects receiving lactulose (*right*), the pH of the colonic contents is reduced, the equilibrium is shifted to the right, and ammonia diffuses into the lumen (*heavy arrow*). (From Conn HO, Liberthal MM. The hepatic coma syndromes and lactulose. Baltimore: Williams & Wilkins, 1979:261.)

hemorrhage. Oral antibiotics have been successful in the treatment of early hepatic encephalopathy. Tetracycline is used in adult subjects but is not appropriate for use in children. Neomycin has been used commonly in children. In subjects with and without encephalopathy, neomycin decreases ammonia production, presumably by directly suppressing ammonia-forming bacteria [247,248]. Long-term use of neomycin has resulted in deafness and renal tubular disease [249,250]. The adult dosage of neomycin is 4–6 g/d. In children, a starting dose of 1 g is recommended.

Lactulose (β-galactosidofructose), a semisynthetic disaccharide, is a mainstay of treatment for hepatic encephalopathy [251,252]. If taken by mouth, this disaccharide reaches the colon intact, where colonizing bacteria metabolize it to its component sugars – galactose and fructose – and further metabolize the sugars to lactic acid, acetic acid, and various organic acids [253]. The acidified fecal contents trap ammonia, making it unavailable for absorption [254] (Figure 6.8). Lactulose also has been shown to alter the colonic flora, resulting in an increase in *Lactobacillus* species [255]. Although the actual mode of action is not certain, it clear is that acidification of the fecal stream is necessary for successful treatment. Acidifying enemas (lactitol or lactose) are much more effective in treating encephalopathy than nonacidifying enemas such as tap water [256]. Although treatment with lactulose results in reversal of encephalopathy and lowering of serum ammonia, stool levels of ammonia are not always increased [257]. The adult dosage of lactulose is 10–30 mL of the standard syrup (10 g lactulose/15 mL) three times each day. Pediatric dosages are 0.3–0.4 mL/kg two or three times per day. The dose should be sufficient to acidify the stools (pH less than 6.0) but should not necessarily result in diarrhea.

Lactitol (β-galactoside sorbitol) is another synthetic disaccharide used in the treatment of encephalopathy. Its mode of action is identical to that of lactulose. Its main advantage is that it is supplied in a powder form and is therefore less sweet and more convenient to use than lactulose. In addition, it is not contaminated (as is lactulose syrup) with lactose, galactose, and other sugars, so it is more acceptable in patients who are lactose intolerant. It appears to be as effective as lactulose in the treatment of acute and chronic hepatic encephalopathy and has been shown to have a more rapid effect than lactose [258].

Therapy with lactulose or with neomycin alone is successful in reducing encephalopathy in a majority of patients. Some, however, do not improve after treatment with a single agent [253]. In these patients, combination therapy with lactulose (or lactitol) and neomycin has been tried, with varying results. Either drug may interfere, in theory, with the mode of action of the other. The efficacy of lactulose relies on the presence of colonic bacteria capable of metabolizing it into its constituent sugars. Neomycin alters the gut flora and may render lactulose ineffective. On the other hand, neomycin is more effective in a pH-neutral environment, and its efficacy might be reduced in the acidified milieu produced by lactulose [259]. In spite of these theoretic concerns, it appears that neomycin preferentially inhibits bacteria that are poor degraders of lactulose, such as enterobacteria, enterococcus, and staphylococcus. One in vitro study showed that in fecal bacteria cultures, the addition of lactitol increased the inhibitory effect of neomycin on ammonia production by 25–50%. In limited clinical trials, combined therapy with lactulose and neomycin has been successful in some subjects, but usually only if the stool pH remains low, suggesting that lactulose metabolism is ongoing even in the presence of neomycin [260,261]. Combination therapy may be tried in patients who have not responded to either regimen alone.

Because the ratio of the serum concentration of aromatic amino acids – phenylalanine, tyrosine, and tryptophan – to the serum concentration of branched-chain amino acids (BCAAs) – leucine, isoleucine, and valine – is increased in subjects with cirrhosis and hepatic encephalopathy, there have been attempts to reverse encephalopathy by giving BCAAs, either intravenously [262,263] or orally [264]. In progressive cirrhosis, amino acids are released on hepatocyte necrosis and from skeletal muscle breakdown. The excess aromatic amino acids are not cleared by the liver because of either impaired hepatocyte function or increased collateral circulation. BCAAs, on the other hand, can be oxidized by a variety of tissues and therefore are not increased in the serum [265,266].

Brain and plasma accumulation of aromatic amino acids may result in an alteration of the synthesis of brain neurotransmitters such as norepinephrine, dopamine, and serotonin [223]. In dogs, large intravenous doses of the aromatic amino acids tryptophan and phenylalanine have caused coma; the combined infusion of tryptophan, phenylalanine, and BCAAs failed to cause coma [266]. BCAAs might treat hepatic encephalopathy successfully by reducing muscle protein breakdown or by normalizing the serum amino acid profile. A placebo-controlled study of adult patients with chronic portosystemic encephalopathy demonstrated a decreased recurrence of acute hepatic encephalopathy in those subjects receiving diets with a BCAA supplement [264,267]; other reports have not shown any effect, however [262,268]. A recent attempt to employ a meta-analytic technique to review the efficacy of BCAAs in the treatment of hepatic encephalopathy was able to conclude only that large long-term multicenter studies are required to provide reliable evidence of the efficacy of this treatment [269,270]. BCAAs have been used as an enteral protein supplement in children with advanced cirrhosis and malnutrition. All children showed improvement in anthropometric indices, and none experienced encephalopathy as a result of the diet. Although this study did not explore the use of BCAAs in the treatment of hepatic encephalopathy in children, it demonstrated the safety of using BCAA in the diets of children with liver disease [271].

Benzodiazepine antagonists recently have gained increasing use in the therapy of hepatic encephalopathy. Because encephalopathy is associated with increased neural inhibition by activation of GABA-benzodiazepine inhibitory neurotransmission systems, direct inhibition of these systems with competitive antagonists might ameliorate the symptoms. Flumazenil, a benzodiazepine antagonist, has been tried in a limited and unblinded fashion in the treatment of hepatic encephalopathy. Case reports document dramatic improvements in encephalopathic symptoms shortly after starting flumazenil, with prompt relapse of symptoms after discontinuing its use [272]. Larger studies have provided conflicting results. Several published series have demonstrated improvements in observable behavior and somatosensory testing after treatment with flumazenil [272,273]; others have failed to show significant improvement after treatment with flumazenil [274]. Controlled blinded studies may confirm the usefulness of benzodiazepine antagonists in the treatment of acute and chronic hepatic encephalopathy.

Because of the decrease in brain dopamine levels in patients with cirrhosis and encephalopathy, there has been interest in treatment aimed at directly replenishing dopamine in such patients. Because dopamine does not cross the blood–brain barrier, its precursor, levodopa, has been given to subjects with encephalopathy. Levodopa has been shown to reverse acute and chronic encephalopathy temporarily, but only in a minority of subjects [275]. Bromocriptine, a dopamine agonist, also has been used in the treatment of cirrhosis and encephalopathy. It has been most successful in subjects with extensive portosystemic shunting and good liver function [276]. As in levodopa therapy, improvement has not been sustained [277].

In subjects with a portacaval anastomosis, surgical or balloon shunt occlusion can reverse the encephalopathy secondary to portosystemic shunting of blood. Reversal or partial occlusion of a TIPS also may result in amelioration of the encephalopathic state [278]. Hepatic transplantation should be considered in patients with intractable or progressive encephalopathy, because such encephalopathy signifies almost complete liver failure.

COAGULOPATHIES

If vessel injury occurs, platelets adhere to the damaged endothelium or subendothelium. The clotting cascade is initiated, either by contact with the subendothelium (intrinsic clotting pathway) or by the release of tissue factors (extrinsic clotting pathway). The clotting cascade ultimately results in the generation of thrombin, which cleaves fibrinogen to fibrin; the fibrin polymerizes into a fibrin clot, which is stabilized by cross-linking by factor XIIIa. Plasminogen activating factor, released by local endothelial cells, activates plasminogen, forming plasmin that degrades the fibrin clot. Coagulation regulators, such as proteins C and S and antithrombin III, also contain the clotting process. Under usual conditions, hemostasis is maintained by a complex balance among coagulation, fibrinolysis, and direct inhibition of coagulation.

The liver plays an important role in the maintenance of all aspects of this balance. All the coagulation factors, except for factor VIII, are synthesized primarily by the liver [279]. Most of the inhibitors of the coagulation system, including plasminogen, α_2-plasmin inhibitor, α_1-antitrypsin, α_2-macroglobulin, and the most important inhibitor, antithrombin III, also are liver derived [280]. Liver reticuloendothelial cells remove and degrade fibrin degradation products (FDPs) and coagulation factors in their active forms [281]. It long has been recognized that chronic liver disease often is accompanied by imbalances in hemostasis [282]. Coagulation disorders associated with liver disease may occur directly, as a result of hepatocellular damage (coagulation factor deficiencies), or indirectly (thrombocytopenia secondary to hypersplenism) or may be complex and multifactorial, as seen in DIC.

Platelets

Platelet number and function can be affected by liver disease. In the setting of cirrhosis and portal hypertension, thrombocytopenia may result from splenic sequestration. In healthy people, the spleen stores 30% of the platelet pool; in those with portal hypertension, 90% of platelets may be sequestered in the spleen [283]. Patients with low platelet counts are more likely to have major gastrointestinal hemorrhage than those with normal platelet counts [284]. Thrombocytopenia also may occur as a result of antiplatelet-associated immunoglobulin G in chronic active hepatitis, or secondary to platelet consumption in DIC. In addition, the platelets of patients with cirrhosis are small, suggesting that the platelets are older, as a result of either decreased platelet production or decreased clearance by the reticuloendothelial system [285]. Platelet adhesion, as measured by adherence to glass beads or by adenosine diphosphate–induced aggregation, is abnormal in cirrhotic patients [286]. These abnormalities may be caused by alterations in plasma and platelet lipids and low platelet concentrations of arachidonic acid [287].

Coagulation Proteins

The hepatic-derived coagulation proteins have half-lives ranging from 6 hours for factor VII to 4 days for fibrinogen. All of these are considerably shorter than that of albumin; therefore, measurable deficiencies in these proteins are a more sensitive indicator of synthetic failure. Still, many such coagulation factors (e.g., fibrinogen, prothrombin, and factors V, IX, and X) have reserve synthetic capacity, so clinically significant serum deficiencies of these proteins are seen only in advanced cirrhosis or fulminant liver failure.

Fibrinogen is altered both quantitatively and qualitatively in liver disease. Low serum levels of fibrinogen appear to be caused by the combination of decreased synthesis and increased consumption [288]. Increased FDPs in patients with cirrhosis are evidence that either fibrinogen is being consumed at an increased rate or the FDPs are being cleared slowly by a diseased liver [289]. In increased concentrations, FDPs can prolong the thrombin time, interfere with fibrinogen polymerization, and prolong the bleeding time through direct interaction with platelets. Fibrinogen not only is decreased in chronic liver disease but also appears in a variant form in cirrhosis. This "acquired dysfibrogenemia," present in up to 80% of patients with chronic liver disease [290], is characterized by fibrinogen that is altered posttranscriptionally by the addition of increased numbers of sialic acid residues on the α and β chains [291]. This altered fibrinogen is not able to polymerize normally. Removal of the excess sialic acid results in fibrinogen capable of normal polymerization [292].

The vitamin K–dependent factors (II, VII, IX, and X) often are more severely depressed in cirrhosis than are the non–vitamin K dependent factors. Factor VII, with its short half-life of 6 hours, is most reflective of hepatocellular damage and has prognostic value in FHF. Patients with factor VII levels less than 8% of normal have an extremely poor prognosis; those with levels greater than this usually survive [140,288]. Factor V also [288] has been shown to have prognostic value in acute hepatic failure [142,293]. One study found that factor V levels less than 50% of normal were associated with spontaneous hemorrhage and a poor prognosis [294].

Factor VIII is synthesized in the liver and in various extrahepatic sites, such as in lymph tissue [295]. Its cofactor, the von Willebrand factor, also is synthesized extrahepatically in vascular endothelial cells. In cirrhosis, factor VIII usually is found in high concentrations [296]. Factor VIII levels can be helpful in distinguishing the coagulopathy of cirrhosis from that of DIC.

Inhibitors of Coagulation

Coagulation is controlled by hepatic clearance of the active forms of clotting factors and by coagulation inhibitors, many of which, like clotting factors, are made in the liver. Several inhibitors of coagulation, such as α_2-macroglobulin and plasminogen activator inhibitor, are acute phase reactants and are found in increased quantities in liver disease. Even these liver-derived proteins are found in low concentrations in advanced liver disease. Other inhibitors, such as antithrombin III, C1 inhibitor, and α_1-antitrypsin, typically are found in decreased concentrations in chronic liver disease. Antithrombin III, the most important inhibitor of the coagulation cascade, acts with heparin to bind to and inactivate thrombin and other coagulation factors. Low serum concentrations of antithrombin III also are associated with poor prognosis [281,282]. As with all clotting and inhibition factors, the low serum concentrations may result from either low synthetic output or increased consumption. Low concentrations of antithrombin III are thought to contribute to the perpetual stimulation of the clotting cascade in DIC [288]. Further disruptions of hemostasis, unrelated to synthetic deficiencies, are seen in subjects with cirrhosis and portal hypertension if blood is shunted away from the liver. In this setting, activated forms of clotting factors persist in the circulation and may cause or promote the low-grade DIC often seen in chronic liver disease.

Disseminated Intravascular Coagulation

It may be difficult to differentiate DIC from the coagulopathy of liver disease because many of the serum markers of both processes are identical. The complex interdependence of clotting factors and inhibitors also makes cause and effect difficult to determine. For example, the low serum levels of antithrombin III observed in cirrhotics may be caused by decreased hepatic synthesis or by increased consumption of that protein. Low levels of antithrombin III may contribute to the continued activation of coagulation in DIC.

The primary biochemical abnormality in DIC is diffuse thrombosis, which results from inappropriate stimulation of coagulation, often by damaged epithelium or toxin release [297]. In cirrhosis, the signal for thrombosis has not been discovered, although it has been postulated that necrosed liver cells release a procoagulant [298]. Fibrinolysis, either coincident or secondary, also is stimulated in DIC [299]. Both DIC and cirrhosis can be associated with thrombocytopenia, low serum clotting factors and inhibitor concentrations, and clinical instability. In cirrhosis, the abnormalities result mainly from decreased synthesis or altered clearance of active coagulation metabolites; in DIC the abnormalities are caused by increased consumption of the factors and inhibitors. Although a large body of literature supports the suggestion that DIC often contributes to the coagulopathy of cirrhosis, many studies are limited by the various laboratory techniques employed or by the types of patients selected for study.

Several laboratory studies can aid in determining the extent that DIC plays in the coagulopathy of a particular patient. Because factor VIII is produced extrahepatically (in the spleen and lymph nodes), it can be helpful in determining the extent to which low factor levels are a result of failure of hepatic synthesis. If factor VIII levels are normal or high, as is often the case in cirrhosis, the coagulopathy can be attributed to hepatocellular failure; low factor VIII levels signal an ongoing consumptive process. Increased levels of FDPs also are suggestive of DIC, although in the setting of liver failure they may be present in high serum concentrations as a result of decreased hepatic clearance. Further information can be obtained by measuring serum levels of D dimer, which is a degradation fragment of cross-linked fibrin and is related specifically to DIC. The formation of D dimers requires the presence of both activated thrombin and plasmin, a key to DIC. The presence of D dimer in a patient with increased FDP and low factor VIII levels is considered diagnostic of DIC [300]. A single measurement of fibrinogen, FDP, and D dimer levels usually does not give as much information as serial samples taken over several days. For example, falling fibrinogen levels in the face of stable liver function are evidence of ongoing DIC [301].

New biochemical markers of coagulation recently have been developed to aid in the diagnosis of DIC. Nonfunctional fragments cleaved from factors during activation provide information regarding the hepatic output of clotting factors. Prothrombin factor F^{1+2} and factor X activation fragment are both present in the circulation in high concentrations in DIC and in low concentrations in the setting of hepatocellular failure [302,303]. One study found that in patients with cirrhosis, if a wide array of hemostatic function tests are employed – including the euglobulin lysis test, protamine sulfate test, and measurement of serum plasminogen levels – the diagnosis of DIC is confirmed more often than if only "conventional" screening is done [304]. Hepatic cofactor II and extrinsic pathway inhibitor are newly discovered coagulation inhibitors. Hepatic cofactor II is liver derived and is present in low concentrations in both DIC and hepatocellular failure. Extrinsic pathway inhibitor, however, is synthesized in vascular endothelial cells and is present in normal concentrations in liver disease but in decreased concentrations in DIC. Low levels of both inhibitors are strong evidence of ongoing DIC [300,305,306]. These tests are not widely available but hold the promise of further improvements for the diagnostic accuracy of DIC in the setting of cirrhosis.

Acute gastrointestinal bleeding is a major complication of cirrhosis and contributes to death in many patients [284]. A prompt response to bleeding is urgent because acute gastrointestinal bleeding often precipitates or intensifies hepatic encephalopathy. The treatment of the coagulopathy of liver disease consists of neutralization of gastric acid, parenteral vitamin K administration, blood product administration as indicated, and prompt treatment of bleeding with vasoconstrictors and directed therapy for specific sites of bleeding. Even in the face of prompt and aggressive treatments, some patients will continue to experience ongoing bleeding problems with adverse outcomes. In such patients, there has been increasing experience with the use of recombinant factor VIIa (rFVIIa) [307,308]. These treatments may be effective and may also provide their benefit with small volume infusions, rather than the repeated large infusions necessary when fresh frozen plasma is administered. In one recent study, four children with liver failure and severe coagulopathy benefited from the administration of rFVIIa. The doses used ranged from 0.067–0.3 mg/kg. All four patients had failed to respond to standard therapy, and all four patients demonstrated laboratory improvements such as improvement in the international normalized ratio. More importantly, bleeding was stopped promptly, even within 10 minutes of administration of the rFVIIa in all patients [309].

The value of giving H_2-receptor antagonists to patients in acute liver failure to prevent upper gastrointestinal bleeding has been established in controlled clinical trials [310]. Patients receiving H_2-blockers have a lower incidence of acute bleeding and a decreased need for blood and blood products. The value of H_2-blocker prophylaxis in chronic liver disease has not been established as clearly. Patients with decompensated cirrhosis may be placed on an H_2-blocker such as cimetidine (20–40 mg/kg/d divided into four doses) or ranitidine (4 mg/kg/d divided into two doses).

Parenteral vitamin K should be given to any patient with liver disease accompanied by a prolonged prothrombin time. The standard dose (5–10 mg in the older child and 1–2 mg in the infant) is given intravenously or intramuscularly each day for up to 3 days. If the coagulopathy is caused by vitamin K deficiency, it is corrected promptly. Fresh frozen plasma and platelets are effective in correcting most cases of cirrhosis-associated coagulopathy transiently. Because these blood products provide only brief correction of bleeding disorders, they are reserved for use in the setting of acute bleeding. If the only sign of coagulopathy is an isolated increase in the prothrombin time, many invasive procedures (including lumbar puncture, paracentesis, and central line placement) are safe even without infusion of blood products such as fresh frozen plasma [311]. Platelets should be given to any patient with a count of less than 60,000 cells/mm^3 who is bleeding actively. Even if there is no bleeding, a patient with a platelet count of less than 50,000 cells/mm^3 should be given a platelet transfusion if an invasive procedure such as a liver biopsy is planned [312]. A patient with persistent thrombocytopenia should be evaluated for DIC, hypersplenism, and antiplatelet antibodies.

Compulsive efforts should be made to determine the site of bleeding and to control it. Bleeding esophageal varices should undergo sclerosis or banding. Gastric or duodenal ulcer hemorrhage should be controlled through endoscopic cauterization or through surgical ligation if necessary. Diffuse gastritis may be treated with antacids, H_2-blockers, proton pump inhibitors, or sucralfate. Several other therapies are available if bleeding is intractable or the site of bleeding is unclear. Intravenous vasopressin, or its analogue, desmopressin, produces several-fold increases in levels of von Willebrand's factor and factor VIII. It has proven efficacy in reducing bleeding time in patients with hemophilia, congenital platelet dysfunction, and uremia. It also has shown promise in controlling bleeding and shortening the prothrombin time and bleeding time in patients with cirrhosis [313–315]. Vasopressin and desmopressin are not effective in patients with thrombocytopenia [314]. Infusions of antithrombin III concentrate have shown efficacy in patients with DIC and FHF. Some subjects given antithrombin III to levels 50–80% of normal showed reduced platelet consumption and decreased mortality rate [316,317].

SPONTANEOUS BACTERIAL PERITONITIS

Spontaneous bacterial peritonitis occurs in 8–19% of adults with cirrhosis and ascites [318,319]. The wide range in reported incidence is partly a result of disparities among studies in patient selection and definition of SBP. Some definitions required positive cultures; others required only an elevated white blood cell count in the peritoneal fluid. Nevertheless, it is clearly a common complication of ascites and cirrhosis, and the possibility of SBP must be entertained in any patient with ascites, especially if there is a sudden clinical deterioration.

Spontaneous bacterial peritonitis refers to bacterial peritonitis not associated with gut perforation or any other "secondary" source. The diagnosis depends on a positive ascitic fluid culture, without an apparent surgically treatable source of infection [320]. It generally is agreed that SBP occurs in the setting of transient bacteremia in patients with "susceptible" ascites. Patients with severe liver disease have many immunologic deficits that predispose them to frequent and prolonged bacteremia, including defects in the reticuloendothelial system [112], abnormalities in neutrophil function [113], and complement deficiencies [117,118]. In one retrospective study, it was shown that SBP (in children with chronic liver disease) occurred in association with low serum C3 and C4 levels [321]. Similar studies in adults have shown no such differences [322]. Portosystemic shunting also prolongs bacteremia [121,182,323]. Patients with ascites with low protein concentrations seem to be at higher risk for SBP. In one study, 15% of patients with ascitic fluid protein concentrations of less than 1.0 g/dL developed SBP, whereas only 1.5% of patients with protein concentrations greater than this developed SBP [324]. Ascitic C3 levels of less than 15 μg/mL also predispose patients to SBP [322,325]. The opsonic activity of ascites correlates well with protein (and C3) concentration [326]; it appears that SBP occurs in patients with ascitic fluid that is unable to carry out an effective immune response. Other factors predisposing to SBP include gastrointestinal hemorrhage, urinary tract infections, indwelling bladder catheters, intravascular catheters, and repeated large-volume paracentesis [327].

Table 6.7: Indications for Diagnostic Paracentesis

New onset ascites
Cirrhotic patients with ascites upon admission
Cirrhotic patients with ascites, with clinical signs of infection
Cirrhotic patients with ascites with unexplained clinical deterioration

Spontaneous bacterial peritonitis is monomicrobial in almost all instances. Most episodes of SBP are caused by bacteria that normally reside in the intestine. However, sources other than the gastrointestinal tract occasionally are implicated, including the urinary tract [328] and the lungs [329]. Gram-negative enteric bacteria are isolated in 60–80% of all adult patients and include most commonly *Escherichia coli, Klebsiella* species, and *Enterococcus faecalis.* Streptococcal and staphylococcal species also often have been reported. Other bacteria are isolated occasionally, including *Listeria monocytogenes* and mycobacteria. The few studies involving children suggest that a different spectrum of organisms may be responsible for SBP, particularly in young children. In one study, *Streptococcus pneumoniae* was isolated from 9 of 12 children with SBP [321]. Other bacterial species recovered from children include *Hemophilus influenzae* and *Neisseria meningitides* [330]. Anaerobes are isolated only occasionally. Polymicrobial infections suggest bowel perforation and secondary peritonitis. Blood cultures also often are positive, especially in symptomatic SBP.

The hallmark of SBP is ascites. SBP should be suspected in a patient with ascites with concurrent fever, abdominal pain, or elevated peripheral white blood cell count. Other signs and symptoms of SBP include hypotension, shock, and worsening of hepatic encephalopathy. It should be remembered that the symptoms can be very subtle. Common symptoms in children also include increasing abdominal distention, pyrexia, abdominal pain, vomiting, and diarrhea. In infants, the symptoms may include poor feeding and lethargy [331]. The physical examination often reveals abdominal tenderness with rebound tenderness and decreased or absent bowel sounds [321]. Several studies have shown, however, that a substantial number of patients with SBP are asymptomatic. In one study, 224 adult patients with cirrhosis and ascites underwent routine abdominal paracentesis, revealing SBP in 27. One third (9) of these 27 subjects had "asymptomatic" SBP [332]. All patients with abrupt onset of ascites or with a sudden increase in ascites should be considered for abdominal paracentesis. Gastrointestinal bleeding has been highly associated with SBP and represents a clear indication for abdominal paracentesis [333]. Indications for diagnostic paracentesis are reviewed in Table 6.7.

Abdominal paracentesis is safe, even in patients with a coagulopathy. The presence of a coagulopathy may be a sign of sepsis or SBP itself. Runyon [334,335], citing 38 years of experience performing more than 1000 abdominal paracenteses per year, emphasizes that prophylactic transfusions of fresh frozen plasma or platelets are not necessary, particularly if the paracentesis is done along the midline. The one exception to this is the setting of DIC, in which hematologic complications are more common [336]. Finally, paracentesis does not predispose the patient to SBP [182,335].

Ascitic fluid obtained at paracentesis should be inoculated into blood culture bottles at the bedside. This has been shown to increase the positive culture "yield" substantially, from approximately 50% using traditional culture methods to approximately 80% [337–339]. The bacterial concentration in infected ascitic fluid is usually low (only about two bacteria per milliliter) [181]. If a 2- or 3-mL sample of ascitic fluid is allowed to sit for several hours during transport and inoculation, the few bacteria likely will perish. Inoculation of a large (10-mL) sample into blood culture bottles at the bedside increases the diagnostic yield substantially and shortens the time to identification of the bacterial species [340].

An ascitic fluid polymorphonuclear neutrophil leukocyte count of greater than 250 cells/mm^3 also is suggestive of SBP and mandates empiric antibiotic therapy. Protein levels of the ascitic fluid also should be measured because low protein concentrations indicate an increased susceptibility to SBP. Glucose and lactate dehydrogenase levels also should be measured. The ascitic fluid of patients with bacterial peritonitis is characterized by a total protein level of greater than 1 g/dL, a glucose level of less than 50 mg/dL, a lactate dehydrogenase level greater than that normal for serum, and a polymorphonuclear neutrophil leukocyte count greatly elevated above 250 cells/mm^3. Any of these findings in a patient with suspected peritonitis also should prompt an investigation for gut perforation [341,342]. When treated only with intravenous antibiotics, gut perforation is almost uniformly fatal whereas unnecessary surgical procedures in patients with SBP may also be associated with high mortality rates [343]. Table 6.8 reviews the findings in ascitic fluid in patients with SBP compared with those with gut perforation. IL-6 and tumor necrosis factor-α have been found in substantially higher concentrations in the serum and ascitic fluid of subjects with SBP than in comparable patients without SBP [344]. As tests for these monokines become widely available, they may be helpful in the early detection of SBP. The pH of the ascitic fluid is usually not helpful because it is related directly to the polymorphonuclear neutrophil leukocyte count [341].

Empiric treatment in patients with an elevated ascitic polymorphonuclear neutrophil leukocyte count is indicated in most patients. Repeated paracenteses in patients suspected of having SBP show that most patients do not clear the infection spontaneously, and in most the bacterial and polymorphonuclear neutrophil leukocyte counts increase without treatment [345]. The ascitic fluid cell count is usually available in hours; the culture result might take days to become determinate. Delaying treatment could result in an overwhelming infection [184]. Broad-spectrum antibiotic treatment is warranted until specific culture and sensitivity results are available. Cefotaxime is the antibiotic of choice in most patients because it covers those organisms most likely to cause SBP [184,346]. Although gentamicin and ampicillin were the recommended antibiotics in the past, the distribution volume of gentamicin in ascites is unpredictable, and aminoglycosides are unduly nephrotoxic, especially in patients with cirrhosis and ascites. Combination therapy with amoxicillin and clavulanic acid also is effective, well tolerated, and associated with a low rate of resistant organisms [347]. The final choice of antibiotic is dictated by the isolation and sensitivity pattern of bacteria from the infected ascitic fluid. Five days of antibiotic therapy is as effective as 10 days in the important outcome variables of clearance of bacteria and mortality and recurrence rates [348].

Table 6.8: Differential Ascitic Fluid Findings in Spontaneous Bacterial Peritonitis and Secondary Peritonitis

	Spontaneous Bacterial Peritonitis	*Secondary Peritonitis*
Polymorphonuclear cell count	>250 cells/mm^3	>250 cells/mm^3
Total protein	<1 g/dL	>1 g/dL
Glucose	>50 mg/dL	<50 mg/dL
Lactate dehydrogenase	Serum levels	>Serum levels
Culture results	Single bacterial organism	Polymicrobial

The use of oral antibiotics for the treatment of SBP has been investigated and appears to be encouraging. One study compared "standard" treatment of 7 days of intravenous ciprofloxacin to a treatment regimen of 2 days of intravenous therapy followed by 5 days of oral medication. Both groups of approximately 40 patients did similarly well [349]. Another study compared oral ofloxacin to intravenous cefotaxime in a group of more than 120 patients with SBP but not in shock. The two groups had almost identical success rates (84% vs. 85%, respectively) [350]. Both studies were carried out entirely in adults. Intravenous albumin has been shown in one study to promote survival, probably because of decreased renal impairment in cirrhotic patients with SBP [351]. Octreotide has also been used in patients with renal impairment and SBP with apparent success and safety. This will be considered more completely in the discussion of the hepatorenal syndrome.

The mortality rate associated with SBP is high. In adults with unstable liver disease, it is estimated to be as high as 55% [352]. One report of SBP in children revealed that 7 of 11 children with newly diagnosed SBP died of complications of severe liver disease despite appropriate antibiotic therapy [321]. The mortality rate decreases with earlier diagnosis and aggressive treatment.

Still, a large percentage of patients with SBP die within several years of the first episode of SBP, often with complications associated with chronic liver disease, such as hemorrhage. Because the recurrence rate for SBP is high (up to 69% after 1 year) [353], efforts should be made to minimize the risk of SBP. Diuresis of ascitic fluid increases the protein concentration many times [354], so aggressive diuresis theoretically may reduce the risk of SBP, although this has never been demonstrated. Many of those most susceptible to SBP (those with high-volume, low-protein ascites), however, are refractory to diuretic therapy and obtain no benefit from aggressive diuresis. Because *S. pneumoniae* appears to be a common pathogen in SBP in children, immunization with the pneumococcal antigen vaccine or prophylactic use of penicillin may provide protection, although prospective studies have not been done.

After it was shown that oral nonabsorbable antibiotics prevent SBP in patients with acute gastrointestinal hemorrhage [323], other forms of bacterial prophylaxis have been considered. Selective intestinal decontamination (the inhibition of gram-negative flora of the gut with preservation of other flora, such as anaerobic bacteria) employing norfloxacin resulted in higher ascitic fluid complement and protein levels [355]. A prospective placebo-controlled, double-blind study of norfloxacin prophylaxis of recurrent SBP demonstrated a substantial reduction of recurrence over 6 months from 68–20% among those taking norfloxacin [356]. Another study reported that the administration of norfloxacin to patients with a high risk of developing SBP (ascitic fluid with low protein content) after admission to the hospital for ascites decreased the incidence of all infections during the hospitalization, including SBP [357]. In neither of these studies were other outcome issues regarding long-term use of antibiotics, such as patient survival, emergence of resistant organisms, and cost-effectiveness, addressed.

HEPATORENAL SYNDROME

Hepatorenal syndrome is defined as a progressive renal insufficiency of unknown cause in a patient with severe liver disease. Although it initially was described in adult patients with alcoholic cirrhosis, it is associated with cirrhosis of any cause. It is a serious complication of cirrhosis and carries a grave prognosis [358,359]. It is almost always accompanied by ascites. Although the pathogenesis of HRS is poorly understood, it is characterized by corticomedullary redistribution of renal blood flow. Selective renal arteriography and xenon-113 washout studies demonstrate a marked reduction in renal cortical blood flow [151,360].

There are two forms of HRS [361]. In some patients, the progression of renal failure is rapid and the overall prognosis is poor. This is termed type 1 HRS. It is characterized by a doubling of the serum creatinine within a 2-week period. In adults, it can also be defined as the finding of a serum creatinine level above 2.5 mg/dL [362,363]. Type I HRS is associated with many complications of chronic liver disease, including SBP and gastrointestinal bleeding. Type II HRS is more subtle than type I and is used to describe patients with a milder and more slowly progressive form of renal impairment. In adults it is associated with serum creatinine levels of 1.5–2.0 mg/dL [364].

Histologic changes are minimal, however, leading to the conclusion that HRS is a "functional" renal impairment. Although autopsy findings in subjects who have undergone liver transplantation show a universal occurrence of glomerular changes including glomerulosclerosis and membranoproliferative glomerulonephritis [365], the changes of HRS are reversible after orthotopic liver transplantation or if the primary liver disease is treated successfully [366,367]. Furthermore, postmortem renal angiography demonstrates complete reversal of the abnormalities seen in HRS, and kidneys from patients who have died with HRS function well after transplantation to patients without liver disease [368].

The cause of the renal cortical vasoconstriction in HRS is unknown. One theory relates the cortical vasoconstriction to the decreased extrarenal plasma volume in patients with cirrhosis [369]. The kidney responds with increased renin release and increased generation of angiotensin II, which lead to decreased glomerular filtration rate, a cycle that ends in oliguric renal failure. High renin levels are seen in patients with cirrhosis, and those with renal failure have higher levels still [370]. Recent studies have demonstrated systemic and regional hemodynamic changes in patients with HRS. Patients with cirrhosis but not HRS have systemic vasodilation; those with HRS have evidence of peripheral vasoconstriction with possible pooling of splanchnic blood, resulting in decreased renal blood flow [371]. Administration of 8 ornithine vasopressin [372] or ornipressin [373], agents known to cause splanchnic vasoconstriction, results in a number of improvements of the vascular abnormalities seen in patients with cirrhosis. These include beneficial increases in mean arterial pressure, renal blood flow, and the glomerular filtration rate in patients with cirrhosis and renal dysfunction [372].

There is also evidence that HRS is caused by an imbalance of locally produced vasodilators and vasoconstrictors. Renal synthesis of the vasodilatory prostaglandins PGE_2, produced by the kidneys in response to vasoconstriction and ischemia, and PGE_1 is increased in patients with cirrhosis but is decreased significantly if cirrhosis is complicated by HRS [370,374]. In animal models, renal vasoconstriction occurs after cyclooxygenase inhibitors are given, again suggesting that the vasoconstriction seen in HRS may be caused by decreased prostaglandin production [375]. It also has been observed that patients with cirrhosis and HRS have large increases in urinary thromboxane B_2, an inactive metabolite of the potent vasoconstrictor thromboxane A_2, and a large decrease in the urinary PGE_2 concentration compared with patients with cirrhosis with no HRS. HRS, therefore, may be caused either by an increase in the production of vasoconstrictive thromboxane B_2 or a decrease in vasodilatory PGE_2, or by an imbalance between the two [376,377]. Calcitonin gene–related peptide, a potent dilator of the splanchnic vascular bed, also has been found in high concentrations in patients with cirrhosis. Patients with and without HRS have increased serum levels of calcitonin gene–related peptide, although those with

Table 6.9: Important Differential Urinary Findings in Acute Azotemia in Patients with Liver Disease

	Prerenal Azotemia	*Hepatorenal Syndrome*	*Acute Tubular Necrosis*
Urinary sodium concentration	<10 mEq/L	<10 mEq/L	>30 mEq/L
Urinary osmolality	>100 mOsm, >plasma osmolality	>100 mOsm, >plasma osmolality	Equal to plasma osmolality
Urine/plasma creatine	>30:1	>30:1	<20:1
Fractional excretion of sodium	<1%	<1%	>2%
Urinary sediment	Normal	Normal	Casts, debris
Response to volume expansion	Sustained diuresis	Brief or no diuresis	No diuresis

HRS have higher levels. It is unclear whether calcitonin gene–related peptide is a mediator of HRS or the high levels seen in cirrhosis are merely reflective of impaired hepatic clearance [378]. The role of the highly potent endothelium-dependent vasoactive substance NO has also been studied in the setting of HRS. Overproduction of NO has been demonstrated in patients with advanced liver disease, and some studies have shown that patients with the highest levels of NO_2 and NO_3 also have some degree of renal failure [379].

The clinical presentation of HRS varies in both rapidity of onset and severity. Its incidence in children has not been well described. One study found that HRS occurred in 20% of adult patients with cirrhosis and ascites within 1 year of presentation and in 39% within 5 years [380]. The HRS usually presents in one of two forms. Type I HRS is characterized by a drop of at least 50% of creatinine clearance and a twofold increase in serum creatinine levels within a 2-week period. Type II HRS is milder. It describes patients with mild renal insufficiency and is characterized by ascites that is resistant to diuretics [381,382].

The hallmark of HRS is progressive renal failure in a patient (usually hospitalized) with cirrhosis and ascites. Typically the renal failure is oliguric, with a benign urinary sediment. The five criteria for the diagnosis of HRS are listed in Table 6.9.

Although patients in severe hepatic failure are at risk for developing HRS, no clinical characteristics or laboratory findings predict the onset of HRS. Although most patients have preexisting mild renal abnormalities, the onset of renal failure is characteristically abrupt and may be precipitated by gastrointestinal hemorrhage, aggressive diuresis, or rarely, large-volume abdominal paracentesis [358]. SBP has also been described as a precipitant for HRS [351,383]. Laboratory findings include increased blood urea nitrogen and creatinine concentrations, although the degree of elevation may not be as high as expected based on the degree of renal failure. This may be partly because of the interference in measuring serum creatinine caused by elevated serum bilirubin levels [384,385]. Blood urea measurements also may be unreliable because of impaired hepatic urea synthesis [386]. Both urea and creatinine production may be decreased in cirrhotic patients because of decreased muscle mass and poor nutritional intake. The mild initial increase in blood urea nitrogen or creatinine may thus be missed entirely. Hypokalemia may be present, usually as a result of gastrointestinal losses (vomiting or diarrhea) or diuretic use. Hyponatremia is secondary to a decrease in free water clearance. The urinary sediment is usually unremarkable. The urine sodium concentration is typically very low and is usually less than 10 mEq/L, with urinary osmolarity 100 mOsm higher than that of serum. The fractional extraction of sodium is less than 1%, and the ratio of urinary to serum creatinine is greater than 30. Although these findings are consistent with intravascular volume deficit, the pulmonary capillary wedge pressure is normal, and there is little or only transient response to fluid challenge. Table 6.9 reviews the findings associated with HRS and acute tubular necrosis.

Hepatorenal syndrome should be considered in any patient with cirrhosis with the onset of oliguric or nonoliguric renal failure. Acute renal failure of any cause may occur in patients with chronic liver disease, although the most common causes include acute tubular necrosis, prerenal azotemia, and HRS. In some patients, especially those with liver failure, renal failure may have several causes. The laboratory findings of acute tubular necrosis include a fractional extraction of sodium of greater than 2%, a urine sodium concentration of greater than 10 mEq/L, and a low urinary osmolarity. On the other hand, patients with prerenal azotemia have findings nearly identical to those of HRS, except that they have a low pulmonary capillary wedge pressure. Pulmonary capillary wedge pressure measurements may be difficult to interpret in patients with tense ascites, which often is seen in HRS. More importantly, patients with prerenal azotemia have a marked and sustained improvement in renal function after replenishment of intravascular volume.

Because there is no known effective therapy for HRS (other than liver transplantation), the most important principles underlying its management include avoidance of agents and conditions known to precipitate HRS and discovery and aggressive treatment of reversible causes of renal failure, especially prerenal azotemia and urinary tract obstruction. Nephrotoxic drugs such as aminoglycosides should be avoided in patients with severe liver failure; infections such as SBP should be treated with cefotaxime or other antibiotics unlikely to aggravate kidney function. Dehydration, gastrointestinal hemorrhage, and septicemia should be addressed promptly to minimize the ensuing increased risk of HRS. Diuresis of tense ascites should be performed carefully to avoid an intravascular fluid deficit. A loop diuretic, muzolimine, appears to promote diuresis more gradually and with less urinary potassium loss and less stimulation of renin activity than furosemide [387]. Although large-volume paracentesis has been avoided in patients with tense ascites, recent studies have confirmed its safety if used in conjunction with replacement of albumin [194,388]. Abdominal paracentesis has improved the status of patients with HRS transiently, but long-term improvements do not occur [389].

If HRS is suspected and acute tubular necrosis is not present, volume expansion should be tried carefully. Even if no prerenal azotemia exists, short-term improvement of HRS has been reported after volume expansion [390]. Supportive measures routinely recommended for acute renal failure, including administration of a low-protein diet and correction of serum electrolyte abnormalities, should be considered. Hemodialysis can help correct fluid and electrolyte imbalances and provide time for expected liver transplantation but does not otherwise improve the outcome of HRS. Because patients with HRS have some degree of hypotension, the use of continuous arteriovenous hemofiltration or ultrafiltration may be preferable [391,392]. These have been used successfully in children with HRS [393].

Portacaval shunts have been used in HRS with limited success. The high operative mortality rate and severe side effects associated with the procedure limit its practicality [394]. Uncontrolled studies have shown that peritoneovenous shunts improve the renal function and urine output in isolated patients with less severe forms of liver disease [395,396]. Experience with peritoneovenous shunts in children remains very limited, although case reports document its successful use in pediatric patients with FHF [397]. TIPS placement has been tried in adult patients with HRS and has been associated with some improvement in renal function [278]. Brensing et al. [398] treated 16 patients with advanced cirrhosis and HRS, all of whom were ineligible for transplant (most were active alcoholics) with TIPS. After 2 weeks, all showed striking reductions in serum urea and creatinine clearance, and glomerular filtration improved gradually over the subsequent 6–8 weeks. Although seven of these patients died from either progressive liver disease or events that were not liver-related, the improvement in HRS persisted for at least 3 months in the majority of the survivors. Randomized controlled trials of TIPS in patients with HRS are still lacking.

Midodrine (a selective α_1-adrenergic agonist) and octreotide (a somatostatin analogue) have been used in combination in patients with HRS. Midodrine is a potent vasoconstrictor, and octreotide inhibits vasodilation. A combination of the two may result in improvements in systemic vascular resistance and renal blood flow [399]. In one study, among five subjects given these medications, three survived hospitalization (one after liver transplant) whereas seven of eight patients receiving dopamine without midodrine or octreotide died within 2 weeks of presentation. All patients receiving the combination therapy had improvements in kidney function, even those who did not subsequently survive [400]. Further confirmatory studies need to be conducted, but this therapy has successfully treated HRS patients without resorting to liver transplant. Treatment with octreotide alone has not shown beneficial effect [401].

Because of the alterations in renal blood flow in HRS, drugs that alter the renal vascular tone theoretically have value in its treatment. The administration of the vasodilatory prostaglandins PGE_1 and PGA_1 had no effect on patients with HRS [402,403]. An uncontrolled and nonrandomized trial of a synthetic form of PGE_2, misoprostol, in four patients with HRS resulted in increased urinary volume and a decrease in serum creatinine concentration. Three of the four patients died within 40 days, although not from renal failure [404]. Inhibition of the potent vasoconstrictor thromboxane with dazoxiben has resulted in a decrease of urinary thromboxane B_2, but no change in creatinine clearance [405]. Another inhibitor of thromboxane A_2 synthesis, OKY140, increases furosemide-induced natriuresis in patients with cirrhosis [406] but has not yet been tried therapeutically in patients with HRS. Finally, dopamine in subpressor doses promotes increased blood flow to the kidneys and may be useful in the prevention of HRS but not in its treatment [407].

If renal and hepatic function do not improve with medical management, the only reliable treatment for HRS is orthotopic liver transplantation [408,409] because progressive, irreversible multiorgan failure ultimately ensues. There is good evidence that orthotopic hepatic transplantation is tolerated similarly in patients with and without HRS. In one large study, Gonwa et al. [367] showed that patients with HRS have the same 90-day (approximately 87%) and similar 2-year survival rates. Glomerular filtration rate was similar in the two groups 1 month after transplantation. In another study, at 24 weeks after transplantation there was no difference in serum creatinine between the two groups [410]. It has been shown, however, that approximately 10% of patients with HRS experience end-stage renal failure after transplantation; only approximately 1% of patients without HRS have similar renal disease [367], and more patients with HRS require hemodialysis after transplantation than do those without HRS.

MALNUTRITION AND CHRONIC LIVER DISEASE

Chronic liver disease may interfere with a patient's nutrition status by either interrupting a key metabolic process or allowing a metabolic imbalance to persist. The liver plays a key role in the homeostasis of various serum proteins, such as albumin and coagulation factors; gluconeogenesis and thus the maintenance of safe blood glucose levels; lipid balance, as an important site of cholesterol synthesis, by controlling the metabolism of fatty acids and by contributing to fat absorption through the production and secretion of bile; and protein balance, because the liver is a major site for protein metabolism and urea synthesis. All these processes require energy, substrate, and control mechanisms. An interruption of any of these processes may result in a diminished state of nutrition.

Malnutrition is common in children with chronic liver disease and may result from a variety of factors. Most obvious is fat malabsorption, seen most commonly in patients with cholestasis. Such patients may present with weight loss or failure to thrive, or they may present with symptoms specific to fat-soluble vitamin deficiency, such as coagulopathy or hypocalcemia. Many patients with cirrhosis suffer from anorexia, nausea, and vomiting and may fail to ingest adequate calories. Clinically stable cirrhotic patients might be in a state of energy balance but still fail to take in optimal amounts of protein or calories. Increasing the caloric density of the diets of such patients has been shown to improve nitrogen balance [411]. In addition to poor caloric intake, dietary recall studies have shown that patients with cirrhosis often fail to meet daily recommended allowances for thiamine, folic acid, vitamin D, vitamin E, magnesium, and zinc [412].

Metabolic studies conducted in patients with cirrhosis have shown that patients with mild or compensated cirrhosis have a variety of subclinical abnormalities, including hypermetabolism, increased lipid utilization, and insulin resistance, even patients with normal anthropometric measurements [413]. Patients with cirrhosis also may have defective glucose storage, enhanced thermogenesis, and negative energy balance [414]. The clinical significance of these changes has not been addressed, although there is some evidence to suggest that reducing the hyperinsulinemic state of patients with cirrhosis (through limitation of dietary carbohydrate) can improve insulin sensitivity in these patients [415].

Children with liver disease should be weighed and measured carefully at each clinic visit, and any changes in anthropometrics should prompt a careful reevaluation of the patient's nutritional state. Because children need to grow and because an impaired nutritional state may result in increased morbidity and mortality rates after transplantation, growth assessment plays a primal role in the care and evaluation of chronic liver disease. Although adult patients may restrict salt at the first sign of fluid imbalance or may restrict protein before any sign of hepatic encephalopathy develops, pediatric patients must be on a palatable diet that supports growth. For example, a child might not find a strict salt-sparing diet to be palatable, thus such a patient may depend on diuretics to a greater degree than would a similar adult patient. Metabolic studies have shown a "nibbling" diet, characterized by an early breakfast, late evening meal, and frequent snacks, to be associated with less fluctuation of the respiratory quotient as well as reduced nighttime catabolic rate as measured by nocturnal amino acid breakdown, thus improving nitrogen balance [416–418].

Although the specific benefits of improved dietary intake may be hard to measure without large randomized trials, there is evidence that improved nutrition may result in an overall improved state of health. Administration of enteral feedings to hospitalized patients with cirrhosis has been well tolerated and associated with a reduction in mortality rate (during that hospitalization) from 47–12% [419]. Hirsch et al. [420] showed that in patients with alcoholic cirrhosis, daily supplementation of protein and calorie intake resulted in specific improvements of host defenses in these patients. Their study, however, does not measure rates of hospitalization or antibiotic use, effects on longevity, or progression to transplantation. The type of protein ingested may have an impact on the manifestations of cirrhosis. Because the administration of BCAAs has been associated with improvements in hepatic encephalopathy, efforts have been made to provide patients with cirrhosis with diets high in these amino acids. Because vegetable protein has lower concentrations of aromatic amino acids and high concentrations of BCAAs, vegetarian diets have been encouraged in patients with cirrhosis and hepatic encephalopathy with some success [421]. The improvements, however, did not result in a complete resolution of the encephalopathy. In children, the emphasis again should be on providing adequate protein to support growth in a culturally palatable diet.

Most children with cirrhosis develop deficiencies in the fat-soluble vitamins. Supplementation with these vitamins as well as medium-chain triglycerides may be necessary to achieve optimal growth. Polyunsaturated lecithin (polyenylphosphatidylcholine) has been shown to be useful in animal models of cirrhosis [422]. It has been shown to attenuate alcohol-induced liver changes and fibrosis in rats [423,424]. Evidence suggests that its use might result in decreased activation of hepatic stellate cells, which control the hepatic ECM [425]. It has not yet been used widely enough in human trials to evaluate its efficacy.

If a child is unable to take adequate protein and calories, supplementation with high-calorie drinks and then nighttime nasogastric tube feeding should be considered [426]. Parenteral nutrition support usually is reserved for acutely ill and hospitalized patients. The nutritional assessment and care of children with cirrhosis may be complicated; a multidisciplinary approach including a pediatric dietitian, liaison nurse, and feeding psychologist is often necessary [427].

SUMMARY

Cirrhosis, both static and progressive, is a potential consequence of many acute and chronic liver disorders affecting the pediatric patient. The pathogenesis of cirrhosis is becoming clearer as the molecular biology of fibrogenesis becomes better understood. The markers and complications of cirrhosis are those of chronic liver disease and dysfunction, with or without cirrhosis. The complications of advancing liver disease are at least partially understood, and the management of these infants and children can be planned on a rational basis. Ultimately, the compromised hepatic function that accompanies cirrhosis leads to hepatic transplantation for many of these patients. It is possible that newer agents that control fibrogenesis and drugs that manage the complications of advanced liver disease will change the irreversibility of the course for many of these patients.

REFERENCES

1. Anthony PP, Ishak KG, Nayak NC. The morphology of cirrhosis: definition, nomenclature, and classification. Bull WHO 1977; 55:521–40.
2. Ruben E, Krus S, Popper H. Pathogenesis of postnecrotic cirrhosis in alcoholics. Arch Pathol 1962;73:288–99.
3. Fauerholdt L, Schlichting P, Christensen E, et al. Conversion of micronodular cirrhosis into macronodular cirrhosis. Hepatology 1983;3:928–31.
4. Poppor H, Berk PD. Lessons from the study of cirrhosis and other fibrotic disease of the liver. In: Berk PD, Wasserman LR, eds. Myelofibrosis and the biology of connective tissue. New York: Alan R. Liss, 1984:405–24.
5. Popper H, Schaffner F. Chronic hepatitis: taxonomic, etiologic and therapeutic problems. In: Schaffner F, Popper H, eds. Progress in liver disease. Vol. 5. New York: Grune and Stratton, 1976:535.
6. Silverman A, Roy CC. Chronic active hepatitis. In: Roy CC, Silverman A, eds. Pediatric clinical gastroenterology. St. Louis: Mosby, 1983.
7. Maddrey WL, Boitnott JK. Drug induced chronic liver disease. Gastroenterology 1977;72:1348–53.
8. Geoffrey L. Dynamic state of collagen: pathways of collagen degradation in vivo and their possible role in regulation of collagen mass. Am J Physiol 1987;252:1–9.
9. Martin GR, Kleinman HK. The extracellular matrix component in development and disease. Semin Liver Dis 1985;5:147–56.
10. Biagini G, Ballardini G. Liver fibrosis and extracellular matrix. J Hepatol 1989;8:115–24.
11. Hascall V. Proteoglycans: structure and function. In: Ginsberg V, ed. Biology of carbohydrates. New York: John Wiley & Sons, 1981:1–49.
12. Hynes R. Molecular biology of fibronectin. Annu Rev Cell Biol 1985;1:67–90.
13. Clark R. Potential roles of fibronectin in cutaneous wound repair. Arch Dermatol 1987;3:57–85.
14. Bitterman PB, Wewers MD, Rennard SI, et al. Modulation of alveolar macrophage-driven fibroblast proliferation by alternative macrophage mediators. J Clin Invest 1986;77:700–8.
15. Aumanailley M, Nurcombe V, Edgar D, et al. The cellular interactions of laminin fragments: cell adhesion correlations with two fragment-specific high affinity binding sites. J Biol Chem 1987;262:11532–8.
16. Martin GR, Timpl R. Laminin and other basement membrane components. Annu Rev Cell Biol 1987;3:57–85.
17. Bissell DM, Stamatoglou SC, Nermut MV, et al. Interactions of rat hepatocytes with type IV collagen, fibronectin and laminin matrices: distinct matrix-controlled models of attachment and spreading. Eur J Cell Biol 1986;40:72–8.
18. Hahn EG, Schuppan D. Ethanol and fibrogenesis in the liver. In: Seitz HK, Kommerell B, eds. Alcohol related disease in gastroenterology. Berlin: Springer Verlag, 1985:124–53.
19. Hahn E, Wick G, Pencev D, Timpl R. Distribution of basement membrane proteins in normal and fibrotic human liver: collagen type IV, laminin and fibronectin. Gut 1980;21:63–71.
20. Preaux AM, Mallat A, Van Nhieu JT, et al. Matrix metalloproteinase-2 activation in human hepatic fibrosis regulation by cell-matrix interactions. Hepatology 1999;30:944–50.
21. Blaheta RA, Kronenberger B, Woitaschek D, et al. Dedifferentiation of human hepatocytes by extracellular matrix proteins in vitro: quantitative and qualitative investigation of cytokeratin 7, 8, 18, 19 and vimentin filaments. J Hepatol 1998;28: 677–90.
22. Bianchi FB, Biagini G, Ballardini G, et al. Basement membrane production by hepatocytes in chronic liver disease. Hepatology 1984;4:1167–72.
23. Schaffner F, Poper H. Capillarization of hepatic sinusoids in man. Gastroenterology 1963;44:239–42.
24. Arthur MJ. Reversibility of liver fibrosis and cirrhosis following treatment for hepatitis C. Gastroenterology 2002;122:1525–8.
25. Issa R, Zhou X, Constandinou CM, et al. Spontaneous recovery from micronodular cirrhosis: evidence for incomplete resolution associated with matrix cross-linking. Gastroenterology 2004;126:1795–808.
26. Pares A, Caballeria J, Bruguera M, et al. Histological course of alcoholic hepatitis. Influence of abstinence, sex and extent of hepatic damage. J Hepatol 1986;2:33–42.
27. Dixon JB, Bhathal PS, Hughes NR, et al. Nonalcoholic fatty liver disease: improvement in liver histological analysis with weight loss. Hepatology 2004;39:1647–54.
28. Knodell RG, Ishak KG, Black WC, et al. Formulation and application of a numerical scoring system for assessing histological activity in asymptomatic chronic active hepatitis. Hepatology 1981;1:431–5.
29. Ishak K, Baptista A, Bianchi L, et al. Histological grading and staging of chronic hepatitis. J Hepatol 1995;22:696–9.
30. Bedossa P, Poynard T. An algorithm for the grading of activity in chronic hepatitis C. The METAVIR Cooperative Study Group. Hepatology 1996;24:289–93.
31. Plebani M, Burlina A. Biochemical markers of hepatic fibrosis. Clin Biochem 1991;24:219–39.
32. Niernela O, Ristcli J, Blake JE, et al. Markers of fibrogenesis and basement membrane formation in alcoholic liver disease: relation to severity, presence of hepatitis, and alcohol intake. Gastroenterology 1990;98:1612–19.
33. Schneider M, Voss B, Hogemann B, et al. Evaluation of serum laminin pl, procollagen-III peptides, and n-acetyl-B-glucosaminidase for monitoring the activity of liver fibrosis. Hepatogasteroenterology 1989;36:506–10.
34. Gressner AM, Tittor W, Negwer A, et al. Serum concentrations of laminin and propeptide of type III collagen in relation to the portal venous pressure of fibrotic liver disease. Clin Chem Acta 1986;161:249–58.
35. Gressner AM, Tittor W, Negwer A. Serum concentrations of N-terminal propeptide of type III procollagen and laminin in the outflow of fibrotic livers. Hepatogasteroenterology 1986;33: 191–5.
36. Bahr MJ, Boker KH, Horn W, et al. Serum laminin P1 levels do not reflect critically elevated portal pressure in patients with liver cirrhosis. Hepatogasteroenterology 1997;44:1200–5.
37. Korner T, Kropf J, Gressner AM. Serum laminin and hyaluronan in liver cirrhosis: markers of progression with high prognastic value. J Hepatol 1996;25:684–8.

38. Murawaki Y, Kusakabe Y, Hirayama C. Serum lysyl oxidase activity in chronic liver disease in comparison with serum levels of prolyl hydroxylase and laminin. Hepatology 1991;14: 1167–73.
39. Misaki M, Shima T, Yano Y, et al. Basement membrane-related and type III procollagen-related antigens in serum of patients with chronic viral liver disease. Clin Chem 1990;36:522–4.
40. Ji X, Li S, Kong X, et al. Clinical significance of serum 7s collagen and type VI collagen levels for the diagnosis of hepatic fibrosis. Chin Med J (Engl) 1997;110:198–201.
41. Babbs C, Smith A, Hunt LP, et al. Type III procollagen peptide: a marker of disease activity and prognosis in primary biliary cirrhosis. Lancet 1988;1:1021–4.
42. Oberti F, Valsesia E, Pilette C, et al. Noninvasive diagnosis of hepatic fibrosis or cirrhosis. Gastroenterology 1997;113: 1609–16.
43. Gregorio GV, Portmann B, Karani J, et al. Autoimmune hepatitis/sclerosing cholangitis overlap syndrome in childhood: a 16-year prospective study. Hepatology 2001;33:544–53.
44. Saile B, Matthes N, Knittel T, et al. Transforming growth factor beta and tumor necrosis factor alpha inhibit both apoptosis and proliferation of activated rat hepatic stellate cells. Hepatology 1999;30:196–202.
45. Li D, Friedman SL. Liver fibrogenesis and the role of hepatic stellate cells: new insights and prospects for therapy. J Gastroenterol Hepatol 1999;14:618–33.
46. Lieber CS. New concepts of the pathogenesis of alcoholic liver disease lead to novel treatments. Curr Gastroenterol Rep 2004;6:60–5.
47. Lieber CS, Leo MA, Cao Q, et al. Silymarin retards the progression of alcohol-induced hepatic fibrosis in baboons. J Clin Gastroenterol 2003;37:336–9.
48. Tilg H, Kaser A. Treatment strategies in nonalcoholic fatty liver disease. Nat Clin Pract Gastroenterol Hepatol 2005;2: 148–55.
49. Yokohama S, Yoneda M, Haneda M, et al. Therapeutic efficacy of an angiotensin II receptor antagonist in patients with nonalcoholic steatohepatitis. Hepatology 2004;40:1222–5.
50. Rimola A, Londono MC, Guevara G, et al. Beneficial effect of angiotensin-blocking agents on graft fibrosis in hepatitis C recurrence after liver transplantation. Transplantation 2004;78: 686–91.
51. Sakaida I, Terai S, Yamamoto N, et al. Transplantation of bone marrow cells reduces CCl4-induced liver fibrosis in mice. Hepatology 2004;40:1304–11.
52. Fausto N, Mead J. Regulation of liver growth: protooncogenes and transforming growth factors. Lab Invest 1989;60:4–13.
53. Smuckler EA, James JL. Irreversible cell injury [abstract]. Pharmacol Rev 1984;36:77S–91S.
54. Higgins GM, Anderson RM. Experimental pathology of the liver: 1. Restoration of the liver of the white rat following surgical removal. Arch Pathol 1931;12:186–202.
55. Andus T, Bauer J, Gerok W. Effects of cytokines on the liver. Hepatology 1991;13:364–75.
56. Waterfield M. Epidermal growth factors and related molecules. Lancet 1989;i:1243–6.
57. Skov-Olsen P, Boesby S, Kirkegaard P, et al. Influence of epidermal growth factor on liver regeneration after partial hepatectomy in rats. Hepatology 1988;8:992–6.
58. Ekberg S, Carlsson L, Carlsson B, et al. Plasma growth hormone pattern regulates epidermal growth factor (EGF) receptor messenger ribonucleic acid levels and EGF binding in the rat liver. Endocrinology 1989;125:2158–66.
59. Francavilla A, Ove P, Polimeno L, et al. Different response to epidermal growth factor of hepatocytes in cultures isolated from male or female rat liver: inhibitor effect of estrogen on binding and mitogenic effect of epidermal growth factor. Gastroenterology 1987;93:597–605.
60. Napoli J, Prentice D, Niinami C, et al. Sequential increases in the intrahepatic expression of epidermal growth factor, basic fibroblast growth factor, and transforming growth factor beta in a bile duct ligated rat model of cirrhosis. Hepatology 1997;26:624–33.
61. Hashimoto M, Kothary PC, Eckhauser FE, Raper SE. Treatment of cirrhotic rats with epidermal growth factor and insulin accelerates liver DNA synthesis after partial hepatectomy. J Gastroenterol Hepatol 1998;13:1259–65.
62. Nakayama H, Tsubouchi H, Gohda E, et al. Stimulation of DNA synthesis in adult rat hepatocytes in primary culture by sera from patients with fulminant hepatic failure. Biomed Res 1985;6:231–7.
63. Tsubouchi H, Hirono S, Gohda E, et al. Clinical significance of human hepatocyte growth factor in blood from patients with fulminant hepatic failure. Hepatology 1989;9:875–81.
64. Gohda E, Tsubouchi H, Nakayama H, et al. Purification and partial characterization of hepatocyte growth factor from plasma of a patient with fulminant hepatic failure. J Clin Invest 1988; 81:414–19.
65. Tashiro K, Hagiya M, Nishizawa T, et al. Deduced primary structure of rat hepotocyte growth factor and expression of the mRNA in rat tissue. Proc Natl Acad Sci U S A 1990;87: 3200–4.
66. Gohda E, Hayashi Y, Kawaida A, et al. Hepatotrophic factor in blood of mice treated with carbon tetrachloride. Life Sci 1990;46:1801–8.
67. Tsubouchi H, Hirono S, Gohda E, et al. Human hepatocyte growth factor in blood of patients with fulminant hepatic failure: I. Clinical aspects. Dig Dis Sci 1991;36:780–4.
68. Shimizu I, Ichihara A, Nakamura T. Hepatocyte growth factor in ascites from patients with cirrhosis. J Biochem (Tokyo) 1991;109:14–18.
69. Gauldie J, Richards C, Harnish D, et al. Interferon beta2/B-cell stimulatory factor type 2 shares identity with monocyte-derived hepatocyte-stimulating factor and regulates the major acute phase protein response in liver cells. Proc Natl Acad Sci U S A 1987;84:7251–5.
70. Mead JE, Fausto N. Transforming growth factor a may be a physiological regulator of liver regeneration by means of an autocrine mechanism. Proc Natl Acad Sci U S A 1989;86: 1558–62.
71. Castilla A, Prieto J, Fausto N. Transforming growth factors B1 and a in a chronic liver disease: effects of interferon alpha therapy. N Engl J Med 1991;324:933–40.
72. Brenner DA, Koch KS, Leffert HL. Transforming growth factor alpha stimulates proto-oncogene cejun expression and a mitogenic program in primary cultures of adult rat hepatocytes. DNA 1989;8:279–85.
73. Harada K, Shiota G, Kawasaki H. Transforming growth factor-alpha and epidermal growth factor receptor in chronic liver disease and hepatocellular carcinoma. Liver 1999;19:318–25.
74. Wollenberg GK, Semple E, Quinn BA, Hayes MA. Inhibition of proliferation of normal preneoplastic and neoplastic rat

hepatocytes by transforming growth factor-beta. Cancer Res 1987;46:6595–9.
75. Nakatsukasa H, Evarts RP, Hsia CC, et al. Transforming growth factor-beta 1 and type 1 procollagen transcripts during regeneration and early fibrosis of rat liver. Lab Invest 1990;63: 171–80.
76. Nagy P, Schaff Z, Lapis K. Immunohistochemical detection of transforming growth factor-beta 1 in fibrotic liver diseases. Hepatology 1991;14:269–73.
77. Czaja M, Weiner FR, Flanders KC, et al. In vitro and in vivo association of transforming growth factor-beta 1 with hepatic fibrosis. J Cell Biol 1989;108:2477–82.
78. Armendariz-Borunda J, Seyer JM, Kang AH, et al. Regulation of TGF beta gene expression in rat liver intoxicated with carbon tetrachloride. FASEB J 1990;4:215–21.
79. Roberts AB, Sporn MB, Assoian RK, et al. Transforming growth factor type beta: rapid induction of fibrosis and angiogenesis in vivo and stimulation of collagen formation in vitro. Proc Natl Acad Sci U S A 1986;83:4167–71.
80. Gressner AM, Weiskirchen R, Breitkopf K, et al. Roles of TGF-beta in hepatic fibrosis. Front Biosci 2002;7:d793–807.
81. Flanders KC. Smad3 as a mediator of the fibrotic response. Int J Exp Pathol 2004;85:47–64.
82. Burgess WH, Maciag T. The heparin-binding (fibroblast) growth factor family of proteins. Annu Rev Biochem 1989;58: 575–606.
83. Presta M, Statuto M, Rusnati M, et al. Characterization of a Mr 25,000 basic fibroblast growth factor form in adult, regenerating, and fetal rat liver. Biochem Biophys Res Commun 1989;164:1182–9.
84. Ikebuchi K, Wong GG, Clark SC, et al. Interleukin-6 enhancement of interleukin-3 dependent proliferation of multipotential hemopoietic progenitors. Proc Natl Acad Sci U S A 1987;84:9035–9.
85. Sharon N, Bird G, Goka J, et al. Elevated plasma IL-6 and increased severity and mortality in alcoholic hepatitis. Clin Exp Immunol 1991;84:449–53.
86. West MA, Billiar TR, Curran RD, et al. Evidence that rat Kupffer cells stimulate and inhibit hepatocyte protein synthesis in vitro by different mechanisms. Gastroenterology 1989;96:1572–82.
87. Goss J, Mangino MJ, Flye MW. Prostaglandin E2 production during hepatic regeneration downregulates Kupffer cell IL-6 production. Ann Surg 1992;215:253–60.
88. Hayakawa T, Kondo T, Shibata T, et al. Serum insulin-like growth factor II in chronic liver disease. Dig Dis Sci 1989;34: 338–42.
89. Wu JC, Daughaday WH, Lee SD, et al. Radioimmunoassay of serum IGF-I and IGF-II in patients with chronic liver diseases and hepatocellular carcinoma with or without hypoglycemia. J Lab Clin Med 1988;112:589–94.
90. Assy N, Hochberg Z, Amit T, et al. Growth hormone-stimulated insulin-like growth factor I and IGF-binding protein-3 in liver cirrhosis. J Hepatol 1997;27:796–802.
91. Caufriez A, Reding P, Urbain D, et al. Insulin-like growth factor I: a good indicator of functional hepatocellular capacity in alcoholic liver cirrhosis. J Endocrinol Invest 1991;14:317–21.
92. Shaarawy M, Fikry MA, Massoud BA, Lotfy S. Insulin-like growth factor binding protein-3: a novel biomarker for the assessment of the synthetic capacity of hepatocytes in liver cirrhosis. J Clin Endocrinol Metab 1998;83:3316–19.
93. Sherlock S. Diseases of the liver and biliary system. Boston: Blackwell, 1985:339.
94. Haellen J, Norden J. Liver cirrhosis unsuspected during life. A series of 79 cases. J Chronic Dis 1964;17:951–8.
95. Attali P, Ink O, Pelletier G, et al. Dupuytren's contracture, alcohol consumption, and chronic liver disease. Arch Intern Med 1987;147:1065–7.
96. Phillips MM, Ramsey GR, Conn HO. Portacaval an anastomosis and peptic ulcer: a nonassociation. Gastroenterology 1975;68:121–31.
97. Bouchier I. Postmortem study of the frequency of gallstones in patients with cirrhosis of the liver. Gut 1969;10:705–10.
98. Nicholas P, Rinaudo PA, Conn HO. Increased incidence of cholelithiasis in Laénnec's cirrhosis. Gastroenterology 1972;63: 112–21.
99. Vlahcevic ZR, Yoshida T, Juttijudata P, et al. Bile acid metabolism in cirrhosis: III. Biliary lipid secretion in patients with cirrhosis and its relevance to gallstone formation. Gastroenterology 1973;64:298–303.
100. Keren G, Boichis H, Zwas TS, Frand M. Pulmonary arteriovenous fistulae in hepatic cirrhosis. Arch Dis Child 1983;58: 302–4.
101. Hall GH, Laidlaw CD. Further experimental evidence implicating reduced ferritin as a cause of digital clubbing. Clin Sci 1963;24:121–6.
102. Tobin CE, Zariquiey MO. Arteriovenous shunts in the human lung. Proc Soc Exp Biol Med 1950;75:827–9.
103. Sheehy TW, Berman A. The anemia of cirrhosis. J Lab Clin Med 1960;56:72–82.
104. Roberts HR, Cederbaum AI. The liver and blood coagulation: physiology and pathology. Gastroenterology 1972;63: 297–320.
105. Pirovino M, Linder R, Boss C, et al. Cutaneous spider nevi in liver cirrhosis: capillary microscopical and hormonal investigations. Klin Wochenschr 1988;66:298–302.
106. Erlinger S, Bircher J. Cirrhosis: clinical aspects. In: Bircher J, Mcintyre N, Rizzetto M, Rodes J, eds. Oxford textbook of clinical hepatology. Oxford: Oxford University Press, 1991:380.
107. Fitzpatrick T, Johnson R, Polano M. Color atlas and synopsis of clinical dermatology: common and serious diseases. 2nd ed. New York: McGraw Hill, 1994.
108. Bannayan GA, Hajdu SI. Gynecomastia: clinicopathologic study of 351 cases. Am J Clin Pathol 1972;57:431–7.
109. Van Thiel DH, Gavaler JS, Schade RR. Liver disease and the hypothalamic pituitary gonadal axis. Semin Liver Dis 1985;5: 35–45.
110. Horton R, Tait JF. Androstenedione production and interconversion rates measured in peripheral blood and studies on the possible site of its conversion to testosterone. J Clin Invest 1966; 45:301–13.
111. Burack WR, Hollister RM. Tuberculous peritonitis: a study of forty-seven proved cases encountered by a general medical unity in twenty-five years. Am J Med 1960;28:510–23.
112. Rimola A, Soto R, Bory F, et al. Reticuloendothelial system phagocytic activity in cirrhosis and its relation to bacterial infections and prognosis. Hepatology 1984;4:53–8.
113. Rajkovic IA, Williams R. Abnormalities of neutrophil phagocytosis, intracellular killing, and metabolic activity in alcoholic cirrhosis and hepatitis. Hepatology 1986;6:252–62.
114. Hassner A, Kletter Y, Shlag D, et al. Impaired monocyte function in liver cirrhosis. Br J Med 1981;282:1262–3.

115. Wyke RJ, Rajkovic IA, Williams R. Impaired opsonization by serum from patients with chronic liver disease. Clin Exp Immunol 1983;51:91–8.

116. Yousif-Kadaru AG, Rajkovic IA, Wyke RJ, et al. Defects in serum attractant activity in different types of chronic liver diseases. Gut 1984;25:79–84.

117. Kourilsky O, Leroy C, Peltier AP. Complement and liver cell function in 53 patients with liver disease. Am J Med 1973;55: 574–678.

118. Fox RA, Dudley FJ, Sherlock S. The serum concentration of the third component of complement beta-1C-beta-1A in liver disease. Gut 1971;12:574–8.

119. Potter BJ, Trueman AM, Jones EA. Serum complement in chronic liver disease. Gut 1973;14:451–6.

120. Deviere J, Denys C, Schandene L, et al. Decreased proliferation activity associated with activation markers in patients with alcoholic liver cirrhosis. Clin Exp Immunol 1988;72:377–82.

121. Rutenburg AM, Sonnenblick E, Koven I, et al. Comparative response of normal and cirrhotic rats to intravenously injected bacteria. Proc Soc Exp Biol 1959;101:279–81.

122. Kerr DN, Pearson DT, Read AE. Infection of the ascitic fluid in patients with cirrhosis. Gut 1963;4:394–8.

123. Sokol R. Medical management of the infant or child with chronic liver disease. Semin Liver Dis 1987;7:166–7.

124. Sokol RJ, Stall C. Anthropometric evaluation of children with chronic liver disease. Am J Clin Nutr 1990;52:203–8.

125. Chin SE, Shepherd RW, Thomas BJ, et al. The nature of malnutrition in children with end-stage liver disease awaiting orthotopic liver transplantation. Am J Clin Nutr 1992;56:164–8.

126. Kaufman SS, Murray ND, Wood RP, et al. Nutritional support for the infant with extrahepatic biliary atresia. J Pediatr 1987;110:679–86.

127. Reichling JJ, Kaplan MM. Clinical use of serum enzymes in liver disease. Dig Dis Sci 1988;33:1601–14.

128. St Louis P. Biochemical studies: liver and intestine. In: Walker WA, Durie PR, Hamilton JR, et al., eds. Pediatric gastroenterology and nutrition. Philadelphia: BC Decker, 1991;1363–73.

129. Kaplan M. Alkaline phosphatase. Gastroenterology 1972;62: 452–68.

130. Astin T. Systemic reaction to bromsulphthalein. Br Med J 1965; 2:1433.

131. Balistreri WF, Setchell K. Newer liver function tests. Front Gastro Res 1989;16:220–45.

132. Schoeller DA, Schneider JF, Solomons NW, et al. Clinical diagnosis with the stable isotope 13C in CO2 breath tests: methodology and fundamental considerations. J Lab Clin Med 1977;90: 412–21.

133. Schneider JF, Baker AL, Haines NW, et al. Aminopyrine N-demethylation: a prognostic test of liver function in patients with alcoholic liver disease. Gastroenterology 1980;79:1145–50.

134. Renner E, Wietholtz H, Huguenin P, et al. Caffeine: a model compound for measuring liver function. Hepatology 1984;4: 38–46.

135. Jost G, Wahllander A, von Mandach U, et al. Overnight salivary caffeine clearance: a liver function test suitable for routine use. Hepatology 1987;7:338–44.

136. Post J, Patek A. Serum proteins in cirrhosis of the liver. Arch Intern Med 1942;169:67–82.

137. Hasch E, Jarnum S, Tygstrup N. Albumin synthesis rate as a measure of liver function in patients with cirrhosis. Acta Med Scand 1967;182:83–92.

138. Rothschild MA, Oratz M, Zimmon D, et al. Albumin synthesis in cirrhotic subjects with ascites studied with carbonate 14-C. J Clin Invest 1969;48:344–50.

139. Haider M, Haider SQ. Assessment of protein-calorie malnutrition. Clin Chem 1984;30:1286–99.

140. Dymock IW, Tucker JS, Woolf IL, et al. Coagulation studies as a prognostic index in acute liver failure. Br J Haematol 1975; 29:385–95.

141. Bernuau J, Goudeau A, Poynard T, et al. Multivariate analysis of prognostic factors in fulminant hepatitis B. Hepatology 1986;6:648–51.

142. Biland L, Duckert F, Prisender S, et al. Qualitative estimation of coagulation factors in liver disease: the diagnostic and prognostic value of factor XIII, factor V, and plasminogens. Thromb Haemost 1978;39:646–56.

143. Schlichting P, Christensen E, Andersen PK, et al. Prognostic factors in cirrhosis identified by Cox's regression model. Hepatology 1983;6:889–95.

144. Malatack JJ, Schaid DJ, Urbach AH. Choosing a pediatric recipient I-or orthotopic liver transplantation. J Pediatr 1987; 111:479–89.

145. Starling E. On the absorption of fluids from the connective tissue spaces. J Physiol (Lond) 1896;19:312.

146. Gines P, Arroyo V, Rodes J. Pathophysiology, complications, and treatment of ascites. Clin Liver Dis 1997;1:129–55.

147. Morali GA, Sniderman KW, Deitel KM, et al. Is sinusoidal portal hypertension a necessary factor for the development of hepatic ascites? J Hepatol 1992;16:249–50.

148. Arroyo V, Rodes J. A rational approach to the treatment of ascites. Postgrad Med 1975;51:558–62.

149. Gines P, Arroyo V, Rodes J. Disorders of renal function in cirrhosis. In: Boyer T, Zakim D, eds. Hepatology: a textbook of liver disease. Philadelphia: BC Decker, 1996:659–64.

150. Gines P, Fernandez-Esparrach G, Arroyo V, et al. Pathogenesis of ascites in cirrhosis. Semin Liver Dis 1997;17:175–89.

151. Epstein M, Berk DP, Hollenberg NK, et al. Renal failure in the patient with cirrhosis: the role of active vasoconstriction. Am J Med 1970;49:175–85.

152. Schrier R. Pathogenesis of sodium and water retention in high-output and low-output cardiac failure, nephrotic syndrome, cirrhosis, and pregnancy, parts I-II. N Engl J Med 1988;9:1127–34.

153. Lieberman FL, Reynolds TB. Plasma volume in cirrhosis of the liver; its relation to portal hypertension, ascites, and renal failure. J Clin Invest 1967;46:1297–308.

154. Lieberman FL, Denison EK, Reynolds TB. The relationship of volume, portal hypertension, ascites, and renal sodium retention in cirrhosis: the overflow theory of ascites formation. Ann NY Acad Sci 1970;170:202–12.

155. Anderson RJ, Cronin RE, McDonald KM, et al. Mechanisms of portal hypertension-induced alterations in renal hemodynamics, renal water excretion, and renin secretion. J Clin Invest 1976;58:964–70.

156. Levy M. Observation on real function and ascites formation in dogs with experimental portal cirrhosis. In: Epstein M, ed. The kidney in liver disease. New York: Elsevier, 1978:131–42.

157. Levy M, Allotey JB. Temporal relationships between urinary salt retention and altered systemic hemodynamics in dogs with experimental cirrhosis. J Lab Clin Med 1978;92:560–9.

158. Levy M, Wexler MJ. Renal sodium retention and ascites formation on dogs with experimental cirrhosis but without portal

hypertension or increased splanchnic vascular capacity. J Lab Clin Med 1978;91:520–36.

159. Rosoff L Jr, Zia P, Reynolds T, et al. Studies of renin and aldosterone in cirrhotic patients with ascites. Gastroenterology 1975;69:698–705.
160. Epstein M. Hepatorenal syndrome. In: Epstein M, ed. The kidney in liver disease. New York: Elsevier Biomedical, 1983:377.
161. Levy M. Pathophysiology of ascites formation. In: Epstein M, ed. The kidney in liver disease. New York: Elsevier Biomedical, 1983:245.
162. Klepetko W, Muller C, Hartter E, et al. Plasma atrial natriuretic factor in cirrhotic patients with ascites: effect of peritoneovenous shunt implantation. Gastroenterology 1988;95:764–70.
163. Bichet DG, Van Putten VJ, Schrier RW. Potential role of increased sympathetic activity impaired sodium and water excretion in cirrhosis. N Engl J Med 1982;307:552–7.
164. Floras JS, Legault L, Morali GA, et al. Increased sympathetic outflow in cirrhosis and ascites: direct evidence from intraneural recordings. Ann Intern Med 1991;114:373–80.
165. Schrier RW, Arroyo V, Bernardi M, et al. Peripheral arterial vasodilation hypothesis: a proposal for the initiation of renal sodium and water retention in cirrhosis. Hepatology 1988;8: 1151–7.
166. Claria J, Jimenez W, Arroyo V, et al. Effects of V1-vasopressin receptor blockade on arterial pressure in conscious rats with cirrhosis and ascites. Gastroenterology 1991;100:494–501.
167. Pariente E, Bataille C, Bercoff E, et al. Acute effects of captopril on systemic and renal hemodynamics and on renal functions in cirrhotic patients with ascites. Gastroenterology 1985;88: 1255–9.
168. Guevara M, Gines P, Fernandez-Esparrach G. Effects of normalization of vasoconstrictor systems on renal functions in cirrhotic patients with hepatorenal syndrome. J Hepatol 1996;25:71.
169. Vorobioff J, Bredfeldt JE, Groszmann RJ. Increased blood flow through the portal system in cirrhotic rats. Gastroenterology 1984;87:1120–6.
170. Groszmann RJ. Hyperdynamic circulation of liver disease 40 years later: pathophysiology and clinical consequences. Hepatology 1994;20:1359–63.
171. Guarner C, Soriano G, Tomas A, et al. Increased serum nitrite and nitrate levels in patients with cirrhosis: relationship to endotoxemia. Hepatology 1993;18:1139–43.
172. Sieber CC, Lopez-Talavera JC, Groszmann RJ. Role of nitric oxide in the in vitro splanchnic vascular hyporeactivity in ascitic cirrhotic rats. Gastroenterology 1993;104:1750–4.
173. Sieber CC, Groszmann RJ. Nitric oxide mediates hyporeactivity to vasopressors in mesenteric vessels of portal hypertensive rats. Gastroenterology 1992;103:235–9.
174. Battista S, Fusco B, Mengozzi G. Systemic and portal nitric oxide and endothelin-1 levels in cirrhotic patients. Hepatology 1995;23(suppl 1):73A.
175. Vallance P, Moncada S. Hyperdynamic circulation in cirrhosis: a role for nitric oxide? Lancet 1991;337:776–8.
176. Cattau EL Jr, Benjamin SB, Knuff TE, et al. The accuracy of the physical examination in the diagnosis of suspected ascites. JAMA 1982;247:1164–6.
177. Dinkel E, Lehnart R, Troger J, et al. Sonographic evidence of intraperitoneal fluid: an experimental study and its clinical implications. Pediatr Radiol 1984;14:299–303.
178. Franken EJ. Ascites in infants and children: roentgen diagnosis. Radiology 1972;102:393–8.
179. Griscom NT, Colodny AH, Rosenberg HK, et al. Diagnostic aspects of neonatal ascites: report of 27 cases. Am J Roentgenol 1977;128:961–9.
180. Runyon BA, Montano AA, Akriviadis EA, et al. The serum-ascites albumin gradient is superior to the exudate-transudate concept in the differential diagnosis of ascites. Ann Intern Med 1992;117:215–20.
181. Runyon BA, Canawati HN, Akriviadis EA. Optimization of ascitic fluid culture technique. Gastroenterology 1988;95: 1351–5.
182. Hoefs JC, Runyon BA. Spontaneous bacterial peritonitis. Dis Mon 1985;31:1–48.
183. Pokros PJ, Reynolds TB. Rapid diuresis in patients with ascites from chronic liver disease: the importance of peripheral edema. Gastroenterology 1986;90:1827–33.
184. Runyon BA. Management of adult patients with ascites caused by cirrhosis. Hepatology 1998;27:264–72.
185. Fogel MR, Sawhney VK, Neal EA, et al. Diuresis in the ascitic patient: a randomized controlled trial of three regimens. J Clin Gastroenterol 1981;3:73–80.
186. Perez-Ayuso RM, Arroyo V, Planas R, et al. Randomized comparative study of efficacy of furosemide versus spironolactone in nonazotemic cirrhosis with ascites. Relationship between the diuretic response and the activity of the renin-aldosterone system. Gastroenterology 1983;84:961–8.
187. Gregory PB, Broekelschen PH, Hill MD, et al. Complications of diuresis in the alcoholic patient with ascites: a controlled trial. Gastroenterology 1977;73:534–8.
188. Moult PJ, Lunzer MR, Trash DB, et al. Use of bumetanide in the treatment of ascites due to liver disease. Gut 1974;15:988–92.
189. Arroyo V, Bosch J, Casamitjana R, et al. Use of piretanide, a new loop diuretic, in cirrhosis with ascites: relationship between the diuretic response and the plasma aldosterone level. Gut 1980;21:855–9.
190. Lebrec D, Hillon P, Munoz C, et al. The effect of propranolol on portal hypertension in patients with cirrhosis: a hemodynamic study. Hepatology 1982;2:523–7.
191. Buhler FR, Laragh JH, Baer L, et al. Propranolol inhibition of renin secretion. A specific approach to diagnosis and treatment of renin-dependent hypertensive diseases. N Engl J Med 1972;287:1209–14.
192. Wilkinson SP, Bernardi M, Smith IK, et al. Effect of beta-adrenergic blocking drugs on the renin-aldosterone system, sodium excretion and renal hemodynamics. Gastroenterology 1977;73:659–63.
193. Rector WG Jr, Reynolds TB. Propranolol in the treatment of cirrhotic ascites. Arch Intern Med 1984;144:1761–3.
194. Gines P, Arroyo V, Quintero E, et al. Comparison between paracentesis and diuretics in the treatment of cirrhotics with tense ascites: results of a randomized study. Gastroenterology 1987;93:234–41.
195. Pinto PC, Amerian J, Reynolds TB. Large-volume paracentesis in nonedematous patients with tense ascites: its effect on intravascular volume. Hepatology 1988;8:207–10.
196. Gines P, Tito L, Arroyo V, et al. Randomized comparative study of therapeutic paracentesis with and without intravenous albumin in cirrhosis. Gastroenterology 1988;94:1493–502.
197. Tito L, Gines P, Arroyo V, et al. Total paracentesis associated with intravenous albumin management patients with cirrhosis and ascites. Gastroenterology 1990;98:146–51.

198. Smart HL, Triger DR. A randomized prospective trial comparing daily paracentesis and intravenous albumin with recirculation in diuretic refractory ascites. J Hepatol 1990;10:191–7.
199. Wilde JT, Cooper P, Kennedy HJ, et al. Coagulation disturbances following ascites recirculation. J Hepatol 1990;10: 217–22.
200. Quiroga J, Sangro B, Nunez M, et al. Transjugular intrahepatic portal-systemic shunt in the treatment of refractory ascites: effect on clinical, renal, humoral, and hemodynamic parameters. Hepatology 1995;21:986–94.
201. Ochs A, Rossle M, Haag K, et al. The transjugular intrahepatic portosystemic stent-shunt procedure for refractory ascites. N Engl J Med 1995;332:1192–7.
202. Stanley MM, Ochi S, Lee KK, et al. Peritoneovenous shunting as compared with medical treatment in patients with alcoholic cirrhosis and massive ascites. Veterans Administration Cooperative Study on Treatment of Alcoholic Cirrhosis with Ascites. N Engl J Med 1989;321:1632–8.
203. Hassall E, Benson L, Hart M, et al. Hepatic encephalopathy after portacaval shunt in a noncirrhotic child. J Pediatr 1984;105: 439–41.
204. Zaki AE, Ede RJ, Davis M, et al. Experimental studies of blood brain barrier permeability in acute hepatic failure. Hepatology 1984;4:359–63.
205. Zaki AE, Wardle EN, Canalese J, et al. Potential toxins of acute liver failure and their effects on blood–brain barrier permeability. Experientia 1983;39:988–91.
206. Roy S, Pomier-Layrargues G, Butterworth RF, et al. Hepatic encephalopathy in cirrhotic and portacaval shunted dogs: lack of changes in brain GABA uptake, brain GABA levels, brain glutamic acid decarboxylase activity and brain postsynaptic GABA receptors. Hepatology 1988;8:845–9.
207. Jalan R, Hayes PC. Hepatic encephalopathy and ascites. Lancet 1997;350:1309–15.
208. Walker CO, Schenker S. Pathogenesis of hepatic encephalopathy – with special reference to the role of ammonia. Am J Clin Nutr 1970;23:619–32.
209. Nance FC, Kaufman HJ, Kline DG. Role of urea in the hyperammonemia of germ-free Eck fistula dogs. Gastroenterology 1974;66:108–12.
210. Snodgrass PJ, DeLong GR. Urea-cycle enzyme deficiencies and an increased nitrogen load producing hyperammonemia in Reye's syndrome. N Engl J Med 1976;294:855–60.
211. Bessman SP, Bradley JE. Uptake of ammonia by muscle; its implications in ammoniagenic coma. N Engl J Med 1955;253: 1143–7.
212. Uribe M, Marquez MA, Garcia Ramos G, et al. Treatment of chronic portal systemic encephalopathy with vegetable and animal protein diets: a controlled cross-over study. Dig Dis Sci 1982;27:1109–16.
213. Pappas SC, Ferenci P, Schafer DF, et al. Visual evoked potentials in a rabbit model of hepatic encephalopathy. II. Comparison of hyperammonemic encephalopathy, postictal coma, and coma induced by synergistic neurotoxins. Gastroenterology 1984;86:546–51.
214. Cole M, Rutherford RB, Smith FO. Experimental ammonia encephalopathy in the primate. Arch Neurol 1972;26:130–6.
215. MacGillilray B. EEG monitoring in metabolic liver disease. In: Glaser G, ed. Handbook of electroencephalography and clinical neurophysiology. Vol 15: Metabolic endocrine and toxi diseases. New York: Elsevier Scientific Publishing, 1975:5–26.
216. Phear EA, Ruebner B, Sherlock S, et al. Methionine toxicity in liver disease and its prevention by chlortetracycline. Clin Sci (Lond) 1956;15:93–117.
217. Challenger F, Walshe JM. Foetor hepaticus. Lancet 1955;268: 1239–41.
218. Zieve L, Doizaki WM, Zieve J. Synergism between mercaptans and ammonia or fatty acids in the production of coma: a possible role for mercaptans in the pathogenesis of hepatic coma. J Lab Clin Med 1974;83:16–28.
219. McClain CJ, Zieve L, Doizaki WM, et al. Blood methanethiol in alcoholic liver disease with and without hepatic encephalopathy. Gut 1980;21:318–23.
220. Chen S, Mahadevan V, Zieve L. Volatile fatty acids in the breath of patients with cirrhosis of the liver. J Lab Clin Med 1970;75:622–7.
221. Linscheer WG, Castell DO, Platt RR. A new method for evaluation of portasystemic shunting. The rectal octanoate tolerance test. Gastroenterology 1969;57:415–23.
222. Zieve L. Coma production with ammonia: synergistic factors. Gastroenterology 1980;78:1327A.
223. Fisher JE, Baldessarini RJ. False neurotransmitters and hepatic failure. Lancet 1971;ii:75–80.
224. Borg J, Warter JM, Schlienger JL, et al. Neurotransmitter modifications in human cerebrospinal fluid and serum during hepatic encephalopathy. J Neurol Sci 1982;57:343–56.
225. Cuilleret G, Pomier-Layrargues G, Pons F, et al. Changes in brain catecholamine levels in human cirrhotic hepatic encephalopathy. Gut 1980;21:565–9.
226. Hirayama C. Tryptophan metabolism in liver disease. Clin Chim Acta 1971;32:191–7.
227. Record CO, Chase RA, Alberti KG, et al. Disturbances in glucose metabolism in patients with liver damage due to paracetamol overdose. Clin Sci Mol Med 1975;49:473–9.
228. Schafer DF, Fowler JM, Jones EA. Colonic bacteria: a source of gamma-aminobutyric acid in blood. Proc Soc Exp Biol Med 1981;167:301–3.
229. Schafer DF, Jones EA. Hepatic encephalopathy and the gamma-aminobutyric-acid neurotransmitter system. Lancet 1982;1: 18–20.
230. Ferenci P, Covell D, Schafer DF, et al. Metabolism of the inhibitory neurotransmitter gamma-aminobutyric acid in a rabbit model of fulminant hepatic failure. Hepatology 1983; 3:507–12.
231. Ferenci P, Schafer DF, Kleinberger G, et al. Serum levels of gamma-aminobutyric-acid-like activity in acute and chronic hepatocellular disease. Lancet 1983;2:811–14.
232. Schafer DF, Fowler JM, Munson PJ, et al. Gamma-aminobutyric acid and benzodiazepine receptors in an animal model of fulminant hepatic failure. J Lab Clin Med 1983;102:870–80.
233. Blitzer BL, Waggoner JG, Jones EA, et al. A model of fulminant hepatic failure in the rabbit. Gastroenterology 1978;74: 664–71.
234. Smiaowski A. The effect of intrahippocampal administration of gamma-aminobutyric acid (GABA). In. Fonnum E, ed. Amino acids as chemical transmitters. New York: Plenum Press, 1978:1977.
235. Lavoie J, Giguere JF, Layrargues GP, et al. Amino acid changes in autopsied brain tissue from cirrhotic patients with hepatic encephalopathy. J Neurochem 1987;49:692–7.
236. Butterworth RF, Lavoie J, Giguere JF, et al. Affinities and densities of high-affinity [3H]muscimol (GABA-A) binding sites and

of central benzodiazepine receptors are unchanged in autopsied brain tissue from cirrhotic patients with hepatic encephalopathy. Hepatology 1988;8:1084–8.
237. Record C. Neurochemistry of hepatic encephalopathy. Gut 1991;32:1261–3.
238. Baraldi M, Zeneroli ML, Ventura E, et al. Supersensitivity of benzodiazepine receptors in hepatic encephalopathy due to fulminant hepatic failure in the rat: reversal by a benzodiazepine antagonist. Clin Sci (Lond) 1984;67:167–75.
239. Olasmaa M, Guidotti A, Rothstein JD. Naturally occurring benzodiazepines in CSF of patients with hepatic encephalopathy. Sjoc Nekurosci Abs 1988;15:199.8.
240. Scolo-Levizzaire G, Steinmann E. Reversal of hepatic coma by benzodiazepine antagonist. Lancet 1985;i:1324–5.
241. Pomier-Layrargues G, Giguere JF, Butterworth RF. Clinical trials of the efficacy of fluamzenil in hepatic coma. J Hepatol 1990; 10:S13.
242. Jones EA, Basile AS. Does ammonia contribute to increased GABA-ergic neurotransmission in liver failure? Metab Brain Dis 1998;13:351–60.
243. Faloon WW, Evans GL. Precipitating factors in genesis of hepatic coma. N Y State J Med 1970;70:2891–6.
244. Cadranel JF, Lebiez E, Di Martino V, et al. Focal neurological signs in hepatic encephalopathy in cirrhotic patients: an underestimated entity? Am J Gastroenterol 2001;96:515–18.
245. Watanabe A. Cerebral changes in hepatic encephalopathy. J Gastroenterol Hepatol 1998;13:752–60.
246. Kostler H. Proton magnetic resonance spectroscopy in portal-systemic encephalopathy. Metab Brain Dis 1998;13:291–301.
247. Dawson AM, McLaren J, Sherlock S. Neomycin in the treatment of hepatic coma. Lancet 1957;273:1262–8.
248. Atterbury CE, Maddrey WC, Conn HO. Neomycin-sorbitol and lactulose in the treatment of acute portal-systemic encephalopathy. A controlled, double-blind clinical trial. Am J Dig Dis 1978; 23:398–406.
249. Berk DP, Chalmers T. Deafness complicating antibiotic therapy of hepatic encephalopathy. Ann Intern Med 1970;73:393–6.
250. Cabrera J, Arroyo V, Ballesta AM, et al. Aminoglycoside nephrotoxicity in cirrhosis. Value of urinary beta 2-microglobulin to discriminate functional renal failure from acute tubular damage. Gastroenterology 1982;82:97–105.
251. Elkington SG, Floch MH, Conn HO. Lactulose in the treatment of chronic portal-systemic encephalopathy. A double-blind clinical trial. N Engl J Med 1969;281:408–12.
252. Conn HO, Leevy CM, Vlahcevic ZR, et al. Comparison of lactulose and neomycin in the treatment of chronic portal-systemic encephalopathy. A double blind controlled trial. Gastroenterology 1977;72(4 pt 1):573–83.
253. Conn HO, Lieberthal MM. The hepatic coma syndromes and lactulose. Baltimore: Williams & Wilkins, 1979:261.
254. Bircher J, Haemmerli UP, Trabert E, et al. The mechanism of action of lactulose in portal-systemic encephalopathy. Nonionic diffusion of ammonia in the canine colon. Rev Eur Etud Clin Biol 1971;16:352–7.
255. Vince A, Zeegen R, Drinkwater JE, et al. The effect of lactulose on the faecal flora of patients with hepatic encephalopathy. J Med Microbiol 1974;7:163–8.
256. Uribe M, Campollo O, Vargas F, et al. Acidifying enemas (lactitol and lactose) vs. nonacidifying enemas (tap water) to treat acute portal-systemic encephalopathy: a double-blind, randomized clinical trial. Hepatology 1987;7:639–43.
257. Vince A, Killingley M, Wrong OM. Effect of lactulose on ammonia production in a fecal incubation system. Gastroenterology 1978;74:544–9.
258. Morgan MY, Hawley KE. Lactitol vs. lactulose in the treatment of acute hepatic encephalopathy in cirrhotic patients: a double-blind, randomized trial. Hepatology 1987;7:1278–84.
259. Sabath LD, Toftegaard I. Rapid microassays for clindamycin and gentamicin when present together and the effect of pH and of each on the antibacterial activity of the other. Antimicrob Agents Chemother 1974;6:54–9.
260. Weber F. Combination therapy with lactulose and antibiotics. In: Seeff LB, Conn H, eds. Hepatic encephalopathy: management with lactulose a and related carbohydrates. East Lansing, MI: Medi Ed Press, 1988:207–17.
261. Pirotte G, Guffens JM, Devos J. Comparative study of basal arterial ammonemia of orally-induced hyperammonemia of chronic portal systemic encephalopathy, treated with neomycin, lactulose, and an association of neomycin and lactulose. Digestion 1974;10:435–44.
262. Eriksson LS, Persson A, Wahren J. Branched-chain amino acids in the treatment of chronic hepatic encephalopathy. Gut 1982;23:801–6.
263. Wahren J, Denis J, Desurmont P, et al. Is intravenous administration of branched chain amino acids effective in the treatment of hepatic encephalopathy? A multicenter study. Hepatology 1983;3:475–80.
264. Horst D, Grace ND, Conn HO, et al. Comparison of dietary protein with an oral, branched chain-enriched amino acid supplement in chronic portal-systemic encephalopathy: a randomized controlled trial. Hepatology 1984;4:279–87.
265. Cascino A, Cangiano C, Calcaterra V, et al. Plasma amino acids imbalance in patients with liver disease. Am J Dig Dis 1978; 23:591–8.
266. Rossi-Fanelli F, Freund H, Krause R, et al. Induction of coma in normal dogs by the infusion of aromatic amino acids and its prevention by the addition of branched-chain amino acids. Gastroenterology 1982;83:664–71.
267. Rossi-Fanelli F, Riggio O, Cangiano C, et al. Branched-chain amino acids vs lactulose in the treatment of hepatic coma: a controlled study. Dig Dis Sci 1982;27:929–35.
268. McGhee A, Henderson JM, Millikan WJ Jr, et al. Comparison of the effects of Hepatic-Aid and a Casein modular diet on encephalopathy, plasma amino acids, and nitrogen balance in cirrhotic patients. Ann Surg 1983;197:288–93.
269. Riordan SM, Williams R. Treatment of hepatic encephalopathy. N Engl J Med 1997;337:473–9.
270. Fabbri A, Magrini N, Bianchi G, et al. Overview of randomized clinical trials of oral branched-chain amino acid treatment in chronic hepatic encephalopathy. JPEN J Parenter Enteral Nutr 1996;20:159–64.
271. Charlton CP, Buchanan E, Holden CE, et al. Intensive enteral feeding in advanced cirrhosis: reversal of malnutrition without precipitation of hepatic encephalopathy. Arch Dis Child 1992;67:603–7.
272. Ferenci P, Grim G, Meryn S. Benzodiazepine antagonists in the treatment of human hepatic encephalopathy. In: Santiago G, ed. Cirrhosis, hepatic encephalopathy and ammonium toxicity. New York: Plenum Press, 1990:255–65.
273. Gyr K, Meier R. Flumazenil in the treatment of portal systemic encephalopathy – an overview. Intensive Care Med 1991; 17(suppl 1):S39–42.

274. Ferenci P, Herneth A, Steindl P. Newer approaches to therapy of hepatic encephalopathy. Semin Liver Dis 1996;16:329–38.
275. Lunzer M, James IM, Weinman J, et al. Treatment of chronic hepatic encephalopathy with levodopa. Gut 1974;15:555–61.
276. Morgan MY, Jakobovits AW, James IM, et al. Successful use of bromocriptine in the treatment of chronic hepatic encephalopathy. Gastroenterology 1980;78:663–70.
277. Uribe M, Farca A, Marquez MA, et al. Treatment of chronic portal systemic encephalopathy with bromocriptine: a double-blind controlled trial. Gastroenterology 1979;76:1347–51.
278. Rossle M, Siegerstetter V, Huber M, et al. The first decade of the transjugular intrahepatic portosystemic shunt (TIPS): state of the art. Liver 1998;18:73–89.
279. Dodds WJ, Hoyer LW. Coagulation activities in perfused organs: regulation by addition of animal plasmas. Br J Haematol 1974;26:497–509.
280. Saito H, Hamilton SM, Tavill AS, et al. Synthesis and release of Hageman factor (Factor XII) by the isolated perfused rat liver. J Clin Invest 1983;72:948–54.
281. Deykin D, Cochios F, DeCamp G, et al. Hepatic removal of activated factor X by the perfused rabbit liver. Am J Physiol 1968;214:414–19.
282. Duetsch D. Blood coagulation changes in liver disease. Prog Liver Dis 1965;2:69–83.
283. Aster R. Production, distribution, life-span, and fate of platelets. In: Beutler E, Williams WJ, eds. Hematology. New York: McGraw-Hill, 1977:1210.
284. Gazzard BG, Portmann B, Murray-Lyon IM, et al. Causes of death in fulminant hepatic failure and relationship to quantitative histological assessment of parenchymal damage. Q J Med 1975;44:615–26.
285. Weston MJ, Langley PG, Rubin MH, et al. Platelet function in fulminant hepatic failure and effect of charcoal haemoperfusion. Gut 1977;18:897–902.
286. Ingeberg S, Jacobsen P, Fischer E, et al. Platelet aggregation and release of ATP in patients with hepatic cirrhosis. Scand J Gastroenterol 1985;20:285–8.
287. Owen JS, Hutton RA, Day RC, et al. Platelet lipid composition and platelet aggregation in human liver disease. J Lipid Res 1981;22:423–30.
288. O'Grady JG, Langley PG, Isola LM, et al. Coagulopathy of fulminant hepatic failure. Semin Liver Dis 1986;6:159–63.
289. Hughes RD, Lane DA, Ireland H, et al. Fibrinogen derivatives and platelet activation products in acute and chronic liver disease. Clin Sci (Lond) 1985;68:701–7.
290. Francis JL, Armstrong DJ. Acquired dysfibrinogenaemia in liver disease. J Clin Pathol 1982;35:667–72.
291. Soria J, Soria C, Ryckewaert JJ, et al. Study of acquired dysfibrinogenaemia in liver disease. Thromb Res 1980;19:29–41.
292. Martinez J, Palascak JE, Kwasniak D. Abnormal sialic acid content of the dysfibrinogenemia associated with liver disease. J Clin Invest 1978;61:535–8.
293. Ekindjian OG, Devanlay M, Duchassaing D, et al. Multivariate analysis of clinical and biological data in cirrhotic patients: application to prognosis. Eur J Clin Invest 1981;11:213–20.
294. Nanji AA, Blank DW. Clinical status as reflected in biochemical tests on patients with chronic alcoholic liver disease. Clin Chem 1983;29:992–3.
295. Wion KL, Kelly D, Summerfield JA, et al. Distribution of factor VIII mRNA and antigen in human liver and other tissues. Nature 1985;317:726–9.
296. Kelly DA, Summerfield JA. Hemostasis in liver disease. Semin Liver Dis 1987;7:182–91.
297. Colman RW, Robboy SJ, Minna JD. Disseminated intravascular coagulation (DIC): an approach. Am J Med 1972;52:679–89.
298. Verstraete M, Vermylen J, Collen D. Intravascular coagulation in liver disease. Annu Rev Med 1974;25:447–55.
299. Colman RW, Marder V, Salzman EW. Overview of hemostasis. In: Hirsh J, Colman RW, Marder VJ, eds. Hemostasis and thrombosis: basic principles and clinical practice. Philadelphia: JB Lippincott, 1987:3–18.
300. Carr JM. Disseminated intravascular coagulation in cirrhosis. Hepatology 1989;10:103–10.
301. Cioni G, Cristani A, Mussini C, et al. Incidence and clinical significance of elevated fibrin(ogen) degradation product and/or D-dimer levels in liver cirrhosis patients. Ital J Gastroenterol 1990;22:70–4.
302. Bauer KA, Rosenberg RD. Thrombin generation in acute promyelocytic leukemia. Blood 1984;64:791–6.
303. Bauer KA, Bednarek M. Detection of factor X activation in humans. Thromb Haemost 1987;58:280A.
304. Ho CH, Hou MC, Lin HC, et al. Can advanced hemostatic parameters detect disseminated intravascular coagulation more accurately in patients with cirrhosis of the liver? Zhonghua Yi Xue Za Zhi (Taipei) 1998;61:332–8.
305. Tollefsen DM, Blank MK. Detection of a new heparin-dependent inhibitor of thrombin in human plasma. J Clin Invest 1981;68:589–96.
306. Sanders NL, Bajaj SP, Zivelin A, et al. Inhibition of tissue factors/factor VIIa activity in plasma requires factor X and an additional plasma component. Blood 1985;66:204–12.
307. Bernstein DE, Jeffers L, Erhardtsen E, et al. Recombinant factor VIIa corrects prothrombin time in cirrhotic patients: a preliminary study. Gastroenterology 1997;113:1930–7.
308. Shami VM, Caldwell SH, Hespenheide EE, et al. Recombinant activated factor VII for coagulopathy in fulminant hepatic failure compared with conventional therapy. Liver Transpl 2003;9:138–43.
309. Atkison PR, Jardine L, Williams S, et al. Use of recombinant factor VIIa in pediatric patients with liver failure and severe coagulopathy. Transplant Proc 2005;37:1091–3.
310. Macdougall BR, Bailey RJ, Williams R. H2-receptor antagonists and antacids in the prevention of acute gastrointestinal haemorrhage in fulminant hepatic failure. Two controlled trials. Lancet 1977;1:617–19.
311. Friedman EW, Sussman II. Safety of invasive procedures in patients with the coagulopathy of liver disease. Clin Lab Haematol 1989;11:199–204.
312. Sharma P, McDonald GB, Banaji M. The risk of bleeding after percutaneous liver biopsy: relation to platelet count. J Clin Gastroenterol 1982;4:451–3.
313. Agnelli G, Berrettini M, De Cunto M, et al. Desmopressin-induced improvement of abnormal coagulation in chronic liver disease. Lancet 1983;1:645.
314. Mannuccio PM, Vicente V, Vianello L, et al. Controlled trial of desmopressin in liver cirrhosis and other conditions associated with a prolonged bleeding time. Blood 1986;67:1148–53.
315. Burroughs AK, Matthews K, Qadiri M, et al. Desmopressin and bleeding time in patients with cirrhosis. Br Med J (Clin Res Ed) 1985;291:1377–81.

316. Burghard R, Leititis JU, Rossi R, et al. Treatment of severe coagulation disturbances as a condition of improved prognosis in fulminant liver failure. Arch Dis Child 1985;60:167–70.
317. Fujiwara K, Ono K, Akamatsu K, et al. Treatment with antithrombin III concentrate in fulminant hepatic failure. Hepatology 1987;7:1067A.
318. Conn HO, Fessel JM. Spontaneous bacterial peritonitis in cirrhosis: variations on a theme. Medicine (Baltimore) 1971;50: 161–97.
319. Almdal TP, Skinhoj P. Spontaneous bacterial peritonitis in cirrhosis. Incidence, diagnosis, and prognosis. Scand J Gastroenterol 1987;22:295–300.
320. Guarner C, Runyon BA. Spontaneous bacterial peritonitis: pathogenesis, diagnosis, and management. Gastroenterologist 1995;3:311–28.
321. Larcher VF, Manolaki N, Vegnente A, et al. Spontaneous bacterial peritonitis in children with chronic liver disease: clinical features and etiologic factors. J Pediatr 1985;106: 907–12.
322. Rabinovitz M, Gavaler JS, Kumar S, et al. Role of serum complement, immunoglobulins, and cell-mediated immune system in the pathogenesis of spontaneous bacterial peritonitis (SBP). Dig Dis Sci 1989;34:1547–52.
323. Rimola A, Bory F, Teres J, et al. Oral, nonabsorbable antibiotics prevent infection in cirrhotics with gastrointestinal hemorrhage. Hepatology 1985;5:463–7.
324. Runyon BA. Low-protein-concentration ascitic fluid is predisposed to spontaneous bacterial peritonitis. Gastroenterology 1986;91:1343–6.
325. Such J, Guarner C, Enriquez J, et al. Low C3 in cirrhotic ascites predisposes to spontaneous bacterial peritonitis. J Hepatol 1988;6:80–4.
326. Runyon BA, Morrissey RL, Hoefs JC, Wyle FA. Opsonic activity of human ascitic fluid: a potentially important protective mechanism against spontaneous bacterial peritonitis. Hepatology 1985;5:634–7.
327. Guarner C, Soriano G. Spontaneous bacterial peritonitis. Semin Liver Dis 1997;17:203–17.
328. Ho H, Guerra LG, Zuckerman MJ. Urinary tract infection: a predisposing factor for spontaneous bacterial peritonitis. Gastroenterology 1990;98:A593.
329. Barnes PF, Arevalo C, Chan LS, et al. A prospective evaluation of bacteremic patients with chronic liver disease. Hepatology 1988;8:1099–103.
330. Leggiadro RJ, Lazar LF. Spontaneous bacterial peritonitis due to Neisseria meningitidis serogroup Z in an infant with liver failure. Clin Pediatr (Phila) 1991;30:350–2.
331. Clark JH, Fitzgerald JF, Kleiman MB. Spontaneous bacterial peritonitis. J Pediatr 1984;104:495–500.
332. Pinzello G, Simonetti RG, Craxi A, et al. Spontaneous bacterial peritonitis: a prospective investigation in predominantly nonalcoholic cirrhotic patients. Hepatology 1983;3:545–9.
333. Such J, Runyon BA. Spontaneous bacterial peritonitis. Clin Infect Dis 1998;27:669–74; quiz 675–6.
334. Runyon BA. Spontaneous bacterial peritonitis: an explosion of information. Hepatology 1988;8:171–5.
335. Runyon BA. Paracentesis of ascitic fluid. A safe procedure. Arch Intern Med 1986;146:2259–61.
336. Grabau CM, Crago SF, Hoff LK, et al. Performance standards for therapeutic abdominal paracentesis. Hepatology 2004;40: 484–8.
337. Runyon BA, Umland ET, Merlin T. Inoculation of blood culture bottles with ascitic fluid. Improved detection of spontaneous bacterial peritonitis. Arch Intern Med 1987;147:73–5.
338. Runyon BA, Antillon MR, Akriviadis EA, et al. Bedside inoculation of blood culture bottles with ascitic fluid is superior to delayed inoculation in the detection of spontaneous bacterial peritonitis. J Clin Microbiol 1990;28:2811–12.
339. Castellote J, Xiol X, Verdaguer R, et al. Comparison of two ascitic fluid culture methods in cirrhotic patients with spontaneous bacterial peritonitis. Am J Gastroenterol 1990;85:1605–8.
340. Siersema PD, de Marie S, van Zeijl JH, et al. Blood culture bottles are superior to lysis-centrifugation tubes for bacteriological diagnosis of spontaneous bacterial peritonitis. J Clin Microbiol 1992;30:667–9.
341. Runyon BA, Hoefs JC. Ascitic fluid analysis in the differentiation of spontaneous bacterial peritonitis from gastrointestinal tract perforation into ascitic fluid. Hepatology 1984;4: 447–50.
342. Akriviadis EA, Runyon BA. Utility of an algorithm in differentiating spontaneous from secondary bacterial peritonitis. Gastroenterology 1990;98:127–33.
343. Garrison RN, Cryer HM, Howard DA, et al. Clarification of risk factors for abdominal operations in patients with hepatic cirrhosis. Ann Surg 1984;199:648–55.
344. Deviere J, Content J, Crusiaux A, et al. IL-6 and TNF alpha in ascitic fluid during spontaneous bacterial peritonitis. Dig Dis Sci 1991;36:123–4.
345. McHutchison JG, Runyon BA. Spontaneous bacterial peritonitis. In: Owen RL, Surawica CM, eds. Gastrointestinal and hepatic infections. Philadelphia: WB Saunders, 1994:455–75.
346. Felisart J, Rimola A, Arroyo V, et al. Cefotaxime is more effective than is ampicillin-tobramycin in cirrhotics with severe infections. Hepatology 1985;5:457–62.
347. Grange JD, Amiot X, Grange V, et al. Amoxicillin-clavulanic acid therapy of spontaneous bacterial peritonitis: a prospective study of twenty-seven cases in cirrhotic patients. Hepatology 1990;11:360–4.
348. Runyon BA, McHutchison JG, Antillon MR, et al. Short-course versus long-course antibiotic treatment of spontaneous bacterial peritonitis. A randomized controlled study of 100 patients. Gastroenterology 1991;100:1737–42.
349. Terg R, Cobas S, Fassio E, et al. Oral ciprofloxacin after a short course of intravenous ciprofloxacin in the treatment of spontaneous bacterial peritonitis: results of a multicenter, randomized study. J Hepatol 2000;33:564–9.
350. Navasa M, Follo A, Llovet JM, et al. Randomized, comparative study of oral ofloxacin versus intravenous cefotaxime in spontaneous bacterial peritonitis. Gastroenterology 1996;111: 1011–17.
351. Sort P, Navasa M, Arroyo V, et al. Effect of intravenous albumin on renal impairment and mortality in patients with cirrhosis and spontaneous bacterial peritonitis. N Engl J Med 1999;341:403–9.
352. Garcia-Tsao G. Spontaneous bacterial peritonitis. Gastroenterol Clin North Am 1992;21:257–75.
353. Tito L, Rimola A, Gines P, et al. Recurrence of spontaneous bacterial peritonitis in cirrhosis: frequency and predictive factors. Hepatology 1988;8:27–31.
354. Runyon BA, Van Epps DE. Diuresis of cirrhotic ascites increases its opsonic activity and may help prevent spontaneous bacterial peritonitis. Hepatology 1986;6:396–9.

355. Such J, Guarner C, Soriano G, et al. Selective intestinal decontamination increases serum and ascitic fluid C3 levels in cirrhosis. Hepatology 1990;12:1175–8.
356. Gines P, Rimola A, Planas R, et al. Norfloxacin prevents spontaneous bacterial peritonitis recurrence in cirrhosis: results of a double-blind, placebo-controlled trial. Hepatology 1990;12 (4 pt 1):716–24.
357. Soriano G, Guarner C, Teixido M, et al. Selective intestinal decontamination prevents spontaneous bacterial peritonitis. Gastroenterology 1991;100:477–81.
358. Ring-Larsen H, Palazzo U. Renal failure in fulminant hepatic failure and terminal cirrhosis: a comparison between incidence, types, and prognosis. Gut 1981;22:585–91.
359. Punukollu RC, Gopalswamy N. The hepatorenal syndrome. Med Clin North Am 1990;74:933–43.
360. Kew MC, Brunt PW, Varma RR, et al. Renal and intrarenal blood-flow in cirrhosis of the liver. Lancet 1971;2:504–10.
361. Arroyo V, Gines P, Gerbes AL, et al. Definition and diagnostic criteria of refractory ascites and hepatorenal syndrome in cirrhosis. International Ascites Club. Hepatology 1996;23:164–76.
362. Gines P, Cardenas A, Arroyo V, et al. Management of cirrhosis and ascites. N Engl J Med 2004;350:1646–54.
363. Cardenas A. Hepatorenal syndrome: a dreaded complication of end-stage liver disease. Am J Gastroenterol 2005;100:460–7.
364. Kramer L, Horl WH. Hepatorenal syndrome. Semin Nephrol 2002;22:290–301.
365. Crawford DH, Endre ZH, Axelsen RA, et al. Universal occurrence of glomerular abnormalities in patients receiving liver transplants. Am J Kidney Dis 1992;19:339–44.
366. Iwatsuki S, Popovtzer MM, Corman JL, et al. Recovery from "hepatorenal syndrome" after orthotopic liver transplantation. N Engl J Med 1973;289:1155–9.
367. Gonwa TA, Morris CA, Goldstein RM, et al. Long-term survival and renal function following liver transplantation in patients with and without hepatorenal syndrome – experience in 300 patients. Transplantation 1991;51:428–30.
368. Koppel MH, Coburn JW, Mims MM, et al. Transplantation of cadaveric kidneys from patients with hepatorenal syndrome. Evidence for the functional nature of renal failure in advanced liver disease. N Engl J Med 1969;280:1367–71.
369. Ring-Larsen H, Hesse B, Stigsby B. Effect of portal-systemic anastomosis on renal haemodynamics in cirrhosis. Gut 1976; 17:856–60.
370. Guarner C, Colina I, Guarner F, et al. Renal prostaglandins in cirrhosis of the liver. Clin Sci (Lond) 1986;70:477–84.
371. Fernandez-Seara J, Prieto J, Quiroga J, et al. Systemic and regional hemodynamics in patients with liver cirrhosis and ascites with and without functional renal failure. Gastroenterology 1989;97:1304–12.
372. Lenz K, Hortnagl H, Druml W, et al. Beneficial effect of 8-ornithine vasopressin on renal dysfunction in decompensated cirrhosis. Gut 1989;30:90–6.
373. Lenz K, Hortnagl H, Druml W, et al. Ornipressin in the treatment of functional renal failure in decompensated liver cirrhosis. Effects on renal hemodynamics and atrial natriuretic factor. Gastroenterology 1991;101:1060.
374. Zipser RD, Hoefs JC, Speckart PF, et al. Prostaglandins: modulators of renal function and pressor resistance in chronic liver disease. J Clin Endocrinol Metab 1979;48:895–900.
375. Zambraski EJ, Dunn MJ. Importance of renal prostaglandins in control of renal function after chronic ligation of the common bile duct in dogs. J Lab Clin Med 1984;103:549–59.
376. Zipser RD, Radvan GH, Kronborg IJ, et al. Urinary thromboxane B2 and prostaglandin E2 in the hepatorenal syndrome: evidence for increased vasoconstrictor and decreased vasodilator factors. Gastroenterology 1983;84:697–703.
377. Moore K, Ward PS, Taylor GW, et al. Systemic and renal production of thromboxane A2 and prostacyclin in decompensated liver disease and hepatorenal syndrome. Gastroenterology 1991;100:1069–77.
378. Gupta S, Morgan TR, Gordan GS. Calcitonin gene–related peptide in hepatorenal syndrome. A possible mediator of peripheral vasodilation? J Clin Gastroenterol 1992;14:122–6.
379. Epstein M, Goligorsky MS. Endothelin and nitric oxide in hepatorenal syndrome: a balance reset. J Nephrol 1997;10:120–35.
380. Gines A, Escorsell A, Gines P, et al. Incidence, predictive factors, and treatment of the hepatorenal syndrome with ascites. Gastroenterolgoy 1993;105:229–36.
381. Gines P, Arroyo V. Hepatorenal syndrome. J Am Soc Nephrol 1999;10:1833–9.
382. Wong F, Blendis L. New challenge of hepatorenal syndrome: prevention and treatment. Hepatology 2001;34:1242–51.
383. Follo A, Llovet JM, Navasa M, et al. Renal impairment after spontaneous bacterial peritonitis in cirrhosis: incidence, clinical course, predictive factors and prognosis. Hepatology 1994;20: 1495–501.
384. Nanji AA, Halstead AC. Spurious decrease in serum creatinine in patients with hyperbilirubinemia. Dig Dis Sci 1982;27:1051.
385. Papadakis MA, Arieff AI. Unpredictability of clinical evaluation of renal function in cirrhosis. Prospective study. Am J Med 1987;82:945–52.
386. Rudman D, DiFulco TJ, Galambos JT, et al. Maximal rates of excretion and synthesis of urea in normal and cirrhotic subjects. J Clin Invest 1973;52:2241–9.
387. Bernardi M, De Palma R, Trevisani F, et al. Effects of a new loop diuretic (muzolimine) in cirrhosis with ascites: comparison with furosemide. Hepatology 1986;6:400–5.
388. Simon DM, McCain JR, Bonkovsky HL, et al. Effects of therapeutic paracentesis on systemic and hepatic hemodynamics and on renal and hormonal function. Hepatology 1987;7:423–9.
389. Epstein M. Hepatorenal syndrome. In: Epstein M, ed. The kidney in liver disease. Baltimore: Williams & Wilkins, 1988:89–97.
390. Tristani FE, Cohn JN. Systemic and renal hemodynamics in oliguric hepatic failure: effect of volume expansion. J Clin Invest 1967;46:1894–906.
391. Golper TA. Continuous arteriovenous hemofiltration in acute renal failure. Am J Kidney Dis 1985;6:373–86.
392. Kaplan AA, Longnecker RE, Folkert VW. Continuous arteriovenous hemofiltration. A report of six months' experience. Ann Intern Med 1984;100:358–67.
393. Alarabi AA, Danielson BG, Wikstrom B, et al. Artificial renal and liver support in a severe hepatorenal syndrome of childhood. Acta Paediatr 1992;81:75–8.
394. Schroeder ET, Anderson GH Jr, Smulyan H. Effects of a portacaval or peritoneovenous shunt on renin in the hepatorenal syndrome. Kidney Int 1979;15:54–61.
395. Linas SL, Schaefer JW, Moore EE, et al. Peritoneovenous shunt in the management of the hepatorenal syndrome. Kidney Int 1986;30:736–40.

396. Pladson TR, Parrish RM. Hepatorenal syndrome. Recovery after peritoneovenous shunt. Arch Intern Med 1977;137:1248–9.
397. Gillam GL, Stokes KB, McLellan J, et al. Fulminant hepatic failure with intractable ascites due to an echovirus 11 infection successfully managed with a peritoneo-venous (LeVeen) shunt. J Pediatr Gastroenterol Nutr 1986;5:476–80.
398. Brensing KA, Textor J, Strunk H, et al. Transjugular intrahepatic portosystemic stent-shunt for hepatorenal syndrome. Lancet 1997;349:697–8.
399. Kalambokis G, Economou M, Fotopoulos A, et al. The effects of chronic treatment with octreotide versus octreotide plus midodrine on systemic hemodynamics and renal hemodynamics and function in nonazotemic cirrhotic patients with cirrhosis. Am J Gastroenterol 2005;100:879–85.
400. Angeli P, Volpin R, Gerunda G, et al. Reversal of type 1 hepatorenal syndrome with the administration of midodrine and octreotide. Hepatology 1999;29:1690.
401. Pomier-Layrargues G, Paquin SC, Hassoun Z, et al. Octreotide in hepatorenal syndrome: a randomized, double-blind, placebo-controlled, crossover study. Hepatology 2003;100:879.
402. Arieff AI, Chidsey CA. Renal function in cirrhosis and the effects of prostaglandin A. Am J Med 1974;56:695–703.
403. Zusman RM, Axelrod L, Tolkoff-Rubin N. The treatment of the hepatorenal syndrome with intra-renal administration of prostaglandin E1. Prostaglandins 1977;13:819–30.
404. Fevery J, Van Cutsem E, Nevens F, et al. Reversal of hepatorenal syndrome in four patients by peroral misoprostol (prostaglandin E1 analogue) and albumin administration. J Hepatol 1990;11:153–8.
405. Zipser RD, Kronborg I, Rector W, et al. Therapeutic trial of thromboxane synthesis inhibition in the hepatorenal syndrome. Gastroenterology 1984;87:1228–32.
406. Pinzani M, Laffi G, Meacci E, et al. Intrarenal thromboxane A2 generation reduces the furosemide-induced sodium and water diuresis in cirrhosis with ascites. Gastroenterology 1988;95:1081–7.
407. Polson RJ, Park GR, Lindop MJ, et al. The prevention of renal impairment in patients undergoing orthotopic liver grafting by infusion of low dose dopamine. Anaesthesia 1987;42:15–19.
408. Arroyo V, Guevara M, Gines P. Hepatorenal syndrome in cirrhosis: pathogenesis and treatment. Gastroenterology 2002;122:1658–76.
409. Badalamenti S, Graziani G, , Salerno F, Ponticelli C. Hepatorenal syndrome: new perspectives in pathogenesis and treatment. Arch Intern Med 1993;153:1957–63.
410. Seu P, Wilkinson AH, Shaked A, et al. The hepatorenal syndrome in liver transplant recipients. Am Surg 1991;57:806–9.
411. Nielsen K, Kondrup J, Martinsen L, et al. Long-term oral refeeding of patients with cirrhosis of the liver. Br J Nutr 1995;74:557–67.
412. Nielsen K, Kondrup J, Martinsen L, et al. Nutritional assessment and adequacy of dietary intake in hospitalized patients with alcoholic liver cirrhosis. Br J Nutr 1993;69:665–79.
413. Greco AV, Mingrone G, Benedetti G, et al. Daily energy and substrate metabolism in patients with cirrhosis. Hepatology 1998;27:346–50.
414. Muller MJ, Fenk A, Lautz HU, et al. Energy expenditure and substrate metabolism in ethanol induced liver cirrhosis. Am J Physiol 1991;260(3 pt 1):E338–44.
415. Cabre E, Gassull MA. Nutritional issues in cirrhosis and liver transplantation. Nutrition in chronic liver disease and liver transplantation. Curr Opin Clin Nutr Metab Care 1999;2:373–80.
416. Swart GR, Zillikens MC, van Vuure JK, et al. Effect of a late evening meal on nitrogen balance in patients with cirrhosis of the liver. BMJ 1989;299:1202–3.
417. Verboeket-van de Venne WP, Westerterp KR, van Hoek B, et al. Energy expenditure and substrate metabolism in patients with cirrhosis of the liver: effects of the pattern of food intake. Gut 1995;36:110–16.
418. Yamanaka H, Genjida K, Yokota K, et al. Daily pattern of energy metabolism in cirrhosis. Nutrition 1999;15:749–54.
419. Cabre E, Gonzalez-Huix F, Abad-Lacruz A, et al. Effect of total enteral nutrition on the short-term outcome of severely malnourished cirrhotics. A randomized controlled trial. Gastroenterology 1990;98:715–20.
420. Hirsch S, de la Maza MP, Gattas V, et al. Nutritional support in alcoholic cirrhotic patients improves host defenses. J Am Coll Nutr 1999;18:434–41.
421. Bianchi GP, Marchesini G, Fabbri A, et al. Vegetable versus animal protein diet in cirrhotic patients with chronic encephalopathy. A randomized cross-over comparison. J Intern Med 1993;233:385–92.
422. Aleynik SI, Leo MA, Ma X, et al. Polyenylphosphatidylcholine prevents carbon tetrachloride induced lipid peroxidation while it attenuates liver fibrosis. J Hepatol 1997;27:554–61.
423. Navder KP, Baraona E, Lieber CS. Polyenylphosphatidylcholine attenuates alcohol-induced fatty liver and hyperlipemia in rats. J Nutr 1997;127:1800–6.
424. Ma X, Zhao J, Lieber CS. Polyenylphosphatidylcholine attenuates non-alcoholic hepatic fibrosis and accelerates its regression. J Hepatol 1996;24:604–13.
425. Poniachik J, Baraona E, Zhao J, et al. Dilinoleoylphosphatidylcholine decreases hepatic stellate cell activation. J Lab Clin Med 1999;133:342–8.
426. Lochs H, Plauth M. Liver cirrhosis: rationale and modalities for nutritional support – the European Society of Parenteral and Enteral Nutrition consensus and beyond. Curr Opin Clin Nutr Metab Care 1999;2:345–9.
427. Protheroe SM. Feeding the child with chronic liver disease. Nutrition 1998;14:796–800.

7

Portal Hypertension

Benjamin L. Shneider, M.D.

A portal system is one, which by definition, begins and ends with capillaries. The major portal system in humans is one in which the capillaries originate in the mesentery of the intestines and spleen and end in the hepatic sinusoids. Capillaries of the superior mesenteric and splenic veins supply the portal vein with a nutrient- and hormone-rich blood supply (Figure 7.1). The partially oxygenated portal venous blood supplements the oxygenated hepatic arterial flow to give the liver unique protection against hypoxia. Blood flow from the hepatic artery and portal vein is well coordinated to maintain consistent flow and explains the ability of the liver to withstand thrombosis of either of these major vascular structures. This well-regulated blood flow in conjunction with the very low resistance found in the portal system results in a low baseline portal pressure in healthy individuals.

Portal hypertension, defined as an elevation of portal blood pressure above 5 mm Hg, is one of the major causes of morbidity and mortality in children with liver disease (Table 7.1). The high prevalence of biliary tract disease in pediatric liver disorders (e.g., biliary atresia), as compared with adult liver disorders, predisposes to the expression of portal hypertension earlier in the clinical course of liver disease relative to the manifestation of the sequelae of hepatic insufficiency. Portal hypertension is a complication of a wide variety of pediatric liver disorders (Table 7.1). Its complications are some of the leading indications for liver transplantation. Systematic investigations of the pathophysiology and treatment of portal hypertension have been limited almost exclusively to adults. Since the previous version of this chapter, increased numbers of anecdotal reports of the natural history of and therapy in children with portal hypertension have been published. The first randomized trials have been reported [1,2]. As before, caution needs to be exercised in the extrapolation of the results of randomized trials in adults to the care of children. Current approaches to the care of children with portal hypertension appear to be variable and are extrapolated from experience in adults [3].

Portal hypertension in general is the result of a combination of increased portal resistance and/or increased portal blood flow. The signs and symptoms of portal hypertension are primarily a result of decompression of this supraphysiologic venous pressure via portosystemic collaterals and can be best understood by examination of the portal venous anatomy (Figure 7.1). Splenomegaly and its associated hypersplenism result from splenic congestion, whereas esophageal and rectal varices form from decompression through portosystemic collaterals. Hemorrhage from esophageal varices is the major cause of morbidity and mortality associated with portal hypertension. Decompression of portal hypertension via portosystemic collaterals by definition leads to portosystemic shunting and results in related complications, including primarily hepatic encephalopathy and hepatopulmonary syndrome. Portal hypertension plays a key role in the pathogenesis of the development of ascites and complications related to ascites, including bacterial peritonitis and hepatorenal syndrome (see Chapter 6). This chapter reviews experimental models of portal hypertension, the pathophysiology of portal hypertension, its clinical presentation, and strategies for evaluation and treatment of its sequelae. Where appropriate, important differences between adult and pediatric disease will be highlighted.

EXPERIMENTAL MODELS OF PORTAL HYPERTENSION

Animal models of portal hypertension have been critical in the study of the pathophysiology of portal hypertension. The clinical applicability of the results of these studies may be directly dependent on the experimental method used to induce the portal hypertension. Two commonly used techniques are bile duct ligation and partial stenosis of the portal vein. Bile duct ligation involves ligation and transsection of the common bile duct [4]. Transsection is essential because of the finding of recanalization of the common bile duct when simple ligation is performed. Bile duct ligation would appear to be most applicable to diseases characterized by high-grade cholestasis, especially biliary atresia. An important proviso is the fact that bile duct ligation models are relatively short term secondary to the degree of illness of the animal. The portal vein stenosis model involves ligature constriction of the portal vein to a set diameter (usually based on a catheter size) and is akin to portal vein obstruction

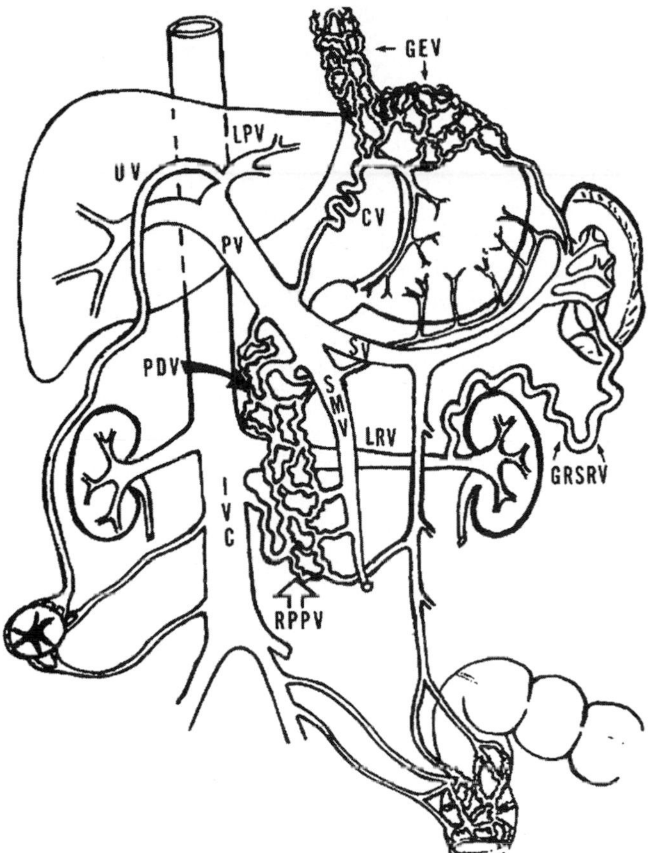

Figure 7.1. Portal venous anatomy and common portosystemic collaterals. PV, portal vein; IVC, inferior vena cava; SMV, superior mesenteric vein; SV, splenic vein; LPV, left branch of the portal vein; UV, umbilical vein (to caput medusae); CV, coronary vein plus short gastric veins lead to GEV, gastroesophageal varices; GRSRV, gastrorenal-splenorenal veins; RPPV, retroperitoneal-paravertebral veins; PDV, pancreaticoduodenal veins. Internal rectal hemorrhoids are unlabeled at the bottom of the diagram. (Reprinted from Subramanyam B, Balthazar E, Madamba M, et al. Sonography of portosystemic venous collaterals in portal hypertension. Radiology 1983;146:161–6; with permission.)

Table 7.1: Pediatric Diseases Associated with Portal Hypertension

Extrahepatic Disorders	*Caroli's Disease*
Venous obstruction	Hepatocellular disease
Splenic vein thrombosis	Autoimmune hepatitis
Portal vein thrombosis/ cavernous transformation	Hepatitis B and C
Budd–Chiari syndrome	Wilson's disease
Inferior vena cava obstruction	α_1-antitrypsin deficiency
Miscellaneous	Glycogen storage type IV
Chronic congestive heart failure	Toxins
Arteriovenous fistula	Ethanol
Splenomegaly	Methotrexate
Intrahepatic disorders	6-Mercaptopurine
Biliary tract disease	Vitamin A
Extrahepatic biliary atresia	Arsenic
Cystic fibrosis	Vinyl chloride
Choledochal cyst	Miscellaneous
Sclerosing cholangitis	Histiocytosis X
Intrahepatic cholestasis syndromes	Veno-occlusive disease
Alagille syndrome	Schistosomiasis
Byler's disease	Gaucher's disease
Bile duct hypoplasia	Hepatoportal sclerosis
Congenital hepatic fibrosis	Peliosis
	Idiopathic portal hypertension

[5]. Varying the size of the catheter permits generation of graded degrees of portal hypertension. Other techniques of generating animal models of portal hypertension include hepatotoxin (e.g., carbon tetrachloride) exposure and infection with *Schistosoma mansoni* [6,7]. In all these approaches, in vivo monitoring is performed with pressure gauges and thermodilution catheters, and by radioactive microsphere distribution. This allows for accurate direct measurement of important parameters of portal hypertension, including heart rate, arterial and portal blood pressures, portal venous and hepatic artery blood flow, and portosystemic shunting [8]. Cardiac output and systemic and portal resistances can be calculated from these direct measurements. The role of endogenous physiologic mediators and the effect of a variety of pharmacologic agents on these parameters can thus be carefully assessed. Application of these models to genetically modified mice has permitted assessment of individual gene products in the pathophysiology of portal hypertension [9,10].

PATHOPHYSIOLOGY OF PORTAL HYPERTENSION

Fluid mechanics are useful in understanding the pathophysiology of portal hypertension. Pressure is directly proportional to both blood flow through the portal system and resistance to that flow. In most circumstances, it appears that the initial abnormality in the development of portal hypertension is an increase in the vascular resistance to flow of blood between the splanchnic bed and the right atrium. The etiology of this increased resistance is variable but usually involves compromise of the vascular lumen [11]. Because resistance is inversely related to the radius of the lumen raised to the fourth power, small changes in the vasculature may result in large changes in pressure. The anatomic level of the vascular change may be prehepatic, intrahepatic, or posthepatic. It is clear that changes in resistance cannot completely explain the picture of portal hypertension. Portosystemic shunting should decompress the system and return portal pressures toward normal, yet this is not the case. A hyperdynamic state is clinically apparent in most patients with portal hypertension and has been well documented in a variety of animal models of portal hypertension [4,5,8]. This is manifested by tachycardia and decreased systemic vascular resistance and was first identified in adults in the 1950s [12]. These hemodynamic changes lead to an overall increase in portal venous flow and thus maintenance of portal hypertension. Decreased responsiveness of the mesenteric vasculature to physiologic levels of endogenous vasoconstrictors contributes to the overall increase in portal blood flow. A variety of hypotheses exist to explain the development of the hyperdynamic circulation that occurs in advanced liver disease. The changes in vascular resistance and hemodynamic state are also referred to as the backward and forward flow theories of portal hypertension and in some combination account for the increased portal blood pressure seen in advanced liver disease.

Increased Vascular Resistance

The portal and hepatic venous systems are low-resistance systems in healthy individuals. It is useful to divide the increased vascular resistance seen in portal hypertension into intra- and extrahepatic sources. Longstanding passive congestion of blood in the liver has been associated with the development of cirrhosis, which leads to increased resistance by other mechanisms. The suprahepatic vena cava and/or hepatic veins may be partially or totally obstructed by membranes or thrombosis, leading to a syndrome often referred to as Budd–Chiari syndrome. This can be an acute or chronic process. The pathophysiology of the obstruction is typically related to compression by a mass, often a tumor or thrombosis related to myeloproliferative disease or a hypercoagulable state [13,14]. Vasculopathies like Behçet's syndrome can also predispose to thrombosis of the hepatic veins [15]. The pediatric manifestations of Budd–Chiari syndrome have been reviewed [16]. Portal pressure was elevated in 19 of 20 children studied, and esophageal varices were present in 11. A clear etiology for the obstruction could be demonstrated in only 5 of the children. A seemingly distinct entity of hepatic vein obstruction in Egyptian children has been described that results in similar but more acute complications of portal hypertension [17].

One of the more common pediatric causes of increased extrahepatic resistance is obstruction of the portal vein. In a review of the treatment of esophageal varices at a major referral center, 33% of the children had portal vein obstruction [18]. Although the etiology is obscure in most instances, neonatal umbilical vein catheterization, omphalitis, or trauma has been associated with portal vein obstruction [19]. A variety of congenital malformations also have been associated with portal vein obstruction, including cardiac and urinary tract anomalies [19]. As in Budd–Chiari syndrome, hypercoagulable states may predispose to the development of portal vein thrombosis [20,21]. These conditions include deficiencies in protein S, protein C, and antithrombin III, and specific mutations in factor V, factor II, and methyltetrahydrofolate reductase. Systemic conditions such as paroxysmal nocturnal hemoglobinuria also can contribute. Cavernous transformation is the appearance of the recanalization of or collaterals around a thrombosed portal vein. These lesions lead to portal hypertension directly because portal resistance is markedly elevated. Compression of the biliary system by the cavernoma may lead to biliary disease [22]. In general, hepatic function is intact and the major morbidity and mortality are a direct result of complications stemming from the associated portal hypertension, particularly esophageal varix hemorrhage. Effective management of these complications may be especially rewarding because of the relative absence of ongoing liver disease. Results of the study of the portal vein stenosis model of portal hypertension may be particularly applicable to this subgroup of pediatric patients. Splenic vein obstruction may result in portal hypertension, although this is uncommon in children. Identification of splenic vein thrombosis as the cause of portal hypertension is very important because splenectomy can be curative [23].

Intrahepatic causes of increased portal resistance constitute the remainder of the diseases associated with pediatric portal hypertension. The mechanisms of increased resistance are more varied than the extrahepatic etiologies. In many pediatric forms of chronic liver disease, resistance is increased secondary to impingement on the intrahepatic portal venule lumen as opposed to sinusoidal effects seen in adults. Hepatocyte swelling and hyperplasia in combination with portal tract inflammation and fibrosis are the major factors involved [24]. Collagen deposition in the space of Disse also may contribute to increased intrahepatic resistance, although this has not been well studied in pediatric diseases [25]. One of the major clinical differences from the extrahepatic etiologies of portal hypertension, especially in portal vein obstruction, is the presence of ongoing hepatocellular injury. Biliary tract disease is a common cause of significant liver disease in children. Biliary atresia and its sequelae after hepatoportoenterostomy make up a large percentage of clinical series of advanced pediatric liver disease [18]. Other relatively common pediatric disorders that primarily involve the biliary tract include cystic fibrosis, choledochal cysts, sclerosing cholangitis, total parenteral hyperalimentation–related cholestasis, Alagille syndrome, chronic rejection, Caroli's disease/biliary disease associated with autosomal recessive polycystic kidney disease, and the progressive intrahepatic cholestasis syndromes (especially BSEP [bile salt export pump] and MDR3 [multidrug resistance protein 3] disease). These diseases, which primarily involve the biliary system, lead to bile duct proliferation, portal inflammation, and fibrosis. These processes all result in compromise of the portal venules and with more advanced disease compromise of the sinusoidal lumen (akin to adult primarily hepatocellular disease), leading to increased resistance to portal flow. Early in the course of disease, hepatocyte function is preserved, resulting in the expression of manifestations of portal hypertension to a greater extent and at an earlier time than the manifestations related to hepatocellular dysfunction. Thus, therapeutic interventions directed at preventing complications of portal hypertension in children with biliary disease may be relatively more meaningful, given the potential long-term function of the liver. In fact, successful management of variceal hemorrhage in children with biliary atresia may postpone the need for liver transplantation for extended periods of time [26]. This is in contrast to adults, where variceal hemorrhage is often a harbinger of poor short-term prognosis [27]. The greater prevalence of biliary tract disease in children (e.g., biliary atresia) relative to adults (e.g., alcoholic liver disease and hepatitis C) makes the complications of portal hypertension relatively more significant in pediatric versus adult liver disease. Adult therapeutic approaches should not necessarily be directly applied to children because of the difference in underlying liver function and the different pathophysiologies of the underlying diseases relative to the development of portal hypertension. Bile duct obstruction models of portal hypertension may be more applicable to the majority of pediatric diseases, although the utility of this model is significantly compromised by the clinical instability and shortened life span of animals with complete bile duct obstruction. Genetic models of biliary disease (e.g., Alagille syndrome, cystic fibrosis, autosomal recessive polycystic kidney disease, MDR3) may be interesting new systems for the study of portal hypertension [28–31].

In most types of liver disease, vasoactive substances may play an important role in regulating intrahepatic resistance to blood flow. In contrast to the peripheral vasodilatation seen in cirrhosis, intrahepatic resistance is increased. The ability of the hepatic sinusoidal endothelial cells to secrete and respond to vasodilators is impaired [32,33]. Local levels of nitric oxide (NO) may be reduced in the liver and novel means of increasing these levels may yield new avenues for the treatment of portal hypertension [34]. Levels of endothelin-1, a potent vasoconstrictor, have been found to be elevated in chronic liver disease associated with cirrhosis [35,36]. Liver injury appears to induce increased release of endothelin-1 from either endothelial or stellate cells in the liver [37]. This endothelin acts locally to cause vasoconstriction of the preterminal portal venules and thus cause significant elevations in portal pressure [38]. Pharmacologic blockade of the specific receptors for endothelin-1 in the liver represents an exciting future prospect for the treatment of portal hypertension [39].

Primarily hepatocellular disorders are also common in children and can lead to portal hypertension. Included in this group of diseases are chronic hepatitis (particularly autoimmune and hepatitis B and C), Wilson's disease, α_1-antitrypsin deficiency, and a variety of metabolic and toxin-related disorders. In these disorders, changes in hepatic architecture and cirrhotic nodule formation lead to increases in portal resistance. In addition, in disorders characterized by significant portal inflammation (e.g., autoimmune hepatitis and Wilson's disease), the portal tract inflammation may lead to a pathophysiology similar to that seen in primary biliary tract disease. The ultimate effect is a compromise of the sinusoidal lumen. In addition, postsinusoidal resistance is most likely increased because of fibrosis and architectural changes. The end result is more similar to chronic liver diseases in adults as there is a greater degree of liver dysfunction present at the time of the manifestation of portal hypertension. Therefore, for these diseases, extrapolations of the results of adult clinical series are more realistic.

A variety of rare disorders exist that lead to portal hypertension but do not fit into the schema of intrahepatic (primary biliary tract or hepatocellular) or extrahepatic etiologies of portal hypertension. These diseases are not common in children and are included as examples of other pathophysiologies involved in the development of portal hypertension. The theory that increased portal inflow alone can lead to portal hypertension is supported by the finding of portal hypertension in patients with splanchnic arteriovenous fistulas or splenomegaly [40]. Veno-occlusive disease of the hepatic venule and hepatoportal sclerosis may increase portal resistance by sclerosis of the venous vessels as opposed to extrinsic compression [41,42]. Veno-occlusive disease is most commonly associated with chemotherapy but has been reported to be reversible when it is related to pyrrolizidine-containing tea [43]. Specific therapies to prevent chemotherapy-related veno-occlusive disease have reduced the prevalence of this problem [44]. Hepatoportal sclerosis is an enigmatic disorder that is manifest by portal hypertension in the face of normal to near-normal liver function test results, patent hepatic and portal veins, and portal fibrosis without evidence of either cirrhosis or nodule formation [45,46]. Experience at our center has led to the identification of a number of children with hepatoportal sclerosis who also had evidence of immune-mediated liver disease. In these patients, portal hypertension was the predominant clinical problem despite relative quiescence of the autoimmune liver disease. Schistosomiasis, one of the leading causes of portal hypertension in the world, is uncommon in the pediatric age range [47]. Portal tract inflammation results from the host response to the parasitic egg in the hepatic venule, leading to compromise of the intrahepatic portal vein lumen. The degree of fibrosis seen in schistosomiasis may have a genetic basis. Pharmacologic treatment of the schistosomiasis also may ameliorate the related portal hypertension [47].

Hemodynamic Changes

Increased resistance to portal blood flow may be the primary event in the development of portal hypertension, but it is clear that a variety of hemodynamic changes contribute to and amplify the increased portal blood pressure that is observed [48]. Both clinical studies and animal models have demonstrated the hemodynamic events that occur. Most of these investigations have not been performed in children or pediatric models, so the findings should be interpreted with caution. In fact, the hyperdynamic circulation has not been well characterized in any cohorts of pediatric patients. The hyperdynamic circulatory state is characterized by increased cardiac output, decreased splanchnic arteriolar tone, and decreased splanchnic vascular vasoconstrictor responsiveness. The net result is increased portal inflow, which directly contributes to portal hypertension. A variety of factors may be involved in the development of this hyperdynamic state, and dissection of their relative contributions to the resulting hyperdynamic circulation is important but difficult at best.

Increased cardiac output in advanced liver disease is the result of increased venous return to the heart and diminished cardiac afterload. Arteriolar vasodilatation is one of the key elements of this process. Parabiotic models indicate that humoral mediators are involved. When the output of the carotid artery of a portal hypertensive rat is infused into the superior mesenteric vein of a normal rat, total vascular resistance of the mesentery is reduced in the recipient rat [49]. Similar studies in which the donated blood is subjected to hepatic metabolism do not show this effect [50]. Thus, portosystemic shunting may be important for the development of this vasodilatation.

A variety of mediators have been proposed to contribute to this vasodilatation, although the focus recently has been primarily on the role of NO. Glucagon causes vasodilatation and is increased in advanced liver disease. This is partly the result of portosystemic shunting and bypassing of normal hepatic metabolism, but in addition, pancreatic output of glucagon is elevated [51]. Bile acids also have been proposed to cause vasodilatation, although experimental models have yielded contradictory results. It is clear that very high levels of bile acids will result in vasodilatation, but these levels may only be seen in severe cholestasis [52]. In a portal vein stenosis model of portal hypertension, cholestyramine therapy, which reduced serum bile acid levels to normal, did not affect portal pressure [53]. In a similar study, bile acid levels were reduced to subphysiologic levels by bile duct diversion. This led to an increase in splanchnic resistance and a decrease in both portal venous inflow and pressure [54]. Neither of these studies is particularly relevant to cholestatic disorders, in which serum bile acids are much higher. It is also important to realize that in cholestasis, luminal concentrations of bile salts are often diminished. Thus, the issue of the role of bile acids remains speculative. Prostaglandins, adenosine, calcitonin gene–related peptide, carbon monoxide, and endocannabinoids also have been thought to mediate the vasodilation in cirrhosis [55–60].

One of the most important mediators of vasodilatation may be NO, which used to be referred to as endothelium-derived relaxing factor [61]. N^G-monomethyl-L-arginine (L-NMMA), an inhibitor of NO production, decreased cardiac output and increased splanchnic and peripheral vascular resistance in a portal vein stenosis model. Portal venous inflow was thus decreased, but portocollateral resistance was increased, yielding an end result of no change in portal pressure. Sieber and Groszmann [62] have demonstrated that N^ω-nitro-L-arginine, another NO synthetase blocker, corrects the vascular hyporeactivity observed in portal hypertensive rats. In the portal vein ligation model, one of the first responses to the portal hypertension is actually vasoconstriction of the superior mesenteric artery. This leads to sheer stresses with subsequent release of NO by endothelial nitric oxide synthase [63]. The effects of NO in the splanchnic bed are dominant and ultimately lead to vasodilatation. There are likely to be multiple pathways that mediated this effect, since mice that lack both inducible and endothelial NO synthase still develop a hyperdynamic state in portal hypertensive models [9]. Although NO synthetase blockers would not appear to be a useful agent to treat portal hypertension, their effect suggests a role of NO in the generation of the vasodilatation associated with portal hypertension. NO release in severe liver diseases may be mediated in part through the effects of elevated levels of tumor necrosis factor-α (TNF-α). Thalidomide, which inhibits TNF-α production, ameliorated the hyperdynamic circulation in rats with portal vein ligation–induced portal hypertension [64]. An expanded intravascular volume is also an important part of the pathophysiology of the hyperdynamic circulation, via an increase in venous return and preload. Vasodilatation alone or associated with advanced liver disease is primarily responsible for increased sodium retention and increased vascular volume. This is the result of the renal response to vasodilatation and effective diminished perfusion. Sodium restriction in a portal vein stenosis model decreased plasma volume and thus normalized cardiac output and decreased portal pressure [65]. Therefore, sodium restriction and/or diuretic therapy might be useful in the management of all patients with significant portal hypertension.

It has recently become clear that in addition to the factors described above, alterations in serotonergic and sympathetic tone play a part in the pathogenesis of portal hypertension. Clonidine, a central α-adrenergic antagonist, decreases postsinusoidal resistance and thus decreases portal blood pressure [66]. Two serotonergic antagonists have been studied for effects on portal hypertension. Ketanserin, a serotonin and α-adrenergic antagonist, reduced portal pressure to an extent greater than its α-adrenergic blockade [66]. Ritanserin, a more specific serotonergic blocker, decreased portal pressure without affecting mean arterial pressure [67]. It is hypothesized that this effect was secondary to a decrease in portocollateral resistance. Although the side effects of hypotension and encephalopathy may limit their clinical usefulness, the effects of these antagonists suggest a role for abnormal serotonergic tone in the pathophysiology of portal hypertension. Decreased responsiveness of the mesenteric vasculature to endogenous vasoconstrictors plays an additional important role in the pathogenesis of portal hypertension.

Overall, a complex cycle of events leads to the hyperdynamic circulation, which is responsible for the forward flow portion of the pathophysiology of portal hypertension. A baseline state of liver disease and increased portal resistance initiates the process. Hepatocellular dysfunction and portosystemic shunting result in the generation of a variety of humoral factors, which lead to vasodilatation, enhanced cardiac output, and increased plasma volume. Splanchnic arteriolar vasodilatation and mesenteric venodilatation lead to increased portal inflow and elevated portal pressure, which lead to further portosystemic shunting and increased levels of circulating vasodilators and may lead to worsened hepatocellular injury. The self-perpetuating cycle of portal hypertension and portosystemic shunting continues until

Table 7.2: Initial Manifestations of Portal Hypertension

Reference	[112]	[68]	[69]	[18]	[74]
Total number of patients	70	33	27	108	97
Percentage with extrahepatic portal vein obstruction	100	67	74	100	100
Percentage presenting with					
Hemorrhage	80	97	85	46	55
Splenomegaly	99	24	100	94	>24
Ascites	17	21	?	8	7

a state of equilibrium is reached, which consists of increased portal pressure and a hyperdynamic circulation. Ultimately, this results in decreased portal perfusion of the injured liver. Intriguing studies in rabbits, whose liver disease is induced by a high-cholesterol diet, appear to indicate that mechanical augmentation of portal blood flow paradoxically reduced portal pressures and vascular resistance [67]. Liver function apparently was also improved and was related to an increase in hepatic oxygenation.

CLINICAL MANIFESTATIONS

The clinical presentation of portal hypertension can be dramatic because it may be the first symptom of longstanding silent liver disease. In several large series of children with portal hypertension, approximately two thirds of the children presented with hematemesis or melena, usually from rupture of an esophageal varix (Table 7.2). Gastrointestinal hemorrhage also may be associated with bleeding from portal hypertensive gastropathy, gastric antral vascular ectasia, or gastric, duodenal, peristomal, or rectal varices. Variceal hemorrhage is the result of increased pressure within the varix, which leads to changes in the diameter of the varix and increased wall tension.

When the wall tension exceeds the variceal wall strength, physical rupture of the varix occurs. Given the high blood flow and pressure in the portosystemic collateral system coupled with the lack of a natural mechanism to tamponade variceal bleeding, the rate of hemorrhage can be striking and life threatening. Almost all the patients reported in the series had splenomegaly at the time of hemorrhage; thus, the combination of gastrointestinal hemorrhage and splenomegaly should be suggestive of portal hypertension until proven otherwise. The sentinel bleeding episode in these children occurred at a wide range of ages, starting as early as 2 months of age. No particular peak age of presentation has been demonstrated. Many of the episodes of hemorrhage that have been reported have been associated with upper respiratory tract infections, fever, or aspirin ingestion [68,69]. It is possible that increases in abdominal pressure from coughing associated with respiratory infections and increases in cardiac output from the tachycardia associated with fever may result in increases in portal pressure and increased tendency to hemorrhage. Aspirin ingestion is associated with platelet dysfunction and gastrointestinal mucosal damage, both of which would predispose to hemorrhage. Other physiologic factors have been associated with increased portal pressures, which might increase the risk of variceal hemorrhage. These factors include physical exercise, blood or food in the stomach, and normal circadian rhythms [70–73].

The next most common presentation of portal hypertension is splenomegaly. In many instances, this is first discovered on routine physical examination. Many patients will have been aware of a vague fullness in the left upper quadrant for many years. Occasionally manifestations of hypersplenism, including thrombocytopenia, leukopenia, petechiae, or ecchymoses, will prompt evaluation, leading to the discovery of portal hypertension. Extensive hematologic evaluations, including bone marrow biopsies, may have been undertaken before portal hypertension is considered. Thus, the hematologist should include a liver profile and potentially Doppler ultrasonography in the evaluation of any child with thrombocytopenia, especially if there is the simultaneous finding of leukopenia. Rarely will the associated cytopenias lead to clinically relevant disease. Although splenomegaly is a common finding in patients with portal hypertension, splenic size does not seem to correlate well with portal pressure [74–76].

Certain cutaneous vascular patterns are specific to portal hypertension. Prominent vascular markings on the abdomen are the result of portocollateral shunting through subcutaneous vessels. The direction of flow through these veins may be indicative of the site of obstruction. When the inferior vena cava is occluded, drainage is usually cephalad, although it is caudad below the umbilicus if the inferior vena cava is patent. Decompression of portal hypertension through the umbilical vein results in prominent periumbilical collaterals, which have been referred to as caput medusae. An audible venous hum, the Cruveilhier-Baumgarten murmur, may occasionally be appreciated through these vessels. Caput medusae are rarely seen in children, partly because of the high prevalence of portal vein obstruction associated with umbilical vein obliteration. Portal hypertensive rectopathy or rectal varices may be more common than generally appreciated [77]. In children with short gut syndrome, stomal varices, which are a site of low resistance, are often easily observed and a common site of hemorrhage [78].

Hepatopulmonary syndrome (pulmonary arteriovenous shunting) is an important clinical manifestation of portal hypertension. In this condition, there is intrapulmonic right-to-left shunting of blood, which results in systemic desaturation. The mechanisms involved in the development of hepatopulmonary syndrome are unknown, but they are likely to include many of the vasoactive substances involved in the genesis of the hyperdynamic circulation, including NO and endothelin-1 [79–83]. One of the best-described animal models of hepatopulmonary syndrome is bile duct ligation, which is especially relevant given the high prevalence of this problem in biliary atresia. Interestingly, hepatopulmonary syndrome can occur in the absence of intrinsic liver disease and has been described as a sequela of congenital portosystemic shunting [84]. Thus portosystemic shunting may be the key pathologic event leading to hepatopulmonary syndrome. The prevalence of hepatopulmonary syndrome in chronic pediatric liver disease is not well characterized and depends on the method of diagnosis. Symptomatic hepatopulmonary syndrome (e.g., shortness of breath, exercise intolerance, and digital clubbing) is typically a late manifestation, thus series that depend on symptomatic presentation likely underestimate the true prevalence of this complication. Agitated saline echocardiography is a very sensitive measure of intrapulmonic shunting and can easily detect asymptomatic disease [85,86]. Positive echocardiographic studies were reported in 64% of children with biliary atresia who were prospectively studied [87]. The clinical relevance of this finding is not known as the natural history of mild shunting is not well described. Macroaggregated albumin scanning may be used to quantify the degree of shunting, which can be useful in clinical decision making and in follow-up of hepatopulmonary syndrome. In a large pediatric series, 26 of 1116 children with chronic liver disease had clinically significant pulmonary arteriovenous shunting [88]. A variety of medical treatments have not been shown to be effective in treating this unusual complication of portal hypertension, although encouraging pilot studies of garlic have been reported [89,90]. Liver transplantation is very effective in reversing hepatopulmonary syndrome but theoretically may have limited efficacy in children with very severe disease. Full reversal of the shunting may take many months. Efficacy of transplantation is primarily limited by the ability of a particular patient to tolerate the perioperative cardiopulmonary stress of surgery. Screening for hepatopulmonary syndrome should be included in the evaluation and treatment of any child with cirrhosis and/or portal hypertension. In light of the orthodeoxia associated with this condition, measurement of peripheral oxygen saturation in children who are upright at the time of testing should be an effective screen [91,92]. Any children with oxygen saturations below 96% should undergo further testing, including agitated saline echocardiography and/or macroaggregated albumin scanning, to assess the presence or absence of hepatopulmonary syndrome and its severity [85,90].

Pulmonary hypertension is pathophysiologically related to hepatopulmonary syndrome. It is an unusual but worrisome manifestation of pediatric liver disease. The exact pathophysiology of the development of this pulmonary hypertension is unclear, but it seems to be associated with the presence of portal hypertension [93–95]. Decreased hepatic clearance and portosystemic shunting of humoral mediators is hypothesized to be involved in this process. Routine screening for this rare complication is recommended in adults but not typically in children, although it has been described both in adults and in children [96,97]. Endothelin-1 receptor antagonists, prostacyclin analogues, and sildenafil may be effective in some cases of portopulmonary hypertension [98–102]. In addition, liver transplantation may need to be considered as an urgent intervention in order to prevent the development of irreversible disease [103]. Severe portopulmonary hypertension, defined by a pulmonary artery pressure greater than 50 mm Hg, is a contraindication to liver transplantation because of perioperative mortality. Unlike hepatopulmonary syndrome, portopulmonary hypertension does not typically reverse after isolated liver transplantation, although anecdotal reports of reversal in children have been reported [104]. This is likely owing to the fact that the disease is the result of obliteration of the lumen of the pulmonary artery. Definitive treatment for severe portopulmonary hypertension may need to include liver, heart, and lung transplantation [105].

The other major manifestations of portal hypertension affect the kidney and brain. Renal-related complications include ascites and hepatorenal syndrome. Sodium retention, which is probably initiated by the already discussed systemic vasodilatation, may lead to ascites as an initial presentation of portal hypertension [106]. The elevated portal blood pressure increases the Starling forces, which drive fluids out of the intravascular space into the peritoneum. In addition, impaired lymphatic drainage contributes to the development of ascites. Portal hypertension predisposes to bacterial translocation in the intestine and bacterial peritonitis [107]. Very-late-stage cirrhosis is associated with enhanced free-water retention and hyponatremia. Hepatorenal syndrome is a particularly ominous complication of the renal disease associated with portal hypertension [108]. Type 1 hepatorenal syndrome is an acute form of renal failure that cannot be ascribed to other causes of renal failure (e.g. infection, nephrotoxic medications, shock, or other forms of nephropathy). Short-term mortality is very high in patients with acute hepatorenal syndrome, although recently described treatment strategies have improved this outlook somewhat [109]. There is little published experience with the diagnostic criteria and management of hepatorenal syndrome in children [110,111]. Hepatic encephalopathy is a complication associated with portosystemic shunting typically in the setting of advanced liver disease and relatively significant hepatocellular dysfunction (Chapter 6). Subtle hepatic encephalopathy may exist in children with portal vein thrombosis, in which there is minimal liver dysfunction. Thus the clinician needs to consider this problem in children with chronic liver disease and behavioral disorders. Diagnosis of hepatic encephalopathy in children, especially in its milder forms, is problematic at best.

NATURAL HISTORY

An accurate description of the natural history of portal hypertension in children is essential for a rigorous assessment of the efficacy of traditional and novel forms of therapy. A variety of complex and relatively accurate modeling systems of portal hypertension in adults have been developed [27]. Unfortunately, the natural history of pediatric portal hypertension is difficult to accurately assess because of the wide range of disorders that result in portal hypertension in children. Many of these disorders have unique pathophysiologies and clinical courses. The most confounding problem in attempting to describe the natural history of portal hypertension in children retrospectively is the wide variety of therapeutic interventions that have been applied in a noncontrolled manner. In addition, there are few distinct diagnostic entities in which the prevalence of portal hypertension is high enough to generate clinically significant series. Extrahepatic portal vein obstruction and biliary atresia represent two entities in which clinically meaningful series of untreated patients exist and can be used as a guide to the natural history of pediatric portal hypertension.

Extrahepatic Portal Vein Obstruction

Portal vein obstruction is a useful example of the natural history of portal hypertension in the setting of slowly progressive liver disease. The presentation in children is usually one of gastrointestinal hemorrhage or the incidental discovery of splenomegaly. In two retrospective series, 167 patients presented from the ages of 10 days to 75 years [74,112]. In most cases, it was not possible to date the event leading to portal vein obstruction. As a result, it is unclear if the wide age range can be used as evidence for longstanding clinically benign disease. In 21 cases of presumed neonatal portal venous obstruction, presentation by hemorrhage was gradual over periods as long as 12 years. Although the vast majority of the patients at some time in their life experienced gastrointestinal hemorrhage, a significant number of patients never bled. Four patients had fatal first hemorrhage episodes, although three of these instances were blamed on insufficient blood supplies. Sixty-one patients received medical management alone. Four described above died during their initial bleeding episode. Of the remainder, eight (13%) subsequently died of gastrointestinal hemorrhage. A minority of patients had no further episodes of hemorrhage. Most had several more episodes of bleeding, with a general observation of decreased frequency and severity after puberty. This phenomenon of apparently "outgrowing" portal hypertension may be the result of recanalization of the portal vein or the development of collaterals and spontaneous portosystemic shunts through sites other than the gastroesophageal varices. Ascites and end-stage liver disease are unusual in portal vein thrombosis. Subtle hepatic encephalopathy may be more prevalent than previously thought (personal communication Peter F. Whitington, Children's Memorial Hospital, Chicago IL). Failure to thrive, pubertal delay, and a form of biliary disease that has cystic features and manifestations akin to sclerosing cholangitis have been reported in long-term follow-up [22,113,114]. It has been hypothesized that the biliary disease is the result of partial bile duct obstruction from the cavernoma associated with the portal vein obstruction. In summary, portal vein obstruction is associated with potentially, but not usually, life-threatening gastrointestinal hemorrhage. The time from portal vein obstruction to hemorrhage appears to be quite variable, as does the clinical course. The relatively reduced underlying hepatic injury makes portal vein obstruction a relatively more benign form of portal hypertension. Treatment recommendations must be tailored to the individual on a case-by-case basis with an understanding of the expertise of the treating center and physicians. Recent reports of the success of mesentericoportal bypass (meso-Rex bypass) surgery needs to be incorporated into the clinical decision making in the management of individuals with portal vein thrombosis [115–117]. In light of the fact that this procedure results in physiologic restoration of normal portal flow, this procedure may become the treatment of choice for children with a cavernoma and portal vein thrombosis even prior to the onset of complications.

Extrahepatic Biliary Atresia

Biliary atresia is the leading cause of significant pediatric liver disease and the leading reason for referral for liver transplantation [118]. Unlike portal vein obstruction, biliary atresia is an example of a disease in which portal hypertension is associated with ongoing and progressive liver disease. Biliary atresia is universally fatal in childhood unless operative intervention is undertaken. At the time of portoenterostomy, portal hypertension has been documented, and its subsequent natural history is complicated by the variable results of portoenterostomy [119]. In general, the complications of portal hypertension are more prevalent in patients with poor biliary drainage or postoperative cholangitis [119]. Variceal hemorrhage is a common problem in children with biliary atresia and may occur as early as the first year of life [26,120–125]. The importance of bile flow, as manifest by total serum bilirubin, in the prognosis after variceal hemorrhage is reflected in reported experiences from Denver and Hong Kong [26,124]. Survival without liver transplantation after first variceal hemorrhage is significantly greater in children with total serum bilirubin below 4 mg/dL [26]. The technique of creating a stoma for biliary drainage, which may lead to potentially fatal stoma-related variceal hemorrhage, is largely being abandoned [126]. In most circumstances, variceal bleeding appears to be life threatening and recurrent unless some intervention is undertaken. In Miyato's early series, 26 of 44 patients died, 20 of them as a direct result of complications of portal hypertension [119]. Variceal hemorrhage in these patients requires intervention, which must be tempered with the prospect of possible liver transplantation in the future. Given the progressive nature of portal hypertension associated with biliary atresia, the effects of interventions, both medical and surgical, are more easily discerned.

DIAGNOSTIC EVALUATIONS

Portal hypertension should be suspected in any child with significant gastrointestinal hemorrhage or unexplained splenomegaly. Physical examination should be directed at assessing for evidence of chronic liver disease. Care should be taken to look for growth failure or cutaneous lesions consistent with chronic liver disease (e.g., telangiectasia, palmar erythema). The combination of gastrointestinal hemorrhage and splenomegaly is highly suggestive of portal hypertension until proved otherwise. Laboratory studies should be aimed at evaluation of liver function. In addition, white blood cell and platelet counts may give evidence of hypersplenism. In children with portal vein thrombosis or Budd–Chiari syndrome, investigation of thrombophilia or myeloproliferative disease is potentially indicated.

A wide variety of diagnostic tests are available to document and quantify portal hypertension. Most have been well studied in adult but not pediatric age groups. Many of the quantitative studies are invasive and most useful in a research setting to study response to treatment and, in some cases, to predict risk of gastrointestinal hemorrhage. In the pediatric age range, a combination of ultrasonography and flexible fiberoptic endoscopy can usually determine if portal hypertension or esophageal varices are present or absent. More invasive radiologic imaging is reserved for documentation of vascular anatomy.

Ultrasonography

Advances in ultrasonography, most specifically Doppler flow studies, have made this the investigation of choice in children. Its noninvasive nature is ideally suited for this age group. A great deal of data can be obtained in a 30- to 60-minute investigation. As with many other procedures, the information that is obtained is directly dependent on the skill and experience of the operator. An abdominal survey can yield important information, including hepatic size and echogenicity. A small liver in the setting of portal hypertension is a potentially worrisome finding. Increased echogenicity is commonly seen in cirrhosis. Intrahepatic bile ducts can be assessed for evidence of dilatation consistent with extrahepatic obstruction or Caroli's disease. Spleen size can be easily measured and will give indirect evidence about the presence or absence of portal hypertension. Unfortunately, spleen size does not appear to correlate directly with portal pressure [75]. Renal abnormalities, associated with portal vein thrombosis and congenital hepatic fibrosis/Caroli's disease, can easily be detected. Finally, ascites, which may not be evident on physical examination, can be demonstrated.

Doppler insonation of the hepatic and mesenteric vasculature affords an even greater amount of important information. The presence or absence of vessels can be determined in addition to vessel diameter, direction of blood flow in the vessel, and the presence or absence of echogenic material within the blood vessel. Vascular anomalies are usually readily detected. In children, normal nonfasting portal blood flow as assessed by Doppler examination is hepatopetal at 10–30 cm/sec [127,128]. Portal vein velocity decreases in severe portal hypertension as intrahepatic resistance increases. Hepatofugal flow in the left gastric, paraduodenal, or paraumbilical veins is consistent with portal hypertension, although this may be a relatively late finding. Reversal of flow in the superior mesenteric vein or splenic vein may be indicative of spontaneous mesentericocaval or splenorenal shunts, respectively. Hepatic arterial flow is often increased in portal hypertension as part of the normal compensation for diminished portal venous inflow [129]. In selected studies, careful analysis of either portal venous blood flow or superior mesenteric artery flow velocity has revealed a correlation with portal pressure [128,130]. Unfortunately, these quantitative ultrasound studies have not been universally useful and have not been characterized in children.

Ultrasound has been demonstrated to be very effective in detecting the presence of esophageal varices [131,132]. Esophageal varices are formed by portosystemic shunting via the left gastric vein through the lesser omentum into the azygous vein tributary system in the lower esophagus (Figure 7.1). As a result, if significant esophageal varices exist, substantial blood flow must pass through the lesser omentum. In children, this can be measured between the posterior surface of the liver and the aorta at the level of the celiac axis. Normal values for the ratio of the width of the lesser omentum (LO) and the diameter of the aorta (AD) have been described in children. The LO/AD ratio in 150 normal children was less than 1.7 [131]. The LO/AD ratio was examined in 28 children who had chronic liver disease or gastrointestinal hemorrhage [132]. The presence of esophageal varices was determined in these children by flexible fiberoptic endoscopy. The LO/AD ratio was significantly increased in children with varices, and its magnitude correlated with the size of those varices.

Endoscopy

Flexible fiberoptic endoscopy can be used for the definitive determination of the presence of esophageal varices (Figure 7.2). This examination is especially useful in determining if gastrointestinal hemorrhage in a child with chronic liver disease is secondary to variceal rupture. The differential diagnosis includes gastric or duodenal ulcers, gastritis, Mallory–Weiss tears, and portal hypertensive gastropathy. Eight of 22 children with cirrhosis and upper gastrointestinal hemorrhage had gastric or duodenal ulcers [133]. In adults, the endoscopic appearance of varices may be predictive of the risk of future hemorrhage. The red wale sign and cherry-red spot are particularly associated with increased risk of hemorrhage [133]. Variceal size may be the most important prognostic finding [134]. These findings have not been systematically assessed in the pediatric age range. In addition, studies have been performed assessing intravariceal pressure by upper endoscopy [135]. These studies require a very cooperative patient and, once again, have not

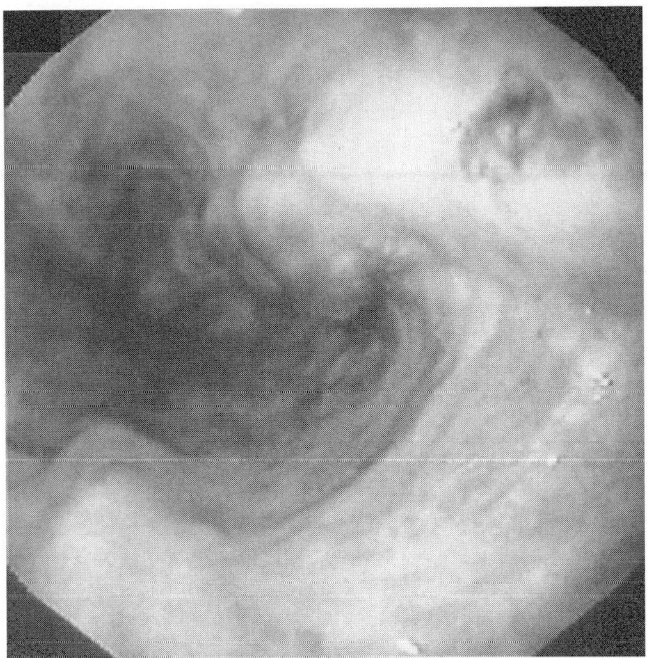

Figure 7.2. Endoscopic view of varices. Three columns of varices are seen.

been performed in children. Indirect variceal pressure measurement using an endoscopic pressure gauge might be more plausible for investigation in children [135–137]. In fact, this technique may even be useful in predicting the risk of future variceal hemorrhage [138]. Capsule endoscopy may be used to look for esophageal varices, although the cost-effectiveness and feasibility of this approach with current equipment/approaches is an open question [139,140].

Other Investigations

A variety of other diagnostic investigations exist for the assessment of portal hypertension. Most of these studies have not been extensively characterized in children secondary to their invasive nature. Selective angiography of the celiac axis, superior mesenteric artery, and splenic vein may be especially useful in assessing the extrahepatic vascular anatomy. In particular, these studies are helpful in cases of suspected portal vein thrombosis and are essential for surgical decompression of this lesion [141]. These studies may be essential for the diagnosis and appropriate therapy of splenic vein thrombosis. A combination of ultrasonography, inferior cavography, computed tomographic scanning with intravenous contrast, and magnetic resonance venography may be used to document the vascular lesions associated with Budd–Chiari syndrome [16,142]. Portal pressure can be directly measured by examination of splenic pulp pressure during splenoportography, although this is primarily a historical technique. In general, this is a procedure with appreciable risks that are not usually offset by significant benefits in the pediatric age group, although a number of pediatric patients have been studied in this manner [143]. The hepatic venous pressure gradient (HVPG) is one of the classic measurements used in assessing portal hypertension in adult patients. A balloon-tipped catheter is inserted into the antecubital vein and advanced to the hepatic vein, where free and wedged hepatic vein pressures can be measured. The wedged hepatic vein pressure is usually a good index of portal vein pressure when the main lesion in the hepatic vasculature is limited to the sinusoidal area. The difference between the free and wedged hepatic vein pressures is the HVPG. An HVPG of greater than 12 mm Hg appears to be needed for variceal hemorrhage to occur [144]. In addition, the HVPG is a reproducible measurement for studying the effects of a variety of medical and surgical interventions. Growing evidence in adults indicates the potential importance of HVPG measurements [145,146]. Responses of HVPG to pharmacotherapy may be predictive of future chances of recurrent variceal hemorrhage [147]. Given the relatively invasive nature of this measurement, no well-documented pediatric measurements of HVPG exist outside the experience at the time of placement of transjugular intrahepatic portosystemic shunts (TIPSs). In addition, HVPG measurements are not as accurate in presinusoidal liver disease, which is the case for many of the prevalent pediatric forms of chronic liver disease (e.g., biliary atresia, portal vein thrombosis). Given the growing data that indicate that assessment of portal pressures is predictive of both the risk of hemorrhage and the potential response to therapy, development of a practical and reliable pediatric measure is of great importance. The noninvasive nature of Doppler evaluation of portal hypertension has the greatest potential for these types of measurements in children [148].

THERAPY

The therapy of portal hypertension is primarily directed at the management of its most dramatic manifestation, variceal hemorrhage. Variceal hemorrhage is a medical emergency, and patients with chronic liver disease should be instructed to seek immediate medical attention for any signs or symptoms of variceal hemorrhage. The management of variceal hemorrhage can be divided into preprimary prophylaxis, prophylaxis (primary) of the first episode of bleeding, emergency therapy, and prophylaxis (secondary) of subsequent bleeding episodes. As with many other aspects of the science of portal hypertension, almost all the modes of therapy are based on trials in adults. Many of these trials are well-controlled randomized double-blinded studies, and comprehensive meta-analyses of these trials have been performed [149–152]. The literature of the management of pediatric variceal hemorrhage is mostly descriptive or anecdotal. There have been only two randomized trials of therapies for portal hypertension in children [1,2].

Preprimary Prophylaxis

The concept of preprimary prophylaxis is that early treatment of portal hypertension has the potential to delay or prevent the development of esophageal varices or other manifestations of portal hypertension. In an *S. mansoni* mouse model of portal hypertension, the administration of propranolol 5 weeks into the infection resulted in a significant reduction in the development of portal hypertension, portosystemic shunting, and portal venous inflow [7]. A randomized trial of timolol, a nonselective β-blocker, on the development of varices in adults unfortunately did not show a significant effect [153]. Thus at present, preprimary prophylaxis remains an interesting concept but one that is not applicable in clinical practice.

Primary Prophylaxis

The issue of prophylaxis of the first episode of variceal hemorrhage in children is controversial and is predicated on experience with adults who primarily have alcoholic cirrhosis. Surveillance endoscopy in children with liver disease and stigmata of portal hypertension is primarily justified if the clinician anticipates recommending a prophylactic regimen, although there may be value in surveillance for patients who live in remote areas far from medical care. Given the unpredictability of the timing of the first episode of variceal hemorrhage, primary prophylaxis regimens need to be associated with relatively low potential morbidity and mortality. As such, β-blockade has been much more extensively used in this setting. The improved risk–benefit ratio of endoscopic ligation therapy relative to sclerotherapy has led to reassessment of its role in primary prophylaxis [154–156]. The technical details of endoscopic ligation therapy are discussed later in this chapter. Uncontrolled preliminary pediatric experience with the use of propranolol in the primary prophylaxis of variceal hemorrhage has recently been reported [143,157–159].

β-Blocker therapy of portal hypertension is optimal with nonselective agents. The primary effect may be β_2-blockade of the splanchnic bed, leaving unopposed α-adrenergic stimulation and thus decreased splanchnic and portal perfusion. An additional important mechanism involves decreasing heart rate by β_1-adrenoreceptor blockade, thus lowering cardiac output and portal perfusion. Finally, evidence exists for a specific effect of propranolol that decreases collateral circulation (e.g., azygous venous blood flow). Therapeutic doses in adults are expected to decrease the pulse rate by at least 25%, although these guidelines are somewhat problematic in children, in whom baseline measures may be difficult. A wide dosing range (0.6–8.0 mg/kg/d divided into two to four doses per day) has been required in children in order to observe a "therapeutic effect" [143,158]. The major adverse effects associated with the use of propranolol are heart block and exacerbation of asthma. β-Blockade will inhibit β-adrenergic treatment of asthma. β-Blockade also has the potential to interfere in the physiologic response to hypoglycemia; thus, this agent should be avoided in children with diabetes.

β-Blockers have been consistently shown to reduce the frequency of bleeding episodes, and in some trials they have improved long-term survival in patients with esophageal varices. Initial randomized trials demonstrated efficacy in patients who had a previous bleeding episode [160]. Subsequently, propranolol was shown to be effective in patients with varices who had never bled. In a study of 230 patients randomized to propranolol or placebo, the incidence of hemorrhage and mortality over a 14-month period was reduced by almost 50% [161]. The successful results of numerous trials of propranolol have been summarized by meta-analyses [149,162]. It is clear that a goal of at least a 25% reduction in resting heart rate needs to be achieved to see these effects. In patients in whom HVPG drops below 12 mm Hg, subsequent variceal hemorrhage appears to be unlikely [147]. Unfortunately, propranolol often does not reduce HVPG below 12 mm Hg, a possible threshold for hemorrhage [144]. Therefore, combinations of β-blockade and vasodilation therapy are now under investigation. Isosorbide-5-mononitrate, a long-acting vasodilator, may potentiate the effects of propranolol on the HVPG [163,164]. Combinatorial pharmacologic agents, such as carvedilol, may have enhanced efficacy [165,166]. Unfortunately, there is little if any prospective data on the safety or feasibility of β-blockade in children with portal hypertension. Furthermore, there are scant data indicating that β-blockade is effective for primary prophylaxis in children. As such, this approach should be considered investigational in children.

Endoscopic band ligation therapy has been used with greater frequency in adults with high-risk varices [167,168]. As with β-blockade, endoscopic band ligation therapy cannot be recommended for routine use in children with varices. In fact, a small randomized trial of prophylactic endoscopic sclerotherapy in children showed no survival benefit [1]. Given the invasive nature of the technique, selected application of this approach may be appropriate only in children who have apparently high-risk varices and who live in remote locations.

Emergency Therapy of Variceal Hemorrhage

The initial management of variceal hemorrhage is stabilization of the patient. Vital signs, particularly tachycardia or hypotension, can be especially helpful in assessing blood loss. Patients on β-blocker therapy may not manifest the usual compensatory tachycardia and are at higher risk of developing hemodynamically significant hypotension. Fluid resuscitation in the form of crystalloid initially, followed by red blood cell transfusion, is critical. One needs to administer these fluids carefully to avoid overfilling the intravascular space and increasing portal pressure. Optimal hemoglobin levels in adults with variceal hemorrhage are between 7 and 9 g/dL [169]. Nasogastric tube placement is safe and may be an essential part of the management of these patients. It allows for documentation of the rate of ongoing bleeding and removal of blood, a protein source that may precipitate encephalopathy. In addition, blood in the stomach increases splanchnic blood flow and potentially could worsen portal hypertension and ongoing hemorrhage [71]. Platelets should be administered for levels less than 50×10^9/L, and coagulopathy should be corrected with vitamin K or fresh frozen plasma, especially in patients with cholestasis. There may be value to the use of recombinant factor VIIa in severe coagulopathy as the fluid requirements of fresh frozen plasma administration may be diminished [170]. Intravenous antibiotic therapy should be strongly considered for all patients with variceal hemorrhage in light of the high risk of potentially fatal infectious complications [171,172]. Once the patient is stabilized, endoscopy should be performed to document that the hemorrhage is indeed from variceal rupture. Signs of recent hemorrhage include visualization of ongoing hemorrhage, the presence of a fresh clot, or the presence of varices with fresh blood in the stomach and no other source of bleeding. Continued hemorrhage at the time of diagnostic endoscopy is a finding that portends a poor prognosis. Care should be taken to avoid disrupting fresh clot formation. A significant percentage of both children and adults with chronic liver disease and gastrointestinal hemorrhage will have sources of bleeding other than varices, including duodenal or gastric ulceration [133,144,173]. As such, diagnostic endoscopy is an integral part of the emergent management of acute gastrointestinal hemorrhage in the child with portal hypertension. Pharmacotherapy of acute hemorrhage need not be withheld until endoscopy can be performed. In fact, adequate pharmacotherapy may facilitate an endoscopic approach. At the time of diagnostic endoscopy, initial management in the form of sclerotherapy or ligation can commence.

Many episodes of variceal hemorrhage will spontaneously terminate, and supportive therapy is all that is required. Unfortunately, some episodes may become life threatening and require urgent therapy. Acute measurement of HVPG in adults may predict which patients will have an eventful evolution after the initial bleeding episode [174]. Hemorrhage that persists for more than 6 hours or requires more than one red blood cell transfusion necessitates further intervention. A wide range of potential therapeutic approaches exist. Documentation of their efficacy in adults is fairly convincing, whereas the data in children are scanty at best [149,175]. In general, a clinical decision is made that the risk of further blood product administration and potential hemodynamic compromise outweighs the side effects associated with further therapy. As in children in general, the most benign therapies are frequently the most favorable initial modalities of treatment.

Emergency Therapy: Pharmacologic

The pharmacologic therapy of acute variceal bleeding typically consists of the use of vasopressin or somatostatin (or their respective analogues) (Table 7.3). Vasopressin has the longest history of usage and acts by increasing splanchnic vascular tone and thus decreasing portal blood flow. Its use is often limited by the side effects of this vasoconstriction, which include left ventricular failure, bowel ischemia, angina, and chest and abdominal pain [173]. Only a limited number of studies have compared vasopressin therapy with supportive care alone. In these studies, vasopressin led to more rapid control of gastrointestinal hemorrhage, but no significant effect on mortality was seen [149]. Of 215 children with acute variceal hemorrhage, 184 had bleeding arrested by the combined use of fluid support and vasopressin [18,173,176]. Vasopressin has a half-life of 30 minutes and is usually administered as a bolus followed by a continuous infusion. The recommended dosage for children is 0.33 U/kg as a bolus over 20 minutes followed by a continuous infusion of the same amount hourly or a continuous infusion of 0.2 U/1.73 m^2/min [176,177]. The continuous infusion may be increased to up to three times its initial rate. These recommendations are apparently empiric, based on clinical practice, and most likely derived from extrapolation of adult dosages. Nitroglycerin, a potent venodilator, increases the effectiveness of vasopressin and ameliorates some of its side effects [178]. Nitroglycerin has been administered to adults to reduce systolic blood pressure to less than 100 mm Hg. The efficacy of this approach in children remains untested. Terlipressin, a long-acting synthetic analogue of vasopressin, has shown similar effects and does not require continuous infusion [179]. Side effects appear to be reduced relative to vasopressin. A potential significant advantage of terlipressin is its favorable effect on both control of hemorrhage and mortality [150]. Unfortunately, terlipressin has not been approved for use in the United States, and there are no data regarding its use in children.

Table 7.3: Acute Management of Esophageal Varix Hemorrhage

Pharmacologic
Vasopressin
Somatostatin
Endoscopic
Sclerotherapy
Ligation
Mechanical
Sengstaken–Blakemore tube
Surgical
Esophageal transection
Emergent portosystemic shunt
Esophageal devascularization
Orthotopic liver transplantation
Other
Transjugular intrahepatic portosystemic shunting

Alternatives to vasopressin have been investigated because of vasopressin's poor side-effect profile. Somatostatin and its synthetic homologue octreotide also have been shown to decrease splanchnic blood flow. This effect is presumably mediated by blockade of secretion of vasoactive peptides by the intestine. Its effects on acute variceal hemorrhage appear to be similar to those of vasopressin, with fewer side effects [180,181]. Like vasopressin, the dosing of these agents in children is empiric. Our own unpublished experience and the published experience in other pediatric centers indicate that intravenous octreotide appears to be relatively well tolerated by sick infants and children [182–185]. Continuous infusions of 1–5 μg/kg/hr of octreotide appear to be effective but may need to be initiated by the administration of a bolus of 1 hour's worth of the infusion. There is a critical need for better safety and efficacy data on these agents in infants and children. New longer-acting somatostatin analogues are currently under investigation [186].

Emergency Therapy: Endoscopic

As noted previously, approximately 15% of pediatric patients will have persistent hemorrhage despite conservative management plus some form of splanchnic vasoconstriction. The most commonly used second approach is endoscopic sclerotherapy or endoscopic band ligation. This therapy is very effective in controlling bleeding, although it may be technically challenging in the individual with rapid hemorrhage. An extensive experience with emergency sclerotherapy exists in children, and it is rare for additional therapy to be required [18,176,187]. A variety of methods are used that chemically cause the varices to clot off and fibrose. Sclerosants, chemically irritating compounds such as ethanolamine or tetradecyl sulfate, are injected either intra- or paravariceally, until bleeding has stopped (Figure 7.3). Sclerotherapy is associated with a series of complications of its own, which will be discussed later. In the setting of emergency sclerotherapy it is important to be aware of the significant incidence of associated bacteremia and to consider prophylaxis in nearly all patients [188]. The major drawback of an endoscopic approach to treating acute hemorrhage is that the bloody field that is frequently encountered makes the procedure technically challenging. Endoscopic band ligation of varices may be

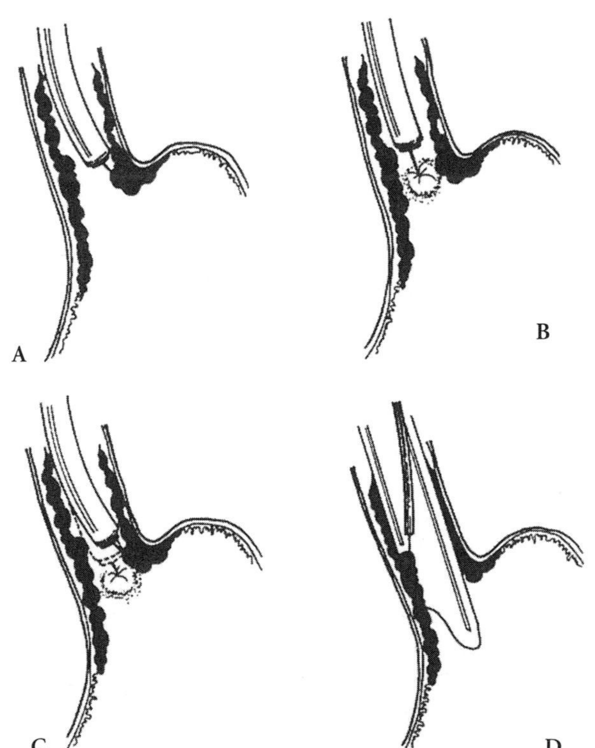

Figure 7.3. Technique of injection sclerotherapy. A flexible endoscope is used for intravariceal injection (**A**), paravariceal injection (**B**), and combined paravariceal and intravariceal injection (**C**), whereas a rigid endoscope with a slot is used for intravariceal injection (**D**). (Reprinted from Terblanche et al. [230], with permission.)

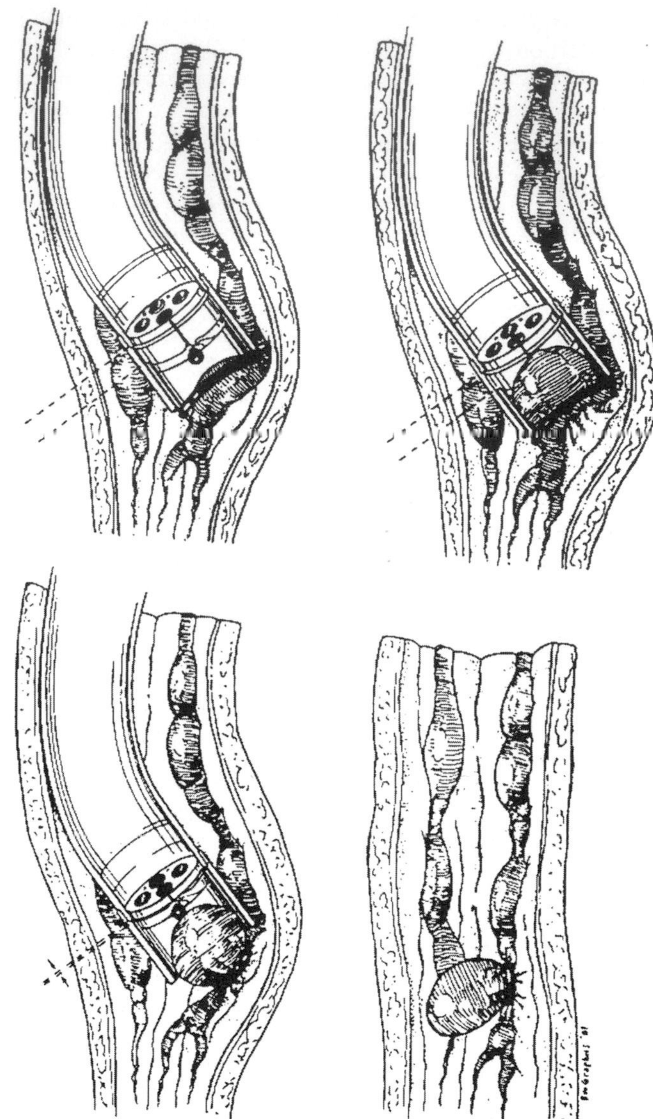

Figure 7.4. Technique of endoscopic ligation of esophageal varices. The endoscopic tip is positioned over a variceal column in the distal esophagus (*upper left*). Suction is applied to draw the esophageal mucosa and varix up into the dead space with the ligating device (*upper right*). The tripwire is pulled and the O-ring slipped around the aspirated tissue (*lower left*). (Reprinted from Van Stiegmann [189], with permission.)

a preferable approach because it is easier and safer to perform in an obscured field [189,190]. In this approach the entire varix is drawn into the endoscope and an elastic band snares the vessel (Figures 7.4 and 7.5). This technique is a variation on ligation of rectal hemorrhoids. A randomized trial of ligation versus sclerotherapy in adults demonstrated similar control of active bleeding and recurrence of hemorrhage with significantly lower overall complications and mortality in the patients treated with endoscopic ligation [191]. A potential concern in the application of this technique to small children, whose esophageal wall is thinner than that of adults, is entrapment of the full thickness of the esophageal wall by the rubber band and subsequent

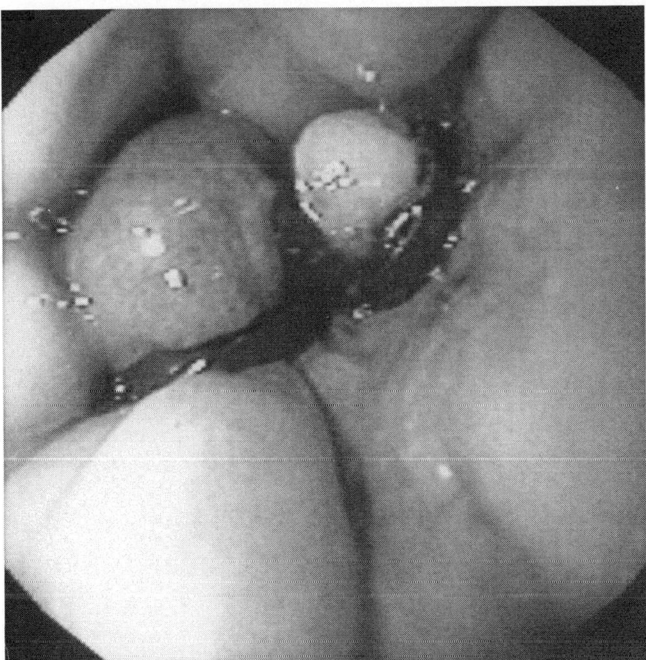

Figure 7.5. Endoscopic view of banded varices. Two bands are seen after placement on a varix.

ischemic necrosis and perforation. In addition, there may be technical difficulties in performing band ligation in children less than 2 years of age because of difficulties in passing the endoscope. In most cases, a combination of conservative management, splanchnic vasoconstriction, and endoscopic sclerotherapy or band ligation will stop acute variceal hemorrhage. In one series, 152 children with varices were managed without additional therapy, whereas 5 of 33 children in a different series required additional therapy [18,176,187].

Emergency Therapy: Mechanical

The Sengstaken–Blakemore tube (SSBT) was designed to stop hemorrhage by mechanically compressing esophageal and gastric varices. The device consists of a rubber tube with at least two balloons. It is passed into the stomach, where the first balloon is inflated and pulled up snug against the gastroesophageal junction (Figure 7.6). Once the tube is secured in place, the second balloon is inflated in the esophagus at a pressure (60–70 mm Hg) that compresses the varices without necrosing the esophagus. A channel in the rubber tube allows gastric contents to be sampled for evidence of bleeding. This therapy is very effective in controlling hemorrhage acutely [192,193]. Unfortunately, it is associated with a significant number of complications and a high incidence of rebleeding when the tube is removed. Most patients find this treatment uncomfortable, and its use in children requires significant sedation [192]. Blockage of the esophagus by the SSBT increases the risk of aspiration pneumonia, which can be a devastating complication in an individual with liver failure. Rebleeding has been reported in 33–60% of patients. Given these problems, the SSBT is reserved for severe uncontrollable hemorrhage and generally serves as a temporizing measure until a more definitive procedure can be performed. Intubation and heavy sedation are typically recommended for children requiring this approach.

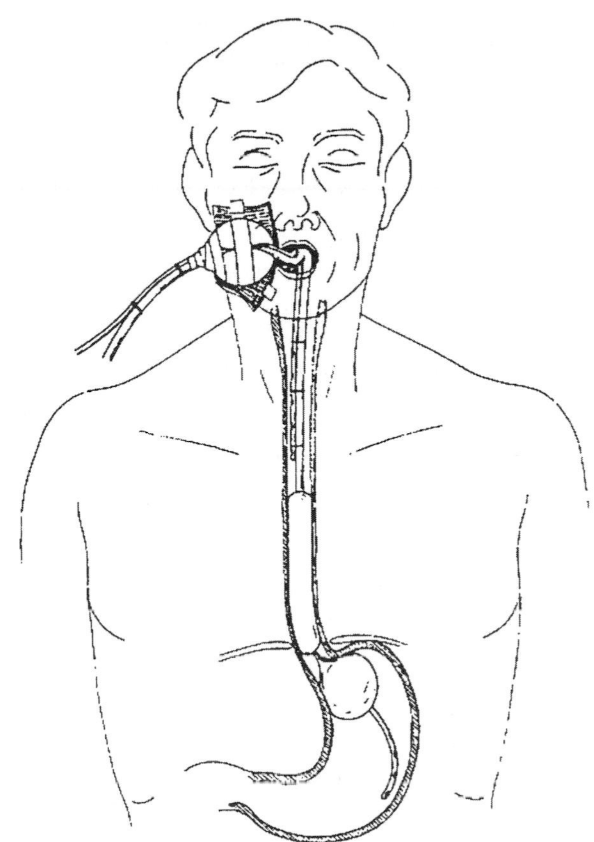

Figure 7.6. Modified Sengstaken–Blakemore tube. A double-balloon catheter is inserted into the esophagus and stomach. The gastric balloon is inflated and pulled up snug against the gastric fundus, compressing the gastric varices. The tube is secured in place by taping it to the side of the patient's face. The esophageal balloon is then inflated to compress the esophageal varices. An additional tube is inserted to aspirate the contents above the esophageal balloon and avoid aspiration into the lungs. Finally, a third tube is inserted through a channel in the Sengstaken–Blakemore tube to allow for sampling of the gastric contents. (Reprinted from Terblanche J, Bornman P, Kirsch R. Sclerotherapy for bleeding esophageal varices. Ann Rev Med 1984;35:83; with permission.)

Emergency Therapy: Surgical and Interventional Radiologic

Surgical therapy is usually a last-resort approach to acute variceal hemorrhage. Many of the patients with recalcitrant hemorrhage will be found to have gastric varices [194]. The reluctance to perform emergency surgery partly stems from its associated high mortality but also from concerns of increased incidence of encephalopathy and greater difficulty of subsequent liver transplantation. The variety of surgical procedures that have been performed for intractable hemorrhage can be divided into transsection, devascularization, and portosystemic shunting. Portosystemic shunting will be discussed in greater detail later in this chapter. The techniques of esophageal

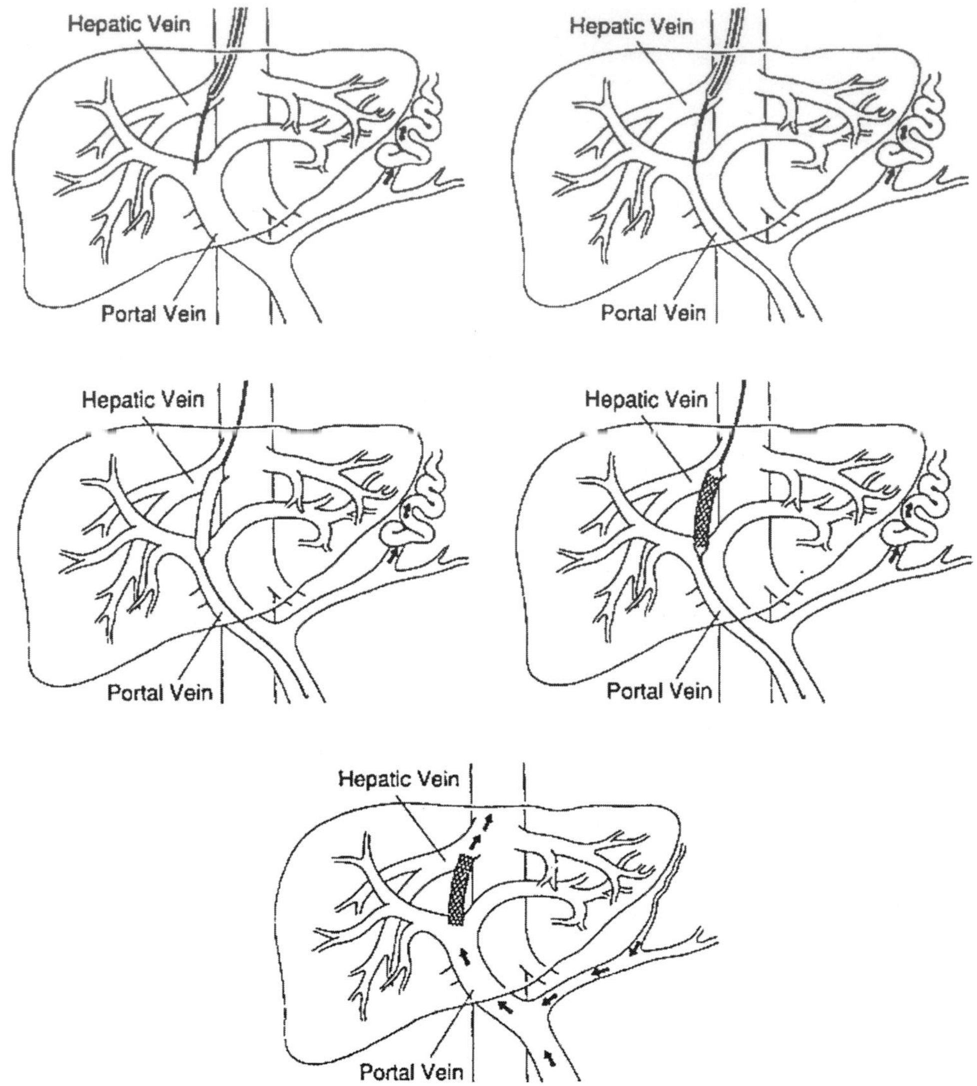

Figure 7.7. Technique of transjugular intrahepatic portosystemic shunting (TIPS). A catheter is inserted into the jugular vein and is advanced into the hepatic vein, where a needle is used to form a tract between the portal vein and the hepatic vein. This tract is expanded with a balloon angioplasty catheter, and a stent is then placed, forming the permanent portosystemic shunt. (Reprinted from Zemel G, Katzen BT, Becker GJ. Percutaneous transjugular portosystemic shunt. JAMA 1991;266:390–3; with permission.)

transection and devascularization are rarely used and work by interrupting blood flow through the esophagus. Obviously, significant morbidity may be associated with esophageal transection. Orthotopic liver transplantation may be an effective means of treating esophageal varix hemorrhage if an acceptable organ can be procured quickly enough [195]. Esophageal varix embolization via a percutaneous transhepatic or transsplenic approach has been advocated by some as another method of controlling acute hemorrhage [196,197]. TIPS placement may be the optimal approach for intractable hemorrhage. TIPS does not require surgery or puncture of an organ that is predisposed to hemorrhage. A catheter is inserted into the jugular vein and is advanced into the hepatic vein, where a needle is used to form a tract between the portal vein and the hepatic vein (Figure 7.7). This tract is expanded with a balloon angioplasty catheter, and a stent is then placed, forming the permanent portosystemic shunt. The experience with this procedure in children as an emergency procedure is somewhat limited [198,199]. Given the high risks associated with either SSBT or emergent surgical approaches, TIPS may be the treatment of choice in this setting, especially when liver transplantation is imminent. Size limitations and local expertise may be the limiting factors in some cases.

In summary, the approach to acute variceal hemorrhage in the pediatric patient is a stepwise progression from least invasive to most invasive (Table 7.3). An adequate trial of conservative medical management is recommended, although evidence of significant bleeding (i.e., requiring transfusion of >10 mL/kg to maintain a hemoglobin >8 g/dL) is an indication for more aggressive treatment. Pharmacotherapy in the acute setting includes vasopressin, somatostatin, or octreotide. Endoscopic sclerotherapy or band ligation is generally effective in the few patients who remain unresponsive and/or should be implemented soon after control of bleeding as part of secondary prophylaxis (see below). TIPS should be reserved for patients with unresponsive hemorrhage and serves as an excellent bridge to transplantation. The ultimate long-term prognosis for the patient and the particular strengths of the team caring for the patient are key factors in the particular approach for a given patient in a given institution.

Secondary Prophylaxis

The decision making in the long-term management of the patient with portal hypertension and a previous episode of variceal hemorrhage is very complex. The first level of consideration involves the natural history of portal hypertension. As discussed earlier, there are significant differences in the natural history of portal hypertension in the setting of minimal and inactive versus active and progressive hepatic disease. As a result, certain individuals may have the possibility of outgrowing their portal hypertension through the development of spontaneous portosystemic shunts, whereas others might be expected to develop end-stage liver disease and ultimately be candidates for liver transplantation. The second issue stems from the great diversity in therapeutic modalities. The physiologic goal of pharmacologic therapy varies from program to program (i.e., change in heart rate, hepatic portal venous gradient pressure, etc.). Sclerotherapy may be administered with a wide variety of sclerosing agents and by two different techniques (e.g., intra- or paravariceal). Endoscopic band ligation offers an important and generally safer alternative to sclerotherapy. Finally, at least six different portosystemic shunting procedures have been described, all with their own advantages and disadvantages. The third level of complexity results from the varying results of randomized and nonrandomized trials in adult patients [149,150]. The trials are difficult enough to compare with one another in adults and cannot necessarily be extrapolated to children, in whom alcoholic liver disease and end-stage hepatitis C are rare. Given these complex issues, the major modalities of long-term secondary prophylactic therapy of portal hypertension –endoscopic therapy, portosystemic shunting, and liver transplantation – will be reviewed. The rationale for β-blockade has been discussed as a possible primary prophylaxis. It may also be used for secondary prophylaxis or as an adjunctive approach to endoscopic therapy. In particular, the rationale, effectiveness, and complications of these treatments will be stressed. Randomized trials will be reviewed and the pediatric experiences highlighted.

Secondary Prophylaxis: Sclerotherapy and Ligation Therapy

Sclerotherapy and band ligation therapy work by physical obliteration of esophageal varices. Hemorrhage may occur during the several weeks required to complete the obliteration, and there is a tendency for the vessels to recanalize. Most importantly, the principal problem of portal hypertension is not addressed, and there is the risk of bleeding from varices elsewhere in the gastrointestinal tract, notably the stomach. Despite these problems, endoscopic therapy has been a mainstay of the treatment of esophageal varices. In addition, there is a significant amount of clinical experience with these approaches in children [1,2,18,176,190,200–205].

Table 7.4: Major Complications of Endoscopic Sclerotherapy in Children

Bleeding before obliteration	39%
Esophageal ulceration	29%
Stricture formation	16%
Recurrent varices	8%

Adapted from Howard et al. [18], with permission.

The effectiveness of sclerotherapy has been studied both for the prevention of initial and subsequent bleeding episodes. Sclerotherapy, which has in general been supplanted by band ligation, is reviewed here for completeness. In addition, in very young children band ligation therapy may not be feasible and sclerotherapy may be required. Intravariceal, paravariceal, and some combination injection protocols have been used. A wide variety of sclerosant agents have been used without a clear-cut difference in their efficacy or adverse effects [206]. Several randomized trials have demonstrated that sclerotherapy, initiated after the first bleeding episode, reduces long-term morbidity and mortality [207,208]. A meta-analysis of seven studies and 748 patients revealed mortality rates of 47% in the sclerotherapy group and 61% in the conservatively managed group [209]. Promising results of sclerotherapy in children have been reported, although no randomized trials have shown survival benefits in pediatrics [18,176,187,210,211].

A variety of complications are associated with sclerotherapy. The complications of a large group of pediatric sclerotherapy patients are displayed in Table 7.4. Retrosternal pain, bacteremia, and fever post treatment are common. Esophageal ulceration may occur after sclerotherapy, and the associated symptoms may be ameliorated with sucralfate (Carafate) slurry therapy [212]. Stricture formation can be managed by dilatation therapy. As previously noted, the primary problem of portal hypertension is not addressed by this therapy, and recurrent varices are not unexpected. Occasional reports of esophageal perforation, aspiration pneumonia, spinal cord paralysis, mediastinitis, septicemia, bronchoesophageal fistulas, and cardiac tamponade exist [213–217]. In pediatric patients, abnormal esophageal manometry may be seen after sclerotherapy [218].

The range of potential complications associated with endoscopic sclerotherapy has prompted the development of alternative endoscopic methods of treatment, including variceal ligation and clipping therapy [190,219]. Endoscopic ligation therapy is a derivative of rubber band ligation of hemorrhoids. The technique involves suctioning of a varix into the end of an endoscope so that a rubber band can be placed around the varix leading to thrombosis (Figures 7.4 and 7.5). Multiple

Table 7.5: Comparison of Pediatric Endoscopic Sclerotherapy and Ligation Therapy

Type of Treatment	*Sclerotherapy*	*Band Ligation*
Number of patients	268	53
References	[18,176,201,202]	[200,203–205]
Number of sessions	5.4	3.3
Percentage eradication	89	78
Percentage rebleeding during therapy	38	23

ligators have circumvented early problems of repeated esophageal intubations [205,220]. Direct comparisons of endoscopic sclerotherapy and variceal ligation in adult patients have yielded results in favor of ligation [191,220–222]. Similar findings have been reported in a randomized trial of sclerotherapy versus ligation therapy in children [2]. The major advantage of variceal ligation is avoidance of needle injection of varices, which appears to reduce the rate of complications. In addition, variceal ligation apparently leads to obliteration in fewer sessions and is associated with a lower rate of early rebleeding. The latter fact may be related to milder esophageal ulcers in ligation compared with sclerotherapy. Review of uncontrolled published pediatric experience and the single randomized pediatric study with these techniques appears to indicate that these principles apply to children (Table 7.5). Endoscopic variceal ligation using a clipping apparatus is an approach that involves application of metal clips as opposed to rubber bands. The technique has the advantage of using a standard endoscope and does not require multiple intubations, because the clips can be passed through the biopsy channel. Published experience with this apparatus in children is limited [219].

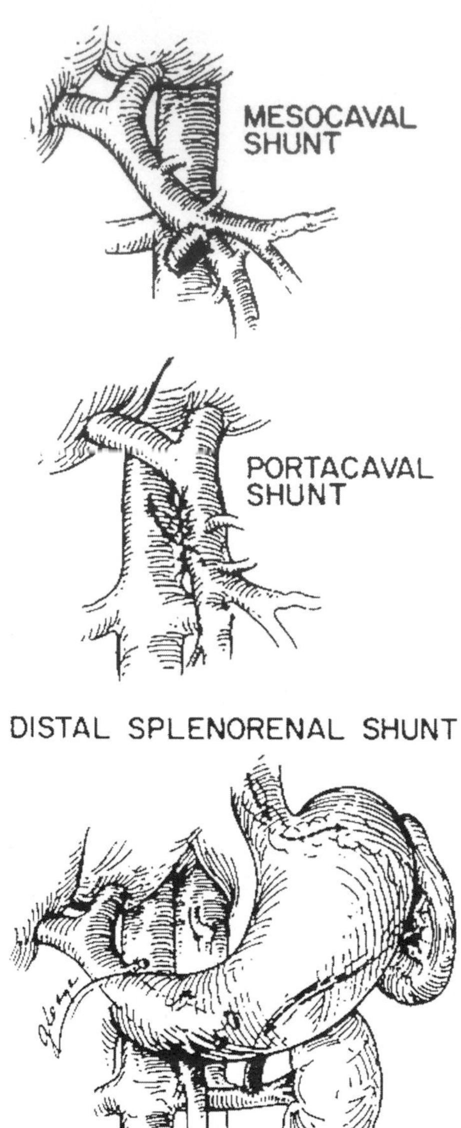

Figure 7.8. Portosystemic shunting procedures. (*Top*) Mesocaval shunt formed with insertion of a graft between the superior mesenteric vein and the inferior vena cava. (*Middle*) Portacaval shunt formed by side-to-side anastomosis of the portal vein and the inferior vena cava. (*Bottom*) Distal splenorenal shunt formed by end-to-side anastomosis of the splenic vein and the left renal vein. (Reprinted from Brems J, Hiatt JR, Klein AS. Effect of a prior portasystemic shunt on subsequent liver transplantation. Ann Surg 1989;209: 51–6; with permission.)

Secondary Prophylaxis: Portosystemic Shunting

A variety of procedures have been used to divert portal blood flow and decrease portal blood pressure (Figure 7.8). The portacaval shunt diverts nearly all the portal blood flow into the subhepatic inferior vena cava. This very effectively decompresses the portal system but also diverts a significant amount of blood from its normal hepatic metabolism, predisposing to the development of hepatic encephalopathy. Decreased hepatic blood flow theoretically also may lead to worsening of underlying liver disease. An intermediate shunt can be made by placing a graft between the mesenteric or portal vein and the vena cava. This decompresses the portal system while allowing a greater amount of portal blood to flow into the liver. The use of grafts unfortunately is associated with increased risk of thrombosis and many times with worsening retrograde flow in the portal vein and greater diversion of portal flow through the shunt. Another approach involves diversion of splenic blood flow into the left renal vein, which can be done nonselectively (central) or semiselectively (distal splenorenal shunt).

A substantial pediatric experience with surgical portosystemic shunting has been accumulated over the past 20 years [223–228]. The results are clearly different in patients with extra- or intrahepatic portal hypertension (Table 7.6). The two sets of data in the extrahepatic disease groups are from a retrospective review of several series and the experience of a single institution. Clearly there is a disparity in the incidence of rebleeding, but mortality is low in both studies. The incidence of hepatic encephalopathy is quite low in the second series and absent in the first. The major morbidity associated with

Table 7.6: Results of Portosystemic Shunting in Children

Type of Portal Hypertension [Ref.]	*Number of Patients*	*Rebleeding (%)*	*Mortality (%)*
Extrahepatic [224]	76	4	0
Extrahepatic [223]	216	45	5
Intrahepatic [223]	76	50	53

portosystemic shunting in extrahepatic portal vein obstruction is shunt thrombosis and the need for second operations. In general, like other surgical procedures, the results of this approach are directly dependent on the skill of the surgeon. The promising results of portosystemic shunting in this group must be tempered by the understanding of the generally good prognosis of children with portal vein thrombosis and the incidence of spontaneous portosystemic shunting.

An alternative shunting procedure for children with extrahepatic portal vein thrombosis is the meso-Rex bypass (Figure 7.9). This procedure involves placement of an autologous venous graft from the mesenteric vasculature to the left intrahepatic portal vein. The procedure was originally devised to treat portal vein thrombosis seen in pediatric liver transplant recipients [115]. It was subsequently applied to treat patients with extrahepatic portal vein thrombosis [116]. One of the major advantages of this approach is the restoration of normal portal blood flow, which eliminates the risk of hepatic encephalopathy and should preserve hepatic function. Recent unpublished studies indicate that children with extrahepatic portal vein thrombosis may have subtle features of encephalopathy, which are ameliorated by the meso-Rex bypass. As such, the criteria for candidacy for this procedure, both from the perspective of clinical indication and surgical feasibility are not clear, and some have advocated that this procedure be considered in all children with portal vein thrombosis and a cavernoma [229]. Standard diagnostic imaging studies may not clearly indicate whether there is patency of the intrahepatic portal vein [117]. Three children in this series of five, who had an apparent absence of the intrahepatic portal vein by angiography, underwent successful placement of a meso-Rex bypass. The potential for hypercoagulable states in these children must be kept in mind, especially in light of the risk for postoperative thrombosis [20,21].

In stark contrast to these excellent results in portal vein thrombosis are the generally poor results of portosystemic shunting in children with decompensated liver disease secondary to intrahepatic diseases. The incidence of recurrent bleeding and death (both from recurrent hemorrhage and progressive liver dysfunction) in this group approaches 50%. Hepatic encephalopathy is a serious and not infrequent complication of portosystemic shunting in decompensated liver disease. The prevalence of this complication in pediatric patients with intrahepatic disease is not well documented. Finally, portosystemic shunting has not been shown to improve long-term

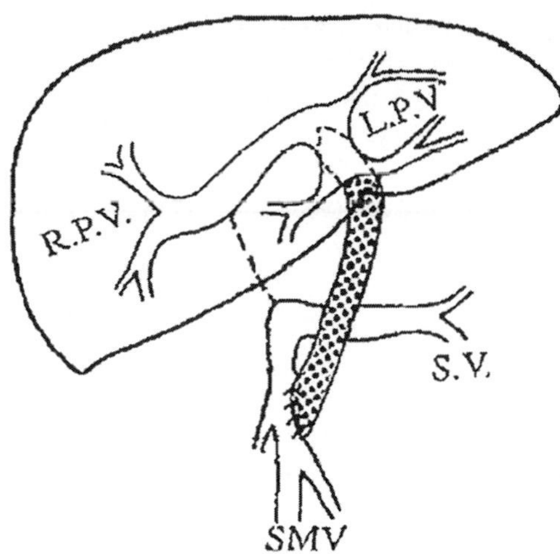

Figure 7.9. Meso-Rex bypass. A graft (stippled) is interposed between the superior mesenteric vein (SMV) and the intrahepatic left portal vein (LPV). SV, splenic vein; RPV, right portal vein. (Reprinted from de Ville de Goyet et al. [116], with permission.)

survival in patients with intrahepatic disease [230]. Ultimately, most children with decompensated progressive liver disease and medically resistant esophageal varices will need to undergo orthotopic liver transplantation. In a group of 85 children who underwent transplantation for advanced liver disease and had a clear history of esophageal varix bleeding, long-term survival was far better than with any other available mode of therapy [195]. Prior portosystemic shunting may make orthotopic liver transplantation technically more difficult, requiring a significantly greater number of transfusions [154]. In addition, prior splenectomy may increase the risk of sepsis; therefore, appropriate immunizations against encapsulated organisms should be considered for children who may require splenectomy. Overall, surgical portosystemic shunting is an excellent approach to the long-term management of children with intractable variceal hemorrhage in the setting of compensated cirrhosis. In addition, significant gastric variceal hemorrhage in children may be an indication to consider surgical shunting, since there is little if any data on the safety and efficacy of endoscopic injection of *N*-butyl-cyanoacrylate in children [231,232]. TIPS may be an alternative shunting procedure for children with refractory variceal hemorrhage and serves as an effective bridge to transplantation [233,234]. The procedure is typically feasible, with published success in children as small as 14 kg, although special procedural modifications must be undertaken for small children [235]. Long-term problems with shunt occlusion limit the overall application of this efficacious therapy, although newer data with coated stents may improve the long-term patency rates for TIPS [236].

SUMMARY OF THE CLINICAL APPROACH TO PORTAL HYPERTENSION

Management of the child with clinical stigmata of portal hypertension who has not experienced variceal hemorrhage is complex and unclear at the present time [237]. Surveillance endoscopy is predicated on the availability of an efficacious primary prophylactic therapy. β-Blocker therapy is accepted as such in adults, and endoscopic ligation therapy is also gaining acceptance. Pilot data in children appear to indicate that this approach is feasible, but sufficient data do not exist to make a firm recommendation in favor of primary prophylaxis. Therefore, surveillance endoscopy and primary prophylaxis do not generally appear to be indicated in children with portal hypertension who have not had variceal hemorrhage. Certain special medical and social circumstances in which an initial bleeding episode is particularly risky would justify application of adult approaches, including annual to biannual surveillance endoscopy and prophylactic β-blocker therapy. The question of primary prophylaxis is one of the most important areas for future investigative trials in pediatric hepatology.

Management of acute variceal hemorrhage is more straightforward. Initial interventions should include stabilization of the patient, placement of a nasogastric tube, and institution of intravenous antibiotic therapy. Diagnostic or therapeutic endoscopy should be scheduled as soon as it is safe and feasible. In the interim, pharmacologic treatment with either vasopressin or octreotide is indicated and may facilitate endoscopic therapy. Intractable and severe hemorrhage should be treated by TIPS.

The long-term approach to prevention of recurrent variceal hemorrhage in children must be adapted for the type of liver disease, the needs of a specific patient, and the particular skills of the institution. The approach to extrahepatic portal vein obstruction is evolving. In general, the unpredictability of the timing of the sentinel bleeding episode and the low incidence of fatality associated with that episode make prophylactic therapy inadvisable. Enthusiasm for utilization of the meso-Rex bypass is increasing because of the physiologic nature of the procedure. It may be possible that this procedure should be considered for all children with portal vein thrombosis and a cavernoma [238]. Certainly, in the patient with persistent problems with variceal hemorrhage, bypass is the procedure of choice. Endoscopic approaches and distal splenorenal shunting may need to be considered in patients in whom bypass is not feasible. The long-term management of portal hypertension in the child with biliary atresia is more complex. In patients with incomplete bile drainage, liver transplantation appears to be inevitable and should be the major focus of therapeutic intervention. Temporizing measures for these children may include band ligation therapy or TIPS. Patients who have a more successful response to portoenterostomy, as manifest by improvement in serum total bilirubin levels, have a more favorable long-term outlook. Variceal hemorrhage may be followed by relatively long-term survival with medical intervention. The potential risks and benefits of β-blocker therapy are unknown and should be the subject of a multicenter trial. Endoscopic therapy in this group is an excellent initial approach. Recurrent hemorrhage might be amenable to portosystemic shunting as opposed to transplantation.

The approach to patients with more slowly progressive intrahepatic diseases is more difficult to generalize. The approach to patients with slowly progressive disease and compensated cirrhosis should be similar to that for the child with biliary atresia and a functioning hepatoportoenterostomy. The child with more rapidly progressive disease and/or decompensated cirrhosis will likely need to be considered for liver transplantation, with either endoscopic treatment or TIPS as a temporizing measure.

The study of portal hypertension has become very sophisticated in adults but is in its infancy in children. Well-conceived multicenter trials are required to determine whether the principles that have been developed in adults can be extrapolated to children. Particular care will be required in choosing a homogenous and representative patient population with a significant risk of complications of portal hypertension.

REFERENCES

1. Goncalves ME, Cardoso SR, Maksoud JG. Prophylactic sclerotherapy in children with esophageal varices: long-term results of a controlled prospective randomized trial. J Pediatr Surg 2000; 35:401–5.
2. Zargar SA, Javid G, Khan BA, et al. Endoscopic ligation compared with sclerotherapy for bleeding esophageal varices in children with extrahepatic portal venous obstruction. Hepatology 2002;36:666–72.
3. Shneider B. Approaches to the management of pediatric portal hypertension: Results of an informal survey. In: Groszmann R, Tygat N, Bosch J, eds. Portal hypertension in the 21st century. Boston: Kluwer Academic Publishers, 2004.
4. Ohllson E, Rutherford R, Boitnott J. Changes in portal circulation after biliary obstruction in dogs. Am J Surg 1970;120:16–22.
5. Chojkier M, Groszmann RJ. Measurement of portal-systemic shunting in the rat by using gamma-labeled microspheres. Am J Physiol 1981;240:G371–5.
6. Okudaira M, Kume H, Ohku M. Experimental portal fibrosis induced by chronic feeding of aflatoxin-B1. In: Sarin SK, ed. Animal models of portal hypertension. New Delhi: Kunj Publishing, 1988:135–41.
7. Sarin SK, Groszmann R, Mosca PG, et al. Propranalol ameliorates the development of portal-systemic shunting in a chronic murine schistosomiasis model of portal hypertension. J Clin Invest 1991;87:1032–6.
8. Vorobioff J, Bredfeldt JE, Groszmann RJ. Increased blood flow through the portal system in cirrhotic rats. Gastroenterology 1984;87:1120–6.
9. Iwakiri Y, Cadelina G, Sessa WC, Groszmann RJ. Mice with targeted deletion of eNOS develop hyperdynamic circulation associated with portal hypertension. Am J Physiol Gastrointest Liver Physiol 2002;283:G1074–81.
10. Biecker E, Neef M, Sagesser H, et al. Nitric oxide synthase 1 is partly compensating for nitric oxide synthase 3 deficiency in nitric oxide synthase 3 knock-out mice and is elevated in murine and human cirrhosis. Liver Int 2004;24:345–53.
11. McIndoe A. Vascular lesions of portal cirrhosis. Arch Pathol 1928;5:23–32.
12. Kowalski HJ, Abelmann WH. The cardiac output at rest in Laennec's cirrhosis. J Clin Invest 1953;32:1025–33.
13. Janssen HL, Garcia-Pagan JC, Elias E, et al. Budd–Chiari syndrome: a review by an expert panel. J Hepatol 2003;38:364–71.

14. Menon KV, Shah V, Kamath PS. The Budd–Chiari syndrome. N Engl J Med 2004;350:578–85.
15. Bayraktar Y, Balkanci F, Bayraktar M, Calguneri M. Budd–Chiari syndrome: a common complication of Behcet's disease. Am J Gastroenterol 1997;92:858–62.
16. Gentil-Kocher S, Bernard O, Brunelle F, et al. Budd–Chiari syndrome in children: report of 22 cases. J Pediatr 1988;113 (1 pt 1):30–8.
17. Safouh M, Shehata AH. Hepatic vein occlusion disease of Egyptian children. J Pediatr 1965;67:415–22.
18. Howard ER, Stringer MD, Mowat AP. Assessment of injection sclerotherapy in the management of 152 children with oesophageal varices. Br J Surg 1988;75:404–8.
19. Alvarez F, Bernard O, Brunelle F, et al. Portal obstruction in children. I. Clinical investigation and hemorrhage risk. J Pediatr 1983;103:696–702.
20. Ahuja V, Marwaha N, Chawla Y, Dilawari JB. Coagulation abnormalities in idiopathic portal venous thrombosis. J Gastroenterol Hepatol 1999;14:1210–11.
21. Denninger MH, Chait Y, Casadevall N, et al. Cause of portal or hepatic venous thrombosis in adults: the role of multiple concurrent factors. Hepatology 2000;31:587–91.
22. Gauthier-Villars M, Franchi S, Gauthier F, et al. Cholestasis in children with portal vein obstruction. J Pediatr 2005;146: 568–73.
23. Sutton JP, Yarborough DY, Richards JT. Isolated splenic vein occlusion. Review of literature and report of an additional case. Arch Surg 1970;100:623–6.
24. Colman JC, Britton RS, Orrego H, et al. Relation between osmotically induced hepatocyte enlargement and portal hypertension. Am J Physiol 1983;245:G382–7.
25. Orrego H, Blendis LM, Crossley IR, et al. Correlation of intrahepatic pressure with collagen in the Disse space and hepatomegaly in humans and in the rat. Gastroenterology 1981;80: 546–56.
26. Miga D, Sokol RJ, Mackenzie T, et al. Survival after first esophageal variceal hemorrhage in patients with biliary atresia. J Pediatr 2001;139:291–6.
27. D'Amico G, De Franchis R. Upper digestive bleeding in cirrhosis. Post-therapeutic outcome and prognostic indicators. Hepatology 2003;38:599–612.
28. Durie PR, Kent G, Phillips MJ, Ackerley CA. Characteristic multiorgan pathology of cystic fibrosis in a long-living cystic fibrosis transmembrane regulator knockout murine model. Am J Pathol 2004;164:1481–93.
29. Moser M, Matthiesen S, Kirfel J, et al. A mouse model for cystic biliary dysgenesis in autosomal recessive polycystic kidney disease (ARPKD). Hepatology 2005;41:1113–21.
30. McCright B, Lozier J, Gridley T. A mouse model of Alagille syndrome: Notch2 as a genetic modifier of Jag1 haploinsufficiency. Development 2002;129:1075–82.
31. Smit JJ, Schinkel AH, Oude Elferink RP, et al. Homozygous disruption of the murine mdr2 P-glycoprotein gene leads to a complete absence of phospholipid from bile and to liver disease. Cell 1993;75:451–62.
32. Gupta TK, Toruner M, Chung MK, Groszmann RJ. Endothelial dysfunction and decreased production of nitric oxide in the intrahepatic microcirculation of cirrhotic rats. Hepatology 1998;28:926–31.
33. Dudenhoefer AA, Loureiro-Silva MR, Cadelina GW, et al. Bioactivation of nitroglycerin and vasomotor response to nitric oxide are impaired in cirrhotic rat livers. Hepatology 2002;36: 381–5.
34. Zafra C, Abraldes JG, Turnes J, et al. Simvastatin enhances hepatic nitric oxide production and decreases the hepatic vascular tone in patients with cirrhosis. Gastroenterology 2004;126: 749–55.
35. Moore K, Wendon J, Frazer M, et al. Plasma endothelin immunoreactivity in liver disease and the hepatorenal syndrome. N Engl J Med 1992;327:774–8.
36. Martinet JP, Legault L, Cernacek P, et al. Changes in plasma endothelin-1 and Big endothelin-1 induced by transjugular intrahepatic portosystemic shunts in patients with cirrhosis and refractory ascites. J Hepatol 1996;25:700–6.
37. Rockey D. The cellular pathogenesis of portal hypertension: stellate cell contractility, endothelin, and nitric oxide. Hepatology 1997;25:2–5.
38. Kaneda K, Ekataksin W, Sogawa M, et al. Endothelin-1-induced vasoconstriction causes a significant increase in portal pressure of rat liver: localized constrictive effect on the distal segment of preterminal portal venules as revealed by light and electron microscopy and serial reconstruction. Hepatology 1998;27: 735–47.
39. Kojima H, Yamao J, Tsujimoto T, et al. Mixed endothelin receptor antagonist, SB209670, decreases portal pressure in biliary cirrhotic rats in vivo by reducing portal venous system resistance. J Hepatol 2000;32:43–50.
40. Donovan A, Reynolds T, Mikkelson W. Systemic-portal arteriovenous fistulas: pathologic and hemodynamic observations in two patients. Surgery 1969;66:474–82.
41. Griner P, Elbadani A, Packman C. Veno-occlusive disease of the liver after chemotherapy of acute leukemia. Ann Intern Med 1976;85:578–82.
42. Maksoud JG, Mies S, da Costa Gayotto LC. Hepatoportal sclerosis in childhood. Am J Surg 1986;151:484–8.
43. Sperl W, Stuppner H, Gassner I, et al. Reversible hepatic veno-occlusive disease in an infant after consumption of pyrrolizidine-containing herbal tea. Eur J Pediatr 1995;154:112–6.
44. Corbacioglu S, Greil J, Peters C, et al. Defibrotide in the treatment of children with veno-occlusive disease (VOD): a retrospective multicentre study demonstrates therapeutic efficacy upon early intervention. Bone Marrow Transplant 2004;33: 189–95.
45. Okuda K, Kono K, Ohnishi K, et al. Clinical study of eighty-six cases of idiopathic portal hypertension and comparison with cirrhosis with splenomegaly. Gastroenterology 1984;86:600–10.
46. Bioulac-Sage P, Le Bail B, Bernard PH, Balabaud C. Hepatoportal sclerosis. Semin Liver Dis 1995;15:329–39.
47. Schwerdtfeger E, Abdel-Rahim I, Kardoff R. Ultrasonic invesigation of periportal fibrosis in children with *Schistoma mansoni* infection: reversibility of morbidity twenty-three years after treatment with praziquantel. Am J Trop Med Hyg 1992; 46:409–15.
48. Vorobioff J, Bredfeldt JE, Groszmann RJ. Hyperdynamic circulation in portal-hypertensive rat model: a primary factor for maintenance of chronic portal hypertension. Am J Physiol 1983;244:G52–7.
49. Benoit JN, Barrowman JA, Harper SL, et al. Role of humoral factors in the intestinal hyperemia associated with chronic portal hypertension. Am J Physiol 1984;247(5 pt 1):G486–93.
50. Sikuler E, Groszmann RJ. Hemodynamic studies in a parabiotic model of portal hypertension. Experientia 1985;41:1323–4.

51. Silva G, Navasa M, Bosch J, et al. Hemodynamic effects of glucagon in portal hypertension. Hepatology 1990;11:668–73.
52. Kvietys PR, McLendon JM, Granger DN. Postprandial intestinal hyperemia: role of bile salts in the ileum. Am J Physiol 1981;241:G469–77.
53. Genecin P, Polio J, Colombato LA, et al. Bile acids do not mediate the hyperdynamic circulation in portal hypertensive rats. Am J Physiol 1990;259(1 pt 1):G21–5.
54. Thomas SH, Joh T, Benoit JN. Role of bile acids in splanchnic hemodynamic response to chronic portal hypertension. Dig Dis Sci 1991;36:1243–8.
55. Sitzmann JV, Bulkley GB, Mitchell MC, Campbell K. Role of prostacyclin in the splanchnic hyperemia contributing to portal hypertension. Ann Surg 1989;209:322–7.
56. Lee SS, Chilton EL, Pak JM. Adenosine receptor blockade reduces splanchnic hyperemia in cirrhotic rats. Hepatology 1992;15:1107–11.
57. Moller S, Bendtsen F, Schifter S, Henriksen JH. Relation of calcitonin gene-related peptide to systemic vasodilatation and central hypovolaemia in cirrhosis. Scand J Gastroenterol 1996;31:928–33.
58. Fernandez M, Bonkovsky HL. Increased heme oxygenase-1 gene expression in liver cells and splanchnic organs from portal hypertensive rats. Hepatology 1999;29:1672–9.
59. Batkai S, Jarai Z, Wagner JA, et al. Endocannabinoids acting at vascular CB1 receptors mediate the vasodilated state in advanced liver cirrhosis. Nat Med 2001;7:827–32.
60. Ros J, Claria J, To-Figueras J, et al. Endogenous cannabinoids: a new system involved in the homeostasis of arterial pressure in experimental cirrhosis in the rat. Gastroenterology 2002; 122:85–93.
61. Pizcueta MP, Pique JM, Bosch J, et al. Effects of inhibiting nitric oxide biosynthesis on the systemic and splanchnic circulation of rats with portal hypertension. Br J Pharmacol 1992;105: 184–90.
62. Sieber CC, Groszmann RJ. In vitro hyporeactivity to methoxamine in portal hypertensive rats: reversal by nitric oxide blockade. Am J Physiol 1992;262(6 pt 1):G996–1001.
63. Tsai MH, Iwakiri Y, Cadelina G, et al. Mesenteric vasoconstriction triggers nitric oxide overproduction in the superior mesenteric artery of portal hypertensive rats. Gastroenterology 2003;125:1452–61.
64. Lopez-Talavera JC, Cadelina G, Olchowski J, et al. Thalidomide inhibits tumor necrosis factor alpha, decreases nitric oxide synthesis, and ameliorates the hyperdynamic circulatory syndrome in portal-hypertensive rats. Hepatology 1996;23:1616–21.
65. Genecin P, Polio J, Groszmann RJ. Na restriction blunts expansion of plasma volume and ameliorates hyperdynamic circulation in portal hypertension. Am J Physiol 1990;259(3 pt 1): G498–503.
66. Willett IR, Esler M, Jennings G, Dudley FJ. Sympathetic tone modulates portal venous pressure in alcoholic cirrhosis. Lancet 1986;2:939–43.
67. Mastai R, Rocheleau B, Huet PM. Serotonin blockade in conscious, unrestrained cirrhotic dogs with portal hypertension. Hepatology 1989;9:265–8.
68. Pinkerton JA, Holcomb GW Jr, Foster JH. Portal hypertension in childhood. Ann Surg 1972;175:870–86.
69. Spence RA, Johnston GW, Odling-Smee GW, Rodgers HW. Bleeding oesophageal varices with long term follow up. Arch Dis Child 1984;59:336–40.
70. Garcia-Pagan JC, Feu F, Castells A, et al. Circadian variations of portal pressure and variceal hemorrhage in patients with cirrhosis. Hepatology 1994;19:595–601.
71. Chen L, Groszmann RJ. Blood in the gastric lumen increases splanchnic blood flow and portal pressure in portal-hypertensive rats. Gastroenterology 1996;111:1103–10.
72. Lee SS, Hadengue A, Moreau R, et al. Postprandial hemodynamic responses in patients with cirrhosis. Hepatology 1988; 8:647–51.
73. Garcia-Pagan JC, Santos C, Barbera JA, et al. Physical exercise increases portal pressure in patients with cirrhosis and portal hypertension. Gastroenterology 1996;111:1300–6.
74. Webb LJ, Sherlock S. The aetiology, presentation and natural history of extra-hepatic portal venous obstruction. Q J Med 1979;48:627–39.
75. Shah SH, Hayes PC, Allan PL, et al. Measurement of spleen size and its relation to hypersplenism and portal hemodynamics in portal hypertension due to hepatic cirrhosis. Am J Gastroenterol 1996;91:2580–3.
76. Westaby S, Wilkinson SP, Warren R, Williams R. Spleen size and portal hypertension in cirrhosis. Digestion 1978;17:63–8.
77. Yachha SK, Dhiman RK, Gupta R, Ghoshal UC. Endosonographic evaluation of the rectum in children with extrahepatic portal venous obstruction. J Pediatr Gastroenterol Nutr 1996;23:438–41.
78. Weinberg GD, Matalon TA, Brunner MC, et al. Bleeding stomal varices: treatment with a transjugular intrahepatic portosystemic shunt in two pediatric patients. J Vasc Interv Radiol 1995;6:233–6.
79. Fallon MB, Abrams GA, Luo B, et al. The role of endothelial nitric oxide synthase in the pathogenesis of a rat model of hepatopulmonary syndrome. Gastroenterology 1997;113: 606–14.
80. Zhang M, Luo B, Chen SJ, et al. Endothelin-1 stimulation of endothelial nitric oxide synthase in the pathogenesis of hepatopulmonary syndrome. Am J Physiol 1999;277(5 pt 1):G944–52.
81. Shah V, Kamath PS. Nitric oxide in liver transplantation: pathobiology and clinical implications. Liver Transpl 2003;9: 1–11.
82. Hoeper MM, Krowka MJ, Strassburg CP. Portopulmonary hypertension and hepatopulmonary syndrome. Lancet 2004; 363:1461–8.
83. Fallon MB. Mechanisms of pulmonary vascular complications of liver disease: hepatopulmonary syndrome. J Clin Gastroenterol 2005;39(4 suppl 2):S138–42.
84. Kinane TB, Westra SJ. Case records of the Massachusetts General Hospital. Weekly clinicopathological exercises. Case 31–2004. A four-year-old boy with hypoxemia. N Engl J Med 2004;351: 1667–75.
85. Abrams GA, Jaffe CC, Hoffer PB, et al. Diagnostic utility of contrast echocardiography and lung perfusion scan in patients with hepatopulmonary syndrome. Gastroenterology 1995;109: 1283–8.
86. Santamaria F, Sarnelli P, Celentano L, et al. Noninvasive investigation of hepatopulmonary syndrome in children and adolescents with chronic cholestasis. Pediatr Pulmonol 2002;33: 374–9.
87. Yonemura T, Yoshibayashi M, Uemoto S, et al. Intrapulmonary shunting in biliary atresia before and after living-related liver transplantation. Br J Surg 1999;86:1139–43.

88. Barbe T, Losay J, Grimon G, et al. Pulmonary arteriovenous shunting in children with liver disease. J Pediatr 1995;126:571–9.
89. Caldwell SH, Jeffers LJ, Narula OS, et al. Ancient remedies revisited: does Allium sativum (garlic) palliate the hepatopulmonary syndrome? J Clin Gastroenterol 1992;15:248–50.
90. Abrams GA, Nanda NC, Dubovsky EV, et al. Use of macroaggregated albumin lung perfusion scan to diagnose hepatopulmonary syndrome: a new approach. Gastroenterology 1998;114:305–10.
91. Lange PA, Stoller JK. The hepatopulmonary syndrome. Ann Intern Med 1995;122:521–9.
92. Krowka MJ, Cortese DA. Hepatopulmonary syndrome. Current concepts in diagnostic and therapeutic considerations. Chest 1994;105:1528–37.
93. Lebrec D, Capron JP, Dhumeaux D, Benhamou JP. Pulmonary hypertension complicating portal hypertension. Am Rev Respir Dis 1979;120:849–56.
94. Budhiraja R, Hassoun PM. Portopulmonary hypertension: a tale of two circulations. Chest 2003;123:562–76.
95. Krowka MJ, Mandell MS, Ramsay MA, et al. Hepatopulmonary syndrome and portopulmonary hypertension: a report of the multicenter liver transplant database. Liver Transpl 2004;10:174–82.
96. Schuijtvlot ET, Bax NM, Houwen RH, Hruda J. Unexpected lethal pulmonary hypertension in a 5-year-old girl successfully treated for biliary atresia. J Pediatr Surg 1995;30:589–90.
97. Soh H, Hasegawa T, Sasaki T, et al. Pulmonary hypertension associated with postoperative biliary atresia: report of two cases. J Pediatr Surg 1999;34:1779–81.
98. Hoeper MM, Halank M, Marx C, et al. Bosentan therapy for portopulmonary hypertension. Eur Respir J 2005;25:502–8.
99. Minder S, Fischler M, Muellhaupt B, et al. Intravenous iloprost bridging to orthotopic liver transplantation in portopulmonary hypertension. Eur Respir J 2004;24:703–7.
100. Halank M, Kolditz M, Miehlke S, et al. Combination therapy for portopulmonary hypertension with intravenous iloprost and oral bosentan. Wien Med Wochenschr 2005;155:376–80.
101. Makisalo H, Koivusalo A, Vakkuri A, Hockerstedt K. Sildenafil for portopulmonary hypertension in a patient undergoing liver transplantation. Liver Transpl 2004;10:945–50.
102. Chua R, Keogh A, Miyashita M. Novel use of sildenafil in the treatment of portopulmonary hypertension. J Heart Lung Transplant 2005;24:498–500.
103. Losay J, Piot D, Bougaran J, et al. Early liver transplantation is crucial in children with liver disease and pulmonary artery hypertension. J Hepatol 1998;28:337–42.
104. Laving A, Khanna A, Rubin L, et al. Successful liver transplantation in a child with severe portopulmonary hypertension treated with epoprostenol. J Pediatr Gastroenterol Nutr 2005;41:466–8.
105. Pirenne J, Verleden G, Nevens F, et al. Combined liver and (heart-)lung transplantation in liver transplant candidates with refractory portopulmonary hypertension. Transplantation 2002;73:140–2.
106. Albillos A, Colombato LA, Groszmann RJ. Vasodilatation and sodium retention in prehepatic portal hypertension. Gastroenterology 1992;102:931–5.
107. Thalheimer U, Triantos CK, Samonakis DN, et al. Infection, coagulation, and variceal bleeding in cirrhosis. Gut 2005;54:556–63.
108. Alessandria C, Ozdogan O, Guevara M, et al. MELD score and clinical type predict prognosis in hepatorenal syndrome: relevance to liver transplantation. Hepatology 2005;41:1282–9.
109. Wong F, Pantea L, Sniderman K. Midodrine, octreotide, albumin, and TIPS in selected patients with cirrhosis and type 1 hepatorenal syndrome. Hepatology 2004;40:55–64.
110. Ellis D, Avner ED. Renal failure and dialysis therapy in children with hepatic failure in the perioperative period of orthotopic liver transplantation. Clin Nephrol 1986;25:295–303.
111. Wood RP, Ellis D, Starzl TE. The reversal of the hepatorenal syndrome in four pediatric patients following successful orthotopic liver transplantation. Ann Surg 1987;205:415–19.
112. Mitra SK, Kumar V, Datta DV, et al. Extrahepatic portal hypertension: a review of 70 cases. J Pediatr Surg 1978;13:51–7.
113. Sarin SK, Agarwal SR. Extrahepatic portal vein obstruction. Semin Liver Dis 2002;22:43–58.
114. Chiu B, Superina R. Extrahepatic portal vein thrombosis is associated with an increased incidence of cholelithiasis. J Pediatr Surg 2004;39:1059–61.
115. de Ville de Goyet J, Gibbs P, Clapuyt P, et al. Original extrahilar approach for hepatic portal revascularization and relief of extrahepatic portal hypertension related to later portal vein thrombosis after pediatric liver transplantation. Long term results. Transplantation 1996;62:71–5.
116. de Ville de Goyet J, Alberti D, Clapuyt P, et al. Direct bypassing of extrahepatic portal venous obstruction in children: a new technique for combined hepatic portal revascularization and treatment of extrahepatic portal hypertension. J Pediatr Surg 1998;33:597–601.
117. Bambini DA, Superina R, Almond PS, et al. Experience with the Rex shunt (mesenterico-left portal bypass) in children with extrahepatic portal hypertension. J Pediatr Surg 2000;35:13–8; discussion 8–9.
118. Utterson EC, Shepherd RW, Sokol RJ, et al. Biliary atresia: clinical profiles, risk factors, and outcomes of 755 patients listed for liver transplantation. J Pediatr 2005;147:180–5.
119. Kasai M, Okamoto A, Ohi R, et al. Changes of portal vein pressure and intrahepatic blood vessels after surgery for biliary atresia. J Pediatr Surg 1981;16:152–9.
120. Miyata M, Satani M, Ueda T, Okamoto E. Long-term results of hepatic portoenterostomy for biliary atresia: special reference to postoperative portal hypertension. Surgery 1974;76:234–7.
121. Ohi R, Mochizuki I, Komatsu K, Kasai M. Portal hypertension after successful hepatic portoenterostomy in biliary atresia. J Pediatr Surg 1986;21:271–4.
122. Lilly JR, Stellin G. Variceal hemorrhage in biliary atresia. J Pediatr Surg 1984;19:476–9.
123. Uflacker R, Pariente DM. Angiographic findings in biliary atresia. Cardiovasc Intervent Radiol 2004;27:486–90.
124. van Heurn LW, Saing H, Tam PK. Portoenterostomy for biliary atresia: long-term survival and prognosis after esophageal variceal bleeding. J Pediatr Surg 2004;39:6–9.
125. Sasaki T, Hasegawa T, Shimizu Y, et al. Portal hypertensive gastropathy after surgery for biliary atresia. Surg Today 2005;35:385–8.
126. Smith S, Wiener ES, Starzl TE, Rowe MI. Stoma-related variceal bleeding: an under-recognized complication of biliary atresia. J Pediatr Surg 1988;23:243–5.
127. Patriquin H, Lafortune M, Weber A, et al. Surgical portosystemic shunts in children: assessment with duplex Doppler US. Work in progress. Radiology 1987;165:25–8.

128. Iwao T, Oho K, Sakai T, et al. Noninvasive hemodynamic measurements of superior mesenteric artery in the prediction of portal pressure response to propranolol. J Hepatol 1998;28: 847–55.
129. Annet L, Materne R, Danse E, et al. Hepatic flow parameters measured with MR imaging and Doppler US: correlations with degree of cirrhosis and portal hypertension. Radiology 2003;229:409–14.
130. Taourel P, Blanc P, Dauzat M, et al. Doppler study of mesenteric, hepatic, and portal circulation in alcoholic cirrhosis: relationship between quantitative Doppler measurements and the severity of portal hypertension and hepatic failure. Hepatology 1998;28:932–6.
131. De Giacomo C, Tomasi G, Gatti C, et al. Ultrasonographic prediction of the presence and severity of esophageal varices in children. J Pediatr Gastroenterol Nutr 1989;9:431–5.
132. Patriquin H, Tessier G, Grignon A, Boisvert J. Lesser omental thickness in normal children: baseline for detection of portal hypertension. AJR Am J Roentgenol 1985;145:693–6.
133. Sokal EM, Van Hoorebeeck N, Van Obbergh L, et al. Upper gastro-intestinal tract bleeding in cirrhotic children candidates for liver transplantation. Eur J Pediatr 1992;151:326–8.
134. Zoli M, Merkel C, Magalotti D, et al. Evaluation of a new endoscopic index to predict first bleeding from the upper gastrointestinal tract in patients with cirrhosis. Hepatology 1996;24:1047–52.
135. Bosch J, Bordas JM, Rigau J, et al. Noninvasive measurement of the pressure of esophageal varices using an endoscopic gauge: comparison with measurements by variceal puncture in patients undergoing endoscopic sclerotherapy. Hepatology 1986;6:667–72.
136. Brensing KA, Neubrand M, Textor J, et al. Endoscopic manometry of esophageal varices: evaluation of a balloon technique compared with direct portal pressure measurement. J Hepatol 1998;29:94–102.
137. Ueno K, Hashizume M, Ohta M, et al. Noninvasive variceal pressure measurement may be useful for predicting effect of sclerotherapy for esophageal varices. Dig Dis Sci 1996;41:191–6.
138. El Atti EA, Nevens F, Bogaerts K, et al. Variceal pressure is a strong predictor of variceal haemorrhage in patients with cirrhosis as well as in patients with non-cirrhotic portal hypertension. Gut 1999;45:618–21.
139. Eisen GM, Eliakim R, Zaman A, et al. The accuracy of PillCam ESO capsule endoscopy versus conventional upper endoscopy for the diagnosis of esophageal varices: a prospective three-center pilot study. Endoscopy 2006;38:31–5.
140. Lapalus MG, Dumortier J, Fumex F, et al. Esophageal capsule endoscopy versus Esophagogastroduodenoscopy for evaluating portal hypertension: a prospective comparative study of performance and tolerance. Endoscopy 2006;38:36–41.
141. Bismuth H, Franco D, Alagille D. Portal diversion for portal hypertension in children. The first ninety patients. Ann Surg 1980;192:18–24.
142. Baert AL, Fevery J, Marchal G, et al. Early diagnosis of Budd–Chiari syndrome by computed tomography and ultrasonography: report of five cases. Gastroenterology 1983;84:587–95.
143. Ozsoylu S, Kocak N, Yuce A. Propranolol therapy for portal hypertension in children. J Pediatr 1985;106:317–21.
144. Groszmann RJ, Bosch J, Grace ND, et al. Hemodynamic events in a prospective randomized trial of propranolol versus placebo in the prevention of a first variceal hemorrhage. Gastroenterology 1990;99:1401–7.
145. Vorobioff J, Groszmann RJ, Picabea E, et al. Prognostic value of hepatic venous pressure gradient measurements in alcoholic cirrhosis: a 10-year prospective study. Gastroenterology 1996;111:701–9.
146. Groszmann RJ. The hepatic venous pressure gradient: has the time arrived for its application in clinical practice? Hepatology 1996;24:739–41.
147. Feu F, Garcia-Pagan JC, Bosch J, et al. Relation between portal pressure response to pharmacotherapy and risk of recurrent variceal haemorrhage in patients with cirrhosis. Lancet 1995;346:1056–9.
148. Piscaglia F, Gaiani S, Donati G, et al. Doppler evaluation of the effects of pharmacological treatment of portal hypertension. Ultrasound Med Biol 1999;25:923–32.
149. D'Amico G, Pagliaro L, Bosch J. The treatment of portal hypertension: a meta-analytic review. Hepatology 1995;22:332–54.
150. D'Amico G, Pagliaro L, Bosch J. Pharmacological treatment of portal hypertension: an evidence-based approach. Semin Liver Dis 1999;19:475–505.
151. Imperiale TF, Chalasani N. A meta-analysis of endoscopic variceal ligation for primary prophylaxis of esophageal variceal bleeding. Hepatology 2001;33:802–7.
152. Banares R, Albillos A, Rincon D, et al. Endoscopic treatment versus endoscopic plus pharmacologic treatment for acute variceal bleeding: a meta-analysis. Hepatology 2002;35:609–15.
153. Groszmann RJ, Garcia-Tsao G, Bosch J, et al. Beta-blockers to prevent gastroesophageal varices in patients with cirrhosis. N Engl J Med 2005;353:2254–61.
154. Gotoh Y, Iwakiri R, Sakata Y, et al. Evaluation of endoscopic variceal ligation in prophylactic therapy for bleeding of oesophageal varices: a prospective, controlled trial compared with endoscopic injection sclerotherapy. J Gastroenterol Hepatol 1999;14:241–4.
155. Sarin SK, Lamba GS, Kumar M, et al. Comparison of endoscopic ligation and propranolol for the primary prevention of variceal bleeding. N Engl J Med 1999;340:988–93.
156. Schepke M, Kleber G, Nurnberg D, et al. Ligation versus propranolol for the primary prophylaxis of variceal bleeding in cirrhosis. Hepatology 2004;40:65–72.
157. de Kolster CC, Rapa de Higuera M, Carvajal A, et al. [Propranolol in children and adolescents with portal hypertension: its dosage and the clinical, cardiovascular and biochemical effects]. G E N 1992;46:199–207.
158. Shashidhar H, Langhans N, Grand RJ. Propranolol in prevention of portal hypertensive hemorrhage in children: a pilot study. J Pediatr Gastroenterol Nutr 1999;29:12–17.
159. Ozsoylu S, Kocak N, Demir H, et al. Propranolol for primary and secondary prophylaxis of variceal bleeding in children with cirrhosis. Turk J Pediatr 2000;42:31–3.
160. Lebrec D, Poynard T, Bernuau J, et al. A randomized controlled study of propranolol for prevention of recurrent gastrointestinal bleeding in patients with cirrhosis: a final report. Hepatology 1984;4:355–8.
161. Pascal JP, Cales P. Propranolol in the prevention of first upper gastrointestinal tract hemorrhage in patients with cirrhosis of the liver and esophageal varices. N Engl J Med 1987;317:856–61.
162. Hayes PC, Davis JM, Lewis JA, Bouchier IA. Meta-analysis of value of propranolol in prevention of variceal haemorrhage. Lancet 1990;336:153–6.

163. Garcia-Pagan JC, Feu F, Bosch J, Rodes J. Propranolol compared with propranolol plus isosorbide-5-mononitrate for portal hypertension in cirrhosis. A randomized controlled study. Ann Intern Med 1991;114:869–73.
164. Merkel C, Marin R, Enzo E, et al. Randomized trial of nadolol alone or with isosorbide mononitrate for primary prophylaxis of variceal bleeding in cirrhosis. Gruppo-Triveneto per L'ipertensione portale (GTIP). Lancet 1996;348:1677–81.
165. Forrest EH, Bouchier IA, Hayes PC. Acute haemodynamic changes after oral carvedilol, a vasodilating beta-blocker, in patients with cirrhosis. J Hepatol 1996;25:909–15.
166. Banares R, Moitinho E, Matilla A, et al. Randomized comparison of long-term carvedilol and propranolol administration in the treatment of portal hypertension in cirrhosis. Hepatology 2002;36:1367–73.
167. Lui HF, Stanley AJ, Forrest EH, et al. Primary prophylaxis of variceal hemorrhage: a randomized controlled trial comparing band ligation, propranolol, and isosorbide mononitrate. Gastroenterology 2002;123:735–44.
168. Chalasani N, Boyer TD. Primary prophylaxis against variceal bleeding: beta-blockers, endoscopic ligation, or both? Am J Gastroenterol 2005;100:805–7.
169. Elizalde JI, Moitinho E, Garcia-Pagan JC, et al. Effects of increasing blood hemoglobin levels on systemic hemodynamics of acutely anemic cirrhotic patients. J Hepatol 1998;29: 789–95.
170. Romero-Castro R, Jimenez-Saenz M, Pellicer-Bautista F, et al. Recombinant-activated factor VII as hemostatic therapy in eight cases of severe hemorrhage from esophageal varices. Clin Gastroenterol Hepatol 2004;2:78–84.
171. Hou MC, Lin HC, Liu TT, et al. Antibiotic prophylaxis after endoscopic therapy prevents rebleeding in acute variceal hemorrhage: a randomized trial. Hepatology 2004;39:746–53.
172. Rolando N, Gimson A, Philpott-Howard J, et al. Infectious sequelae after endoscopic sclerotherapy of oesophageal varices: role of antibiotic prophylaxis. J Hepatol 1993;18:290–4.
173. Terblanche J, Burroughs AK, Hobbs KE. Controversies in the management of bleeding esophageal varices (1). N Engl J Med 1989;320:1393–8.
174. Moitinho E, Escorsell A, Bandi JC, et al. Prognostic value of early measurements of portal pressure in acute variceal bleeding. Gastroenterology 1999;117:626–31.
175. McKiernan PJ. Treatment of variceal bleeding. Gastrointest Endosc Clin N Am 2001;11:789–812, viii.
176. Hill ID, Bowie MD. Endoscopic sclerotherapy for control of bleeding varices in children. Am J Gastroenterol 1991;86: 472–6.
177. Mowat AP. Liver disorders in childhood. 2nd ed. London: Buttersworth, 1987.
178. Bosch J, Groszmann RJ, Garcia-Pagan JC, et al. Association of transdermal nitroglycerin to vasopressin infusion in the treatment of variceal hemorrhage: a placebo-controlled clinical trial. Hepatology 1989;10:962–8.
179. Walker S, Stiehl A, Raedsch R, Kommerell B. Terlipressin in bleeding esophageal varices: a placebo-controlled, double-blind study. Hepatology 1986;6:112–5.
180. Kravetz D, Bosch J, Teres J, et al. Comparison of intravenous somatostatin and vasopressin infusions in treatment of acute variceal hemorrhage. Hepatology 1984;4:442–6.
181. Burroughs AK, McCormick PA, Hughes MD, et al. Randomized, double-blind, placebo-controlled trial of somatostatin for variceal bleeding. Emergency control and prevention of early variceal rebleeding. Gastroenterology 1990;99: 1388–95.
182. Eroglu Y, Emerick KM, Whitingon PF, Alonso EM. Octreotide therapy for control of acute gastrointestinal bleeding in children. J Pediatr Gastroenterol Nutr 2004;38:41–7.
183. Heikenen JB, Pohl JF, Werlin SL, Bucuvalas JC. Octreotide in pediatric patients. J Pediatr Gastroenterol Nutr 2002;35: 600–9.
184. Zellos A, Schwarz KB. Efficacy of octreotide in children with chronic gastrointestinal bleeding. J Pediatr Gastroenterol Nutr 2000;30:442–6.
185. Siafakas C, Fox VL, Nurko S. Use of octreotide for the treatment of severe gastrointestinal bleeding in children. J Pediatr Gastroenterol Nutr 1998;26:356–9.
186. Mottet C, Sieber CC, Nauer A, et al. Hemodynamic effects of the somatostatin analog lanreotide in humans: placebo-controlled, cross-over dose-ranging echo-Doppler study. Hepatology 1998;27:920–5.
187. Thapa BR, Mehta S. Endoscopic sclerotherapy of esophageal varices in infants and children. J Pediatr Gastroenterol Nutr 1990;10:430–4.
188. Ho H, Zuckerman MJ, Wassem C. A prospective controlled study of the risk of bacteremia in emergency sclerotherapy of esophageal varices. Gastroenterology 1991;101:1642–8.
189. Van Stiegmann G. Endoscopic ligation of esophageal varices. Am J Surg 1988;156(3 pt 2).9B–12B.
190. Hall RJ, Lilly JR, Stiegmann GV. Endoscopic esophageal varix ligation: technique and preliminary results in children. J Pediatr Surg 1988;23:1222–3.
191. Stiegmann GV, Goff JS, Michaletz-Onody PA, et al. Endoscopic sclerotherapy as compared with endoscopic ligation for bleeding esophageal varices. N Engl J Med 1992;326:1527–32.
192. Panes J, Teres J, Bosch J, Rodes J. Efficacy of balloon tamponade in treatment of bleeding gastric and esophageal varices. Results in 151 consecutive episodes. Dig Dis Sci 1988;33: 454–9.
193. Novis BH, Duys P, Barbezat GO, et al. Fibreoptic endoscopy and the use of the Sengstaken tube in acute gastrointestinal haemorrhage in patients with portal hypertension and varices. Gut 1976;17:258–63.
194. Millar AJ, Brown RA, Hill ID, et al. The fundal pile: bleeding gastric varices. J Pediatr Surg 1991;26:707 9.
195. Iwatsuki S, Starzl TE, Todo S, et al. Liver transplantation in the treatment of bleeding esophageal varices. Surgery 1988;104: 697–705.
196. Rasinska G, Wermenski K, Rajszys P. Percutaneous transsplenic embolization of esophageal varices in a 5-year-old child. Acta Radiol 1987;28:299–301.
197. L'Hermine C, Chastanet P, Delemazure O, et al. Percutaneous transhepatic embolization of gastroesophageal varices: results in 400 patients. AJR Am J Roentgenol 1989;152:755–60.
198. Johnson SP, Leyendecker JR, Joseph FB, et al. Transjugular portosystemic shunts in pediatric patients awaiting liver transplantation. Transplantation 1996;62:1178–81.
199. Cao S, Monge H, Semba C, et al. Emergency transjugular intrahepatic portosystemic shunt (TIPS) in an infant: a case report. J Pediatr Surg 1997;32:125–7.
200. Price MR, Sartorelli KH, Karrer FM, et al. Management of esophageal varices in children by endoscopic variceal ligation. J Pediatr Surg 1996;31:1056–9.

201. Maksoud JG, Goncalves ME, Porta G, et al. The endoscopic and surgical management of portal hypertension in children: analysis of 123 cases. J Pediatr Surg 1991;26:178–81.
202. Yachha SK, Sharma BC, Kumar M, Khanduri A. Endoscopic sclerotherapy for esophageal varices in children with extrahepatic portal venous obstruction: a follow-up study. J Pediatr Gastroenterol Nutr 1997;24:49–52.
203. Fox VL, Carr-Locke DL, Connors PJ, Leichtner AM. Endoscopic ligation of esophageal varices in children. J Pediatr Gastroenterol Nutr 1995;20:202–8.
204. Sasaki T, Hasegawa T, Nakajima K, et al. Endoscopic variceal ligation in the management of gastroesophageal varices in postoperative biliary atresia. J Pediatr Surg 1998;33:1628–32.
205. McKiernan PJ, Beath SV, Davison SM. A prospective study of endoscopic esophageal variceal ligation using a multiband ligator. J Pediatr Gastroenterol Nutr 2002;34:207–11.
206. Sarin SK, Kumar A. Sclerosants for variceal sclerotherapy: a critical appraisal. Am J Gastroenterol 1990;85:641–9.
207. Sclerotherapy after first variceal hemorrhage in cirrhosis. A randomized multicenter trial. The Copenhagen Esophageal Varices Sclerotherapy Project. N Engl J Med 1984;311:1594–600.
208. Westaby D, Macdougall BR, Williams R. Improved survival following injection sclerotherapy for esophageal varices: final analysis of a controlled trial. Hepatology 1985;5:827–30.
209. Infante-Rivard C, Esnaola S, Villeneuve JP. Role of endoscopic variceal sclerotherapy in the long-term management of variceal bleeding: a meta-analysis. Gastroenterology 1989;96:1087–92.
210. Vane DW, Boles ET Jr, Clatworthy HW Jr. Esophageal sclerotherapy: an effective modality in children. J Pediatr Surg 1985;20:703–7.
211. Hassall E, Berquist WE, Ament ME, et al. Sclerotherapy for extrahepatic portal hypertension in childhood. J Pediatr 1989; 115:69–74.
212. Polson RJ, Westaby D, Gimson AE, et al. Sucralfate for the prevention of early rebleeding following injection sclerotherapy for esophageal varices. Hepatology 1989;10:279–82.
213. Seidman E, Weber AM, Morin CL, et al. Spinal cord paralysis following sclerotherapy for esophageal varices. Hepatology 1984;4:950–4.
214. Helpap B, Bollweg L. Morphological changes in the terminal oesophagus with varices, following sclerosis of the wall. Endoscopy 1981;13:229–33.
215. Gerhartz HH, Sauerbruch T, Weinzierl M, Ruckdeschel G. Nosocomial septicemia in patients undergoing sclerotherapy for variceal hemorrhage. Endoscopy 1984;16:129–30.
216. Carr-Locke DL, Sidky K. Broncho-oesophageal fistula: a late complication of endoscopic variceal sclerotherapy. Gut 1982;23: 1005–7.
217. Tabibian N, Schwartz JT, Smith JL, Graham DY. Cardiac tamponade as a result of endoscopic sclerotherapy: report of a case. Surgery 1987;102:546–7.
218. Greenholz SK, Hall RJ, Sondheimer JM, et al. Manometric and pH consequences of esophageal endosclerosis in children. J Pediatr Surg 1988;23(1 pt 2):38–41.
219. Ohnuma N, Takahashi H, Tanabe M, et al. Endoscopic variceal ligation using a clipping apparatus in children with portal hypertension. Endoscopy 1997;29:86–90.
220. Saeed ZA. The Saeed Six-Shooter: a prospective study of a new endoscopic multiple rubber-band ligator for the treatment of varices. Endoscopy 1996;28:559–64.
221. Laine L, Cook D. Endoscopic ligation compared with sclerotherapy for treatment of esophageal variceal bleeding. A meta-analysis. Ann Intern Med 1995;123:280–7.
222. Sarin SK, Govil A, Jain AK, et al. Prospective randomized trial of endoscopic sclerotherapy versus variceal band ligation for esophageal varices: influence on gastropathy, gastric varices and variceal recurrence. J Hepatol 1997;26:826–32.
223. Fonkalsrud EW. Surgical management of portal hypertension in childhood: long-term results. Arch Surg 1980;115:1042–5.
224. Alvarez F, Bernard O, Brunelle F, et al. Portal obstruction in children. II. Results of surgical portosystemic shunts. J Pediatr 1983;103:703–7.
225. Mitra SK, Rao KL, Narasimhan KL, et al. Side-to-side lienorenal shunt without splenectomy in noncirrhotic portal hypertension in children. J Pediatr Surg 1993;28:398–401; discussion 402.
226. Prasad AS, Gupta S, Kohli V, et al. Proximal splenorenal shunts for extrahepatic portal venous obstruction in children. Ann Surg 1994;219:193–6.
227. Evans S, Stovroff M, Heiss K, Ricketts R. Selective distal splenorenal shunts for intractable variceal bleeding in pediatric portal hypertension. J Pediatr Surg 1995;30:1115–18.
228. Shun A, Delaney DP, Martin HC, et al. Portosystemic shunting for paediatric portal hypertension. J Pediatr Surg 1997;32:489–93.
229. Dasgupta R, Roberts E, Superina RA, Kim PC. Effectiveness of Rex shunt in the treatment of portal hypertension. J Pediatr Surg 2006;41:108–12; discussion 112.
230. Terblanche J, Burroughs AK, Hobbs KE. Controversies in the management of bleeding esophageal varices (2). N Engl J Med 1989;320:1469–75.
231. Huang YH, Yeh HZ, Chen GH, et al. Endoscopic treatment of bleeding gastric varices by N-butyl-2-cyanoacrylate (Histoacryl) injection: long-term efficacy and safety. Gastrointest Endosc 2000;52:160–7.
232. Greenwald BD, Caldwell SH, Hespenheide EE, et al. N-2-butyl-cyanoacrylate for bleeding gastric varices: a United States pilot study and cost analysis. Am J Gastroenterol 2003;98:1982–8.
233. Heyman MB, LaBerge JM, Somberg KA, et al. Transjugular intrahepatic portosystemic shunts (TIPS) in children. J Pediatr 1997;131:914–19.
234. Hackworth CA, Leef JA, Rosenblum JD, et al. Transjugular intrahepatic portosystemic shunt creation in children: initial clinical experience. Radiology 1998;206:109–14.
235. Heyman MB, LaBerge JM. Role of transjugular intrahepatic portosystemic shunt in the treatment of portal hypertension in pediatric patients. J Pediatr Gastroenterol Nutr 1999;29:240–9.
236. Vignali C, Bargellini I, Grosso M, et al. TIPS with expanded polytetrafluoroethylene-covered stent: results of an Italian multicenter study. AJR Am J Roentgenol 2005;185:472–80.
237. Shneider B, Emre S, Groszmann R, et al. Portal hypertension in children: expert pediatric opinion on the report of the Baveno IV consensus workshop on the methodology of diagnosis and therapy in portal hypertension. Pediatr Transplant 2006;10:893–907.
238. Superina R, Shneider B, Emre S, et al. Surgical guidelines for the management of extra-hepatic portal vein obstruction. Pediatr Transplant 2006;10:908–13.

8

Laboratory Assessment of Liver Function and Injury in Children

Vicky Lee Ng, M.D., F.R.C.P.C.

The liver is a multifunctional organ that is involved in a number of critical excretory, synthetic, and metabolic functions. Biochemical assessment of these functions in children is undertaken by utilizing a number of tests performed in clinical laboratories. Many of the most commonly used serum chemistry tests, such as aminotransferase and alkaline phosphatase levels, are often referred to as liver function tests (LFTs), which is a misnomer as they do not actually measure or indicate liver function. Rather, these tests should be referred to as liver enzyme tests, with the term *LFTs* reserved to refer to measures of hepatocyte synthetic function such as serum albumin and prothrombin time (PT). Any single biochemical test provides limited information, which must be placed in the context of the entire clinical and historic picture. Currently available laboratory evaluative tests of the liver are used to (1) screen for and document liver injury; (2) identify the type or pattern of liver disorder and the site of injury; (3) prognosticate and follow up children with chronic liver disease; and (4) serially monitor the course of liver disease, evaluate the response to treatment, and adjust a treatment regimen when appropriate.

The widespread availability and frequent use of serum chemistry tests in children have resulted in an increase in the number of both normal and abnormal liver chemistry test values that must be evaluated by physicians. However, some limitations of liver biochemical tests must be recognized [1]. First, screening laboratory tests may lack sensitivity; that is, if a liver chemistry test is normal, it does not ensure that the patient is free of liver disease [2]. Children with chronic liver disease may have normal serum aminotransferase levels. Second, these tests are not specific for liver dysfunction. For example, aminotransferase levels may be elevated in patients with a nonhepatic disorder such as a musculoskeletal condition or cardiomyopathy. Finally, liver chemistry tests rarely provide a specific diagnosis; rather, they suggest a general category of liver disorder. For example, these tests do not distinguish viral hepatitis from autoimmune hepatitis or delineate intrahepatic from extrahepatic etiologies of cholestasis.

The sensitivity and specificity of screening laboratory tests in the detection of liver disease may be increased when used as a battery [3,4]. When more than one test run within a battery is serially abnormal, then the probability of liver disease is higher. When all test results within the battery are normal, the probability of missing occult liver disease is lower. Ultimately, the clinical significance of any liver chemistry test abnormality in a child must be interpreted in the context of the clinical setting.

Tests to evaluate liver disease can be divided into five categories (Table 8.1):

1. *Tests that detect liver injury* are based on measurement of the serum level of endogenous substances released from damaged hepatocytes, including alanine aminotransferase (ALT), aspartate aminotransferase (AST), and lactate dehydrogenase (LDH).
2. *Tests that detect impaired bile flow or cholestasis* are based on measurement of the serum level of endogenous substances released from damaged tissue, such as alkaline phosphatase (AP), γ-glutamyltransferase (GGT), and 5′-nucleotidase (5′-NT).
3. *Tests of liver synthetic capacity* include the serum levels of albumin, the PT, and partial thromboplastin time (PTT), and individual clotting factors (such as factor VII and factor V). Triglyceride, cholesterol, lipid, and lipoprotein synthesis also occur in the liver.
4. *Tests of hepatic excretory function* are based on measurement of serum concentrations of substances metabolized and transported by the liver, including endogenously produced compounds such as bilirubin and serum bile acids, as well as the determination of the rate of clearance of exogenously administered dyes or drugs, such as indocyanine green, caffeine, lidocaine and para-aminobenzoic acid (PABA).
5. *Tests of hepatic metabolic function* reflect the liver's central role in metabolic and regulatory pathways, including the detoxification and clearance of endogenous metabolites such as ammonia. Multiple metabolic abnormalities due to specific inherited deficiencies of enzymes that reside almost exclusively in the liver, such as the urea cycle defects, can have a primary or secondary effect on the liver.

Table 8.1: Tests of Liver Function and Injury

Tests based on substances *released* from damaged tissue
Endogenous substances released by damaged hepatocytes
Alanine aminotransferase (ALT)
Aspartate aminotransferase (AST)
Lactic dehydrogenase (LDH)
Endogenous substances reflecting impaired bile flow (cholestasis)
γ-Glutamyltransferase (GGT)
Alkaline phosphatase (AP)
5′-nucleotidase (5′-NT)
Leucine aminopeptidase (LAP)
Tests based on substances *synthesized* by the liver
Albumin
Coagulation factors
Serum lipids and lipoproteins
Triglycerides
Cholesterol
Tests based on substances *metabolized and transported* by the liver
Endogenous substances
Serum bilirubin
Serum bile acids
Urobilinogen
Exogenous substances
Lidocaine
Caffeine
Aminopyrine
Para-aminobenzoic acid
Tests based on substances *detoxified and cleared* by the liver
Endogenous substances (ammonia)
Miscellaneous specific serum tests
Serum immunoglobulins
Autoantibodies
Plasma and urine amino acids

In this chapter, the tests most frequently used in assessing liver function and injury in children are discussed.

TESTS BASED ON SUBSTANCES RELEASED FROM INJURED LIVER

Aminotransferases

The serum aminotransferases (formerly known as transaminases), aspartate aminotransferase (AST) and alanine aminotransferase (ALT), are the liver chemistry tests most commonly used to assess injury to hepatocytes and to identify patients with liver disease [1,3].

Aspartate aminotransferase is an enzyme that catalyzes the reversible transfer of the amino group from aspartic acid to the α-keto group of α-ketoglutaric acid to form oxaloacetic acid plus glutamic acid (hence, AST's former name – serum glutamic oxaloacetate transaminase [SGOT]). Similarly, ALT is the enzyme that catalyzes the reversible α-amino group transfer from the amino acid alanine to the α-keto group of α-ketoglutaric acid to yield pyruvic acid plus glutamic acid (hence, ALT's former name – serum glutamic pyruvic transaminase [SGPT]).

Both serum aminotransferases are normally present in serum in low concentrations in the healthy population [5]. A recent multivariate analysis of 6835 first-time acceptable blood-donor candidates showed a strong correlation of serum ALT levels with body mass index (BMI) and laboratory indicators of abnormal lipid or carbohydrate metabolism. A review of 3927 subsequent donors receiving no medications and with normal BMI and normal serum cholesterol, triglyceride, and glucose levels led to the recommendation to decrease the upper range of normal serum ALT level [6]. However, the gain of a few additional asymptomatic patients with conditions without reported efficacious therapy (such as fatty liver or chronic hepatitis C) was felt to be strongly outweighed by the cost of a great increase in health care dollars required to evaluate these otherwise healthy people [7].

Aspartate transaminase is present as both cytosolic and mitochondrial isoenzymes and is found in high concentrations in many tissues, including liver, heart muscle, skeletal muscle, kidney, brain, pancreas, lung, leukocytes, and red blood cells. ALT is a cytosolic enzyme that is present in highest concentrations in the liver. Elevation of enzyme activities in serum results from damage to or destruction of tissues rich in the aminotransferases or to a change in cell membrane permeability allowing AST and/or ALT to leak from damaged cells into serum. However, because of the wide tissue distribution of AST, the hepatic origin of an isolated serum AST level elevation should be confirmed by obtaining a serum ALT level. Differentiation of tissue sources by isoenzyme analysis is not routinely clinically available and typically not needed. Ratios of the mitochondrial and cytosolic isoenzymes have been proposed as a diagnostic tool but are rarely used in clinical practice.

A disproportionately isolated increase in serum AST level should prompt a search for evidence of hemolysis (including difficult venipuncture attempts), acute rhabdomyolysis (such as seen during a systemic viral illness), a myopathic process [8,9], myocardial disease (including undiagnosed cardiomyopathy), and recent vigorous physical activity (such as long-distance running or weight lifting). Results of specific biochemical tests (such as serum haptoglobin, lactate dehydrogenase, creatine phosphokinase, or aldolase levels) may verify hemolysis or myopathy/muscle disease as the underlying etiology of a disproportionately elevated AST level. Spuriously high serum levels of AST can be caused by a macro-AST formed by the enzyme complexing with an immunoglobulin, usually immunoglobulin G [10,11], leading to decreased clearance, similar to the confusion that may occur in the case of macroamylasemia in the assessment of pancreatic diseases.

The value of an increased AST:ALT ratio in adults as a noninvasive indicator of cirrhosis in patients with chronic hepatitis C and to recognize undisclosed alcoholic liver disease is often debated. In patients with cirrhosis, impairment of functional hepatic blood flow results in a decrease in hepatic sinusoidal uptake of AST [12]. Alcoholic patients, often deficient in pyridoxal 5′-phosphate, the coenzyme needed for ALT synthesis, have increased serum AST:ALT ratios, reflecting altered synthesis ratios in the liver [13]. Pediatric experience with AST:ALT ratios is very limited; in a retrospective review of 73 infants with chronic liver disease, a single center demonstrated an increase in AST:ALT ratio over a 13-month period of follow-up in those with a worse clinical outcome [14]. An AST:ALT ratio of more than 4 in the appropriate clinical setting is highly suggestive of fulminant Wilson's disease [15].

An elevated serum ALT level is more specific for the presence of liver disease because ALT is present in relatively low concentrations in tissues other than the liver, but it does not provide a specific etiology. Increased serum aminotransferase levels may be the only manifestation of celiac disease. In one study, serum ALT was elevated in 4.3% of children with gluten-sensitive enteropathy at presentation [16]. In another pediatric study of 425 consecutive children evaluated at a tertiary pediatric institution for the investigation of isolated elevated aminotransferase levels without typical symptoms or signs, an underlying genetic disease was found in 12% of cases, including diagnoses of Wilson's disease, α_1-antitrypsin deficiency, Alagille syndrome, hereditary fructose intolerance, glycogen storage disease, and ornithine transcarbamylase deficiency [17]. Nonalcoholic fatty liver disease is becoming increasingly common as a pediatric diagnosis [18] and may present with an isolated increase in serum ALT level [19]. The differential diagnosis of elevated aminotransferase level in a transplanted allograft mandates consideration of the time from transplantation surgery and prompt attention to the possibilities of rejection (hyperacute, acute cellular, or chronic), de novo autoimmune hepatitis, infection (hepatitis or intercurrent systemic), and biliary or vascular complications [20]. After blunt abdominal trauma, parallel elevations in aminotransferase levels may provide an early clue to liver injury [21]. In chronic liver diseases or in biliary obstruction (both intrahepatic and extrahepatic), AST and ALT elevations are usually less marked. A differential rise or fall in AST and ALT levels may, however, provide useful information. In acute hepatitis, the rise in ALT may be greater than the rise in AST. In fulminant echovirus infection, alcohol-induced liver injury, and various metabolic diseases, more predominant rises in AST have been reported.

Aminotransferases are one of the important means of following the clinical activity of acute hepatitis from viral or autoimmune etiology in children and evaluating the response to immune suppression therapy in chronic hepatitis or acute cellular rejection after liver transplantation. Serial measurements of serum aminotransferase levels are also used in detecting drug-induced hepatotoxicity and monitoring for progression or regression of liver injury [22]. Further understanding of the susceptibility to drug-induced liver injury requires further understanding of relevant mechanisms, the genetic and environmental factors influencing such mechanisms, and advances in toxicogenomics and proteomics [23].

Some of the highest AST and ALT levels (elevations >15 times normal) are seen following an acute episode of hypoxia or hypoperfusion (shock liver) and during the course of acute viral hepatitis, medication- or toxin-induced hepatotoxicity, and autoimmune hepatitis. Ischemic and hypoxic acute liver damage is more likely in patients with concomitant clinical conditions such as sepsis or low-flow hemodynamic states. However, there is a poor correlation between serum elevations of aminotransferases and the extent of liver cell necrosis seen on liver biopsy. Accordingly, serum AST and ALT elevations alone have limited prognostic value. Nevertheless, a rapid decline in aminotransferase levels, reflecting massive destruction and loss of viable hepatocytes, in association with increasing bilirubin levels and a coagulopathy portends a poor prognosis in the setting of the child with acute liver failure.

Lactate Dehydrogenase

Lactate dehydrogenase is a cytoplasmic enzyme present in many tissues. There are five isoenzymes of LDH present in the serum, which can be separated using electrophoretic techniques. The slowest migrating band predominates in the liver. The differential diagnoses of elevated serum LDH levels include skeletal or cardiac muscle injury, hemolysis, stroke, and renal infarction as well as acute and chronic liver disease [24]. Because of limited specificity, serum LDH levels rarely add information to that obtained from the aminotransferases alone. Uncommon clinical situations in which serum LDH levels may be diagnostically useful include the massive and transient elevation characteristic of ischemic hepatitis and the sustained elevation accompanying elevated serum AP levels suggesting malignant infiltration of the liver.

ENZYMES THAT DETECT IMPAIRED BILE FLOW OR CHOLESTASIS

Alkaline Phosphatase

Alkaline phosphatase is a group of isoenzymes originating in different tissues in the body that hydrolyze organic phosphate esters at alkaline pH, generating inorganic phosphate and an organic radical. The APs are true isoenzymes because they all catalyze this reaction, with differences in physicochemical properties.

Alkaline phosphatases are found in several tissues, including the canalicular membrane of hepatocytes, bone osteoblasts, the brush border of enterocytes in the small intestine, proximal convoluted tubules of the kidney, the placenta, and white blood cells. Although the bone AP isoenzyme appears to be involved with calcification, the precise function of the liver AP isoenzyme is not known, although some postulate that it may participate in transport processes [25].

Alkaline phosphatase activity is normally demonstrable in serum, with the most likely sources being the liver and bone. The serum level of AP varies considerably with age. Normal growing children and rapidly growing adolescents, in particular, have elevations of serum AP of bone origin. Therefore, an isolated increase in AP does not indicate hepatic or biliary disease if other liver biochemical tests are normal. Mean serum AP activity is higher in males 15–50 years of age; levels in females greater than age 60 years equal or exceed those of age-matched males. The reasons for these differences are not known. In children, serum AP activity is considerably increased in both sexes and correlates well with the rate of bone growth that causes influx of enzyme from osteoid tissues. Serum AP in healthy adolescent males may reach mean levels three times greater than those in healthy adults without implying the presence of underlying hepatobiliary disease [26,27].

When an elevation of serum AP is detected, it must be interpreted in the clinical setting. Initial management may involve repeating the test or confirming the hepatic origin with another liver chemistry test, such as the GGT or 5′-NT (discussed in the next section). The mechanism by which hepatobiliary disease leads to an elevated serum AP level is the result of increased de novo synthesis of AP (induced and mediated by the action of bile acids) in the liver and leakage into the systemic circulation occurring because of disruption of organelles and solubilization of phosphates bound to plasma membranes [28].

Biliary obstruction results in levels greater than four times normal in over 75% of patients. However, up to 20% of adults without extrahepatic obstruction and with viral hepatitis will have AP values more than four times normal [1]. AP levels up to three times normal are relatively nonspecific and occur in a variety of different liver diseases. The extent of the abnormal elevation does not differentiate or discriminate intrahepatic from extrahepatic causes nor do values differ significantly among various extrahepatic obstructive disorders, such as choledochal cyst, bile duct stenosis, and sclerosing cholangitis. Similarly, values do not discriminate among various intrahepatic causes, such as primary biliary cirrhosis, drug-induced hepatitis, and liver transplant rejection [29]. Markedly increased AP levels are seen predominantly with infiltrative liver disorders (such as primary or metastatic tumor) or biliary obstruction. Conversely, serum AP levels may be normal despite extensive hepatic metastasis or despite documented large duct obstruction.

The differential diagnoses of increased serum AP levels in the absence of liver disease include pregnancy, familial inheritance, chronic renal failure, blood group type B or O, and transient hyperphosphatemia of infancy (THI). THI is an apparently benign condition characterized by a marked transient increase in serum AP lasting several weeks in the absence of any clinical, radiologic, or biochemical evidence of bone or liver pathology [30,31]. The rise in AP is quite dramatic, often exceeding ten times the upper limit for the laboratory, with return to normal levels within 8–12 weeks. Awareness of this condition will curtail unnecessary extensive investigations for hepatobiliary disease. During pregnancy, serum AP levels may double because of increased activity from the placental isoenzyme. Adults with malignant tumors without apparent liver involvement have been found to have an enzyme that is indistinguishable from the placental form, the so-called Regan isoenzyme [25]. Increased measured activity of the intestinal isoenzyme may be caused by hepatic disease, such as alcoholic cirrhosis in adults [32]. Also, patients with blood groups O and B, who are ABH secretors and Lewis antigen positive, may have increased amounts of serum intestinal AP activity, especially after a fatty meal [33]. Measurement of AP in the fasting patient eliminates or reduces this elevated activity. Unexplained elevation of AP activity was found to be familial, occurring in several healthy members of one family in an autosomal dominant inheritance pattern in the absence of bone or hepatic diseases [34]. Macro-APs formed by the complexing of AP from liver or bone with immunoglobulin are demonstrated as slow-moving forms on electrophoresis, but their significance is uncertain [30].

A low serum AP level is seen in zinc deficiency and Wilson's disease. Because zinc is a cofactor for the AP, the measured activity of the enzyme in serum will be low owing to zinc deficiency states accompanying intestinal disorders such as acrodermatitis enteropathica and Crohn's disease. Serum AP activity may be low in the fulminant presentation of Wilson's disease.

In summary, because normal growing children have significant elevations of serum AP activity originating from influx into serum of the bone isoenzyme, this determination is of less value in the assessment of cholestasis in children, particularly in rapidly growing adolescents. The tissue origin of elevated AP activity can be determined by polyacrylamide gel electrophoresis, but this is not routinely available in most clinical laboratories. Heat denaturation of the enzyme in serum takes advantage of the fact that the liver isoenzyme is more resistant to denaturation than the bone form, but this method is unreliable [24]. The most practical method most clinicians use to determine if an elevation of total serum AP activity signifies hepatic disease is to measure another enzyme that increases in cholestatic conditions and which is more specific to the liver, such as GGT or 5′-NT.

γ-Glutamyltransferase

γ-Glutamyltransferase is a microsomal enzyme that catalyzes the transfer of γ-glutamyl groups from peptides such as glutathione to other amino acids. GGT is present in the cell membranes of multiple body organs, including the kidney, pancreas, liver, spleen, brain, breast, and small intestine. Because the enzyme is found in so many tissues, including the biliary epithelium and hepatocyte, the usefulness of an elevated GGT level is limited by its lack of specificity [35]. However, GGT does not increase in the serum of patients with bone disease or children with active bone growth. Thus, GGT is helpful in confirming the hepatic origin of an elevated AP level.

γ-Glutamyltransferase is present in normal human serum. The newborn may have very high levels of GGT, up to five to eight times the upper limit of normal for adults [35]. In premature infants, in the first few days of life the values of GGT may be even higher than in the full-term infant. Serum values then decline rapidly in both the full-term and premature infant and reach adult normal levels by 6–9 months of age [35,36]. Table 8.2 shows normal values of GGT by age used at

Table 8.2: Reference Normal Values for Serum γ-Glutamyltransferase by Patient Age

Patient Age	*Sex*	*U/L*
<1 mo	M, F	<385
1–2 mo	M, F	<225
2–4 mo	M, F	<135
4–7 mo	M, F	<75
7 mo–15 yr	M, F	<45
>15 yr	M	<75
>15 yr	F	<55

From the Hospital for Sick Children [37]; used with permission.

the Hospital for Sick Children in Toronto, Canada, using the Eastman Kodak Ektachem 700 analyzer, a spectrophotometric method in common use in pediatric laboratory facilities because of the microliter quantities of serum required for analysis [37].

As with other microsomal enzymes, GGT activity is inducible by certain drugs. Hence, elevated GGT levels are often found in children taking anticonvulsants such as phenobarbital and phenytoin. Valproic acid may not induce an increase in serum GGT levels, except in cases of true hepatotoxicity, making this biochemical test a good candidate for monitoring for liver injury during therapy with this anticonvulsant [38].

γ-Glutamyltransferase is elevated in up to 90% of cases of primary liver disease, and hence is not of great value in considering the differential diagnosis. The highest levels of GGT are found in biliary obstruction, but extremely high levels are also found in intrahepatic cholestatic disorders, such as Alagille syndrome. The presence of increased serum GGT levels in both intrahepatic and extrahepatic cholestasis is variable and cannot be used to differentiate between them. In one study of 398 children (268 with cholestatic liver disease, 120 children with noncholestatic disease, and 10 control children without evidence of liver disease), GGT was normal in all 10 controls, 19 of 19 children with portal vein obstruction, and 10 of 12 children with congenital hepatic fibrosis. Serum GGT was high in all children with biliary atresia, sclerosing cholangitis, and paucity of intrahepatic bile ducts and in cholestatic patients with α_1-antitrypsin deficiency [39].

Normal or decreased serum GGT levels in the clinical setting of persistent jaundice are used as a test to distinguish among the different subtypes of genetic cholestatic syndromes [40]. *Progressive familial intrahepatic cholestasis* (PFIC) is a general term encompassing a group of illnesses characterized by persistent and profound cholestasis without extrahepatic pathology, typically presenting in the neonatal or infancy period, and with a progressive clinical course to cirrhosis. Although not typically correlated with genotype data, elevated serum levels of GGT are thought to distinguish PFIC type 3 (also known as MDR3 – multidrug resistance gene 3) disease from the normal to low serum GGT levels more typical of PFIC type 1 (also known as Byler's disease) and PFIC type 2 (also known as BSEP – bile salt export pump) disease. Recent scientific advances have helped clarify the molecular basis of many of these disorders [41].

While one report suggests that a normal GGT in infants with idiopathic cholestasis defined a group with poor prognosis [42], a normal or low GGT also occurs in infants with benign recurrent intrahepatic cholestasis (BRIC) with a good long-term prognosis [43]. As considered in detail in Chapter 31, BRIC is an autosomal recessive liver disease characterized by intermittent attacks of cholestasis, which start at any age and last for several weeks to months. Characteristically, the serum GGT is low and normal liver structure is preserved. BRIC shares a locus (chromosome 18q21) with PFIC type 1. Four patients diagnosed early in life with the clinical and histopathologic characteristics of BRIC and with low serum GGT were reported to progress to PFIC type 1 [44], suggesting a continuum for causes of low GGT in the setting of cholestasis.

γ-Glutamyltransferase activity is depressed by female sex hormones, which may interfere with release of GGT from the liver. In addition, the in vitro measured activity of serum GGT is artificially low in some assays when concomitant hyperbilirubinemia is present [45].

Elevations in GGT have been described in adults with a wide range of clinical conditions, including chronic alcoholism, exocrine pancreatic disease, myocardial infarction, renal failure, chronic obstructive pulmonary disease, and diabetes. Although measurement of serum GGT levels provides a sensitive indicator of the presence or absence of hepatobiliary disease, the usefulness of this biochemical test is limited by its lack of specificity. Measurement of serum GGT levels is probably best used in combination to evaluate the meaning of elevations in other serum liver biochemical tests.

5′-Nucleotidase

5′-Nucleotidase catalyzes the hydrolysis of nucleotides such as adenosine-5′-phosphate or inosine-5′-phosphate, which are unique for having the phosphate group attached to the 5′ position of a pentose sugar moiety. 5′-NT is found in the liver, intestines, brain, heart, blood vessels, and endocrine pancreas. Despite this widespread tissue distribution, marked serum elevations of 5′-NT are found almost exclusively in the setting of liver disease. In the liver, 5′-NT is located in both sinusoidal and canalicular membranes, but its precise physiologic purpose is not known. Serum 5′-NT levels are substantially lower in children than in adults, increase gradually with adolescence, and reach a plateau after 50 years of age [46].

Serum 5′-NT levels are elevated in hepatobiliary diseases such as biliary obstruction, cholestasis of various etiologies, and hepatic infiltration. The spectrum of abnormal 5′-NT values may parallel that of serum AP levels, probably because both enzymes have similar locations within the hepatocyte. However, unlike AP, serum 5′-NT levels typically do not increase in the presence of bone disease. Elevated 5′-NT levels in the presence of high ALT and AST suggest both hepatic and biliary tree involvement as in patients with sickle cell disease [47]. The main value of 5′-NT is its specificity for hepatobiliary disease when it is elevated in the nonpregnant patient, especially with a concomitantly increased serum AP level. Pregnancy also causes an increased value. Occasionally, the 5′-NT may be normal while the AP is elevated, yet the phosphatase may still be of hepatic origin [46].

Leucine Aminopeptidase

Leucine aminopeptidase (LAP) catalyzes the hydrolysis of amino acids from the N-terminus of peptides and proteins, but its physiologic function is not known. The name derives from the fact that LAP reacts most readily with peptides containing leucine. LAP is found widely in human tissues, but its activity is especially high in liver, particularly in biliary epithelium. Activity is increased in both pregnancy and hepatobiliary diseases but not in bone disease. Values are the same in children and adults [48]. LAP appears to be as sensitive in detecting obstructive biliary disease as 5′-NT and AP but also cannot differentiate among intrahepatic and extrahepatic causes of cholestasis [49]. Because of the common availability of AP, 5′-NT, and GGT, LAP has not found its way into common clinical use.

TESTS OF LIVER SYNTHETIC FUNCTION

Albumin

Albumin, the principal serum protein, is synthesized only in the liver. The serum albumin level at any point in time reflects the rate of synthesis, rate of degradation, and volume of distribution. Albumin is synthesized in the rough endoplasmic reticulum of hepatocytes at a rate of 150 mg/kg/d and has a half-life in the serum of approximately 20 days. Albumin synthesis is regulated by changes in nutritional status, osmotic pressure, systemic inflammation, and hormone levels. The major functions of albumin are to maintain intravascular colloid osmotic pressure and to bind and serve as a carrier for a variety of compounds in serum, including bilirubin, inorganic ions such as calcium, and many drugs [50].

As serum albumin has a long half-life, low serum albumin levels are often taken as a sign of chronic liver disease rather than acute injury. However, a patient with compensated chronic liver disease may demonstrate an abrupt decrease in serum albumin concentration during an acute illness such as sepsis or even a flulike minor illness. This is caused partly by an acute decrease in synthesis below that already present because of the parenchymal liver disease, possibly regulated by cytokines such as tumor necrosis factor and interleukin-1. Hypoalbuminemia is not specific for liver disease because it also occurs in the setting of protein-losing enteropathy, chronic infection, and nephrotic syndrome. In the absence of other nonhepatic etiologies, serum albumin levels may be useful in assaying hepatic synthetic function. Chronic inflammation, chronic liver disease, and protein malnutrition can inhibit albumin synthesis, whereas the presence of ascites causes an increased volume of distribution.

Coagulation Disorders in Liver Disease

Abnormal hemostasis is a common complication of liver disease. Mechanisms resulting in these defects include (1) diminished hepatic synthesis of coagulation factors V, VII, IX, X, and XI, prothrombin, and fibrinogen (reflected in prolongation of the PT); (2) dietary vitamin K deficiency due to inadequate intake or malabsorption (based on intrahepatic or extrahepatic cholestasis and intestinal malabsorption); (3) dysfibrinogenemia; (4) enhanced fibrinolysis due to decreased synthesis of α_2-plasmin inhibitor; (5) disseminated intravascular coagulation (DIC); and (6) thrombocytopenia due to hypersplenism [51,52]. Because of the large functional reserve of the liver, failure of hemostasis may not be a complication of every liver disease and may not arise as a complication except in severe or chronic liver diseases. Thus, testing for a coagulation defect is not a screening procedure. Rather, it serves as a means of following the progress of the liver disease or for assessing the risk of bleeding before an invasive and traumatic diagnostic procedure is undertaken [53]. As storage capacity of vitamin K in the liver is limited, depletion occurs quickly when absorption is impaired, and the PT increases above normal ranges.

The PT is a measure of the time it takes for prothrombin (factor II) to be converted into thrombin in the presence of tissue extract (thromboplastin), calcium ions, and activated clotting factors V, VII, and X. There follows then a secondary reaction involving the polymerization of fibrinogen (factor I) to fibrin by thrombin. The result of the initial reaction that produced thrombin is expressed in seconds or as a ratio of the plasma PT time to a control PT time. This reaction evaluates the extrinsic pathway of coagulation and is prolonged if any of the involved factors (I, II, V, VII, and X) are deficient, either individually or in combination.

A prolonged PT is not specific for liver disease because it is seen in various congenital deficiencies of coagulation factors and in acquired conditions such as consumption of clotting factors (as in DIC) and ingestion of drugs that affect the PT complex. Factor VIII, being made in nonhepatic tissues, is helpful in differentiating the depression of clotting factor activity and prolongation of hemostasis caused by severe liver disease alone (normal factor VIII) from that caused by accompanying DIC (depressed factor VIII activity from consumption). DIC is more common in children with end-stage liver failure because of the increased risk of infection from general debilitation and synthetic deficiencies of plasma proteins such as complement and opsonins normally made by the liver.

In the presence of normal factor VIII activity, prolongation of the PT indicates plasma clotting factor deficiency from impaired hepatic synthesis or secondary to vitamin K deficiency. Recent intake of antibiotics that alter the intestinal flora should be queried. Because the plasma half-life of several of the clotting factors is short (such as 3–5 hours for factor VII), the PT will rapidly reflect changes in hepatic synthetic function, such as may occur in acute liver failure, and thereby provides a good indicator of ultimate prognosis [54]. Most patients with extrahepatic obstruction respond promptly to parenterally administered vitamin K. In patients with jaundice, the type of response to vitamin K is therefore of some value in differential diagnosis, especially because it can be surmised that parenchymal function is good if the PT returns to normal within 24 hours after a single parenteral injection of vitamin K. In some inherited metabolic diseases in the newborn, such as tyrosinemia, there may be profound prolongations of both PT and PTT that may appear out of proportion to other parameters of liver dysfunction [55].

The PT test is not a sensitive index of chronic liver disease because even in severe cirrhosis, levels may be normal or only slightly prolonged. On the other hand, the PT test has high prognostic value, particularly for patients with acute hepatocellular disease. A persistently abnormal PT in a previously well child can be the single laboratory test that draws attention to the possibility of the development of acute liver failure. However, not all patients with prolonged PTs prove to have evidence of acute liver failure. In children with chronic cholestatic liver disease, an abnormal PT level refractory to maximal vitamin K therapy and decreasing serum albumin should raise for consideration the merits of a referral to a liver transplantation center for assessment.

Specific assays of clotting factors and other proteins involved in the hemostatic process may supply additional information in assessing patients with liver disease. Although fibrinogen levels are usually normal in hepatic disease because it is made both in the liver and in extrahepatic sites, increased catabolism of fibrinogen has been noted in patients with acute and chronic liver disease. Low levels of fibrinogen are seen in liver disease accompanied by DIC when there is consumption of fibrinogen and other clotting factors. Conversely, high levels of fibrinogen may be seen in patients with hepatic diseases because fibrinogen is an acute phase reactant or because of elevations described specifically in cholestatic disease. Finally, some patients with liver disease develop a dysfibrinogenemia with an abnormal fibrin monomer aggregate, which is manifested by a normal measured fibrinogen level in serum together with prolonged thrombin time.

Nearly all the above data are derived from studies in adults because of the considerable lag in knowledge of the unique aspects of the hemostatic system in full-term and preterm infants and the young child. Some of the distinctions that have been recently recognized include differences in the concentration of clotting factors, differences in the ability to generate thrombin (i.e., the very process measured by the PT), and the ability to inhibit the activity of thrombin once it is formed [56]. Many of the clotting factors, including the vitamin K–dependent factors II, VII, IX, and X, are less than 70% of adult levels in both full-term and preterm newborns. It is now clear that the hemostatic system of the neonate is dynamic and still evolving toward that of the normal adult.

Therefore, in assessing liver dysfunction in young infants based on prolongation of the PT, normal values specific to the gestational age at term and the postnatal age need to be considered [57,58] (Table 8.3). Despite these prolongations in PT and activated PTT, clinical evidence indicates that the healthy infant is not at an increased risk of bleeding. By contrast, in the sick infant, further reductions in clotting factors will further decrease the production of prothrombin, which may then result in bleeding observed in sick newborns with liver disease.

Table 8.3: Reference Values for Prothrombin Time (PT) and Activated Partial Thromboplastin Time (PTT) in the Healthy Premature (30–36 Weeks' Gestation) Infant During the First 6 Months of Life

Postnatal Age	*PT, Sec**	*Activated PTT, Sec**
Day 1	13.0 (10.6–16.2)	53.6 (27.5–79.4)
Day 5	12.5 (10.0–15.3)	50.5 (26.9–74.1)
Day 30	11.8 (10.0–13.6)	44.7 (26.9–62.5)
Day 90	12.3 (10.0–14.6)	39.5 (28.3–50.7)
Day 180	12.5 (10.0–15.0)	37.5 (21.7–53.3)
Adult	12.4 (10.8–13.9)	33.5 (26.6–40.3)

*Values in parentheses are normal ranges.

Lipids and Lipoproteins

The liver plays a central role in production and degradation of lipoproteins [59]. Lipoprotein abnormalities are common in chronic cholestatic disorders of either intrahepatic or extrahepatic etiology [60]. Marked elevations in the plasma levels of cholesterol and phospholipids occur because of the regurgitation into plasma of biliary phospholipids that produce secondary effects leading to an increase in plasma cholesterol because of enhanced hepatic synthesis of cholesterol. The cholesterol is transported in the blood in lipoprotein X, an unusual vesicular form of lipoprotein specific to cholestasis [61]. However, in noncholestatic liver diseases, declining lipoprotein cholesterol may also reflect deteriorating liver function and may be an indicator of prognosis [62], supporting earlier studies that the decrease in cholesterol observed in advanced cirrhosis is a prognostic marker of poor outcome in a multivariate analysis of children under consideration for liver transplantation [63].

In acute hepatocellular injury, levels of hepatic enzymes such as lecithin-cholesterol acyltransferase (LCAT) and triglyceride lipase (TGL) are decreased. Patients with acute liver disease have increased levels of plasma triglycerides, a decreased percentage of cholesterol esters, and abnormal electrophoretic lipoprotein patterns. Mild hypertriglyceridemia is characteristic of acute hepatocellular injury, with accumulation of triglyceride-rich low-density lipoprotein levels. Deficiency of hepatic TGL may account for the increased LDL triglyceride levels seen in acute hepatitis [64].

Attempts to correlate blood lipid and apolipoprotein levels with specific causes of liver dysfunction have been unsuccessful [64]. Some investigators advocate analyses of multiple apolipoproteins and subclasses, particularly apo A-II, as a more sensitive index of liver dysfunction [65]. In one study, lipoprotein parameters in plasma obtained from infants and children with biliary atresia (n = 15), Alagille syndrome (n = 10), and PFIC type 1 (n = 10) were helpful in discriminating among the three cholestatic disorders [66].

TESTS BASED ON SUBSTANCES METABOLIZED AND TRANSPORTED BY THE LIVER

Bilirubin

A more detailed discussion of the biochemistry and physiology of bilirubin metabolism is found in Chapter 13.

Bilirubin is a yellow tetrapyrrole pigment produced from the breakdown of ferriprotoporphyrin IX (heme), an integral part of heme-containing proteins. Approximately 75% of total bilirubin produced comes from the heme moiety of hemoglobin released from senescent erythrocytes destroyed in the reticuloendothelial cells of the liver, spleen, and bone marrow. The remaining bilirubin is produced from the premature destruction of red blood cell precursors in the bone marrow (i.e., ineffective erythropoiesis) and from the turnover and catabolism of other heme-containing proteins, such as myoglobin, cytochromes, and peroxidases.

Unconjugated bilirubin must be taken up into the hepatocyte and conjugated into the glucuronide form by the endoplasmic reticulum enzyme bilirubin uridine diphosphate (UDP)-glucuronyltransferase (bilirubin-UGT); the water-soluble bilirubin mono- and diglucuronides are then secreted across the canalicular membrane into bile. The molecular mechanisms of these processes have been delineated, with many excellent recent reviews [41,67].

When hepatic excretion of bilirubin glucuronides is impaired, serum levels of bilirubin glucuronides increase. Bilirubin glucuronides covalently bound to serum albumin form a fourth form of bilirubin, known as δ bilirubin; δ bilirubin is identified in the fourth fraction (the first three forms of bilirubin being α, β, and γ, corresponding to unconjugated, monoconjugated and diconjugated species, respectively) to elute when bilirubin is fractionated by high-pressure liquid chromatography [68]. In both children and adults, the appearance of δ bilirubin is associated with elevations of conjugated bilirubin and not with those disorders producing unconjugated bilirubin. Albumin-bound δ bilirubin has a prolonged half-life of approximately 14 days compared with the 4-hour half-life of bilirubin. The prolonged half-life of albumin-bound δ bilirubin explains why some children with reversible hepatobiliary diseases have serum bilirubin levels that decline slower than one might expect during an otherwise satisfactory clinical recovery. The increase in δ bilirubin accompanying the decrease in total serum bilirubin levels during recovery from an obstructive hepatobiliary disorder likely reflects decreased clearance of δ bilirubin because of its protein-bound nature and larger size. The percentage of δ bilirubin in jaundiced neonates is low compared with icteric adults, which may reflect delayed maturation of the enzymatic processes that produce protein-bound bilirubin from elevated conjugated bilirubin in serum.

Clinical laboratories still use spectrophotometry to measure serum bilirubin as direct-reacting or indirect-reacting fractions [69]. In this method, some bilirubin in the serum of jaundiced patients reacts directly with Ehrlich's diazo reagent (direct bilirubin), whereas some bilirubin requires alcohol as an accelerator for the reaction to proceed to a color product (indirect bilirubin). The value of indirect bilirubin is then calculated as the difference between the total value measured with the accelerator and the direct value obtained without the accelerator (direct fraction). In this method, protein-bound δ bilirubin is not detected as a separate species and is present in the direct fraction. Many clinical laboratories now measure and report separate true values for conjugated, unconjugated, and total bilirubin. δ Bilirubin value can then be calculated as the difference between total bilirubin and the sum of the conjugated and unconjugated fractions. High-performance liquid chromatography can precisely quantitate separate fractions of conjugated, unconjugated, and protein-bound or δ bilirubin, but the method is not generally available for routine clinical use.

Unconjugated hyperbilirubinemia may result from hemolysis or genetic diseases such as Crigler–Najjar syndrome, a rare genetic disease that presents shortly after birth and is characterized by a severe or total impairment of bilirubin conjugation by the liver [70] due to a deficiency of bilirubin-UGT. Diminished expression of the same enzyme is also the defect that causes Gilbert's syndrome, a benign, unconjugated hyperbilirubinemia occurring in up to 5% of the normal population. The term *physiologic jaundice* is used to describe the frequently observed jaundice in otherwise completely normal neonates and is the result of a number of factors involving increased bilirubin production and decreased excretion. These entities are discussed in further detail in Chapter 13.

Conjugated hyperbilirubinemia (>15% of the total bilirubin) indicates hepatobiliary disease and is always pathologic. It is usually accompanied by bilirubin in the urine, the presence of which can be tested quickly and cheaply using a urine dipstick. The presence of bilirubin in the urine confirms the presence of conjugated hyperbilirubinemia because unconjugated bilirubin is not excreted in urine. Bilirubinuria may appear before overt clinical jaundice. Further diagnostic evaluations in this setting should never be delayed, with an approach focused on the age-specific onset of diseases affecting the developing liver. The merits of quickly diagnosing causes amenable to specific medical therapies (such as galactosemia, tyrosinemia, hypopituitarism, sepsis) or to early surgical interventions (such as biliary atresia or choledochal cyst) must be emphasized. Various infectious, metabolic, toxic, genetic, and anatomic causes of a mechanical obstruction to bile flow or a functional impairment of any of the many processes involved in hepatic excretory function and bile secretion must be meticulously sought [71].

Although serum bilirubin levels increase in cholestatic disorders, the magnitude of the increase does not help differentiate between intrahepatic and extrahepatic biliary disorders. Both conjugated and unconjugated bilirubins are retained in these disorders, and a wide range of elevated serum concentrations of each form of bilirubin may be observed. Identification of the altered expression of several hepatocellular transport proteins in human cholestatic disease is bridging the gap between basic science and clinical medicine. New insight provided with the cloning and functional characterization of transport proteins involved in bile formation and secretion has led to a more precise characterization of a number of intrahepatic etiologies for conjugated hyperbilirubinemia [67].

Urobilinogen

Urobilinogen refers to a group of three colorless tetrapyrroles formed when unconjugated bilirubin (formed after the bilirubin glucuronides secreted into the upper small intestine are hydrolyzed to the unconjugated pigment) is reduced by the anaerobic intestinal microbial flora. Up to 20% of the urobilinogens produced daily are then reabsorbed from the intestine and undergo enterohepatic recirculation. The majority of the reabsorbed urobilinogen is taken up by the liver and then re-excreted into bile. A small amount is also excreted in the urine. In the lower intestinal tract, the urobilinogen tetrapyrroles spontaneously oxidize to produce the major color pigments of stool.

The formation of urobilinogen is decreased in all conditions in which biliary excretion of bilirubin is impaired. In the presence of hepatic dysfunction, more urobilinogen escapes hepatic uptake and biliary-enteric excretion and, thus, appears in the urine. As biliary obstruction becomes more complete, delivery of bilirubin to the intestinal tract is limited and urine as well as stool urobilinogen excretion decreases to very low concentrations.

Some confounding factors must be considered in the measurement and interpretation of urinary urobilinogen. Excretion has some diurnal variation, with peak urinary output between 12:00 and 16:00 hours. Urinary excretion of urobilinogen depends strongly on urinary pH; tubular reabsorption increases and urobilinogen stability decreases as pH decreases. Urobilinogen production and hence urinary excretion decrease with antibiotic treatment and diarrhea. These changes in urobilinogen unrelated to altered hepatobiliary function need to be considered when interpreting urinary urobilinogen values.

Bile Acid Tests

Bile acids are a class of endogenous organic anions synthesized from cholesterol exclusively in the hepatocytes, conjugated to glycine or taurine, and then secreted into bile (reviewed in Chapter 31). Alterations in hepatic bile acid synthesis, intracellular metabolism, excretion, intestinal absorption, and plasma extraction are reflected in derangements in bile acid metabolism. A disease that affects any of these functions should thereby theoretically affect serum bile acid levels and allow some quantification of the functional reserve of hepatocyte function.

Serum bile acid tests are disproportionately elevated in certain cholestatic diseases, such as primary sclerosing cholangitis and PFIC syndromes (subtypes 1, 2, and 3) in children, and primary biliary cirrhosis and pregnancy in adults. Serum bile acid levels are elevated in patients with liver biopsy–proven acute and chronic liver disease, even when the serum bilirubin is normal [72]. However, levels of serum bile acids do not provide specific information on the type of liver disease [73]. Nevertheless, serum bile acids may be a sensitive test for detecting early cirrhosis [74] in adults and a useful marker in predicting survival [75]. The abnormal serum bile acid levels in cirrhosis of any cause are the result of the decreased liver cell mass, decreased bile excretion, and portosystemic shunting usually present in chronic liver disease. Measuring serum bile acids may not be as useful a test in children because of the presence of a relative physiologic cholestasis in neonates, which results in baseline elevations of serum levels even in healthy babies [76,77]. These baseline elevations decrease within the first year of life, indicating a maturation of the bile acid transport processes [78]. Attempts to employ serum bile acid measurements to differentiate biliary atresia from other, nonobstructive causes of neonatal cholestasis have not been successful [79]. The same measurements also fail to offer prognostic information in children with α_1-antitrypsin deficiency [80].

Several methods to measure serum concentrations of bile acids are available, including enzymatic assays, in which the bacterial enzyme 3α-hydroxysteroid dehydrogenase is coupled to either fluorimetric or bioluminescence techniques; gas-liquid chromatography; radioimmunoassay; or a highly specific assay that combines gas–liquid chromatography and mass spectrometry [81]. The development of the technique of fast atom bombardment mass spectrometry in a handful of specialized laboratories has allowed the rapid screening of urine samples from infants and older children with suspected bile acid synthetic disorders using microliter amounts of sample directly, without requiring time-consuming sample preparation (see Chapter 31). Mass spectra are generated and indicate whether bile acid conjugates are present in an abnormal profile [81]. These newer techniques of precise bile acid analysis have delineated several inborn metabolic defects of bile acid synthesis involving modification of the cholesterol steroid nucleus [82].

TESTS BASED ON SUBSTANCES CLEARED FROM PLASMA BY THE LIVER

Ammonia

The concentration of ammonia in the blood is regulated by the balance of its production and clearance. Production is mainly in the large intestine by the action of bacterial urease on dietary protein and amino acids. Clearance of ammonia under normal circumstances occurs mainly in the liver via transformation of ammonia into urea via the urea cycle and into glutamine by transamination of α-ketoglutarate to glutamate and then to glutamine. The liver ordinarily removes 80% of the portal venous ammonia in a single pass.

In chronic liver diseases, disturbed urea cycle function caused by parenchymal liver cell destruction and portosystemic shunts permit large amounts of ammonia (and other putative toxins) to bypass the liver and exert their effects on the central nervous system [83]. Some ammonia is also made by the kidney and small intestine, a fact that becomes important when a patient is taking certain drugs, such as the anticonvulsant valproic acid, which can cause an increase in serum ammonia independent of any hepatotoxicity because of the drug-induced ammonia production by the kidney [84].

Advanced liver disease is the most commonly encountered acquired cause of hyperammonemia. Any cause of severe liver failure can lead to a significant impairment of normal ammonia metabolism. Hepatic encephalopathy, which develops in patients with cirrhosis, may be precipitated by an episode of gastrointestinal bleeding, which enhances ammonia production by bacterial metabolism of the blood proteins in the colon. However, in children, levels of encephalopathy and serum ammonia have a poor correlation [85]. Other metabolites elevated in liver disease, such as cerebrospinal fluid glutamine, correlate better with the clinical level of encephalopathy [86].

Patients with advanced cirrhosis may have normal fasting levels of ammonia. Conversely, nonfasting values of ammonia may be elevated even in a patient with mild liver disease. Therefore, fasting serum levels should be determined to reflect accurately the clearance of ammonia in blood. Serial measurements are useful because an increasing trend of fasting ammonia values has more value in assessing the development of advancing liver disease and hepatic encephalopathy than a single measurement in time.

Other causes of elevated blood ammonia include portosystemic shunts (either those created surgically or those of congenital origin); inherited defects of the urea cycle enzymes, such as ornithine carbamoyltransferase deficiency; defects in mitochondrial fatty acid β-oxidation; and Reye's syndrome. When cirrhosis is accompanied by impaired venous drainage from the intestinal tract into the liver via the portal vein, venous anastomoses develop. These collateral vessels shunt ammonia of intestinal origin away from the liver and into the general systemic circulation and cause increases in blood ammonia. Impaired renal function also often accompanies severe liver disease, with decreasing urinary output leading to increasing blood urea concentration, and increased excretion of urea into the intestine, where it is converted to ammonia. Finally, the patient with compensated liver disease and normal or near normal ammonia levels may develop the sudden onset of encephalopathy and increased serum ammonia levels if presented with a large protein load. This may occur during the setting of a large blood loss into the gastrointestinal tract with or without the catabolic stress of sepsis, both of which are common events in patients with chronic liver disease.

Exogenous Substances Used in Tests to Assess Quantitative Liver Function

The tests for quantitative liver function or true dynamic liver function are based on uptake, metabolism, and excretion of a determinate substance. The ideal test would be inexpensive, be easy to perform and analyze, be safe, have a single pharmacokinetic profile with minimal drug interactions, have a high predictive value, and provide quick results [87]. No single test has yet met these ideal performance characteristics.

Dynamic function tests can be classified in two categories: those using elimination of a substrate for testing (e.g., indocyanine green clearance, caffeine clearance, and galactose elimination) and studies that detect metabolites of the substance administered (e.g., aminopyrine breath test, monoethylglycinexylidide [MEGX] test, and PABA test].

In the MEGX test, exogenously administered lidocaine is metabolized by oxidative de-ethylation (within the hepatic cytochrome P450 system) to MEGX; analysis of MEGX by common laboratory instrumentation makes rapid evaluation of liver function possible. However, because the rate of MEGX production declines significantly with age, results of the MEGX test must be interpreted for age [88]. MEGX testing may have the most clinical utility in evaluating liver function to determine the suitability of the donor liver for transplant and to measure graft function post transplantation [89].

The use of PABA as a probe drug to quantify hepatic function has been reported to be a promising prognostic test for children with both chronic liver disease and fulminant liver failure [90,91]. PABA is a nontoxic, inexpensive, and orally administered probe drug that is readily absorbed from the gastrointestinal tract [92] and undergoes biotransformation to three metabolites independent of phase I cytochrome P450 biotransformation reactions. Through phase II conjugation reactions, PABA combines with either glycine (to form para-aminohippuric acid [PAHA]); acetyl–coenzyme A (CoA) (to form para-acetamidobenzoic acid [PAABA]); or both glycine and acetyl CoA (to form para-acetamidohippuric acid [PAAHA] [93]. With extensive hepatocellular damage, glycine conjugation and hepatic acetylation of PABA is rapidly lost. The measurement of a serum PAHA of 0 mol/L at 30 minutes after oral administration by high-performance liquid chromatography was the most reliable early prognostic marker of outcome in 24 children with acute liver failure or acute severe hepatitis, with a sensitivity of 92% and negative predictive value of 92% compared with a sensitivity of 54% and a negative predictive value of 63% with King's College criteria [91]. Further multicenter studies are needed to confirm the promising results of this pilot work.

OTHER LABORATORY TESTS TO ASSESS FOR LIVER DISEASE IN CHILDREN

Serum Globulins

The serum globulin level can be quickly determined by subtracting the albumin concentration from the total protein level. Serum globulins can be further separated by using serum protein electrophoresis into α_1, α_2, β, and γ fractions. Within each of these fractions is a heterogenous collection of different serum proteins. The α_1 fraction is composed principally of α_1-antitrypsin, ceruloplasmin, and orosomucoid (an α_1-acid glycoprotein), all of which are acute-phase reactants and increase in response to liver disease and many inflammatory disorders.

Haptoglobin makes up a large part of the α_2 fraction and is also an acute-phase reactant. Transferrin and β-lipoprotein make up a major portion of the β fraction. The principal constituents of the γ fraction are the immunoglobulins, particularly IgG, IgA, and IgM. Abnormalities may occur in the serum protein electrophoresis profile in various liver diseases, such as hypergammaglobulinemia seen in autoimmune hepatitis and low α_1 peak in α_1-antitrypsin deficiency. Few of these abnormalities are of great specific diagnostic aid. Serum immunoglobulins are produced by stimulated B lymphocytes. Thus, measurement of these substances is not a direct test of liver function or hepatocyte injury.

Plasma and Urine Amino Acids

Measures of amino acids in the blood and urine may provide specific information critical to or supportive of the diagnosis of an inborn error of intermediary metabolism, such as hereditary tyrosinemia, methylmalonic acidemia, and defects of ureagenesis. These are discussed in further detail in Chapter 22.

CONCLUSIONS

The initial evaluation of a serum liver chemistry value in a child must be assessed in the context of the findings of a detailed history and physical examination. A reliable literature to make unequivocal recommendations for the diagnostic evaluation of children with abnormal liver chemistry tests is lacking. In the individual patient care setting, additional serologic, radiologic, and histopathologic tests may well be warranted. Advances in laboratory medicine have made possible increasingly sophisticated analysis of compounds in body fluids related to the liver function in both healthy and diseased states. These analyses provide the clinician with valuable diagnostic as well as, on occasion, prognostic information. Some tests still are not widely available for routine clinical use. Others continue to lack the diagnostic sensitivity and specificity clinicians seek for the ideal liver injury and function tests. Further advances in our knowledge of the physiology and biochemistry of the normal and diseased liver will contribute to the fulfillment of this goal.

ACKNOWLEDGMENTS

This chapter is revised and updated from Chapter 7 written by Drs. L. Arturo Batres and Eric S. Maller in *Liver Disease in Children, Second Edition,* edited by F. J. Suchy, R. J. Sokol, and W. F. Balistreri, Lippincott Williams & Wilkins, Philadelphia © 2001.

REFERENCES

1. Green RM, Flamm S. American Gastroenterological Association technical review on the evaluation of liver chemistry tests. Gastroenterology 2002;123:1367–84.
2. Kim HC, Nam CM, Jee SH, et al. Normal serum aminotransferase concentration and risk of mortality from liver disease: prospective cohort study. BMJ 2004;328:983.
3. Giannini EG, Testa R, Savarino V. Liver enzyme alteration: a guide for clinicians. Can Med Assoc Journal 2005;172:367–79.
4. Adams PC, Arthur MJ, Boyer TD, et al. Screening in liver disease: report of an AASLD clinical workshop. Hepatology 2004;39:1204–12.
5. Clark JM, Brancati FL, Diehl AM. The prevalence and etiology of elevated aminotransferase levels in the United States. Am J Gastroenterol 2003;98:960–7.
6. Prati D, Taioli E, Zanella A, et al. Updated definitions of healthy ranges for serum alanine aminotransferase levels. Ann Intern Med 2002;137:1–9.
7. Kaplan MM. Alanine transferase levels: what's normal. Ann Intern Med 2002;137:49–50.
8. Kohli R, Harris DC, Whitington PF. Relative elevations of serum alanine and aspartate aminotransferase in muscular dystrophy. J Pediatr Gastroenterol Nutr 2005;41:121–4.
9. Morse RP, Rosman NP. Diagnosis of occult muscular dystrophy: importance of the "chance" finding of elevated serum aminotransferase activities. J Pediatr 1993;122:254–6.
10. Triester SL, Douglas DD. Development of macro-aspartate aminotransferase in a patient undergoing specific allergen injection immunotherapy. Am J Gastroenterol 2005;100:243–5.
11. Wiltshire EJ, Crooke M, Grimwood K. Macro-AST: a benign cause of persistently elevated aspartate aminotransferase. J Pediatr Child Health 2004;40:642–3.
12. Giannini E, Risso D, Botta F, et al. Validity and clinical utility of the aspartate aminotransferase–alanine aminotransferase ratio in assessing disease severity and prognosis in patients with hepatitis c virus – related chronic liver disease. Arch Intern Med 2003;163:218–24.
13. Diehl AM, Potter J, Boitnott J, et al. Relationship between pyridoxal 5′-phosphate deficiency and aminotransferase levels in alcoholic hepatitis. Gastroenterology 1984;86:632–6.
14. Rosenthal P, Haight M. Aminotransferase as a prognostic index in infants with liver disease. Clin Chem 1990;36:346–8.
15. Berman DH, Leventhal RI, Gavaler JS, et al. Clinical differentiation of fulminant Wilsonian hepatitis from other causes of hepatic failure. Gastroenterology 1991;100:1129.
16. Farre C, Esteve M, Curcoy A, et al. Hypertransaminasemia in pediatric celiac disease patients and its prevalence as a diagnostic clue. Am J Gastroenterol 2002;97:3176–81.
17. Iorio R, Sepe A, Giannattasio A, et al. Hypertransaminasemia in childhood as a marker of genetic liver disorders. J Gastroenterol 2005;40:820–6.
18. Mager DR, Roberts EA. Nonalcoholic fatty liver disease in children. Clin Liver Dis 2006;10:109–31.
19. Iannou GN, Weiss NS, Boyko EJ, et al. Contribution of metabolic factors to alanine aminotransferase activity in person with other causes of liver disease. Gastroenterology 2005;128:627–35.
20. Tiao G, Ryckman FC. Pediatric liver transplantation. Clin Liver Dis 2006;10:169–97.
21. Keller MS, Coln CE, Trimble JA, et al. The utility of routine trauma laboratories in pediatric trauma resuscitations. Am J Surg 2004;188:671–8.
22. Kaplowitz N. Drug-induced liver injury. Clin Infect Dis 2004;38(suppl 2):S44–8.

23. Russo MW, Watkins PB. Are patients with elevated liver tests at increased risk of drug-induced liver injury? Gastroenterology 2004;126:1477–80.
24. Chopra S, Griffin PH. Laboratory tests and diagnostic procedures in evaluation of liver disease. Am J Med 1985;79:221–30.
25. Kaplan MM. Alkaline phosphatase. Gastroenterology 1972;62: 452–68.
26. Clarke LC, Beck E. Plasma "alkaline" phosphatase activity. I. Normative data for growing children. J Pediatr 1950;36:335–41.
27. Salz JL, Daum F, Cohen MI. Serum alkaline phosphatase activity during adolescence. J Pediatr 1973;82:536–7.
28. Seetharam S, Sussman NL, Komoda T, Alpers DH. The mechanism of elevated alkaline phosphatase activity after bile duct ligation in the rat. Hepatology 1986;6:374.
29. Crofton PM. Biochemistry of alkaline phosphatase isoenzymes. CRC Crit Rev Clin Lab Sci 1982;16:161–94.
30. Posen S, Lee C, Vines R, et al. Transient hyperphosphatasemia of infancy – an insufficiently recognized syndrome. Clin Chem 1977;23(2 pt 1):292–4.
31. Kraut JR, Metrick M, Maxwell NR, Kaplan MM. Isoenzyme studies in transient hyperphosphatasemia of infancy: ten new cases and a review of the literature. Am J Dis Child 1985;139:736–40.
32. Warnes TW, Hine P, Kay G. Intestinal alkaline phosphatase in the diagnosis of liver disease. Gut 1977;18:274–80.
33. Bamford KF, Harris H, Luffman JE, et al. Serum alkaline phosphatase and the ABO blood groups. Lancet 1965;1:530–1.
34. McEvoy M, Skrabanek P, Wright E, et al. Family with raised alkaline phosphatase activity in the absence of disease. BMJ 1981; 282:1272–5.
35. Cabrera-Abreu JC, Green A. Gamma-glutamyltransferase: value of its measurement in paediatrics. Ann Clin Biochem 2002;39: 22–5.
36. Huang YC, Chen HL, Tsai KS, et al. Serum gamma-glutamyl transpeptidase activity and bile acids in normal Taiwanese infants. Acta Paediatr Taiwan 2002;43:245–8.
37. Reference values and SI unit information. Toronto, ON: Hospital for Sick Children, 1993.
38. Deutsch J, Fritsch G, Golles J, Semmelrock HJ. Effects of anticonvulsive drugs on the activity of gamma-glutamyltransferase and aminotransferases in serum. J Pediatr Gastroenterol Nutr 1986;5:542–8.
39. Maggiore G, Bernard O, Hadchouel M, et al. Diagnostic value of serum gamma-glutamyl transpeptidase activity in liver diseases in children. J Pediatr Gastroenterol Nutr 1991;12:21–6.
40. Jansen PL, Sturm E. Genetic cholestasis, causes and consequences for hepatobiliary transport. Liver Int 2003;23:315–22.
41. Carlton VE, Pawlikowska L, Bull LN. Molecular basis of intrahepatic cholestasis. Ann Med 2004;36:606–17.
42. Maggiore G, Bernard O, Riely CA, et al. Normal serum gamma-glutamyl-transpeptidase activity identifies groups of infants with idiopathic cholestatis with poor prognosis. J Pediatr 1987;111: 251–2.
43. Lachaux A, Loras-Duclaux I, Bouvier R, et al. Benign recurrent cholestasis with normal gamma-glutamyl-transpeptidase activity. J Pediatr. 1992;121:78–80.
44. van Ooteghem NA, Klomp LW, van Berge-Henegouwen GP, Houwen RH. Benign recurrent intrahepatic cholestasis progressing to progressive intrahepatic cholestasis: low GGT cholestasis is a clinical continuum. J Hepatol 2002;36:439–43.
45. Combes B, Shore GM, Cunningham FG, et al. Serum gamma-glutamyl transpeptidase activity in viral hepatitis: suppression in pregnancy and by birth control pills. Gastroenterology 1977;72: 271–4.
46. Hill PG, Sammons HG. An assessment of 5′-nucleotidase as a liver-function test. Q J Med 1967;36:457–68.
47. Ahn H, Li CS, Wang W. Sickle cell hepatopathy: clinical presentation, treatment, and outcome in pediatric and adult patients. Pediatr Blood Cancer 2005;45:184–90.
48. Rutenburg AM, Pineda EP, Goldberg JA, et al. Serum leucine aminopeptidase activity: in normal infants, in biliary atresia and in other diseases. Am J Dis Child 1962;103:47–54.
49. Banks BM, Pineda EP, Goldberg JA, Rutenburg AM. Clinical value of serum leucine aminopeptidase determinations. N Engl J Med 1960;263:1277–81.
50. Doumas BT, Peters T. Serum and urine albumin: a progress report on their measurement and clinical significance. Clin Chim Acta 1997;258:3–20.
51. Amitrano L, Guardascione MA, Brancaccio V, Balzano A. Coagulation disorders in liver disease. Semin Liver Dis 2002;22:83–96.
52. Kaul VV, Munoz SJ. Coagulopathy of liver disease. Curr Treat Options Gastroenterol 2002;3:433–8.
53. Segal JB, Dzik WH. Transfusion Medicine/Hemostasis Clinical Trials Network. Paucity of studies to support that abnormal coagulation test results predict bleeding in the setting of invasive procedures: an evidence-based review. Transfusion 2005;45: 1413–25.
54. Kujovich JL. Hemostatic defects in end stage liver disease. Crit Care Clin 2005;21:563–87.
55. Croffie JM, Gupta SK, Chong SK, Fitzgerald JF. Tyrosinemia type 1 should be suspected in infants with severe coagulopathy even in the absence of other signs of liver failure. Pediatrics 1999;103: 675–8.
56. Andrew M, Paes B, Johnston M. Development of the hemostatic system in the neonate and young infant. Am J Pediatr Hematol Oncol 1990;12:95–104.
57. Andrew M, Paes B, Milner R, et al. The development of the human coagulation system in the fullterm infant. Blood 1987;72: 165–72.
58. Andrew M, Paes B, Milner R, et al. Development of the coagulation system in the healthy preterm infant. Blood 1988;72: 1651–7.
59. Dixon JL, Ginsberg HN. Hepatic synthesis of lipoproteins and apolipoproteins. Semin Liver Dis 1992;12:364–72.
60. Miller JP. Dyslipoproteinemia of liver disease. Baillieres Clin Endocrinol Metab 1990;4:807–32.
61. Sabesin SM. Cholestatic lipoproteins: their pathogenesis and significance. Gastroenterology 1982;83:704–9.
62. Habib A, Anastasios AM, Abou-Assi SG, et al. High-density lipoprotein cholesterol as an indicator of liver function and prognosis in noncholestatic cirrhosis. Gastroenterol Hepatol 2005; 3:286–91.
63. Malatack JJ, Schald DJ, Urbach AH, et al. Choosing a pediatric recipient of orthotopic liver transplantation. J Pediatr 1987; 111:479–89.
64. Seidel D. Lipoproteins in liver diseases. J Clin Chem Clin Biochem 1987;25:541–51.
65. Lontie JF, Dubois DY, Malmendier CL, et al. Plasma lipids and apolipoproteins in end-stage liver disease. Clin Chim Acta 1990;195:91–4.
66. Bojanovski M, Lukermann R, Schulz-Falten J, et al. Parameters of lipoprotein metabolism and cholestasis in healthy and cholestatic infants and children. Prog Lipid Res 1991;30:295–300.

67. Trauner M, Wagner M, Fickert P, Zollner G. Molecular regulation of hepatobiliary transport systems: clinical implications for understanding and treating cholestasis. J Clin Gastroenterol 2005;39(4 suppl 2):S111–24.
68. Weiss JS, Gautam A, Lauff JJ, et al. The clinical importance of a protein-bound fraction of serum bilirubin in patients with hyperbilirubinemia. N Engl J Med 1983;309:147–50.
69. van den Bergh AAH, Muller P. Uber eine direkte und eine indirekte Diazoreaktion auf Bilirubin. Biochem Z 1916;77:90–103.
70. Turkey RH, Strassburg CP. Human UDP-glucuronosyltransferases: metabolism, expression, and disease. Annu Rev Pharmacol Toxicol 2000;40:581–616.
71. Moyer V, Freese DK, Whitington PF, et al. North American Society for Pediatric Gastroenterology, Hepatology and Nutrition. Guideline for the evaluation of cholestatic jaundice in infants: recommendations of the North American Society for Pediatric Gastroenterology, Hepatology and Nutrition. J Pediatr Gastroenterol Nutr 2004;39:115–28.
72. Ferraris R, Colombatti G, Forentini MT, et al. Diagnostic value of serum bile acids and routine liver function tests in hepatobiliary disease: sensitivity, specificity, and predictive value. Dig Dis Sci 1983;28:129–36.
73. Festi D, Morselli Labate AM, Roda A, et al. Diagnostic effectiveness of serum bile acids in liver diseases as evaluated by multivariate statistical methods. Hepatology 1983;3:707–13.
74. Mannes GA, Stellaard F, Paumgartner G. Increased serum bile acids in cirrhosis with normal transaminases. Digestion 1982;25: 217–21.
75. Mannes GA, Thieme C, Stellaard F, et al. Prognostic significance of serum bile acids in cirrhosis. Hepatology 1986;6:50–3.
76. Heubi J. Serum bile acids as markers of liver disease in childhood. J Pediatr Gastroenterol Nutr 1982;1:457–8.
77. Suchy FJ, Balistreri WF, Heubi JE, et al. Physiologic cholestasis: elevation of the primary serum bile acid concentrations in normal infants. Gastroenterology 1981;80:1037–41.
78. Balistreri WF. Immaturity of hepatic excretory function and the ontogeny of bile acid metabolism. J Pediatr Gastroenterol Nutr 1983;2(suppl):207–14.
79. Javitt NB, Keating JP, Grand RJ, Harris RC. Serum bile acid patterns in neonatal hepatitis and extrahepatic biliary atresia. J Pediatr 1977;90:736–9.
80. Nemeth A, Samuelason K, Strandvik B. Serum bile acids as markers of juvenile liver disease in alpha-1-antitrypsin deficiency. J Pediatr Gastroenterol Nutr 1982;1:469–78.
81. Setchell KDR, O'Connell NC. Bile acid synthesis and metabolism. In: Walker WA, Goulet O, Kleinman RE, et al., eds. Pediatric gastrointestinal disease: pathophysiology, diagnosis, management. Vol 2. Philadelphia: BC Decker, 2004:1308–43.
82. Bove KE, Heubi JE, Balistreri WF, Setchell KD. Bile acid synthetic defects and liver disease: a comprehensive review. Pediatr Dev Pathol 2004;7:315–34.
83. Bachmann C. Mechanisms of hyperammonemia. Clin Chem Lab Med 2002;40:653–62.
84. Panda S, Radhakrishnan K. Two cases of valproate-induced hyperammonemic encephalopathy without hepatic failure. J Assoc Physicians India 2004;52:746–8.
85. Cohn RM, Roth KS. Hyperammonemia, bane of the brain. Clin Pediatr (Phila) 2004;43:683–9.
86. Hourani BT, Hamlin EM, Reynolds TB. Cerebrospinal fluid glutamine as a measure of hepatic encephalopathy. Arch Intern Med 1971;127:1033–6.
87. Burra P, Masier A. Dynamic tests to study liver function. Eur Rev Med Pharmacol Sci 2004;8:19–21.
88. Orlando R, Palatini P. The effect of age on plasma MEGX concentrations. Br J Clin Pharmacol 1997;44:206–8.
89. Tanaka E, Inomata S, Yasuhara H. The clinical importance of conventional and quantitative liver function tests in liver transplantation. J Clin Pharmacol Ther 2000;25:411–19.
90. Lebel S, Nakamachi Y, Hemming A, et al. Glycine conjugation of para-aminobenzoic acid (PABA): a pilot study of a novel prognostic test in acute liver failure in children. J Pediatr Gastroenterol Nutr 2003;36:62–71.
91. Furuya KN, Duric PR, Roberts EA, et al. Glycine conjugation of para-aminobenzoic acid (PABA): a quantitative test of liver function. Clin Biochem 1995;28:531–40.
92. Weizman Z, Forstner GG, Gaskin KJ, et al. Bentiromide test for assessing pancreatic dysfunction using analysis of para aminobenzoic acid in plasma and urine. Gastroenterology 1985; 89:596 604.
93. Gunawardhana L, Barr J, Weir AJ, et al. The N-acetylation of sulfamethazine and p aminobenzoic acid by human liver slices in dynamic organ culture. Drug Metab Dispos 1991;19:648 53.

Section II: Cholestatic Liver Diseases

9

Approach to the Infant with Cholestasis

Frederick J. Suchy, M.D.

Jaundice sometimes appears at birth, indicated by the dark yellow color of the countenance and arising from obstructions of the liver. Cases are generally incurable [1].

– Eli Ives of Yale University, America's first academic pediatrician, circa 1829

Cholestasis may be defined physiologically as a measurable decrease in bile flow, pathologically as the histologic presence of bile pigment in hepatocytes and bile ducts, and clinically as the accumulation in blood and extrahepatic tissues of substances normally excreted in bile (e.g., bilirubin, bile acids, and cholesterol). The process occurs as a result of impaired bile formation by the hepatocyte or from obstruction to the flow of bile through the intrahepatic and extrahepatic biliary tree [2,3]. In the neonate, the clinical and laboratory features of the many liver diseases presenting with cholestasis are quite similar. An important focus of the pediatric hepatologist is to differentiate intrahepatic from extrahepatic cholestasis and, if possible, establish a specific diagnosis [4]. Strategies for the treatment of metabolic or infectious liver disease and for the surgical management of biliary anomalies require early diagnosis. Even when treatment is not available or effective, infants with progressive liver disease usually benefit from optimal nutritional support and medical management of medical complications of cholestasis and possibly cirrhosis until liver transplantation is done.

This chapter presents an overview of the approach to the infant with cholestatic liver disease. The diagnostic evaluation of these patients is emphasized. The incidence and scope of the problem are placed in perspective, and the differential diagnosis is reviewed, but the large number of specific disorders are not discussed here in detail. These disorders are covered comprehensively in subsequent chapters.

INCIDENCE

The overall incidence of neonatal liver disease, most cases manifesting clinical or biochemical evidence of cholestasis, may be as high as 1 in 2500 live births. Idiopathic neonatal hepatitis, the most common diagnosis in older series, had an incidence of 1 in 4800 to 1 in 9000 live births [5,6]. Reliable figures do not exist regarding the current incidence, but, as will be discussed later, newer and more accurate diagnostic methods have markedly decreased the number of infants labeled as having idiopathic neonatal hepatitis. The estimated incidence of biliary atresia ranges from 1 in 8000 to 1 in 21,000 live births, with cases occurring more frequently in Far Eastern than in Western countries [7]. In a prospective study conducted over 25 years in Atlanta, Georgia, the calculated incidence of biliary atresia was 0.73 cases per 10,000 live births, with a higher prevalence in African-American children than in white children [8]. Table 9.1 details the diagnoses of 1086 consecutive infants with conjugated hyperbilirubinemia referred over a 20-year period to King's College Hospital, a tertiary-care center serving the majority of England. The high percentage of patients with biliary atresia in this impressive series in part reflects the interest and expertise of these physicians in the diagnosis and surgical correction of biliary tract disorders. In another prospective study of 790,385 Australian infants by Danks et al. [6], 55 cases of biliary atresia (1 in 14,000 live births), 11 cases of intrahepatic biliary hypoplasia (1 in 70,000), and 99 cases of idiopathic neonatal hepatitis (1 in 8000) were observed [6]. The time sequence of births for patients with neonatal hepatitis was fairly even in this study, but there was a suggestion of time–space clustering for some cases of biliary atresia. However, there is a considerable disagreement between studies in regard to seasonal clustering of cases [8,9]. In a recent study of 207 infants from Australia, the etiology of the cholestasis was idiopathic in 25%, metabolic/genetic in 23%, biliary obstruction in 20%, parenteral nutrition in 20%, infection in 9%, and bile duct hypoplasia in 3% [10].

DIFFERENTIAL DIAGNOSIS OF NEONATAL CHOLESTASIS

Liver dysfunction in the neonate, regardless of the etiology, is commonly associated with a failure of bile secretion and conjugated hyperbilirubinemia [11]. Jaundice is a frequent and early presenting feature of liver disease during early life rather than

Table 9.1: Infants with Conjugated Hyperbilirubinemia Referred to King's College Hospital Between 1970 and 1990

Diagnosis	*Number*	*Percentage*
Biliary atresia	377	34.7
Idiopathic neonatal hepatitis	331	30.5
α_1-Antitrypsin deficiency	189	17.4
Other hepatitis	94	8.7
Alagille syndrome	61	5.6
Choledochal cyst	34	3.1

Modified from Mieli-Vergani et al. [32], with permission.

a late manifestation of advanced disease, as is seen in the older child or adult [11]. Owing to an immaturity of hepatic excretory function, a susceptibility to infection during the perinatal period, and the initial effects of congenital malformations and inborn errors of metabolism, the number of distinct disorders presenting with cholestasis is greater in the neonate than at any other time of life. A conceptually useful overview of the differential diagnosis of neonatal cholestasis is presented in Table 9.2. Although the origin or the predominating form of liver damage may be traced primarily to the level of the hepatocyte or to the biliary apparatus, there is considerable overlap between disorders in their clinical features as well as in the subsequent sites of injury [12,13]. For example, injury to the biliary epithelium may be a prominent finding in neonatal infection with cytomegalovirus, α_1-antitrypsin deficiency, and some inborn errors of bile acid metabolism. Moreover, mechanical obstruction of the common bile duct invariably results in liver dysfunction and intrahepatic injury, which may include in the neonate significant giant cell transformation of hepatocytes [14]. It is unclear in this setting whether giant cells, which appear to be a frequent, nonspecific manifestation of neonatal liver injury, reflect the noxious effects of biliary obstruction or whether the hepatocytes as well as the biliary epithelium are damaged by a common insult such as a virus or toxin with tropism for both types of cells.

The term *neonatal hepatitis* refers to the histologic finding of extensive giant cell transformation of hepatocytes. The term is misleading because it implies an infectious process involving the liver (such as the numerous forms of viral hepatitis), but has been used to describe virtually all forms of liver disease after structural disorders of the biliary tree, such as biliary atresia and choledochal cysts, have been excluded. Because of improved imaging techniques, advances in virology, and the application of sophisticated biochemical and molecular methods to the diagnosis of inborn errors of metabolism, there are fewer infants whose liver disease may be classified as idiopathic or cryptogenic. A disorder should now be designated as neonatal hepatitis only if an infectious agent can be documented or suspected on the basis of other clinical features associated with congenital infection. An increasing number of infections have been associated with neonatal hepatitis, including parvovirus B19, human herpesvirus 6, and the human immunodeficiency virus [15,16]. The percentage of cases that can be classified as idiopathic will also be influenced by referral patterns, the prevalence of certain infections within a population, and the availability of specialized diagnostic techniques and biochemical assays.

Spontaneously resolving forms of neonatal cholestasis may result from the association of several factors, including immaturity of bile secretion and perinatal disease leading to hepatic hypoxia or ischemia [17]. In a recent study, histologic examination, performed in 70 affected infants, showed moderate portal and lobular fibrosis, multinucleated giant hepatocytes, and hematopoietic foci; findings in follow-up liver biopsy specimens from 15 children were normal or improved [17]. The occurrence of so-called neonatal hepatitis in babies with other serious disorders, such as Down's syndrome, hemolytic disease of the newborn, and congenital heart disease, also suggests that systemic disease may either increase susceptibility to agents capable of causing hepatitis or exacerbate further an underlying immaturity of hepatic excretory function to the point of producing pathologic cholestasis.

In approximately 10% of patients with a familial form of neonatal hepatitis, which usually carries a poor prognosis, there is increasing evidence for cellular defects in metabolism and substrate transport pathways as the basis for liver injury. For example, multiple inherited defects in the biosynthetic pathway for bile acids have been described that cause cholestasis and progressive liver injury [18]. Moreover, the genes for several forms of progressive familial intrahepatic cholestasis (PFIC) have recently been identified and encode proteins critically important for bile formation [19,20]. Giant cell transformation of hepatocytes is the predominant histologic feature in type 2 PFIC because of mutations in the gene encoding the bile salt excretory pump [21].

Another feature often accompanying neonatal cholestasis is bile ductular paucity, a histologic finding implying a diminution in the number of interlobular bile ducts [22]. The abnormality may be of primary importance in patients with so-called syndromic paucity of interlobular bile ducts (PILBD) but also may occur occasionally in many other disorders, including cytomegalovirus and rubella infections, α_1-antitrypsin deficiency, and bile acid synthetic defects [23]. The finding may not be present or may be difficult to recognize in the neonate. Serial liver biopsies may demonstrate injury to bile ductular epithelial cells, a variable amount of associated inflammation, and a progressive decrease in the number of bile ductules per portal tract.

MANIFESTATIONS OF CHOLESTATIC LIVER DISEASE IN THE NEONATE

Jaundice is the most overt physical sign of liver disease and occurs more commonly in the neonatal period than at any

Table 9.2: Classification of Cholestatic Disorders

Neonatal hepatitis
Idiopathic
Viral
Cytomegalovirus
Herpes (simplex, zoster, human type 6)
Rubella
Reovirus type 3
Adenovirus
Enteroviruses
Parvovirus B19
Hepatitis B
Human immunodeficiency virus
Syncytial giant cell hepatitis with paramyxovirus-like inclusions
Bacterial and parasitic
Bacterial sepsis
Urinary tract infection
Syphilis
Listeriosis
Tuberculosis
Toxoplasmosis
Malaria
Bile duct obstruction
Cholangiopathies
Biliary atresia
Choledochal cysts
Nonsyndromic PILBD
Alagille syndrome
Neonatal sclerosing cholangitis (**with**/without ichthyosis)
Spontaneous perforation of common bile duct
Caroli's disease
Congenital hepatic fibrosis
Bile duct stenosis
Williams syndrome
Other
Inspissated bile/mucous plug
Cholelithiasis
Tumors/masses (intrinsic and extrinsic)
Cholestatic syndromes
PFIC caused by transport defects
Type 1 (Byler's disease, defect in a P-type ATPase)
Type 2 (defect in canalicular bile acid pump)
Type 3 (defect in MDR3, a canalicular phospholipid transporter)
Hereditary cholestasis with lymphedema (Aagenaes syndrome)
Cholestasis of North American Indians
Nielsen syndrome (Greenland Eskimos)
Benign recurrent cholestasis (defect in same gene as PFIC type 1)
Neonatal Dubin–Johnson syndrome (MRP2 deficiency)
Arthrogryposis, renal dysfunction, and cholestasis syndrome
Metabolic disorders
α_1-antitrypsin deficiency
Cystic fibrosis
Neonatal iron storage disease
Endocrinopathies
Hypopituitarism (septo-optic dysplasia)
Hypothyroidism
McCune–Albright syndrome
HNF1β mutations with type 5 maturity-onset diabetes of the young
Donahue syndrome (leprechaunism)
Amino acid disorders
Tyrosinemia
Hypermethionemia
Storage disorders
Niemann–Pick disease
Gaucher's disease
Wolman's disease
Farber's disease
Cholesterol ester storage disease
Mucolipidosis type II (I cell disease)
Mucopolysaccharidosis type VII
Glycogen storage disease type IV
Urea cycle disorders (arginase deficiency)
Carbohydrate disorders
Galactosemia
Fructosemia

(*continued*)

Table 9.2 (*continued*)

Mitochondrial disorders	Toxic
Respiratory chain defects	Drugs
GRACILE syndrome (growth retardation, aminoaciduria, cholestasis, iron overload, lactic acidosis, early death)	Parenteral nutrition
Citrin deficiency	Aluminum
β-oxidation defects	Fetal alcohol syndrome
Short-chain acyl-CoA dehydrogenase deficiency	Ceftriaxone lithiasis
Long-chain acyl-CoA dehydrogenase deficiency	**Cardiovascular disorders**
Peroxisomal disorders	Shock/hypoperfusion
Zellweger's syndrome	Congestive heart failure
Infantile Refsum's disease	Perinatal asphyxia
Other enzymopathies	Veno-occlusive disease
Bile acid synthetic defects	Extracorporeal membrane oxygenation
3β-Hydroxy $\Delta^5 C_{27}$ steroid dehydrogenase isomerase	Fetal arrhythmia
δ^{4-}3-Oxosteroid 5β-reductase	Budd–Chiari syndrome
Oxysterol 7α-hydroxylase	**Chromosomal disorders**
Sterol 27-hydroxylase	**Autosomal trisomies**
2-methyl-CoA-racemase CoA/amino acid *N*-acyltransferase	**Turner syndrome**
Defects in cholesterol biosynthesis	**Miscellaneous associations**
Smith–Lemli–Opitz syndrome (7-dehydrocholesterol reductase)	Neonatal leukemia
Lathosterolosis (3-β-hydroxysteroid-Δ^5-desaturase)	Histiocytosis X
Mevalonate kinase deficiency	Neonatal lupus erythematosus
	Indian childhood cirrhosis
	Graft-versus-host disease
	Erythrophagocytic lymphohistiocytosis
	Erythroblastosis fetalis
	Systemic juvenile xanthogranuloma
	Pseudo-TORCH syndrome

The genetic defect has been identified and genetic testing is either feasible or available for disorders shown in bold.
ATPase, adenosine triphosphatase; CoA, coenzyme A; HNF1β, hepatocyte nuclear factor-1β; MDR3, multidrug resistance protein 3; MRP2, multidrug resistance–related protein 2; TORCH, toxoplasmosis, other, rubella, cytomegalovirus, and herpes (congenital infections).

other time of life [24]. Unconjugated hyperbilirubinemia in the older patient is usually harmless, but in the neonate with an immature blood–brain barrier, it may be associated with deposition of free bilirubin in neuronal tissue and brain damage. In contrast, conjugated bilirubin is not toxic, but an elevated level is the most common presenting feature of liver disease in the neonate. Unconjugated jaundice is first appreciated in the head and progresses caudally to the palms and soles as the serum bilirubin increases. Jaundice becomes clinically apparent in the older child when the serum bilirubin concentration reaches 2–3 mg/dL, but the neonate may not appear icteric until the bilirubin level is over 5 mg/dL. A serum conjugated (direct) bilirubin concentration of greater than 1 mg/dL with a total bilirubin of less than 5 mg/dL or over 20% of the total bilirubin concentration if the total is more than 5 mg/dL is abnormal and requires evaluation [25]. Many clinical laboratories now employ the Ektachem method that specifically measures direct bilirubin. A serum conjugated bilirubin concentration greater than 1 mg/dL is abnormal using this assay.

The majority of infants with cholestatic liver disease present during the first month of life [11]. Differentiation of cholestatic jaundice from the common physiologic hyperbilirubinemia of the neonate or the prolonged jaundice occasionally associated with breast-feeding is essential. The initial goal of the physician must be to exclude rapidly life-threatening but potentially treatable disorders such as gram-negative infection, endocrinopathies (such as panhypopituitarism), galactosemia, and inborn errors of bile acid metabolism. Prompt identification of cholestatic infants is also required to minimize the risk of hemorrhage from vitamin K deficiency [26]. Unfortunately, some cholestatic infants may escape detection until the first well-baby examination at 6–8 weeks of age. The possibility of liver or biliary tract disease must be considered in any neonate jaundiced beyond 2 weeks of age. Between 2.4% and 15% of newborns will still be jaundiced at 2 weeks of age; the majority are breast fed. These infants should be evaluated for cholestasis by measurement of total and conjugated serum bilirubin. However, with reliable follow up, this testing may be deferred in jaundiced breast-fed infants until 3 weeks of age if stool color, urine color, and physical examination are normal. In one study, the incidence of jaundice in breast-fed babies at 4 weeks was 9%, but none had liver disease [27]. The utility of screening for neonatal liver disease remains unsettled. In a community-based study in which 27,654 neonates were tested for a serum conjugated bilirubin concentration greater than 18 μmol/L using the Ektachem method [28], a positive result requiring further testing was found in 107 babies. Gross hemolysis or insufficient sample size precluded analysis in 15.3% of the cases. Twelve babies had persistently elevated values on repeat testing, 11 of whom had confirmed liver disease including neonatal hepatitis (n = 6), biliary atresia (n = 2), hypopituitarism (n = 1), α_1-antitrypsin deficiency (n = 1), and Alagille syndrome (n = 1). The sensitivity and specificity of the test was 100% and 99.6%, respectively. General application of this approach will likely require methods to measure conjugated bilirubin on dried blood spots.

The vast majority of infants with biliary atresia appear entirely well during the first 4–6 weeks of life apart from mild jaundice. However, the apparent well-nourished appearance of infants with biliary atresia may be a factor in a delay of diagnosis. Thorough anthropometric studies show that infants with biliary atresia have significantly decreased fat stores and lean body mass [29]. The added weight of an enlarged liver and spleen and the occasional finding of subclinical ascites may account for a relatively normal weight for age and weight for length on standardized growth curves [30].

Stools of a patient with biliary atresia are acholic, but early in the course of incomplete or evolving obstruction, stools may appear normally pigmented or only intermittently pigmented. Similarly, fluctuating levels of serum bilirubin do not rule out biliary atresia [31]. Liver disease also must be suspected in a jaundiced infant whose urine is dark yellow as opposed to colorless. Mieli-Vergani et al. [32] recently reported factors contributing to delayed referral of infants with biliary atresia. Lack of follow-up of neonatal jaundice, inadequate investigation of hemorrhagic disease, misdiagnosis of breast milk jaundice, and being misled by pigmented stools or a decrease in serum bilirubin were cited as reasons for late referral. In this study, surgical relief of biliary obstruction was successful in 12 of 14 babies (86%) referred at less than 8 weeks of age but in only 13 of 36 (36%) of those over 8 weeks of age.

A number of clinical features may provide clues about the etiology of neonatal cholestasis [4,11]. Idiopathic neonatal hepatitis occurs more commonly in males, especially those born prematurely or with low birth weight; there is a familial incidence of approximately 10–15%. A second disease, possibly predisposing to liver injury, may present in up to 40% of patients without affected siblings. In contrast, biliary atresia is more common in females of normal birth weight; familial cases are rare.

A stepwise discriminant analysis by Alagille [33] of many clinical and biochemical findings identified several variables that were useful in evaluating the cholestatic infant. In a series of 288 patients, the following features occurred more commonly in infants with intrahepatic cholestasis than in those with biliary atresia: male gender (66% vs. 45%), low birth weight (2680 g vs. 3230 g), later onset of jaundice (mean, 23 days vs. 11 days), and later onset of acholic stools (mean, 30 days vs. 16 days). An enlarged liver with a firm or hard consistency was present in 53% of those with intrahepatic compared with 87% of those with extrahepatic cholestasis. The addition of another variable (progressive or irregular course of the jaundice) did not improve the results of the analysis. Thus, this study indicates that, although clinical features are useful, there are no details in the history or physical examination that can identify all cases of biliary atresia [29].

The spectrum of illness is remarkably wide in infants with cholestatic jaundice [4]. Acholic stools are a cardinal feature of biliary obstruction but also may occur as a result of severe bile secretory failure at the level of the hepatocyte [29]. The affected infant may appear remarkably well, particularly during the evolution of biliary obstruction, or may manifest hepatic failure at birth. These infants also may be small for gestational age and fail to thrive. Congenital infection may be associated with low birth weight, microcephaly, purpura, and chorioretinitis. Dysmorphic facies may be observed in association with chromosomal aberrations and with syndromatic PILBD [34]. Congenital malformations, including cardiac anomalies, polysplenia, intestinal malrotation, and situs inversus viscerum, may be found in almost a third of infants with biliary atresia [35,36]. Hepatomegaly is often a presenting feature of neonatal liver disease; in cases of large duct obstruction, the liver is firm or even hard to palpation. In the polysplenia syndrome, a midline liver may be palpable in the hypogastrium. The spleen may be enlarged with infection or as a result of advanced prenatal liver disease and fibrosis but is usually of normal size early in the course of biliary tract disease. A mass in the right upper quadrant may be felt in approximately 50% of patients with a choledochal cyst. Pruritus and xanthomata, cutaneous manifestations of chronic cholestasis, are not observed in the neonate.

Irritability, poor feeding, vomiting, and lethargy are frequent symptoms in metabolic disorders such as galactosemia and tyrosinemia [37]. Ascites, edema, and coagulopathy may be present at birth or evolve rapidly during the first weeks of life after massive loss of hepatocytes through necrosis or apoptosis [38]. A profound impairment of hepatic synthetic function, often in excess of that expected for the degree of cholestasis, may be an early indication of metabolic liver disease, such as neonatal iron storage disease or tyrosinemia. Neurologic abnormalities in the infant with liver disease may be primary symptoms, as found in mitochondrial disorders and Zellweger's syndrome, or they may be secondary to hypoglycemia, hyperammonemia, or intracranial hemorrhage [39].

EVALUATION OF THE CHOLESTATIC NEONATE

An algorithm for the investigation of the cholestatic infant is presented in Figure 9.1. The order in which this assessment proceeds may vary depending on the clinical findings that may strongly suggest a diagnosis. Table 9.3 lists the individual studies that are often used in this evaluation [40]. The optimal diagnostic strategy demands a cooperative medical and surgical effort at a center prepared to investigate and manage potentially correctable abnormalities of the biliary tree as well as hepatocellular disorders [29]. The initial assessment should confirm rapidly that cholestasis is present, provide a baseline assessment of the severity of liver dysfunction, and exclude potentially treatable infectious and metabolic disorders. Next, to establish a specific diagnosis, a comprehensive plan for investigation is outlined, which should be guided by the initial history and physical examination. Because of the frequent lack of specific clinical features and overlap of many diagnostic studies, most cholestatic infants require a stepwise, comprehensive evaluation. However, at any point during the process, a serologic test or imaging study may establish the probable cause of the liver disease. For example, ultrasonography may promptly demonstrate a choledochal cyst in a jaundiced infant, obviating the need to search for an

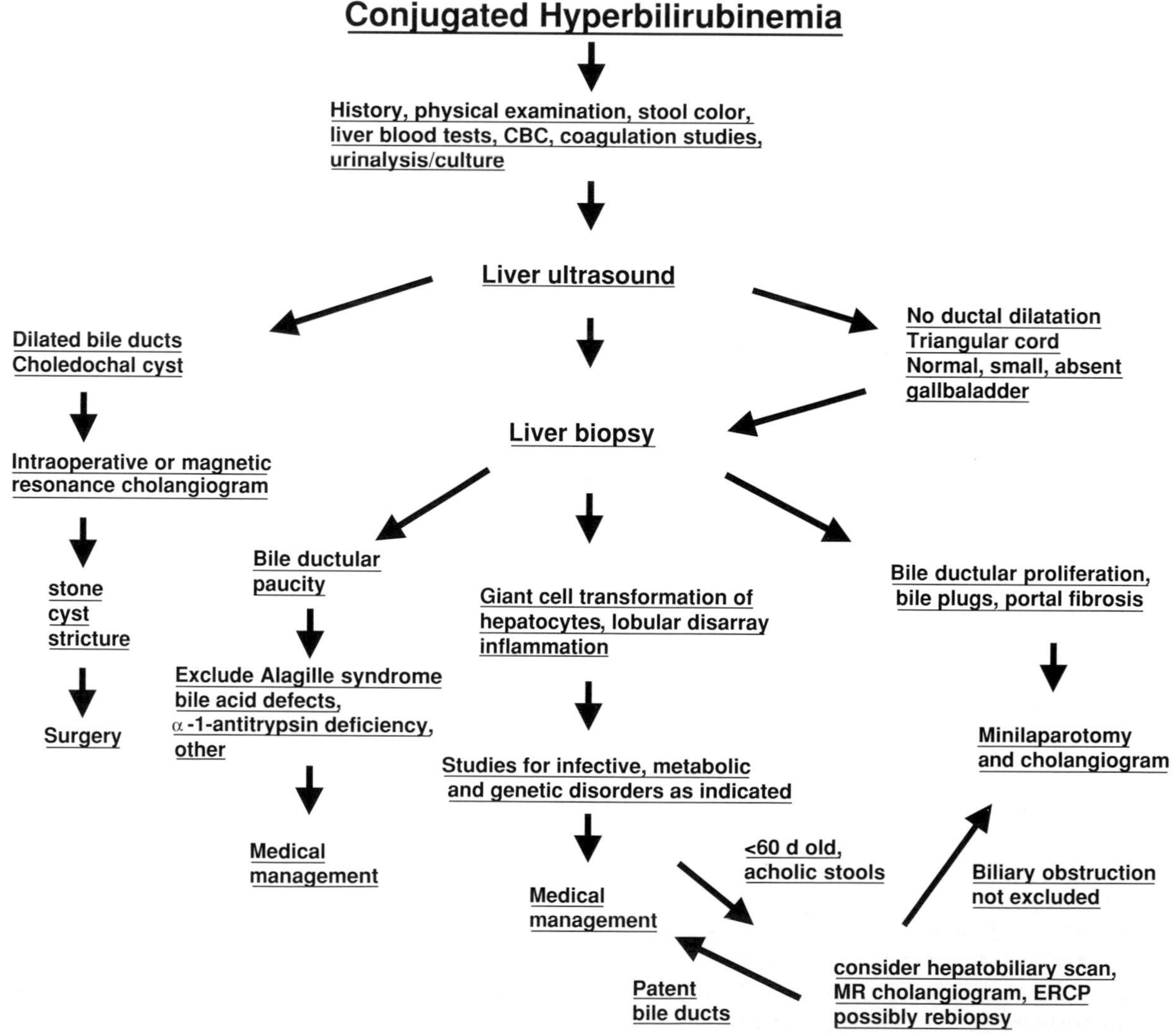

Figure 9.1. Algorithm for evaluation of neonatal cholestasis.

Table 9.3: Evaluation of the Infant with Cholestasis

Initial investigations: to establish the presence of cholestasis, define the severity of the liver disease, and detect readily treatable disorders.

- History, physical examination (including details of family history, pregnancy, early neonatal course, presence of extrahepatic anomalies, extrahepatic disease, stool color)
- Fractionated serum bilirubin analysis
- Serum tests for liver injury (ALT, AST, alkaline phosphatase, 5′-nucleotidase, γGTP)
- Tests of liver function (prothrombin time, partial thromboplastin time, coagulation factors, serum albumin, serum ammonia, serum cholesterol, serum glucose)
- Complete blood count, including platelet count
- Bacterial cultures of blood, urine, other as indicated
- Paracentesis if ascites (examine for bile and infection)

Investigations to establish a specific diagnosis

- Ultrasonography (MRC in selected cases)
- Serum α_1-antitrypsin level and phenotype
- Serologies for infectious disorders (HBsAg, TORCH, EB virus, parvovirus B19, human herpesvirus 6, HIV, other)
- Sweat chloride analysis
- Metabolic screen (urine and serum amino acids, urine organic acids)
- Serum thyroid hormone, thyroid-stimulating hormone (evaluation for hypopituitarism as indicated)
- Serum iron and ferritin
- Urine and serum analysis for bile acid and bile acid precursors
- Red blood cell galactose-1-phosphate uridyl transferase
- Viral cultures
- Genetic testing for Alagille syndrome, three forms of PFIC, other
- Hepatobiliary scintigraphy
- Radiographs of skull and long bones for congenital infection and bone dysplasia and of the chest for lung and heart disease
- Bone marrow examination and skin fibroblast culture for suspected storage disease
- Percutaneous or endoscopic retrograde cholangiography (rarely indicated)
- Percutaneous liver biopsy (routine histology, immunohistochemistry, electron microscopy, viral culture, and enzymology as required)
- Exploratory laparotomy and intraoperative cholangiogram

ALT, alanine amino transferase; AST, aspartate transaminase; EB, Epstein–Barr; γGTP, γ-guanosine triphosphate; HBsAg, hepatitis B surface antigen; HIV, human immunodeficiency virus; TORCH, toxoplasmosis, other, rubella, cytomegalovirus, herpes.
Adapted from Suchy FJ, Shneider BI. Neonatal jaundice and cholestasis. In: Kaplowitz N, ed. Liver and biliary diseases. Baltimore: Williams & Wilkins, 1992:446; with permission.

infectious or metabolic basis for the liver disease. Increasing numbers of infants will be identified as a result of neonatal screening programs. Some states are using tandem mass spectroscopy with other methods to detect as many as 40 inherited disorders, some of which may present as cholestasis in the neonate, including hypothyroidism, cystic fibrosis, and galactosemia [41].

Numerous biochemical and imaging studies have been used in an effort to distinguish between infants with intrahepatic versus obstructive cholestasis and thus avoid unnecessary surgical exploration [42]. Standard liver biochemical tests show nonspecific and variable elevation of serum direct bilirubin, aminotransferases, alkaline phosphatase, 5′-nucleotidase, and lipids [42,43]. Poor hepatic function at birth, including hypoglycemia and coagulopathy unresponsive to vitamin K, may reflect the prenatal effects of an inborn error of metabolism or an intrauterine infection. Because loss of hepatocyte mass in some metabolic disorders occurs by apoptosis rather than cell necrosis, serum aminotransferase values may be normal or only modestly elevated. Low or normal serum γ-glutamyl transpeptidase activity is found in the serum of patients with PFIC (Byler's disease), some inborn errors of bile acid metabolism, and benign recurrent cholestasis compared with other cholestatic patients [20,44]. However, no single biochemical test or imaging study or even combination of noninvasive tests has proved to be of sufficient discriminatory value in excluding extrahepatic obstruction because approximately 10% of infants with intrahepatic cholestasis have clinical and laboratory studies that overlap with results from patients with biliary atresia. The presence of bile pigment in stools is sometimes cited as evidence against complete biliary obstruction, but the physician may be misled by historical information about stool color, by feces colored by bile-stained secretions and shed epithelial cells, and by the gradual evolution of bile duct obstruction. Aspiration and visual inspection of duodenal secretions for bile pigment or measurement of radioactivity in duodenal fluid after scintigraphy have been used by some workers to distinguish intrahepatic from extrahepatic cholestasis [45].

A variety of newer diagnostic tests are becoming part of the armamentarium of the hepatologist. Any infant with intrahepatic cholestasis of obscure etiology should be evaluated for a possible inborn error of bile acid metabolism by analysis of a urine sample for abnormal bile acid metabolites by fast atom bombardment mass spectroscopy [18]. Identification of these infants is critical because some of these disorders are treatable by oral bile acid replacement. The genes for three distinct forms of PFIC and for Alagille syndrome have recently been cloned. Genetic tests for these disorders will become more readily available once the range of mutations is better defined [19].

Ultrasonography is often the most useful initial imaging modality for providing information about liver structure, size, and composition. A high-frequency, real-time examination can assess gallbladder size, detect gallstones and sludge in the bile ducts and gallbladder, demonstrate ascites, and define cystic or obstructive dilatation of the biliary tree. Extrahepatic anomalies also may be detected. Common bile duct dilatation is not a feature of biliary atresia; either the duct is not visualized or a portion of the duct appears to be of normal caliber. There may sometimes be slight dilatation of the intrahepatic bile ducts, and the gallbladder may be absent or reduced to a remnant in biliary atresia. However, these findings cannot be reliably used to diagnose biliary atresia. A triangular or tubular echogenic density or triangular cord (TC) representing a fibrous cone of tissue at the porta hepatis on a transverse or longitudinal scan has been proposed as a specific ultrasonographic finding for biliary atresia [46]. The TC sign was present in 16 of 20 patients (80%) with biliary atresia and in 1 of 66 patients with neonatal hepatitis. Use of 4-mm thickness as the criterion for TC sign resulted in a sensitivity of 80%, specificity of 98%, and positive and negative predictive values of 94% for the diagnosis of biliary atresia [47]. Absence of the gallbladder or a gallbladder with an irregular shape or wall is found in some infants with biliary atresia [48]. The sensitivity and specificity of a small or absent gallbladder in detecting biliary atresia varies from 73% to 100% and 67% to 100%, respectively, when data are compiled from several studies [25].

Computed tomography provides information similar to that obtained by ultrasonography but is usually less useful in infants because of a paucity of intra-abdominal fat for contrast and the need for heavy sedation or general anesthesia.

Magnetic resonance cholangiography (MRC), performed with T2-weighted turbo spin-echo sequences, is being widely used to assess the biliary tract in all age groups, with visualization previously possible only with transhepatic or endoscopic retrograde cholangiography (ERCP). In several pilot studies, MRC reliably demonstrated the common bile duct and gallbladder in normal neonates. Nonvisualization of the common bile duct and demonstration of a small gallbladder characterized MRC findings in a small number of patients with biliary atresia [49]. For example, in one study MRC accuracy was 82% (19 of 23); sensitivity, 90% (9 of 10); and specificity, 77% (10 of 13) for the detection of extrahepatic biliary atresia, with a positive predictive value of 75% (9 of 12) and a negative predictive value of 91% (10 of 11) [50]. Further advances will be required before reliability of MRC in evaluating the cholestatic infant can be established.

Hepatobiliary scintigraphy, using the technetium Tc 99m iminodiacetic acid derivatives, has been used to help differentiate biliary atresia from other causes of neonatal cholestasis [51]. Unfortunately, a recent study showed that 50% of patients with PILBD but no extrahepatic obstruction failed to show biliary excretion of radionuclide. Twenty-five percent of patients with idiopathic neonatal hepatitis demonstrated no biliary excretion [52]. However, the modality remains useful for assessing cystic duct patency in a patient with a hydropic gallbladder or with cholelithiasis.

Percutaneous transhepatic cholangiography or cholecystocholangiography may be required to visualize the biliary tract in selected patients [53]. However, these techniques are more difficult to perform in infants because of the small size of the intrahepatic bile ducts and because most of the disorders in this age group do not result in dilatation of the intrahepatic bile ducts.

Endoscopic retrograde cholangiography may be useful in the evaluation of selected infants with obstructive cholestasis [54,55]. In a recent study, ERCP was performed successfully under general anesthesia in 43 of 50 infants (86%) with prolonged cholestasis. Six of seven infants in whom ERCP failed had biliary atresia diagnosed by exploratory laparotomy. The other patient had a choledochal cyst. Twenty-nine of the 43 patients in whom complete visualization of the biliary tree was not achieved had biliary atresia diagnosed by exploratory laparotomy. Complete visualization of the biliary tree was obtained in 14 patients, including 9 with neonatal hepatitis, 2 with PILBD, and 3 with a choledochal cyst. ERCP also provides detailed information on anomalous arrangement of the pancreaticobiliary junction in patients with choledochal cysts. Considerable technical expertise is necessary for a successful examination in infants. Most require general anesthesia for a satisfactory examination. The greater availability of specially designed pediatric duodenoscopes will facilitate the use of ERCP in infants with obstructive cholestasis.

Percutaneous liver biopsy remains one of the important diagnostic steps in evaluating the cholestatic infant and may be performed in even the smallest infants using only local anesthesia and sedation. In several studies, a diagnosis of biliary atresia was possible in 90–95% of cases. A recent report found that liver biopsy was 100% sensitive and 76% specific in detecting biliary atresia [56]. The characteristic features of large duct obstruction include bile duct proliferation, bile plugs in small bile ducts, and portal tract edema and fibrosis [57]. The basic lobular architecture is usually intact. However, these findings require time to develop and may not all be present in biopsy samples taken in the first weeks of life. Thus, serial assessment, possibly a repeat liver biopsy, may be required until a specific diagnosis is established or extrahepatic obstruction is clearly excluded [58]. In patients with intrahepatic disease, diffuse cellular swelling and giant cell transformation of hepatocytes, variable inflammation, and focal hepatocellular necrosis are commonly observed. Fibrosis, bile ductular injury, and even bile duct paucity may be present. Pseudoacinar arrangement of hepatocytes and steatosis suggest a metabolic liver disease. Abnormal storage of material in hepatocytes or Kupffer cells and viral inclusions also may be found. Electron microscopy and immunohistochemical methods may aid in the identification and localization of these abnormalities. Liver tissue also may be frozen for later biochemical or molecular analysis.

Lai et al. [59] have studied the diagnostic efficacy of many of the approaches that have been covered individually in this chapter and that were used in a 3-day evaluation. One hundred twenty-six infants, including 84 with neonatal hepatitis (age 65.1 ± 24.1 days) and 42 with biliary atresia (age 60.3 ± 31.1 days), were studied prospectively. The diagnostic accuracy of various methods was as follows: liver histology, 96.8%; color of duodenal juice, 91.6%; peak radioisotope count in duodenal juice, 84.2%; ultrasonographic examination of the hepatobiliary system, 80.2%; and persistence of clay-colored stool, 80.2%. After stepwise logistic regression, the diagnostic methods of significance were liver biopsy, color of duodenal juice, abdominal ultrasonography, and stool color. However, stool color and the onset of jaundice could not differentiate severe neonatal hepatitis from biliary atresia. The diagnostic methods of significance then were liver biopsy and duodenal juice color. With this 3 day protocol, an overall diagnostic accuracy of 96.8% was attained. No cases of biliary atresia were missed, although four cases of neonatal hepatitis were misdiagnosed, resulting in unnecessary laparotomy.

In cases consistent with a diagnosis of biliary atresia or in the small number of cases in which doubt persists about the diagnosis after review of the imaging studies and liver biopsy, the patency of the biliary tree should be directly examined at the time of a minilaparotomy and intraoperative cholangiogram [29]. The adverse effects of a diagnostic laparotomy are minimal. High-risk patients with features of liver failure including uncorrectable coagulopathy, hepatic encephalopathy, and ascites do not have biliary atresia and do not require surgical exploration. The surgeon should avoid transecting a biliary tree that is patent but small in diameter because of biliary hypoplasia or a low rate of bile flow associated with severe intrahepatic cholestasis [60]. Moreover, the dynamic nature of the neonatal obstructive cholangiopathies is exemplified by rare cases in which the patency of the extrahepatic bile ducts was initially proved on cholangiopathy but evolution to biliary atresia was later documented at autopsy or laparotomy.

REFERENCES

1. Pearson HA. Lectures on the diseases of children by Eli Ives, MD, of Yale and New Haven: America's first academic pediatrician. Pediatrics 1986;77:680–6.
2. Trauner M, Meier PJ, Boyer JL. Molecular pathogenesis of cholestasis. N Engl J Med 1998;339:1217–27.
3. Koopen NR, Muller M, Vonk RJ, et al. Molecular mechanisms of cholestasis: causes and consequences of impaired bile formation. Biochim Biophys Acta 1998;22:1–17.
4. Suchy FJ. Neonatal cholestasis. Pediatr Rev 2004;25:388–96.
5. Dick MC, Mowat AP. Hepatitis syndrome in infancy – an epidemiological survey with 10 year follow up. Arch Dis Child 1985; 60:512–16.
6. Danks DM, Campbell PE, Jack I, et al. Studies of the aetiology of neonatal hepatitis and biliary atresia. Arch Dis Child 1977; 52:360–7.
7. Nio M, Ohi R, Miyano T, et al. Five- and 10-year survival rates after surgery for biliary atresia: a report from the Japanese Biliary Atresia Registry. J Pediatr Surg 2003;38:997–1000.
8. Yoon PW, Bresee JS, Olney RS, et al. Epidemiology of biliary atresia: a population-based study. Pediatrics 1997;99: 376–82.
9. Fischler B, Haglund B, Hjern A. A population-based study on the incidence and possible pre- and perinatal etiologic risk factors of biliary atresia. J Pediatr 2002;141:217–22.
10. Stormon MO, Dorney SF, Kamath KR, et al. The changing pattern of diagnosis of infantile cholestasis. J Paediatr Child Health 2001;37:47–50.
11. Bezerra JA, Balistreri WF. Cholestatic syndromes of infancy and childhood. Semin Gastrointest Dis 2001;12:54–65.
12. Landing BH. Considerations of the pathogenesis of neonatal hepatitis, biliary atresia and choledochal cyst – the concept of infantile obstructive cholangiopathy. Prog Pediatr Surg 1974;6: 113–39.
13. Lefkowitch JH. Biliary atresia. Mayo Clin Proc 1998;73:90–5.

14. Davenport M, Betalli P, D'Antiga L, et al. The spectrum of surgical jaundice in infancy. J Pediatr Surg 2003;38:1471–9.
15. Metzman R, Anand A, DeGiulio PA, et al. Hepatic disease associated with intrauterine parvovirus B19 infection in a newborn premature infant. J Pediatr Gastroenterol Nutr 1989;9:112–14.
16. Ozaki Y, Tajiri H, Tanaka-Taya K, et al. Frequent detection of the human herpesvirus 6–specific genomes in the livers of children with various liver diseases. J Clin Microbiol 2001;39:2173–7.
17. Jacquemin E, Lykavieris P, Hadchouel M, et al. Transient neonatal cholestasis: origin and outcome. J Pediatr 1998;133:563–7.
18. Bove KE, Heubi JE, Balistreri WF, Setchell KD. Bile acid synthetic defects and liver disease: a comprehensive review. Pediatr Dev Pathol 2004;7:315–34.
19. Emerick KM, Whitington PF. Molecular basis of neonatal cholestasis. Pediatr Clin North Am 2002;49:221–35.
20. Carlton VE, Pawlikowska L, Bull LN. Molecular basis of intrahepatic cholestasis. Ann Med 2004;36:606–17.
21. Thompson R, Strautnieks S. BSEP: function and role in progressive familial intrahepatic cholestasis. Semin Liver Dis 2001;21:545–50.
22. Kahn E. Paucity of interlobular bile ducts. Arteriohepatic dysplasia and nonsyndromic duct paucity. Perspect Pediatr Pathol 1991;14:168–215.
23. Yehezkely-Schildkraut V, Munichor M, Mandel H, et al. Nonsyndromic paucity of interlobular bile ducts: report of 10 patients. J Pediatr Gastroenterol Nutr 2003;37:546–9.
24. Balistreri WF. Intrahepatic cholestasis. J Pediatr Gastroenterol Nutr 2002;35(suppl 1):S17–23.
25. Moyer V, Freese DK, Whitington PF, et al. Guideline for the evaluation of cholestatic jaundice in infants: recommendations of the North American Society for Pediatric Gastroenterology, Hepatology and Nutrition. J Pediatr Gastroenterol Nutr 2004;39:115–28.
26. Vorstman EB, Anslow P, Keeling DM, et al. Brain haemorrhage in five infants with coagulopathy. Arch Dis Child 2003;88:1119–21.
27. Crofts DJ, Michel VJ, Rigby AS, et al. Assessment of stool colour in community management of prolonged jaundice in infancy. Acta Paediatr 1999;88:969–74.
28. Powell JE, Keffler S, Kelly DA, Green A. Population screening for neonatal liver disease: potential for a community-based programme. J Med Screen 2003;10:112–16.
29. Sokol RJ, Mack C, Narkewicz MR, Karrer FM. Pathogenesis and outcome of biliary atresia: current concepts. J Pediatr Gastroenterol Nutr 2003;37:4–21.
30. Sokol RJ, Stall C. Anthropometric evaluation of children with chronic liver disease. Am J Clin Nutr 1990;52:203–8.
31. Davenport M. Biliary atresia. Semin Pediatr Surg 2005;14:42–8.
32. Mieli-Vergani G, Howard ER, Portman B, Mowat AP. Late referral for biliary atresia – missed opportunities for effective surgery. Lancet 1989;1:421–3.
33. Alagille D. Cholestasis in the first three months of life. Prog Liver Dis 1979;6:471–85.
34. Kamath BM, Piccoli DA. Heritable disorders of the bile ducts. Gastroenterol Clin North Am 2003;32:857–75, vi.
35. Carmi R, Magee CA, Neill CA, et al. Extrahepatic biliary atresia and associated anomalies: etiologic heterogeneity suggested by distinctive patterns of associations. Am J Med Genet 1993;45:683–93.
36. Sokol RJ, Mack C. Etiopathogenesis of biliary atresia. Semin Liver Dis 2001;21:517–24.
37. Kelly DA, McKiernan PJ. Metabolic liver disease in the pediatric patient. Clin Liver Dis 1998;2:1–30.
38. van den Anker JN, Sinaasappel M. Bleeding as presenting symptom of cholestasis. J Perinatol 1993;13:322–4.
39. Goncalves I, Hermans D, Chretien D, et al. Mitochondrial respiratory chain defect: a new etiology for neonatal cholestasis and early liver insufficiency. J Hepatol 1995;23:290–4.
40. Suchy FJ. Clinical problems with developmental anomalies of the biliary tract. Semin Gastrointest Dis 2003;14:156–64.
41. Rinaldo P, Tortorelli S, Matern D. Recent developments and new applications of tandem mass spectrometry in newborn screening. Curr Opin Pediatr 2004;16:427–33.
42. Balistreri WF, A-Kader HH, Setchell KD, et al. New methods for assessing liver function in infants and children. Ann Clin Lab Sci 1992;22:162–74.
43. Rosenthal P. Assessing liver function and hyperbilirubinemia in the newborn. National Academy of Clinical Biochemistry. Clin Chem 1997;43:228–34.
44. Maggiore G, Bernard O, Hadchouel M, et al. Diagnostic value of serum gamma-glutamyl transpeptidase activity in liver diseases in children. J Pediatr Gastroenterol Nutr 1991;12:21–6.
45. Rosenthal P, Miller JH, Sinatra FR. Hepatobiliary scintigraphy and the string test in the evaluation of neonatal cholestasis. J Pediatr Gastroenterol Nutr 1989;8:292–6.
46. Kanegawa K, Akasaka Y, Kitamura E, et al. Sonographic diagnosis of biliary atresia in pediatric patients using the "triangular cord" sign versus gallbladder length and contraction. AJR Am J Roentgenol 2003;181:1387–90.
47. Lee HJ, Lee SM, Park WH, Choi SO. Objective criteria of triangular cord sign in biliary atresia on US scans. Radiology 2003;229:395–400.
48. Farrant P, Meire HB, Mieli-Vergani G. Ultrasound features of the gall bladder in infants presenting with conjugated hyperbilirubinaemia. Br J Radiol 2000;73:1154–8.
49. Ryeom HK, Choe BH, Kim JY, et al. Biliary atresia: feasibility of mangafodipir trisodium-enhanced MR cholangiography for evaluation. Radiology 2005;235:250–8.
50. Norton KI, Glass RB, Kogan D, et al. MR cholangiography in the evaluation of neonatal cholestasis: initial results. Radiology 2002;222:687–91.
51. Johnson K, Alton HM, Chapman S. Evaluation of mebrofenin hepatoscintigraphy in neonatal-onset jaundice. Pediatr Radiol 1998;28:937–41.
52. Gilmour SM, Hershkop M, Reifen R, et al. Outcome of hepatobiliary scanning in neonatal hepatitis syndrome. J Nucl Med 1997;38:1279–82.
53. Meyers RL, Book LS, O'Gorman MA, et al. Percutaneous cholecysto-cholangiography in the diagnosis of obstructive jaundice in infants. J Pediatr Surg 2004;39:16–18.
54. McKiernan PJ. Neonatal cholestasis. Semin Neonatol 2002;7:153–65.
55. Iinuma Y, Narisawa R, Iwafuchi M, et al. The role of endoscopic retrograde cholangiopancreatography in infants with cholestasis. J Pediatr Surg 2000;35:545–9.

56. Zerbini MC, Gallucci SD, Maezono R, et al. Liver biopsy in neonatal cholestasis: a review on statistical grounds. Mod Pathol 1997;10:793–9.
57. Finegold MJ. Common diagnostic problems in pediatric liver pathology. Clin Liver Dis 2002;6:421–54.
58. Kahn E. Biliary atresia revisited. Pediatr Dev Pathol 2004;7:109–24.
59. Lai MW, Chang MH, Hsu SC, et al. Differential diagnosis of extrahepatic biliary atresia from neonatal hepatitis: a prospective study. J Pediatr Gastroenterol Nutr 1994;18:121–7.
60. Markowitz J, Daum F, Kahn EI, et al. Arteriohepatic dysplasia. I. Pitfalls in diagnosis and management. Hepatology 1983;3:74–6.

10

Medical and Nutritional Management of Cholestasis in Infants and Children

Andrew P. Feranchak, M.D., and Ronald J. Sokol, M.D.

When first encountering an infant or child with cholestatic liver disease, it is essential that diagnostic evaluation be conducted promptly in order to (i) recognize disorders amenable either to specific medical therapy (e.g., galactosemia, tyrosinemia, hypothyroidism, urinary tract infection) or to early surgical intervention (e.g., biliary atresia, choledochal cyst), (ii) institute treatment directed toward enhancing bile flow, and (iii) prevent and treat the varied medical, nutritional, and emotional consequences of chronic liver disease. Because many of the treatable causes require early diagnosis and prompt institution of therapy, the evaluation of the cholestatic infant should never be delayed. Although "physiologic cholestasis" (hypercholemia, or elevated bile acids) may be present in the infant, there is no state of "physiologic conjugated hyperbilirubinemia." For the jaundiced infant, historical and clinical information such as color of the stools, birth weight, and presence of hepatomegaly may provide important clues as to the etiology of cholestasis. Consanguinity or liver disease in siblings suggests the possibility of metabolic, familial, or genetic disease. Review of the prenatal and postnatal course may reveal intrauterine infection, occurrence of hypoglycemia or seizures, and exposure to toxins/drugs (i.e., total parenteral nutrition [TPN]). Careful physical examination may reveal features of typical disorders or syndromes. For the older child and adolescent, a history of exposure to drugs/toxins (e.g., acetaminophen), the presence of vascular insufficiency, and the presence of underlying disease (e.g., inflammatory bowel disease) provide helpful clues. The diagnostic evaluation of the infant with cholestasis is detailed in Chapter 9.

Once the diagnosis is made, a limited number of disorders are amenable to specific treatments. Although less than 10% of infants with neonatal cholestasis are found to have treatable medical disorders, the individual patient will derive important benefits from early diagnosis and treatment. Those infants found to require surgical correction of anatomic causes of cholestasis likewise require early identification and therapy for optimal outcome [1]. A classification scheme relating the availability of specific therapy to the individual causes of prolonged neonatal cholestasis is listed in Table 10.1. In the majority of cases in which there is no "curable" etiology or in which surgical correction of biliary atresia is unsuccessful, medical management is largely supportive; directed at inducing choleresis, optimizing growth and nutrition, minimizing discomfort and disability, and aiding the child and his family in coping with the stress, social, and emotional effects of chronic liver disease. The success of therapeutic intervention, however, is limited by the residual functional capacity of the liver and by the rate of progression of the underlying liver disease. Because orthotopic liver transplantation (OLT) in children has become standard therapy for end-stage liver disease, it is increasingly important to optimize the care, growth, and development of children with chronic liver disease in order to enhance their chances for successful liver transplantation.

The ultimate prognosis for an affected child is related to the severity of the complications resulting from chronic cholestasis. These complications are attributable directly or indirectly to diminished bile flow and reflect (i) retention of substances normally excreted in bile (bile acids, bilirubin, cholesterol, and trace elements) with resultant hepatocyte apoptosis and necrosis and induction of portal fibrosis progressing to portal hypertension, cirrhosis, and liver failure; (ii) transfer of constituents of bile into the systemic circulation, leading to pruritus, fatigue, hypercholesterolemia, and xanthoma formation; and (iii) reduced delivery of bile to the small bowel with decreased intraluminal bile acid concentrations, leading to malabsorption of fat and fat-soluble vitamins. These departures from normal physiology lead to discomfort, failure to thrive, specific nutrient deficiencies, and psychological/behavioral problems in the developing child. A summary of medical treatment options for cholestasis, including medications, doses, and toxicity, is found in Table 10.2 [2–43].

RETENTION OF BILE CONSTITUENTS

Hepatocellular Injury

Pathogenesis of Cholestatic Injury

The retention of endogenous bile acids in the hepatocyte during cholestasis is believed to be involved in the pathogenesis of progressive liver injury and may lead to perpetuation

Table 10.1: Treatable Causes of Neonatal Cholestasis

Disease	*Liver Involvement*	*Treatment*	*References*
Congenital infectious hepatitis			
Herpes simplex virus	Coagulative necrosis	Intravenous (IV) acyclovir	[2]
Syphilis	Hepatitis, periportal and interlobular fibrosis	IV penicillin G (50,000 units/kg/d for 10–14 d)	[3,4]
Listeria monocytogenes infection	Granulomatous hepatitis	IV ampicillin (neonatal doses)	[5,6]
Tuberculosis	Granulomatous hepatitis	Consult neonatal infectious disease expert	[7]
Toxoplasmosis	Cholestasis	Pyrimethamine (1 mg/kg every 2–4 d) and sulfadiazine (50–100 mg/kg/d) for 21 d	[8,9]
HIV	Cholestasis	Consult neonatal infectious disease expert	
Metabolic diseases			
Galactosemia	Cholestasis, steatosis, fibrosis, cirrhosis	Galactose-free diet	[10,11]
Hereditary tyrosinemia	Steatosis, fibrosis, cirrhosis	Low tyrosine/phenylalanine diet, NTBC	[12–18]
Hereditary fructose intolerance	Steatosis, fibrosis	Fructose/sucrose-free diet	[19,20]
Hypothyroidism/hypopituitarim	Cholestasis	Thyroid, adrenal, growth hormone replacement	[21]
Cystic fibrosis	Biliary mucus plugging, cholestasis, focal biliary cirrhosis, multilobular cirrhosis, cholelithiasis	Oral pancreatic enzyme replacement, pulmonary therapy, fat-soluble vitamin supplements, UDCA	[22,23]
Bile acid synthesis defects:			
Δ^4-3-oxosteroid-5β-reductase def.	Cholestasis, giant-cell hepatitis	UDCA and cholic acid	[24,25]
3β-hydroxysteroid dehydrogenase/isomerase def.	Cholestasis, giant-cell hepatitis	UDCA	[26,27]
Neonatal iron storage disease	Cholestasis, fibrosis, cirrhosis	Antioxidant therapy,* liver transplantation	[28]
Drugs and toxins			
Drugs	Variable	Discontinue drug	[29]
Bacterial endotoxin (sepsis, urinary tract infections, etc.)	Cholestasis, hepatocyte necrosis	Appropriate IV antibiotic therapy	[6,30,31]
TPN-associated	Cholestasis, steatosis, bile duct proliferation, portal fibrosis, cirrhosis	Institute early enteral feedings, avoid excessive (IV) calories and protein, use neonatal amino acid solutions, ursodeoxycholic acid (?)	[32–36]
Anatomic lesions			
Extrahepatic biliary atresia	Cholestasis, bile duct proliferation, fibrosis, cirrhosis	Hepatoportoenterostomy	[1,37–39]
Choledochal cyst	Cholestasis, fibrosis, cirrhosis	Choledochoenterostomy	[40]
Spontaneous perforation of common bile duct	Peritonitis, ascites, cholestasis	Surgical drainage	[41]
Inspissated bile/calculi in common bile duct	Cholestasis, bile duct proliferation, fibrosis, cirrhosis	Biliary tract irrigation	[42,43]

*Vitamin E (TPGS) 25 IU/kg/d oral; desferrioxamine 15 mg/kg/h IV continuous infusion until ferritin <500 μg/L; selenium 2–3 μg/kg/d IV (in TPN); *N*-acetylcysteine 70 mg/kg/dose every 4 hr via nasogastric tube or IV for 20 doses.

NTBC, 2-(2-nitro-4-trifluoromethylbenzoyl)-1,3-cyclohexanedione; TPGS, tocopherol polyethylene glycol-1000 succinate; TPN, total parenteral nutrition; UDCA, ursodeoxycholic acid.

Reproduced with permission from Sokol RJ. Medical management of neonatal cholestasis. In: Balistreri WF, Stocker JT, eds. Pediatric hepatology. Philadelphia: Hemisphere Publishing Corporation, 1990:43.

Table 10.2: Medical Treatment Options for Cholestasis

Treatment	*Indications*	*Dosage*	*Toxicity*
Bile acid–binding agents: cholestyramine, colestipol, aluminum hydroxide antacids, sucralfate (?)	Hypercholesterolemia Xanthoma Pruritus Hypercholemia (?)	250–500 mg/kg/d (cholestyramine and colestipol)	Constipation Hyperchloremic acidosis Binding of drugs Increased steatorrhea Intestinal obstruction
Naltrexone	Pruritus	50 mg/d (adults)	Nausea, headache Hepatotoxicity (?) Opioid withdrawal reactions
Phenobarbital	Hypercholesterolemia Pruritus Hypercholemia (?)	3–10 mg/kg/d	Drowsiness Behavior changes Interference with vitamin D metabolism Risk for suicide and suicidal behavior
Rifampicin	Pruritus	10 mg/kg/d	Hepatotoxicity Drug interactions Hemolytic anemia Renal failure
Ursodeoxycholic acid	Pruritus Hypercholesterolemia Cholestasis Cystic fibrosis liver disease	20–30 mg/kg/d	Diarrhea Increased pruritus Hepatotoxicity (?)
Antihistamines	Pruritus	Diphenhydramine, 5–10 mg/kg/d Hydroxyzine, 2–5 mg/kg/d	Drowsiness
Ultraviolet B light	Pruritus		Skin burn
Carbamazepine	Pruritus	20–40 mg/kg/d	Hepatotoxicity, bone marrow suppression, fluid retention, behavioral changes

Reproduced with permission from Sokol RJ. Medical management of neonatal cholestasis. In: Balistreri WF, Stocker JT, eds. Pediatric hepatology. Philadelphia: Hemisphere Publishing Corporation, 1990:48–9.

of cholestasis [44]. It has been shown that the hydrophobic bile acids (i.e., monohydroxy and dihydroxy bile acids) are more hepatotoxic than the hydrophilic bile acids (trihydroxy bile acids and ursodeoxycholic acid [UDCA]) [45]. These differences in hepatotoxicity may be related to effects on membrane properties, inhibition of microsomal enzymes, generation of free radicals, stimulation of cellular death receptors on the plasma membrane, activation of protein kinase signaling pathways, and induction of pathologic mitochondrial permeability [46–48]. The mitochondrial permeability transition is caused by opening of a large channel in the inner mitochondrial membrane, with subsequent mitochondrial swelling, impaired oxidative phosphorylation, and release of cytochrome *c* into the cytosol, and is believed to be a key event triggering hepatocyte necrosis and apoptosis. Hydrophobic bile acids (e.g., conjugates of chenodeoxycholic acid) stimulate the permeability transition and cause necrosis of hepatocytes at high concentrations [48] and induce apoptosis at lower concentrations [49,50], both of which appear to involve oxidant stress. Antioxidants and UDCA appear to protect the mitochondria from the bile acid–induced permeability transition [51]. In the pathogenesis of cholestatic liver injury, it appears that hydrophobic bile acids play an important role in activation of death receptors, induction of the mitochondrial permeability transition, and various intracellular pathways of apoptosis and cellular necrosis.

To counteract the effects of retained toxic bile acids, several agents have been proposed to improve choleresis. Choleretic agents such as UDCA, tauroursodeoxycholic acid (TUDCA), and phenobarbital may potentially minimize the toxic effects of bile acids by enhancing hepatocyte excretion of bile acids into bile, improving bile acid–independent bile flow, stabilizing hepatocyte membranes, and protecting hepatocyte mitochondria from the permeability transition [51–54]. In addition, UDCA and TUDCA may be hepatoprotective by displacing toxic bile acids in the bile acid pool [55–57] and by producing a bicarbonate-rich hypercholeresis [58]. Phenobarbital induces hepatic microsomal enzymes and increases bile acid–independent bile flow [59–61].

Treatment with Choleretic Agents

Ursodeoxycholic Acid

Ursodeoxycholic acid is the major bile acid of the black bear and has been used for centuries in traditional Chinese and Japanese medicine for the treatment of gallbladder and liver disease [62–64]. UDCA ($3\alpha,7\beta$-dihydroxy-5β-cholan-24-oic acid), which normally occurs in only small quantities (<3%) in human bile, is formed by 7β-epimerization of the primary bile salt, chenodeoxycholic acid, through the action of colonic bacteria. The difference in the position of the hydroxyl group (β instead of α) confers the marked hydrophilicity of UDCA as compared with chenodeoxycholic acid.

Several mechanisms have been proposed to explain the potential beneficial effects of UDCA in the treatment of cholestatic liver diseases. Because intracellular retention of hydrophobic bile acids is thought to lead to liver cell injury, replacement of these compounds with a nontoxic hydrophilic bile acid such as UDCA should theoretically reduce injury. UDCA may be hepatoprotective by displacing toxic bile acids from both the bile acid pool [65] and hepatocellular membranes [65]. In vitro studies have demonstrated that UDCA has a direct hepatoprotective effect on cultured hepatocytes exposed to toxic, hydrophobic bile acids [52–54]. In addition, UDCA has been shown to improve mitochondrial oxidative phosphorylation [66] and prevent the mitochondrial membrane permeability transition, a key signaling pathway in both apoptotic and necrotic cell death [47]. In vivo studies in the rat have also shown that administration of UDCA (either enterally or parenterally) ameliorates the effects of hydrophobic bile acid–induced cholestasis [57,67]. Although this cytoprotective effect may be the result of direct stabilization of the hepatocyte membrane, UDCA may also work by altering the bile salt pool with a decrease in hydrophobic bile salts. UDCA is poor at micelle formation and solubilization and is poorly absorbed from the proximal intestine [68,69]. Therefore, a large amount of orally administered UDCA reaches the terminal ileum, where it interferes with the absorption of endogenous, more hydrophobic, and toxic bile acids [68]. Studies have demonstrated a significant increase in serum UDCA concentration (from 2–40%) during UDCA therapy, with a corresponding decrease in serum chenodeoxycholic and cholic acid levels [70]. In addition to its effects on the bile salt pool composition, UDCA has a direct hypercholeretic effect. In rats, unconjugated UDCA secreted by the liver becomes protonated in the biliary ductule. The protonated UDCA is very lipophilic and is rapidly reabsorbed by biliary epithelial cells before reaching the small intestine, transported back to the liver, and secreted again [68,71,72]. This "cholehepatic shunt" mechanism leads to a significant hypercholeresis [68,73]. Recently, identification of bile acid transporters on both the cholangiocyte apical (luminal) and basolateral membranes has provided a more mechanistic understanding of this process [74,75]. In addition to the effect on bile salt–dependent bile flow, UDCA also increases bile salt–independent flow through a direct effect on cholangiocyte Ca^{2+}-activated Cl^- secretion [58], resulting in bicarbonate-rich choloresis [76]. Lastly, UDCA may have an important immunomodulatory role, reducing immunologic injury associated with some cholestatic liver diseases [77,78]. Whereas normal hepatocytes do not express human leukocyte antigen (HLA) class 1 or 2, cholestasis may induce abnormal HLA class 1 expression in these cells, resulting in cytotoxic T cell–mediated lysis and further liver injury [78–80]. In vivo studies in the mouse [81] and patients with primary biliary cirrhosis (PBC) [82,83] have shown that UDCA therapy leads to a reduction in the expression of abnormal HLA class 1 proteins on hepatocytes.

The observation that some patients with chronic active hepatitis demonstrated improvement in biochemical markers of liver injury when treated for gallstones with UDCA led to trials of UDCA for a wide variety of cholestatic liver diseases. The evidence supporting use of UDCA for the treatment of specific cholestatic liver diseases is reviewed in the following sections.

PRIMARY BILIARY CIRRHOSIS

The therapeutic efficacy of UDCA has been best demonstrated in the treatment of the cholestatic adult disease PBC, an autoimmune fibrosing cholangiopathy. UDCA treatment markedly improves serum liver tests as shown by four large randomized, double blind, placebo controlled trials of adults treated with doses of 10–15 mg/kg/d for 2 years [84–87]. More importantly, UDCA treatment has been shown to improve pruritus [84–87] and histologic features of liver injury and fibrosis [84,85], reduce the development of esophageal varices [88], and increase liver transplant–free survival [89,90]. In one study, transplant-free survival increased by approximately 25% in patients treated with UDCA (13–15 mg/kg/d) compared with placebo after 48 months of therapy [89]. The most significant effect was demonstrated in those patients with cirrhosis or higher serum bilirubin levels. Recently, the cost-effectiveness of UDCA in the treatment of PBC has also been established [91]. Therefore, UDCA is safe, efficacious, and cost-effective in the treatment of adults with PBC, although it does not prevent progressive disease in all patients. Unfortunately, the data establishing the effectiveness of UDCA in other adult and childhood cholestatic disorders have not been as definitive.

PRIMARY SCLEROSING CHOLANGITIS

In randomized, controlled studies, UDCA has been shown to improve serum liver tests [92,93], improve liver histology [92], and decrease HLA class 1 expression on hepatocytes [94] in adults with primary sclerosing cholangitis (PSC). Although there was an improvement of symptoms (pruritis, fatigue) in several uncontrolled studies, this was not observed in larger, controlled studies [92,95,96]. In addition, there was exacerbation of pruritus and worsening biochemical parameters when UDCA was discontinued. UDCA has not been shown to significantly affect long-term survival [93], and no reliable data are available regarding the effect of UDCA on possible delay to liver transplantation, development of cholangiocarcinoma, or cost-effectiveness. Also it is not clear if there is any effect of UDCA on the activity of ulcerative colitis, often accompanying PSC. Diarrhea is a rare side effect of UDCA, which may complicate any associated colitis. The use of UDCA in PSC initially appeared promising; however, long-term controlled trials have yet to demonstrate that therapy alters the natural progression of the disease. Clinical trials using larger doses of UDCA in PSC are currently in progress. No controlled trials have been conducted in pediatric patients with PSC.

CYSTIC FIBROSIS

The best data demonstrating a therapeutic effect of UDCA in pediatric cholestatic disorders are in the treatment of cystic fibrosis (CF). Clinically significant liver disease develops in 10–20% of patients with CF, and 5–10% develop cirrhosis by adolescence [97,98]. The pathogenesis of CF-associated liver disease remains speculative. One model suggests that liver injury is the result of the retention of hepatotoxic bile salts secondary to obstruction of bile ducts by inspissated secretions and viscid mucus [23]. This provides a logical rationale for the use of UDCA as a potential cytoprotective agent and stimulator of bicarbonate-rich bile flow. Prospective clinical trials of UDCA in pediatric patients with CF liver disease at doses of 10–20 mg/kg/d for 6–12 months have shown significant improvement in alanine aminotransferase (ALT), alkaline phosphatase, and γ-glutamyltransferase (GGT) [22,99–101] and demonstrated that these effects persist even after 2 years of treatment [99]. A double-blind multicenter trial demonstrated improved biochemical and clinical parameters (as measured by the Shwachman score) after 1 year of treatment with UDCA (15 mg/kg/d) [22]. Several studies have reported a dose-response for UDCA in CF liver disease with maximal effect at a dosage of 20 mg/kg/d, suggesting that higher doses of UDCA may be necessary in CF compared with other forms of cholestasis [100,102]. In addition to improvement of liver blood tests in CF liver disease, radionuclide hepatobiliary scintigraphy documented improved hepatobiliary excretory function and presumably bile secretion after treatment with 15–20 mg/kg/d of UDCA for 10–12 months [103]. In a 2-year uncontrolled study, UDCA therapy improved the liver histology, with less inflammation and bile duct proliferation, in seven of ten patients with CF-related liver disease [104]. Lastly, UDCA may improve the nutritional status of patients with CF-related liver disease, including rises in serum essential fatty acid [105], retinol [105], and vitamin E levels [106]. Despite the improved biochemical, biliary excretory, and perhaps histologic data, it remains to be seen whether UDCA alters the natural course of liver disease in patients with CF. Although there is a need for long-term pediatric studies, it appears prudent to use UDCA in CF patients with evidence of liver disease as recommended by the Cystic Fibrosis Foundation Hepatobiliary Disease Consensus Group [23].

ALAGILLE SYNDROME

In a study of 31 patients with Alagille syndrome, Balistreri et al. [107–109] demonstrated a decrease in serum ALT and cholesterol levels and a marked improvement in pruritus during UDCA therapy. Fifteen of the 31 patients had an initial clinical response with a decrease in pruritus after 1 month of therapy (15–30 mg/kg/d). Eleven of the 16 initial nonresponders showed improvement with an increase in the dose of UDCA (45 mg/kg/d). Several case studies have also reported an improvement in pruritus and serum liver enzyme, cholesterol, triglyceride, and phospholipid levels [110,111]. However, although there was complete resolution of cutaneous xanthomas in one patient, UDCA did not prevent the progression of liver disease [111]. Although further studies are desirable, these preliminary reports suggest that the use of UDCA in Alagille syndrome is warranted. However, there are no data available as to alteration of the natural history of Alagille syndrome by UDCA therapy.

PROGRESSIVE FAMILIAL INTRAHEPATIC CHOLESTASIS

Progressive familial intrahepatic cholestasis (PFIC) is a group of childhood cholestatic diseases with at least three different subtypes: PFIC type 1, or Byler's disease, caused by mutations in the gene *FIC-1* (*ATP8B1*, associated with normal serum GGT levels); PFIC type 2, resulting from a defect in the canalicular bile salt export pump (BSEP) (*ABCB11*, associated with normal GGT levels); and PFIC type 3, or multidrug resistance protein 3 (MDR3) deficiency (*ABCB4*, associated with elevated GGT levels). Jacquemin et al. [26] used UDCA (20–30 mg/kg/d) in 39 patients divided into two groups based on serum GGT levels (Group 1 had normal GGT and Group 2, elevated GGT). After 2–4 years of therapy, liver tests normalized in 32%, improved in 20%, and worsened in 48% in Group 1, whereas in Group 2, liver tests normalized in 50%, improved in 29%, and worsened in 21% [26]. In an open trial of UDCA in 27 patients with PFIC, Balistreri et al. [108,109] noted an improvement in liver tests and pruritus in 85% of patients during UDCA treatment (15 mg/kg/d). Although long-term data are lacking, empiric therapy with UDCA appears worthwhile in patients with PFIC. UDCA has not been effective in patients with benign recurrent intrahepatic cholestasis (BRIC) [112,113].

BILE ACID SYNTHESIS DEFECTS

Several distinct abnormalities in primary bile salt synthesis have been described including Δ^4–3-oxosteroid-5β-reductase deficiency and 3β-hydroxysteroid dehydrogenase/isomerase deficiency. In these inherited defects, primary bile acid synthesis is absent or markedly impaired. Δ^4–3-Oxosteroid-5β-reductase deficiency results in increased synthesis of abnormal oxo-bile acids and neonatal liver failure. Patients with this defect have demonstrated a dramatic response to combined UDCA and cholic acid therapy with suppression of oxo-bile synthesis, normalization of liver blood tests, marked improvement in liver histology, and long-term survival of a presumably fatal disorder [24,25]. 3β-Hydroxysteroid dehydrogenase/isomerase deficiency is clinically similar to PFIC, with low GGT; however, patients do not have pruritus. The failure of normal bile acid synthesis and the accumulation of atypical bile acids in this disorder presumably account for the progressive liver injury.

Treatment with UDCA alone results in a dramatic improvement and a return to completely normal liver function [24,27,114], although most patients also receive cholic acid therapy.

BILIARY ATRESIA

Although initial reports suggested that UDCA might be beneficial in biliary atresia after portoenterostomy, a preliminary report of a randomized, double-blinded, placebo-controlled trial failed to demonstrate any benefit of UDCA [115]. However, other reports suggested that UDCA therapy improved bile flow [116], reduced episodes of cholangitis [117], and resulted in improved weight gain [116–119] in these children. Further studies are needed to determine whether subgroups of patients with biliary atresia (e.g., those with recurrent cholangitis after the establishment of bile flow) will benefit from UDCA therapy. Clearly, when portoenterostomy is unsuccessful or has not been performed, UDCA is of no benefit in biliary atresia.

TPN-ASSOCIATED CHOLESTASIS

Ursodeoxycholic acid has been shown to improve bile flow and decrease serum bilirubin levels in an animal model of TPN-associated cholestasis [35]. Spagnuolo et al. [36] reported seven children with cholestasis while on long-term TPN that responded to oral therapy with UDCA with a decrease in liver tests. One limitation to the use of UDCA in patients at risk for the development of TPN-associated cholestasis is poor intestinal absorption of UDCA in patients with short gut. However, Schwarzenberg and Bundy [120] have suggested that UDCA may bind bacterial endotoxin in the gut lumen and prevent its absorption, thereby reducing activation of Kupffer cells, inhibiting tumor necrosis factor (TNF) generation, and reducing liver injury. This mechanism could explain a beneficial effect of UDCA therapy in children with short gut syndrome and bacterial overgrowth of the small bowel.

Recently a controlled study of enteral supplementation with TUDCA was conducted of 22 infants with short bowel syndrome and cholestasis. TUDCA (30 mg/kg/d) was given in one group, which was compared with a concurrent untreated group. There were no differences in liver blood tests or total and conjugated bilirubin for up to 120 days of TPN administration [121]. Concerns were raised about the poor biliary enrichment of the TUDCA, most likely as a consequence of poor intestinal absorption. Thus, oral treatment with UDCA is, likewise, unlikely to yield a benefit in infants with short bowel syndrome and cholestasis.

CHRONIC VIRAL HEPATITIS

Ursodeoxycholic acid has been studied in a number of randomized placebo-controlled trials for the treatment of chronic hepatitis C infection. Although the addition of UDCA to interferon therapy significantly prolonged the normalization of ALT [122,123], UDCA failed to affect the elimination rate of viral RNA [122,124] or improve liver histology [122,125]. Further studies are needed to determine if UDCA has any role in the long-term therapy of chronic viral hepatitis.

REJECTION FOLLOWING ORTHOTOPIC LIVER TRANSPLANTATION

Given the role of UDCA as an immunomodulator [82,126,127] and its ability to alter HLA expression on hepatocytes during cholestasis [79,80], the use of UDCA as adjunctive therapy with immunosuppression has been evaluated. Although two large studies have not detected an effect of UDCA on the incidence of acute allograft rejection [128,129], a third study demonstrated fewer patients with multiple rejection episodes [130]. The present data, therefore, do not support the routine use of UDCA in most patients after OLT.

HEPATIC VENO-OCCLUSIVE DISEASE AND GRAFT-VERSUS-HOST DISEASE

Ursodeoxycholic acid has been used both prophylactically and in the treatment of hepatic complications related to bone marrow transplantation. Compared with a historical control group, prophylactic treatment with UDCA decreased serum bilirubin levels, reduced the incidence of veno-occlusive disease (VOD), and improved survival after bone marrow transplantation [131]. In an open-label study, marked improvement of serum liver tests was observed in patients with graft-versus-host disease (GVHD) of the liver. However, biochemical abnormalities returned after discontinuation of UDCA [132]. Although further data are desirable, UDCA may be considered for the treatment of liver GVHD and in the prevention of VOD following bone marrow transplantation, particularly in patients at high risk because of the type of chemotherapy used.

In summary, the use of UDCA has proven long-term benefit in adult PBC and childhood bile acid synthesis defects. Although further studies are needed, it appears prudent to use UDCA in the treatment of PSC, CF-associated liver disease, Alagille syndrome, PFIC, GVHD, and VOD. There has been no proven benefit of its use in TPN-associated cholestasis, biliary atresia, chronic hepatitis, or OLT. It must be pointed out that, at present, no UDCA trials in children with cholestasis have shown that UDCA therapy has altered the ultimate course of the underlying liver disease or survival, with the exception of bile acid synthesis defects [133]. However, most experience shows that it is safe to use in infants and children who do not have fixed obstruction to bile flow.

Tauroursodeoxycholic Acid

Concerns regarding the long-term use of UDCA have included its poor enteral absorption during cholestasis [134], poor biliary enrichment of the unconjugated form [134], and increased biotransformation to more hydrophobic bile acids, such as lithocholic acid [135,136]. Several recent studies have therefore focused on other hydrophilic bile acids, including TUDCA, the taurine conjugate of UDCA. TUDCA has been shown in vitro and in vivo to have greater cytoprotective effects than UDCA [57,137–139]. Possible mechanisms of its hepatoprotective action include membrane enrichment and stability [140], enhanced Kupffer cell phagocytosis [141], and calcium homeostasis and hepatocyte exocytosis [49,142]. Data from animal studies [143,144] and from preliminary trials in patients with PBC [137,145,146] suggest that TUDCA is better absorbed, induces more favorable changes in the composition of the bile salt pool, and undergoes less biotransformation to hydrophobic species when compared with UDCA. Preliminary, short-term studies in adults with PBC demonstrated that TUDCA was equally as beneficial as UDCA, with comparable doses (500 mg/d), in lowering serum liver enzyme levels. However, higher TUDCA doses (1000 and 1500 mg/d) resulted in greater bile pool enrichment with hydrophilic bile acids, both UDCA and TUDCA, and a significant decrease in both total and high-density lipoprotein (HDL) cholesterol [138,146]. These preliminary studies are encouraging, and further long-term adult trials and investigational trials in pediatric cholestatic disorders appear warranted. As stated previously, TUDCA does not appear to be effective in treating TPN-associated cholestasis in the infant with short bowel syndrome.

Phenobarbital

Phenobarbital therapy has been used for years as a choleretic and antipruritic agent for many cholestatic liver diseases. By increasing the bile acid–independent fraction of bile flow [59], enhancing bile acid synthesis [60], inducing hepatic microsomal enzymes [147], and increasing hepatic Na-K-ATPase activity [148], it has been used in cholestasis to decrease serum bilirubin, lower circulating serum bile acids, and, by its hepatic microsomal stimulation and excretory enhancement, possibly help in the elimination of a pruritogenic substance. The usual dose of phenobarbital is 3–10 mg/kg/d, aimed at achieving a serum level of approximately 10–20 μg/mL [148–150]. High-dose phenobarbital therapy may be associated with sedation, and alterations in the metabolism of a wide variety of drugs, including vitamin D, may occur [151]. One long-term study [152], however, showed that phenobarbital did not impede the response to vitamin D supplements for treatment of concomitant rickets. More importantly, chronic phenobarbital therapy in children with seizure disorders has been associated with poor self-esteem, labile moods, neurotic symptoms, frank depression, and an increased risk for suicide and suicidal behavior [153–155]. In a small cohort of epileptic patients who developed depression while on phenobarbital therapy, discontinuation of phenobarbital use was associated with resolution of depression [156]. A modest decline in social competency among these children was also observed [156], but this was thought to be attributed to the underlying chronic epilepsy. Although detailed study has not been conducted on the effects of phenobarbital on cognitive and behavior functions in children with chronic cholestasis, with the availability of other medications that reduce pruritus and stimulate bile flow, phenobarbital treatment is now used rarely for the treatment of cholestasis.

Glucocorticoids

Although steroids have not been used as long-term choleretic agents, high-dose "bursts" of intravenous methylprednisolone have been shown to be effective in stimulating bile flow during episodes of refractory cholangitis after hepatic portoenterostomy treatment for extrahepatic biliary atresia [157]. It should be pointed out that this report was generated before the availability of more potent antibiotics that have broad spectra against enteric organisms and reach good bile levels. Short-term intravenous corticosteroid therapy is frequently used routinely in Asia following portoenterostomy for biliary atresia. One recent U.S. study demonstrated an improvement in conjugated bilirubin levels and transplant-free survival in a group of patients with biliary atresia following portoenterostomy when treated with high-dose steroids in conjunction with antibiotics and UDCA compared with those who did not receive steroid treatment [158]. However, the lack of randomization confounds the interpretation of this and other reports of steroid use following portoenterostomy. Several controlled randomized studies are now in progress. There have not been any studies to suggest a beneficial effect of long-term steroid administration in cholestatic disorders; in view of the many complications of chronic steroid therapy, its use for chronic cholestasis is not warranted.

Cholecystokinin

Cholecystokinin (CCK), a peptide hormone secreted by the intestine in response to a meal, stimulates gallbladder contraction, relaxes the sphincter of Oddi, and increases intestinal motility. A synthetic CCK-octapeptide (sincalide) has been developed and is believed to be of potential benefit in treating cholestasis associated with abnormal gallbladder function, such as TPN-associated cholestasis, in which lack of enteral nutrition is associated with a decrease in endogenous CCK secretion. Several small trials of sincalide have been conducted in the pediatric population. In a study of eight postoperative infants with TPN-associated cholestasis, administration of a lyophilized porcine preparation of CCK caused a rapid decline in serum conjugated bilirubin levels and resolution of acholic stools [159]. In another uncontrolled study of 11 surgical infants (9 were premature) with TPN-associated cholestasis, sincalide treatment reduced serum bilirubin levels; however, no significant improvement in serum aminotransferases was observed [160]. Lastly, a small study suggests that prophylactic sincalide treatment may potentially decrease the development of TPN-associated cholestasis in infants on parenteral nutrition; however, some benefit in the treatment group may have been the result of the institution of enteral feeds [161]. In a recently completed large multicenter randomized, controlled trial of sincalide in infants at risk for TPN-associated cholestasis, 243 infants were enrolled and received twice-daily CCK-octapeptide or placebo [162]. CCK did not affect conjugated bilirubin levels, sepsis incidence, time to achieve 50% and 100% energy intake enterally, morality rate, incidence of cholelithiasis, or number of intensive care unit and hospital days. Based on these results, sincalide should not be recommended for prevention of TPN-associated cholestasis in infants at risk.

Nuclear Receptor Agonists

The identification of the proteins involved in hepatic bile acid uptake, transport, and excretion has provided a more mechanistic model of liver transport functions in both health and disease. Identification of these transport proteins has provided insight into the pathogenesis of many cholestatic liver disorders while advancing our basic knowledge of normal liver transport functions. One exciting area has been the identification of the regulatory pathways involved in the transcription and expression of these transport proteins [163], which involve the binding of ligands to specific nuclear receptors that regulate transcription. Several nuclear receptors have been identified that regulate bile acid transport proteins and enzymes involved in bile acid synthesis, including the farnesoid X receptor (FXR), the constitutive androstane receptor (CAR), and the pregnane X receptor (PXR). Identification of these nuclear receptors suggests a new category of agents to treat cholestasis, namely, specific receptor activators that will alter the expression of bile acid transporters directly.

Farnesoid X receptor is highly expressed in the liver and activated by bile acids such as the hydrophobic bile acid, chenodeoxycholic acid (CDCA) [163]. Binding of bile acids to FXR up-regulates transcription of genes coding for BSEP, MDR3, and multidrug resistance–related protein 2 (MRP2), proteins responsible for the export of bile acids from the hepatocyte. FXR activation also inhibits the transcription of CYP7A and CYP8B, both involved in bile acid synthesis, and hence provides feedback inhibition of bile acid synthesis. There has, therefore, been considerable interest in developing agonists of FXR to harness these potential hepatoprotective pathways. Recently, a synthetic FXR agonist, GW4064, was shown to reduce liver damage in a rat model of cholestasis [164]. Another FXR agonist, 6-ethyl chenodeoxycholic acid, has been shown to protect rats from ethinyl estradiol–induced cholestasis by increasing expression of BSEP and MRP2 and decreasing synthesis of the Na^+/taurocholate cotransporter (Ntcp) [165].

Consititutive androstane receptor is another nuclear receptor found in liver and plays an important role in the detoxification of bile acids as well as mediating the response to phenobarbital. CAR appears to abrogate the hepatotoxicity associated with lithocholic acid [166]. CAR agonists, including the herbal medicine Yin Zhi Huang and phenobarbital, have been shown to reduce bile acid levels in adults with PBC as well as bilirubin levels in neonates [167]. Another nuclear receptor, PXR, is closely related to CAR and regulates genes in the pathways affecting hepatic oxidation, conjugation, and transport [168,169]. Interestingly, rifampicin is a ligand for PXR; therefore, the antipruritic effects of this drug may be by direct modulation of bile acid synthesis and transport activity [170].

Clearly the area of transcriptional regulation of the enzymes and proteins involved in bile acid synthesis and transport warrant further study. In the future, the use of nuclear receptor agonists may provide another useful therapeutic strategy in the treatment of cholestasis.

Progressive Fibrosis and Cirrhosis

Pathogenesis of Liver Fibrosis

The long-term survival of children with chronic cholestatic liver disease will ultimately depend on the residual functional capacity of the liver and the rate of progression of the underlying disorder. Chronic cholestatic liver disease is, with rare exception, associated with hepatic fibrosis, a complex process that involves changes in the amounts of extracellular matrix (ECM) components, activation of cells capable of producing matrix materials (e.g., hepatic stellate cells, fibroblasts), cytokine release, and tissue remodeling [171–173]. One result of the matrix protein accumulation is an imbalance in the relationship between the hepatic parenchymal cells and their blood supply, ultimately leading to increased intrahepatic vascular resistance, microcirculatory ischemia, and consequent portal hypertension, which are the hallmarks of hepatic cirrhosis. Although recent research has led to a greater understanding of the biologic importance of the major macromolecules of the ECM in the pathogenesis of excessive collagen deposition, disturbances in hepatocyte growth, and regeneration and repair during progressive hepatic fibrosis, there is no established therapy to attenuate hepatic fibrogenesis. Current antifibrotic therapy is directed toward (a) modulation of inflammatory mediators that stimulate hepatic stellate cells to proliferate and increase collagen production and (b) stimulation of collagenase and other proteinases.

Treatment

Several antifibrotics have been evaluated in clinical trials. Colchicine is an antifibrogenic drug that suppresses collagen biosynthesis directly by inhibiting polymerization of microtubules and blocking transcellular movement of procollagen [174,175]. In addition, it has inhibitory effects on anti-inflammatory cells, reducing their ability to stimulate production of ECM components [176] and accelerating breakdown of collagen by stimulating collagenase activity [177]. Clinical trials of colchicine in adults with various types of cirrhosis have variably shown improvement in biochemical liver tests [178–180] and improvement in liver biopsy histologic patterns [180]. More recent long-term studies in adults report no influence of colchicine therapy on progression of disease in patients with PBC [181] and no improvement in hepatic histology in patients who have been treated for 8 years [182]. A recent large placebo-controlled, double-blinded trial of colchicine for 2–6 years in 549 adults with alcohol-induced cirrhosis has been completed and found no effect of colchicine on mortality, complications of portal hypertension, or liver fibrosis [183]. Thus, this drug cannot be recommended for adults with cirrhosis until there is evidence supporting its use.

In a pilot trial of colchicine involving 17 children with a variety of neonatal cholestatic disorders followed over 5–10 years, colchicine did not appear to significantly prevent hepatic failure or portal hypertension or alter outcome [182]. The small numbers of patients with individual liver diseases make interpretation of these results difficult. Hatziioannidou et al. [184] reported the preliminary findings of a randomized, double-blind trial of colchicine in children with biliary atresia. A dose of 25 μg/kg/d for 4 years was not associated with any difference in need for liver transplantation or measures of morbidity. The colchicine was well tolerated. Further study of colchicine in other cholestatic disorders associated with significant hepatic fibrosis is indicated.

Two other antifibrogenic agents that have been studied in adults with liver disease are d-penicillamine and glucocorticoids. The use of D-penicillamine in conditions of hepatic fibrogenesis was suggested by its inhibition of intra- and intermolecular collagen cross-linking [185,186] in addition to its cupruretic activity [187]. Prospective trials of D-penicillamine in patients with PBC, however, failed to show any significant clinical or histologic benefit or improvement in survival [188–190]. Significant toxicity (bone marrow suppression, rash, dysgeusia) was observed relatively frequently in these trials. Thus, D-penicillamine is not used as an antifibrogenic agent in adults. In addition to their anti-inflammatory effects, glucocorticoids are believed to decrease collagen synthesis by different mechanisms [191–194]. However, the unacceptable systemic effects of long-term glucocorticoid therapy (including osteoporosis) preclude its aggressive use to treat hepatic fibrogenesis. Antioxidants (e.g., vitamin E) have been shown to reduce fibrogenesis in animal models of cirrhosis induced by chemical agents [195], possibly by the reduction of lipid peroxide products that can stimulate collagen synthesis in hepatic stellate cells [196,197]. Preliminary studies in adults with hepatitis C viral infection suggest a reduction in stellate cell activation and extracellular matrix during vitamin E therapy [198]. Further evaluation of the potential use of antioxidants in cholestatic liver disease is in progress.

Finally, a number of herbal preparations and combinations may reduce hepatic fibrosis in animal models and are under study in humans [199].

Understanding the role of the hepatic stellate cell in the progressive fibrosis associated with many cholestatic disorders may lead to new treatment strategies to prevent ongoing cellular injury and interrupt fibrogenesis [200]. Although a number of antifibrogenic agents that target stellate cells are in the development phase and may prove to be beneficial in the future, the role of antifibrotic agents in the treatment of cholestatic disorders requires further study. The development of new agents to reduce fibrogenesis based on the molecular mechanisms of fibrogenesis will hopefully lead to more effective medical therapy to prevent progression to cirrhosis.

TRANSFER OF BILE CONSTITUENTS INTO SYSTEMIC CIRCULATION

Defective hepatocyte canalicular transport results in hepatocyte retention of components of bile, with leakage or transport of these substances into the hepatic sinusoid, raising serum levels of bile acids, bilirubin, and triglycerides. Additionally, transfer of biliary phospholipids into plasma may lead to increased circulating levels of cholesterol and triglycerides. Other mechanisms contributing to elevated systemic concentrations of bile acids, cholesterol, and triglycerides include decreased uptake of bile acids by the hepatocyte [201], down-regulation of basolateral bile acid transporters [202,203], and alterations in cholesterol synthesis and metabolism. Evidence suggests that during cholestasis, hepatocytes demonstrate decreased uptake of bile acids due to down-regulation of Ntcp on the basolateral membrane [203]. Although this altered uptake may play a hepatoprotective role, by preventing further accumulation of toxic bile acids in the hepatocyte, it further contributes to the systemic elevation of bile acids. Although the mechanisms underlying elevated serum levels of bile acids, cholesterol, and triglyceride may be complex, the end result leads to significant and debilitating complications, including pruritus, fatigue, hyperlipidemia, and cutaneous xanthomas.

Pruritus

Pruritus is a distressing manifestation of both intrahepatic and extrahepatic cholestasis. Its severity varies from mild, with no interference of normal activities, to moderate, with disturbance of sleep, to severe and intractable [204]. Because of incessant scratching, the resulting open skin lesions may predispose to secondary bacterial skin infections (especially staphylococcal and streptococcal) and disfiguring scars. Interference with sleep at night and the inability to concentrate and be attentive at school may impair normal development and school performance. In adults, severe pruritus has driven some patients with primary biliary cirrhosis to contemplate suicide. Unremitting, severe pruritus may in itself be an indication for liver transplantation [205]. Usually, the pruritus is generalized, with the palms and soles, extensor surfaces of the extremities, face and ears, and upper trunk most severely affected. Children with paucity of interlobular bile duct disorders, PFIC, unsuccessful or failing portoenterostomy for treatment of biliary atresia, PSC, cholestatic forms of autoimmune chronic hepatitis, and BRIC appear to be most severely affected with pruritus. Patients with bile acid synthesis and metabolism defects generally do not experience pruritus.

Pathogenesis

The pathogenesis of the pruritus of cholestasis is poorly understood. Penicillate intraepidermal nerve endings, which arise from unmyelinated subepidermal free nerve endings, have been implicated as the sensors that mediate general pruritus [206]; however, the mediators that stimulate these nerve endings during cholestasis are still unknown. Earlier studies suggested that elevated serum and skin concentration of bile acids were responsible [207,208], but a direct causal relationship between itching and bile acid levels in skin and/or serum has not been confirmed [209–211]. Other evidence refuting the role of bile acids in pruritus is the reduction of pruritus in patients with uremia [212] and polycythemia vera [213], disease states not associated with bile acid retention, by cholestyramine treatment. However, the absence of pruritus in children with bile acid synthesis defects and those with low serum concentrations of bile acids despite significant cholestasis argues for a role of circulating bile acids [24,114].

More recent evidence suggests that a significant component of the pruritus may be of central neurogenic origin, possibly involving the opiate receptor system [204,214,215]. This is based on the observation that pruritus is a recognized side effect of morphine [216,217] and other opiate receptor agonists [218,219]. Indeed, physicians who use meperidine for sedation before procedures are familiar with the "itching of the nose" behavior associated with the administration of this medication [220]. This opioid-associated pruritus is reversed by opiate receptor antagonists, such as naloxone [218,219,221], but not by antihistamines [216,218,222]. The central effect of opiates is mediated via opiate receptors in the brain. Bergasa et al. [223] injected serum from patients with PBC into the medullary dorsal horn of monkeys and induced itching, which was blocked by the opioid receptor antagonist naloxone. In addition, Bergasa and colleagues have shown, in a rat model of cholestasis, that binding of a selective μ-opioid receptor ligand to μ-opioid receptors is altered in cholestasis. These μ-opioid receptors were observed to be down-regulated, suggesting that cholestasis may be associated with chronically elevated levels of endogenous opioids [224]. In a study of patients with chronic cholestatic liver disease, nalmefene, a specific oral opiate receptor antagonist, produced symptoms strikingly similar to the "withdrawal reaction" of opiate addiction [225,226]. This observation suggests that patients with cirrhosis and impaired hepatocellular function were chronically exposed to increased levels of endogenous opiate receptor agonists [204], and is further supported by the finding of elevated levels of the endogenous opiate ligands methionine enkephalin and leucine enkephalin in these patients [214,227]. Furthermore, other evidence suggests that these elevated plasma levels of pentapeptide enkephalins allow them to cross the blood–brain barrier [228–230]. Preliminary reports on the beneficial effects of opiate receptor antagonists (naloxone and nalmefene) [214,222,231] in the pruritus of cholestasis likewise support the concept that increased availability of endogenous opiate ligands at central opiate receptors may stimulate the pruritus of cholestasis.

Treatment

The therapeutic agents most commonly used for pruritus in cholestasis are oral bile acid–binding resins (cholestyramine or colestipol) [209,232–234], phenobarbital [59–61,147, 148,150,152,235], rifampicin [235–239], UDCA, [78,84,240, 241], and carbamazepine [242]. Cool baths, moisturizers, topical steroid creams, topical anesthetics, antihistamines, and sedatives have offered little long-term relief, although they may be of temporary benefit in individual patients. In small children, fingernails should be trimmed, long-sleeve nightshirts worn, and occasionally the hands covered securely with stockings at night to minimize the effects of scratching. Plasmapheresis and ultraviolet light treatment have improved pruritus in adults with PBC [243–247]. The possible use of opioid antagonists is being explored. Finally, partial biliary diversion, ileal exclusion, and liver transplantation are considered when all other therapeutic options have been exhausted.

NONABSORBABLE ION EXCHANGE RESINS

Cholestyramine, colestipol, and colesevelam hydrochloride are nonabsorbable anion exchange resins that bind bile acids, cholesterol, many drugs, and presumably other toxic agents in the intestinal lumen, thereby increasing fecal excretion of these substances. These bile acid–binding agents interrupt the enterohepatic circulation of bile acids, decreasing the negative feedback to the liver, enhancing conversion of cholesterol to bile acids, and possibly stimulating a choleresis. Because of the possible long-term benefit of reducing hepatic accumulation of potentially toxic bile acids [233], these agents are recommended for long-term management of intrahepatic cholestatic disorders [232,234]. Because cholestyramine relieves pruritus without causing a change in serum bile acids [248], it is possible that it also removes other anionic molecules that may be contributing to pruritus [209].

Cholestyramine and colestipol are usually administered mixed with juice or water at a dosage of 0.25–0.50 g/kg/d, given either before and after breakfast, when bile flow is maximal, or less commonly divided among two or three daily meals. Colestipol appears to be better tolerated than cholestyramine; however, cholestyramine bars are now available and are more palatable [249]. No other medications or vitamins should be given orally for the 2 hours preceding or following administration of these resins because of the risk of binding to the resin and impaired absorption. Several other factors limit the use of cholestyramine and colestipol: the unpalatable nature of the compounds (which may lead to poor compliance); increased steatorrhea and fat-soluble vitamin deficiency due to further reduction in the already low concentrations of free bile acids in the intestinal lumen; constipation; intestinal obstruction due to inspissation of the drug; and hyperchloremic metabolic acidosis. These compounds are generally contraindicated in the infant with biliary atresia and a Roux-en-Y portoenterostomy because of the risk that the compound may accumulate in and obstruct the reconstructed biliary intestinal conduit, leading to ascending cholangitis.

RIFAMPICIN

Studies suggest that rifampicin, an antibiotic for tuberculosis, is an effective treatment for severe pruritus in primary biliary cirrhosis [235,236,238,239] and in children with chronic cholestatic liver disease [237,250]. In a comparison of rifampicin with phenobarbitone for treatment of pruritus in biliary cirrhosis [236], 19 of 21 patients who completed a 2-week course of rifampicin (10 mg/kg/d) had significant relief from pruritus compared with only 8 of 18 who took phenobarbitone (3 mg/kg/d). For both drugs, relief of pruritus occurred after the first week of administration, and both had similar effects in lowering serum aminotransferase levels and in inducing hepatic microsomal function. Rifampicin, however, reduced alkaline phosphatase, γ-glutamyl transpeptidase, and serum bile acid levels that did not respond to phenobarbitone. A reduction in severe pruritus with rifampicin treatment was also observed in a double-blind crossover randomized trial of rifampicin (300–450 mg/d) versus placebo in adults; however, no significant changes in serum alkaline phosphatase or serum bile acid levels were seen [235]. Cynamon et al. [237] conducted a double-blind crossover study of five children with chronic cholestatic liver disease using a dosage of 10 mg/kg/d (maximum = 300 mg/d) of rifampicin. Rifampicin proved effective in all five children compared with placebo, and its effectiveness was maintained for 6 months. As in the adult study [235], no significant changes in serum aminotransferase, bilirubin, or total bile acid levels were observed throughout the study. One patient developed transient elevation of his ALT, which did not appear to be related to rifampicin treatment.

Recently, Yerushalmi et al. [250] treated 24 children with cholestasis with rifampicin (10 mg/kg/d in two divided doses). After an average of 18 months of therapy, 10 patients had a complete response and 12 patients had a partial response as assessed by a clinical scoring system. Treatment was associated with a reduction in GGT, and no clinical or biochemical toxicity of rifampicin was observed. Complete response was more common in children with extrahepatic cholestasis (e.g., biliary atresia) than intrahepatic cholestasis (64% vs. 10%). In a study by Gregorio et al. [251] using a slightly lower average dosage of rifampicin (5 mg/kg/d; range, 4–10 mg/kg/d), complete response was observed in 15% and a partial response in 36% of patients with chronic cholestasis. The lower response rate may reflect the large number of patients with intrahepatic cholestasis in this study, who may not respond as favorably to treatment [250].

The precise mechanisms of rifampicin action on pruritus are unknown. By enhancing hepatic microsomal enzyme activities [252] and inhibiting bile acid uptake into the hepatocyte [253], it is believed to facilitate metabolism and urinary excretion of dihydroxy and monohydroxy bile acids [239] and toxic bile acids such as hyocholate and ω-muricholate [254]. Rifampicin is also a ligand for the nuclear receptor PXR; activation of downstream target genes of PXR that control bile acid metabolism may explain the action of rifampicin. Despite the apparent amelioration of pruritus with rifampicin and the lack of toxicity noted in three pediatric series [237,250,251], its propensity for toxic hepatitis [255,256] requires careful monitoring. The other potential adverse effects associated with its use are drug interactions [257,258], hemolytic anemia [236], and renal failure [236,259]. We have been very pleased with the response of children with a variety of cholestatic disorders to rifampicin treatment.

OPIOID ANTAGONISTS

Given the theory that cholestasis-associated pruritus may be caused by centrally mediated increased opioid tone, the use of several opioid antagonists, including naloxone, nalmefene, and naltrexone, has been investigated. Bernstein and Swift [222] with the use of naloxone first reported relief of pruritus in a woman with PBC unresponsive to conventional therapies. Following this, a small cross-over study in eight patients with PBC and a larger double-blind, controlled crossover trial in 29 patients with liver diseases of various causes demonstrated marked improvement in pruritus during intravenous 24-hour naloxone infusions compared with placebo [260]. Mild neuropsychiatric disturbances, described as "ill-defined anxiety," were reported in four patients in the larger study and no patients in the pilot study. This complication may be explained by a mild opiate withdrawal effect in the presence of chronic increased opioid tone postulated to exist in patients with cholestasis [215,261]. Because of the opioid receptor specificity of the action of naloxone, these findings support the hypothesis that a mechanism underlying the pruritus of cholestasis is modulated by endogenous opioids. Although effective, naloxone has several limitations for long-term use, including a short half-life and large first-pass metabolism, which necessitate intravenous administration.

Nalmefene, another opioid antagonist, has a longer duration of action compared with naloxone and can be given orally; however, at the present time it is only available in the United States as a parenteral product [261,262]. In an initial report of 11 patients with cirrhosis, nalmefene therapy (starting at a dosage of 5 mg/d and gradually increasing to a maximum of 20–40 mg three times daily) resulted in a significant reduction in patients' pruritus scores and sense of fatigue [214]. Distressingly, all 11 patients experienced withdrawal reactions consisting of nausea, abdominal pain, diaphoresis, tremor, and occasional hallucinations. Larger doses of nalmefene (up to 300 mg) given to healthy subjects have not produced withdrawal reactions [262], once again supporting the theory of increased opioid tone in patients with cholestasis-associated pruritus. A recent open-label trial of oral nalmefene also demonstrated a beneficial effect in relieving pruritus, but with fewer adverse reactions reported [263]. In this study of 14 adult patients with cholestasis, the initial starting dosage was 2 mg twice a day and was gradually increased over 2–4 weeks until a satisfactory clinical response was achieved (average maintenance dosage was 60 mg/d, with a range of 20–240 mg/d) and continued for 2–26 months. Only 5 patients experienced withdrawal-like reactions, which did not preclude continuation of therapy. A significant decrease in visual analogue scores was noted in 13 patients, and a decrease in scratching activity was noted in 12 patients. Possible tolerance occurred in 3 patients, and 3 patients experienced a marked exacerbation of pruritus after therapy was suddenly discontinued. This uncontrolled study suggests that orally administered nalmefene is of benefit to patients with cholestasis-associated pruritus and is associated with fewer withdrawal reactions with the lower starting dose.

The opioid antagonists investigated to date have severe limitations. Naloxone has a short half-life and can only be administered parenterally, whereas nalmefene treatment is associated with a severe opiate withdrawal reaction and is not currently licensed for clinical use. These limitations have prompted investigation of other opioid antagonists. Naltrexone is an opiate receptor antagonist with a bioavailability and half-life that lie between those of naloxone and nalmefene and can be administered orally. It is a structural analogue of naloxone and nalmefene that undergoes extensive first-pass metabolism; however, the main metabolite, 6β-naltrexol, reaches higher plasma levels than does the parent drug and exerts long-lasting opiate antagonist activity [264]. An initial trial of oral naltrexone (50 mg/d for 1 week) decreased pruritus scores in three of five patients with cholestasis. Two patients withdrew from the study because of severe nausea and emesis [265]. A larger double-blind, placebo-controlled study demonstrated significant decreases in both daytime and nighttime itching (as recorded by the patient using the visual analogue scale) [264]. In this study, 16 adult patients with cholestasis were randomized to receive oral naltrexone (50 mg/d for 4 weeks, n = 8) or placebo (n = 8). Compared with the placebo group, the naltrexone-treated group had significantly decreased pruritus scores at the end of treatment, with associated improvement in sleep satisfaction and less fatigue compared with baseline scores before treatment. Withdrawal reactions were noted in four patients in the treatment group but were generally transient, with the exception of one patient who required discontinuation of treatment. Naltrexone may be an effective alternative therapy for patients with cholestasis-associated pruritus unresponsive to other antipruritics; however, larger, long-term studies are needed. The initial concern over possible hepatotoxicity of naltrexone in studies of alcoholism was not validated in a review of adult patients who received naltrexone for 12 weeks [266]. Nausea (9%) and headaches (6%) were the most common side effects of naltrexone in this study.

The use of opioid antagonists may provide an effective alternative treatment for patients with severe pruritus unresponsive to other therapies; however, the significant side effects and withdrawal reactions may severely limit the general use of these medications. Further placebo-controlled trials are needed to determine safety, proper dosage, and long-term efficacy in pediatric patients with cholestatic liver disease. Concerns of the effects of chronic opioid antagonism in the developing brain will need to be addressed as well.

PHENOBARBITAL

In addition to its choleretic effects, phenobarbital therapy has been beneficial in improving cholestasis-associated pruritus [61]. The mechanism of action in ameliorating pruritus is not entirely clear. The antipruritic action of phenobarbital has been demonstrated without corresponding decreases in circulating levels of bile acids, suggesting that the effect of phenobarbital may not be entirely explained by a decrease in bile acid levels. However, through microsomal enzyme stimulation and excretory enhancement, phenobarbital may eliminate another, as of yet unidentified, pruritogenic substance. The beneficial effect of phenobarbital in relieving cholestasis-associated pruritus has been demonstrated in a number of cholestatic disorders, including adults with PBC [61] and children with intrahepatic cholestasis [235,267]. However, studies comparing the efficacy of phenobarbital to other antipruritics have not been as favorable. Rifampicin appeared to improve cholestasis-associated pruritus to a greater degree and with fewer side effects than did phenobarbital [236]. As previously mentioned, the sedative effects, irritability, and altered performance associated with phenobarbital therapy are undesirable and limit its chronic use in children.

URSODEOXYCHOLIC ACID

As previously described, UDCA is a potent choleretic and has been shown to improve biochemical parameters associated with several cholestatic disorders. Preliminary data in children with chronic intrahepatic cholestasis suggest that UDCA administration may similarly result in significant improvement in refractory pruritus [133,268,269]. Of 24 patients with Alagille syndrome with uncontrolled itching given UDCA, sustained amelioration or complete disappearance of refractory pruritus occurred in 21 (88%); 15 patients received UDCA at a dosage of 15 mg/kg/d, whereas 6 required a dosage of 30 mg/kg/d [268]. Among 27 patients with idiopathic intrahepatic cholestasis, 24 (89%) experienced significant improvement in pruritus; all but 1 patient responded to a dosage of 15 mg/kg/d [269]. However, in infants with biliary atresia and poor bile drainage following portoenterostomy, administration of UDCA may worsen pruritus and possibly lead to a significant worsening of liver dysfunction [270]. The other side effect reported in children has been occasional diarrhea.

PARTIAL BILIARY DIVERSION AND ILEAL EXCLUSION

Partial external diversion of bile has been proposed as a treatment for refractory pruritus in children with severe intrahepatic cholestasis [268,269,271,272]. This surgical procedure consists of the construction of a 10–15-cm jejunal conduit from the dome of the gallbladder to the abdominal wall. The gallbladder is anastomosed end-to-side to the blind proximal portion of a jejunal conduit, with the distal end of the conduit brought out to the skin as a permanent cutaneous stoma [271]. Others have described using the appendix as a conduit between the gallbladder and skin [273,274]. The bile collected in the stoma appliance is discarded. Of six patients with refractory pruritus who were diverted, four with progressive intrahepatic cholestasis had complete clinical remission from pruritus within 48 hours of surgery and had no recurrence of itching in the 3–8 years of follow-up [271]. There was also significant reversal of biochemical markers of cholestasis in these four children. The two patients with Alagille syndrome, in contrast, showed partial clinical improvement after 1–2 weeks and had mild, persistent itching since surgery [271]. Partial external biliary diversion has been combined with UDCA therapy in two children with Alagille syndrome and one child with idiopathic intrahepatic cholestasis, and has provided relief after failure of UDCA therapy alone [268,269]. In two small studies, partial biliary diversion led to resolution of pruritus, serum markers of cholestasis, and decreased progression of hepatic fibrosis in children with PFIC (Byler's disease) after a follow-up of 1–13 years [272,275]. Our own experience in five patients with PFIC has also been very favorable, with resolution of pruritus, normalization of liver blood tests, reversal of portal fibrosis, and improved growth following partial biliary diversion. Surprisingly, the characteristic granular inclusions ("Byler's bile") in canaliculi disappeared in electron micrographs of liver biopsies following the operation [276].

The mechanism by which this procedure produces these results is poorly understood. It is not known if a toxin in bile is discarded, if hepatic bile acid metabolism is altered, or if another process is taking place. Recently, it has been shown that the ileal bile acid transporter is up-regulated in PFIC 1 (*Familial Intrahepatic Cholestasis 1 FIC1* disease) [277], providing an explanation for the significant cholestasis and elevated bile acids in this disorder as well as providing a rationale for the use of biliary diversion. Partial external biliary diversion or ileal exclusion is an option that should be considered in planning the management of children with progressive intrahepatic cholestasis, particularly those with intractable pruritus uncontrolled by medical therapy.

Ileal exclusion is a surgical internal ileal colonic bypass of the distal ileum, which results in an interruption of the enterohepatic circulation of bile acids by the failure of bile acids to be actively transported in the terminal ileum. In patients who have undergone cholecystectomy, ileal exclusion has been suggested as an alternative for increasing fecal excretion of bile acids and reduction of pruritus [278]. Others have now used this surgery as primary therapy. Initial studies suggest that ileal exclusion may be as effective as partial biliary diversion (and cosmetically more acceptable to the child and family); however, its benefits may diminish over time [279]. Further experience comparing these two procedures will be needed in order to develop solid recommendations.

Recently, nasobiliary drainage has been employed to effectively reduce pruritus in patients with exacerbations of BRIC, a milder form of FIC1 and BSEP diseases [280].

OTHER THERAPIES

Tegretol (carbamazepine), at a dose of 20–40 mg/kg/d, has been suggested as another medication to help reduce pruritus because of its effect on neuralgia and other painful conditions [242]. Its major side effects are hepatotoxicity, bone marrow suppression, fluid retention, and behavioral changes. The other modes of therapy that may be beneficial in patients who are unresponsive to conventional treatment include phototherapy with either ultraviolet (UV) A or B (UVB) radiation, and plasma perfusion or plasmapheresis. Although UVB radiation has provided significant relief in adults with PBC [243–245], its use in children has not been investigated. The various theories advanced to account for the effects of UV radiation on pruritus have been reviewed by Garden et al. [209]. Plasma perfusion or plasmapheresis has provided temporary improvement for intractable pruritus in PBC, presumably by removal of a circulating "pruritogenic factor" [246,247]. The pruritus may not disappear completely and may gradually return to its preperfusion intensity within several weeks following the procedure. Other medications that have been tried primarily in adults with PBC are intravenous naloxone [231], terfenadine [281], androgenic steroids [282,283], systemic corticosteroids (prednisone and triamcinolone) [284], azathioprine [285,286], ondansetron [287], and propofol [288]. Glucocorticoid admininstration for pruritus in neonatal liver disease is discouraged because of its unproved benefits and risks for osteoporosis and immune suppression. However, high-dose "bursts" of intravenous methylprednisolone have been shown to be effective in stimulating bile flow during episodes of refractory cholangitis after hepatic portoenterostomy treatment for biliary atresia [157].

Fatigue

It has long been appreciated that significant fatigue is associated with chronic cholestatic liver disease, particularly in adults, often out of proportion to that explained by chronic illness alone. Indeed, fatigue is the most common symptom reported by patients with PBC (in up to 80%) [289]. In addition, fatigue has been shown to adversely affect job performance and family life and has been significantly associated with depression in PBC [290]. The mechanism underlying fatigue in chronic cholestasis is unknown. Altered behavioral state has been linked to hepatic function as demonstrated by hepatic encephalopathy, in which altered neurotransmission may play a role. The recent evidence that increased central opioid tone may play a role in cholestasis-associated pruritus suggests that altered central neurotransmission may play a role in other behavioral manifestations of cholestasis, such as fatigue. Two studies by Swain and Maric [291,292] suggest that this may in fact be the case. In the first, the authors showed that an abnormal pattern of behavior and altered function of the hypothalamic–pituitary–adrenal axis coexist in rats with cholestasis secondary to bile duct ligation [291] and postulated that this might be implicated in the mediation of fatigue. It is interesting to note that an alteration of hypothalamic function has also been postulated to contribute to the hyperpigmentation in patients with PBC [293]. In the second study, the authors demonstrated that cholestatic rats [294], as compared with sham-operated controls, were more easily fatigued and spent a significantly longer time floating (as opposed to active swimming) when placed in a swim tank [292]. The administration of LY293284, a 5-hydroxytryptamine$_{1A}$ (5-HT$_{1A}$) receptor agonist [292], did not affect floating times in controls but corrected the prolonged floating times in cholestatic rats. This finding was interpreted as suggesting that the abnormal behavior state was attributable to altered transmission in serotonin neural pathways on which 5-HT$_{1A}$ receptors are located and that it could be corrected by enhancing neurotransmission in these pathways. To test this postulated mechanism in humans, Jones [295] administered ondansetron to a patient with chronic hepatitis C and fatigue and found marked improvement in her energy level and ability to work, further supporting the hypothesis that altered central serotoninergic neurotransmission contributes to the fatigue complicating chronic liver disease. The preliminary studies regarding serotonin neurotransmission are novel and will require further investigation. Other factors that may be involved in the fatigue associated with cholestatic liver disease include altered sleep patterns caused by pruritus, chronic disease, depression, chronic anemia, and poor nutritional status. The clinical manifestations of fatigue are more difficult to delineate in children with cholestasis; however, following liver transplantation, parents frequently report that their child is more energetic, participates in new activities, and demonstrates improved school performance.

Hyperlipidemia/Xanthomas

Hyperlipidemia and xanthomas are common consequences of severe intrahepatic cholestasis (e.g., Alagille syndrome) but are less severe in biliary atresia. With increasing impairment of bile flow during cholestasis, the plasma concentration of circulating lipoproteins and individual lipids increases. The primary event is the regurgitation into plasma of biliary phospholipids that produce secondary effects leading to an increase in plasma cholesterol, perhaps because of enhanced hepatic synthesis of cholesterol [296]. The cholesterol is transported in the blood in lipoprotein X (LPX), an unusual vesicular form of lipoprotein specific to cholestasis [297]. Lecithin-cholesterol acyltransferase activity is also diminished during cholestasis, further altering lipoprotein metabolism [296]. These pertubations may cause severe hypercholesterolemia (serum cholesterol 1000–2000 mg/dL), leading to cholesterol deposition in skin, mucous membranes, and arteries. The disfiguring effect of xanthomas on fine motor function of affected fingers and on self-image (Figure 10.1) should not be underestimated in young, developing children. The risk for atherosclerosis in children with chronic cholestasis is unknown; however, severe hypercholesterolemia in Alagille syndrome has been associated with renal lipidoses, causing renal failure [298], and with atheromatous plaque deposition in the aorta within the first few years of life [299]. Atherosclerosis has been reported in adults with hypercholesterolemia caused by cholestasis [300]; however, there does not appear to be an increased risk of atherosclerosis in women with PBC compared with healthy women [301]. With longer survival in children with chronic cholestasis and hyperlipidemia associated with immunosuppressive drugs after liver transplantation, more attention may need to be focused in the future on measures to reduce serum cholesterol levels in children with cholestatic disorders.

Treatment is directed at increasing conversion of cholesterol to bile acids, reducing biliary regurgitation into the systemic circulation, and enhancing the elimination of bile acids and cholesterol. In general, the efficacy of therapeutic agents depends on generating increased bile flow and, therefore, requires a patent biliary tract. In some conditions, such as Alagille syndrome, spontaneous improvement in bile flow after age 2–3 years may lead to reduction of serum lipids.

Nonabsorbable Ion Exchange Resins

Cholestyramine, colestipol, and colesevelam hydrochloride interrupt the enterohepatic circulation of bile acids by binding to intraluminal bile acids and increasing fecal excretion, thus decreasing negative feedback to the liver mediated through FXR, thereby enhancing conversion of cholesterol to bile acids. The up-regulation of low-density lipoprotein (LDL) receptors may also increase clearance of circulating LDL [302]. Although these bile acid–binding resins effectively lower serum bile acid concentrations in most patients, a similar effect on serum cholesterol is not noted as frequently [303]. The dosage used and side effects are the same as for the treatment of pruritus mentioned previously.

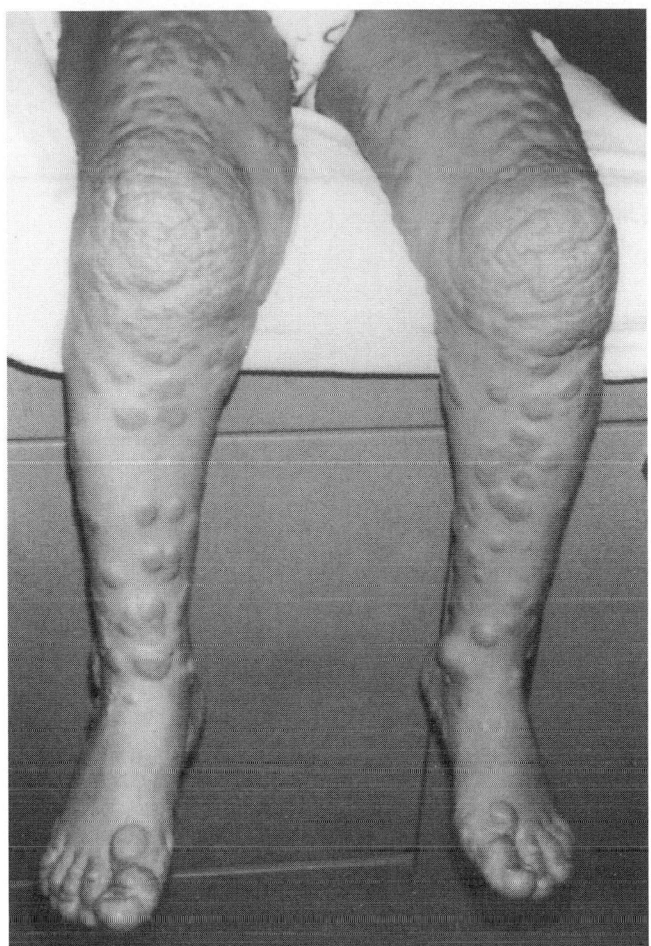

Figure 10.1. Extensive cutaneous xanthomas in a 4-year-old child with Alagille syndrome whose serum cholesterol levels were between 1000 and 2000 mg/dL.

Ursodeoxycholic Acid

Ursodeoxycholic acid affects cholesterol and lipoprotein metabolism in several ways. UDCA directly stimulates receptor-dependent LDL uptake in the liver and decreases 3-hydroxy-3-methylglutaryl coenzyme A (HMG-CoA) reductase activity [304–306] and indirectly decreases cholesterol absorption from the intestine by causing a marked reduction in the secretion of cholesterol into the bile [307]. In a preliminary report [268], the effect of UDCA therapy (15 mg/kg/d) on hypercholesterolemia in 24 children with Alagille syndrome was studied. After 1 month of UDCA therapy, baseline serum cholesterol concentrations significantly decreased. In 8 of the 24 who had marked hypercholesterolemia (1098 mg/dL ± 100), the level dropped almost 40% after 1 month of therapy and continued to decline during follow-up visits [268]. Similar encouraging results have been seen in children with idiopathic intrahepatic cholestasis [308]. Parallel xanthoma resolution has been documented with

UDCA therapy [111]. These data suggest that UDCA therapy may significantly reduce hypercholesterolemia in children with chronic intrahepatic cholestasis. However, the resulting serum cholesterol levels are still higher than those in the normal population.

Cholesterol Synthesis Blocking Agents

Cholesterol synthesis blocking agents (e.g., lovastatin, simvastatin) are effective in lowering serum cholesterol in familial heterozygous and nonfamilial hypercholesterolemia. The mechanism of action of these drugs centers on inhibition of HMG-CoA reductase, the rate-limiting enzyme in cholesterol synthesis [309,310]. Recent studies have also demonstrated that lovastatin and simvastatin have a synergistic effect with UDCA in reducing biliary cholesterol output and binary cholesterol saturation index but have no effects on bile acid metabolism [311–313]. Because these agents do little to the underlying pathophysiology in cholestasis and because of potential hepatotoxicity, they currently play little role in treating hypercholesterolemia in pediatric cholestasis.

Diet and Other Agents

Low-cholesterol and low–saturated fat diets have been ineffective in reducing serum cholesterol in cholestatic patients unresponsive to bile acid–binding resins and phenobarbital. Moreover, restriction of fat in the diet will make the diet less palatable and lower dietary caloric content, thereby exacerbating the malnutrition common in cholestatic children. Other cholesterol-lowering agents (e.g., L-thyroxine, clofibrate) have likewise been unsuccessful in our experience. The serum lipid–lowering effect of phenobarbital appears to be modest [61,314,315], thus its use must be counterbalanced by its effects of sedation, irritability, and drug interaction. Future studies may determine whether plasmapheresis [316] or partial ileal bypass [317,318] therapies that have successfully lowered serum cholesterol in adult patients with familial and nonfamilial hypercholesterolemia will be effective in cholestasis and whether these therapies are practical in selected cases. Partial biliary diversion and ileal exclusion have successfully reduced serum lipids in selected cases of Alagille syndrome (i.e., in patients without bridging fibrosis or cirrhosis on liver biopsy) [319]. Lastly, liver transplantation has been successful in relieving hypercholesterolemia and reversing xanthomas in refractory cases [320,321].

REDUCED DELIVERY OF BILE TO THE INTESTINE CAUSING MALABSORPTION

Steatorrhea, Malnutrition, and Growth Failure

Bile acids are important amphipathic molecules that aid in the solubilization of dietary fat, allowing the interaction between pancreatic lipase and colipase that is essential for hydrolysis of dietary lipids [322]. The monoglycerides and free fatty acids produced are then incorporated into mixed micelles, formed in the presence of bile acids and transported across the aqueous luminal environment into the intestinal epithelium (Figure 10.2). The decreased delivery of bile acids to the duodenum during cholestasis may lead to intraluminal bile acid concentrations that are inadequate for the formation of micelles [323], resulting in the malabsorption of dietary lipids and the fat-soluble vitamins. Because of this defect in the intraluminal phase of fat digestion, steatorrhea is invariably present in children with severe cholestasis and is one important cause of malnutrition. In addition, other factors that contribute to the malnutrition of chronic cholestasis include abnormalities in amino acid [324,325] and glucose metabolism [326], increased resting energy expenditure [327,328], recurrent infections [299,329], anorexia [327,330], and early satiety, gastroesophageal reflux, or vomiting secondary to compression of abdominal viscera by the enlarged liver, spleen, or ascites [299].

Recent evidence suggests that children with liver disease have alterations in the growth hormone axis. The liver is an important endocrine organ producing factors such as insulin-like growth factor I (IGF-I) and IGF binding proteins 1, 2, and 3 in response to stimulation by growth hormone (GH). Most of circulating IGF-I is derived from liver and appears to mediate

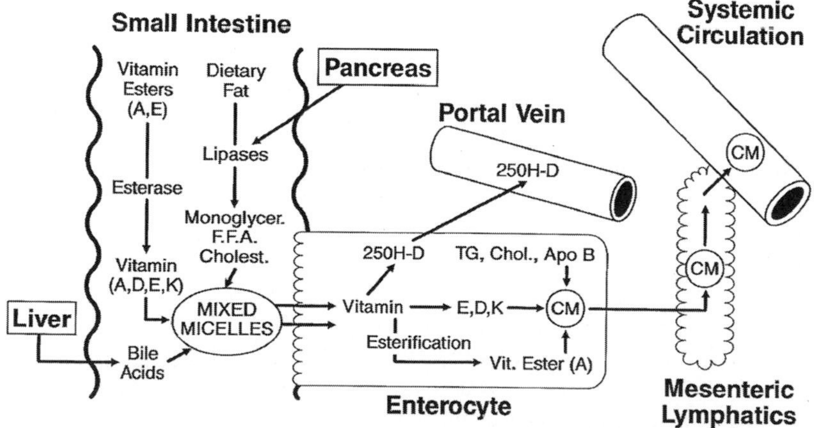

Figure 10.2. Pathways of absorption of dietary fat and the fat-soluble vitamins. FFA, free fatty acids; monoglycer, monoglycerides; TG, triglycerides; Apo B, apolipoprotein B; chol, cholesterol; CM, chylomicrons.

the anabolic actions of GH. The production of normal levels of IGF-I depends on normal liver function. In children with end-stage liver disease, IGF-I levels fall to undetectable levels and serum GH levels are increased [331]. Additionally, IGF binding proteins 1 and 2 are elevated, whereas binding protein 3 is low [332–334]. The low levels of IGF-I and IGF binding protein 3 despite high GH levels suggests that GH resistance is present in chronic liver failure. Additionally, treatment of children with end-stage liver disease awaiting transplant with recombinant human GH did not appear to improve body composition or growth [335].

Aside from the debilitation attributed to generalized and specific nutrient deficiencies, malnutrition has been associated with decreased brain growth [336,337], impairment of mental development [337,338], and decreased immunocompetence with increased susceptibility of infection [329]. For example, the severity of malnutrition and poor growth in children with biliary atresia before liver transplantation is predictive of cognitive performance years after transplantation [339]. Thus, to improve neurocognitive outcomes, an aggressive approach to nutritional support is essential in the care of the pediatric patient with chronic liver disease. A summary of nutritional assessment, therapies, and potential side effects of the therapies are listed in Table 10.3.

Nutritional Assessment

Nutritional assessment should be initiated at the first visit of the cholestatic child and used to monitor effects of nutritional rehabilitation. Although helpful in following growth and development of normal children, serial weight for age, height for age, and weight for height measurements are less reliable for children with chronic liver disease [336,340,341]. Weight gain may result from hepatosplenomegaly and ascites [340,341] and from excessive tissue sequestration of water because of poor intravascular colloid osmotic status, renal retention of salt and water, and hyperaldosteronism [327]. Thus, weight-for-age and weight-for-height measurements may incorrectly indicate better nutritional status than is present. The utility of serial height-for-age plots is likewise reduced in some infants and children with chronic cholestasis if the underlying disease (e.g., Alagille syndrome, familial cholestasis) influences growth independent of nutritional status [298]. Instead, serial estimates of body fat using triceps and subscapular skinfold thickness and of body protein using midarm muscle circumference compared with age- and height-matched normal values are a better estimation of nutritional status during chronic liver disease [327,336,340,341]. Other means of assessing body composition (e.g., dual electron x-ray absorptiometry [DEXA]) may provide additional information; however, these methods are most useful in a research setting. Measurement of visceral protein status (serum albumin, prealbumin, retinol-binding protein [RBP], and transferrin) may also be helpful; however, liver synthetic failure and vitamin A deficiency may confound interpretation of these tests [340]. RBP and prealbumin, with half-lives of 12 hours and 2 days, respectively, respond rapidly and are useful parameters to follow during nutritional repletion [342,343]. Indirect calorimetry may be used to estimate oxygen consumption and caloric requirements if weight gain is poor despite seemingly adequate caloric intake.

Nutritional Therapy

Energy

In the presence of steatorrhea and increased energy expenditure, the goal for caloric intake should be approximately 125% of the recommended dietary allowance (RDA) based on ideal body weight (50th percentile of weight for height). Additional calories may be needed to provide for catch-up growth if a significant deficit in weight is present. The infant formula can be mixed with less water to provide 24 or 27 kcal/oz. Alternatively, glucose polymers (8 cal/teaspoon [Polycose powder; Ross Laboratories, Columbus, OH]) or MCT (medium-chain triglyceride) oil (7.7 cal/mL [Mead Johnson, Evansville, IN]) can be added to the standard 20 cal/oz dilution of the formula. Whenever possible, oral feeding is preferred, but with increasing anorexia and debilitation secondary to progressive liver disease, supplemental nocturnal nasogastric infusions may be required to meet caloric and fluid requirements and prevent or reverse inadequate weight gain, particularly in children awaiting liver transplantation. The use of narrow-bore, soft, weighted Silastic or polyurethane feeding tubes is generally well tolerated, with minimal risk of aspiration or upper gastrointestinal hemorrhage [344–346]. Compared with bolus gavage feeding techniques, continuous formula infusion leads to better energy balance [346,347] and reduces the hazard of significant regurgitation [348]. Nocturnal nasogastric feedings can be safely administered in the home. Because of portal hypertensive gastropathy and the development of gastric varices, gastrostomy tubes are not used in this setting. Occasionally, parenteral nutrition through an indwelling central venous catheter is required to assure adequate weight gain while a child is bridged to liver transplantation.

Fat

In general, infant formulas containing significant quantities of MCTs, C-8 to C-12 fatty acids, will provide better energy balance during cholestasis. Unlike long-chain triglycerides (LCTs), which require bile acid micelles for solubilization [336], MCTs are relatively water soluble and directly absorbed into the portal circulation. For this reason, MCT oil–containing diets have been used successfully to reduce steatorrhea, improve energy balance, and promote growth in children with chronic cholestasis [150,299,322,330,349,350]. Pregestimil (Mead Johnson, Evansville, IN) and Alimentum (Ross Laboratories, Columbus, OH) are MCT oil–predominant formulas frequently used in cholestasis and contain approximately 60% and 50% of fat calories as MCT oil, respectively. Breast-fed infants with chronic cholestasis should be supplemented with these formulas if growth is not adequate. It is not unusual, however, for unremitting steatorrhea in the breast-fed cholestatic infant to require weaning to an MCT oil–containing

Table 10.3: Guidelines for Nutritional Management in Chronic Cholestasis

Nutritional Factor	*Index of Assessment*	*Treatment Options*	*Toxicity*
Energy	Anthropometrics Triceps & subscapular skinfold thickness	Caloric goal: 125% of RDA based on weight for height at 50th percentile	
	Serial measurements of weight/height Indirect calorimetry Fat malabsorption	Glucose polymers (Polycose powder or solution) to ↑ to 24–27 cal/oz formula	
		Supplemental nighttime nasogastric drip feedings	
		MCT infant formulas (Pregestimil, Alimentum)	Financial burden EFA deficiency
		MCT oil supplements: 1–2 mL/kg/d in 2–4 doses	Aspiration pneumonia
EFA	EFA deficiency Triene:tetraene ratio >0.3, ↓ linoleic acid	Corn oil or oral lipid emulsions IV lipid emulsions	
Protein	Mid-arm muscle circumference	Protein intake 2–3 g/kg/d in infants	
	Serum albumin, prealbumin, RBP, transferrin		
		Protein intake 0.5–1.0 g/kg/d – hepatic encephalopathy	
		Branched-chain amino acid supplements	Unknown
Fat soluble vitamins			
Vitamin A	Vit. A deficiency: Retinol:RBP molar ratio <0.8 or serum retinol, 20 μg/dL RDR CIC Xerosis, Bitot spots, etc.	5000–25,000 U/d orally of water-miscible preparation of vit. A	Hepatotoxicity Pseudotumor cerebri Bone lesions Hypercalcemia
Vitamin D	Vit. D deficiency: 25-OH-D <14 ng/mL	Vit. D (Drisdol), 3–10× RDA for age	
	Rickets	25-OHD (Calderol), 3–5 μg/kg/d	Hypercalcemia
	Osteomalacia	1,25-OH_2-D (Rocaltrol), 0.05–0.2 μg/kg/d	Hypercalcemia Nephrocalcinosis
Vitamin E	Vit. E deficiency: Vit. E:total lipid ratio: <0.6 mg/g (age <1 yr) <0.8 mg/g (age >1 yr)	α-Tocopherol (acetate), 25–200 IU/kg/d TPGS (Liqui E), 15–25 IU/kg/d	Potentiation of vit. K deficiency coagulopathy Diarrhea Hyperosmolality (TPGS)
Vitamin K	Vit. K deficiency: Prolonged prothrombin time	Mephyton, 2.5 mg twice/wk to 5.0 mg/d	
	Elevated PIVKA-II	AquaMEPHYTON (IM) 2–5 mg every 4 wk	
Water-soluble vitamins		Prevent deficiency of water-soluble vitamins Dose: 1–2× RDA	Fat-soluble vitamin toxicity
Mineral & trace elements			
Calcium	Calcium deficiency due to steatorrhea despite corrected vit. D status	25–100 mg/kg/d up to 800–1200 mg/d	Hypercalcemia Hypercalciuria
Phosphorus	Low serum phosphorus despite corrected vit. D & calcium status	25–50 mg/kg/d up to 500 mg/d	Gastrointestinal intolerance

Nutritional Factor	*Index of Assessment*	*Treatment Options*	*Toxicity*
Magnesium	Magnesium deficiency: Serum Mg <1.4 mEq/L	Magnesium oxide, 1–2 mEq/kg/d orally or 50% solution of $MgSO_4$, 0.3–0.5 mEq/kg IV over 3 hr (max. 3–6 mEq)	Respiratory depression Lethargy Coma
Zinc	Zinc deficiency: Plasma zinc <60 μg/dL	Zinc SO_4 solution (10 mg elemental zinc/mL) 1 mg/kg/d orally for 2–3 mo	↓ Intestinal absorption of copper and iron
Selenium	Selenium deficiency: Plasma Se <40 μg/L	1–2 μg/kg/d of oral Na selenite or 1–2 μg/kg/d Se in TPN	Dermatologic changes (skin eruptions, pathologic nails, hair loss), dyspepsia, diarrhea, anorexia
Iron	Iron deficiency: ↓ Serum iron ↑ TIBC Iron saturation index <16%	5–6 mg/kg/d of elemental iron	Teeth staining Hemorrhagic gastroenteritis Metabolic acidosis Coma Liver failure

↑, increased; ↓, decreased; CIC, conjunctival impression cytology; EFA, essential fatty acids; IM, intramuscularly; IV, intravenous; MCT, medium-chain triglyceride; PIVKA II, protein induced in vitamin K absence; RBP, retinol-binding protein; RDA, recommended daily allowance; RDR, relative dose response; TIBC, total iron-binding capacity; TPGS, tocopherol polyethylene glycol-1000 succinate; TPN, total parenteral nutrition.

formula as the only means of attaining adequate weight gain and growth if total fluid intake is limited by the child's appetite or because of ascites or organomegaly.

Protein

It is essential that adequate protein intake be preserved (2–3 g/kg/d in small infants) while delivering optimal energy intake. Plasma aminograms of patients with chronic cholestasis and cirrhosis are often abnormal, with low levels of branched-chain amino acids (BCAAs) and an elevated ratio of aromatic amino acids to BCAAs [325]. These abnormalities reflect disturbed amino acid kinetics and relate to increased BCAA utilization in muscle, where under the influence of hyperinsulinemia they provide an alternative substrate source for gluconeogenesis, and to impaired hepatic enzymatic processing of aromatic amino acids. There is some evidence to suggest that diets relatively rich in BCAAs may confer significant advantages in nutritional therapy for chronic liver disease. In an animal model of cholestasis, oral supplementation with BCAAs improved nitrogen retention, body composition, and growth [351]. Additionally, a randomized study in children with end-stage liver disease demonstrated improved nutritional status and body composition in those who were fed the BCAA-enriched formula [352]. However, MCT-containing complete BCAA formulas are rather expensive and not readily available (e.g., Hepatic Formula Complete; Scientific Hospital Supplies, Liverpool, UK). If hepatic encephalopathy occurs, dogma is that protein intake may need to be limited to 0.5–1.0 g/kg/d. However, it has been recently shown that nutritional rehabilitation using enteral drip feedings (140% of recommended caloric intake, 4 g/kg/d of protein) in children with severe chronic liver disease awaiting liver transplant led to improved nutritional status without hyperammonemia or adverse clinical and biochemical effects [353]. This relatively large amount of protein was well tolerated, although it did contain 31% of protein calories as BCAAs. However, stable levels of plasma ammonia were not accompanied by any significant change in amino acid profiles during therapy [353]. Our own clinical experience indicates that similar protein intakes of MCT oil–containing formulas are well tolerated without hyperammonemia or signs of hepatic encephalopathy unless liver failure is advanced.

Essential Fatty Acids

The combination of malabsorption of LCTs and inadequate intake of energy may lead to essential fatty acid (EFA) deficiency. The EFAs are fatty acids that cannot be generated in mammalian organisms by desaturation and elongation of shorter fatty acids. Linoleic acid ($C_{18:2\,\omega\text{-}6}$) and linolenic acid ($C_{18:3\,\omega\text{-}3}$) are the two main EFAs. Arachidonic acid ($C_{20:4\,\omega\text{-}6}$), derived from linoleic acid, should also be considered an EFA. Deficiency of EFAs may produce growth impairment, a dry scaly rash, and thrombocytopenia; impair immune function; and inhibit eicosanoid pathways [354–358]. These long-chain fatty acids are poorly absorbed if bile flow is diminished, as in chronic cholestasis. Because infants have small linoleic acid stores [359], fat malabsorption in cholestasis places them at a higher risk of developing EFA deficiency. In addition, ingested linoleic and linolenic acids may be preferentially oxidized for energy if caloric intake and absorption are inadequate [360]. Importantly, Pregestimil and Alimentum contain only 7–14% of calories, respectively, as linoleic acid. It is generally accepted that the minimum amount of linoleic acid necessary to prevent EFA deficiency is 3–4% of dietary calories. If 30–40% of dietary fat is malabsorbed during cholestasis, the absorbed amount of linoleic acid may be only borderline adequate using these infant formulas. Several reports document biochemical evidence (low linoleic acid levels, triene:tetraene ratio >0.3) [361] of EFA deficiency in infants with cholestasis receiving these types of formulas [362–365]. Clearly, other formulas containing 85% of fat calories as MCT oil and under 3% of calories as EFAs (e.g., Portagen, Mead Johnson) may induce EFA deficiency and should not be used in chronic cholestasis [364]. Corn oil or safflower oil, with 5.4 and 7.2 g linoleic acid/mL, respectively, may be added to foods, and lipid emulsions (0.40 g linoleic acid/mL [e.g., Microlipid; Novartis Medical Nutrition, Fremont, MI]) may be added to formula to provide additional linoleic acid, if needed. Linoleic acid levels and the plasma triene:tetraene ratio should be measured in the cholestatic child with poor growth to evaluate for the possibility of EFA deficiency and the need for EFA supplementation.

Fat-Soluble Vitamins

The intestinal absorption of vitamins A, D, E, and K is strongly dependent on adequate hepatic secretion of bile acids into the intestinal lumen (Figure 10.2). When intraluminal bile acid concentrations are below the critical micellar concentration of 1.5–2.0 mmol/L, malabsorption of fat-soluble vitamins is common. The use of bile acid–binding agents (e.g., cholestyramine) as treatment for cholestasis may further impair absorption [366]. In addition, vitamin A and vitamin E esters require hydrolysis before intestinal absorption by an intestinal esterase that is bile acid dependent. When cholestasis begins in infancy, depletion of meager body stores present at birth occurs rapidly, resulting in biochemical and clinical features of fat-soluble vitamin deficiency as early as age 4–12 months if supplementation is not initiated. The frequency of biochemical evidence of fat-soluble vitamin deficiency despite "routine" vitamin supplementation is approximately 35–50% for vitamin A, 66% for vitamin D, 50–75% for vitamin E, and 25% for vitamin K [367]. Evaluation of vitamin status, supplemental doses, and monitoring differ for each vitamin and will be considered separately.

VITAMIN A

The term *vitamin A* refers to retinol and derivatives that have the same β-ionone ring and qualitatively similar biologic activities. The principal vitamin A compounds – retinol, retinal (retinaldehyde), retinoic acid, and retinyl esters – differ in the terminal C-15 group at the end of the side chain. Vitamin A is present in the diet as retinyl esters derived almost exclusively from animal sources (liver and fish liver oils, dairy products, kidney, and eggs) and provitamin A carotenoids (mainly β-carotene) that are distributed widely in green and yellow vegetables. The RDA is 375 μg RE (retinol equivalents) for 0–1 year of age, 400 μg RE for 1–3 years, 500 μg RE for 4–6 years, and 700–1000 μg RE for older children and adults (1 μg RE = 3.3 IU vitamin A) [368]. The functions of vitamin A are maintenance of proper vision, epithelial cell integrity, and regulation of glycoprotein synthesis and cell differentiation.

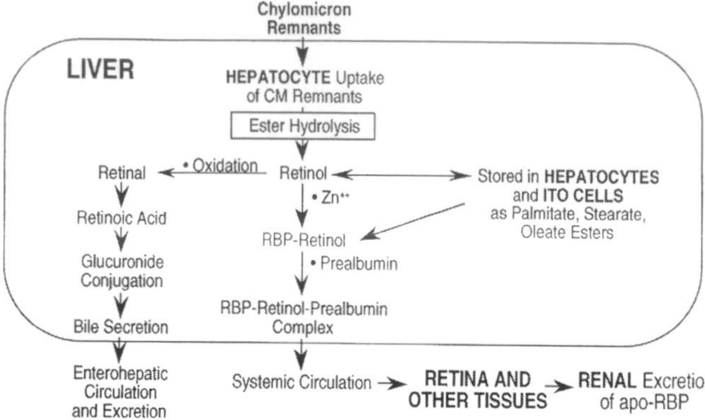

Figure 10.3. Processes involved in hepatic metabolism of vitamin A. CM, chylomicrons; Zn, zinc; RBP, retinol-binding protein.

Following micellar solubilization and hydrolysis by pancreatic esterase in the intestinal lumen, retinol is absorbed into the enterocyte, undergoes re-esterification with palmitate, stearate, or oleate, and is then incorporated into newly synthesized chylomicrons or very-low-density lipoproteins (VLDLs) for transport into the mesenteric lymphatics (Figure 10.2). Upon reaching the bloodstream, the triglyceride content of the chylomicra is hydrolyzed and the retinyl ester–rich chylomicron remnants are taken up by the liver. In the hepatocyte (Figure 10.3), retinyl esters may be hydrolyzed, releasing the free retinol, which can be transported into the sinusoids bound in a 1:1 molar ratio with RBP in a ternary complex with prealbumin (transthyretin). Circulating RBP-retinol is the transport form that delivers retinol to target tissues such as the retina. Alternatively, retinyl esters may be stored in the hepatocyte or transported as RBP-bound retinol from the hepatocyte to hepatic stellate cells (lipocytes, Ito cells), the storage site of over 80% of hepatic vitamin A under normal conditions [369].

Several alterations in hepatic metabolism of vitamin A occur in chronic cholestasis, and deficiency of vitamin A has been observed in 35–69% of children with chronic cholestatic liver disease [367,370,371]. Intraluminal solubilization of vitamin A and other carotenoids is compromised by lack of bile flow, resulting in malabsorption of vitamin A [372]. If protein malnutrition, zinc deficiency, or depressed hepatic synthetic function is present, hepatic synthesis and secretion of RBP is diminished, leading to low plasma levels of retinol and impaired delivery of retinol to target tissues [373,374].

The evaluation of vitamin A status in cholestasis is confounded by a reportedly poor correlation between serum and hepatic vitamin A concentrations [372,375]. In patients without liver disease, serum retinol levels below 20 μg/dL generally correlate with deficient hepatic stores of vitamin A. However, in children with cholestatic liver disease, previous reports suggest that serum retinol may not correlate with hepatic stores of vitamin A [372].

Because of these inaccuracies in using serum retinol alone to define vitamin A status, other potential indices have been proposed for the evaluation of vitamin A status during cholestasis, including the relative dose response (RDR) [376], retinol: RBP ratio [377], and ocular measures including conjunctival impression cytology (CIC) [378,379], ophthalmologic slit-lamp examination [380], and the rapid darkfield adaptation test [381].

The RDR, considered the best noninvasive test of vitamin A status, is based on the observation that when hepatic stores of vitamin A are normal, plasma retinol concentration does not change significantly following administration of a small oral loading dose of exogenous vitamin A. However, when hepatic vitamin A reserves are low, the plasma retinol concentration increases markedly after the administration of an exogenous vitamin A dose, reaching a peak several hours after the vitamin A dose. This paradoxic effect observed during vitamin A deficiency is most likely the result of rapid mobilization of hepatic RBP bound to incoming retinol in an attempt to redistribute the absorbed vitamin A to peripheral tissues. The standardized RDR is expressed as the percentage increase in plasma retinol 5 hours after an oral loading dose of vitamin A. However, use of the oral RDR test in cholestasis is potentially problematic because of poor absorption of the oral dose of vitamin A [382]. We have recently studied an RDR using an intramuscular injection (IM-RDR) of vitamin A (Aquasol A; Astra Pharmaceuticals, Westborough, MA) [383]. In a study of 23 patients with cholestatic liver disease and 10 patients with noncholestatic liver disease (controls), vitamin A deficiency was identified in 10 of the cholestatic patients and none of the control patients using the IM-RDR (Figure 10.4). Comparing other tests to the IM-RDR revealed that serum retinol alone was a good screening measure with a sensitivity of 90% and a specificity of 78% to detect vitamin A deficiency [383] (Table 10.4).

It has been proposed that the molar ratio of serum retinol to RBP may reflect hepatic stores more accurately. Mourey et al. [375] showed that the molar ratio of retinol:RBP was 0.62 ± 0.15 in vitamin A–deficient patients but was 1.04 ± 0.06 in vitamin A–repleted cholestatic patients. This ratio differentiated all but one vitamin A–deficient patient from the vitamin A–sufficient patients, whereas plasma retinol did not. However, in a larger controlled study, the ratio of retinol to RBP did not improve the detection of vitamin A deficiency over serum retinol level alone [383].

Another measure used in assessing vitamin A status is CIC [379,384–387]. In this test, a small piece of filter paper is applied to the bulbar conjunctiva after local anesthesia, patted gently, and peeled off slowly. After fixation and staining, the morphology of adherent epithelial cells is evaluated histologically for abnormalities in epithelial cell morphology, decreased number of goblet cells, and mucin spots covering less than 25% of the sample, all of which are consistent with vitamin A deficiency [384]. One study [385] showed that CIC correctly identified the vitamin A status of 16 children with chronic cholestasis. However, the test may have a lower specificity, especially in Western or developed nations [386]. In fact, in our study CIC had a sensitivity of only 44% and a specificity of 48% to detect vitamin A deficiency [383]. Likewise, ophthalmologic examination was also a poor discriminator of vitamin A deficiency in this population. Direct measures of visual acuity and darkfield adaptation

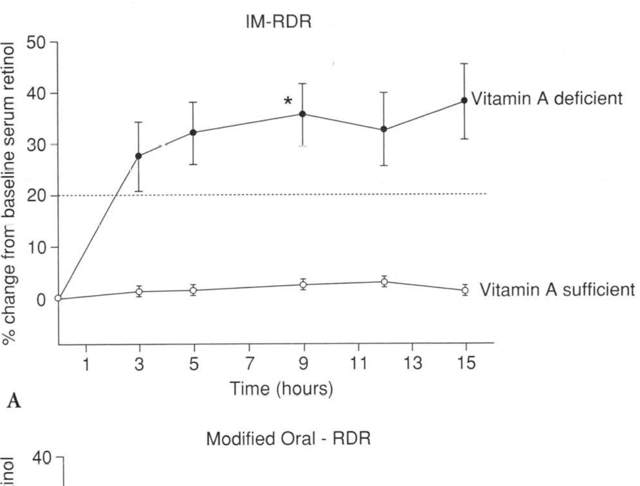

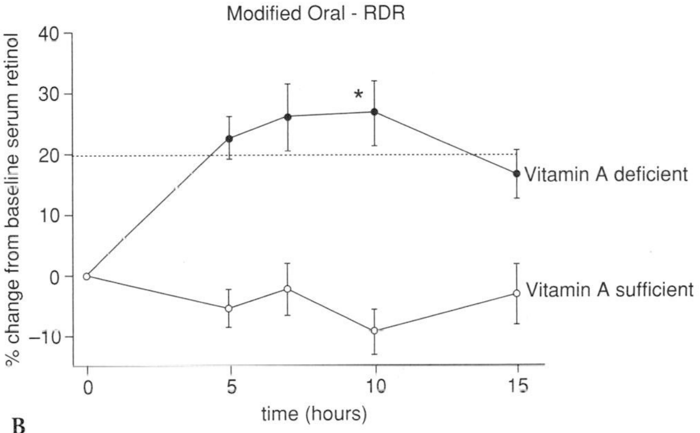

Figure 10.4. Relative dose response (RDR) tests for the detection of vitamin A deficiency. (**A**) Modified intramuscular RDR. Percent rise in serum retinol level from baseline following intramuscular injection of vitamin A. Mean values ± SEM are shown at each time point. A rise of greater than 20% at 9 hours is considered abnormal and indicative of vitamin A deficiency. All patients with vitamin A deficiency had a greater than 20% rise in serum retinol by 9 hours (*closed circles*). Conversely, all patients with vitamin A sufficiency had no significant rise in serum retinol following the injection (normal response, *open circles*). (**B**) Modified oral RDR. Percent rise in serum retinol level from baseline following an oral dose of vitamin A (1500 IU) given concurrently with vitamin E (25 IU/kg of TPGS). A rise of greater than 20% at 10 hours is considered abnormal. Mean values ± SEM are shown at each time point. *Closed circles* represent vitamin A–deficient and *open circles* vitamin A–sufficient patients (defined by the IM RDR). IM, intramuscular; SEM, standard error of the mean; TPGS, tocopherol polyethylene glycol succinate. (Reproduced with permission from Feranchak et al. [383].)

have been used to assess vitamin A deficiency but may not be feasible in younger children.

We subsequently developed a modified version of the RDR by the oral co-administration of tocopherol polyethylene glycol succinate (TPGS) vitamin E and retinyl palmitate, with the TPGS promoting solubilization and absorption of oral vitamin A, thus mitigating against the need for parenteral (intravenous or intramuscular) RDR to assess vitamin A status [388]. In fact, the oral RDR had a sensitivity of 80% and a specificity of 100% to detect vitamin A deficiency in this group of patients with chronic cholestasis [383] (Figure 10.4). Based on these findings, serum retinol level as an initial screen followed by confirmation

Table 10.4: Comparison of Indices of Vitamin A Status in Cholestasis

	*Sensitivity (%)**	*Specificity (%)**
Retinol	90	78
RBP	40	91
Retinol:RBP ratio	60	74
Oral RDR	80	100
CIC	44	48
Slit lamp	20	66

*For the detection of vitamin A deficiency.
CIC, conjunctival impression cytology; RBP, retinol-binding protein; RDR, relative dose response.
From Feranchak et al. [383].

with a modified oral RDR test may be the most effective means of identifying vitamin A deficiency in these patients.

It is important to detect vitamin A deficiency in children with chronic cholestatic liver disease as deficiency may lead to xerophthalmia, keratomalacia, and irreversible damage to the cornea as well as night blindness and pigmentary retinopathy. Although these ocular findings are rare in children with chronic cholestasis, the potential for impairment of vision exists. Vitamin A deficiency may also potentially put patients at risk for infection and abnormalities in biliary epithelialization of Roux-en-Y conduits following hepatic portoenterostomy. The effect of vitamin A deficiency on immune function during cholestasis has not been evaluated.

The recommended oral supplements of vitamin A range from 5000–25,000 IU per day of water-miscible preparations of vitamin A (e.g., Aquasol A) [149,330,389]. Alagille et al. [150] recommended intramuscular injections of 100,000 IU (33,000 μg) of an aqueous preparation of retinyl palmitate every 2 months for at least 6 months in patients who have vitamin A deficiency, in line with recommendations for vitamin A–deficient children in developing countries. The water-soluble form of vitamin E, TPGS, has been shown to solubilize and improve intestinal absorption of other lipid-soluble molecules (cyclosporin [390] and vitamin D [391]) during cholestasis. Thus oral co-administration of vitamin A supplements with TPGS may improve absorption of vitamin A during cholestasis and would most likely result in the need for smaller dosages of vitamin A (e.g., 5000–10,000 IU/d).

Because of the known hepatotoxicity of vitamin A, careful monitoring during vitamin A repletion and supplementation is mandatory [392–395]. In a recent report, Geubel et al. [393] found that in adults, as little as 25,000 IU of vitamin A for 6 years may lead to cirrhosis. Similar doses have been administered to children with chronic cholestasis. Vitamin A toxicity is also manifested by increased intracranial pressure in children, painful bone lesions, precocious bone growth, and desquamative dermatitis [395–400]. To monitor for vitamin A toxicity during high-dose vitamin A therapy, serum retinyl esters, normally not present, should be monitored. Elevated retinyl esters are associated with hepatotoxicity [401]. Plasma levels of retinol and RBP are not reliable means of detecting vitamin A toxicity [373,374]. Whether other indices of vitamin A status, such as the molar ratio of serum retinol to RBP, will be useful in assessing toxicity in children with chronic cholestasis is currently not known.

VITAMIN D

Vitamin D (calciferol) refers to two secosteroids, vitamin D_2 (ergocalciferol) and vitamin D_3 (cholecalciferol). They differ in their side chains; vitamin D_2 has a methyl group at C-24 and a double bond at C 22 to C 23. Vitamin D_2 is derived from plants and fungi and is added to vitamin D–supplemented cow's milk. The RDA is 300 IU (7.5 μg cholecalciferol) in infants (<6 months) and 400 IU (10 μg cholecalciferol) in older children and adults [368]. The absorption of vitamin D_2 is dependent on micellar solubilization, thus vitamin D_2 malabsorption has been observed in cholestasis (see Figure 10.2). Vitamin D_3 is synthesized in the skin from 7-dehydrocholesterol upon exposure to sunlight. Dietary vitamin D is absorbed in the jejunum and ileum and is then either transported into the lymphatics in chylomicrons (vitamins D_2 and D_3) or absorbed directly into the portal system (25-hydroxyvitamin D). In the blood, vitamin D is transported primarily bound to a vitamin D–binding protein (DBP) synthesized in the liver. Vitamins D_2 and D_3 subsequently undergo 25-hydroxylation in the liver to form 25-hydroxyvitamin D (25-OH-D, calcifidiol), which is the major circulating form of vitamin D (Figure 10.5). From the liver, 25-OH-D bound to DBP is transported to the kidney for 1α-hydroxylation to form 1,25-dihydroxyvitamin D (1,25-OH_2-D, calcitriol). Calcitriol is the biologically active form of vitamin D that stimulates intestinal absorption of calcium and phosphorus, renal reabsorption of filtered calcium, and mobilization of calcium and phosphorus from bone. In the presence of low serum calcium, increased levels of parathormone activate 1α-hydroxylase in the kidney, increasing circulating levels of calcitriol and thus stimulating calcium absorption. A 24-hydroxylation step in the kidney may result in the synthesis of 24,25-dihydroxyvitamin D that appears necessary for adequate bone mineralization [369].

The primary manifestations of vitamin D deficiency are related to the effects of 1,25-OH_2-D on calcium metabolism.

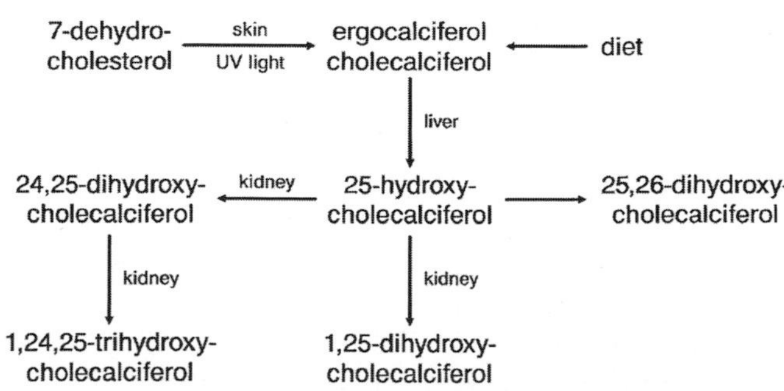

Figure 10.5. Schema of vitamin D metabolism.

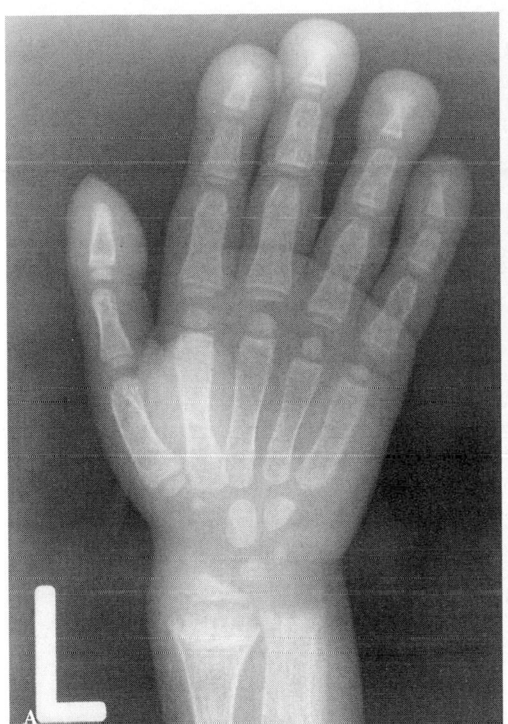

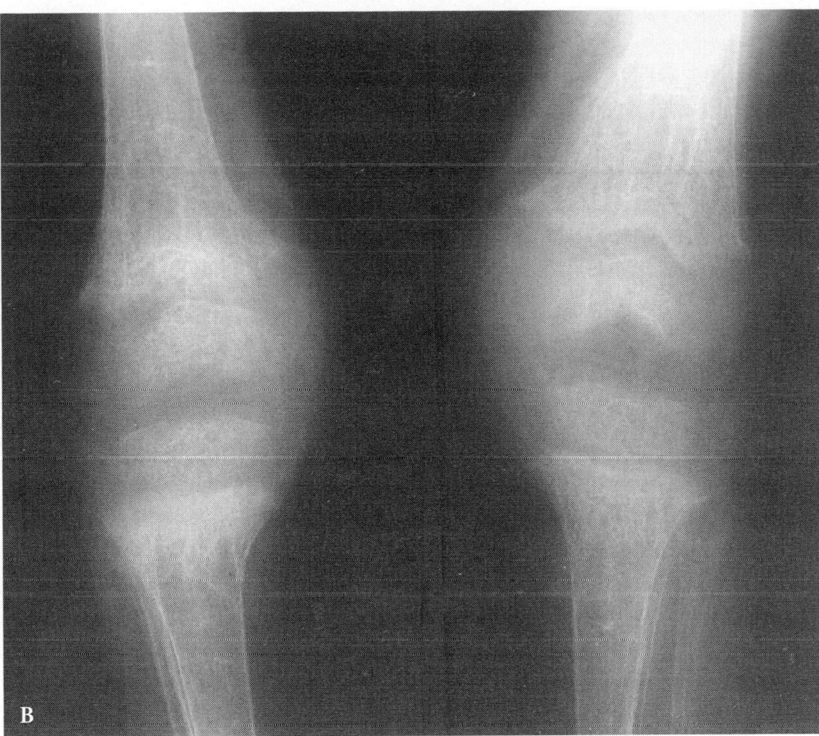

Figure 10.6. Extensive rickets caused by prolonged vitamin D deficiency in a 6-year-old child with biliary atresia and a nonfunctioning portoenterostomy who did not receive vitamin D supplements. (**A**) Radiograph of the wrist shows that the provisional zones of calcification at the distal ends of the radius and ulna are extensively frayed, cupped, and irregularly mineralized. The carpal and metacarpal bones and the distal shafts of the radius and ulna are diffusely osteopenic and coarse in texture (osteomalacia). This patient also had a markedly delayed bone age. Note the pronounced flattening and rounding of the soft tissues surrounding the terminal phalanges consistent with severe digital clubbing. (**B**) Bone films of the same patient's legs demonstrate marked osteopenia in the shafts. The metaphyses of the distal femur and proximal tibia and fibula are poorly calcified, widened, and frayed, denoting advanced rickets.

Hypocalcemia, hypophosphatemia, tetany, osteomalacia, and rickets are the most common clinical features.

During cholestasis, several factors predispose to vitamin D deficiency. Absorption of ingested vitamin D_2 is impaired [391,402], although 25-hydroxylation in the liver is intact [403,404]. Hepatic secretion of DBP may be reduced in liver disease, leading to lower levels of bound 25-OH-D. Consequently, the photosynthesized vitamin D_3 becomes a more important source of vitamin D. However, because of chronic debilitation, many children with chronic cholestatic liver disease are not exposed to adequate sunlight, thus decreasing the cutaneous synthesis of vitamin D_3. Phenobarbital therapy during cholestasis has also been shown to alter vitamin D metabolism, resulting in rickets [405]. Before the development of newer vitamin D analogues, approximately 29% of children with cholestasis had radiographic evidence of rickets (Figure 10.6) [406] whereas up to 80% had decreased bone mineral density based on iodohippurate sodium I 131 photon absorptiometry [407]. It has been shown that although patients with chronic cholestasis may normalize vitamin D status with therapy, they may continue to show evidence of metabolic bone disease. Using stable isotope technology, it was demonstrated that calcium absorption is not impaired in children with chronic cholestasis [408]. Furthermore, calcium balance was positive in four of five cholestatic children studied, despite diminished bone density. These data suggest that factors other than calcium malabsorption and decreased serum 25-OH-D levels contribute to the osteopenia commonly observed in children with chronic cholestasis. Recently, Heubi et al. [409] proposed that magnesium deficiency may play a role in the development of this bone disease. The role of circulating cytokines has not been investigated.

The clinical evaluation of vitamin D status in cholestatic children is performed initially by measuring serum 25-OH-D blood levels. Serum calcium, magnesium, phosphorus, alkaline phosphatase, and parathyroid hormone (PTH) levels, as well as bone radiography or bone densitometry may be used to identify osteomalacia, osteopenia, or rickets. A serum level of 25-OH-D below 14–15 ng/mL is indicative of vitamin D deficiency. The serum level of 1,25-OH_2-D is more indicative of calcium than of vitamin D status, with a high level indicative of calcium deficiency, and is not essential for routine monitoring for vitamin D deficiency.

It is currently recommended that children with chronic cholestasis have periodic monitoring of serum 25-OH-D levels along with adequate sunlight exposure and normal intake of calcium and phosphorus in the diet [299]. If vitamin D deficiency is present, oral vitamin D_3 (Drisdol; Winthrop-Breon Laboratories, New York, NY) may be administered in a dosage three to ten times the RDA for a child of that age per day;

however, close monitoring of serum 25-OH-D levels is required. If vitamin D is provided in a multiple vitamin supplement, it should be accounted for in the daily vitamin D dose. Intestinal absorption of these supplements may be improved by the co-administration of oral TPGS vitamin E as a solubilizing agent [391]. If patients fail to respond, have significant bony changes, or have severe cholestasis, supplementation with 1,25-OH_2-D (Rocaltrol; Roche Laboratories, Nutley, NJ) at a dosage of 0.05–0.2 μg/kg/d should be administered. This requires monitoring (including 1,25-OH_2-D levels) because there is no physiologic regulation of this compound [410]. Rocaltrol is expensive and is available in North America only in capsule form, thus the contents should be aspirated into a syringe to allow for proper dosing (given with meals) in small children. Serum concentrations of 25-OH-D (or 1,25-OH_2-D if Rocaltrol is used) should be rechecked in 1–2 months until normalization and every 3–6 months thereafter. Monitoring for vitamin D toxicity should include urine calcium:creatinine ratio, serum calcium and phosphorus, and serum 25-OH-D (or 1,25-OH_2-D). The principal manifestations of vitamin D intoxication are hypercalcemia leading to depression of the central nervous system and ectopic calcification, and hypercalciuria leading to nephrocalcinosis and nephrolithiasis. Recently, bisphosphonate drugs have been used to prevent and treat osteoporosis associated with PBC in adults [411]. The use of these agents in cholestatic children requires further study.

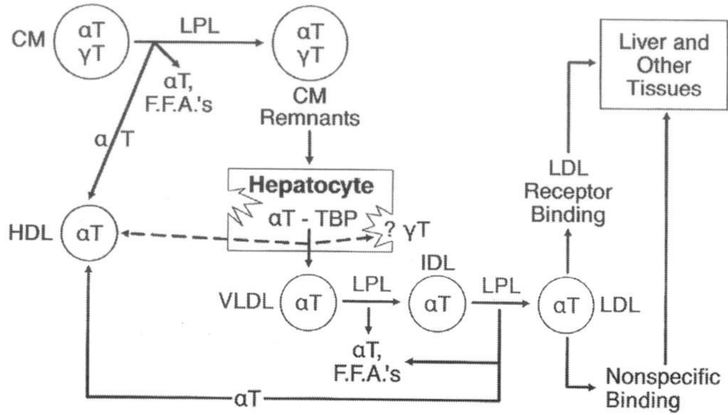

Figure 10.7. Proposed lipoprotein transport and delivery of vitamin E to the liver and peripheral tissues. TBP, tocopherol-binding protein; LPL, lipoprotein lipase; αT, α-tocopherol; γT, γ-tocopherol; FAs, fatty acids.

VITAMIN E

The term *vitamin E* refers to a group of eight compounds called the tocopherols and the tocotrienols, which consist of substituted hydroxylated chromanol ring systems linked to an isoprenoid side chain [412]. The four major forms of vitamin E (α, β, δ, and γ) differ by the number and position of the methyl group substitutions on the chromanol ring and in their bioactivity. α-Tocopherol has the highest biologic activity and is the predominant form in foodstuffs with the exception of soy and other vegetable oils that contain high levels of γ-tocopherol. The common dietary sources of vitamin E are the oil-containing grains, plants, and vegetables. The RDA is approximately 12–15 mg d-α-tocopherol per day in adults and less in children (4–15 mg per day) depending on age [368] (1 mg d-α-tocopherol = 1 tocopherol equivalent [TE]; 1 mg dl-α-tocopheryl acetate = 1 IU).

The ingested vitamin E requires solubilization by bile acids into mixed micelles and hydrolysis by pancreatic or intestinal esterases (bile acid dependent) before traversing the unstirred water layer in the intestinal lumen into the enterocyte [412,413] (see Figure 10.2). Absorption occurs by a nonsaturable, non–carrier-mediated passive diffusion process. Absorbed α- and γ-tocopherol are then incorporated in the enterocyte into chylomicrons and VLDL and are secreted into the mesenteric lymphatics, finally reaching the systemic circulation. Upon reaching the blood, vitamin E is transported predominantly in LDL and high-density lipoprotein (HDL). The α- and γ-tocopherol remaining in chylomicrons are taken up by the hepatocyte. α-Tocopherol (particularly d-α or the R-R-R stereoisomer) is preferentially resecreted as a component of hepatic-derived VLDLs and perhaps HDLs (Figure 10.7). γ- and δ-tocopherols as well as nonnatural stereoisomers of α-tocopherol are metabolized or excreted by the liver. The hepatic tocopherol-transfer protein (TTP) appears to play a role in the hepatic discrimination process by which R-R-R α-tocopherol is incorporated into lipoproteins and other forms of vitamin E are not [413]. The delivery of vitamin E to peripheral tissues involves lipoprotein lipase hydrolysis of chylomicrons [414] and LDL binding to cell receptors [415].

The impaired secretion of bile acids during cholestasis results in malabsorption of vitamin E [413]. Vitamin E is the most hydrophobic of the fat-soluble vitamins and therefore has the greatest requirement for intraluminal bile acids for absorption. Vitamin E absorption, measured by the oral vitamin E tolerance test, is profoundly depressed in cholestatic children who were vitamin E deficient [413]. Co-administration of bile acids enhances the absorption of vitamin E [413]. The frequency of vitamin E deficiency in children with chronic cholestasis is 49–77% [367,413,416,417] despite the administration of "routine" oral supplements.

The physiologic role of vitamin E in the maintenance of structure and function of the human nervous system and skeletal muscle was recognized by the discovery of a progressive degenerative neuromuscular disorder associated with vitamin E deficiency during cholestasis and other states of fat malabsorption [413,416–419]. Involved regions include the spinocerebellar tracts; cranial nerve nuclei III and IV; large-caliber myelinated axons in peripheral nerves, the posterior columns of the spinal cord, and gracilis and cuneatus nuclei in the brainstem; skeletal muscle; and the ocular retina [420] (Figure 10.8). Clinical manifestations of vitamin E deficiency appear as hyporeflexia at approximately 18–24 months of age in children with prolonged neonatal cholestatic disorders and may be accompanied by sural nerve lesions even before 1 year of age [421]. Uncorrected vitamin E deficiency during childhood leads to sequential development of neurologic symptoms, including

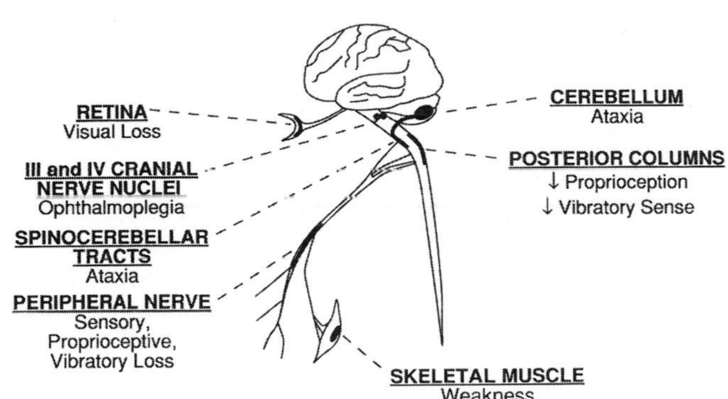

Figure 10.8. Sites of neuromuscular involvement of vitamin E deficiency and corresponding clinical manifestations.

truncal and limb ataxia, depressed vibratory and position sensation, impairment in balance and coordination, peripheral neuropathy, proximal muscle weakness, ophthalmoplegia, and retinal dysfunction [417]. Significant cognitive and behavioral abnormalities have been described in association with prolonged vitamin E deficiency as well [337,422–424]. The neurologic lesions may be irreversible to a substantial degree if vitamin E deficiency remains untreated [418,425]. Studies in the United States [418] and France [425] have demonstrated reversal or prevention of neurologic degeneration if vitamin E deficiency is corrected before age 3–4 years, whereas older children with more severe neurologic symptoms show a more limited response to therapy; thus aggressive evaluation and normalization of vitamin E status early in the course of chronic cholestasis in children are required. Deficiency of vitamin E has also been associated with hemolytic anemia in premature infants fed a diet high in polyunsaturated fatty acids [426]; however, this has not been reported in cholestasis.

The major function of vitamin E is its role as an antioxidant, protecting cell membrane polyunsaturated fatty acids and thiol-rich proteins from oxidant damage initiated by free radical reactions [427,428]. Vitamin E has also recently been shown to be an agonist for the PXR nuclear receptor [429]. The possibility that vitamin E deficiency may worsen cholestatic liver injury has been proposed based on the observation that lipid peroxidation increases in the cholestatic rat liver and that vitamin E deficiency combined with a diet containing over 30% of calories as fat may exacerbate cholestatic hepatic injury in the rat [294]. In addition, pro-oxidants, such as copper and manganese, which accumulate during cholestasis, increase free radical generation and the requirement for vitamin E and other antioxidants [430]. Vitamin E deficiency may impair immune function as well [431,432].

The assessment of vitamin E status during cholestasis should utilize the ratio of the serum vitamin E concentration to total serum lipid concentration (E:lipid) [433,434]. Elevated circulating lipid levels during cholestasis cause vitamin E to partition into the plasma lipoproteins and may increase the serum vitamin E concentration into the normal range (5–20 μg/mL) in a vitamin E–deficient patient [435]. Calculation of the ratio of E:lipid (mg/g) compensates for this phenomenon [433,434]. Vitamin E deficiency is indicated by a ratio of less than 0.6 mg/g in children less than 1 year of age and less than 0.8 mg/g in older children [433–435]. For vitamin E repletion of deficient patients, we aim to achieve an E:lipid ratio of >0.8–1.0 mg/g. Measurement of vitamin E in adipose tissue assesses vitamin E stores; however, it requires adipose biopsies and few laboratories perform this analysis. Other functional assays for vitamin E status include red blood cell (RBC) hydrogen peroxide hemolysis [436] and the RBC malondialdehyde release test [437], which depend on the ability of the RBCs to resist an oxidant stress. With the former test, vitamin E deficiency is suggested if more than 10% of RBCs hemolyze when exposed to hydrogen peroxide [436]. However, because selenium deficiency and other nutritional factors (e.g., polyunsaturated fatty acid status) also affect hydrogen peroxide hemolysis, this test is not specific for vitamin E deficiency. Increased amounts of malondialdehyde, a lipid peroxidation product, released by RBCs exposed to hydrogen peroxide is another indicator of vitamin E depletion but is open to the same problems as hydrogen peroxide hemolysis.

To prevent the development of vitamin E deficiency, routine supplementation with vitamin E is indicated in all infants and young children with chronic cholestasis. In older children and adults, vitamin E stores will maintain adequacy of vitamin E status for at least 6–12 months. Infants newly diagnosed with cholestatic disorders are treated with 25–50 IU/kg/d of vitamin E (α-tocopherol, α-tocopheryl acetate, α-tocopheryl succinate, or α-tocopheryl nicotinate) or 15–25 IU/kg/d of the liquid preparation of the water-soluble ester of vitamin E, d-α-tocopheryl polyethylene glycol-1000 succinate (TPGS) (Liqui-E [26.6 IU/mL]; Twin Laboratories, Ronkonkoma, NY; or Aqua-E [20 IU/mL]; Yasoo Health Inc., Johnson City, TN). The vitamin E is given as a single morning dose with breakfast (when bile flow is maximal) or at least 2 hours apart from medications that may interfere with its absorption (e.g., cholestyramine, iron). Alternatively, capsules of vitamin E (100–400 IU) can be slit open and the oil carefully squeezed into the infant's or child's mouth followed by formula or breast-feeding, or into solid food in order to deliver these large doses in an inexpensive manner. If TPGS is used, 25 IU/kg/d is almost always effective in normalizing vitamin E status. If other forms of vitamin E are used, doses are increased by 25–50 IU/kg/d up to a 100–200 IU/kg/d maximum if there is no response in serum E:lipid ratio in 3–4 weeks. If vitamin E status fails to normalize (E:lipid ratio >0.8 mg/g) after several months of therapy with 100 IU/kg/d of the standard vitamin E preparations, either TPGS or intramuscular injections of vitamin E (Ephynal [50 mg/mL]; Hoffman LaRoche, Basel, Switzerland) will need to be instituted. The effective dose for this parenteral form of vitamin E is 0.5–1.0 IU/kg/d given as 0.5–1.0-mL intramuscular injections every 3–10 days to provide the calculated dose [418]. In a U.S. multicenter trial, all 60 vitamin E–deficient children with cholestasis who failed to respond to large doses of standard vitamin E responded to 15–30 IU/kg/d of TPGS without detectable side effects [438]. Therefore, intramuscular vitamin E is used only in the rare instances of TPGS failure.

Vitamin E therapy is monitored by obtaining trough E:lipid ratios every 2–3 months and by performing serial neurologic examinations. Attempts are made to keep serum vitamin E levels below 25–30 μg/mL; however, to achieve an E:lipid ratio above 0.8 mg/g, it is occasionally necessary to allow serum vitamin E to exceed this range in the severely hyperlipidemic child. Once normalization of the serum E:lipid ratio has been achieved, these levels are repeated every 6 months during continued vitamin E supplementation, unless there is a major change in the severity of cholestasis. If profound neurologic deficits are present, serial visual evoked response or somatosensory evoked response measurements may be helpful in documenting neurologic improvement. Vitamin E toxicity is rare. Normal adults appear to tolerate oral doses of 100–800 mg/d without clinical signs or biochemical evidence of toxicity [439,440]. Because up to 3–4% of the polyethylene glycol contained in TPGS may be absorbed [438], there is a small risk of inducing a hyperosmolar state if glomerular filtration rate is decreased because of renal failure or dehydration. Therefore, TPGS should be administered cautiously in these circumstances. One additional concern is the potential exacerbation of vitamin K–deficient coagulopathy. Adults without liver disease who received very large doses of vitamin E (>1000–1500 IU/d) in conjunction with warfarin therapy had significantly prolonged prothrombin time beyond that expected from the warfarin alone [441,442]. Presumably the excess vitamin E inhibited the γ-carboxylation reaction of vitamin K. Thus, to prevent this occurrence in cholestatic children receiving large doses of vitamin E, vitamin K status should be corrected, prothrombin time monitored, and excessively high serum vitamin E levels avoided. In addition, large parenteral doses of vitamin E that achieved extremely high serum vitamin E levels (>40–50 μg/mL) in preterm infants (without significant liver disease) were associated with an increased incidence of bacterial and fungal sepsis, presumably as a result of inhibition of neutrophil function (generation of free radicals) [443]. Proper monitoring of serum vitamin E levels in cholestatic patients should prevent this possible complication. Finally, intravenous use of an untested form of α-tocopheryl acetate solubilized in polysorbate (Eferol) led to fatal liver injury in a number of preterm infants [444]. It was most likely the polysorbate and not the vitamin E that was toxic. This product was promptly removed from the market when this toxicity was recognized.

VITAMIN K

Vitamin K belongs to the family of 2-methyl-1,4-naphthoquinones and exists as three forms [445,446]. Phylloquinone (vitamin K_1) is obtained from leafy vegetables, soybean oil, fruits, seeds, and cow's milk. Menaquinone (vitamin K_2), which has 60% of the activity of vitamin K_1, is synthesized by intestinal bacteria. Menadione (vitamin K_3) is not a natural form but is synthesized chemically and has better water solubility than the two natural forms. The RDA for infants is 5 μg of phylloquinone or menaquinone for the first 6 months, 10 μg during the second 6 months, and 1 μg/kg body weight for older children [368].

The absorption of vitamin K requires bile and pancreatic secretions and is therefore impaired during cholestasis. Small intestinal absorption of vitamin K_1 is by a saturable process requiring metabolic energy, whereas K_2 absorption occurs by passive diffusion. The absorbed vitamin K is incorporated in the enterocyte into chylomicrons and is transported to the blood via the lymph (see Figure 10.2). In the liver, vitamin K is taken up in chylomicron remnants and incorporated into VLDL and ultimately into LDL for transport to tissues. Little vitamin K is stored in the liver.

Vitamin K is necessary for the posttranslational γ-carboxylation of glutamic acid residues of the vitamin K–dependent coagulation proteins (factors II, VII, IX, and X, protein C, and protein S) [447]. Carboxylation allows these proteins to bind calcium, thus leading to activation of the clotting factors. In addition, there is a family of other vitamin K–dependent proteins ("Gla proteins") found in all tissues, the function of which are largely unknown. Osteocalcin is one such Gla protein involved in bone mineralization [448,449]. Recent studies in adults suggest that vitamin K status may impact bone mineralization [450,451]. Vitamin K deficiency causes a coagulopathy that may present in infancy with intracranial bleeding [452,453]. Malabsorption of vitamin K, as well as frequent antibiotic suppression of intestinal floral production of vitamin K, predisposes to deficiency during cholestasis. In one study [454], 23% of 43 patients with biliary atresia who had undergone portoenterostomy were found to be vitamin K deficient.

Vitamin K status is clinically evaluated by measuring the prothrombin time/international normalized ratio (INR), which is dependent on the vitamin K–dependent clotting factors. If the prothrombin time/INR is prolonged in comparison to the partial thromboplastin time, then this most likely represents vitamin K deficiency. Response in prothrombin time to intramuscular injection of vitamin K is the most accurate means of diagnosing deficiency. A more sensitive measure of vitamin K status is analysis of plasma levels of protein induced in vitamin K absence (PIVKA II) [455]. Factor II, VII, IX, and X assays offer no real advantage over the prothrombin time and are not only costly but are also unavailable in many laboratories. Serum vitamin K levels can be measured but do not represent vitamin K stores, are only available in research laboratories, and may not correlate with prothrombin time/INR measurements.

Because children with chronic liver disease have other risk factors for bleeding (e.g., development of esophageal varices, portal hypertensive gastropathy, platelet dysfunction, thrombocytopenia, and diminished hepatic synthesis of other coagulation factors), vitamin K deficiency should be routinely prevented. Oral forms of vitamin K supplements of 2.5–5.0 mg two to seven times a week should be given to all children with chronic cholestasis [149,299,389,456]. Vitamin K_1 (Mephyton; Merck, Sharpe, and Dohme, West Point, PA) is preferred because it lacks toxicity if given in excess [455]. Co-administration of Mephyton with TPGS may also theoretically enhance its absorption. Vitamin K_3 (Synkayvite; Roche Laboratories, Nutley, NJ), more water-soluble and thus better absorbed, may be needed if there is no response to vitamin K_1. However, large doses of vitamin K_3 have the potential for hepatotoxicity if completely absorbed [457]. In addition, massive hemolysis in glucose 6-phosphate dehydrogenase–deficient infants has been reported [457]. Synkayvite is currently not available in North America. If oral vitamin K supplementation is unsuccessful, intramuscular or intravenous injection of vitamin K (AquaMEPHYTON; Merck & Co., Whitehouse Station, NJ) every 3–4 weeks at a dose of 2–5 mg prevents and reverses vitamin K deficiency–induced coagulopathy.

Water-Soluble Vitamins

Little is known about the nutritional status of water-soluble vitamins during chronic childhood cholestasis. In adults with chronic liver disease, however, deficiencies of vitamins B_1, B_6, and C and folic acid have been described [458]. Therefore, it seems prudent to supplement the vitamins normally present in the diet with an additional one to two times the RDA of water-soluble vitamins contained in standard pediatric multivitamin supplements (one to two per day). Because these supplements also contain additional amounts of the fat-soluble vitamins, these should be taken into account when calculating supplemental doses for each vitamin, particularly for vitamins A and D.

Calcium and Phosphate

Fat malabsorption during cholestasis decreases the intestinal absorption of calcium and phosphate as the result of formation of insoluble soaps. Mineral deficiency may develop and potentially contribute to bone disease unresponsive to normalization of vitamin D status. In addition to encouraging high-calcium and -phosphate food (Table 10.4), enteral supplements of 25–100 mg/kg/d of elemental calcium and of 25–50 mg/kg of phosphorus may be necessary to reverse bone abnormalities. Calcium may be administered as inexpensive chewable calcium-carbonate antacid tablets (e.g., Tums, Rolaids). Serum calcium and phosphorus concentrations, urine calcium:creatinine ratio, and the fractional excretion of phosphate should be used to monitor supplementation with these minerals [330].

Magnesium

Hypomagnesemia has been described in adults and children with cirrhosis [459–461]. The mechanism for the low plasma magnesium is believed to be related to malabsorption [459], hyperaldosteronism leading to increased renal excretion of magnesium [460], hepatic fibrosis, decreased albumin:γ-globulin ratio [461], and chronic malnutrition [462]. Like serum zinc, serum magnesium may be normal in the presence of depleted total body stores or be low with normal stores. Isolated magnesium deficiency is actually rare because of very effective control of magnesium homeostasis by the kidney. But if magnesium depletion is present, it may lead to hypocalcemia [463] as a result of decreased synthesis [464] and secretion [465] of PTH. Studies in magnesium-deficient humans have shown inappropriately low immunoreactive PTH levels for the degree of hypocalcemia and a normal target tissue response to exogenous PTH [466,467], supporting the postulated impaired secretion of immunoreactive PTH in the magnesium-deficient state. As a consequence, impaired 1α-hydroxylation of vitamin D occurs [468,469], which may worsen hypocalcemia and lead to rickets. Acquired resistance to therapy with active metabolites of vitamin D during magnesium deficiency has also been observed [468,470].

It has been postulated that negative magnesium balance may be a contributing factor to the metabolic bone disease of chronic liver disease. In a small group of children with cholestasis, all were found to be magnesium depleted, with significantly reduced serum PTH levels [409]. Furthermore, reduced bone mineral density in children with chronic cholestasis was associated with reduced urinary excretion of an intravenous loading dose of magnesium, indicating magnesium deficiency [409]. Supplementation with magnesium oxide for at least 12 months led to improvement in bone mineral density in these children. These data need to be corroborated to delineate the role of magnesium in cholestatic metabolic bone disease. Magnesium deficiency is treated with 1–2 mEq/kg/d of oral magnesium oxide. Acute states of magnesium depletion may be treated with 0.3–0.5 mEq/kg/dose (3–6 mEq maximum) of a 50% solution of magnesium sulfate given intravenously over 3 hours and repeated over the remainder of the 24-hour period. Magnesium excess may cause respiratory depression, lethargy, and coma.

Zinc

Zinc is an essential trace metal, present in more than 100 zinc metalloenzymes and a range of transcription proteins. The RDA for infants and children is 5–10 mg/d [368]. Deficiency of zinc leads to poor linear growth, hypogeusia, anorexia, impaired immune function, and an erythematous vesicular eruption on the face and distal extremities. Delayed recovery from infectious diarrheal states has also been reported. Low plasma zinc is common in infants with chronic cholestasis [371,459,471]. In a series of 27 children awaiting liver transplantation, 42% were reported to have low plasma zinc concentrations [371]. The reduced zinc concentrations may be related to poor intake of zinc-containing foods, malabsorption of zinc, reduced levels of serum albumin available for binding and transport of zinc, compartmentation of zinc into the liver as part of the acute phase response, or increased zinc excretion in urine [471,472]. Inappropriately elevated urinary zinc excretion rapidly reverses after liver transplantation [473]. Unfortunately, plasma zinc concentrations do not correlate well with total body zinc status. For example, in children with cirrhosis, normal plasma zinc levels have been observed in the presence of diminished hepatic zinc concentrations [459]. Thus, identifying infants and children with chronic zinc deficiency may be difficult. If infants are growing poorly with inadequate oral intake or if plasma zinc concentration is low (<60 μg/dL), we recommend supplementation with 1 mg/kg/d of elemental zinc as a zinc sulfate solution (10 mg zinc/mL) for 2–3 months as a therapeutic trial. Further study of zinc balance and the effects of zinc deficiency in cholestasis is needed.

Selenium

As part of the enzyme glutathione peroxidase, selenium functions as an antioxidant catalyzing the reduction of hydrogen peroxide to water and of lipid hydroperoxides. Other selenoproteins have also been discovered recently. The RDA for selenium is 10 μg/d in infants and 15–50 μg/d in children and adolescents [368]. The plasma selenium concentrations of the majority of healthy infants and children fall within the range of 50–150 μg/L, with the mean around 100 μg/L [474]. Selenium deficiency may cause a cardiomyopathy [475,476] and a skeletal myopathy [477] manifested by weakness and muscle pain. Keshan disease is an endemic form of cardiomyopathy caused by selenium deficiency found in China. Milder selenium deficiency is associated with macrocytosis of erythrocytes and loss of hair pigment [478]. Plasma selenium levels less than 40 μg/L (0.5 mmol/L) indicate mild selenium deficiency and those less than 10 μg/L (0.12 mmol/L), severe selenium deficiency [479]. Levander [480] reported selenium deficiency in a child with biliary atresia whose expired ethane gas did not normalize after correction of vitamin E deficiency. Plasma selenium was found to be 62 μg/L (normal: 90–170 in their laboratory). After oral selenium supplementation, plasma levels rose to 95 μg/L and breath ethane became undetectable. Subsequently, 13–33% of children with chronic cholestasis were found to have plasma selenium levels below 20 μg/L [251,363]; however, clinical manifestations of selenium deficiency were not detected in these children. Whether selenium deficiency potentiates the skeletal myopathy of vitamin E–deficient children is unknown. Although definite recommendations cannot be made, it seems prudent to monitor plasma selenium levels periodically in children with severe cholestasis, particularly those with poor growth. Consumption of selenium-rich foods such as cereals, meat, eggs, and dairy products should be encouraged. If serum selenium levels are low, supplementation with 1–2 μg/kg body weight per day of oral sodium selenite should be considered. For infants and children on parenteral nutrition, an intravenous dose of 2 μg/kg body weight per day is recommended for repletion therapy followed by 1 μg/kg/d for long-term TPN maintenance [478,480]. Plasma selenium levels should be monitored during and after supplementation, with the goal of 50–150 μg/L [474].

Iron

Iron deficiency results from a combination of decreased intake and chronic blood loss from esophageal varices, portal hypertensive gastropathy, and prolonged bleeding from other sites because of coagulopathy and thrombocytopenia. A 32% incidence of iron-deficiency anemia has been reported in children with end-stage liver disease [371]. Low serum iron, increased total iron-binding capacity, and a saturation index less than 16% suggest a diagnosis of iron deficiency. Treatment is elemental iron at a dose of 5–6 mg/kg/d during deficiency and 1–2 mg/kg/d to compensate for ongoing blood loss. Correction of vitamin E deficiency, if present, should be performed concomitantly with iron therapy to prevent precipitation of hemolysis. The role of iron deficiency in the developmental delays and psychological and emotional problems encountered during chronic cholestasis has not been investigated.

Copper, Manganese, and Aluminum

Copper accumulates in the liver during all forms of cholestasis because its major excretory pathway is through the biliary route. To compensate for this impaired excretion of copper, liver synthesis and secretion of ceruloplasmin are increased, leading to elevated serum concentrations of ceruloplasmin and copper during cholestasis. Extraordinarily elevated hepatic copper concentrations, sometimes well within the range found in patients with Wilson's disease, have been observed in children with various forms of cholestasis [481] and in adults with PBC [482]. Although there has been no convincing demonstration of toxicity of copper during childhood cholestasis, the possible interaction between copper, a pro-oxidant capable of stimulating the generation of free radicals [483], especially in the face of depletion of antioxidants (such as vitamin E, selenium, and glutathione), in an already injured liver deserves further attention [430]. Two small uncontrolled trials of the copper chelator D-penicillamine in children with chronic cholestasis failed to demonstrate any improvement in liver function or histology, although copper chelation was achieved [484,485]. However, all children had advanced liver disease at the time of chelation therapy and no attempts were made to correct antioxidant deficiencies. Similar results have been described in adults with PBC [486,487]. Currently, copper chelation is not recommended for childhood cholestatic disorders that are not inborn errors of copper metabolism. Low-copper diets and removal or lowering of copper supplements from parenteral nutrition infusates administered to cholestatic children are recommended [488,489] but have not been thoroughly investigated.

Manganese is another trace element that is excreted primarily in bile [490] and accumulates in the liver in infants with biliary atresia [491]. The major toxicity of manganese appears to be related to the central nervous system, where it may accumulate in the globus pallidus and subthalamic nuclei during cholestasis, causing basal ganglia injury [492,493]. Increasing evidence suggests that manganese deposition is responsible for the T1-weighted magnetic resonance imaging (MRI) signal hyperintensity observed in the globus pallidus of cirrhotic patients and correlates with elevated blood manganese levels [494,495]. Both chronic liver disease and the presence of portosystemic shunting have been significantly associated with brain manganese accumulation [496,497]. In a study of autopsy specimens, globus pallidal manganese concentrations were significantly higher in patients with a history of chronic liver disease who died of hepatic coma as compared with controls [496]. The association of extrapyramidal symptoms in patients with cirrhosis and hyperintense pallidal signaling on MRI suggests a role for manganese in hepatic encephalopathy [498–500]. In a report of a child with Alagille syndrome, dystonia, and tremor, whole blood manganese levels were associated with symmetric hyperintense globus pallidi on T1-weighted MRI [326]. Following liver transplantation, neurologic function improved, blood manganese levels normalized, and the MRI signal abnormality completely resolved.

Additionally, rats injected with high doses of manganese simultaneously with bilirubin developed cholestatic liver disease [501], raising concern for possible hepatotoxicity of manganese during cholestasis. Pending further investigation, it is recommended that manganese supplements be withheld from parenteral nutrition solutions administered to infants and children with cholestasis [488,489,502]. Furthermore, because intravenous nutrition solutions are contaminated with variable amounts of manganese [502,503], plasma manganese levels should be monitored in cholestatic patients receiving TPN. Furthermore, intestinal absorption of both iron and manganese are increased during iron deficiency; therefore, iron deficiency may increase the susceptibility to manganese toxicity [504]. Patients with chronic liver disease should avoid manganese supplements without concurrent iron supplementation.

Aluminum is commonly found in aluminum hydroxide antacids and sucralfate and as a contaminant in many TPN constituents [505–507] and other common intravenous products (e.g., calcium gluconate, albumin, potassium phosphate) [508,509]. This metal appears to have hepatotoxic effects in large doses [510]. Because biliary excretion is an important route of elimination of orally absorbed aluminum [511], it is possible that cholestasis may lead to accumulation of aluminum in the liver [512]. Consequently, the use of aluminum-containing medications should be discouraged in cholestasis unless absolutely necessary until more is known about the hepatic metabolism and potential hepatotoxicity of aluminum.

GENERAL PEDIATRIC CARE

The long-term management of the child with chronic liver disease is directed not only toward the medical treatment of the varied complications of the underlying liver disease but in optimizing growth and development, alleviating psychological/emotional problems in the developing child, and helping the family cope with the emotional and financial stresses resulting from raising a child with a chronic disease.

Growth and Development

Deficits in both growth and mental development observed in children with chronic liver disease are believed to arise from a combination of the following factors: prolonged illness, repeated hospitalizations, and malnutrition and nutrient deficiencies associated with the underlying liver disease [337,422, 513]. Children with early-onset liver disease (<12 months of age) score significantly lower on verbal, performance, and full-scale IQ testing [337]. Furthermore, in contrast to children with a later onset of liver disease (>12 months of age), those with early onset are more compromised in linear growth and head circumference and have lower serum vitamin E levels [337], consistent with the results of earlier studies [422]. Although it is generally difficult to predict cognitive outcomes accurately based on testing in the first 2 years of life [514–518], developmental testing (McCarthy Scales of Children's Abilities) in seven children who had undergone portoenterostomy 4–7 years earlier demonstrated slight mental delay and learning disabilities in all of them [513]. Although the number of children studied was small, these findings once again emphasize the importance of aggressive nutritional management and correction of malnutrition and micronutrient deficiencies (e.g., vitamin E), particularly in children who develop chronic cholestatic liver disease within the first year of life. It has also been suggested that delaying transplantation in children with biliary atresia and poor growth may compromise their eventual intellectual development [339]. Periodic testing of cognitive and motor development will help identify those children at risk for developmental delay and learning disabilities so that appropriate intervention can be initiated early.

For the adolescent, chronic liver disease has many frustrating complications, including primary or secondary amenorrhea and delayed puberty [519]. Adolescent females with severe liver disease often have amenorrhea that resolves as the liver disease abates. However, the use of spironolactone, frequently used as a diuretic in the treatment of patients with ascites, has been associated with primary or secondary amenorrhea in adolescents with chronic liver disease [520]. The mechanism of action is believed to be the suppression of estrogen or androgen synthesis by spironolactone or binding at estrogen or androgen receptors, resulting in negative feedback regulation of gonadotropins [520]. In the reported cases, regular menses began shortly after discontinuation of spironolactone. It is therefore recommended that if amenorrhea develops during spironolactone therapy, alternative treatments, such as triamterene, should be considered.

Immunizations

In general, children with chronic liver disease should receive routine childhood immunizations, with the exception of patients who have recently undergone portoenterostomy for biliary atresia and those who have had a liver transplantation. For patients who have recently undergone a hepato portoenterostomy, diphtheria-pertussis-tetanus (DPT) vaccination may be delayed temporarily following surgery. The occurrence of fever and irritability that is common following DPT immunization is difficult to differentiate clinically from cholangitis and would necessitate admission into the hospital for treatment of presumed cholangitis. In addition, dehydration and decreased bile flow secondary to poor intake and fever following DPT vaccination may predispose to bile stasis and cholangitis. Vaccines with live viruses are generally contraindicated in children who have undergone liver transplantation. Thus, it is recommended that children who are scheduled to receive a liver transplant and who are older than 12 months should be given measles, mump, and rubella and varicella vaccines, preferably at least 1 month before transplantation. Only inactivated polio vaccine (Salk) should be given to transplant recipients and their household contacts because the attenuated virus in oral polio vaccine can spread from person to person in a household. Immunization with influenza and pneumococcal vaccines should be encouraged as well in the absence of contraindications. Passive immunization with immunoglobulin should be employed for postexposure prophylaxis for other infections (e.g., varicella-zoster immune globulin for varicella). Hepatitis A and B vaccines should be routinely administered at the earliest recommended ages.

Dental Hygiene

Discoloration of teeth and dental caries are common in children with chronic liver disease. The yellow-green staining of primary teeth in infants with chronic cholestasis is attributed to exposure of the developing dentin and enamel to hemosiderin, biliverdin, and bilirubin [521]. The degree of pigment deposition may be proportionate to the serum concentration of bilirubin [522]. Unless the child continues to have severe cholestasis through 8 years of age, when formation of permanent teeth is completed, permanent teeth are unlikely to be affected [521]. On the other hand, surface discoloration of teeth may occur in all ages and may result from oral bacteria causing black or green stains as a result of poor oral hygiene, use of sweetened acidic iron preparations leaving black iron sulfide deposits, dental caries, and ingested food products. The numerous oral medications taken by children with chronic liver disease usually contain sweeteners and have a syrupy consistency [25], increasing the risk for development of dental caries. The poor absorption of calcium, phosphorus, and vitamin D due to chronic cholestasis may likewise lead to decreased integrity of dental structures and increased susceptibility to development of dental caries. Restriction of sugar-containing medications, stressing good oral hygiene, and frequent dental examinations and surveillance will aid in the prevention of dental caries, gingivitis, or abscesses, which may develop into severe infections in this group of relatively immunocompromised patients. Lastly, cosmetic treatment of discolored teeth may become necessary for self-esteem as the child grows older.

Family Support

Chronic liver disease presents an enormous stress not only on the affected child but on the family as well. Parental fear that the child might die, guilt over having "caused" the liver disease in some way, parenting inadequacy to fulfill the child's "special needs," pain from seeing their child frequently experience discomfort and physical pain (e.g., medical procedures), financial concerns, uncertainty and fear of the future, lack of control and taking control, and strained relationships among family members are stresses identified by families caring for a child with chronic liver disease [523]. In addition, because many children with chronic liver disease are hospitalized frequently, families are often separated for long and indefinite periods of time, disrupting normal routines. Early identification of these stresses and attention to these aspects of the child's care should help improve the quality of life for the child and his family. Establishing friendships and communication among patients, parents, and the medical team as well as patient and family education offer invaluable support in dealing with the emotional stress and turmoil associated with living with chronic liver disease. Organizing family and patient support groups locally is recommended. National foundations and patient advocacy groups can also supply families with useful information, contacts with other families, and "chat rooms" on the Internet.

CONCLUSION

Cholestatic liver disease in infancy and childhood is heterogeneous in etiology and natural history. Because specific medical/surgical therapy is available for many cholestatic disorders, prompt diagnosis is imperative before irreversible liver damage occurs. Anticipation and recognition of the varied medical, nutritional, emotional, and psychological consequences of chronic cholestasis will optimize growth and development and minimize discomfort and disability. For children who will eventually require OLT, supportive medical care including aggressive nutritional therapy may enhance their chances for a successful operation as well as normal growth and development following transplantation. An improved understanding of the molecular and cellular mechanisms causing liver injury and fibrosis in cholestasis is needed. It is hoped that new biotechnologic and translational approaches will lead to the development of newer treatment strategies designed to prevent, reverse, and treat these disorders.

ACKNOWLEDGMENTS

This chapter was supported in part by USPHS grant (M01-RR00069) from the General Clinical Research Centers Branch, National Center for Research Resources, National Institutes of Health (NIH); National Institute of Diabetes, Digestive and Kidney Diseases, NIH: K08 DK 61480 (APF) and R01 DK 38446, U54 DK 078377, UO1-DK062453- (RJS); the Abby Bennett Liver Research Fund, and the Cystic Fibrosis Foundation.

REFERENCES

1. Kasai M. Treatment of biliary atresia with special reference to hepatic portoenterostomy and its modifications. Prog Pediatr Surg 1974;6:5.
2. Whitley RJ, Nahmias AJ, Soong SJ, et al. Vidarabine therapy of neonatal herpes simplex virus infection. Pediatrics 1980 Oct;66:495–501.
3. Ingall D, Musher D. Infectious diseases of the fetus and newborn infant. In: Remington JS, Klein JO, eds. Syphilis. Philadelphia: Saunders, 1983:335.
4. Wright DJ, Berry CL. Letter: liver involvement in congenital syphilis. Br J Vener Dis 1974;50:241.
5. Ray CG, Wedgwood RJ. Neonatal listeriosis. Six case reports and a review of the literature. Pediatrics 1964;34:378–92.
6. Seelinger H, Finger H. Infectious diseases of the fetus and newborn infant. In: Remington JS, Klein JO, eds. Listeriosis. Philadelphia: Saunders, 1983:264.

7. Huber GL. Tuberculosis. In: Remington J, Klein J, eds. Tuberculosis. Philadelphia: Saunders, 1983:570.
8. Couvreur J, Desmonts G. Congenital and maternal toxoplasmosis. A review of 300 congenital cases. Dev Med Child Neurol 1962;4:519–30.
9. Remington JS, Desmonts G. Infectious diseases of the fetus and newborn infant. In: Remington JS, Klein JO, eds. Toxoplasmosis. Philadelphia: Saunders, 1983:143.
10. Applebaum MN, Thaler MM. Reversibility of extensive liver damage in galactosemia. Gastroenterology 1975;69:496–502.
11. Komrower GM, Lee DH. Long-term follow-up of galactosaemia. Arch Dis Child 1970;45:367–73.
12. Hill A, Nordin PM, Zaleski WA. Dietary treatment of tyrosinosis. J Am Diet Assoc 1970;56:308–12.
13. Hostetter MK, Levy HL, Winter HS, et al. Evidence for liver disease preceding amino acid abnormalities in hereditary tyrosinemia. N Engl J Med 1983;308:1265–7.
14. Lindblad B, Lindstedt S, Steen G. On the enzymic defects in hereditary tyrosinemia. Proc Natl Acad Sci U S A 1977;74:4641–5.
15. Starzl TE, Zitelli BJ, Shaw BW Jr, et al. Changing concepts: liver replacement for hereditary tyrosinemia and hepatoma. J Pediatr 1985;106:604–6.
16. Weinberg AG, Mize CE, Worthen HG. The occurrence of hepatoma in the chronic form of hereditary tyrosinemia. J Pediatr 1976;88:434–8.
17. Lindstedt S, Holme E, Lock EA, et al. Treatment of hereditary tyrosinaemia type I by inhibition of 4-hydroxyphenylpyruvate dioxygenase. Lancet 1992;340:813–17.
18. Holme E, Lindstedt S, Lock E. Treatment of tyrosinemia type I with an enzyme inhibitor (NTBC). Int Pediatr 1995;10:41–3.
19. Mock DM, Perman JA, Thaler M, Morris RC Jr. Chronic fructose intoxication after infancy in children with hereditary fructose intolerance. A cause of growth retardation. N Engl J Med 1983;309:764–70.
20. Odievre M, Gentil C, Gautier M, Alagille D. Hereditary fructose intolerance in childhood. Diagnosis, management, and course in 55 patients. Am J Dis Child 1978;132:605–8.
21. Herman SP, Baggenstoss AH, Cloutier MD. Liver dysfunction and histologic abnormalities in neonatal hypopituitarism. J Pediatr 1975;87(6 pt 1):892–5.
22. Colombo C, Battezzati PM, Podda M, et al. Ursodeoxycholic acid for liver disease associated with cystic fibrosis: a double-blind multicenter trial. The Italian Group for the Study of Ursodeoxycholic Acid in Cystic Fibrosis. Hepatology 1996;23:1484–90.
23. Sokol RJ, Durie PR. Recommendations for management of liver and biliary tract disease in cystic fibrosis. Cystic Fibrosis Foundation Hepatobiliary Disease Consensus Group. J Pediatr Gastroenterol Nutr 1999;28(suppl 1):S1–13.
24. Balistreri WF. Inborn errors of bile acid metabolism: clinical and therapeutic aspects. In: Hofmann A, Paumgartner G, Stiehl A, eds. Bile acids in gastroenterology: basic and clinical advances (proceedings of the 13th International Bile Acid Symposium). London: Kluwer Academic Publishers, 1995:333–53.
25. Daugherty CC, Setchell KD, Heubi JE, Balistreri WF. Resolution of liver biopsy alterations in three siblings with bile acid treatment of an inborn error of bile acid metabolism (delta 4–3-oxosteroid 5 beta-reductase deficiency). Hepatology 1993;18:1096–101.
26. Jacquemin E, Hermans D, Myara A, et al. Ursodeoxycholic acid therapy in pediatric patients with progressive familial intrahepatic cholestasis. Hepatology 1997;25:519–23.
27. Setchell K, O'Connell N. Inborn errors of bile acid biosynthesis: update on biochemical aspects. In: Hofmann A, Paumgartner G, Stiehl A, eds. Bile acids in gastroenterology: basic and clinical advances. London: Kluwer Academic Publishers, 1995:129–36.
28. Shamieh I, Kibort P, Suchy F, Freese D. Antioxidant therapy for neonatal iron storage disease. Pediatr Res 1993;33:109A.
29. Zimmerman H. Hepatotoxicity. New York: Appleton-Century-Crofts, 1978.
30. Levy HL, Sepe SJ, Shih VE, et al. Sepsis due to *Escherichia coli* in neonates with galactosemia. N Engl J Med 1977;297:823–5.
31. Ng SH, Rawstron JR. Urinary tract infections presenting with jaundice. Arch Dis Child 1971;46:173–6.
32. Cooke RJ, Whitington PF, Kelts D. Effect of taurine supplementation on hepatic function during short-term parenteral nutrition in the premature infant. J Pediatr Gastroenterol Nutr 1984;3:234–8.
33. Graham M, Tavill A, Halpin T, Louis L. The effect of amino acids on bile flow and sodium taurocholate excretion in the isolated perfused rat liver. Gastroenterology 1981;80:1334.
34. Vileisis RA, Inwood RJ, Hunt CE. Prospective controlled study of parenteral nutrition-associated cholestatic jaundice: effect of protein intake. J Pediatr 1980;96:893–7.
35. Duerksen DR, Van Aerde JE, Gramlich L, et al. Intravenous ursodeoxycholic acid reduces cholestasis in parenterally fed newborn piglets. Gastroenterology 1996;111:1111–17.
36. Spagnuolo MI, Iorio R, Vegnente A, Guarino A. Ursodeoxycholic acid for treatment of cholestasis in children on long-term total parenteral nutrition: a pilot study. Gastroenterology 1996;111:716–19.
37. Lilly JR, Altman RP, Schroter G, et al. Surgery of biliary atresia. Current status. Am J Dis Child 1975;129:1429–32.
38. Lilly JR, Karrer FM, Hall RJ, et al. The surgery of biliary atresia. Ann Surg 1989;210:289–94.
39. Laurent J, Gauthier F, Bernard O, et al. Long-term outcome after surgery for biliary atresia. Study of 40 patients surviving for more than 10 years. Gastroenterology 1990;99:1793–7.
40. Barlow B, Tabor E, Blanc WA, et al. Choledochal cyst: a review of 19 cases. J Pediatr 1976;89:934–40.
41. Lilly JR, Weintraub WH, Altman RP. Spontaneous perforation of the extrahepatic bile ducts and bile peritonitis in infancy. Surgery 1974;75:664–73.
42. Lilly JR. Common bile duct calculi in infants and children. J Pediatr Surg 1980;15:577–80.
43. Rickham PP, Lee EY. Neonatal jaundice: surgical aspects. Clin Pediatr (Phila) 1964;71:197–208.
44. Scholmerich J, Becher MS, Schmidt K, et al. Influence of hydroxylation and conjugation of bile salts on their membrane-damaging properties – studies on isolated hepatocytes and lipid membrane vesicles. Hepatology 1984;4:661–6.
45. Greim H, Trulzsch D, Roboz J, et al. Mechanism of cholestasis. 5. Bile acids in normal rat livers and in those after bile duct ligation. Gastroenterology 1972;63:837–45.
46. DeLange RJ, Glazer AN. Bile acids: antioxidants or enhancers of peroxidation depending on lipid concentration. Arch Biochem Biophys 1990;276:19–25.
47. Botla R, Spivey JR, Aguilar H, et al. Ursodeoxycholate (UDCA) inhibits the mitochondrial membrane permeability transition

induced by glycochenodeoxycholate: a mechanism of UDCA cytoprotection. J Pharmacol Exp Ther 1995;272:930–8.

48. Sokol RJ, Devereaux M, Khandwala R, O'Brien K. Evidence for involvement of oxygen free radicals in bile acid toxicity to isolated rat hepatocytes. Hepatology 1993;17:869–81.
49. Faubion WA, Guicciardi ME, Miyoshi H, et al. Toxic bile salts induce rodent hepatocyte apoptosis via direct activation of Fas. J Clin Invest 1999;103:137–45.
50. Patel T, Gores GJ. Apoptosis and hepatobiliary disease. Hepatology 1995;21:1725–41.
51. Rodrigues CM, Fan G, Wong PY, et al. Ursodeoxycholic acid may inhibit deoxycholic acid-induced apoptosis by modulating mitochondrial transmembrane potential and reactive oxygen species production. Mol Med 1998;4:165–78.
52. Heuman DM, Pandak WM, Hylemon PB, Vlahcevic ZR. Conjugates of ursodeoxycholate protect against cytotoxicity of more hydrophobic bile salts: in vitro studies in rat hepatocytes and human erythrocytes. Hepatology 1991;14:920–6.
53. Galle PR, Theilmann L, Raedsch R, et al. Ursodeoxycholate reduces hepatotoxicity of bile salts in primary human hepatocytes. Hepatology 1990;12(3 pt 1):486–91.
54. Hillaire S, Ballet F, Franco D, et al. Effects of ursodeoxycholic acid and chenodeoxycholic acid on human hepatocytes in primary culture. Hepatology 1995;22:82–7.
55. Lillienau J, Crombie DL, Munoz J, et al. Negative feedback regulation of the ileal bile acid transport system in rodents. Gastroenterology 1993;104:38–46.
56. Hofmann AF. Pharmacology of ursodeoxycholic acid, an enterohepatic drug. Scand J Gastroenterol Suppl 1994;204:1–15.
57. Kitani K, Ohta M, Kanai S. Tauroursodeoxycholate prevents biliary protein excretion induced by other bile salts in the rat. Am J Physiol 1985;248(4 pt 1):G40#1–27.
58. Shimokura GH, McGill JM, Schlenker T, Fitz JG. Ursodeoxycholate increases cytosolic calcium concentration and activates Cl- currents in a biliary cell line. Gastroenterology 1995; 109:965–72.
59. Berthelot P, Erlinger S, Dhumeaux D, Preaux AM. Mechanism of phenobarbital-induced hypercholeresis in the rat. Am J Physiol 1970;219:809–13.
60. Miller NE, Nestel PJ. Altered bile acid metabolism during treatment with phenobarbitone. Clin Sci Mol Med Suppl 1973; 42:257–62.
61. Bloomer JR, Boyer JL. Phenobarbital effects in cholestatic liver diseases. Ann Intern Med 1975;82:310–17.
62. Makino I, Shinozaki K, Yoshino K, Nakagawa S. [Dissolution of cholesterol gallstones by long-term administration of ursodeoxycholic acid]. Nippon Shokakibyo Gakkai Zasshi 1975;72:690–702.
63. Bachrach WH, Hofmann AF. Ursodeoxycholic acid in the treatment of cholesterol cholelithiasis. Part I. Dig Dis Sci 1982;27: 737–61.
64. Ichida F. Clinical experience with ursodeoxycholic acid (S-urso) for chronic hepatitis. Diagn Treat 1961;36:388.
65. Hofmann AF, Popper H. Ursodeoxycholic acid for primary biliary cirrhosis. Lancet 1987;2:398–9.
66. Krahenbuhl S, Fischer S, Talos C, Reichen J. Ursodeoxycholate protects oxidative mitochondrial metabolism from bile acid toxicity: dose-response study in isolated rat liver mitochondria. Hepatology 1994;20:1595–1601.
67. Heuman DM, Mills AS, McCall J, et al. Conjugates of ursodeoxycholate protect against cholestasis and hepatocellular necrosis caused by more hydrophobic bile salts. In vivo studies in the rat. Gastroenterology 1991;100:203–11.
68. Hofmann A. Targeting drugs to the enterohepatic circulation: lessons from bile acids and other endobiotics. J Controlled Release 1985;2:3–11.
69. Aldini R, Montagnani M, Roda A, et al. Intestinal absorption of bile acids in the rabbit: different transport rates in jejunum and ileum. Gastroenterology 1996;110:459–68.
70. Batta AK, Arora R, Salen G, et al. Characterization of serum and urinary bile acids in patients with primary biliary cirrhosis by gas-liquid chromatography-mass spectrometry: effect of ursodeoxycholic acid treatment. J Lipid Res 1989;30:1953–62.
71. Yoon YB, Hagey LR, Hofmann AF, et al. Effect of side-chain shortening on the physiologic properties of bile acids: hepatic transport and effect on biliary secretion of 23-nor-ursodeoxycholate in rodents. Gastroenterology 1986;90:837–52.
72. Elsing C, Sagesser H, Reichen J. Ursodeoxycholate-induced hypercholeresis in cirrhotic rats: further evidence for cholehepatic shunting. Hepatology 1994;20(4 pt 1):1048–54.
73. Knyrim K, Vakil N, Pfab R, Classen M. The effects of intraduodenal bile acid administration on biliary secretion of ionized calcium and carbonate in man. Hepatology 1989;10:134–42.
74. Lazaridis KN, Tietz P, Wu T, et al. Alternative splicing of the rat sodium/bile acid transporter changes its cellular localization and transport properties. Proc Natl Acad Sci U S A 2000;97:11092–7.
75. Lazaridis KN, Pham L, Tietz P, et al. Rat cholangiocytes absorb bile acids at their apical domain via the ileal sodium-dependent bile acid transporter. J Clin Invest 1997;100:2714–21.
76. Erlinger S, Dumont M. Influence of UDCA on bile secretion. In: Paumgartner G, Stiehl A, Barbara L, Roda E, eds. Strategies for the treatment of hepatobiliary disease. Dordrecht: Kluwer Academic Publishers, 1990:35–42.
77. Spengler U, Pape GR, Hoffmann RM, et al. Differential expression of MHC class II subregion products on bile duct epithelial cells and hepatocytes in patients with primary biliary cirrhosis. Hepatology 1988;8:459–62.
78. Calmus Y, Gane P, Rouger P, Poupon R. Hepatic expression of class I and class II major histocompatibility complex molecules in primary biliary cirrhosis: effect of ursodeoxycholic acid. Hepatology 1990;11:12–15.
79. Calmus Y, Arvieux C, Gane P, et al. Cholestasis induces major histocompatibility complex class I expression in hepatocytes. Gastroenterology 1992;102(4 pt 1):1371–7.
80. Innes GK, Nagafuchi Y, Fuller BJ, Hobbs KE. Increased expression of major histocompatibility antigens in the liver as a result of cholestasis. Transplantation 1988;45:749–52.
81. Calmus Y, Weill B, Ozier Y, et al. Immunosuppressive properties of chenodeoxycholic and ursodeoxycholic acids in the mouse. Gastroenterology 1992;103:617–21.
82. Kurktschiev D, Subat S, Adler D, Schentke KU. Immunomodulating effect of ursodeoxycholic acid therapy in patients with primary biliary cirrhosis. J Hepatol 1993;18:373–7.
83. Terasaki S, Nakanuma Y, Ogino H, et al. Hepatocellular and biliary expression of HLA antigens in primary biliary cirrhosis before and after ursodeoxycholic acid therapy. Am J Gastroenterol 1991;86:1194–9.
84. Poupon RE, Balkau B, Eschwege E, Poupon R. A multicenter, controlled trial of ursodiol for the treatment of primary biliary cirrhosis. UDCA-PBC Study Group. N Engl J Med 1991;324: 1548–54.

85. Heathcote EJ, Cauch-Dudek K, Walker V, et al. The Canadian Multicenter Double-blind Randomized Controlled Trial of ursodeoxycholic acid in primary biliary cirrhosis. Hepatology 1994;19:1149–56.
86. Lindor KD, Dickson ER, Baldus WP, et al. Ursodeoxycholic acid in the treatment of primary biliary cirrhosis. Gastroenterology 1994;106:1284–90.
87. Combes B, Carithers RL Jr, Maddrey WC, et al. A randomized, double-blind, placebo-controlled trial of ursodeoxycholic acid in primary biliary cirrhosis. Hepatology 1995;22:759–66.
88. Lindor KD, Jorgensen RA, Therneau TM, et al. Ursodeoxycholic acid delays the onset of esophageal varices in primary biliary cirrhosis. Mayo Clin Proc 1997;72:1137–40.
89. Poupon RE, Lindor KD, Cauch-Dudek K, et al. Combined analysis of randomized controlled trials of ursodeoxycholic acid in primary biliary cirrhosis. Gastroenterology 1997;113:884–90.
90. Lindor K, Therneau T, Jorgensen R, et al. Effects of ursodeoxycholic acid on survival in patients with primary biliary cirrhosis. Gastroenterology 1994;110:1515–18.
91. Pasha T, Heathcote J, Gabriel S, et al. Cost-effectiveness of ursodeoxycholic acid therapy in primary biliary cirrhosis. Hepatology 1999;29:21 6.
92. Beuers U, Spengler U, Kruis W, et al. Ursodeoxycholic acid for treatment of primary sclerosing cholangitis: a placebo-controlled trial. Hepatology 1992;16:707–14.
93. Lindor KD. Ursodiol for primary sclerosing cholangitis. Mayo Primary Sclerosing Cholangitis-Ursodeoxycholic Acid Study Group. N Engl J Med 1997;336:691–5.
94. Broome U, Glaumann H, Hultcrantz R, Forsum U. Distribution of HLA-DR, HLA-DP, HLA-DQ antigens in liver tissue from patients with primary sclerosing cholangitis. Scand J Gastroenterol 1990;25:54–8.
95. O'Brien CB, Senior JR, Rora-Mirchandani R, et al. Ursodeoxycholic acid for the treatment of primary sclerosing cholangitis: a 30-month pilot study. Hepatology 1991;14:838–47.
96. Chazouilleres O, Poupon R, Capron JP, et al. Ursodeoxycholic acid for primary sclerosing cholangitis. J Hepatol 1990;11:120–3.
97. Feigelson J, Anagnostopoulos C, Poquet M, et al. Liver cirrhosis in cystic fibrosis – therapeutic implications and long term follow up. Arch Dis Child 1993;68:653–7.
98. Sinaasappel M. Hepatobiliary pathology in patients with cystic fibrosis. Acta Paediatr Scand Suppl 1989;363:45–50.
99. Cotting J, Lentze MJ, Reichen J. Effects of ursodeoxycholic acid treatment on nutrition and liver function in patients with cystic fibrosis and longstanding cholestasis. Gut 1990;31:918–21.
100. Colombo C, Setchell KD, Podda M, et al. Effect of UDCA on liver disease associated with cystic fibrosis. J Ped 1990;117:412–19.
101. Galabert C, Montet JC, Lengrand D, et al. Effects of ursodeoxycholic acid on liver function in patients with cystic fibrosis and chronic cholestasis. J Pediatr 1992;121:138–41.
102. van de Meeberg PC, Houwen RH, Sinaasappel M, et al. Low-dose versus high-dose ursodeoxycholic acid in cystic fibrosis-related cholestatic liver disease. Results of a randomized study with 1-year follow-up. Scand J Gastroenterol 1997;32:369–73.
103. Colombo C, Castellani MR, Balistreri WF, et al. Scintigraphic documentation of an improvement in hepatobiliary excretory function after treatment with ursodeoxycholic acid in patients with cystic fibrosis and associated liver disease. Hepatology 1992;15:677–84.
104. Lindblad A, Glaumann H, Strandvik B. A two-year prospective study of the effect of ursodeoxycholic acid on urinary bile acid excretion and liver morphology in cystic fibrosis-associated liver disease. Hepatology 1998;27:166–74.
105. Lepage G, Paradis K, Lacaille F, et al. Ursodeoxycholic acid improves the hepatic metabolism of essential fatty acids and retinol in children with cystic fibrosis. J Pediatr 1997;130:52–8.
106. Thomas PS, Bellamy M, Geddes D. Malabsorption of vitamin E in cystic fibrosis improved after ursodeoxycholic acid. Lancet 1995;346:1230–1.
107. Bittner P, Posselt H, Sailor T, et al. The effect of treatment with ursodeoxycholic acid in cystic fibrosis and hepatopathy: results of a placebo-controlled study. In: Paumgartner G, Stiehl A, Gerok W, eds. Bile acids as therapeutic agents: from basic science to clinical practice. Lancaster: Kluwer Academic Publishers, 1991:345–8.
108. Balistreri WF, A-Kader H, Setchell K, and the Ursodeoxycholic Acid Study Group. Ursodeoxycholic acid therapy in pediatric patients with chronic cholestasis. In: Lentze M, Reichen J, eds. Paediatric cholestasis: novel approaches to treatment. Lancaster, England: Kluwer Academic Press, 1997:333–44.
109. Balistreri WF. Ursodeoxycholic acid in the treatment of pediatric liver disease. In: Fromm H, Leuschner U, eds. Proceedings of the Falk Symposium 84: Advances in basic and clinical bile acid research. London: Kluwer Acad Publishers, 1995;327–42.
110. Levy E, Bendayan M, Thibault L, et al. Lipoprotein abnormalities in two children with minimal biliary excretion. J Pediatr Gastroenterol Nutr 1995;20:432–9.
111. Krawinkel MB, Santer R, Oldigs HD. Ursodesoxycholic acid: effect on xanthomas in Alagille-Watson syndrome. J Pediatr Gastroenterol Nutr 1994;19:476–7.
112. Bijleveld CM, Vonk RJ, Kuipers F, et al. Benign recurrent intrahepatic cholestasis: altered bile acid metabolism. Gastroenterology 1989;97:427–32.
113. Crosignani A, Podda M, Bertolini E, et al. Failure of ursodeoxycholic acid to prevent a cholestatic episode in a patient with benign recurrent intrahepatic cholestasis: a study of bile acid metabolism. Hepatology 1991;13:1076–83.
114. Jacquemin E, Setchell KD, O'Connell NC, et al. A new cause of progressive intrahepatic cholestasis: 3 beta-hydroxy-C27-steroid dehydrogenase(isomerase deficiency. J Pediatr 1994;125: 379–84.
115. A-Kader H, Santangelo J, Setchell K, et al. The effects of ursodeoxycholic acid (UDCA) therapy in biliary atresia (BA): a double blind randomized, placebo controlled trial. Ped Res 1993;33:97A.
116. Nittono H, Tokita A, Hayashi M, et al. Ursodeoxycholic acid therapy in the treatment of biliary atresia. Biomed Pharmacother 1989;43:37–41.
117. A-Kader H, Heubi J, Setchell K, et al. The effects of UDCA therapy in children with EHBA. Gastroenterology 1990;98:A564.
118. Ullrich D, Rating D, Schroter W, et al. Treatment with ursodeoxycholic acid renders children with biliary atresia suitable for liver transplantation. Lancet 1987;2:1324.
119. Nittono H, Tokita A, Hayashi M, et al. Ursodeoxycholic acid in biliary atresia. Lancet 1988;1:528.
120. Schwarzenberg SJ, Bundy M. Ursodeoxycholic acid modifies gut-derived endotoxemia in neonatal rats. Pediatr Res 1994;35: 214–17.
121. Heubi JE, Wiechmann DA, Creutzinger V, et al. Tauroursodeoxycholic acid (TUDCA) in the prevention of total parenteral nutrition-associated liver disease. J Pediatr 2002;141: 237–42.

122. Boucher E, Jouanolle H, Andre P, et al. Interferon and ursodeoxycholic acid combined therapy in the treatment of chronic viral C hepatitis: results from a controlled randomized trial in 80 patients. Hepatology 1995;21:322–7.
123. Takano S, Ito Y, Yokosuka O, et al. A multicenter randomized controlled dose study of ursodeoxycholic acid for chronic hepatitis C. Hepatology 1994;20:558–64.
124. Angelico M, Gandin C, Pescarmona E, et al. Recombinant interferon-alpha and ursodeoxycholic acid versus interferon-alpha alone in the treatment of chronic hepatitis C: a randomized clinical trial with long-term follow-up. Am J Gastroenterol 1995;90:263–9.
125. Bellentani S, Podda M, Tiribelli C, et al. Ursodiol in the long-term treatment of chronic hepatitis: a double-blind multicenter clinical trial. J Hepatol 1993;19:459–64.
126. Lacaille F, Paradis K. The immunosuppressive effect of ursodeoxycholic acid: a comparative in vitro study on human peripheral blood mononuclear cells. Hepatology 1993;18:165–72.
127. Yoshikawa M, Tsujii T, Matsumura K, et al. Immunomodulatory effects of ursodeoxycholic acid on immune responses. Hepatology 1992;16:358–64.
128. Keiding S, Hockerstedt K, Bjoro K, et al. The Nordic multicenter double-blind randomized controlled trial of prophylactic ursodeoxycholic acid in liver transplant patients. Transplantation 1997;63:1591–4.
129. Pageaux GP, Blanc P, Perrigault PF, et al. Failure of ursodeoxycholic acid to prevent acute cellular rejection after liver transplantation. J Hepatol 1995;23:119–22.
130. Barnes D, Talenti D, Cammell G, et al. A randomized clinical trial of ursodeoxycholic acid as adjuvant treatment to prevent liver transplant rejection. Hepatology 1997;26:853–7.
131. Essell JH, Thompson JM, Harman GS, et al. Pilot trial of prophylactic ursodiol to decrease the incidence of veno-occlusive disease of the liver in allogeneic bone marrow transplant patients. Bone Marrow Transplant 1992;10:367–72.
132. Fried RH, Murakami CS, Fisher LD, et al. Ursodeoxycholic acid treatment of refractory chronic graft-versus-host disease of the liver. Ann Intern Med 1992;116:624–9.
133. Narkewicz MR, Smith D, Gregory C, et al. Effect of ursodeoxycholic acid therapy on hepatic function in children with intrahepatic cholestatic liver disease. J Pediatr Gastroenterol Nutr 1998;26:49–55.
134. Balistreri WF. Bile acid therapy in pediatric hepatobiliary disease: the role of ursodeoxycholic acid. J Pediatr Gastroenterol Nutr 1997;24:573–89.
135. Cowen AE, Korman MG, Hofmann AF, et al. Metabolism of lithocholate in healthy man. II. Enterohepatic circulation. Gastroenterology 1975;69:67–76.
136. Hirano S, Masuda N, Oda H. In vitro transformation of chenodeoxycholic acid and ursodeoxycholic acid by human intestinal flora, with particular reference to the mutual conversion between the two bile acids. J Lipid Res 1981;22:735–43.
137. Invernizzi P, Setchell KD, Crosignani A, et al. Differences in the metabolism and disposition of ursodeoxycholic acid and of its taurine-conjugated species in patients with primary biliary cirrhosis. Hepatology 1999;29:320–7.
138. Setchell KD, Rodrigues CM, Podda M, Crosignani A. Metabolism of orally administered tauroursodeoxycholic acid in patients with primary biliary cirrhosis. Gut 1996;38:439–46.
139. Kitani K, Kanai S. Tauroursodeoxycholate prevents taurocholate induced cholestasis. Life Sci 1982;30:515–23.
140. Miyake H, Tazuma S, Miura H, et al. Partial characterization of mechanisms of cytoprotective action of hydrophilic bile salts against hydrophobic bile salts in rats: relation to canalicular membrane fluidity and packing density. Dig Dis Sci 1999;44:197–202.
141. Funaoka M, Komatsu M, Toyoshima I, et al. Tauroursodeoxycholic acid enhances phagocytosis of the cultured rat Kupffer cell. J Gastroenterol Hepatol 1999;14:652–8.
142. Beurs U, Nathanson M, Isales C, Boyer J. Tauroursodeoxycholic acid stimulates hepatocellular exocytosis and mobilizes extracellular Ca^{++} mechanisms defective in cholestasis. Clin Invest 1993;92:2984–93.
143. Kinbara S, Ishizaki K, Sakakura H, et al. Improvement of estradiol-17 beta-D-glucuronide-induced cholestasis by sodium tauroursodeoxycholate therapy in rats. Scand J Gastroenterol 1997;32:947–52.
144. Roda A, Piazza F, Baraldini M, et al. Taurohyodeoxycholic acid protects against taurochenodeoxycholic acid-induced cholestasis in the rat. Hepatology 1998;27:520–5.
145. Larghi A, Crosignani A, Battezzati PM, et al. Ursodeoxycholic and tauro-ursodeoxycholic acids for the treatment of primary biliary cirrhosis: a pilot crossover study. Aliment Pharmacol Ther 1997;11:409–14.
146. Crosignani A, Battezzati PM, Setchell KD, et al. Tauroursodeoxycholic acid for treatment of primary biliary cirrhosis. A dose-response study. Dig Dis Sci 1996;41:809–15.
147. Capron JP, Dumont M, Feldmann G, Erlinger S. Barbiturate-induced choleresis: possible independence from microsomal enzyme induction. Digestion 1977;15:556–65.
148. Simon FR, Sutherland E, Accatino L. Stimulation of hepatic sodium and potassium-activated adenosine triphosphatase activity by phenobarbital. Its possible role in regulation of bile flow. J Clin Invest 1977;59:849–61.
149. Sinatra FR. Cholestasis in infancy and childhood. Curr Probl Pediatr 1982;12:1–54.
150. Alagille D. Management of chronic cholestasis in childhood. Semin Liver Dis 1985;5:254–62.
151. Hahn TJ, Hendin BA, Scharp CR, Haddad JG Jr. Effect of chronic anticonvulsant therapy on serum 25-hydroxycalciferol levels in adults. N Engl J Med 1972;287:900–4.
152. Ghent CN, Bloomer JR, Hsia YE. Efficacy and safety of long-term phenobarbital therapy of familial cholestasis. J Pediatr 1978;93:127–32.
153. Ferrari M, Barabas G, Matthews WS. Psychologic and behavioral disturbance among epileptic children treated with barbiturate anticonvulsants. Am J Psychiatry 1983;140:112–13.
154. Brent DA, Crumrine PK, Varma RR, et al. Phenobarbital treatment and major depressive disorder in children with epilepsy. Pediatrics 1987;80:909–17.
155. Brent DA. Overrepresentation of epileptics in a consecutive series of suicide attempters seen at a children's hospital, 1978–1983. J Am Acad Child Psychiatry 1986;25:242–6.
156. Brent DA, Crumrine PK, Varma R, et al. Phenobarbital treatment and major depressive disorder in children with epilepsy: a naturalistic follow-up. Pediatrics 1990;85:1086–91.
157. Karrer FM, Lilly JR. Corticosteroid therapy in biliary atresia. J Pediatr Surg 1985;20:693–5.
158. Meyers RL, Book LS, O'Gorman MA, et al. High-dose steroids, ursodeoxycholic acid, and chronic intravenous antibiotics improve bile flow after Kasai procedure in infants with biliary atresia. J Pediatr Surg 2003;38:406–11.

159. Rintala RJ, Lindahl H, Pohjavuori M. Total parenteral nutrition-associated cholestasis in surgical neonates may be reversed by intravenous cholecystokinin: a preliminary report. J Pediatr Surg 1995;30:827–30.
160. Teitelbaum DH, Han-Markey T, Schumacher RE. Treatment of parenteral nutrition-associated cholestasis with cholecystokinin-octapeptide. J Pediatr Surg 1995;30:1082–5.
161. Teitelbaum DH, Han-Markey T, Drongowski RA, et al. Use of cholecystokinin to prevent the development of parenteral nutrition-associated cholestasis. JPEN J Parenter Enteral Nutr 1997;21:100–3.
162. Teitelbaum DH, Tracy TF Jr, Aouthmany MM, et al. Use of cholecystokinin-octapeptide for the prevention of parenteral nutrition-associated cholestasis. Pediatrics 2005;115:1332–40.
163. Wagner M, Trauner M. Transcriptional regulation of hepatobiliary transport systems in health and disease: implications for a rationale approach to the treatment of intrahepatic cholestasis. Ann Hepatol 2005;4:77–99.
164. Liu Y, Binz J, Numerick MJ, et al. Hepatoprotection by the farnesoid X receptor agonist GW4064 in rat models of intra- and extrahepatic cholestasis. J Clin Invest 2003;112:1678–87.
165. Fiorucci S, Clerici C, Antonelli E, et al. Protective effects of 6-ethyl chenodeoxycholic acid, a farnesoid X receptor ligand, in estrogen-induced cholestasis. J Pharmacol Exp Ther 2005;313:604–12.
166. Saini SP, Sonoda J, Xu L, et al. A novel constitutive androstane receptor-mediated and CYP3A-independent pathway of bile acid detoxification. Mol Pharmacol 2004;65:292–300.
167. Huang W, Zhang J, Moore DD. A traditional herbal medicine enhances bilirubin clearance by activating the nuclear receptor CAR. J Clin Invest 2004;113:137–43.
168. Stedman CA, Liddle C, Coulter SA, et al. Nuclear receptors constitutive androstane receptor and pregnane X receptor ameliorate cholestatic liver injury. Proc Natl Acad Sci U S A 2005;102:2063–8.
169. Zhang J, Huang W, Qatanani M, et al. The constitutive androstane receptor and pregnane X receptor function coordinately to prevent bile acid-induced hepatotoxicity. J Biol Chem 2004;279:49517–22.
170. Marschall HU, Wagner M, Zollner G, et al. Complementary stimulation of hepatobiliary transport and detoxification systems by rifampicin and ursodeoxycholic acid in humans. Gastroenterology 2005;129:476–85.
171. Friedman SL. Cytokines and fibrogenesis. Semin Liver Dis 1999;19:129–40.
172. Li D, Friedman SL. Liver fibrogenesis and the role of hepatic stellate cells: new insights and prospects for therapy. J Gastroenterol Hepatol 1999;14:618–33.
173. Siegelmann R, Peterkofsky B. Inhibition of collagen secretion from bone and culture fibroblasts by microtubular disruptive drugs. Proc Natl Acad Sci U S A 1972;69:892–6.
174. Scherft JP, Heersche JN. Accumulation of collagen-containing vacuoles in osteoblasts after administration of colchicine. Cell Tissue Res 1975;157:353–65.
175. Dinarello CA, Chusid MJ, Fauci AS, et al. Effect of prophylactic colchicine therapy on leukocyte function in patients with familial Mediterranean fever. Arthritis Rheum 1976;19:618–22.
176. Gordon S, Werb Z. Secretion of macrophage neutral proteinase is enhanced by colchicine. Proc Natl Acad Sci U S A 1976;73:872–6.
177. Warnes TW, Smith A, Lee FI, et al. A controlled trial of colchicine in primary biliary cirrhosis. Trial design and preliminary report. J Hepatol 1987;5:1–7.
178. Kaplan MM, Alling DW, Zimmerman HJ, et al. A prospective trial of colchicine for primary biliary cirrhosis. N Engl J Med 1986;315:1448–54.
179. Kershenobich D, Vargas F, Garcia-Tsao G, et al. Colchicine in the treatment of cirrhosis of the liver. N Engl J Med 1988;318:1709–13.
180. Klion FM, Fabry T, Zifroni A, Schaffner F. Progression of PBC with and without colchicine therapy. Hepatology 1990;12:420.
181. Zifroni A, Schaffner F. Long-term follow-up of patients with primary biliary cirrhosis on colchicine therapy. Hepatology 1991;14:990–3.
182. Collins J, Morecki R, McPhillips J, Gartner L. Colchicine treatment of paediatric chronic cholestatic liver disease. In: Lentze M, Reichen J, eds. Pediatric cholestasis: novel approaches to treatment. Dordrecht, The Netherlands: Kluwer Academic Publishers, 1992:305–8.
183. Morgan TR, Weiss DG, Nemchausky B, et al. Colchicine treatment of alcoholic cirrhosis: a randomized, placebo-controlled clinical trial of patient survival. Gastroenterology 2005;128:882–90.
184. Hatziioannidou A, Cheesman P, Trivedi P, et al. Double blind controlled trial of colchicine versus placebo in extrahepatic biliary atresia: interim results. Hepatology 1992;16:60A.
185. Nimni ME, Bavetta LA. Collagen defect induced by penicillamine. Science 1965;150:905–7.
186. Deshmukh K, Nimni ME. A defect in the intramolecular and intermolecular cross-linking of collagen caused by penicillamine. II. Functional groups involved in the interaction process. J Biol Chem 1969;244:1787–95.
187. Walshe JM. Wilson's disease; new oral therapy. Lancet 1956;270:25–6.
188. Neuberger J, Christensen E, Portmann B, et al. Double blind controlled trial of d-penicillamine in patients with primary biliary cirrhosis. Gut 1985;26:114–19.
189. Bodenheimer HC Jr, Schaffner F, Sternlieb I, et al. A prospective clinical trial of D-penicillamine in the treatment of primary biliary cirrhosis. Hepatology 1985;5:1139–42.
190. Dickson ER, Fleming TR, Wiesner RH, et al. Trial of penicillamine in advanced primary biliary cirrhosis. N Engl J Med 1985;312:1011–15.
191. Oikarinen AI, Vuorio EI, Zaragoza EJ, et al. Modulation of collagen metabolism by glucocorticoids. Receptor-mediated effects of dexamethasone on collagen biosynthesis in chick embryo fibroblasts and chondrocytes. Biochem Pharmacol 1988;37:1451–62.
192. Oikarinen AI, Uitto J, Oikarinen J. Glucocorticoid action on connective tissue: from molecular mechanisms to clinical practice. Med Biol 1986;64:221–30.
193. Weiner FR, Czaja MJ, Giambrone MA, et al. Transcriptional and posttranscriptional effects of dexamethasone on albumin and procollagen messenger RNAs in murine schistosomiasis. Biochemistry 1987;26:1557–62.
194. Jefferson DM, Reid LM, Giambrone MA, et al. Effects of dexamethasone on albumin and collagen gene expression in primary cultures of adult rat hepatocytes. Hepatology 1985;5:14–20.
195. Zhang M, Song G, Minuk GY. Effects of hepatic stimulator substance, herbal medicine, selenium/vitamin E, and ciprofloxacin on cirrhosis in the rat. Gastroenterology 1996;110:1150–5.

196. Chojkier M, Houglum K, Lee KS, Buck M. Long- and short-term D-alpha-tocopherol supplementation inhibits liver collagen alpha1(I) gene expression. Am J Physiol 1998; 275 (6 pt 1):G1480–5.
197. Houglum K, Brenner DA, Chojkier M. d-Alpha-tocopherol inhibits collagen alpha 1(I) gene expression in cultured human fibroblasts. Modulation of constitutive collagen gene expression by lipid peroxidation. J Clin Invest 1991;87:2230–5.
198. Houglum K, Venkataramani A, Lyche K, Chojkier M. A pilot study of the effects of d-alpha-tocopherol on hepatic stellate cell activation in chronic hepatitis C. Gastroenterology 1997;113:1069–73.
199. Stickel F, Brinkhaus B, Krahmer N, et al. Antifibrotic properties of botanicals in chronic liver disease. Hepatogastroenterology 2002;49:1102–8.
200. Rockey DC. Antifibrotic therapy in chronic liver disease. Clin Gastoenterol Hepatol 2005;3:95–107.
201. Gartung C, Matern S. Molecular regulation of sinusoidal liver bile acid transporters during cholestasis. Yale J Biol Med 1997; 70:355–63.
202. Koopen NR, Wolters H, Voshol P, et al. Decreased Na^+-dependent taurocholate uptake and low expression of the sinusoidal Na^+-taurocholate cotransporting protein (Ntcp) in livers of mdr2 P-glycoprotein-deficient mice. J Hepatol 1999;30: 14–21.
203. Gartung C, Ananthanarayanan M, Rahman MA, et al. Down-regulation of expression and function of the rat liver Na^+/bile acid cotransporter in extrahepatic cholestasis. Gastroenterology 1996;110:199–209.
204. Jones EA, Bergasa NV. The pruritus of cholestasis: from bile acids to opiate agonists. Hepatology 1990;11:884–7.
205. Maddrey WC, Van Thiel DH. Liver transplantation: an overview. Hepatology 1988;8:948–59.
206. Cauna N. Fine morphological changes in the penicillate nerve endings of human hairy skin during prolonged itching. Anat Rec 1977;188:1–11.
207. Herndon JH Jr. Pathophysiology of pruritus associated with elevated bile acid levels in serum. Arch Intern Med 1972;130:632–7.
208. Schoenfield L. The relationship of bile acids to pruritus in hepatobiliary disease. In: Schiff L, Carey J, Dietschy J, eds. Bile salt metabolism. Springfield, IL: Charles C Thomas Publisher, 1969:257–65.
209. Garden JM, Ostrow JD, Roenigk HH Jr. Pruritus in hepatic cholestasis. Pathogenesis and therapy. Arch Dermatol 1985;121:1415–20.
210. Ghent CN, Bloomer JR, Klatskin G. Elevations in skin tissue levels of bile acids in human cholestasis: relation to serum levels and topruritus. Gastroenterology 1977;73:1125–30.
211. Freedman MR, Holzbach RT, Ferguson DR. Pruritus in cholestasis: no direct causative role for bile acid retention. Am J Med 1981;70:1011–16.
212. Silverberg DS, Iaina A, Reisin E, et al. Cholestyramine in uraemic pruritus. Br Med J 1977;1:752–3.
213. Chanarin I, Szur L. Letter: relief of intractable pruritis in polycythaemia rubra vera with cholestyramine. Br J Haematol 1975;29:669–70.
214. Thornton JR, Losowsky MS. Opioid peptides and primary biliary cirrhosis. BMJ 1988;297:1501–4.
215. Swain MG, Rothman RB, Xu H, et al. Endogenous opioids accumulate in plasma in a rat model of acute cholestasis. Gastroenterology 1992;103:630–5.
216. Reiz S, Westberg M. Side-effects of epidural morphine. Lancet 1980;2:203–4.
217. Ballantyne JC, Loach AB, Carr DB. Itching after epidural and spinal opiates. Pain 1988;33:149–60.
218. Bernstein JE, Grinzi RA. Butorphanol-induced pruritus antagonized by naloxone. J Am Acad Dermatol 1981;5:227–8.
219. Justins DM, Reynolds F. Intraspinal opiates and itching: a new reflex? Br Med J (Clin Res Ed) 1982;284:1401.
220. Graham-Smith D, Aronson J. Narcotic analgesics. In: Graham-Smith D, Aronson J, eds. Oxford textbook of clinical pharmacology and drug therapy. 2nd ed. New York: Oxford, 1992:641–4.
221. Jaffe J, Martin W. Opioid analgesics and antagonists. In: Gilman A, Goodman L, Rall T, Marad F, eds. The pharmacologic basis of therapeutics. 7th ed. New York: MacMillan Publishing Co., 1985:491–531.
222. Bernstein JE, Swift R. Relief of intractable pruritus with naloxone. Arch Dermatol 1979;115:1366–7.
223. Bergasa NV, Thomas DA, Vergalla J, et al. Plasma from patients with the pruritus of cholestasis induces opioid receptor-mediated scratching in monkeys. Life Sci 1993;53:1253–7.
224. Bergasa NV, Rothman RB, Vergalla J, et al. Central mu-opioid receptors are down-regulated in a rat model of cholestasis. J Hepatol 1992;15:220–4.
225. Gold MS, Redmond DE Jr, Kleber HD. Clonidine blocks acute opiate-withdrawal symptoms. Lancet 1978;2:599–602.
226. Charney DS, Heninger GR, Kleber HD. The combined use of clonidine and naltrexone as a rapid, safe, and effective treatment of abrupt withdrawal from methadone. Am J Psychiatry 1986;143:831–7.
227. Thornton JR, Losowsky MS. Plasma methionine enkephalin concentration and prognosis in primary biliary cirrhosis. BMJ 1988;297:1241–2.
228. Kastin AJ, Nissen C, Schally AV, Coy DH. Blood-brain barrier, half-time disappearance, and brain distribution for labeled enkephalin and a potent analog. Brain Res Bull 1976;1:583–9.
229. Rapoport SI, Klee WA, Pettigrew KD, Ohno K. Entry of opioid peptides into the central nervous system. Science 1980;207: 84–6.
230. Banks WA, Kastin AJ, Fischman AJ, et al. Carrier-mediated transport of enkephalins and N-Tyr-MIF-1 across blood-brain barrier. Am J Physiol 1986;251(4 pt 1):E477–82.
231. Summerfield JA. Naloxone modulates the perception of itch in man. Br J Clin Pharmacol 1980;10:180–3.
232. Sharp HL, Carey JB Jr, White JG, Krivit W. Cholestyramine therapy in patients with a paucity of intrahepatic bile ducts. J Pediatr 1967;71:723–36.
233. Palmer RH. Bile acids, liver injury, and liver disease. Arch Intern Med 1972;130:606–17.
234. Levy JS, Gelb AM, Stenger RJ, Javitt NB. Prolonged neonatal cholestasis: bile acid pattern and response to cholestyramine. Mt Sinai J Med 1979;46:169–73.
235. Ghent CN, Carruthers SG. Treatment of pruritus in primary biliary cirrhosis with rifampin. Results of a double-blind, crossover, randomized trial. Gastroenterology 1988;94:488–93.
236. Bachs L, Pares A, Elena M, et al. Comparison of rifampicin with phenobarbitone for treatment of pruritus in biliary cirrhosis. Lancet 1989;1:574–6.
237. Cynamon HA, Andres JM, Iafrate RP. Rifampin relieves pruritus in children with cholestatic liver disease. Gastroenterology 1990;98:1013–16.

238. Podesta A, Lopez P, Terg R, et al. Treatment of pruritus of primary biliary cirrhosis with rifampin. Dig Dis Sci 1991;36:216–20.
239. Bachs L, Pares A, Elena M, et al. Effects of long-term rifampicin administration in primary biliary cirrhosis. Gastroenterology 1992;102:2077–80.
240. Chretien Y, Poupon R, Gherardt M, et al. Bile acid glycine and taurine conjugates in serum of patients with PBC: effect of ursodeoxycholic acid treatment. Gut 1990;30:1110–15.
241. Stiehl A, Rudolph G, Raedsch R, et al. Ursodeoxycholic acid-induced changes of plasma and urinary bile acids in patients with primary biliary cirrhosis. Hepatology 1990;12(3 pt 1): 492–7.
242. Rail T, Schleifer L. Drugs effective in the therapy of epilepsies. In: Gilman A, Goodman L, Rail T, Murod F, eds. The pharmacologic basis of therapeutics. New York: MacMillan, 1985: 457.
243. Hanid MA, Levi AJ. Phototherapy for pruritus in primary biliary cirrhosis. Lancet 1980;2:530.
244. Perlstein SM. Phototherapy for primary biliary cirrhosis. Arch Dermatol 1981;117:608.
245. Person JR. Ultraviolet A (UV A) and cholestatic pruritus. Arch Dermatol 1981;117:684.
246. Lauterburg BH, Pineda AA, Dickson ER, et al. Plasmaperfusion for the treatment of intractable pruritus of cholestasis. Mayo Clin Proc 1978;53:403–7.
247. Lauterburg BH, Pineda AA, Burgstaler E. Treatment of pruritus of cholestasis by plasma perfusion thru USP-charcoal coated glass beads. Lancet 1990;2:53–5.
248. Datta DV, Sherlock S. Treatment of pruritus of obstructive jaundice with cholestyramine. Br Med J 1963;5325:216–19.
249. Sweeney MF, Fletcher BJ, Rice CR, et al. Efficacy and compliance with cholestyramine bar versus powder in the treatment of hyperlipidemia. Am J Med 1991;90:469–73.
250. Yerushalmi B, Sokol RJ, Narkewicz MR, et al. Use of rifampin for severe pruritus in children with chronic cholestasis. J Pediatr Gastroenterol Nutr 1999;29:442–7.
251. Gregorio GV, Ball CS, Mowat AP, Mieli-Vergani G. Effect of rifampicin in the treatment of pruritus in hepatic cholestasis. Arch Dis Child 1993;69:141–3.
252. Ohnhaus EE, Gerber-Taras E, Park BK. Enzyme-inducing drug combinations and their effects on liver microsomal enzyme activity in man. Eur J Clin Pharmacol 1983;24:247–50.
253. Galeazzi R, Lorenzini I, Orlandi F. Rifampicin-induced elevation of serum bile acids in man. Dig Dis Sci 1980;25:108–12.
254. Nakashima T, Sano A, Seto Y, et al. Unusual trihydroxy bile acids in the urine of patients treated with chenodeoxycholate, ursodeoxycholate or rifampicin and those with cirrhosis. Hepatology 1990;11:255–60.
255. Hollins PJ, Simmons AV. Jaundice associated with rifampicin. Tubercle 1970;51:328–32.
256. Scheuer PJ, Summerfield JA, Lal S, Sherlock S. Rifampicin hepatitis. A clinical and histological study. Lancet 1974;1:421–5.
257. Miguet JP, Mavier P, Soussy CJ, Dhumeaux D. Induction of hepatic microsomal enzymes after brief administration of rifampicin in man. Gastroenterology 1977;72(5 pt 1):924–6.
258. Brodie MJ, Boobis AR, Dollery CT, et al. Rifampicin and vitamin D metabolism. Clin Pharmacol Ther 1980;27:810–14.
259. Rothwell DL, Richmond DE. Hepatorenal failure with self-initiated intermittent rifampicin therapy. Br Med J 1974;2: 481–2.
260. Bergasa NV, Alling DW, Talbot TL, et al. Effects of naloxone infusions in patients with the pruritus of cholestasis. A double-blind, randomized, controlled trial. Ann Intern Med 1995;123: 161–7.
261. Terra SG, Tsunoda SM. Opioid antagonists in the treatment of pruritus from cholestatic liver disease. Ann Pharmacother 1998;32:1228–30.
262. Gal TJ, DiFazio CA, Dixon R. Prolonged blockade of opioid effect with oral nalmefene. Clin Pharmacol Ther 1986;40:537–42.
263. Bergasa NV, Schmitt JM, Talbot TL, et al. Open-label trial of oral nalmefene therapy for the pruritus of cholestasis. Hepatology 1998;27:679–84.
264. Wolfhagen FH, Sternieri E, Hop WC, et al. Oral naltrexone treatment for cholestatic pruritus: a double-blind, placebo-controlled study. Gastroenterology 1997;113:1264–9.
265. Carson KL, Tran TT, Cotton P, et al. Pilot study of the use of naltrexone to treat the severe pruritus of cholestatic liver disease. Am J Gastroenterol 1996;91:1022–3.
266. Croop RS, Faulkner EB, Labriola DF. The safety profile of naltrexone in the treatment of alcoholism. Results from a multicenter usage study. The Naltrexone Usage Study Group. Arch Gen Psychiatry 1997;54:1130–5.
267. Sharp HL, Mirkin BL. Effect of phenobarbital on hyperbilirubinemia, bile acid metabolism, and microsomal enzyme activity in chronic intrahepatic cholestasis of childhood. J Pediatr 1972;81:116–26.
268. Balistreri WF, A-Kader H, Setchell K. UDCA therapy in patients with Alagille syndrome (syndromic paucity of intrahepatic bile ducts): results of a multicenter pilot trial. Pediatr Res 1991;29:A99.
269. Balistreri WF, A-Kader H, Ryckman F, et al. Biochemical and clinical response to UDCA administration in pediatric patients with chronic cholestasis. In: Paumgartner G, Stiehl A, Gerok W, eds. Bile acids as therapeutic agents. Lancaster: Kluwer Academic Publishers, 1991:323–33.
270. Paradis K, Weber A. Sudden liver deterioration in infants receiving UDCA. Gastroenterology 1992;102:866.
271. Whitington PF, Whitington GL. Partial external diversion of bile for the treatment of intractable pruritus associated with intrahepatic cholestasis. Gastroenterology 1988;95:130–6.
272. Emond JC, Whitington PF. Selective surgical management of progressive familial intrahepatic cholestasis (Byler's disease). J Pediatr Surg 1995;30:1635–41.
273. Gauderer MW, Boyle JT. Cholecystoappendicostomy in a child with Alagille syndrome. J Pediatr Surg 1997;32:166–7.
274. Rebhandl W, Felberbauer FX, Turnbull J, et al. Biliary diversion by use of the appendix (cholecystoappendicostomy) in progressive familial intrahepatic cholestasis. J Pediatr Gastroenterol Nutr 1999;28:217–19.
275. Ng VL, Ryckman FC, Porta G, et al. Long-term outcome after partial external biliary diversion for intractable pruritus in patients with intrahepatic cholestasis. J Pediatr Gastroenterol Nutr 2000;30:152–6.
276. Kurbegov AC, Setchell KD, Haas JE, et al. Biliary diversion for progressive familial intrahepatic cholestasis: improved liver morphology and bile acid profile. Gastroenterology 2003; 125:1227–34.
277. Chen F, Ananthanarayanan M, Emre S, et al. Progressive familial intrahepatic cholestasis, type 1, is associated with decreased farnesoid X receptor activity. Gastroenterology 2004;126:756–64.

278. Whitington P, Freese D, Alonso E, et al. Surgery for treatment of Pediatric Cholestasis. In: Schoelmerich J, Sraub R, Lentntze MJ, Reichen J, eds. Pediatric cholestasis: novel approaches to treatment. London: Kluwer Academic Publishers, 1992:173.
279. Kalicinski PJ, Ismail H, Jankowska I, et al. Surgical treatment of progressive familial intrahepatic cholestasis: comparison of partial external biliary diversion and ileal bypass. Eur J Pediatr Surg 2003;13:307–11.
280. Stapelbroek JM, van Erpecum KJ, Klomp LW, et al. Nasobiliary drainage induces long-lasting remission in benign recurrent intrahepatic cholestasis. Hepatology 2006;43:51–53.
281. Duncan JS, Kennedy HJ, Triger DR. Treatment of pruritus due to chronic obstructive liver disease. Br Med J (Clin Res Ed) 1984; 289:22.
282. Alva J, Iber FL. Relief of the pruritus of jaundice with methandrostenolone and speculations on the nature of pruritus in liver disease. Am J Med Sci 1965;250:60–5.
283. Walt RP, Daneshmend TK, Fellows IW, Toghill PJ. Effect of stanozolol on itching in primary biliary cirrhosis. Br Med J (Clin Res Ed) 198827;296:607.
284. Osborn EC, Wootton ID, da Silva SL, Sherlock S. Serum-bile-acid levels in liver disease. Lancet 1959;2:1049–53.
285. Fischer JA, Schmid M. Treatment of primary biliary cirrhosis with azothioprine. Lancet 1967;1:421–4.
286. Arcon-Segovia D, Mayorga-Cortes A, Wolpert E. Primary biliary cirrhosis. Prompt relief of pruritus with azathioprine treatment. JAMA 1970;214:367–8.
287. Schworer H, Hartmann H, Ramadori G. Relief of cholestatic pruritus by a novel class of drugs: 5-hydroxytryptamine type 3 (5-HT3) receptor antagonists: effectiveness of ondansetron. Pain 1995;61:33–7.
288. Borgeat A, Wilder-Smith OH, Mentha G. Subhypnotic doses of propofol relieve pruritus associated with liver disease. Gastroenterology 1993;104:244–7.
289. Witt-Sullivan H, Heathcote J, Cauch K, et al. The demography of primary biliary cirrhosis in Ontario, Canada. Hepatology 1990;12:98–105.
290. Cauch-Dudek K, Abbey S, Stewart D, Heathcote EJ. Fatigue and quality of life in primary biliary cirrhosis. Hepatology 1995; 22:108A.
291. Swain MG, Maric M. Defective corticotropin-releasing hormone mediated neuroendocrine and behavioral responses in cholestatic rats: implications for cholestatic liver disease-related sickness behaviors. Hepatology 1995;22:1560–4.
292. Swain MG, Maric M. Improvement in cholestasis-associated fatigue with a serotonin receptor agonist using a novel rat model of fatigue assessment. Hepatology 1997;25:291–4.
293. Bergasa NV, Vergalla J, Turner ML, et al. Alpha-melanocyte-stimulating hormone in primary biliary cirrhosis. Ann N Y Acad Sci 1993;680:454–8.
294. Sokol RJ, Devereaux M, Khandwala RA. Effect of dietary lipid and vitamin E on mitochondrial lipid peroxidation and hepatic injury in the bile duct-ligated rat. J Lipid Res 1991;32: 1349–57.
295. Jones EA. Relief from profound fatigue associated with chronic liver disease by long-term ondansetron therapy. Lancet 1999;354:397.
296. Sabesin SM. Cholestatic lipoproteins – their pathogenesis and significance. Gastroenterology 1982;83:704–9.
297. Seidel D. Lipoproteins in liver disease. J Clin Chem Clin Biochem 1987;25:541–51.
298. Alagille D, Estrada A, Hadchouel M, et al. Syndromic paucity of interlobular bile ducts (Alagille syndrome or arteriohepatic dysplasia): review of 80 cases. J Pediatr 1987;110:195–200.
299. Sokol RJ. Medical management of neonatal cholestasis. In: Balistreri WF, Stocker J, eds. Pediatric hepatology. Philadelphia: Hemisphere Publishing, 1990:41–76.
300. Thannhauser SJ. Hypercholesterolemic zanthomatosis secondary to liver disease. Lipidosis. New York: Oxford University Press, 1950:143.
301. Crippin JS, Lindor KD, Jorgensen R, et al. Hypercholesterolemia and atherosclerosis in primary biliary cirrhosis: what is the risk? Hepatology 1992;15:858–62.
302. Shepherd J, Packard CJ, Bicker S, et al. Cholestyramine promotes receptor-mediated low-density-lipoprotein catabolism. N Engl J Med 1980;302:1219–22.
303. Schaffner F, Klion FM, Latuff AJ. The long term use of cholestyramine in the treatment of primary biliary cirrhosis. Gastroenterology 1965;48:293–8.
304. Armstrong MJ, Carey MC. The hydrophobic-hydrophilic balance of bile salts. Inverse correlation between reverse-phase high performance liquid chromatographic mobilities and micellar cholesterol-solubilizing capacities. J Lipid Res 1982;23:70–80.
305. Carulli N, Loria P, Bertolotti M, et al. Effects of acute changes of bile acid pool composition on biliary lipid secretion. J Clin Invest 1984;74:614–24.
306. Fromm H. Bile acid-lipoprotein interactions: effects of ursodeoxycholic acid (ursodiol). Dig Dis Sci 1989;34(12 suppl): 21S–23S.
307. Hawton K, Fagg J, Marsack P. Association between epilepsy and attempted suicide. J Neurol Neurosurg Psychiatry 1980;43:168–70.
308. Balistreri WF, A-Kader H, Heubi JE, et al. UDCA decreases serum cholesterol levels, ameliorates symptoms and improves biochemical parameters in pediatric patients w/chronic intrahepatic cholestasis. Gastroenterology 1990;96:A566.
309. Mol MJ, Erkelens DW, Leuven JA, et al. Effects of synvinolin (MK-733) on plasma lipids in familial hypercholesterolaemia. Lancet 1986;2:936–9.
310. Grundy SM. HMG-CoA reductase inhibitors for treatment of hypercholesterolemia. N Engl J Med 1988;319:24–33.
311. Duane WC, Hunninghake DB, Freeman ML, et al. Simvastatin, a competitive inhibitor of HMG-CoA reductase, lowers cholesterol saturation index of gallbladder bile. Hepatology 1988;8:1147–50.
312. Logan GM, Duane WC. Lovastatin added to ursodeoxycholic acid further reduces biliary cholesterol saturation. Gastroenterology 1990;98:1572–6.
313. Mazzella G, Parini P, Festi D, et al. Effect of simvastatin, ursodeoxycholic acid and simvastatin plus ursodeoxycholic acid on biliary lipid secretion and cholic acid kinetics in nonfamilial hypercholesterolemia. Hepatology 1992;15:1072–8.
314. Linarelli LG, Hengstenberg FH, Drash AL. Effect of phenobarbital on hyperlipemia in patients with intrahepatic and extrahepatic cholestasis. J Pediatr 1973;83:291–8.
315. Becker M, von Bergmann K, Rotthauwe HW, Leiss O. Effects of phenobarbital on biliary lipid metabolism in children with chronic intrahepatic cholestasis. Eur J Pediatr 1984;143:41–44.
316. Matsubara S, Abe Y, Blasutig E, et al. Treatment for cholestatic liver disease (CLD): plasma sorption and filtration for improved bilirubin removal. Trans Am Soc Artif Intern Organs 1983;29:693–7.

317. Buchwald H, Fitch L, Campos C. Partial ileal bypass in the treatment of hypercholesterolemia. J Fam Practice 1992;35:69–76.
318. Hollands CM, Rivera-Pedrogo FJ, Gonzalez-Vallina R, et al. Ileal exclusion for Byler's disease: an alternative surgical approach with promising early results for pruritus. J Pediatr Surg 1998; 33:220–4.
319. Emerick KM, Whitington PF. Partial external biliary diversion for intractable pruritus and xanthomas in Alagille syndrome. Hepatology 2002;35:1501–6.
320. Buckley DA, Higgins EM, du Vivier AW. Resolution of xanthomas in Alagille syndrome after liver transplantation. Pediatr Dermatol 1998;15:199–202.
321. Cardona J, Houssin D, Gauthier F, et al. Liver transplantation in children with Alagille syndrome – a study of twelve cases. Transplantation 1995;60:339–42.
322. Watkins J. Fat digestion in cholestasis. In: Adcock EI, Lester R, eds. Neonatal cholestasis: causes, syndromes, therapies. Report of the 87th Ross Conference in Pediatric Research. Columbus, OH: Ross Laboratories, 1984:94.
323. Badley BW, Murphy GM, Bouchier IA, Sherlock S. Diminished micellar phase lipid in patients with chronic nonalcoholic liver disease and steatorrhea. Gastroenterology 1970;58:781–9.
324. Freund H, Dienstag J, Lehrich J, et al. Infusion of branched-chain enriched amino acid solution in patients with hepatic encephalopathy. Ann Surg 1982;196:209–20.
325. Weisdorf SA, Freese DK, Fath JJ, et al. Amino acid abnormalities in infants with extrahepatic biliary atresia and cirrhosis. J Pediatr Gastroenterol Nutr 1987;6:860–4.
326. Devenyi AG, Barron TF, Mamourian AC. Dystonia, hyperintense basal ganglia, and high whole blood manganese levels in Alagille's syndrome. Gastroenterology 1994;106:1068–71.
327. Goulet OJ, de Ville de GJ, Otte JB, Ricour C. Preoperative nutritional evaluation and support for liver transplantation in children. Transplant Proc 1987;19:3249–55.
328. Pierro A, Koletzko B, Carnielli V, et al. Resting energy expenditure is increased in infants and children with extrahepatic biliary atresia. J Pediatr Surg 1989;24:534–8.
329. O'Keefe SJ, El-Zayadi AR, Carraher TE, et al. Malnutrition and immuno-incompetence in patients with liver disease. Lancet 1980;2(8195 pt 1):615–17.
330. Kaufman SS, Murray ND, Wood RP, et al. Nutritional support for the infant with extrahepatic biliary atresia. J Pediatr 1987;110:679–86.
331. Bucuvalas JC, Cutfield W, Horn J, et al. Resistance to the growth-promoting and metabolic effects of growth hormone in children with chronic liver disease. J Pediatr 1990;117:397–402.
332. Maes M, Sokal E, Otte JB. Growth factors in children with end-stage liver disease before and after liver transplantation: a review. Pediatr Transplant 1997;1:171–5.
333. Holt RI, Baker AJ, Jones JS, Miell JP. The insulin-like growth factor and binding protein axis in children with end-stage liver disease before and after orthotopic liver transplantation. Pediatr Transplant 1998;2:76–84.
334. Holt RI, Baker AJ, Miell JP. The pathogenesis of growth failure in paediatric liver disease. J Hepatol 1997;27:413–23.
335. Greer RM, Quirk P, Cleghorn GJ, Shepherd RW. Growth hormone resistance and somatomedins in children with end-stage liver disease awaiting transplantation. J Pediatr Gastroenterol Nutr 1998;27:148–54.
336. Sokol RJ, Stall C. Anthropometric evaluation of children with chronic liver disease. Am J Clin Nutr 1990;52:203–8.
337. Stewart SM, Uauy R, Kennard BD, et al. Mental development and growth in children with chronic liver disease of early and late onset. Pediatrics 1988;82:167–72.
338. Stewart SM, Uauy R, Waller DA, et al. Mental and motor development, social competence, and growth one year after successful pediatric liver transplantation. J Pediatr 1989;114(4 pt 1):574–81.
339. Wayman KI, Cox KL, Esquivel CO. Neurodevelopmental outcome of young children with extrahepatic biliary atresia 1 year after liver transplantation. J Pediatr 1997;131:894–8.
340. Merritt RJ, Suskind RM. Nutritional survey of hospitalized pediatric patients. Am J Clin Nutr 1979;32:1320–5.
341. Hehir DJ, Jenkins RL, Bistrian BR, Blackburn GL. Nutrition in patients undergoing orthotopic liver transplant. JPEN J Parenter Enteral Nutr 1985;9:695–700.
342. Tuten MB, Wogt S, Dasse F, Leider Z. Utilization of prealbumin as a nutritional parameter. JPEN J Parenter Enteral Nutr 1985;9:709–11.
343. Meritt R, Blackburn G. In: Suskind R, ed. Textbook of pediatric nutrition. New York: Raven, 1981:294.
344. Moreno LA, Gottrand F, Hoden S, et al. Improvement of nutritional status in cholestatic children with supplemental nocturnal enteral nutrition. J Pediatr Gastroenterol Nutr 1991;12:213–16.
345. Smith J, Horowitz J, Henderson JM, Heymsfield S. Enteral hyperalimentation in undernourished patients with cirrhosis and ascites. Am J Clin Nutr 1982;35:56–72.
346. Fuchs IG. Enteral support of the hospitalized child. In: Suskind R, Lewinter-Suskind L, eds. Textbook of pediatric nutrition. 2nd ed. New York: Raven, 1993:239–48.
347. Parker P, Stroop S, Greene H. A controlled comparison of continuous versus intermittent feeding in the treatment of infants with intestinal disease. J Pediatr 1981;99:360–4.
348. Ferry GD, Selby M, Pietro TJ. Clinical response to short-term nasogastric feeding in infants with gastroesophageal reflux and growth failure. J Pediatr Gastroenterol Nutr 1983;2:57–61.
349. Weber A, Roy CC. The malabsorption associated with chronic liver disease in children. Pediatrics 1972;50:73–83.
350. Cohen MI, Gartner LM. The use of medium-chain triglycerides in the management of biliary atresia. J Pediatr 1971;79: 379–84.
351. Sokal EM, Baudoux MC, Collette E, et al. Branched chain amino acids improve body composition and nitrogen balance in a rat model of extra hepatic biliary atresia. Pediatr Res 1996;40:66–71.
352. Chin SE, Shepherd RW, Thomas BJ, et al. Nutritional support in children with end-stage liver disease: a randomized crossover trial of a branched-chain amino acid supplement. Am J Clin Nutr 1992;56:158–63.
353. Charlton CP, Buchanan E, Holden CE, et al. Intensive enteral feeding in advanced cirrhosis: reversal of malnutrition without precipitation of hepatic encephalopathy. Arch Dis Child 1992;67:603–7.
354. Wene JD, Connor WE, DenBesten L. The development of essential fatty acid deficiency in healthy men fed fat-free diets intravenously and orally. J Clin Invest 1975;56:127–34.
355. Marcus AJ. The role of lipids in platelet function: with particular reference to the arachidonic acid pathway. J Lipid Res 1978;19:793–826.
356. Barr LH, Dunn GD, Brennan MF. Essential fatty acid deficiency during total parenteral nutrition. Ann Surg 1981;193:304–11.

357. Hansen A, Wiese H, Boelshe A, et al. Role of linoleic acid in infant nutrition. Pediatr 1963;31:171–92.
358. Caldwell MD, Jonsson HT, Othersen HB Jr. Essential fatty acid deficiency in an infant receiving prolonged parenteral alimentation. J Pediatr 1972;81:894–8.
359. Clandinin MT, Chappell JE, Heim T, et al. Fatty acid utilization in perinatal de novo synthesis of tissues. Early Hum Dev 1981;5:355–66.
360. Swart G, Frenkel M, Van der Berg J. Minimum protein requirements in advanced liver disease: a metabolic ward study of the effects of BCAA. In: Walser M, Williamson R, eds. Metabolism and clinical implications of branched chain amino and ketoacids. New York: Elsevier North Holland, 1981:427–32.
361. Holman R. EFA deficiency in humans. In: Rechcigl M, ed. CRC handbook series in nutrition and food: section E, nutritional disorders. West Palm Beach, FL: CRC Press, 1978:335–68.
362. Gourley GR, Farrell PM, Odell GB. Essential fatty acid deficiency after hepatic portoenterostomy for biliary atresia. Am J Clin Nutr 1982;36:1194–9.
363. Miyano T, Yamashiro Y, Shimizu T, et al. Essential fatty acid deficiency in congenital biliary atresia: successful treatment to reverse deficiency. J Pediatr Surg 1986;21:277–81.
364. Pettei MJ, Daftary S, Levine JJ. Essential fatty acid deficiency associated with the use of a medium-chain-triglyceride infant formula in pediatric hepatobiliary disease. Am J Clin Nutr 1991;53:1217–21.
365. Socha P, Koletzko B, Swiatkowska E, et al. Essential fatty acid metabolism in infants with cholestasis. Acta Paediatr 1998;87: 278–83.
366. Thompson G. Absorption of fat-soluable vitamins and sterols. J Clin Pathol 1971;24(suppl 5):85.
367. Book L. Fat soluble vitamins in cholestasis. In: Adcock EI, Lester R, eds. Neonatal cholestasis: causes, syndromes, therapies. Report of the Eighty-Seventh Ross Conference in Pediatric Research. Columbus, OH: Ross Laboratories, 1984:104–10.
368. The National Research Council Recommended Dietary Allowances. 10th ed. Washington, DC: National Research Council, 1989.
369. Blomhoff R, Wake K. Perisinusoidal stellate cells of the liver: important roles in retinol metabolism and fibrosis. FASEB J 1991;5:271–7.
370. Andrews WS, Pau CM, Chase HP, et al. Fat soluble vitamin deficiency in biliary atresia. J Pediatr Surg 1981;16:284–90.
371. Chin SE, Shepherd RW, Thomas BJ, et al. The nature of malnutrition in children with end-stage liver disease awaiting orthotopic liver transplantation. Am J Clin Nutr 1992;56:164–8.
372. Amedee-Manesme O, Furr HC, Alvarez F, et al. Biochemical indicators of vitamin A depletion in children with cholestasis. Hepatology 1985;5:1143–8.
373. Mobarhan S, Russell RM, Underwood BA, et al. Evaluation of the relative dose response test for vitamin A nutriture in cirrhotics. Am J Clin Nutr 1981;34:2264–70.
374. McClain CJ, Van Thiel DH, Parker S, et al. Alterations in zinc, vitamin A, and retinol-binding protein in chronic alcoholics: a possible mechanism for night blindness and hypogonadism. Alcohol Clin Exp Res 1979;3:135–41.
375. Mourey MS, Siegenthaler G, Amedee-Manesme O. Regulation of metabolism of retinol-binding protein by vitamin A status in children with biliary atresia. Am J Clin Nutr 1990;51:638–43.
376. Amedee-Manesme O, Mourey MS, Hanck A, Therasse J. Vitamin A relative dose response test: validation by intravenous injection in children with liver disease. Am J Clin Nutr 1987;46: 286–9.
377. Ong DE, Amedee-Manesme O. Liver levels of vitamin A and cellular retinol-binding protein for patients with biliary atresia. Hepatology 1987;7:253–6.
378. Carlier C, Coste J, Etchepare M, Amedee-Manesme O. Conjunctival impression cytology with transfer as a field-applicable indicator of vitamin A status for mass screening. Int J Epidemiol 1992;21:373–80.
379. Natadisastra G, Wittpenn JR, West KP Jr, et al. Impression cytology for detection of vitamin A deficiency. Arch Ophthalmol 1987;105:1224–8.
380. Sommer A, Sugana T. Corneal xerophthalmia and keratomalacia. Arch Ophthalmol 1982;100:404–11.
381. Solomons NW, Russell RM, Vinton E, et al. Application of a rapid dark adaptation test in children. J Pediatr Gastroenterol Nutr 1982;1:571–4.
382. Russell RM, Iber FL, Krasinski SD, Miller P. Protein-energy malnutrition and liver dysfunction limit the usefulness of the relative dose response (RDR) test for predicting vitamin A deficiency. Hum Nutr Clin Nutr 1983;37:361–71.
383. Feranchak AP, Gralla J, King R, et al. Comparison of indices of vitamin A status in children with chronic liver disease. Hepatology 2005;42:782–92.
384. Scheffer C, Tseng G. Staging of conjunctival squamous metaplasia by impression cytology. J Ophthalmol 1985;92:728–33.
385. Amedee-Manesme O, Luzeau R, Wittepen JR, et al. Impression cytology detects subclinical vitamin A deficiency. Am J Clin Nutr 1988;47:875–8.
386. Kjolhede CL, Gadomski AM, Wittpenn J, et al. Conjunctival impression cytology: feasibility of a field trial to detect subclinical vitamin A deficiency. Am J Clin Nutr 1989;49:490–4.
387. Gadomski AM, Kjolhede CL, Wittpenn J, et al. Conjunctival impression cytology (CIC) to detect subclinical vitamin A deficiency: comparison of CIC with biochemical assessments. Am J Clin Nutr 1989;49:495–500.
388. Feranchak A, Ramirez R, Shivaram K, et al. Assessment of vitamin A status in children with cholestasis liver disease using a modified oral relative dose response test. J Pediatr Gastro and Nutr 1996;23:A351.
389. Balistreri WF. Neonatal cholestasis. J Pediatr 1985;106:171–84.
390. Sokol RJ, Johnson KE, Karrer FM, et al. Improvement of cyclosporin absorption in children after liver transplantation by means of water-soluble vitamin E. Lancet 1991;338:212–14.
391. Argao EA, Heubi JE, Hollis BW, Tsang RC. d-Alpha-tocopheryl polyethylene glycol-1000 succinate enhances the absorption of vitamin D in chronic cholestatic liver disease of infancy and childhood. Pediatr Res 1992;31:146–50.
392. Russell RM, Boyer JL, Bagheri SA, Hruban Z. Hepatic injury from chronic hypervitaminosis a resulting in portal hypertension and ascites. N Engl J Med 1974;291:435–40.
393. Geubel AP, De Galocsy C, Alves N, et al. Liver damage caused by therapeutic vitamin A administration: estimate of dose-related toxicity in 41 cases. Gastroenterology 1991 Jun;100:1701–9.
394. Minuk GY, Kelly JK, Hwang WS. Vitamin A hepatotoxicity in multiple family members. Hepatology 1988;8:272–5.
395. Rubin E, Florman AL, Degnan T, Diaz J. Hepatic injury in chronic hypervitaminosis A. Am J Dis Child 1970;119:132–8.
396. Lippe B, Hensen L, Mendoza G, et al. Chronic vitamin A intoxication. A multisystem disease that could reach epidemic proportions. Am J Dis Child 1981;135:634–6.

397. Oliver TK Jr. Chronic vitamin A intoxication; report of a case in an older child and review of the literature. AMA J Dis Child 1958;95(1 part 1):57–68.
398. Mahoney CP, Margolis MT, Knauss TA, Labbe RF. Chronic vitamin A intoxication in infants fed chicken liver. Pediatrics 1980,65.893–7.
399. Fisher G, Skillern PG. Hypercalcemia due to hypervitaminosis A. JAMA 1974;227:1413–14.
400. Frame B, Jackson CE, Reynolds WA, Umphrey JE. Hypercalcemia and skeletal effects in chronic hypervitaminosis A. Ann Intern Med 1974;80:44–8.
401. Smith FR, Goodman DS. Vitamin A transport in human vitamin A toxicity. N Engl J Med 1976;294:805–8.
402. Heubi JE, Hollis BW, Specker B, Tsang RC. Bone disease in chronic childhood cholestasis. I. Vitamin D absorption and metabolism. Hepatology 1989;9:258–64.
403. Skinner R, Long R, Sherlock S, Willis M. 25hydroxylation of vitamin D in PBC. Lancet 1972;1:720–1.
404. Plourde V, Gascon-Barre M, Willems B, Huet PM. Severe cholestasis leads to vitamin D depletion without perturbing its C-25 hydroxylation in the dog. Hepatology 1988;8:1577–85.
405. Bouillon R, Reynaert J, Claes JH, et al. The effect of anticonvulsant therapy on serum levels of 25-hydroxy-vitamin D, calcium, and parathyroid hormone. J Clin Endocrinol Metab 1975;41:1130 5.
406. Holda ME, Ryan JR. Hepatobiliary rickets. J Pediatr Orthop 1982;2:285–7.
407. Roberts C, Book L, Chan G, et al. Rickets in children with cholestatic liver disease: evaluation and treatment. Pediatr Res 1981;15:544.
408. Bucuvalas JC, Heubi JE, Specker BL, et al. Calcium absorption in bone disease associated with chronic cholestasis during childhood. Hepatology 1990;12:1200–5.
409. Heubi JE, Higgins JV, Argao EA, et al. The role of magnesium in the pathogenesis of bone disease in childhood cholestatic liver disease: a preliminary report. J Pediatr Gastroenterol Nutr 1997;25:301–6.
410. Heubi JE, Tsang RC, Steichen JJ, et al. 1,25-Dihydroxyvitamin D3 in childhood hepatic osteodystrophy. J Pediatr 1979;94:977–82.
411. Vleggaar FP, Van Buuren HR, Wolfhagen FH, et al. Prevention and treatment of osteoporosis in primary biliary cirrhosis. Eur J Gastroenterol Hepatol 1999;11:617–21.
412. Norman A, Miller B. Vitamin D. In: Machlin J, ed. Handbook of vitamins — nutritional, biochemical and clinical aspects. New York: Marcel-Dekker, Inc., 1984:45–98.
413. Sokol RJ, Heubi JE, Iannaccone S, et al. Mechanism causing vitamin E deficiency during chronic childhood cholestasis. Gastroenterology 1983;85:1172–82.
414. Traber MG, Olivecrona T, Kayden HJ. Bovine milk lipoprotein lipase transfers tocopherol to human fibroblasts during triglyceride hydrolysis in vitro. J Clin Invest 1985;75:1729–34.
415. Traber MG, Kayden HJ. Vitamin E is delivered to cells via the high affinity receptor for low-density lipoprotein. Am J Clin Nutr 1984;40:747–51.
416. Guggenheim MA, Jackson V, Lilly J, Silverman A. Vitamin E deficiency and neurologic disease in children with cholestasis: a prospective study. J Pediatr 1983;102:577–9.
417. Sokol RJ, Guggenheim MA, Heubi JE, et al. Frequency and clinical progression of the vitamin E deficiency neurologic disorder in children with prolonged neonatal cholestasis. Am J Dis Child 1985;139:1211–15.
418. Sokol RJ, Guggenheim MA, Iannaccone ST, et al. Improved neurologic function after long-term correction of vitamin E deficiency in children with chronic cholestasis. N Engl J Med 1985;313:1580–6.
419. Sokol RJ. Vitamin E deficiency and neurologic disease. Annu Rev Nutr 1988;8:351–73.
420. Rosenblum JL, Keating JP, Prensky AL, Nelson JS. A progressive neurologic syndrome in children with chronic liver disease. N Engl J Med 1981;304:503–8.
421. Sokol RJ, Bove KE, Heubi JE, Iannaccone ST. Vitamin E deficiency during chronic childhood cholestasis: presence of sural nerve lesion prior to 2 1/2 years of age. J Pediatr 1983;103:197–204.
422. Stewart SM, Uauy R, Waller DA, et al. Mental and motor development correlates in patients with end-stage biliary atresia awaiting liver transplantation. Pediatrics 1987;79:882–8.
423. Satel SL, Riely CA. Vitamin E deficiency and neurologic dysfunction in children. N Engl J Med 1986;314:1389–90.
424. Arria AM, Tarter RE, Warty V, Van Thiel DH. Vitamin E deficiency and psychomotor dysfunction in adults with primary biliary cirrhosis. Am J Clin Nutr 1990;52:383–90.
425. Alvarez F, Landrieu P, Feo C, et al. Vitamin E deficiency is responsible for neurologic abnormalities in cholestatic children. J Pediatr 1985;107:422–5.
426. Oski FA, Barness LA. Vitamin E deficiency: a previously unrecognized cause of hemolytic anemia in the premature infant. J Pediatr 1967;70:211–20.
427. Tappel A. Vitamin E as the biological lipid antioxidant. Vitam Horm 1962;20:493–510.
428. Burton GW, Joyce A, Ingold KU. Is vitamin E the only lipid-soluble, chain-breaking antioxidant in human blood plasma and erythrocyte membranes? Arch Biochem Biophys 1983;221:281–90.
429. Traber MG. Vitamin E, nuclear receptors and xenobiotic metabolism. Arch Biochem Biophys 2004;423:6–11.
430. Sokol RJ, Devereaux M, Mierau GW, et al. Oxidant injury to hepatic mitochondrial lipids in rats with dietary copper overload. Modification by vitamin E deficiency. Gastroenterology 1990;99:1061–71.
431. Sokol R, Harris R, Heubi J. Effect of vitamin E on neutrophil chemotasis in chronic childhood cholestasis. Hepatology 1984;4:1048.
432. Kowdley KV, Mason JB, Meydani SN, et al. Vitamin E deficiency and impaired cellular immunity related to intestinal fat malabsorption. Gastroenterology 1992;102:2139–42.
433. Horwitt MK, Harvey CC, Dahm CH Jr, Searcy MT. Relationship between tocopherol and serum lipid levels for determination of nutritional adequacy. Ann N Y Acad Sci 1972;203:223–36.
434. Sokol RJ, Heubi JE, Iannaccone ST, et al. Vitamin E deficiency with normal serum vitamin E concentrations in children with chronic cholestasis. N Engl J Med 1984;310:1209–12.
435. Farrell PM, Levine SL, Murphy MD, Adams AJ. Plasma tocopherol levels and tocopherol-lipid relationships in a normal population of children as compared to healthy adults. Am J Clin Nutr 1978;31:1720–6.
436. Gordon HH, Nitowsky HM, Cornblath M. Studies of tocopherol deficiency in infants and children. I. Hemolysis of erythrocytes in hydrogen peroxide. AMA Am J Dis Child 1955;90:669–81.
437. Cynamon HA, Isenberg JN, Nguyen CH. Erythrocyte malondialdehyde release in vitro: a functional measure of vitamin E status. Clin Chim Acta 1985;151:169–76.

438. Sokol RJ, Butler-Simon N, Conner C, et al. Multicenter trial of d-alpha-tocopheryl polyethylene glycol 1000 succinate for treatment of vitamin E deficiency in children with chronic cholestasis. Gastroenterology 1993;104:1727–35.
439. Bendich A, Machlin LJ. Safety of oral intake of vitamin E. Am J Clin Nutr 1988;48:612–19.
440. Farrell PM, Bieri JG. Megavitamin E supplementation in man. Am J Clin Nutr 1975;28:1381–6.
441. Corrigan JJ Jr, Marcus FI. Coagulopathy associated with vitamin E ingestion. JAMA 1974;230:1300–1.
442. Corrigan JJ Jr. The effect of vitamin E on warfarin-induced vitamin K deficiency. Ann N Y Acad Sci 1982;393:361–8.
443. Johnson L, Bowen FW Jr, Abbasi S, et al. Relationship of prolonged pharmacologic serum levels of vitamin E to incidence of sepsis and necrotizing enterocolitis in infants with birth weight 1,500 grams or less. Pediatrics 1985;75:619–38.
444. Lorch V, Murphy D, Hoersten LR, et al. Unusual syndrome among premature infants: association with a new intravenous vitamin E product. Pediatrics 1985;75:598–602.
445. Suttie J. Vitamin K. In: Diplock A, ed. Fat soluble vitamins. Lancaster, PA: Technomic Publishing Co., 1985:225.
446. Olson RE. The function and metabolism of vitamin K. Annu Rev Nutr 1984;4:281–337.
447. Shah DV, Suttie JW. The vitamin K dependent, in vitro production of prothrombin. Biochem Biophys Res Commun 1974;60:1397–402.
448. Price PA, Williamson MK, Lothringer JW. Origin of the vitamin K-dependent bone protein found in plasma and its clearance by kidney and bone. J Biol Chem 1981;256:12760–6.
449. Price PA, Parthemore JG, Deftos LJ. New biochemical marker for bone metabolism. Measurement by radioimmunoassay of bone GLA protein in the plasma of normal subjects and patients with bone disease. J Clin Invest 1980;66:878–83.
450. Vermeer C, Knapen MH, Schurgers LJ. Vitamin K and metabolic bone disease. J Clin Pathol 1998;51:424–6.
451. Feskanich D, Weber P, Willett WC, et al. Vitamin K intake and hip fractures in women: a prospective study. Am J Clin Nutr 1999;69:74–9.
452. Verity C, Carswell F, Scott G. Vitamin K deficiency causing infantile intracranial hemorrhage after the neonatal period. Lancet 1983;i:1439–40.
453. Bancroft J, Cohen MB. Intracranial hemorrhage due to vitamin K deficiency in breast-fed infants with cholestasis. J Pediatr Gastroenterol Nutr 1993;16:78–80.
454. Yanofsky RA, Jackson VG, Lilly JR, et al. The multiple coagulopathies of biliary atresia. Am J Hematol 1984;16:171–80.
455. Lane PA, Hathaway WE. Vitamin K in infancy. J Pediatr 1985;106: 351–9.
456. Silverman A, Roy C. Pediatric clinical gastroenterology. St. Louis: C.V. Mosby, 1983:526.
457. Zinkham WH. Peripheral blood and bilirubin values in normal full-term primaquine-sensitive Negro infants: effect of vitamin K. Pediatrics 1963;31:983–95.
458. Rossouw JE, Labadarios D, Davis M, Williams R. Water-soluble vitamins in severe liver disease. S Afr Med J 1978;54:183–6.
459. Goksu N, Ozsoylu S. Hepatic and serum levels of zinc, copper, and magnesium in childhood cirrhosis. J Pediatr Gastroenterol Nutr 1986;5:459–62.
460. Cohen MI, McNamara H, Finberg L. Serum magnesium in children with cirrhosis. J Pediatr 1970;76:453–5.
461. Kaya G, Ozsoylu S. Serum magnesium levels in children with cirrhosis. Acta Paediatr Scand 1972;161:442–4.
462. Stutzman FL, Matuzio DS. Blood serum magnesium in portal cirrhosis and diabetes mellitus. J Lab Clin Med 1953;41:215–19.
463. Zelikovic I, Dabbagh S, Friedman AL, et al. Severe renal osteodystrophy without elevated serum immunoreactive parathyroid hormone concentrations in hypomagnesemia due to renal magnesium wasting. Pediatrics 1987;79:403–9.
464. Wiegmann T, Kaye M. Hypomagnesemic hypocalcemia. Early serum calcium and late parathyroid hormone increase with magnesium therapy. Arch Intern Med 1977;137:953–5.
465. Anast CS, Winnacker JL, Forte LR, Burns TW. Impaired release of parathyroid hormone in magnesium deficiency. J Clin Endocrinol Metab 1976;42:707–17.
466. Rude RK, Oldham SB, Sharp CF Jr, Singer FR. Parathyroid hormone secretion in magnesium deficiency. J Clin Endocrinol Metab 1978;47:800–6.
467. Duran MJ, Borst GC 3rd, Osburne RC, Eil C. Concurrent renal hypomagnesemia and hypoparathyroidism with normal parathormone responsiveness. Am J Med 1984;76:151–4.
468. Ralston S, Boyle IT, Cowan RA, et al. PTH and vitamin D responses during treatment of hypomagnesaemic hypoparathyroidism. Acta Endocrinol (Copenh) 1983;103:535–8.
469. Rude RK, Adams JS, Ryzen E, et al. Low serum concentrations of 1,25-dihydroxyvitamin D in human magnesium deficiency. J Clin Endocrinol Metab 1985;61:933–40.
470. Medalle R, Waterhouse C, Hahn TJ. Vitamin D resistance in magnesium deficiency. Am J Clin Nutr 1976;29:854–8.
471. Hambidge KM, Krebs NF, Lilly JR, Zerbe GO. Plasma and urine zinc in infants and children with extrahepatic biliary atresia. J Pediatr Gastroenterol Nutr 1987;6:872–7.
472. Committee on Nutrition. Zinc. Pediatrics 1978;62:408–12.
473. Narkewicz MR, Krebs N, Karrer F, et al. Correction of hypozincemia following liver transplantation in children is associated with reduced urinary zinc loss. Hepatology 1999;29:830–3.
474. Litov RE, Combs GF Jr. Selenium in pediatric nutrition. Pediatrics 1991;87:339–51.
475. Collipp PJ, Chen SY. Cardiomyopathy and selenium deficiency in a two-year-old girl. N Engl J Med 1981;304:1304–5.
476. Fleming CR, Lie JT, McCall JT, et al. Selenium deficiency and fatal cardiomyopathy in a patient on home parenteral nutrition. Gastroenterology 1982;83:689–93.
477. Brown MR, Cohen HJ, Lyons JM, et al. Proximal muscle weakness and selenium deficiency associated with long term parenteral nutrition. Am J Clin Nutr 1986;43:549–54.
478. Vinton NE, Dahlstrom KA, Strobel CT, Ament ME. Macrocytosis and pseudoalbinism: manifestations of selenium deficiency. J Pediatr 1987;111:711–17.
479. Hambidge K, Krebs N. Normal childhood nutrition and its disorders. In: Hathaway W, Hay W, Groothius J, Paisley J, eds. Current pediatric diagnosis and treatment. 11th ed. Norwalk, CT: Appleton & Lange, 1993:244.
480. Levander OA. The importance of selenium in total parenteral nutrition. Bull N Y Acad Med 1984;60:144–55.
481. Evans J, Newman S, Sherlock S. Liver copper levels in intrahepatic cholestasis of childhood. Gastroenterology 1978;75:875–8.
482. Benson GD. Hepatic copper accumulation in primary biliary cirrhosis. Yale J Biol Med 1979;52:83–8.
483. Hochstein P, Kumar KS, Forman SJ. Lipid peroxidation and the cytotoxicity of copper. Ann N Y Acad Sci 1980;355:240–8.

484. Jones M, Grand K, Perrault J, Dickson E. Clinical response to penicillamine in cholestatic liver disease. In: Daum F, ed. Extrahepatic biliary atresia. New York: Marcel-Dekker, 1983:227.
485. Evans J, Zerpa H, Nuttall L, et al. Copper chelation therapy in intrahepatic cholestasis of childhood. Gut 1983;24:42–8.
486. Dickson ER, Fleming TR, Wiesner RH, et al. Trial of penicillamine in advanced primary biliary cirrhosis. N Engl J Med 1985;312:1011–15.
487. Matloff DS, Alpert E, Resnick RH, Kaplan MM. A prospective trial of D-penicillamine in primary biliary cirrhosis. N Engl J Med 1982;306:319–26.
488. Sinatra R. Does total parenteral nutrition produce cholestasis? Neonatal cholestasis. Proceedings of the 87th Ross Conference on Pediatric Research. Columbus, OH: Ross Laboratories, 1984:85.
489. Farrell MK, Balistreri WF, Suchy FJ. Serum-sulfated lithocholate as an indicator of cholestasis during parenteral nutrition in infants and children. JPEN J Parenter Enteral Nutr 1982;6: 30–3.
490. Underwood E. Manganese. In: Underwood E (ed). Trace elements in human and animal nutrition. 4th ed. New York: Academic Press, 1977:170–95.
491. Bayliss EA, Hambidge KM, Sokol RJ, et al. Hepatic concentrations of zinc, copper and manganese in infants with extrahepatic biliary atresia. J Trace Elem Med Biol 1995;9:40–3.
492. Plaa GL, de Lamirande E, Lewittes M, Yousef IM. Liver cell plasma membrane lipids in manganese-bilirubin-induced intrahepatic cholestasis. Biochem Pharmacol 1982;31:3698–701.
493. Fell JM, Reynolds AP, Meadows N, et al. Manganese toxicity in children receiving long-term parenteral nutrition. Lancet 1996;347:1218–21.
494. Spahr L, Butterworth RF, Fontaine S, et al. Increased blood manganese in cirrhotic patients: relationship to pallidal magnetic resonance signal hyperintensity and neurological symptoms. Hepatology 1996;24:1116–20.
495. Hauser RA, Zesiewicz TA, Martinez C, et al. Blood manganese correlates with brain magnetic resonance imaging changes in patients with liver disease. Can J Neurol Sci 1996;23:95–8.
496. Rose C, Butterworth RF, Zayed J, et al. Manganese deposition in basal ganglia structures results from both portal-systemic shunting and liver dysfunction. Gastroenterology 1999;117:640–4.
497. Morgan MY. Cerebral magnetic resonance imaging in patients with chronic liver disease. Metab Brain Dis 1998;13:273–90.
498. Layrargues GP, Rose C, Spahr L, et al. Role of manganese in the pathogenesis of portal-systemic encephalopathy. Metab Brain Dis 1998;13:311–17.
499. Krieger D, Krieger S, Jansen O, et al. Manganese and chronic hepatic encephalopathy. Lancet 1995;346:270–4.
500. Layrargues GP, Shapcott D, Spahr L, Butterworth RF. Accumulation of manganese and copper in pallidum of cirrhotic patients: role in the pathogenesis of hepatic encephalopathy? Metab Brain Dis 1995;10:353–6.
501. Ayotte P, Plaa GL. Biliary excretion in Sprague-Dawley and Gunn rats during manganese-bilirubin-induced cholestasis. Hepatology 1988;8:1069–78.
502. Hambidge KM, Sokol RJ, Fidanza SJ, Goodall MA. Plasma manganese concentrations in infants and children receiving parenteral nutrition. JPEN J Parenter Enteral Nutr 1989;13:168–71.
503. Kurkus J, Alcock NW, Shils ME. Manganese content of large-volume parenteral solutions and of nutrient additives. JPEN J Parenter Enteral Nutr 1984;8:254–7.
504. Malecki EA, Devenyi AG, Barron TF, et al. Iron and manganese homeostasis in chronic liver disease: relationship to pallidal T1-weighted magnetic resonance signal hyperintensity. Neurotoxicology 1999;20:647–52.
505. Klein GL, Alfrey AC, Miller NL, et al. Aluminum loading during total parenteral nutrition. Am J Clin Nutr 1982;35:1425–9.
506. Klein GL, Ott SM, Alfrey AC, et al. Aluminum as a factor in the bone disease of long-term parenteral nutrition. Trans Assoc Am Physicians 1982;95:155–64.
507. Popinska K, Kierkus J, Lyszkowska M, et al. Aluminum contamination of parenteral nutrition additives, amino acid solutions, and lipid emulsions. Nutrition 1999;15:683–6.
508. Sedman AB, Klein GL, Merritt RJ, et al. Evidence of aluminum loading in infants receiving intravenous therapy. N Engl J Med 1985;312:1337–43.
509. Milliner DS, Shinaberger JH, Shuman P, Coburn JW. Inadvertent aluminum administration during plasma exchange due to aluminum contamination of albumin-replacement solutions. N Engl J Med 1985;312:165–7.
510. Klein G, Heyman M, Lee T, Alfrey A. Intravenous aluminum loading induces cholestasis. Hepatology 1986;6:1127.
511. Williams JW, Vera SR, Peters TG, et al. Biliary excretion of aluminum in aluminum osteodystrophy with liver disease. Ann Intern Med 1986;104:782–5.
512. Andersen KJ, Nordgaard K, Julshamn K, Schjoensby H. Increased serum aluminum in patients with jaundice. N Engl J Med 1979;301:728–9.
513. Burgess DB, Martin HP, Lilly JR. The developmental status of children undergoing the Kasai procedure for biliary atresia. Pediatrics 1982;70:624–9.
514. Bayley N. The value and limitation of infant testing. Children 1958;5:129.
515. Escalona SK, Moriarty A. Prediction of schoolage intelligence from infant tests. Child Dev 1961;32:597–605.
516. Thomas H. Some problems of studies concerned with evaluating the predictive validity of infant tests. J Child Psychol Psychiatry 1967;8:197.
517. Lewis M, McGurk H. Evaluation of infatn intelligence. Science 1972;178:1174.
518. Matheny R. Testing infant intelligence. Science 1973;182:734.
519. Conn H, Atterbury C. Cirrhosis. In: Schiff L, Schiff E, eds. Diseases of the liver. Philadelphia: JB Lippincott, 1987:725–864.
520. Potter C, Willis D, Sharp HL, Scharzenberg SJ. Primary and secondary amenorrhea associated with spironolactone therapy in chronic liver disease. J Pediatr 1992;121:141–3.
521. Rosenthal P, Ramos A, Mungo R. Management of children with hyperbilirubinemia and green teeth. J Pediatr 1986;108:103–5.
522. Eisenberg E. Anomalies of the teeth with stains and discolorations. J Prev Dent 1975;2:7–20.
523. Simon NB, Smith D. Living with chronic pediatric liver disease: the parents' experience. Pediatr Nurs 1992;18:453–8, 489.

11

Neonatal Hepatitis and Congenital Infections

Philip Rosenthal, M.D.

Neonatal hepatitis refers to a heterogeneous group of disorders that result in a somewhat similar morphologic change in the liver of an infant less than 3 months of age in response to various insults. The term *neonatal hepatitis* has been used at times to include all causes of cholestasis in infancy in which extrahepatic biliary obstruction is excluded. Although in the majority of cases an etiology cannot be found, specific infectious and metabolic causes have been identified that may present as neonatal hepatitis. At final diagnosis, neonatal hepatitis is responsible for approximately 40% of the cases of infants with cholestasis and is the most frequently encountered liver disorder of early infancy. Males usually predominate over females (two to one). Additionally, some familial cases have been reported, suggesting either a maternal environmental factor or autosomal recessive inheritance.

Histologically, there is a loss of the lobular architecture with preservation of the zonal distribution of portal tracts and central veins. There is ballooning degeneration of hepatocytes with fusion of hepatocyte membranes and nuclear transformation into multinucleated giant cells. These multinucleated giant cells are believed to be the response of immature hepatocytes to most forms of injury and are a nonspecific finding in neonatal liver biopsy samples. There may be abundant extramedullary hematopoiesis and variable inflammation (Figure 11.1). Cholestasis may be marked because the newborn already is in a relative state of physiologic cholestasis. Finding cytoplasmic inclusions, steatosis, or storage material or elucidating a positive family history may aid in distinguishing metabolic, viral, and familial causes of neonatal hepatitis.

This chapter reviews known causes of neonatal hepatitis with intrahepatic cholestasis, concentrating in particular on associated congenital infections. It has become increasingly clear that the term *neonatal hepatitis* is too vague and is no longer clinically or therapeutically appropriate. Hepatitis in a neonate caused by a known etiologic agent that may be amenable to therapy needs to be differentiated from idiopathic neonatal hepatitis, in which etiologic agents are unknown and probably multiple. This becomes increasingly important as new therapeutic regimens are developed.

ROUTES OF INFECTION

The newborn may acquire infection transplacentally in utero, during delivery, or after birth. The study of transplacental infection has been hampered by the latency of many viruses. It has been well established that transplacental passage may result in congenital syphilis, toxoplasmosis, rubella, and cytomegalovirus (CMV) infections. The secondary liver abnormalities at birth may be inactive because of remote in utero infection, with the consequent scarred, cirrhotic liver, or relatively new, with an acute hepatitis. An essential factor in the transmission of the infection from the mother to the fetus is the time of maternal infection during the pregnancy. In general, infectious agents cross the placenta best during the third trimester. This is particularly true for syphilis, toxoplasmosis, and hepatitis B virus (HBV).

Perinatal acquisition of infection may be the result of the upward spread of bacterial agents from vaginitis, endometritis, or placentitis. Inhalation or swallowing of infected amniotic fluid may transmit the infection to the fetus. During labor and delivery, direct contact with pathogens in vaginal or uterine secretions or contaminated blood may result in neonatal infection. *Listeria,* herpes simplex, and CMV may be transmitted by this route and can cause neonatal hepatitis.

Postnatal infection less frequently results in neonatal hepatitis. Close contact with maternal infecting secretions (oral, nasal, breast milk) is possible. Blood or blood product transfusions may contain agents that could result in a neonatal hepatitis.

ETIOLOGIC AGENTS

Bacterial Infections

The reticuloendothelial system in the liver and spleen is responsible for effectively clearing bacteria from the bloodstream. However, in the neonate, the reticuloendothelial system is often immature and there may be diminished amounts of complement and opsonins, which impair the neonate's ability to handle

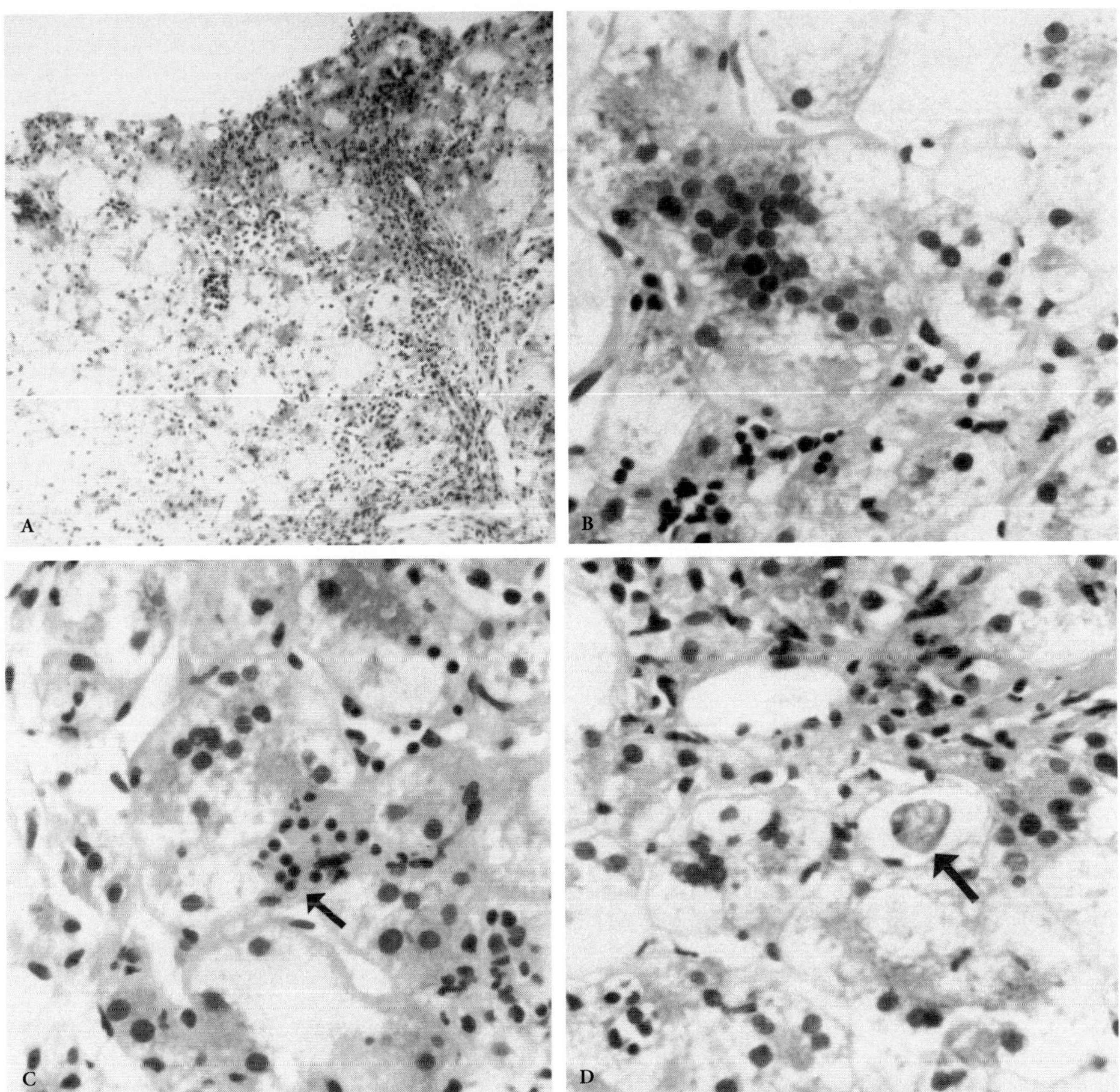
Figure 11.1. Neonatal hepatitis; needle biopsy at 6 weeks of age. (**A**) Portal area with inflammation at top and parenchymal lobular disarray below. (Hematoxylin and eosin [H&E], original magnification 40×.) (**B**) Ballooned hepatocytes and multinucleated giant cell. (**C**) Extramedullary hematopoiesis (*arrow*). (**D**) Necrotic hepatocyte (Councilman body, *arrow*). (**B**, **C**, and **D**, H&E, original magnification 450×.)

bacterial infections adequately. Hepatic injury from systemic bacterial infections may result from direct invasion of hepatocytes and Kupffer cells, from circulating toxins, or as a result of fever or hypoxia.

Hepatomegaly and jaundice may be clinical signs of neonatal sepsis with hepatic involvement [1]. Both gram-positive and gram-negative organisms have been implicated, with gram-negative bacteria being the most frequent etiologic agents reported [2]. Hepatotoxicity is believed to be secondary to circulating endotoxin from the bacterial cell walls and secondary to cholestasis [3]. Endotoxin is known to diminish bile flow in isolated perfused liver preparations [4].

Laboratory studies in infants with bacterial infection often reveal a leukocytosis, conjugated hyperbilirubinemia, and elevated alkaline phosphatase levels. Serum aminotransferase levels are only slightly to moderately elevated. A prolonged prothrombin time and abnormal clotting factors may be related to a coexisting disseminated intravascular coagulopathy.

Percutaneous liver biopsies are rarely performed in infants with sepsis because of the accompanying abnormal coagulation parameters and because the findings are often nonspecific [5]. There may be bile stasis, focal hepatocyte necrosis, a polymorphonuclear portal infiltrate, giant cell transformation, and Kupffer cell hyperplasia. Occasionally, culture of the hepatic tissue may be positive.

The most frequent bacterial organism isolated resulting in a neonatal hepatitis is *Escherichia coli. Streptococcus* group B is rarely implicated. *Listeria monocytogenes* infection invariably results in hepatic manifestations.

Liver abscesses, the result of hepatic injury from umbilical catheterization, are uncommonly observed [6]. When present, *E. coli* and *Staphylococcus aureus* are the most common pathogens isolated and are presumed secondary to colonization of the umbilical stump.

Urinary Tract Infection

Neonatal bacterial infections associated with jaundice have frequently been associated with the urinary tract [7]. They commonly present between the second and eighth weeks of postnatal life. These infections are rarely associated with fever or urinary symptoms. There may be a history of lethargy, irritability, poor feeding, and, occasionally, vomiting or diarrhea. Males are more frequently affected than females. Anatomic abnormalities of the genitourinary tract are infrequent. Hepatomegaly is frequently apparent. Laboratory studies reveal a conjugated hyperbilirubinemia, mildly increased aminotransferase levels, and leukocytosis with an increase in polymorphonuclear cells. Urinalysis shows pyuria, and urine culture usually reveals *E. coli.* Blood cultures may be transiently positive. Hepatic pathology is relatively benign, with nonspecific findings of bile stasis, periportal inflammation, and Kupffer cell hyperplasia.

Treatment consists of appropriate antibiotic therapy to avoid significant morbidity and mortality. Resolution of the jaundice may be delayed despite successful bacterial eradication because of the formation of bilirubin–protein conjugates in the serum. An underlying metabolic disease (e.g., galactosemia) must be considered in all infants with cholestasis and gram-negative bacterial infections.

Congenital Syphilis

Despite penicillin and routine maternal screening, congenital syphilis remains a problematic perinatal infection. In utero, transplacental transmission of *Treponema pallidum* spirochetes to the fetus may result in a mild to severe range of symptoms [8]. Severe infections may result in prematurity, apnea, hepatosplenomegaly, jaundice, hydrops fetalis, skin and mucosal lesions, rhinitis, osteochondritis, osteomyelitis, periostitis, and pseudoparalysis. Findings may be present at birth or may develop over days to weeks. Milder cases may present with anicteric hepatitis, poor weight gain, or purulent nasal discharge. Laboratory abnormalities include a conjugated hyperbilirubinemia and elevated serum aminotransferase levels.

Liver histology classically reveals an intralobular dissecting fibrosis with centrilobular mononuclear infiltration. Silver stains may demonstrate spirochetes. In milder cases or cases presenting late, the histologic features may not be typical. There may be portal fibrosis and portal inflammation, which are nonspecific signs of hepatitis. Unless the clinical history is obtained, the diagnosis could easily be missed. Occasionally, congenital syphilis may lead to fulminant hepatic failure with subsequent liver calcifications [9].

Congenital syphilis should be entertained in the differential diagnosis of any neonate with hepatitis. A definitive diagnosis can be made if spirochetes are identified in skin or mucosal lesions. Serologic testing of serum and cerebrospinal fluid analysis using specific treponemal antibody tests (e.g., microhemagglutination test for *T. pallidum*, fluorescent treponemal antibody absorption) and nonspecific nontreponemal reagin and flocculation tests (e.g., Venereal Disease Research Laboratory [VDRL], rapid plasma reagin [RPR], automated reagin test [ART]) may be required to distinguish syphilis from other spirochetal diseases. Serology may be positive in normal unaffected infants for up to 3 months after birth because of passively acquired maternal antibodies confounding the diagnosis.

Treatment includes parenteral penicillin therapy. Erythromycin and ceftriaxone are reserved for penicillin allergy, but efficacy has not been proved and penicillin desensitization is preferable. Tetracycline or doxycycline, although useful in adults, should not be used in pregnant mothers or infants because of effects on developing teeth and bones. If penicillin G cannot be administered, alternate treatment recommendations can be found at the Centers for Disease Control and Prevention (CDC) website (http://www.cdc.gov/nchstp/dstd/penicillinG.htm). After appropriate therapy, serology may remain positive for up to 2 years. Serum aminotransferase levels may remain elevated after onset of therapy for a prolonged period. Prognosis may ultimately depend on the extent of hepatic damage before the institution of therapy. Chronic liver disease has not been reported in infants appropriately treated for congenital syphilis.

Tuberculous Hepatitis

Neonatal infection of the liver with tuberculosis is exceedingly rare. Infection may occur by way of placental spread from miliary tuberculosis in the mother or by inhalation with pulmonary involvement or by aspiration of contaminated amniotic fluid. Usually, respiratory symptoms predominate. Hepatic lesions have caseating necrosis with surrounding giant cells and epithelioid cells with tubercle bacilli [10]. The clinical course is usually rapidly fatal. If a newborn is suspected of having congenital tuberculosis, a Mantoux skin test (5 tuberculin units of purified protein derivative [TUPPD]), chest radiographs, lumbar puncture, and cultures should be obtained rapidly. Regardless of the skin test results, which are frequently negative in congenital tuberculosis, treatment should be initiated promptly with isoniazid, pyrazinamide, rifampin, and streptomycin or kanamycin.

Toxoplasmosis

Maternal infection with the intracellular protozoan parasite is usually acquired by contact with the oocytes excreted in cat feces or ingestion of inadequately cooked meat (lamb, beef, or pork). Maternal infection may be asymptomatic or mild but is a prerequisite for the development of congenital toxoplasmosis during gestation [11]. The majority of infected newborns may be asymptomatic [12]. Hepatitis may be the only indicator of infection. Serious disease is primarily related to hepatic and central nervous system involvement [13]. Manifestations of congenital infection with *Toxoplasma gondii* may include purpura, microcephaly, chorioretinitis, intracranial calcification, meningoencephalitis, and psychomotor retardation. Most infants with congenital toxoplasmosis have hepatosplenomegaly, but jaundice may be variable.

Liver biopsy may show a generalized hepatitis with areas of necrosis. Intracellular bile stasis and periportal infiltration with histiocytes, lymphocytes, granulocytes, and eosinophils may accompany hepatocyte necrosis. *Toxoplasma* organisms may be seen in the liver using fluorescent antibody staining. Plain abdominal roentgenograms may show hepatic microcalcifications, the result of calcification of necrotic lesions.

Diagnosis may be made prenatally by detection of the parasite in fetal blood or amniotic fluid or from the placenta, cord, or infant's peripheral blood using mouse inoculation or polymerase chain reaction (PCR) of its genomic material. Serologic diagnosis can be made by immunoglobulin M (IgM) or IgA or persistent (over 12 months) IgG anti-*Toxoplasma* antibody tests determined in the infant's blood. A case of congenital toxoplasmosis diagnosed by the use of exfoliative cytology of neonatal ascites has been reported [14]. Mothers known to be infected during pregnancy may be treated with sulfadiazine and pyrimethamine or spiramycin (an investigational drug) in an attempt to prevent congenital infection. Infants with documented infection may be treated with pyrimethamine and sulfadiazine with folinic acid added to prevent hematologic toxicity of therapy. Although further cellular invasion may be prevented, preexisting damage and intracellular organisms may not be influenced by this regimen.

Viral Infections

Cytomegalovirus

Cytomegalovirus may be acquired transplacentally, at delivery, or postnatally from infected secretions (saliva or breast milk) or from transfusion of blood products [15]. Significant congenital CMV disease has been reported in the offspring of liver transplant recipients [16]. Most congenitally infected infants remain asymptomatic. The minority (5–10%) develop clinically apparent infection, but, unfortunately, these may include low birth weight, microcephaly, periventricular cerebral calcifications, chorioretinitis, thrombocytopenia, purpura, deafness, and psychomotor retardation. Hepatosplenomegaly and conjugated hyperbilirubinemia are often seen in neonatal CMV infection [17,18]. The hepatosplenomegaly may be secondary to significant extramedullary hematopoiesis.

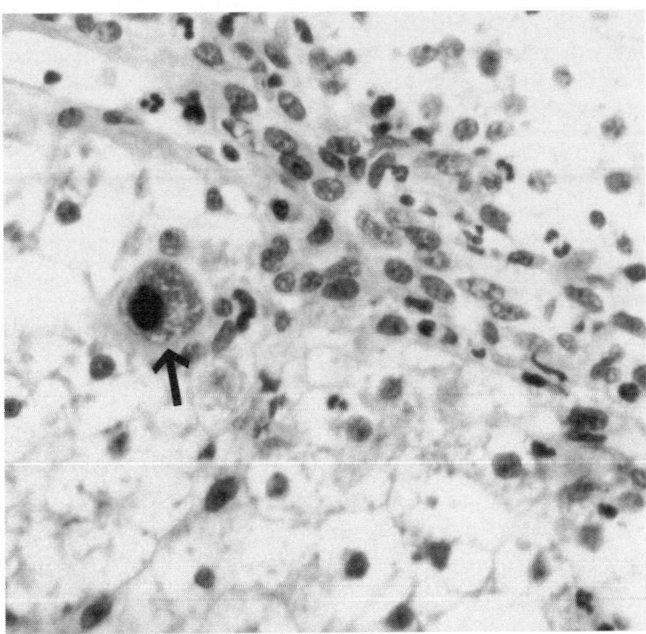

Figure 11.2. Cytomegalovirus infection. Large hard-appearing intranuclear inclusion. Adjacent portal tract has acute and chronic inflammatory infiltrate. (H&E, original magnification 450×.)

Liver biopsy may reveal significant giant cell transformation. The presence of large intranuclear inclusion bodies in bile duct epithelium and occasionally in hepatocytes or Kupffer cells, and intracytoplasmic inclusion bodies in hepatocytes, confirms the diagnosis (Figure 11.2) [17]. Bile stasis, inflammation, fibrosis, and bile duct proliferation are also featured.

Diagnosis of CMV infection includes culture of the nasopharynx, saliva, and urine. Culture of the liver may yield positive results, but the yield is usually not as good as from the urine [19]. The detection of CMV in hepatic tissue can be improved with the use of electron microscopy, viral DNA by PCR, and monoclonal antibody techniques [20,21]. Serologic tests are also useful for CMV diagnosis. IgM CMV-specific antibodies can be monitored.

Long-term follow-up of congenital CMV-infected patients may show resolution of hepatomegaly but development of portal hypertension despite the absence of cirrhosis [22,23]. Treatment for congenital CMV infection includes use of the antiviral drug ganciclovir and CMV immunoglobulin intravenously. Foscarnet may be used as an alternative drug in cases of ganciclovir-resistant virus or in patients unable to tolerate ganciclovir therapy. Liver transplantation also has been used rarely for infants with severe hepatic involvement. Prognosis is poor for infants with severe infection, with neurologic sequelae frequently occurring.

Herpes Hepatitis

Hepatitis from herpes simplex may present as part of a generalized disease in the newborn [24]. Symptoms may not appear until 4–8 days of age, which coincides with the incubation period for herpes. Congenital herpes infection may present with microcephaly and necrotic, ulcerative, vesicular, or purpuric lesions on the mucosal surfaces or the skin. Although the liver may be mildly affected, more often there is jaundice, hepatosplenomegaly, and abnormal coagulation factors. Gastrointestinal bleeding, coagulopathy, encephalitis, and seizures may be present in severe cases. Diagnosis may be confirmed by typical cutaneous lesions, by identification of the virus in skin lesions using direct fluorescent antibody staining or enzyme immunoassay detection of herpes antigens, cell culture, and PCR of herpes simplex viral DNA [25]. Acute and convalescent sera may be tested for increases in herpes simplex antibody titers to confirm acute infection, but serologic diagnosis is less helpful than viral isolation, which has become the more rapid diagnostic procedure of choice.

An asymptomatic maternal genital lesion is often the cause of the neonatal infection, with herpes simplex type 2 accounting for the majority of congenital herpes infections. Fetal scalp monitoring, prolonged rupture of membranes, prematurity, and low birth weight may contribute to the risk of infection. Infection in the newborn can be avoided by cesarean section delivery. Other less common sources of neonatal infection include transmission from a parent from a nongenital infection (e.g., from the hands or mouth) or postnatal infection from another infected infant in the nursery, probably from the hands of personnel caring for the infants.

Liver histology reveals necrosis (either multifocal or generalized) with characteristic intranuclear acidophilic inclusions in hepatocytes. Multinucleated giant cells also may be present (Figure 11.3). Culture of liver tissue may confirm the diagnosis but may take up to a week to be positive. Morphologic demonstration of herpesvirus is usually faster. Immunohistochemical staining using commercially available antisera can demonstrate herpesvirus in tissue [26]. The closely related varicella-zoster virus, which can produce an identical histologic appearance in the liver, can be distinguished by the difference in cutaneous rash. CMV intranuclear inclusions are much larger than those of herpesvirus intranuclear inclusions, and there may be bile duct cell involvement in CMV infection, aiding in the diagnosis [27]. Herpes simplex viral DNA may be detected by PCR.

Without treatment, the outcome invariably is death. The use of antiviral therapy (acyclovir) in conjunction when necessary with liver transplantation has significantly improved the outlook for herpes-infected neonates with severe disease limited to the liver [25,28]. Acyclovir has become the drug of choice because of its ease of administration and lower toxicity. Prophylactic use of acyclovir in exposed newborns is not recommended because of potential drug toxicity and the low risk of disease to most newborns.

Rubella

The incidence of congenital rubella has diminished because of the widespread use of rubella vaccine [29]. Hepatic involvement in congenital rubella is common [30,31]. Hepatomegaly is always found, and splenomegaly, jaundice, and cholestasis with a conjugated hyperbilirubinemia and elevated serum alkaline phosphatase and aminotransferases also may be concomitantly featured. Congenital rubella is associated with ophthalmologic (cataracts, microphthalmia, glaucoma, chorioretinitis), cardiac (patent ductus arteriosus, peripheral pulmonic stenosis, atrial or ventricular septal defects), auditory (sensorineural deafness), and neurologic (microcephaly, meningoencephalitis, retardation) anomalies. Growth retardation, thrombocytopenia, and purpuric skin lesions (blueberry muffin) may be observed.

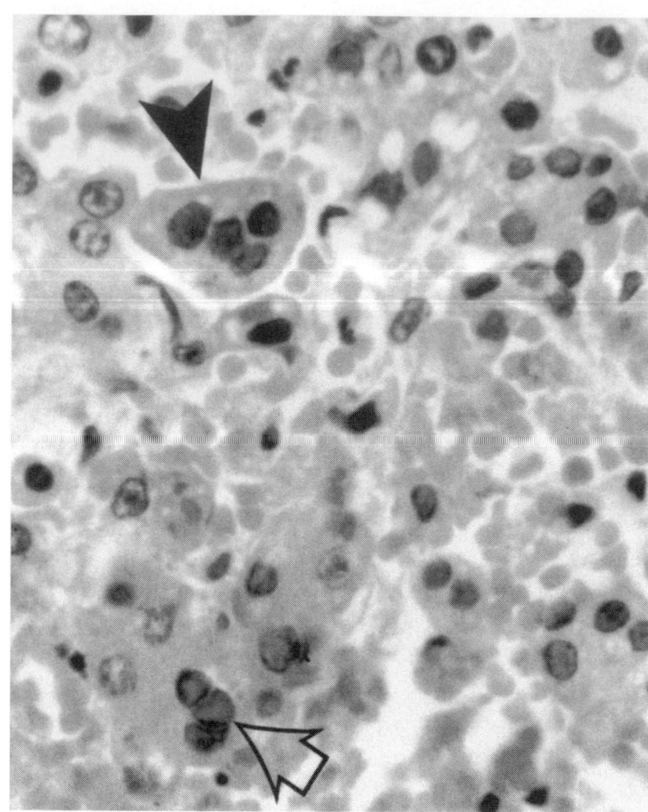

Figure 11.3. Herpesvirus infection. Viable hepatocytes adjacent to areas of necrosis. A multinucleated giant cell (*solid arrow*) and pale intranuclear inclusions with rim of chromatin (*open arrow*) are noted. (H&E, original magnification 450×.)

Humans are the sole source of rubella infection. Postnatal rubella is transmitted by direct or droplet contact with nasopharyngeal secretions. Congenitally infected infants may shed rubella virus in nasopharyngeal secretions and urine for up to 1 year and transmit infection to contacts.

Liver histology reveals mononuclear infiltrates of the portal zones with intralobular fibrosis and extramedullary hematopoiesis (Figure 11.4). There may be giant cell transformation, focal areas of necrosis, cholestasis, and evidence of bile duct proliferation. An increased incidence of biliary atresia has been reported in these infants [18].

Diagnosis may be made by isolation of virus from the nose by inoculation of appropriate tissue culture. Throat swabs, urine, blood, and cerebrospinal fluid may yield positive cultures, especially in congenitally infected infants. Serologic testing is also useful in confirming the diagnosis. Specific rubella IgM antibody is indicative of recent postnatal or congenital infection. The use of PCR for prenatal and postnatal diagnosis

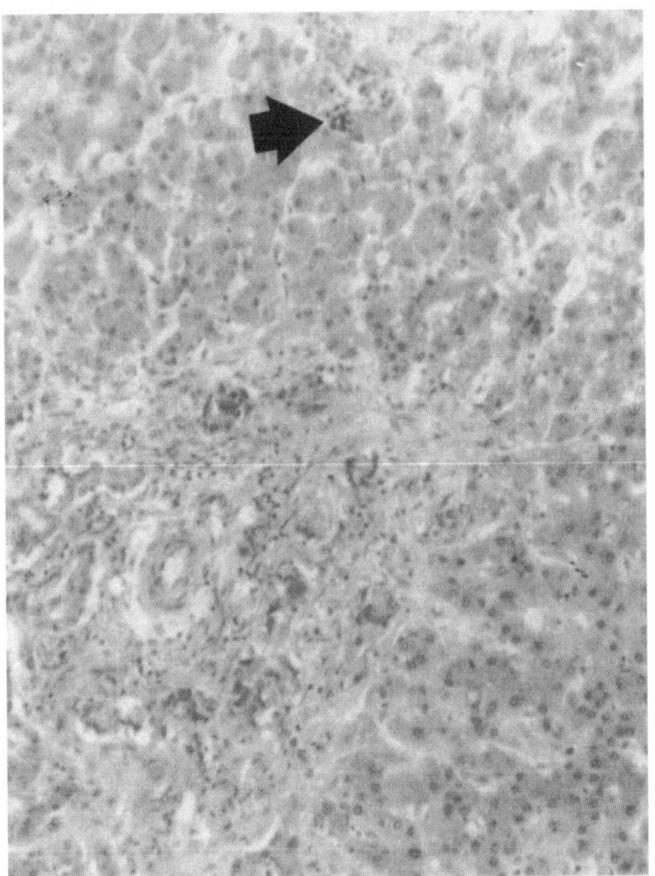

Figure 11.4. Congenital rubella infection. Portal and periportal fibrosis and extramedullary hematopoiesis (*arrow*). (H&E, original magnification 100×.)

of congenital rubella is being used successfully in research laboratories.

Treatment is supportive. Control of rubella has been attempted by the routine immunization of all infants and the testing of all women for evidence of protective antibody to rubella before marriage. Infants with congenital rubella usually recover from the hepatitis without the development of hepatic failure. However, significant morbidity and mortality in these infants usually are the result of the cardiac lesions or hemorrhage.

Hepatitis A

Although hepatitis A virus (HAV) is a frequent cause of hepatitis in childhood, it is not a frequent cause of hepatitis in the newborn [32]. Acquisition of HAV by blood transfusions has been reported in the neonatal period [33]. Most of these neonates developed serologic evidence of acute HAV infection but were clinically and biochemically asymptomatic. Though rare, neonatal cholestasis resulting from vertical transmission of hepatitis A infection has been reported [34,35].

In general, HAV is spread by the orofecal route. Infection occurs at a younger age in lower socioeconomic groups and is endemic in developing countries. Children usually are anicteric and have a milder course than do adults. No HAV carrier state exists, and chronic hepatitis A does not occur.

Serologic testing for IgM- and IgG-specific anti-HAV antibodies is commercially available. Recent infection is denoted by an elevated titer of IgM anti-HAV.

Treatment is supportive. Enteric precautions should be observed. If the mother is not jaundiced, no special care of the infant is recommended. Breast-feeding may occur as long as proper hygiene is practiced. If the mother is jaundiced, immunoglobulin is recommended, although its efficacy in this situation is not proven. Limited data exist on the use of the HAV vaccine in infants; the currently available vaccines in the United States are approved for children over 1 year of age.

Hepatitis B

Overall in the United States, hepatitis B is an uncommon cause of neonatal hepatitis. However, in certain regions of the United States and parts of the world, it is common for perinatal transmission of HBV to occur from a chronic hepatitis B carrier mother or the mother with acute hepatitis B during the third trimester of pregnancy [36]. Perinatal transmission of hepatitis B is also more likely if the mother is positive for hepatitis Be antigen (HBeAg) and thus has hepatitis B viral DNA circulating in the bloodstream. If the infant does not acquire hepatitis B infection at birth, close contact with other family members places the infant at high risk for acquisition of the virus, making preexposure hepatitis B immunization imperative.

The majority of infants who develop hepatitis B through vertical transmission show evidence of hepatitis B surface antigen (HBsAg) positivity between 4 and 16 weeks of age and become asymptomatic carriers. However, some infants develop a chronic active form of hepatitis B, and others, with time, develop cirrhosis and hepatocellular carcinoma. A coinfection or superinfection with delta hepatitis (hepatitis D) is also possible. It is rare for perinatally acquired hepatitis B to result in an acute icteric hepatitis [37]. These infants may have a benign course, with the development of anti-HBsAg and loss of HBsAg, or uncommonly may progress to a rapidly fulminant and fatal hepatitis.

All mothers with the potential for hepatitis B infection should be screened for HBsAg. In many states, the law requires that all pregnant women have their hepatitis B status investigated during their pregnancy. For infants whose mothers are found to be HBsAg positive, immunoprophylaxis should be instituted at birth. Neonates born to mothers who are HBsAg positive should be bathed carefully soon after birth to remove potentially infected maternal blood or secretions. Hepatitis B immunoglobulin (HBIG) should be administered intramuscularly (0.5 mL) as soon as possible after birth and preferably within 12 hours. Efficacy of HBIG after 12 hours and before 48 hours is presumed but unproved. At another distant injection site, hepatitis B vaccine (0.5 mL) should be administered intramuscularly using a different syringe at the same time as HBIG. The second and third doses of vaccine are given at 1–2 and 6 months after the first. For preterm infants who weigh less than 2 kg at birth born to HBsAg-positive mothers, the initial vaccine dose should not be counted in the required three doses to complete the immunization series, so these preterm infants receive a total of four doses. The need for booster doses of hepatitis B vaccine for children and adults with a normal immune system is not recommended as immune memory remains intact for 15 years or more. The Infectious Disease Advisory Committee of the American Academy of Pediatrics recommends routine immunization with hepatitis B vaccine of all infants regardless of risk factors or maternal hepatitis B status. Although the cost benefits of this approach will not be immediate, it is anticipated that within 10–20 years of this practice, hepatitis B infection could be effectively controlled and potentially eliminated as a significant cause of liver disease within the United States.

Diagnosis of hepatitis B uses commercially available serologic tests for hepatitis B antigens (HBsAg and HBeAg) and antibodies to HBsAg, hepatitis B core antigen (HBcAg), and HBeAg. In acute infection, HBsAg positivity detects the great majority of cases. However, because HBsAg is also positive in chronic infection, IgM anti-HBcAg presence can be used to establish acute or recent hepatitis B infection. Quantitative tests of serum hepatitis B virus DNA by PCR or branched-chain DNA methods are commercially available and useful in the selection and monitoring of patients for therapy.

Liver biopsy is seldom necessary for the diagnosis of acute hepatitis B. Focal or single-cell necrosis with clear cells, balloon cells, and acidophilic bodies is usually evident. There may be centrilobular necrosis with surrounding mononuclear infiltrate as well as bile stasis and Kupffer cell enlargement.

There is no specific treatment for acute hepatitis B. For chronic hepatitis B in childhood, interferon alfa-2b therapy and lamivudine have been approved for use in children with evidence of viral replication (HBV DNA or HBeAg positivity) and increased serum aminotransferase levels [38]. Interferon therapy requires an injection three times a week for 24 weeks. Lamivudine requires 52 weeks of daily oral administration. With interferon, 26% of children became HBeAg negative and 10% lost HBsAg. With lamivudine, 23% had HBeAg seroconversion and only 2% lost HBsAg. Currently, trials are under way using the orally administered drug adefovir dipivoxil for children with chronic hepatitis B.

Hepatitis C

The signs and symptoms of hepatitis C are similar to those of hepatitis A and B. Acute disease is associated with jaundice in only 25% of patients, and abnormalities in serum liver function tests occur less frequently than with hepatitis B infection. Most infections are asymptomatic. Transmission of hepatitis C virus (HCV) can occur by way of parenteral administration of blood or blood products, but the majority of cases in the United States are not associated with blood transfusion. High-risk groups for hepatitis C include parenteral drug users, persons transfused with blood or blood products, health care workers who are frequently exposed to blood, and persons with household or sexual contact with an infected person. Perinatal transmission of HCV has been demonstrated [39]. Seroprevalence among pregnant women in the United States is estimated at 1–2%, with maternal–fetal transmission at about 5%. Maternal coinfection with human immunodeficiency virus (HIV) has been associated with an increased risk of perinatal transmission of HCV. Vertical transmission of HCV may depend on the hepatitis C genotype and the serum titer of maternal viral RNA. Serum HCV antibody and HCV RNA have been detected in breast milk, but HCV transmission to infants by breast-feeding has not been demonstrated [40]. The rate of vertical transmission of HCV is identical in breast-fed and bottle-fed infants. A key feature of hepatitis C is its propensity to progress to chronic hepatitis and more severe hepatic dysfunction. About 60–80% of children with hepatitis C progress to chronicity, and cirrhosis develops in at least 20% of these [41,42]. Hepatitis C has been associated with the development of hepatocellular carcinoma [43].

The two major tests currently available for the laboratory diagnosis of HCV infections are antibody assays for HCV and those for detecting and quantitating HCV RNA. The initial antibody test involves a screening enzyme-linked immunosorbent assay. If positive, confirmation is made by a recombinant immunoblot assay. Both assays detect IgG antibodies; no IgM assays are available. Highly sensitive PCR assays for detection and quantitation of HCV RNA and a nucleic acid–based amplification test (bDNA) are commercially available. These tests are costly, but they may be useful for monitoring patients undergoing therapy and identifying infection early in infants because maternal antibody can cross the placenta and interfere with the ability to detect antibody produced by the infant.

Interferon, pegylated interferon, and pegylated interferon in combination with ribavirin have been found to be safe and efficacious in the treatment of chronic hepatitis C in adults [44,45]. Combination therapy (interferon with ribavirin) was shown to result in higher rates of sustained virologic, biochemical, and histologic response then interferon alone. The effectiveness of interferon therapy for hepatitis C in children appears similar to that in adults [46,47]. A large-scale trial of pegylated interferon with and without ribavirin in children with chronic hepatitis C is currently in progress, with small pilot studies suggesting very good results [48].

The use of immunoglobulin for postexposure prophylaxis against HCV infection is not recommended based on the lack of clinical efficacy in humans and animal laboratory studies. Furthermore, immunoglobulin is manufactured from plasma documented to be negative for anti-HCV antibodies.

Delta Hepatitis (Hepatitis D)

Delta hepatitis virus (HDV) requires infection with HBV because the outer coat of the complete HDV is HBsAg. If HDV infection occurs at the same time as hepatitis B infection, this is referred to as a coinfection. If HDV infection occurs in a person who is already chronically infected with hepatitis B, this is referred to as a superinfection. Delta hepatitis can be transmitted by parenteral, percutaneous, or mucous membrane inoculation. Delta hepatitis may be transmitted by blood or blood products, intravenous drug use, or sexual contact if HBsAg is present in the person's blood. Transmission of HDV from mother to newborn infant is unusual. Delta hepatitis also may be spread among families with HBsAg carriers. Delta hepatitis is most commonly found in southern Italy, eastern Europe, South America, Africa, and the Middle East. Although there is a high prevalence of hepatitis B infection in the Far East, delta hepatitis is uncommon there. In the United States, delta hepatitis is found most frequently in intravenous drug abusers, hemophiliacs, and immigrants from endemic areas.

Diagnosis of delta hepatitis can be made using a commercially available anti-HDV antibody test. IgM-specific anti-HDV and delta antigen tests are available investigationally. Differentiation of HDV coinfection from superinfection can be established by use of IgM anti-HBcAg, which is present only with acute hepatitis B infection.

Treatment of delta hepatitis is supportive. Use of interferon therapy in limited trials has been disappointing [49]. Because delta hepatitis cannot be transmitted in the absence of hepatitis B, care in avoiding HDV should be taken by hepatitis B–positive individuals. Successful immunization with hepatitis B vaccine affords protection from HDV infection.

Hepatitis E (Enterically Transmitted Non-A, Non-B Hepatitis)

Transmission of this virus is by the orofecal route. The disease is more common in adults than children and is associated with a significantly high incidence of mortality in pregnant women. Cases have been reported in epidemics and have usually been traced to contaminated water. Endemic enterically transmitted non-A, non-B hepatitis has been reported in the United States, but most reported cases have occurred among travelers to endemic regions.

Diagnosis is established by exclusion of other known causes of acute hepatitis (i.e., hepatitis A, B, C, and D). Serologic tests that detect antibody (IgM) to the hepatitis E virus and hepatitis E viral RNA detection by PCR of stool or serum are available to confirm the diagnosis by commercial and research laboratories, but none is licensed by the Food and Drug Administration.

Treatment is supportive. Passive immunoprophylaxis with immunoglobulin prepared in the United States has not been effective.

GB Virus C (Hepatitis G)

Two viruses belonging to the Flaviviridae family, GB virus C and hepatitis G virus (HGV), are variants of the same viral species and distantly related to HCV. Although there is considerable evidence demonstrating persistent viral infection, this virus has not been demonstrated to cause disease in humans or other primates. An association with posttransfusion hepatitis has been reported, but most infected children remain asymptomatic. Mother-to-infant transmission of HGV has been documented, resulting in a high viral persistence rate and lack of immune response to the virus [50,51]. In mothers coinfected with either HIV or HCV and HGV, HGV transmission is more frequent and occurs at a higher rate than that for HCV. HGV may be transmitted by blood or blood products, injection drug use, or sexual contact.

No serologic test is commercially available. An indirect immunoassay, which uses the E2 (envelope) protein as an antigenic target, is available for research purposes. GB virus C RNA can be detected in serum samples using a reverse-transcription, PCR method.

Because the virus has not been demonstrated to cause either persistent hepatitis or symptomatic disease, treatment is supportive. Although HGV has been demonstrated to be sensitive to treatment with interferon therapy, the infection frequently recurs once therapy is terminated [52].

Transfusion-Transmitted Virus

This unenveloped, single-stranded DNA virus has been implicated as a cause of posttransfusion hepatitis [53]. Transfusion-transmitted virus (TTV) has been found to contaminate blood and blood product transfusions and has been found in the feces [54]. No data have been published on maternal–neonatal transmission of this virus. Coinfection with HCV has been noted. Like HGV, TTV does not seem to be linked to biochemical signs of liver disease.

No serologic test is currently available. The viral DNA has been detected by use of PCR using seminested primers [55]. In preliminary studies in adults coinfected with HCV and TTV, interferon therapy seemed useful in TTV eradication.

Enteroviral Hepatitis

Although many viruses may produce disease in the newborn, only a few viruses are frequently encountered. Among the less frequent viruses, which may on occasion result in nursery epidemics of significant clinical illness, are viruses within the enterovirus classification. These generally include nonpolio enteroviruses, including coxsackieviruses, echoviruses, and enteroviruses. Transmission may have occurred during the prenatal, intrapartum, or perinatal period. A maternal history of a viral syndrome or fever just before delivery may be elicited. Initially the infant may appear healthy and vigorous. However, poor feeding, fever, lethargy, diarrhea, jaundice, and skin rash signal clinical infection. These nonspecific signs, however, do not help distinguish these viruses from other bacterial or viral etiologies. In the majority of cases, these infections are benign and self-limited. However, there are reports of death resulting from enteroviral infections in neonates [56,57]. Fatal and massive hepatic necrosis with failure has been reported with infections of Coxsackie group B virus and echovirus groups 6, 9, 11, 14, and 19. These patients demonstrated jaundice, markedly elevated serum aminotransferases, disseminated intravascular coagulation, and progressive hepatic failure.

Diagnosis is made by viral isolation from the throat, rectum, or other sites of clinical involvement or biopsy material. Tissue culture techniques may not be adequate for viral isolation, and suckling mouse inoculation may be required to isolate the offending virus. Sera for antibody testing during the acute and convalescent periods should be collected and stored because an increase in titer for an isolated virus suggests a causal role. Because no common enterovirus antigen is available, serologic screening without viral isolation is generally not performed. PCR testing for the presence of enteroviral RNA in cerebrospinal fluid is available in several research laboratories.

There is no specific approved therapy for enteroviral infections. Good supportive care, attention to bleeding problems, and treatment of secondary bacterial infections are important considerations. Intravenous immunoglobulin has been used in life-threatening neonatal enteroviral infections in hope of the presence of a high antibody titer to the infecting virus. Pleconaril is an investigational drug that inhibits viral attachment to host cell receptors and uncoating of viral nucleic acid. It has potent anti-enterovirus activity and has shown promise in treatment of neonatal echovirus and Coxsackie B virus infections including severe hepatitis [57a].

Parvovirus Hepatitis

Parvovirus B19 is most often associated with erythema infectiosum (fifth disease) and is usually manifested by mild systemic symptoms, fever, and the distinctive "slapped cheek" rash. However, parvovirus B19 has been reported to cause liver disease ranging from an acute hepatitis to fulminant hepatitis with an associated aplastic anemia [58,59].

Laboratory diagnosis can be made by testing for B19 parvovirus IgM antibody. IgG serum antibody indicates prior infection and immunity. Commercial, research, and state health department laboratories provide assays using the PCR or nucleic acid hybridization techniques that are useful for detecting chronic infection.

Treatment with monoclonal anti-CD52 antibodies has been successful in a few cases [59]. In immunodeficient patients with chronic infection, intravenous immunoglobulin therapy should be considered.

Human Herpesvirus 6 Infection

Human herpesvirus 6 (HHV-6) infection has been identified as the etiologic agent for roseola infantum (exanthema subitum, sixth disease). Young children usually present with an acute febrile illness for several days, with rapid defervescence followed by an erythematous maculopapular rash lasting 1–2 days. Acute liver failure and chronic hepatitis in an infant associated with HHV-6 has been reported [60]. The presence of HHV-6 DNA in liver tissue was confirmed by both in situ hybridization and PCR.

Reovirus 3 Infection

The concept of infantile obstructive cholangiopathy postulated by Landing [61] suggests a common etiologic agent for several neonatal liver diseases, including biliary atresia and neonatal hepatitis. Reovirus 3 has been proposed as a candidate virus serving as an etiologic agent for biliary atresia and neonatal hepatitis. Infection of weanling mice results in hepatic lesions similar to those observed in neonates with neonatal hepatitis. Several early studies suggested elevated reovirus 3 antibody titers in the sera of infants with biliary atresia and neonatal hepatitis. Reovirus type 3 was also detected in the porta hepatis of an infant with biliary atresia and in a monkey infected with reovirus that developed biliary atresia. However, this association has not been confirmed. Studies using molecular techniques have yielded mixed results [62,63]. If reovirus type 3 infection results in biliary atresia or neonatal hepatitis in human newborns, only some of the cases may be attributed to its presence.

Paramyxovirus Infection

Ten patients with an unusual form of giant cell hepatitis associated with a severe clinical course have been reported [64]. Two of the patients were infants 5 months and 7 months of age. Both infants had features of autoimmune chronic active hepatitis, and one infant also had evidence of autoimmune hemolytic anemia. Histopathologic and electron microscopic evaluation of the liver biopsy samples from these infants showed the presence of syncytial multinucleated giant cells replacing hepatocyte cords most prominently in the centrilobular region, as well as severe acute and chronic hepatitis with bridging necrosis of hepatocytes, ballooning, and dropout of hepatocytes, cholestasis, and small round cell inflammation within the lobule. Ultrastructural studies revealed the presence of viruslike structures within the giant cells resembling the nucleocapsids of paramyxoviruses. Inoculation from one of the patients into two chimpanzees failed to induce biochemical or histologic evidence of hepatitis. However, in one animal, an increase in titer of antibodies to measles virus and parainfluenza 4 was found. The giant cells in these infants were larger and of different morphology than the giant cells usually encountered in neonatal hepatitis and biliary atresia. Paramyxoviruses should be considered in patients with severe sporadic hepatitis.

Human Immunodeficiency Virus Infection

Human immunodeficiency virus infection in children is associated with a broad spectrum of disease and a varied clinical course. Acquired immunodeficiency syndrome (AIDS) represents the most severe form. The great majority of cases of AIDS in children are the result of vertical transmission from an infected mother. Other infections (e.g., hepatitis B and C) may be transmitted to the newborn more efficiently when the mother is coinfected with HIV. Other routes of HIV transmission include sexual contact with an infected individual and exposure to infected blood or blood products. Clinical manifestations of HIV infection often involve the gastrointestinal tract and the liver and include generalized lymphadenopathy, hepatomegaly, splenomegaly, failure to thrive, oral candidiasis, recurrent diarrhea, parotitis, cardiomyopathy, hepatitis, nephropathy, central nervous system disease, lymphoid interstitial pneumonia, recurrent invasive bacterial infections, opportunistic infections, and malignancies.

Although liver involvement is frequently observed in HIV infection, whether the liver lesions are primary or secondary to opportunistic infection in an immunosuppressed host is difficult to determine. Children with HIV infection have demonstrated hepatosplenomegaly and elevated serum aminotransferases. Histology has revealed both lobular and portal changes with lymphocytic infiltration, piecemeal necrosis, hepatocellular and bile duct damage, sinusoidal cell hyperplasia, and endothelialitis [65]. In adults with HIV infection with abnormal liver test abnormalities or fever greater then 2 weeks or hepatomegaly who undergo liver biopsy, the most common biopsy-derived diagnosis has been *Mycobacterium avium* complex [66]. Other frequently diagnosed infections have included *Mycobacterium tuberculosis,* other *Mycobacterium* species, and other opportunistic infections. Biliary tract abnormalities, including papillary stenosis and sclerosing cholangitis, have been observed. The most common neoplasm has been lymphoma. The efficacy of liver biopsy in HIV-infected persons is still unknown. Liver biopsy may be a helpful diagnostic tool in HIV-positive patients with fever, hepatomegaly, or liver test abnormalities.

Diagnosis of HIV infection is made by serum antibody tests (enzyme immunoassays), except in children less than 18 months of age because of passive maternal antibody acquisition across the placenta. Western blot or immunofluorescent antibody tests should be used for confirmation of positive results. In young children (18 months), the preferred tests are HIV culture and detection of HIV genomic sequences by PCR.

Antiretroviral therapy is the standard of care for HIV-infected children. Therapeutic strategies are rapidly changing in this field, so consultation with an expert or enrollment of an HIV-infected child into an available clinical trial is recommended.

Neonatal Lupus Erythematosus

Hepatic involvement expressed as neonatal cholestasis has been associated with neonatal lupus erythematosus [67,68]. Hepatomegaly and splenomegaly have been noted in 20–40% of reported cases. Several infants with neonatal lupus erythematosus have been reported with liver histology demonstrating giant cell transformation, ductal obstruction, and extramedullary hematopoiesis. It is postulated that maternal autoantibodies by way of a transplacental mechanism result in an immune response in the infant that results in hepatic injury. This is an extension of the theory that maternal autoantibodies to Sjögren's syndrome antigen A (Ro-SSA) and Sjögren's syndrome antigen B (La-SSB) cause congenital heart block in infants with neonatal lupus erythematosus whose initial pathologic lesion is myocardial inflammation. Clearly, a prospective study investigating maternal autoantibodies and the incidence of liver involvement in neonatal lupus erythematosus is required before this hypothesis can be proved.

Chromosomal Disorders

Both neonatal hepatitis and biliary atresia have been associated with trisomy 17–18 syndrome (trisomy E) and trisomy 21 (Down's syndrome) [69,70]. Intrahepatic cholestasis and variable combinations of hepatocellular and portal tract involvement have been observed. Giant cell transformation and focal obliteration of bile ducts have been seen. Diffuse lobular fibrosis surrounding proliferating ductular elements and residual hepatocytes, which proved fatal, was observed in a group of Down's syndrome infants. The possibility of a viral etiology for the hepatic lesions observed was not sufficiently excluded. Whether the chromosomal defects directly contribute to the hepatic dysfunction observed in these infants is unknown.

Familial Intrahepatic Cholestatic Syndromes

These syndromes are discussed in detail in Chapters 14 and 15. Affected children often present in infancy or early childhood because of their propensity to develop cholestasis, thus have often been classified under the umbrella of neonatal hepatitis. These children may have disease limited to the liver or have abnormalities often striking in other organs. Laboratory findings vary widely depending on the condition. Typical obstructive cholestasis with jaundice, pruritus, and hypercholesterolemia may dominate the picture, although certain syndromes are atypical, with normal serum cholesterol levels, normal γ-glutamyl transpeptidase levels, and cholestasis.

Among these syndromes are conditions that are fatal in childhood, whereas others are essentially benign. Investigation of many of the conditions in this group has led to clear identification and characterization within the past few years [71–74].

Pseudo-TORCH Syndrome (Baraitser–Reardon Syndrome)

Intracranial calcifications may be observed in neonates with environmental or metabolic disturbances. The predominant environmental factors associated with intracranial calcifications are congenital infections with toxoplasmosis, rubella, CMV, herpes, and others (TORCH). Yet, there are infants in whom all confirmatory tests for congenital infection are negative. Reports of more then one affected child within a sibship has led to the recognition of an autosomal recessive congenital infection-like syndrome called pseudo-TORCH syndrome [75,76,76a]. In addition to the intracranial calcifications, microcephaly, seizures, neurologic delay, hepatomegaly, splenomegaly, raised serum aminotransferases (aspartate aminotransferase, alanine aminotransferase) and thrombocytopenia have been observed [77]. A liver biopsy performed at 2 months of age in a child with this syndrome showed preserved liver architecture without any sign of inflammation or focal necrosis. Abundant iron pigmentary accumulations were observed within many hepatocytes in association with features of cholestasis. Aicardi–Goutieres syndrome shares many of the features of pseudo-TORCH syndrome but differs by the presence of cerebrospinal fluid lymphocytosis with raised levels of interferon alfa. Two boys of consanguineous parents demonstrating the phenotypic overlap of Aicardi-Goutieres and pseudo-TORCH syndromes have been reported.

Coombs-Positive Giant Cell Hepatitis

Although giant cell hepatitis is a frequent pattern of injury in the neonate, it is unusual after infancy. Coombs-positive giant cell hepatitis is a rare disease of early childhood with unknown etiology and a variable response to immunosuppressive therapy [78]. An immune dysregulation mechanism is postulated. Liver histology reveals severe giant cell transformation with cholestasis, marked inflammation, clusters of neutrophils, spotty hepatocyte necrosis, and fibrosis. Many reports in the literature suggest this disorder is distinct and has an aggressive course. Liver transplantation for giant cell hepatitis with autoimmune Coombs-positive hemolytic anemia has had inconsistent success, with reports of recurrence of disease in the graft [79].

DIFFERENTIAL DIAGNOSIS

A diverse group of disorders may present in the neonate as cholestasis with a conjugated hyperbilirubinemia. A logical, well-organized, and rapid evaluation of the infant with conjugated hyperbilirubinemia is mandatory. Although the differential list is long and may be intimidating, the work-up is relatively straightforward. The initial evaluation should determine the severity of the hepatic dysfunction. It should identify specific metabolic, infectious, endocrinologic, toxic, or surgically correctable disorders amenable to therapy. The initial evaluation should identify recognizable genetic or congenital disorders and determine the need for further investigation. Statistically, approximately 75% of all cases of neonatal cholestasis are the result of biliary atresia or neonatal hepatitis. Neonatal hepatitis is the most common diagnosis of infants with neonatal cholestasis. Epidemiologic data suggest two categories of neonatal hepatitis: a sporadic form and a familial form. The increased incidence of neonatal hepatitis within some families suggests that a metabolic or genetic cause is responsible. Unfortunately, no etiologic factor has been identified in these cases. Some of these familial cases may have forms of progressive familial intrahepatic cholestasis.

Discriminating among the several forms of familial intrahepatic cholestasis may be aided by a comparison of several factors. These include birth weight; age of onset of cholestasis; associated anomalies of the heart, eyes, bones, or kidneys; pattern of cholestasis (episodic or continuous); laboratory parameters; biopsy findings; outcome; and presumed inheritance pattern.

CLINICAL PRESENTATION

Differentiating extrahepatic from intrahepatic cholestasis remains the challenge for the clinician because early recognition of extrahepatic obstruction may be amenable to surgical intervention. Furthermore, avoiding unnecessary and potentially harmful surgery is always warranted. Unfortunately, there is no pathognomonic symptom to distinguish biliary atresia from neonatal hepatitis. Infants in both groups present with jaundice and acholic stools. Observation of the stools by an experienced individual is an inexpensive and highly useful procedure. Verbal reports of stool pigment from the parents in my experience are notoriously inaccurate. Pruritus does not occur until later in the course. The liver is enlarged on physical examination. Clinical features may be useful in helping to discriminate between biliary atresia and neonatal hepatitis.

Biliary atresia is more common in girls with normal birth weight, whereas neonatal hepatitis is more common in boys [79,80]. Familial occurrence favors neonatal hepatitis. An associated polysplenia syndrome favors BA. Intermittent pigmentation of stools favors intrahepatic cholestasis, whereas consistently acholic stools favor a diagnosis of BA. Unfortunately, severe intrahepatic cholestasis also may result in acholic stools. With neonatal hepatitis, jaundice may persist after the first week of physiologic jaundice of the newborn, so jaundice may already be observed as abnormal during the second week of life. In contrast, a jaundice-free interval between the disappearance of physiologic jaundice and the onset of pathologic obstructive jaundice may be seen in patients with BA.

Pathologic jaundice requires biochemical confirmation with fractionation of the serum bilirubin. A conjugated hyperbilirubinemia with elevated serum aminotransferase levels, alkaline phosphatase, and γ-glutamyl transpeptidase is seen. Although many attempts have been made to discriminate intrahepatic from extrahepatic cholestasis based on biochemical profiles, overlap between groups has significantly hampered this approach.

Ultrasonographic examination of the liver, radionuclide hepatobiliary imaging, collection of duodenal fluid by a tube or string device, endoscopic retrograde cholangiopancreatography, percutaneous transhepatic cholangiography, and percutaneous liver biopsy all provide valuable information to aid in discrimination of intrahepatic and extrahepatic cholestasis. The combination of procedures performed depends on the results, skills, and expertise of the institution. However, there will still be cases in which an intraoperative cholangiogram is necessary. Use of new therapeutic regimens (i.e., ursodeoxycholic acid) should not be instituted until a definitive diagnosis has been made. Early surgical intervention is the preferred treatment for biliary atresia.

HISTOPATHOLOGY

In neonatal hepatitis, alterations in the parenchyma of the liver are more prominent than alterations in the portal zone [81–85] (Figure 11.5, color plate). Giant cells are usually more prominent than in biliary atresia and may be ballooned or may show degeneration [84,85]. Necrosis of giant cells in the parenchyma

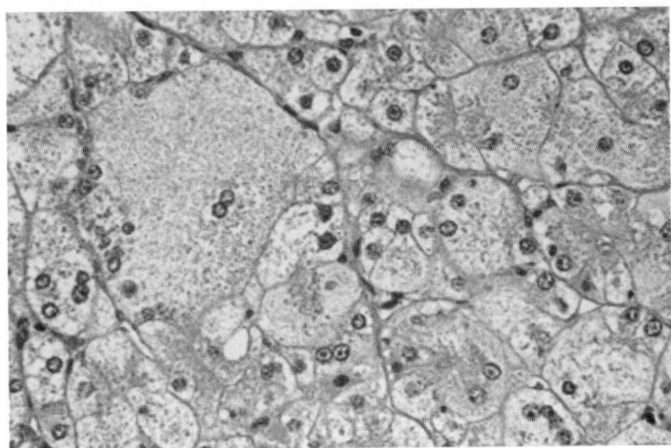

Figure 11.5. Neonatal hepatitis with giant cell transformation. Centrizonal region shows enlarged giant hepatocytes and scattered lobular sinusoidal mononuclear infiltrates. (H&E, original magnification 100×.) For color reproduction, see Color Plate 11.5.

may result in neutrophil infiltration. Extramedullary hematopoiesis and hemosiderin deposition in parenchymal and Kupffer cells are generally more prominent in neonatal hepatitis than in biliary atresia. Intralobular inflammation and Kupffer cell hyperplasia are usually apparent in neonatal hepatitis, whereas portal and periportal inflammation is more apparent in biliary atresia. Cholestasis may be variable in neonatal hepatitis with pigment granules in parenchymal and Kupffer cells and intercellular bile plugs present. With severe cholestasis in neonatal hepatitis, bile plugs may be seen in portal ductules but usually not to the extent seen in biliary atresia. Bile ductular proliferation may occasionally be observed in neonatal hepatitis but is usually much more prominent in cases of biliary atresia.

By light and electron microscopic studies, the multinucleated giant cells in neonatal hepatitis appear to be of parenchymal origin. The number of nuclei in the giant cells may vary, as may their positions centrally or peripherally within the cytoplasm. By hematoxylin and eosin staining, the cytoplasm of multinucleated giant cells seen in neonatal hepatitis is pale. This may be the result of glycogen content or hydropic changes. Brownish pigment granules present in the giant cells may be a combination of bilirubin, hemosiderin, or lipofuscin deposition. Histochemical analysis of multinucleated giant cells in neonatal hepatitis reveals intense periodic acid–Schiff staining with diastase digestion, signifying glycogen presence [84]. Additionally, there is intense staining for glucose-6-phosphatase, succinic dehydrogenase, nicotinamide adenine dinucleotide, and nicotinamide adenine dinucleotide phosphate diaphorases. Inclusions that are acid phosphatase positive are numerous, and there is increased alkaline phosphatase staining at the sinusoidal border.

Electron microscopic evaluation of multinucleated giant cells in neonatal hepatitis reveals well-preserved nuclei, mitochondria, endoplasmic reticulum, and plasma membranes [84,85]. Numerous intracytoplasmic vacuoles, bilirubin deposits, and nuclei are present. The formative mechanisms of giant cells have been debated, although fusion of several mononuclear hepatocytes to form a giant cell appears to be the most plausible explanation [84]. The mechanism whereby there is loss of giant cells spontaneously with time is also unknown. Giant cells appear to have a life span of several months, and their disappearance seems to parallel resolution of cholestasis. Their presence seems to be a nonspecific response of the immature liver to injury [82]. Their biologic significance is unknown, and although they are more commonly seen in the newborn, they also may be seen on occasion in the livers of adults with various viral or drug-induced hepatic disorders [64]. A case of neonatal hepatitis progressing to cirrhosis and hepatocellular carcinoma by 28 months of age in a girl has been reported [86].

PROGNOSIS

Prognosis of patients with neonatal hepatitis may be variable and depends on the extent of parenchymal injury and fibrosis [87–91]. In general, patients with neonatal hepatitis have a better prognosis than infants with biliary atresia or metabolic liver diseases, which are not amenable to diet therapy. Sporadic cases of neonatal hepatitis have a better prognosis than familial cases or cases with associated conditions such as α_1-antitrypsin deficiency. Quoted recovery rates from neonatal hepatitis are in the 60–80% range for sporadic cases, whereas for familial cases the recovery rate is in the 20–40% range. However, the impact of early recognition and intervention with diet therapy, vitamin supplementation, choleretic agents, and hepatic transplantation on the prognosis for neonatal hepatitis awaits further study.

ACKNOWLEDGMENTS

I thank Samuel H. Pepkowitz of the Department of Pathology and Laboratory Medicine, Cedars-Sinai Medical Center, and Linda Ferrell of the Department of Pathology, University of California, San Francisco, for help with photographing the figures and creating the legends.

REFERENCES

1. Hamilton JR, Sass-Kortsak A. Jaundice associated with severe bacterial infection in young infants. J Pediatr 1963;63:121–32.
2. Zimmerman HJ, Fang M, Utili R, et al. Jaundice due to bacterial infection. Gastroenterology 1979;77:362–74.
3. Andres JM, Walker WA. Effect of *Escherichia coli* endotoxin on the developing rat liver. I. Giant cell induction and disruption in protein metabolism. Pediatr Res 1979;13:1290–3.
4. Bolder U, Ton-Nu HT, Schteingart CD, et al. Hepatocyte transport of bile acids and organic anions in endotoxemic rats: impaired uptake and secretion. Gastroenterology 1997;112:214–25.

5. Borges MAG, DeBrito T, Borges JMG. Hepatic manifestations in bacterial infections of infants and children. Clinical features, biochemical data and morphologic hepatic changes. Acta Hepatogastroenterol 1972;19:328–44.
6. Lam HS, Li AM, Chu WCW, et al. Mal-positioned umbilical venous catheter causing liver abscess in a preterm infant. Biol Neonate 2005;88:54–6.
7. Garcia FJ, Nager AL. Jaundice as an early diagnostic sign of urinary tract infection in infancy. Pediatrics 2002;109:846–51.
8. Hoarau C, Ranivoharimina V, Chavet-Queru MS, et al. Congenital syphilis: update and perspectives. Sante 1999;9:38–45.
9. Herman TE. Extensive hepatic calcification secondary to fulminant neonatal syphilitic hepatitis. Pediatr Radiol 1995;25:120–2.
10. Kumar R, Gupta N, Sabharwal A, Shalini. Congenital tuberculosis. Indian J Pediatr 2005;72:631–3.
11. Montoya JG, Rosso F. Diagnosis and management of toxoplasmosis. Clin Perinatol 2005;32:705–26.
12. Desmonts G, Couvreur J. Congenital toxoplasmosis. A prospective study of 378 pregnancies. N Engl J Med 1974;290:1110–16.
13. Schmidt DR, Hogh B, Andersen O, et al. Treatment of infants with congenital toxoplasmosis: tolerability and plasma concentrations of sulfadiazine and pyrimethamine. Eur J Pediatr 2005;165:19–25.
14. Nicol KK, Geisinger KR. Congenital toxoplasmosis: diagnosis by exfoliative cytology. Diagn Cytopathol 1998;18:357–61.
15. Munro SC, Trincado D, Hall B, Rawlinson WD. Symptomatic infant characteristics of congenital cytomegalovirus disease in Australia. J Paediatr Child Health 2005;41:449–52.
16. Laifer SA, Ehrlich GD, Huff DS, et al. Congenital cytomegalovirus infection in offspring of liver transplant recipients. Clin Infect Dis 1995;20:52–5.
17. Zuppan CW, Bui HD, Grill BG. Diffuse hepatic fibrosis in congenital cytomegalovirus infection. J Pediatr Gastroenterol Nutr 1986;5:489–91.
18. Watkins JB, Sunaryo FP, Berezin SH. Hepatic manifestations of congenital and perinatal disease. Clin Perinatol 1981;8:467–80.
19. Weller TH, Hanshaw JB. Virologic and clinical observations on cytomegalic inclusion disease. N Engl J Med 1962;266:1233–44.
20. Snover DC, Horwitz CA. Liver disease in cytomegalovirus mononucleosis: a light microscopical and immunoperoxidase study of six cases. Hepatology 1984;3:408–12.
21. Greenfield C, Sinickas V, Harrison LC. Detection of cytomegalovirus by the polymerase chain reaction. A simple, rapid and sensitive non-radioactive method. Med J Aust 1991;154:383–5.
22. Berenberg W, Nankervis G. Long-term followup of cytomegalic inclusion disease of infancy. Pediatrics 1970;46:403–10.
23. Dressler S, Linder D. Noncirrhotic portal fibrosis following neonatal cytomegalic inclusion disease. J Pediatr 1978;93:887–8.
24. Hanshaw JB. Herpes virus hominis infections in the fetus and newborn. Am J Dis Child 1973;126:546–55.
25. Twagira M, Hadzic N, Smith M, et al. Disseminated neonatal herpes simplex virus (HSV) type 2 infection diagnosed by HSV DNA detection in blood and successfully managed by liver transplantation. Eur J Pediatr 2004;163:166–9.
26. Nakamura Y, Yamamoto S, Tanaka S, et al. Herpes simplex viral infection in human neonates: an immunohistochemical and electron microscopic study. Human Pathol 1985;16:1091–7.
27. Raga J, Chrystal V, Coovadia HM. Usefulness of clinical features and liver biopsy in diagnosis of disseminated herpes simplex infection. Arch Dis Child 1984;59:820–4.
28. Egawa H, Inomata Y, Nakayama S, et al. Fulminant hepatic failure secondary to herpes simplex virus infection in a neonate: a case report of successful treatment with liver transplantation and perioperative acyclovir. Liver Transplant Surg 1998;4:513–15.
29. Schluter WW, Reef SE, Redd SC, et al. Changing epidemiology of congenital rubella syndrome in the United States. J Infect Dis 1998;178:636–41.
30. Monif GRG, Asofsky R, Sever JL. Hepatic dysfunction in the congenital rubella syndrome. BMJ 1966;1:1086–8.
31. Strauss L, Bernstein J. Neonatal hepatitis in congenital rubella. Arch Pathol 1968;86:317–27.
32. Duff P. Hepatitis in pregnancy. Semin Perinatol 1998;22:277–83.
33. Noble RC, Kane MA, Reeves SA, et al. Posttransfusion hepatitis A in a neonatal intensive care unit. JAMA 1984;252:2711–15.
34. Renge RL, Dani VS, Chitambar SD, Arankalle VA. Vertical transmission of hepatitis A. Indian J Pediatr 2002;69:535–6.
35. Leikin E, Lysikiewicz A, Garry D, Tejani N. Intrauterine transmission of hepatitis A virus. Obstet Gynecol 1996;88:690–1.
36. Poland GA, Jacobson RM. Prevention of hepatitis B with the hepatitis B vaccine. N Eng J Med 2004;351:2832–8.
37. Tang JR, Hsu HY, Lin HH, et al. Hepatitis B surface antigenemia at birth: a long-term follow-up study. J Pediatr 1998;133:374–7.
38. Suskind DL, Rosenthal P. Chronic viral hepatitis. Adolesc Med Clinic 2004;15:145–58.
39. Granovsky MO, Minkoff HL, Tess BH, et al. Hepatitis C virus infection in the mothers and infants cohort study. Pediatrics 1998;102:355–9.
40. Kumar RM, Shahul S. Role of breast-feeding in transmission of hepatitis C virus to infants of HCV-infected mothers. J Hepatol 1998;29:191–7.
41. Chang MH. Chronic hepatitis virus infection in children. J Gastroenterol Hepatol 1998;13:541–8.
42. Realdi G, Alberti A, Rugge M, et al. Long-term follow-up of acute and chronic non-A, non-B post-transfusion hepatitis: evidence of progression to liver cirrhosis. Gut 1982;23:270–5.
43. Hasan F, Jeffers LJ, De Medina M, et al. Hepatitis-C associated hepatocellular carcinoma. Hepatology 1990;12:589–91.
44. McHutchison JG, Gordon SC, Schiff ER, et al. Interferon alfa-2b alone or in combination with ribavirin as initial treatment for chronic hepatitis C. Hepatitis Interventional Therapy Group. N Engl J Med 1998;339:1485–92.
45. Fried MW, Shiffman ML, Reddy KR, et al. Peginterferon alfa-2a plus ribavirin for chronic hepatitis C virus infection. N Engl J Med 2002;347:975–82.
46. Gonzalez-Peralta RP. Treatment of chronic hepatitis C in children. Pediatr Transplantation 2004;8:639–43.
47. Bortolotti F, Iorio R, Nebbia G, et al. Interferon treatment in children with chronic hepatitis C: long-lasting remission in responders, and risk for disease progression in non-responders. Dig Liver Dis 2005;37:336–41.
48. Kowala-Piaskowska A, Sluzewski W, Figlerowicz M, Mozer-Lisewska I. Factors influencing early virological response in

children with chronic hepatitis C treated with pegylated interferon and ribavirin. Hep Res 2005;32:224–6.
49. Dalekos GN, Galanakis E, Zervou E, et al. Interferon-alpha treatment of children with chronic hepatitis D virus infection: the Greek experience. Hepatogastroenterology 2000;47:1072–6.
50. Chen HL, Chang MH, Lin HH, et al. Antibodies to E2 protein of hepatitis G virus in children: different responses according to age at infection. J Pediatr 1998;133:382–5.
51. Zanetti AR, Tanzi E, Romano L, et al. Multicenter trial on mother-to-infant transmission of GBV-C virus. The Lombardy Study Group on Vertical/Perinatal Hepatitis Viruses Transmission. J Med Virol 1998;54:107–12.
52. Woelfle J, Berg T, Keller KM, et al. Persistent hepatitis G virus infection after neonatal transfusion. J Pediatr Gastroenterol Nutr 1998;26:402–7.
53. Naoumov NV, Petrova EP, Thomas MG, et al. Presence of a newly described human DNA virus (TTV) in patients with liver disease. Lancet 1998;352:195–7.
54. Okamoto H, Akahane Y, Ukita M, et al. Fecal excretion of a nonenveloped DNA virus (TTV) associated with posttransfusion non-A-G hepatitis. J Med Virol 1998;56:128–32.
55. Koidl C, Michael B, Berg J, et al. Detection of transfusion transmitted virus DNA by real-time PCR. J Clin Virol 2004;29: 277–81.
56. Abzug MJ. Prognosis for neonates with enterovirus hepatitis and coagulopathy. Pediatr Infect Dis J 2001;20:758–63.
57. Kawashima H, Ryou S, Nishimata S, et al. Enteroviral hepatitis in children. Pediatr Int 2004;46:130–4.
57a. Abzug MJ. Presentation, diagnosis, and management of enterovirus infections in neonates. Paediatr Drugs 2004;6:1–10.
58. Pardi DS, Romero Y, Mertz LE, et al. Hepatitis-associated aplastic anemia and acute parvovirus B19 infection: a report of two cases and a review of the literature. Am J Gastroenterol 1998;93: 468–70.
59. Granot E, Miskin H, Aker M. Monoclonal anti-CD52 antibodies: a potential mode of therapy for parvovirus B19 hepatitis. Transplant Proc 2001;33:2151–3.
60. Tajiri H, Tanaka-Taya K, Ozaki Y, et al. Chronic hepatitis in an infant, in association with human herpesvirus-6 infection. J Pediatr 1997;131:473–5.
61. Landing BH. Considerations of the pathogenesis of neonatal hepatitis, biliary atresia and choledochal cyst: the concept of infantile obstructive cholangiopathy. Prog Pediatr Surg 1974;4:113–39.
62. Steele MI, Marshall CM, Lloyd RE, et al. Reovirus 3 not detected by reverse transcriptase-mediated polymerase chain reaction analysis of preserved tissue from infants with cholestatic liver disease. Hepatology 1995;21:697–702.
63. Tyler KL, Sokol RJ, Oberhaus SM, et al. Detection of reovirus RNA in hepatobiliary tissues from patients with extrahepatic biliary atresia and choledochal cysts. Hepatology 1998;27: 1475–82.
64. Phillips MJ, Blendis LM, Poucell S, et al. Syncytial giant-cell hepatitis: sporadic hepatitis with distinctive pathological features, a severe clinical course, and paramyxoviral features. N Engl J Med 1991;324:455–60.
65. Kahn E, Greco MA, Daum F, et al. Hepatic pathology in pediatric acquired immunodeficiency syndrome. Human Pathol 1991;22:1111–19.
66. Poles MA, Dieterich DT, Schwarz ED, et al. Liver biopsy findings in 501 patients infected with human immunodeficiency virus (HIV). J AIDS Hum Retrovirol 1996;11:170–7.
67. Laxer RM, Roberts EA, Gross KR, et al. Liver disease in neonatal lupus erythematosus. J Pediatr 1990;116:238–42.
68. Lee LA, Sokol RJ, Buyon JP. Hepatobiliary disease in neonatal lupus: prevalence and clinical characteristics in cases enrolled in a national registry. Pediatrics 2002;109:E11.
69. Alpert LI, Strauss L, Hirschhorn K. Neonatal hepatitis and biliary atresia associated with trisomy 17–18 syndrome. N Engl J Med 1969;280:16–20.
70. Schwab M, Niemeyer C, Schwarzer U. Down syndrome, transient myeloproliferative disorder, and infantile liver fibrosis. Med Pediatr Oncol 1998;31:159–65.
71. Pratt DS. Cholestasis and cholestatic syndromes. Curr Opin Gastroenterol 2005;21:270–4.
72. van Mil SW, Houwen RH, Klomp LW. Genetics of familial intrahepatic cholestasis syndromes. J Med Genet 2005;42:449–63.
73. Krantz ID, Piccoli DA, Spinner NB. Alagille syndrome. J Med Genet 1997;34:152–7.
74. Bull LN, van Eijk MJ, Pawlikowska L, et al. A gene encoding a P-type ATPase mutated in two forms of hereditary cholestasis. Nat Genet 1998;18:219–24.
75. Vivarelli R, Grosso S, Cioni M, et al. Pseudo-TORCH syndrome or Baraitser-Reardon syndrome: diagnostic criteria. Brain Dev 2001;23:18–23.
76. Sanchis A, Cervero L, Bataller A, et al. Genetic syndromes mimic congenital infections. J Pediatr 2005;146: 701–5.
76a. Knoblauch H, Tyennstedt C, Brueck W, et al. Two brothers with findings resembling congenital intrauterine infection-like syndrome (pseudo-TORCH syndrome). Am J Med Genet A 2003;120:261–5.
77. Hadzic N, Portmann B, Lewis I, Mieli-Vergani G. Coombs positive giant cell hepatitis-a new feature of Evans' syndrome. Arch Dis Child 1998;78:397–8.
78. Akylidiz M, Karasu Z, Arikan C, et al. Successful liver transplantation for giant cell hepatitis and Coombs-positive haemolytic anemia: a case report. Pediatr Transplant 2005;9:630–3.
79. Balistreri WF, Grand R, Hoofnagle JH, et al. Biliary atresia: current concepts and research directions. Summary of a symposium. Hepatology 1996;23:1682–92.
80. Bates MD, Bucuvalas JC, Alonso MH, et al. Biliary atresia: pathogenesis and treatment. Semin Liver Dis 1998;18:281–93.
81. Tazawa Y, Abukawa D, Maisawa S, et al. Idiopathic neonatal hepatitis presenting as neonatal hepatic siderosis and steatosis. Dig Dis Sci 1998;43:392–6.
82. Shet TM, Kandalkar BM, Vora IM. Neonatal hepatitis — an autopsy study of 14 cases. Ind J Pathol Microbiol 1998;41: 77–84.
83. Nishinomiya F, Abukawa D, Takada G, et al. Relationships between clinical and histological profiles of non-familial idiopathic neonatal hepatitis. Acta Paediatr Jpn 1996;38:242–7.
84. Ruebner B, Thaler MM. Giant-cell transformation in infantile liver disease. In: Javitt NB, ed. Neonatal hepatitis and biliary atresia. DHEW publication no. (NIH) 79–1296. Bethesda, MD: U.S. Department of Health, Education and Welfare, 1979: 299–314.
85. Park WH, Kim SP, Park KK, et al. Electron microscopic study of the liver with biliary atresia and neonatal hepatitis. J Pediatr Surg 1996;31:367–74.

86. Moore L, Bourne AJ, Moore DJ, et al. Hepatocellular carcinoma following neonatal hepatitis. Pediatr Pathol Lab Med 1997; 17:601–10.
87. Suita S, Arima T, Ishii K, et al. Fate of infants with neonatal hepatitis: pediatric surgeons' dilemma. J Pediatr Surg 1992;27: 696–9.
88. Dick MC, Mowat AP. Hepatitis syndrome in infancy – an epidemiological survey with 10 year follow up. Arch Dis Child 1985;60:512–16.
89. Lee PI, Chang MH, Chen DS, et al. Prognostic implications of serum alpha-fetoprotein levels in neonatal hepatitis. J Pediatr Gastroenterol Nutr 1990;11:27–31.
90. Chang MH, Hsu HC, Lee CY, et al. Neonatal hepatitis: a follow-up study. J Pediatr Gastroenterol Nutr 1987;6: 203–7.
91. Deutsch J, Smith AL, Danks DM, et al. Long-term prognosis for babies with neonatal liver disease. Arch Dis Child 1985;60: 447–51.

12

BILIARY ATRESIA AND OTHER DISORDERS OF THE EXTRAHEPATIC BILE DUCTS

William F. Balistreri, M.D., Jorge A. Bezerra, M.D., and Frederick C. Ryckman, M.D.

Biliary atresia and related disorders of the biliary tract, such as choledochal cysts, must be considered in the differential diagnosis of prolonged conjugated hyperbilirubinemia in the newborn (neonatal cholestasis). In this chapter, we review the current status of diagnosis and management of these disorders, as well as advances in the intriguing quest for an understanding of their pathogenesis.

OVERVIEW

Neonatal hepatobiliary diseases, including biliary atresia, choledochal cysts, and "idiopathic" neonatal hepatitis, have historically been viewed as a continuum – a gradation of manifestations of a basic underlying disease process in which giant cell transformation of hepatocytes is strongly associated with inflammation at any level of the hepatobiliary tract. These disease entities may be polar end points of a common initial insult, as originally stated in the unifying hypothesis of Landing [1]. The end result represents the sequela of the inflammatory process at the primary site of injury. Landing suggested that this inflammatory process may injure bile duct epithelial cells, leading to either duct obliteration (*biliary atresia*) or weakening of the bile duct wall with subsequent dilatation (*choledochal cyst*). The lesions may be dependent on the stage of fetal development when the injury occurs and the site within the developing hepatobiliary tree at which the injury occurs [1,2]. A relationship of the pathogenesis of these obstructive cholangiopathies of infancy to the process of development is suggested by the association with disorders of situs determination such as the polysplenia syndrome and the observation of the so-called ductal plate malformation within the liver of a few patients with biliary atresia. The ductal plate malformation is postulated to represent either a primary developmental anomaly or disruption of a developmental sequence early in fetal life, resulting in incomplete regression of the immature bile ducts [2]. In contrast, most patients with biliary atresia have the late-onset type, which probably occurs after maturation of the intra- and extrahepatic bile ducts; this represents injury (destruction) of fully formed structures [2]. The dynamic nature of the underlying process has been further suggested by an apparent postnatal evolution of patent to atretic ducts: patients initially shown to have neonatal hepatitis with a patent biliary system subsequently were found to have acquired biliary atresia. The overlap concept is additionally supported by the frequent documentation of *intrahepatic* ductal injury in patients with *extrahepatic* biliary atresia [3,4]. Depletion of intrahepatic bile ducts is observed regularly at autopsy in children with biliary atresia who were never subjected to a biliary drainage procedure [5].

In biliary atresia, the initial insult and the sustaining mechanisms remain undefined. For example, although viral infection is a postulated initial insult, no specific viral agent has been reproducibly detected in tissue from affected infants, nor is there conclusive serologic evidence of their presence [6]. Other theories (discussed below) include defective embryogenesis or an altered immune response to injury. Further studies are warranted; biliary atresia and related disorders continue to offer clinicians and scientists stimulating challenges.

BILIARY ATRESIA

Biliary atresia is the end result of a destructive, idiopathic, inflammatory process that affects intra- and extrahepatic bile ducts, leading to fibrosis and obliteration of the biliary tract and eventual development of biliary cirrhosis [6]. This disorder should be of interest to all individuals involved in basic and clinical studies of diseases of the liver; the rapidly progressive fibro-obliterative process may represent a paradigm for other forms of hepatobiliary injury, perhaps reflecting an interrelationship between genetic predisposition and environmental exposure [6].

Biliary atresia is the most common cause of chronic cholestasis in infants and children, and because of the high frequency of progression to end-stage liver disease, it is the most frequent indication for liver transplantation in the pediatric age group. There is general agreement that the older theory that biliary atresia was caused by failure of recanalization of embryonic bile ducts should be abandoned. The lesion, in most patients, is not a true congenital malformation but seems to be acquired in late gestation or after birth [6–8]. Recent studies of liver samples obtained from patients with biliary atresia at the time of diagnosis revealed unique proinflammatory features [9,10]; how the inflammatory process produces complete or partial sclerosis of the extrahepatic (and intrahepatic) biliary ducts is now the subject of ongoing studies [6,11–13]. This idiopathic process leads to obliteration or discontinuity of the hepatic or common bile ducts at any point from the porta hepatis to the duodenum. In most patients, cordlike remnants of the extrahepatic ducts are encountered at surgery.

Incidence

Biliary atresia occurs worldwide, affecting an estimated 1 in 8000–12,000 live births [7,12–14]. There is a slight female predominance in most series. One population-based birth defects surveillance system for infants with biliary atresia in metropolitan Atlanta calculated an incidence rate of 0.73 per 10,000 live births [15]. There was significant seasonal clustering of the disease, with rates three times higher in infants born between December and March. Rates were significantly higher among nonwhite infants. The demonstration of significant seasonal clustering in this and other studies supports the theory that biliary atresia may be caused by environmental exposure (consistent with a viral cause) during the perinatal period [6].

Clinical Forms

Schweizer [16] has postulated the existence of at least two different forms of biliary atresia, with disparate pathogenesis: a *fetal* or *embryonic* form, and a *peri-* or *postnatal* form. In patients with the less common fetal form (10–35% of all patients), cholestasis is present from birth, with no jaundice-free interval. Bile duct remnants may not be detectable in the hepatic hilum, and there is a high frequency (10–20%) of associated malformations such as the "polysplenia syndrome," which may include cardiovascular defects, asplenia or abdominal situs inversus, intestinal malrotation, and positional anomalies of the portal vein and hepatic artery [17] (Table 12.1). The fetal form of biliary atresia may represent a true malformation syndrome (defective embryogenesis). In contrast, the postnatal form, in which there are no associated congenital abnormalities, may be the result of an acquired obliteration. These two forms have not been distinguished on the basis of histology of porta hepatis specimens; both forms may have inflamed and obliterated bile duct segments in this resected tissue mass.

In the series of Davenport et al. [17] of 308 patients with biliary atresia, 23 (7.5%) had polysplenia, 2 had double spleens, and 2 had asplenia. All 27 had anomalies that may occur in the polysplenia syndrome; the investigators used the term *biliary atresia splenic malformation syndrome* to describe all such infants [17]. In this series, infants with this syndrome had a lower birth weight and a higher incidence of maternal diabetes compared with nonsyndromic cases. The extrahepatic anatomy of the biliary tract also reportedly was different, including instances of what they termed *biliary agenesis.* These findings suggest that either the timing or the nature of the lesion of this "fetal" subgroup may differ from that of the more usual "postnatal" case. We believe that the postnatal form of biliary atresia may be the result of the sporadic occurrence of a virus-induced or virus-initiated progressive obliteration of the bile ducts, with some degree of intrahepatic bile duct injury [6,7,18]. Biliary atresia in both subtypes appears to involve an ongoing inflammatory process that produces complete or partial sclerosis of extrahepatic bile ducts and progression to cirrhosis [17,19]; whether the lesion noted in intrahepatic bile ducts results from an extension of the extrahepatic lesion or is a consequence of cholestasis is not defined. It is believed that ductal plate malformation and segmental agenesis of bile ducts in porta hepatis specimens are identified more commonly in the fetal form, but this has not been studied systematically.

There is no proven difference in histologic features of the liver between infants with and without congenital anomalies.

Table 12.1: Extrahepatic Anomalies Reported in Patients with Biliary Atresia

Splenic anomalies
Polysplenia
Double spleen
Asplenia
Portal vein anomalies
Preduodenal
Absence
Cavernomatous transformation
Situs inversus
Malrotation
Cardiac anomalies
Annular pancreas
Immotile cilia syndrome (Kartagener's syndrome)
Duodenal atresia
Esophageal atresia
Renal anomalies (polycystic kidney, etc.)
Cleft palate
Jejunal atresia

Modified from Davenport et al. [17], with permission.

Clinical Features

Despite the postulated variant cause and pathogenesis, there is consistency in the clinical features of biliary atresia: affected infants present with jaundice (conjugated hyperbilirubinemia) and acholic stools; the presence of hepatomegaly, failure to thrive, pruritus, and coagulopathy depends on the level of progression of disease. Affected infants usually are born at term and are of normal birth weight; weight gain is appropriate early in the course. Patients with biliary atresia occasionally present with bleeding as a result of vitamin K deficiency. Examination may reveal hepatomegaly and splenomegaly. Ascites and wasting may be seen as late manifestations if biliary cirrhosis has supervened. At present, an increased awareness to ensure early diagnosis and development of methods to prevent progressive hepatic fibrosis are needed. Early recognition of babies who have biliary atresia is especially critical for optimal intervention; ideally, biliary atresia should be identified by the time of the first well-baby visit after discharge from the hospital. The importance of a prompt and precise diagnosis must be stressed to all pediatric health care providers. In the United Kingdom, an educational effort (the Yellow Alert campaign) was established to indicate the significance of jaundice persisting after 14 days of age. Population screening also has been considered [20,21]. The ultimate goals are to define the pathogenesis of biliary atresia and establish preventive strategies.

Cause and Pathogenesis of Biliary Atresia

Although our understanding of the cause and pathogenesis of biliary atresia has remained unchanged for several decades, there is now increasing interest with resultant studies investigating mechanisms of this disease. Theoretic considerations of the cause of biliary atresia have been based on epidemiologic and clinical features. Two critical clinical features offer potential clues about chief biologic processes. The first is the onset of disease restricted to the perinatal or immediate postnatal period (<4 months). The second is inflammation and fibrosis of the extrahepatic bile ducts. In the "typical" patient, the structural changes present in the hepatobiliary tract suggest a progression of the lesion from acute cholangitis to fibrotic obliteration of the ducts (Figure 12.1). The dynamic nature of the obliterative process is illustrated by the fact that atresia has been found at autopsy or reexploration in infants previously shown to have patent extrahepatic ducts or "neonatal hepatitis" [6,12,13].

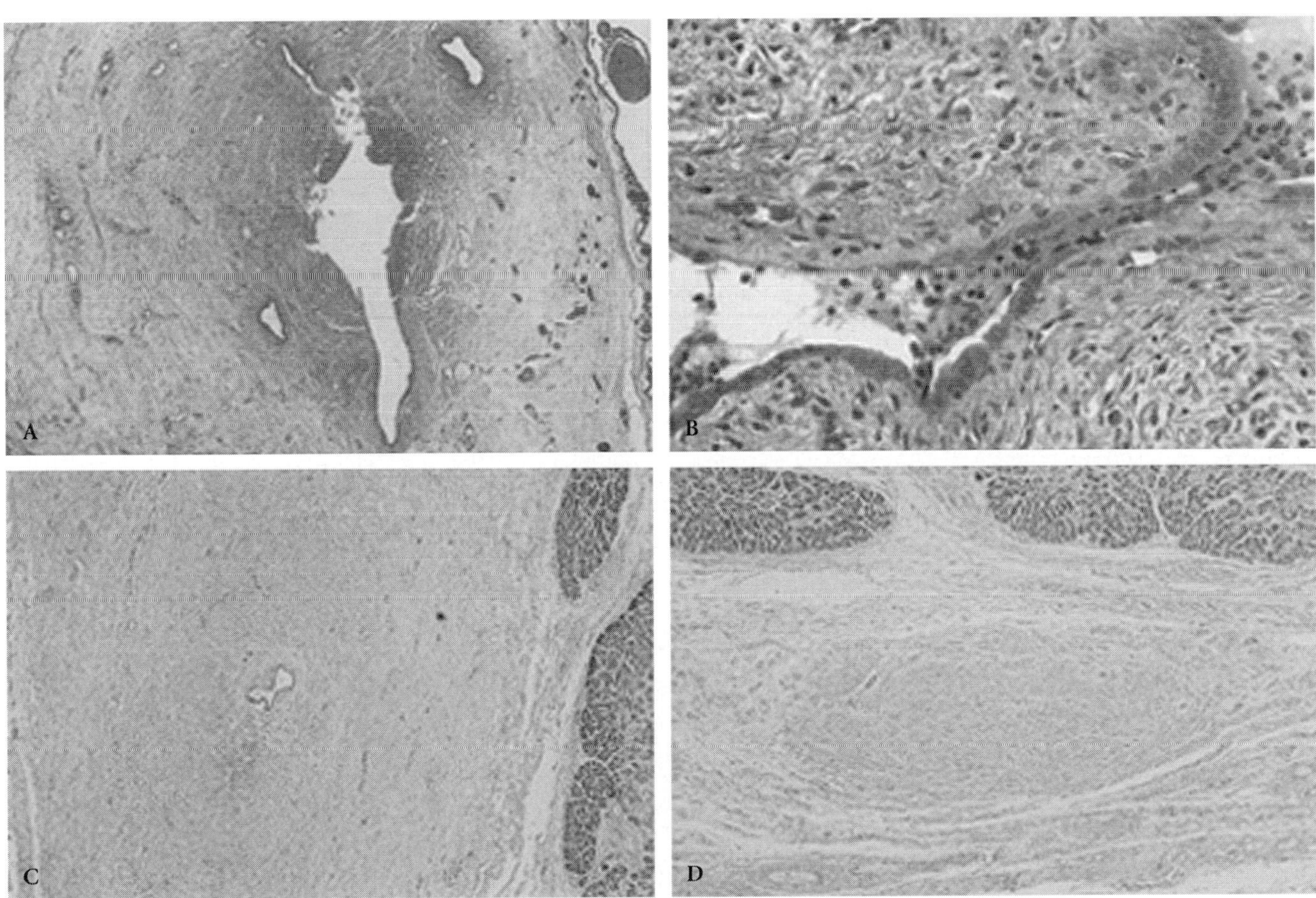

Figure 12.1. Stages of biliary atresia. (**A**) Patent bile duct in a specimen from porta hepatis exhibits periductal inflammation and epithelial erosion; elsewhere in this case, the duct was obliterated by reactive tissue. (**B**) Detail of eroded bile duct shows regressive epithelial change, periductal edema, and mild inflammation. (**C**) At the autopsy of a patient with biliary atresia, a minute remnant of common bile duct has intact epithelium. (**D**) Minute fibrous cord represents the final stage of biliary atresia. In many patients, the atretic duct is not visible to the naked eye. (Hematoxylin and eosin [H&E] staining; [**A**] 37×, [**B**] 250×, and [**C** and **D**] 100× magnification.)

Multiple studies have focused on normal and altered bile duct morphogenesis and the role of various factors (infectious or toxic agents and metabolic insults) in isolation or in combination with a genetic or immunologic susceptibility to biliary atresia [6]. Biliary atresia is not thought to be inherited in the majority of patients. The absence of documented recurrence in siblings of infants with biliary atresia and reports of dizygotic and monozygotic twins discordant for biliary atresia appears to exclude simple Mendelian genetic causes [22–24]. The concept that an acquired obliterative process underlies biliary atresia is attractive and suggests that a virus-related inflammation may initiate the sequence that leads to fibrosis and luminal obstruction [1,19,25,26]. In support of this concept, giant multinucleate hepatocytes have been noted in up to 40% of liver biopsy samples obtained early from patients with biliary atresia [6].

Viral Infection

A favored theory implicates occult viral infection as the inciting mechanism [15,27–34]. The demonstration of significant seasonal clustering provides support for the theory that biliary atresia may be caused by environmental exposure (consistent with a viral cause) during the perinatal period [15]. Multiple potential etiopathogenic viruses have been ruled out as "suspects." Hepatitis A, B, and C virus infections are not related to biliary atresia [6], and there was no apparent increase in the incidence of biliary atresia during rubella epidemics. Cytomegalovirus (CMV), which characteristically infects the biliary epithelium, has been suggested as a cause of biliary atresia [34–37]. For example, a Swedish study showed a higher prevalence of CMV antibodies in mothers of infants with biliary atresia, and CMV DNA was present in livers from 9 of 18 infants with biliary atresia [37]. An important role for CMV in the pathogenesis of biliary atresia, however, seems unlikely because examination of porta hepatis specimens by in situ hybridization and polymerase chain reaction (PCR) using CMV DNA probes was negative [36]. Drut et al. [38] reported a high prevalence of human papillomavirus DNA in archived liver tissue of 16 of 18 Argentinean children with biliary atresia compared with none of 30 controls or age-matched autopsy specimens from patients without liver disease. Human papillomavirus DNA also was detected in cervical swabs from mothers of four patients with biliary atresia, and the types of papillomavirus were concordant between infants and mothers. There is no animal model, however, demonstrating the consequences of human papillomavirus infection in an immature liver, nor have these findings been confirmed elsewhere. Mason et al. [39] detected retroviral antibody reactivity in patients with biliary atresia attributable either to an autoimmune response to antigenically related cellular proteins or to an immune response to uncharacterized viral proteins that share antigenic determinants with these retroviruses. Further studies are needed.

The viral agents most frequently implicated in the pathogenesis of biliary atresia include reovirus and rotavirus. Morecki et al. [27,28] found evidence for serologic reactivity to reovirus type 3 in several children with biliary atresia [27] and for localization of reovirus particles in the porta hepatis of one infant [28]. It had been known for some time that this virus could cause an obliterative cholangiopathy in weanling mice; a similarity exists between the hepatitis with biliary tract inflammation induced by reovirus type 3 infection in this weanling mouse model and the progressive postnatal fibrotic obliteration of the extrahepatic bile ducts and liver cell injury noted in biliary atresia [27–29]. Reovirus type 3 infection therefore has been implicated as the initial insult in the sequence of events resulting in the observed lesions [7,18,27–29,40]. Murine reovirus infection may lead to necrosis of bile duct epithelium and hepatocytes, inflammatory infiltration, and possibly identifiable viral inclusions in bile duct epithelial cells [29,40]. Pathologic changes in reovirus-infected mice, including distal stenosis of the common bile duct and dilation of the proximal bile duct, remain after infectious virus or viral antigens can no longer be detected [41]. Previous attempts to show an association between reoviruses and human hepatobiliary disease have yielded conflicting results. Spontaneous biliary atresia was documented in a nonhuman primate; sequential serum samples showed persistently high reovirus type 3 titers [42]. A disease resembling human biliary atresia was reported in an infant monkey after natural reovirus infection [42]. Reoviruses have not been isolated from human hepatobiliary tissue, but reovirus antigen was detected in the bile duct remnant resected from an infant with biliary atresia, and reovirus-like virion particles were seen in this tissue by electron microscopy [27,28]. This case remains unique, however, because reovirus antigen could not be detected in any specimens of extrahepatic biliary tissue removed at the time of portoenterostomy in another series of eight patients with biliary atresia [43]. Two studies have examined hepatobiliary tissues from infants with biliary atresia for evidence of reovirus infection. Steele et al. [44] failed to detect reovirus RNA in preserved tissues using nested reverse transcription PCR. Tyler et al. [41], however, subsequently reported finding PCR evidence of reovirus infection in fresh frozen liver or bile duct tissue from 11 of 20 patients with the perinatal form of biliary atresia, in 0 of 3 patients with the fetal form, and in only 8–15% of autopsy control or other liver disease control subjects younger than 1 year. The discrepancies between these two studies may lie in the methods of preparation of the tissue (frozen vs. archived fixed tissue), different methods of RNA isolation, and the use of probes for different genes. A recent study of reovirus type 3 infection in the immediate postnatal period did not show extrahepatic obstruction [45].

Riepenhoff-Talty et al. [30] have reported the development of extrahepatic biliary obstruction in newborn mice orally inoculated with group A rotavirus. These investigators also have presented evidence for PCR amplification of group C rotavirus sequences from livers of patients with biliary atresia, for immunoreactivity to group C rotavirus in serum of patients with biliary atresia, and for group C rotavirus particles in the stool of patients with biliary atresia [31]. Additional studies in newborn mice have clearly shown the lesion to reside in the biliary epithelium; the obstructive phenotype is present only when rotavirus infection occurs in the first few days of life [46–48]. In one study, prophylactic treatment with interferon prevented biliary atresia induced by rotavirus in susceptible newborn mice, which also supports a viral etiology [32]. This model of rotavirus-induced biliary injury may offer a unique opportunity to study the mechanisms of biliary atresia because it recapitulates two consistent clinical features of the disease in humans: the onset of disease in the immediate neonatal period and the progressive cholangiopathy.

Additional studies are needed to further investigate a relationship between reovirus, rotavirus, or any other virus in the pathogenesis of biliary atresia [33,34]. Investigation into the contribution of virus-initiated immune or autoimmune mechanisms of hepatobiliary injury in these disorders may yield information essential for development of treatment or prevention strategies. It is unlikely, however, that antiviral therapy alone would alter the natural history of biliary atresia if the pathologic process is an immunologic reaction to a preceding viral injury, without ongoing viral replication [6,41].

Defect in Morphogenesis

The hypothesis that a defect in morphogenesis of the biliary tract is a mechanism for the pathogenesis of biliary atresia is appealing [6], especially considering the coexistence of other anomalies, particularly anomalies of visceral organ symmetry (Table 12.1), that occur in 10–30% of infants with biliary atresia. Tan et al. [49] compared the developing biliary system of normal human embryos and fetuses with the resected extrahepatic biliary remnants from 205 patients with biliary atresia. At the porta hepatis level, the primary biliary ductal plate underwent a specific sequence of remodeling between 11 and 13 weeks after fertilization, resulting in the formation of large tubular bile ducts surrounded by thick mesenchyme. Luminal continuity with the extrahepatic biliary tree was maintained throughout gestation. Contrary to previous speculation, no "solid phase" was documented during the development of the extrahepatic bile duct. Examination of the biliary remnants in biliary atresia showed that the porta hepatis was encased in fibrous tissue, with a variable pattern of obliteration of the common hepatic and common bile ducts. There were similarities on anticytokeratin immunostaining between the abnormal ductules within the porta hepatis in biliary atresia and the normal developing bile ducts during the first trimester. The investigators proposed that biliary atresia may be caused by failure of the remodeling process at the hepatic hilum, with persistence of fetal bile ducts poorly supported by mesenchyme [49]. They further postulated that, as bile flow increases perinatally, bile leakage from these abnormal ducts may trigger an intense inflammatory reaction, with subsequent obliteration of the biliary tree. Alternatively, an underlying infectious or immune injury could interfere with the normal remodeling process at the hepatic hilum and with ductal plates within the liver.

Anomalies of visceral organ symmetry, including complete abdominal situs inversus, severe jaundice, and death within the first week of life, have been reported in transgenic mice that have a recessive insertional mutation (*inv*) in the proximal region of mouse chromosome 4 and deletion of the inversin gene [50,51]. Presumably, the gene mutated in this *inv* mouse ordinarily directs a critical phase in the morphogenetic program for establishing visceral symmetry and for early development of the extrahepatic biliary tree. Mazziotti et al. [51] further examined the pathogenesis of jaundice in this *inv* mouse. Cholestasis with conjugated hyperbilirubinemia, failure to excrete solute from the liver into the small intestine, and lack of continuity between the extrahepatic biliary tree and the small intestine were demonstrated by trypan blue cholangiography. Hepatic histology was indicative of extrahepatic biliary obstruction with negligible inflammation and necrosis within the hepatic parenchyma. Lectin histochemical staining of biliary epithelial cells in serial sections suggested the presence of several different anomalies in the architecture of the extrahepatic biliary system. These results suggest that the inversin gene plays an essential role in the morphogenesis of the hepatobiliary system. The degree to which this gene may participate in the pathogenesis of biliary atresia remains to be determined in view of the inability to detect abnormalities of the inversin gene in children with laterality defects and biliary atresia [52].

An interesting series of observations clarified the morphogenesis and differentiation of the intrahepatic bile ducts [2,53]. Using human liver from different stages of fetal development and immunostaining with anticytokeratin antibodies specific for bile duct epithelial cells, it was shown that bile ducts arise within the mesenchyme surrounding portal vein radicals. Presumed primitive hepatic precursor cells differentiate into a single layer of cytokeratin-staining cells and then form a double layer. At focal points, these cells then scatter and remodel as a single layer around a lumen. In livers from some infants with biliary atresia, there was evidence for an arrest in remodeling such that lumens are not formed (ductal plate malformation) [2,53]. The *c-met* oncogene was suggested to play a potential role in mediating differentiation of mesenchymal tissue into epithelial cells, scattering and remodeling these epithelial cells in a manner that results in formation of a lumen [6,54]. However, no biliary abnormality was reported in mice with targeted inactivation of the receptor [55,56]. In contrast, abnormalities in the biliary tract have been reported in mice with genetic mutations in *Hes1*, *Hnf6*, *Hnf1b*, and *Foxm1b*, and raise questions about the potential role of these genes as susceptibility factors or modifiers of disease in humans [57–61].

Disordered Immunologic Mechanisms

An abnormality in the immune or inflammatory response in patients with biliary atresia has been proposed. Biliary atresia may be the result of a "multiple hit" phenomenon [62]. The theory holds that a viral or toxic insult to the biliary epithelium leads to newly expressed antigens on the surface of bile duct epithelia, which in the proper genetically determined immunologic milieu (e.g., major histocompatibility molecules) are recognized by circulating T lymphocytes that elicit a cellular immune injury, resulting in inflammation and fibrosis of the bile duct [62]. In support of this notion, Silveira et al. [63] reported an association of the human leukocyte antigen (HLA)-B12 allele and haplotypes A9-B5 and A28-B35 with biliary atresia. The increase in HLA-B12 was most evident in infants with biliary atresia who did not have other associated congenital anomalies, making an immune mechanism plausible. Jurado et al. [64], however, could not replicate these findings. Another study suggested a relationship to HLA-Cw4/7 and associations with A33, B44, and DR6 [65]. There has not been a consistent segregation of HLA type in biliary atresia patients from different areas of the world, possibly because of ethnic differences.

Also consistent with an immune mechanism in the pathogenesis of biliary atresia was the finding of aberrant expression of HLA-DR [65–67] and immune cell adhesion molecule 1 (ICAM-1) [66] in biliary epithelia of liver biopsy specimens from patients with biliary atresia, but not from the tissue of patients with other forms of cholestatic disease or from normal liver. The report of *TNF2* gene polymorphisms associated with primary sclerosing cholangitis (PSC) raises the possibility of another potential immunologic genetic predisposition to biliary injury, which should be investigated in patients with biliary atresia [68].

Histologic and immunostaining analyses of the liver and extrahepatic remnants suggest that lymphocytes and Kupffer cells may play key roles in the regulation of inflammation and destruction of bile ducts in infants with biliary atresia. For example, lymphocytes have been associated with epithelial cell pyknoses within intrahepatic portal tracts, porta hepatis, and common bile duct remnants [69–71]. The expression of CD8+ and CD4+ markers and the expression of interleukin-2 receptor, tumor necrosis factor-α, and interferon gamma in portal tracts of livers from patients with biliary atresia are in keeping with the existence of a proinflammatory circuit within the hepatic environment [9,65,72–74]. This has been further validated in a large-scale gene expression study, which revealed a profile of differential lymphocyte activation, with an increased expression of cytokines at the time of diagnosis when compared with age-matched infants with intrahepatic cholestasis [9]. Among the cytokines, interferon gamma emerged as a key soluble factor controlling the inflammatory obstruction of the neonatal extrahepatic bile duct in the mouse model of rotavirus-induced experimental biliary atresia [75]. Using this model, the loss of interferon gamma completely prevented duct obstruction and increased long-term survival. Future studies are necessary to determine whether inactivation of interferon gamma may constitute a therapeutic tool to halt disease progression in children with biliary atresia.

Environmental Toxic Exposure

Despite the apparent existence of time–space clustering of cases of biliary atresia, there is no conclusive evidence of a link between maternal drug ingestion or environmental exposure and the subsequent development of biliary atresia in the newborn.

Vascular Abnormalities

Developmental abnormalities in the position of the portal vein and in hepatic artery anatomy at the porta hepatis are common in patients with biliary atresia. There are no consistent experimental data, however, to confirm the hypothesis that a vascular basis, such as ischemia, is a cause of the progressive duct injury seen in biliary atresia [76]. In utero devascularization or ligation of the extrahepatic bile duct has been attempted in some animal models, and lesions similar to the less common "correctable" variants of biliary atresia have been produced [77]; however, other studies have been inconclusive [78].

Table 12.2: Evaluation of Infants with Cholestasis

General evaluation

1. Clinical evaluation (family and gestational history, feeding history, physical examination, assessment of stool color)
2. Index of hepatic synthetic function (prothrombin time)
3. Cultures (blood, urine, spinal fluid) as indicated
4. Determination of serum bile acid levels (followed by *qualitative analysis* of urinary bile acid profile if abnormal)
5. γ-Glutamyl transpeptidase
6. Serum electrolytes (to exclude acidosis)

Specific evaluation (to exclude or confirm a specific diagnosis)

1. α-Antitrypsin phenotype
2. Thyroxine and thyroid-stimulating hormone
3. Sweat chloride–mutational analysis (to exclude cystic fibrosis)
4. Ferritin–transferrin concentration and saturation (to exclude neonatal iron storage disease)
5. Metabolic screen (urine-reducing substances, urine/serum amino acids, organic acids, succinyl acetone)
6. Hepatitis B surface antigen, anti-HIV, and Venereal Disease Research Laboratory (VDRL) titers (in selected, high-risk patients)
7. Abdominal ultrasonography
8. Hepatobiliary *scintigraphy* or duodenal intubation for bilirubin content
9. Liver biopsy

Diagnosis of Biliary Atresia

Various laboratory tests, imaging methods, and biopsy samples have been utilized in attempts to establish the diagnosis of biliary atresia, particularly in differentiating it from various forms of intrahepatic cholestasis (idiopathic neonatal hepatitis) [6]. In our experience, the most reliable information is obtained by review of hepatic histopathology followed by direct visualization of obliterated extrahepatic bile ducts (intraoperative cholangiography). Percutaneous liver biopsy has a diagnostic accuracy of 95% if a sample of adequate size, containing five to seven portal spaces, is obtained and carefully interpreted.

Evaluation

Our approach to the work-up of an infant with cholestasis is shown in Table 12.2. We recommend the following sequential approach: (1) Prompt recognition of cholestasis is essential. Jaundice in an infant must not be attributed erroneously to physiologic hyperbilirubinemia or to breast-feeding; fractionation of the serum bilirubin usually separates out these conditions, which cause a predominant elevation (>80%) of unconjugated bilirubin levels. In addition, the serum bile acid concentration in blood obtained during the first 10 days of life is elevated significantly in infants with cholestasis [20]; this may offer a potential screening method. (2) Procedures should be expeditiously performed to rule out potentially devastating illnesses such as sepsis, endocrine disorders, and nutritional hepatotoxicity attributable to metabolic disease (e.g., galactosemia). Definitive detection is usually straightforward, and institution of appropriate treatment may prevent further liver injury. Early recognition of specific, treatable primary causes of neonatal cholestasis then is attempted. Early in the evaluation of any infant with cholestasis, other clinical issues need to be addressed. Hypoprothrombinemia may be present regardless of the cause of cholestasis; administration of vitamin K may prevent spontaneous, life-threatening bleeding, such as intracranial hemorrhage. (3) "Idiopathic" neonatal hepatitis must be differentiated from biliary atresia because the prognosis and management differ significantly. In infants with biliary atresia, progressive fibrosis rapidly occurs; therefore, significant delay in diagnosis or treatment must be avoided.

No single test is entirely satisfactory in discriminating neonatal hepatitis (intrahepatic cholestasis) from biliary atresia; however, historical and clinical features may aid in the differential diagnosis. Neonatal hepatitis is reported to have a familial incidence of 15–20%; the intrafamilial recurrence risk is negligible for biliary atresia [8,79–81]. Infants with biliary atresia may look well, become clinically jaundiced at 3–6 weeks of age, and have slowly progressive elevation of serum bilirubin levels but seldom have pruritus or skin xanthoma. The liver is enlarged and firm; splenomegaly occurs as cirrhosis develops. Stools are acholic at presentation, but early in the course, during the evolving process of bile duct obliteration, they may contain some bile pigment. Acholic stools, an important clue to the presence of biliary atresia, are either intermittent or delayed in onset in one fourth of patients and are present in some patients with neonatal hepatitis. The consistent presence of pigmented stools rules out biliary atresia; however, acholic stools may be intermittent in evolving cases.

Duodenal fluid may be obtained to assess the bilirubin content; if bile-stained fluid is collected, biliary atresia is excluded [7,18,79]. Hepatobiliary scintigraphy using iminodiacetic acid analogues has been used to provide discriminatory data [82]. In biliary atresia, hepatocyte function is intact early in the disease; therefore, uptake of the imaging agent is unimpaired, but excretion into the intestine is absent [83,84]. Conversely, in neonatal hepatitis, tracer uptake is sluggish or impaired but excretion into the bile and intestine eventually occurs. Oral administration of phenobarbital, 5 mg/kg/d, for 5 days before the study may enhance biliary excretion of the isotope and therefore the sensitivity of the procedure [7,18,83]. Techniques that are used extensively in evaluation of adults with cholestatic disease, such as percutaneous transhepatic and endoscopic retrograde cholangiography, are not of proven value in children [85]. The role of magnetic resonance cholangiography is undefined [86–88]. Ultrasonography may detect dilation of the biliary tract, the presence of a choledochal cyst, or, in patients with biliary atresia, absence of the gallbladder. Choi et al. [89] identified a sonographic finding known as a *triangular cord*, a fibrous cone of tissue at the bifurcation of the portal vein, in nine patients, all of whom had evidence of biliary atresia on biopsy and intraoperatively [89]. All but one of the patients without a triangular cord had neonatal hepatitis seen in biopsy samples.

Numerous diagnostic algorithms incorporating these features have been proposed in an attempt to select those infants who are surgical candidates and to avoid unnecessary surgery. Discriminatory analysis of clinical, biochemical, and histologic data obtained from 288 infants younger than 3 months presenting with neonatal cholestasis allowed for an accurate differentiation in 85% of the patients studied [90]. In infants with intrahepatic disease, the following features occurred significantly more frequently than in infants with biliary atresia: male gender, low birth weight, later onset of jaundice (mean of 23 vs. 11 days of age), later onset of acholic stools (mean of 30 vs. 16 days), and pigmented stools within 10 days after admission (79% vs. 26%). Patients with biliary atresia more frequently had hepatomegaly, and the liver usually had a firm or hard consistency [90]. Despite the use of scoring systems such as this, about 10% of infants with intrahepatic disease (neonatal hepatitis) cannot be distinguished from those with biliary atresia [12,91]. Unnecessary explorations are, of course, to be avoided; however, delay in establishing a diagnosis also is unwarranted because the data suggest that the success rate for surgical management of patients with biliary atresia rapidly declines with age [11–13,92–94].

Role of Liver Biopsy

In our experience, clinical examination, careful and repeated examination of the stool, and needle biopsy of the liver correctly identify a large majority of patients with biliary atresia. In most patients, biopsy can be performed safely using the Menghini technique of percutaneous aspiration with local anesthesia [7,18,95]. An accurate, biopsy-based diagnosis is possible in up to 95% of patients and avoids unnecessary surgery in patients with intrahepatic disease. Early in the progression of biliary atresia, the liver shows preservation of the basic hepatic architecture, with bile ductular proliferation, canalicular and cellular bile stasis, and portal or perilobular edema and fibrosis (Figure 12.2). Bile plugs in the portal ducts are relatively specific but are found in only 40% of biopsy specimens. Portal fibrosis with wide swaths of connective tissue extending into the liver substance develops in older infants but may be established as early as 3 months after birth. Approximately 25–40% of infants have portal inflammatory infiltration and hepatocyte giant cell transformation indistinguishable from neonatal hepatitis. These portal tract findings contrast with those of neonatal hepatitis, in which variable, often severe intralobular cholestasis may be accompanied by focal hepatocellular necrosis

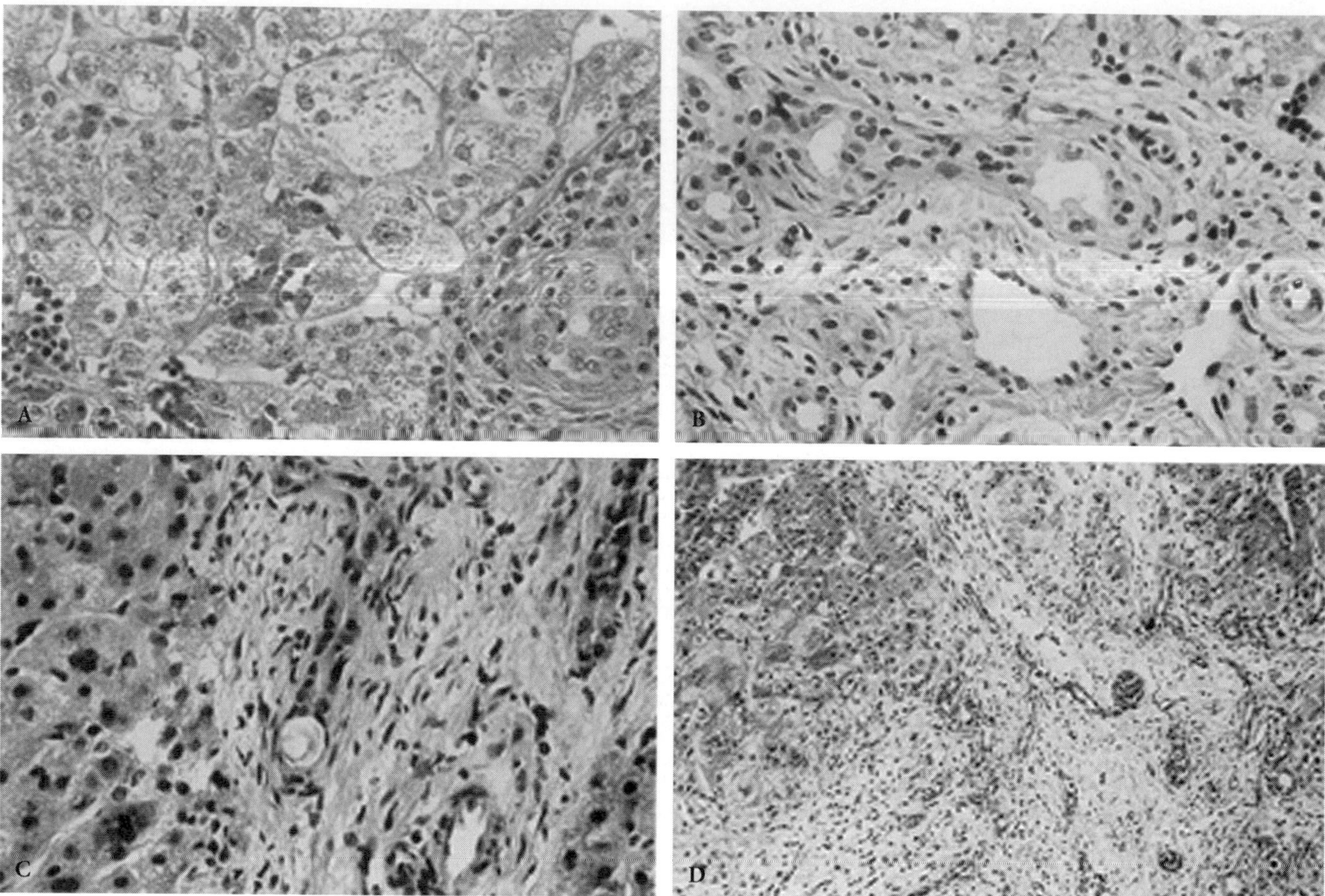

Figure 12.2. Intrahepatic changes in biliary atresia. (**A**) Giant cell transformation of hepatocytes, sinusoidal erythropoiesis, and slight bile duct proliferation may overlap with neonatal hepatitis. (**B** and **C**) Histologic changes that are diagnostic of biliary obstruction include unequivocal proliferation of interlobular bile ducts, portal stromal edema, and bile concretions in ducts. (**D**) Advanced changes in this liver biopsy specimen suggest transition to biliary cirrhosis, which is unusual before 3 months after birth. (H&E staining; [**A**, **B**, and **C**] 250× and [**D**] 100× magnification.)

(Figure 12.3). Bile ducts show little or no alteration in neonatal hepatitis. Portal inflammatory infiltrates are present in both conditions and tend to be more prominent in neonatal hepatitis. Portal area stroma is more likely to show edema in patients with biliary atresia. In the series of Alagille [90], bile ductular proliferation was present in only 30% of the patients with neonatal hepatitis compared with 86% of those with biliary atresia. Giant cell transformation and extramedullary hematopoiesis, especially sinusoidal erythropoiesis, are found in a high percentage of infants with either condition and have no diagnostic specificity. In very young infants, the initial biopsy may be inconclusive; rebiopsy after 7–14 days may resolve the issue.

Zerbini et al. [96] assessed a scoring system to improve the accuracy of the histopathologic diagnosis in the differential diagnosis between obstructive and nonobstructive forms of neonatal cholestasis. The accuracy, sensitivity, and specificity rates were all 94%. The model then was applied to a new sample of 74 needle liver biopsy specimens. The accuracy, sensitivity, and specificity rates were 91%, 100%, and 76%, respectively. This suggests that if extrahepatic obstruction cannot be ruled out, limited exploration with cholangiography and repeat needle or wedge biopsy of the liver should be performed; if atresia is apparent, the biliary tract can be explored further.

Role of Surgical Exploration

When the suspicion of biliary obstruction has been sufficiently established, operative exploration should be performed to document the presence and the site of obstruction and to direct attempts at surgical drainage [11,13]. Cholangiography and meticulous exploration of the entire biliary tree should be carried out. The decision made at the operating table may be aided by observations of features usually associated with biliary atresia, such as consistency (coarse, fibrotic) and color (green) of the liver, and the presence of subcapsular telangiectasia (early vascular obstruction secondary to fibrosis). The presence of biliary epithelium and the size of residual ducts can be evaluated in frozen sections of the transected porta hepatis.

The approach outlined here is not without pitfalls; caution should be exercised in interpretation of certain studies, especially in very young infants. In four patients reported by Markowitz et al. [97], scintigraphic evidence of biliary atresia was present, and intraoperative cholangiography failed to

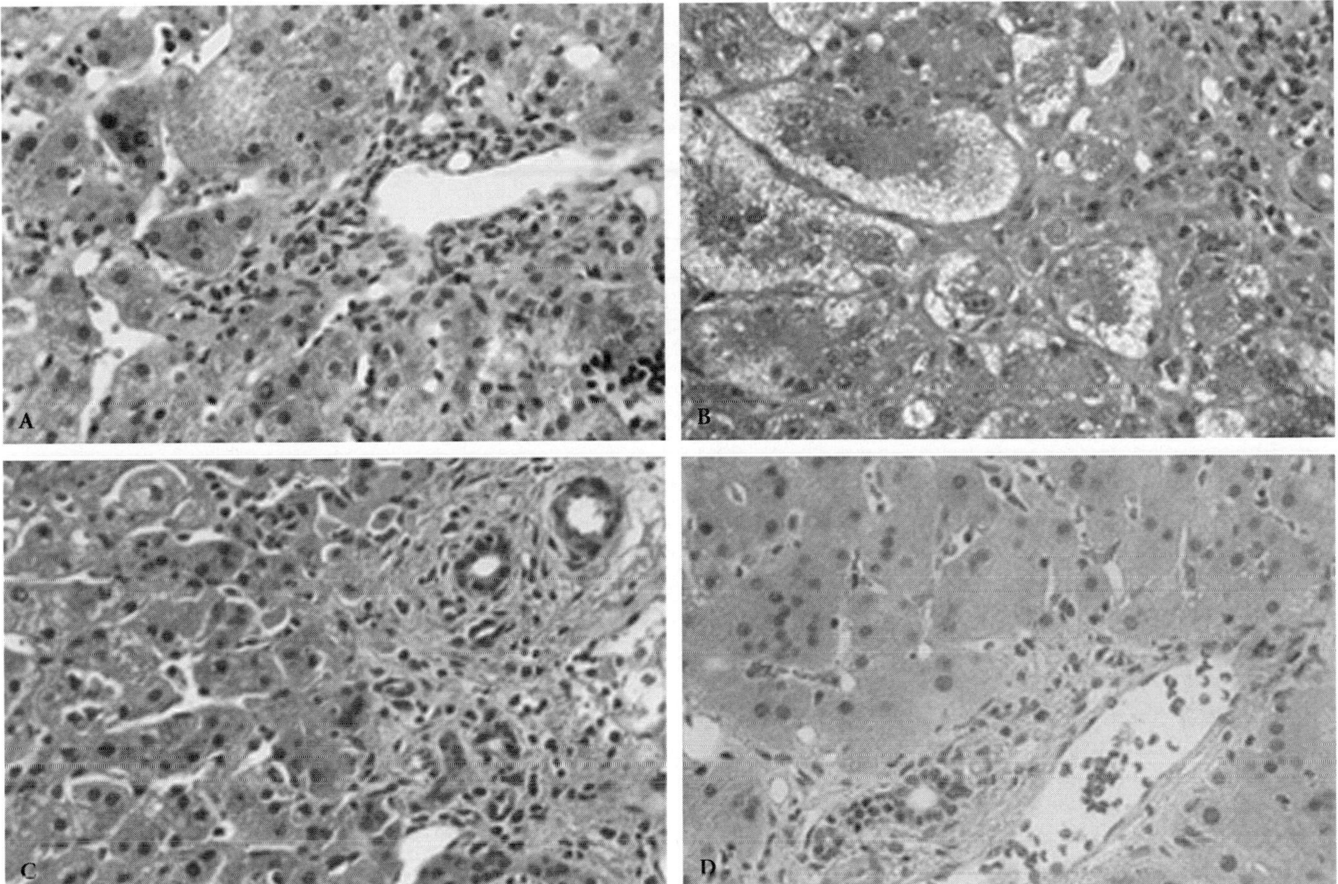

Figure 12.3. Neonatal hepatitis. Inflammation is typically mild. Giant cell transformation is variable in severity and extent in these four examples. Interlobular bile ducts may be inconspicuous (**A**), slightly proliferative (**B**), or normal (**C** and **D**). Pseudotubular metaplasia of zone 1 hepatocytes may occur along fibrotic portal zone margins (**C**). Mild cholestasis and giant cell transformation of hepatocytes (**D**) may linger for months, as in this 3-month-old infant who eventually recovered. (H&E staining, 250× magnification.)

demonstrate any proximal intrahepatic biliary radicals; therefore, hepatoportoenterostomy was performed. There was inadequate postoperative drainage with cholangitis, development of cirrhosis in two, and death from hepatic failure in one infant. Subsequently, a histologic and clinical diagnosis of intrahepatic cholestasis (Alagille syndrome) was made in each of the four patients. The progression of the hepatic disease in these patients demonstrated that portoenterostomy had severely and adversely altered the course of their disease. During cholangiography, an absence of retrograde flow into the proximal intrahepatic ducts does not exclude the presence of a patent, albeit hypoplastic, extrahepatic biliary duct system in a patient with intrahepatic disease. The liver disease in intrahepatic cholestasis syndromes (e.g., Alagille syndrome) is not amenable to surgical correction, and portal dissection should not be attempted.

Management of Biliary Atresia

At present, there is no specific medical therapy for biliary atresia. The first breakthrough in the surgical therapy of patients with biliary atresia occurred in the late 1950s. Kasai and associates [92,98,99], investigating the pathology of the intrahepatic and extrahepatic bile ducts in patients with biliary atresia, showed that over the first 10–12 months of life there was progressive destruction of the intralobular bile ducts, with a gradual diminution of the degree of pseudoductular proliferation of the portal tracts. They also described microscopic bile ducts within the fibrous remnant of the atretic biliary tree at the porta hepatis. This led to the critical observation that if the extrahepatic bile ducts were removed at a time at which there was continuity between the microscopic ducts in the ductal plate at the porta hepatis and the intrahepatic biliary system, the progression of biliary atresia could be arrested. This operation, the *Kasai hepatoportoenterostomy (HPE)*, has become the current standard surgical approach [6,100,101]. As experience has grown, there have been minor though significant technical improvements in the HPE. For example, extension of the dissection beyond the portal vein bifurcation incorporates a larger amount of biliary remnants and improves bile flow [101].

The principles of contemporary surgical management for biliary atresia are based, in part, on the conclusions of the 1983 National Institutes of Health Consensus Conference on Liver Transplantation: (a) HPE should be the primary surgical therapy for biliary atresia; (b) transplantation is appropriate therapy for patients with biliary atresia who fail primary HPE; (c) liver transplantation should be delayed as long as possible to permit maximum growth; (d) transplantation should be deferred until progressive cholestasis, hepatocellular decompensation, or severe portal hypertension supervenes; and (e) multiple attempts to revise an unsuccessful Kasai procedure are not warranted because they can make liver transplantation more difficult and dangerous [102].

Surgical Management

Sequential surgical therapy for biliary atresia is divided into two steps: the establishment of a secure diagnosis, then the construction of the portoenterostomy [11]. The importance of establishing an unequivocal diagnosis before proceeding to HPE cannot be overstated. The initial step in the exploration should both confirm the diagnosis of biliary atresia and exclude other diagnoses not improved by operative intervention, such as various forms of intrahepatic cholestasis. This can be done through direct observation and definition of the distal biliary ductal anatomy using direct cholecystocholangiography. The liver in patients with biliary atresia is firm and shows a cholestatic brown-green discoloration often accompanied by multiple subcapsular telangiectasias. The gallbladder remnant is usually fibrotic but may contain a small amount of clear mucoid secretions. Early in the course of the disease, the hilar structures and the biliary ductal remnant may show a considerable amount of edema. In older children, these structures are fibrotic and more difficult or impossible to identify. If these findings are accompanied by a fibrotic gallbladder, cholangiography is not necessary and biliary atresia is confirmed. If the gallbladder is not obliterated, gentle cholecystocholangiography is undertaken to further define the operative course. Because of the small gallbladder volume and minimal ductal size in infants, the cholangiogram should be visualized from its onset using fluoroscopy to avoid overdistention and extravasation, which preclude successful visualization of ductal structures. If the ductal system is normal or the bile ducts are small but patent, a generous wedge and needle biopsy is obtained; however, biliary reconstruction should be specifically avoided. If flow into the distal biliary tract is seen but no proximal flow is documented, a light spring-loaded vascular occlusion clamp should be placed on the supraduodenal biliary structures before additional attempts to visualize the proximal ductal system. The Kasai HPE should be undertaken if no proximal patency is documented.

Anatomic Variants of Biliary Atresia

The anatomy of the abnormal extrahepatic bile ducts in patients with biliary atresia is variable. The currently accepted classification of anatomic variants of biliary atresia is based on that proposed by the Japanese Society of Pediatric Surgeons, which divides cases into three principal types [100]: *type 1*, atresia of the common bile duct; *type 2*, atresia of the common hepatic duct; and *type 3*, atresia of the right and left hepatic ducts. Further subdivisions include the variable morphology of the gallbladder and the distal common bile duct [100]. Absence of the proximal biliary tree has been termed *biliary agenesis* [103]. "Correctable" lesions – having distal common bile duct atresia but a patent portion of the extrahepatic duct up to the porta hepatis and joining the intrahepatic ducts – allow direct drainage into a Roux-en-Y anastomosis [92,98,99]. The most commonly encountered lesion (seen in 75–85%), however, is obliteration of all of the ducts throughout the porta hepatis, presenting an apparently "noncorrectable" type of atresia. Kasai et al. [99] observed that minute bile duct remnants or residual channels are present in the fibrous tissue within the porta hepatis. These channels are often in continuity with the intrahepatic ductal system and therefore should provide drainage [93,99,104]. If flow is not established rapidly in these ducts, progressive obliteration ensues. Biliary drainage is attempted by excision of the obliterated extrahepatic ducts and apposition of the resected surface of the transected porta hepatis to the bowel mucosa in the Roux-en-Y loop (HPE) – the Kasai procedure [11–13,94,98,100,105]. The unusual patient with "agenesis" in porta hepatis specimens does not respond to Kasai drainage procedures [17,103].

Hepatoportoenterostomy

When the diagnosis of biliary atresia is secure, the second phase of the operative procedure, the Kasai HPE, is begun. The traditional dissection of the portal fibrous mass begins by transecting the distal duct remnant above the duodenal margin, mobilizing the gallbladder remnant from its hepatic bed, and dissecting this fibrous remnant from the anterior portal vein wall. It is important to emphasize that in biliary atresia, the bile ducts are not absent but rather replaced by fibrous tissue. The anatomic course of the ductal remnants follows the normal biliary position within the portal triad to reach the liver hilum. As emphasized by Ohi et al. [100,104], the fibrous remnant then proceeds posteriorly and passes superior to but within the bifurcation of the portal vein to reach the capsular surface of the liver. Individual small portal vein branches passing directly into the fibrous mass must be divided. This allows downward displacement of the portal vein bifurcation, which facilitates full dissection of the fibrous triangular mass before its transection at the level of the liver capsule (Figure 12.4).

In the original Kasai HPE, the fibrous triangle was dissected and divided between the right and left branches of the portal vein at the level of the posterior surface of the portal vein. Further revision of this technique has shown that meticulous dissection of the lateral fibrous triangle tissues allows more of the segmental biliary structures to be included in the divided hilar tissue. On the right, the dissection is carried to the dorsal aspect of the anterior portal branch and over the bifurcation of the anterior and posterior portal vein branches. The left portal vein is also dissected to the umbilical point, which often requires division of the parenchymal bridge surrounding the round ligament between segments 3 and 4 of the liver [106–108]. The fibrous remnant tissue is divided sharply along a plane parallel to and at the level of the hepatic capsule. Deeper dissections into the hepatic parenchyma have not led to improved results [109]. Hemostasis at the transected remnant is achieved

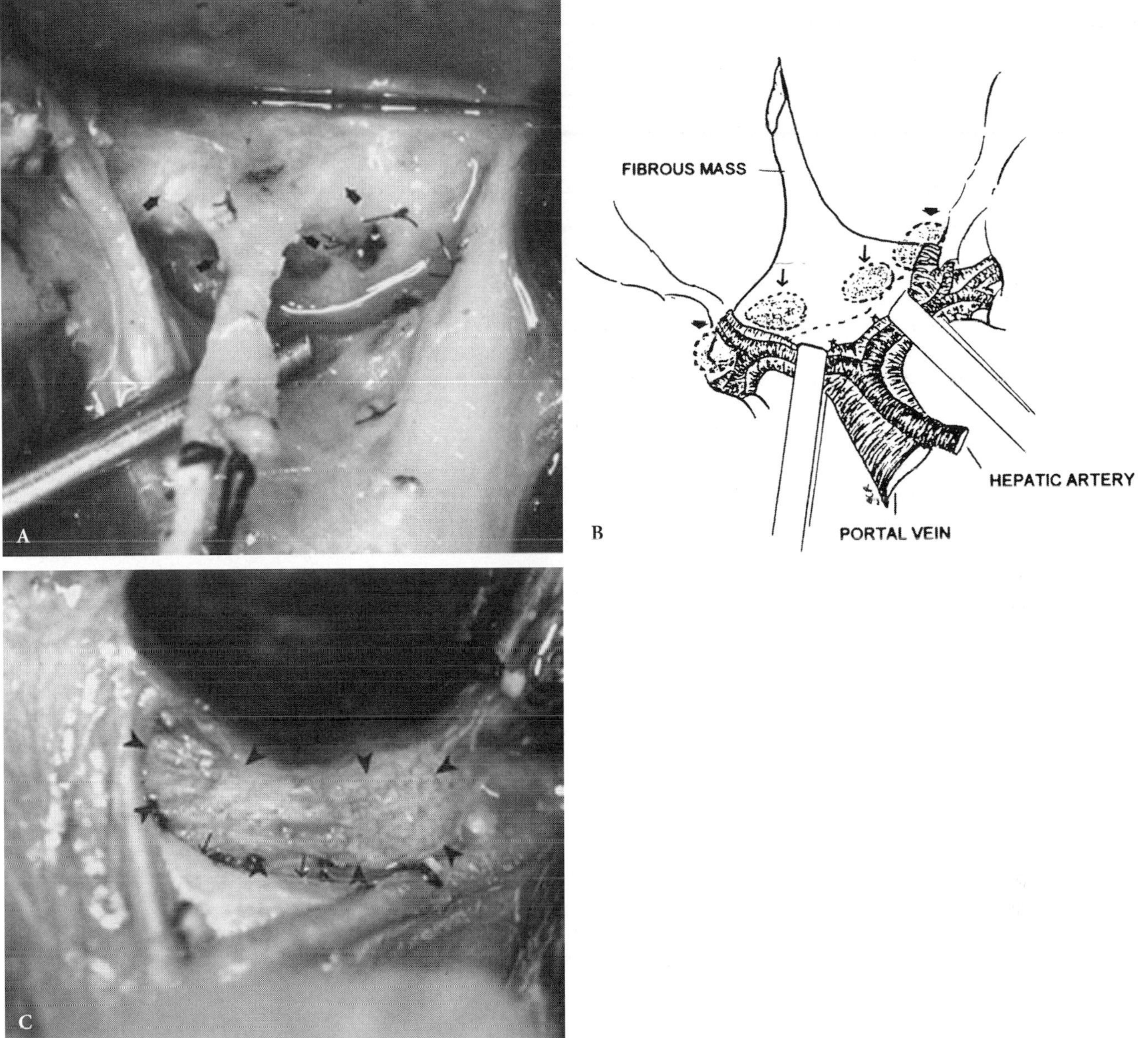

Figure 12.4. The Kasai hepatoportoenterostomy. (**A**) Division site. Fibrous triangle (*arrows*) dissected superior to the bifurcation of the portal vein before division. The portal vein must be retracted inferiorly to visualize the posterior surface of the fibrous mass and the liver capsule. (**B**) Kasai procedure. Schematic representation of fibrous triangular mass before its division and the location (stippled areas) of the primary biliary remnants within the classic dissection limits (*small arrows*) and within the extended dissection areas (*broad arrows*). (**C**) Completed hilar dissection. The fibrous mass is divided parallel and at the level of the liver capsule within the bifurcation of the portal vein (*small arrows*). (Divided fibrous mass margins outlined with *arrowheads*).

by warm irrigation and direct pressure. Suture ligation and electrocautery are discouraged because they may damage the small ductal remnants critical for success. Roux-en-Y drainage using a 35- to 40-cm isoperistaltic retrocolic jejunal limb is preferred because this limb may be used for later transplantation if necessary. This limb should be fashioned from the most proximal portion of the jejunum, allowing bile to return to the proximal intestine, improving nutrient and medication absorption. The Roux-en-Y hilar anastomosis should be undertaken using absorbable monofilament suture material to avoid the presence of a nidus for later infection. This suture margin is placed just outside of the divided hilar tissue margin to avoid transfixing any ductal remnants. The anastomotic suture line should surround or invaginate the vascular branches, incorporating all the fibrous tissue within the lumen. This technique excludes the portal vein wall from the cut surface and inhibits its attachment to and scarring of the potential ductal drainage area. Antireflux valves are not recommended, but the anastomosis is fashioned to inhibit enteric flow into the drainage limb.

In patients in whom cholangiography indicates distal patency of the common bile duct with good luminal caliber and proximal biliary ductal atresia, a hepatic portocholecystostomy (*gallbladder Kasai*) procedure is an alternative to conventional HPE. In this procedure, the gallbladder is mobilized from its hepatic fossa, protecting the cystic arterial supply. The distal gallbladder is transected, and an opening is sutured to the biliary hilum, replacing the Roux-en-Y drainage limb. In these patients, drainage through the distal biliary structure and intact sphincter of Oddi virtually eliminates ascending cholangitis in the postoperative period, so long as the distal biliary structures are large enough to accommodate normal bile flow [94].

Prognosis

A proportion of patients with biliary atresia derives long-term benefit from HPE [6,11–13,16,98,99,105,110–115]. In most patients, however, variable degrees of hepatic dysfunction persist, often because of severe intrahepatic cholangiopathy [13,116–118]. The long-term prognosis is related directly to the establishment of successful bile flow and the disappearance of jaundice, as suggested by a retrospective study showing increased long-term survival with the native liver in children with serum bilirubin less than 1 mg/dL within 3 months of HPE [119]. Ten-year survival rates ranging from 73–92% have been reported for infants in whom jaundice has cleared [6,12,13]. In those patients in whom jaundice remains and bile flow is inadequate, the 3-year survival rate decreases to 20%. Even in patients with transient bile flow whose jaundice does not resolve, some benefit, namely growth to a size sufficient for transplantation, is often achievable.

The variable prognosis after HPE is related to several factors; one of these factors is age at operation. With the Kasai procedure, the timing of the surgery correlates with outcome. In several series, it has been reported that bile flow has been reestablished in more than 80% of infants who were referred for surgery within 60 days after birth [6,13,99,113,116–119]. The success rate drops dramatically, to under 20%, in those older than 90 days at the time of operation. Thus performance of the Kasai procedure after 3 months of age may be justified, but only in selected cases [120,121]. A second factor is size of the ducts visualized in tissue from the porta hepatis. Microscopic patency of more than 150 μmol/L should determine successful postoperative bile flow [122,123], although this concept is not universally recognized. For those patients with smaller or no identifiable epithelial-lined structures in fibrous tissue, the success rate was low [122,123]. Prognosis after portoenterostomy procedures may also be correlated with the degree or proliferation of the periductular glands; the hilar biliary plexus may act as a drainage route for bile in these patients [124]. A third determinant is the experience and operative technique of the surgeon [12,13,98,99,113]. Another factor attracting attention of clinicians and investigators alike is the potential use of corticosteroid as an adjuvant therapy following HPE. Analyses of individual or combined centers' experience have suggested improved bile drainage and survival in infants receiving corticosteroids after HPE [125–129]. The retrospective nature of these studies and the lack of adequate controls limit the validity of the data. These variables can be best addressed by prospective double-blind, placebo-controlled trials that are statistically powered to determine efficacy and carefully monitor for short- and long-term adverse events of corticosteroids in infants with biliary atresia.

The rate of progression of the liver disease may be the overall limiting factor; a nearly universal finding is the presence of a persistent intrahepatic inflammatory process [3,4], which may partially account for the poor results and the development of portal hypertension. The continuing nature of the disease process may be caused by persistence of an infectious agent, an immunologically mediated injury, or the presence of an undefined metabolic aberration. Markers of hepatic fibrogenesis, such as serum hyaluronic acid and procollagen propeptides, may be useful in establishing the prognosis in biliary atresia [130]. Another factor affecting prognosis is prevention of secondary postoperative complications, namely bacterial cholangitis, which is a constant threat and may lead to reobstruction [6,93,110,122,131–133]. Patients who previously had good bile excretion may have repeated episodes of fever, increased jaundice, leukocytosis, and evidence of contamination with intestinal flora. Intrahepatic portal vein thrombosis can aggravate preexisting presinusoidal resistance caused by progressive parenchymal fibrosis, which is the end result of intrahepatic inflammation or recurrent bouts of ascending cholangitis [134]. Hepatic artery resistance index has been measured by Doppler ultrasonography and has been found to predict rapid deterioration and death in children with biliary atresia [135,136]. Intrahepatic biliary cysts have been noted in about 20% of patients with biliary atresia [137]. Episodes of cholangitis may precede discovery of the cysts.

Role of Reoperation Following Hepatoportoenterostomy

Several series have emphasized the potential value of reoperation in patients with cessation of bile flow after initial success or in patients with refractory cholangitis. In many patients, debridement or revision of the scarred area was associated with the reestablishment of bile flow [12,13,93]. Ohi et al. [93] were successful in obtaining bile drainage after reoperation in 13 of 15 patients in whom flow had been initially established but cessation of flow developed. If a patient had poor bile flow initially, reoperation is usually unsuccessful in establishing flow. Reoperation should be limited to infants in whom active bile drainage is achieved after their initial operative procedures, leading to an anicteric state followed by abrupt cessation of bile excretion. These infants should have favorable hepatic histology and biliary ductal remnants at their initial operation. Reconstitution of suitable bile flow following debridement or revision of the scarred hilar area is successful in more than half the patients undergoing reoperation using these highly selective criteria [100,104]. Infants with inadequate or no initial bile flow are poor candidates for reoperation and should not be reexplored [100,138]. Subsequent tertiary reexploration should be limited to patients with established bile drainage with suspected mechanical obstruction originating in the intestinal conduit. The increased intraperitoneal and perihepatic adhesions that complicate subsequent liver transplantation are most often the consequence of repetitive but misdirected attempts to reoperate on poorly selected candidates with a poor prognosis for improvement or recurrent episodes of bacterial peritonitis.

Outcome

Progressive biliary cirrhosis and hepatic failure may occur despite apparent success in achieving bile drainage [6]. Factors that contribute to failure include stenosis of the anastomosis, ascending cholangitis, and progressive loss of intrahepatic bile ducts that may have been injured before the drainage procedure. Liver transplantation is necessary in infants with a failed HPE, manifest by progressive hepatocellular decompensation, jaundice, refractory growth failure with hepatic synthetic dysfunction and the development of a coagulopathy, or intractable portal hypertension with recurrent gastrointestinal hemorrhage or hypersplenism [13,139,140]. Children with biliary atresia have a variable prognosis that has been shown to correlate with total serum bilirubin concentration. In a review of 134 patients with biliary atresia who underwent portoenterostomy between 1973 and 1992, it was noted that 29% had esophageal variceal hemorrhage (EVH) [139]. The risk of death or need for liver transplantation was 50% at 6 years after the initial episode of EVH. Patients with a serum bilirubin concentration of 4 mg/dL or less at the first episode of EVH had a transplant-free survival rate of more than 80% for 4 years after this episode, those with bilirubin levels greater than 4–10 mg/dL had 50% survival at 1 year, and those with bilirubin levels greater than 10 mg/dL had 50% survival at 4 months. Thus, compared with the risk for an age-matched child who did not have EVH, the risk of death or transplant for a child with EVH was 12-fold greater when the total serum bilirubin level was greater than 10 mg/dL, sevenfold when the level was 4–10 mg/dL, and 0.6-fold when the level was 4 mg/dL or less.

The interim medical management of the child with biliary atresia and chronic cholestasis is similar to that prescribed for all patients with chronic cholestasis, with attention devoted to nutritional support [6,141]. Ursodeoxycholic acid therapy (15–20 mg/kg/d divided into two or three doses orally) has been suggested as a means of inducing or improving bile flow, preventing cholangitis, and fostering growth in patients with biliary atresia [6,141,142]. As mentioned previously, controversy exists regarding the effect of corticosteroids on bile flow after Kasai portoenterostomy [143]. Each of these medical approaches needs further study. A late complication of biliary atresia–associated portal hypertension is the hepatopulmonary syndrome (HPS), defined as intrapulmonary vascular dilatation with shunting and arterial desaturation. This syndrome is associated with decreased exercise tolerance and digital clubbing and seems to correlate with the presence of cutaneous spider telangiectasia. HPS may be reversed by liver transplantation [144]; however, patients with HPS are more susceptible to postoperative complications [7,12,18,90,145]. Portopulmonary hypertension (PPHTN), another of the pulmonary vascular disorders complicating chronic liver disease, is defined as pulmonary arterial hypertension associated with severe liver disease or portal hypertension [146]. PPHTN, when left untreated, is fatal; mean survival in adults is 15 months. The criteria for PPHTN include an elevated mean pulmonary arterial pressure (>25 mm Hg at rest), increased pulmonary vascular resistance, and normal pulmonary capillary wedge pressure in the presence of portal hypertension. A recently reported series of children who developed PPHTN demonstrated that clinical symptoms are subtle and thus may be overlooked [146]. Children with portal hypertension who develop a new heart murmur, dyspnea, or syncope or who are being evaluated for liver transplantation require evaluation for PPHTN [146]. Electrocardiography and chest radiography are insensitive screening tests for PPHTN, hence an echocardiogram and cardiology evaluation may be needed to confirm the diagnosis [146].

Although the success rate for biliary enteric anastomosis in patients with biliary atresia cannot be predicted, it remains the most reasonable initial approach [6,13]. A retrospective study was carried out to define the long-term outcome of children who have undergone surgery for biliary atresia [112]. Of 122 children, 38% were alive after 10 years; however, firm hepato- and splenomegaly were present in about 75%. Normal liver function tests and an absence of portal hypertension were observed in only 9% of the children. These results suggest that although HPE may be helpful, about 80% of such children eventually require liver transplantation [112]. In our series, of all children with biliary atresia who underwent HPE before 3 months of age, 65% eventually required transplantation [6,13].

Liver Transplantation

Biliary atresia remains the primary indication for liver transplantation in the pediatric age population [13,147–149]. Patients with biliary atresia constitute about 50% of the pediatric candidates for transplantation [6,13,147,148]. Liver transplantation should be delayed as long as possible to permit maximal growth. Repeated attempts at revision of the HPE or portosystemic shunting, however, may be ineffective and render eventual transplantation more difficult.

Pediatric patients undergoing liver replacement today can expect survival rates approaching 90% as a result of improved techniques of preoperative management, resolution of major intraoperative technical problems associated with microvascular reconstruction of the hepatic vasculature, and precise postoperative immunosuppression and management of infectious diseases [147,148]. The remaining factor that limits widespread application and prevents access by all pediatric candidates to transplantation is the *scarcity* of adequate donor organs. The surgical techniques necessary to allow all variations of whole, split liver, and living donor transplantation were developed in an attempt to meet this desperate need, yet increasing numbers of potential recipients overwhelm these resources. The disparity in size-matched pediatric donors is compounded by the preponderance of children with biliary atresia among the candidates for liver transplantation in the pediatric population; 55% of deaths in children from liver diseases occur before 2 years of age. In these patients, liver replacement is necessary at a very young age and small size, in view of the rapid progression of the hepatic disease and poor nutritional status [147,148,150]. This creates an "epidemiologic disparity" because most pediatric donors are of school age or older. Consequently there may be an increased death rate in pediatric patients awaiting liver transplantation; alternatively, suboptimal donor organs may be accepted in a desperate attempt to address recipient needs [150]. The use of reduced-size liver transplantation as an initial strategy was successful in both improving patient survival and decreasing the waiting-list mortality rate [150,151]. Since the institution of segmental transplantation at Cincinnati Children's Hospital Medical Center, the number of deaths while awaiting donor organ availability and the incidence of hepatic artery thrombosis have been reduced dramatically. Before the introduction of reduced-size liver transplantation at our center, 29% of children listed for transplantation died because of the lack of donor organ availability [147,150]. After the implementation of reduced-size liver transplant techniques, the waiting-list mortality rate has been reduced to 2% in our center, with similar reductions in other centers [150]. Although 45% of children still undergo transplantation with a status of high medical urgency, the wider range of donors available using reduced-size allografts has allowed the selection of donors with improved hemodynamic stability and liver function. These procedures established the successful techniques needed to advance both living donor and split liver transplantation, both of which increase the donor pool rather then redistributing the resources. However, these procedures encompass increased perioperative risks to the recipient (and living donor) [150–156]. Broader use of the current wave of innovative techniques is needed to ensure equitable stewardship [157]. Reduced-size liver transplantation is not the ideal solution; however, expansion of the donor pool may be possible through extension of the surgical techniques used to prepare reduced-size allografts. The need for orthotopic liver transplantation in small pediatric patients stimulated the development of other innovative operative procedures based on the concept of reduced-size allografts; these include split liver transplantation and the use of living, related organ donors. Liver transplantation survival rates for living donor, split, and reduced-size transplantation are similar to those with whole-organ graft transplantation in children older than 2 years [147,148,150]. Recent data have suggested that living donor transplantation is best performed in recipients 1–2 years of age.

Despite the high overall success rate of liver transplantation in children, multiple challenges remain, including improvement of methods of preoperative management to address the problems of malnutrition, improvement of methods of immune suppression to prevent graft loss and avoid lymphoproliferative disease and other infectious complications, and development of protocols to avoid growth suppression [13,147,148,158]. Children are particularly sensitive to the consequences of both under-immunosuppression (rejection) and over-immunosuppression (posttransplantation lymphoproliferative disease, renal insufficiency, infection). The latter is complicated by the fact that children appear to be more immunoresponsive than adults. A careful balance is sought throughout the posttransplantation period. We also must strive to provide services in a cost-effective manner.

Liver Transplantation as Primary Therapy for Biliary Atresia

Those who propose primary transplantation as the procedure of choice for children with biliary atresia cite several potential advantages, including the lack of adhesions in a previously undisturbed abdomen leading to a decreased need for blood products [159]. In the past, survival of children less than 1 year of age was compromised; however, experienced transplant centers now report 1-year survival of more than 85%, even in these critical infants [160]. However, the most compelling argument against primary transplantation centers on inadequate donor resources. Mortality awaiting transplantation is highest in the over-1-year-old group, and an influx of biliary atresia infants would further increase the disparity and mortality. Selection of candidates for primary transplantation is not well accepted, except possibly in patients in whom liver disease is so advanced (advanced age and cirrhosis) that bile flow cannot be restored. Conservative decision making should be practiced in this regard, knowing that even partial return of bile flow may delay transplantation to an age at which prognosis is more favorable and a donor organ more readily available.

The limitations and potential pitfalls of primary liver transplantation have led to adaptation of a *sequential approach* in the management of biliary atresia (Figure 12.5). HPE would obviate the need for transplantation for patients in whom the procedure was a long-term success and delay transplantation in another significant proportion. The cost benefits of this strategy have been discussed [14]. In our opinion, therefore, sequential surgical therapy for biliary atresia should begin with creation of

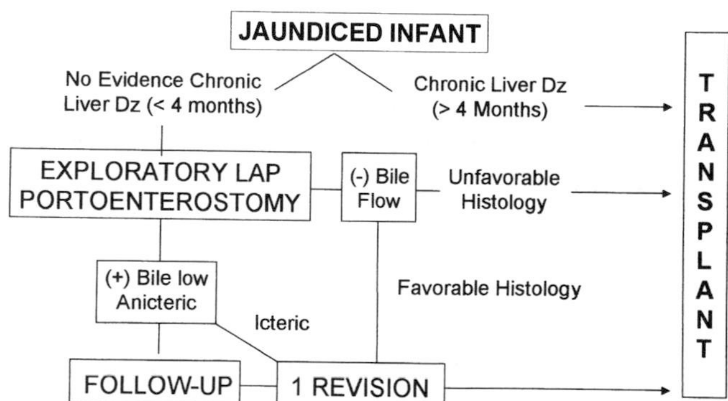

Figure 12.5. Flow chart for patients with biliary atresia. Management strategy indicating success rates following sequential Kasai hepatoportoenterostomy procedure followed, when needed, by liver transplantation.

an HPE. Infants with poor response will undergo transplantation within the first 2 years. Children with initially "successful" drainage but with progressive liver disease with portal hypertension, hypersplenism, variceal hemorrhage, and malnutrition will need orthotopic liver transplantation at a later date. Occasionally, long-term survivors may not require transplantation.

Chardot et al. [161] reviewed all patients with biliary atresia living in France and born between the years 1986 and 1996. A total of 472 patients were identified; the 10-year overall survival rate was 68%. Independent prognostic factors for overall survival were the performance of the Kasai operation, age at operation, anatomic pattern of extrahepatic bile ducts, polysplenia syndrome, and experience of the managing center. Survival with native liver depended on the same independent prognostic factors. These data support the concepts that the Kasai operation should remain the first-line treatment of biliary atresia and that early performance of this operation and treatment in an experienced center should reduce the need for liver transplantation in infancy and childhood and provide children with the best chance of survival [101]. High survival rates for patients with biliary atresia can be achieved through the complementary and sequential utilization of early primary therapy with the Kasai portoenterostomy followed by liver transplantation if necessary [6,14,159,162]. The series of Chardot et al. [161] also emphasizes the value of "center experience" in achieving these high success rates. The Kasai procedure is technically difficult, and success in achieving bile flow is related to the skill with which this procedure is performed. The need for primary transplantation is not well accepted, except possibly in those patients in whom liver disease is so advanced that bile flow cannot be restored. Studies such as this argue for conservative decision making in this regard, knowing that even partial return of bile flow may delay transplantation to an age at which prognosis is more favorable. Optimizing the outcome of the HPE can be obtained by addressing the controllable factors involved in the prognosis: early diagnosis and referral to a center experienced in the care of children with this disorder.

Outcome of Orthotopic Liver Transplantation in Children

The most important factor determining survival at our center is the severity of the patient's illness at the time of transplantation [147,148,163]. Survival in infants has improved with increasing experience. Infants younger than 1 year now have 1-year survival rates greater than 85%, an improvement over previously reported rates of 50–60% [147,148,150,164–168]. This increase in survival results from technical operative improvements and experienced care management. A major challenge is the high frequency of virus-related disease in children, especially CMV- and Epstein–Barr virus–related. As the survival rates following orthotopic liver transplantation in children have increased, health care providers have begun to measure the overall health status of liver transplant recipients (functional outcome) as a complement to traditional measures of medical outcomes. The overriding objective of hepatic transplantation in children is complete rehabilitation with improved quality of life [147,148,168]. Factors contributing to the attainment of this goal include improved nutritional status with appropriate growth and development as well as enhanced motor and cognitive skills, allowing social reintegration.

FUTURE

The ultimate goal is to prevent biliary atresia; to accomplish that objective, a multicenter, multifaceted effort is necessary. The National Institutes of Health have recently established a consortium – The Biliary Atresia Clinical Research Consortium (BARC) – consisting of ten pediatric clinical research centers in the United States [169] (see http://www.barcnetwork.org). The individual centers and a data coordinating center will accelerate advances in the understanding, diagnosis, and clinical management of biliary atresia and related pediatric liver diseases. Their goals are to:

1. determine the etiology of the disorder
2. develop rapid and sensitive means for diagnosis
3. define the natural history of biliary atresia
4. determine the optimal medical and surgical treatment strategies
5. identify risk factors for progression of the disease

The consortium has developed a prospective clinical database and a repository of tissue, serum, and plasma samples and has recently reported an analysis of the outcomes of infants with biliary atresia. This database will be a valuable resource in the quest to achieve the goals outlined here and thus clearly represents an important first step in our fight against this disease.

CHOLEDOCHAL CYST

Choledochal cysts are considered to be congenital anomalies of the biliary tract characterized by varying degrees of cystic dilatation at various segments of the biliary tract (extrahepatic or intrahepatic). The frequency of choledochal cysts is about 1 in 15,000 live births in Western countries and as high as 1 in 1000 live births in Japan. There is a marked female predominance (four to one) regardless of the racial origin. A choledochal cyst (or congenital bile duct cyst) may be detected at any age and in any portion of the bile duct [170–173]. Todani [173] has proposed classification of choledochal cysts into five subtypes (Figure 12.6, Table 12.3). Although cysts are uncommonly present in the neonatal period, this consideration must be included in the differential diagnosis of neonatal cholestasis; antenatal diagnosis has been described [174]. Cysts are present in up to 2% of infants with obstructive jaundice. Infants present in a manner simulating biliary atresia and, if unrecognized, may have progressive disease. Prolonged obstruction results in biliary cirrhosis, portal hypertension resulting from cirrhosis, and pressure on the portal vein by the distended cyst; recurrent pancreatitis is an unusual complication of the malformation [173].

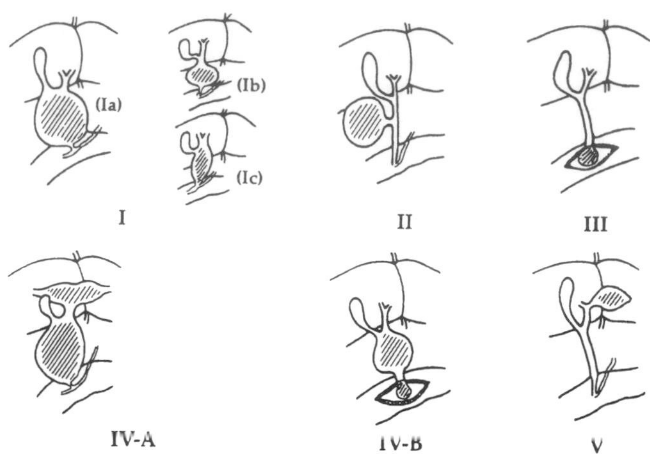

Figure 12.6. Classification of congenital bile duct cysts (according to Todani [173]); see Table 12.3 for descriptions of each type.

Clinical Features

The classic triad of intermittent abdominal pain, jaundice, and right epigastric mass varies in incidence; this triad is usually not present in infants and indeed is uncommon in older children, occurring in about 20% [170,173]. Jaundice (conjugated hyperbilirubinemia) is the common manifestation. Abdominal pain may be a presenting symptom, often with elevated serum amylase levels. The lesion may be detected at any age, with 18% appearing before 1 year. Older children may have mild chronic liver disease, which may reflect variable degrees of common bile duct obstruction. In certain patients, the lesion appears to be a true congenital malformation and is associated with other anomalies of the biliary tree, such as double common duct, double gallbladder, and accessory hepatic ducts, as well as polycystic and hypoplastic kidneys [173]. Complete distal biliary obstruction also may be seen in infants, with no detectable biliary remnant at the site of the distal common bile duct. In these infants, the histologic changes in the liver are indistinguishable from biliary atresia or constitute a distinct clinical subgroup [175]. Adults with choledochal cyst disease commonly have acute biliary tract or pancreatic symptoms [170,176]. It is possible that the variability in age and clinical course represents two distinct entities: congenital disease (in infants) versus acquired disease (in older children) [177].

Spontaneous perforation of a choledochal cyst in infancy is not a rare event. Of 187 patients with infantile choledochal cyst treated at one hospital, 13 cases of spontaneous perforation were encountered; 8 patients were found to have biliary peritonitis, and 5 had sealed perforation [178]. The cause of the perforation is postulated to be biliary epithelial irritation as a result of reflux of pancreatic juice caused by pancreaticobiliary malunion associated with mural immaturity, rather than an abnormal rise in ductal pressure or congenital mural weakness at a certain point.

Pathogenesis

The pathogenesis of choledochal cysts is undetermined; there are several theories. Cysts may represent (1) anomalous union of the common bile duct and the pancreatic duct proximal to the sphincter of Oddi, which may permit reflux of pancreatic enzymes into the common bile duct with resultant inflammation, localized weakness, and dilation [179]; (2) congenital segmental weakness of the common bile duct wall; or (3) obstruction of the distal common bile duct leading to dilatation. Further research is needed.

Table 12.3: Classification of Bile Duct Cysts

Type I: cystic dilatation of the common bile duct
- a. Large saccular cystic dilatation
- b. Small localized segmental dilatation
- c. Diffuse (cylindric) fusiform dilatation

Type II: diverticulum of the common bile duct and/or the gallbladder

Type III: choledochocele

Type IV: multiple cysts
- a. Intrahepatic and extrahepatic*
- b. Extrahepatic only

Type V: fusiform intrahepatic dilatations (relation to Caroli's disease?)

*Most common form.
Modified from Todani [173], with permission.

Diagnosis of Choledochal Cysts

In most infants, the diagnosis is suggested if noninvasive imaging studies are undertaken for vague right upper quadrant symptoms (Figure 12.7). Ultrasonography should be the initial procedure in the evaluation of suspected choledochal cyst [180]. Radiographs of the upper gastrointestinal tract may

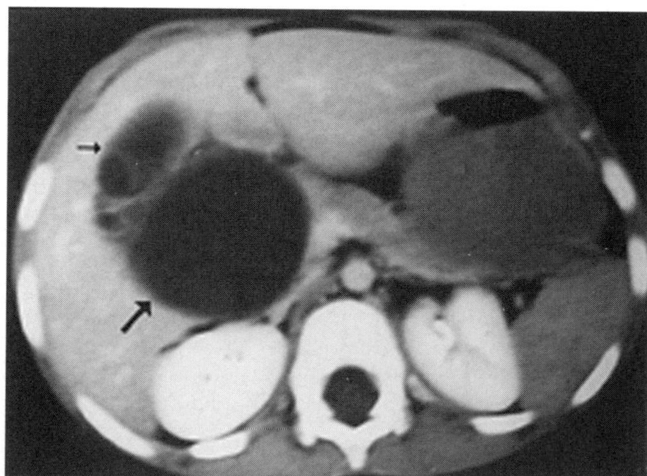

Figure 12.7. Computed tomographic scan of an infant with a type I choledochal cyst. A *large arrow* indicates the cyst, a *small arrow* the gallbladder.

outline the mass as it displaces the first and second portion of the duodenum but are unnecessary. Mebrofenin scintigraphy is accurate in confirming the presence of a choledochal cyst and in refuting the diagnosis of biliary atresia [82].

Ultrasonography also may be helpful in the preoperative differential diagnosis of choledochal cysts in neonates and infants. Cysts are larger, intrahepatic ducts are dilated, and gallbladders are not atretic in patients with choledochal cysts compared with patients with biliary atresia [180].

The accuracy of antenatal ultrasonography in the diagnosis of choledochal cysts is not known [181–183]. We detected choledochal cysts in five patients through antenatal ultrasonography (at 17–35 weeks' gestational age) [174]. All had cystic dilatation of the common bile duct (type I cysts). All those with distal obstruction by operative cholangiography had varying degrees of fibrosis. Each improved following surgical excision and porto- or choledochoenterostomy. Redkar et al. [184] studied 13 patients with proven biliary disease who had abnormal antenatal scans at a mean of 20 weeks. Two infants had type I cystic biliary atresia, and one had a noncommunicating segmental dilatation of the bile duct in a type 3 biliary atresia. The remainder had choledochal cysts and included two patients with intrahepatic cysts. The correct diagnosis was made antenatally in only two patients (15%). Of the remaining patients, seven were diagnosed with intra-abdominal cysts of unknown cause, three with duodenal atresia, and one with an ovarian cyst. Antenatal diagnosis offers the possibility of early definitive surgery for uncomplicated choledochal dilatation and the chance for improved outcome for surgically treated biliary atresia.

Treatment of Choledochal Cysts

The goal is complete surgical excision of the cyst mucosa, with a Roux-en-Y choledochojejunostomy proximal to the most distal lesion [11,173,185 189]. This allows direct bile duct mucosa–to–bowel mucosa anastomosis, with the lowest risk of stenosis or stricture. This strategy has evolved from historical attempts at aspiration and external drainage, internal decompression and drainage into the duodenum (cyst duodenostomy), or direct anastomosis of the cyst to a jejunal Roux-en-Y loop. Each of these drainage techniques retained the wall of the cyst with its abnormal mucosa. Poor drainage leading to stasis and persistent cyst inflammation resulted in stricture formation, biliary lithiasis, and an increased risk of malignant evolution within the cyst wall. The recommended treatment currently includes elimination of the entire cyst mucosal wall by complete excision of the extrahepatic cyst and excision and reconstruction of the extrahepatic biliary tree to a retrocolic, isoperistaltic, 35- to 45-cm jejunal Roux-en-Y loop. Internal or external biliary transanastomotic stents rarely are needed because of the large size of the anastomosis (Figure 12.8).

In patients in whom prolonged or recurrent inflammation within and surrounding the cyst has complicated identification of the portal vasculature, the cyst can be transected along its anterolateral wall, allowing complete excision of the mucosa while retaining the fibrous cyst wall overlying the hepatic artery and portal vein. This protects the critical portal vascular structures and allows excision of all of the abnormal lining of the cyst [190].

The distal remnant of the common bile duct should be closed through the open base of the choledochal cyst, taking great care not to injure the often ectopically located pancreatic duct junction. Failure to remove this distal, often retroduodenal, portion of the cyst may lead to recurrence.

It is important to define the extent of any intrahepatic cystic disease at the time of choledochal cyst excision. This is best undertaken with an intraoperative cholangiogram or through preoperative percutaneous transhepatic or endoscopic retrograde cholangiography. If the cystic disease is in continuity with the primary bile duct cyst and no intervening strictures leading to stasis are present, reconstruction at the hepatic hilum is appropriate therapy. If intrahepatic cystic disease with interposed areas of stenosis (Caroli's disease) is present, such decompressive methods are not applicable. Segmental multifocal cystic disease isolated to a single hepatic lobe can be treated successfully by cyst excision and hepatic lobectomy. If the intrahepatic disease is diffuse and involves all hepatic lobes, liver transplantation may be necessary if complete and successful decompressive drainage is not possible.

Complications and Outcome

Cholangitis may occur in up to 15% of patients following surgery, even with the Roux-en-Y procedure, but is much less common than with direct anastomosis to the duodenum; the latter procedure is not advisable [191]. The high rate of stricture (73%) after cyst enterostomy is also preventable by total cyst excision and Roux-en-Y reconstruction. Pancreatitis is uncommon but may occur secondary to proximal pancreatic duct or sphincter stenosis or stones.

Malignancy in Choledochal Cysts

Carcinoma has been reported in residual cystic tissue in up to 26% of patients [171,173,192,193], an incidence that is 20 times greater than that in the general population. The typical malignancy is adenocarcinoma of the bile duct or gallbladder; less commonly squamous cell carcinoma and cholangiocarcinoma have been described. The risk of developing malignancy increases with age, making complete excision of the cyst and proximal bile duct mucosa an essential component of the operation in older patients. Malignant change also may occur in areas of the biliary tree remote from the cyst. The increased risk of malignant degeneration and the dismal prognosis once cancer has developed warrant complete cyst excision, even in asymptomatic patients, including those with prior cyst enterostomies [171].

SPONTANEOUS PERFORATION OF THE COMMON BILE DUCT

Spontaneous perforation of the common bile duct is a rare curiosity; about 60 cases have been reported [194–197]. The

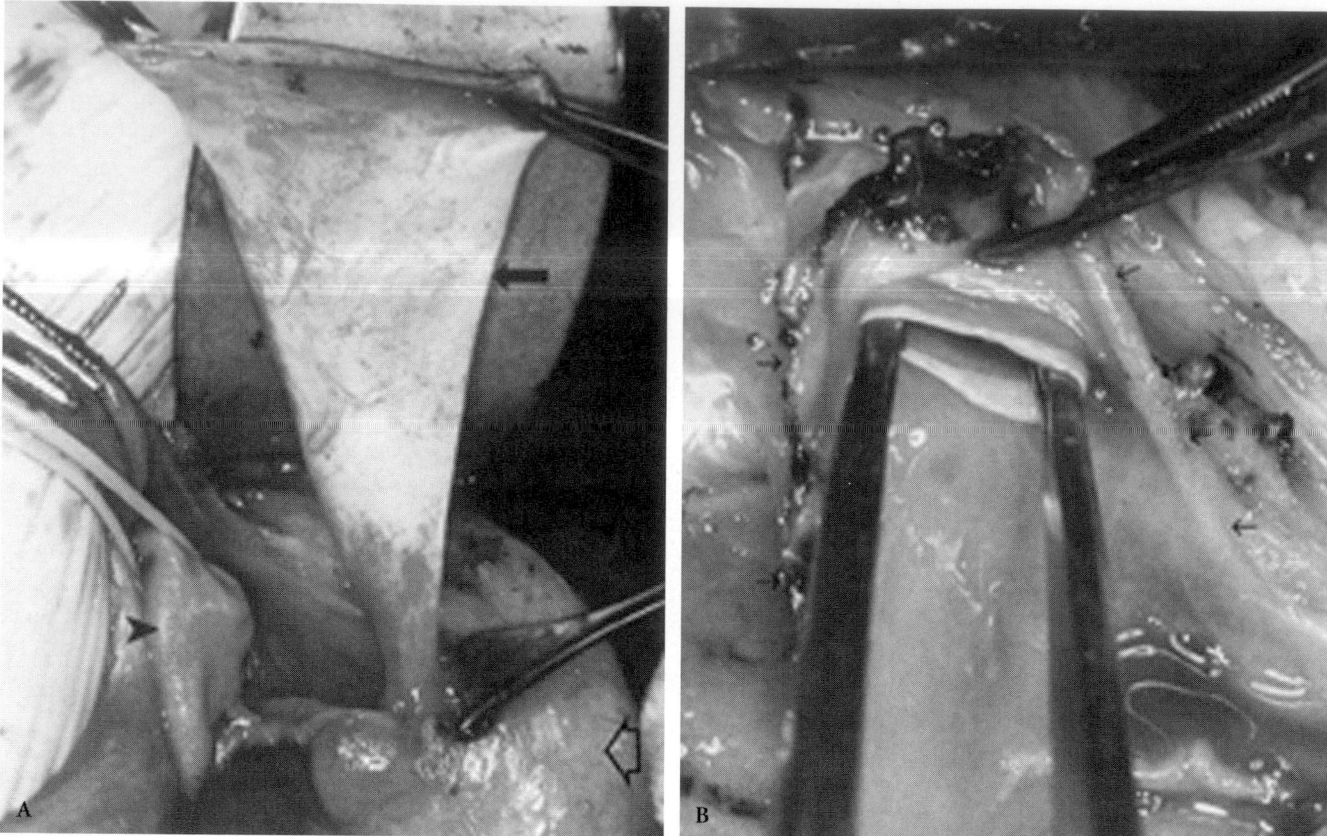

Figure 12.8. Surgical management of choledochal cyst. (**A**) Operative photograph of the "Lilly" dissection showing the inflammatory wall of the proximal choledochal cyst separated from the internal lining "mucosa" (*arrow*). The distal cyst wall is identified by the *arrowhead.* (**B**) Transection of the mucosal dissection just proximal to the proper hepatic duct bifurcation and prepared for reconstruction as an end-to-side choledochojejunostomy using an isoperistaltic jejunal Roux-en-Y loop. *Arrows* outline the retained outer wall of the choledochal cyst.

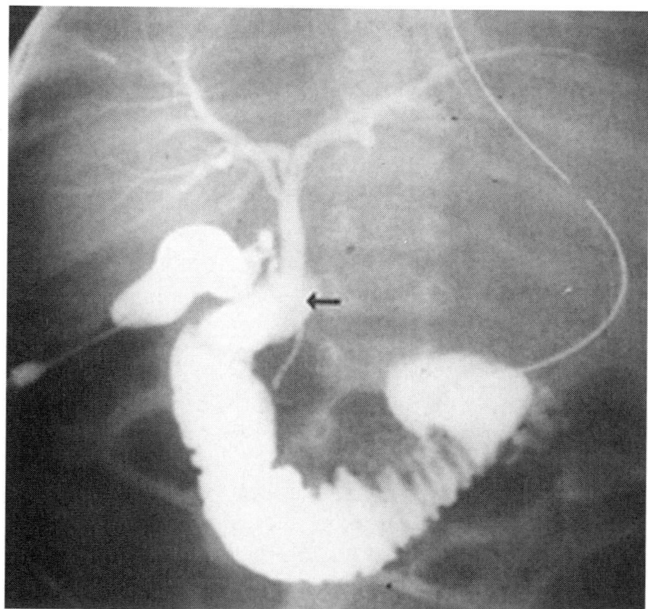

Figure 12.9. An infant with a bile duct stricture at the junction of the cystic duct with the proper hepatic duct (*arrow*). The hypoplastic distal common bile duct is seen. The patient was treated with a choledochojejunostomy into an isoperistaltic jejunal Roux-en-Y loop.

typical onset of symptoms (mild jaundice, ascites, acholic stools, poor weight gain, and vomiting) occurs before 3 months of age. Progressive abdominal distention occurs, with bile staining of umbilical and inguinal hernias and of the abdominal wall. The diagnosis is suggested by the relatively modest degree of conjugated hyperbilirubinemia with minimal elevation of aminotransferase levels in association with acholic stools. Sonography may reveal ascites or loculated fluid around the gallbladder [195], and hepatobiliary scintigraphy may demonstrate evidence of activity outside the biliary tract [198]. Abdominal paracentesis yields clear, bile-stained ascitic fluid. Histologically, the liver manifests cholestasis with a normal lobular pattern. Operative cholangiography usually demonstrates the presence of the perforation, frequently in association with obstruction at the distal end of the common bile duct, secondary to stenosis, segmental atresia, or inspissated bile. The rather constant location of the perforation at the junction of the cystic and common bile ducts is highly suggestive of a developmental weakness at this site (Figure 12.9). Drainage with suture closure of the perforation may be a satisfactory treatment. Internal diversion through a Roux-en-Y loop of jejunum may be used for drainage in some infants.

REFERENCES

1. Landing BH. Considerations of the pathogenesis of neonatal hepatitis, biliary atresia and choledochal cyst: the concept of infantile obstructive cholangiopathy. Prog Pediatr Surg 1974;6:113–39.
2. Desmet VJ. Congenital diseases of intrahepatic bile ducts: variations on the theme "ductal plate malformation." Hepatology 1992;16:1069–83.
3. Ito T, Horisawa M, Ando H. Intrahepatic bile ducts in biliary atresia: a possible factor determining the prognosis. J Pediatr Surg 1983;18:124.
4. Raweily EA, Gibson AAM, Burt AD. Abnormalities of intrahepatic bile ducts in extrahepatic biliary atresia. Histopathology 1990;17:521–7.
5. Landing BH, Wells TR, Ramicone E. Time course of the intrahepatic lesion of extrahepatic biliary atresia: a morphometric study. Pediatr Pathol 1985;4:309.
6. Balistreri WF, Grand R, Suchy FJ, et al. Biliary atresia: current concepts and research directions. Hepatology 1996;23:1682–92.
7. Balistreri WF. Neonatal cholestasis: medical progress. J Pediatr 1985;106:171.
8. Danks DM, Campbell PE, Smith AL, et al. Studies of the aetiology of neonatal hepatitis and biliary atresia. Arch Dis Child 1977;52:360.
9. Bezerra JA, Tiao G, Ryckman FC, et al. Genetic induction of proinflammatory immunity in children with biliary atresia. Lancet 2002;360:1653–9.
10. Mack CL, Tucker RM, Sokol RJ, et al. Biliary atresia is associated with CD4+ Th1 cell-mediated portal tract inflammation. Pediatr Res 2004;56:79–87.
11. Ryckman FC, Noseworthy J. Neonatal cholestatic conditions requiring surgical reconstruction. Semin Liver Dis 1987;7:134–54.
12. Ohi R. Biliary atresia. In: Balistreri WF, Ohi R, Todani T, et al., eds. Hepatobiliary, pancreatic and splenic disease in children: medical and surgical management. Amsterdam: Elsevier Science, 1997:231–60.
13. Ryckman FC, Fisher RA, Pedersen SH, et al. Improved survival in biliary atresia patients in the present era of liver transplantation. J Pediatr Surg 1993;28:382–6.
14. Rudolph JA, Balistreri WF. Optimal treatment of biliary atresia: "halfway" there! [editorial]. Hepatology 1999;30:808–10.
15. Yoon PW, Bresee JS, Olney RS, et al. Epidemiology of biliary atresia: a population-based study. Pediatrics 1997;99:376–82.
16. Schweizer P. Treatment of extrahepatic bile duct atresia: results and long-term prognosis after hepatic portoenterostomy. Pediatr Surg 1986;1:30–6.
17. Davenport M, Savage M, Mowat AP, et al. Biliary atresia splenic malformation syndrome. Surgery 1993;113:662–8.
18. Balistreri WF. Neonatal cholestasis: lessons from the past, issues for the future. Semin Liver Dis 1987;7:1–3.
19. Perlmutter DH, Shepherd RW. Extrahepatic biliary atresia: a disease or a phenotype? Hepatology 2002:35:1298–304.
20. Matsui A, Fujimoto T, Takazawa Y, et al. Serum bile acid levels in patients with extrahepatic biliary atresia and neonatal hepatitis during the first 10 days of life. J Pediatr 1985;107:255.
21. Mushtaq I, Logan S, Morris M, et al. Screening of newborn infants for cholestatic hepatobiliary disease with tandem mass spectrometry. BMJ 1999;319:471–7.
22. Hyams JS, Glaser GH, Leichtner AM, et al. Discordance for biliary atresia in two sets of monozygotic twins. J Pediatr 1985;107:420.
23. Schweizer P, Kerremans J. Discordant findings in extrahepatic bile duct atresia in 6 sets of twins. Z Kinderchir 1988;43:72–5.
24. Strickland AD, Shannon K, Coln CD, et al. Biliary atresia in two sets of twins. J Pediatr 1985;107:418.
25. Gautier M. Morphologic study of 98 biliary remnants. Arch Pathol Lab Med 1981;105:397.
26. Hadchouel M. Immunoglobulin deposits in the biliary remnants of extrahepatic biliary atresia: a study by immunoperoxidase staining in 128 infants. Histopathology 1981;5:217.
27. Morecki R, Glaser JH, Cho S, et al. Biliary atresia and reovirus type 3 infection. N Engl J Med 1982;307:481.
28. Morecki R, Glaser JH, Johnson AB, et al. Detection of reovirus type 3 in the porta hepatis of an infant with extrahepatic biliary atresia: ultrastructural and immunocytochemical study. Hepatology 1984;4:1137.
29. Glaser JH, Morecki R. Reovirus type 3 and neonatal cholestasis. Semin Liver Dis 1987;7:100–7.
30. Riepenhoff-Talty M, Shaekel K, Clark HF, et al. Group A rotaviruses produce extrahepatic biliary obstruction in orally inoculated newborn mice. Pediatr Res 1993;33:394–9.
31. Riepenhoff-Talty M, Gouvea V, Evans MJ, et al. Detection of group C rotavirus in infants with extrahepatic biliary atresia. J Infect Dis 1996;174:8–15.
32. Petersen C, Bruns E, Kuske M, et al. Treatment of extrahepatic biliary atresia with interferon-a in a murine infectious model. Pediatr Res 1997;42:623–8.
33. Bobo L, Ojeh C, Chiu D, et al. Lack of evidence for rotavirus by polymerase chain reaction/enzyme immunoassay of hepatobiliary samples from children with biliary atresia. Pediatr Res 1997;41:229–34.
34. Oppenheimer E, Esterly JR. Cytomegalovirus infection: a possible cause of biliary atresia. Am J Pathol 1973;72:2a.
35. Finegold MJ, Carpenter RJ. Obliterative cholangitis due to cytomegalovirus: a possible precursor of paucity of intrahepatic bile ducts. Hum Pathol 1982;13:662–5.
36. Jevon GP, Dimmick JE. Biliary atresia and cytomegalovirus infection: a DNA study. Pediatr Dev Pathol 1999;2:11–14.
37. Fischler B, Ehrnst A, Forsgren M, et al. The viral association of neonatal cholestasis in Sweden: a possible link between cytomegalovirus infection and extrahepatic biliary atresia. J Pediatr Gastroenterol Nutr 1998;27:57–64.
38. Drut R, Drut RM, Gomez MA, et al. Presence of human papillomavirus in extrahepatic biliary atresia. J Pediatr Gastroenterol Nutr 1998;27:530–5.
39. Mason AL, Xu L, Guo L, et al. Detection of retroviral antibodies in primary biliary cirrhosis and other idiopathic biliary disorders. Lancet 1998;351:1620–4.
40. Glaser JH, Balistreri WF, Morecki R. The role of reovirus type 3 in persistent infantile cholestasis. J Pediatr 1984;105:912–15.
41. Tyler KL, Sokol RJ, Oberhaus SM, et al. Detection of reovirus RNA in hepatobiliary tissues from patients with extrahepatic biliary atresia and choledochal cysts. Hepatology 1998;27:1475–82.
42. Rosenberg DP, Morecki R, Lollini LO, et al. Extrahepatic biliary atresia in a rhesus monkey (*Macaca mulatta*). Hepatology 1983;3:377–80.

43. Brown WR, Sokol RJ, Levin MJ, et al. Lack of correlation between infection with reovirus 3 and extrahepatic biliary atresia or neonatal hepatitis. J Pediatr 1988;113:670–6.
44. Steele MI, Marshall CM, Lloyd RE, et al. Reovirus 3 not detected by reverse transcriptase-mediated polymerase chain reaction analysis of preserved tissue from infants with cholestatic liver disease. Hepatology 1995;21:697–702.
45. Szavay PO, Leonhardt J, Czech-Schmidt, Petersen C. The role of reovirus type 3 infection in an established murine model for biliary atresia. Eur J Pediatr Surg 2002;12:248–50.
46. Petersen C, Biermanns D, Kuske M, et al. New aspects in a murine model for extrahepatic biliary atresia. J Pediatr Sur 1997;32:1190–5.
47. Petersen C, Grasshoff Sabine, Luciano L. Diverse morphology of biliary atresia in an animal model. J Hepatol 1998;28:603–7.
48. Czech-Schmidt G, Verhagen W, Szavay P, et al. Immunological gap in the infectious animal model of biliary atresia. J Surg Res 2001;101:62–7.
49. Tan CEL, Davenport M, Driver M, et al. Does the morphology of the extrahepatic biliary remnants in biliary atresia influence survival? A review of 205 cases. J Pediatr Surg 1994;29:1459–64.
50. Yokoyama T, Copeland NG, Jenkins NA, et al. Reversal of left-right asymmetry: a situs inversus mutation. Science 1993;260:679–82.
51. Mazziotti MV, Willis LK, Heuckeroth RO, et al. Anomalous development of the hepatobiliary system in the *Inv* mouse. Hepatology 1999;30:372–8.
52. Schon P, Tsuchiya K, Lenoir D, et al. Identification, genomic organization, chromosomal mapping and mutation analysis of the human INV gene, the ortholog of a murine gene implicated in left-right axis development and biliary atresia. Hum Genet 2002;110:157–65.
53. Desmet VJ. Intrahepatic bile ducts under the lens. J Hepatol 1985;1:545–59.
54. Schmidt C, Bladt F, Goedecke S, et al. Scatter factor/hepatocyte growth factor is essential for liver development. Nature 1995; 373:699–702.
55. Borowiak M, Garratt AN, Wustefeld T, et al. Met provides essential signals for liver regeneration. Proc Natl Acad Sci U S A 2004; 101:10608–13.
56. Huh CG, Factor VM, Sanchez A, et al. Hepatocyte growth factor/c-met signaling pathway is required for efficient liver regeneration and repair. Proc Natl Acad Sci U S A 2004;101: 4477–82.
57. Clotman F, Lannoy VJ, Reber M, et al. The onecut transcription factor HNF6 is required for normal development of the biliary tract. Development 2002;129:1819–28.
58. Sumazaki R, Shiojiri N, Isoyama S, et al. Conversion of biliary system to pancreatic tissue in Hes1-deficient mice. Nat Genet 2004;36:83–7.
59. Mahlapuu M, Ormestad M, Enerback S, Carlsson P. The forkhead transcription factor Foxf1 is required for differentiation of extra-embryonic and lateral plate mesoderm. Development 2001;128:155–66.
60. Coffinier C, Gresh L, Fiette L, et al. Bile system morphogenesis defects and liver dysfunction upon targeted deletion of HNF1beta. Development 2002;129:1829–38.
61. Krupczak-Hollis K, Wang X, Kalinichenko VV, et al. The mouse Forkhead Box m1 transcription factor is essential for hepatoblast mitosis and development of intrahepatic bile ducts and vessels during liver morphogenesis. Dev Biol 2004;276:74–88.
62. Schreiber RA, Kleinman RE. Genetics, immunology, and biliary atresia: an opening or a diversion? J Pediatr Gastroenterol Nutr 1993;16:111–13.
63. Silveira TR, Salzano FM, Donaldson PT, et al. Association between HLA and extrahepatic biliary atresia. J Pediatr Gastroenterol Nutr 1993;16:114–17.
64. Jurado A, Jara P, Camarena C, et al. Is extrahepatic biliary atresia an HLA-associated disease? J Pediatr Gastroenterol Nutr 1997;25:557–8.
65. Nakada M, Nakada K, Kawaguchi F, et al. Immunologic reaction and genetic factors in biliary atresia. Tohoku J Exp Med 1997;181:41–7.
66. Broome U, Nemeth A, Hultcrantz R, et al. Different expression of HLA-DR and ICAM-1 in livers from patients with biliary atresia and Byler's disease. J Hepatol 1997;26:857–62.
67. Kobayashi H, Puri P, O'Brian DS, et al. Hepatic overexpression of MHC class II antigens and macrophage-associated antigens (CD68) in patients with biliary atresia of poor prognosis. J Pediatr Surg 1997;32:590–3.
68. Bernal W, Moloney M, Underhill J, et al. Association of tumor necrosis factor polymorphism with primary sclerosing cholangitis. J Hepatol 1999;30:237–41.
69. Bill AH, Haas JE, Foster GL. Biliary atresia: histopathologic observations and reflections upon its natural history. J Pediatr Surg 1977;12:977–82.
70. Gosseye S, Otte JB, De Meyer R, Maldague P. A histological study of extrahepatic biliary atresia. Acta Paediatrica Belgica 1977;30:85–90.
71. Ohya T, Fujimoto T, Shimomura H, Miyano T. Degeneration of intrahepatic bile duct with lymphocyte infiltration into biliary epithelial cells in biliary atresia. J Pediatr Surg 1995;30: 515–18.
72. Ahmed AF, Ohtani H, Nio M, et al. CD8+ T cells infiltrating into bile ducts in biliary atresia do not appear to function as cytotoxic T cells: a clinicopathological analysis. J Pathol 2001;193: 383–9.
73. Dillon PW, Belchis D, Minnick K, Tracy T. Differential expression of the major histocompatibility antigens and ICAM-1 on bile duct epithelial cells in biliary atresia. Tohoku J Exper Med 1997;181:33–40.
74. Carvalho E, Liu C, Shivakumar P, et al. Analysis of biliary transcriptome in experimental biliary atresia. Gastroenterology 2005;129:713–17.
75. Shivakumar P, Campbell KM, Sabla GE, et al. Obstruction of extrahepatic bile ducts by lymphocytes is regulated by IFN-gamma in experimental biliary atresia. J Clin Invest 2004;114: 322–9.
76. Klippel CH. A new theory of biliary atresia. J Pediatr Surg 1972; 7:651–4.
77. Spitz L. Ligation of the common bile duct in the fetal lamb: an experimental model for the study of biliary atresia. Pediatr Res 1980;14:740–8.
78. Holder T, Ashcraft KW. The effects of bile duct ligation and inflammation in the fetus. J Pediatr Surg 1967;2:35–40.
79. Mowat AP, Psacharopoulos HT, Williams R. Extrahepatic biliary atresia versus neonatal hepatitis: review of 137 prospectively investigated infants. Arch Dis Child 1976;51:763.
80. Danks D, Bodian M. A genetic study of neonatal obstructive jaundice. Arch Dis Child 1963;38:378.
81. Danks DM, Campbell PE, Smith AL, et al. Prognosis of babies with neonatal hepatitis. Arch Dis Child 1977;52:368.

82. Johnson K, Alton HM, Chapman S. Evaluation of mebrofenin hepatoscintigraphy in neonatal-onset jaundice. Pediatr Radiol 1998;28:937–41.
83. Gerhold JP, Klingensmith WC 3rd, Kuni CC, et al. Diagnosis of biliary atresia with radionuclide hepatobiliary imaging. Radiology 1983;146:499.
84. Spivak W, Sarkar S, Winter D, et al. Diagnostic utility of hepatobiliary scintigraphy with 99mTc-DISIDA in neonatal cholestasis. J Pediatr 1987;110:855–61.
85. Wilkinson ML, Mieli-Vergani G, Ball C, et al. Endoscopic retrograde cholangiopancreatography in infantile cholestasis. Arch Dis Child 1991;66:121–3.
86. Jaw TS, Kuo YT, Liu GC, et al. MR cholangiography in the evaluation of neonatal cholestasis. Radiology 1999;212:249–56.
87. Peng SS, Li YW, Chang MH, et al. Magnetic resonance cholangiography for evaluation of cholestatic jaundice in neonates and infants. J Formos Med Assoc 1998;97:698–703.
88. Guibaud L, Lachaud A, Touraine R, et al. MR cholangiography in neonates and infants: feasibility and preliminary applications. AJR Am J Roentgenol 1998;170:27–31.
89. Choi SO, Park WH, Lee HJ, et al. "Triangular cord": a sonographic finding applicable in the diagnosis of biliary atresia. J Pediatr Surg 1996;31:363–6.
90. Alagille D. Cholestasis in the first three months of life. In: Popper H, Schaffner F, eds. Progress in liver disease. New York: Grune & Stratton, 1979:471.
91. Hays DM, Woolley MM, Snyder WH Jr, et al. Diagnosis of biliary atresia: relative accuracy of percutaneous liver biopsy, open liver biopsy and operative cholangiography. J Pediatr 1967;71:598.
92. Kasai M. Treatment of biliary atresia with special reference to hepatic portoenterostomy and its modifications. Prog Pediatr Surg 1974;6:5–52.
93. Ohi R, Hanamatsu M, Mochizuki I, et al. Reoperation in patients with biliary atresia. J Pediatr Surg 1985;20:256.
94. Karrer FM, Price MR, Bensard DD, et al. Long-term results with the Kasai operation for biliary atresia. Arch Surg 1996;131: 493–6.
95. Hong R, Schubert WK. Menghini needle biopsy of the liver. Am J Dis Child 1960;100:42.
96. Zerbini MC, Gallucci SD, Maezono R, et al. Liver biopsy in neonatal cholestasis: a review on statistical grounds. Mod Pathol 1997;10:793–9.
97. Markowitz J, Daum F, Kahn EI, et al. Arteriohepatic dysplasia: I. pitfalls in diagnosis and management. Hepatology 1983;3:74.
98. Kasai M, Kimura S, Asakura Y. Surgical treatment of biliary atresia. J Pediatr Surg 1968;3:665–75.
99. Kasai M, Watanabe I, Ohi R. Follow-up studies of long-term survivors after hepatic portoenterostomy for "noncorrectable" biliary atresia. J Pediatr Surg 1975;10:173.
100. Ohi R, Ibrahim M. Biliary atresia. Semin Liver Dis 1992;1: 115–24.
101. Ryckman FC, Alonso MH, Bucuvalas JC, et al. Biliary atresia: surgical management and treatment options as they relate to outcome. Liver Transplant Surg 1998;4:S24–33.
102. National Institutes of Health Consensus Development Conference statement: liver transplantation. June 20–23, 1983. Hepatology 1983;4:107S–110S.
103. Schwartz MZ, Hall RJ, Reubner B, et al. Agenesis of the extrahepatic bile ducts: report of five cases. J Pediatr Surg 1990;25:805–7.
104. Ohi R, Hanamatsu M, Mochizuki I, et al. Progress in the treatment of biliary atresia. World J Surg 1985;9:285–93.
105. Lilly JR, Karrer FM, Hall RJ, et al. The surgery of biliary atresia. Ann Surg 1989;210:289–96.
106. Endo M, Katsumata K, Yokoyama J, et al. Extended dissection of the portahepatis and creation of an intussuscepted ileocolic conduit for biliary atresia. J Pediatr Surg 1983;18:784 93.
107. Hashimoto T, Otobe Y, Shimizu Y, et al. A modification of hepatic portoenterostomy (Kasai operation) for biliary atresia. J Am Coll Surg 1997;185:548–53.
108. Toyosaka A, Okamoto E, Okasora T, et al. Extensive dissection at the porta hepatis for biliary atresia. J Pediatr Surg 1994;29: 896–9.
109. Kimura K, Tsugawa C, Kubo M, et al. Technical aspects of hepatic portal dissection in biliary atresia. J Pediatr Surg 1979;14: 27–32.
110. Davenport M, De Ville de Goyet J, Stringer MD, et al. Seamless management of biliary atresia in England and Wales (1999–2002). Lancet 2004;363:1354–7.
111. Kasai M, Mochizuki I, Ohkohchi N, et al. Surgical limitations for biliary atresia: indication for liver transplantation. J Pediatr Surg 1989;24:851–4.
112. Laurent J, Gauthier F, Bernard O, et al. Long-term outcome after surgery for biliary atresia: study of 40 patients surviving for more than 10 years. Gastroenterology 1990;99:1793–7.
113. McClement JW, Howard ER, Mowat AP. Results of surgical treatment for extrahepatic biliary atresia in United Kingdom 1980–2. Br Med J 1985;290:345.
114. Lykavieris P, Chardot C, Sokhn M, et al. Outcome in adulthood of biliary atresia: a study of 63 patients who survived for over 20 years with their native liver. Hepatology 2005;41:366–71.
115. Nio M, Ohi R, Hayashi Y, et al. Current status of 21 patients who have survived more than 20 years since undergoing surgery for biliary atresia. J Pediatr Surg 1996;31:381–4.
116. Grosfeld JL, Fitzgerald JF, Predaina R, et al. The efficacy of hepatoportoenterostomy in biliary atresia. Surgery 1989;106:692–701.
117. Lally KP, Kanegaye J, Matsumura M, et al. Perioperative factors affecting the outcome following repair of biliary atresia. Pediatrics 1989;83:723–6.
118. Mieli-Vergani G, Howard ER, Portmann B, et al. Later referral for biliary atresia: missed opportunity for effective surgery. Lancet 1989;i:421–3.
119. Ohhama Y, Shinkai M, Fujita S, et al. Early prediction of long-term survival and the timing of liver transplantation after the Kasai operation. J Pediatr Surg 2000;1031–4.
120. Chardot C, Carton M, Spire-Bendelac N, et al. Is the Kasai operation still indicated in children older than 3 months diagnosed with biliary atresia? J Pediatr 2001;138:224–8.
121. Davenport M, Puricelli V, Farrant P, et al. The outcome of the older ($\geq$100 days) infant with biliary atresia. J Pediatr Surg 2004;39:575–81.
122. Chandra RS, Altman RP. Ductal remnants in extrahepatic biliary atresia: a histopathologic study with clinical correlation. J Pediatr 1978;93:196.
123. Ohya T, Miyano T, Kimura K. Indication for portoenterostomy based on 103 patients with Suruga II modification. J Pediatr Surg 1990;25:801–4.
124. Yamamoto K, Fisher MM, Phillips MJ. Hilar biliary plexus in human liver: a comparative study of the intrahepatic bile ducts in man and animals. Lab Invest 1985;52:103.
125. Karrer F, Lilly JR. Corticosteroid therapy in biliary atresia. J Pediatr Surg 1985;20:693–5.

126. Dillon P, Owings E, Cilley R, et al. Immunosuppression as adjuvant therapy for biliary atresia. J Pediatr Surg 2001;36:80–5.
127. Meyers R, Book L, O'Gorman M, et al. High-dose steroids, ursodeoxycholic acid, and chronic intravenous antibiotics improve bile flow after Kasai procedure in infants with biliary atresia. J Pediatr Surg 2003;38:406–11.
128. Tatekawa Y, Muraji T, Tsugawa C. Glucocorticoid receptor alpha expression in the intrahepatic biliary epithelium and adjuvant steroid therapy in infants with biliary atresia. J Pediatr Surg 2005;40:1574–80.
129. Escobar MA, Jay CL, Brooks RM, et al. Effect of corticosteroid therapy on outcomes in biliary atresia after Kasai portoenterostomy. J Pediatr Surg 2006;41:99–103; discussion 99–103.
130. Trivedi P, Dhawan A, Risteli J, et al. Prognostic value of serum hyaluronic acid and type I and III procollagen propeptides in extrahepatic biliary atresia. Pediatr Res 1995;38:568–73.
131. Lunzmann K, Schweizer P. The influence of cholangitis on the prognosis of extrahepatic biliary atresia. Eur J Pediatr Surg 1999;9:19–23.
132. Ecoffey C, Rothman E, Barnard O, et al. Bacterial cholangitis after surgery for biliary atresia. J Pediatr 1987;111:824–9.
133. Gottrand F, Bernard O, Hadchouel M, et al. Late cholangitis after successful surgical repair of biliary atresia. Am J Dis Child 1991;145:213–15.
134. Cuffari C, Seidman E, DuBois J, et al. Acute intrahepatic portal vein thrombosis complicating cholangitis in biliary atresia. Eur J Pediatr 1997;156:186–9.
135. Broide E, Farrant P, Reid F, et al. Hepatic artery resistance index can predict early death in children with biliary atresia. Liver Transpl Surg 1997;3:604–10.
136. Kardorff R, Klotz M, Melter M, et al. Prediction of survival in extrahepatic biliary atresia by hepatic duplex sonography. J Pediatr Gastroenterol Nutr 1999;28:411–17.
137. Takahashi A, Tsuchida Y, Suzuki N, et al. Incidence of intrahepatic biliary cysts in biliary atresia after hepatic portoenterostomy and associated histopathologic findings in the liver and porta hepatis at diagnosis. J Pediatr Surg 1999;34:1364–8.
138. Ibrahim M, Ohi R, Chiba T, et al. Indications and results of reoperation for biliary atresia. In: Ohi R, ed. Biliary atresia. Tokyo: Icom Associates, 1998:96–100.
139. Miga D, Sokol RJ, MacKenzie T, et al. Survival after first esophageal variceal hemorrhage in patients with biliary atresia. J Pediatr 2001;139:291–6.
140. Okazaki T, Kobayashi H, Yamataka A, et al. Long-term postsurgical outcome of biliary atresia. J Pediatr Surg 1999;34:312–5.
141. Balistreri WF. Bile acid therapy in pediatric hepatobiliary disease: the role of ursodeoxycholic acid. J Pediatr Gastroenterol Nutr 1997;24:573–89.
142. Ernest van Heurn LW, Saing Htut, Tam PK. Cholangitis after hepatic portoenterostomy for biliary atresia: a multivariate analysis of risk factors. J Pediatr 2003;142:566–71.
143. Escobar MA, Jay CL, Brooks RM, et al. Effect of corticosteroid therapy on outcomes in biliary atresia after Kasai portoenterostomy. J Pediatr Surg 2006;41:99–103.
144. Yonemura T, Yoshibayashi M, Uemoto S, et al. Intrapulmonary shunting in biliary atresia before and after living-related liver transplantation. Br J Surg 1999;86:1139–43.
145. Egawa H, Kasahara M, Inomata Y, et al. Long-term outcome of living related liver transplantation for patients with intrapulmonary shunting and strategy for complications. Transplantation 1999;67:712–17.
146. Condino AA, Ivy DD, O'Connor JA, et al. Portopulmonary hypertension in pediatric patients. J Pediatr 2005;147:20–6.
147. Ryckman FC, Fisher RA, Pedersen SH, et al. Liver transplantation in children. Semin Pediatr Surg 1992;1:162–72.
148. Whitington PF, Balistreri WF. Liver transplantation in pediatrics: indications, contraindications, and pre-transplant management. J Pediatr 1991;118:169–77.
149. Goss JA, Shackleton CR, Swenson K, et al. Orthotopic liver transplantation for congenital biliary atresia: an 11-year, single-center experience. Ann Surg 1996;224:276–87.
150. Ryckman FC, Flake AW, Fisher RA, et al. Segmental orthotopic hepatic transplantation as means to improve patient survival and diminish waiting-list mortality. J Pediatr Surg 1991;26:422–8.
151. Broelsch CE, Emond JC, Thistlewaite JR, et al. Liver transplantation, including the concept of reduced-size liver transplants in children. Ann Surg 1988;208:410–20.
152. Langnas AN, Marujo WC, Inagaki M, et al. The results of reduced-size liver transplantation, including split livers, in patients with end-stage liver disease. Transplantation 1992;53:387–91.
153. Kawarasaki H, Makuuchi M, Kawasaki S. Liver transplantation from living donors. In: Balistreri WF, Ohi R, Todani T, et al., eds. Hepatobiliary, pancreatic and splenic disease in children: medical and surgical management. Amsterdam: Elsevier Science, 1997:433–46.
154. Tanaka K, Uemoto S, Tokunaga Y, et al. Living related liver transplantation in children. Am J Surg 1994;168:41–8.
155. Rogiers X, Malago M, Gawad K, et al. In situ splitting of cadaveric livers. Ann Surg 1996;224:331–41.
156. Fujita S, Tanaka K, Tokunaga Y, et al. Living-related liver transplantation for biliary atresia. Clin Transplant 1993;7:571–7.
157. Strom SC, Fisher RA, Thompson MT, et al. Hepatocyte transplantation as a bridge to orthotopic liver transplantation in terminal liver failure. Transplantation 1997;63:559–69.
158. Balistreri WF, Bucuvalas JC, Ryckman FC. The effect of immunosuppression on growth and development. Liver Transpl Surg 1995;S1:64–73.
159. Visser BC, Suh I, Hirose S, et al. The influence of portoenterostomy on transplantation for biliary atresia. Liver Transpl 2004;10:1279–86.
160. Tiao GM, Alonso M, Bezerra J, et al. Liver transplantation in children younger than 1 year – the Cincinnati experience. J Pediatr Surg 2005;40:268–73; discussion 273.
161. Chardot C, Carton M, Spire-Bendelac N, et al. Prognosis of biliary atresia in the era of liver transplantation: French national study from 1986 to 1996. Hepatology 1999;30:606–11.
162. Utterson EC, Shepherd RW, Sokol RJ, et al.; The Split Research Group. Biliary atresia: clinical profiles, risk factors, and outcomes of 755 patients listed for liver transplantation. J Pediatr 2005;147:180–5.
163. Ryckman FC, Alonso MH, Bucuvalas JC, et al. Long-term survival after liver transplantation. J Pediatr Surg 1999;34:845–9.
164. Cacciarelli TV, Esquivel CO, Moore DH, et al. Factors affecting survival after orthotopic liver transplantation in infants. Transplantation 1997;64:242–8.
165. Fouquet V, Alves A, Branchereau S, et al. Long-term outcome of pediatric liver transplantation for biliary atresia: a 10-year follow-up in a single center. Liver Transpl 2005;11:152–60.

166. Hung PY, Chen CC, Chen WJ, et al. Long-term prognosis of patients with biliary atresia: a 25 year summary. J Pediatr Gastroenterol Nutr 2006;42:190–5.
167. Barshes NR, Lee TC, Balkrishnan R, et al. Orthotopic liver transplantation for bililary atresia: the US experience. Liver Transpl 2005;11:1193–200.
168. Zitelli BJ, Miller JW, Gartner J, et al. Changes in life-style after liver transplantation. Pediatrics 1988;82:173–80.
169. Hoofnagle JH. Biliary Atresia Research Consortium (BARC). Hepatology. 2004;39:891.
170. Lipsett PA, Pitt HA, Colombani PM, et al. Choledochal cyst disease: a changing pattern of presentation. Ann Surg 1994;220:644–52.
171. Stain SC, Guthrie CR, Yellin A, et al. Choledochal cyst in the adult. Ann Surg 1995;222:128–33.
172. Stringer MD, Dhawan A, Davenport M, et al. Choledochal cysts: lessons from a 20 year experience. Arch Dis Child 1995;73:528–31.
173. Todani T. Choledochal cysts and pancreatobiliary maljunction. In: Balistreri WF, Ohi R, Todani T, et al., eds. Hepatobiliary, pancreatic and splenic disease in children: medical and surgical management. Amsterdam: Elsevier Science, 1997:231–60.
174. Bancroft JD, Bucuvalas JC, Ryckman FC, et al. Antenatal diagnosis of choledochal cyst. J Pediatr Gastroenterol Nutr 1994;18:142–5.
175. De Matos V, Erlichman J, Russo PA, Haber BA. Does "cystic" biliary atresia represent a distinct clinical and etiological subgroup? A series of three cases. Pediatr Dev Pathol 2005;8:725–31.
176. Weyant MJ, Maluccio MA, Bertagnolli MM, et al. Choledochal cysts in adults: a report of two cases and review of the literature. Am J Gastroenterol 1998;93:2580–3.
177. Watanatittan S, Niramis R. Choledochal cyst: review of 74 pediatric cases. J Med Assoc Thai 1998;81:586–95.
178. Ando K, Miyano T, Kohno S, et al. Spontaneous perforation of choledochal cyst: a study of 13 cases. Eur J Pediatr Surg 1998;8:23–5.
179. Okada A, Nakamura T, Higaki J, et al. Congenital dilatation of the bile duct in 100 instances and its relationship with anolalous junction. Surg Gynecol Obstet 1990;171:291–8.
180. Kim WS, Kim IO, Yeon KM, et al. Choledochal cyst with or without biliary atresia in neonates and young infants: US differentiation. Radiology 1998;209:465–9.
181. Gallivan EK, Crombleholme TM, D'Alton ME. Early prenatal diagnosis of choledochal cyst. Prenat Diagn 1996;16:934–7.
182. Benhidjeb T, Chaoui R, Kalache K, et al. Prenatal diagnosis of a choledochal cyst: a case report and review of the literature. Am J Perinatol 1996;13:207–10.
183. Hamada Y, Tanano A, Sato M, et al. Rapid enlargement of a choledochal cyst: antenatal diagnosis and delayed primary excision. Pediatr Surg Int 1998;13:419–21.
184. Redkar R, Davenport M, Howard ER. Antenatal diagnosis of congenital anomalies of the biliary tract. J Pediatr Surg 1998;33:700–4.
185. Yamataka A, Ohshiro K, Okada Y, et al. Complications after cyst excision with hepaticoenterostomy for choledochal cysts and their surgical management in children versus adults. J Pediatr Surg 1997;32:1097–102.
186. Miyano T, Yamataka A, Kato Y, et al. Hepaticoenterostomy after excision of choledochal cyst in children: a 30-year experience with 180 cases. J Pediatr Surg 1996;31:1417–21.
187. Saing H, Han H, Chan KL, et al. Early and late results of excision of choledochal cysts. J Pediatr Surg 1997;32:1563–6.
188. Chaudhary A, Dhar P, Sachdev A. Reoperative surgery for choledochal cysts. Br J Surg 1997;84:781–4.
189. Chen HM, Jan YY, Chen MF, et al. Surgical treatment of choledochal cyst in adults: results and long-term follow-up. Hepatogastroenterology 1996;43:1492–9.
190. Lilly JR. The surgical treatment of choledochal cyst. Surg Gynecol Obstet 1979;149:36–42.
191. Fonkalsrud EW, Boles T. Choledochal cysts in infancy and childhood. Surg Gynecol Obstet 1965;121:733.
192. Watanabe Y, Toki A, Todani T. Bile duct cancer developed after cyst excision for choledochal cyst. J Hepatobiliary Pancreat Surg 1999;6:207–12.
193. Bismuth H, Krissat J. Choledochal cystic malignancies. Ann Oncol 1999;10(suppl 4):94–8.
194. Chilukuri S, Bonet V, Cobb M. Antenatal spontatneous perforation of the extrahepatic biliary tree. Am J Obstet Gynecol 1990;163:1201–2.
195. Haller JO, Condon VR, Berdon WE, et al. Spontaneous perforation of the common bile duct in children. Radiology 1989;172:621–4.
196. Hammoudi SM, Alauddin A. Idiopathic perforation of the biliary tract in infancy and childhood. J Pediatr Surg 1988;23:185–7.
197. Johnston JH. Spontaneous perforation of the common bile duct in infancy. Br J Surg 1961;48:532.
198. So SKS, Lindahl JA, Sharp HL, et al. Bile ascites during infancy: diagnosis using disofenin Tc 99m sequential scintiphotography. Pediatrics 1983;71:402.

13

Neonatal Jaundice and Disorders of Bilirubin Metabolism

Glenn R. Gourley, M.D.

Elevation of the serum bilirubin level is a common if not universal finding during the first week of life. This can be a transient phenomenon that will resolve spontaneously. Alternatively, hyperbilirubinemia may signify a serious or even potentially life-threatening condition. There are many causes of hyperbilirubinemia, and each has its own therapeutic and prognostic implications. Independent of the cause, elevated serum bilirubin levels may be potentially toxic to the newborn infant. This chapter begins with a review of perinatal bilirubin metabolism. Assessment, etiology, toxicity, and therapy for neonatal jaundice are then addressed. Finally, the diseases in which there is a primary disorder in the metabolism of bilirubin are reviewed regarding their clinical presentation, pathophysiology, diagnosis, and treatment. Other pertinent reviews have been published [1–3].

BILIRUBIN METABOLISM

Production and Circulation

In 1864, Städeler [4] used the term *bilirubin*, derived from Latin (*bilis*, "bile"; *ruber*, "red"), for the red-colored bile pigment. Bilirubin is formed from the degradation of heme-containing compounds (Figure 13.1). The largest source for the production of bilirubin is hemoglobin. However, other heme-containing proteins are also degraded to bilirubin, including the cytochromes, catalases, tryptophan pyrrolase, and muscle myoglobin [5].

The formation of bilirubin is initiated by cleaving the tetrapyrrole ring of protoheme (protoporphyrin IX), which results in a linear tetrapyrrole (biliverdin). The first enzyme system involved in the formation of bilirubin is microsomal heme oxygenase (HO). Two major forms of HO have been identified [6]. HO1, the inducible form, is located in the spleen and liver. HO2, the constitutive form, is located in brain, testes, and pancreatic islets [7,8]. HO results in reduction of the porphyrin iron (Fe^{III} to Fe^{II}) and hydroxylation of the α methine ($=$C$-$) carbon. This α carbon is then oxidatively excised from the tetrapyrrole ring, yielding carbon monoxide (CO). This excision opens the ring structure and is associated with oxygenation of the two carbons adjacent to the site of cleavage. The cleaved α carbon is excreted as CO, which also functions as a neurotransmitter [9,10]. The iron released by HO can be reutilized by the body. The resultant linear tetrapyrrole is biliverdin IXα. The *IX* designation is a result of Fischer's grouping the protoporphyrin isomers, group IX being the physiologic source of bilirubin [11]. The stereospecificity of the enzyme produces cleavage almost exclusively at the α carbon of the tetrapyrrole. This is unlike in vitro chemical oxidation, which results in cleavage at any of the four carbons (α, β, γ, and δ; see Figure 13.1, structure 1) linking the four pyrrole rings and produces equimolar amounts of the α, β, γ, and δ isomers [12]. In utero, bilirubin IXβ is the first bile pigment seen and can be found in bile or meconium by 15 weeks' gestation [13]. Small amounts of bilirubin IXβ are also found in adult human bile [14]. The central carbon (C-10) on biliverdin IXα is then reduced from a methine to a methylene group ($-CH_2-$), thus forming bilirubin IXα. This is accomplished by the cytosolic enzyme biliverdin reductase [15]. The proximity of this enzyme results in very little biliverdin ever being present in the circulation. Bilirubin formation can be assessed by measurement of carbon monoxide production [16,17]. Such assessments indicate that the daily production rate of bilirubin is 6–8 mg/kg/24 hr in healthy term infants and 3–4 mg/kg/24 hr in healthy adults [18,19]. In mammals, approximately 80% of bilirubin produced daily originates from hemoglobin [20–23]. Degradation of hepatic and renal heme appears to account for most of the remaining 20%, reflecting the very rapid turnover of certain of these heme proteins. Although the precise fate of myoglobin heme is unknown, its turnover appears to be so slow as to be relatively insignificant [24]. Catabolism of hemoglobin occurs very largely from the sequestration of erythrocytes at the end of their life span (120 days in adult humans, 90 days in newborns, 50–60 days in rats). A small fraction of newly synthesized hemoglobin is degraded in the bone marrow. This process, termed *ineffective erythropoiesis*, normally represents less than 3% of daily bilirubin production but may be substantially increased in persons with hemoglobinopathies, vitamin deficiencies, and heavy metal intoxication [25–27]. Infants produce more bilirubin per unit body weight because red blood cell (RBC) mass is greater and RBC life span is shorter in infants.

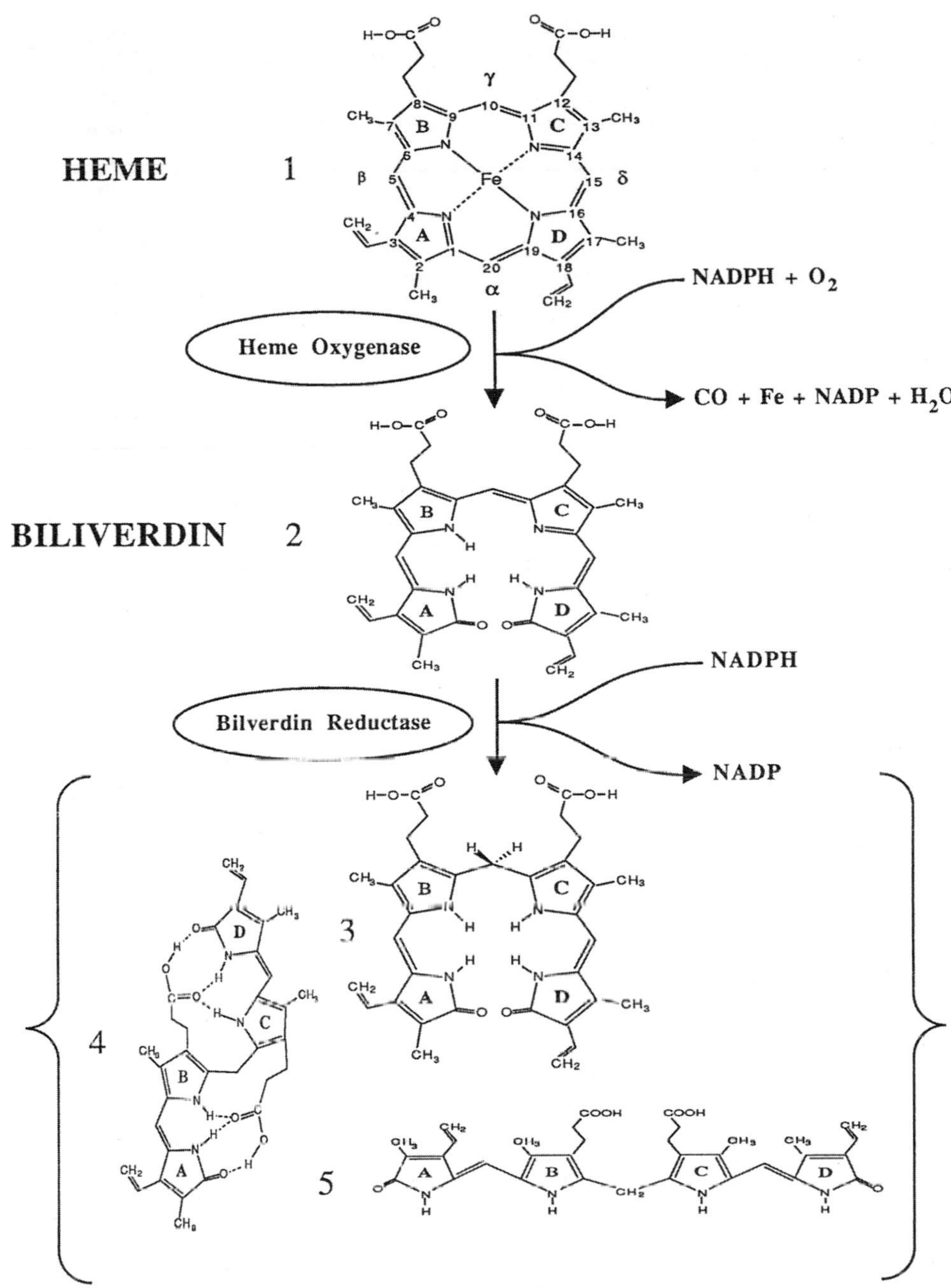

Figure 13.1. Chemical structures depicting the conversion of heme to bilirubin. Bilirubin is frequently represented by any of the three structures (3–5) shown at the bottom. NADP, nicotinamide adenine dinucleotide phosphate; NADPH, NADP oxidase.

Additionally, hepatic heme proteins represent a larger fraction of total body weight in infants. Although bilirubin has long been thought of solely as a waste product of heme catabolism, there are data to suggest that some mild degree of hyperbilirubinemia may be helpful because of the antioxidant capacity of bilirubin and its potential role as a free radical scavenger and cytoprotectant [28].

Bilirubin is poorly soluble in aqueous solvents and thus requires biotransformation to more water-soluble derivatives for excretion from the body. This poor solubility is related to the structure of bilirubin [29]. Rather than being linear (structure 5, Figure 13.1), bilirubin undergoes extensive internal hydrogen bonding (structure 4, Figure 13.1). This occurs because the saturated middle carbon (C-10) permits the two halves of the bilirubin molecule to rotate such that the pyrrole nitrogens and lactam oxygen of one half form hydrogen bonds with the carboxyl groups of the propionic acid side chain on the other half. This shields the polar propionic acid side chains and makes bilirubin very nonpolar and lipophilic. The carbon–carbon double bonds at positions 4–5 and 15–16 can assume two different configurations (similar to "cis" and "trans") depending on whether the higher priority atoms or groups (based on atomic number) are on the same (Z, *zusammen*; German, "together") or opposite (E, *entgegen*; German, "opposite") sides of the double bond. The naturally occurring form of bilirubin, 4Z,15Z-bilirubin IXα, can be represented by any of the three structures (3–5) depicted at the bottom of Figure 13.1. Knowledge of this stereochemistry is important in understanding phototherapy, which will be discussed later. The internal hydrogen bonding of bilirubin makes the molecule very hydrophobic and insoluble in aqueous media.

This poor aqueous solubility makes a carrier molecule necessary for bilirubin transport from its sites of production in the reticuloendothelial system to the liver for excretion (Figure 13.2). Albumin is this carrier [30]. Each albumin molecule possesses a single high-affinity ($K_a = 7 \times 10^7$ M^{-1}) binding site for one molecule of bilirubin [31]. A binding affinity of this magnitude implies that, at normal serum bilirubin levels, all bilirubin will be transported to the liver bound to albumin, with negligible amounts free to diffuse into other tissues. Secondary binding sites of lesser affinity also exist on albumin. Albumin also serves as a carrier for other compounds, such as xenobiotics and fatty acids. It is important to remember that albumin from each animal species has different binding characteristics for various ligands [32].

Hepatocyte Uptake

The structure of the liver is well suited for the uptake of bilirubin by individual hepatocytes. Cords of hepatocytes are arranged radially so that adjacent sinusoids border all hepatocytes. The flow of blood through the sinusoids is slower than that of other capillary beds because it is generated by portal venous pressure rather than arterial pressure. There is easy passage of albumin-bound bilirubin from the plasma into the tissue fluid space (space of Disse) between the endothelium and the hepatocyte. This is so because the sinusoidal endothelium of the liver lacks the basal laminae that are found in other organ capillary systems [33,34]. The pores of the endothelium allow direct contact with the plasma membrane of the hepatocyte.

A hepatocyte with a schematic illustration of bilirubin metabolism is shown in Figure 13.2. In the first step, bilirubin dissociates from its albumin carrier [35] and enters the hepatocyte via a membrane receptor-carrier that facilitates entry into the hepatocyte. Carrier-mediated transport into the hepatocyte has been demonstrated for several organic anions, including bilirubin, bromsulfophthalein (BSP), and indocyanine green (ICG) [36], though bilirubin has been shown to be able to pass through membranes by simple passive diffusion [37]. Evidence suggests that bilirubin, BSP, and ICG share the same hepatocyte receptor-carrier because they exhibit competitive inhibition when injected simultaneously. This finding cannot be explained by subsequent intrahepatic metabolism because these anions are handled differently by the hepatocyte: bilirubin is conjugated with glucuronic acid in the endoplasmic reticulum (ER), BSP is conjugated with glutathione in the cytosol, and ICG is excreted directly, without biotransformation. Data from rat hepatocytes suggest that the anion-binding receptor-carrier is a dimeric protein with a subunit molecular weight of 55,000 daltons [38–40]. Antibody studies confirm the expected location in the plasma membrane [39] and demonstrate blocking of uptake [40]. Organic anion transporting polypeptide 2 (OATP2) has shown high-affinity uptake of bilirubin in the presence of albumin and is a member of the OATP family, transporter symbol SLC21 A [41,42].

Carrier-mediated transport of bilirubin into the hepatocyte is necessary because of differences in protein binding inside and outside the hepatocyte. Outside the hepatocyte, bilirubin is bound to albumin (affinity constant, $\sim 10^8$; concentration, 0.6 mM) [31]. Inside the hepatocyte, bilirubin is bound to glutathione S-transferase B (GST), historically known as ligandin or the Y protein (affinity constant, $\sim 10^6$; concentration, 0.04 mM) [43,44]. GST constitutes a family of proteins that exhibit important functions both as enzymes and as intracellular binding proteins for nonsubstrate ligands such as bilirubin [45]. Carrier-mediated uptake helps generate a concentration gradient for bilirubin uptake despite the difference in affinity between albumin and GST. GST is important in the intracellular storage of bilirubin and bilirubin conjugates and reduces efflux from the hepatocyte back into plasma [44].

Conjugation

Inside the hepatocyte, bilirubin is conjugated with glucuronic acid [46]. This process occurs in the endoplasmic reticulum (ER, microsomes). The glucuronic acid donor is uridine diphosphate glucuronic acid (UDPGA). The conjugation results in an ester linkage formed with either or both of the propionic acid side chains on the B and C pyrrole rings of bilirubin (Figure 13.3). The enzyme responsible for this esterification is bilirubin UDP-glucuronosyltransferase (BUGT; Online Mendelian Inheritance in Man [OMIM] *191740). BUGT is distinct from the other glucuronosyltransferase isoforms that catalyze the conjugation of thyroxine, steroids, bile acids, and xenobiotics [47–51]. BUGT is embedded in the lipid environment of the microsomal membrane, and perturbations of this environment greatly affect in vitro measurements of BUGT activity. Because BUGT is located on the interior of the ER, the existence of a permease has been hypothesized to facilitate the transport of UDPGA from the cytosol across the lipid layers of the ER. The permease has been proposed because uridine diphosphate glucose (UDPG) is present in the cytosol in higher concentrations, yet UDPGA serves as the preferred donor for bilirubin conjugation [52]. Uridine diphosphate *N*-acetylglucosamine (UDPNAG) is considered to be a natural regulator of BUGT [53] because UDPNAG can increase in vitro BUGT activity threefold. The mechanism for this is unknown and could possibly involve facilitation of the permease UDPGA transporter [54]. After providing glucuronic acid for conjugation, UDP can be converted to uridine and inorganic pyrophosphate by a nucleoside diphosphatase (NDPase), which is also located on the interior of the ER [55] and prevents the reverse reaction.

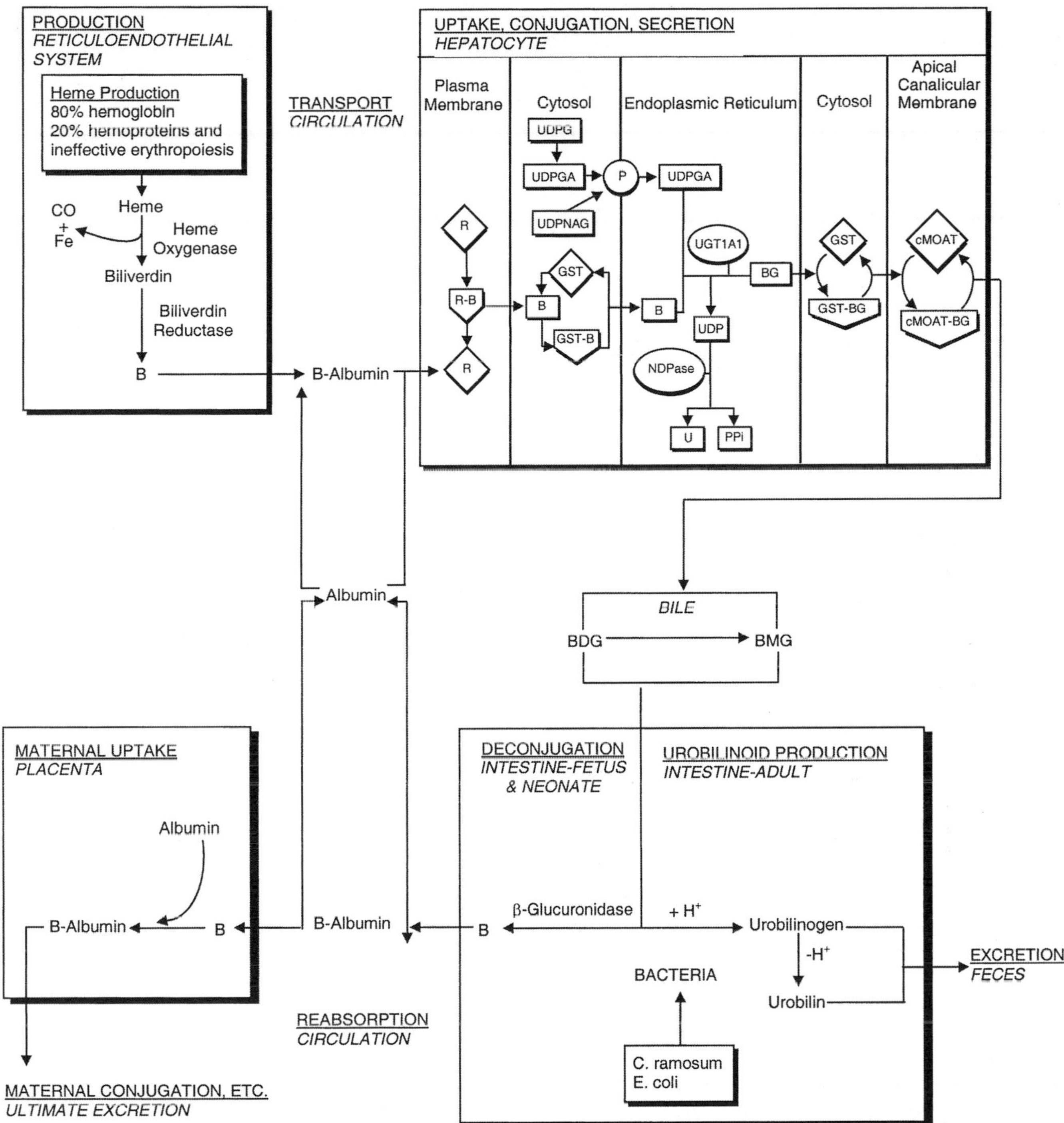

Figure 13.2. A schematic overview of bilirubin (B) metabolism in the fetus, neonate, and adult. R, membrane carrier; GST, glutathione S-transferase (ligandin); UDPG, uridine diphosphate glucose; UDPGA, uridine diphosphate glucuronic acid; UDPNAG, uridine diphosphate *N*-acetylglucosamine; P, permease; UGT1A1, bilirubin glucuronosyltransferase; NDPase, nucleoside diphosphatase; PPi, inorganic pyrophosphate; BDG/BMG, bilirubin di- or monoglucuronide; cMOAT, canalicular multispecific organic anion transporter (also known as MRP2 or ABCC2); BG, bilirubin glucuronide.

The specific isoform responsible for bilirubin conjugation is UGT1A1 (trivial name, HUG-Br1; EC 2.4.1.17) [56]. This is part of the UDP-glycosyltransferase superfamily of enzymes encoded by the *UGT* gene complex on chromosome 2 [57] that is involved with metabolism of many xenobiotic and endogenous substances. The *UGT1* gene encodes several isoforms and has a complex structure consisting of four common exons (2–5) and 13 variable exons encoding different isoforms (Figure 13.4) [58,59]. At least 30 different *UGT1* mutant alleles have been described that cause Gilbert's syndrome (GS) and

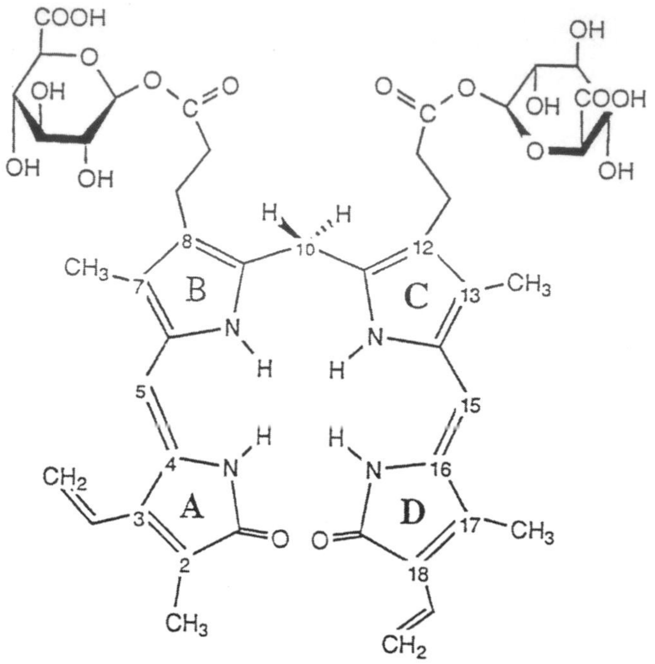

Figure 13.3. Bilirubin diglucuronide. In bilirubin monoglucuronide, only one propionic acid side chain (C-8 or C-12) is glucuronidated.

Crigler–Najjar syndromes I (CNI) and II (CNII) [60]. UGT1A1 catalyzes the formation of both bilirubin mono- and diglucuronides [61–65] but also metabolizes other hormones and drugs, so mutations may be involved in carcinogenesis and adverse drug reactions [66]. In normal adult humans, the majority of bilirubin conjugates are excreted in the bile as bilirubin diglucuronides (~80%) [67–72] (Figure 13.5, *middle panel*). Lesser amounts of bilirubin monoglucuronides (~15%) are also excreted along with very small amounts of unconjugated bilirubin and other bilirubin conjugates (e.g., glucose, xylose, and mixed diesters). In infants, because there is lower UGT1A1 activity, bile contains less bilirubin diglucuronide and more bilirubin monoglucuronide than that of the adult (Figure 13.6, *middle panel*).

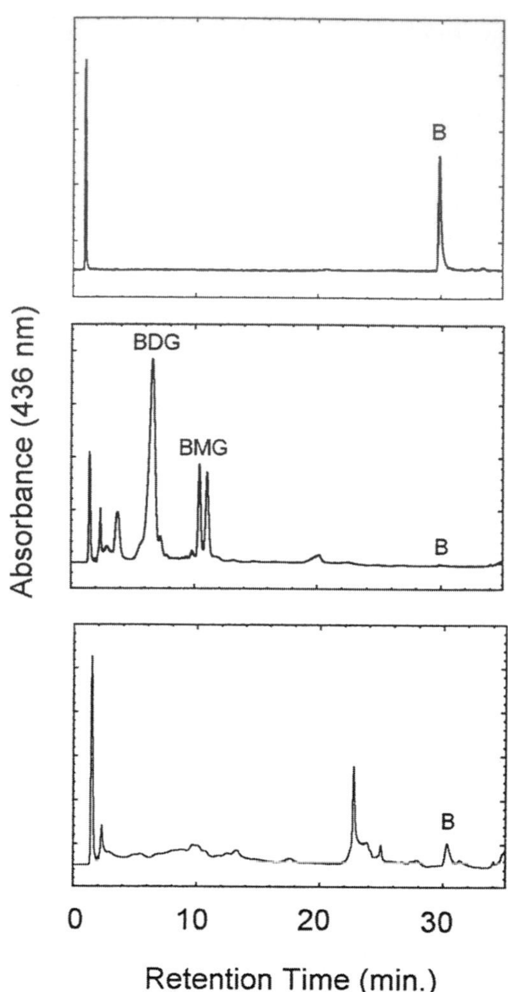

Figure 13.5. Bile pigment excretion in the adult human as assessed by high-performance liquid chromatography. Chromatograms represent analysis of serum (20 μL, *top*), duodenal bile (20 μL, *middle*), and stool extract (equivalent to 50 mg of wet stool, *bottom*) from a normal man. Scale of *y*-axes varies. Serum bile pigments are almost all bilirubin. The bilirubin di- and monoglucuronides (BDG, BMG) that predominate in adult bile are not present in adult feces because of metabolism by intestinal bacteria.

Secretion of Bilirubin Conjugates

Following conjugation, bilirubin conjugates are excreted against a concentration gradient from the hepatocyte through the canalicular membrane into the bile. Data from purified canalicular membrane vesicles of rat liver suggest that bilirubin diglucuronide transport through the canalicular membrane is carrier mediated, electrogenic, and stimulated by HCO_3^-

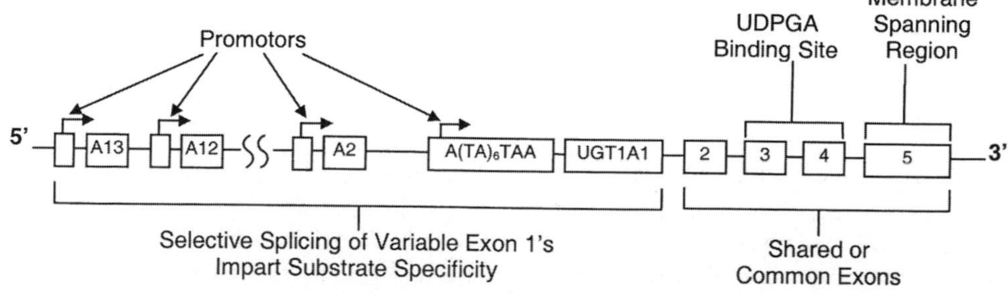

Figure 13.4. The human uridine diphosphate glucuronosyltransferase 1 gene (*UGT1*).

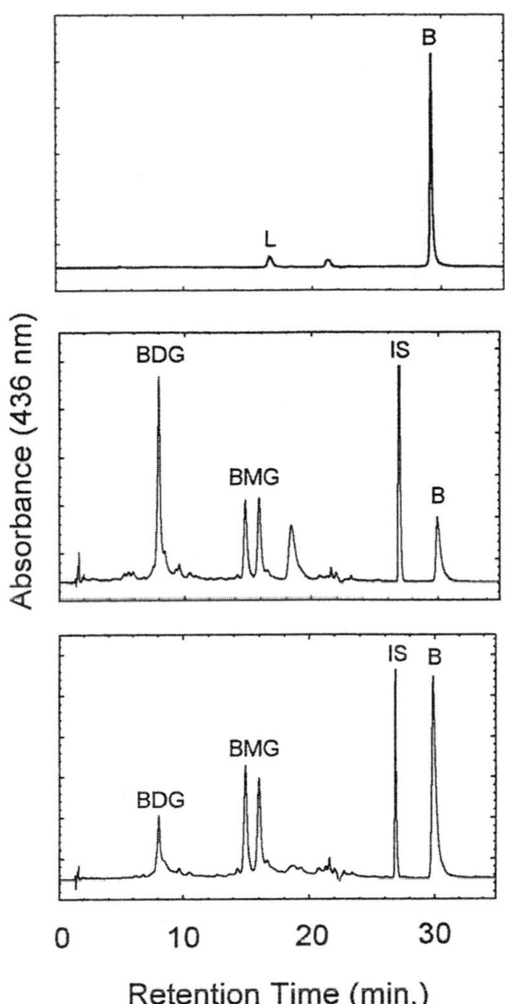

Figure 13.6. Bile pigment excretion in the newborn human as assessed by high-performance liquid chromatography. Chromatograms represent analysis of serum (20 μL, *top*) of an infant receiving phototherapy in the first week of life and duodenal bile (20 μl, *middle*) and stool extract (equivalent to 50 mg of wet stool, *bottom*) from a normal full-term, formula-fed female infant on day 3 of life. Serum bile pigments include lumirubin (L). Scale of *y*-axes varies. Neonates lack an intestinal bacterial flora, hence large quantities of bilirubin di- and monoglucuronides (BDG, BMG) and bilirubin (B) are present in feces.

[73]. Similar data also suggest that bilirubin glucuronides are transported across the canalicular membrane by both adenosine triphosphate (ATP)-dependent and membrane potential–dependent transport systems and that in the normal rat, these systems are additive [74]. The ATP-dependent transporter responsible for bilirubin glucuronide passage from the hepatocyte through the canalicular membrane is canalicular multispecific organic anion transporter (cMOAT). cMOAT is a member of the ATP-binding cassette (ABC) transporter superfamily and is homologous to the multidrug resistance–related protein (MRP2) [75,76] and is also known as ABCC2 because it is encoded by the *ABCC2* gene [77]. cMOAT/MRP2/ABCC2 is involved with ATP-dependent transport across the apical canalicular membrane of a variety of endogenous compounds and xenobiotics [78], including both bilirubin mono- and diglucuronides [79]. cMOAT has previously been described as the non-bile acid organic anion transporter, the glutathione S-conjugate export pump, or the leukotriene export pump [80]. Genetic mutations that alter these ABC transporters cause diseases that include cystic fibrosis, hyperinsulinemia, adrenoleukodystrophy, multidrug resistance [81] and, as discussed later in this chapter, Dubin–Johnson syndrome (DJS). This mechanism can be saturated with increasing amounts of bilirubin or bilirubin conjugates [82–84]. Many other organic anions (e.g., BSP, ICG) share this same canalicular membrane excretion mechanism [85]. Simultaneous infusions of BSP and ICG will decrease the maximal canalicular excretion of bilirubin, and vice versa [86,87]. The canalicular excretion mechanism for bilirubin and BSP is different from that of bile salts. Biliary excretion of conjugated bilirubin and BSP is decreased in individuals with DJS [88], though bile salt excretion is not impaired. However, bile salt and bilirubin conjugate excretion by the canalicular membrane is not completely independent because infusion of bile salts does increase the maximal excretion of bilirubin conjugates [89]. A similar effect is seen with phenobarbital [90]. Conversely, the maximal excretion of bilirubin conjugates can be decreased by cholestatic agents like estrogens and anabolic steroids [91,92].

Under normal conditions, there is evidence that bilirubin conjugates equilibrate across the sinusoidal membrane of hepatocytes [93–95]. This results in small amounts of bilirubin conjugates being present in the systemic circulation. If there is diminished hepatic glucuronidation of bilirubin (e.g., in the neonate), there will be a decreased amount of bilirubin conjugates present in the serum [93,94,96]. Data show that in full-term newborns, there is an increase in the serum level of bilirubin diconjugates (0.55 $\pm$ 0.25% on days 2–4 to 1.62 $\pm$ 0.99% on days 9–13) that is consistent with the maturation of bilirubin glucuronidation [97]. In contrast, in premature infants less than 33 weeks' gestation, bilirubin diconjugates are very low and remain so, suggesting a more severe immaturity of the glucuronidation process.

In many pathologic circumstances, bilirubin mono- and diglucuronides are not excreted from the hepatocyte fast enough to prevent significant reflux back into the circulation. The resulting elevation of serum bilirubin conjugate levels results in the transesterification of bilirubin glucuronide with an amino group on albumin, producing a covalent bond between albumin and bilirubin [98]. This product is formed spontaneously and is known as delta bilirubin or bilirubin-albumin [99]. Similar nonenzymatic reactions have been demonstrated between albumin and various drugs [98,100–102]. Delta bilirubin is not formed in hyperbilirubinemic conditions unless there is elevation of the conjugated bilirubin fraction. Both delta bilirubin and bilirubin conjugates are direct reacting, which explains a situation that has long confounded clinicians. The direct bilirubin may continue to be elevated in patients who otherwise are recovering from a hepatic insult because the delta

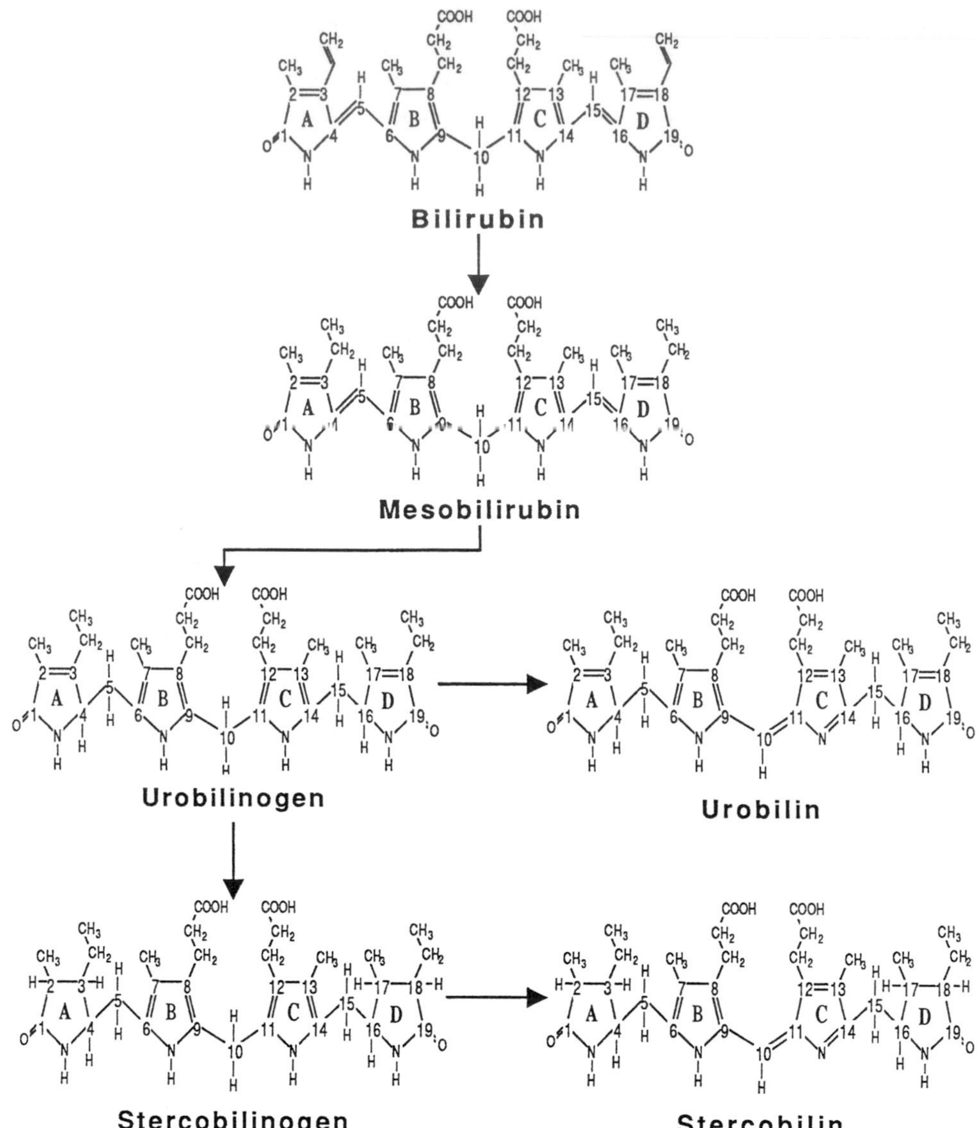

Figure 13.7. The reduction and oxidation of bilirubin to a family of related compounds known collectively as urobilinoids. Only several examples are given of this much larger family.

bilirubin formed lingers because of the long (~20 day [103]) half-life of albumin.

Enterohepatic Circulation

When bilirubin conjugates enter the intestinal lumen (see Figure 13.2), several possibilities for further metabolism arise. In adults, the normal bacterial flora hydrogenates various carbon double bonds in bilirubin to produce assorted urobilinogens (Figure 13.7). Subsequent oxidation of the middle carbon (C-10) produces the related urobilins. Because there are a large number of unsaturated bonds in bilirubin, there are many compounds formed by reduction and oxidation of these bonds. This large family of related reduction–oxidation products of bilirubin is known as urobilinoids [104] and excreted in the feces. The most important bacterium for the production of urobilinoids is *Clostridium ramosum* [105], and synergy has been demonstrated with *Escherichia coli* [106]. The conversion of bilirubin conjugates to urobilinoids is important because it blocks the intestinal absorption of bilirubin, known as the enterohepatic circulation [107,108]. Neonates lack an intestinal bacterial flora and are more likely to absorb bilirubin from the intestine. This difference in bile pigment excretion between adults and neonates is demonstrated by comparing Figures 13.5 and 13.6 (*lower panels*).

Bilirubin conjugates in the intestine may also act as substrate for either bacterial [109–111] or endogenous tissue [112] β-glucuronidase. This enzyme hydrolyzes glucuronic acid from bilirubin glucuronides. The unconjugated bilirubin produced is more rapidly absorbed from the intestine [113]. In the fetus, tissue β-glucuronidase is detectable by 12 weeks' gestation and is believed to play an important role in facilitating intestinal bilirubin absorption that enables bilirubin to be cleared via the placenta. Following birth, increased intestinal β-glucuronidase can increase the neonate's likelihood of experiencing higher serum bilirubin levels [114]. The ability of endogenous tissue β-glucuronidase to deconjugate bilirubin glucuronides has been demonstrated in germ-free animals [115]. Breast milk may contain high levels of β-glucuronidase, and it has been suggested that this is one factor related to the higher jaundice levels seen in breast-fed infants [116]. Feeding specific nutritional ingredients that inhibit β-glucuronidase, such as L-aspartic acid [117], has been shown to result in increased fecal bilirubin excretion and lower levels of jaundice [118].

JAUNDICE ASSESSMENT

Jaundice and *icterus* both refer to the yellow discoloration of the tissues (skin, sclerae, etc.) caused by deposition of bilirubin. *Jaundice* originates from the French *jaune*, which means "yellow." *Icterus* is derived from the Greek word for jaundice (*ikteros*). Jaundice is a sign that hyperbilirubinemia exists (i.e., total serum bilirubin $>\sim 1.4$ mg/dL after 6 months of age; 1 mg/dL = 17 μmol/L). The degree of yellow is directly related to the level of serum bilirubin and the related amount of bilirubin deposition into the extravascular tissues. Hypercarotenemia may impart a yellow hue to the skin, but the sclerae remain white. There are many conditions associated with neonatal jaundice. Some of these states are so commonly recognized as to be termed "physiologic." Alternatively, jaundice may be a sign of severe hemolysis, infection, or liver failure.

Measurement of the total serum bilirubin concentration allows quantitation of jaundice. Such measurements are very common in the newborn nursery and in one study, were made at least once in 61% of term newborn infants [119]. Two components of total serum bilirubin can be routinely measured in the clinical laboratory: conjugated bilirubin ("direct" reacting because in van den Bergh's test, color development takes place directly without adding methanol) and unconjugated bilirubin ("indirect" fraction). Although the terms *direct* and *indirect* are used equivalently with conjugated and unconjugated bilirubin, it is now known that this is not quantitatively correct because the direct fraction includes both conjugated bilirubin and delta bilirubin [120]. Elevation of either of these fractions can result in jaundice. There is a long history of undesirable variability in the measurement of serum bilirubin fractions [121]. The automated laboratory methods now used to measure serum bilirubin have been reviewed elsewhere [120,122–124]. The Jendrassik–Grof procedure is the method of choice for total bilirubin measurement, though this method also has problems [125]. When the total serum bilirubin level is high, factitious elevation of the direct fraction has been reported [126].

Three newer methods have been developed that can more accurately determine the various bilirubin fractions (unconjugated, monoconjugated, diconjugated, and albumin bound or delta): high-performance liquid chromatography (HPLC) [127], multilayered slides [128,129], and use of bilirubin oxidase [130]. HPLC analysis is superior but too expensive and time consuming for the clinical laboratory [120]. HPLC analysis of serum from normal human neonates in the first 4 days of life [131] showed that unconjugated and conjugated bilirubin levels rose in parallel, with the conjugated fraction making up only 1.2–1.6% of total pigment (3.6% in adults). Although the absolute concentration of conjugates was two to six times higher in neonates, only 20% were diconjugates (54% in adults). These sensitive HPLC data are consistent with the increased bilirubin production and relatively deficient glucuronidation seen in the neonate. Analysis with automated multilayered slide technology (Vitros; Johnson & Johnson) is currently available and in use in some clinical laboratories. This allows measurement of specific conjugated and unconjugated bilirubin fractions without inclusion of delta bilirubin. The conjugated bilirubin measurement is an earlier indicator of relief from biliary cholestasis than is direct bilirubin because of the long half-life of delta bilirubin [132]. A comparison of the bilirubin oxidase method concluded that determinations of total bilirubin in neonatal serum were not advanced by this method [133].

There are conflicting data regarding the accuracy of capillary versus venous serum bilirubin levels [134,135]. However, as Maisels [136] has pointed out, the literature regarding kernicterus, phototherapy, and exchange transfusion is based on bilirubin measurements in capillary samples.

Noninvasive methods to measure jaundice levels also exist and have been shown to be particularly useful in neonates. Current commercially available methods available include the BiliCheck (Respironics, Pittsburgh, PA) [137,138] and the Minolta/Hill-Rom Air-Shields Transcutaneous Jaundice Meter 103 (Air Shields, Hatboro, PA) [139]. The device is touched to the skin in a painless manner, with the immediate resulting point-of-care measurement of transcutaneous bilirubin that correlates highly with transcutaneous serum bilirubin (TSB). Some suggest that the yellow color of the skin is a better risk indicator of bilirubin-dependent brain damage than is the serum bilirubin level [140]. A less technical method to quantitate jaundice that uses a Plexiglas color chart pressed against the baby's nose (Ingram icterometer; Thos. A. Ingram and Co. Ltd, Birmingham, UK) has been found to be useful in assessing jaundice [141,142] and much less expensive [143].

NEONATAL JAUNDICE

In general, infants are not jaundiced at the moment of birth, even if significant hemolysis existed in utero. This is because of the impressive ability of the placenta to clear bilirubin from the fetal circulation. However, within the next few days, most if not all infants will develop elevated serum bilirubin levels (>1.4 mg/dL). As the serum bilirubin rises, the skin becomes more jaundiced in a cephalocaudal manner [144]. Icterus is first observed in the head and progresses caudally to the palms and soles. Kramer [145] found the following serum indirect bilirubin levels as jaundice progressed: head and neck, 4–8 mg/dL;

upper trunk, 5–12 mg/dL; lower trunk and thighs, 8–16 mg/dL; arms and lower legs, 11–18 mg/dL; and palms and soles, greater than 15 mg/dL [145]. Hence, when the bilirubin was greater than 15 mg/dL, the entire body was icteric. However, darker skin tones may make jaundice difficult to estimate visually [146]. Jaundice is best observed by blanching the skin with gentle digital pressure under well-illuminated (white light) conditions. At least one third of infants develop visible jaundice. A combined analysis of several large studies involving thousands of infants during the first week of life showed that moderate jaundice (bilirubin >12 mg/dL) occurs in at least 12% of breast-fed infants and 4% of formula-fed infants whereas severe jaundice (>15 mg/dL) occurs in 2% and 0.3% of these respective feeding groups [147].

In recent years, changes in perinatal care have made severe neonatal jaundice a larger problem and there has been a reemergence of kernicterus [148–150]. Possible reasons for this include [150,151] (a) early hospital discharge (before the extent of jaundice is known and signs of impending brain damage have appeared) [152]; (b) lack of adequate concern for the risks of severe jaundice in healthy term and near-term newborns [149]; (c) an increase in breast-feeding [153]; (d) medical care cost constraints; (e) paucity of educational materials to enable parents to participate in safeguarding their newborns; (f) limitations within health care systems to monitor the outpatient progression of jaundice [154]; (g) difficulty in estimating the degree of jaundice, particularly in dark-skinned infants [155]; and (h) demonstration of bilirubin being an antioxidant [28]. Newborn infants are now being described who are discharged early, develop severe hyperbilirubinemia (30–40 mg/dL) at home, and go on to develop classic signs of kernicterus [1,146,149,156–159]. This has been reported in otherwise healthy breast-fed infants with no other identified etiology for their jaundice [160–162]. Although early postpartum discharge has advantages, one disadvantage is the risk associated with delayed diagnosis of severe hyperbilirubinemia. The American Academy of Pediatrics (AAP) has recommended that infants discharged at less than 48 hours of age be seen in follow-up within 48 hours of discharge [163]. Many physicians do not follow these recommendations [146,164] despite the serious impact that a short hospital stay has on the jaundiced newborn [165]. The AAP updated their 1994 guidelines [166] for the management of hyperbilirubinemia in newborn infants in 2004 [146].

Jaundice may be caused by increased bilirubin production, decreased bilirubin excretion, or combinations of these mechanisms (see Table 13.1 for specific examples). Figure 13.8 presents one possible clinical approach to assess these diagnoses. An approach to management of jaundice in the newborn nursery has been published elsewhere [146]. Although Newman et al. [167] found that obtaining a direct bilirubin measurement was seldom helpful because of low yield and poor specificity, others advocate measurement of an early conjugated bilirubin as a population screening test that could lead to the earlier diagnosis of neonatal liver disease [168]. Bhutani et al. [169,170] advocated universal bilirubin measurement before hospital discharge to identify infants at risk for severe neonatal hyperbilirubinemia on the basis of a predischarge hour-specific total serum bilirubin measurement (Figure 13.9). This universal predischarge screening is now recommended by the AAP [146]. Despite the large number of etiologies for neonatal jaundice, no cause for the jaundice could be identified in nearly half the infants evaluated during one study of 447 infants [119] and in one third of the infants in a kernicterus registry [162].

Table 13.1: Causes of Neonatal Hyperbilirubinemia

Increased production of bilirubin
Fetal–maternal blood group incompatibilities
Extravascular blood in body tissues
Polycythemia
Red blood cell abnormalities (hemoglobinopathies, membrane and enzyme defects)
Induction of labor
Decreased excretion of bilirubin
Increased enterohepatic circulation of bilirubin
Breast-feeding
Inborn errors of metabolism
Hormones and drugs
Prematurity
Hepatic hypoperfusion
Cholestatic syndromes
Obstruction of the biliary tree
Combined increased production and decreased excretion of bilirubin
Sepsis
Intrauterine infection
Congenital cirrhosis

The term *physiologic jaundice* has been used to describe the frequently observed jaundice in otherwise completely normal neonates. However, physiologic jaundice is merely the result of a number of factors involving increased bilirubin production and decreased excretion. Jaundice should always be considered a sign of possible disease and not routinely explained as physiologic. Specific characteristics of neonatal jaundice to be considered abnormal until proven otherwise include (1) development before 36 hours of age, (2) persistence beyond 10 days of age, (3) serum bilirubin greater than 12 mg/dL at any time, and (4) elevation of the direct reacting fraction of bilirubin (>2 mg/dL or 30% of the total serum bilirubin) at any time.

There are a number of epidemiologic risk factors related to neonatal jaundice that have been reviewed elsewhere [146,171–174]. Some of the factors associated with increased neonatal bilirubin levels are male sex, low birth weight, prematurity, certain races (Asian, American Indian, Greek), maternal medications (e.g., oxytocin, promethazine hydrochloride), premature rupture of the membranes, increased weight loss after birth, delayed meconium passage, breast-feeding, and neonatal infection. Delivery with the vacuum extractor increases the risk

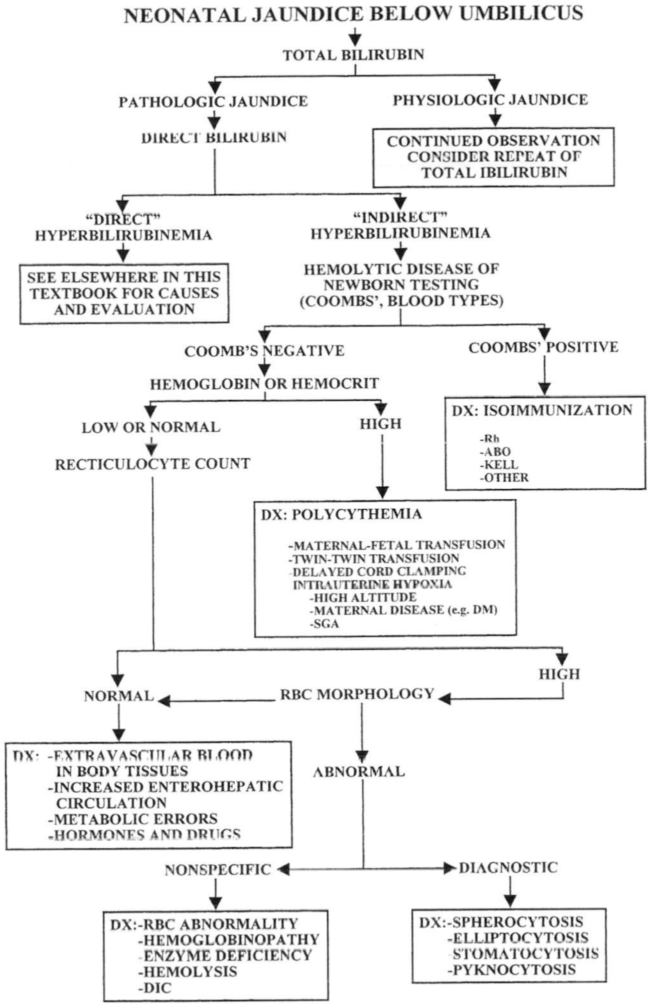

Figure 13.8. One possible approach to the clinical evaluation of neonatal jaundice. DIC, disseminated intravascular coagulation; SGA, small for gestational age.

of cephalohematoma and neonatal jaundice [175]. Data suggest that pancuronium is associated with an increased risk of hyperbilirubinemia [176]. There is a close correlation between umbilical cord serum bilirubin level and subsequent hyperbilirubinemia [177,178]. Maternal serum bilirubin level at the time of delivery and transplacental bilirubin gradient also correlate positively with neonatal serum bilirubin concentrations [178]. Other factors are associated with decreased neonatal bilirubin levels [146,179] and include black race, exclusive formula feeding, gestational age of 41 weeks, maternal smoking, and certain drugs given to the mother (e.g., phenobarbital).

Neonatal Jaundice Caused by Increased Production of Bilirubin

The most common cause of severe early jaundice is fetal–maternal blood group incompatibility with resulting isoimmunization. Maternal immunization develops when erythrocytes leak from fetal to maternal circulation. Fetal erythrocytes carrying different antigens are recognized as foreign by the maternal immune system that forms antibodies against them (maternal sensitization). These antibodies (IgG immunoglobulins) cross the placental barrier into the fetal circulation and bind to fetal erythrocytes. In Rh incompatibility, sequestration and destruction of the antibody-coated erythrocytes take place in the reticuloendothelial system of the fetus. In ABO incompatibility, hemolysis is intravascular, complement mediated, and usually not as severe as in Rh disease [180]. Significant hemolysis may also result from incompatibilities between minor blood group antigens (e.g., Kell) [181]. Although hemolysis is predominantly associated with elevation of unconjugated bilirubin, the conjugated fraction may also be elevated [182].

Rh incompatibility problems do not usually develop until the second pregnancy. Thus, prenatal blood typing and serial testing of Rh-negative mothers for the development of Rh antibodies provide important information to guide possible intrauterine care. If maternal Rh antibodies develop during pregnancy, potentially helpful measures include serial amniocentesis (with bilirubin measurement) [183,184], ultrasound assessment of the fetus [185,186], intrauterine transfusion [187,188], and premature delivery. The prophylactic administration of anti-D γ-globulin [189] has been most helpful in preventing Rh sensitization. The newborn infant with Rh incompatibility presents with pallor, hepatosplenomegaly, and rapidly developing jaundice in the first hours of life. If the problem is severe, the infant may be born with generalized edema (fetal hydrops). Laboratory findings in the neonate's blood include reticulocytosis, anemia, a positive direct Coombs' test, and a rapidly rising serum bilirubin level. Exchange transfusion continues to be an important therapy for seriously affected infants [190]. Intravenous γ-globulin has been shown to reduce the need for exchange transfusions in both Rh and ABO hemolytic disease [191–194]. ABO incompatibility usually presents clinically with the first pregnancy. ABO hemolytic disease is largely limited to blood group A or B infants born to group O mothers [195]. ABO hemolytic disease is relatively rare in type A or B mothers. Development of jaundice is not as rapid as with Rh disease, and a serum bilirubin greater than 12 mg/dL on day 3 of life would be typical. Laboratory abnormalities include reticulocytosis (>10%) and a weakly positive direct Coombs' test, though this is sometimes negative. Anti-A or anti-B antibodies may be seen in the serum of the newborn if examined within the first few days of life, before they rapidly disappear. Spherocytes are the most prominent feature seen in the peripheral blood smear with ABO incompatibility.

Extravascular blood within the body may be rapidly metabolized to bilirubin by tissue macrophages. Examples of this increased bilirubin production include cephalohematoma, ecchymoses, petechiae, and hemorrhage. Although the diagnosis can often be made on physical examination, occult intracranial, intestinal, or pulmonary hemorrhage may also produce hyperbilirubinemia. Similarly, swallowed blood may be converted to bilirubin by the heme oxygenase of intestinal epithelium. The Apt test may be used to distinguish blood of

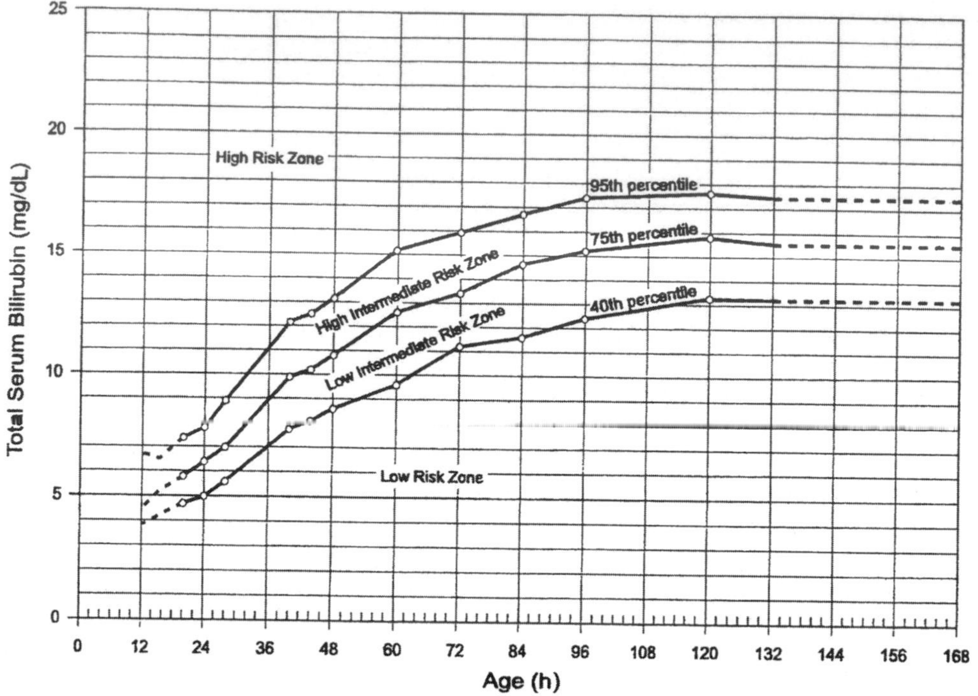

Figure 13.9. Risk designation of term and near-term well newborns based on their hour-specific serum bilirubin values. (Reproduced with permission from Pediatrics 2004;114:297–316; Copyright © 2004 by the AAP.)

maternal or infant origin because of differences in alkali resistance between fetal and adult hemoglobin [196,197].

Polycythemia can cause hyperbilirubinemia because the absolute increase in red cell mass results in elevated bilirubin production through normal rates of erythrocyte breakdown. A number of mechanisms may result in neonatal polycythemia (usually defined by venipuncture hematocrits >65%), as reviewed by Danish [198]. During placental separation at the time of birth, bleeding may occur from the maternal circulation into the fetus (maternal–fetal transfusion) or because of a delay in cord clamping [199]. Twin–twin transfusions may also result in polycythemia. Similarly, intrauterine hypoxia and maternal diseases such as diabetes mellitus [200] may result in neonatal polycythemia. Therapy for symptomatic polycythemia is partial exchange transfusion, though therapy for asymptomatic polycythemia remains controversial [199,201].

A number of specific abnormalities related to the RBC may result in neonatal jaundice, including hemoglobinopathies and RBC membrane and enzyme defects. Hereditary spherocytosis is not usually a neonatal problem, but hemolytic crises may occur and present with a rising bilirubin level and a falling hematocrit [202]. A family history of spherocytosis, anemia, or early gallstone disease (before age 40) is helpful in suggesting this diagnosis. The characteristic spherocytes seen in the peripheral blood smear may be impossible to distinguish from those seen with ABO hemolytic disease. Other hemolytic anemias associated with neonatal jaundice include drug-induced hemolysis, deficiencies of the erythrocyte enzymes (glucose-6-phosphate dehydrogenase [G6PD] deficiency [203–205], pyruvate kinase deficiency, and others), and hemolysis induced by vitamin K or bacteria. α-Thalassemia may result in severe hemolysis and lethal hydrops fetalis [206]. $\gamma\beta$-Thalassemia may also present with hemolysis and severe neonatal hyperbilirubinemia [207]. There are a wide variety of clinical findings associated with the thalassemias, extending from profound intrauterine hydrops and death, to mild neonatal jaundice and anemia, to no jaundice or anemia. Southeast Asian ovalocytosis has been associated with severe hyperbilirubinemia [208]. These RBC abnormalities are more likely to result in hyperbilirubinemia in the presence of GS, as described later in this chapter. Drugs or other substances responsible for hemolysis may be passed to the fetus across the placenta or to the neonate via the breast milk.

Induction of labor with oxytocin has been shown to be associated with neonatal jaundice. There is a significant association between hyponatremia and jaundice in infants of mothers who received oxytocin to induce labor [209,210]. The vasopressin-like action of oxytocin prompts electrolyte and water transport such that the erythrocyte swells and increased osmotic fragility and hyperbilirubinemia may result. Steroid administration at the initiation of oxytocin and 4 hours later may be helpful in preventing this hyperbilirubinemia [211].

Neonatal Jaundice Caused by Decreased Excretion of Bilirubin

Increased enterohepatic circulation of bilirubin is believed to be an important factor in neonatal jaundice. As previously reviewed, neonates are at risk for the intestinal absorption of bilirubin because (1) their bile contains increased levels of bilirubin monoglucuronide, which allows easier conversion to bilirubin; (2) they have significant amounts of β-glucuronidase within the intestinal lumen, which hydrolyzes bilirubin conjugates to bilirubin, which is more easily absorbed from the intestine; (3) they lack an intestinal flora to convert bilirubin conjugates to urobilinoids; and (4) meconium, the intestinal contents accumulated during gestation, contains significant amounts of bilirubin [212]. Conditions that prolong meconium passage (e.g., Hirschsprung's disease, meconium ileus, meconium plug syndrome) are associated with hyperbilirubinemia [213,214]. Earlier passage of meconium has been shown to be associated with lower serum bilirubin levels [215,216]. This may be facilitated by rectal temperature measurement during the neonatal period [217]. The enterohepatic circulation of bilirubin may be blocked by the enteral administration of compounds that bind bilirubin, such as agar [107,218–220], charcoal [221], and cholestyramine [222]. Breast-feeding has been clearly identified as a factor related to neonatal jaundice [147], and this subject has been reviewed elsewhere [153,223–225]. Breast-fed infants have been shown to have significantly higher serum bilirubin levels than formula-fed infants on each of the first 5 days of life [226], and this unconjugated hyperbilirubinemia may persist for weeks [227] to months [228,229]. Jaundice during the first week of life is sometimes described as "breast-feeding jaundice" to differentiate it from "breast milk jaundice syndrome," which occurs after the first week of life [230–232]. The former is frequently associated with inadequate breast milk intake, whereas the later generally occurs in otherwise thriving infants. There is probably an overlap between these conditions and physiologic jaundice. Early reports linking breast-milk and neonatal jaundice with a steroid (pregnane-3(α),20(β)-diol) in some milk samples [233] have not been confirmed by more recent, larger studies using more sensitive methods [234]. There are also conflicting data regarding efforts to attribute this jaundice to increased lipase activity in the breast milk, resulting in elevated levels of free fatty acids, which could inhibit hepatic glucuronosyltransferase [235–239]. It has been suggested that the enterohepatic circulation of bilirubin can be facilitated by the presence of β-glucuronidase [114,240] or some other substance in human milk [241]. Other factors possibly related to jaundice in breast-fed infants include caloric intake, fluid intake, weight loss, delayed meconium passage, intestinal bacterial flora, and inhibition of bilirubin glucuronosyltransferase by an unidentified factor in the milk [116]. Lascari [231] suggests that a healthy breast-fed infant with unconjugated hyperbilirubinemia, normal hemoglobin concentration, reticulocyte count, blood smear, no blood group incompatibility, and no other abnormalities on physical examination may be presumed to have early breast-feeding jaundice. Because there is no specific laboratory test to confirm a diagnosis of breast milk jaundice, it is important to rule out treatable causes of jaundice before ascribing the hyperbilirubinemia to breast milk. Some infants with presumed breast milk jaundice exhibit elevated serum bile acid levels, suggesting mild hepatic dysfunction or cholestasis [242], though in general this is not the case. Maisels and Gifford [243] suggest waiting until the serum bilirubin level reaches 15 mg/dL before evaluating an otherwise well-appearing breast-fed infant. The author believes 12 mg/dL is more appropriate given the delays in practice. Breast-fed infants who are fed specific nutritional ingredients that inhibit β-glucuronidase, such as L-aspartic acid [117], excrete more fecal bilirubin and have lower levels of jaundice [118] than do breast-fed infants who receive no supplements. No commercial preparations of these specific ingredients are presently available.

Several inborn errors of metabolism may present with neonatal hyperbilirubinemia. Perhaps the most impressive of these is the Crigler–Najjar syndrome (CN), or congenital nonhemolytic jaundice [244], which is characterized by a hereditary deficiency of hepatic bilirubin glucuronosyltransferase [245,246]. Without the ability to conjugate and, hence, excrete bilirubin, affected infants develop an intense persistent jaundice in the first few days of life despite otherwise normal liver function tests. Serum bilirubin levels of 25–35 mg/dL may result without treatment, and there is a severe risk of kernicterus. Three types of CN have been described. Types I and II are distinguished by treatment with phenobarbital. Type I shows no response to this therapy, and no significant amounts of bilirubin conjugates are seen in bile [247]. Type I patients require lifelong treatment with nocturnal phototherapy and blockage of the enterohepatic circulation. In type II, or Arias' syndrome [248], phenobarbital produces an enhanced biliary excretion of bilirubin mono- and diglucuronides [70,249]. Although this is associated with some decrease in the serum bilirubin, significant jaundice persists (~15 mg/dL). Type III [250] resembles type I in that there is no biliary excretion of bilirubin glucuronide. However, type III patients do excrete mono- and diglucoside conjugates of bilirubin. Although not as severe as CN, GS is also associated with increased neonatal jaundice. Both of these conditions are further described later in this chapter.

Various hormones may cause development of neonatal unconjugated hyperbilirubinemia. Congenital hypothyroidism may present with serum bilirubin greater than 12 mg/dL before the development of other clinical findings [251]. Prolonged jaundice is seen in one third of infants with congenital hypothyroidism [252]. Similarly, hypopituitarism and anencephaly may be associated with jaundice caused by inadequate thyroxine, which is necessary for hepatic clearance of bilirubin.

Certain drugs may affect the metabolism of bilirubin and result in hyperbilirubinemia or displacement of bilirubin from albumin. Such displacement increases the risk of kernicterus and may be caused by sulfonamides [253], moxalactam [254], and ceftriaxone [255] (independent of its sludge-producing effect [256]). The popular Chinese herb Chuen-Lin, given to 28–51% of Chinese newborn infants, has been shown to have a significant effect in displacing bilirubin from albumin [257]. Pancuronium bromide [176] and chloral hydrate [258] have been suggested as causes of neonatal hyperbilirubinemia.

Infants of diabetic mothers have higher peak bilirubin levels and a greater frequency of hyperbilirubinemia compared with normal neonates [259]. These patients have shown a positive correlation between total bilirubin and hematocrit, thus implicating polycythemia as one possible mechanism [259]. Other potential reasons for this hyperbilirubinemia include prematurity, substrate deficiency for glucuronidation (secondary to hypoglycemia), and poor hepatic perfusion (secondary to either respiratory distress, persistent fetal circulation, or cardiomyopathy).

The Lucey–Driscoll syndrome [260] consists of neonatal hyperbilirubinemia within families in whom there is in vitro inhibition of glucuronosyltransferase by both maternal and infant serum. It is presumed that this is caused by gestational hormones.

Prematurity is frequently associated with unconjugated hyperbilirubinemia in the neonatal period. Hepatic UDP-glucuronosyltransferase activity is markedly decreased in premature infants and rises steadily from 30 weeks' gestation until reaching adult levels 14 weeks after birth [261]. In addition, there may be deficiencies for both uptake [262] and secretion [263]. Bilirubin clearance improves rapidly following birth [264].

Hepatic hypoperfusion may result in neonatal jaundice. Inadequate perfusion of the hepatic sinusoids may not allow sufficient hepatocyte uptake and metabolism of bilirubin. Causes include patent ductus venosus (e.g., with respiratory distress syndrome), congestive heart failure, and portal vein thrombosis. Other specific liver diseases, as listed in Table 13.1 and described elsewhere in this text, may result in neonatal jaundice.

Neonatal Jaundice Caused by Both Increased Production and Decreased Excretion of Bilirubin

In neonatal diseases with jaundice caused by increased production of bilirubin and decreased excretion, both conjugated and unconjugated bilirubin fractions may be elevated. Bacterial sepsis increases bilirubin production by producing erythrocyte hemolysis due to hemolysins released by bacteria. Endotoxins released by bacteria may also decrease canalicular bile formation.

Toxicity of Neonatal Jaundice

Reviews of neonatal bilirubin toxicity have been published elsewhere [1,265,266]. Kernicterus (German, *kern* – "nucleus"; *icterus* – "yellow") is the neuropathologic finding associated with severe unconjugated hyperbilirubinemia and is named for the yellow staining of certain regions of the brain, particularly the basal ganglia, hippocampus, cerebellum, and nuclei of the floor of the fourth ventricle [265,267]. Clinical findings associated with kernicterus, termed *bilirubin encephalopathy,* include sluggish Moro reflex, opisthotonos, hypotonia, vomiting, high-pitched cry, hyperpyrexia, seizures, paresis of gaze ("setting-sun sign"), oculogyric crisis, and death. Long-term findings include spasticity, choreoathetosis, and sensorineural hearing loss. Milder forms of bilirubin encephalopathy include cognitive dysfunction and learning disabilities [268,269]. In 17-year-old males, the risk of having an IQ score less than 85 was found to be significantly higher among full-term subjects with neonatal serum bilirubin levels above 20 mg/dL [270]. The mechanisms of bilirubin cytotoxicity are complex and have been reviewed elsewhere [265,266,271,272]. Though the neonatal period is the most common time for bilirubin-related brain damage, the neurotoxicity of bilirubin has also been documented in older children and adults with CNI [273,274].

The absolute level of serum bilirubin has not been a good predictor of the risk of severe neonatal jaundice. However, it has long been known that kernicterus is likely with serum unconjugated bilirubin levels greater than 30 mg/dL and unlikely with levels less than 20 mg/dL [275–277]. In one study, 90% of the patients who had a bilirubin level greater than 35 mg/dL either died or had cerebral palsy or physical retardation [277]. Alternatively, no developmental retardation was found in 129 infants with bilirubin levels less than 20 mg/dL. Albumin concentration is an important variable because of the high-affinity binding with bilirubin, and the ratio of bilirubin to albumin is a risk factor that has been included in the most recent AAP guidelines [146]. Drugs and organic anions also bind to albumin and can displace bilirubin, thereby increasing the free bilirubin that can diffuse into cells and cause toxicity [278,279]. The most notable example of this is the kernicterus that occurred with low bilirubin levels when sulfisoxazole was given to premature infants [280]. Walker [266] has reviewed neonatal bilirubin toxicity and drug-induced bilirubin displacement. There is considerable debate at present regarding the risk of bilirubin encephalopathy in otherwise healthy full-term infants, with the suggestion that such infants are not at risk until the serum bilirubin level rises well over 20 mg/dL [276]. Although it has been acknowledged that total serum bilirubin may not be the most important factor related to risk, there are, at present, no other generally accepted tests (e.g., albumin saturation, reserve bilirubin-binding capacity, or free bilirubin) that are more helpful in identifying infants at risk for bilirubin encephalopathy. Recently, Ahlfors and Wennberg [281] reviewed the basics of bilirubin–albumin binding, the reasons it has not been integrated into mainstream clinical management of newborn jaundice, recent evidence suggesting that measuring free bilirubin would be useful in the clinical care of jaundiced newborns, and strategies for determining whether and how free bilirubin measurements should be incorporated into clinical care. Ahlfors et al. [282] recently described how to use zone fluidics to measure free bilirubin and overcome some of the existing problems with unbound (free) bilirubin measurement.

Another approach aimed at measuring early changes in the central nervous system (CNS) caused by bilirubin has assessed brainstem auditory evoked potentials (BAEP) [283–286]. Abnormalities in the BAEP have been demonstrated in jaundiced infants and shown to improve after exchange transfusion [287–290]. Data have shown that even moderate hyperbilirubinemia (mean $\pm$ SD: 14.3 $\pm$ 2.8 mg/dL) affects the BAEP, specific components of the Brazelton Neonatal Behavioral Assessment Scale [291], and cry characteristics [292]. Gunn rat data suggest that binaural difference waves (the difference between the sum of the two monaural BAEP waves and the binaural BAEP) may be a sensitive method for detecting bilirubin toxicity [293]. Somatosensory evoked potentials

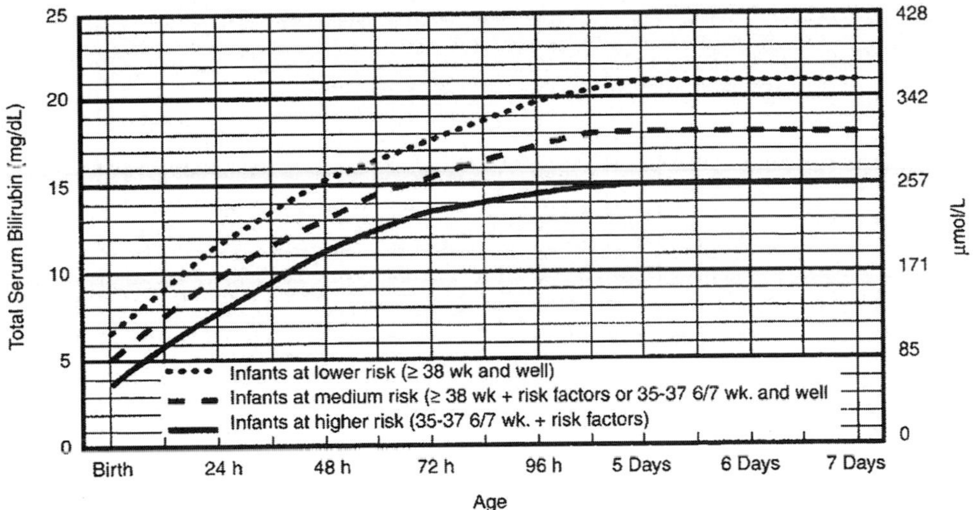

Figure 13.10. Guidelines for phototherapy in hospitalized infants of 35 or more weeks' gestation. These guidelines are based on limited evidence, and the levels shown are approximations. The guidelines refer to the use of intensive phototherapy, which should be used when the TSB exceeds the line indicated for each category. "Intensive phototherapy" implies irradiance in the blue-green spectrum (wavelengths of approximately 430–490 nm) of at least 30 $\mu W/cm^2/nm$ (measured at the infant's skin directly below the center of the phototherapy unit) and delivered to as much of the infant's surface area as possible. If the total serum bilirubin does not decrease or continues to rise in an infant who is receiving intensive phototherapy, this strongly suggests the presence of hemolysis. Infants who receive phototherapy and have an elevated direct-reacting or conjugated bilirubin level (cholestatic jaundice) may develop the bronze-baby syndrome. Use total bilirubin; do not subtract direct reacting or conjugated bilirubin. Risk factors are isoimmune hemolytic disease, G6PD deficiency, asphyxia, significant lethargy, temperature instability, sepsis, acidosis, and albumin less than 3.0 g/dL. For well infants 35–37 6/7 weeks old, adjust TSB levels for intervention around the medium-risk line. It is an option to intervene at lower TSB levels for infants closer to 35 weeks and at higher TSB levels for those closer to 37 6/7 weeks. It is an option to provide conventional phototherapy in the hospital or at home at TSB levels 2–3 mg/dL (35–50 μmol/L) below those shown, but home phototherapy should not be used in any infant with risk factors. (Reproduced with permission from Pediatrics 2004;114:297–316; Copyright © 2004 by the AAP.)

(SEP), which have their pathway through the region of the basal ganglia, an area commonly affected by kernicterus, also show abnormalities with jaundice and have been suggested as another method of monitoring the CNS effects of bilirubin [294]. At present, neither BAEP nor SEP is measured routinely to assess the potential toxicity of bilirubin.

Another reported toxicity of neonatal jaundice relates not to the CNS of the jaundiced infant, but rather to the attitude of that infant's parents. Mothers of jaundiced infants more frequently exhibited behavior suggesting the "vulnerable child syndrome" [295,296], including inappropriate visits to the physician because of unrealistic perceptions of illness, separation difficulties, and early termination of breast-feeding. Another study showed, however, that hyperbilirubinemia and/or phototherapy during the neonatal period are not associated with impaired mother–child attachment after the first year of life [297].

Management of Neonatal Jaundice

Hyperbilirubinemia is the most frequent reason infants are readmitted to the hospital in the first weeks of life [152,298,299]. The management of neonatal jaundice has been reviewed elsewhere [146] (Figures 13.10 and 13.11). The most important step in treatment of jaundice is determination of the primary etiology. However, independent of the etiology of the jaundice, elevation of the serum unconjugated bilirubin fraction prompts concern about possible kernicterus. As previously reviewed [266,279], when the unconjugated bilirubin fraction is elevated, care must be taken to avoid administration of agents that bind to albumin and displace bilirubin, thus promoting kernicterus. Although historically sulfonamides are the most well-known bilirubin-displacing agents, drugs such as ceftriaxone and ibuprofen are also strong bilirubin displacers, with a potential for inducing bilirubin encephalopathy [255,300]. Therapeutic options to lower unconjugated bilirubin levels include phototherapy, exchange transfusion, interruption of the enterohepatic circulation, enzyme induction, and alteration of breast-feeding. Research into these and other modalities continues actively. The outcomes of rational therapeutic guidelines for unconjugated hyperbilirubinemia during the first 7 days of life have been published elsewhere [301].

Phototherapy consists of irradiation of the jaundiced infant with light and has been recently reviewed [302,303]. Photon

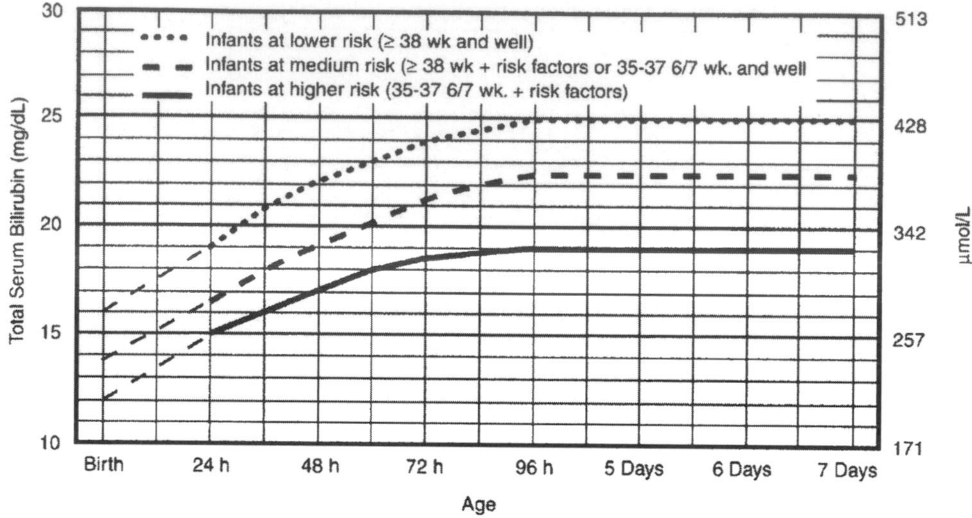

Figure 13.11. Guidelines for exchange transfusion in infants 35 or more weeks' gestation. These suggested levels are based on limited evidence, and the levels shown are approximations. During birth hospitalization, exchange transfusion is recommended if the TSB rises to these levels despite intensive phototherapy. For readmitted infants, if the TSB level is above the exchange level, repeat TSB measurement every 2–3 hours and consider exchange if the TSB remains above the levels indicated after intensive phototherapy for 6 hours. The *dashed lines* for the first 24 hours indicate uncertainty caused by a wide range of clinical circumstances and a range of responses to phototherapy. Immediate exchange transfusion is recommended if the infant shows signs of acute bilirubin encephalopathy (hypertonia, arching, retrocollis, opisthotonos, fever, high-pitched cry) or if TSB is 5 mg/dL (85 μmol/L) or more above these lines. Risk factors are isoimmune hemolytic disease, G6PD deficiency, asphyxia, significant lethargy, temperature instability, sepsis, and acidosis. Use total bilirubin; do not subtract direct reacting of conjugated bilirubin. If the infant is well and 35–37 6/7 weeks old (median risk), individualize TSB levels for exchange based on actual gestational age. (Reproduced with permission from Pediatrics 2004;114:297–316; Copyright © 2004 by the AAP.)

energy derived from light changes the structure of the bilirubin molecule in two ways (Figure 13.12), allowing bilirubin to be excreted into bile or urine without the usual requirement for hepatic glucuronidation. One change involves a 180° rotation around the double bonds between either the A and B or C and D rings [304], converting the normal Z configuration to the E configuration. 4Z,15E bilirubin is preferentially formed and can spontaneously reisomerize to native bilirubin. More importantly, a new seven-member ring structure may be formed between rings A and B, resulting in "lumirubin" [305] or "cyclobilirubin" [306]. It now appears that formation of lumirubin occurs via the 4E,15Z-isomer intermediate [307]. Both changes interfere with the internal hydrogen bonding of native bilirubin and by exposing the propionic acid groups, result in a more polar compound. Thus, the lumirubin and E isomers can be excreted directly into bile. Lumirubin appears to be the major route by which bilirubin is eliminated with phototherapy [308,309]. The choice of light for phototherapy is a subject about which there are many conflicting data [302]. Special blue light (or Super Blue, but not regular blue) appears to be better than white or green light, though white is less disturbing to nursery personnel [310]. New phototherapy devices using woven fiberoptic pads are currently available [311] that are effective (comparable to conventional phototherapy) and safe, eliminate the need for eye patches, and permit greater time for maternal–infant bonding [312–314]. Proposed guidelines for phototherapy have been published elsewhere [315–317]. In general, phototherapy is used to prevent serum bilirubin concentrations from reaching levels necessitating exchange transfusion (see Figure 13.10). Phototherapy is now frequently done at home [318,319], a practice accepted and recommended by the AAP [320]. Despite documented complications [321–323], phototherapy is widely used and generally safe [324]. Although phototherapy does affect cardiac output and blood flow to other organs (e.g., increased cerebral blood flow) and may be associated with opening of the ductus arteriosus, these effects are generally not problematic [325,326]. In extremely premature infants (<800 g birth weight), prolonged phototherapy and low peak serum bilirubin levels (<9.4 mg/dL) were shown in one study to be independently associated with blindness [327]. This could possibly be related to direct effects of light on the unshielded immature eye or decreased antioxidant protection by low serum bilirubin levels. Phototherapy should not be employed without prior diagnostic evaluation of the cause of the jaundice. The shielding of phototherapy units should never be removed because of the ultraviolet radiation hazards that may result [328]. Although it has been recommended that the infant's position be changed every 6 hours during

4Z,15Z-BILIRUBIN

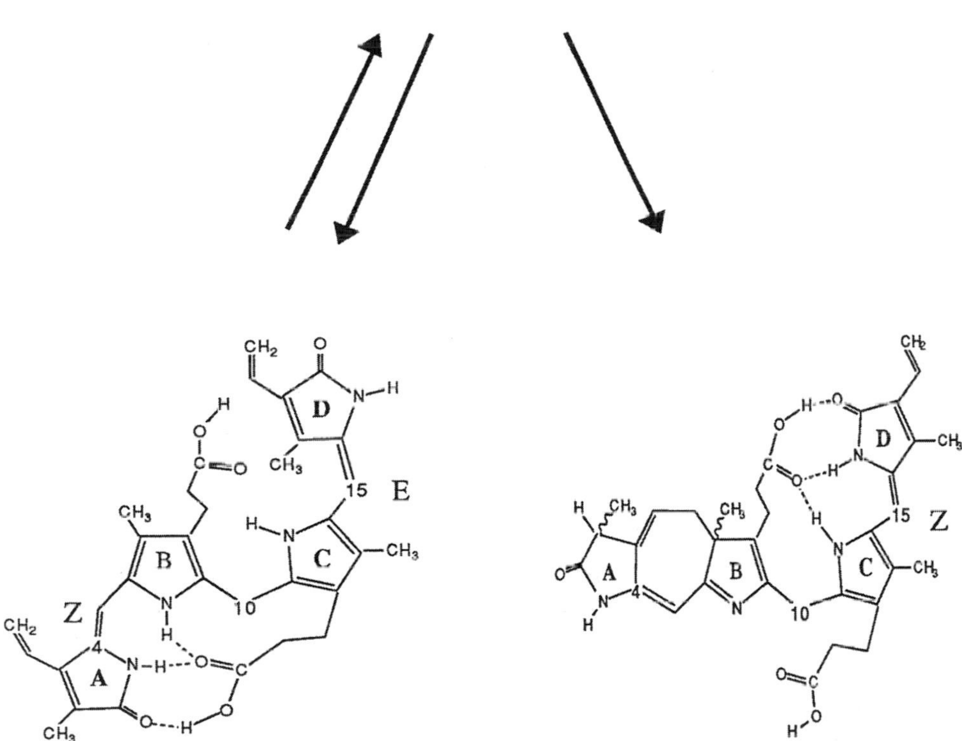

4Z,15E-BILIRUBIN

LUMIRUBIN

Figure 13.12. The major products of phototherapy. Light induces an isomerization of 4Z,15Z-bilirubin to produce the configurational isomer 4Z,15E-bilirubin and the structural isomer lumirubin. Both isomers interrupt the internal hydrogen bonding and expose the propionic acid side chains, thus increasing the polarity of the compound and allowing excretion in bile without hepatic glucuronidation.

phototherapy [329], data from one study showed position change made no difference in serum bilirubin levels [330]. One study of 264 neonates (some with hemolytic jaundice) who completed an average of 121 hours of phototherapy, indicated that significant rebound hyperbilirubinemia did not occur [331]. Similarly, no significant rebound hyperbilirubinemia occurred in 163 healthy full-term infants with nonhemolytic jaundice (including those receiving breast milk, formula, and mixed feedings) receiving an average of 54–65 hours [332]. In healthy term newborns, phototherapy may be stopped when the serum bilirubin level falls below 14–15 mg/dL, and hospital discharge need not be delayed to observe for rebound [166].

Exchange transfusion is the most rapid method to acutely lower the serum bilirubin concentration. Indications for exchange transfusion vary, have been published elsewhere [316, 321,333,334] (see Figure 13.11), and may be related to either anemia or an elevated serum bilirubin level. In neonatal hemolytic disease, suggested indications for transfusion include (a) anemia (hematocrit <45%), positive direct Coombs' test, and bilirubin greater than 4 mg/dL in the cord blood; (b) postnatal rise of the serum bilirubin concentration that exceeds 1 mg/dL/hr for more than 6 hours; (c) progressive anemia and rate of increase in serum bilirubin of greater than 0.5 mg/dL/hr; and (d) continuing progression of anemia despite control of hyperbilirubinemia. Sometimes exchange transfusion for hemolytic disease can be avoided through the use of high-dose intravenous immunoglobulin therapy [335]. Suggested indications for exchange transfusion because of hyperbilirubinemia alone include (a) bilirubin concentration greater than 15 mg/dL for more than 48 hours; (b) salicylate saturation index greater than 8.0 or HABA binding less than 50% on two successive determinations 4 hours apart; (c) ratio of total serum bilirubin (milligrams per deciliter) divided by total serum protein (grams per deciliter) greater than 3.7; and (d) molar concentration ratio of serum bilirubin to serum albumin of greater than 0.7 [321]. Although there are many well-described risks with exchange transfusion, mortality should be low (<0.6%) if it is performed properly [264,336,337].

There are a number of pharmacologic approaches to the prevention and treatment of neonatal hyperbilirubinemia that have been recently reviewed [338]. The enterohepatic circulation may be interrupted by enteral administration of agents that bind bilirubin in the intestine and prevent reabsorption. Such agents include agar [107,219,220], cholestyramine [222], activated charcoal [221], and calcium phosphate [339–341]. Increased intestinal peristalsis would be expected to allow less time for bilirubin absorption. Frequent feedings [342] and rectal stimulation [217] are associated with lower serum bilirubin levels. Enteral feedings of bilirubin oxidase, an enzyme that degrades bilirubin to biliverdin, dipyrrols, and other unidentified products [343], are an additional method to block the enterohepatic circulation that remains experimental at present [344]. Another experimental approach uses intravenous bilirubin oxidase [345,346].

Because neonatal hepatic BUGT activity has been shown to be low in neonates [261], it is not surprising that induction of hepatic BUGT results in lower serum bilirubin levels. Such induction in the neonate may be accomplished with prenatal maternal use of phenobarbital or diphenylhydantoin [347,348]. Even very low–birth weight infants (<2000 g) have been shown to respond to in utero phenobarbital therapy with significantly increased serum levels of conjugated bilirubin and decreased need for phototherapy [349]. In the postnatal period, use of phenobarbital by the neonate has the same bilirubin-lowering effect [350]. Clofibrate is advocated by French workers as a simple, nontoxic pharmacologic treatment that induces BUGT and is used increasingly in France to prevent and treat neonatal jaundice [351].

Optimization of breast-feeding in the perinatal period is important [352]. If the bilirubin level is rising, published recommendations support encouraging mothers to breast-feed more frequently [166,171,224], with an average suggested interval between feeds of 2 hours and no feeding supplements [353] or at least eight to ten feedings per 24 hours [166]. A strong dose-response relationship has been shown between feeding frequency and a decreased incidence of hyperbilirubinemia [354]. More frequent nursing may not increase intake but has been suggested to increase peristalsis and stool frequency, thus promoting bilirubin excretion [316]. Frequency of breast-feeding during the first 24 hours of life has been shown to be correlated significantly with the frequency of meconium passage [354]. The serum bilirubin level at which breast feeding should be discontinued is controversial; recommendations include 14 [355], 15 [231], 16–17 [171], and 18–20 mg/dL [353]. When breast-feeding is interrupted, formula feeding may be initiated for 24–48 hours, or breast- and formula-feeding can be alternated with each feeding [166]. No studies have addressed the cost-effectiveness of various formulas in their jaundice-lowering effects, though two independent studies have shown that infants exclusively fed Nutramigen (a casein hydrolysate formula made by Mead Johnson) have lower jaundice levels than infants fed routine formula [356,357]. Supplementing breast-fed infants with small volumes of specific nutritional ingredients has been shown to result in increased fecal bilirubin excretion and lower transcutaneous bilirubin levels [118], though no commercial preparations of these ingredients are currently available. Feeding heated expressed breast milk is also said to reduce serum bilirubin levels [353]. A fall in the serum bilirubin level of 2–5 mg/dL [316] is consistent with a diagnosis of breast milk jaundice. Breast-feeding may then be resumed, with the acknowledgment that serum bilirubin levels may rise for several days but will gradually level off and decline [224,231]. If breast-feeding is to be resumed following the interruption, it is important to preserve lactation with the use of a breast pump. In one study, interruption of breast-feeding for approximately 50 hours (during which time a formula was given) was shown to have the same bilirubin-lowering effect as a similar duration of phototherapy [358]. Interruptions of breast-feeding for 24–48 hours have been shown to be successful at lowering serum bilirubin levels and avoiding the need for phototherapy in 81 of 87 jaundiced infants [355]. Formula feedings to Asian neonates receiving phototherapy resulted in a greater decrease of serum bilirubin levels than in infants who were exclusively breast-fed [332]. Careful counseling and support can prevent the interruption of breast-feeding from becoming a permanent discontinuance of nursing [355].

An alternative approach to treating neonatal hyperbilirubinemia is to block the first enzyme responsible for the production of bilirubin, heme oxygenase. This can be accomplished by several different metalloporphyrins [359,360]. Sn-protoporphyrin has been used successfully in the experimental management of jaundice in neonates with ABO incompatibility

Table 13.2: Comparison of Disorders of Unconjugated Hyperbilirubinemia

		Gilbert's Syndrome	*Crigler–Najjar Type 1*	*Crigler–Najjar Type 2*
Prevalence		3%	Rare	Rare
Inheritance		Autosomal dominant or recessive	Autosomal recessive	Autosomal recessive, rarely dominant
Genetic defect		*UGT1A1* gene	*UGT1A1* gene	*UGT1A1* gene
Hepatocyte defect site		Microsomes +/– plasma membrane	Microsomes	Microsomes
Deficient hepatocyte function		Glucuronidation +/– uptake	Glucuronidation	Glucuronidation
BUGT activity		5–53% of controls	Severely decreased	2–23% of controls
Hepatocyte uptake		Decreased in 20–30%	Normal	Normal
Serum total bilirubin level (mg/dL)		0.8–4.3	15–45	8–25
Serum bilirubin decrease with phenobarbital (%)		70	0	77
HPLC serum bilirubin composition (%)	Normal			
Unconjugated	92.6	98.8	~100	99.1
Diglucuronide	6.2	1.1	0	0.6
Monoglucuronide	0.5	0	0	0
Bile bilirubin conjugates (%)	Normal			
Diglucuronide	~80	60	0 to trace	5–10
Monoglucuronide	~15	30	Predominant if measurable	90–95
Other routine liver function tests		Normal	Normal	Normal
Prognosis		Benign	Kernicterus common	Occasional kernicterus

+, with; –, without

[361]. Treatment of neonatal jaundice with heme oxygenase inhibition remains experimental at this point in time, though clinical trials appear promising. Two studies with Sn-mesoporphyrin (Sn-MP) showed that phototherapy could be abolished by using Sn-MP [362,363]. In addition to inhibiting bilirubin production, metalloporphyrins are photosensitizers that can accelerate the destruction of bilirubin by light but also cause other unwanted side effects [364]. Because CO is now suggested to be a significant neurotransmitter, blocking heme oxygenase activity early in life may not be a completely benign process. Thus, a major concern about metalloporphyrins is the lack of detailed long-term follow-up studies addressing safety issues [365].

Another experimental therapy for neonatal hyperbilirubinemia is hemoperfusion. Research into this method has employed hemoperfusion with ion exchange [366], bilirubin oxidase [367], and sorbents [368,369]. Sodium benzoate–augmented hemoperfusion has shown encouraging results in dogs [370].

DISORDERS OF BILIRUBIN METABOLISM

The disorders described in this section, summarized in Tables 13.2 and 13.3, are those in which there is a primary abnormality in bilirubin metabolism without other liver disease [371]. The disorders can best be understood in the context of the normal pathway in which bilirubin is cleared from the circulation (Figure 13.2). Defects in these metabolic steps are responsible for the disorders described in the final section of this chapter.

Gilbert's Syndrome

Clinical Presentation

Gilbert's syndrome (OMIM #143500) was first described in 1901 by Gilbert and Lereboullet [372]. It is characterized by a hereditary chronic or recurrent, mild unconjugated hyperbilirubinemia with otherwise normal liver function tests (for reviews see references [373–375]). The serum unconjugated

Table 13.3: Comparison of Disorders of Conjugated Hyperbilirubinemia

	Rotor's Syndrome	*Dubin–Johnson Syndrome*
Prevalence	Rare	Rare
Inheritance	Autosomal recessive	Autosomal recessive
Genetic defect	Unknown	*cMOAT/MRP2/ABCC2* gene
Hepatocyte defect site	GST	Apical canalicular membrane
Deficient hepatocyte function	Intracellular binding of bilirubin and conjugates	Cannalicular secretion of bilirubin conjugates
Brown-black liver	No	Yes
Serum total bilirubin level (mg/dL)	2–7	1.5–6.0
Serum conjugated bilirubin (%)	>50	>50
Other routine liver function tests	Normal	Normal
Oral cholecystogram	Usually visualizes	Usually does not visualize
^{99m}Tc-HIDA cholescintigraphy: liver gall bladder	Poor to no visualization	Intense, prolonged visualization Delayed or no visualization
BSP clearance test	Serum BSP levels elevated (delayed clearance)	Serum BSP levels normal at 45 min but elevated at 90–120 min
ICG clearance test	Delayed clearance	Normal
Response to estrogens or pregnancy	No change	Increased jaundice
Total urinary coproporphyrin excretion (isomers I + III)	2.5–5 times increased	Normal
Urinary coproporphyrin isomer I composition (normal = 25%)	Usually <80% of total	>80% of total
Prognosis	Benign (asymptomatic)	Benign (occasional abdominal complaints; probably incidental)

^{99m}Tc-HIDA, technetium Tc 99m hepatic iminodiacetic acid.

bilirubin elevation is variable and usually ranges from 1–4 mg/dL (17 μmol/L = 1 mg/dL). Frequently, patients are first identified when an elevated serum bilirubin is found on screening blood chemistry or mild jaundice (perhaps only scleral icterus) is noted during a period of fasting associated with a nonspecific viral illness or religious activities [376]. Icteric plasma from a blood donor may suggest GS [377]. Alternatively, hyperbilirubinemia post liver transplantation may be a sign that the donor had GS [378–381]. GS is generally associated with no negative implications for health or longevity; however, a large variety of common symptoms have been reported by patients with GS [382,383]. These symptoms include vertigo, headache, fatigue, abdominal pain, nausea, diarrhea, constipation, and loss of appetite. The possible relationship of these symptoms to GS was evaluated in a group of 2395 Swedish subjects [384]. The only symptom that was more common in GS was diarrhea in men aged 57–67 years. The authors suggested that this was most likely a type 1 error because of the large number of comparisons made and concluded that there was no higher prevalence of symptoms associated with GS. There are limited reports suggesting that GS is a risk factor for chronic fatigue syndrome [385,386].

In two large surveys of normal individuals, approximately 3% of the population had serum bilirubin levels greater than 1.0 mg/dL [387,388]. If the normal upper limit of serum bilirubin is defined as 1.4 mg/dL, then there is a strong male predominance (approximately four to one). This finding might be related to the observation that females clear bilirubin better than males [389]. GS may be inherited in either an autosomal dominant [390–393] or recessive [394] fashion.

Although GS is a congenital disorder, it rarely becomes clinically apparent until after puberty. The reasons for this are unknown but have been suggested to be related to the hormonal changes of puberty. Steroid hormones can suppress hepatic bilirubin clearance [92]. During pregnancy, increased estrogen levels are associated with impaired clearance of exogenous bilirubin [395]. Gonadectomy has been shown to alter BUGT activity [396]. Odell [397] speculated that some infants with nonhemolytic neonatal jaundice are manifesting GS. Use of genetic markers (see below) has allowed investigation of the

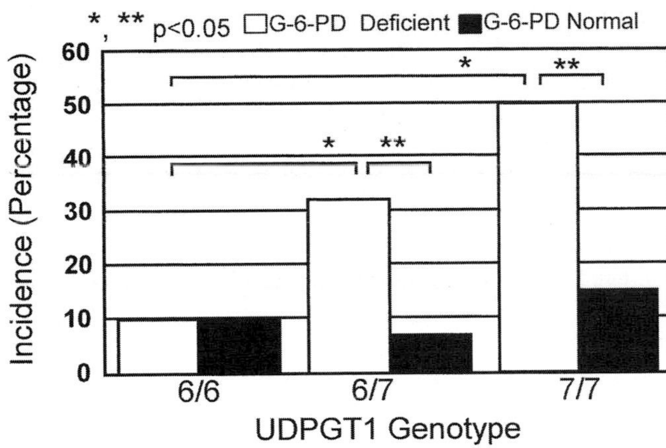

Figure 13.13. Incidence (percentage) of hyperbilirubinemia (serum total bilirubin $\geq$257 μmol/L) in G6PD-deficient neonates and normal controls, stratified for the three genotypes of the UGT1A1 promoter. (Reprinted from Kaplan et al. [404]. Copyright © 1997, with permission from the National Academy of Sciences, USA.)

role GS plays in neonatal jaundice. Individuals carrying such markers have been shown to have a more rapid rise in their jaundice levels during the first two days of life [398], a predisposition to prolonged or severe neonatal hyperbilirubinemia [399,400], and variably increased jaundice when the GS polymorphism occurs with pyloric stenosis [401,402] or is coinherited with hematologic abnormalities such as G6PD deficiency [403,404], β-thalassemia [403,405–407], or hereditary spherocytosis [408]. Thus, studies from several different parts of the world indicate that GS, as detected by *UGT1A1* analysis, does play some role in neonatal jaundice. In their study, Kaplan et al. [404] noted that neither G6PD deficiency nor the GS type UDPGT1 promoter polymorphism (also known as UGT1A1*28) alone increased the incidence of hyperbilirubinemia, but both in combination did (Figure 13.13). They speculated that this gene interaction may serve as a paradigm of the interaction of benign genetic polymorphisms in the causation of disease; that is, it may take two genetic abnormalities to produce disease symptoms.

Pathophysiology

Gilbert's syndrome is a heterogeneous group of disorders, all of which share at least a 50% decrease in hepatic BUGT activity [409–412]. Based on plasma clearance of other organic anions (BSP and ICG) that share the same hepatocyte uptake receptor-carrier, there appear to be at least four subtypes of GS [413,414]. In GS type I, clearance of BSP and ICG is normal. In GS type II, there is delayed BSP clearance but ICG clearance is normal. Because BSP uptake is normal in type II, delayed clearance must be related to subsequent intrahepatic metabolism or canalicular excretion [415]. In GS type III, clearance of both BSP and ICG is delayed. The delay in the initial rate of disappearance from the plasma suggests a defect in uptake at the hepatocyte plasma membrane [415]. Those with GS type IV have delayed uptake of ICG but not BSP. Thus, some individuals with GS have delayed uptake of bilirubin into the hepatocyte, others have delayed biotransformation, and others demonstrate both abnormalities [72,416–418]. Immunohistochemical staining for UDP-glucuronosyltransferase shows a clear reduction throughout the hepatic lobule in specimens from individuals with GS when compared with normals [419].

The elucidation of the structure of the *UGT1* gene, which encodes human bilirubin, phenol, and other UDP-glucuronosyltransferase isozymes [57,420], leads to the discovery of *UGT1A1* mutations or polymorphisms associated with GS. In Caucasian populations, the homozygous finding of an additional TA repeat in the promoter region, or so-called TATA box [i.e., $(TA)_7TAA$ rather than $(TA)_6TAA$], of the *UGT1A1* gene has been shown to be a necessary though not sufficient condition for GS [421–423]. Individuals who are heterozygous for seven TA repeats have significantly higher serum bilirubin levels than the homozygous wild-type six repeats [421]. In Asian populations, the $(TA)_7TAA$ mutation is relatively rare [424], but several different *UGT1A1* mutations have been associated with GS [393,425,426]. These Asian mutations involve exon 1 of the *UGT1A1* gene rather than the TATA promoter region. One of the most common mutations in Asians, a Gly71Arg mutation in exon 1, has also linked GS and severe neonatal hyperbilirubinemia [400]. It has been reported that although within Caucasians promoter TA repeat number and bilirubin level are strongly positively correlated, in other ethnic groups [e.g., Africans, in whom two other variants $(TA)_5$ and $(TA)_8$ have been identified] there is a negative correlation [427]. Thus, the ethnic implications of these genetic polymorphisms of the *UGT1A1* gene require further analysis.

Although decreased hepatic BUGT activity is universal in GS, there is poor correlation between measured enzyme activity in liver and serum bilirubin level [428]. This may be explained by the increased bilirubin production associated with the decreased red cell half-life seen in as many as 40% of patients with GS [392,418]. Unlike other conditions with increased bilirubin production (e.g., sickle cell disease), there is no induction of BUGT activity in GS [429]. Even phenobarbital produces little if any BUGT induction in GS [410]. Hepatic BUGT activity in GS is generally higher than that seen in CNII; however, there is significant overlap [412].

Related to the decreased BUGT activity is the observation that duodenal bile from individuals with GS contains a decreased amount of bilirubin diglucuronides and an increased amount of bilirubin monoglucuronides compared with normals [69,72,412,430] (Figure 13.14). This distribution is similar to that seen in infants [431]. Despite the observations noted above regarding poor BUGT induction, administration of phenobarbital has been shown to normalize the bile pigment profile in duodenal fluid [72], lower plasma bilirubin levels, and increase hepatic clearance of bilirubin [432,433]. Clofibrate and glutethimide also normalize serum bilirubin concentrations but do not normalize the duodenal bile pigment profile [434]. In animals, clofibrate is an inducer of BUGT but does not affect BSP uptake or GST [435].

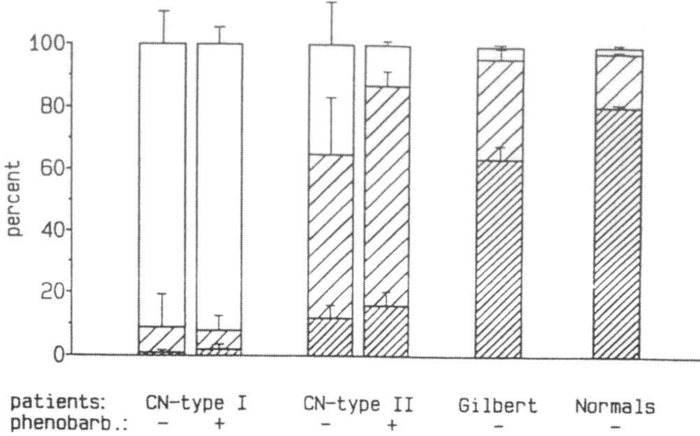

Figure 13.14. Bile pigment composition in bile from normal (n = 8), Crigler–Najjar (CN) type I (n = 3), CN type II (n = 3), and Gilbert's syndrome (n = 16) patients receiving (+) or not receiving (−) phenobarbital. Relative bile pigment composition is indicated in the vertical columns as percentage of total ± standard deviation. Shading: white, unconjugated bilirubin; intermediate, bilirubin monoconjugate; dark, bilirubin diconjugate. (Reprinted from Sinaasappel and Jansen [69]. Copyright © 1991, with permission from the American Gastroenterological Association.)

An additional unexplained phenomenon in GS is the exaggerated rise in serum bilirubin associated with fasting [436–439]. Although normal individuals can double their serum bilirubin level in response to fasting, in GS a more pronounced rise occurs. This is not related to decreased hepatic blood flow because ICG clearance is not affected [437]. Although fasting may reduce BUGT activity [439] and increase heme oxygenase (the enzyme responsible for bilirubin production) activity [440], neither of these effects is believed to explain the fasting hyperbilirubinemia of GS [432,441]. Enhanced enterohepatic circulation of bilirubin is suggested to be a major factor in the pathogenesis of fasting-induced hyperbilirubinemia [442]. Intraluminal noncalorie food-bulk can blunt the bilirubin rise [443].

Diagnosis and Treatment

Generally, a diagnosis of Gilbert's syndrome can be made when there is a mild, fluctuating unconjugated hyperbilirubinemia, the rest of the liver function tests are normal, and there is no hemolysis. Hemolysis can add confusion because it may result in similar findings and it is not unusual in GS. Hence, other tests are sometimes used to aid in diagnosis.

One test sometimes used to aid in diagnosing GS involves the intravenous administration of nicotinic acid (niacin) with assessment of the subsequent rise in serum bilirubin concentration [444]. Nicotinic acid is usually administered to adults in a dose of 50 mg [445–447] over 30 seconds, though results were similar with 300-mg injections in one study [448]. Nonconjugated serum bilirubin is then measured every 30–60 minutes for the next 4–5 hours. Nicotinic acid produces a rise in serum unconjugated bilirubin in normal individuals and in those with GS. However, in GS the bilirubin rise is higher and clearance is delayed longer than in normals [444,448–451]. Nicotinic acid causes increased osmotic fragility and hemolysis of RBCs with sequestration in the spleen. Splenic heme oxygenase is also induced, with rapid conversion of heme to bilirubin [450]. Nicotinic acid–induced hemolysis produces a rise in serum iron that is similar in healthy controls and those with GS [451]. Hence, the prolonged serum bilirubin levels are related to delayed hepatic clearance of bilirubin. Nicotinic acid infusion has been suggested to be a better method to diagnose GS than a 400-kcal fast because delayed bilirubin clearance was seen after nicotinic acid in GS subjects who otherwise had normal serum bilirubin levels [445]. The nicotinic acid test is not useful in differentiating GS from chronic liver disease, as both groups showed positive tests [452].

Another test suggested to aid in the diagnosis of GS involves fractionation of the total serum bilirubin using alkaline methanolysis and thin-layer chromatography [96,182]. This allows precise measurement of the conjugated and unconjugated bilirubin levels. This approach has shown that in GS, approximately 6% of the total serum bilirubin was conjugated compared with approximately 17% in normals and those with chronic hemolysis. Individuals with chronic persistent hepatitis had 28% of their total bilirubin present as conjugates. Fasting did not change the percentage of conjugates in GS, despite the rise in total serum bilirubin concentration. An overlap of only three individuals was seen among the 77 with GS and 60 normal subjects [182]. Other studies support these findings [453]. In patients with GS, fractionation of the total serum bilirubin by HPLC showed significantly decreased bilirubin monoglucuronides (1.1% vs. 6.2% in normals) and increased unconjugated bilirubin (98.8% vs. 92.6% in normals) [454].

Monaghan et al. [399] have suggested GS genetic screening for the *UGT1A1* TA repeat as a simple, useful additional test in the investigation of very prolonged neonatal jaundice in North American, African, and European populations and for the Gly71Arg mutation in Asians. However, the value of such a genetic test cannot be fully determined until accurate data regarding the prevalence and penetrance of the GS genotype are known [455]. Thus, genetic testing for GS cannot be routinely recommended [455].

Gilbert's syndrome has no significant negative implications regarding morbidity or mortality. In general, drug metabolism studies have revealed no major dangers [453,456], although there appears to be an increased incidence of slow acetylators [457,458] and lorazepam clearance is 20–40% decreased [459]. Concurrent genetic deficiencies in other xenobiotic pathways may put individuals with GS at increased risk of drug toxicity from compounds such as acetaminophen [460,461], cancer chemotherapeutic agents CPT-11 (irinotecan) [462] and TAS-103 [463], and the viral protease inhibitor indinavir [371,464]. For this reason, Bosma [371] suggests that screening for GS is of clinical importance. No specific treatment is necessary for GS, though phenobarbital has been shown to lower serum bilirubin levels [465]. If the well-documented antioxidant effect of bilirubin [466] provides a biological advantage [467], then the mild hyperbilirubinemia of GS might actually be a significant benefit against such things as vascular disease [468,469], in which free radicals are involved in pathogenesis. Bosma [371] concluded that a selective advantage in GS because of the antioxidant capacity of bilirubin seems unlikely.

Crigler–Najjar Syndrome

Clinical Presentation

In 1952, Crigler and Najjar [244] described seven infants with congenital familial nonhemolytic jaundice who developed severe unconjugated hyperbilirubinemia shortly after birth and died from kernicterus within months. These infants were from three related families. The serum bilirubin concentration reached 25–35 mg/dL despite a lack of hemolytic disease. Other liver function tests were normal. Liver histology was normal except for the deposition of bile pigments. Subsequent reports have documented that the main risk for patients with CN is kernicterus [1]. An excellent review of the neurologic perspectives of CN has been published [470]. Although some patients survive into the second decade with normal development [471], the possibility of developing late kernicterus is always a concern, even in adulthood [245,247,472,473]. Serum bilirubin levels vary from approximately 15 to 45 mg/dL.

In 1969, Arias et al. [248] described a second, more frequent type of severe nonhemolytic hyperbilirubinemia. The previous syndrome was termed CNI (OMIM #218800), whereas the new findings were termed CNII or Arias' syndrome (OMIM #606785) [248]. Hyperbilirubinemia is less severe in type II patients and varies from approximately 8 to 25 mg/dL. Hence, these individuals have a much lower incidence of kernicterus, though such damage occurs [249,474].

Pathophysiology

Both CNI and CNII are generally inherited in an autosomal recessive manner, though one case of autosomal dominant inheritance of CNII has been reported [475]. CNI and CNII result from mutations to the *UGT* gene complex (see Clarke et al. [58]). Patients with one normal allele demonstrate normal metabolism of bilirubin [476]. The genetic details determine the severity of clinical disease. In CNI there is a complete absence of functional UGT1A1, whereas in CNII UGT1A1 activity is markedly reduced [477]. In CNI, 18 of 23 described mutations of the *UGT1* gene are found in the common exons 2–5 (see Figure 13.4) and thus affect many UGT1 enzymes [58,478]. Intronic mutations causing CNI have also been reported [479]. However, in CNII, four of nine known mutations are found in exon 1A1. There is some overlap in classification of mild CNII and GS (e.g., Gly71Arg) that relate to differences in definitions based on serum bilirubin levels [58]. The TATA box TA_7 repeat mutation seen in GS can be seen along with other mutations resulting in either CNI or CNII [480].

In both CNI and CNII, assays of liver tissue from affected patients demonstrate negligible or very low BUGT activity [69,70,245,246,248,412,481]. Hence, patients with these disorders experience a profound block in bilirubin excretion because they lack the ability to conjugate bilirubin with UDPGA. Thus, liver biopsy is not helpful in differentiating CNI and CNII. Study of the resected livers from four patients with CNI undergoing liver transplantation showed that there was heterogeneous glucuronidation of various substrates other than bilirubin [482]. Hence, several in the family of glucuronosyltransferase isoenzymes can be affected in the same patient. There is considerable overlap of hepatic BUGT activity between CNII and GS [412] (see Table 13.3).

In family studies of CNI patients [483,484], partial deficiencies have been found in the glucuronidation of salicylate and menthol among siblings, parents, and grandparents. Hence, it has generally been accepted that this represents an autosomal recessive inheritance [483].

In family studies of CNII patients, the original report by Arias et al. [248] found abnormalities of glucuronidation (menthol) in only one parent, suggesting autosomal dominant inheritance. Subsequent studies of siblings or parents have often found elevated serum bilirubin levels (1.2–4 mg/dL), delayed bilirubin clearance tests, and decreased hepatic BUGT activity as would be seen in GS [245,248,249,433,485,486]. These findings in both parents [433,485] suggest that CNII may represent homozygous GS. However, if CNII is truly the homozygous form of GS, one would expect many more affected individuals because GS occurs in at least 3% of the population. Pertinent genetic data have been reviewed elsewhere [487], and the inheritance of CNII is now believed to be autosomal recessive.

The major differentiating characteristic between CNI and CNII is the response to drugs that stimulate hyperplasia of the ER. When CNII patients received phenobarbital or diphenylhydantoin, there was a significant decline in the serum bilirubin level, increased hepatic clearance of radiolabeled bilirubin [248,433,474,488–491], and increased biliary levels of bilirubin diglucuronides [69,249] (see Figure 13.14). In a study of five CNII patients, the magnitude of the phenobarbital-induced decrease in serum bilirubin ranged from 2.1–12.1 mg/dL (27–72%), with pre- and postphenobarbital serum bilirubin levels ranging from 7.8–16.9 and 4.7–10.1 mg/dL, respectively [69]. Summarizing data from seven earlier studies [248,433,474,488–491] regarding the response of CNII patients to oral phenobarbital treatment revealed the following: 11 females and 13 males had a total serum bilirubin of 15.7 ± 13.8 (mean ± SD) prior to phenobarbital. After doses ranging from 90–390 mg/d, or alternatively 4 mg/kg/d, the serum bilirubin decreased 12.0 ± 4.0 mg/dL (77 ± 13%). The lowest total serum bilirubin following phenobarbital therapy was 5.9 mg/dL. In contrast, CNI patients show neither a decrease in serum bilirubin nor significantly increased biliary bilirubin conjugates in response to drugs [69,247] (see Figure 13.14). The response to phenobarbital is the criterion used to differentiate between these two disorders [492]. Bile analysis has also been suggested as another method to differentiate CNI and CNII [69]. In CNI, bile contains insignificant bilirubin conjugates (<10%) and unconjugated bilirubin predominates. In CNII, bile contains small amounts of bilirubin conjugates, and those present are predominantly bilirubin monoglucuronides (>60%) [412].

Recently, two cousins with CN were described with unique features that raise the possibility of a new variant of this syndrome (type III) [250]. This new variant resembled CNI in that there was no biliary excretion of bilirubin di- or monoglucuronide. However, the type III patients did excrete mono- and diglucoside conjugates of bilirubin. It has been speculated that type III patients lack the long-proposed permease [54] that has been hypothesized to transport UDP-glucuronic acid to the luminal side of the ER, where glucuronosyltransferase is located. This absence is suggested to force utilization of a very inefficient substrate for conjugation to bilirubin, UDP-glucose.

Diagnosis and Treatment

Although CN can be diagnosed during the prenatal period [493,494], evaluation of infants with CN more typically begins during the first days of life, when serum bilirubin levels exceed 20 mg/dL. The conjugated fraction will not be elevated, except possibly for the factitious elevation sometimes seen when the total serum bilirubin level is very high [126]. Evaluation of such infants will eliminate hemolysis, hypothyroidism, infection, and other more common causes of jaundice. Formula feedings will help identify those infants with jaundice related to human milk. During this period of testing, the magnitude of the serum bilirubin elevation will prompt use of phototherapy to avoid kernicterus [265]. Exchange transfusion may be necessary. Yet despite these efforts, CN patients will have persistent jaundice. There is currently no widely available simple clinical test to confirm a diagnosis of CN. CN can be excluded by finding significant amounts of bilirubin conjugates in neonatal stools, if collected before establishment of sufficient intestinal bacteria that convert bilirubin conjugates to urobilinoids [1]. HPLC analysis of duodenal bile will show that in CNI, there are negligible bilirubin di- or monoglucuronides, whereas in CNII, these conjugates are present but in low concentration [58,69]. An easy method to collect such fluid for analysis utilizes the pediatric Enterotest capsule [430]. This approach to diagnosis is much less invasive than performing a liver biopsy to confirm negligible BUGT activity with in vitro assay. The ratio of serum bilirubin conjugates (as determined by alkaline methanolysis with thin-layer chromatography) to total bilirubin, although abnormally low, does not allow differentiation of CN patients from those with GS [182]. Similar overlap occurs with HPLC fractionation of serum bilirubin conjugates [454]. DNA analysis can be very helpful in establishing the correct diagnosis [495] and in the future, it is expected that DNA array technology will allow rapid screening for known mutations.

A world registry of patients with CNI aimed at developing management guidelines has been published [496]. Phenobarbital (4 mg/kg/d in infants) should be used when there is concern about deficiency of BUGT. Within 48 hours, CNII patients may demonstrate a significant decrease in serum bilirubin levels (as detailed above) and an increased biliary excretion of bilirubin di- and monoglucuronides [70,249], whereas the CNI patients will show no significant response. Occasionally, CNII patients do not respond to the first trial of phenobarbital therapy, but subsequent trials months later will demonstrate the significant decrease in serum bilirubin level [492]. However, despite the decrease in serum bilirubin in response to phenobarbital, CNII patients will usually continue to manifest a significant hyperbilirubinemia (approximately 5–15 mg/dL). Phototherapy for 6–12 hours daily has been the primary modality to keep serum bilirubin levels below 20 mg/dL during the first several months of life [497], since CNI patients can excrete all bilirubin photoisomers [498]. CNI patients will require lifelong treatment with phototherapy until more definitive therapy such as liver transplantation. Phototherapy has been found to be least intrusive when given at night, and improvements have been made in effectiveness and comfort [499,500]. Although phototherapy is very helpful in infancy, in adolescence, social inconvenience and compliance problems may bring increased risk of kernicterus [496].

Other therapeutic considerations involve the oral administration of binding agents, such as agar or cholestyramine, or calcium phosphate [219,222,339]. These agents bind to bilirubin in the intestinal lumen because of phototherapy or through direct intestinal permeation [501]. They prevent the enterohepatic circulation of bilirubin. Problems associated with the use of cholestyramine include cost, taste, and concern about bile salt depletion and fat malabsorption. Problems regarding agar include significant variation in bilirubin binding affinity among various preparations and batches [219,220,245]. During acute episodes of severe hyperbilirubinemia after the first year of life, plasmapheresis has been shown to rapidly decrease serum bilirubin levels [245,502]. Peritoneal dialysis and exchange transfusion have not been helpful in this setting [247]. Repeated intramuscular injections of tin-protoporphyrin, a heme oxygenase inhibitor that blocks bilirubin formation, have been used in one CNI patient, with data suggesting a decreased need for phototherapy [503]. Two patients with CNI were treated with Sn-mesoporphyrin to block bilirubin formation and also received daily phototherapy and intermittent plasmapheresis over a 400-day period [504]. They developed an iron deficiency anemia believed to be the result of the porphyrin therapy [505], but Sn-mesoporphyrin (stannsoporfin; 2–4 μmol/kg) [506] is suggested to offer a promising though still experimental additional therapy for controlling episodes of acute, severe jaundice [507]. Drugs that bind to albumin and potentially displace bilirubin should be avoided at all times [508].

Because patients with CN have good hepatic function other than conjugating bilirubin, they are ideal candidates for auxiliary liver transplantation. This option has recently become clinically available [509–511]. More commonly, orthotopic liver transplantation has been performed [512–519], and this represents the only true cure for the hyperbilirubinemia of CNI. Ideally the timing of transplantation would precede irreversible neurologic injury [520]. Transplantation of other BUGT-containing tissues (e.g., segments of small intestine [521,522], kidneys [523], or hepatocytes [524]) remains experimental. Successful cloning of the gene responsible for bilirubin glucuronosyltransferase activity offers the hope of future gene therapy to correct this deficiency based on studies in Gunn rats, the congenitally jaundiced model for CNI [520,525–527].

Rotor's Syndrome

Clinical Presentation

Rotor's syndrome (RS; OMIM%237450), first described in 1948, is a familial disorder that involves chronic elevation of both the conjugated and unconjugated serum bilirubin fractions [528,529]. Half or more of the total serum bilirubin is conjugated, and total bilirubin levels usually range from 2–7 mg/dL but occasionally may reach 20 mg/dL [530]. Liver function tests are otherwise normal, and there is no evidence of hemolysis. Liver histology is normal when examined with both light and electron microscopy. Oral cholecystograms reveal normal gallbladder opacification. This disorder may present in early childhood [531] or possibly the first months of life if coinherited with G6PD deficiency or heterozygous β-thalassemia [532] and manifests no gender predisposition. Family studies suggest an autosomal recessive mode of inheritance [528,529,533].

Pathophysiology

The primary abnormality in RS is listed in OMIM as unknown but appears to be a deficiency in the intracellular storage capacity of the liver for binding anions [534,535], which can be demonstrated by constant infusions of BSP and ICG [536]. Patients with RS demonstrate a delayed plasma clearance of both BSP and ICG, and heterozygotes show delayed BSP clearance with values intermediate between normals and those with homozygous RS [534]. GST serves as an intracellular carrier protein for certain organic molecules, acting as an intracellular equivalent to albumin in blood plasma [537]. A patient with RS has been shown to have a deficiency of hepatic GST [538], and this would be consistent with observations regarding the pathogenesis of this disorder. Deficiency of GST would result in impaired uptake of bilirubin within the cytosol. In addition, because bilirubin conjugates are bound to GST while awaiting excretion from the hepatocyte via the canalicular membrane [539], deficient intracellular storage would result in leakage of bilirubin conjugates back into the circulation. Serum elevations of both conjugated and nonconjugated bilirubin result.

Another important observation in RS relates to the urinary excretion of coproporphyrin. In normal, healthy individuals, only the I and III isomers of coproporphyrin are excreted in the urine. In RS, there is a marked increase in urinary coproporphyrin excretion, and usually, less than 80% of the total (I + III) is isomer I. Heterozygotes demonstrate urinary coproporphyrin values that are intermediate between normals and homozygotes [540]. Urinary excretion of coproporphyrin is believed to be increased because biliary excretion is impaired, similar to findings in other liver diseases [541].

Diagnosis and Treatment

A diagnosis of RS should be considered in all individuals having elevation of both conjugated and nonconjugated serum bilirubin fractions along with otherwise normal liver function tests. The diagnosis can be confirmed by measuring urinary coproporphyrin levels that are 2.5 to 5 times higher than normal levels [540]. Of the total urinary coproporphyrin isomers I plus III, isomer I constitutes less than 80% of the total in RS [542]. Technetium Tc 99m hepatic iminodiacetic acid cholescintigraphy has also been shown to be useful in diagnosing RS and demonstrates poor to no visualization of the liver [543,544].

Patients with RS require no specific therapy and are asymptomatic. Although jaundice is a lifelong finding, it is associated with no morbidity or mortality.

Dubin–Johnson Syndrome

Clinical Presentation

Dubin–Johnson syndrome (OMIM #237500), first described in 1954 [545], involves elevation of both the conjugated and unconjugated serum bilirubin fractions [546]. More than half of the total serum bilirubin conjugated and total bilirubin levels usually range from 1.5–6 mg/dL, though have been reported as high as 25 mg/dL during intercurrent illness [547]. It is not unusual for patients with DJS to report vague abdominal complaints, though this is not believed to reflect serious pathology. Although hepatomegaly is sometime seen, liver function tests are otherwise normal, including bile acids [548], and there is no evidence of hemolysis [545,546,549]. Although this syndrome occurs in both sexes, males predominate and present at an earlier age. It occurs in all races; however, Iranian Jews have an increased incidence [550,551]. It is usually diagnosed after puberty, though cases have also been reported in neonates [552–555], at which time cholestasis may be significant [554,556–559]. DJS is inherited as an autosomal recessive trait, with heterozygotes manifesting normal serum bilirubin levels [550,560,561]. This syndrome is far more common than RS, and jaundice may be worsened by pregnancy and oral contraceptives [562]. Often patients with DJS do not visualize the gallbladder when undergoing oral cholecystogram [546].

A striking characteristic of DJS is the brown to black discoloration of the liver. There is still debate about the identity of this pigment, which is located in the lysosomes [563]. Although originally thought to be lipofuscin, more recent data provide conflicting evidence for a relationship to melanin [564–566] or polymerized epinephrine or other metabolites [567,568] that accumulate in the lysosomes. It is hypothesized that these pigments accumulate in the liver because of impaired secretion of various metabolites from the hepatocyte into the bile [568]. This pigment disappears from the liver during acute viral hepatitis, with subsequent reappearance [569]. Other than this striking pigmentation, the liver is histologically normal. Recently, a black liver was reported in an individual who did not have DJS [570].

Pathophysiology

The primary defect in the DJS is deficient hepatic excretion of non–bile salt organic anions at the apical canalicular membrane, by the ABC transport system known variously as cMOAT, MRP2, or ABCC2 (OMIM *601107) [571,572]. cMOAT is encoded by a single-copy gene located on chromosome 10q24 [573]. Mutations of this gene have been shown to produce a highly defective cMOAT that is associated with DJS

[81,571,572,574–577]. Similar findings made in the homologous *cMOAT* gene of two rat models of hyperbilirubinemia (transport deficient [TR−] and Eisai) have been very helpful in understanding DJS in humans [81].

Although hepatic BSP clearance tests are no longer performed, they nicely demonstrate the effect of deficient transport via the canalicular membrane, characteristic of DJS [578]. Initially the clearance rate of intravenously administered BSP from the circulation is rapid and results in a BSP retention that is often normal at 45 minutes. However, a subsequent rise in serum BSP concentration occurs at 90 and 120 minutes because the conjugated BSP cannot be excreted and thus refluxes out of the hepatocyte back into the circulation [578–581]. Data suggest that BSP hepatic storage is normal, but there is a 90% decrease in the BSP excretory transport maximum [562,580]. Other substances (e.g., ICG, rose bengal, and dibromosulfophthalein) have also been shown to have a decreased excretory transport maximum, though these substances do not require hepatic biotransformation and do not show the late rise in plasma levels during clearance tests [582]. Hence, in DJS, deficient excretion of bilirubin glucuronides at the canalicular membrane in the presence of otherwise normal intrahepatic metabolism results in reflux of conjugated bilirubin back into the circulation.

An important observation in DJS patients relates to the urinary excretion of coproporphyrins [583,584]. Patients with this disorder have an increase in the urinary excretion of coproporphyrin I with a concomitant decrease in the excretion of coproporphyrin III. This results in a total coproporphyrin excretion (I + III) that is normal or only slightly increased but that consists of greater than 80% coproporphyrin I (normal, 25%) [584–587]. In heterozygotes, the coproporphyrin I/III ratios are intermediate between normals and homozygotes [584,586,587], though there is some overlap between heterozygotes and normals. The explanation for these findings regarding urinary coproporphyrin excretion is unclear. Several pathogenetic mechanisms have been suggested [584]. Fecal coproporphyrin levels are normal [584]. Healthy neonates have been shown to have impressive elevations of urinary coproporphyrin levels, with more than 80% isomer I during the first 2 days of life [588]. By day 10, levels fall to overlap normal adult values.

Diagnosis and Treatment

A diagnosis of DJS should be considered in all individuals having elevation of conjugated bilirubin in the serum along with otherwise normal liver function tests. The diagnosis can be confirmed by measuring urinary coproporphyrin levels of isomers I and III. Although the total coproporphyrin level will be approximately normal, more than 80% will be isomer I. This finding is pathognomonic for DJS when congenital erythropoietic porphyria [589] or arsenic poisoning [590] have been excluded. Although oral cholecystogram may fail to visualize the gallbladder, ultrasound examination will show a normal biliary tree. Cholescintigraphy demonstrates prolonged intense visualization of the liver with delayed appearance of the gallbladder and only faint or nonvisualization of the biliary ducts [544,591,592]. Computed tomography of the liver has shown increased attenuation in one report [593]. Because cMOAT transport of leukotrienes into bile is defective in DJS, there is increased excretion of leukotriene metabolites into urine, and this has been suggested to be a new approach to the noninvasive diagnosis of this disease [594]. Another proposed diagnostic tool for DJS involves micro–positron emission tomographic imaging of a copper complex studied in normal and cMOAT-deficient (TR−) rats [595]. In normal rats, the radioactive copper complex was cleared quickly from the liver into the intestine, whereas radioactivity accumulated continuously in the liver of TR− rats and was not excreted into the small intestine.

Patients with DJS require no specific therapy. Although jaundice is a lifelong finding, it is associated with no morbidity or mortality, as demonstrated in a 30-year follow-up of ten Japanese individuals [577]. Avoidance of oral contraceptives has been recommended [596] because they can increase jaundice. Anticipatory guidance regarding pregnancy [562] is appropriate. Increased fetal wastage has been reported in one study [597]. In one case report of neonatal DJS with severe cholestasis, phenobarbital significantly decreased serum levels of bilirubin and bile acids [556], though chronic phenobarbital therapy is not recommended [598].

ELECTRONIC DATABASE INFORMATION

Online Mendelian Inheritance in Man (OMIM) is located at http://www.ncbi.nlm.nih.gov/entrez/query.fcgi?db=OMIM.

REFERENCES

1. Gourley GR. Bilirubin metabolism and kernicterus. Advances in pediatrics. Adv Pediatr 1997;44:173–229.
2. Bhutani VK, Johnson LH, Keren R. Diagnosis and management of hyperbilirubinemia in the term neonate: for a safer first week. Pediatr Clin North Am 2004;51:843–61, vii.
3. Maisels MJ. Jaundice. In: MacDonald MG, Seshia MMK, Mullett MD, eds. Avery's neonatology: pathophysiology & management of the newborn. 6th ed. Philadelphia: JB Lippincott Company, 2005:768–846.
4. Städeler G. Ueber die farbstoffe der galle. Justus Liebigs Ann Chem 1864;132:323–54.
5. Schmid R, McDonagh AF. The enzymatic formation of bilirubin. Ann N Y Acad Sci 1975;244:533–52.
6. Maines MD. The heme oxygenase system: a regulator of second messenger gases. Annu Rev Pharmacol Toxicol 1997;37:517–54.
7. Ewing JF, Maines MD. Histochemical localization of heme oxygenase-2 protein and MRNA expression in rat brain. Brain Res Brain Res Protoc 1997;1:165–74.
8. Henningsson R, Alm P, Ekstrom P, Lundquist I. Heme oxygenase and carbon monoxide: regulatory roles in islet hormone release: a biochemical, immunohistochemical, and confocal microscopic study. Diabetes 1999;48:66–76.
9. Zakhary R, Poss KD, Jaffrey SR, et al. Targeted gene deletion of heme oxygenase 2 reveals neural role for carbon monoxide. Proc Natl Acad Sci U S A 1997;94:14848–53.
10. Ryter SW, Otterbein LE. Carbon monoxide in biology and medicine. Bioessays 2004;26:270–80.

11. Fischer H, Orth H. Die chemie des pyrrols. Leipzig: Akademische Verlagsgesellschaft M.B.H., 1937:626.
12. O'Carra P, Colleran E. Methine bridge selectivity in haem-cleavage reactions: relevance to the mechanism of haem catabolism. Biochem Soc Trans 1976;4:209–14.
13. Blumenthal SG, Stucker T, Rassmussen RD, et al. Changes in bilirubins in human prenatal development. Biochem J 1980;186:693–700.
14. Blumenthal SG, Taggart DB, Ikeda R, et al. Conjugated and unconjugated bilirubins in bile of human and rhesus monkeys – structure of adult human and rhesus monkey bilirubins compared with dog bilirubins. Biochem J 1977;167:535–48.
15. Colleran E, O'Carra P. Enzymology and comparative physiology of biliverdin reduction. In: Berk PD, Berlin NE, eds. International symposium on chemistry and physiology of bile pigments. Washington, DC: U.S. Government Printing Office, 1977:69.
16. Bartoletti AL, Stevenson DK, Ostrander CR, Johnson JD. Pulmonary excretion of carbon monoxide in the human infant as an index of bilirubin production. I. Effects of gestational age and postnatal age and some common neonatal abnormalities. J Pediatr 1979;94:952–5.
17. Stevenson DK, Ostrander CR, Cohen RS, et al. Pulmonary excretion of carbon monoxide in the human infant as an index of bilirubin production. IIb. Evidence for the possible effect of maternal prenatal glucose metabolism on postnatal bilirubin production in a mixed population of infants. Eur J Pediatr 1981;137:255–9.
18. Maisels MJ, Pathak A, Nelson NM, et al. Endogenous production of carbon monoxide in normal and erythroblastotic infants. J Clin Invest 1971;50:1–8.
19. Bloomer JR, Berk PD, Howe RB, et al. Comparison of fecal urobilinogen excretion with bilirubin production in normal volunteers and patients with increased bilirubin production. Clin Chim Acta 1970;29:463.
20. Whipple GH, Hooper CW. Bile pigment metabolism. VII. Bile pigment output influenced by hemoglobin injections, anemia and blood regeneration. Am J Physiol 1917;43:258–74.
21. London IM. Conversion of hematin to bile pigment. J Biol Chem 1950;184:373–6.
22. Ostrow JD, Jandle JG, Schmid R. The formation of bilirubin from hemoglobin in vivo. J Clin Invest 1962;41:1628–37.
23. Coburn RF, Kane PB. Maximal erythrocyte and hemoglobin catabolism. J Clin Invest 1968;47:1435–46.
24. Daly JS, Little JM, Troxler RF, Lester R. Metabolism of 3H-myoglobin. Nature 1967;216:1030–1.
25. London IM, West R. The formation of bile pigment in pernicious anemia. J Biol Chem 1950;184:359–64.
26. Gray CH, Scott JJ. The effect of haemorrhage on the incorporation [α-C^{14}] glycine into stercobilin. J Biochem 1959;71:38–42.
27. Robinson SH, Tsong M, Brown BW, and et al. The sources of bile pigment in the rat: studies of early labeled fraction. J Clin Invest 1966;45:1569–86.
28. Sedlak TW, Snyder SH. Bilirubin benefits: cellular protection by a biliverdin reductase antioxidant cycle. Pediatrics 2004;113:1776–82.
29. Bonnett R, Davies JE, Hursthouse MB. Structure of bilirubin. Nature 1976;262:327–8.
30. Bennhold H. Uber die vehikelfunktion der serumeiweisskorper. Ergebnisse Inneren Medizin Kinderheilkunde 1932;42:273–375.
31. Jacobsen J. Binding of bilirubin to human serum albumin – determination of the dissociation constants. FEBS Lett 1969;5:112–14.
32. Robertson A, Karp W, Brodersen R. Comparison of the binding characteristics of serum albumins from various animal species. Dev Pharmacol Ther 1990;15:106–11.
33. Vracko R. Basal lamina scaffold. Anatomy and significance for maintenance of orderly tissue structure. Am J Pathol 1974;77:314–38.
34. Schaffner F, Popper H. Capillarization of hepatic sinusoids in man. Gastroenterology 1963;44:239–42.
35. Bloomer JR, Berk PD, Vergalla J, Berlin NI. Influence of albumin on the hepatic uptake of unconjugated bilirubin. Clin Sci Mol Med 1973;45:505–16.
36. Scharschmidt BF, Waggoner JG, Berk PD. Hepatic organic anion uptake in the rat. J Clin Invest 1975;56:1280–92.
37. Zucker SD, Goessling W, Hoppin AG. Unconjugated bilirubin exhibits spontaneous diffusion through model lipid bilayers and native hepatocyte membranes. J Biol Chem 1999;274:10852–62.
38. Wolkoff AW, Chung CT. Identification, purification and partial characterization of an organic anion binding protein from rat liver plasma membrane. J Clin Invest 1980;65:1152–61.
39. Wolkoff AW, Sosiak A, Greenblutt HC, et al. Immunologic studies on an organic anion-binding protein isolated from rat liver cell plasma membrane. J Clin Invest 1985;76:454–9.
40. Stremmel W, Gerber M, Glezerov V, et al. Physiochemical and immunohistological studies of a sulfobromophthalein- and bilirubin-binding protein from rat liver plasma membranes. J Clin Invest 1983;71:1796–805.
41. Cui Y, Konig J, Leier I, et al. Hepatic uptake of bilirubin and its conjugates by the human organic anion transporter SLC21A6. J Biol Chem 2001;276:9626–30.
42. Cui Y, Walter B. Influence of albumin binding on the substrate transport mediated by human hepatocyte transporters OATP2 and OATP8. J Gastroenterol 2003;38:60–8.
43. Wolkoff AW, Weisiger RA, Jakoby WB. The multiple roles of the glutathione transferases (ligandin). Prog Liver Dis 1979;6:213–24.
44. Wolkoff AW, Goresky CA, Sellin J, et al. Role of ligandin in transfer of bilirubin from plasma into liver. Am J Physiol 1979; 236:E638–48.
45. Boyer TD. The glutathione S-transferases: an update. Hepatology 1989;9:486–96.
46. Dutton GJ. The biosynthesis of glucuronides. In: Dutton GJ, ed. Glucuronic acid, free and combined: chemistry, biochemistry, pharmacology and medicine. London: Academic Press, 1966: 186–299.
47. Burchell B. Substrate specificity and properties of uridine diphosphate glucuronyltransferase purified to apparent homogeneity from phenobarbital-treated rat liver. Biochem J 1978;173:749–57.
48. Bock KW, Josting D, Lilienblum W, Pfeil H. Purification of rat liver microsomal UDP-glucuronyltransferase. Separation of two enzyme forms inducible by 3-methylcholanthrene or phenobarbital. Eur J Pediatr 1979;98:19–26.
49. Falany CN, Tephly TR. Separation, purification and characterization of three isozymes of UDP-glucuronyltransferase from rat liver microsomes. Arch Biochem Biophys 1983;227:248–58.
50. Matern H, Matern S, Gerok W. Isolation and characterization of rat liver microsomal UDP-glucuronsyltransferase activity

toward chenodeoxycholic acid and testosterone as a single form of enzyme. J Biol Chem 1982;257:7422–9.

51. Roy Chowdhury N, Gross F, Moscioni AD, et al. Isolation of multiple normal and functionally defective forms of uridine diphosphate-glucuronosyl-transferase from inbred Gunn rats. J Clin Invest 1987;79:327–34.
52. Senafi SB, Clarke DJ, Burchell B. Investigation of the substrate specificity of a cloned expressed human bilirubin UDP-glucuronosyltransferase: UDP-sugar specificity and involvement in steroid and xenobiotic glucuronidation. Biochem J 1994;303(pt 1):233–40.
53. Pogell BM, LeLoir LF. Nucleotide activation of liver microsomal glucuronidation. J Biol Chem 1961;236:293–8.
54. Berry C, Hallinan T. Summary of a novel, three-component regulatory model for uridine diphosphate glucuronyltransferase. Biochem Soc Trans 1976;4:650–2.
55. Kuriyama T. Studies on microsomal nucleoside diphosphatase of rat hepatocytes. Its purification, intramembranous location and turnover. J Biol Chem 1972;247:2979–88.
56. Bosma PJ, Seppen J, Goldhoorn B, et al. Bilirubin UDP-glucuronosyltransferase 1 is the only relevant bilirubin glucuronidating isoform in man. J Biol Chem 1994;269:17960–4.
57. Ritter JK, Chen F, Sheen Y, et al. A novel complex locus *UGT1* encodes human bilirubin, phenol, and other UDP-glucuronosyltransferase isozymes with identical carboxyl termini. J Biol Chem 1992;267:3257–61.
58. Clarke DJ, Moghrabi N, Monaghan G, et al. Genetic defects of the UDP-glucuronosyltransferase-1 (*UGT1*) gene that cause familial non-haemolytic unconjugated hyperbilirubinaemias. Clin Chim Acta 1997;266:63–74.
59. Gong QH, Cho JW, Huang T, et al. Thirteen UDPglucuronosyltransferase genes are encoded at the human *UGT1* gene complex locus. Pharmacogenetics 2001;11:357–68.
60. Mackenzie PI, Owens IS, Burchell B, et al. The UDP glycosyltransferase gene superfamily: recommmended nomenclature update based on evolutionary divergence. Pharmacogenetics 1997;7:255–69.
61. Blanckaert N, Gollan J, Schmid R. Bilirubin diglucuronide synthesis by a UDP-glucuronic acid-dependent enzyme system in rat liver microsomes. Proc Natl Acad Sci U S A 1979;76:23037–41.
62. Gordon ER, Meier PJ, Goresky CA, Boyer JL. Mechanism and subcellular site of bilirubin diglucuronide formation in rat liver. J Biol Chem 1984;259:5500–6.
63. Hauser SC, Ziurys JC, Gollan JL. Regulation of bilirubin glucuronide synthesis in primate (*Macaca fascicularis*) liver – kinetic analysis of microsomal bilirubin uridine diphosphate glucuronyltransferase. Gastroenterology 1986;91:287–96.
64. Burchell B, Blanckaert N. Bilirubin mono- and diglucuronide formation by purified rat liver microsomal bilirubin UDP-glucuronyltransferase. Biochem J 1984;223:461–5.
65. Chowdhury NR, Arias IM, Lederstein M, Chowdhury JR. Substrates and products of purified rat liver bilirubin UDP-glucuronsyltransferase. Hepatology 1986;6:123–8.
66. Maruo Y, Iwai M, Mori A, et al. Polymorphism of UDP-glucuronosyltransferase and drug metabolism. Curr Drug Metab 2005; 6:91–9.
67. Fevery J, Van Damme B, Mechiel R, et al. Bilirubin conjugates in bile of man and rat in the normal state and in liver disease. J Clin Invest 1972;51:2482–92.
68. Gordon ER, Goresky CA, Chan TH, Perlin AS. The isolation and characterization of bilirubin diglucuronide, the major bilirubin conjugate in dog and human bile. Biochem J 1976;155: 477–86.
69. Sinaasappel M, Jansen PL. The differential diagnosis of Crigler–Najjar disease, types 1 and 2, by bile pigment analysis. Gastroenterology 1991;100:783–9.
70. Fevery J, Blanckaert N, Heirwegh KPM, et al. Unconjugated bilirubin and an increased proportion of bilirubin monoconjugates in the bile of patients with Gilbert's syndrome and Crigler–Najjar disease. J Clin Invest 1977;60:970–9.
71. Fevery J, Blanckaert N, Leroy P, et al. Analysis of bilirubins in biological fluids by extraction and thin-layer chromatography of the intact tetrapyrrole: application to bile of patients with Gilbert's syndrome, hemolysis, or cholelithiasis. Hepatology 1983;3:177–83.
72. Goresky CA, Gordon ER, Shaffer EA, et al. Definition of a conjugation dysfunction in Gilbert's syndrome: studies of the handling of bilirubin loads and of the pattern of bilirubin conjugates secreted in bile. Clin Sci 1978;55:63–71.
73. Adachi Y, Kobayashi H, Kurumi Y, et al. Bilirubin diglucuronide transport by rat liver canalicular membrane vesicles: stimulation by biocarbonate ion. Hepatology 1991;14:1251–8.
74. Nishida T, Gatmaitan Z, Roy-Chowdhry J, Arias IM. Two distinct mechanisms for bilirubin glucuronide transport by rat bile canalicular membrane vesicles. Demonstration of defective ATP-dependent transport in rats (TR-) with inherited conjugated hyperbilirubinemia. J Clin Invest 1992;90:2130–5.
75. Paulusma CC, Oude, Elferink RP. The canalicular multispecific organic anion transporter and conjugated hyperbilirubinemia in rat and man. J Mol Med 1997;75:420–8.
76. Keppler D, Konig J. Hepatic canalicular membrane 5: expression and localization of the conjugate export pump encoded by the MRP2 (CMRP(CMOAT) gene in liver. FASEB J 1997;11:509–16.
77. Chandra P, Brouwer KL. The complexities of hepatic drug transport: current knowledge and emerging concepts. Pharm Res 2004;21:719–35.
78. Paulusma CC, Bosma PJ, Zaman GJ, et al. Congenital jaundice in rats with a mutation in a multidrug resistance-associated protein gene. Science 1996;271:1126–8.
79. Kamisako T, Leier I, Cui Y, et al. Transport of monoglucuronosyl and bisglucuronosyl bilirubin by recombinant human and rat multidrug resistance protein 2. Hepatology 1999;30:485–90.
80. Keppler D, Leier I, Jedlitschky G, et al. The function of the multidrug resistance proteins (MRP and CMRP) in drug conjugate transport and hepatobiliary excretion. Adv Enzyme Regul 1996;36:17–29.
81. Wada M, Toh S, Taniguchi K, et al. Mutations in the canilicular multispecific organic anion transporter (CMOAT) gene, a novel ABC transporter, in patients with hyperbilirubinemia II(Dubin-Johnson syndrome. Hum Mol Genet 1998;7:203–7.
82. Erlinger S. Physiology of bile flow. Prog Liver Dis 1975;4:63–82.
83. Weinbren K, Billing BH. Hepatic clearance of bilirubin as an index of cellular function in the regenerating rat liver. Br J Exper Pathol 1956;37:199–204.
84. Natzschka JC, Odell GB. The influence of albumin on the distribution and excretion of bilirubin in jaundiced rats. Pediatrics 1966;37:51–61.
85. Albert S, Mosher M, Shanske A, Arias IM. Multiplicity of hepatic excretory mechanisms for organic anions. J Gen Physiol 1969;53:238–47.

86. Hargreaves T, Lathe GH. Inhibitory aspects of bile secretion. Nature 1963;200:1172–6.
87. Clarenburg R, Kao CC. Shared and separate pathways for biliary excretion of bilirubin and BSP in rats for biliary excretion of bilirubin and BSP in rats. Am J Physiol 1973;225:192–200.
88. Schoenfield LJ, McGill DB, Hunton DB, et al. Studies of chronic idiopathic jaundice (Dubin-Johnson syndrome). I. Demonstration of hepatic excretory defect. Gastroenterology 1963;44:101–11.
89. Goresky CA, Haddad HH, Kluger WS, et al. The enhancement of maximal bilirubin excretion with taurocholate-induced increments in bile flow. Can J Physiol Pharmacol 1974;52:389–403.
90. Roberts RJ, Plaa GS. Effect of phenobarbital on the excretion of an exogenous bilirubin load. Biochem Pharmacol 1967;16: 827–35.
91. Gallagher TF, Mueller MN, Kappas A. Estrogen pharmacology. IV. Studies on the structural basis for estrogen-induced impairment of liver function. Medicine 1966;45:471–9.
92. Zimmerman HJ. Hormonal derivatives and other drugs used to treat endocrine disease. In: Hepatotoxicity. The adverse effects of drug and other chemicals on the liver. New York: Appleton, Crofts, 1978:436–67.
93. Fevery J, Blanckaert N. Review. What can we learn from analysis of serum bilirubin? J Hepatol 1986;2:113–21.
94. Muraca M, Fevery J, Blanckaert N. Relationships between serum bilirubins and production and conjugation of bilirubin – studies in Gilbert's syndrome, Crigler-Najjar disease, hemolytic disorders, and rat models. Gastroenterology 1987;92:309–17.
95. Van Steenbergen W, Fevery J. Effects of uridine diphosphate glucuronosyltransferase activity on the maximal secretion rate of bilirubin conjugates in the rat. Gastroenterology 1990;99:488–99.
96. Sieg A, Stiehl A, Raedsch R, et al. Gilbert's syndrome: diagnosis by typical serum bilirubin pattern. Clin Chim Acta 1986;154: 41–7.
97. Ullrich D, Fevery J, Sieg A, et al. The influence of gestational age on bilirubin conjugation in newborns. Eur J Clin Invest 1991;21:83–9.
98. Weiss JS, Guatam A, Lauff JJ, et al. The clinical importance of a protein-bound fraction of serum bilirubin in patients with hyperbilirubinemia. N Engl J Med 1983;309:147–50.
99. Brett EM, Hicks JM, Powers DM, Rand RN. Delta bilirubin in serum of pediatric patients: correlations with age and disease. Clin Chem 1984;30:1561–4.
100. Van Breemen RB, Fenselau C. Acylation of albumin by 1-O-acyl glucuronides. Drug Metab Dispos 1985;13:318–20.
101. Stogniew M, Fenselau C. Electrophilic reactions of acyl-linked glucuronides-formation of clofibrate mercapturate in humans. Drug Metab Dispos 1982;10:609–13.
102. Van Breemen RB. Electrophilic reactions of 1-*O*-acyl glucuronides [dissertation]. Baltimore: Johns Hopkins University, 1985.
103. Berson SA, Yalow RS, Schreiber SS. Tracer experiments with I^{131} labeled human serum albumin: distribution and degradation studies. J Clin Invest 1953;32:746–68.
104. Billing BH. Intestinal and renal metabolism of bilirubin including enterohepatic circulation. In: Ostrow JD. Bile pigments and jaundice. New York: Marcel Dekker, 1986;255–69.
105. Midtvedt T, Gustafsson BE. Microbial conversion of bilirubin to urobilins in vitro and in vivo. Acta Pathol Microbiol Immunol Scand [B] 1981;89:57–60.
106. Fahmy K, Gray CH, Nicholson DC. The reduction of bile pigments by faecal and intestinal bacteria. Biochim Biophys Acta 1972;264:85–97.
107. Poland RL, Odell GB. Physiologic jaundice: the enterohepatic circulation of bilirubin. NEngl J Med 1971;284:1–6.
108. Vitek L, Zelenka J, Zadinova M, Malina J. The impact of intestinal microflora on serum bilirubin levels. J Hepatol 2005;42:238–43.
109. Hawksworth G, Drasar BS, Hill MJ. Intestinal bacteria and the hydrolysis of glycosidic bonds. J Med Microbiol 1971;4:451–9.
110. Kent TH, Fischer LJ, Marr R. Glucuronidase activity in intestinal contents of rat and man and relationship to bacterial flora. Proc Soc Exp Biol Med 1972;140:590–4.
111. Nanno M, Morotomi M, Takayama H, et al. Mutagenic activation of biliary metabilites of benzo(a)pyrene by beta-glucuronidase-positive bacteria in human faeces. J Med Microbiol 1986;22:351–5.
112. Musa BU, Doe RP, Seal US. Purification and properties of human liver β-glucuronidase. J Biol Chem 1965;240:2811–16.
113. Lester R, Schmid R. Intestinal absorption of bile pigments. I. The enterohepatic circulation of bilirubin in the cat. J Clin Invest 1963;42:736–46.
114. Gourley GR, Arend RA. β-glucuronidase and hyperbilirubinemia in breast-fed and formula-fed babies. Lancet 1986;i:644–6.
115. Saxerholt H, Skar V, Midtvedt T. HPLC separation and quantification of bilirubin and its glucuronide conjugates in faeces and intestinal contents of germ-free rats. Scand J Clin Lab Invest 1990;50:487–95.
116. Gourley GR. Pathophysiology of breast-milk jaundice. In: Polin RA, Fox WW, eds. Fetal and neonatal physiology. 2nd ed. Philadelphia: WB Saunders Company, 1998:1499–505.
117. Kreamer BL, Siegel FL, Gourley GR. A novel inhibitor of β-glucuronidase: L-aspartic acid. Pediatr Res 2001;50:460–6.
118. Gourley GR, Li Z, Kreamer BL, Kosorok MR. A controlled, randomized, double-blind trial of prophylaxis against jaundice among breastfed newborns. Pediatrics 2005;116:385–91.
119. Newman TB, Easterling MJ, Goldman ES, Stevenson DK. Laboratory evaluation of jaundice in newborns – frequency, cost and yield. Am J Dis Child 1990;144:364–8.
120. Rutledge JC, Ou CN. Bilirubin and the laboratory. Advances in the 1980s, considerations for the 1990s. Pediatr Clin North Am 1989;36:189–97.
121. Schreiner RL, Glick MR. Interlaboratory bilirubin variability. Pediatrics 1982;69:277–81.
122. Rosenthal P, Keefe MT, Henton D, et al. Total and direct-reacting bilirubin values by automated methods compared with liquid chromatography and with manual methods for determining delta bilirubin. Clin Chem 1990;36:788–91.
123. Westwood A. The analysis of bilirubin in serum. Ann Clin Biochem 1991;28:119–30.
124. Vreman HJ, Verter J, Oh W, et al. Interlaboratory variability of bilirubin measurements. Clin Chem 1996;42:869–73.
125. Schlebusch H, Axer K, Schneider C, et al. Comparison of five routine methods with the candidate reference method for the determination of bilirubin in neonatal serum. J Clin Chem Clin Biochem 1990;28:203–10.
126. Mair B, Klempner LB. Abnormally high values for direct bilirubin in the serum of newborns as measured with the DuPont Aca. Am J Clin Pathol 1987;87:642–4.
127. Blanckaert N, Kabra PM, Farina FA. Measurement of bilirubin and its monoconjugates and diconjugates in human serum by

alkaline methanolysis and high-performance liquid chromatography. J Lab Clin Med 1980;96:198–212.
128. Wu TW, Dappen GM, Powers DM. The Kodak EKTACHEM clinical chemistry slide for measurement of bilirubin in newborns: principles and performance. Clin Chem 1982;28:2366–72.
129. Wu TW, Dappen GM, Spayd RW. The EKTACHEM clinical chemistry slide for simultaneous determination of unconjugated and sugarconjugated bilirubin. Clin Chem 1984;30:1304–9.
130. Mullon C, Langer R. Determination of conjugated and total bilirubin in serum of neonates, with use of bilirubin oxidase. Clin Chem 1987;33:1822–5.
131. Muraca M, Rubaltelli FF, Blanckaert N, Fevery J. Unconjugated and conjugated bilirubin pigments during perinatal development. II. Studies on serum of healthy newborns and of neonates with erythroblastosis fetalis. Biol Neonate 1990;57:1–9.
132. Arvan D, Shirey TL. Conjugated bilirubin: a better indicator of impaired hepatobiliary excretion than direct bilirubin. Ann Clin Lab Sci 1985;15:252–9.
133. Schlebusch H, Schneider C. Enzymatic determination of bilirubin in serum of newborns – any advantage over previous methods? Ann Clin Biochem 1991;28:290–6.
134. Leslie GI, Phillips JB, Cassady G. Capillary and venous bilirubin values: are they really different? Am J Dis Child 1987;141:1199–200.
135. Eidelman AI, Schimmel MS. Capillary and venous bilirubin values: they are different – and how! Am J Dis Child 1989;143:642.
136. Maisels MJ. Capillary vs. venous bilirubin values. Am J Dis Child 1990;144:521–2.
137. Bhutani VK, Gourley GR, Adler S, et al. Noninvasive measurement of total serum bilirubin in a multiracial predischarge newborn population to assess the risk of severe hyperbilirubinemia. Pediatrics 2000;106:e17.
138. Rubaltelli FF, Gourley GR, Loskamp N, et al. Transcutaneous bilirubin measurement: a multi-centre evaluation of a new device. Pediatrics 2001;107:1264–71.
139. Maisels MJ, Ostrea EM Jr, Touch S, et al. Evaluation of a new transcutaneous bilirubinometer. Pediatrics 2004;113:1628–35.
140. Knudsen A, Brodersen R. Skin color and bilirubin in neonates. Arch Dis Child 1989;64:605–9.
141. Schumacher RE, Thornbery JM, Gutcher GR. Transcutaneous bilirubinometry: a comparison of old and new methods. Pediatrics 1985;76:10–14.
142. Gossett IH, Oxon BM. A perspex icterometer for neonates. Lancet 1960;i:87–8.
143. Bilgen H, Ince Z, Ozek E, et al. Transcutaneous measurement of hyperbilirubinaemia: comparison of the Minolta jaundice meter and the Ingram icterometer. Ann Trop Paediatr 1998;18:325–8.
144. Knudsen A. The cephalocaudal progression of jaundice in newborns in relation to the transfer of bilirubin from plasma to skin. Early Hum Dev 1990;22:23–8.
145. Kramer LI. Advancement of dermal icterus in the jaundiced newborn. Am J Dis Child 1969;118:454–8.
146. American Academy of Pediatrics Subcommittee on Hyperbilirubinemia. Management of hyperbilirubinemia in the newborn infant 35 or more weeks of gestation. Pediatrics 2004;114:297–316.
147. Schneider AP. Breast milk jaundice in the newborn – a real entity. JAMA 1986;255:3270–4.
148. Johnson L, Brown AK. A pilot registry for acute and chronic kernicterus in term and near-term infants. Pediatrics 1999;104:736.
149. Brown AK, Johnson L. Loss of concern about jaundice and the re-emergence of kernicterus in full term infants in the era of managed care. In: Fanaroff A, Klaus M. Yearbook of neonatal and perinatal medicine. St. Louis: Mosby, 1996:xvii–xxviii.
150. Ebbesen F. Recurrence of kernicterus in term and near-term infants in Denmark. Acta Paediatr 2000;89:1213–17.
151. Bhutani VK, Johnson LH. Newborn jaundice and kernicterus – health and societal perspectives. Indian J Pediatr 2003;70:407–16.
152. Liu LL, Clemens CJ, Shay DK, et al. The safety of newborn early discharge. The Washington State experience. JAMA 1997;278:293–8.
153. Gourley GR. Breast-feeding, neonatal jaundice and kernicterus. Semin Neonatol 2002;7:135–41.
154. Salem-Schatz S, Peterson LE, Palmer RH, et al. Barriers to first-week follow-up of newborns: findings from parent and clinician focus groups. Jt Comm J Qual Saf 2004;30:593–601.
155. Szabo P, Wolf M, Bucher HU, et al. Detection of hyperbilirubinaemia in jaundiced full-term neonates by eye or by bilirubinometer? Eur J Pediatr 2004;163:722–7.
156. Shell ER. The hospital hustle. Parenting 1990;4:57–61.
157. Johnson L. Hyperbilirubinemia in the term infant: when to worry, when to treat. N Y State J Med 1991;91:483–7.
158. Joint Commission on Accreditation of Healthcare Organizations. Kernicterus threatens healthy newborns. Sentinel Event Alert, issue 18, April 2001.
159. Anonymous. Kernicterus in full-term infants – United States, 1994–1998. MMWR 2001;50:491–4.
160. Maisels MJ, Newman TB. Kernicterus in otherwise healthy, breast-fed term newborns. Pediatrics 1995;96:730–3.
161. American Academy of Pediatrics Subcommittee on Neonatal Hyperbilirubinemia. Neonatal jaundice. Pediatrics 2001;108:763–5.
162. Johnson LH, Bhutani VK, Brown AK. System-based approach to management of neonatal jaundice and prevention of kernicterus. J Pediatr 2002;140:396–403.
163. Committee on Fetus and Newborn. Hospital stay for healthy newborns. Pediatrics 1995;96:788–90.
164. Madlon-Kay DJ. Evaluation and management of newborn jaundice by Midwest family physicians. J Fam Pract 1998;47:461–4.
165. Maisels MJ, Newman TB. Jaundice in full-term and near-term babies who leave the hospital within 36 hours. The pediatrician's nemesis. Clin Perinatol 1998;25:295–302.
166. American Academy of Pediatrics. Practice parameter: management of hyperbilirubinemia in the healthy term newborn. Pediatrics 1994;94:558–65.
167. Newman TB, Hope S, Stevenson DK. Direct bilirubin measurements in jaundiced term newborns. A reevaluation. Am J Dis Child 1991;145:1305–9.
168. Keffler S, Kelly DA, Powell JE, Green A. Population screening for neonatal liver disease: a feasibility study. J Pediatr Gastroenterol Nutr 1998;27:306–11.
169. Bhutani VK, Johnson L, Sivieri EM. Predictive ability of a predischarge hour-specific serum bilirubin for subsequent significant hyperbilirubinemia in healthy term and near-term newborns. Pediatrics 1999;103:6–14.
170. Johnson L, Bhutani VK. Guidelines for management of the jaundiced term and near-term infant. Clin Perinatol 1998;25:555–74.

171. Maisels MJ. Neonatal jaundice. In: Avery GB, ed. Neonatology – pathophysiology and management of the newborn. Philadelphia: JB Lippincott, 1987:534–629.
172. Linn S, Schoenbaum SC, Monson RR, et al. Epidemiology of neonatal hyperbilirubinemia. Pediatrics 1985;75:770–4.
173. Bracci R, Buonocore G, Garosi G, et al. Epidemiologic study of neonatal jaundice – a survey of contributing factors. Acta Paediatr Scand Suppl 1989;360:87–92.
174. Johnson CA, Liese BS, Hassanein RE. Factors predictive of heightened third-day bilirubin levels: a multiple stepwise regression analysis. Fam Med 1989;21:283–7.
175. Meyer L, Mailloux J, Blanchet P, et al. Maternal and neonatal morbidity in instrumental deliveries with the Kobayashi vacuum extractor and low forceps. Acta Obstet Gynecol Scand 1987;66:643–7.
176. Freeman J, Lesko SM, Mitchell AA, et al. Hyperbilirubinemia following exposure to pancuronium bromide in newborns. Dev Pharmacol Ther 1990;14:209–15.
177. Knudsen A. Prediction of the development of neonatal jaundice by increased umbilical cord blood bilirubin. Acta Paediatr Scand 1989;78:217–21.
178. Knudsen A, Lebech M. Maternal bilirubin, cord bilirubin, and placenta function at delivery and the development of jaundice in mature newborns. Acta Obstet Gynecol Scand 1989;68:719–24.
179. Diwan VK, Vaughan TL, Yang CY. Maternal smoking in relation to the incidence of early neonatal jaundice. Gynecol Obstet Invest 1989;27:22–5.
180. Zipursky A. Mechanisms of hemolysis. Mead Johnson Symp Perinat Dev Med 1982;17–24.
181. Wenk RE, Goldstein P, Felix JK. Kell alloimmunization, hemolytic disease of the newborn, and perinatal management. Obstet Gynecol 1985;66:473–6.
182. Sieg A, Konig R, Ullrich D, Fevery J. Subfractionation of serum bilirubins by alkaline methanolysis and thin-layer chromatography. An aid in the differential diagnosis of icteric diseases. J Hepatol 1990;11:159–64.
183. Bevis DCA. The antenatal prediction of hemolytic disease of the newborn. Lancet 1952;i:395–8.
184. Odell GB. Evaluation of fetal hemolysis. N Engl J Med 1970; 282:1204–5.
185. Frigoletto FD, Greene MF, Benacerraf BR, et al. Ultrasonographic fetal surveillance in the management of the isoimmunized pregnancy. N Engl J Med 1986;315:430–2.
186. Vintzileos AM, Campbell WA, Storlazzi E, et al. Fetal liver ultrasound measurements in isoimmunized pregnancies. Obstet Gynecol 1986;62:162–7.
187. Grannum PA, Copel JA, Plaxe SC, et al. In utero exchange transfusion by direct intravascular injection in severe erythroblastosis fetalis. N Engl J Med 1986;314:1431–4.
188. Queenan JT. Erythroblastosis fetalis: closing the circle. N Engl J Med 1986;314:1448–9.
189. Clarke CA. Prevention of Rh-hemolytic disease. Br Med J 1967; 4:484–5.
190. Allen FH Jr, Diamond LK. Erythroblastosis fetalis, including exchange transfusion technique. Boston: Little, Brown and Co., 1958.
191. Gottstein R, Cooke RW. Systematic review of intravenous immunoglobulin in haemolytic disease of the newborn. Arch Dis Child Fetal Neonatal Ed 2003;88:F6–10.
192. Sato K, Hara T, Kondo T, et al. High-dose intravenous gammaglobulin therapy for neonatal immune haemolytic jaundice due to blood group incompatibility. Acta Paediatr Scand 1991;80:163–6.
193. Rubo J, Albrecht K, Lasch P, et al. High-dose intravenous immune globulin therapy for hyperbilirubinemia caused by Rh hemolytic disease. J Pediatr 1992;121:93–7.
194. Hammerman C, Kaplan M, Vreman HJ, Stevenson DK. Intravenous immune globulin in neonatal ABO isoimmunization: factors associated with clinical efficacy. Biol Neonate 1996;70:69–74.
195. Feng CS, Wan CP, Lau J, et al. Incidence of ABO haemolytic disease of the newborn in a group of Hong Kong babies with severe neonatal jaundice. J Paediatr Child Health 1990;26: 155–7.
196. Apt L, Downey WS. Melena neonatorum: the "swallowed blood syndrome." J Pediatr 1955;47:6–12.
197. Jacobs DS, Kasten BL, Demott WR, Wolfson WL. APT test. Laboratory test handbook with DRG index. St. Louis: Mosby/Lexi-Comp, 1984:277.
198. Danish EH. Neonatal polycythemia. In: Brown EB, ed. Progress in hematology. Vol. 14. New York: Grune and Stratton, 1986:55–98.
199. Oh W. Neonatal polycythemia and hyperviscosity. Pediatr Clin North Am 1986;33:523–32.
200. Mimouni F, Miodovnik M, Siddiqi TA, et al. Neonatal polycythemia in infants of insulin-dependent diabetic mothers. Obstet Gynecol 1986;68:370–2.
201. Schimmel MS, Bromiker R, Soll RF. Neonatal polycythemia: is partial exchange transfusion justified? Clin Perinatol 2004;31:545–53.
202. Wong WY, Powars DR, Abdalla C, Wu PY. Phototherapy failure in jaundiced newborns with hereditary spherocytosis. Acta Paediatr Scand 1990;79:568–9.
203. Owa JA. Relationship between exposure to icterogenic agents, glucose-6-phosphate dehydrogenase deficiency and neonatal jaundice in Nigeria. Acta Paediatr Scand 1989;78:848–52.
204. Kaplan M, Hammerman C. Severe neonatal hyperbilirubinemia. A potential complication of glucose-6-phosphate dehydrogenase deficiency. Clin Perinatol 1998;25:575–90.
205. Anonymous. Glucose-6-phosphate dehydrogenase deficiency. WHO Working Group. Bull World Health Organ 1989;67:601–11.
206. Liang ST, Wong VCW, So WW, et al. Homozygous α-thalassemia: clinical presentation, diagnosis and management: a review of 46 cases. Br J Obstet Gynaecol 1985;92:680–4.
207. Kan YW, Forget BG, Nathan DG. Gamma-beta thalassemia: a cause of hemolytic disease of the newborn. N Engl J Med 1972; 286:129–34.
208. Laosombat V, Dissaneevate S, Peerapittayamongkol C, Matsuo M. Neonatal hyperbilirubinemia associated with southeast asian ovalocytosis. Am J Hematol 1999;60:136–9.
209. Singhi S, Chookang E, Hall JSE. Intrapartum infusion of aqueous glucose solution, transplacental hyponatraemia, and risk of neonatal jaundice. Br J Obstet Gynaecol 1984;99:1014–18.
210. D'Souza SW, Lieberman B, Cadman J, Richards B. Oxytocin induction of labour: hyponatraemia and neonatal jaundice. Eur J Obstet Gynecol Reprod Biol 1986;22:309–17.
211. Leylek OA, Ergur A, Senocak F, et al. Prophylaxis of the occurrence of hyperbilirubinemia in relation to maternal oxytocin infusion with steroid treatment. Gynecol Obstet Invest 1998;46:164–8.

212. Odell GB. Normal metabolism of bilirubin during neonatal life. In: Neonatal hyperbilirubinemia. New York: Grune & Stratton, 1980:35–49.
213. Boggs TR Jr, Bishop H. Neonatal hyperbilirubinemia associated with high obstruction of the small bowel. J Pediatr 1965;66:349–56.
214. Porto SO. Jaundice in congenital malrotation of the intestine. Am J Dis Child 1969;117:684–8.
215. Clarkson JE, Cowan JO, Herbison GP. Jaundice in full-term healthy neonates – a population study. Aust Paediatr J 1984; 20:303–8.
216. Rosta J, Makoi Z, Kertesz A. Delayed meconium passage and hyperbilirubinemia. Lancet 1986;2:1138.
217. Cottrell BH, Anderson GC. Rectal or axillary temperature measurement: effect on plasma bilirubin and intestinal transit of meconium. J Pediatr Gastroenterol Nutr 1984;3:734–9.
218. Poland RL, Odell GB. The binding of bilirubin to agar. Proc Soc Exp Biol Med 1974;146:1114–18.
219. Odell GB, Gutcher GR, Whitington PF, Yang G. Enteral administration of agar as an effective adjunct to phototherapy of neonatal hyperbilirubinemia. Pediatr Res 1983;17:810–4.
220. Kemper K, Horwitz RI, McCarthy P. Decreased neonatal serum bilirubin with plain agar: a meta-analysis. Pediatrics 1988;82: 631–8.
221. Ulstrom RA, Eisenklam E. The enterohepatic shunting of bilirubin in the newborn infant: I. use of oral activated charcoal to reduce normal serum bilirubin values. J Pediatr 1964;65:27–37.
222. Arrowsmith WA, Payne RB, Littlewood JM. Comparison of treatments for congenital nonobstructive nonhaemolytic hyperbilirubinemia. Arch Dis Child 1975;50:197–201.
223. Gourley GR. The pathophysiology of breast milk jaundice. In: Polin RA, Fox WW, eds. Fetal and neonatal physiology. Philadelphia: WB Saunders, 1992:1173–9.
224. Gartner LM, Auerbach KG. Breast milk and breastfeeding jaundice. In: Barness LA, ed. Advances in pediatrics. Vol. 34. Chicago: Yearbook Medical Publishers, 1987:249–74.
225. Leung AK, Sauve RS. Breastfeeding and breast milk jaundice. J R Soc Health 1989;6:213–17.
226. Saigal S, Lunyk O, Bennett KJ, Patterson MC. Serum bilirubin levels in breast- and formula-fed infants in the first 5 days of life. Can Med Assoc J 1982;127:985–9.
227. Kivlahan C, James EJP. The natural history of neonatal jaundice. Pediatrics 1984;74:364–70.
228. Gartner LM, Arias IM. Studies of prolonged neonatal jaundice in the breast-fed infant. J Pediatr 1966;68:54–66.
229. Grunebaum E, Amir J, Merlob P, et al. Breast milk jaundice: natural history, familial incidence and late neurodevelopmental outcome of the infant. Eur J Pediatr 1991;150:267–70.
230. Behrman RE, Kliegman JM. Jaundice and hyperbilirubinemia in the newborn. In: Behrman RE, Vaughan VC 3rd, Nelson WE. Nelson textbook of pediatrics. 12th ed. Philadelphia: WB Saunders Co., 1983:378–81.
231. Lascari AD. "Early" breast-feeding jaundice: clinical significance. J Pediatr 1986;108:156–8.
232. Orlowski JP. Breast milk jaundice – early and late. Cleve Clin Q 1983;50:339.
233. Arias IM, Gartner LM, Seifter S, Furman M. Prolonged neonatal unconjugated hyperbilirubinemia associated with breast feeding and a steroid, pregnane-3(alpha), 20(beta)-diol in maternal milk that inhibits glucuronide formation in vitro. J Clin Invest 1964;43:2037–47.
234. Murphy JF, Hughs I, Verrier Jones ER, et al. Pregnanediols and breast-milk jaundice. Arch Dis Child 1981;56:474–6.
235. Bevan BR, Holton JB. Inhibition of bilirubin conjugation in rat liver slices by free fatty acids, with relevance to the problem of breast-milk jaundice. Clin Chim Acta 1972;41:101–7.
236. Poland RL, Schultz GE, Gayatri G. High milk lipase activity associated with breast-milk jaundice. Pediatr Res 1980;14:1328–31.
237. Hernell O. Breast-milk jaundice. J Pediatr 1982;99:311–14.
238. Constantopoulos A, Messaritakis J, Matsanoitis N. Breast-milk jaundice: the role of lipoprotein lipase and the free fatty acids. Eur J Pediatr 1980;134:35–8.
239. Forsyth JS, Donnet L, Ross PE. A study of the relationship between bile salts, bile salt-stimulated lipase, and free fatty acids in breast milk: normal infants and those with breast milk jaundice. J Pediatr Gastroenterol Nutr 1990;11:205–10.
240. Gaffney PT, Buttenshaw RL, Ward M, Diplock RD. Breast milk β-glucuronidase and neonatal jaundice. Lancet 1986;i:1161–2.
241. Alonso EM, Whitington PM, Whitington SH, et al. Enterohepatic circulation of nonconjugated bilirubin in rats fed with human milk. J Pediatr 1991;118:425–30.
242. Tazawa Y, Abukawa D, Watabe M, et al. Abnormal results of biochemical liver function tests in breast-fed infants with prolonged indirect hyperbilirubinaemia. Eur J Pediatr 1991;150: 310–13.
243. Maisels MJ, Gifford K. Normal serum bilirubin levels in the newborn and the effect of breast-feeding. Pediatrics 1986;78:837–43.
244. Crigler JF, Najjar VA. Congenital familial nonhemolytic jaundice with kernicterus. Pediatrics 1952;10:169–80.
245. Blaschke TF, Berke PD, Scharschmidt BF, et al. Crigler-Najjar syndrome: an unusual course with development of neurological damage at age eighteen. Pediatr Res 1974;8:573–90.
246. Duhamel G, Blanckaert N, Metreau JM, et al. An unusual case of Crigler-Najjar disease in the adult. Classification into types I and II revisited. J Hepatol 1985;1:47–53.
247. Blumenschein SD, Kallen RJ, Storey B, et al. Familial nonhemolytic jaundice with late onset of neurologic damage. Pediatrics 1968;42:786–92.
248. Arias IM, Gartner LM, Cohen M, et al. Chronic nonhemolytic unconjugated hyperbilirubinemia with glucuronyl transferase deficiency. Am J Med 1969;47:395–409.
249. Gordon ER, Shaffer EA, Sass-Kortsak A. Bilirubin secretion and conjugation in the Crigler-Najjar syndrome type II. Gastroenterology 1976;70:761–5.
250. Odell GB, Whitington PF. Crigler-Najjar syndrome, type III: a new variant of hereditary non-hemolytic, non-conjugated hyperbilirubinemia. Hepatology 1990;12:871.
251. Thompson GN, McCrossin RB, Penfold JL, et al. Management and outcome of children with congenital hypothyroidism detected on neonatal screening in South Australia. Med J Aust 1986;145:18–22.
252. Lafranchi S. Diagnosis and treatment of hypothyroidism in children. Compr Therapy 1987;13:20–30.
253. Odell GB. Studies in kernicterus. I. Protein binding of bilirubin. J Clin Invest 1959;38:823.
254. Stutman HR, Parker KM, Marks MI. Potential of moxalactam and other new antimicrobial agents for bilirubin-albumin displacement in neonates. Pediatrics 1985;75:294–8.
255. Brodersen R, Robertson A. Ceftriaxone binding to human serum albumin: competition with bilirubin. Mol Pharmacol 1989;36:478–83.

256. Park HZ, Lee SP, Suchy AL. Ceftriaxone-associated gallbladder sludge. Identification of calcium-ceftriaxone salt as a major component of gallbladder precipitate. Gastroenterology 1991;100:1665–70.
257. Yeung CY, Lee FT, Wong HN. Effect of a popular chinese herb on neonatal bilirubin protein binding. Biol Neonate 1990;58: 98–103.
258. Lambert GH, Muraskas J, Anderson CL, Myers TF. Direct hyperbilirubinemia associated with chloral hydrate administration in the newborn. Pediatrics 1990;86:277–81.
259. Jahrig D, Jahrig K, Stiete S, et al. Neonatal jaundice in infants of diabetic mothers. Acta Paediatr Scand 1989;360(suppl):101–7.
260. Arias IM, Wolfson S, Lucey JF, McKay RJ Jr. Transient familial neonatal hyperbilirubinemia. J Clin Invest 1965;44:1442–50.
261. Kawade N, Onishi S. The prenatal and postnatal development of UDP-glucuronyltransferase activity towards bilirubin and the effect of premature birth on this activity in the human liver. Biochem J 1981;196:257–60.
262. Obrinsky W, Denley ML, Brauer RW. Sulfobromophthalein sodium excretion test as a measure of liver function in premature infants. Pediatrics 1952;9:421–38.
263. Vest M, Rossier R. Detoxification in the newborn: the ability of the newborn infant to form conjugates with glucuronic acid, glycine, acetate and glutathione. Ann N Y Acad Sci 1963;111: 183–98.
264. Boggs TR Jr, Westphal MD Jr. Mortality of exchange transfusions. Pediatrics 1960;26:745–55.
265. Odell GB, Schutta HS. Bilirubin encephalopathy. In: McCandless DW, ed. Cerebral energy metabolism and metabolic encephalopathy. New York: Plenum Publishing Corp, 1985:229–61.
266. Walker PC. Neonatal bilirubin toxicity – a review of kernicterus and the implications of drug-induced bilirubin displacement. Clin Pharmacokinet 1987;13:26–50.
267. Claireaux AE. Pathology of human kernicterus. In: Sass-Kortsak A, ed. Kernicterus: a report based on a symposium held at the IX International Congress of Paediatrics. Toronto: University of Toronto Press, 1961:140.
268. Odell GB, Storey GNB, Rosenberg LA. Studies in kernicterus. III. The saturation of serum proteins with bilirubin during neonatal life and its relationship to brain damage at five years. J Pediatr 1970;76:12–21.
269. Johnson L, Boggs TR Jr. Bilirubin-dependent brain damage: incidence and indication for treatment. In: Odell GB, Schaffer R, Simopoulous AP, eds. Phototherapy in the newborn: an overview. Washington, DC: National Academy of Sciences, 1974:122–49.
270. Seidman DS, Paz I, Stevenson DK, et al. Neonatal hyperbilirubinemia and physical and cognitive performance at 17 years of age. Pediatrics 1991;88:828–33.
271. Brodersen R, Stern L. Deposition of bilirubin acid in the central nervous system – a hypothesis for the development of kernicterus. Acta Paediatr Scand 1990;79:12–19.
272. Brito MA, Brites D, Butterfield DA. A link between hyperbilirubinemia, oxidative stress and injury to neocortical synaptosomes. Brain Res 2004;1026:33–43.
273. Gardner WA Jr, Konigsmark BW. Familial nonhemolytic jaundice: bilirubinosis and encephalopathy. Pediatrics 1969;43:365–76.
274. Rubboli G, Ronchi F, Cecchi P, et al. A neurophysiological study in children and adolescents with Crigler-Najjar syndrome type I. Neuropediatrics 1997;28:281–6.
275. Hsia DYY, Allen FH Jr, Gellis SS, Diamond LK. Erythroblastosis fetalis. VIII. Studies of serum bilirubin in relation to kernicterus. N Engl J Med 1952;247:668–71.
276. Newman TB, Maisels MJ. Does hyperbilirubinemia damage the brain of healthy full-term infants? Clin Perinatol 1990;17:331–58.
277. Ose T, Tsuruhara T, Araki M, et al. Follow-up study of exchange transfusion for hyperbilirubinemia in infants in Japan. Pediatrics 1967;40:196–201.
278. Odell GB. The dissociation of bilirubin from albumin and its clinical implications. J Pediatr 1959;55:268–79.
279. Wadsworth SJ, Suh B. In vitro displacement of bilirubin by antibiotics and 2-hydroxybenzoylglycine in newborns. Antimicrob Agents Chemother 1988;32:1571–5.
280. Harris RC, Lucey JF, MacLean JR. Kernicterus in premature infants associated with low concentrations of bilirubin in the plasma. Pediatrics 1958;21:875–84.
281. Ahlfors CE, Wennberg RP. Bilirubin-albumin binding and neonatal jaundice. Semin Perinatol 2004;28:334–9.
282. Ahlfors CE, Marshall GD, Wolcott DK, et al. Measurement of unbound bilirubin by the peroxidase test using zone fluidics. Clin Chim Acta 2006;365:78–85.
283. Lenhardt ML, McArtor R, Bryant B. Effects of neonatal hyperbilirubinemia on the brainstem electric response. J Pediatr 1984;104:281–4.
284. Nakamura H, Takada S, Shimabuku R, et al. Auditory nerve and brainstem responses in newborn infants with hyperbilirubinemia. Pediatrics 1985;75:703–8.
285. Hung K. Auditory brainstem responses in patients with neonatal hyperbilirubinemia and bilirubin encephalopathy. Brain Dev 1989;11:297–301.
286. Gupta AK, Mann SB. Is auditory brainstem response a bilirubin neurotoxicity marker? Am J Otolaryngol 1998;19:232–6.
287. Perlman M, Fainmesser P, Sohmer H, et al. Auditory nerves–brainstem evoked responses in hyperbilirubinemic neonates. Pediatrics 1983;72:658–64.
288. Nwaesei CG, VanAerde J, Boyden M, Perlman M. Changes in auditory brainstem responses in hyperbilirubinemic infants before and after exchange transfusion. Pediatrics 1984;74: 800–3.
289. Wennberg RP, Ahlfors CE, Bickers R. Abnormal auditory brainstem response in a newborn infant with hyperbilirubinemia: improvement with exchange transfusion. J Pediatr 1982;100:624–6.
290. Deliac P, Demarquez JL, Barberot JP, et al. Brainstem auditory evoked potentials in icteric fullterm newborns: alterations after exchange transfusion. Neuropediatrics 1990;21:115–18.
291. Vohr BR, Karp D, O'Dea C, et al. Behavioral changes correlated with brain-stem auditory evoked responses in term infants with moderate hyperbilirubinemia. J Pediatr 1990;117:288–91.
292. Vohr BR, Lester B, Rapisardi G, et al. Abnormal brain-stem function (brain-stem auditory evoked response) correlates with acoustic cry features in term infants with hyperbilirubinemia. J Pediatr 1989;115:303–8.
293. Shapiro SM. Binaural effects in brainstem auditory evoked potentials of jaundiced Gunn rats. Hear Res 1991;53:41–8.
294. Bongers-Schokking JJ, Colon EJ, Hoogland RA, et al. Somatosensory evoked potentials in neonatal jaundice. Acta Paediatr Scand 1990;79:148–55.
295. Kemper K, Forsyth B, McCarthy P. Jaundice, terminating breast-feeding, and the vulnerable child. Pediatrics 1989;84:773–8.

296. Kemper KJ, Forsyth BW, McCarthy PL. Persistent perceptions of vulnerability following neonatal jaundice. Am J Dis Child 1990;144:238–41.
297. Schedle A, Fricker HS. Impact of hyperbilirubinaemia and transient mother-child separation in the neonatal period on mother-child attachment in the 1st year of life. Eur J Pediatr 1990;149:587–91.
298. Britton JR, Britton HL, Beebe SA. Early discharge of the term newborn: a continued dilemma. Pediatrics 1994;94:291–5.
299. Soskolne EL, Schumacher R, Fyock C, et al. The effect of early discharge and other factors on readmission rates of newborns. Arch Pediatr Adolesc Med 1996;150:373–9.
300. Ahlfors CE. Effect of ibuprofen on bilirubin-albumin binding. J Pediatr 2004;144:386–8.
301. Cockington RA, Drew JH, Eberhard A. Outcomes following the use of rational guidelines in the management of jaundiced newborn infants. Aust Paediatr J 1989;25:346–50.
302. Ennever JF. Blue light, green light, white light, more light: treatment of neonatal jaundice. Clin Perinatol 1990;17:467–81.
303. Pratesi R, Agati G, Fusi F. Phototherapy for neonatal hyperbilirubinemia. Photodermatol 1989;6:244–57.
304. McDonagh AF, Lightner DA. 'Like a shrivelled blood orange' – bilirubin, jaundice and phototherapy. Pediatrics 1985;75:443–5.
305. McDonagh AF, Palma LA, Lightner DA. Phototherapy for neonatal jaundice: stereospecific and regioselective photoisomerization of bilirubin bound to human serum albumin and NMR characterization of intramolecular cyclized photoproducts. J Am Chem Soc 1982;104:6867–9.
306. Itoh S, Onishi S, Manabe M, Yamakawa T. Wavelength dependence of the geometric and structural photoisomerization of bilirubin bound to human serum albumin. Biol Neonate 1987; 51:10–17.
307. Ennever JF, Dresing TJ. Quantum yields for the cyclization and configurational isomerization of 4e,15Z-bilirubin. Photochem Photobiol 1991;53:25–32.
308. Onishi S, Isobe K, Itoh S, et al. Metabolism of bilirubin and its photoisomers in newborn infants during phototherapy. J Biochem (Toyko) 1986;100:789–95.
309. Ennever JF, Costarino AT, Polin RA, et al. Rapid clearance of a structural isomer of bilirubin during phototherapy. J Clin Invest 1987;79:1674–8.
310. Tan KL. Efficacy of fluorescent daylight, blue, and green lamps in the management of nonhemolytic hyperbilirubinemia. J Pediatr 1989;114:132–7.
311. Rosenfeld W, Twist P, Concepcion L. A new device for phototherapy. Pediatr Res 1989;25:227A.
312. Rosenfeld W, Twist P, Concepcion L. A new device for phototherapy treatment of jaundiced infants. J Perinatol 1990;10: 243–8.
313. Gale R, Dranitzki Z, Dollberg S, Stevenson DK. A randomized, controlled application of the Wallaby phototherapy system compared with standard phototherapy. J Perinatol 1990;10:239–42.
314. van Kaam AH, van Beek RH, Vergunst-van Keulen JG, et al. Fibre optic versus conventional phototherapy for hyperbilirubinaemia in preterm infants. Eur J Pediatr 1998;157:132–7.
315. Fetus and Newborn Committee and Canadian Paediatric Society. Use of phototherapy for neonatal hyperbilirubinemia. Can Med Assoc J 1986;134:1237–45.
316. Cashore WJ, Stern L. The management of hyperbilirubinemia. Clin Perinatol 1984;11:339–57.
317. Polin RA. Management of neonatal hyperbilirubinemia: rational use of phototherapy. Biol Neonate 1990;58(suppl 1): 32–43.
318. Grabert BE, Wardwell C, Harburg SK. Home phototherapy. An alternative to prolonged hospitalization of the full-term, well newborn. Clin Pediatr 1986;25:291–4.
319. Ludwig MA. Phototherapy in the home setting. J Pediatr Health Care 1990;4:304–8.
320. Greenwald JL. Hyperbilirubinemia in otherwise healthy infants. Am Fam Physician 1988;38:151–8.
321. Gourley GR, Odell GB. Bilirubin metabolism in the fetus and neonate. In: Lebenthal E, ed. Human gastrointestinal development. New York: Raven Press, 1989:581–621.
322. De Curtis M, Guandalini S, Fasano A, et al. Diarrhea in jaundiced neonates treated with phototherapy: a role of intestinal secretion. Arch Dis Child 1989;64:1161–4.
323. Drew JH, Marriage KJ, Bayle V. Phototherapy. Short and long-term complications. Arch Dis Child 1976;51:454–8.
324. Scheidt PC, Bryla DA, Nelson KB, et al. Phototherapy for neonatal hyperbilirubinemia: six-year follow-up of the National Institute of Child Health and Human Development Clinical Trial. Pediatrics 1990;85:455–63.
325. Benders MJ, van Bel F, Van de Bor M. The effect of phototherapy on cerebral blood flow velocity in preterm infants. Acta Paediatr 1998;87:786–91.
326. Benders MJ, van Bel F, Van de Bor M. Haemodynamic consequences of phototherapy in term infants. Eur J Pediatr 1999;158: 323–8.
327. Yeo KL, Perlman M, Hao Y, Mullaney P. Outcomes of extremely premature infants related to their peak serum bilirubin concentrations and exposure to phototherapy. Pediatrics 1998;102:1426–31.
328. Gies HP, Roy CR. Bilirubin phototherapy and potential UVR hazards. Health Phys 1990;58:313–20.
329. Poland RL, Ostrea EM. Care of the high risk neonate. In: Klaus MH, Fanaroff AA, eds. Neonatal hyperbilirubinemia. 3rd ed. Philadelphia: Ardmore Medical Bools, an imprint of WB Saunders Company, 1986:238–61.
330. Yamauchi Y, Kasa N, Yamanouchi I. Is it necessary to change the babies' position during phototherapy. Early Hum Dev 1989; 20:221–7.
331. Yetman RJ, Parks DK, Huseby V, et al. Rebound bilirubin levels in infants receiving phototherapy. J Pediatr 1998;133:705–7.
332. Tan KL. Decreased response to phototherapy for neonatal jaundice in breast-fed infants. Arch Pediatr Adolesc Med 1998;152: 1187–90.
333. Odell GB. Treatment of neonatal hyperbilirubinemia. In: Neonatal hyperbilirubinemia. New York: Grune and Stratton, 1980:117.
334. Gartner LM, Lee K-S. Jaundice and liver disease. Part I. Unconjugated hyperbilirubinemia. In: Fanaroff AA, Martin RJ, eds. Behrman's neonatal-perinatal medicine. 3rd ed. St. Louis: CV Mosby, 1983:754–70.
335. Alpay F, Sarici SU, Okutan V, et al. High-dose intravenous immunoglobulin therapy in neonatal immune haemolytic jaundice. Acta Paediatr 1999;88:216–19.
336. Shapiro M. Safer exchange transfusions with ACD blood. Bibl Haematol 1965;23:883–6.
337. Weldon VV, Odell GB. Mortality risk of exchange transfusion. Pediatrics 1968;41:797–801.

338. Valaes TN, Harvey-Wilkes K. Pharmacologic approaches to the prevention and treatment of neonatal hyperbilirubinemia. Clin Perinatol 1990;17:245–73.
339. van der Veere CN, Jansen PL, Sinaasappel M, et al. Oral calcium phosphate: a new therapy for Crigler-Najjar disease? Gastroenterology 1997;112:455–62.
340. van der Veere CN, Schoemaker B, van der Meer R, et al. Rapid association of unconjugated bilirubin with amorphous calcium phosphate. J Lipid Res 1995;36:1697–707.
341. van der Veere CN, Schoemaker B, Bakker C, et al. Influence of dietary calcium phosphate on the disposition of bilirubin in rats with unconjugated hyperbilirubinemia. Hepatology 1996;24:620–6.
342. De Carvalho M, Klaus MH, Merkatz RB. Frequency of breastfeeding and serum bilirubin concentration. Am J Dis Child 1982;136:737–8.
343. Wu T-W, Li GS. A new bilirubin-degrading enzyme from orange peels. Biochem Cell Biol 1988;66:1248.
344. Johnson L, Dworanczyk R, Jenkins D. Bilirubin oxidase (BOX) feedings at varying time intervals and enzyme concentrations in infant Gunn rats. Pediatr Res 1989;25:116A.
345. Kimura M, Matsumura Y, Miyauchi Y, Maeda H. A new tactic for the treatment of jaundice: an injectable polymer-conjugated bilirubin oxidase. Proc Soc Exp Biol Med 1988;188:364–9.
346. Kimura M, Matsumura Y, Konno T, et al. Enzymatic removal of bilirubin toxicity by bilirubin oxidase in vitro and excretion of degradation products in vivo. Proc Soc Exp Biol Med 1990;195:64–9.
347. Gartner LM, Lee KS, Vaisman L, et al. Development of bilirubin transport and metabolism in the newborn rhesus monkey. J Pediatr 1977;90:513–31.
348. Waltman R, Nigrin G, Bonura F, et al. Ethanol in prevention of hyperbilirubinaemia in the newborn. Lancet 1969;ii:1265–7.
349. Rayburn W, Donn S, Piehl E, Compton A. Antenatal phenobarbital and bilirubin metabolism in the very low birth weight infant. Am J Obstet Gynecol 1988;159:1491–3.
350. Stern L, Khanna NN, Levy G, et al. Effect of phenobarbital on hyperbilirubinemia and glucuronide formation in newborns. Am J Dis Child 1970;120:26–31.
351. Gabilan JC, Benattar C, Lindenbaum A. Clofibrate treatment of neonatal jaundice. Pediatrics 1990;86:647–8.
352. Neifert MR. The optimization of breast-feeding in the perinatal period. Clin Perinatol 1998;25:303–26.
353. Gartner LM. Breast milk jaundice. In: Levine RL, Maisels MJ. Hyperbilirubinemia in the newborn. Report of the 85th Ross Conference on Pediatric Research. Columbus: Ross Laboratories, 1983:75–86.
354. Yamauchi Y, Yamanouchi I. Breast-feeding frequency during the first 24 hours after birth in full-term neonates. Pediatrics 1990;86:171–5.
355. Osborn LM, Bolus R. Breast feeding and jaundice in the first week of life. J Fam Pract 1985;20:475.
356. Gourley GR, Kreamer B, Arend R. The effect of diet on feces and jaundice during the first 3 weeks of life. Gastroenterology 1992;103:660–7.
357. Gourley GR, Kreamer B, Cohnen M, Kosorok MR. Neonatal jaundice and diet. Arch Pediatr Adolesc Med 1999;153:184–8.
358. Amato M, Howald H, von Muralt G. Interruption of breast-feeding versus phototherapy as treatment of hyperbilirubinemia in full-term infants. Helv Paediatr Acta 1985;40:127–31.
359. Stevenson DK, Rodgers PA, Vreman HJ. The use of metalloporphyrins for the chemoprevention of neonatal jaundice. Am J Dis Child 1989;143:353–6.
360. Rodgers PA, Stevenson DK. Developmental biology of heme oxygenase. Clin Perinatol 1990;17:275–91.
361. Kappas A, Drummond GS, Manola T, et al. Sn-protoporphyrin use in the management of hyperbilirubinemia in term newborns with direct Coombs-positive ABO-incompatibility. Pediatrics 1988;81:485–97.
362. Martinez JC, Garcia HO, Otheguy LE, et al. Control of severe hyperbilirubinemia in full-term newborns with the inhibitor of bilirubin production Sn-mesoporphyrin. Pediatrics 1999;103:1–5.
363. Valaes T, Drummond GS, Kappas A. Control of hyperbilirubinemia in glucose-6-phosphate dehydrogenase-deficient newborns using an inhibitor of bilirubin production, Sn-mesoporphyrin. Pediatrics 1998;101:E1.
364. Vreman HJ, Stevenson DK. Metalloporphyrin-enhanced photodegradation of bilirubin in vitro. Am J Dis Child 1990;144:590–4.
365. Cooke RW. New approach to prevention of kernicterus. Lancet 1999;353:1814–15.
366. Mor L, Thaler I, Brandes JM, Sideman S. In vivo hemoperfusion studies of bilirubin removal from jaundiced dogs. Int J Artif Organs 1981;4:192–8.
367. Mullon CJ, Tosone CM, Langer R. Simulation of bilirubin detoxification in the newborn using an extracorporeal bilirubin oxidase reactor. Pediatr Res 1989;26:452–7.
368. Brian BF, Dorson WJ, Pizziconi VB. Augmented hemoperfusion for hyperbilirubinemia. Trans Am Soc Artif Intern Organs 1988;34:585–9.
369. Denizli A, Kocakulak M, Piskin E. Bilirubin removal from human plasma in a packed-bed column system with dye-affinity microbeads. J Chromatogr 1998;707:25–31.
370. Miles DR, Dorson WJ, Brandon TA, et al. An efficient method for removing bilirubin. ASAIO Trans 1990;36:M611–15.
371. Bosma PJ. Inherited disorders of bilirubin metabolism. J Hepatol 2003;38:107–17.
372. Gilbert A, Lereboullet P. La cholemie simple familiale. Sem Medicale 1901;21:241–3.
373. Odell GB, Gourley GR. Hereditary hyperbilirubinemia. In: Lebenthal E, ed. The textbook of gastroenterology and nutrition in infancy. 2nd ed. New York: Raven Press, 1989.949–67.
374. Watson KJ, Gollan JL. Gilbert's syndrome. Baillieres Clin Gastroenterol 1989;3:337–55.
375. Berk PD, Noyer C. The familial unconjugated hyperbilirubinemias. Semin Liver Dis 1994;14:356–85.
376. Ashraf W, van Someren N, Quigley EM, et al. Gilbert's syndrome and Ramadan: exacerbation of unconjugated hyperbilirubinemia by religious fasting. J Clin Gastroenterol 1994;19:122–4.
377. Naiman JL, Sugasawara EJ, Benkosky SL, Mailhot EA. Icteric plasma suggests Gilbert's syndrome in the blood donor. Transfusion 1996;36:974–8.
378. Lachaux A, Aboufadel A, Chambon M, et al. Gilbert's syndrome: a possible cause of hyperbilirubinemia after orthotopic liver transplantation. Transpl Proc 1996;28:2846.
379. Jansen PL, Bosma PJ, Bakker C, et al. Persistent unconjugated hyperbilirubinemia after liver transplantation due to an abnormal bilirubin UDP-glucuronosyltransferase gene promoter sequence in the donor. J Hepatol 1997;27:1–5.

380. Gates LK Jr, Wiesner RH, Krom RA, et al. Etiology and incidence of unconjugated hyperbilirubinemia after orthotopic liver transplantation. Am J Gastroenterol 1994;89:1541–3.
381. Arnold JC, Otto G, Kraus T, et al. Gilbert's syndrome – a possible cause of hyperbilirubinemia after orthotopic liver transplantations. J Hepatol 1992;14:404.
382. Wilding P, Rollason JG, Robinson D. Patterns of change for various biochemical constituents detected in well population screening. Clin Chim Acta 1972;41:375–87.
383. Sieg A, Schlierf G, Stiehl A, Kommerell B. Die prävalenz des Gilbert-syndromes in Deutschland. Dtsch Med Wochenschr 1987;112:1206–8.
384. Olsson R, Bliding Å, Jagenburg R, et al. Gilbert's syndrome – does it exist? Acta Med Scand 1988;244:485–90.
385. Cleary KJ, White PD. Gilbert's and chronic fatigue syndromes in men. Lancet 1993;341:842.
386. Valesini G, Conti F, Priori R, Balsano F. Gilbert's syndrome and chronic fatigue syndrome. Lancet 1993;341:1162–3.
387. Owens D, Evans J. Population studies on Gilbert's syndrome. J Med Genet 1975;12:152–6.
388. Bailey A, Robinson D, Dawson AM. Does Gilbert's disease exist? Lancet 1977;1:931–3.
389. Berk PD, Howe RB, Bloomer JR, Berlin NI. Studies of bilirubin kinetics in normal adults. J Clin Invest 1969;48:2176–90.
390. Alwall N, Laurell CB, Nilsby I. Studies on hereditary in cases of "nonhemolytic bilirubinemia without direct Van Den Bergh reaction" (hereditary, nonhemolytic bilirubinemia). Acta Med Scand 1946;124:114–25.
391. Foulk WT, Butt HR, Owen CA, et al. Constitutional hepatic dysfunction (Gilbert's disease): its natural history and related syndromes. Medicine 1959;38:25–46.
392. Powell LW, Hemingway E, Billing BH, Sherlock S. Idiopathic unconjugated hyperbilirubinemia (Gilbert's syndrome). A study of 42 families. N Engl J Med 1967;277:1108–12.
393. Aono S, Adachi Y, Uyama E, et al. Analysis of genes for bilirubin UDP-glucuronosyltransferase in Gilbert's syndrome. Lancet 1995;345:958–9.
394. Bosma P, Chowdhury JR, Jansen PH. Genetic inheritance of Gilbert's syndrome. Lancet 1995;346:314–15.
395. Soffer LJ. Bilirubin excretion as a test for liver function during normal pregnancy. Bull Johns Hopkins Hosp 1933;52:365–75.
396. Muraca M, Fevery J. Influence of sex and sex steroids on bilirubin uridine diphosphate-glucuronsyltransferase activity of rat liver. Gastroenterology 1984;87:308–13.
397. Odell GB. The estrogenation of the newborn. In: Neonatal hyperbilirubinemia. New York: Grune & Stratton, 1980:39–41.
398. Bancroft JD, Kreamer B, Gourley GR. Gilbert syndrome accelerates development of neonatal jaundice. J Pediatr 1998;132:656–60.
399. Monaghan G, McLellan A, McGeehan A, et al. Gilbert's syndrome is a contributory factor in prolonged unconjugated hyperbilirubinemia of the newborn. J Pediatr 1999;134:441–6.
400. Akaba K, Kimura T, Sasaki A, et al. Neonatal hyperbilirubinemia and a common mutation of the bilirubin uridine diphosphate-glucuronosyltransferase gene in Japanese. J Hum Genet 1999;44:22–5.
401. Trioche P, Chalas J, Francoual J, et al. Jaundice with hypertrophic pyloric stenosis as an early manifestation of Gilbert syndrome. Arch Dis Child 1999;81:301–3.
402. Hua L, Shi D, Bishop PR, et al. The role of UGT1A1*28 mutation in jaundiced infants with hypertrophic pyloric stenosis. Pediatr Res 2005;58:881–4.
403. Sampietro M, Lupica L, Perrero L, et al. The expression of uridine diphosphate glucuronosyltransferase gene is a major determinant of bilirubin level in heterozygous beta-thalassaemia and in glucose-6-phosphate dehydrogenase deficiency. Br J Haematol 1997;99:437–9.
404. Kaplan M, Renbaum P, Levy-Lahad E, et al. Gilbert syndrome and glucose-6-phosphate dehydrogenase deficiency: a dose-dependent genetic interaction crucial to neonatal hyperbilirubinemia. Proc Natl Acad Sci U S A 1997;94:12128–32.
405. Galanello R, Cipollina MD, Dessi C, et al. Co-inherited Gilbert's syndrome: a factor determining hyperbilirubinemia in homozygous beta-thalassemia. Haematologica 1999;84:103–5.
406. Galanello R, Perseu L, Melis MA, et al. Hyperbilirubinaemia in heterozygous beta-thalassaemia is related to co-inherited Gilbert's syndrome. Br J Haematol 1997;99:433–6.
407. Tzetis M, Kanavakis E, Tsezou A, et al. Gilbert syndrome associated with beta-thalassemia. Pediatr Hematol Oncol 2001;18:477–84.
408. Sharma S, Vukelja SJ, Kadakia S. Gilbert's syndrome co-existing with and masking hereditary spherocytosis. Ann Hematol 1997;74:287–9.
409. Black M, Billing BH. Hepatic bilirubin UDP-glucuronyl transferase activity in liver disease. N Engl J Med 1969;280:1266–71.
410. Felsher BF, Craig JR, Carpio N. Hepatic bilirubin glucuronidation in Gilbert's syndrome. J Lab Clin Med 1973;81:829–37.
411. Auclair C, Hakim J, Boivin H, et al. Bilirubin and paranitrophenol glucuronyl transferase activities of the liver in patients with Gilbert's syndrome. An attempt at a biochemical breakdown of the Gilbert's syndrome. Enzyme 1976;21:97–107.
412. Adachi Y, Yamashita M, Nanno T, Yamamoto T. Proportion of conjugated bilirubin in bile in relation to hepatic bilirubin UDP-glucuronyltransferase activity. Clin Biochem 1990;23:131–4.
413. Martin JF, Vierling JM, Wolkoff AW, et al. Abnormal hepatic transport of indocyanine green in Gilbert's syndrome. Gastroenterology 1976;70:385–91.
414. Ohkubo H, Okuda K, Jida S. A constitutional unconjugated hyperbilirubinemia combined with indocyanine green intolerance: a new functional disorder. Hepatology 1981;1:319–24.
415. Berk PD, Blaschke TF, Waggoner JG. Defective bromosulfophthalein clearance in patients with constitutional hepatic dysfunction (Gilbert's syndrome). Gastroenterology 1972;63:472–81.
416. Billing BH, Williams R, Richards TG. Defects in hepatic transport of bilirubin in congenital hyperbilirubinemia: an analysis of plasma bilirubin disappearance curves. Clin Sci 1964;27:245–57.
417. Berk PD, Bloomer JR, Hower RB, Berlin NI. Constitutional hepatic dysfunction (Gilbert's syndrome): a new definition based on kinetic studies with unconjugated radiobilirubin. Am J Med 1970;49:296–305.
418. Okoliesanyi L, Ghidini O, Orlando R, et al. An evaluation of bilirubin kinetics with respect to the diagnosis of Gilbert's snydrome. Clin Sci Mol Med 1978;54:539–47.
419. Debinski HS, Lee CS, Dhillon AP, et al. UDP-glucuronosyltransferase in Gilbert's syndrome. Pathology 1996;28:238–41.
420. Jansen PL, Bosma PJ, Chowdhury JR. Molecular biology of bilirubin metabolism. Prog Liver Dis 1995;13:125–50.

421. Bosma PJ, Chowdhury JR, Bakker C, et al. The genetic basis of the reduced expression of bilirubin UDP-glucuronosyltransferase 1 in Gilbert's syndrome. N Engl J Med 1995;333:1171–5.
422. Sampietro M, Lupica L, Perrero L, et al. TATA-box mutant in the promoter of the uridine diphosphate glucuronosyltransferase gene in Italian patients with Gilbert's syndrome. Ital J Gastroenterol Hepatol 1998;30:194–8.
423. Monaghan G, Ryan M, Seddon R, et al. Genetic variation in bilirubin UPD-glucuronosyltransferase gene promoter and Gilbert's syndrome. Lancet 1996;347:578–81.
424. Ando Y, Chida M, Nakayama K, et al. The UGT1A1*28 allele is relatively rare in a Japanese population. Pharmacogenetics 1998; 8:357–60.
425. Koiwai O, Nishizawa M, Hasada K, et al. Gilbert's syndrome is caused by a heterozygous missense mutation in the gene for bilirubin UDP-glucuronosyltransferase. Hum Mol Genet 1995;4:1183–6.
426. Maruo Y, Sato H, Yamano T, et al. Gilbert syndrome caused by a homozygous missense mutation (tyr486asp) of bilirubin UDP-glucuronosyltransferase gene. J Pediatr 1998;132:1045–7.
427. Beutler E, Gelbart T, Demina A. Racial variability in the UDP-glucuronosyltransferase 1 (UGT1A1) promoter: a balanced polymorphism for regulation of bilirubin metabolism? Proc Natl Acad Sci U S A 1998;95:8170–4.
428. Metreau JM, Yvart J, Dhumeaux D, Berthelot P. Role of bilirubin overproduction in revealing Gilbert's syndrome: is dyserythropoiesis an important factor? Gut 1978;19:838–43.
429. Maddrey WC, Cukier JO, Maglalang AC, et al. Hepatic bilirubin UDP-glucuronyltransferase in patients with sickle cell anemia. Gastroenterology 1978;74:193–5.
430. Gourley GR, Siegel FL, Odell GB. A rapid method for collection and analysis of bile pigments in humans. Gastroenterology 1984;86:1322A.
431. Onishi S, Itoh S, Kawade N, et al. An accurate and sensitive analysis by high-pressure liquid chromatography of conjugated and unconjugated bilirubin IX-α in various biological fluids. Biochem J 1980;185:281–4.
432. Blaschke TF, Berk PD, Rodkey FL, et al. Drugs and the liver. I. Effects of glutethimide and phenobarbital on hepatic bilirubin clearance, plasma bilirubin turnover and carbon monoxide production in man. Biochem Pharmacol 1974;23:2795–806.
433. Black M, Fevery J, Parker D, et al. Effect of phenobarbitone on plasma [^{14}C] bilirubin clearance in patients with unconjugated hyperbilirubinemia. Clin Sci Mol Med 1974;46:1–17.
434. Kutz K, Kandler H, Gugler R, Fevery J. Effect of clofibrate on metabolism of bilirubin, bromosulphophthalein and indocyanine green and on the biliary lipid composition in Gilbert's syndrome. Clin Sci 1984;66:389–97.
435. Foliot A, Drocourt JL, Etienne JP, et al. Increase in the hepatic glucuronidation of bilirubin in clofibrate-treated rats. Biochem Pharmacol 1977;26:547–9.
436. Felsher BF, Richard D, Redeker AG. The reciprocoal relation between caloric intake and the degree of hyperbilirubinemia in Gilbert's syndrome. N Engl J Med 1970;283:170–2.
437. Bloomer JR, Barrett PV, Rodkey FL, Berlin NI. Studies of the mechanisms of fasting hyperbilirubinemia. Gastroenterology 1971;61:479–87.
438. Whitmer DI, Gollan JL. Mechanisms and significance of fasting and dietary hyperbilirubinemia. Semin Liver Dis 1983;3:42–51.
439. Owens D, Sherlock S. Diagnosis of Gilbert's syndrome: role of reduced caloric intake test. Br Med J 1973;3:559–63.
440. Bakken AF, Thaler MM, Schmid R. Metabolic regulation of heme catabolism and bilirubin production. I. Hormonal control of hepatic heme oxygenase activity. J Clin Invest 1972;51:530–6.
441. Kirshenbaum G, Shames DM, Schmid R. An expanded model of bilirubin kinetics; effect of feeding, fasting and phenobarbital in Gilbert's syndrome. J Pharmacokinet Biopharm 1976;4:115–55.
442. Gartner U, Goeser T, Wolkoff AW. Effect of fasting on the uptake of bilirubin and sulfobromophthalein by the isolated perfused liver. Gastroenterology 1997;113:1707–13.
443. Ricci GL, Ricci RR. Effect of an intraluminal food-bulk on low calorie induced hyperbilirubinemia. Clin Sci 1984;66:493–6.
444. Fromke VL, Miller D. Constitutional hepatic dysfunction (CHD; Gilbert's syndrome): a review with special reference to a characteristic increase and prolongation of the hyperbilirubinemic response to nicotinic acid. Medicine 1972;51:451–64.
445. Rollinghoff W, Paumgartner G, Preisig R. Nicotinic acid test in the diagnosis of Gilbert's syndrome: correlation with the bilirubin clearance. Gut 1981;22:663–8.
446. Gentile S, Orzes N, Persico M, et al. Comparison of nicotinic acid and caloric restriction induced hyperbilirubinemia in the diagnosis of Gilbert's syndrome. J Hepatol 1985;1:537–45.
447. Gentile S, Rubba P, Persico M, et al. Improvement of the nicotinic acid test in the diagnosis of Gilbert's syndrome by pretreatment with indomethacin. Hepatogastroenterology 1985;33: 267–9.
448. Gentile S, Marmo R, Persico M, et al. Dissociation between vascular and metabolic effects of nicotinic acid in Gilbert's syndrome. Clin Physiol 1990;10:171–8.
449. Davidson AR, Rojas Bueno A, Thompson RPH, Williams R. Reduced caloric intake test and nicotinic acid provocation test in the diagnosis of Gilbert's syndrome. Br Med J 1975;2:480.
450. Ohkubo H, Musha H, Okuda K. Studies on nicotinic acid interaction with bilirubin metabolism. Dig Dis Sci 1979;24:700–4.
451. Gentile S, Tiribelli C, Persico M, et al. Dose dependence of nicotinic acid-induced hyperbilirubinemia and its dissociation from hemolysis in Gilbert's syndrome. J Lab Clin Med 1986;107: 166–71.
452. Dickey W, McAleer JJ, Callender ME. The nicotinic acid provocation test and unconjugated hyperbilirubinaemia. Ulster Med J 1991;60:49–52.
453. Ullrich D, Sieg A, Blume R, et al. Normal pathways for glucuronidation, sulphation and oxidation of paracetamol in Gilbert's syndrome. Eur J Clin Invest 1987;17:237–40.
454. Adachi Y, Katoh H, Fuchi I, Yamamoto T. Serum bilirubin fractions in healthy subjects and patients with unconjugated hyperbilirubinemia. Clin Biochem 1990;23:247–51.
455. Rudenski AS, Halsall DJ. Genetic testing for Gilbert's syndrome: how useful is it in determining the cause of jaundice? Clin Chem 1998;44(8 pt 1):1604–9.
456. Berk PB, Isola LM. Specific defects in hepatic storage and clearance of bilirubin. In: Ostrow JD, ed. Bile pigments and jaundice: molecular, metabolic and medical aspects. New York: Marcel Dekker, 1986:279–316.
457. Evans DA. Survey of the human acetylator polymorphism in spontaneous disorders. J Med Genet 1984;21:243–53.
458. Siegmund W, Fengler JD, Franke G, et l. N-acetylation and debrisoquine hydroxylation polymorphisms in patients with Gilbert's syndrome. Br J Clin Pharmacol 1991;32:467–72.
459. Herman RJ, Chaudhary A, Szakacs CB. Disposition of lorazepam in Gilbert's syndrome: effects of fasting, feeding, and enterohepatic circulation. J Clin Pharmacol 1994;34:978–84.

460. de Morais SM, Uetrecht JP, Wells PG. Decreased glucuronidation and increased bioactivation of acetaminophen in Gilbert's syndrome. Gastroenterology 1992;102:577–86.
461. Esteban A, Perez-Mateo M. Gilbert's disease: a risk factor for paracetamol overdosage? J Hepatol 1993;18:257–8.
462. Wasserman E, Myara A, Lokiec F, et al. Severe CPT-11 toxicity in patients with Gilbert's syndrome: two case reports. Ann Oncol 1997;8:1049–51.
463. Ewesuedo RB, Iyer L, Das S, et al. Phase I clinical and pharmacogenetic study of weekly TAS-103 in patients with advanced cancer. J Clin Oncol 2001;19:2084–90.
464. Zucker SD, Qin X, Rouster SD, et al. Mechanism of indinavir-induced hyperbilirubinemia. Proc Natl Acad Sci U S A 2001; 98:12671–6.
465. Black M, Sherlock S. Treatment of Gilbert's syndrome with phenobarbitone. Lancet 1970;1:1359–61.
466. Stocker R, McDonagh AF, Glazer AN, Ames BN. Antioxidant activities of bile pigments: biliverdin and bilirubin. Meth Enzymol 1990;186:301–9.
467. McDonagh AF. Is bilirubin good for you? Clin Perinatol 1990; 17:359–69.
468. Breimer LH, Wannamethee G, Ebrahim S, Shaper AG. Serum bilirubin and risk of ischemic heart disease in middle-aged British men. Clin Chem 1995;41:1504–8.
469. Schwertner HA, Jackson WG, Tolan G. Association of low serum concentration of bilirubin with increased risk of coronary artery disease. Clin Chem 1994;40:18–23.
470. Shevell MI, Majnemer A, Schiff D. Neurologic perspectives of Crigler-Najjar syndrome type I. J Child Neurol 1998;13: 265–9.
471. Childs B, Najjar VA. Familial nonhemolytic jaundice with kernicterus. A report of two cases without neurologic damage. Pediatrics 1956;18:369–77.
472. Labrune PH, Myara A, Francoual J, et al. Cerebellar symptoms as the presenting manifestations of bilirubin encephalopathy in children with Crigler-Najjar type I disease. Pediatrics 1992;89 (4 pt 2):768–70.
473. Chalasani N, Chowdhury NR, Chowdhury JR, Boyer TD. Kernicterus in an adult who is heterozygous for Crigler-Najjar syndrome and homozygous for Gilbert-type genetic defect. Gastroenterology 1997;112:2099–103.
474. Gollan JL, Huang SM, Billing B, Sherlock S. Prolonged survival in 3 brothers with severe type II Crigler-Najjar syndrome: ultrastructural and metabolic studies. Gastroenterology 1975;68:1543–55.
475. Koiwai O, Aono S, Adachi Y, et al. Crigler-Najjar syndrome type II is inherited both as a dominant and as a recessive trait. Hum Mol Genet 1996;5:645–7.
476. Burchell B, Coughtrie MW, Jansen PL. Function and regulation of UDP-glucuronosyltransferase genes in health and liver disease: report of the Seventh International Workshop on Glucuronidation, September 1993, Pitlochry, Scotland. Hepatology 1994;20:1622–30.
477. Seppen J, Bosma PJ, Goldhoorn BG, et al. Discrimination between Crigler-Najjar type I and II by expression of mutant bilirubin uridine diphosphate-glucuronosyltransferase. J Clin Invest 1994;94:2385–91.
478. Labrune P, Myara A, Hadchouel M, et al. Genetic heterogeneity of Crigler-Najjar syndrome type I: a study of 14 cases. Hum Genet 1994;94:693–7.
479. Gantla S, Bakker CT, Deocharan B, et al. Splice-site mutations: a novel genetic mechanism of Crigler-Najjar syndrome type 1. Am J Hum Genet 1998;62:585–92.
480. Ciotti M, Chen F, Rubaltelli FF, Owens IS. Coding defect and a TATA box mutation at the bilirubin UDP-glucuronosyltransferase gene cause Crigler-Najjar type I disease. Biochim Biophys Acta 1998;1407:40–50.
481. Szabo L, Kovács Z, Ebrey PB. Crigler-Najjar syndrome. Acta Paediatr Hung 1962;3:49–70.
482. van Es HHG, Goldhoorn BG, Paul-Abrahamse M, et al. Immunochemical analysis of uridine diphosphate-glucuronosyltransferase in four patients with Crigler-Najjar syndrome type I. J Clin Invest 1990;85:1199–205.
483. Childs B, Sidbury JB, Migeon CJ. Glucuronic acid conjugation by patients with familial nonhemolytic jaundice and their relatives. Pediatrics 1959;23:903–13.
484. Szabo L, Ebrey P. Studies on the inheritance of Crigler-Najjar's syndrome by the menthol test. Acta Paediatr Hung 1963;4: 153–9.
485. Hunter JO, Thompson PH, Dunn PM, Williams R. Inheritance of type 2 Crigler-Najjar hyperbilirubinemia. Gut 1973;14:46–9.
486. Labrune P, Myara A, Hennion C, et al. Crigler-Najjar type II disease inheritance: a family study. J Inherit Metab Dis 1989; 12:302–6.
487. Okolicsanyi L, Nassauto G, Muraca M, et al. Epidemiology of unconjugated hyperbilirubinemia: revisited. Semin Liver Dis 1988;8:179–82.
488. Ertel IJ, Newton WA Jr. Therapy in congenital hyperbilirubinemia: phenobarbital and diethylnicotinamide. Pediatrics 1969;44:43–8.
489. Crigler JF, Gold NI. Effect of phenobarbital on bilirubin metabolism in an infant with congenital, nonhemolytic, unconjugated hyperbilirubinemia, and kernicterus. J Clin Invest 1969; 48:42–55.
490. Yaffe SJ, Levy G, Matsuzawa T, Baliah T. Enhancement of glucuronide-conjugating capacity in a hyperbilirubinemic infant due to apparent enzyme induction by phenobarbital. N Engl J Med 1966;275:1461–6.
491. Kreek MJ, Sleisenger MH. Reduction of serum-unconjugated bilirubin with phenobarbitone in adult nonhaemolytic unconjugated hyperbilirubinaemia. Lancet 1968;2:73–8.
492. Rubaltelli FF, Novello A, Zancan L, et al. Serum and bile bilirubin pigments in the differential diagnosis of Crigler-Najjar disease. Pediatrics 1994;94:553–6.
493. Francoual J, Trioche P, Mokrani C, et al. Prenatal diagnosis of Crigler-Najjar syndrome type I by single-strand conformation polymorphism (SSCP). Prenat Diagn 2002;22:914–16.
494. Ciotti M, Obaray R, Martin MG, Owens IS. Genetic defects at the UGT1 locus associated with Crigler-Najjar type I disease, including a prenatal diagnosis. Am J Med Genet 1997;68:173–8.
495. Moghrabi N, Clarke DJ, Burchell B, Boxer M. Cosegregation of intragenic markers with a novel mutation that causes Crigler-Najjar syndrome type I: implication in carrier detection and prenatal diagnosis. Am J Hum Genet 1993;53:722–9.
496. van der Veere CN, Sinaasappel M, McDonagh AF, et al. Current therapy for Crigler-Najjar syndrome type 1: report of a world registry. Hepatology 1996;24:311–15.
497. Gorodischer R, Levy G, Krasner J, Jaffe SJ. Congenital nonobstructive, nonhemolytic jaundice. effect of phototherapy. N Engl J Med 1970;282:375–80.

498. Agati G, Fusi F, Pratesi S, et al. Bilirubin photoisomerization products in serum and urine from a Crigler-Najjar type I patient treated by phototherapy. J Photochem Photobiol 1998;47:181–9.
499. Job H, Hart G, Lealman G. Improvements in long term phototherapy for patients with Crigler- Najjar syndrome type I. Phys Med Biol 1996;41:2549–56.
500. Nydegger A, Bednarz A, Hardikar W. Use of daytime phototherapy for Crigler-Najjar disease. J Paediatr Child Health 2005;41:387–9.
501. Kotal P, van der Veere CN, Sinaasappel M, et al. Intestinal excretion of unconjugated bilirubin in man and rats with inherited unconjugated hyperbilirubinemia. Pediatr Res 1997;42:195–200.
502. Sherker AH, Heathcote J. Acute hepatitis in Crigler-Najjar syndrome. Am J Gastroenterol 1987;82:883–5.
503. Rubaltelli FF, Guerrini P, Reddi E, Jori G. Tin-protoporphyrin in the management of children with Crigler-Najjar disease. Pediatrics 1989;84:728–31.
504. Galbraith RA, Drummond GS, Kappas A. Suppression of bilirubin production in the Crigler-Najjar type I syndrome: studies with the heme oxygenase inhibitor tin-mesoporphyrin. Pediatrics 1992;89:175–82.
505. Kappas A, Drummond GS, Galbraith RA. Prolonged clinical use of a heme oxygenase inhibitor: hematological evidence for an inducible but reversible iron-deficiency state. Pediatrics 1993;91:537–9.
506. Rubaltelli FF. Current drug treatment options in neonatal hyperbilirubinaemia and the prevention of kernicterus. Drugs 1998;56:23–30.
507. Drummond GS, Kappas A. Chemoprevention of severe neonatal hyperbilirubinemia. Semin Perinatol 2004;28:365–8.
508. Prager MC, Johnson KL, Ascher NL, Roberts JP. Anesthetic care of patients with Crigler-Najjar syndrome. Anesth Analg 1992;74:162–4.
509. Whitington PF, Emond JC, Heffron T, Thistlethwaite JR. Orthotopic auxiliary liver transplantation for Crigler-Najjar syndrome type 1. Lancet 1993;342:779–80.
510. Rela M, Muiesan P, Andreani P, et al. Auxiliary liver transplantation for metabolic diseases. Transpl Proc 1997;29:444–5.
511. Rela M, Muiesan P, Vilca-Melendez H, et al. Auxiliary partial orthotopic liver transplantation for Crigler-Najjar syndrome type I. Ann Surg 1999;229:565–9.
512. Kaufman SS, Wood RP, Shaw BW Jr, et al. Orthotopic liver transplantation for type 1 Crigler-Najjar syndrome. Hepatology 1986;6:1259–62.
513. Shevell MI, Bernard B, Adelson JW, et al. Crigler-Najjar syndrome type I: treatment by home phototherapy followed by orthotopic hepatic transplantation. J Pediatr 1987;110:429–31.
514. Sokal EM, Silva ES, Hermans D, et al. Orthotopic liver transplantation for Crigler-Najjar type I disease in six children. Transplantation 1995;60:1095–8.
515. McDiarmid SV, Millis MJ, Olthoff KM, So SK. Indications for pediatric liver transplantation. Pediatr Transpl 1998;2:106–16.
516. Rela M, Muiesan P, Heaton ND, et al. Orthotopic liver transplantation for hepatic-based metabolic disorders. Transpl Int 1995;8:41–4.
517. Mowat AP. Orthotopic liver transplantation in liver-based metabolic disorders. Eur J Pediatr 1992;151(suppl 1):S32–8.
518. Gridelli B, Lucianetti A, Gatti S, et al. Orthotopic liver transplantation for Crigler-Najjar type I syndrome. Transpl Proc 1997;29:440–1.
519. Pratschke J, Steinmuller T, Bechstein WO, et al. Orthotopic liver transplantation for hepatic associated metabolic disorders. Clin Transpl 1998;12:228–32.
520. Toietta G, Mane VP, Norona WS, et al. Lifelong elimination of hyperbilirubinemia in the Gunn rat with a single injection of helper-dependent adenoviral vector. Proc Natl Acad Sci U S A 2005;102:3930–5.
521. Jaffe BM, Burgos AA, Martinez-Noack M. The use of jejunal transplants to treat a genetic enzyme deficiency. Ann Surg 1996;223:649–56.
522. Medley MM, Hooker RL, Rabinowitz S, et al. Correction of congenital indirect hyperbilirubinemia by small intestinal transplantation. Am J Surg 1995;169:20–7.
523. Kokudo N, Takahashi S, Sugitani K, et al. Supplement of liver enzyme by intestinal and kidney transplants in congenitally enzyme-deficient rat. Microsurgery 1999;19:103–7.
524. Ambrosino G, Varotto S, Strom SC, et al. Isolated hepatocyte transplantation for Crigler-Najjar syndrome type 1. Cell Transpl 2005;14:151–7.
525. Bellodi-Privato M, Aubert D, Pichard V, et al. Successful gene therapy of the Gunn rat by in vivo neonatal hepatic gene transfer using murine oncoretroviral vectors. Hepatology 2005;42:431–8.
526. Jia Z, Danko I. Single hepatic venous injection of liver-specific naked plasmid vector expressing human UGT1A1 leads to long-term correction of hyperbilirubinemia and prevention of chronic bilirubin toxicity in Gunn rats. Hum Gene Ther 2005;16:985–95.
527. Thummala NR, Ghosh SS, Lee SW, et al. A non-immunogenic adenoviral vector, coexpressing CTLA4Ig and bilirubin-uridine-diphosphoglucuronateglucuronosyltransferase permits long-term, repeatable transgene expression in the Gunn rat model of Crigler-Najjar syndrome. Gene Ther 2002;9:981–90.
528. Rotor AB, Manahan L, Florentin A. Familial nonhemolytic jaundice with direct Van Den Bergh reaction. Acta Med Phil 1948;5:37–49.
529. Namihisa T, Yamaguchi K. The constitutional hyperbilirubinemia in Japan: studies on 139 cases reported during the period 1963–1969. Gastroenterol Jpn 1973;8:311–21.
530. Wolkoff AW. Inheritable disorders manifested by conjugated hyperbilirubinemia. Semin Liver Dis 1983;3:65–72.
531. Vest MF, Kaufmann JH, Fritz E. Chronic nonhaemolytic jaundice with conjugated bilirubin in the serum and normal histology: a case study. Arch Dis Child 1960;36:600–4.
532. Fretzayas A, Koukoutsakis P, Moustaki M, et al. Coinheritance of rotor syndrome, G-6-PD deficiency, and heterozygous beta thalassemia: a possible genetic interaction. J Pediatr Gastroenterol Nutr 2001;33:211–13.
533. Pascasio FM, de la Fuenta D. Rotor-Manahan-Florentin syndrome: clinical and genetic studies. Phil J Int Med 1969;7:151–7.
534. Wolpert E, Pascasio FM, Wolkoff AW. Abnormal sulfobromophthalein metabolism in Rotor's syndrome and obligate heterozygotes. N Engl J Med 1977;296:1099–101.
535. Dhumeaux D, Berthelot P. Chronic hyperbilirubinemia associated with hepatic uptake and storage impairment. Gastroenterology 1975;69:988–93.

536. Wheeler HO, Meltzer JI, Bradley SE. Biliary transport and hepatic storage of sulfobromophthalein sodium in the unanesthetized dog, in normal man, and in patients with hepatic disease. J Clin Invest 1960;39:1131–44.
537. Tipping E, Ketterer B. The role of intracellular proteins in the transport and metabolism of lipophilic compounds. In: Blaver G, Sund H, eds. Transport by proteins. Berlin: Walter de Gruyter & Co., 1978;369.
538. Adachi Y, Yamamoto T. Partial defect inhepatic glutathionine S-transferase activity in a case of Rotor's syndrome. Gastroenterology 1987;22:34–8.
539. Wolkoff AW, Ketley JN, Waggoner JG, et al. Hepatic accumulation and intracellular binding of conjugated bilirubin. J Clin Invest 1978;61:142–9.
540. Wolkoff AW, Wolpert E, Pascasio FN, Arias IM. Rotor's syndrome. A distinct inheritable pathophysiologic entity. Am J Med 1976;60:173–9.
541. Aziz MA, Schwartz S, Watson CJ. Studies on coproporphyrin VIII. Reinvestigation of the isomer distribution in jaundice and liver diseases. J Lab Clin Med 1964;63:596–604.
542. Shimizu Y, Naruto H, Ida S, Kohakura M. Urinary coproporphyrin isomers in Rotor's syndrome: a study in eight families. Hepatology 1981;1:173–8.
543. Fretzayas AM, Garoufi AI, Moutsouris CX, Karpathios TE. Cholescintigraphy in the diagnosis of Rotor syndrome. J Nucl Med 1994;35:1048–50.
544. Bar-Meir S, Baron J, Seligson U, et al. 99mTc-HIDA cholescintigraphy in Dubin-Johnson and Rotor syndromes. Radiology 1982;142:743–6.
545. Dubin IN, Johnson FB. Chronic idiopathic jaundice with unidentified pigment in liver cells: a new clincopathologic entity with a report of 12 cases. Medicine 1954;33:155–97.
546. Dubin IN. Chronic idiopathic jaundice. A review of fifty cases. Am J Med 1958;24:268–92.
547. Gustein SL, Alpert L, Arias IM. Studies of hepatic excretory function. IV. Biliary excretion of sulfobromophthalein sodium in a patient with Dubin-Johnson syndrome and a biliary fistula. Isr J Med Sci 1968;4:36–40.
548. Javitt NB, Kondo T, Kuchiba, K. Bile acid excretion in Dubin-Johnson syndrome. Gastroenterology 1978;75:931–2.
549. Sprinz H, Nelson RS. Persistent nonhemolytic hyperbilirubinemia associated with lipochrome-like pigment in liver cells: report of four cases. Ann Intern Med 1954;41:952–62.
550. Shani M, Seligsohn V, Gilon E, et al. Dubin-Johnson syndrome in Israel. I. Clinical, laboratory and genetic aspects of 101 cases. Q J Med 1970;39:549–67.
551. Zlotogora J. Hereditary disorders among Iranian Jews. Am J Med Genet 1995;58:32–7.
552. Kondo T, Yagi R. Dubin-Johnson syndrome in a neonate. N Engl J Med 1975;292:1028–9.
553. Nakata F, Oyanagi K, Fujiwara M, et al. Dubin-Johnson syndrome in a neonate. Eur J Pediatr 1979;132:299–301.
554. Haimi-Cohen Y, Merlob P, Marcus-Eidlits T, Amir J. Dubin-Johnson syndrome as a cause of neonatal jaundice: the importance of coproporphyrins investigation. Clin Pediatr 1998;37:511–13.
555. Tsai WH, Teng RJ, Chu JS, et al. Neonatal Dubin-Johnson syndrome. J Pediatr Gastroenterol Nutr 1994;18:253–4.
556. Kimura A, Ushijima K, Kage M, et al. Neonatal Dubin-Johnson syndrome with severe cholestasis: effective phenobarbital therapy. Acta Paediatr Scand 1991;80:381–5.
557. Shieh CC, Chang MH, Chen CL. Dubin-Johnson syndrome presenting with neonatal cholestasis. Arch Dis Child 1990;65:898–9.
558. Haimi-Cohen Y, Amir J, Merlob P. Neonatal and infantile Dubin-Johnson syndrome. Pediatr Radiol 1998;28:900.
559. Kimura A, Yuge K, Kosai KI, et al. Neonatal cholestasis in two siblings: a variant of Dubin-Johnson syndrome? J Paediatr Child Health 1995;31:557–60.
560. Kondo T, Kuchiba K, Ohtsuka Y, et al. Clinical and genetic studies on Dubin-Johnson syndrome in a cluster area in Japan. Jpn J Hum Genet 1974;18:378–92.
561. Edwards RH. Inheritance of the Dubin-Johnson-Sprinz syndrome. Gastroenterology 1975;63:734–49.
562. Cohen L, Lewis C, Arias IM. Pregnancy, oral contraceptives and chronic familial jaundice with predominantly con jugated hyperbilirubinemia (Dubin-Johnson syndrome). Gastroenterology 1972;62:1182–90.
563. Muscatello U, Mussini I, Agnolucci MT. Dubin-Johnson syndrome: an electron microscopic study of the liver cell. Acta Hepatosplenol 1967;14:162–70.
564. Ehrlich JC, Novikoff AB, Platt R, et al. Hepatocellular lipofuscin and the pigment of chronic idiopathic jaundice. Bull N Y Acad Med 1960;36:488–91.
565. Swartz HM, Sarna, Varma RR. On the nature and excretion of the hepatic pigment in the Dubin-Johnson syndrome. Gastroenterology 1979;76:958–64.
566. Swartz HM, Chen K, Roth JA. Further evidence that the pigment in the Dubin-Johnson syndrome is not melanin. pigment cell research. 1987;1:69–75.
567. Arias IM, Blumberg W. The pigment in Dubin-Johnson syndrome. Gastroenterology 1979;77:820–1.
568. Kitamura T, Alroy J, Gatmaitan Z, et al. Defective biliary excretion of epinephrine metabolites in mutant (TR-) rats: relation to the pathogenesis of black liver in the Dubin-Johnson syndrome and Corriedale sheep with an analogous excretory defect. Hepatology 1992;15:1154–9.
569. Hunter FM, Sparks RD, Flinner RL. Hepatitis with resulting mobilization of hepatic pigment in a patient with Dubin-Johnson syndrome. Gastroenterology 1964;47:631–5.
570. Kobayashi Y, Ishihara T, Wada M, et al. Dubin-Johnson-like black liver with normal bilirubin level. J Gastroenterol 2004;39:892–5.
571. Paulusma CC, Kool M, Bosma PJ, et al. A mutation in the human canalicular multispecific organic anion transporter gene causes the Dubin-Johnson syndrome. Hepatology 1997;25:1539–42.
572. Toh S, Wada M, Uchiumi T, et al. Genomic structure of the canalicular multispecific organic anion-transporter gene (*MRP2/CMOAT*) and mutations in the ATP-binding-cassette region in Dubin-Johnson syndrome. Am J Hum Genet 1999;64:739–46.
573. van Kuijck MA, Kool M, Merkx GF, et al. Assignment of the canalicular multispecific organic anion transporter gene (*CMOAT*) to human chromosome 10q24 and mouse chromosome 19d2 by fluorescent in situ hybridization. Cytogenet Cell Genet 1997;77:285–7.
574. Kajihara S, Hisatomi A, Mizuta T, et al. A splice mutation in the human canalicular multispecific organic anion transporter gene causes Dubin-Johnson syndrome. Biochem Biophys Res Commun 1998;253:454–7.
575. Tsujii H, König J, Rost D, et al. Exon-intron organization of the human multidrug-resistance protein 2 (MRP2) gene mutated

in Dubin-Johnson syndrome. Gastroenterology 1999;117:653–60.

576. Materna V, Lage H. Homozygous mutation Arg768Trp in the ABC-transporter encoding gene MRP2/CMOAT/ABCC2 causes Dubin-Johnson syndrome in a caucasian patient. J Hum Genet 2003;48:484–6.
577. Machida I, Wakusawa S, Sanae F, et al. Mutational analysis of the *MRP2* gene and long-term follow-up of Dubin-Johnson syndrome in Japan. J Gastroenterol 2005;40:366–70.
578. Mendema E, DeFraiure WH, Nieweg HO, et al. Familial chronic idiopathic jaundice. Am J Med 1960;28:42–50.
579. Charbonnier A, Brisbois P. Etude chromatographique de la BSP au cours de l'epreuve clinique d'epuration plasmatique de ce colorant. Rev Int Hepatol. 1960;10:1163–213.
580. Shani M, Gilon E, Ben-Ezzer J, Sheba C. Sulfobromophthalein tolerance test in patients with Dubin-Johnson syndrome and their relatives. Gastroenterology 1970;59:842–7.
581. Abe H, Okuda K. Biliary excretion of conjugated sulfobromophthalein (BSP) in constitutional conjugated hyperbilirubinemias. Digestion 1975;13:272–83.
582. Erlinger S, Dhumeaux D, DesJeux JF, Benhamou JP. Hepatic handling of unconjugated dyes in the Dubin-Johnson syndrome. Gastroenterology 1973;64:106–10.
583. Koskelo P, Toivonen I, Aldercreutz H. Urinary coproporphyrin isomer distribution in Dubin-Johnson syndrome. Clin Chem 1967;13:1006–9.
584. Frank M, Doss M, de Carvalho DG. Diagnostic and pathogenetic implications of urinary coproporphyrin excretion in the Dubin-Johnson syndrome. Hepatogastroenterology 1990;37:147–51.
585. Ben-Ezzer J, Seligson U, Shani M, et al. Abnormal excretion of the isomers of urinary coproporphyrin by patients with Dubin-Johnson syndrome in Israel. Clin Sci 1971;40:17–30.
586. Wolkoff AW, Cohen LE, Arias IM. Inheritance of the Dubin-Johnson syndrome. N Engl J Med 1973;288:113–17.
587. Kondo T, Kuchiba K, Shimizu Y. Coporporphyrin isomers in Dubin-Johnson syndrome. Gastroenterology 1976;70:1117–20.
588. Rocchi F, Balli F, Gibertini P, et al. Coproporphyrin excretion in health newborn babies. J Pediatr Gastroenterol Nutr 1984;3:402–7.
589. Kappas A, Sassa S, Anderson KE,et al. The metabolic basis of inherited disease. New York: McGraw-Hill, 1983:1299–384.
590. Garcia-Vargas GG, Del Razo LM, Cebrian ME, et al. Altered urinary porphyrin excretion in a human population chronically exposed to arsenic in Mexico. Hum Exp Toxicol 1994;13:839–47.
591. Kladchareon N, Suwannakul P, Bauchum V. Dubin-Johnson syndrome: report of two siblings with Tc-99 m IODIDA cholescintigraphic findings. J Med Assoc Thai 1988;71:640–2.
592. Pinós T, Constansa JM, Palacin A, Figueras C. A new diagnostic approach to the Dubin-Johnson syndrome. Am J Gastroenterol 1990;85:91–3.
593. Shimizu T, Tawa T, Maruyama T, et al. A case of infantile Dubin-Johnson syndrome with high CT attenuation in the liver. Pediatr Radiol 1997;27:345–7.
594. Mayatepek E, Lehmann WD. Defective hepatobiliary leukotriene elimination in patients with the Dubin-Johnson syndrome. Clin Chim Acta 1996;249:37–46.
595. Yoo J, Reichert DE, Kim J, et al. A potential Dubin-Johnson syndrome imaging agent: synthesis, biodistribution, and microPET imaging. Mol Imaging 2005;4:18–29.
596. Lindberg MC. Hepatobiliary complications of oral contraceptives. J Gen Intern Med 1992;7:199–209.
597. Di Zoglio JD, Cardillo E. Dubin-Johnson syndrome and pregnancy. Obstet Gynecol 1973;42:560–3.
598. Berk PD, Noyer C. The familial conjugated hyperbilirubinemias. Semin Liver Dis 1994;14:386–94.

14

Familial Hepatocellular Cholestasis

Frederick J. Suchy, M.D., and Benjamin L. Shneider, M.D.

Inherited cholestasis of hepatocellular origin has long been described in the neonate or during the first year of life [1]. Many of these infants were categorized as having idiopathic neonatal hepatitis after biliary atresia, metabolic diseases, and congenital infections were excluded [2,3]. The prognosis in familial cases was poor compared with sporadic cases that sometimes had an identifiable etiology. As the clinical and genotypic heterogeneity of these inherited disorders has become apparent, it is now recognized that patients may present initially and progress to end-stage liver disease at ages ranging from infancy to adulthood [4]. There may be significant overlap in clinical features such as intense pruritus and a low serum concentration of γ-glutamyl transpeptidase (γGT). The histopathology, immunohistochemical staining, and hepatic ultrastructure may provide additional diagnostic clues as to the underlying defect. However, the identification of the genes responsible for several of these disorders now allows a specific diagnosis in many cases, may suggest therapy with varying success based on the genotype of the patient, and has advanced our understanding of molecular mechanisms of bile secretion and acquired cholestasis. It is not surprising that, so far, mutations in three genes encoding adenosine triphosphate (ATP)-dependent transport proteins localized to the canalicular membrane that result in progressive cholestasis and liver injury have been discovered. The features of these disorders are compared in Table 14.1. Other genes encoding proteins involved in membrane transport, vesicular trafficking, and integrity of the cell junction may also be mutated in some patients. Owing to an immaturity of hepatic excretory function, cholestasis may occasionally occur in inherited diseases because of systemic illness rather than a primary defect in the liver (see Table 9.1). These disorders will not be considered in this review.

PROGRESSIVE FAMILIAL INTRAHEPATIC CHOLESTASIS TYPE 1 (PFIC1 – FIC1 DISEASE)

The diseases that are now known to be caused by defects in the *FIC1* (*ATP8B1*) gene, namely Byler's disease and benign recurrent intrahepatic cholestasis (BRIC), were some of the first clinically well-described forms of familial intrahepatic cholestasis [5,6]. Most of the published literature regarding these disorders predates the molecular genetics of these diseases, so completely accurate genotype/phenotype correlation is not possible. BRIC, first described in 1959, is an intermittent form of intrahepatic cholestasis characterized by variable periods of intense pruritus often associated with jaundice [7]. The age of onset is variable, but it typically occurs during childhood or adolescence. The severity and duration of attacks also vary, and triggering features are not well known. The benign designation of BRIC refers to the general lack of progressive liver disease, although the pruritus is far from benign during an intense episode.

Byler's disease was initially described in direct descendents of Jacob Byler [5,6]. Unlike BRIC and despite an intermittent nature of the disease at its onset, the pruritus and liver disease in Byler's disease are eventually persistent and progressive. The clinical spectrum between BRIC and Byler's disease may be a continuum, thus the historical nomenclature of Byler's disease and BRIC may be outdated [8]. PFIC1 has also been described in the Inuit populations of Greenland and Canada [9,10]. Many clinicians now refer to all these diseases in a general sense as FIC1 disease.

Clinical Features

PFIC1 is an autosomal recessive liver disease characterized by unremitting cholestasis with pruritus and jaundice that usually starts before the age of 1 year and progresses to cirrhosis and liver failure [6,11]. Serum γGT activity is normal. The average age at onset is 3 months, but some patients are affected as neonates and rarely cholestasis may not be manifest until adolescence [12,13]. Diarrhea, malabsorption, and failure to thrive are common in the first months of life. Fat-soluble vitamin malabsorption commonly leads to bleeding diathesis from vitamin K deficiency, rickets from vitamin D deficiency, and neuromuscular dysfunction from vitamin E deficiency. Hepatosplenomegaly eventually develops. Pancreatitis has been reported. The disorder may rapidly progress to end-stage liver disease during early childhood or evolve gradually to cirrhosis in the second decade of life.

Table 14.1: Progressive Familial Intrahepatic Cholestasis

	PFIC1	*PFIC2*	*PFIC3*
Transmission	Autosomal recessive	Autosomal recessive	Autosomal recessive
Chromosome	18q21-22	2q24	7q21
Gene	*ATP8B1/FIC1*	*ABCB11/BSEP*	*ABCB4/MDR3*
Protein	FIC1	BSEP	MDR3
Location	Hepatocyte, colon, intestine, pancreas: on apical membranes	Hepatocyte canalicular membrane	Hepatocyte canalicular membrane
Function	ATP-dependent aminophospholipid flippase; unknown effects on intracellular signaling	ATP-dependent bile acid transport	ATP-dependent phosphatidylcholine translocation
Phenotype	Progressive cholestasis, diarrhea, steatorrhea, growth failure, severe pruritus	Rapidly progressive cholestatic giant cell hepatitis, growth failure, pruritus	Later-onset cholestasis, portal hypertension, minimal pruritus, intraductal and gallbladder lithiasis
Histology	Initial bland cholestasis; coarse, granular canalicular bile on EM	Neonatal giant cell hepatitis, amorphous canalicular bile on EM	Bile ductular proliferation, periportal fibrosis, eventually biliary cirrhosis
Biochemical features	Normal serum γGT; high serum, low biliary bile acid concentrations	Normal serum γGT; high serum, low biliary bile acid concentrations	Elevated serum γGT; low to absent biliary PC; absent serum LPX; normal biliary bile acid concentrations
Treatment	Biliary diversion, ileal exclusion, liver transplantation – but post-OLT diarrhea, steatorrhea, fatty liver	Biliary diversion, liver transplantation	UDCA if residual PC secretion; liver transplantation

EM, electron microscopy; OLT, orthotopic liver transplantation; PC, phosphatidylcholine

Few patients with early onset of cholestasis have survived into the third decade without treatment. Several patients have also been described with recurrent attacks of cholestasis beginning in infancy, which eventually became permanent as adults [8].

Pruritus is the dominant feature of cholestasis in the majority of patients and is often out of proportion to the level of jaundice [12]. It may initially vary in intensity and may be exacerbated during intercurrent illness. Pruritus may not be noticed until 6 months of age because the neural pathways necessary for concerted scratching are not fully developed. However, affected infants often are irritable and fretful and sleep poorly with onset of cholestasis. Scratching is usually evident first as digging at the ears and eyes, which are the first areas to show evidence of excoriation. By 1 year of age, patients may show generalized mutilation of skin, usually most severe on the extensor surfaces of the arms and legs and on the flanks of the back. The pruritus is very disabling and often responds poorly to medical therapies. In contrast to other cholestatic disorders, these patients do not develop xanthomas.

Growth failure is another major feature of PFIC1. Most patients have short stature (less than the fifth percentile), although their weight for height is often normal, giving a stocky appearance [11]. Delayed onset of puberty and sexual development is characteristic of patients surviving until adolescence without treatment. Patients receiving effective treatment experience normal sexual development, and several have borne normal children. Intellectual development and school performance are generally normal in patients receiving effective treatment but often are delayed before treatment, probably as a result of constant pruritus.

FIC1 disease is associated with a variety of extrahepatic manifestations, which we now understand may be the result of the wide tissue distribution of *FIC1* gene expression. Many of these problems persist and may even worsen after liver transplantation, supporting the notion that they are the result of *FIC1* expression in organs other than the liver. The more commonly described extrahepatic manifestations include recurrent pancreatitis, diarrhea that is independent of cholestasis, sensorineural hearing loss, chronic cough/wheezing, somatic short stature, and posttransplantation steatosis [14].

A form of benign recurrent intrahepatic cholestasis (BRIC1) is characterized by attacks of jaundice and pruritus separated by symptom-free intervals [7,12]. Patients may also experience fatigue, anorexia, steatorrhea, dark-colored urine, and weight loss. Progression to cirrhosis and long-term complications of chronic liver disease do not occur. The disorder is caused by mutations in the *FIC1* gene and is inherited as an autosomal recessive trait

The age of presentation of the first attack of jaundice ranges from 1–50 years, but jaundice usually occurs before the age of 20 years [13]. Attacks usually are preceded by a minor illness and consist of a preicteric phase of 2–4 weeks (characterized by malaise, anorexia, and pruritus) and an icteric phase that may last from 1–18 months. In some patients, hormonal factors such as the use of oral contraceptives and pregnancy have been associated with precipitation of an attack [15]. Patients may have severe coughing during episodes, as is seen sometimes in patients with PFIC1 [16].

During the icteric phase, the concentrations of serum bile acid, bilirubin, and alkaline phosphatase are increased. Serum γGT concentration, however, remains low. Liver biopsy results are very benign, often showing no pathologic change even during an episode. Some specimens show hepatocellular cholestasis and cholate injury, mostly centrilobular. During the asymptomatic period, all parameters are normal: clinical, laboratory, and liver histology.

Laboratory Findings

The laboratory findings in PFIC1 and BRIC1 are remarkable for the presence of low serum γGT and normal or near normal serum cholesterol levels, even in the presence of severe cholestasis [11]. Patients may have γGT levels greater than 100 IU/L while receiving microsomal inducers such as phenobarbital. Serum concentrations of alkaline phosphatase, bilirubin, and bile salts are not different from those seen in several other cholestatic disorders and may be normal or near normal early in the course of the disease. Serum aminotransferase levels are usually no higher than twice normal values. Patients with PFIC1 or a prolonged episode of BRIC1 frequently develop complications of cholestasis, including fat-soluble vitamin deficiency. Sweat chloride and sodium levels may be elevated. With progressive liver injury, features of hepatic failure and portal hypertension develop that are similar to those of any other end-stage liver disease.

A low serum γGT level is highly unusual in the presence of cholestasis. It should suggest the possibility of one of the forms of PFIC or BRIC. However, the differential diagnosis should include inborn errors of bile acid synthesis [17]. In PFIC and BRIC, serum concentrations of primary bile acids are markedly elevated, whereas in bile synthetic defects, the serum contains abnormal bile acid precursors but no primary bile acids. Pruritus is an uncommon manifestation in bile acid synthetic defects.

The mechanism for the low serum concentration of γGT in PFIC and BRIC is not clear [11,18]. γGT is normally bound to the canalicular membrane by a glycosyl phosphatidyl inositol (GPI) anchor. In obstructive cholestasis, when excessive amounts of bile salts accumulate in the canalicular lumen under increased pressure, γGT is released from the membrane by detergent action and refluxes back into serum, possibly via leaky intercellular junctions. However, in PFIC and BRIC, the reduced concentrations of biliary bile acids preserve canalicular γGT localization. This explanation is not entirely satisfactory as serum γGT is elevated in most other forms of intrahepatic cholestasis in which biliary bile acid levels are low. Preliminary studies indicate that some canalicular proteins, including γGT and carcinoembryonic antigen (CEA), are poorly expressed at the canaliculus in PFIC1 [19]. It is possible that low serum γGT levels result from the lack of canalicular γGT available for elution as well as from the inadequate concentrations of intracanalicular bile acids to act as detergents.

Consistent with severe cholestasis, total serum bile acid concentrations are markedly elevated (usually >200 μmol/L; normal, <10 μmol/L) with an elevated ratio of chenodeoxycholic acid to cholic acid conjugates, usually greater than 10:1 [11]. The total biliary bile acid concentrations are generally low (0.1–0.3 μmol/L; normal, >20 μmol/L), with a predominance of cholic acid conjugates. These findings have suggested a defect in biliary excretion, particularly of chenodeoxycholic acid conjugates [20].

Histopathology

A bland hepatocellular and canalicular cholestasis with some pseudo acinar transformation are the most uniform histologic findings early in the course of the disease (Figure 14.1) [21]. Minimal giant cell formation and ballooning of hepatocytes also may be found. Giant cells are present more often during infancy and may regress with age. Bile duct damage is minimal in infants but may be more prominent later, leading to ductal paucity. The degenerating biliary epithelium shows apoptotic changes consisting of small hyperchromatic nuclei, attenuated cytoplasm, and loss of duct lumina, but inflammation is absent. The typical progression of fibrosis starts early, with 76% of patients having some fibrosis by 2 years of age, and fibrosis may

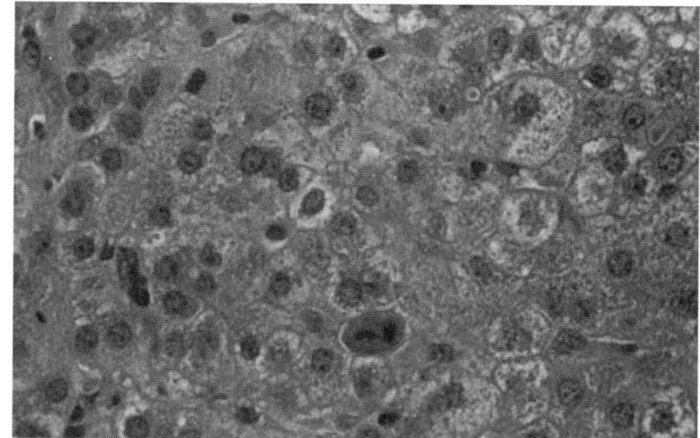

Figure 14.1. Histopathology in PFIC1. Liver biopsy from a 2-year-old patient showing swelling of hepatocytes, a bland hepatocellular and canalicular cholestasis, and occasional necrotic hepatocytes. (Courtesy of Dr. Kevin Bove.) For color reproduction, see Color Plate 14.1.

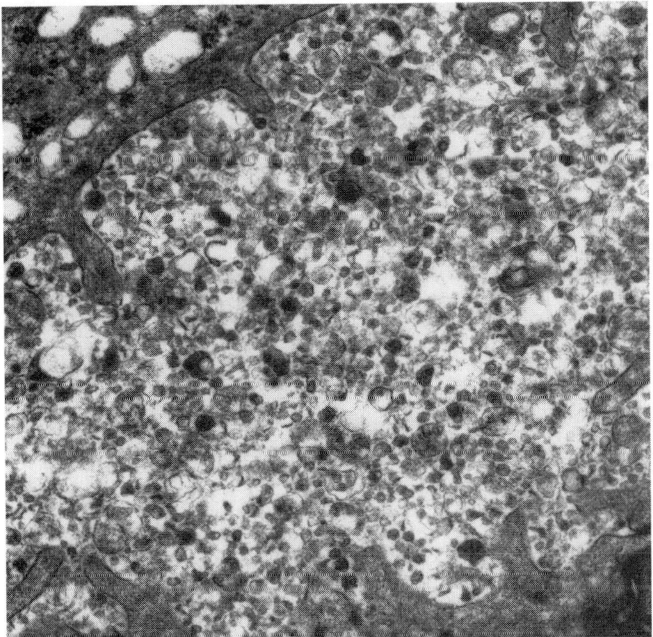

Figure 14.2. Ultrastructural pathology of PFIC1. Electron microscopy of liver from a patient with PFIC1 shows distended bile canaliculi with microvilli that are reduced in number and length. Bile canaliculi contain unusually coarse and granular bile (so-called Byler's bile). (Courtesy of Dr. Alex Knisely.)

appear initially either as pericentral sclerosis or portal fibrosis, or sometimes both. Portal to central bridging then develops in association with lacy lobular fibrosis and eventually leads to cirrhosis [21]. Proliferating bile ductules are observed at the edge of the portal tracts in patients with significant fibrosis. The rate of progression of the fibrosis is highly variable but correlates loosely with the severity of the clinical disease. Mallory hyaline and hepatocellular carcinoma may be seen with very advanced disease.

Unfortunately, well-characterized and clinically useful antibodies against the FIC1 protein do not exist, so routine histochemical analysis cannot be performed to diagnose FIC1 disease.

Electron microscopy on liver samples from patients who are not receiving ursodeoxycholic acid (UDCA) shows distended bile canaliculi with microvilli that are reduced in number and length (Figure 14.2) [12,22,23]. Bile canaliculi contain unusually coarse and granular bile (so-called Byler's bile). In some confirmed cases of PFIC1, aggregated vesicles of membranous material rather than coarse granular bile are observed. Bile is retained in hepatocytes and Kupffer cells and is predominantly periportal in localization. The pericanalicular ectoplasm is often thickened. These ultrastructural abnormalities are highly suggestive of but are not absolutely specific for PFIC1 [22].

Genetics

Gene linkage analysis of BRIC and Byler's disease indicated that the same gene is involved in both of these diseases, and it was mapped to chromosome 18q21. Refined linkage analysis and gene sequencing of patients with well-characterized disease ultimately led to the discovery that defects in the P-type ATPase, *ATP8B1*, are responsible for FIC1 disease [24,25]. *ATP8B1* contains 28 exons, spans at least 77 kilobases (kb), and yields no alternatively spliced transcripts [26]. The FIC1 protein (ATP8B1) consists of 1251 amino acids and has 10 predicted membrane-spanning domains typical of P-type ATPases. A recent report of mutation analyses in 130 families with PFIC1 and 50 families with BRIC1 identified 54 distinct disease mutations, including 10 mutations predicted to disrupt splicing, 6 nonsense mutations, 11 small insertion or deletion mutations predicted to induce frameshifts, 1 large genomic deletion, 2 small in-frame deletions, and 24 missense mutations [26]. *ATP8B1* mutations were detected in 30% and 41%, respectively, of the PFIC and BRIC families screened. Most mutations were rare, occurring in one to three families, or were limited to specific populations. Compound heterozygotes were commonly observed (9 in 39 with PFIC1 and 12 in 20 with BRIC1). There was also a correlation with the type of mutation and clinical severity. Based on sequence analysis and the predicted effects of specific mutations, it is hypothesized that BRIC-like disease is the result of functionally less severe mutations in the *FIC1* gene. Missense mutations were more common in BRIC1 (58% vs. 38% in PFIC1), whereas nonsense, frameshifting, and large deletion mutations were more common in PFIC1 (41% vs. 16% in BRIC1) [26]. Fourteen of 16 patients with BRIC1 were either homozygous or compound heterozygous for the I661T mutation, which was frequently found in European patients [26]. Nonsense mutations at the 5′ end of the FIC1 coding region are typically associated with severe disease, whereas mutations at the 3′ end are associated with milder and intermittent disease. Because there is no functional assay for FIC1, direct testing of this hypothesis has not been possible. It was surprising that in some circumstances, the same mutations led to a wide range of phenotypes, from PFIC to BRIC, or even no clinical disease.

Pathophysiology

FIC1 disease appears to be the result of abnormalities in the enterohepatic circulation of bile acids. In vivo clearance of radiolabeled bile acids in patients with Byler's disease and careful examination of biliary bile acids suggest that there is reduced hepatic canalicular excretion of bile salts [20,27]. Clinical response to partial biliary diversion or ileal exclusion indicates that enhanced intestinal reabsorption of bile acids may also be involved in the disease process. Animal models of Byler's disease have not yielded a clear picture of the molecular events involved in FIC1 disease [1]. The genetic mutation initially described in the Byler's kindred, G308V, was introduced into mice. Adult *Atp8b1*$^{G308V/G308V}$ mice expressed FIC1 mRNA but not protein. The mice were normal appearing, although serum aspartate aminotransferase (AST) and bile salts were elevated compared with wild-type littermate controls. Paradoxically, bile flow and hepatic excretion of bile salts were enhanced in the Byler mice. Cholate feeding of the *Atp8b1*$^{G308V/G308V}$ mice exacerbated the pathology and suggests that abnormal regulation of bile acid homeostasis is operative in the pathogenesis of FIC1 disease. The combination of an enlarged bile salt pool with normal hepatic transport and markedly down-regulated expression of bile salt–synthetic enzymes probably results from increased bile salt intestinal reabsorption in the mutant mice.

Thus at present, the exact molecular pathophysiology of FIC1 disease is uncertain. This is in contrast to defects in the bile salt export pump (BSEP) and multidrug resistance 3 (MDR3) protein, in which the presumed pathophysiology follows directly from protein function. Based on sequence and homology analysis, it has been presumed that the FIC1 protein is a P-type ATPase that functions as an aminophospholipid flippase, transferring aminophospholipids from the outer to inner hemi-leaflet of cell membranes [25,28]. Aminophospholipid translocase activity has been demonstrated in rat liver canalicular membrane vesicles that contained FIC1 protein [29]. Transfection of CHOK1 cells with *ATP8B1* cDNA resulted in the expression of FIC1 in membrane preparations and energy-dependent translocation of a fluorescent analogue of phosphatidylserine. These data provide indirect evidence that FIC1 is an aminophospholipid transporter that helps maintain the distribution of aminophospholipids between the inner and outer leaflets of the plasma membrane. It is unknown how this proposed function is related to bile salt transport. Asymmetry of aminophospholipids in lipid bilayers may play a role in regulating important lipid-dependent signaling pathways and the activity of membrane receptors and transport proteins [30,31]. FIC1 protein is expressed at the canalicular membrane of the hepatocyte and at the apical membrane of bile duct epithelial cells and enterocytes [29,32,33]. It is abundant along the entire length of the gastrointestinal tract from the stomach to the colon and is also expressed in the pancreas. Yet, there is no clear linkage of the presumed function(s) of FIC1 and alterations in bile formation. In Madin–Darby canine kidney (MDCK) cell culture systems, expression of normal or mutant forms of FIC1 had no effect on bile acid transport mediated by either the intestinal apical sodium-dependent bile acid transporter or the hepatic canalicular BSEP [34]. However, there is preliminary evidence in the *Atp8b1*$^{G308V/G308V}$ mouse that the canalicular membrane becomes unstable when Atp8b1 (FIC1) is lacking, resulting in shedding of lipid vesicles that contain ectoenzymes into bile and impairment of bile secretion [35].

FIC1 expression may influence posttranslational modification of the farnesoid X receptor (FXR), leading to enhancement of its nuclear localization and transcriptional activity [36]. The FXR is a nuclear protein that is integral to the bile acid responsiveness of a variety of genes involved in bile acid biosynthesis and transport. Preliminary studies (Figure 14.3) indicate that FIC1 deficiency in humans is associated with diminished FXR activity, leading to reduced expression of the canalicular BSEP and increased expression of the ileal apical sodium-dependent bile acid transporter [36,37]. The net effect of these changes would be enhanced reabsorption of intestinal bile acids coupled with diminished hepatic excretion of bile acids, yielding marked hypercholanemia and diminished hepatic bile acid secretion.

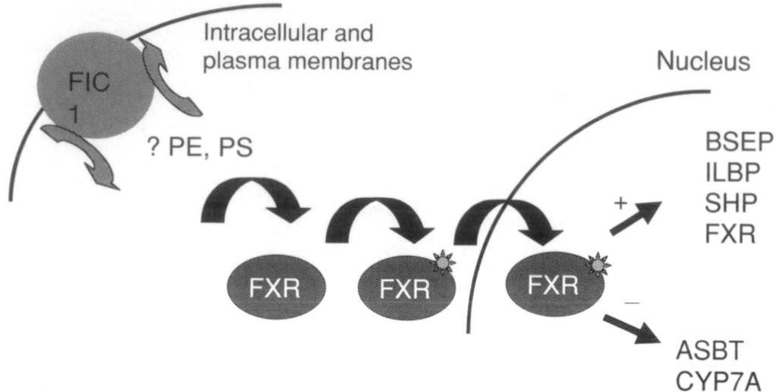

Figure 14.3. Hypothetical model of the effect of FIC1. FIC1 is a membrane protein that alters membrane aminophospholipid asymmetry and transduces an unknown signaling pathway (*curved arrows*). This leads to a posttranslational modification of FXR, possibly through some type of phospholipid-dependent signaling pathway (indicated by the attached star). The posttranslational modification is necessary for nuclear translocation of FXR. FXR in the nucleus then activates itself (FXR), the ileal lipid-binding protein (ILBP), the inhibitory transcription factor, the short heterodimer partner (SHP), and the bile salt export pump (BSEP). FXR, via the effect of SHP, inhibits the expression of the apical sodium-dependent bile acid transporter (ASBT) and cholesterol 7α-hydroxylase (CYP7A). (Modified from Chen et al. [36].)

PROGRESSIVE FAMILIAL INTRAHEPATIC CHOLESTASIS TYPE 2 (PFIC2 – BSEP DEFICIENCY)

Following the identification of the gene underlying PFIC1 and better delineation of its clinical features, it became clear that there was genetic and clinical heterogeneity in PFIC patients with low serum γGT [38]. A second locus for PFIC was then mapped to 2q24 by homozygosity mapping and linkage analysis in six consanguineous families of Middle Eastern origin [39]. Mutations were defined later in a liver-specific gene of unknown function, initially called the *sister of P-glycoprotein*, that was found within this region [40]. Further studies revealed that this gene's protein, a member of the ATP-binding cassette family of transporters, was located exclusively on the canalicular membrane of hepatocytes and functioned as an ATP-dependent BSEP [4,41,42]. Numerous mutations in the *BSEP(ABCB11)* gene have been defined in patients with the form of PFIC (now named PFIC2) linked to 2q24. The phenotype of these patients is consistent with defective bile salt excretion at the hepatocyte canalicular membrane. BSEP mutations have also been detected in some patients with BRIC [40].

Clinical Features

Patients with PFIC2 usually present in the neonatal period with progressive cholestasis [43]. In general, these patients lack the relapsing course seen in the early stages of PFIC1 and instead have a more rapid progression to cirrhosis without therapy [44]. Irritability and bleeding related to vitamin K deficiency are commonly seen. Failure to thrive related to fat malabsorption and poor intake occurs. The majority of patients have hepatomegaly; significant splenomegaly implies portal hypertension related to advanced fibrosis or cirrhosis [11]. Cholelithiasis may occur owing to impaired bile acid secretory function and supersaturation of bile with cholesterol [44]. Similar to patients with PFIC1, these patients do not have xanthomas. Extrahepatic features may help distinguish PFIC1 and 2. Watery diarrhea, pancreatitis, and impaired hearing occur in PFIC1 but not in PFIC2 patients [44].

Pruritus is the dominant feature of the disorder in the majority of patients before complications of cirrhosis develop [43]. Pruritus is often out of proportion to the level of jaundice and is not clinically evident in the first months of life.

Patients with PFIC2 are at risk for developing hepatocellular carcinoma and cholangiocarcinoma [45]. Malignancy may occur as early as 10 months of age and in patients with normalized liver tests following biliary diversion.

Patients fitting the phenotype of BRIC have recently been described with mutations in *BSEP* [46]. These patients had at least two recurrent episodes of cholestasis and were clinically healthy and biochemically normal between attacks. The age of onset and total number of recurrent episodes were highly variable. Cholelithiasis occurred in 7 of 11 patients with BRIC2. Several patients had a relatively early onset of the disease and developed permanent cholestasis as adults after initial periods of recurrent attacks.

There has been a recent association of single-nucleotide polymorphisms of the *BSEP* gene with intrahepatic cholestasis of pregnancy [47]. A patient with transient neonatal cholestasis has also been reported with a small heterozygous deletion in the long arm of chromosome 2 [48].

Laboratory Findings

Patients with PFIC2 have low serum γGT and normal or near normal serum cholesterol levels [49]. The serum γGT concentration may increase to greater than 100 IU/L in patients receiving microsomal inducers such as phenobarbital and rifampicin. Serum concentrations of alkaline phosphatase, bilirubin, and bile salts are not different from those seen in many other cholestatic disorders. In contrast to patients with PFIC1, serum aminotransferase levels are usually elevated to at least five times normal values. Patients frequently develop complications of cholestasis, including fat-soluble vitamin malabsorption steatorrhea.

Histopathology

Liver morphology in PFIC2 shows a neonatal hepatitis with giant cell transformation of hepatocytes and lobular cholestasis that may persist beyond infancy [21,23,44]. Canalicular cholestasis is prominent, particularly in zone 3. Balloon cholestasis of hepatocytes and isolated hepatocyte necrosis may be found. Injury to hepatocytes results in perivenular, pericellular, and periportal fibrosis with progression to cirrhosis. There is mild ductular proliferation and scattered polymorphonuclear leukocytes in portal tracts. The interlobular bile ducts are normal.

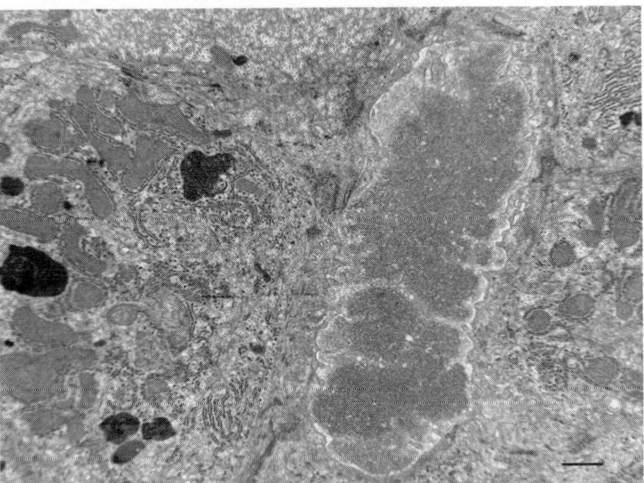

Figure 14.4. Ultrastructural pathology of PFIC2. Amorphous bile is observed in the canaliculus of this 2-year-old patient with absent hepatic BSEP immunostaining and low-γGT cholestasis. Bile canaliculi are distended, and microvilli are reduced in number and length. (Magnification 8000×, bar = 1.25 μ.) (Image courtesy of Ronald Gordon, Mount Sinai School of Medicine.)

Electron microscopy (Figure 14.4) demonstrates effaced microvilli and dilated bile canaliculi that contain finely granular or filamentous bile [43].

Genetics

PFIC2 is inherited as an autosomal recessive trait. The *BSEP* (*ABCB11*) gene is located on chromosome 2q24. Numerous mutations have been defined in patients with PFIC2 and BRIC2. In PFIC2, about half the mutations resulted in an early stop codon or a frameshift in the encoded protein [50]. The other PFIC2 mutations and all BRIC2 mutations were nonsynonymous. In a 2001 report describing the genetic analysis of 194 patients with low-γGT PFIC, 103 mutant *BSEP* alleles were found in 63 families [43]. In this group, there were 5 different nonsense mutations, 19 different missense mutations, 8 different 1- or 2-base pair insertions or deletions, 2 major gene rearrangements, and 1 complete gene deletion. Two mutations, E297G and D482G, were found in approximately 30% of patients of European descent with PFIC2. In 22 of these families, the affected patients were homozygotes; in 41 families, the affected individuals were compound heterozygotes.

Of a group of patients with *BSEP* gene mutations, 10 of 11 showed no BSEP expression on the canalicular membrane by immunohistochemical staining [44]. These patients had a variety of abnormalities in the *BSEP* gene, including missense, nonsense, and deletional mutations. Protein expression could not be reliably assessed in one patient. No *BSEP* mutations were found in any of the eight patients with positive canalicular BSEP staining. This suggests that in the majority of PFIC2 patients, the gene defect is severe enough to produce no product or a protein that cannot be inserted into the canalicular membrane. Immunolocalization may provide a means of diagnosing PFIC2 in the clinical setting [51].

Van Mil et al. [46] recently screened all coding regions, including intron–exon boundaries of *ABCB11* for mutations in patients with BRIC in whom *ATP8B1* mutations had been excluded. Apparent homozygous *ABCB11* mutations were found in seven patients from five families. Three patients from two families were compound heterozygotes. There was only one heterozygous mutation in another family. A total of seven different missense and one putative splice site mutation were detected. One mutation (E297G) had previously been associated with PFIC2, but no other nonsense, frameshift, or missense mutations that should severely impair BSEP expression and/or function were found.

Pathophysiology

The clinical implications of defective canalicular BSEP expression are quite clear; there will be markedly diminished bile salt secretion and progressive cholestasis. In patients studied by Jansen et al. [44], biliary bile salt concentrations were 0.2 ± 0.2 mmol/L (<1% of normal) in patients with PFIC2 versus 18.1 ± 9.9 mmol/L (~40% of normal) in patients with other forms of PFIC [44]. Both biliary cholesterol and phospholipid secretion were also markedly reduced. A bile salt kinetic study in one BSEP-deficient patient showed a dramatic decrease in bile salt secretion, with most of the bile salt pool confined to a "central compartment" consisting of liver, blood, and the extracellular space. Owing to bile secretory failure, bile salts and other biliary constituents are retained in the hepatocyte and lead to progressive liver damage. Seven patients studied by Jansen et al. [44] were treated with UDCA but were able to excrete very low amounts of UDCA into bile. These findings indicate that in addition to secretion of the primary bile salts, cholic acid, and chenodeoxycholic acid, BSEP is largely responsible for canalicular transport of UDCA.

Targeted inactivation of *bsep* in mice has yielded some surprising results [52]. The *bsep*$^{-/-}$ mice were growth retarded but exhibited no signs of overt cholestasis or abnormalities in serum liver biochemical tests. As expected, the secretion of cholic acid in mutant mice was greatly reduced (6% of wild-type), but total bile salt output in mutant mice was about 30% of wild-type. Expression of the mdr1 p-glycoprotein was enhanced in these mice and provided an alternative but incomplete mechanism for bile salt secretion [53]. Secretion of a large amount of tetrahydroxylated bile acids occurred in mutant but not wild-type mice. These results suggest that hydroxylation and an alternative canalicular transport mechanism for bile acids compensate for the absence of bsep function and protect the mutant mice from severe cholestatic damage. However, feeding of mutant mice with a more hydrophobic bile salt, cholic acid, led to severe cholestasis characterized by jaundice, weight loss, elevated plasma bile acid concentrations, elevated serum aminotransferases, cholangiopathy (with proliferation of bile ductules and cholangitis), liver necrosis, and high mortality [54].

Wang et al. [55] examined the effects in vitro of a number of missense mutations in *BSEP* that have been associated with PFIC2. Five mutations, G238V, E297G, G982R, R1153C, and R1268Q, prevented the protein from trafficking to the apical membrane, and E297G, G982R, R1153C, and R1268Q also abolished taurocholate transport activity, possibly by causing BSEP to misfold. C336S may not be a disease-causing mutation as it had no effect on transport activity or apical trafficking of BSEP. D482G did not affect the apical expression but partially decreased the transport activity of BSEP. Mutant G238V was rapidly degraded in both MDCK and Sf9 cells, and a proteasome inhibitor resulted in intracellular accumulation of this and other mutants, suggesting proteasome-mediated degradation is involved in processing of BSEP mutants. These studies provide useful information on amino acid residues that are critical for BSEP function.

Hayashi et al. [56] studied the consequences of the E297G and D482G mutants. E297G and D482G are missense mutations involving the second intracellular loop and the first ATP-binding domain, respectively. Introduction of these mutations into the human BSEP resulted in a significantly reduced BSEP expression in kidney cell lines. Most of the D482G and some of the E297G BSEP was retained intracellularly, probably in the endoplasmic reticulum in an immature, core-glycosylated form. However, the transport function of the BSEP mutants assessed in membrane vesicles isolated from transfected HEK 293 cells was normal [56]. These studies indicate that impaired membrane trafficking is the abnormality produced by the E297G and D482G mutations. As a strategy to treat certain forms of PFIC2, it may be feasible to develop agents that can induce trafficking of BSEP mutants that retain transport activity to the canalicular membrane.

Treatment of PFIC and BRIC

The treatment of PFIC includes standard measures related to the management of chronic cholestasis and specific approaches to these forms of intrahepatic cholestasis. Fat-soluble vitamin supplementation and monitoring are necessary for all forms of chronic cholestasis. Nutritional supplementation with medium-chain triglycerides may be necessary for adequate caloric assimilation. The most difficult therapeutic issue in PFIC relates to management of pruritus. Conventional therapies with antihistamines and UDCA are of limited efficacy in this patient population. Opioid antagonists are problematic to administer and not terribly efficacious. Variable and typically temporary response may be observed with rifampicin [57]. Thus, most common medical approaches to the intractable pruritus associated with cholestasis are often ineffective in PFIC1 and 2.

Interruption of the enterohepatic circulation has yielded excellent clinical, biochemical, and histologic response in a number of children with progressive intrahepatic cholestasis [58–64]. The exact mechanism(s) by which this intervention works is unclear, although it is likely that there is a significant change in the composition of the bile acid pool. At present, it is unclear if these approaches are optimal for specific genetic forms of PFIC. It is possible that these interventions may be best for severe PFIC1 (FIC1 disease) and milder phenotypic variants of PFIC2 (BSEP disease). There are two major surgical techniques to permanently interrupt the enterohepatic circulation, namely partial cutaneous external biliary diversion and internal ileal exclusion. In the first procedure, one end of an intestinal conduit is anastamosed to the dome of the gallbladder, whereas the other is used to form a cutaneous ostomy. Bile in the gallbladder then flows either out of the ostomy or into the intestine. Typically 30–50% of bile drains out of the ostomy and is discarded. This procedure, first described by Whitington and Whitington [58], yields excellent clinical responses in a significant percentage of patients with low-γGT intrahepatic cholestasis (presumed FIC1 disease in many cases). The response often includes complete amelioration of pruritus and importantly biochemical and histologic stabilization and possible improvement. Interestingly, the response may be transiently diminished in females near the time of puberty.

An alternative, though less commonly used, surgical approach to interrupting the enterohepatic circulation of bile acid involves internal ileal exclusion. The vast majority of intestinal bile salts are reabsorbed in the distal ileum, that is, the distal 20–25% of the small intestine. Therefore, exclusion of this segment of intestine may lead to bile acid wasting, as has been extensively demonstrated in the surgical treatment of hypercholesterolemia [65]. The small intestine is transected at a point that demarcates the distal 15% of the small intestine, and a blind loop is formed with the distal ileal segment. The proximal loop of the intestine is sewn end-to-side to the cecum, completing the internal bypass of the distal ileum. There is limited experience with this surgical approach in PFIC, although some success has been reported [60,63]. Avoidance of an ostomy is attractive for many patients and their families. Accurate assessment of the appropriate amount of ileum for bypass is likely to be critical; too little is unlikely to be therapeutic and too much is likely to yield bile acid–induced diarrhea. At present, it is not clear if there will be compensatory responses in the intestine that will ultimately diminish the long-term effectiveness of ileal exclusion in PFIC [63].

The evidence base for the efficacy of surgical treatments of PFIC is inadequate. A review of published studies reveals a relatively small number of noncirrhotic patients (<100) with low-γGT PFIC who were treated with one of several different procedures, including partial external biliary diversion, ileal exclusion, and cholecystoappendicostomy. Patients were usually referred for intractable pruritus. Approximately 75% of patients in these studies were reported to have improved, but the end points were highly variable and included improved pruritus, liver tests, and growth. In some cases, progression of liver disease decreased and there was even regression of fibrosis and ultrastructural abnormalities [63]. Genotyping was done in only a few patients, so it was often not possible to know whether PFIC1, PFIC2, or some other disorder was being treated. Further studies are needed to correlate the outcome of surgical therapy with the genotype of the patient. Mutational analysis may be used eventually to predict which patients are most likely to benefit from surgery.

Pharmacologic interruption of the enterohepatic circulation using bile acid transport inhibitors or potent bile acid sequestrants is a theoretical alternative to these surgical approaches [66]. Temporary endoscopic nasobiliary drainage was used to induce longstanding remissions in three adults with BRIC1 who had been refractory to medical therapies [67]. Pruritus disappeared within 24 hours, with normalization of serum bile acid concentrations.

Ursodeoxycholic acid is frequently given to patients with PFIC1 and 2 in a dosage of 10–20 mg/kg/d [68]. Liver tests may improve, but the drug has little benefit in patients with severe pruritus. Moreover, there is no evidence that UDCA alters the natural history of these disorders, including the need for biliary diversion or liver transplantation, or shortens the duration or frequency of episodes of BRIC.

Liver transplantation remains an option for the management of end-stage liver disease in PFIC and as an alternative approach in patients with refractory and severe pruritus. In BSEP and MDR3 disease, in which the disease is hepatocyte specific, liver transplantation appears to be a definitive approach. In contrast, in FIC1 disease, liver transplantation is potentially fraught with a number of potential complications related to the extrahepatic expression of the *FIC1* gene. The most prominent posttransplantation problems include intractable diarrhea, hepatic steatosis, poor growth, and recurrent pancreatitis [69,70]. Therefore, in FIC1 disease, nontransplantation surgical approaches should be considered the preferred first-line of therapy.

PROGRESSIVE FAMILIAL INTRAHEPATIC CHOLESTASIS TYPE 3 (PFIC3)

PFIC3 is an autosomal recessive disease that may have some clinical features that overlap with PFIC1 and 2, particularly with presentation in early life, but can be distinguished from these disorders by an elevation in the serum concentration of γGT and by histologic findings of bile ductular proliferation, portal fibrosis, and inflammation with patency of the intra- and extrahepatic bile ducts [1,71]. These patients have a defect in biliary phospholipid secretion related to mutations in *MDR3*. The spectrum of disease associated with this genetic defect has expanded to include distinct presentations in older children and adults.

Clinical Features

Patients may present in infancy with jaundice, hepatomegaly, and acholic stools. However, the age of onset is extremely broad, ranging from 1 month to more than 20 years (mean age, ~3.5 years). In a series of 31 patients reported by Jacquemin et al. [72,73], clinical signs of cholestasis were uncommon in the neonate but were manifest by 1 year of age in about one third of patients. Pruritus occurs less frequently than in the other types of PFIC and is usually mild. Height and weight may be below normal as the disease progresses. Liver disease tends to evolve slowly to biliary cirrhosis with or without overt cholestatic jaundice. Splenomegaly reflecting portal hypertension was detected in 27 of 31 children at a mean age of 5.5 years (range, 8 months to 20.5 years). Esophageal varices were found in 19 patients at a mean age of 9 years (range, 5–20.5 years) and led to variceal hemorrhage in 9 children at a mean age of 11.5 years (range, 5–20.5 years). In 10 patients, liver transplantation was required at a mean of 7.5 years (range, 2–12.5 years) because of complications of portal hypertension, liver failure, or severe cholestasis [73]. Asymptomatic disease leading to cirrhosis, portal hypertension, and variceal bleeding in adolescent and young adults has also been reported. Cholangiography performed in a limited number of cases has been normal [73].

Mutations in *MDR3* have also been described in children and adults with symptomatic intrahepatic and gallbladder cholesterol cholelithiasis [74]. The adult patients also had mild chronic cholestasis, recurrence of symptoms after cholecystectomy, and prevention of recurrence by treatment with ursodeoxycholate [75]. Consistent with a defect in *MDR3*, bile analysis showed supersaturation with cholesterol together with a low phospholipid concentration. A predisposition to develop gallstones in these patients is not surprising as phospholipids are the main carrier and solvent of cholesterol in hepatic bile [74,76].

Some cases of intrahepatic cholestasis of pregnancy (ICP) have been associated with heterozygous mutations in *MDR3* [77,78]. These women developed generalized pruritus with or without jaundice, which was exacerbated near term. Serum ALT values and serum bile acid concentrations are increased. The serum γGT level remained within normal limits or was increased. The occurrence of ICP carries a risk to the fetus because of premature delivery or sudden fetal death. Pruritus may cause severe discomfort for the mother. Cholestasis frequently recurs in subsequent pregnancies and rarely during administration of oral contraceptives [77].

LABORATORY STUDIES

The serum concentration of γGT is elevated in PFIC3, often more than ten times the normal value. This distinguishes the disorder from the other forms of PFIC but not from other inherited and acquired cholestatic liver diseases in which the serum γGT is usually elevated. Other commonly used liver tests are variably elevated, including serum aminotransferases, conjugated bilirubin, and alkaline phosphatase. Serum cholesterol concentration is usually normal. The total serum bile acid concentration is elevated to as high as 25 times the normal value, but biliary bile acid concentrations are normal.

The cardinal feature of PFIC3 is markedly reduced concentrations of biliary phospholipids. In nine carefully studied patients with PFIC3, the mean biliary phospholipid concentration was 1.4 mmol/L compared with 29.1 mmol/L in a group of control cholestatic children [73]. Ratios of biliary bile acid to phospholipid and cholesterol to phospholipids were approximately fivefold higher than in control samples.

Because measurement of biliary phospholipids is impractical in the evaluation of most patients, measurement of serum lipoprotein X (LPX) may serve as a surrogate marker for PFIC3 and is available through several commercial clinical laboratories. Serum LPX is absent from the serum of patients with homozygous *MDR3* mutations [72]. This finding explains the normal serum cholesterol levels in patients with PFIC3. LPX is the predominant lipoprotein in the plasma of cholestatic patients. LPX is probably composed of biliary vesicles that are formed at the subapical compartment of the hepatocyte, transcytosed to sinusoidal membrane, and released into plasma [79]. This process is absolutely dependent on MDR3, but the precise mechanism has not been defined.

Histopathology

The morphology of PFIC3 is distinct from that of PFIC1 and 2. Bile ductular proliferation and mixed inflammatory infiltrates (Figure 14.5) are observed in the early stages despite patency of intra- and extrahepatic bile ducts [73]. Cytokeratin immunostaining confirms marked bile ductular proliferation. Cholestasis with slight giant cell transformation and isolated eosinophilic necrotic hepatocytes may also be present. Periductal sclerosis affecting the interlobular bile ducts eventually occurs. Extensive portal fibrosis evolves into biliary cirrhosis in older children. Electron microscopy of liver has not been reported in proven cases.

Bile canalicular immunostaining for MDR3 protein is variable and depends on the type of *MDR3* mutation [72]. Missense mutations or mutations leading to synthesis of a truncated protein show a complete absence of canalicular immunostaining for MDR3 protein. However, some missense mutations have demonstrated faint or normal MDR3 staining. Thus, normal canalicular staining does not exclude the possibility of PFIC3.

Genetics

MDR3 is located on chromosome 7q21. In the largest reported series, 17 different *MDR3* mutations were found in 22 of 31 patients with the PFIC3 phenotype [73,80]. Eleven missense mutations and six mutations predicted to yield a truncated protein were found. Patients with homozygous mutations producing a truncated protein had no immunohistochemical canalicular staining for MDR3 protein and had no biliary phospholipid excretion. In these cases, there may be a rapid breakdown of the truncated protein or the premature stop codon may cause instability and decay of *MDR3* mRNA. In keeping with the latter explanation, there was minimal to undetectable *MDR3* mRNA

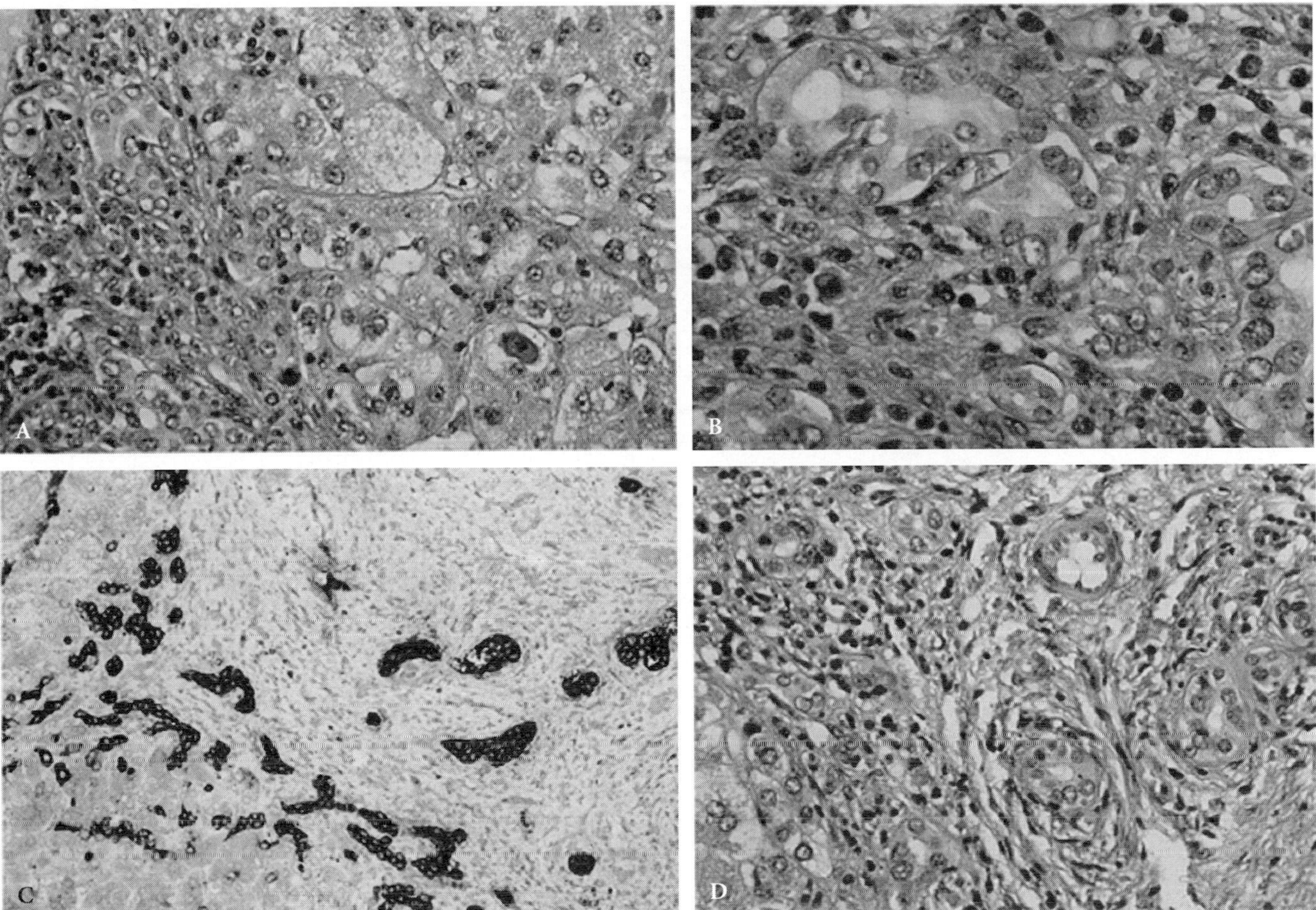

Figure 14.5. Histopathology of liver in a child with PFIC3. (**A**) Cholestatic hepatitis with giant cell transformation and isolated eosinophilic necrotic hepatocyte. Portal zone at the left shows bile ductular proliferation and mild mixed inflammatory infiltrate. (**B**) Bile ducts are increased in number, tortuous, and lined by swollen reactive epithelium. Inflammatory cells include lymphocytes, plasma cells, and occasional polymorphonuclear leukocytes. Bile stasis in ducts is absent. (**C**) A cytokeratin immunostain shows increased numbers of periportal ductules and interlobular bile ducts. (**D**) In PFIC3, progressive bile duct injury is associated with periductal fibroblast proliferation, as shown here, and eventually fibrosis. (Courtesy of Drs. Kevin Bove and James Heubi.) For color reproduction, see Color Plate 14.5.

in the livers of some of these patients. However, MDR3 protein could be demonstrated in some patients with missense mutations and was associated with low but detectable amounts of biliary phospholipids. Owing to residual function of MDR3, these patients had milder disease with later onset and slower progression. Most of the 11 missense mutations were found in the highly conserved Walker A and Walker B motifs essential for ATP binding, so ATPase activity and membrane transport would be disrupted. Other missense mutations located in the transmembrane domains might have effects on substrate binding, transport activity, and intracellular trafficking of MDR3 [77]. In patients with the PFIC3 phenotype and without detection of disease-causing mutations, it is possible that mutations might be located outside the coding region in introns or in the regulatory sequence of the gene. Moreover, because in most studies the search for *MDR3* mutations was done by single-strand conformation polymorphism analysis, it is possible that additional mutations might have been discovered by complete sequencing of the coding region. Alternatively, there is evidence for other genetic defects causing PFIC with elevated serum γGT, leading to biliary cirrhosis [81].

Pathophysiology

The function of MDR3 was suggested by studies in mice with homozygous disruption of the *mdr2* gene (homologue of human *MDR3*) [82]. The $mdr^{-/-}$ mice developed a cholangiopathy characterized histologically by bile ductular proliferation, portal inflammation, and progressive fibrosis. Hepatocellular carcinoma developed in mice surviving over 1 year. These mice had low to absent concentrations of biliary phosphatidylcholine but maintained normal bile salt secretion. Both MDR3 and mdr2 (Figure 14.6) are members of the ATP-binding cassette family of transporters that serve as phospholipid flippases essential for biliary phospholipid secretion. These transporters are located exclusively on the canalicular membrane of the hepatocyte and work in conjunction with the BSEP. BSEP (ABCB11) pumps bile salts from the hepatocyte into the canalicular lumen.

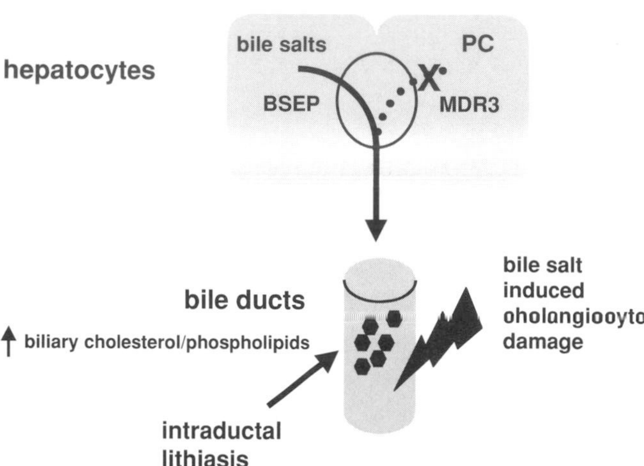

Figure 14.6. Pathophysiology of biliary tract disease in PFIC3 (*MDR3* deficiency). Phosphatidylcholine (PC) in bile normally protects cholangiocytes from bile salt (BS) toxicity by forming mixed micelles. However, a mutation of the *MDR3* gene results in decreased biliary PC secretion (*dotted line*) and high BS-to-PC ratio, leading to bile duct injury (cholangitis and ductular proliferation). A mutation of the *MDR3* gene also results in a decreased biliary PC concentration and high cholesterol (Chol)-to-PC ratio. The high biliary cholesterol saturation index (CSI) promotes crystallization of cholesterol and the lithogenicity of bile.

Phosphatidylcholine is flipped from the cytoplasmic leaflet to the luminal side of the canalicular membrane by mdr2 (ABCB4) or MDR3. Bile salts incorporate phosphatidylcholine that has been flipped to the outer leaflet either directly in contact with mdr2/MDR3 or from projections of phosphatidylcholine from the luminal leaflet into small mixed phosphatidylcholine–bile salt micelles [76]. These micelles interact with the cholesterol transporter (ABCG5G8), which transfers cholesterol partly into the aqueous phase so it can be captured by the micelles. Mixed bile salt/phosphatidylcholine/cholesterol micelles move down the biliary tract into the gallbladder and duodenum. These mixed micelles are thought to protect the canalicular and cholangiocyte membranes from bile acid–induced cell injury.

Fickert et al. [83] recently provided direct evidence for cholangiocyte injury leading to an obliterative cholangitis in $mdr2^{-/-}$ mice. To visualize leakage of bile from the biliary tree, fluorescent-labeled UDCA was injected intravenously. There was disruption of tight junctions and basement membranes, with bile acid leakage into portal tracts of $mdr2^{-/-}$ but not wild-type mice. The bile acid–induced injury led to the induction of a portal inflammatory (CD11b, CD4+) infiltrate and activation of proinflammatory (tumor necrosis factor [TNF]-α, interleukin [IL]-1β) and profibrogenic cytokines (transforming growth factor [TGF]-β1) [83]. These mediators resulted in activation of periductal myofibroblasts, producing periductal fibrosis, the separation of the peribiliary plexus from cholangiocytes, and eventually atrophy and death of the cholangiocytes. Although nonmicellar toxic bile acids may directly produce chemical/detergent damage to bile ducts, these studies indicate that the peribiliary vascular plexus may be displaced from the biliary epithelium by the expanding fibrotic bands, leading to ischemic ductal injury.

Whereas biliary bile salt concentrations are normal in patients with PFIC3, serum bile salt levels are elevated. Downregulation of transporters involved in bile acid uptake, including the sodium-cotransporting peptide (NTCP) and several members of the organic anion-transporting polypeptide family (OATP), explains in part the elevated serum bile acid levels in this disorder [50]. In contrast, the multidrug resistance–related protein 4 (MRP4) is strongly up-regulated at the mRNA and protein level, mediating bile salt efflux into serum. It is unknown how and why bile salts are directed to MRP4 rather than to the canalicular BSEP, which is expressed normally in PFIC3 [51].

Treatment

Patients with PFIC3 should receive nutritional support including supplements of fat-soluble vitamins. Pruritus is usually mild in this condition. Oral administration of UDCA appears to be of value in some patients. The rationale underlying this therapy is that enrichment of bile with this hydrophilic bile acid reduces cytotoxic injury to hepatocytes and bile ducts and stimulates bile flow. In the $mdr2^{-/-}$ mouse model, feeding of UDCA led to significant improvement in liver disease [84]. Jacquemin et al. [73] found that UDCA was effective in some patients with *MDR3* missense mutations and residual biliary phospholipid secretion. However, there was no improvement in patients with nonsense mutations, who have a complete lack of biliary phospholipids. These patients progress to biliary cirrhosis and liver failure at a variable rate and ultimately require liver transplantation.

Transgenic *MDR3*-expressing hepatocytes as well as normal $mdr2^{+/+}$ hepatocytes have been transplanted in $mdr2^{-/-}$ mice [85]. Transplanted hepatocytes partially repopulated the liver, restored phospholipid secretion, and diminished liver pathology. A similar approach may be considered for treatment of patients with PFIC3.

HEREDITARY CHOLESTASIS WITH LYMPHEDEMA

Aagenaes et al. [86,87] described patients of Norwegian decent with intrahepatic cholestasis and lymphedema. The disease is not limited to Norwegians and has been reported in Italian, Japanese, and English children. The cause of this syndrome and the relation between peripheral lymphatic obstruction and cholestatic liver disease remain unknown. It has been suggested that deficiency of intrahepatic lymphatics contributes to the cholestasis. Study of reported cases supports an autosomal recessive mode of inheritance. There is one report, however, of a mother and child with the disease, suggesting autosomal dominant inheritance. The locus (LS1) for the disorder, at least in Norwegian patients, has been mapped to a 6.6-centimorgan interval on chromosome 15q [23]. All Norwegian patients are likely homozygous for the same disease mutation, inherited from a shared ancestor. A second locus has been proposed based on a report of a Serbian-Romanian patient with features atypical of the Norwegian form of the disease [88]. The patient had low serum cholesterol and γGT concentrations and progressed rapidly to end-stage liver disease. The disorder did not map to the *LCS1*, *ATP8B1*, and *ABCB11* loci.

The clinical course in the first months of life is dominated by cholestasis with malabsorption [89]. Jaundice appears in most patients within 2–4 weeks of life and always before 2 months. The stools are usually acholic. Growth and weight gain may be poor during infancy. Lymphedema is rarely present at birth or at the time patients initially are found to be cholestatic. Lymphedema is observed in the lower extremities, usually in early childhood, and has been attributed to lymphatic vessel hypoplasia [86,89].

The cholestatic liver disease tends to improve with age, with most patients having a normal serum bilirubin concentration by 3 or 4 years of age [89]. Serum bile acid concentrations may remain elevated even after jaundice improves. Serum aminotransferase levels may be high during the first year of life but gradually return to the normal range before school age. Serum γGT is increased only modestly in this syndrome, about twice the upper normal value. These patients, however, may have an exaggerated increase in γGT after treatment with phenobarbital [89]. Cholestasis occurs episodically in older children, with cholestatic periods lasting 2–6 months. Puberty and pregnancy seem to be important initiators of cholestatic episodes later in life. The liver disease tends to be mild in most patients, but several older children and adults have progressed to cirrhosis [89]. Two siblings with particularly marked cholestasis, including severe pruritus and hepatic fibrosis, responded well to partial cutaneous biliary diversion (Whitington PF, unpublished observations). Neither has had progression of liver disease in more than 16 years of follow-up.

Liver histopathology in early childhood shows massive giant cell transformation of hepatocytes and intracellular retention of bile pigment [89]. Patients in clinical remission may have liver morphology close to normal. Some patients may have bile plugs and a slight increase in portal fibrosis. Of 26 patients reported by Aagenaes [89], 4 have developed biopsy-proven cirrhosis. A 50-year-old woman with cirrhosis developed hepatocellular carcinoma.

Treatment is limited to avoiding complications of malabsorption during episodes of cholestasis, particularly fat-soluble vitamin deficiency. Lymphedema tends to become the dominant symptom of disease later in life and may be disabling in some patients [89]. It may improve later in life and can be controlled in some patients by symptomatic treatment such as physiotherapy and wrapping of the lower extremities.

ARTHROGRYPOSIS MULTIPLEX CONGENITA, RENAL DYSFUNCTION, AND CHOLESTASIS (ARC) SYNDROME

Severe cholestasis may occur in association with arthrogryposis multiplex congenita and renal disease [90,91]. The neurogenic muscular atrophy is related to rarefaction of the anterior horn cells of the spinal cord. Additional cerebral manifestations may be observed if the patient survives infancy, including severe developmental delay, hypotonia, nerve deafness, poor feeding, microcephaly, and defects of the corpus callosum [91]. An increased risk of bleeding is caused by platelet dysfunction. The cholestatic liver disease is usually present at birth. An unexpected finding in these patients has been the normal serum concentration of γGT. Some patients have cholestasis and pigmentary change in the liver, similar to the Dubin–Johnson syndrome. Other patients have had paucity of intrahepatic bile ducts and giant cell transformation of hepatocytes as the predominant features [92]. Bile duct paucity and lipofuscin disposition may be seen in a wide range of liver diseases and probably represent nonspecific changes resulting from a common insult. Pigmentary change, bile duct paucity, and giant cell transformation may coexist in some patients. The varying liver histology probably represents a spectrum of injury found in the same disorder. With survival beyond infancy, progressive cholestasis and paucity of intrahepatic bile ducts may occur in this disorder, with progression to cirrhosis. Patients also may develop renal tubular cell degeneration with nephrocalcinosis.

The pattern of inheritance deduced from reported cases has been consistent with an autosomal recessive trait. The gene for the disorder was localized to chromosome 15q26.1. Fourteen affected kindreds were then used to identify germline mutations in the gene *VPS33B* [93]. *VPS33B* encodes a homologue of the class C yeast vacuolar protein sorting gene, *Vps33*, that is involved in vacuolar biogenesis and the late stages of protein trafficking from the Golgi to the vacuole [94]. Consistent with the protean manifestations of the disorder, VPS33B is widely expressed in fetal and adult tissues. In liver biopsy specimens from ARC patients, there was a marked disturbance in localization of plasma membrane proteins, including CEA, dipeptidyl peptidase and γGT, suggesting a defect in regulation of intracellular protein trafficking. There is a recent report of a patient with cholestasis, neurologic defects, ichthyosis, and aminoaciduria who was homozygous for a novel *VPS33* mutation but did not have arthrogryposis [95].

NORTH AMERICAN INDIAN CHOLESTASIS

Weber et al. [96] and Drouin et al. [97] described 30 North American Indian children with a severe nonsyndromic form of intrahepatic cholestasis. The disorder is inherited as an autosomal recessive trait. Cholestatic jaundice was present in 21 patients (70%) within the neonatal period. Clinical jaundice disappeared in most patients during the first year of life, but conjugated fraction of bilirubin was elevated in 75% by the age of 1 year. The serum concentration of γGT was also elevated. Other patients presented with no history of jaundice but initially were seen for gastrointestinal bleeding or for hepatomegaly later in childhood. Ongoing cholestasis was associated with chronic pruritus, persistent elevation of serum aminotransferase, serum alkaline phosphatase, and serum bile acid concentrations. Normal or moderately increased serum cholesterol levels were found in most patients. Progression to periportal fibrosis and cirrhosis was typical in childhood and adolescence. Early onset of portal hypertension and variceal hemorrhage necessitated portosystemic shunts in 13 of the children. Ten of 14 deaths were related to chronic liver disease. Liver transplantation is the only effective therapy.

Giant cell hepatitis, bile stasis, and neoductular proliferation characterized histopathology early in the course of the disorder. Later, portal fibrosis became evident and was followed by rapid progression to biliary cirrhosis. The electron microscopic changes were initially thought to be distinctive. Bile canaliculi appeared slightly dilated, with preservation or partial loss of microvilli. There was marked widening of the pericanalicular ectoplasm with abundant pericanalicular microfilaments [96]. Immunofluorescence microscopy confirmed that the prominent pericanalicular filamentous web was composed of actin-containing microfilaments. Because these contractile proteins may be involved in canalicular motility and generation of bile flow, microfilament dysfunction was proposed as the cause of cholestasis in these children. These findings, however, recently have been questioned and now are thought to be nonspecific and secondary to cholestatic injury, perhaps a cholangiopathy. The hepatic ultrastructure cannot be reliably distinguished from other inherited forms of cholestasis [97].

The gene for the disorder was mapped to chromosome 16q22 and recently identified [98]. The product of this gene, called cirhin, is a 686–amino acid protein of unknown function. Cirhin is preferentially expressed in embryonic liver and has been localized to the nucleolus [99]. The disease-causing R565W mutation is thought to change the predicted secondary structure of cirhin but has no effect on its nucleolar localization.

FAMILIAL HYPERCHOLANEMIA

Most patients with familial hypercholanemia are of Amish descent and present with pruritus, malabsorption, poor growth, and in some cases, bleeding and rickets from deficiency of vitamins K and D, respectively [100,101]. The disorder is inherited as an autosomal recessive trait. Serum bile acids are elevated and may fluctuate significantly. Serum bilirubin, γGT, and cholesterol levels are usually normal. Serum aminotransferase levels are normal to slightly increased. Liver histology is available on only a few patients and may be normal or show a mild reactive hepatitis or canalicular cholestasis [102]. Symptoms usually respond to treatment with UDCA.

The phenotype in these patients initially suggested a possible defect in uptake of conjugated bile acids across the basolateral membrane of the hepatocyte. However, expression of mRNA and protein for the human sodium-dependent bile acid transporter (NTCP) was normal in liver biopsy specimens from two affected children [102]. NTCP could also be detected on the basolateral membrane by indirect immunofluorescent microscopy. Moreover, no mutations were found on complete sequencing of the *NTCP* coding regions of both patients.

Recent studies of 17 Amish individuals from 12 families with familial hypercholanemia have identified mutations in genes encoding the tight junction protein 2 (*TPJ2*) and bile acid coenzyme A: amino acid *N*-acyltransferase (*BAAT*) [100]. Eleven patients were homozygous for a mutation in *TPJ2* and five were homozygous for a mutation in *BAAT*. Five individuals who were homozygous for a mutation in *TPJ2* also carried a *BAAT* mutation in one allele. One individual who was homozygous for a mutation in *BAAT* also carried a *TPJ2* mutation in one allele.

TPJ2 is a tight junction protein that participates in the formation of intercellular barriers separating bile from blood and controlling paracellular solute diffusion. It is proposed that mutations in *TPJ2* increase paracellular permeability to bile acids and probably other small molecules. This "short circuiting" with leakage of bile acids into blood is likely to adversely affect bile flow and result in intestinal concentrations of bile acids inadequate for micelle formation and normal absorption of dietary fat and fat-soluble vitamins.

BAAT is an enzyme that mediates conjugation of bile acids with glycine and taurine. Unconjugated bile acids are poor substrates for transport by NTCP and BSEP and for the nuclear receptor FXR that regulates bile acid homeostasis in the liver and intestine [103]. It is proposed that unconjugated bile acids diffuse back into blood and less so into bile, leading to high serum and low biliary bile acid concentrations.

CONCLUSION

The progress made in our understanding of inherited cholestatic liver diseases has been dramatic. New insights into hepatobiliary physiology and the behavior of liver transport proteins in acquired liver disease have also come from studies on PFIC. It is uncertain whether the heterozygous state or polymorphisms in the genes underlying these disorders can be associated with liver disease or affect the outcome of other forms of cholestasis, such as biliary atresia. Moreover, at least 30% of patients with low-γGT forms of PFIC and BRIC have no mutations in *ATP8B1* and *ABCB11*. Additional work is required to discover the genetic basis and define the pathophysiology of these disorders [26,104].

REFERENCES

1. Carlton VE, Pawlikowska L, Bull LN. Molecular basis of intrahepatic cholestasis. Ann Med 2004;36:606–17.
2. Danks DM, Smith AL. Hepatitis syndrome in infancy – an epidemiological survey with 10 year follow up. Arch Dis Child 1985;60:1204.

3. Deutsch J, Smith AL, Danks DM, Campbell PE. Long term prognosis for babies with neonatal liver disease. Arch Dis Child 1985;60:447–51.
4. Elferink RO, Groen AK. Genetic defects in hepatobiliary transport. Biochim Biophys Acta 2002;1586:129–45.
5. Carlton VE, Knisely AS, Freimer NB. Mapping of a locus for progressive familial intrahepatic cholestasis (Byler disease) to 18q21-q22, the benign recurrent intrahepatic cholestasis region. Hum Mol Genet 1995;4:1049–53.
6. Clayton RJ, Iber FL, Ruebner BH, McKusick VA. Byler disease. Fatal familial intrahepatic cholestasis in an Amish kindred. Am J Dis Child 1969;117:112–24.
7. Summerskill WH, Walshe JM. Benign recurrent intrahepatic "obstructive" jaundice. Lancet 1959;2:686–90.
8. van Ooteghem NA, Klomp LW, van Berge-Henegouwen GP, Houwen RH. Benign recurrent intrahepatic cholestasis progressing to progressive familial intrahepatic cholestasis: low GGT cholestasis is a clinical continuum. J Hepatol 2002;36: 439–43.
9. Ornvold K, Nielsen IM, Poulsen H. Fatal familial cholestatic syndrome in Greenland Eskimo children. A histomorphological analysis of 16 cases. Virchows Arch A Pathol Anat Histopathol 1989;415:275–81.
10. Nielsen IM, Eiberg H. Cholestasis Familiaris Groenlandica: an epidemiological, clinical and genetic study. Int J Circumpolar Health 2004;63(suppl 2):192–4.
11. Whitington PF, Freese DK, Alonso EM, et al. Clinical and biochemical findings in progressive familial intrahepatic cholestasis. J Pediatr Gastroenterol Nutr 1994;18:134–41.
12. van Mil SW, Klomp LW, Bull LN, Houwen RH. FIC1 disease: a spectrum of intrahepatic cholestatic disorders. Semin Liver Dis 2001;21:535–44.
13. Jansen PL, Sturm E. Genetic cholestasis, causes and consequences for hepatobiliary transport. Liver Int 2003;23: 315–22.
14. Oshima T, Ikeda K, Takasaka T. Sensorineural hearing loss associated with Byler disease. Tohoku J Exp Med 1999;187:83–8.
15. Mullenbach R, Bennett A, Tetlow N, et al. ATP8B1 mutations in British cases with intrahepatic cholestasis of pregnancy. Gut 2005;54:829–34.
16. Chatila R, Bergasa NV, Lagarde S, West AB. Intractable cough and abnormal pulmonary function in benign recurrent intrahepatic cholestasis. Am J Gastroenterol 1996;91:2215–19.
17. Bove KE, Heubi JE, Balistreri WF, Setchell KD. Bile acid synthetic defects and liver disease: a comprehensive review. Pediatr Dev Pathol 2004;7:315–34.
18. Cabrera-Abreu JC, Green A. Gamma-glutamyltransferase: value of its measurement in paediatrics. Ann Clin Biochem 2002;39(pt 1):22–5.
19. Hanigan MH, Bull LN, Strautnieks SS, et al. Low serum concentrations of γGT activity in progressive familial intrahepatic cholestasis: evidence for different mechanisms in PFIC, type 1(FIC1 disease), and PFIC, type 2 (BSEP disease) [abstract]. Hepatology 2002;36:310.
20. Jacquemin E Dumont M, Bernard O, et al. Evidence for defective primary bile acid secretion in children with progressive familial intrahepatic cholestasis (Byler disease). Eur J Pediatr 1994;153:424–8.
21. Alonso EM, Snover DC, Montag A, et al. Histologic pathology of the liver in progressive familial intrahepatic cholestasis. J Pediatr Gastroenterol Nutr 1994;18:128–33.
22. Phillipps MJ, Poucell S, Patterson J, Valencia P. The liver. An atlas of ultrastructural pathology. New York: Raven Press, 1987.
23. Bull LN, Roche E, Song EJ, et al. Mapping of the locus for cholestasis-lymphedema syndrome (Aagenaes syndrome) to a 6.6-cM interval on chromosome 15q. Am J Hum Genet 2000; 67:994–9.
24. Bull LN, Juijn JA, Liao M, et al. Fine-resolution mapping by haplotype evaluation: the examples of PFIC1 and BRIC. Hum Genet 1999;104:241–8.
25. Bull LN, van Eijk MJ, Pawlikowska L, et al. A gene encoding a P-type ATPase mutated in two forms of hereditary cholestasis. Nat Genet 1998;18:219–24.
26. Klomp LW, Vargas JC, van Mil SW, et al. Characterization of mutations in ATP8B1 associated with hereditary cholestasis. Hepatology 2004;40:27–38.
27. Williams CN, Kaye R, Baker L, et al. Progressive familial cholestatic cirrhosis and bile acid metabolism. J Pediatr 1972; 81:493–500.
28. Tang X, Halleck MS, Schlegel RA, Williamson P. A subfamily of P-type ATPases with aminophospholipid transporting activity. Science 1996;272:1495–7.
29. Ujhazy P, Ortiz D, Misra S, et al. Familial intrahepatic cholestasis 1: studies of localization and function. Hepatology 2001;34 (4 pt 1):768–75.
30. Verkleij AJ, Post JA. Membrane phospholipid asymmetry and signal transduction. J Membr Biol 2000;178:1–10.
31. Paulusma CC, Oude Elferink RP. The type 4 subfamily of P-type ATPases, putative aminophospholipid translocases with a role in human disease. Biochim Biophys Acta 2005;1741: 11–24.
32. Eppens EF, van Mil SW, de Vree JM, et al. FIC1, the protein affected in two forms of hereditary cholestasis, is localized in the cholangiocyte and the canalicular membrane of the hepatocyte. J Hepatol 2001;35:436–43.
33. van Mil SW, van Oort MM, van den Berg IE, et al. Fic1 is expressed at apical membranes of different epithelial cells in the digestive tract and is induced in the small intestine during postnatal development of mice. Pediatr Res 2004;56:981–7.
34. Harris MJ, Kagawa T, Dawson PA, Arias IM. Taurocholate transport by hepatic and intestinal bile acid transporters is independent of FIC1 overexpression in Madin-Darby canine kidney cells. J Gastroenterol Hepatol 2004;19:819–25.
35. Paulusma CC, Groen A, Kunne C, et al. ATP8B1 renders the canalicular membrane resistant to hydrophobic bile salts [abstract]. Hepatology 2005;42:457.
36. Chen F, Ananthanarayanan M, Emre S, et al. Progressive familial intrahepatic cholestasis, type 1, is associated with decreased farnesoid X receptor activity. Gastroenterology 2004;126: 756–64.
37. Alvarez L, Jara P, Sanchez-Sabate E, et al. Reduced hepatic expression of farnesoid X receptor in hereditary cholestasis associated to mutation in ATP8B1. Hum Mol Genet 2004;13: 2451–60.
38. Bull LN, Carlton VE, Stricker NL, et al. Genetic and morphological findings in progressive familial intrahepatic cholestasis (Byler disease [PFIC-1] and Byler syndrome): evidence for heterogeneity. Hepatology 1997;26:155–64.
39. Strautnieks SS, Kagalwalla AF, Tanner MS, et al. Identification of a locus for progressive familial intrahepatic cholestasis PFIC2 on chromosome 2q24. Am J Hum Genet 1997;61:630–3.

40. Strautnieks SS, Bull LN, Knisely AS, et al. A gene encoding a liver-specific ABC transporter is mutated in progressive familial intrahepatic cholestasis. Nat Genet 1998;20:233–8.
41. Kullak-Ublick GA, Stieger B, Meier PJ. Enterohepatic bile salt transporters in normal physiology and liver disease. Gastroenterology 2004;126:322–42.
42. Byrne JA, Strautnieks SS, Mieli-Vergani G, et al. The human bile salt export pump: characterization of substrate specificity and identification of inhibitors. Gastroenterology 2002;123:1649–58.
43. Thompson R, Strautnieks S. BSEP: function and role in progressive familial intrahepatic cholestasis. Semin Liver Dis 2001;21:545–50.
44. Jansen PL, Strautnieks SS, Jacquemin E, et al. Hepatocanalicular bile salt export pump deficiency in patients with progressive familial intrahepatic cholestasis. Gastroenterology 1999;117:1370–9.
45. Knisely AS, Strautnieks S, Scheimann AO, et al. Bile salt export pump (BSEP) deficiency is a significant risk factor for both pediatric and adult hepatobiliary malignancy. Hepatology 2005;42:380A.
46. van Mil SW, van der Woerd WL, van der Brugge G, et al. Benign recurrent intrahepatic cholestasis type 2 is caused by mutations in ABCB11. Gastroenterology 2004;127:379–84.
47. Eloranta ML, Hakli T, Hiltunen M, et al. Association of single nucleotide polymorphisms of the bile salt export pump gene with intrahepatic cholestasis of pregnancy. Scand J Gastroenterol 2003;38:648–52.
48. Hermeziu B, Sanlaville D, Girard M, et al. Heterozygous bile salt export pump deficiency: a possible genetic predisposition to transient neonatal cholestasis. J Pediatr Gastroenterol Nutr 2006;42:114–16.
49. Jacquemin E. Progressive familial intrahepatic cholestasis. Genetic basis and treatment. Clin Liver Dis 2000;4:753–63.
50. Noe J, Kullak-Ublick GA, Jochum W, et al. Impaired expression and function of the bile salt export pump due to three novel ABCB11 mutations in intrahepatic cholestasis. J Hepatol 2005;43:536–43.
51. Keitel V, Burdelski M, Warskulat U, et al. Expression and localization of hepatobiliary transport proteins in progressive familial intrahepatic cholestasis. Hepatology 2005;41:1160–72.
52. Wang R, Salem M, Yousef IM, et al. Targeted inactivation of sister of P-glycoprotein gene (spgp) in mice results in nonprogressive but persistent intrahepatic cholestasis. Proc Natl Acad Sci U S A 2001;98:2011–16.
53. Lam P, Wang R, Ling V. Bile acid transport in sister of P-glycoprotein (ABCB11) knockout mice. Biochemistry 2005;44:12598–605.
54. Wang R, Lam P, Liu L, et al. Severe cholestasis induced by cholic acid feeding in knockout mice of sister of P-glycoprotein. Hepatology 2003;38:1489–99.
55. Wang L, Soroka CJ, Boyer JL. The role of bile salt export pump mutations in progressive familial intrahepatic cholestasis type II. J Clin Invest 2002;110:965–72.
56. Hayashi H, Takada T, Suzuki H, et al. Two common PFIC2 mutations are associated with the impaired membrane trafficking of BSEP/ABCB11. Hepatology 2005;41:916–24.
57. Yerushalmi B, Sokol RJ, Narkewicz MR, et al. Use of rifampin for severe pruritus in children with chronic cholestasis. J Pediatr Gastroenterol Nutr 1999;29:442–7.
58. Whitington PF, Whitington GL. Partial external diversion of bile for the treatment of intractable pruritus associated with intrahepatic cholestasis. Gastroenterology 1988;95:130–6.
59. Emond JC, Whitington PF. Selective surgical management of progressive familial intrahepatic cholestasis (Byler's disease). J Pediatr Surg 1995;30:1635–41.
60. Hollands CM, Rivera-Pedrogo FJ, Gonzalez-Vallina R, et al. Ileal exclusion for Byler's disease: an alternative surgical approach with promising early results for pruritus. J Pediatr Surg 1998;33:220–4.
61. Ismail H, Kalicinski P, Markiewicz M, et al. Treatment of progressive familial intrahepatic cholestasis: liver transplantation or partial external biliary diversion. Pediatr Transplant 1999;3:219–24.
62. Melter M, Rodeck B, Kardorff R, et al. Progressive familial intrahepatic cholestasis: partial biliary diversion normalizes serum lipids and improves growth in noncirrhotic patients. Am J Gastroenterol 2000;95:3522–8.
63. Kalicinski PJ, Ismail H, Jankowska I, et al. Surgical treatment of progressive familial intrahepatic cholestasis: comparison of partial external biliary diversion and ileal bypass. Eur J Pediatr Surg 2003;13:307–11.
64. Kurbegov AC, Setchell KD, Haas JE, et al. Biliary diversion for progressive familial intrahepatic cholestasis: improved liver morphology and bile acid profile. Gastroenterology 2003;125:1227–34.
65. Buchwald H, Varco RL, Matts JP, et al. Effect of partial ileal bypass surgery on mortality and morbidity from coronary heart disease in patients with hypercholesterolemia. Report of the Program on the Surgical Control of the Hyperlipidemias (POSCH). N Engl J Med 1990;323:946–55.
66. Neimark E, Shneider B. Novel surgical and pharmacological approaches to chronic cholestasis in children: partial external biliary diversion for intractable pruritus and xanthomas in Alagille syndrome. J Pediatr Gastroenterol Nutr 2003;36:296–7.
67. Stapelbroek JM, van Erpecum KJ, Klomp LW, et al. Nasobiliary drainage induces long-lasting remission in benign recurrent intrahepatic cholestasis. Hepatology 2006;43:51–3.
68. Jacquemin E, Hermans D, Myara A, et al. Ursodeoxycholic acid therapy in pediatric patients with progressive familial intrahepatic cholestasis. Hepatology 1997;25:519–23.
69. Lykavieris P, van Mil S, Cresteil D, et al. Progressive familial intrahepatic cholestasis type 1 and extrahepatic features: no catch-up of stature growth, exacerbation of diarrhea, and appearance of liver steatosis after liver transplantation. J Hepatol 2003;39:447–52.
70. Egawa H, Yorifuji T, Sumazaki R, et al. Intractable diarrhea after liver transplantation for Byler's disease: successful treatment with bile adsorptive resin. Liver Transpl 2002;8:714–16.
71. Deleuze JF, Jacquemin E, Dubuisson C, et al. Defect of multidrug-resistance 3 gene expression in a subtype of progressive familial intrahepatic cholestasis. Hepatology 1996;23:904–8.
72. Jacquemin E. Role of multidrug resistance 3 deficiency in pediatric and adult liver disease: one gene for three diseases. Semin Liver Dis 2001;21:551–62.
73. Jacquemin E, De Vree JM, Cresteil D, et al. The wide spectrum of multidrug resistance 3 deficiency: from neonatal cholestasis to cirrhosis of adulthood. Gastroenterology 2001;120:1448–58.

74. Rosmorduc O, Hermelin B, Poupon R. MDR3 gene defect in adults with symptomatic intrahepatic and gallbladder cholesterol cholelithiasis. Gastroenterology 2001;120:1459–67.
75. Lucena JF, Herrero JI, Quiroga J, et al. A multidrug resistance 3 gene mutation causing cholelithiasis, cholestasis of pregnancy, and adulthood biliary cirrhosis. Gastroenterology 2003;124:1037–42.
76. Small DM. Role of ABC transporters in secretion of cholesterol from liver into bile. Proc Natl Acad Sci U S A 2003;100:4–6.
77. Dixon PH, Weerasekera N, Linton KJ, et al. Heterozygous MDR3 missense mutation associated with intrahepatic cholestasis of pregnancy: evidence for a defect in protein trafficking. Hum Mol Genet 2000;9:1209–17.
78. Gendrot C, Bacq Y, Brechot MC, et al. A second heterozygous MDR3 nonsense mutation associated with intrahepatic cholestasis of pregnancy. J Med Genet 2003;40:e32.
79. Elferink RP, Ottenhoff R, van Marle J, et al. Class III P-glycoproteins mediate the formation of lipoprotein X in the mouse. J Clin Invest 1998;102:1749–57.
80. van Mil SW, Houwen RH, Klomp LW. Genetics of familial intrahepatic cholestasis syndromes. J Med Genet 2005;42:449–63.
81. Chen HL, Chang PS, Hsu HC, et al. Progressive familial intrahepatic cholestasis with high gamma-glutamyltranspeptidase levels in Taiwanese infants: role of MDR3 gene defect? Pediatr Res 2001;50:50–5.
82. Elferink RP, Groen AK. The mechanism of biliary lipid secretion and its defects. Gastroenterol Clin North Am 1999;28:59–74, vi.
83. Fickert P, Fuchsbichler A, Wagner M, et al. Regurgitation of bile acids from leaky bile ducts causes sclerosing cholangitis in Mdr2 (Abcb4) knockout mice. Gastroenterology 2004;127:261–74.
84. Van Nieuwkerk CM, Elferink RP, Groen AK, et al. Effects of ursodeoxycholate and cholate feeding on liver disease in FVB mice with a disrupted mdr2 P-glycoprotein gene. Gastroenterology 1996;111:165–71.
85. De Vree JM, Ottenhoff R, Bosma PJ, et al. Correction of liver disease by hepatocyte transplantation in a mouse model of progressive familial intrahepatic cholestasis. Gastroenterology 2000;119:1720–30.
86. Aagenaes O, Sigstad H, Bjorn-Hansen R. Lymphoedema in hereditary recurrent cholestasis from birth. Arch Dis Child 1970;45:690–5.
87. Aagenaes O. Hereditary recurrent cholestasis with lymphoedema – two new families. Acta Paediatr Scand 1974;63:465–71.
88. Fruhwirth M, Janecke AR, Muller T, et al. Evidence for genetic heterogeneity in lymphedema-cholestasis syndrome. J Pediatr 2003;142:441–7.
89. Aagenaes O. Hereditary cholestasis with lymphoedema (Aagenaes syndrome, cholestasis-lymphoedema syndrome). New cases and follow-up from infancy to adult age. Scand J Gastroenterol 1998;33:335–45.
90. Nezelof C, Dupart MC, Jaubert F, Eliachar E. A lethal familial syndrome associating arthrogryposis multiplex congenita, renal dysfunction, and a cholestatic and pigmentary liver disease. J Pediatr 1979;94:258–60.
91. Di Rocco M, Callea F, Pollice B, et al. Arthrogryposis, renal dysfunction and cholestasis syndrome: report of five patients from three Italian families. Eur J Pediatr 1995;154:835–9.
92. Horslen SP, Quarrell OW, Tanner MS. Liver histology in the arthrogryposis multiplex congenita, renal dysfunction, and cholestasis (ARC) syndrome: report of three new cases and review. J Med Genet 1994;31:62–4.
93. Gissen P, Johnson CA, Morgan NV, et al. Mutations in VPS33B, encoding a regulator of SNARE-dependent membrane fusion, cause arthrogryposis-renal dysfunction-cholestasis (ARC) syndrome. Nat Genet 2004;36:400–4.
94. Gissen P, Johnson CA, Gentle D, et al. Comparative evolutionary analysis of VPS33 homologues: genetic and functional insights. Hum Mol Genet 2005;14:1261–70.
95. Bull LN, Mahmoodi BS, Baker AJ, et al. VPS33B mutation with ichthyosis, cholestasis, and renal dysfunction but without arthrogryposis: incomplete ARC syndrome phenotype. J Pediatr 2006;148:271–3.
96. Weber AM, Tuchweber B, Yousef I, et al. Severe familial cholestasis in North American Indian children: a clinical model of microfilament dysfunction? Gastroenterology 1981;81:653–62.
97. Drouin E, Russo P, Tuchweber B, et al. North American Indian cirrhosis in children: a review of 30 cases. J Pediatr Gastroenterol Nutr 2000;31:395–404.
98. Chagnon P, Michaud J, Mitchell G, et al. A missense mutation (R565W) in cirhin (FLJ14728) in North American Indian childhood cirrhosis. Am J Hum Genet 2002;71:1443–9.
99. Yu B, Mitchell GA, Richter A. Nucleolar localization of cirhin, the protein mutated in North American Indian childhood cirrhosis. Exp Cell Res 2005;311:218–28.
100. Morton DH, Salen G, Batta AK, et al. Abnormal hepatic sinusoidal bile acid transport in an Amish kindred is not linked to FIC1 and is improved by ursodiol. Gastroenterology 2000;119:188–95.
101. Carlton VE, Harris BZ, Puffenberger EG, et al. Complex inheritance of familial hypercholanemia with associated mutations in TJP2 and BAAT. Nat Genet 2003;34:91–6.
102. Shneider BL, Fox VL, Schwarz KB, et al. Hepatic basolateral sodium-dependent–bile acid transporter expression in two unusual cases of hypercholanemia and in extrahepatic biliary atresia. Hepatology 1997;25:1176–83.
103. Karpen SJ. Nuclear receptor regulation of hepatic function. J Hepatol 2002;36:832–50.
104. Strautnieks S, Byrne J, Knisely AS, et al. There must be a third locus for low GGT PFIC [abstract]. Hepatology 2001;34:240A.

15

Alagille Syndrome

Binita M. Kamath, M.B. B.Chir., Nancy B. Spinner, Ph.D., and
David A. Piccoli, M.D.

Alagille syndrome (AGS) is a highly variable, multisystem, autosomal dominant disorder that primarily affects the liver, heart, eyes, face, and skeleton [1–3]. There is significant variability in the extent to which each of these systems is affected in an individual, if at all [4,5]. AGS has traditionally been diagnosed based on the presence of intrahepatic bile duct paucity on liver biopsy in association with at least three of the major clinical features: chronic cholestasis, cardiac disease (most often peripheral pulmonary stenosis), skeletal abnormalities (typically butterfly vertebrae), ocular abnormalities (primarily posterior embryotoxon), and characteristic facial features [6]. It has an estimated frequency of 1 in 70,000 live births based on the presence of neonatal cholestasis. However, this is an underestimate as molecular testing has demonstrated that many individuals with a disease-causing mutation do not have neonatal liver disease.

Alagille syndrome is caused by mutations in *Jagged1* (*JAG1*), a ligand in the Notch signaling pathway [7,8]. *JAG1* mutations are identified in more than 90% of clinically diagnosed probands [9]. Recently, mutations in *Notch2* have been identified in a few patients with AGS who do not have *JAG1* mutations [10]. This exciting development has enhanced our understanding of the heterogeneity of this disorder, though much remains to be understood about the tremendous variability seen in affected individuals and the likely genetic modifiers involved.

BILE DUCT PAUCITY

Bile duct paucity is present in a diverse group of metabolic, infectious, and inflammatory hepatic disorders in infancy. In some of these disorders, paucity occurs only occasionally, and it may not be the most common histopathologic pattern. In a larger group of disorders, paucity is the final histologic pattern. Patients with many of these diseases may have neonatal hepatitis or even bile duct proliferation in early phases, with the progression to paucity over a period varying from months to years. Paucity may be the predominant pattern for certain disorders, but it cannot be considered an absolute feature of any disease. The observed bile duct–portal tract ratio, by which paucity is defined, varies substantially with gestational and postnatal age, disease course and severity, and even biopsy sample size. It appears that some disorders may have a decrease in number of bile ducts with a concomitant decrease in portal tract number such that a true "paucity" of bile ducts is not reflected adequately by the ratio of ducts to portal tracts. A decrease in the number of bile ducts (and possibly of portal tracts) could be caused by a deficit in development, disuse atrophy, or an active toxic, inflammatory, or infectious destruction. In many of the disorders with paucity, the pathogenesis of the duct deficit is not understood. Finally, in some disorders, the degree of duct paucity does not seem to correlate with extent of liver disease or outcome. Therefore, it is not possible to organize the disorders with paucity into a rational classification scheme. Table 15.1 lists disorders in which paucity seems to be, at least occasionally, a feature.

In 1969, Alagille et al. [11] recognized that some patients with idiopathic bile duct paucity had similar clinical features and that this pattern was common to other family members. In 1975, they extended these observations [1], and Watson and Miller [3] independently recognized this pattern of abnormalities in patients with prominent cardiac disease. Since these descriptions, bile duct paucity has been classified into syndromic and nonsyndromic paucity. The syndromic form has associated cardiac, renal, facial, musculoskeletal, and other features. It is the most common and most important type of paucity. Nonsyndromic paucity is an unrelated and diverse group of disorders, each of which is relatively rare. With the current understanding of the molecular or infectious basis for many of these disorders, the term *nonsyndromic paucity* should no longer be used because it is inappropriate to assign a pathogenesis or outcome to this broad group of disorders. *Syndromic paucity* also has been called *arteriohepatic dysplasia, intrahepatic atresia, biliary hypoplasia, intrahepatic biliary dysgenesis,* and *Watson–Alagille syndrome.* Each of these terms has significant limitations, and currently the term *Alagille syndrome* has achieved nearly uniform acceptance in the hepatic, cardiac, and genetic literature. The most important features of AGS are its multiple organ involvement, the high degree of variability even within families, and the dominant pattern of inheritance

Table 15.1: Causes of Bile Duct Paucity

Genetic disorders
- Alagille syndrome
- Down's syndrome
- Other chromosomal abnormalities

Metabolic disorders
- α_1-antitrypsin deficiency
- Cystic fibrosis
- Hypopituitarism

Infections
- Congenital cytomegalovirus infection
- Congenital rubella infection
- Congenital syphilis

Immunologic disorders
- Graft-versus-host disease
- Chronic hepatic allograft rejection
- Sclerosing cholangitis

Other disorders
- Zellweger syndrome
- Ivemark syndrome

Idiopathic disorders

caused by mutations in *JAG1*. Many infants with AGS do not have duct paucity at the time of presentation, and some parents of affected children and cardiac patients with AGS mutations appear to have no cholestasis or even biochemical hepatic disease. Although the hepatic manifestations are predominant in many patients, the term *Alagille syndrome* serves to shift the focus from the liver to the complicated systemic manifestations of the disorder.

Overview and Definitions

The normal bile duct–portal space ratio is between 0.9 and 1.8. Bile duct paucity is defined histologically in a full-term or older infant as a ratio of bile duct to portal tract that is less than 0.9 (Figure 15.1). It is important to note that bile ductules should not be included. The interlobular bile duct typically is located more centrally in the portal tract; the bile ductule is located peripherally. An adequate number of true portal tracts must be examined to arrive at an accurate ratio. The initial recommendations suggested that 20 portal tracts should be evaluated [1]. This number cannot be achieved with a needle biopsy; wedge biopsies are necessary if the diagnosis of paucity is considered. Subsequently, it has been shown that a reasonably accurate estimation can be made with needle biopsy specimens containing as few as six portal tracts [12]. The bile duct–portal tract ratio in older infants with AGS is usually less than 0.5–0.75 [1,13].

Kahn et al. [14] demonstrated that the number of bile ducts is diminished in the normal fetus and preterm infant. This may represent incomplete terminal differentiation of the bile duct, which starts near the hilus and extends outward to the subcapsular region. The site of the biopsy therefore may have some effect on the apparent ratio in young infants; a wedge biopsy specimen typically contains proportionately more subcapsular hepatic tissue than does a needle biopsy specimen.

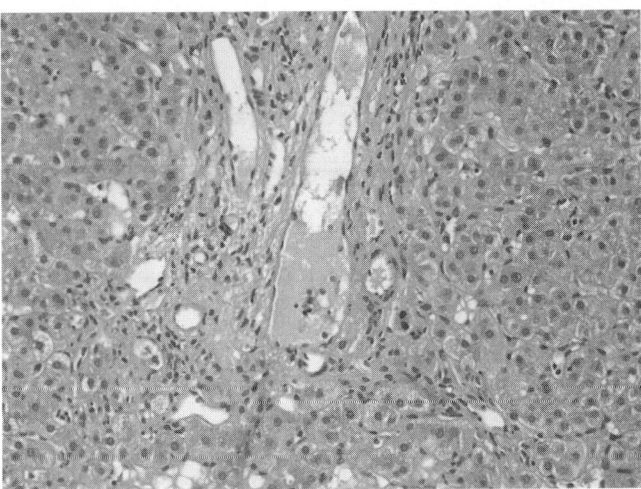

Figure 15.1. Liver specimen from an infant with Alagille syndrome with bile duct paucity. The portal tract is shown without any identifiable interlobular bile duct. (Hematoxylin and eosin [H&E] staining, 200× magnification.) (Courtesy of Pierre A. Russo, M.D.) For color reproduction, see Color Plate 15.1.

Because paucity is not a constant feature of most disorders in which it is seen, including AGS, it seems reasonable to assess duct number with the less invasive needle biopsy techniques. In neonatal cholestasis, the most diagnostically important feature of a biopsy is the presence of true duct proliferation, as opposed to paucity. Bile duct proliferation is consistent with obstruction and certain metabolic disorders but is seen only rarely in AGS (Figure 15.2). If proliferation is identified in a patient with features of AGS, the DISIDA (di-isopropyl iminodiacetic acid) scan and intraoperative cholangiogram should be interpreted with caution. AGS patients with nonexcretion and apparent

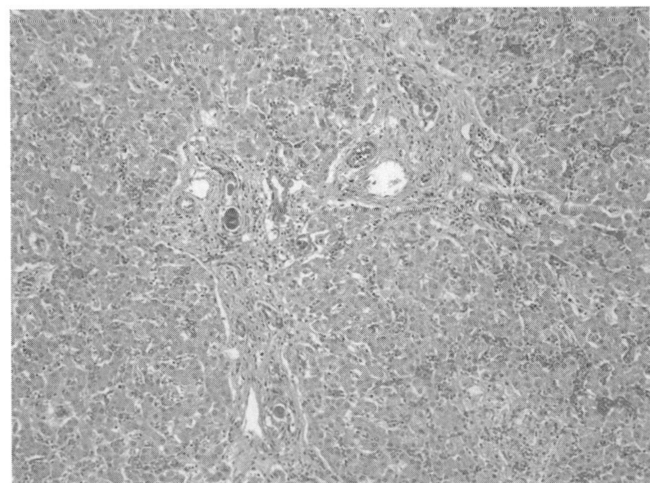

Figure 15.2. Liver specimen from a 1-month-old patient with Alagille syndrome demonstrating marked bile duct proliferation. (H&E staining, 100× magnification.) (Courtesy of Pierre A. Russo, M.D.) For color reproduction, see Color Plate 15.2.

noncommunication may be diagnosed mistakenly as having biliary atresia.

Histopathology in Alagille Syndrome

Bile duct paucity has been considered the most important and constant feature of AGS. This paucity, however, is not present in infancy in many patients ultimately shown to have AGS. Furthermore, a systematic study of adults with mild, noncholestatic AGS has not been performed. Paucity is present in about 89% of patients reported in large series [2,6,15–17]. The frequency of paucity in these series varies in large part with the criteria used to define AGS. Older studies required paucity to consider the diagnosis of syndromic paucity [2]; newer studies focusing on the systemic manifestations or the presence of *JAG1* mutations identify paucity in only 80–85% of patients with AGS [6,15–17].

Several studies of serial liver biopsies have demonstrated that paucity is more common later in infancy and childhood [6,12,18,19]. Emerick et al. [6] found that paucity was present in 60% of 48 infants younger than 6 months of age but in 95% of 40 who underwent biopsy after 6 months. The progression to paucity typically accompanies a worsening of clinical hepatic disease in infancy over a period of months or years. Occasional reports have demonstrated, however, that the progression to paucity is not an absolute feature of AGS. Hypotheses explaining this progression to paucity include a destruction of ducts postnatally and a differential maturation of portal tracts and their incumbent ducts. The original theory that there is a lack of development of interlobular bile ducts was not supported by later studies. The factors that lead to a decrease in the number of ducts are not yet understood, but it is likely that *JAG1* has an integral role in the development of new ducts as the liver enlarges substantially in late fetal and early postnatal development [20].

Several groups have described a reduction in the number of portal tracts in this condition [19,21]. The portal tracts may or may not show an inflammatory infiltrate, and early in life there is minimal or no fibrosis. Fibrosis, if noted early, may be perisinusoidal rather than portal in location. Hashida and Yunis [19] have described epithelial degeneration, concentric mesenchymal layering around ducts, edema, and lymphatic and vascular dilatation in the portal tracts.

Ductular proliferation is present in a small number of infants with AGS, leading to significant potential diagnostic confusion. This is seen most commonly in association with portal inflammation. Cytokeratin stains can help differentiate duct from ductular elements, but at times the biopsy specimen may be misleading. As with any infantile cholestatic condition, giant cell hepatitis may be a predominant feature in the infant with AGS. In part because of the variability in the early histopathology of the liver in AGS, a number of patients have been misdiagnosed as having biliary atresia [6,16,17]. Histologic cholestasis is prominent early, but in many patients this tends to disappear unless there is progression to end-stage liver disease. Ultrastructural studies have demonstrated the apparent retention of bile in hepatocytes at the level of the Golgi apparatus, unusually large amounts of intercellular bile, and relatively normal bile canaliculi [22], but these findings are not absolute and may not be diagnostically useful [23].

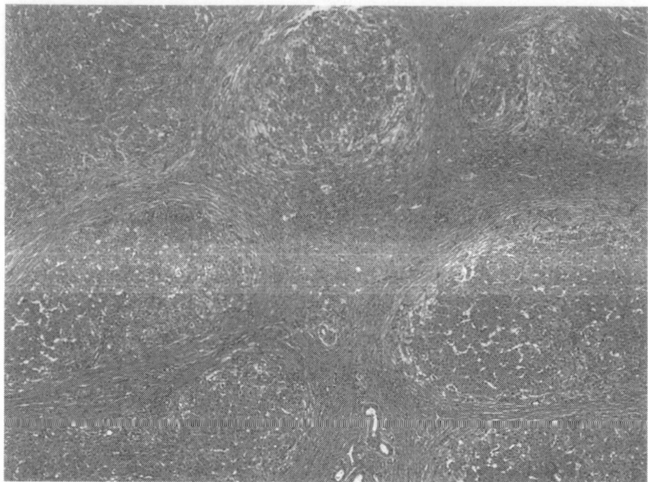

Figure 15.3. Liver specimen from a 16-year-old with Alagille syndrome. There is established cirrhosis. Portal tracts are expanded and fibrotic. There is a complete absence of interlobular bile ducts. (H&E staining, 100× magnification.) (Courtesy of Pierre A. Russo, M.D.) For color reproduction, see Color Plate 15.3.

An interesting characteristic of the hepatic histopathology of AGS is the uncommon progression to cirrhosis (Figure 15.3). Typically, diseases with duct deficit and obstruction manifested by severe cholestasis progress to end-stage liver disease and cirrhosis. Not only does this not occur in most patients with AGS, but the biochemical cholestasis and its clinical manifestations most commonly improve with time, despite the lack of reappearance of interlobular ducts. Progressive liver disease with significant fibrosis or cirrhosis does occur, with reported incidence between 10% and 50% of patients [2,6,15,16].

DIAGNOSIS OF ALAGILLE SYNDROME

In the original descriptions of the disorder, Alagille et al. [1,11] recognized that there was a number of manifestations common to patients with AGS. Initially, the syndrome was defined by bile duct paucity associated with at least three of five major criteria: cholestasis, characteristic facies, vertebral anomalies, ocular anomalies, and a heart murmur. Since that time, a wide range of manifestations in many organs has been associated with AGS. Large series of patients reported by Alagille et al. [2], Deprettere et al. [15], Hoffenberg et al. [16], Emerick et al. [6], and Quiros-Tejeira et al. [17] have demonstrated differing frequencies of the manifestations of AGS (Table 15.2). A comparison of these series is somewhat limited by the retrospective nature and the time period of certain studies and by the lack of uniform evaluation of each organ system potentially involved in AGS.

The list of abnormalities identified in the "major" organ systems and the list of other affected organs have grown appreciably. Renal disease, pancreatic disease, and vascular system involvement are recognized as significant manifestations of AGS, contributing to the injury and deaths it causes. Several

Table 15.2: Features of Alagille Syndrome

	Study					
Feature	*Alagille et al., 1987 [2]*	*Deprettere et al., 1987 [15]*	*Hoffenberg et al., 1995 [16]*	*Emerick et al., 1999 [6]*	*Quiros-Tejeira et al., 1999 [17]*	*Weighted % of all studies*
Patients, n	80	27	26	92	43	
Paucity, % (n)	100 (80)	81 (22)	80 (20)	85 (69)	83 (34)	89
Cholestasis, % (n)	91 (73)	93 (25)	100 (26)	96 (88)	100 (43)	95
Murmur, % (n)	85 (68)	96 (26)	96 (24)	97 (90)	98 (42)	94
Vertebral, % (n)	87 (70)	33 (6)	48 (11)	51 (37)	38 (12)	61
Facies, % (n)	95 (76)	70 (19)	92 (23)	96 (86)	98 (42)	92
Ocular, % (n)	88 (55)	56 (9)	85 (17)	78 (65)	73 (16)	80
Renal, % (n)	73 (17)		19 (5)	40 (28)	50 (15)	44
Other features						
Growth retardation, % (n)		73 (16)		87 (27)	86 (37)	
Mental retardation		0 (0)		2 (2)		
Developmental delay, % (n)		52 (14)		16 (15)		
Pancreatic insufficiency, % (n)				41 (7)		
Intracranial bleeding, % (n)			12 (3)	14 (13)	12 (5)	

of the diagnostic "syndromic" features, however, are seen in normal individuals. Posterior embryotoxon has been estimated to be present in 7–12% of normal individuals, and heart murmurs are present in 6% of all newborns. Cholestasis is common in most individuals with neonatal liver disease. Features such as posterior embryotoxon, complex congenital cardiac disease, and butterfly vertebrae are seen in at least one other genetically determined multisystem disorder, 22q deletion, the velocardiofacial syndrome [24]. Finally, some relatives of AGS probands have few or only one feature of AGS and yet carry a mutation in *JAG1* [25]. It remains to be clarified whether those individuals who carry disease-causing mutations in *JAG1* but are without syndromic features should be classified as having AGS or merely as carriers of a gene defect with minimal expression. Because the genetic risk for progeny is high, the designation of a diagnosis of AGS seems appropriate, even in the absence of an adequate number of syndromic features.

With the advent of molecular testing for AGS (see Genetics), the diagnostic criteria for AGS can be modified significantly. Though mutational analysis is available, the diagnosis remains predominantly a clinical one. For the index case (proband) in the family, it seems reasonable to continue with the original Alagille criteria, requiring bile duct paucity with at least three features from the list of cholestasis, characteristic Alagille facies, posterior embryotoxon, butterfly vertebrae, typical AGS renal disease, and consistent cardiac disease. On this basis, some patients may be assigned the AGS designation incorrectly as a result of the frequency of some of these features. In infants younger than 6 months of age, in whom paucity is not common, three or four features should be adequate to make the diagnosis. In an older child without paucity, AGS is much less likely and other diagnostic considerations should be entertained. In families with one definite proband, other members with two or even one feature are likely to have the gene defect and should be considered as having AGS. A family history is important for patients who have *JAG1* mutations but highly atypical manifestations. Mutational analysis may assist in screening mildly affected relatives. Others with typical AGS manifestations but no mutation in *JAG1* ultimately may be shown to have defects in other Notch or Jagged ligands. Finally, as molecular testing becomes more readily available and requested by cardiologists and nephrologists, it is likely that patients with isolated or limited manifestations in extrahepatic organs will be diagnosed as having AGS through identification of *JAG1* mutations. A revised list of diagnostic criteria is proposed in Table 15.3.

CLINICAL FEATURES AND COMPLICATIONS

Since the original publications by Alagille and Watson, there have been more than 500 patients reported in the literature. A strikingly large number of abnormalities have been associated

Table 15.3: Revised Diagnostic Criteria for the Diagnosis of Alagille Syndrome

AGS Family History	*Paucity*	*JAG1 Defect*	*Number of Criteria Needed**
None (proband)	Present	Not identified	3 or more features†
None (proband)	Absent	Not identified	4 or more features
None (proband)	Absent	Identified	1 or more features
Present	Present	Not identified	1 or more features
Present	Unknown	Not identified	1 or more features
Present	Absent	Identified	Any or no features

*Major clinical criteria include consistent cardiac, renal, or ocular disease; butterfly vertebrae; and characteristic "Alagille" facies of childhood or adulthood.
†A number of index cases with two criteria or even one criterion ultimately will be shown to have AGS by molecular testing, but two criteria should be considered insufficient to establish the diagnosis in a proband.

with AGS. These problems are best organized into those features that are structural defects in the embryogenesis of the fetus or postnatal infant, functional defects resulting from abnormalities of embryogenesis, or complications of longstanding anatomic or biochemical abnormalities. The latter are not truly features of the syndrome, but quite commonly are substantial problems. For example, the hepatic duct deficit is a result of a defect in organogenesis, but the coagulopathy is commonly a complication of fat malabsorption or end-stage liver disease. Structural cardiac disease is caused by an embryopathy, but atheromatous lesions are complications of chronic severe cholestasis. The severe limitations in height seen in many patients may be a feature of the vertebral and skeletal development seen in AGS or a complication of malnutrition. The marked increase in long-bone fractures may result from an intrinsic abnormality of bone structure and development in AGS or be a complication of vitamin D and nutrient malabsorption.

This classification has several implications. Cholestasis should not be considered a "cardinal feature" of the disorder, and it probably adds little to the diagnostic algorithm. Cholestasis is merely a substantial complication of bile duct paucity seen in some patients at some time in development. Features that are caused by defects in embryogenesis are unlikely to be easily corrected with medical, surgical (except transplantation), or genetic interventions or to be prevented in the fetus or infant. Complications may respond to therapy, with substantial improvement in quality and quantity of life.

The large patient series reported by Alagille et al. [2] (n = 80), Deprettere et al. [15] (n = 27), Hoffenberg et al. [16] (n = 26), Emerick et al. [6] (n = 92), and Quiros-Tejeira et al. [17] (n = 43) include patients from different time periods, representing different understandings of the features and complications of the disorder and evolving therapeutic options. Referral bias is present in each study. The tertiary nature of an institution and the availability of liver and cardiac transplantation at those centers influence the apparent severity of the disorder in each of these studies. The reports are weighted with the severely affected index cases in families, and most reports either do not seek or deliberately exclude minimally affected relatives. Kamath et al. [25] studied the feature frequency and morbidity in mutation-positive relatives separately, thereby excluding the severely affected index cases. In mutation-positive relatives, the presence of significant cardiac and hepatic disease was less than in the proband cases. Thus overall, the clinical consequence of carrying a *JAG1* mutation is less severe than previously thought, and the disease certainly seems to have a better outcome. This point is important for genetic counseling.

Hepatic Features and Complications

The majority of symptomatic patients present in the first year of life. The hepatic manifestations typically vary from mild to severe cholestasis. Hepatitis is present in many infants but generally is less important than the cholestasis. Synthetic liver failure is extremely uncommon in the first year of life. Hepatomegaly is recognized in 93–100% of patients with AGS [2,6] and is common in infancy. Splenomegaly is unusual early in the course of the disease but eventually is found in up to 70% of patients [6]. Jaundice is present in the majority of symptomatic patients and typically presents as a conjugated hyperbilirubinemia in the neonatal period. In half of these infants, it is persistent, resolving only in later childhood. The severity of jaundice commonly is increased during intercurrent illnesses. The magnitude of the hyperbilirubinemia is typically less than the degrees of cholestasis and pruritus. The pruritus seen is among the most severe of any chronic liver disease. It rarely is present before 3–5 months of age but is seen in most children by the third year of life, even in some who are anicteric.

Multiple xanthomas are common sequelae of severe cholestasis. The timing for the formation of xanthomas relates to the severity of the cholestasis and correlates with a serum cholesterol level greater than 500 mg/dL. They typically form on the extensor surfaces of the fingers, the palmar creases, the nape of the neck, the ears, the popliteal fossa, the buttocks, and around the inguinal creases. These xanthomas increase in number over the first few years of life and may disappear subsequently as cholestasis improves.

The most striking laboratory abnormalities are in the measures of cholestasis and bile duct damage. Elevations of serum bilirubin up to 30 times normal and serum bile salt elevations of 100 times normal are not uncommon. Bile salt elevations are common, even if the bilirubin concentration is normal. Levels of markers of bile duct damage, including γ-glutamyltransferase and alkaline phosphatase, usually are elevated markedly. The amounts of other substances typically excreted in bile are increased in blood. Cholesterol levels may exceed 1000–2000 mg/dL. Serum and urine copper levels may be elevated. The aminotransferases typically are elevated three- to tenfold but may be normal in some patients with cholestasis. Hepatic synthetic function usually is well preserved. Serum albumin and ammonia levels are normal early in the course of the disease, and coagulopathy generally responds to vitamin K administration.

Of patients who present with liver disease in infancy, 10–50% eventually go on to develop intractable portal hypertension, cirrhosis, or synthetic liver failure. The reported incidence appears to be higher in series with long-term follow-up. The features that lead to synthetic dysfunction are unknown, but prolonged accumulation of toxins and metals in the liver may play a role. The peak level of bilirubin in infancy does not seem to be directly correlated with eventual liver failure [6].

Liver transplantation is eventually necessary in 21–31% of patients [6,16]. Hoffenberg et al. [16] estimated that 50% of patients diagnosed in infancy require transplantation by 19 years of age. Indications for transplantation include one or more problems including synthetic dysfunction, intractable portal hypertension, bone fractures, pruritus, xanthomata, and growth failure. The survival rate of patients with AGS undergoing liver transplantation has significantly improved in recent years with careful selection of transplant candidates and better management of concomitant cardiac disease. Recent studies include 1-year posttransplantation patient survival rates of 90% in 21 patients [26] and 92% in 37 patients [27]. These results show that patients with AGS are good candidates for liver transplantation.

Care must be undertaken in evaluating parents for consideration as living related liver donors [28] because 17–23% of all patients' parents have AGS [29]. Gurkan et al. [30] reported two instances in which apparently unaffected parents underwent donor operations that were unsuccessful because of a paucity of duct structures discovered intraoperatively. Evaluation of a potential living related donor should include a careful physical and biochemical evaluation, an ophthalmologic examination, and a biopsy or cholangiographic procedure. If the *JAG1* gene mutation has been identified in the child, the parent may be screened. If unsuspected bile duct paucity can thus be adequately excluded, living related transplantation remains a viable modality. Kasahara et al. [31] reported 20 patients with AGS who underwent successful living related transplantation, with 80% 5-year patient survival.

There have been many reports of hepatocellular carcinoma in patients with AGS [32–34], including one in a 4-year-old child [35]. These have occurred in the presence and the absence of cirrhosis. A nodular hamartoma resembling focal nodular hyperplasia was seen in one patient with end-stage cirrhosis [36]. Although there have been occasional reports of extrahepatic malignancies in AGS, the overall incidence does not seem to be increased dramatically.

Features of Hepatic Disease at Diagnosis in Infancy

The majority of infants with AGS are evaluated for conjugated hyperbilirubinemia in the first weeks or months of life. The differential diagnosis and general evaluation for conjugated hyperbilirubinemia are discussed in Chapter 9. AGS is most easily confused with extrahepatic disorders such as biliary atresia and metabolic disorders with elevated γ-glutamyltransferase. In these disorders, cholestasis may be the predominant biochemical and clinical feature. AGS occasionally is misdiagnosed as biliary atresia because of the overlap of biochemical, scintigraphic, and operative cholangiographic features. The pattern of histologic involvement of the ducts is significantly different, however, and biopsy must be a routine component of the evaluation. Serum bilirubin, bile acid, and γ-glutamyltransferase levels typically are elevated in each of these disorders. Ultrasound should identify choledochal cysts and cholelithiasis accurately, but both patients with biliary atresia and those with AGS may have small or apparently absent gallbladders. Excretion of nuclear tracer (DISIDA) into the duodenum eliminates biliary atresia from consideration, but nonexcretion of tracer is common in AGS. There was no excretion of scintiscan in 61% of 36 infants with AGS [6]. Excretion was evident only after 24-hour follow-up in another 25% of these 36 patients.

The initial noninvasive evaluation should be followed by a liver biopsy, particularly if the studies suggest noncommunication from the liver to the duodenum. In AGS, paucity is evident in only 60% of infants younger than 6 months but in 95% of older patients [6]. In biliary atresia, bile duct proliferation is the typical histologic lesion and paucity is extremely rare at diagnosis. Unfortunately, there may be a normal number of ducts early in the course of biliary atresia and also in some patients with AGS. In very young infants in whom the percutaneous liver biopsy is not diagnostic, it may be helpful to delay exploration for 1 or 2 weeks and repeat the biopsy (recognizing that the success of therapy for extrahepatic biliary atresia is correlated with surgery before 60 days of age). Giant cell hepatitis has been seen in both disorders.

A cholangiogram is indicated if there is scintigraphic and histologic evidence to support a diagnosis of biliary atresia. Various approaches to cholangiography have been attempted, with varying success. Endoscopic retrograde cholangiography has been performed successfully in infants. Magnetic resonance cholangiography and percutaneous cholangiography are technically more difficult in this setting and age group, although percutaneous gallbladder cholangiography has been successful. An operative cholangiogram provides the most reliable information about the extrahepatic and intrahepatic biliary tree and affords the opportunity to further sample hepatic tissue. Cholangiography of any type, however, is likely to be misleading if interpreted without attention to history, examination, biochemistry, and radiologic evaluation. The extra- and intrahepatic ducts are extremely small in patients with AGS, and the cholangiogram commonly does not demonstrate communication proximally. In 37% of 19 cholangiograms in infants with AGS, there was no opacification of the proximal extrahepatic ducts, and in another 37%, the proximal extrahepatic tree was abnormally small [6]. The intrahepatic ducts were normal in only 10% of 19 infants with AGS, small or hypoplastic in 16%, and not visualized in 74%. Therefore, cholangiography, the final diagnostic study attempting to differentiate AGS from biliary atresia, appears to be the least accurate. As a result, almost every large series includes AGS patients who were diagnosed with biliary atresia and treated with a Kasai portoenterostomy. Although it has been reported that AGS and biliary atresia can occur together, the majority of these patients examined histologically demonstrate extremely hypoplastic but patent extrahepatic biliary ducts.

Hepatoportoenterostomy is inappropriate in AGS and may increase the amount of injury. Patients with AGS who undergo the Kasai procedure seem to do poorly, with increased complications and rate of transplantation. Some problems, such as cholangitis, clearly are related to portoenterostomy [16]. This increased morbidity in childhood and the high rate of transplantation, however, cannot be attributed solely to the surgery itself; it appears likely that portoenterostomy is performed more commonly in patients who are severely cholestatic. Approximately 60% of patients with AGS who undergo a portoenterostomy eventually require transplantation [6,16].

Cardiac Features and Complications

The early reports by Watson and Miller [3] and Greenwood et al. [37] focus on the cardiac manifestations associated with familial liver disease. Watson and Miller [3] recognized the association of cholestatic liver disease, butterfly vertebrae, and particular facies in patients with familial dominant pulmonary arterial stenosis in infancy. In a comprehensive evaluation of 200 AGS subjects, 94% had some cardiac involvement [38]. Pulmonary artery anomalies are the most common abnormality identified and may occur in isolation or in combination with structural intracardiac disease [6,38,39]. Intracardiac lesions were present in 24% of 92 patients with AGS [6]. The most common congenital defect is tetralogy of Fallot (TOF), which occurs in 7–12% [1,6,38,39]. It appears that severe forms of TOF (especially TOF with pulmonary atresia) occur with greater frequency in the AGS population than in the general population of individuals with TOF [6,38]. Approximately 40% of patients with AGS demonstrating TOF have pulmonary atresia. Other cardiovascular lesions include truncus arteriosus, ventricular septal defect complex, atrial septal defect, ventricular septal defect, valvular pulmonic stenosis, and isolated pulmonic stenosis [6,38] (Figure 15.4). Extracardiac vascular lesions in AGS include coarctation of the aorta and patent ductus arteriosus with or without PPS (peripheral pulmonic stenosis).

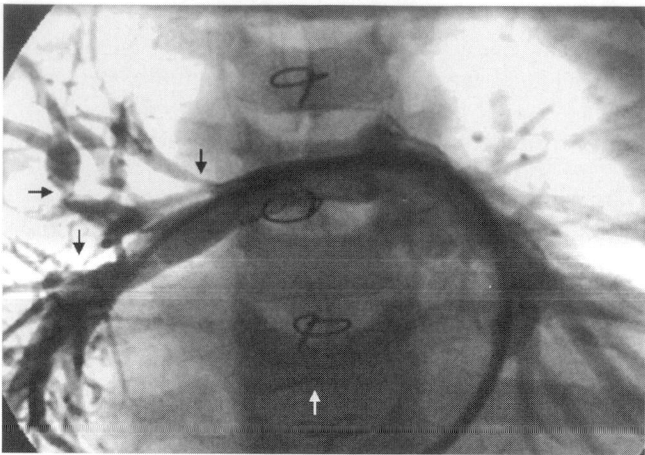

Figure 15.4. Right pulmonary arteriogram demonstrating multiple stenoses (*black arrows*) in a patient with prior surgery for tetralogy of Fallot, peripheral pulmonic stenoses, a butterfly vertebrae (*white arrow*), and a deletion of chromosome 20p12.

Cardiac surgery was performed in infancy in 11% of 92 infants with AGS [6]. The mortality rates were 33% for those with TOF and 75% for those with TOF with pulmonary atresia. The survival of patients with AGS with these lesions is markedly lower than for patients without AGS. This may be a result, in part, of the common presence of significant stenoses in the distal pulmonary artery, or of other systemic manifestations of the syndrome (Figure 15.5).

The exact incidence of severe neonatal cardiac disease is probably underestimated in all series of patients with AGS. It is not uncommon to diagnose AGS in an infant who has a sibling with severe congenital heart disease. With the application of molecular techniques to diagnostic cardiology, Krantz et al. [40] screened cell lines from patients with TOF unassociated with any recognized syndromic features and identified mutations in *JAG1* in 7%. Mutations in *JAG1* also have been identified in patients with multigenerational PPS in the absence of apparent hepatic disease [40]. Loomes et al. [41] demonstrated that the expression of *Jag1* in the mammalian fetal heart correlates with the spectrum of cardiovascular disease seen in AGS. Patients with the 22q deletion syndrome (velocardiofacial syndrome) may have severe intracardiac disease including TOF in association with particular facies, butterfly vertebra, and posterior embryotoxon [24]. Bile duct paucity is not a feature of this disorder. The common embryologic abnormality accounting for this apparent overlap is not yet known, though it has been suggested that members of the Notch signaling pathway may be genetic modifiers of the phenotype in 22q deletion syndrome. Patients with features not typical of AGS should undergo fluorescence in situ hybridization analysis for 22q deletion and a formal genetic evaluation.

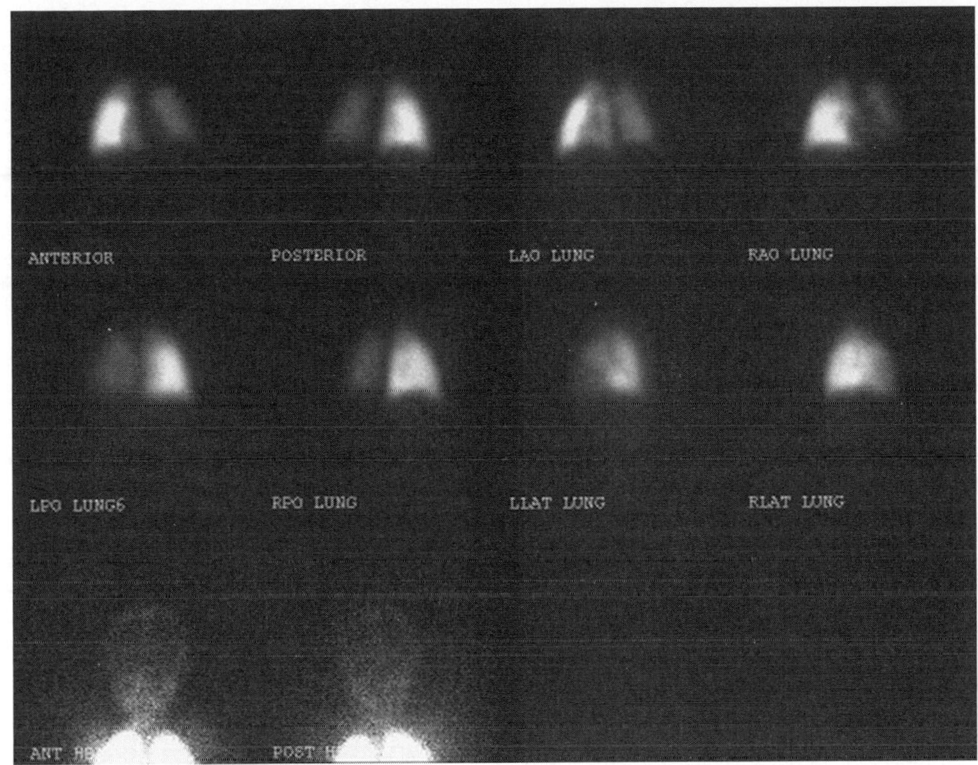

Figure 15.5. Lung perfusion scan from a patient with Alagille syndrome demonstrating differential blood flow within the pulmonary tree. The right lung receives more than 86% of pulmonary blood flow secondary to stenosis of the left pulmonary artery.

Cardiac disease accounts for nearly all the early deaths in AGS. Patients with intracardiac disease have approximately a 40% rate of survival to 6 years of life, compared with a 95% survival rate in patients with AGS without intracardiac lesions [6]. Cardiovascular disease contributes significantly to the injury caused by the disorder and has been implicated in the increased posttransplantation mortality rate seen in some series.

Nonsurgical invasive techniques have been used successfully for patients with AGS, including valvuloplasty, balloon dilatation, and stent implantation [42,43]. Heart–lung transplantation has been performed in combination with liver transplantation in a child with AGS [43a].

Renal Features and Complications

Renal disease is an important feature of AGS. Studies suggest that renal abnormalities occur in 40–50% of patients with AGS [6,17]. A wide variety of structural, functional, and acquired renal disorders have been identified, though they have yet to be characterized. Solitary kidney, ectopic kidney, bifid pelvis, and reduplicated ureter may be identified by ultrasound, tomography, or pyelography. Small kidneys [44,45] and unilateral and bilateral multicystic and dysplastic kidneys [6,46,47], with and without renal failure, have been reported in patients with AGS (Figure 15.6). Renal artery stenosis is a cause of systemic hypertension in patients with AGS [17,48]. Renal tubular acidosis in infancy [6], neonatal renal insufficiency [6], and fatal juvenile nephronophthisis [49] have been reported. In some patients, a characteristic "lipidosis" involves the glomeruli most prominently and apparently reflects prolonged elevations of serum lipid and cholesterol levels [47,50,51]. Tubulointerstitial nephropathy with tubular atrophy and interstitial fibrosis has been reported in patients with AGS [52,53]. Adult-onset renal insufficiency and failure may occur, requiring renal transplantation [17,54].

Renal disease should be considered one of the "major" criteria for the diagnosis of AGS. In fact, recent data suggest that renal disease is a more prominent phenotype in a subset of AGS patients. Individuals carrying a mutation in *Notch2* appear to have a higher prevalence of renal disease compared with those carrying *JAG1* mutations [10]. Functional and structural evaluation of the kidneys should be undertaken in all patients. The role of renal tubular acidosis in early growth failure is unclear, but administration of bicarbonate is necessary in some individuals. Renal function should be reassessed during the evaluation for hepatic transplantation.

Ocular Features and Complications

A large and varied number of ocular abnormalities involving the cornea, iris, retina, and optic disk have been described in patients with AGS. A few of the abnormalities are secondary to

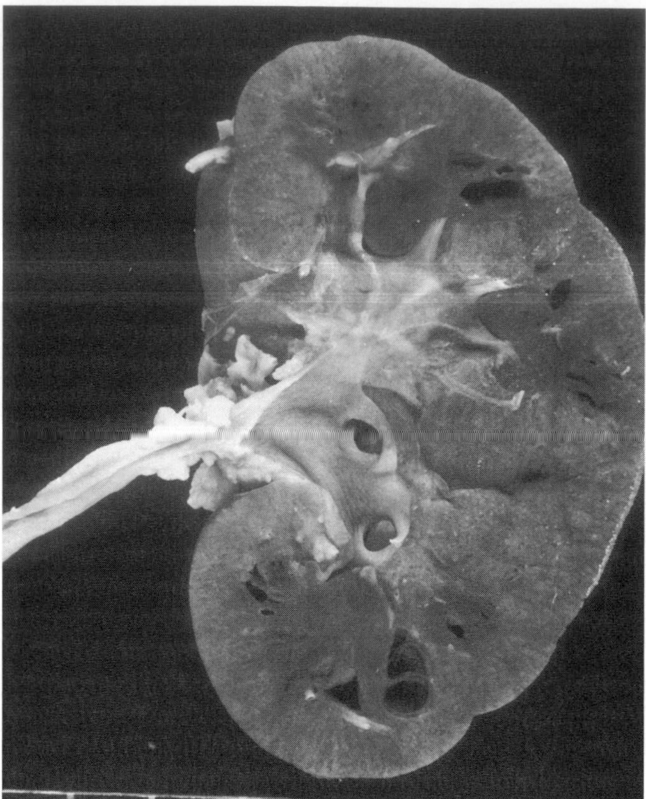

Figure 15.6. Diffuse renal cystic dysplasia in a patient with paucity of bile ducts. (Courtesy of Pierre A. Russo, M.D.)

chronic vitamin deficiencies. Of the primary ocular abnormal ities, posterior embryotoxon is the most important diagnostically. Posterior embryotoxon is a prominent, centrally positioned Schwalbe's ring (or line) at the point at which the corneal endothelium and the uveal trabecular meshwork join (Figure 15.7). Posterior embryotoxon occurs in 56–95% of patients with AGS [2,6,15,16,55]; it occurs in 8–15% of normal eyes. Posterior

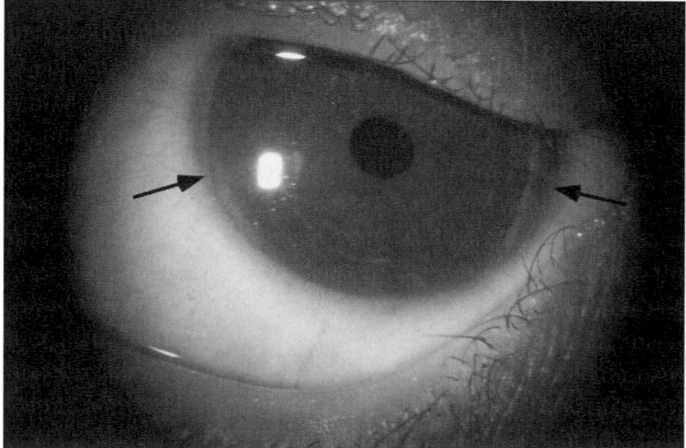

Figure 15.7. Posterior embryotoxon and prominent Schwalbe's line (*arrows*). For color reproduction, see Color Plate 15.7.

embryotoxon also is present in 69% of patients with 22q deletion syndrome [24] and is seen in other multisystem disorders as well. Posterior embryotoxon may be part of an "anterior chamber malformation syndrome" [56]. The malformations fall into three groups of peripheral and central abnormalities. Many of these abnormalities have been reported in patients with AGS. The Axenfeld anomaly, seen in 13% of patients with AGS, is a prominent Schwalbe's ring with attached iris strands. Approximately 50% of normal patients with this anomaly develop glaucoma, which has been reported in patients with AGS [57].The Rieger anomaly (primary mesodermal dysgenesis) is a prominent Schwalbe's ring with attached iris strands and hypoplastic anterior iris stroma. This malformation also has been demonstrated in patients with AGS [58]. Nischal et al. [59] found ultrasound evidence of optic disk drusen in at least one eye in 95% and bilateral disk drusen in 80% of patients with AGS but in none of the liver patients without AGS whom they studied. This is markedly higher than the incidence in the normal population (0.3–2%), suggesting that this newer ophthalmologic sign may be an extremely useful diagnostic tool [59]. A peculiar mosaic pattern of iris stromal hypoplasia is present in many patients [60]. In addition, microcornea, keratoconus, congenital macular dystrophy, shallow anterior chambers, exotropia, ectopic pupil, band keratopathy, cataracts, strabismus, iris hypoplasia, choroidal folds, and anomalous optic disks have been reported [55,61,62]. Other ocular findings, including retinal pigmentary changes, are identified in many patients with cholestasis but are not specific for the syndrome. In a large series of patients with AGS studied systematically, Hingorani et al. [55] identified posterior embryotoxon in 95% of 22 patients, iris abnormalities in 45%, diffuse fundic hypopigmentation in 57%, speckling of the retinal pigment epithelium in 33%, and optic disk abnormalities in 76%. The frequency of these findings, higher than in other reported series, suggests that a formal ophthalmologic examination can provide one of the most crucial clues to the diagnosis of AGS in infancy. Furthermore, these investigators identified at least one of these abnormalities in one parent in 36% of families, a frequency quite similar to the identification of *JAG1* mutations in parents reported by Krantz et al. [29].

Facial Characteristics

Characteristic facial features are described in the original reports of syndromic paucity. These include a prominent forehead, deep-set eyes with moderate hypertelorism, a pointed chin, and a saddle or straight nose with a bulbous tip. The combination of these features gives the face a triangular appearance (Figure 15.8). The facies may be present early in infancy but in general becomes more dramatic with increasing age. Other facial characteristics include a flat appearance of the face in profile and prominent ears. The usefulness of the facies as a major diagnostic criterion has been challenged because of subjectivity and interobserver differences. Kamath et al. [63] presented photographs of patients with AGS and patients with other

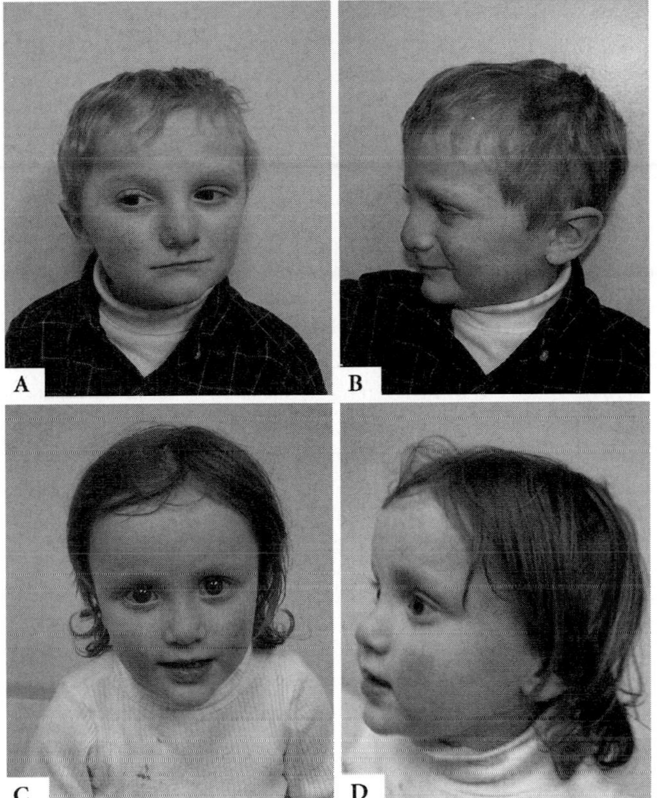

Figure 15.8. Characteristic facies of children with Alagille syndrome. (Courtesy of Ian D. Krantz, M.D.)

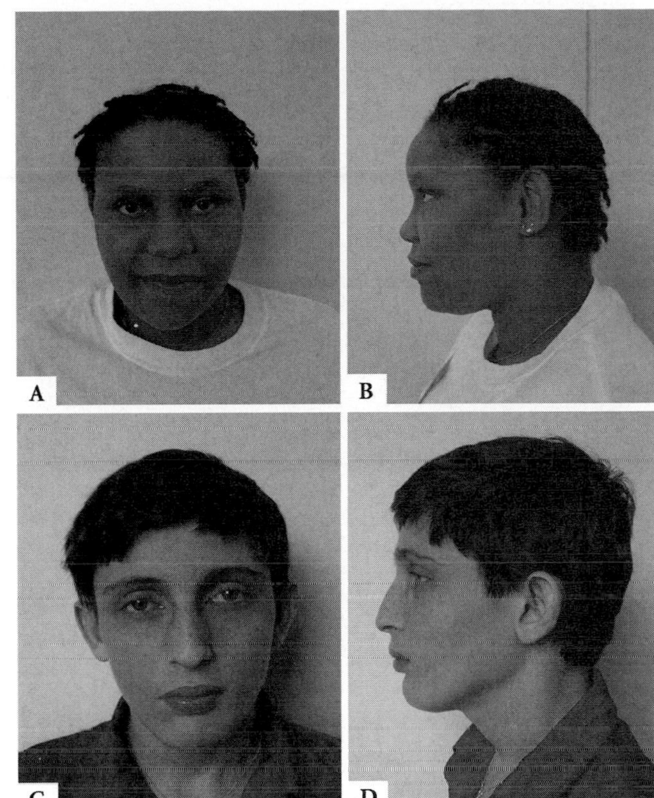

Figure 15.9. Characteristic facies of adults with Alagille syndrome. (Courtesy of Ian D. Krantz, M.D.)

known early-onset liver diseases to dysmorphologists, who were able to correctly identify patients with *JAG1* mutations 79% of the time. The facies in adults were least well identified in this study. They also reported that the facies change with age. The characteristic facies of an adult do not resemble childhood facies, but they do have striking similarities to other adults with AGS or the *JAG1* gene defects [63] (Figure 15.9). In adults, the forehead is much less prominent and the protruding chin is more noticeable. The correct identification of these adults, who commonly have minimal signs and symptoms of AGS, would help physicians in the evaluation of adults with apparently idiopathic cardiac, hepatic, or renal disease.

It has been suggested that the characteristic facies are results of the effects of chronic cholestasis, but they are not seen in other diseases in infancy with severe cholestasis; furthermore, the characteristic facies may be seen in asymptomatic siblings and parents. It is likely that the facial bone formation is directly affected by mutations in *JAG1*, as in situ studies in the mouse show expression of *Jag1* in the facial structures [63]. The terms *cholestatic*, *syndromic*, and *peculiar* facies have decreased in usage because the terms *characteristic* and *particular* facies seem more appropriate.

Other facial and head abnormalities include large ears, recurrent sinusitis, recurrent otitis [17], and a high-pitched voice.

Musculoskeletal Features and Complications

Vertebral abnormalities are described in the initial reports of this syndrome. The most characteristic finding is the sagittal cleft or butterfly vertebrae, which is found in 33–87% of patients with AGS [1,6,15–17] (Figures 15.10 and 15.11). This relatively uncommon anomaly may occur in normal individuals but is seen in other multisystem abnormalities, such as 22q deletion syndrome (in 19%) [24], VATER (vertebral defects, anal atresia, tracheoesophageal fistula, radial and renal defect) syndrome, Crouzon syndrome, MURCS association (Mullerian hypoplasia–aplasia, renal agenesis, cervicothoracic somite dysplasia), Kabuki syndrome, and in Jarcho–Levin spondylocostal dysostosis. The affected vertebral bodies are split sagittally into paired hemivertebrae because of a failure of the fusion of the anterior arches of the vertebrae. Generally, these are asymptomatic and of no structural significance. The mildly affected vertebrae have a central lucency. A fully affected vertebra has a pair of separate triangular hemivertebrae whose apices face each other like the wings of a butterfly. Though these abnormalities are present from birth, they often are unrecognized at the time of evaluation for neonatal hepatitis, only to be identified on spinal radiographs taken later. Other associated skeletal abnormalities include an abnormal narrowing of the adjusted interpedicular space in the lumbar spine in half of the patients [2,64], a pointed anterior process of C1, spina bifida occulta

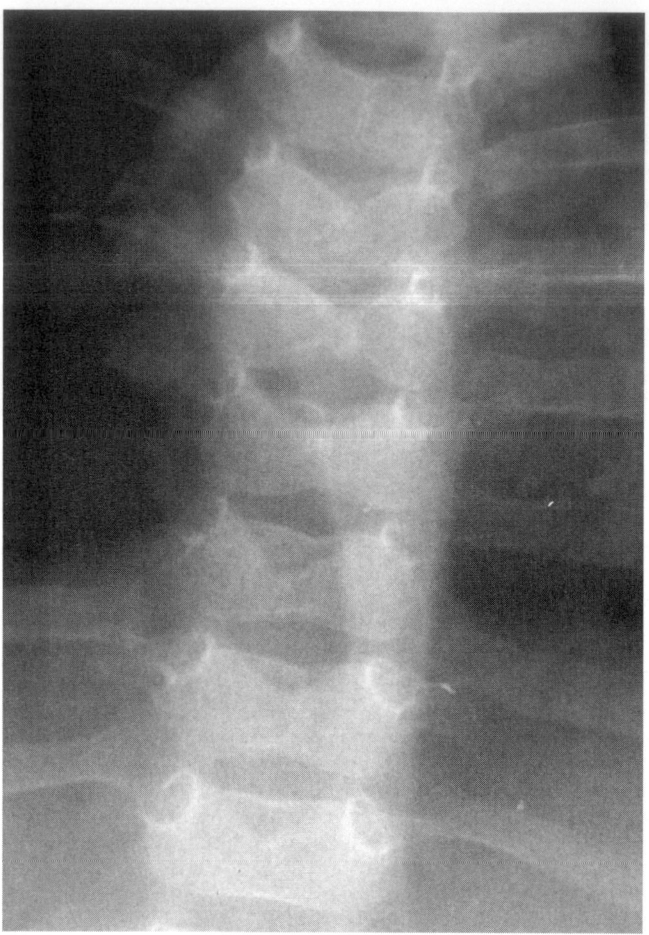

Figure 15.10. Butterfly vertebrae at T5 and T6, with vertebral anomalies at T4, T7, T8, and T9, in an infant with Alagille syndrome.

[65], fusion of the adjacent vertebrae, hemivertebrae [37], the absence of the 12th rib [66], and the presence of a bony connection between ribs [3]. The fingers may seem short, with broad thumbs [64]. Digital clubbing may be evident [15].

Severe metabolic bone disease with osteoporosis and pathologic fractures is common in patients with AGS. Recurrent fractures, particularly of the femur, have been cited as a major indication for hepatic transplantation [16] (Figure 15.12). A number of factors may contribute to osteopenia and fractures, including severe chronic malnutrition, vitamin D and vitamin K deficiency, chronic hepatic and renal disease, magnesium deficiency [67], and pancreatic insufficiency. Aggressive supplementation of calories, vitamin D, and vitamin K is required. Heubi et al. [67] identified magnesium deficiency in eight of eight cholestatic patients with AGS who had normal hepatic synthetic function, despite normal serum magnesium levels. They suggested that oral magnesium supplementation be considered for all cholestatic patients. It is not known whether the cortical or trabecular structure of the long bones is abnormal in patients with AGS. The incidence of fractures seems to be significantly higher in these patients than in those with other liver diseases with onset in infancy. Another inherited defect in the Notch signaling pathway has been identified to cause Jarcho–Levin syndrome, or recessive spondylocostal dysostosis. This disorder is caused by homozygous abnormalities in another Notch ligand, delta-like 3 [68]. The identification of Notch signaling abnormalities in a dysostosis syndrome strongly suggests that intrinsic bone abnormalities eventually will be identified in AGS.

Vascular System Involvement and Complications

Vascular anomalies have been noted in AGS from some of the earliest descriptions of this syndrome [2,3]. Indeed, even the alternative name for the condition, arteriohepatic dysplasia, recognizes the vascular contribution. Pulmonary artery involvement is a hallmark feature of the condition and one of the most common manifestations [6]. However, the literature documents multiple case reports of intracranial vessel abnormalities and other vascular anomalies in AGS.

Unexplained intracranial bleeding is a recognized complication and cause of mortality in AGS. Intracranial bleeds occur in approximately 15% of patients, and in 30–50% of these events, the hemorrhage is fatal [6,16]. There does not seem to be any pattern to the location and/or severity of the intracranial bleeding, which ranges from massive fatal events to asymptomatic cerebral infarcts. Epidural, subdural, subarachnoid, and intraparenchymal bleeding have been reported. The majority of this bleeding has occurred in the absence of significant coagulopathy. Head trauma, typically of a minor degree, has been associated with the bleeding in a number of patients. The majority of cases of bleeding are spontaneous, however, with no clear risk factors. Lykavieris et al. [69] studied a cohort of 174 individuals with AGS and identified 38 patients (22%) who had 49 bleeding episodes. All these hemorrhages occurred in the absence of liver failure, with normal median platelet counts and prothrombin times, suggesting that AGS patients may be at particular risk for bleeding.

Underlying vessel abnormalities in the central nervous system that could explain the occurrence of bleeding and stroke in AGS have been described in some of these patients [16,70]. Aneurysms of the basilar and middle cerebral arteries and various internal carotid artery anomalies have been described. Moyamoya disease (progressive intracranial arterial occlusive disease) also has been previously described in several children with AGS [71–74] (Figure 15.13). Emerick et al. [75] prospectively studied 26 patients with AGS using magnetic resonance imaging (MRI) with angiography of the head. Cerebrovascular abnormalities were detected in 10 of 26 patients (38%). One hundred percent of symptomatic patients had detected abnormalities, and 23% of screened, asymptomatic patients had detected anomalies. These results suggest that MRI with angiography is useful in detecting these lesions and may have a valuable role in screening for treatable lesions such as aneurysms (Figure 15.14). The current recommendation is for all asymptomatic AGS patients to have a screening MRI/magnetic resonance angiography as a baseline and for physicians to have a low threshold for reimaging AGS patients in the event of any symptoms, head trauma, or suspicious neurologic signs.

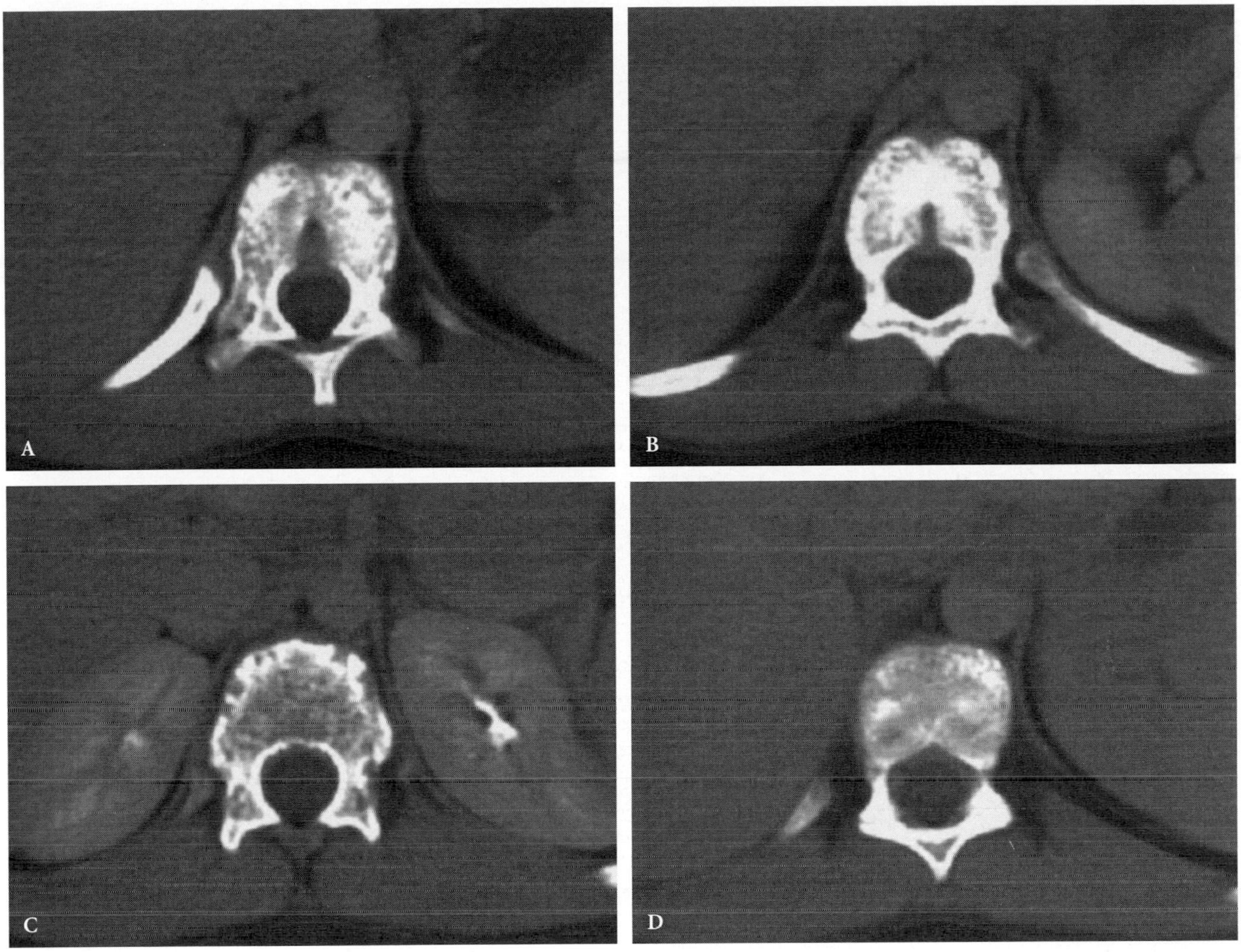

Figure 15.11. Vertebral anomalies in Alagille syndrome. (**A**) Computed tomographic (CT) scan of a butterfly vertebral body. (**B**) CT scan image of a vertebral body with a posterior sagittal cleft. (**C**) CT scan image of a vertebral body with marked cortical irregularity. (**D**) CT scan image of a nearly normal vertebral body.

Systemic vascular abnormalities have also been well documented in AGS. Aortic aneurysms and coarctations, renal artery, celiac artery, superior mesenteric artery, and subclavian artery anomalies have all been described [44,48,72,76,77]. Kamath et al. [72] evaluated a large cohort of AGS patients and identified 9% (25 of 268) with noncardiac vascular anomalies or events. In addition, vascular accidents accounted for 34% of the mortality in this cohort. These findings suggest that vascular abnormalities have been underrecognized as a potentially devastating complication of AGS.

This body of clinical evidence demonstrating arterial involvement in AGS suggests that the Notch signaling pathway plays an important role in vascular development. Notch ligands and receptors are expressed in vascular endothelium or

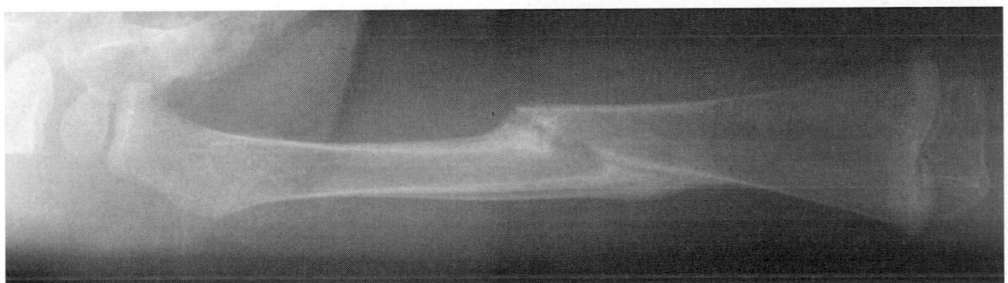

Figure 15.12. Healing spontaneous fracture of the right femur. One of multiple femoral fractures in a 4-year-old with Alagille syndrome.

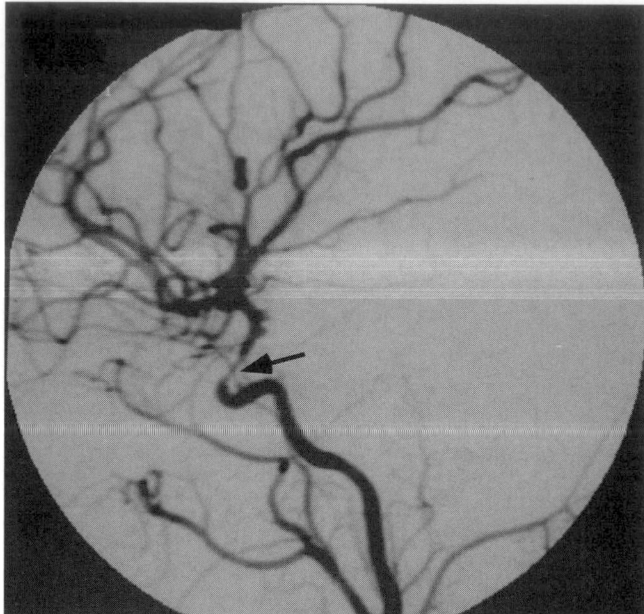

Figure 15.13. Moyamoya in Alagille syndrome. Cerebral angiogram demonstrating multiple areas of vascular stenoses.

supporting cells [78–80], and in particular, studies in mouse embryos show strong expression of *Jag1* in all major arteries [81]. Further evidence of the role of *JAG1* and Notch in vascular development is provided by the phenotype of targeted Notch pathway mutants. Mice homozygous for a mutation in *Jag1* die from hemorrhage during early embryogenesis because of defects in angiogenic vascular remodeling in the yolk sac and embryo [82]. Both *Notch1* mutant and *Notch1/Notch4* double-mutant mouse embryos also display severe defects in angiogenic vascular remodeling [83]. In fact, even activated expression of Notch4 protein leads to similar abnormal vessel structure and patterning and embryonic lethality, demonstrating that appropriate levels and regulation of Notch signaling are critical for proper vascular development [84]. A human model also exists to support a role for the Notch pathway in vascular homeostasis. In adults, CADASIL (cerebral autosomal dominant arteriopathy with subcortical infarcts and leukoencephalopathy), a

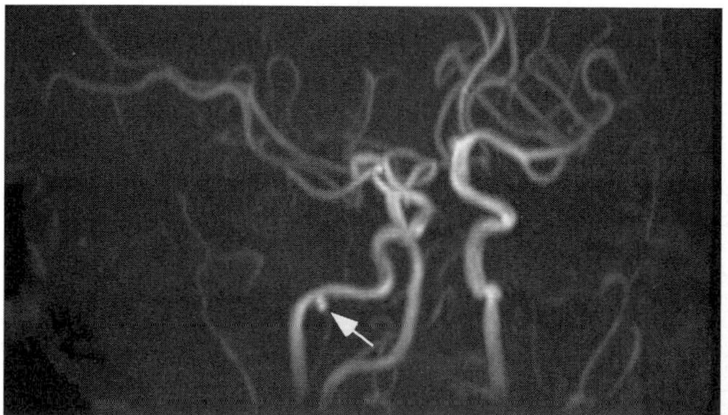

Figure 15.14. Aneurysm of the external carotid artery in a 17-year-old with Alagille syndrome found by routine screening.

degenerative disorder characterized by late-onset strokes and dementia, is caused by mutations in the Notch3 receptor that result in alterations of vascular smooth muscle cells [85].

Neurologic Features and Complications

The initial reports of AGS suggested that significant mental retardation is a prominent feature [2]. Undoubtedly, many of these patients suffered from severe nutritional deficits. Mental retardation currently is uncommon, in part because of earlier diagnosis and more aggressive nutritional therapy. Although only 2% of patients in one series had mental retardation, gross motor delays occurred in 16% [10]. Studies emphasize the impact of chronic liver disease on brain development, regardless of cause [61], and focus on the role of vitamin E supplementation and aggressive nutritional management in improving outcome [62]. Abnormal visual, auditory, and somatosensory evoked potentials have been noted in patients with AGS. Visual evoked potentials return to normal following resolution of the cholestasis with transplantation. Dystonia and tremor associated with elevated whole blood manganese levels were reported in a patient with end-stage liver disease and abnormalities in the globus pallidus on MRI [63]. The symptoms and the imaging findings resolved following transplantation.

Growth Disorders

Severe growth retardation is seen in 50–87% of patients [2,6,16,17]. It is particularly evident in the first 4 years of life. Malnutrition resulting from malabsorption is a major factor in this failure to thrive, and chronic wasting as documented by height, weight, and anthropometry is severe in patients with AGS [86–88]. Rovner et al. [86] assessed growth failure in 26 prepubertal children with AGS and found that more than half the children were less than fifth percentile for weight and height, 96% had steatorrhea, and 20% had a diet poor in calories, fat, and other nutrients. There appear to be limitations to linear growth even if protein-calorie malnutrition is not evident. Olsen et al. [89] evaluated bone status in prepubertal children with AGS and identified significant deficits in bone size and bone mass that were related to fat absorption but not dietary intake. These deficits may result, in part, from long-bone and spine abnormalities associated with AGS, although they do not appear to be directly correlated with butterfly vertebrae. Endocrine abnormalities do not appear to be common in patients with AGS, although deficiencies in thyroid function have been recognized. Patients with growth failure appear to be insensitive to exogenous growth hormone [90]. Many adults appear to have short stature, although a systematic study of adult height in AGS has not been completed.

Pancreatic Features and Complications

The profound steatorrhea seen in patients with AGS initially was attributed solely to decreased intraluminal bile acid concentrations, resulting in diminished micellarization of fats.

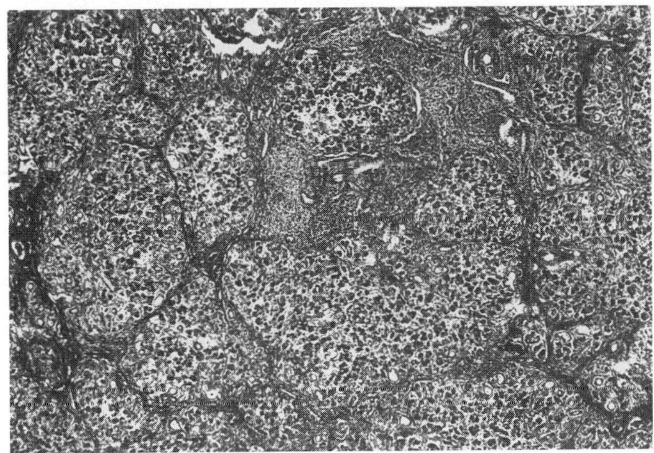

Figure 15.15. Autopsy specimen from a patient with Alagille syndrome. The pancreatic parenchyma is subdivided into nodules by extensive and widespread fibrosis with pockets of chronic inflammation. (Masson trichrome staining, 40× magnification.)

Pancreatic function was assessed by Chong et al. [91] in 13 patients with growth failure and paucity of the interlobular bile ducts. The duodenal aspirate volume, bicarbonate concentration and output, and lipase concentrations were lower in patients with paucity and diarrhea compared with those with paucity without diarrhea or with controls. Other enzyme concentrations and pH were not different. Three children treated with pancreatic enzyme supplementation had reductions in stool frequency, increased appetite, and increased rates of weight gain. Insulin dependent diabetes also has been seen in patients with AGS. At postmortem evaluation, pancreatic fibrosis and ductular abnormalities have been noted incidentally (Figure. 15.15). It is not clear whether pancreatic abnormalities are secondary to chronic cholestasis, altered bile flow or composition, or other toxic factors. Studies have not been undertaken in patients with AGS without cholestasis. It is likely, however, that Jagged1 and Notch signaling play a role in the development and maintenance of pancreatic secretion and duct formation, analogous to their role in hepatic duct formation. There are a number of hepatopancreaticorenal developmental disorders, which suggests common embryologic pathways. The role of pancreatic insufficiency in growth failure, malnutrition, and osteodystrophy has yet to be fully characterized. Clinically, the identification of pancreatic insufficiency is important because therapy with enzyme supplementation is available, with a likely improvement in at least some of these abnormalities.

Other Abnormalities Associated with Alagille Syndrome

Other abnormalities have been associated with AGS, including tracheal and bronchial stenosis, jejunal atresia and stenosis, ileal atresia, malrotation, and microcolon. Otitis media and chronic sinusitis or poor sinus development and macrocephaly have been reported. Hypothyroidism and insulin-dependent diabetes have been seen in patients with AGS. Urethral strictures and agenesis of a Fallopian tube have been noted. One patient had an expanding mandibular cyst and another, a malignant bone tumor. Occasional other nonhepatic tumors also have been noted.

Morbidity and Mortality Rates and Outcome

The mortality rate of AGS is highly variable. Cardiac, hepatic, and vascular systemic disease account for the majority of deaths. The presence of complex intracardiac disease at diagnosis is the only predictor of an excessive early mortality rate, and cardiac disease accounts for nearly all deaths in early childhood. Hepatic complications account for most later deaths, although the recent series demonstrate a significant number of deaths from intracranial bleeding. Most large reports demonstrate a significant overall mortality rate in AGS. Quiros-Tejeira et al. [17] reported a 72% survival rate in 43 patients at a mean follow-up of 8.9 years in a population in which 47% received hepatic transplantation. Hoffenberg et al. [16] estimated the rate of survival to age 19 without transplantation to be approximately 50% in 26 patients, but with transplantation (which in this series had a 100% survival rate), the 20-year survival rate was estimated at 87%. Emerick et al. [6] estimated the 20-year survival rate in 92 patients to be 75% overall, 80% for those not requiring hepatic transplantation and 60% for those requiring transplantation. For patients with structural intracardiac disease, however, the survival rate was only 40% at 7 years.

THERAPY

The therapy for cholestasis and its associated abnormalities is discussed in detail in Chapter 10. Patients with AGS present significant management challenges. Cholestasis commonly is profound. Bile flow may be stimulated with the choleretic ursodeoxycholic acid, but in many patients, the pruritus continues unabated. Care should be taken to keep the skin hydrated with emollients, and fingernails should be trimmed to prevent further damage. Therapy with antihistamines may provide some relief, but many patients require additional therapy with agents such as rifampin or naltrexone [92]. Biliary diversion [93–96] has been successful in a number of patients. Emerick et al. [96] studied nine AGS patients with severe mutilating pruritus who underwent partial external biliary diversion. Mean pruritus scores were significantly lower 1 year after the procedure, and eight of the nine had only mild scratching when not distracted. Three of the nine also had complete resolution of extensive xanthomas. Thus biliary diversion may be offered as a viable therapy before transplantation, which was previously the only option for intractable pruritus.

Malnutrition and growth failure should be treated with aggressive nutritional therapy. The optimal percentage and distribution of fat calories have not been determined systematically. There is significant malabsorption of long-chain fat; therefore, formulas supplemented with medium-chain triglycerides have some nutritional advantage. Essential fatty acid deficiency in patients with AGS has been reported, however, with acral lesions resembling porphyria that responded to parenteral supplementation of essential fatty acids [97]. The increased caloric needs of AGS patients result from malabsorption of fats and fat-soluble vitamins but do not appear to be related to markedly increased basal metabolism [98]. Carbohydrates should be absorbed normally, and supplementation may improve overall caloric deficit. Many patients are unable to eat enough to provide the substantial quantities of energy required for growth and development, and nasogastric or gastrostomy tube feedings can provide necessary supplementation and aid greatly in administration of medication.

Fat-soluble vitamin deficiency is present to a variable degree in most patients with significant AGS. Oral or parenteral supplementation is necessary for prevention of vitamin deficiencies and their sequelae. Multivitamin preparations may not provide the correct ratio of fat-soluble vitamins; vitamins are best administered as individual supplements tailored to the specific needs of the patient. Failure to correct vitamin deficiencies may have substantial sequelae, and frequent laboratory evaluation is necessary, particularly in the first years of life.

GENETICS

Alagille syndrome is inherited in an autosomal dominant manner, with highly variable expressivity [1–3]. AGS is a genetically heterogeneous disorder and may be caused by either mutation in *JAG1* (seen in 94% of clinically diagnosed probands) [8,9,99] or *Notch2* (seen in 0.8%) [10]. Jagged1 is a cell surface protein that serves as a ligand for the four Notch receptors (Notch1, 2, 3, and 4), and together these proteins begin the cascade of events that turn on the Notch signaling pathway. The Notch signaling pathway is involved in the determination of cell fate and as such plays a crucial role in normal development.

Gene Identification and Mutation Analysis

Alagille syndrome was recognized to have an autosomal dominant mode of inheritance in the first reports by Alagille et al. [1] and Watson and Miller [3]. The site of the gene responsible for AGS was first suggested more than ten years later by the identification of visible gene deletions and translocations on the short arm of chromosome 20 [100–103]. Based on the clues provided by the cytogenetics, two groups identified mutations in *JAG1* as the cause of AGS in 1997 [7,8]. Jagged1 is a single-pass transmembrane protein with an extracellular and an intracellular domain. The extracellular domain contains a region conserved among all Notch ligands called the DSL region (for ligands Delta and Serrate from *Drosophila* and Lag-2 from *Caenorhabditis elegans*), 16 epidermal growth factor (EGF)-like repeats, and a cysteine-rich region. There is a transmembrane domain and a small intracellular region. The genomic sequence is composed of 26 exons, and the standard strategy to screen for *JAG1* mutations is to analyze the coding regions of each of the exons in addition to about 20 intronic bases surrounding each exon to identify potential splice site mutations. To date, more than 430 *JAG1* mutations have been identified in patients with AGS. The frequency of mutations has been around 60–70% in most studies [4,29,104–112]. However, recently a cohort of patients was exhaustively studied with sequencing of the genomic coding region and cDNA, and the mutation rate was found to be 94% [9]. The frequency of sporadic mutations (i.e., new in the proband) is approximately 56–70%. Of affected parents with identified mutations, half were male and half were female.

The *JAG1* mutations identified in patients with AGS have been found distributed across the entire coding region, with no real hotspots [111]. The majority of the mutations are predicted to result in premature termination of the protein in the extracellular domain. Approximately 50% of AGS patients have protein-truncating (frameshift or nonsense) mutations [4,9,111]. Approximately 7% have gene deletions, and 9% have splice site mutations. Missense mutations are identified in 9%. Haploinsufficiency, a decrease in the amount of the normal protein, is hypothesized to be the mechanism causing AGS. However, there is evidence to support the role of other potential mechanisms, such as the dominant negative effect of mutant transcripts [5,113].

The Notch2 protein is also a single-pass transmembrane protein. The *Notch2* gene is made up of 34 exons occupying 158,099 base pairs (bp) of genomic DNA, which codes for an 11,433-bp message. Screening of this gene for mutations in AGS patients has been accomplished by sequencing of the genomic DNA. In a recent study, we sequenced the *Notch2* gene of 11 AGS patients who did not have a mutation in *JAG1* and identified mutations in 2 of these patients [10].

Notch Signaling Pathway

The Notch signaling pathway is involved in regulation of cell fate determination, and it functions in many different cell types throughout development to regulate cell fate decisions [114]. The name *Notch* derives from the characteristic notched wing found in flies carrying only one functioning copy of the gene. Homozygous mutations in *Notch* are lethal, and affected flies show hypertrophy of the nervous system, indicating the inability for appropriate cells to adopt an alternative cell fate. Notch signaling is initiated by contact between a cell surface ligand on one cell and a Notch receptor on an adjacent cell. The Notch receptors appear on the cell surface as two associated peptides, one extracellular and the other consisting of the transmembrane segment and intracellular domain. On stimulation of the receptor by a ligand (e.g., Jagged1), the intracellular domain translocates into the nucleus, where it mediates downstream effects in conjunction with intracellular regulatory proteins [115]. The molecular outcome of the initiation of Notch signaling is the transcription of Notch-sensitive genes, which then act to regulate cellular differentiation.

The finding that mutations in *JAG1* and *Notch2* cause AGS indicates that Notch signaling is important in the development of the organ systems affected, namely the liver, heart, skeleton, eye, face, and kidney. Studies of the pattern of expression of the various Notch receptors and ligands confirm that Jagged1 is expressed in the locations and at the times expected for a gene that contributes to the normal development of the organs affected in AGS (heart, liver, skeleton, kidney) [41,63,81,116]. This is also supported by studies in the mouse designed to test the consequences of loss of *Jag1* or *Notch2* [82,117,118]. To date, mutations in seven other Notch signaling pathway genes have been found to cause human disease. Mutations in *Notch1* are associated with congenital cardiac disease [119] and T-cell neoplasms [120]. Mutations in *Notch2* have been recently demonstrated in two families with clinical features of AGS [10], and *Notch3* mutations cause CADASIL, which is characterized by stroke and early dementia, with onset in the fourth or fifth decade [85]. The autosomal recessive disorder spondylocostal dysostosis has been shown to be caused by three different genes in the Notch signaling pathway, delta-like 3 [68], mesoderm posterior 2 [121], and lunatic fringe [122].

Genotype–Phenotype Correlations

JAG1 Mutations

Although the AGS phenotype is highly variable, there is no apparent correlation with *JAG1* genotype in the majority of patients. There is extreme variability of AGS phenotype within families, suggesting other genetic or environmental factors contribute significantly to the clinical manifestations of the disease. A study of 53 *JAG1* mutation–positive relatives of a cohort of AGS probands demonstrated that only 53% met the clinical criteria for a diagnosis of AGS [25], including 11 of 53 with clinical features that would have led to a diagnosis of AGS and 17 of 53 (32%) who had mild features that would have only been apparent on targeted evaluation following the diagnosis of a proband in their family (i.e., discovery of elevation of liver enzymes or posterior embryotoxon in an asymptomatic individual). This study was done in an attempt to select a group of mutation carriers based on criteria other than a diagnosis of AGS, and the frequency of clinical findings stands in contrast to those reported in patients with a clinical diagnosis of AGS, in which clinical features are apparent by definition [25].

The observation that relatives of probands with AGS often have only a partial manifestation of AGS led to the hypothesis that some patients with a *JAG1* mutation will present with apparently isolated heart disease in the absence of a family history of AGS. Multiple patients that fit these criteria have now been reported [40,123,124]. In each of these reports, mutations in the gene were identified that included gene deletion and protein-truncating mutations [40] and missense mutations [123,124]. These patients most likely represent one part of the spectrum for clinical consequences of *JAG1* mutations. One exception to this pattern is a relatively large family with cardiac disease in 14 individuals, which segregated with a *JAG1* missense mutation [123]. This family is remarkable in that none of the mutation-positive individuals was reported to have hepatic features of AGS. Expression and functional studies of this mutant have demonstrated that it is different from all other *JAG1* mutations studied to date in that it is "leaky" [125]; that is, some of the G274D protein molecules are normally processed and transported to the cell surface where they function appropriately while some of them are incorrectly processed and transported [126]. These results suggest that while haploinsufficiency for *JAG1* is associated with the well-characterized phenotype of AGS, the "leaky" G274D mutant, which allows more Jagged1 protein to reach the cell surface, is associated with a cardiac-specific phenotype. Therefore, cardiac development appears to be more sensitive to Jagged1 dosage than does liver development. This is the first *JAG1* mutation identified with a phenotypic correlation. The missense mutation C234Y was also found to be segregating with congenital heart defects (TOF, ventricular septal defects, and peripheral pulmonic stenosis), deafness, and posterior embryotoxon in a single family with eight affected individuals [124]. None of the affected individuals in this family had any evidence of hepatic dysfunction. Results of functional and expression studies have not yet been reported for this mutation. These studies suggest *JAG1* mutations make a significant contribution to cardiac malformations, but the frequency of *JAG1* mutations in patients with apparently isolated cardiac defects is still under investigation.

Notch2 Mutations

To date, only two families (five individuals) have been identified with a *Notch2* mutation [10]. Data from the mouse had implicated the *Notch2* gene in the etiology of clinical features associated with AGS. While the *Jag1* knockout heterozygous mouse did not phenocopy AGS, a *Jag1/Notch2* double heterozygote was found to have liver, cardiac, ocular, and renal manifestations similar to those seen in AGS patients [118]. Additionally, the spatial and temporal expression pattern of Notch2 in tissues involved in AGS made it an excellent candidate to be the Jagged1 interacting receptor [117,118]. This led to screening of a cohort of *JAG1* mutation–negative AGS patients for alterations in *Notch2*. Eleven probands were screened for the coding region (34 exons) of *Notch2*. Mutations were identified in two probands [10]. The first mutation affected the splice consensus sequence of exon 33 and resulted in the splicing out of this 98-bp exon, with a subsequent frameshift and loss of three of the seven ankyrin repeats. This mutation was found in an AGS proband and his affected mother. The second mutation, a loss-of-cysteine mutation in one of the EGF-like repeats of the extracellular domain, was found in a proband, her mildly affected mother, and her grandmother. Both her mother and grandmother had a prominent renal phenotype as their primary manifestation, leading us to hypothesize that *Notch2*-associated AGS may have a different phenotypic profile (increased frequency of renal disease) than *JAG1*-associated AGS [9].

Genetic Testing for Alagille Syndrome

Molecular analysis of the *JAG1* and *Notch2* genes is available to screen for mutations associated with AGS. An evaluation by fluorescence in situ hybridization (FISH) for deletions including the *JAG1* gene will identify these deletions in less than 7% of patients. Molecular testing is now available in several centers for *JAG1*, and hopefully availability of *Notch2* sequencing will follow. The most straightforward approach is direct sequencing of the coding region of these genes, as recent data shows that this approach identifies mutations in close to 95% of patients [9,10]. Once a *JAG1* mutation is identified in a proband, it is relatively simple to test parents and other relatives for the identified mutation. Mutations are inherited from an affected parent in 30–50% of patients, whereas the mutations appear de novo in 50–70% [4,106,111]. If a parental mutation is identified, there is a 50% risk for each future offspring to inherit the *JAG1* mutation. However, it should be emphasized that expressivity of the disorder is highly variable, and it is not currently possible to predict disease severity. If no parental mutation is identified, then the recurrence risk is limited to the chance of germline mosaicism, which for multiple different disorders is estimated at from 1–3%. There have also been cases of parental somatic mosaicism observed in apparently unaffected individuals [106,127]. Prenatal testing may also be carried out in a family once the proband's mutation is identified. Testing can help reassure parents of children with de novo mutations who may be concerned about germline mosaicism. Testing has also aided in the diagnosis of AGS in patients with minor or atypical manifestations and has expanded the spectrum of AGS manifestations.

SUMMARY

Alagille syndrome is a genetically heterogeneous disorder characterized by highly variable expression in multiple organ systems. AGS exemplifies a multisystem embryologic disorder resulting from single gene mutations. The variable expressivity of this disorder has opened the door for further investigation of genetic modifiers. The study of this model will undoubtedly lead to enhanced understanding of the genetic basis of multisystem disease in humans.

REFERENCES

1. Alagille D, Odievre M, Gautier M, et al. Hepatic ductular hypoplasia associated with characteristic facies, vertebral malformations, retarded physical, mental, and sexual development, and cardiac murmur. J Pediatr 1975;86:63–71.
2. Alagille D, Estrada A, Hadchouel M, et al. Syndromic paucity of interlobular bile ducts (Alagille syndrome or arteriohepatic dysplasia): review of 80 cases. J Pediatr 1987;110:195–200.
3. Watson GH, Miller V. Arteriohepatic dysplasia: familial pulmonary arterial stenosis with neonatal liver disease. Arch Dis Child 1973;48:459–66.
4. Crosnier C, Driancourt C, Raynaud N, et al. Mutations in JAGGED1 gene are predominantly sporadic in Alagille syndrome. Gastroenterology 1999;116:1141–8.
5. Crosnier C, Lykavieris P, Meunier-Rotival M, et al. Alagille syndrome. The widening spectrum of arteriohepatic dysplasia. Clin Liver Dis 2000;4:765–78.
6. Emerick KM, Rand EB, Goldmuntz E, et al. Features of Alagille syndrome in 92 patients: frequency and relation to prognosis. Hepatology 1999;29:822–9.
7. Oda T, Elkahloun AG, Pike BL, et al. Mutations in the human *Jagged1* gene are responsible for Alagille syndrome. Nat Genet 1997;16:235–42.
8. Li L, Krantz ID, Deng Y, et al. Alagille syndrome is caused by mutations in human *Jagged1*, which encodes a ligand for Notch1. Nat Genet 1997;16:243–51.
9. Warthen DM, Moore EC, Kamath BM, et al. Jagged1 (JAG1) mutations in Alagille syndrome: increasing the mutation detection rate. Hum Mutat 2006;27:436–43.
10. McDaniell R, Warthen DM, Sanchez-Lara PA, et al. *NOTCH2* mutations cause Alagille syndrome, a heterogeneous disorder of the Notch signaling pathway. Am J Hum Genet 2006;79:169–71.
11. Alagille D, Habib EC, Thomassin N. L'atresie des voies biliaires extrahepatiques permeables chez l'enfant. J Par Pediatr 1969; 301–18.
12. Kahn E. Paucity of interlobular bile ducts. Arteriohepatic dysplasia and nonsyndromic duct paucity. Perspect Pediatr Pathol 1991;14:168–215.
13. Treem WR, Krzymowski GA, Cartun RW, et al. Cytokeratin immunohistochemical examination of liver biopsies in infants with Alagille syndrome and biliary atresia. J Pediatr Gastroenterol Nutr 1992;15:73–80.
14. Kahn E, Markowitz J, Aiges H, et al. Human ontogeny of the bile duct to portal space ratio. Hepatology 1989;10:21–3.
15. Deprettere A, Portmann B, Mowat AP. Syndromic paucity of the intrahepatic bile ducts: diagnostic difficulty; severe morbidity throughout early childhood. J Pediatr Gastroenterol Nutr 1987;6:865–71.
16. Hoffenberg EJ, Narkewicz MR, Sondheimer JM, et al. Outcome of syndromic paucity of interlobular bile ducts (Alagille syndrome) with onset of cholestasis in infancy. J Pediatr 1995;127:220–4.
17. Quiros-Tejeira RE, Ament ME, Heyman MB, et al. Variable morbidity in Alagille syndrome: a review of 43 cases. J Pediatr Gastroenterol Nutr 1999;29:431–7.
18. Dahms BB, Petrelli M, Wyllie R, et al. Arteriohepatic dysplasia in infancy and childhood: a longitudinal study of six patients. Hepatology 1982;2:350–8.
19. Hashida Y, Yunis EJ. Syndromatic paucity of interlobular bile ducts: hepatic histopathology of the early and endstage liver. Pediatr Pathol 1988;8:1–15.
20. Libbrecht L, Spinner NB, Moore EC, et al. Peripheral bile duct paucity and cholestasis in the liver of a patient with Alagille syndrome: further evidence supporting a lack of postnatal bile duct branching and elongation. Am J Surg Pathol 2005;29:820–6.
21. Hadchouel M, Hugon RN, Gautier M. Reduced ratio of portal tracts to paucity of intrahepatic bile ducts. Arch Pathol Lab Med 1978;102:402.
22. Valencia-Mayoral P, Weber J, Cutz E, et al. Possible defect in the bile secretory apparatus in arteriohepatic dysplasia (Alagille's syndrome): a review with observations on the ultrastructure of liver. Hepatology 1984;4:691–8.
23. Witzleben CL, Finegold M, Piccoli DA, et al. Bile canalicular morphometry in arteriohepatic dysplasia. Hepatology 1987;7: 1262–6.
24. McDonald-McGinn DM, Kirschner R, Goldmuntz E, et al. The Philadelphia story: the 22q11.2 deletion: report on 250 patients. Genet Couns 1999;10:11–24.

25. Kamath BM, Bason L, Piccoli DA, et al. Consequences of JAG1 mutations. J Med Genet 2003;40:891–5.
26. Maldini G, Torri E, Lucianetti A, et al. Orthotopic liver transplantation for Alagille syndrome. Transplant Proc 2005;37:1174–6.
27. Englert C, Grabhorn E, Burdelski M, et al. Liver transplantation in children with Alagille syndrome: indications and outcome. Pediatr Transplant 2006;10:154–8.
28. Baker A, Dhawan A, Devlin J, et al. Assessment of potential donors for living related liver transplantation. Br J Surg 1999; 86:200–5.
29. Krantz ID, Colliton RP, Genin A, et al. Spectrum and frequency of jagged1 (JAG1) mutations in Alagille syndrome patients and their families. Am J Hum Genet 1998;62:1361–9.
30. Gurkan A, Emre S, Fishbein TM, et al. Unsuspected bile duct paucity in donors for living-related liver transplantation: two case reports. Transplantation 1999;67:416–18.
31. Kasahara M, Kiuchi T, Inomata Y, et al. Living-related liver transplantation for Alagille syndrome. Transplantation 2003;75: 2147–50.
32. Bhadri VA, Stormon MO, Arbuckle S, et al. Hepatocellular carcinoma in children with Alagille syndrome. J Pediatr Gastroenterol Nutr 2005;41:676–8.
33. Kaufman SS, Wood RP, Shaw BW Jr, et al. Hepatocarcinoma in a child with the Alagille syndrome. Am J Dis Child 1987;141:698–700.
34. Rabinovitz M, Imperial JC, Schade RR, et al. Hepatocellular carcinoma in Alagille's syndrome: a family study. J Pediatr Gastroenterol Nutr 1989;8:26–30.
35. Bekassy AN, Garwicz S, Wiebe T, et al. Hepatocellular carcinoma associated with arteriohepatic dysplasia in a 4-year-old girl. Med Pediatr Oncol 1992;20:78–83.
36. Nishikawa A, Mori H, Takahashi M, et al. Alagille's syndrome. A case with a hamartomatous nodule of the liver. Acta Pathol Jpn 1987;37:1319–26.
37. Greenwood RD, Rosenthal A, Crocker AC, et al. Syndrome of intrahepatic biliary dysgenesis and cardiovascular malformations. Pediatrics 1976;58:243–7.
38. McElhinney DB, Krantz ID, Bason L, et al. Analysis of cardiovascular phenotype and genotype-phenotype correlation in individuals with a JAG1 mutation and/or Alagille syndrome. Circulation 2002;106:2567–74.
39. Silberbach M, Lashley D, Reller MD, et al. Arteriohepatic dysplasia and cardiovascular malformations. Am Heart J 1994;127: 695–9.
40. Krantz ID, Smith R, Colliton RP, et al. Jagged1 mutations in patients ascertained with isolated congenital heart defects. Am J Med Genet 1999;84:56–60.
41. Loomes KM, Underkoffler LA, Morabito J, et al. The expression of Jagged1 in the developing mammalian heart correlates with cardiovascular disease in Alagille syndrome. Hum Mol Genet 1999;8:2443–9.
42. Sugiyama H, Veldtman GR, Norgard G, et al. Bladed balloon angioplasty for peripheral pulmonary artery stenosis. Catheter Cardiovasc Interv 2004;62:71–7.
43. Saidi AS, Kovalchin JP, Fisher DJ, et al. Balloon pulmonary valvuloplasty and stent implantation. For peripheral pulmonary artery stenosis in Alagille syndrome. Tex Heart Inst J 1998;25: 79–82.
43a. Gandhi SK, Reyes J, Webber SA, et al. Case report of combined pediatric heart-lung-liver transplantation. Transplantation 2002;73:1968–9.
44. LaBrecque DR, Mitros FA, Nathan RJ, et al. Four generations of arteriohepatic dysplasia. Hepatology 1982;2:467–74.
45. Wolfish NM, Shanon A. Nephropathy in arteriohepatic dysplasia (Alagille's syndrome). Child Nephrol Urol 1988;9: 169–72.
46. Martin SR, Garel L, Alvarez F. Alagille's syndrome associated with cystic renal disease. Arch Dis Child 1996;74:232–5.
47. Russo PA, Ellis D, Hashida Y. Renal histopathology in Alagille's syndrome. Pediatr Pathol 1987;7:557–68.
48. Berard E, Sarles J, Triolo V, et al. Renovascular hypertension and vascular anomalies in Alagille syndrome. Pediatr Nephrol 1998;12:121–4.
49. Tolia V, Dubois RS, Watts FB, Jr., et al. Renal abnormalities in paucity of interlobular bile ducts. J Pediatr Gastroenterol Nutr 1987;6:971–6.
50. Chung-Park M, Petrelli M, Tavill AS, et al. Renal lipidosis associated with arteriohepatic dysplasia (Alagille's syndrome). Clin Nephrol 1982;18:314–20.
51. Habib R, Dommergues JP, Gubler MC, et al. Glomerular mesangiolipidosis in Alagille syndrome (arteriohepatic dysplasia). Pediatr Nephrol 1987;1:455–64.
52. Oestreich AE, Sokol RJ, Suchy FJ, et al. Renal abnormalities in arteriohepatic dysplasia and nonsyndromic intrahepatic biliary hypoplasia. Ann Radiol (Paris) 1983;26:203–9.
53. Hyams JS, Berman MM, Davis BH. Tubulointerstitial nephropathy associated with arteriohepatic dysplasia. Gastroenterology 1983;85:430–4.
54. Schonck M, Hoorntje S, van Hooff J. Renal transplantation in Alagille syndrome. Nephrol Dial Transplant 1998;13:197–9.
55. Hingorani M, Nischal KK, Davies A, et al. Ocular abnormalities in Alagille syndrome. Ophthalmology 1999;106:330–7.
56. Reese AB, Ellsworth RM. The anterior chamber cleavage syndrome. Arch Ophthalmol 1966;75:307–18.
57. Potamitis T, Fielder AR. Angle closure glaucoma in Alagille syndrome. A case report. Ophthalmic Paediatr Genet 1993;14: 101–4.
58. Johnson BL. Ocular pathologic features of arteriohepatic dysplasia (Alagille's syndrome). Am J Ophthalmol 1990;110: 504–12.
59. Nischal KK, Hingorani M, Bentley CR, et al. Ocular ultrasound in Alagille syndrome: a new sign. Ophthalmology 1997;104: 79–85.
60. Brodsky MC, Cunniff C. Ocular anomalies in the Alagille syndrome (arteriohepatic dysplasia). Ophthalmology 1993;100: 1767–74.
61. Romanchuk KG, Judisch GF, LaBrecque DR. Ocular findings in arteriohepatic dysplasia (Alagille's syndrome). Can J Ophthalmol 1981;16:94–9.
62. Wells KK, Pulido JS, Judisch GF, et al. Ophthalmic features of Alagille syndrome (arteriohepatic dysplasia). J Pediatr Ophthalmol Strabismus 1993;30:130–5.
63. Kamath BM, Loomes KM, Oakey RJ, et al. Facial features in Alagille syndrome: specific or cholestasis facies? Am J Med Genet 2002;112:163–70.
64. Rosenfield NS, Kelley MJ, Jensen PS, et al. Arteriohepatic dysplasia: radiologic features of a new syndrome. AJR Am J Roentgenol 1980;135:1217–23.
65. Berman MD, Ishak KG, Schaefer EJ, et al. Syndromatic hepatic ductular hypoplasia (arteriohepatic dysplasia): a clinical and hepatic histologic study of three patients. Dig Dis Sci 1981;26: 485–97.

66. Berrocal T, Gamo E, Navalon J, et al. Syndrome of Alagille: radiological and sonographic findings. A review of 37 cases. Eur Radiol 1997;7:115–18.
67. Heubi JE, Higgins JV, Argao EA, et al. The role of magnesium in the pathogenesis of bone disease in childhood cholestatic liver disease: a preliminary report. J Pediatr Gastroenterol Nutr 1997;25:301–6.
68. Bulman MP, Kusumi K, Frayling TM, et al. Mutations in the human delta homologue, DLL3, cause axial skeletal defects in spondylocostal dysostosis. Nat Genet 2000;24:438–41.
69. Lykavieris P, Crosnier C, Trichet C, et al. Bleeding tendency in children with Alagille syndrome. Pediatrics 2003;111:167–70.
70. Moreau S, Bourdon N, Jokic M, et al. Alagille syndrome with cavernous carotid artery aneurysm. Int J Pediatr Otorhinolaryngol 1999;50:139–43.
71. Connor SE, Hewes D, Ball C, et al. Alagille syndrome associated with angiographic moyamoya. Childs Nerv Syst 2002;18:186–90.
72. Kamath BM, Spinner NB, Emerick KM, et al. Vascular anomalies in Alagille syndrome: a significant cause of morbidity and mortality. Circulation 2004;109:1354–8.
73. Rachmel A, Zeharia A, Neuman-Levin M, et al. Alagille syndrome associated with moyamoya disease. Am J Med Genet 1989;33:89–91.
74. Woolfenden AR, Albers GW, Steinberg GK, et al. Moyamoya syndrome in children with Alagille syndrome: additional evidence of a vasculopathy. Pediatrics 1999;103:505–8.
75. Emerick KM, Krantz ID, Kamath BM, et al. Intracranial vascular abnormalities in patients with Alagille syndrome. J Pediatr Gastroenterol Nutr 2005;41:99–107.
76. Quek SC, Tan L, Quek ST, et al. Abdominal coarctation and Alagille syndrome. Pediatrics 2000;106:E9.
77. Shefler AG, Chan MK, and Ostman-Smith I. Middle aortic syndrome in a boy with arteriohepatic dysplasia (Alagille syndrome). Pediatr Cardiol 1997;18:232–4.
78. Villa N, Walker L, Lindsell CE, et al. Vascular expression of Notch pathway receptors and ligands is restricted to arterial vessels. Mech Dev 2001;108:161–4.
79. Shutter JR, Scully S, Fan W, et al. Dll4, a novel Notch ligand expressed in arterial endothelium. Genes Dev 2000;14:1313–18.
80. Leimeister C, Schumacher N, Steidl C, et al. Analysis of HeyL expression in wild-type and Notch pathway mutant mouse embryos. Mech Dev 2000;98:175–8.
81. Jones EA, Clement-Jones M, Wilson DI. JAGGED1 expression in human embryos: correlation with the Alagille syndrome phenotype. J Med Genet 2000;37:663–8.
82. Xue Y, Gao X, Lindsell CE, et al. Embryonic lethality and vascular defects in mice lacking the Notch ligand Jagged1. Hum Mol Genet 1999;8:723–30.
83. Krebs LT, Xue Y, Norton CR, et al. Notch signaling is essential for vascular morphogenesis in mice. Genes Dev 2000;14:1343–52.
84. Uyttendaele H, Ho J, Rossant J, et al. Vascular patterning defects associated with expression of activated Notch4 in embryonic endothelium. Proc Natl Acad Sci U S A 2001;98:5643–8.
85. Joutel A, Corpechot C, Ducros A, et al. Notch3 mutations in CADASIL, a hereditary adult-onset condition causing stroke and dementia. Nature 1996;383:707–10.
86. Rovner AJ, Schall JI, Jawad AF, et al. Rethinking growth failure in Alagille syndrome: the role of dietary intake and steatorrhea. J Pediatr Gastroenterol Nutr 2002;35:495–502.
87. Sokol RJ, Stall C. Anthropometric evaluation of children with chronic liver disease. Am J Clin Nutr 1990;52:203–8.
88. Arvay JL, Zemel BS, Gallagher PR, et al. Body composition of children aged 1 to 12 years with biliary atresia or Alagille syndrome. J Pediatr Gastroenterol Nutr 2005;40:146–50.
89. Olsen IE, Ittenbach RF, Rovner AJ, et al. Deficits in size-adjusted bone mass in children with Alagille syndrome. J Pediatr Gastroenterol Nutr 2005;40:76–82.
90. Bucuvalas JC, Horn JA, Carlsson L, et al. Growth hormone insensitivity associated with elevated circulating growth hormone-binding protein in children with Alagille syndrome and short stature. J Clin Endocrinol Metab 1993;76:1477–82.
91. Chong SK, Lindridge J, Moniz C, et al. Exocrine pancreatic insufficiency in syndromic paucity of interlobular bile ducts. J Pediatr Gastroenterol Nutr 1989;9:445–9.
92. Yerushalmi B, Sokol RJ, Narkewicz MR, et al. Use of rifampin for severe pruritus in children with chronic cholestasis. J Pediatr Gastroenterol Nutr 1999;29:442–7.
93. Whitington PF, Whitington GL. Partial external diversion of bile for the treatment of intractable pruritus associated with intrahepatic cholestasis. Gastroenterology 1988;95:130–6.
94. Neimark E, Shneider B. Novel surgical and pharmacological approaches to chronic cholestasis in children: partial external biliary diversion for intractable pruritus and xanthomas in Alagille syndrome. J Pediatr Gastroenterol Nutr 2003;36:296–7.
95. Mattei P, von Allmen D, Piccoli D, et al. Relief of intractable pruritis in Alagille syndrome by partial external biliary diversion. J Pediatr Surg 2006;41:104–7; discussion 104–7.
96. Emerick KM, Whitington PF. Partial external biliary diversion for intractable pruritus and xanthomas in Alagille syndrome. Hepatology 2002;35:1501–6.
97. Poh-Fitzpatrick MB, Zaider E, Sciales C, et al. Cutaneous photosensitivity and coproporphyrin abnormalities in the Alagille syndrome. Gastroenterology 1990;99:831–5.
98. Wasserman D, Zemel BS, Mulberg AE, et al. Growth, nutritional status, body composition, and energy expenditure in prepubertal children with Alagille syndrome. J Pediatr 1999;134:172–7.
99. Novotny NM, Zetterman RK, Antonson DL, et al. Variation in liver histology in Alagille's syndrome. Am J Gastroenterol 1981;75:449–50.
100. Anad F, Burn J, Matthews D, et al. Alagille syndrome and deletion of 20p. J Med Genet 1990;27:729–37.
101. Byrne JL, Harrod MJ, Friedman JM, et al. del(20p) with manifestations of arteriohepatic dysplasia. Am J Med Genet 1986;24:673–8.
102. Krantz ID, Rand EB, Genin A, et al. Deletions of 20p12 in Alagille syndrome: frequency and molecular characterization. Am J Med Genet 1997;70:80–6.
103. Spinner NB, Rand EB, Fortina P, et al. Cytologically balanced t(2;20) in a two-generation family with Alagille syndrome: cytogenetic and molecular studies. Am J Hum Genet 1994;55:238–43.
104. Colliton RP, Bason L, Lu FM, et al. Mutation analysis of Jagged1 (JAG1) in Alagille syndrome patients. Hum Mutat 2001;17:151–2.
105. Crosnier C, Driancourt C, Raynaud N, et al. Fifteen novel mutations in the JAGGED1 gene of patients with Alagille syndrome. Hum Mutat 2001;17:72–3.
106. Giannakudis J, Ropke A, Kujat A, et al. Parental mosaicism of JAG1 mutations in families with Alagille syndrome. Eur J Hum Genet 2001;9:209–16.

107. Heritage ML, MacMillan JC, Colliton RP, et al. Jagged1 (JAG1) mutation detection in an Australian Alagille syndrome population. Hum Mutat 2000;16:408–16.
108. Jurkiewicz D, Popowska E, Glaser C, et al. Twelve novel JAG1 gene mutations in Polish Alagille syndrome patients. Hum Mutat 2005;25:321.
109. Pilia G, Uda M, Macis D, et al. Jagged-1 mutation analysis in Italian Alagille syndrome patients. Hum Mutat 1999;14:394–400.
110. Onouchi Y, Kurahashi H, Tajiri H, et al. Genetic alterations in the JAG1 gene in Japanese patients with Alagille syndrome. J Hum Genet 1999;44:235–9.
111. Spinner NB, Colliton RP, Crosnier C, et al. Jagged1 mutations in Alagille syndrome. Hum Mutat 2001;17:18–33.
112. Yuan ZR, Kohsaka T, Ikegaya T, et al. Mutational analysis of the Jagged 1 gene in Alagille syndrome families. Hum Mol Genet 1998;7:1363–9.
113. Boyer J, Crosnier C, Driancourt C, et al. Expression of mutant JAGGED1 alleles in patients with Alagille syndrome. Hum Genet 2005;116:445–53.
114. Artavanis-Tsakonas S, Rand MD, and Lake RJ. Notch signaling: cell fate control and signal integration in development. Science 1999;284:770–6.
115. Weinmaster G. Notch signal transduction: a real rip and more. Curr Opin Genet Dev 2000;10:363–9.
116. Crosnier C, Attie-Bitach T, Encha-Razavi F, et al. JAGGED1 gene expression during human embryogenesis elucidates the wide phenotypic spectrum of Alagille syndrome. Hepatology 2000;32:574–81.
117. McCright B, Gao X, Shen L, et al. Defects in development of the kidney, heart and eye vasculature in mice homozygous for a hypomorphic Notch2 mutation. Development 2001;128:491–502.
118. McCright B, Lozier J, Gridley T. A mouse model of Alagille syndrome: Notch2 as a genetic modifier of Jag1 haploinsufficiency. Development 2002;129:1075–82.
119. Garg V, Muth AN, Ransom JF, et al. Mutations in NOTCH1 cause aortic valve disease. Nature 2005;437:270–4.
120. Zhu YM, Zhao WL, Fu JF, et al. NOTCH1 mutations in T-cell acute lymphoblastic leukemia: prognostic significance and implication in multifactorial leukemogenesis. Clin Cancer Res 2006;12:3043–9.
121. Whittock NV, Sparrow DB, Wouters MA, et al. Mutated MESP2 causes spondylocostal dysostosis in humans. Am J Hum Genet 2004;74:1249–54.
122. Sparrow DB, Chapman G, Wouters MA, et al. Mutation of the LUNATIC FRINGE gene in humans causes spondylocostal dysostosis with a severe vertebral phenotype. Am J Hum Genet 2006;78:28–37.
123. Eldadah ZA, Hamosh A, Biery NJ, et al. Familial tetralogy of Fallot caused by mutation in the jagged1 gene. Hum Mol Genet 2001;10:163–9.
124. Le Caignec C, Lefevre M, Schott JJ, et al. Familial deafness, congenital heart defects, and posterior embryotoxon caused by cysteine substitution in the first epidermal-growth-factor-like domain of jagged 1. Am J Hum Genet 2002;71:180–6.
125. Lu F, Morrissette JJ, Spinner NB. Conditional JAG1 mutation shows the developing heart is more sensitive than developing liver to JAG1 dosage. Am J Hum Genet 2003;72:1065–70.
126. Morrissette JD, Colliton RP, Spinner NB. Defective intracellular transport and processing of JAG1 missense mutations in Alagille syndrome. Hum Mol Genet 2001;10:405–13.
127. Laufer-Cahana A, Krantz ID, Bason LD, et al. Alagille syndrome inherited from a phenotypically normal mother with a mosaic 20p microdeletion. Am J Med Genet 2002;112:190–3.

16

Diseases of the Gallbladder in Infancy, Childhood, and Adolescence

James E. Heubi, M.D.

EMBRYOLOGIC DEVELOPMENT OF THE GALLBLADDER

The hepatic rudiment appears at approximately day 18 of gestation in the human embryo. By day 25, it can be recognized as an endodermal diverticulum, which projects into the mesenchymal septum transversum. By day 30, the hepatic diverticulum enlarges and divides into the pars hepatica cranially and the pars cystica caudally. The pars hepatica forms parenchymal liver components; the pars cystica differentiates into the gallbladder and cystic ducts (Figure 16.1). The gallbladder primordium is a solid structure that later in development becomes cystic, as found in the adult [1–3].

CONGENITAL ANOMALIES OF THE GALLBLADDER

A variety of structural anomalies of the gallbladder has been described (Table 16.1). Congenital absence of the gallbladder long has been recognized in humans; it was known to Aristotle. Overall, the incidence of agenesis of the gallbladder has been estimated at between 1 in 7500 and 1 in 10,000 among the general population [4,5]. There are a number of mammalian species, including the horse, camel, deer, rat, and dolphin, lacking a gallbladder. Absence of the gallbladder may occur as an isolated anomaly or in association with other malformations. In the isolated form, absence of the gallbladder is of little clinical significance. It is believed to result from failed development of the pars cystica [6]. Rarely, symptoms develop related to calculi formation in the biliary ductal system.

A number of anomalies have been described in association with congenital absence of the gallbladder. Extrahepatic biliary atresia is associated not uncommonly with absence of the gallbladder, situs inversus, asplenia or polysplenia, and complex congenital heart defects frequently accompany this form of biliary atresia. Imperforate anus, genitourinary anomalies, anencephaly, bicuspid aortic valves, and cerebral aneurysms are associated with agenesis of the gallbladder. Absence of the gallbladder also accompanied thalidomide embryopathy [4,6,7].

Hypoplasia of the gallbladder also has been described. As many as one third of patients with cystic fibrosis may have a small, poorly functional gallbladder [8]. Gallbladder hypoplasia is associated with trisomy 18 [4].

Heterotopic tissue may be found within the gallbladder wall, with gastric or hepatic tissue being the most common tissue found [9,10]. Ectopic adrenal, pancreatic, and thyroid tissues also have been found [11–13]. The cause of heterotopia is poorly understood. Because the ectopic tissues are all of foregut, endodermal origin, localized heteroplastic differentiation during organogenesis has been proposed. These ectopic foci within the gallbladder wall are seldom of clinical significance; however, chemical irritation secondary to "gastric" acid secretion has been reported [10].

The incidence of a double gallbladder has been estimated between 0.1 and 0.75 per 1000 in the general population [4]. Gross [6] described 28 patients with gallbladder duplication, which he defined as structures having two separate gallbladder cavities and two cystic ducts. The two cystic ducts may converge into a single duct forming a Y-shaped structure or may enter the biliary ductal system separately. The paired gallbladders may lie in an appropriate position in the gallbladder fossa, or the accessory gallbladder may be located under the left lobe of the liver, draining into the left hepatic ducts. Rarely, it may be found surrounded by hepatic parenchyma [6].

Developmentally, duplicate gallbladders are presumed to arise as diverticula of the embryologic cystic, hepatic, or common duct. Such diverticula commonly are seen in vertebrate embryos. If these ductal buds fail to regress, an accessory gallbladder may form, which drains into the duct from which it originated. The accessory gallbladder may be more prone to pathologic changes than a normal organ [5]. One case report described a double gallbladder draining into the pancreatic duct of Wirsung [14].

A single report of a triple gallbladder has been described in the literature [15].

In contrast to multiple gallbladders, a single gallbladder may be divided into multiple chambers by longitudinal septa, presumably secondary to incomplete resolution of its solid phase. Conversely, small diverticula off the body of the gallbladder may

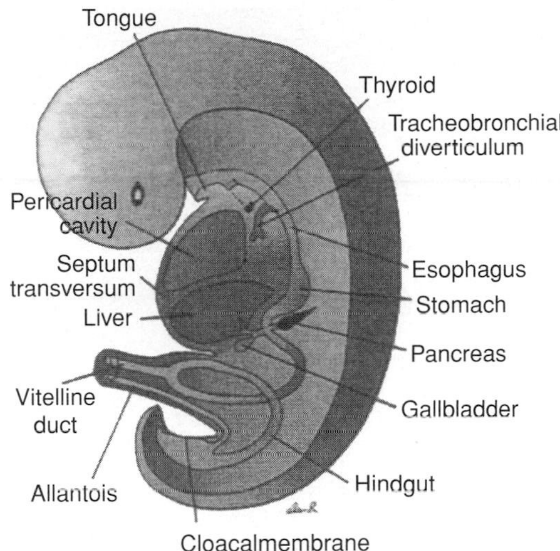

Figure 16.1. Representation of a 9-mm embryo (36 days' gestation) showing the early formation of the bile ducts and gallbladder between the liver and digestive tract. (From Langman [1].)

be seen. Because these diverticula promote bile stasis, gallstones may form.

A normally formed, single gallbladder may be malpositioned. Gallbladders have been described lying beneath the left lobe of the liver, horizontally in the transverse fissure, or embedded within hepatic parenchyma [5]. Malposition of the gallbladder may be caused by one of two mechanisms: Abnormal migration of the pars cystica could result in an aberrant gallbladder location. Alternatively, a ductal diverticulum forming a "second gallbladder," in conjunction with failed genesis of the pars cystica, could result in a single malpositioned gallbladder. Anomalous gallbladder position is clinically silent unless accompanied by cholelithiasis and cholecystitis. An increased frequency of gallstone formation in association with malposition of the gallbladder is suspected, although it has not been studied systematically [5].

An uncommon occurrence that may be of clinical significance is the so-called floating gallbladder. This is a gallbladder with a peritoneal coat suspending it from the undersurface of the liver. The embryogenesis is unknown, but a gallbladder-supporting membrane of this type has been seen in approximately 5% of routine postmortem examinations. This "mesentery" may cover the entire length of the gallbladder, creating a stable structure. On occasion, however, it surrounds only the cystic duct, creating a pendulous gallbladder. With this anatomic arrangement, torsion of the gallbladder may occur [5].

Torsion of the gallbladder is a rare clinical entity but may present a surgical emergency. Elderly women are at greatest risk, although pediatric cases have been reported. The presentation is with abrupt onset of severe, right upper quadrant abdominal pain, with nausea and vomiting. The patient is usually afebrile. On physical examination, there is marked right upper quadrant tenderness and often a palpable mass. Peritoneal signs may be present. Shock may ensue. Surgical intervention reveals an infarcted gallbladder on a twisted pedicle. Rarely has the diagnosis been presumed preoperatively [5,16,17].

Table 16.1: Congenital Anomalies of the Gallbladder

Congenital absence (agenesis) of the gallbladder
Hypoplasia of the gallbladder
Heterotopic tissue in the gallbladder (gastric, hepatic, adrenal, pancreatic, thyroid)
Multiple gallbladder formation (double gallbladder, triple gallbladder)
Septate gallbladder
Diverticula of the gallbladder
Malposition of the gallbladder
Pendulous gallbladder ("floating gallbladder")

ACALCULOUS GALLBLADDER DISEASE

Gallbladder disease in the absence of gallstones is being recognized with increasing frequency with the availability of newer and better techniques of ultrasonography. Classically, acute noncalculous gallbladder disease has been classified as either hydrops or acalculous cholecystitis; the distinction between the two syndromes may be unclear. These conditions may represent a spectrum of disease ranging from transient gallbladder distention with spontaneous resolution to acute acalculous cholecystitis with necrosis of the gallbladder wall [18,19].

Hydrops of the Gallbladder

Acute hydrops is defined by marked gallbladder distention in the absence of calculi, bacterial infection, or congenital gallbladder anomaly associated with a normal caliber extrahepatic biliary ductal system. The absence of a significant inflammatory component and its typically benign prognosis are the features that distinguish hydrops from acalculous cholecystitis [20,21].

Etiology and Pathogenesis

Hydrops most commonly is recognized associated with Kawasaki syndrome. The incidence of gallbladder hydrops complicating Kawasaki syndrome ranges from 5–20%. In the most extensive series, abdominal ultrasonographic images were obtained in 117 children diagnosed with Kawasaki syndrome and hydrops was identified in 16 (13.7%) [22]. The typical presentation includes abdominal pain, vomiting, and right upper quadrant mass superimposed on the clinical features of Kawasaki syndrome (fever for longer than 5 days, conjunctivitis, oral mucosal changes, rash, and cervical adenopathy) [22,23]. A mild, direct hyperbilirubinemia also may be present. Gallbladder hydrops also has been discovered by screening

Table 16.2: Conditions Associated with Gallbladder Hydrops

Infants and children
Kawasaki syndrome
Mesenteric adenitis
Viral hepatitis
Streptococcal pharyngitis
Staphylococcal infection
Henoch–Schönlein purpura
Hypokalemia
Sjögren syndrome
Nephrotic syndrome
Neonates
Sepsis
Total parenteral nutrition
α_1-Antitrypsin deficiency
Fasting

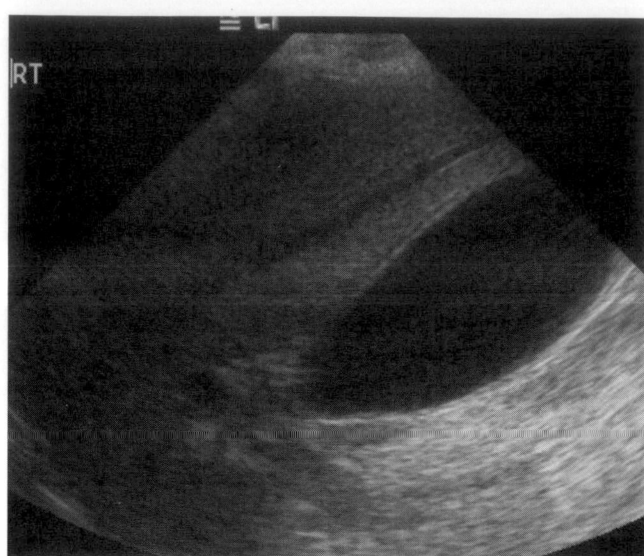

Figure 16.2. Ultrasound depicting a markedly distended gallbladder with minimal intraluminal debris and minimal wall thickening in an 8-year-old presenting with group A beta-hemolytic streptococcal pharyngitis and right upper quadrant pain.

ultrasonography in patients with Kawasaki syndrome in the absence of significant abdominal complaints. In the vast majority of patients, gallbladder distention is self-limited, resolving without surgical intervention [23–26]. Complications of gallbladder necrosis and perforation, however, have been reported in patients with Kawasaki syndrome [27,28]. Serial clinical and ultrasonographic examinations are suggested to monitor for resolution.

The hydrops in this disorder is believed to be secondary to a vasculitic process in the gallbladder wall with cystic duct obstruction. Perivascular leukocytic infiltration with vascular congestion has been described on pathologic examination of a hydropic gallbladder from a child with Kawasaki syndrome. Bile cultures are sterile [29]. Enlarged lymph nodes surrounding, and perhaps obstructing, the cystic duct also have been reported [27]. As depicted in Table 16.2, hydrops of the gallbladder has been reported in association with a variety of disorders.

Hydrops may accompany staphylococcal or streptococcal infection, with associated toxin production [30,31]. A number of cases of gallbladder hydrops have been described in young children with antecedent upper respiratory infection (or no clear antecedent illness) in whom surgical intervention revealed enlarged mesenteric lymph nodes. Whether cystic duct obstruction secondary to adenopathy played a role in the pathogenesis of the hydrops is unclear [32,33].

Single cases of gallbladder hydrops have been reported in infants and children with Sjögren's syndrome, Henoch–Schönlein purpura, viral hepatitis, and hypokalemia secondary to Bartter's syndrome [34–37].

Clinical Features

The child with hydrops of the gallbladder typically presents with abdominal pain and a tender right upper quadrant mass. Vomiting, fever, and stigmata of an associated illness commonly are found. The clinical picture may mimic intussusception or acute appendicitis [18,20].

The diagnosis of hydrops generally is made by ultrasonography demonstrating a markedly distended, echo-free gallbladder and a normal-caliber biliary tree (Figure 16.2). Before the routine use of ultrasonography, the diagnosis typically was encountered as an unsuspected finding at laparotomy.

The mainstay of therapy is supportive, with fluid resuscitation and therapy aimed at an associated illness, if indicated (such as antibiotics for streptococcus). Serial ultrasonographic examination is useful to confirm resolution. Surgery should be reserved for the exceedingly rare complication of gallbladder perforation. Symptomatic abdominal pain may resolve after 1–2 days [38].

Transient gallbladder distention has been recognized with increasing frequency in neonates as well. Typically the presentation is as a right upper quadrant abdominal mass in a sick neonate or premature infant [39,40]. Associated conditions have included sepsis, prolonged fasting, and administration of total parenteral nutrition (TPN), likely related to the reduced cholecystokinin secretion and impaired gallbladder contraction [18,40,41]. Gallbladder distention in neonates with cystic fibrosis (perhaps secondary to inspissation of bile) and α_1-antitrypsin deficiency (perhaps secondary to cystic duct hypoplasia) has been reported [42,43].

Ultrasonography is used to confirm that the abdominal mass is the gallbladder. Typically, with the institution of feeding, transient gallbladder distention of the neonate resolves spontaneously. It is important to remember, however, that a number of cases of culture-proven acalculous cholecystitis in neonates have been documented. Because there are no reliable ultrasonographic criteria for distinguishing inflammation from benign

Table 16.3: Conditions Associated with Acalculous Cholecystitis

Postoperative state

Burns

Systemic infection
- Sepsis
- Leptospirosis
- Rocky Mountain spotted fever
- Typhoid fever

Immunocompromised host
- *Cryptosporidium* infection
- *Giardia* infection
- Cytomegalovirus
- *Candida* infection
- *Aspergillus* infection

Hemophagocytic lymphohistiocytosis

distention (thickening of the gallbladder wall is neither entirely sensitive nor specific for inflammation), failure of the abdominal mass to resolve or clinical deterioration should warrant further investigations. Surgical intervention may be required in some patients.

Acalculous Cholecystitis

Acalculous cholecystitis, characterized by distention and inflammation of the gallbladder, is uncommon in infants and children. It is an important entity to recognize, however, because it may present as an abdominal emergency.

Etiology and Pathogenesis

Acalculous cholecystitis has been reported at all ages from neonates to adolescents [19,44]. Acalculous cholecystitis in adults commonly accompanies serious illness or trauma. Predisposing factors for the development of acalculous cholecystitis have been identified in 50% of pediatric patients and include previous surgical procedure, burns, multiple transfusions, trauma, and systemic infection [19,44–48] (Table 16.3). A case of acalculous cholecystitis in an adolescent male with Crohn's disease has been described [49].

The pathophysiology of acalculous cholecystitis is poorly understood. In the postoperative or severely ill patient, the lack of enteral feeding, the administration of TPN, and the use of opiates result in gallbladder stasis. In some patients, congenital narrowing or local inflammation of the cystic duct has been demonstrated at the time of surgical intervention [19,44]. Obstruction of the cystic duct with gallbladder distention and secondary bacterial invasion may lead to cholecystitis. Episodic ischemia or hypoperfusion also could play a role in the development of acalculous cholecystitis in the patient in intensive care [10].

Acalculous cholecystitis has been described in association with systemic infectious illness. Ternberg and Keating [45] described three patients with leptospirosis presenting as fever, pharyngitis, cervical adenopathy, and rash, in whom tender abdominal masses were found. At laparotomy, an inflamed, distended gallbladder was found in each of the three patients. Therapy included tube cholecystostomy, with good results. In a review of the experience with leptospirosis at St. Louis Children's Hospital, five of nine cases were complicated by acalculous cholecystitis requiring surgical drainage [50].

In a review of neonates with acalculous cholecystitis, eight of ten infants had systemic infection [44]. Bile cultures grew *Escherichia coli*, *Streptococcus viridans*, *Serratia*, and *Pseudomonas*. The two infants in whom there was no evidence of sepsis had congenital anomalies of the biliary tree with cystic duct obstruction [44].

Gallbladder inflammation has been described in Rocky Mountain spotted fever, with rickettsial organisms demonstrated in a surgically resected gallbladder [51]. The course of typhoid fever frequently has been complicated by acalculous cholecystitis; the first cholecystostomy was performed for acute gallbladder inflammation secondary to typhoid fever in 1901 [52]. Children with hemophagocytic lymphohistiocytosis (HLH) may present with a constellation of ultrasound findings, including hepatosplenomegaly, ascites, pleural effusion, periportal echogenicity, and gallbladder wall thickening [53,54].

Associated illness or anomaly is not necessary for the development of acalculous cholecystitis in the pediatric population. None of the seven patients in the series reported by Holcomb et al. [19] had an associated predisposing illness or documented systemic infection. Cholecystectomy was performed in all seven without postoperative complication.

Opportunistic infection may occur in the gallbladder of an immunocompromised host. Adult patients with human immunodeficiency virus (HIV) disease or those who have undergone orthotopic liver transplantation have been reported to have cholecystitis secondary to cytomegalovirus [55]. Fungal infections of the gallbladder with *Candida*, *Torulopsis*, and *Aspergillus* have been described [55,56]. Additionally, parasitic infestation of the gallbladder with *Giardia* and *Cryptosporidium* has occurred in association with HIV infection and other immunodeficiency states [55,57,58].

Clinical Features

Patients with acalculous cholecystitis present with right upper quadrant abdominal pain, nausea, vomiting, and fever. Physical examination reveals right upper quadrant or generalized abdominal tenderness. A mass may be palpable. Leukocytosis is an inconsistent finding. Signs and symptoms may be less readily apparent in the neonate or the severely ill patient. The clinical presentation may be dominated by the findings of an associated illness, such as trauma or a systemic infectious process [19,45,48].

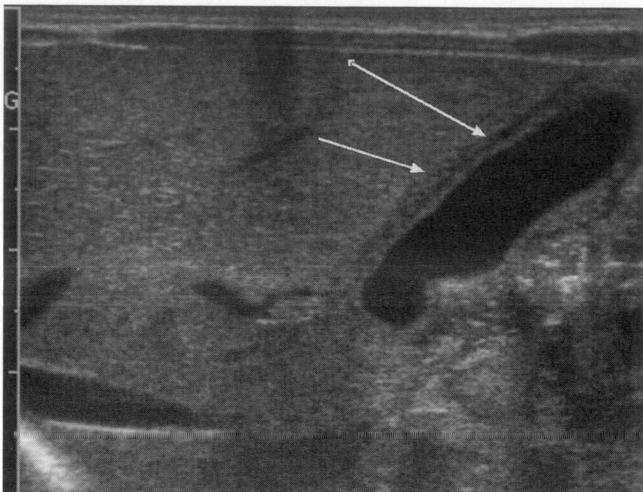

Figure 16.3. Thickening of the gallbladder wall in a 9-year-old child with leukemia and right upper quadrant pain. Longitudinal ultrasound images demonstrate striking thickening of the gallbladder wall (*arrows*) and pericholecystic fluid collections.

The differential diagnosis includes appendicitis, intussusception, infectious hepatitis, choledochal cyst, and diffuse peritonitis. Ultrasonography may demonstrate gallbladder distention, with thickening of the gallbladder wall (Figure 16.3) and echogenic intraluminal debris. Thickening of the gallbladder wall can also be demonstrated by axial computed tomography (CT) scans (Figure 16.4). The reliability of excessive thickness of the gallbladder wall as an indicator of acute inflammation has been questioned. In a report by Sanders [59], a thickened gallbladder wall was present in 45% of adult patients with acute calculous and acalculous cholecystitis studied by ultrasound. In a series of 793 consecutively studied infants and children, Patriquin et al. [60] reported that 20 patients were identified as meeting ultrasound criteria for a thick gallbladder wall (defined as >3 mm). Of these 20 patients, 16 had hypoalbuminemia, 2 had ascites, 1 had physiologic thickening associated with contraction of the gallbladder wall, and 1 had heart disease with associated systemic venous hypertension. None of the patients had clinical findings suggestive of acute cholecystitis. Of five patients with surgically proven acute cholecystitis who underwent ultrasonographic examinations during the study period, none had a thickened gallbladder wall. Most recently, Jeffrey and Sommer [61] evaluated 14 adult patients with clinically suspected acute acalculous cholecystitis but inconclusive initial abdominal ultrasounds. Four of the patients with normal gallbladder walls demonstrated progressive thickening on subsequent studies, and three of these patients had acute acalculous cholecystitis as a surgical finding. Six patients had thickened gallbladder walls at the initial ultrasonographic examination, but only one of these patients required a cholecystectomy after continuing to have symptoms consistent with acute acalculous cholecystitis. These data suggest that repetitive sonography may be helpful in diagnosing acute acalculous cholecystitis. Gallbladder wall thickening may represent a local inflammatory response or may be a reflection of a systemic process; a thickened gallbladder wall depicted by ultrasonography must be interpreted in the context of the clinical setting.

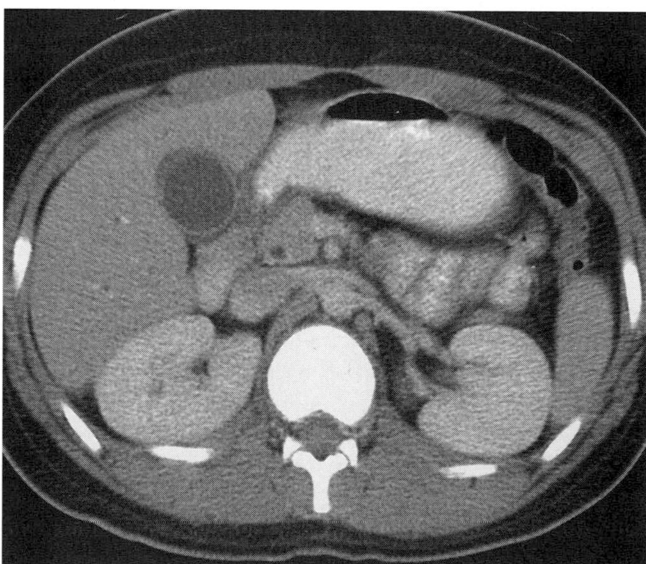

Figure 16.4. Axial CT scan with intravenous contrast demonstrating striking thickening of the gallbladder wall. There is also dilatation of the common bile duct as it traverses the pancreas.

The diagnosis of acute acalculous cholecystitis requires a high index of clinical suspicion. Radiographic techniques can provide strong supportive evidence in the appropriate clinical setting. Ultrasonographic findings consistent with acute acalculous cholecystitis, however, such as gallbladder distention, gallbladder wall thickening, lack of calculi, and a poor response to cholecystokinin, also may be seen in gallbladder hydrops [49]. Radioisotope studies with technetium-labeled mebrofenin may be used to demonstrate patency (or lack thereof) of the cystic duct. Nonfilling of the gallbladder, in the presence of good hepatic uptake and intestinal excretion of radioisotope, suggests cholecystitis. Swayne [62] demonstrated that technetium cholescintigraphy has a high sensitivity for biliary obstruction in a retrospective study of adults with clinically suspected acute acalculous cholecystitis. Another study showed that scintigraphy was not specific compared with both ultrasonography and CT [63]. False-positive scintigraphic results have been seen in alcoholism and in patients receiving parenteral nutrition [64].

Definitive therapy for acalculous cholecystitis remains controversial. Surgical intervention with tube cholecystostomy, or preferably cholecystectomy, is considered prudent to prevent complications such as gangrenous necrosis of the gallbladder wall, perforation, and bile peritonitis [19,44]. In a recently published series of 12 patients, Imamoglu et al. [48] performed cholecystectomy on 3, with resolution without operative intervention in the other 9.

Other Acalculous Entities of the Gallbladder

Another category of acalculous disease that is becoming more commonly diagnosed is gallbladder dyskinesia, also known as *biliary colic*. Patients presenting with this disorder often are female and have a history of right upper quadrant pain and fatty food intolerance that may have been present for longer than 1 year. Often a family history of cholelithiasis is present. Ultrasonography does not show gallstones, and ultrasonography or scintigraphy with cholecystokinin stimulation shows a decreased biliary ejection fraction [65,66]. Dumont and Caniano [67] examined 42 children with abdominal pain and abnormal gallbladder emptying (contractility <50%) diagnosed by either ultrasonography or scintigraphy with cholecystokinin. All patients were treated with cholecystectomies, and all but one improved after surgery after a mean follow-up period of 20 months. Almost half the removed gallbladders had chronic inflammation. A retrospective analysis by Vegunta et al. [68] revealed that among 107 consecutive cholecystectomies in children at a single medical center, 62 were performed for biliary dyskinesia. Short-term relief of symptoms was observed in 85% of patients with a preoperative diagnosis of dyskinesia, and approximately half the removed gallbladders had chronic cholecystitis. Another retrospective study showed a much higher incidence of chronic cholecystitis in such patients [65].

Gallbladder motility has been shown to be impaired in children with Down's syndrome and children and adolescents with type I diabetes mellitus [69,70]. Fasting gallbladder volumes are increased in both conditions, and contraction after a meal stimulus is reduced in Down's syndrome. These abnormalities may predispose to the known increased gallstone formation in both conditions.

Other Inflammatory Lesions of the Gallbladder

Rarely, lesions of the gallbladder accompany other systemic inflammatory disorders. A characteristic granulomatous inflammatory lesion has been demonstrated in the gallbladder wall of a patient with Crohn's disease [71]. Malacoplakia involving the gallbladder, with the formation of Michaelis–Gutmann bodies, has been reported as well [72]. The gallbladder may be affected in patients with polyarteritis nodosa [73].

TUMORS OF THE GALLBLADDER

Neoplastic disorders of the gallbladder occur uncommonly in childhood. Adenoma of the gallbladder, a benign polypoid lesion, has been described in a pediatric patient. It may present with symptoms of biliary colic; ultrasonography may allow visualization of a gallbladder polyp (Figure 16.5). Resection is recommended because of the tumor's potential for malignancy and association with acute acalculous cholecystitis [74,75]. Gallbladder polyps also have been reported in association with Peutz–Jeghers syndrome [76]. Only three cases of adenomyomatosis of the gallbladder have been described in children

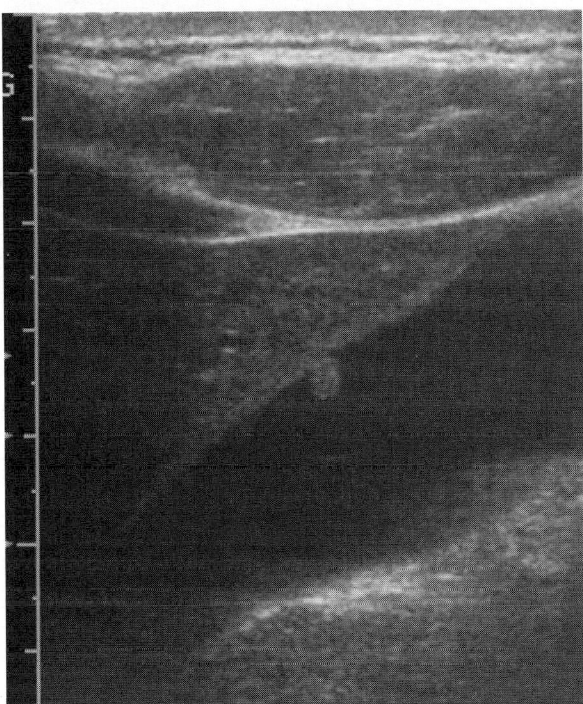

Figure 16.5. Longitudinal ultrasound demonstrating a pedunculated mass hanging from the mucosa of the gallbladder wall. This mass was found to be a polyp when cholecystectomy was performed.

[77–79]. This condition may lead to abdominal pain. Although there is no consensus regarding an association with malignancy, most clinicians would recommend cholecystectomy.

Primary malignant neoplasms of the gallbladder are exceedingly uncommon in the pediatric age group. Presenting as obstructive jaundice, embryonal rhabdomyosarcoma is the most frequently encountered malignancy arising from the gallbladder and biliary tree. Because the tumor is poorly responsive to surgical and chemotherapeutic intervention, the prognosis is dismal [80].

MISCELLANEOUS CONDITIONS

There are a number of disorders characterized by accumulation of lipids or calcium salts intraluminally or intramurally within the gallbladder. These disorders are more common in the adult population.

Porcelain gallbladder, an entity characterized by calcification of the gallbladder wall, occurs in association with chronic inflammation. One case was described that was associated with extrahepatic bile duct obstruction. Cholecystectomy is advised because of the high frequency of gallbladder carcinoma reported in adult patients with porcelain gallbladder [81,82].

A single case of "milk of calcium" bile has been reported in the pediatric literature. For unknown reasons, excessive quantities of calcium carbonate accumulate in gallbladder bile; the gallbladder is radiopaque on plain film, which appears much like a cholecystogram [83].

Cholesterolosis of the gallbladder involves deposition of triglycerides and cholesterol esters in macrophages within the lamina propria of the gallbladder wall. It may occur as a diffuse or localized phenomenon [10].

Gallbladder adenomyosis involves benign hyperplasia of the muscularis mucosa with intramucosal diverticula formation. Adenomyosis has been seen in a 16-year-old whose gallbladder was resected for symptoms of cholecystitis [10,84].

CALCULOUS GALLBLADDER DISEASE

Approximately 20–25 million North American adults have gallstones [85]. Based on the Framingham study, it is estimated that 12 million females and 6 million males have gallstones [86]. Cholelithiasis is relatively uncommon in infancy and childhood; however, gallstones have been detected in utero as early as after 30 weeks' gestation and in newborns [87,88]. One newborn has been described with clinical and ultrasonographic evidence of acute calculous cholecystitis [89].

Few studies have been performed examining the incidence or prevalence of gallstone disease in children. The prevalence of gallstones among 1502 Italian males and females 6–19 years of age screened with ultrasound was 0.13% overall (0.27% in females) [90]. This compares with a prevalence of 2.9% and 1.1% among Italian females and males, respectively, between 18 and 29 years of age [91]. The incidence of gallbladder disease remains negligible in males throughout childhood and adolescence; in females, there is a remarkable increase in incidence between 11 and 13 years of age [92] (Figure 16.6). The true prevalence of gallstones has been evaluated in adult Caucasians by survey with ultrasonography or oral cholecystography (Figure 16.7). For both males and females, there is an increasing prevalence of gallstones with increasing age. At all ages from puberty until menopause, women have a higher frequency of

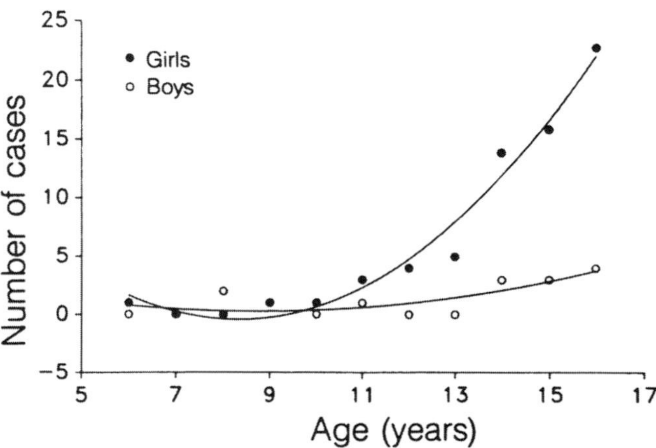

Figure 16.6. Incidence of gallstones among hospitalized Swedish children younger than 16 years. Note the minimal incidence for both boys and girls before 11 years of age, with a sharp increase in incidence in girls and a minimal increase in boys. (From Nilsson [92] as modified by Shaffer [145], with permission.)

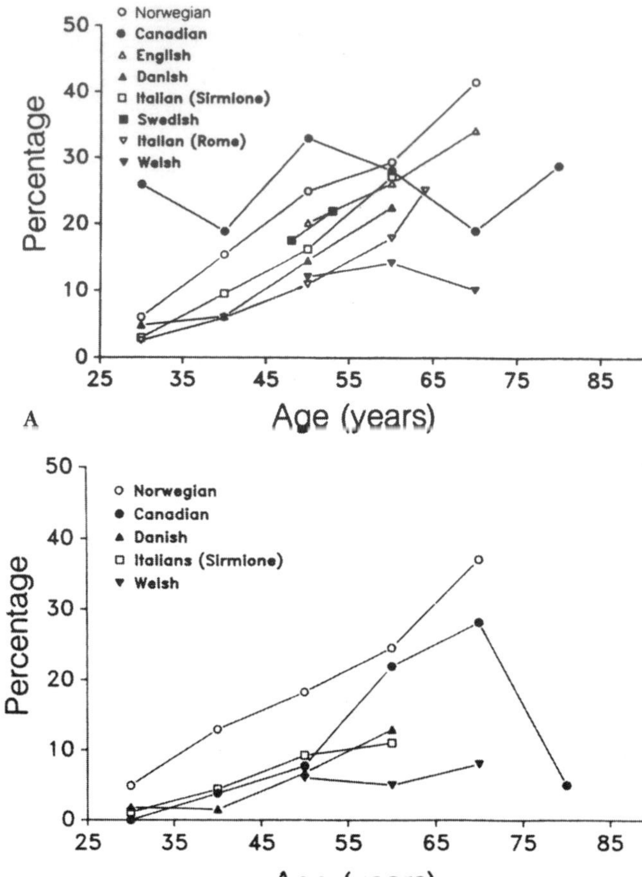

Figure 16.7. Prevalence of gallstones by surveys (from Shaffer [145]) using ultrasonography or oral cholecystography in Caucasian women (**A**) and men (**B**) from Europe and Canada. Gallstones are more common in women and increase in frequency with increasing age.

stones than do men [91,93,94]. Clear differences in gallstone frequency exist among ethnic backgrounds. The frequency is exceedingly low (near 0%) among Canadian Eskimos and East and West African natives; it reaches 30–70% among American Indians, Swedish, and Czechs [94]. The type of stones also varies with geographic region. Cholesterol gallstones predominate in Western cultures; pigment stones are more common among Asian populations.

Classification of Gallstones

Stones may be divided into two major categories (Figure 16.8). Cholesterol stones contain more than 50% cholesterol by weight, with variable amounts of protein and calcium salts. Pigment stones (black and brown) are complex mixtures of insoluble calcium salts including calcium bilirubinate, calcium phosphate, and calcium carbonate. Cholesterol content in pigment stones ranges from less than 10% in black stones to 10–30% in brown pigment stones.

Approximately 25–33% of stones removed during cholecystectomy in adults are pigment stones; as many as 72% in

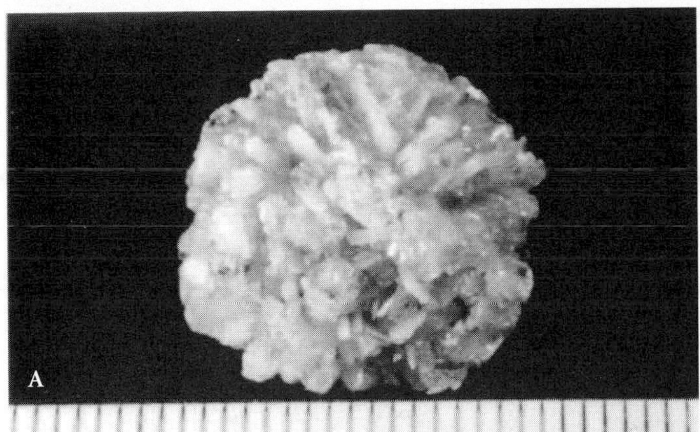

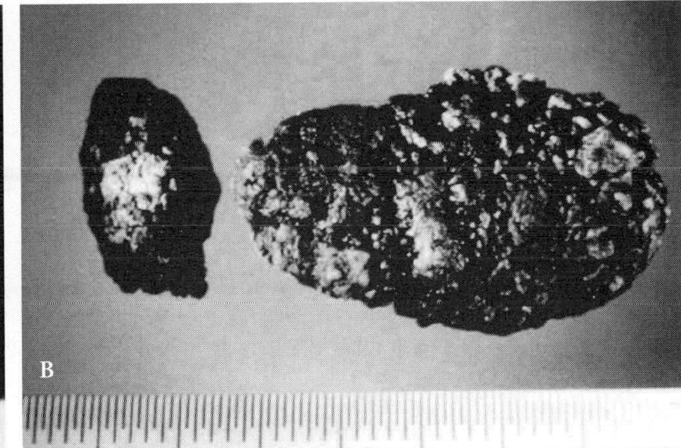

Figure 16.8. Typical appearance of a cholesterol stone with minimal bilirubin staining (**A**) and black pigment stones (**B**) removed from children. (Scale, 10 mm.)

children are pigment stones [85,95]. Less than 10% of gallstones obtained during cholecystectomy during adolescence are pigment stones; by the seventh decade of life, pigment stones are more common than cholesterol stones [92,95–99]. Black and white adults have similar frequencies of pigment stones [100]. Obesity does not appear to predispose to pigment stone formation.

Causes of Gallstones in Children

Several series have reported the causes of gallstones in children and adolescents [19,84,95,96,98,101–111]. Few have addressed carefully the issue of the type of stone associated with certain conditions. Friesen and Roberts [95] reviewed their hospital's experience and a total of 693 cases of pediatric gallstones reported in the literature. Based on their experience, 72% of stones were pigmented, 17% were cholesterol, and in 11% the composition was unknown. Over the entire series, pigment stones predominated in infants and children to the age of 5 years, with cholesterol stones found more commonly between 6 and 21 years of age. Unfortunately, the composition of the stones was unknown in the majority of studies, and determination of composition was based on visual inspection rather than chemical analysis. Hemolytic disease was considered the cause of gallstones in 30% of the entire series. The causes of and conditions associated with stones from the entire series are illustrated in Table 16.4. In a second smaller study, Stringer et al. [96] examined stone type obtained from 20 consecutive cholecystectomies for cholelithiasis in children. Of these 20 patients, 11 had pigment stones, 2 had cholesterol stones, and 7 had calcium carbonate stones. These recent findings suggest that the stone composition in children is different from that in adults, particularly with regard to the finding of calcium carbonate stones. These stones appear to have a similar composition to pigment stones but lack bilirubinate salts. Many, but not all, had received parenteral nutrition, which may provide a potential explanation for the high frequency of calcium carbonate stones in this series.

Pigment Gallstones

There are two major types of pigment stones, "black" and "brown" [112]. In both types, pigment is present as calcium bilirubinates. In black pigment stones, pigment is cross-linked to form a black polymer that is insoluble in all solvents. In contrast, in brown pigment stones, the cross-linked polymers are present in low concentrations and the pigments are soluble in most organic solvents. Black pigment stones are found in sterile gallbladder bile. About 50% of black pigment stones appear to be radiopaque with conventional radiographic techniques [113,114]. Two thirds of all opaque stones are pigment stones because of their high content of calcium carbonates and phosphates. Brown pigment stones generally are found in infected bile in intra- and extrahepatic bile ducts. They are usually radiolucent because they contain smaller amounts of calcium phosphate and carbonate than do black pigment stones. Brown stones contain more cholesterol than do black stones because the bile in which they develop tends to be continuously supersaturated with cholesterol. Black pigment stones are shiny like anthracite chips or dull like asphalt and are relatively hard and spiculated. Brown pigment stones are soft and soaplike or greasy in consistency [115].

Unconjugated bilirubin (UCB) is the major bile pigment in gallstones. Typically the major components of bile are bilirubin diglucuronides and two bilirubin monoglucuronide isomers. The glucuronides generally bind calcium as soluble complexes. UCB ordinarily makes up only a small fraction of normal bile pigment (1%). Most UCB derives from endogenous enzymatic (β-glucuronidase) or nonenzymatic hydrolysis of conjugated bilirubins. Unlike the conjugates, UCB is very sensitive to precipitation with ionized calcium [116]. Although the process is still poorly understood, polymers of cross-linked bilirubin tetrapyrroles are formed in bile that serve as the basis for stone formation. The chemical initiators of the polymerization process are not known. It seems likely that polymerization is initiated by free radicals or singlet oxygen, possibly produced by the liver and secreted in bile or by macrophages or neutrophils in the gallbladder mucosa [117].

Table 16.4: Associated Conditions by Age for 693 Patients with Cholelithiasis Reported in the Literature, Expressed as Percentage of Total Cases in Age Group

0–12 mo	*1–5 yr*	*6–11 yr*
None (36.4)	Hepatobiliary disease (28.6)	Pregnancy (37.2)
TPN (29.1)	Abdominal surgery (21.4)	Hemolytic disease (22.5)
Abdominal surgery (29.1)	Artificial heart valve (14.3)	Obesity (8.1)
Sepsis (14.8)	None (14.3)	Abdominal surgery (5.1)
Bronchopulmonary dysplasia (12.7)	Malabsorption (7.1)	None (3.4)
Hemolytic disease (5.5)		Hepatobiliary disease (2.7)
Malabsorption (5.5)		TPN (2.7)
Necrotizing enterocolitis (5.5)		Malabsorption (2.8)
Hepatobiliary disease (3.6)		

TPN, total parenteral nutrition.
Data from Friesen and Roberts [95].

Calcium carbonate and phosphate are the major components of most black pigment stones; brown pigment stones do not contain appreciable amounts of these substances. Precipitation of these salts is determined by bile pH. Insoluble calcium salt formation is enhanced markedly in alkaline bile, and it is likely that black pigment stones containing calcium carbonates only form in alkaline bile [117]. Fatty acid salts (calcium soaps) are important components of brown pigment stones. Palmitate and stearate are principal Sn1 salts of fatty acids of biliary lecithin. They generally are not found free in bile and are produced by bacterial phospholipase A_1 hydrolysis of lecithin.

Mucin glycoproteins are the framework on which pigment stones grow [118]. Mucin is produced in the gallbladder crypts. Mucin hypersecretion by the gallbladder may play an important role in pigment stone formation.

In black pigment stone disease, bile should be supersaturated with calcium bilirubinates, calcium carbonate, and calcium phosphate. This may result from an absolute increase in the amount of UCB or ionized calcium. Increased biliary UCB may derive from increased pigment production and excretion in bile. In humans, the output and proportion of UCB in bile may increase after a load of hemoglobin or bilirubin. Patients with spontaneous hemolysis have no more than 3% of total biliary bilirubin as UCB. Increased UCB also may result from increased enzymatic (β-glucuronidase) hydrolysis of bilirubin conjugates or reduced amounts of an inhibitor of β-glucuronidase, glutaric acid. Potential causes of increased levels of ionized calcium are increased amounts of plasma-ionized calcium or reduced biliary calcium binders such as micellar bile salts and lecithin–cholesterol vesicles. Increased ionization of normal amounts of UCB and increased CO_3^{2-} occurs in alkaline biliary pH. Decreased biliary bile salts and cholesterol concentrations found in cirrhotic patients may lead to increased levels of ionized calcium in bile as well as reduced levels of micellar bile salt and vesicle deficiency.

Brown pigment stones require both stasis and infection. Bacterially derived β-glucuronidase, phospholipase A_1, and bile salt deconjugase produce UCB, fatty acids, and unconjugated bile acids. All these products are insoluble and precipitate as calcium salts. Ductal precipitation of these compounds together with cholesterol and mucin form soft, greasy stones shaped like the bile ducts.

Conditions Predisposing to Black Pigment Stone Formation

CHRONIC HEMOLYTIC DISEASE

The risk of black pigment stone formation is increased in patients with chronic hemolytic disorders including congenital spherocytosis, sickle cell (S-S and S-C) disease (SCD), thalassemia major and minor, pyruvate kinase deficiency, glucose-6-phosphate dehydrogenase deficiency, and autoimmune hemolytic disease. The prevalence of pigment stones in patients with hemolytic disorders increases with age, as illustrated by the age-related frequencies of gallstones in sickle cell anemia. In children younger than 10 years, the frequency is 14%. In 10- to 20-year-olds, the frequency increases to 36%. At age 22 years, the frequency is 50%, and by age 33 years it is between 60% and 85% [119–121]. Despite the identification of gallstones in more than half of a cohort of patients with SCD, few are symptomatic at the time of ultrasound identification of stones [122]. Elective laparoscopic cholecystectomy is encouraged for patients with SCD who have gallstones identified by ultrasonography. Recent studies have suggested a 12-day reduction in hospital stay with elective laparoscopic cholecystectomy compared with emergent surgery (4 vs. 16 days) [123,124].

TOTAL PARENTERAL NUTRITION

The natural history of TPN-related biliary tract disease has been elucidated recently in both neonates and adults. In a prospective study of 41 neonates performed by Matos et al.

[125], 44% developed gallbladder sludge after a mean of 10 days of TPN. The authors found that the appearance of sludge related to prematurity, lack of enteral nutrition, and duration of TPN. In 12% of the neonates, sludge evolved to "sludge balls," and two developed uncomplicated gallstones. In one of these patients, the stone resolved within 6 months; in the other, the stone was still present after 1.5 years. King et al. [126] studied 84 infants and children treated with TPN and found cholelithiasis in 13%. Patients with cholelithiasis had a mean duration of TPN of 218 days versus 115 days in patients without gallstones. Gallstones were more common in patients who had lost their ileocecal valve, had short bowel syndrome, or had more surgery. Roslyn et al. [127] found gallstones in 43% of 21 children receiving long-term TPN. Children who developed gallstones were treated with TPN more than twice as long as children without gallstones. Seventy-eight percent of children with stones received TPN for longer than 20 months; patients without stones received TPN for a mean of 14 months. Several anecdotal reports have appeared that suggest that a significant proportion of stones formed during TPN remain "silent" or disappear over time [127–130]. In adults treated with TPN studied by Messing et al. [131], biliary sludge was first seen in 6% of subjects in the first 3 weeks of therapy. By 4–6 weeks of treatment, 50% had developed sludge. With increasing duration of therapy, well-circumscribed stones developed in 6 of 14 sludge-positive patients with prolonged TPN. With discontinuation of TPN and resumption of oral feeding, the sludge disappeared from all patients after 5 weeks. Cholecystectomy was required for symptomatic stones in three patients, stones persisted in two, and the stones resolved spontaneously in one. Minimal enteral nutrition or parenteral administration of cholecystokinin or its analogues may allow intermittent gallbladder contraction, reduce gallbladder stasis, and reduce the risk of gallstone formation in patients treated with TPN; however, the benefits of these interventions have been inconsistent [132,133]. In a study of 95 children (mean age, 20 months) reported by Mashako et al. [134], gallbladder sludge appeared in 23% after 1 month and 32% after 3 months of continuous TPN. With the initiation of partial oral feeding, the rate was reduced to 17% after 1 month, and sludge disappeared within 1 month of complete oral feeding. Two subjects developed gallbladder lithiasis, which disappeared with oral feeding. With both partial and total oral feeding, the plasma level of cholecystokinin increased significantly postprandially, and a significant negative correlation ($r = -0.88$) was found between the gallbladder sludge rate and cholecystokinin levels for any of the feeding methods used.

CIRRHOSIS AND CHRONIC CHOLESTASIS

Adults with cirrhosis are at increased risk for pigment gallstone formation. In autopsy studies in adults, pigment stones were more prevalent in patients with primary biliary cirrhosis (30.8%) and all patients with cirrhosis (29.4%) compared with noncirrhotic patients (12.8%) [135,136]. The cause for stone formation currently is unknown; it may be related, however, to hypersplenism and attendant hemolysis. The excess quantities of bilirubin produced may exceed its solubility in bile. In addition, cirrhotic patients also are prone to stone formation because their bile has limited solubilizing capability as a result of reduced concentrations of biliary bile acids [137]. Patients with Wilson's disease may have calcified pigment stones produced because of recurrent episodes of hemolysis. Children with progressive familial intrahepatic cholestasis type 1 (PFIC1) appear prone to gallstone formation [138]. Pigment stones have been identified in gallbladders removed from a number of symptomatic children with cirrhosis at autopsy or at the time of orthotopic liver transplantation at Children's Hospital of Cincinnati. Defective bile acid synthesis as found with inborn errors of bile salt metabolism may lead to decreased bile salt secretion, but because of attendant cholestasis, patients are likely to have pigment rather than cholesterol stones. Despite reductions in biliary bile acid concentrations, the prevalence of cholesterol gallstones does not appear to be increased in cirrhosis, probably because there is a concurrent reduction in cholesterol synthesis, resulting in normal biliary cholesterol–bile acid ratios.

MISCELLANEOUS

A number of disparate conditions appear to be associated with sludge formation and merit discussion. Gallbladder sludge and lithiasis have been noted in infants born to morphine abusers [139]. Ceftriaxone, a third-generation cephalosporin with broad-spectrum antimicrobial activity, is largely excreted in the bile. Up to 46% of children receiving ceftriaxone for treatment of meningitis have been found to develop gallbladder sludge, which characteristically disappears with cessation of therapy [140]. It has been proposed that excess quantities of ceftriaxone in the bile precipitate as a calcium salt–producing sludge [141]. Use of TPN, presence of an ileal conduit, or a history of abdominal surgery places long-term survivors of childhood cancer at an increased risk for gallstone formation [142].

Other conditions may also predispose to cholelithiasis; however, insufficient data are available to classify the stones as either pigment or cholesterol containing. Recent studies have suggested an increased frequency of gallstones in girls with Rhett syndrome, with two thirds of girls and women younger than 43 years having stones; however, the pathophysiology of stones has not been investigated [143]. In one small series, cholelithiasis was observed in 10 of 311 infants and children (3.2%) after heart transplantation [144].

Conditions Predisposing to Brown Pigment Stone Formation

Although common in the Pacific Rim, brown pigment stones are uncommon in the West. In the Pacific Rim, most are associated with biliary infection of infestations with parasites such as *Ascaris lumbricoides.* Most brown pigment stones occur in obstructed bile ducts [145]. They are rare in infants and children. Recently, Treem et al. [146] reported two infants with biliary obstruction caused by brown pigment stones found in infected bile.

Cholesterol Gallstones

Cholesterol gallstone formation results from a number of events, including hepatic secretion of bile supersaturated with cholesterol, nucleation of cholesterol monohydrate crystals in the gallbladder, and impaired emptying of the gallbladder contents. Biliary supersaturation with cholesterol commonly occurs in normal individuals during a portion of the day but occurs almost universally in patients with cholesterol gallstones [147]. Nucleation times appear to differentiate those who develop stones from those who do not.

Bile is an aqueous solution that is relatively enriched with water-insoluble hydrophobic lipids (cholesterol and phospholipids) solubilized in detergents (bile acids). The dissolved solids make up about 3%, by weight, of hepatic bile. Bile salts are the predominant solute, averaging 20–30 mmol/L in hepatic bile. Phospholipid concentrations average 7 mmol/L, and cholesterol averages 2–3 mmol/L. Bilirubin normally is present at concentrations of 0.2 mmol/L. Proteins are present in concentrations of about 0.2% by weight. A fraction of these proteins play an important role in cholesterol crystal nucleation and gallstone formation.

The principal lipid components (phospholipid and cholesterol) are solubilized by bile salt micelles. Bile salts are extremely effective solubilizers of phospholipids. In addition, the presence of phospholipid markedly increases the extent to which bile salts can incorporate cholesterol into micelles. The relative amounts of cholesterol, phospholipid, and bile salt that may coexist in micellar solution have been determined empirically by Admirand and Small [148] and by Carey and Small [149] (Figure 16.9).

The maximum equilibrium solubility of cholesterol in bile can be determined from the molar ratios of cholesterol, phospholipid, and bile acids and is expressed as the cholesterol saturation index. A supersaturated bile is one in which cholesterol concentration exceeds the maximum cholesterol saturation index and from which cholesterol monohydrate crystals precipitate.

Once cholesterol concentrations exceed their maximum equilibrium solubility, multilamellar cholesterol vesicles fuse and aggregate into a cluster that serves as a nidus for crystal formation. Nucleation may be either homogeneous or heterogeneous. Homogeneous nucleation occurs if crystallization occurs without foreign material. Heterogeneous nucleation occurs if crystallization takes place on a foreign surface such as epithelial cells, protein, calcium salts, or a foreign body. Because nucleation occurs rapidly at low levels of cholesterol supersaturation, it most probably occurs through a heterogeneous pathway.

Recently, promoters and inhibitors of cholesterol crystal formation and growth have been identified in human bile. These promoting and inhibiting factors may directly influence the "nucleating time" of bile. Biliary proteins of molecular weight 130 kDa have been proposed as potential pronucleators [150]. In contrast, there are proteins in normal bile that inhibit nucleation. These antinucleating factors may stabilize cholesterol–phospholipid vesicles in "normal" bile and retard crystallization. Potential candidate antinucleating proteins include apolipoproteins A-I and A-II [151].

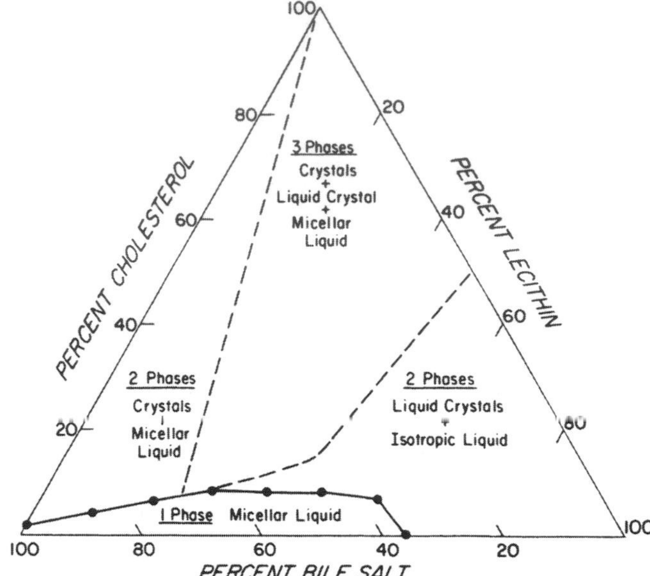

Figure 16.9. Tricoordinate phase diagram representing a single intersecting point for the relative concentrations of cholesterol, phospholipids, and bile salts in bile as proposed by Carey and Small [149]. Note that a clear micellar solution would be present with a composition of bile falling at the lower left of the diagram (micellar liquid). Bile with components that contain crystals would be supersaturated with cholesterol and prone to precipitate out of solution.

Gallbladder mucin also may promote stone formation. Mucin causes a time- and concentration-dependent acceleration of cholesterol crystallization [152]. Lee et al. [153] demonstrated that mucus hypersecretion occurs before gallstone formation in animals fed a gallstone-promoting diet. Inhibition of mucus secretion with aspirin prevents gallstone formation but does not alter the development of diet-induced biliary cholesterol supersaturation.

Current concepts regarding gallstone formation invoke the notion that nucleation of cholesterol crystals occurs in a mucous gel through protein–lipid interactions. The rate of cholesterol crystal nucleation may be influenced by a balance between pro- and antinucleating factors.

Gallbladder stasis facilitates growth of microscopic crystals into macroscopic stones. Animal studies have suggested that a gallbladder motility defect may antedate gallstone formation [154]. In addition, gallbladder motility worsens as stones develop. Biliary stasis complicates treatment with TPN and oral contraceptives and pregnancy [131,155].

Bile supersaturated with cholesterol may result from a deficiency of secretion of bile salts or phospholipids or a disproportionately increased secretion of cholesterol. Cholesterol stones are characteristically more common in women beyond puberty. The differences in prevalence between sexes decline after menopause. Pregnancy, which is associated with biliary cholesterol supersaturation and impaired gallbladder emptying, may

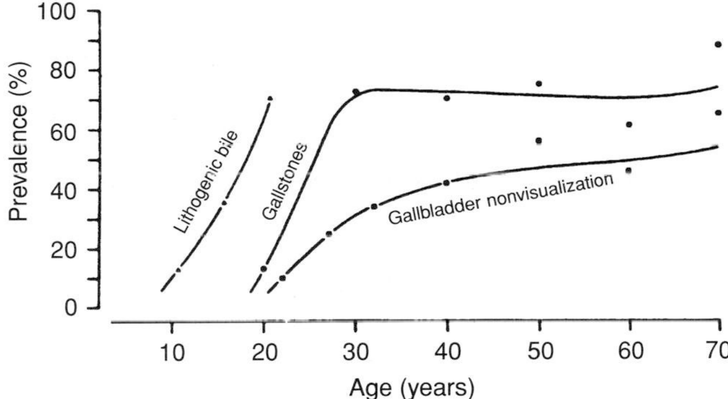

Figure 16.10. Natural history of gallstone disease in female Pima Indians [159]. Lithogenic bile first appears in the second decade of life. The prevalence of gallstones rises approximately 10 years later, followed by nonvisualization of the gallbladder, verified several years later by two consecutive oral cholecystograms without gallbladder opacification.

contribute to the increased frequency of stones in women of childbearing age. Estrogens and oral contraceptives enhance cholesterol saturation of bile and are associated with increases in cholelithiasis. American whites and blacks have a prevalence of cholesterol stones of 9% and 5%, respectively.

Limited information is available regarding biliary lipid composition and cholesterol saturation in normal infants and children. Bile is relatively undersaturated with cholesterol in infants and children compared with adults [156,157]. This finding may be explained by the observation that the bile salt pools expand rapidly after birth, and body size–matched pools in infancy and childhood actually exceed those observed in young adults [158,159]. This may lead to a higher biliary bile salt–cholesterol secretion ratio, with less saturated bile. In the Pima Indians, a population at high risk of cholesterol cholelithiasis in adulthood, biliary lipid composition is already abnormal by 9–12 years of age, and bile becomes very supersaturated in females after puberty [159]. Nearly 90% of Pima Indian women have gallstones by the age of 65 years [160]. The time course of development of biliary cholesterol saturation and gallstones is illustrated for this population in Figure 16.10. In populations at lower risk for cholesterol cholelithiasis and obesity, no significant changes in biliary cholesterol saturation are noted with puberty in males. In contrast, females have undersaturated bile before puberty, which becomes supersaturated after puberty [161]. Enhanced cholesterol secretion may be observed with certain drugs (e.g., estrogens, clofibrate). Most adults with gallstones have a combination of both reduced bile salt secretion and enhanced biliary cholesterol secretion.

Conditions Predisposing to Cholesterol Gallstone Formation

OBESITY

Obese adults have a prevalence of cholesterol gallstones that is almost twice that of the nonobese population. Evidence has accumulated that the biliary secretion of cholesterol is increased relative to bile acid and phospholipid secretion in obese subjects. As a consequence, bile is supersaturated with cholesterol, predisposing to stone formation. Supersaturated bile may develop at puberty in women and often is associated with obesity [162,163]. Unfortunately, little is known about nucleating factors in obesity. With weight loss, the cholesterol saturation actually increases. Once the patient's weight has stabilized at a lower level, the cholesterol saturation tends to decline. Little, if anything, is known about the risk of cholesterol gallstone formation in children with obesity; however, obesity appears to predispose to stone formation in adolescent females [164]. Findings from a recent German study suggest that the prevalence of gallstones could be as high as 2% in obese children and adolescents. Gallstones were more common in the more severely obese and older children, with no prepubertal children having stones [165].

Ileal Resection, Jejunoileal Bypass, or Ileal Crohn's Disease

The development of gallstones when the enterohepatic circulation is interrupted may be multifactorial. With excess fecal loss of bile acids, the pool is reduced, biliary bile acid secretion declines, and bile may become supersaturated with cholesterol. Concurrently, intestinal luminal binding of calcium to fatty acids with formation of fatty acid soaps may preclude bilirubin precipitation in the lumen, thereby allowing its reabsorption in the distal bowel with recirculation and reappearance in bile [165,166]. This may produce conditions conducive to both cholesterol and pigment stone formation. Gallstone prevalence in adults with inflammatory bowel disease affecting the ileum, assessed radiographically, ranges from 28–34%. The increased frequency of gallstones correlates with the duration and extent of ileal disease or the interval following ileal resection [167–169]. Recent studies have suggested that the incidence of gallstone disease was no greater in patients with ileal disease or resection than in appropriately age- and sex-matched control subjects [170]. In children, anecdotal reports have appeared that suggest that children with ileal resection or disease may have an increased incidence of cholelithiasis. In most circumstances, patients have been found to have pigment rather than cholesterol stones, with stone formation associated with conditions requiring prolonged parenteral nutrition and diuretics in the neonatal period [171–173]. Studies of biliary lipids in children with ileal resection or dysfunction have failed to demonstrate cholesterol supersaturation; after puberty, however, biliary cholesterol supersaturation develops [174]. It appears that children with ileal resection or dysfunction are not at increased risk of cholesterol cholelithiasis; after puberty, their biliary lipid composition is similar to that of adults, and they then may be prone to stone formation.

Cystic Fibrosis

Autopsy series have documented the presence of radiolucent gallstones in 12–27.5% of patients with cystic fibrosis. The gallbladder is hypoplastic in approximately 25% of patients, and at autopsy it is filled with clear mucus [175]. More recent prospective annual screening studies have shown a frequency of stones of approximately 5% [176]. Several abnormalities of bile salt metabolism have been identified in cystic fibrosis [177,178]. Initially, it was believed that increased fecal bile acid excretion led to reduced bile acid pools. Children, adolescents, and adults with cystic fibrosis were found to have high biliary cholesterol concentrations relative to bile acids and phospholipids and bile supersaturated with cholesterol [179]. Because of the radiolucency of gallstones and the cholesterol supersaturation of bile in patients with cystic fibrosis, it was assumed that gallstones in this disease were predominantly cholesterol. More recent studies have failed to confirm some of the observations made in the 1970s. The biliary lipid composition and bile acid pools in patients with cystic fibrosis have not been shown to be different from those in control subjects [180,181]. Recent work from Angelico et al. [182] suggests that the radiolucent stones found in cystic fibrosis may be pigment stones in most circumstances. Recent studies have suggested that fasting and residual gallbladder volumes are increased in patients with cystic fibrosis who do not have microgallbladders [183]. This finding, coupled with abnormalities of mucus, may predispose patients to stasis and nidus formation in the gallbladder.

Pregnancy

Women have a higher frequency of gallstones than do men at all ages from puberty to menopause [91,93,95]. This suggests that hormonal influences in women may play an important role in the pathogenesis of cholesterol gallstones. Women have a smaller total bile acid pool and enhanced biliary cholesterol secretion than men, resulting in increased biliary cholesterol saturation [184]. The use of oral contraceptives and pregnancy accentuate these sex-related differences. During pregnancy, the total bile acid pool expands; however, there is enhanced sequestration of the pool in the intestine [185]. Consequently, there is no change or a decline in the biliary bile acid secretion rate. Increases in gallbladder residual volume and fasting volumes and reductions in contractility and rate of emptying make pregnant women and those receiving oral contraceptives particularly susceptible to gallstone formation [186]. In two series of adolescent girls aged 14–20 years reported by Honore [164] and by Buimsohn et al. [187], strong associations were found between the presence of gallstones and parity and obesity. A weak, statistically nonsignificant association was found between oral contraceptive use and gallstones [164,187].

Miscellaneous

Gallstones have been identified in at least one child with familial hypobetalipoproteinemia who presented with obstructive jaundice. In this rare condition, stones may form because of increased biliary cholesterol secretion [188].

Clinical Features of Gallstones

In adults, gallstones may remain asymptomatic for years. The natural history of gallstones has been carefully studied. Gracie and Ransohoff [189] evaluated the outcome of gallstones in adults identified 24 years earlier on preemployment oral cholecystograms. The study population comprised 123 male university faculty members. In 16 subjects identified with asymptomatic or silent gallstones, symptoms developed that were heralded by the appearance of biliary tract pain. Three of 13 developed biliary tract complications, 2 with acute cholecystitis and 1 with pancreatitis. If complications occurred, they were likely to follow previous episodes of biliary colic. Based on this study, it appears that the risk of serious complications associated with silent gallstones is small. Nonelective cholecystectomy is necessary in less than 5% of patients with identified silent gallstones. No studies of this type have been performed in infants and children; however, there is no reason to believe that the risk of complications with silent stones would be higher in children than adults. Nonspecific dyspepsia, fatty food intolerance, and vague epigastric or right upper quadrant discomfort are common in adults with and without gallstones. In children, only recurrent right upper quadrant pain or epigastric pain would suggest gallstone disease. Typically, biliary colic is episodic and characterized by pain that is steady and lasts 1–3 hours, rather than colicky or crampy in nature. Although commonly localized to the right upper quadrant, pain may be localized to the epigastrium. Radiation of pain to the umbilicus may suggest the presence of acute appendicitis. Pain also may radiate to the right shoulder. Nausea and vomiting are common. Fever commonly is present in children younger than 15 years. Episodes of pain may occur irregularly over years, and the severity of attacks may vary.

The mechanism of pain is believed to relate to obstruction of the cystic duct. Pressure in the gallbladder increases in an attempt to contract against the obstruction. During an attack, there may be right upper abdomen or epigastric tenderness. Some guarding may be observed, but rebound is typically absent. Results of the physical examination may even be normal

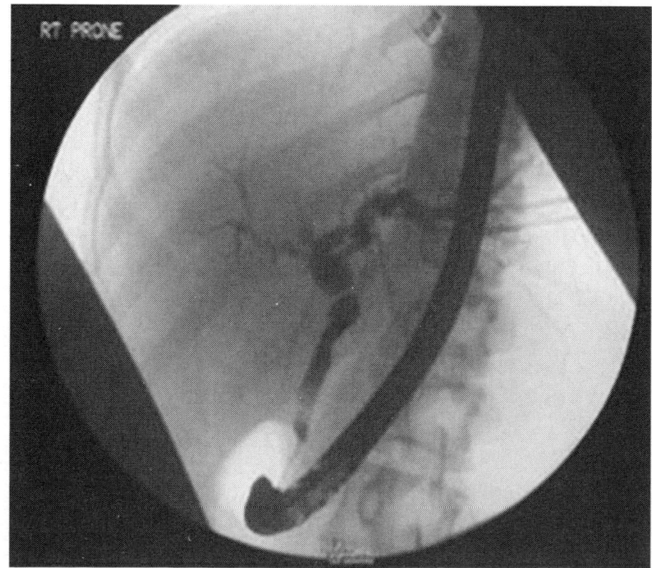

Figure 16.11. Common duct cannulated during endoscopic retrograde cholangiopancreatography. The contrast outlines the common duct stone, with proximal dilatation of the duct.

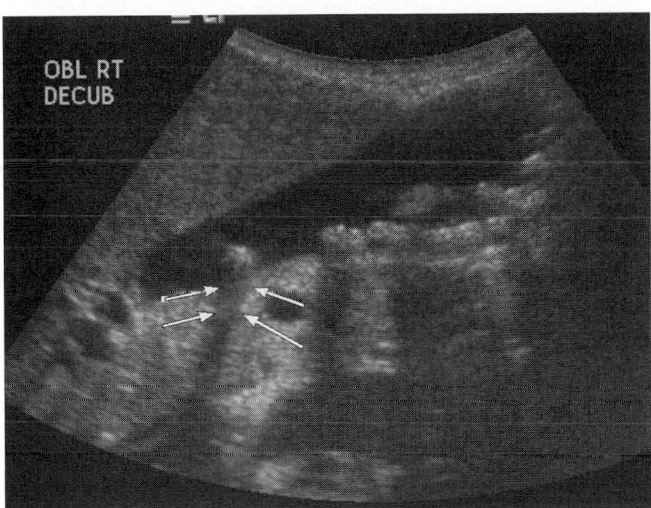

Figure 16.12. Real-time ultrasonogram demonstrating multiple, echogenic stones within the gallbladder with acoustic shadowing (*arrows*).

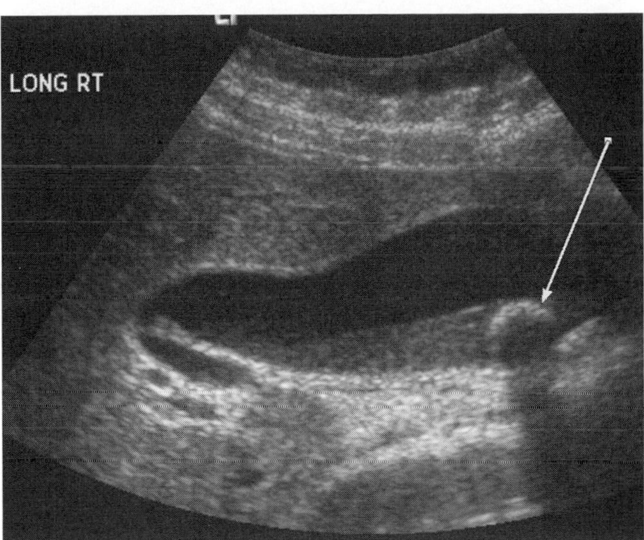

Figure 16.13. Longitudinal ultrasound of the right upper quadrant in a 16-year-old with sickle cell disease abdomen. The image shows echogenic sludge in the gallbladder and a stone with acoustic shadowing (*arrow*).

during an attack. Acute cholecystitis generally subsides spontaneously within a few days. In one third of patients, inflammation leads to necrosis with either perforation or empyema of the gallbladder. Passage of stones into the common bile duct may cause bile duct obstruction (Figure 16.11), cholangitis, and pancreatitis.

Laboratory test results commonly are normal. The white blood cell count may be normal. In a small fraction of patients, there is transient mild elevation of serum bilirubin, aminotransferase, and alkaline phosphatase levels.

Ultrasonography is the safest and most sensitive and specific method for identifying gallstones (Figure 16.12). If a gallbladder can be identified by ultrasound, the stone discovery rate is as high as 98% of that expected [190]. Typically stones appear as echogenic masses with acoustic shadows. Sludge may be identified as echogenic material that layers (Figure 16.13). A thickened gallbladder wall suggests inflammation. Plain abdominal radiographs identify only stones that have a high calcium content (usually about 15% of all stones). Additional diagnostic techniques may be helpful in some circumstances. Oral cholecystography may be helpful in identifying noncalculous causes of gallbladder disease and evaluating function. Cholescintigraphy, using one of the technetium-99m–labeled acetanilide aminodiacetic acid derivatives, is currently the most accurate method for evaluating the patient with acute cholecystitis [190]. Axial CT may also be helpful in demonstrating stones (Figure 16.14). In general, ultrasonographic evaluation is the method of choice for identifying gallstones in children and adolescents complaining of recurrent epigastric or right abdominal pain.

CHRONIC CHOLECYSTITIS OR CHOLELITHIASIS

Generally, some inflammation accompanies cholelithiasis. In some patients, chronic inflammation leads to the development of a fibrotic and shrunken gallbladder. With fibrosis, visualization of the gallbladder and its contents may be difficult with ultrasonography. As with acute cholecystitis, nuclear imaging techniques may prove helpful in diagnosing chronic cholecystitis. Failure of gallbladder visualization should suggest the presence of chronic cholecystitis.

TREATMENT OF CHOLELITHIASIS AND ACUTE AND CHRONIC CHOLECYSTITIS

Cholecystectomy is the definitive treatment for symptomatic stones. The only treatment questions that arise focus on the

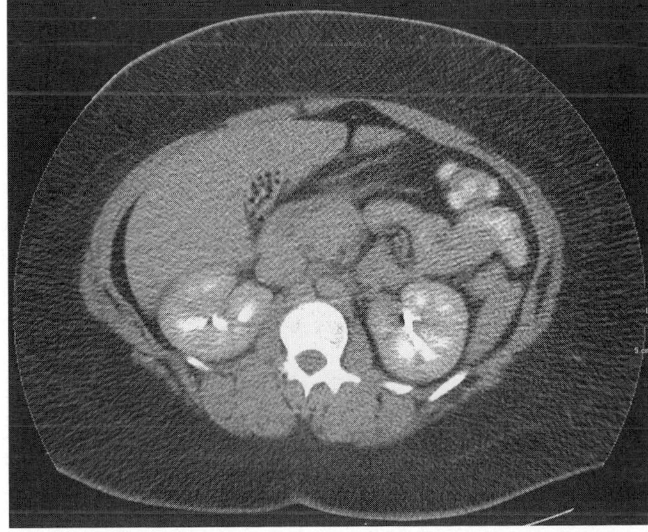

Figure 16.14. Axial CT of the abdomen demonstrating multiple cholesterol stones, which typically have a low attenuation.

timing of surgery and the operative approach. In a study in which patients with gallstones were monitored carefully, 112 patients who had experienced biliary pain in the previous 12 months were followed [191]. Sixty-nine percent developed recurrent pain within 2 years, and 6% required cholecystectomy. Those with recurrent pain are more likely to develop significant complications and should have elective cholecystectomy without prolonged waiting.

With acute cholecystitis, emergency cholecystectomy might be warranted if complications supervene; in most patients, however, cholecystectomy can be delayed safely for between a few days and 2–3 months. The only exception to the use of cholecystectomy for treatment of gallstones might be in patients whose medical conditions make operative cholecystectomy dangerous. In chronically ill children with high-risk conditions such as severe pulmonary compromise in cystic fibrosis, cholecystotomy might be a reasonable therapeutic alternative to cholecystectomy.

Cholecystectomy is one of the most common operations performed in the United States and Britain [192]. Experience with laparoscopic cholecystectomy has demonstrated its advantage over conventional forms of operative cholecystectomy. Indications for this technique in children are the same as for open cholecystectomy, and the gallbladder should be surgically removed from patients with symptomatic cholelithiasis or children with a hemoglobinopathy and asymptomatic cholelithiasis [193]. Several studies have demonstrated the efficacy of this technique in children with cholelithiasis caused by familial hyperlipidemia, hereditary spherocytosis, glucose-6-phosphatase deficiency, thalassemia, glycogen storage disease, and sickle cell anemia [122,123,193–197]. Pediatric laparoscopic cholecystectomy has been modified from the adult procedure because the operating area is considerably smaller and children have a higher risk of having an umbilical hernia adhering to the peritoneal lining [194]. Intraoperative cholangiography is important to rule out common bile duct stones or congenital biliary anomalies. Laparoscopic cholecystectomy allows a short postoperative recovery and is unlikely to have surgical complications [195]. Typically, the length of hospital stay with laparoscopic cholecystectomy is 1 or 2 days in the United States and patients are able to return to work or normal activity in 1–2 weeks. It is believed that approximately 80% of adults requiring cholecystectomy are suitable for the laparoscopic technique. The mortality rate with the technique is less than 1%. In about 5% of patients, the surgeon must perform an open cholecystectomy because of anatomic problems or adhesions. Patients with acute cholecystitis, pancreatitis, or a high probability of upper abdominal adhesions are not considered candidates for this procedure [198]. Reported experiences with laparoscopic cholecystectomy in children are limited. In a report of a 5-year experience from three institutions, including 110 children aged 1–16 years, there were no fatalities and the complication rate was 15.5%. As experience has been gained at most major pediatric centers, laparoscopic cholecystectomy has become the treatment of choice for elective cholecystectomies [199,200].

In adults with cholesterol stones, alternative nonsurgical therapies have been suggested, including dissolution with chenodeoxycholic or ursodeoxycholic acids or combinations of these agents, extracorporal shock wave lithotripsy with continued dissolution of fragments with oral bile acids, or direct instillation of cholesterol solvents into the gallbladder. The efficacies of bile acid, chenodeoxycholic acid, and ursodeoxycholic acid are similar [201]. Because of dose-related side effects associated with the use of chenodeoxycholic acid (diarrhea, increased aminotransferases, and modest hypercholesterolemia), it is not used at all for gallstone dissolution. If drug therapy is used, ursodeoxycholic acid is the drug of choice for oral gallstone dissolution. Dissolution of stones can be achieved in 60% of selected patients with small gallstones [202]. Unfortunately, cessation of therapy is associated with a recurrence rate of 10% per year. Most stones recur within 3–5 years after dissolution therapy [203–205]. The recurrence of stones seriously limits the utility of dissolution therapy in adults and makes it particularly unsuitable for children with gallstones because of the cost of lifelong administration of oral bile acids to prevent recurrence. Only for patients who are at a high surgical risk, including children, is oral therapy a reasonable treatment option.

Lithotripsy using shock waves has been used in the past to disintegrate stones after several hundred to several thousand shocks. Currently few, if any, centers use lithotripsy for stone dissolution, and any discussion is only of historical interest. Patients with solitary stones were the best candidates for this therapy [206]. Varying results have been obtained, depending on the number and size of gallstones found in the gallbladder. Large solitary stones of 2–3 cm may be dissolved in up to 90% of all patients after 13–18 months [207]. The efficacy is reduced with multiple smaller stones, even though the total stone mass may be smaller than with solitary stones. Without concomitant oral bile acid therapy, the gallstone recurrence rate is very high [208].

The management of asymptomatic adults with so-called silent gallstones found incidentally has changed over several decades. Silent stones do not require surgery or medical therapy, because their natural history is benign. Nonsurgical approaches to therapy, including oral bile acid therapy or lithotripsy, should not be considered for individuals with silent gallstones. For children with asymptomatic stones, the guidelines for therapy are not clear. It seems reasonable to assume that the risk of significant complications with silent gallstones in infants and children should be no greater than that observed in adult males in the studies of Gracie and Ransohoff [189]. With this in mind, expectant management would appear appropriate, particularly for otherwise healthy infants and children with stones that are smaller than 2 cm. For patients with smaller stones, serial ultrasonographic examinations appear warranted because spontaneous disappearance of stones may occur. Larger stones are more problematic. Gallstones may play a role in the development of carcinoma of the gallbladder, with larger stones (>2 cm) carrying a greater risk than small ones. Because larger stones are unlikely to disappear spontaneously, one could make a reasonable argument for removing the gallbladder in an otherwise asymptomatic child because of the inherent enhanced risk of gallbladder carcinoma caused by the presence of a stone in the gallbladder over several decades [209].

In infants and children with known hemolytic disease, pigment stone formation will only worsen with increasing age, and cholecystectomy at the time of identification of stones (even though they may be silent) appears warranted. Specifically, in patients with SCD, once stones are identified the gallbladder should be removed. With increasing age, it is clear that gallstone formation and the risk of cholecystitis and attendant adhesions increase. The differentiation between biliary colic and abdominal sickle cell crisis may be more difficult with increasing age, and the risk of operative intervention increases with age, so morbidity and mortality rates are lessened by early operative therapy. In patients with hemolytic disease, laparoscopic cholecystectomy should be considered before the development of chronic cholecystitis and potential attendant adhesions because of the lower operative morbidity rate and the reduced cost compared with operative cholecystectomy. Reports of small case series of laparoscopic cholecystectomy in children suggest that it has complication and mortality rates similar to those found in adults [123,199].

ACKNOWLEDGMENTS

The authors wish to acknowledge the valuable assistance of Lona Pearson for manuscript preparation and Janet Strife, MD, Division of Pediatric Radiology, Children's Hospital Medical Center, for supplying outstanding examples of ultrasonographic and CT examinations to illustrate the text. This work is supported in part by a grant from the National Center for Research Resources of the National Institutes of Health, M01-RR08084 and DK 068463.

REFERENCES

1. Langman J. The digestive system. In: Langman's medical embryology, 3rd ed. Baltimore: Williams & Wilkins, 1981:217–20.
2. Hamilton WJ. The alimentary and respiratory systems. In: Patton B, ed. Human embryology, 3rd ed. New York: McMillan Press, 1981:341.
3. Langman J. In: Langman's medical embryology, 6th ed. Baltimore: Williams & Wilkins, 1990:243.
4. Warkany J. The liver in congenital malformations. Chicago: Yearbook Medical Publishers, 1971:722–3.
5. Vanderpool D, Klinpensmith W, Oles P. Congenital absence of the gallbladder. Am Surgeon 1964;30:324–30.
6. Gross RE. Congenital abnormalities of the gallbladder: a review of one hundred and forty eight cases, with report of a double gallbladder. Arch Surg 1936;32:131–62.
7. Stolkind E. Congenital abnormalities of the gallbladder and extrahepatic ducts: review of two hundred forty five reported cases with report of thirty one unpublished cases. Br J Child Dis 1939;36:115,182,295.
8. Isenberg JN, L'Heureux PR, Warwick WJ, et al. Clinical observations on the biliary system in cystic fibrosis. Am J Gastroenterol 1976;65:134–41.
9. DeSchryver-Kecskemetri K. Gallbladder and biliary ducts. In: Anderson's pathology. 9th ed. St. Louis: Mosby, 1990:1321–45.
10. Williamson R. Acalculous disease of the gallbladder. Gut 1988; 29:860–72.
11. Curtis LE, Sheahan DG. Heterotopic tissues in the gallbladder. Arch Pathol 1969;88:677–83.
12. Busuttil A. Ectopic adrenal within the gallbladder wall. J Pathol 1974;113:231–3.
13. Thorsness ET. An aberrant pancreatic nodule arising on the neck of a human gallbladder from multiple outgrowths of the mucosa. Anat Rec 1940;77:319–33.
14. Ishibashi T, Nagai H, Yasuda T, et al. Pancreatic bladder or double gallbladder draining into the pancreatic duct? J Hepatobiliary Pancreat Surg 1999;6:199–203.
15. Skielboe B. Anomalies of the gallbladder-vesica fellea triplex: report of a case. Am J Clin Pathol 1958;30:252.
16. Greenwood RK. Torsion of the gallbladder. Gut 1963;4:27–9.
17. Shaikh AA, Charles A, Domingo S, Schaub G. Gallbladder volvulus: report of two original cases and review of the literature. Am Surg 2005;71:87–9.
18. Logan GB, Thistle JL. The gallbladder and bile ducts. In: Practice of pediatrics. Vol 5. Philadelphia: Harper and Row, 1986:1–18.
19. Holcomb GW Jr, O'Neill JA, Holcomb GW III. Cholecystitis cholelithiasis and common duct stones in children and adolescents. Ann Surg 1980;191:626–35.
20. Silverman A, Roy CC. Acute and chronic biliary tract disease. In: Pediatric clinical gastroenterology. 3rd ed. St. Louis: Mosby, 1983.
21. Rumley TO, Rodgers BM. Hydrops of the gallbladder in children. J Pediatr Surg 1983;18:138–40.
22. Suddleson EA, Reid B, Woolley MM, et al. Hydrops of the gallbladder associated with Kawasaki syndrome. J Pediatr Surg 1987;22:956–9.
23. Grisoni E, Fisher R, Izant R. Kawasaki syndrome: report of four cases with acute gallbladder hydrops. J Pediatr Surg 1984;19:9–11.
24. Melish ME, Hicks RV, Reddy V. Kawasaki syndrome: an update. Hosp Pract (Off Ed) 1982;17:99–106.
25. Friesen CA, Gamis AS, Riddell LD, et al. Bilirubinemia: an early indicator of gallbladder hydrops associated with Kawasaki disease. J Pediatr Gastroenterol Nutr 1989;8:384–6.
26. Slovis TL, Hight DW, Pilippart AI, et al. Sonography in the diagnosis and management of hydrops of the gallbladder in children with mucocutaneous lymph node syndrome. Pediatrics 1980;65:789–94.
27. Mercer S, Carpenter B. Surgical complications of Kawasaki disease. J Pediatr Surg 1981;16:444–8.
28. Sty JR, Starshak RJ, Gorenstein L. Gallbladder perforation in a case of Kawasaki disease: image correlation. J Clin Ultrasound 1983;11:381–4.
29. Magilavy DB, Speert DP, Silver TM, et al. Mucocutaneous lymph node syndrome: report of two cases complicated by gallbladder hydrops and diagnosed by ultrasound. Pediatrics 1978;61:699–702.
30. Strauss RG. Scarlet fever with hydrops of the gallbladder. Pediatrics 1969;44:741–5.
31. Dickinson SJ, Corley G, Santulli T. Acute cholecystitis as a sequel of scarlet fever. Am J Dis Child 1971;121:331–3.
32. Chamberlain JW, Hight DW. Acute hydrops of the gallbladder in childhood. Surgery 1970;68:899–905.

33. Bloom RA, Swain VAJ. Non-calculous distension of the gallbladder in childhood. Arch Dis Child 1966;41:503–8.
34. Tanaka K, Shimada M, Hattori M, et al. Sjogren's syndrome with abnormal manifestations of the gallbladder and central nervous system. J Pediatr Gastroenterol Nutr 1985;4:148–51.
35. McGahan JJ, Whittinghill JA. Acute idiopathic hydrops of the gallbladder not due to calculi possibly to infectious hepatitis. Pediatrics 1958;21:91–3.
36. McCrindle BW, Wood RA, Nussbaum AR. Henoch-Schonlein Syndrome, unusual manifestations with hydrops of the gallbladder. Clin Pediatr 1988;27:254–6.
37. Goren A, Drachman R, Hadas-Halperin I, et al. Transient gallbladder dilatation associated with hypokalemia in a patient with Bartter syndrome. Eur J Pediatr 1989;149:88–9.
38. Gomezcoe S, Garcia F, Echeverry J, et al. New aspects of gallbladder pathology in children. Cir Pediatr 1989;2:114–16.
39. El-Shafie M, Mah CL. Transient gallbladder distension in sick premature infants: the value of ultrasonography and radionuclide scintigraphy. Pediatr Radiol 1986;16:468–71.
40. Bowen A. Acute gallbladder dilatation in a neonate: emphasis on ultrasonography. J Pediatr Gastroenterol Nutr 1984;3:304–8.
41. Peevy KJ, Wiseman HJ. Gallbladder distension in septic neonates. Arch Dis Child 1982;57:75–6.
42. Longino LA, Martin LW. Abdominal masses in the newborn infant. Pediatrics 1958;21:596–604.
43. Gremse DA, Peevy KJ, Simon N, et al. Neonatal gallbladder enlargement and α_1-antitrypsin deficiency. J Pediatr Gastroenterol Nutr 1987;6:977–9.
44. Traynelis VC, Hrabovsky EE. Acalculous cholecystitis in the neonate. Am J Dis Child 1985;139:893–5.
45. Ternberg JL, Keating JP. Acute acalculous cholecystitis. Arch Surg 1975;110:543–7.
46. Wald M. Gangrenous cholecystitis with bile peritonitis as a complication of burns in a 14 year old boy. Med J Aust 1961;11:553–5.
47. Rice J, Williams H, Lewis MF, et al. Postraumatic acalculous cholecystitis. South Med J 1980;73:14–17.
48. Imamoglu M, Sarihan H, Sari A, Ahmetoglu A. Acute acalculous cholecystitis in children: diagnosis and treatment. J Pediatr Surg 2002;37:36–9.
49. Hyams JS, Baker E, Schwartz AN, et al. Acalculous cholecystitis in Crohn's disease. J Adolesc Health Care 1989;10:151–4.
50. Wong ML, Kaplan S, Dunkle LM, et al. Leptospirosis: a childhood disease. J Pediatr 1977;90:532–7.
51. Walker DH, Leseske HR, Varma VA, et al. Rocky Mountain spotted fever mimicking acute cholecystitis. Arch Intern Med 1985;145:2194–6.
52. Reid MR, Montgomery JC. Acute cholecystitis in children as a complication of typhoid fever. Johns Hopkins Hosp Bull 1920; 347:7–11.
53. Schmidt MH, Sung L, Shuckett BM. Hemophaogcytic lymphohistiocytosis in children: abdominal US findings within 1 week of presentation. Radiology 2004;230:685–9.
54. Chateil J, Brun M, Perel Y, et al. Abdominal ultrasound findings in children with hemophagocytic lymphohistiocytosis. Eur Radiol 1999;9:474–7.
55. Weedon D. Disease of the gallbladder. In: Pathology of the liver. 2nd ed. New York: Churchill Livingstone, 1987:454–77.
56. Schreiber M, Black L, Noah Z, et al. Gallbladder candidiasis in a leukemic child. Am J Dis Child 1982;136:462–3.
57. Reubner B. The gallbladder. In: Diagnostic pathology of the liver and biliary tract. New York: Hemisphere, 1991:454–67.
58. Pitlik SD, Fainstein V, Garza D, et al. Human cryptosporidiosis: spectrum of disease. Arch Intern Med 1983;143:2269–75.
59. Sanders R. The significance of sonographic gallbladder wall thickening. J Clin Ultrasound 1980;8:143–6.
60. Patriquin HB, DiPietro M, Barber FE, et al. Sonography of thickened gallbladder wall: causes in children. AJR 1983;141:57–60.
61. Jeffrey RB Jr, Sommer FG. Follow-up sonography in suspected acalculous cholecystitis: preliminary clinical experience. J Ultrasound Med 1993;12:183–7.
62. Swayne LC. Acute acalculous cholecystitis: sensitivity in detection using technetium-99m imiodiacetic acid cholescintigraphy. Radiology 1986;160:33–8.
63. Mirvis SE, Vainright JR, Nelson AW, et al. The diagnosis of acute acalculous cholecystitis: a comparison of sonography, scintigraphy and CT. AJR 1986;147:1171–5.
64. Shuman WP, Gibbs P, Rudd TG, et al. PIPIDA scintigraphy for cholecystitis: false positives in alcoholism and total parenteral nutrition. AJR 1982;138:1–5.
65. Lugo-Vincente HL. Gallbladder dyskinesia in children. J Soc Laparoendosc Surg 1997;1:61–4.
66. Gollin G, Raschbaum GR, Moorthy C, et al. Cholecystectomy for suspected biliary dyskinesia in children with chronic abdominal pain. J Pediatr Surg 1999;34:854–7.
67. Dumont RC, Caniano DA. Hypokinetic gallbladder disease: a cause of chronic abdominal pain in children and adolescents. J Pediatr Surg 1999;34:858–61.
68. Vegunta RK, Raso M, Pollock J, et al. Biliary dyskinesia: the most common indication for cholecystectomy in children. Surgery 2005;138:726–31.
69. Tasdemir HA, Cetinkaya MC, Polat C, et al. Gallbladder motility in children with Down syndrome. J Pediatr Gastroent Nutr 2004;39:187–91.
70. Arlanoglu I, Unal F, Sagin F, et al. Real-time sonography for screening gallbladder dysfunction in children with type 1 diabetes mellitus. J Pediatr Endocrinol Metab 2001;14:61–9.
71. McClure J, Benerjee SS, Schofield PS. Crohn's disease of the gallbladder. J Clin Pathol 1984;37:516–18.
72. Ranchod M, Kahn LB. Malacoplakia of the GI tract. Arch Pathol 1972;94:90–7.
73. Livolsi VA, Perzin KH, Porter M. Polyarteritis nodosa of the gallbladder presenting as acute cholecystitis. Gastroenterology 1973;65:115–23.
74. Mogilner JG, Dharan M, Siplovich M. Adenoma of the gallbladder in childhood. J Pediatr Surg 1991;26:223–4.
75. Stringel G, Beneck D, Bostwick HE. Polypoid lesions of the gallbladder in children. J Soc Laparoendosc Surg 1997;1:247–9.
76. Foster DR, Foster DBE. Gallbladder polyps in Peutz-Jeghers syndrome. Postgrad Med J 1980;56:373–6.
77. Cetinkursum S, Surer I, Devceci S, et al. Adenomyomatosis of the gallbladder in a child. Dig Dis Sci 2003;48:733–6.
78. Alberti D, Callea F, Camoni G, et al. Adenomyomatosis of the gallbladder in childhood. J Pediatr Surg 1998;33:1411–12.
79. Zani A, Pacilli M, Conforti A, et al. Adenomyomatosis of the gallbladder in childhood: report of a case and review of the literature. Pediatr Dev Path 2005;8:577–80.
80. Ruymann FB, Raney RB, Crist WM, et al. Rhabdomyosarcoma of the biliary tree in childhood: a report from the Intergroup Rhabdomyosarcoma Study. Cancer 1985;56:575–81.
81. Casteel HB, Williamson SL, Golladay ES, et al. Porcelain gallbladder in a child: a case report. J Pediatr Surg 1990;25:1302–3.

82. Snajdauf J, Petru O, Pycha K, et al. Porcelain gallbladder with extrahepatic duct obstruction in a child. Pediatr Surg Int 2006;22:293–6.
83. Beauregard WG, Ferguson WT. Milk of calcium cholecystitis. J Pediatr 1980;96:876–7.
84. Takiff H, Funkalsrud EW. Gallbladder disease in childhood. Am J Dis Child 1984;138:565–8.
85. Strom BL, West SL. The epidemiology of gallstone disease. In: Cohen S, Soloway RD, eds. Gallstones. New York: Churchill Livingstone, 1985.
86. Friedman GD, Kannel WB, Dawber TR. The epidemiology of gallbladder disease: observations in Framingham study. J Chron Dis 1966;19:273–92.
87. Kingensmith WC, Cioffi-Ragan DT. Fetal gallstones. Radiology 1988;167:143–4.
88. Suma V, Marini A, Bucci N, et al. Fetal gallstones: sonographic and clinical observations. Ultrasound Obstet Gynecol 1998;12:439–41.
89. Ghose I, Stringer MD. Successful nonoperative management of neonatal acute calculous cholecystitis. J Pediatr Surg 1999;34: 1029–30.
90. Palasciano G, Portincasa P, Vinciguerra V, et al. Gallstone prevalence and gallbladder volume in children and adolescents: an epidemiological ultrasonographic survey and relationship to body mass index. Am J Gastroenterol 1989;84:1378–82.
91. Barbara L, Sama C, Labate AMM, et al. A population study on the prevalence of gallstone disease: the Sirmione Study. Hepatology 1987;7:913–17.
92. Nilsson S. Gallbladder disease and sex hormones. Acta Chir Scand 1966;132:275–9.
93. Jorgensen T. Prevalence of gallstones in a Danish population. Am J Epidemiol 1987;126:912–21.
94. Shaffer EA, Small DM. Gallstone disease: pathogenesis and management. Curr Probl Surg 1976;13:3–72.
95. Friesen CA, Roberts CC. Cholelithiasis: clinical characteristics in children. Clin Pediatr 1989;7:294–8.
96. Stringer MD, Taylor DR, Soloway RD. Gallstone composition: are children different? J Pediatr 2003;142:435–40.
97. Soderlund S, Zetterstrom B. Cholecystitis and cholelithiasis in children. Arch Dis Child 1962;37:174–80.
98. Sears HF, Golden GT, Horsley JS III. Cholecystitis in adolescents. Arch Surg 1973;106:651–3.
99. Newman HF, Northrup JD. The autopsy incidence of gallstones. Int Abst Surg 1959;109:1–13.
100. Trotman BW, Soloway RD. Pigment vs. cholesterol cholelithiasis: clinical and epidemiological aspects. Am J Dig Dis 1975; 20:735–40.
101. Holcomb GW Jr, Holcomb GW. Cholelithiasis in infants, children and adolescents. Pediatr Rev 1991;11:268–74.
102. Pokorny WJ, Saleem M, O'Gorman RB, et al. Cholelithiasis and cholecystitis in childhood. Am J Surg 1984;148:742–4.
103. MacMillan RW, Schullinger JN, Santulli TV. Cholelithiasis in childhood. Am J Surg 1974;127:689–92.
104. Harned RK, Babbit DP. Cholelithiasis in childhood. Radiology 1975;117:391–3.
105. Andrassy RJ, Treadwell TA, Ratner IA. Gallbladder disease in childhood and adolescents. Am J Surg 1976;132:19–21.
106. Odom FC, Oliver BB, Kline M. Gallbladder disease in patients 20 years of age and younger. South Med J 1976;69:1299–300.
107. Grace N, Rogers B. Cholecystitis in childhood. Clin Pediatr 1977;16:179–81.
108. Reif S, Sloven DG, Lebenthal E. Gallstones in children. Am J Dis Child 1991;145:105–8.
109. Goodman DB. Cholelithiasis in persons under 25 years old. JAMA 1976;236:1731–2.
110. Bailey PV, Connors RH, Tracy TF Jr, et al. Changing spectrum of cholelithiasis and cholecystitis in infants and children. Am J Surg 1989;158:585–8.
111. Strauss RT. Cholelithiasis in childhood. Am J Dis Child 1969; 117:689–92.
112. Trotman BW, Soloway RD. Pigment gallstone disease: summary of the National Institutes of Health – International Workshop. Hepatology 1982;2:879–84.
113. Dolgin SM, Schwartz S, Knessel HS, et al. Identification of patients with cholesterol on pigment stones by discriminant analysis of radiographic features. N Engl J Med 1981;304: 808–11.
114. Trotman BW, Petrella EJ, Soloway RD, et al. Evaluation of radiographic lucency or opaqueness of gallstones as a means of identifying cholesterol or pigment stones. Gastroenterology 1975;68:1563–6.
115. Soloway RD, Trotman BW, Ostrow JD. Pigment gallstones. Gastroenterology 1977;72:167–82.
116. Ostrow JD, Celic L. Bilirubin chemistry, ionization and solubilization by bile salts. Hepatology 1984;4:385–455.
117. Cahalane MJ, Neubrand MW, Carey MC. Physical-chemical pathogenesis of pigment gallstones. Semin Liver Dis 1988;8: 317–28.
118. LaMont JT, Ventola AS, Trotman BW, et al. Mucin glycoprotein content of human pigment gallstones. Hepatology 1983;3: 377–82.
119. Bond LR, Hatty SR, Horn MEC, et al. Gallstones in sickle cell disease in the United Kingdom. Br J Med 1987;295: 234–6.
120. Schubert TT. Hepatobiliary system in sickle cell disease. Gastroenterology 1986;90:2013–21.
121. Sarnaik S, Slovis TL, Corbett DP, et al. Incidence of cholelithiasis in sickle-cell anemia using the ultrasonic gray-scale technique. J Pediatrics 1980;96:1005–8.
122. Walker WM, Hambleton IR, Serjeant GR. Gallstones in sickle cell disease: observations from the Jamaican cohort study. J Pediatr 2000;136:80–5.
123. Suell MN, Horton TM, Dishop MK, et al. Outcomes for children with gallbladder abnormalities and sickle cell disease. J Pediatr 2004;145:617–21.
124. Alonso MH. Gallbladder abnormalities in children with sickle cell disease: management with laparoscopic cholecystectomy. J Pediatr 2004;145:580–1.
125. Matos C, Avni EF, Van Gansbeke D, et al. Total parenteral nutrition (TPN) and gallbladder diseases in neonates. J Ultrasound Med 1987;6:243–8.
126. King DR, Ginn-Pease ME, Lloyd TV, et al. Parenteral nutrition with associated cholelithiasis: another iatrogenic disease of infants and children. J Pediatr Surg 1987;22:593–6.
127. Roslyn JJ, Berquist WE, Pitt HA, et al. Increased risk of gallstones in children receiving total parenteral nutrition. Pediatrics 1983;71:784–9.
128. Jacir NN, Anderson KD, Eichelberger M, et al. Cholelithiasis in infancy: resolution of gallstones in three of four infants. J Pediatr Surg 1986;21:567–9.
129. Keller MS, Markle BM, Laffey PA, et al. Spontaneous resolution of cholelithiasis in infants. Radiology 1985;155:345–8.

130. Schirmer WJ, Grisoni ER, Gauderer WL. The spectrum of cholelithiasis in the first year of life. J Pediatr Surg 1989;24: 1064–7.
131. Messing B, Bories C, Kunstlinger F, et al. Does total parenteral nutrition induce gallbladder sludge formation and lithiasis? Gastroenterology 1983;84:1012–19.
132. Sitzmann JV, Pitt HA, Steinborn PA, et al. Cholecystokinin prevents parenteral nutrition induced biliary sludge in humans. Surg Gynecol Obstet 1990;170:25–31.
133. Tsai S, Strouse PJ, Drongowski RA, et al. Failure of cholecystokinin-octapeptide to prevent TPN-associated gallstone disease. J Pediatr Surg 2005;40:263–7.
134. Mashako NNL, Cezard J-P, Borge N, et al. The effect of artificial feeding on cholestasis, gallbladder sludge and lithiasis in infants: correlation with plasma cholecystokinin levels. Clin Nutr 1991;10:320–7.
135. Nicholas P, Rinaudo PA, Conn CO. Increased incidence of cholelithiasis in Laennec's cirrhosis. Gastroenterology 1972;62: 112–14.
136. Bonchier IAD. Postmortem study of the frequency of gallstones in patients with cirrhosis of the liver. Gut 1969;10:705–10.
137. Angelin B, Einarsson K, Ewerth S, et al. Biliary lipid composition in patients with portal cirrhosis of the liver. Scand J Gastroenterol 1980;15:849–52.
138. Odievre M, Gautier M, Hadchouel M, et al. Severe familial intrahepatic cholestasis. Arch Dis Child 1973;48:806–12.
139. Fiqueroa-Colon R, Tolaymat N, Kao SCS. Gallbladder sludge and lithiasis in an infant born to a morphine user mother. J Pediatr Gastroenterol Nutr 1990;10:234–8.
140. Schaad UB, Suter S, Gianella-Borradovi A, et al. A comparison of ceftriaxone and cefuroxime for the treatment of bacterial meningitis in children. N Engl J Med 1990;522:141–7.
141. Xia Y, Lembert K, Gu JJ, et al. The mechanism of biliary sludge formation during ceftriaxone therapy. Gastroenterology 1989;95:A674.
142. Mahmond H, Schell M, Pui C-H. Cholelithiasis after treatment for childhood cancer. Cancer 1991;67:1439–42.
143. Sakopoulos AG, Gundry S, Razzouk AJ, et al. Cholelithiasis in infant and pediatric heart transplant patients. Pediatr Transplant 2002;6:231–4.
144. Percy AK, Lane JB. Rett syndrome: model of neurodevelopmental disorders. J Clin Neurol 2005;20:718–21.
145. Shaffer EA. Gallbladder disease. In: Walker WA, Durie PR, Hamilton JR, et al., eds. Pediatric gastrointestinal disease. Vol 2. Philadelphia: Mosby, 1991:1152–70.
146. Treem WR, Malet PF, Gourley GR, et al. Bile and stone analysis in two infants with brown pigment gallstones and infected bile. Gastroenterology 1989;96:519–23.
147. Holzbach RT, Marsh M, Olszewski M, et al. Cholesterol solubility in bile: evidence that supersaturated bile is frequent in healthy man. J Clin Invest 1973;52:1467–79.
148. Admirand WH, Small DM. The physico-chemical basis of cholesterol gallstone formation in man. J Clin Invest 1968;47: 1043–52.
149. Carey MC, Small DM. The physical chemistry of cholesterol solubility in bile: relationship to gallstone formation and dissolution in man. J Clin Invest 1978;61:998–1026.
150. Groen AK, Noordam C, Drapers JAG, et al. Isolation of a potent cholesterol nucleation-promoting activity from human gallbladder bile: role in the pathogenesis of gallstone disease. Hepatology 1990;11:525–33.
151. Kibe A, Holzbach RT, LaRusso NF, et al. Inhibition of cholesterol crystal formation by apolipoproteins in supersaturated model bile. Science 1984;25:514–16.
152. Bouchier IAD, Cooperband SR, Aikodsi BM. Mucous substances and viscosity of normal and pathological human bile. Gastroenterology 1965;49:343–53.
153. Lee SP, LaMont JT, Carey MC. Role of gallstone mucous hypersecretion in the evolution of cholesterol gallstone: studies in a prairie dog. J Clin Invest 1981;67:1712–23.
154. Fridhandler TM, Davison JS, Shaffer EA. Defective gallbladder contractility in the ground squirrel and prairie dog during the early stages of cholesterol gallstone formation. Gastroenterology 1983;85:830–6.
155. Kern F Jr, Everson GT, DeMark B, et al. Biliary lipids, bile acids, and gallbladder function in the human female: effects of pregnancy and the ovulatory cycle. J Clin Invest 1981;68:1229–42.
156. Heubi JE, Soloway RD, Balistreri WF. Biliary lipid composition in healthy and diseased infants, children and young adults. Gastroenterology 1982;82:1295–9.
157. von Bergmann J, von Bergmann K, Hadorn B, et al. Biliary lipid composition in early childhood. Clin Chim Acta 1975;64:241–6.
158. Heubi JE, Balistreri WF, Suchy FJ. Bile salt metabolism in first year of life. J Lab Clin Med 1982;100:127–36.
159. Bennion LJ, Knowler WC, Mott DM, et al. Development of lithogenic bile during puberty in Pima Indians. N. Engl J Med 1979;300:873–6.
160. Sampliner RE, Bennett PH, Comess LJ, et al. Gallbladder disease in Pima Indians: demonstration of high prevalence and early onset by cholecystography. N Engl J Med 1970;283:1358–64.
161. von Bergmann K, Becker M, Leiss O. Biliary cholesterol saturation in non-obese women and non-obese men before and after puberty. Eur J Clin Invest 1986;16:531–5.
162. Bennion LJ, Grundy SM. Effects of obesity and caloric intake on biliary lipid metabolism in man. J Clin Invest 1975;56:996–1011.
163. Shaffer EA, Small DM. Biliary lipid secretion in cholesterol gallstone disease: the effect of cholecystectomy and obesity. J Clin Invest 1977;59:828–40.
164. Honore LH. Cholesterol cholelithiasis in adolescent females. Arch Surg 1980;114:62–4.
165. Kaechele V, Wabitsch M, Thiere D, et al. Prevalence of gallbladder stone disease in obese children and adolescents: influence of the degree of obesity, sex and pubertal development. J Pediatr Gastroent Nutr 2006;42:66–70.
166. Dowling RH, Bell GD, White J. Lithogenic bile in patients with ileal dysfunction. Gut 1972;13:415–20.
167. Brink MA, Sors JPM, Keulemans CA, et al. Enterohepatic cycling of bilirubin: a putative mechanism for pigment gallstone formation in Crohn's disase. Gastroenterology 1999;116:1420–7.
168. Heaton KW, Read AE. Gallstones in patients with disorders of the terminal ileum and disturbed bile salt metabolism. Br Med J 1969;3:494–6.
169. Baker AL, Kaplan MM, Norton RA, et al. Gallstones in inflammatory bowel disease. Am J Dig Dis 1974;19:109–12.
170. Cohen S, Kaplan M, Gottlieb L, et al. Liver disease and gallstones in regional enteritis. Gastroenterology 1971;60:237–45.
171. Farkkila MA. Biliary cholesterol and lithogenicity of bile in patients after ileal resection. Surgery 1988;104:18–25.
172. Pellerin D, Bertin P, Nikhoul-Fekete C. Cholelithiasis and ileal pathology in childhood. J Pediatr Surg 1975;10:35–41.

173. Kirks DR. Lithiasis due to interruption of the enterohepatic circulation of bile salts. Am J Radiol 1979;133:383–8.
174. Heubi JE, O'Connell NC, Setchell KDR. Ileal resection/dysfunction in childhood predisposes to lithogenic bile after puberty. Gastroenterology 1992;103:636–40.
175. Esterly J, Oppenheimer E. Observations in cystic fibrosis of the pancreas: 1. the gallbladder. Johns Hopkins Hosp Bull 1962;110: 247–54.
176. Williams SM, Goodman R, Thomson A, et al. Ultrasound evaluation of liver disease in cystic fibrosis as part of an annual assessment clinic: a 9-year review. Clin Radiol 2002;57:365–70.
177. Weber A, Roy C, Morin C, et al. Malabsorption of bile acids in children with cystic fibrosis. N Engl J Med 1973;289:1001–5.
178. Watkins J, Tercyal A, Szcepanik P, et al. Bile salt kinetics in cystic fibrosis: influence of pancreatic enzyme replacement. Gastroenterology 1977;73:1023–8.
179. Roy C, Weber A, Morin C, et al. Abnormal biliary lipid composition in cystic fibrosis. N Engl J Med 1977;297:1301–5.
180. Strandvik B, Angelin B, Einarsson K. Bile acid kinetics and bile lipid composition in cystic fibrosis [abstract]. Scand J Gastroenterol 1988;23(suppl 143):166.
181. Becker M, Staab D, Leiss O, et al. Biliary lipid composition in patients with cystic fibrosis. J Pediatr Gastroenterol Nutr 1989; 8:308–12.
182. Angelico M, Gandin C, Canuzzi P. Gallstones in cystic fibrosis: a critical reappraisal. Hepatology 1991;14:768–75.
183. Santamaria F, Vajro P, Oggero V, et al. Volume and emptying of the gallbladder in patients with cystic fibrosis. J Pediatr Gastroenterol Nutr 1990;10:303–6.
184. Bennion LJ, Drobny E, Knowler WC, et al. Sex differences in the size of bile acid pools. Metabolism 1978;27:961–9.
185. Kern F, Everson GT, DeMark B, et al. Biliary lipids, bile acids, and gallbladder function in the human female: effects of pregnancy and the ovulatory cycle. J Clin Invest 1981;68:1229–42.
186. Braverman DZ, Johnson ML, Kern F Jr. Effects of pregnancy and contraceptive steroids on gallbladder function. N Engl J Med 1980;302:362–4.
187. Buimsohn A, Albu E, Geist PH, et al. Cholelithiasis and teenage mothers. J Adolesc Health Care 1990;11:339–42.
188. Lancellotti S, Zaffanello M, DiLeo E, et al. Pediatric gallstone disease in familial hypobetalipoproteinemia. J Hepatol 2005;43: 188–91.
189. Gracie WA, Ransohoff DF. The natural history of silent gallstones. The innocent gallstone is not a myth. N Engl J Med 1982; 307:798–800.
190. Way LA, Sleisenger MH. Cholelithiasis: chronic and acute cholecystitis in gastrointestinal disease. In: Sleisinger MH, Fordtran JS, eds. Gastrointestinal disease. 4th ed. Philadelphia: WB Saunders, 1989:1691–714.
191. Comfort MW, Gray HK, Wilson JM. The silent gallstone: a ten to twenty year follow-up of 112 cases. Ann Surg 1948;128:931–7.
192. Sauerbruch T, Paumgartner G. Gallbladder stones: management. Lancet 1991;338:1121–4.
193. Simi M, Schietroma M, Carlei F, et al. Is laparoscopic cholecystectomy a safe alternative to open cholecystectomy for pediatric patients with cholelithiasis. Endoscopy 1996;28:312–15.
194. Davidoff AM, Branum GD, Murray EA, et al. The technique of laparoscopic cholecystectomy in children. Ann Surg 1992;215: 186–91.
195. Vinograd I, Halevy A, Klin B, et al. Laparoscopic cholecystectomy: treatment of choice for cholelithiasis in children. World J Surg 1993;17:263–6.
196. Ware RE, Kinney TR, Casey JR, et al. Laparoscopic cholecystectomy in young patients with sickle hemoglobinopathies. J Pediatr 1992;120:58–61.
197. Holcomb GW, Naffis D. Laparoscopic cholecystectomy in infants. J Pediatr Surg 1994;29:86–7.
198. The Southern Surgeons Club. A prospective analysis of 1518 laparoscopic cholecystectomies. N Engl J Med 1991;324:1073–8.
199. Newman KD, Marmon LM, Attorri R, et al. Laparoscopic cholecystectomy in pediatric patients. J Pediatr Surg 1991;26:1184–5.
200. Esposito C, Gonzales Sabin MA, Corcione F, et al. Results and complications of laparoscopic cholecystectomy in childhood. Surg Endosc 2001;15:890–2.
201. Fromm H, Malavolti M. Dissolving gallstones. Adv Intern Med 1988;33:409–30.
202. Podda M, Zuin M, Battezzati PM, et al. Efficacy and safety of a combination of chenodeoxycholic acid and ursodeoxycholic acid for gallstone dissolution: a comparison with ursodeoxycholic acid alone. Gastroenterology 1989;96:222–9.
203. Lancini A, Jazrawi RP, Kupfer RM, et al. Gallstone recurrence after medical dissolution: an overestimated threat? J Hepatol 1986;3:241–6.
204. O'Donnell LDJ, Heaton KW. Recurrence and re-recurrence of gallstones after medical dissolution: a long-term follow up. Gut 1988;29:655–8.
205. Villanova N, Bazzoli F, Taroni F, et al. Gallstone recurrence after successful oral bile acid treatment. Gastroenterology 1989; 97:726–31.
206. Sackman M, Pauletzki J, Sauerbruch T, et al. The Munich gallbladder lithotripsy study: results of the first five years with 711 patients. Ann Intern Med 1991;114:290–6.
207. Schoenfield LJ, Berci G, Carnoval RL, et al. The effect of ursodiol on the efficacy and safety of extracorporeal shock-wave lithotripsy of gallbladder stones: the Dornier National Biliary Lithotripsy Study. N Engl J Med 1990;323:1239–45.
208. Sackmann M, Ippisch E, Sauerbruch T, et al. Early gallstone recurrence rate after successful shock-wave therapy. Gastroenterology 1990;98:392–6.
209. Diehl AK. Gallstone size and the risk of gallbladder cancer. JAMA 1983;250:2323–6.

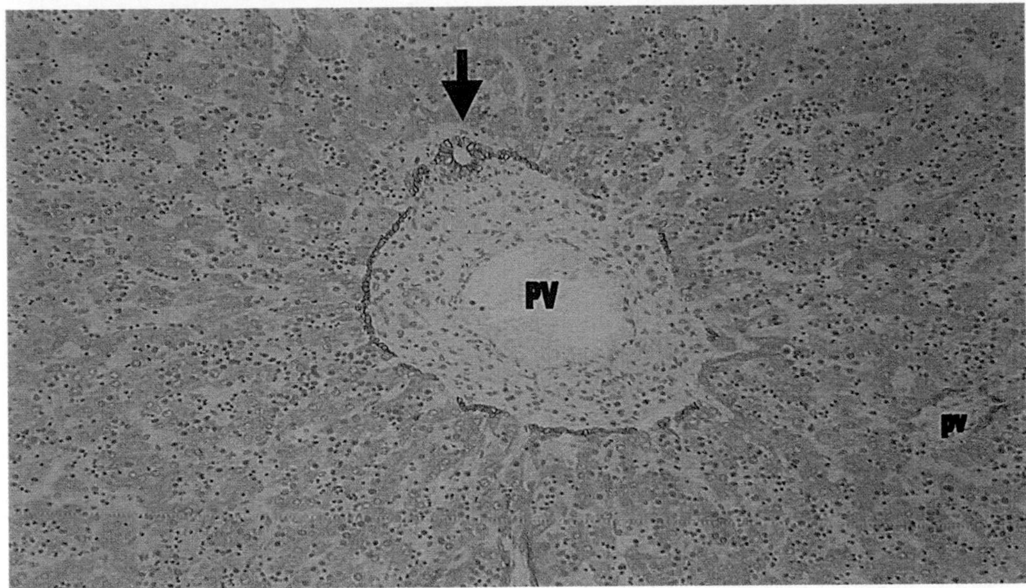

Color Plate 4.1. Autopsy liver specimen from an 18-week-old fetus. The picture shows a primitive portal tract containing a branch of the portal vein and its surrounding mesenchyme. Immediately surrounding the mesenchyme lies a layer of smaller cells with stronger immunoreactivity for cytokeratins. This layer is double over some segments. An early stage of remodeling of this ductal plate is seen at 12 o'clock, with development of a "tubular" lumen, lined by taller cells. (Monoclonal anticytokeratin antibody KL-1 immunostain [Immunotech, Marseille, France], hematoxylin counterstain, 312× magnification.) (Specimen courtesy of Dr. Philippe Moerman, Catholic University of Leuven, Leuven, Belgium.)

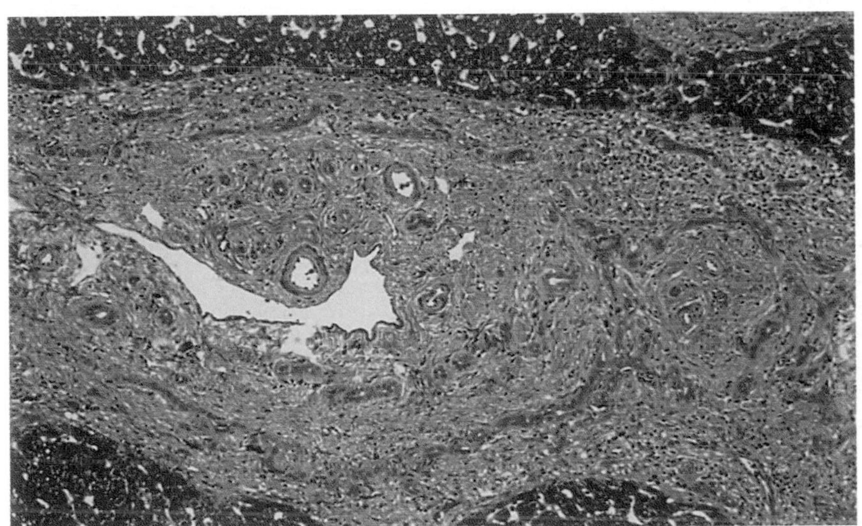

Color Plate 4.6. Follow-up liver biopsy specimen from a child who has undergone hepatic portoenterostomy for early severe biliary atresia, after 4 years of a favorable postoperative course. The liver shows a congenital hepatic fibrosis-like pattern, with perilobular fibrous bands carrying numerous irregular bile duct structures in ductal plate configuration. (Masson trichrome stain, 125× magnification.) (Specimen courtesy of Dr. Francesco Callea, Rome, Italy.)

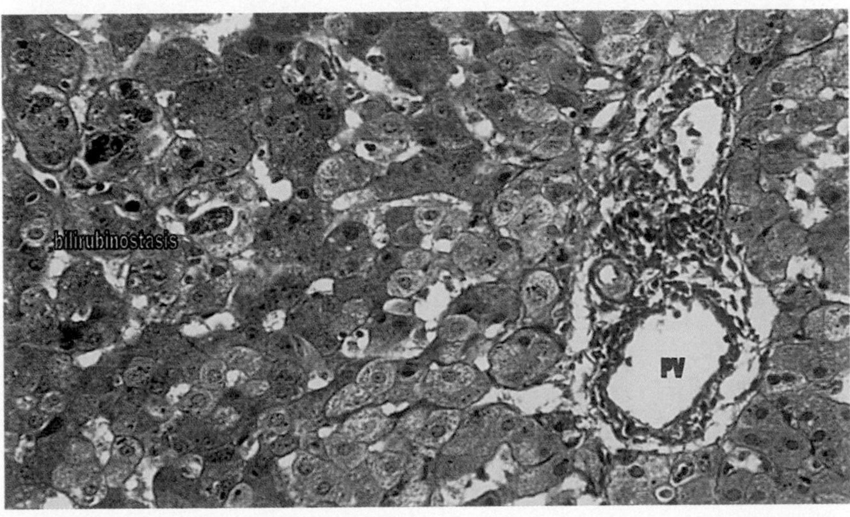

Color Plate 4.7. Detail from a liver biopsy specimen from a 5-year-old child with nonsyndromic paucity of interlobular bile ducts. The portal tract (*right*) is devoid of an interlobular bile duct. Note the bilirubinostasis in the lobular parenchyma at left. PV, portal vein. (Masson trichrome stain, 500× magnification.)

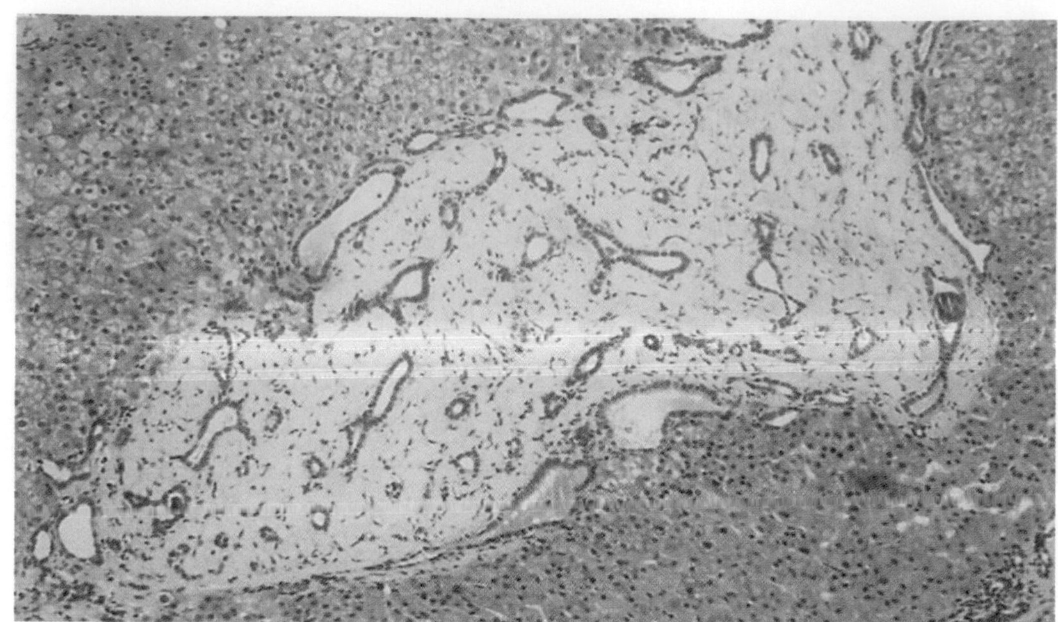

Color Plate 4.10. Liver biopsy specimen from a 6-year-old girl with congenital hepatic fibrosis. The picture shows an enlarged portal tract with numerous bile duct structures. The whole fibrous area can be interpreted as a fusion of several portal tracts containing incompletely remodeled ductal plates (pollard willow pattern). Note the extreme hypoplasia or virtual absence of portal vein branches. The lower right corner displays a more normal-appearing small portal tract. (Hematoxylin and eosin [H&E], 125× magnification.)

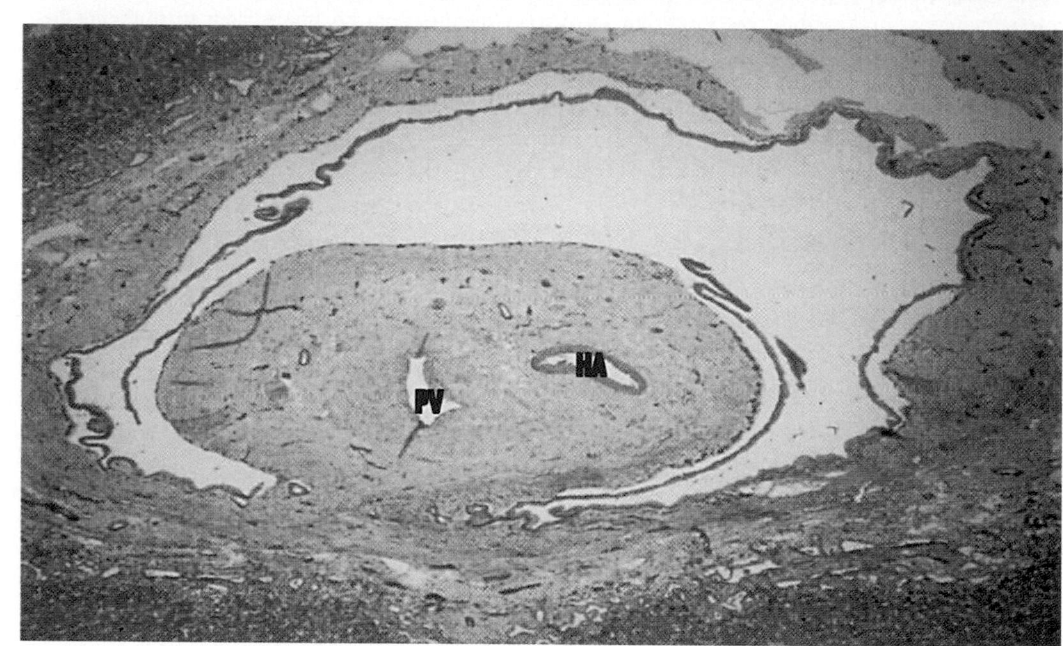

Color Plate 4.11. Low magnification of a cross-section through a dilated hilar bile duct from the liver of a patient with Caroli's disease. Ductal plate malformation with minimal degree of remodeling, appearing as a polypoid projection in the bile duct lumen. PV, portal vein; HA, hepatic artery. (H&E, 1× magnification.) (Specimen courtesy of Dr. Philippe Moerman, Catholic University of Leuven, Leuven, Belgium.)

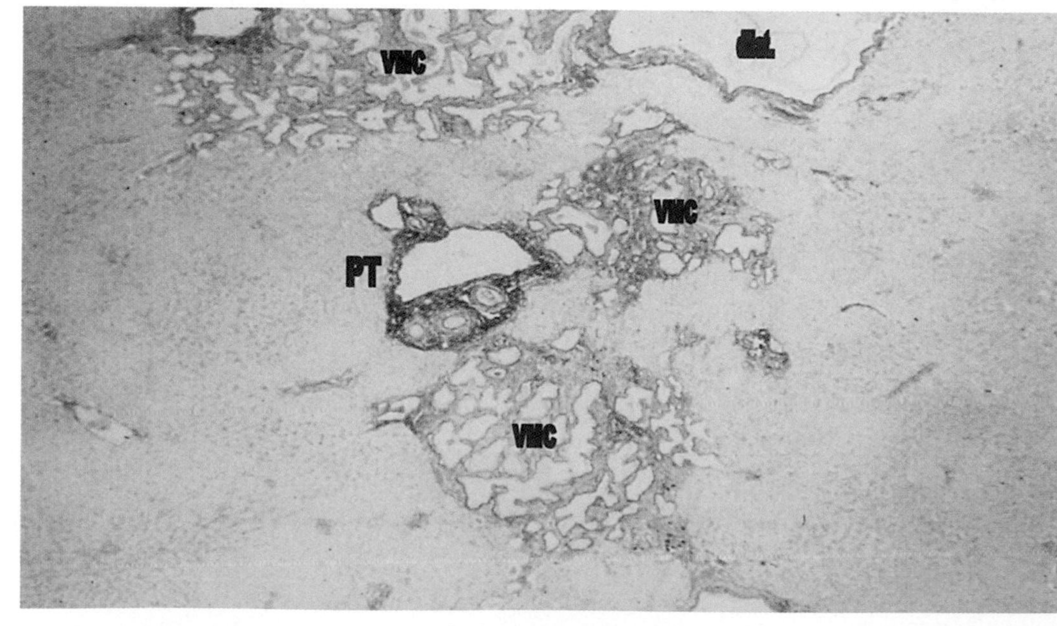

Color Plate 4.13. Liver specimen from a patient with autosomal dominant polycystic kidney disease. The picture shows a portal tract (PT) and three von Meyenburg complexes (VMC). Note the paraportal location of the complexes, and the contrast of their connective tissue matrix with that of the portal tract. One component bile duct structure (dilat.) is dilated. (Orcein stain, 25× magnification.)

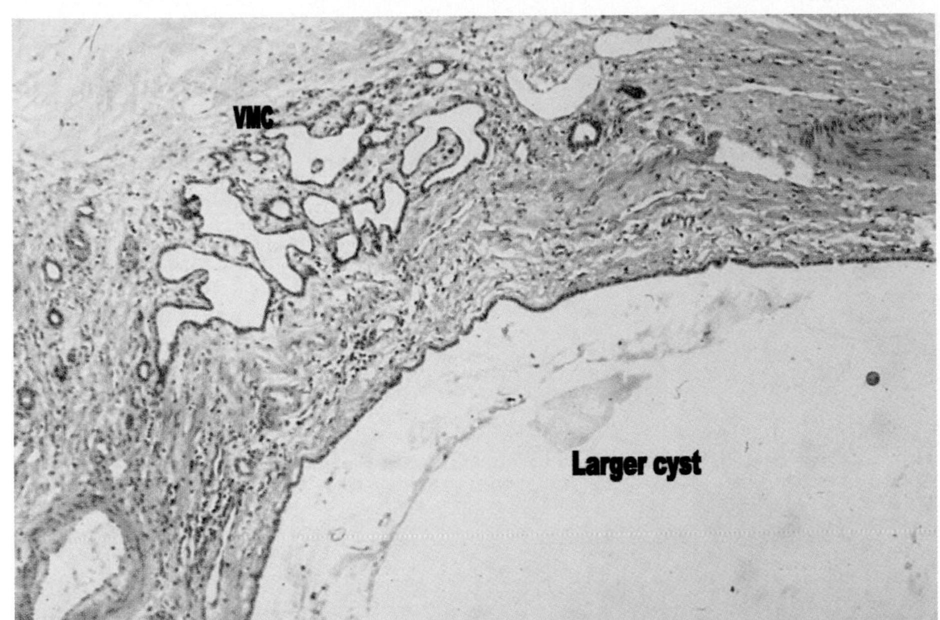

Color Plate 4.14. Liver cyst in autosomal dominant polycystic disease in a male patient 75 years of age. The picture shows a small cyst, lined by bile duct epithelium. The cyst can be viewed as a more dilated component in a cluster of less dilated, smaller bile duct structures of a von Meyenburg complex (*left upper portion*). (H&E, 125× magnification.)

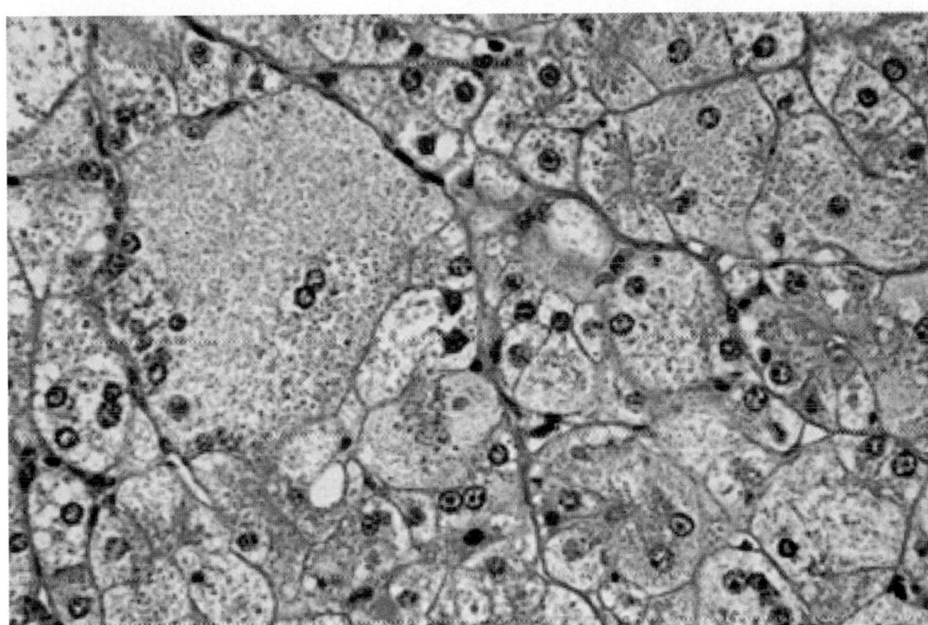

Color Plate 11.5. Neonatal hepatitis with giant cell transformation. Centrizonal region shows enlarged giant hepatocytes and scattered lobular sinusoidal mononuclear infiltrates. (H&E, original magnification 100×.)

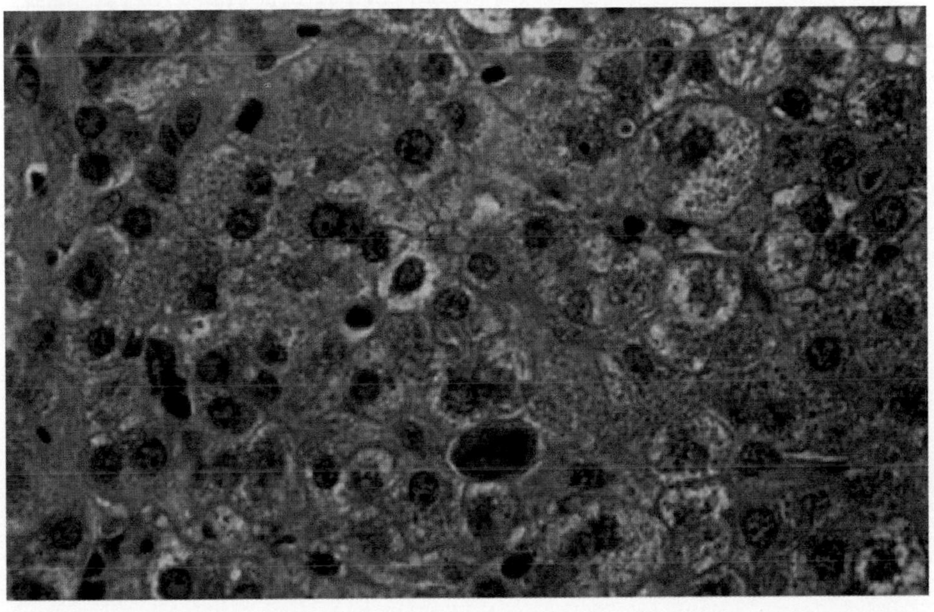

Color Plate 14.1. Histopathology in PFIC1. Liver biopsy from a 2-year-old patient showing swelling of hepatocytes, a bland hepatocellular and canalicular cholestasis, and occasional necrotic hepatocytes. (Courtesy of Dr. Kevin Bove.)

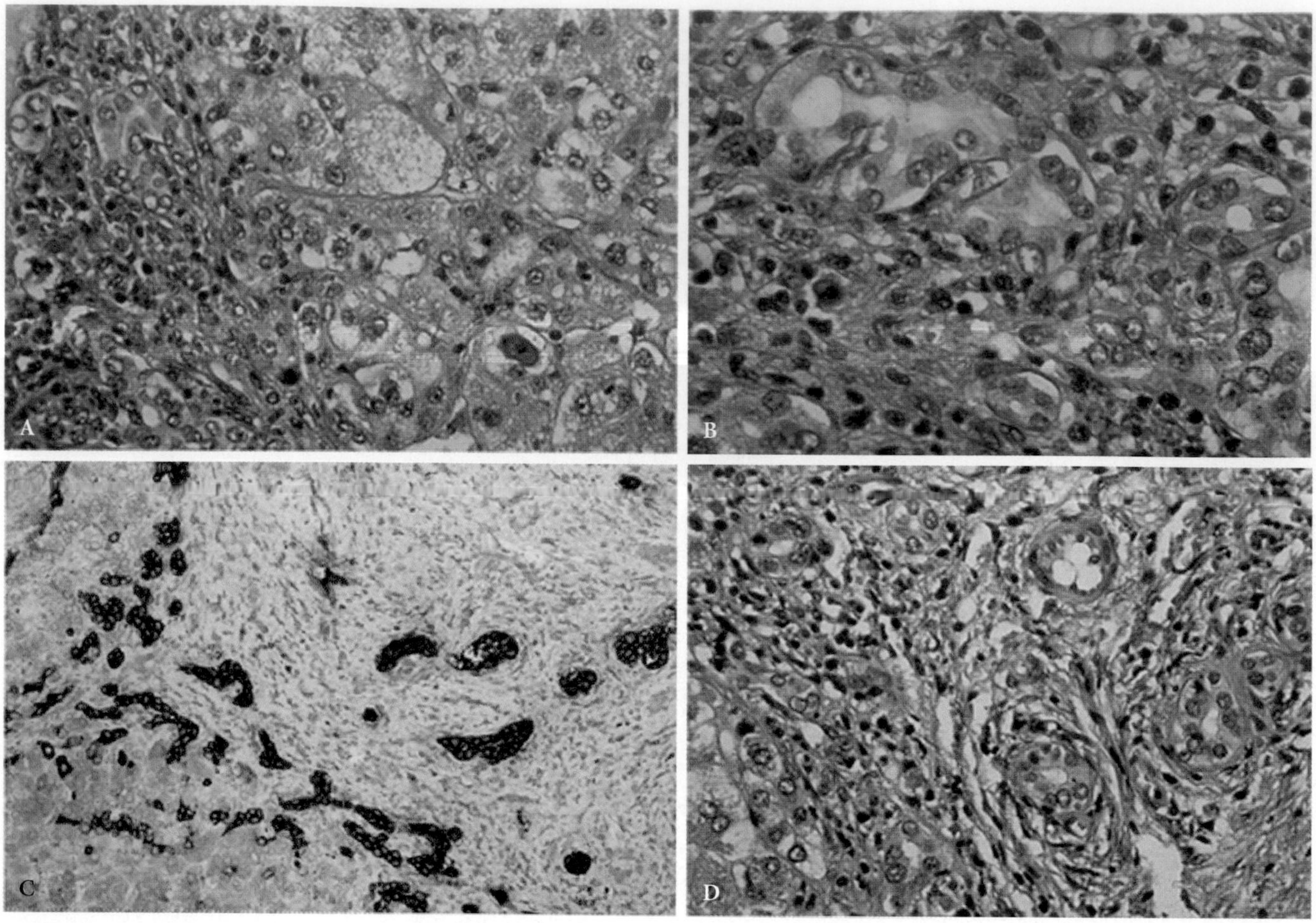

Color Plate 14.5. Histopathology of liver in a child with PFIC3. (**A**) Cholestatic hepatitis with giant cell transformation and isolated eosinophilic necrotic hepatocyte. Portal zone at the left shows bile ductular proliferation and mild mixed inflammatory infiltrate. (**B**) Bile ducts are increased in number, tortuous, and lined by swollen reactive epithelium. Inflammatory cells include lymphocytes, plasma cells, and occasional polymorphonuclear leukocytes. Bile stasis in ducts is absent. (**C**) A cytokeratin immunostain shows increased numbers of periportal ductules and interlobular bile ducts. (**D**) In PFIC3, progressive bile duct injury is associated with periductal fibroblast proliferation, as shown here, and eventually fibrosis. (Courtesy of Drs. Kevin Bove and James Heubi.)

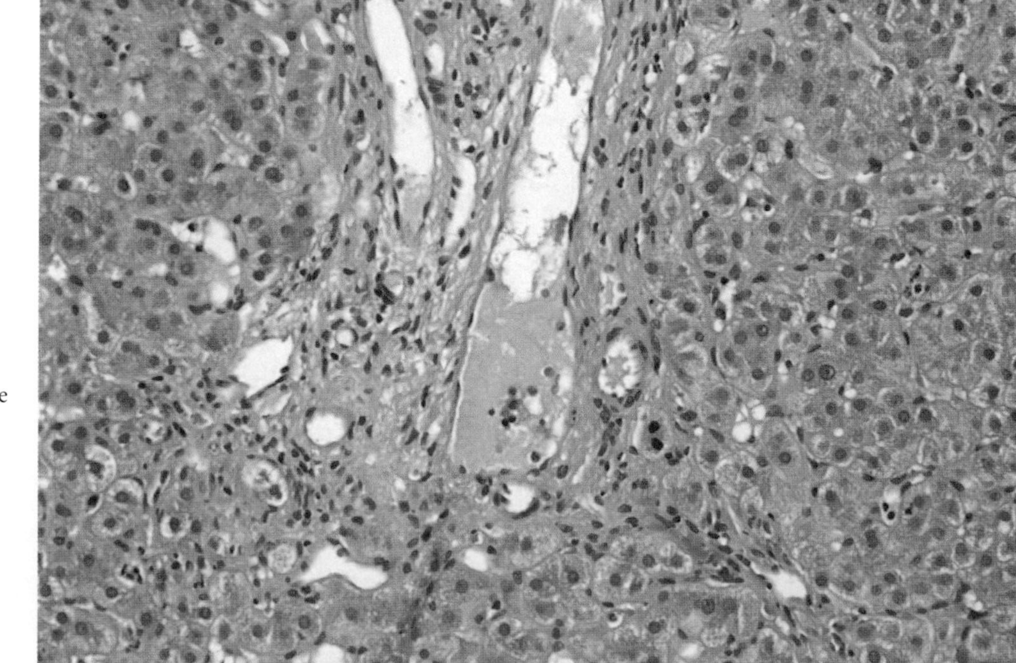

Color Plate 15.1. Liver specimen from an infant with Alagille syndrome with bile duct paucity. The portal tract is shown without any identifiable interlobular bile duct. (H&E staining, 200× magnification.) (Courtesy of Pierre A. Russo, MD.)

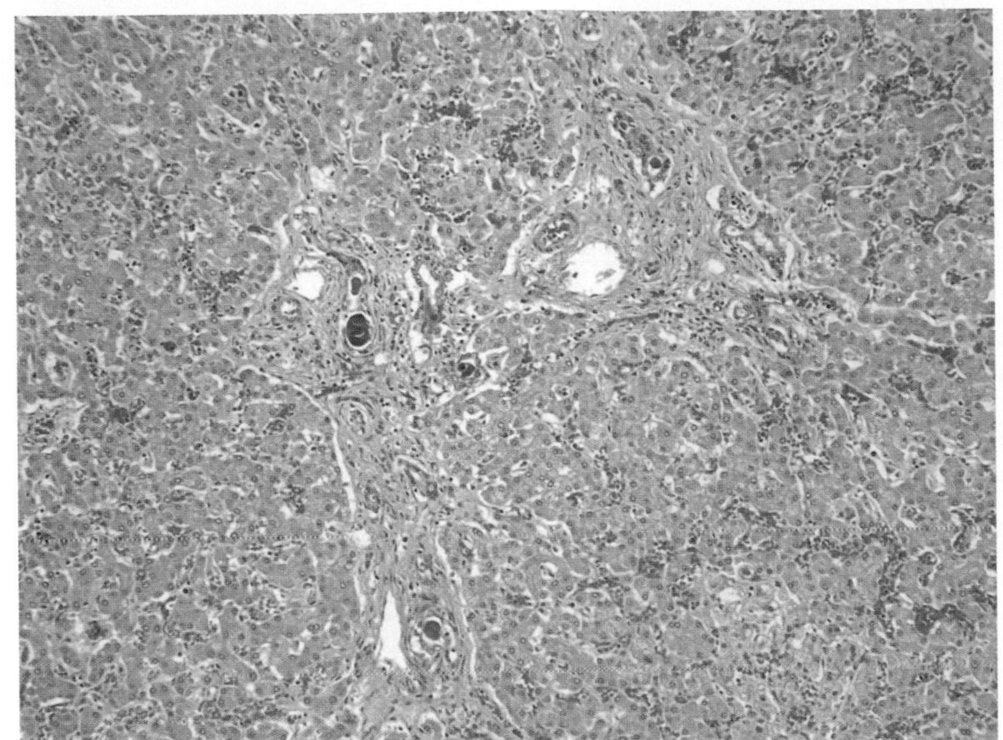

Color Plate 15.2. Liver specimen from a 1-month-old patient with Alagille syndrome demonstrating marked bile duct proliferation. (H&E staining, 100× magnification.) (Courtesy of Pierre A. Russo, MD.)

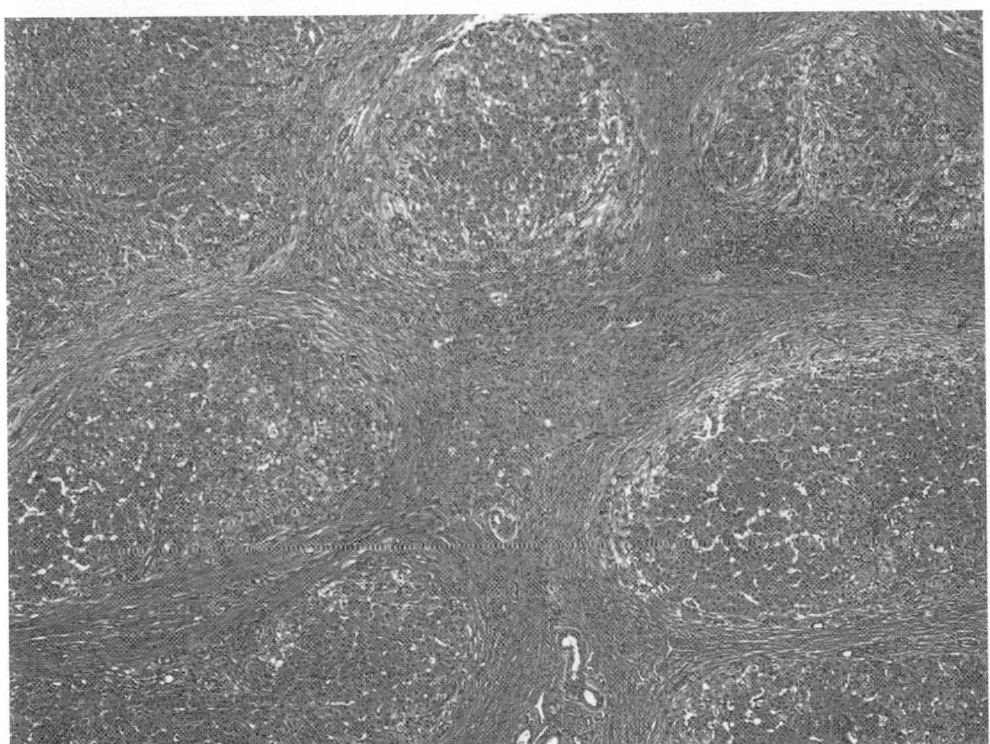

Color Plate 15.3. Liver specimen from a 16-year-old with Alagille syndrome. There is established cirrhosis. Portal tracts are expanded and fibrotic. There is a complete absence of interlobular bile ducts. (H&E staining, 100× magnification.) (Courtesy of Pierre A. Russo, MD.)

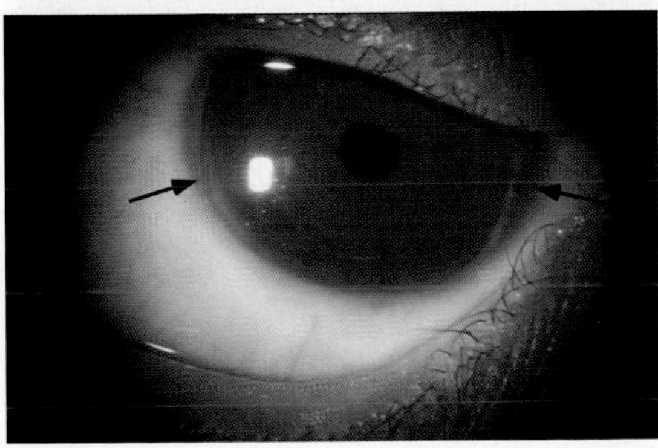

Color Plate 15.7. Posterior embryotoxon and prominent Schwalbe's line (*arrows*).

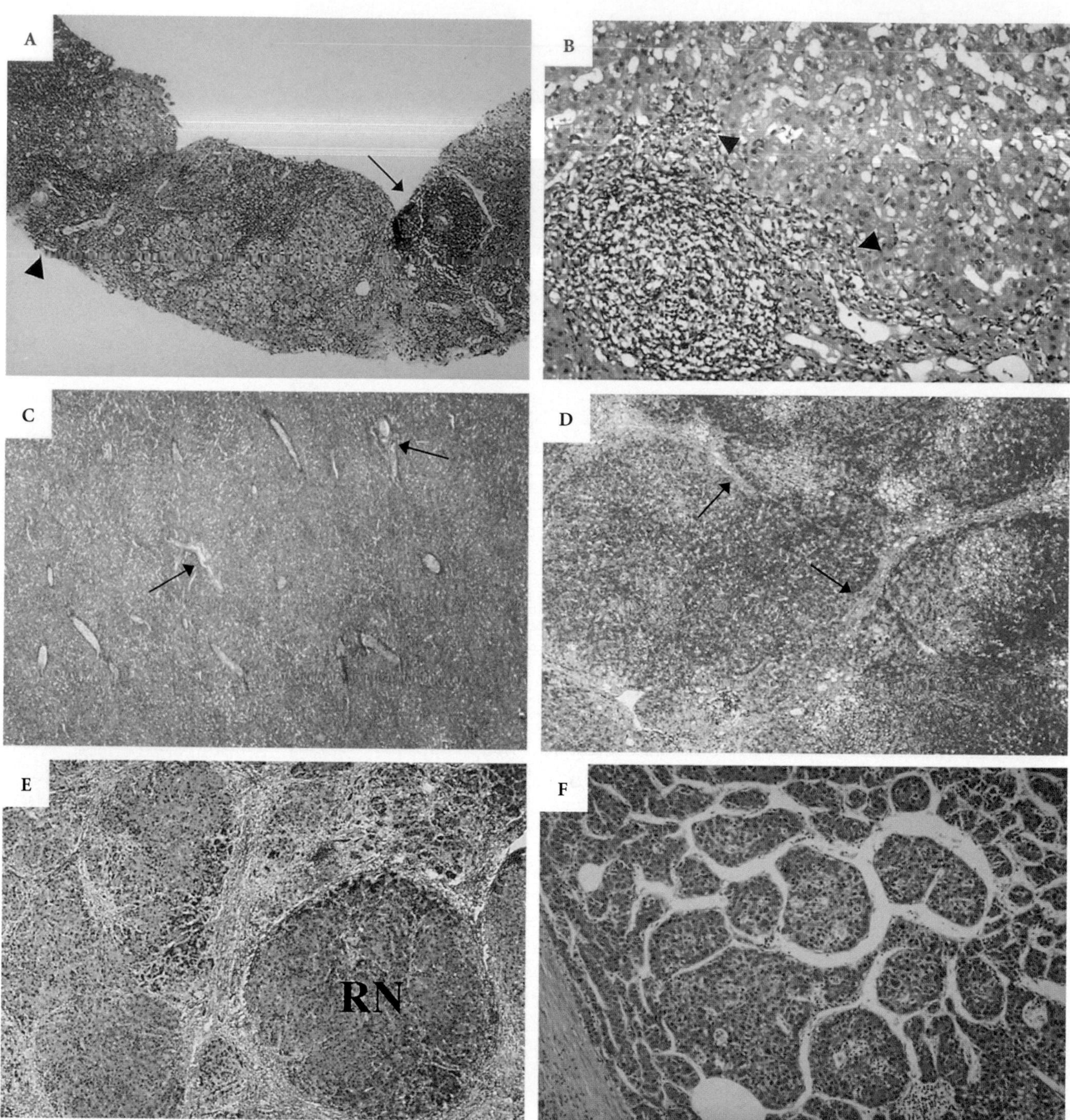

Color Plate 17.21. Histologic stages of hepatitis C virus (HCV) infection. (**A**) A core biopsy specimen from an adult patient chronically infected with HCV shows dense portal lymphocytic infiltrates (*arrow*) and architectural changes (*arrowhead*). (Hematoxylin and eosin [H&E] stain, 10× magnification.) (**B**) The lymphocytes are not limited to the portal tract but extend to the lobules (*arrowheads*). (H&E stain, 100× magnification.) (**C**) Normal liver architecture with scant fibrous tissue (*arrows*) to the portal tracts is evident. (Trichrome stain, 20× magnification.) (**D**) During progressive infections, the fibrotic areas expand and bridging fibrosis develops (*arrows*). (Trichrome stain, 20× magnification.) (**E**) Cirrhosis characterized by marked fibrosis and regenerative nodules (RN) occurs in about 20% of chronically infected persons. (Trichrome stain, 20× magnification.) (**F**) Hepatocellular carcinoma, also a consequence of chronic HCV infection. (H&E stain, 20× magnification.) (Reprinted with permission from Lauer GM, Walker BD. Medical progress: hepatitis C infection. N Engl J Med 2001;345:41–52.

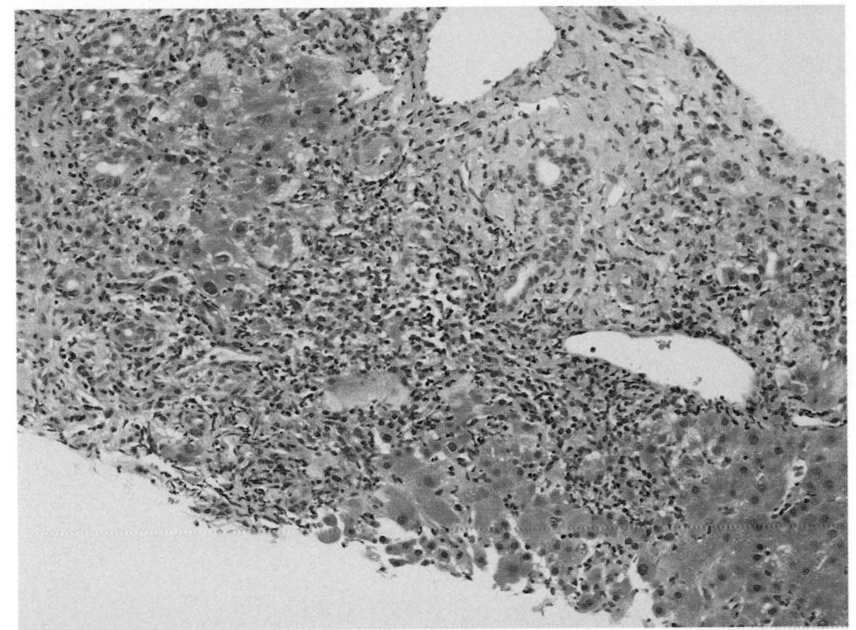

Color Plate 18.1. Portal and periportal lymphocyte and plasma cell infiltrate extending to and disrupting the parenchymal limiting plate (interface hepatitis). Swollen hepatocytes, pyknotic necroses, and acinar inflammation are present. (H&E staining.) (Picture kindly provided by Dr. Alberto Quaglia.)

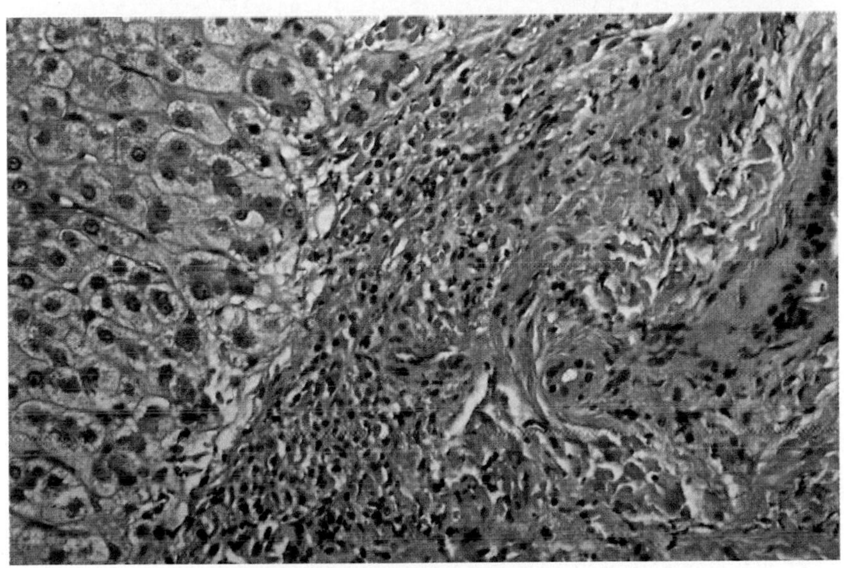

Color Plate 19.2. Liver biopsy in a patient with autoimmune hepatitis and primary sclerosing cholangitis shows periductular stromal edema and inflammation, along with hepatitis along portal margins. (H&E, original magnification ×400.)

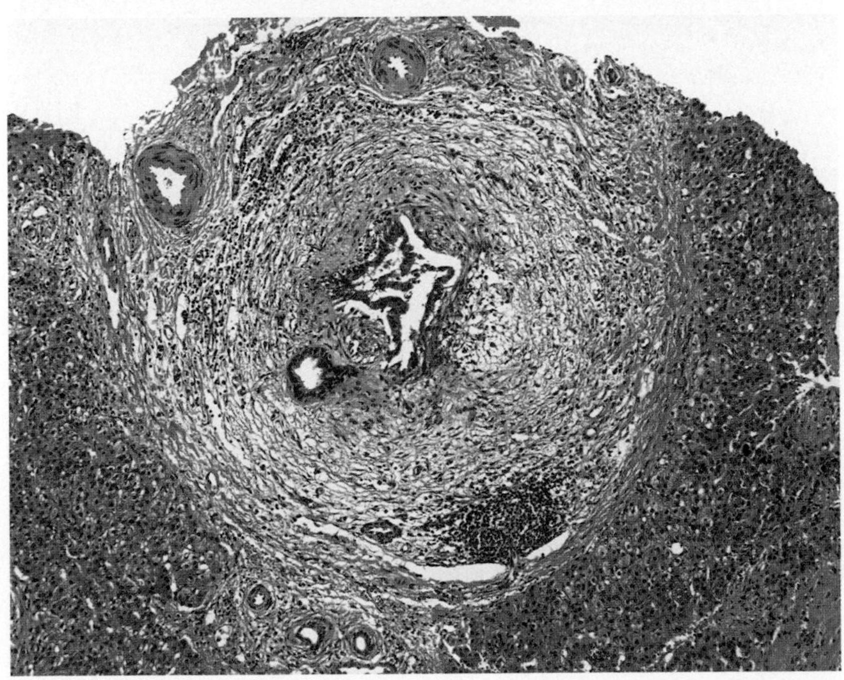

Color Plate 19.5. Classic "onion-skinning" periductular sclerosis in a patient with primary sclerosing cholangitis. (H&E, original magnification ×400.)

Color Plate 23.5. Hepatic histology in homozygous PiZZ α_1-antitrypsin deficiency. (**A**) Micrograph of liver biopsy specimen in α_1-antitrypsin deficiency demonstrating increased fibrous tissue deposition *(arrowheads)* and nodular transformation. (PAS–diastase staining, 4× magnification.) (**B**) Micrograph of liver biopsy in α_1-antitrypsin deficiency demonstrating the PAS-positive, diastase-resistant globules. (Two of the hepatocytes with globules are indicated by *arrows.*) (PAS–diastase staining, 40× magnification.)

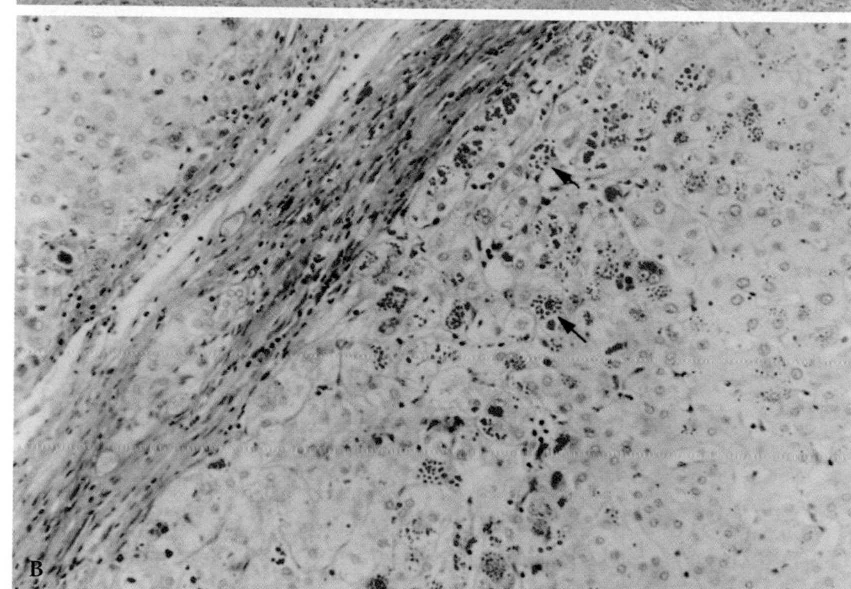

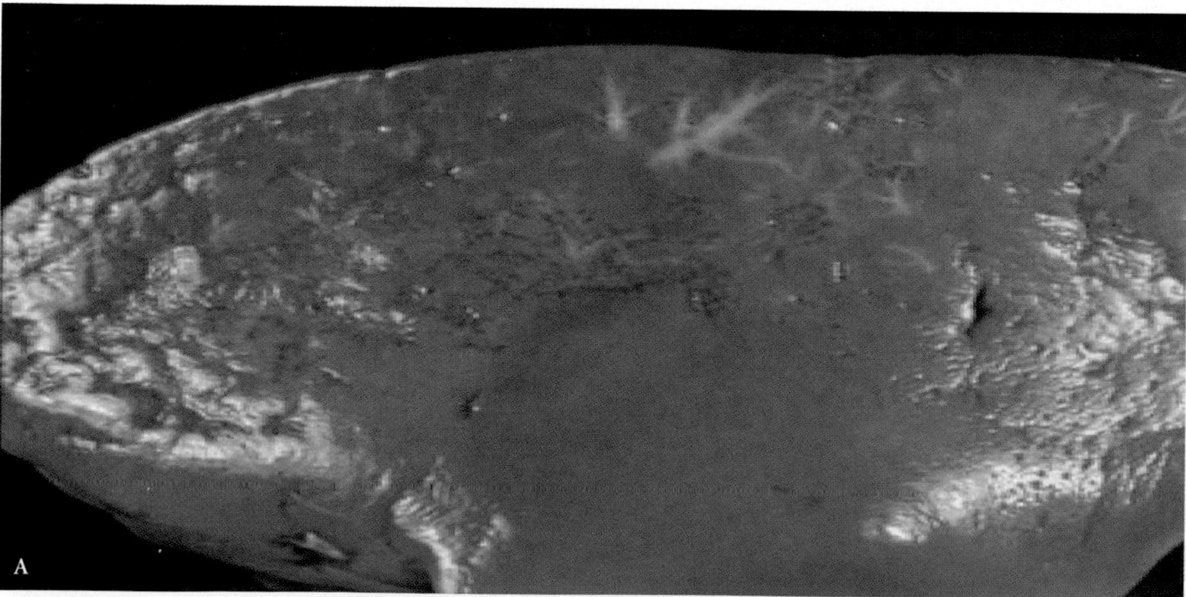

Color Plate 24.6. Focal biliary cirrhosis in cystic fibrosis. (**A**) The surface of the liver displays focal areas of scarring and furrowing. Large areas of normal preserved hepatic architecture are present. (Courtesy of Dr. Arthur Weinberg, University of Texas Southwestern Medical Center, Dallas, Texas.)

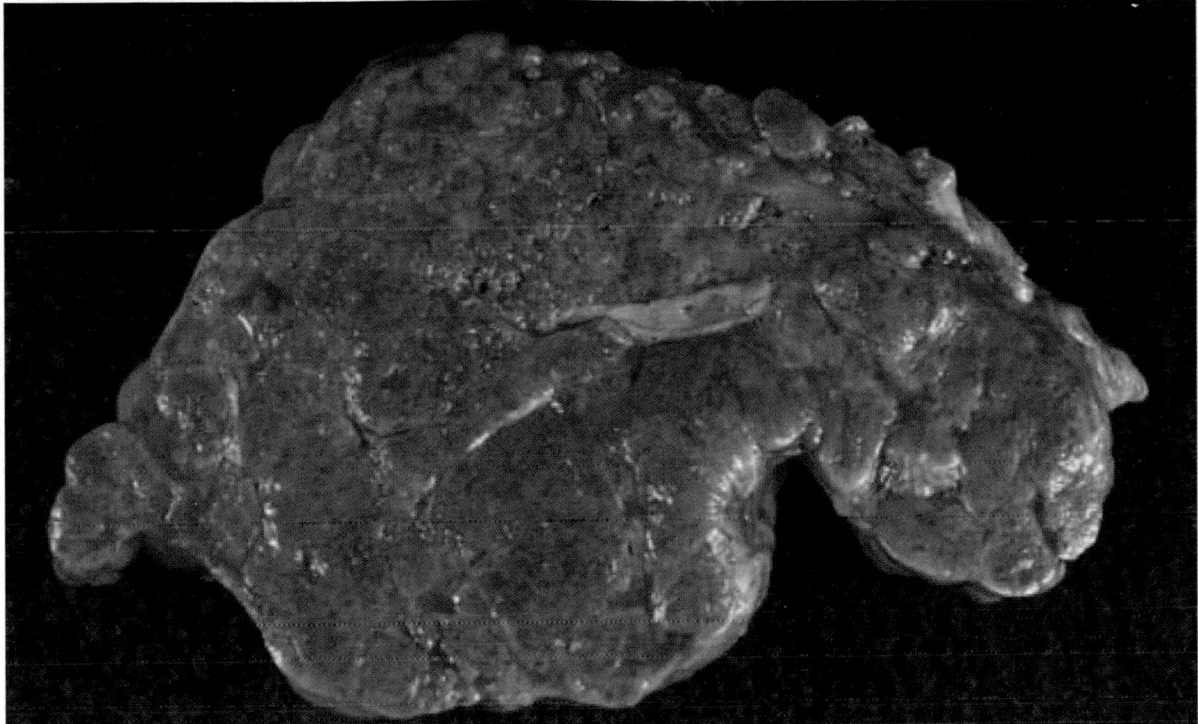

Color Plate 24.7. Multilobular cirrhosis in cystic fibrosis. Cut section of the liver revealing significant lobulation, fibrosis, scarring, and cirrhosis. (Courtesy of Dr. Arthur Weinberg, University of Texas Southwestern Medical Center, Dallas, Texas).

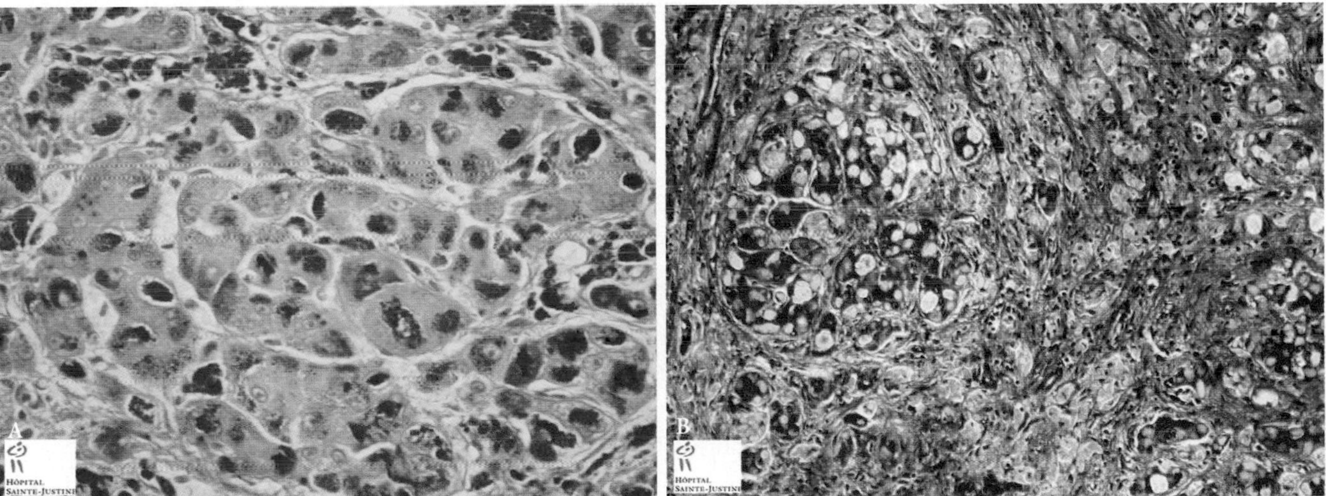

Color Plate 25.11. Glycogen storage disease type IV. (**A**) Periodic acid–Schiff stain positive inclusions in cytoplasm and (**B**) micronodular cirrhosis with hepatocytes containing cytoplasmic inclusions. (Masson trichrome stain.) (Image courtesy of humpath.com.)

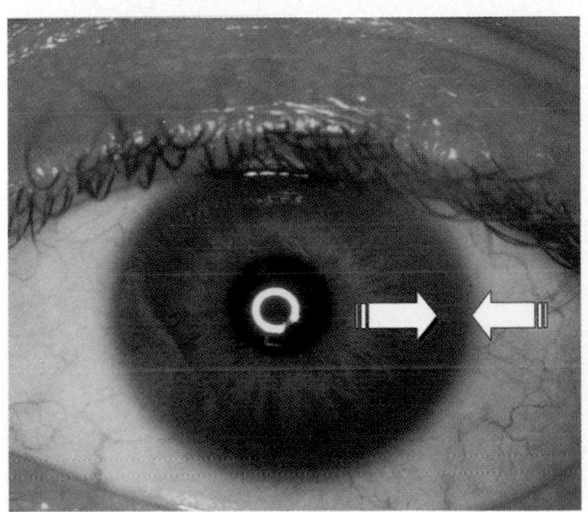

Color Plate 26.5. Kayser–Fleischer ring (noted by *arrows*) in a 30-year-old man with Wilson's disease. (Used by permission from Sokol RJ. Copper storage diseases. In: Kaplowitz N, ed. Liver and biliary diseases. Baltimore: Williams & Wilkins, 1992:322–33.)

Color Plate 26.7. Liver histology of Wilson's disease in a 3-year-old asymptomatic boy diagnosed because his sister presented with fulminant liver failure caused by Wilson's disease. Portal tract mononuclear infiltrate and prominent periportal glycogenated hepatocyte nuclei (*arrows*) are present. Early evidence of portal fibrosis is also present. (H&E stain, 400× magnification.)

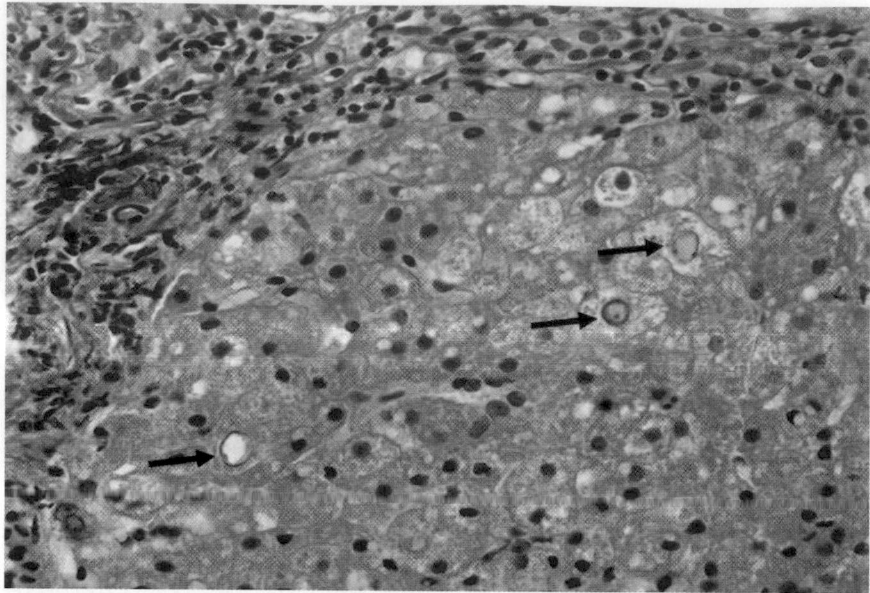

Color Plate 26.8. Liver histology of Wilson's disease in a 16-year-old girl presenting with fulminant liver failure. Macrovesicular steatosis (*arrows*), mononuclear cell portal tract inflammatory infiltrate, bridging fibrosis, and micronodular cirrhosis are present. (Masson trichrome stain, 200× magnification.)

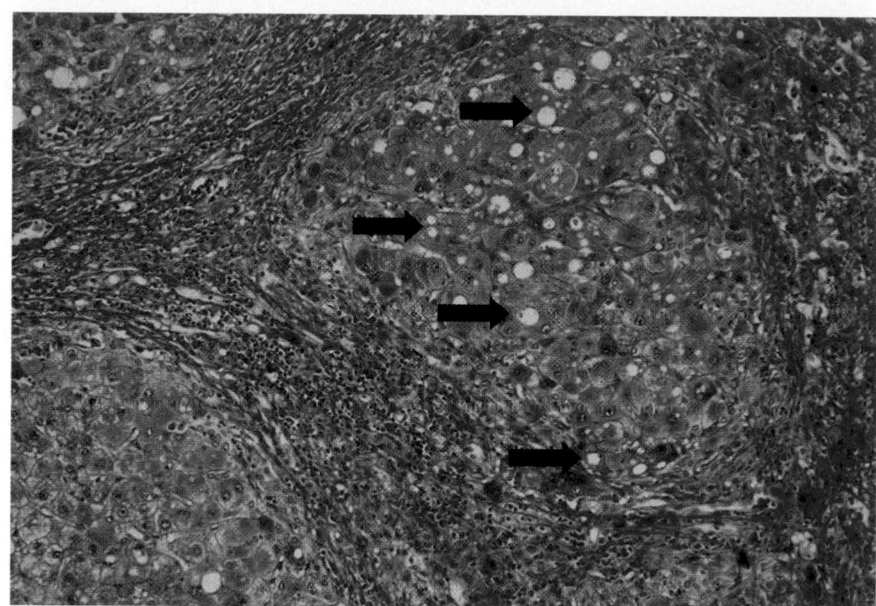

Color Plate 26.9. Liver histology of Wilson's disease in a 13-year-old girl. Bridging fibrosis and both mild micro- and macrovesicular hepatocytic steatosis (*arrows*) are present, with less inflammatory infiltrate than that seen in Color Plate 26.8. (H&E stain, 100× magnification.)

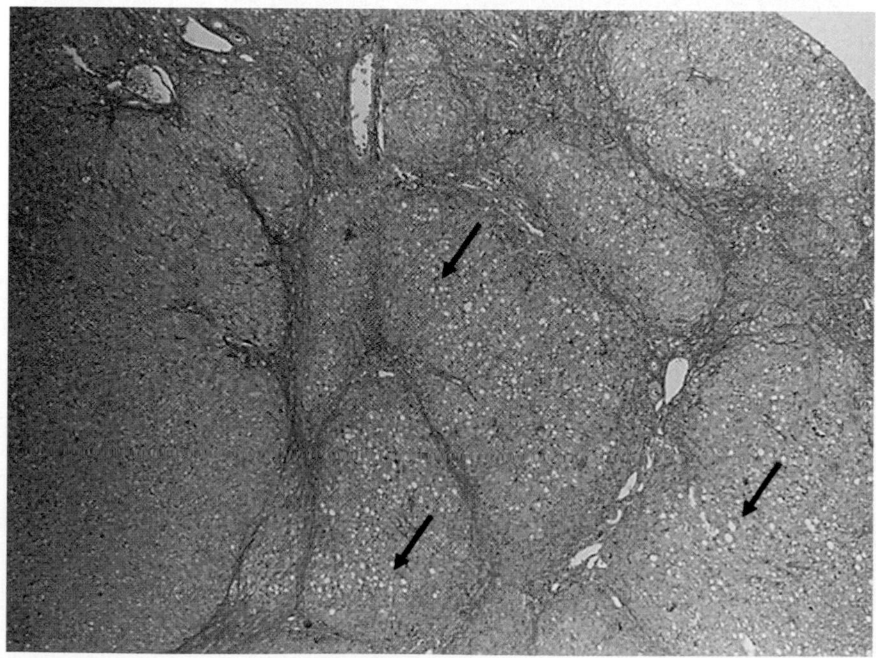

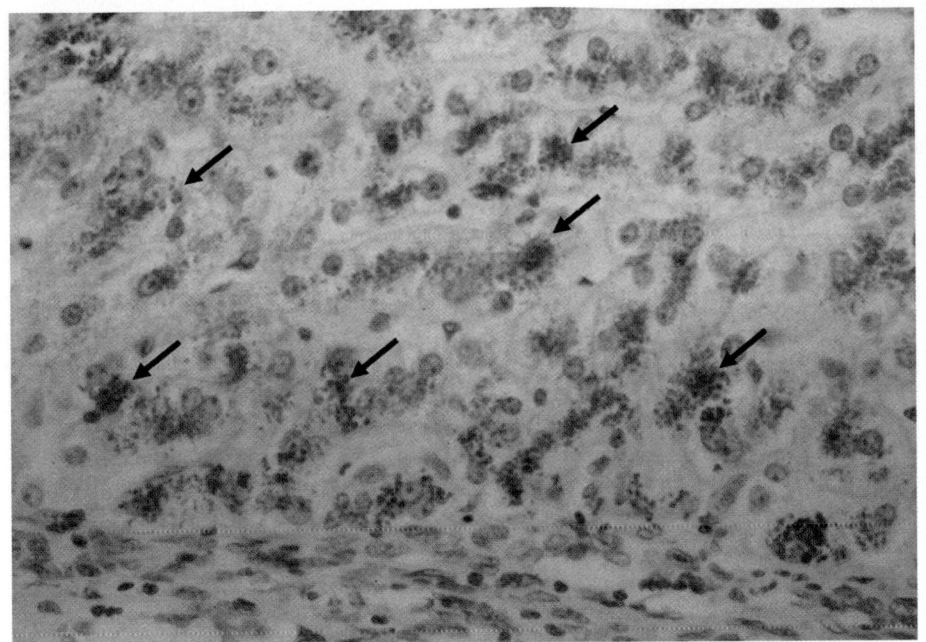

Color Plate 26.10. Copper staining of liver removed at the time of liver transplantation from a 16-year-old girl with fulminant hepatic failure caused by Wilson's disease (see Color Plate 26.8). Staining of copper-associated proteins in multiple hepatocytes (*arrows*) by rhodanine histochemical stain is strongly positive. (1000× magnification.)

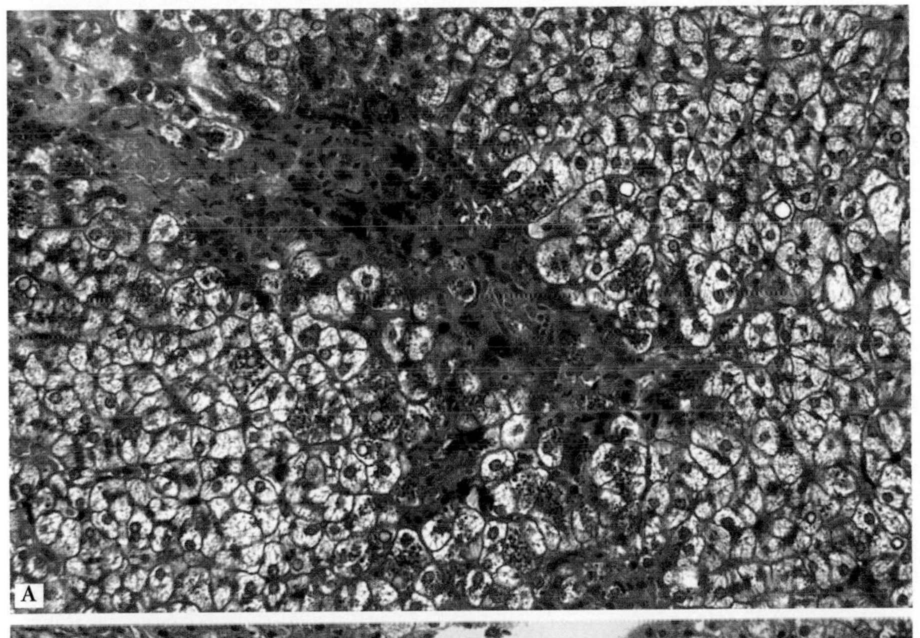

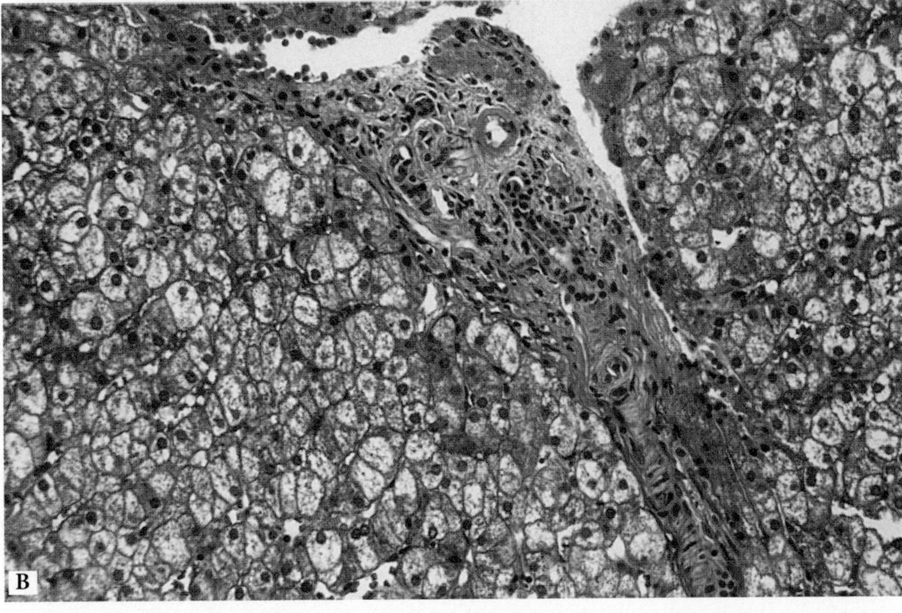

Color Plate 27.8. Effects of intravenous deferoxamine treatment. (**A**) Liver biopsy from a 16-year-old girl with β-thalassemia. Increased stainable iron shown on Prussian blue stain. Quantitative hepatic iron of 15,483 μg/g dry weight. (**B**) Repeat liver biopsy with Prussian blue stain in the same patient following 1 year of daily intravenous deferoxamine (hepatic iron, 669 μg/g dry weight). Note the dramatic reduction in stainable iron.

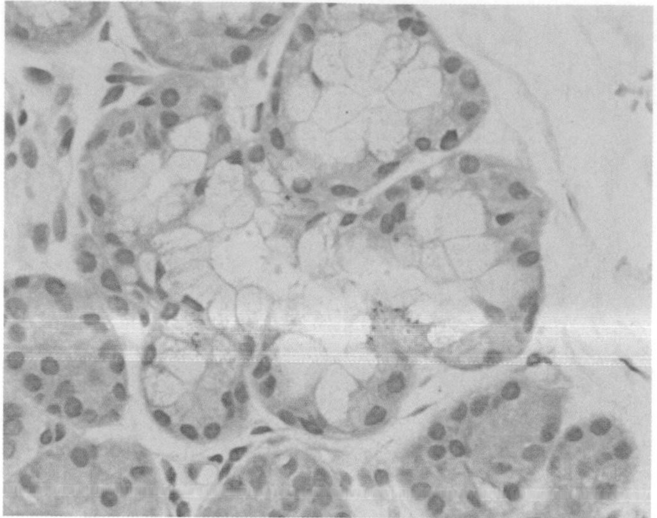

Color Plate 27.9. Buccal biopsy from a patient with neonatal hemochromatosis. Finely granular stainable iron is seen, particularly within mucus cells, in epithelium of a minor salivary gland from the inner aspect of the lower lip. (Prussian blue/nuclear fast red, original magnification 400×.)

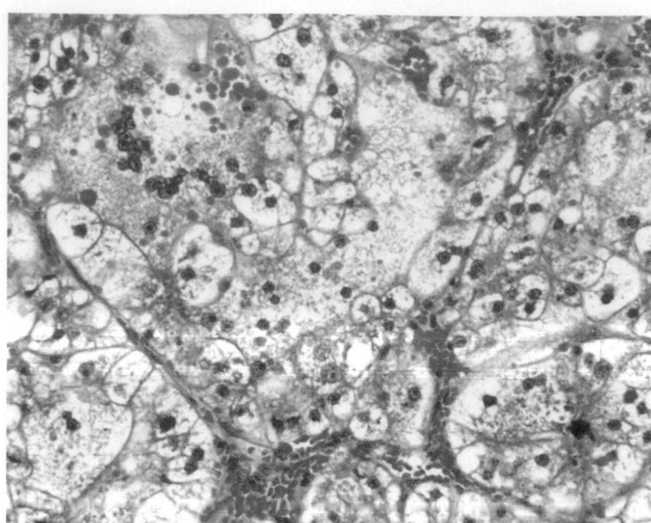

Color Plate 27.10. Liver biopsy from a patient with neonatal hemochromatosis. Edema, pigment accumulation (both bile and hemosiderin), and giant cell change with rosetting are seen in severely injured liver. (H&E stain, original magnification 200×.)

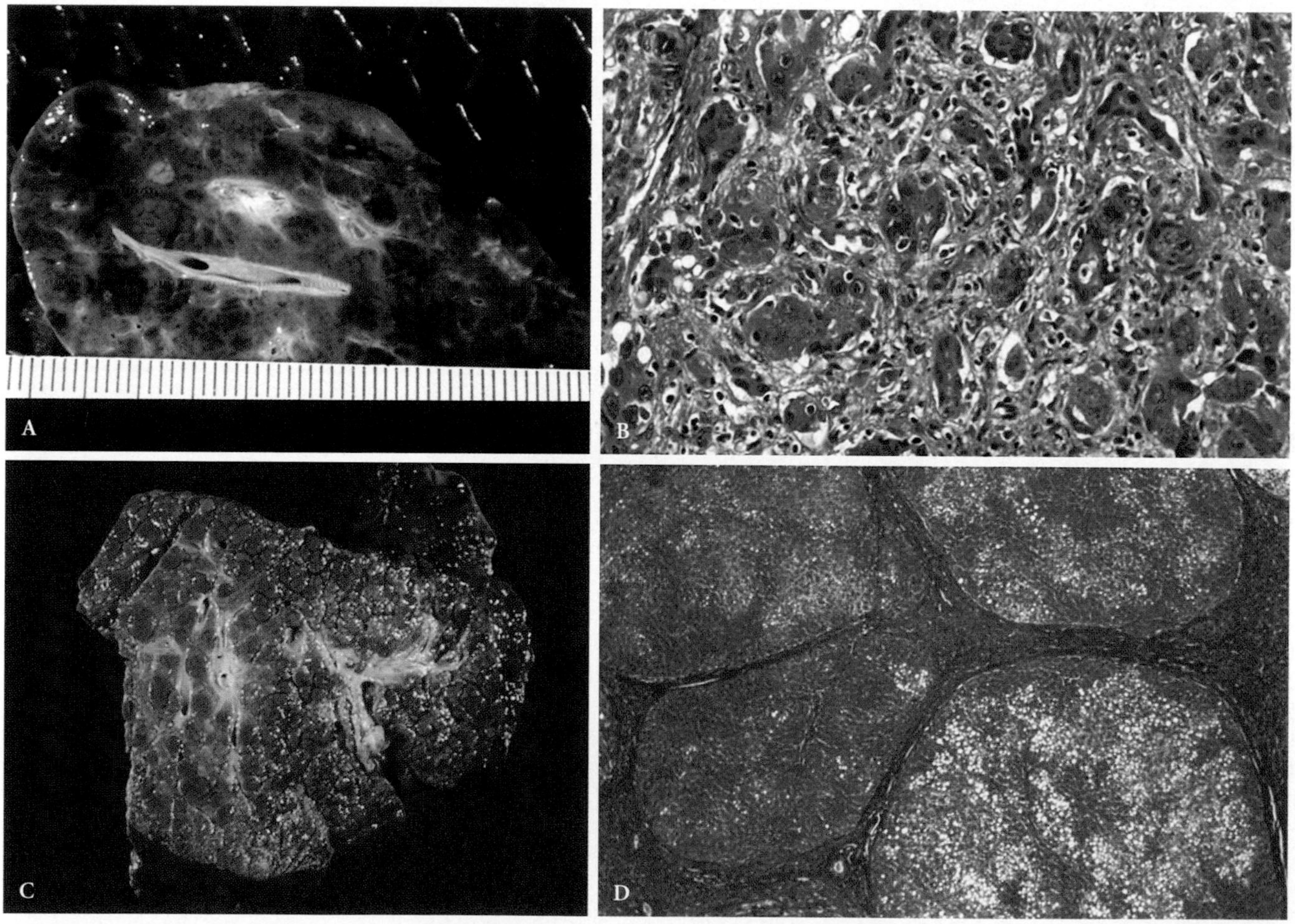

A

B

C

D

Color Plate 29.2. Liver pathology in tyrosinemia. Acute and chronic courses. (**A**) Microscopic appearance of liver from a 3-month-old girl with the acute form of tyrosinemia. The liver was firm, shrunken, and vaguely nodular. (**B**) Histologic examination of the liver revealed massive parenchymal collapse and fibrosis. There is cholangiolar proliferation, and surviving hepatocytes are frequently arranged in a pseudoglandular pattern. There is intracellular cholestasis and hemosiderin deposition as well as a mild, nonspecific chronic inflammatory infiltrate. (Hematoxylin-phloxine-saffron [HPS] stain, original magnification 125×.) (**C**) Enlarged, cirrhotic liver from a 2-year-old boy with a chronic form of the disease reveals a coarsely nodular external and cut surface. (**D**) Low-power histologic examination reveals a mixed macro- and micronodular cirrhosis. The nodules appear histologically heterogenous because of a variable degree of fat content in the hepatocytes. (HPS stain, original magnification 30×.)

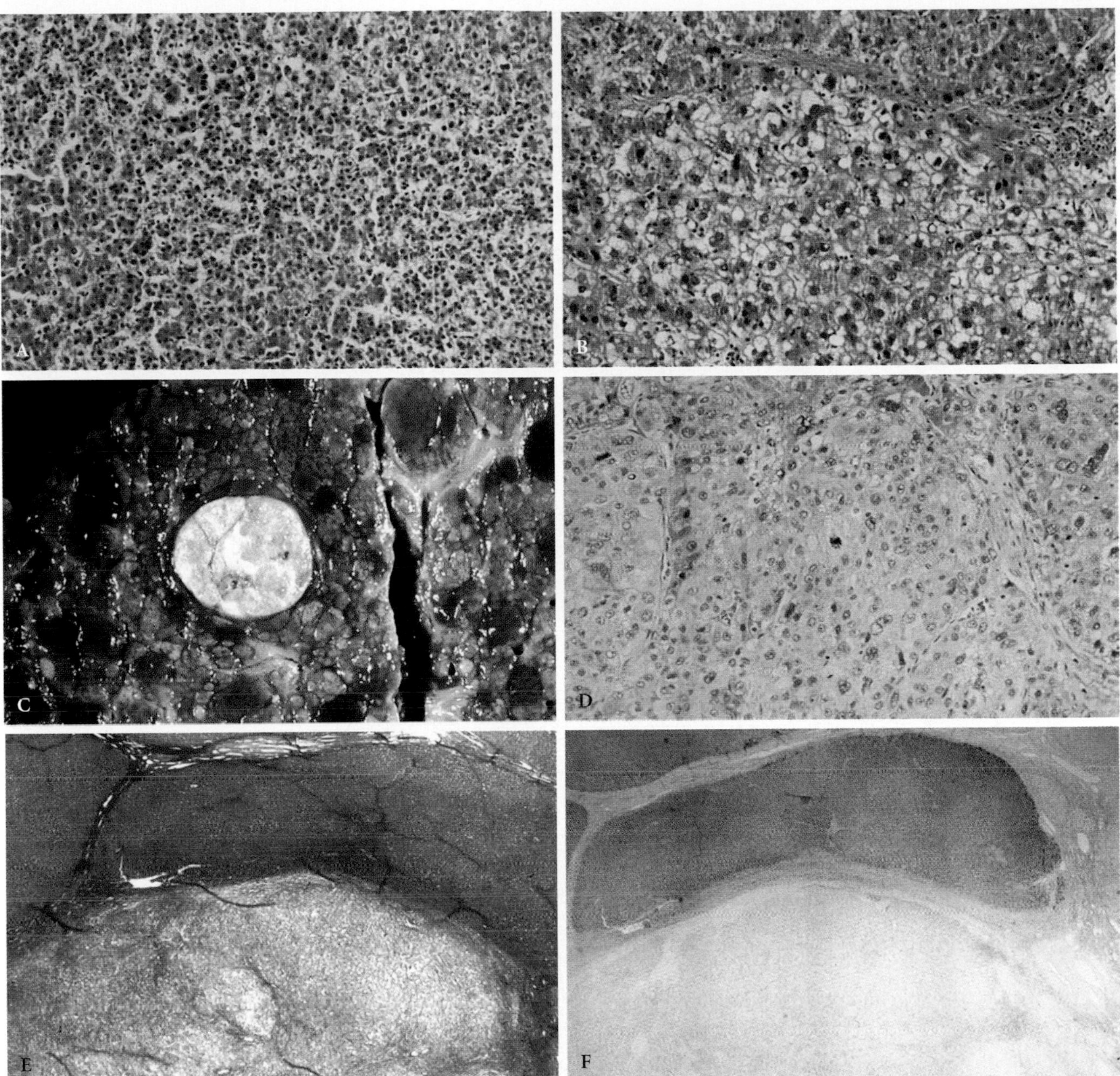

Color Plate 29.3. Dysplasia, carcinoma, and regenerative nodules. (**A**) Histologic examination of native liver from a 1-year-old patient undergoing a liver transplantation revealed multiple foci of dysplasia. This microphotograph shows the small cell variant, composed of fetal hepatocyte-like cells with increased nucleocytoplasmic ratio and hyperchromatic nuclei. (HPS stain, original magnification 200×.) (**B**) In the liver from the same patient, foci of large cell dysplasia are shown, characterized by irregular hyperchromatic nuclei and an increased nucleocytoplasmic ratio. Distinction from a microscopic hepatocellular carcinoma may be very difficult. (HPS stain, original magnification 200×.) (**C**) Native liver from a 4-year-old hepatic transplantation patient showing cirrhosis and one nodule that clearly stood out from the rest of the parenchyma. (**D**) Histologic examination of the nodule in the previous panel revealing hepatocellular carcinoma with extensive nuclear irregularity and many mitoses. (HPS stain, original magnification 200×.) (**E**) Native liver from an 11-year-old liver transplant recipient with extensive macronodular cirrhosis; one large focus of hepatocellular carcinoma was noted (pale staining nodule, lower portion of figure). (HPS stain, original magnification 20×.) (**F**) Immunostaining with an antibody to fumarylacetoacetate hydrolase revealed a positive reaction in many of the regenerating nodules, indicating reacquisition of the missing enzyme by the regenerating hepatocytes, suggesting reversion of the mutation. Note that the carcinomatous nodule remains negative, indicating absence of reversion. (Avidin-biotin-peroxidase technique with hematoxylin counterstaining, original magnification 20×.)

Color Plate 30.2. Bone marrow and liver findings in Gaucher's disease. (**A**) The bone marrow macrophage is typical of the storage cells, that is, Gaucher cells. The typical "crinkled tissue paper" cytoplasmic inclusions are evident. (**B**) Liver slice showing nodules (white/yellow) made up almost entirely of Gaucher cells. (**C**) By light microscopy, only Kupffer cells contain visible storage material, glucosylceramide, whereas the hepatocytes do not. PAS staining is negative in Kupffer cells. (**D**) Electron micrograph showing characteristic tubular storage material of Gaucher's disease cellular inclusions. (Magnification 20,000×.) (Courtesy of D. Witte.)

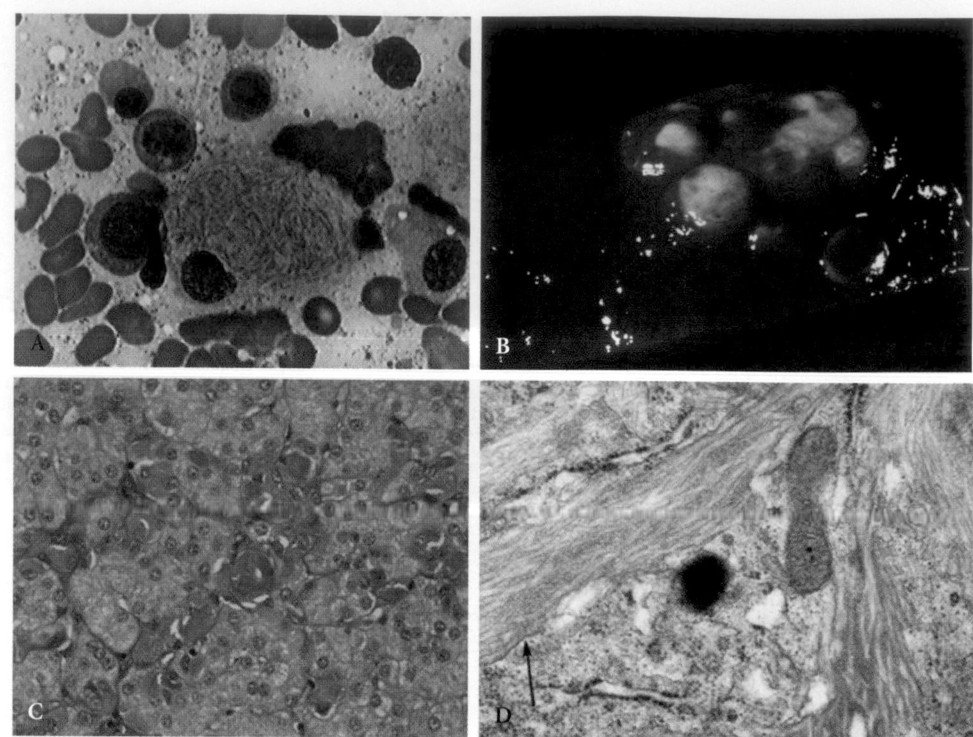

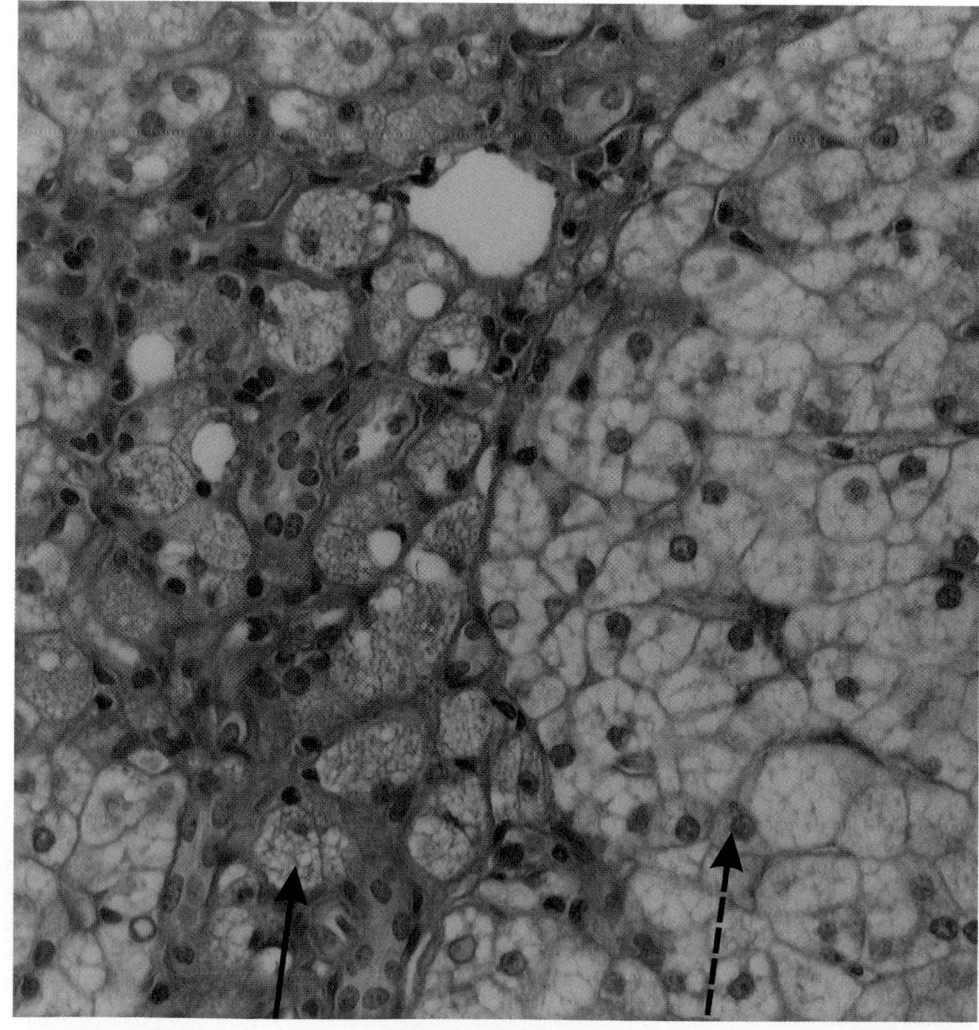

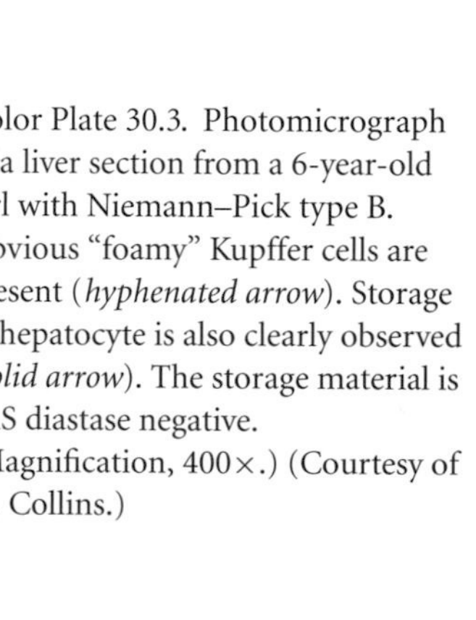

Color Plate 30.3. Photomicrograph of a liver section from a 6-year-old girl with Niemann–Pick type B. Obvious "foamy" Kupffer cells are present (*hyphenated arrow*). Storage in hepatocyte is also clearly observed (*solid arrow*). The storage material is PAS diastase negative. (Magnification, 400×.) (Courtesy of M. Collins.)

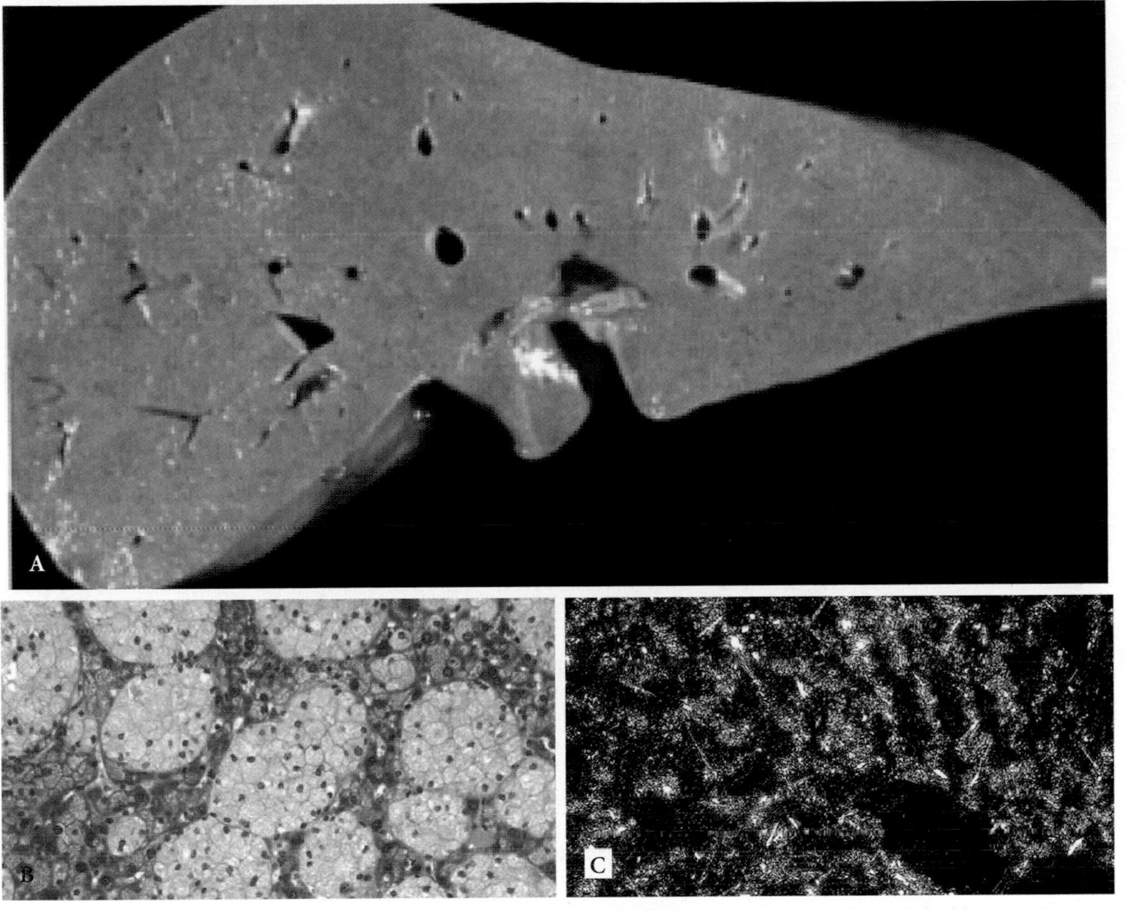

Color Plate 30.5. Liver from a lysosomal acid lipase–deficient human (CESD, **A**) and mouse (**B** and **C**). (**A**) Typical orange-yellow color of the liver from a patient with CESD. (**B**) Clusters of engorged Kupffer cells are evident as is the storage of neutral fats (cholesteryl esters and triglycerides) in hepatocytes. (Magnification 200×.) (**C**) Polarized light micrograph of lysosomal acid lipase–deficient mouse liver section. (Courtesy of H. Du.) Cholesterol crystals are evident as are numerous other birefringent bodies. Livers in patients with Wolman's disease and CESD are similar.

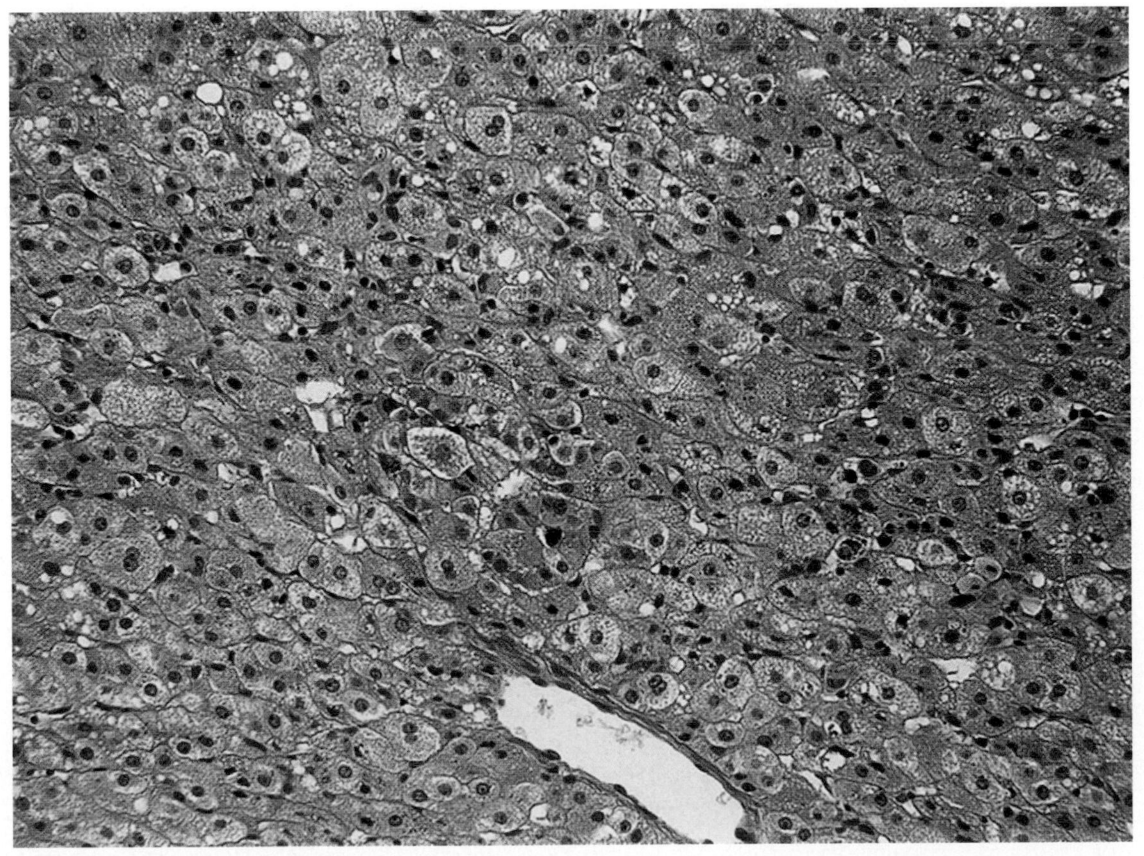

Color Plate 33.2. Liver histology from 11-week-old male infant with mtDNA depletion caused by *POLG* mutation. Biopsy at presentation with diarrhea, weakness, failure to thrive, and elevated AST, ALT, INR, and plasma lactate. Biopsy shows mild hepatocyte swelling with scattered microvesicular steatosis and cholestasis. Portal tracts are normal and there is no fibrosis. (H&E, ×200.)

Color Plate 33.3. Higher power views of liver histology from patient with mtDNA depletion syndrome in Color Plate 33.2, showing microvesicular steatosis (*arrows*) and canalicular cholestasis (*circles*). (PAS positive diastase, ×800.)

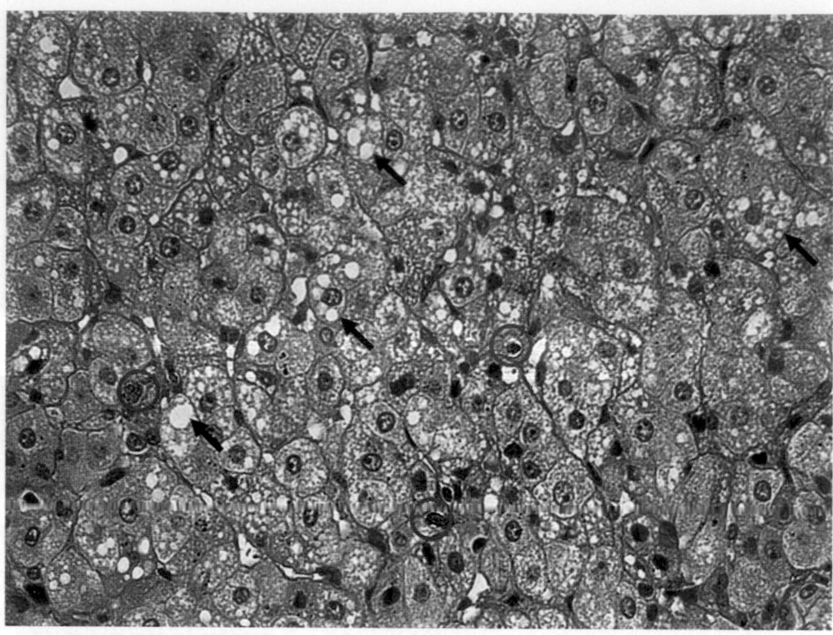

Color Plate 33.4. Oil-red-O stain of frozen section of liver biopsy in Color Plate 33.2, showing marked microvesicular steatosis in most hepatocytes, despite benign appearance of the biopsy in Color Plate 33.2. (Oil-red-O, ×100.)

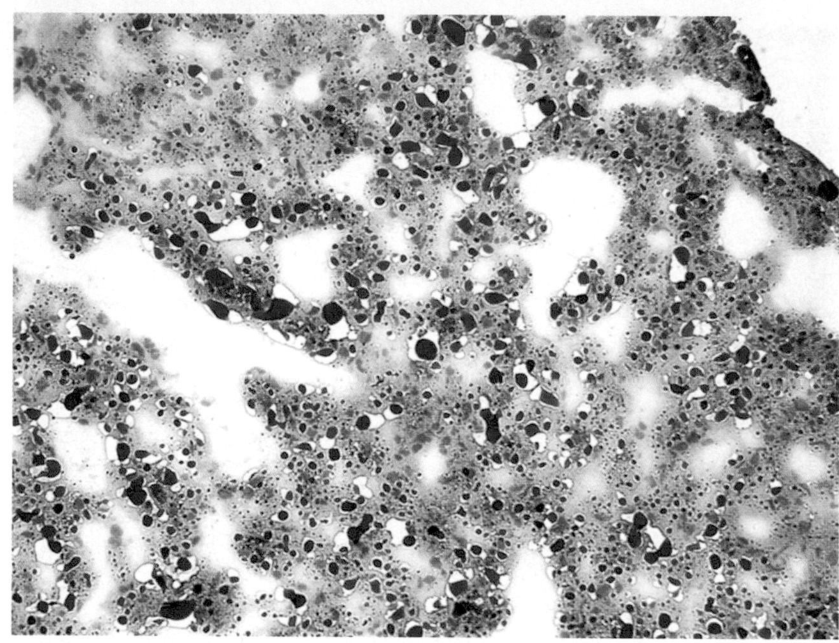

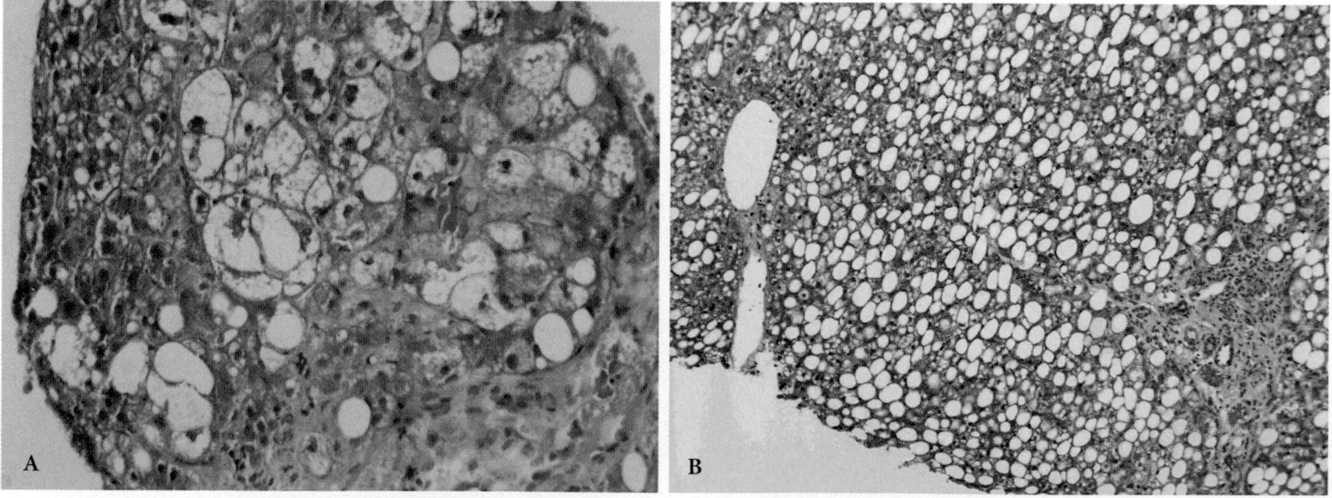

Color Plate 34.1. Histologic patterns of pediatric nonalcoholic steatohepatitis (NASH). Shown are liver biopsies from two children with NASH. (**A**) A biopsy typical of type 1 NASH with ballooning degeneration of hepatocytes and perisinusoidal fibrosis. (**B**) A biopsy typical of type 2 NASH with a normal central vein, no hepatocytes ballooning but with portal inflammation and fibrosis.

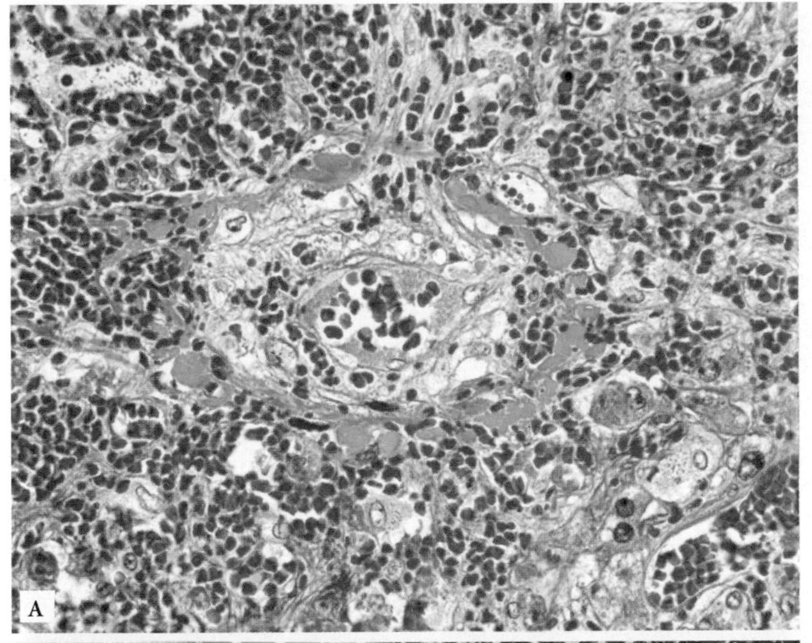

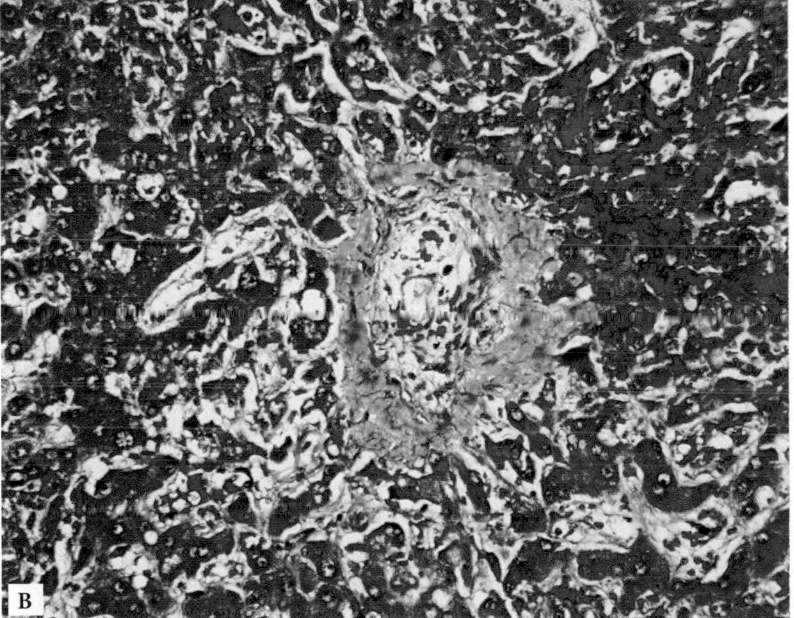

Color Plate 38.1. Pathology of hepatic veno-occlusive following bone marrow transplantation. (**A**) Partial occlusion of hepatic venule shows endothelial proliferation overlying cell debris. The vein wall is fibrotic. Perivenular zone is hemorrhagic because of obstruction. (**B**) Complete obstruction of a hepatic venule with sinusoidal congestion. (H&E stain, original magnification ×350.) (Courtesy of Drs. Howard Shulman and Laurie Deleve.)

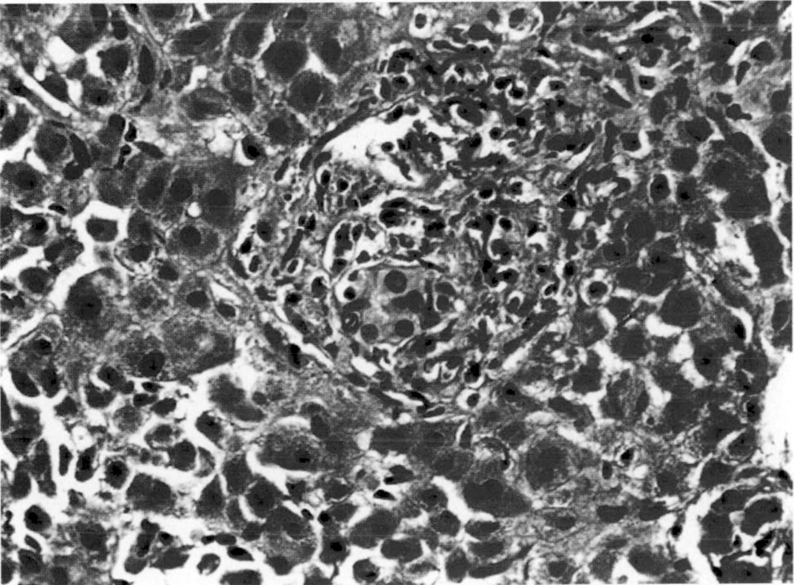

Color Plate 38.2. Pathology of hepatic graft-versus-host disease. Lymphocytic infiltrate in the portal area following allogeneic bone marrow engraftment. The lymphocytic infiltrate is invading the biliary epithelium causing degeneration and necrosis (*arrow*). (H&E stain, original magnification ×400.) (From Barshes NR, Myers GD, Lee D, et al. Liver transplantation for severe hepatic graft-versus-host disease. An analysis of aggregate survival data. Liver Transpl 2005;11:525–31; used with permission.)

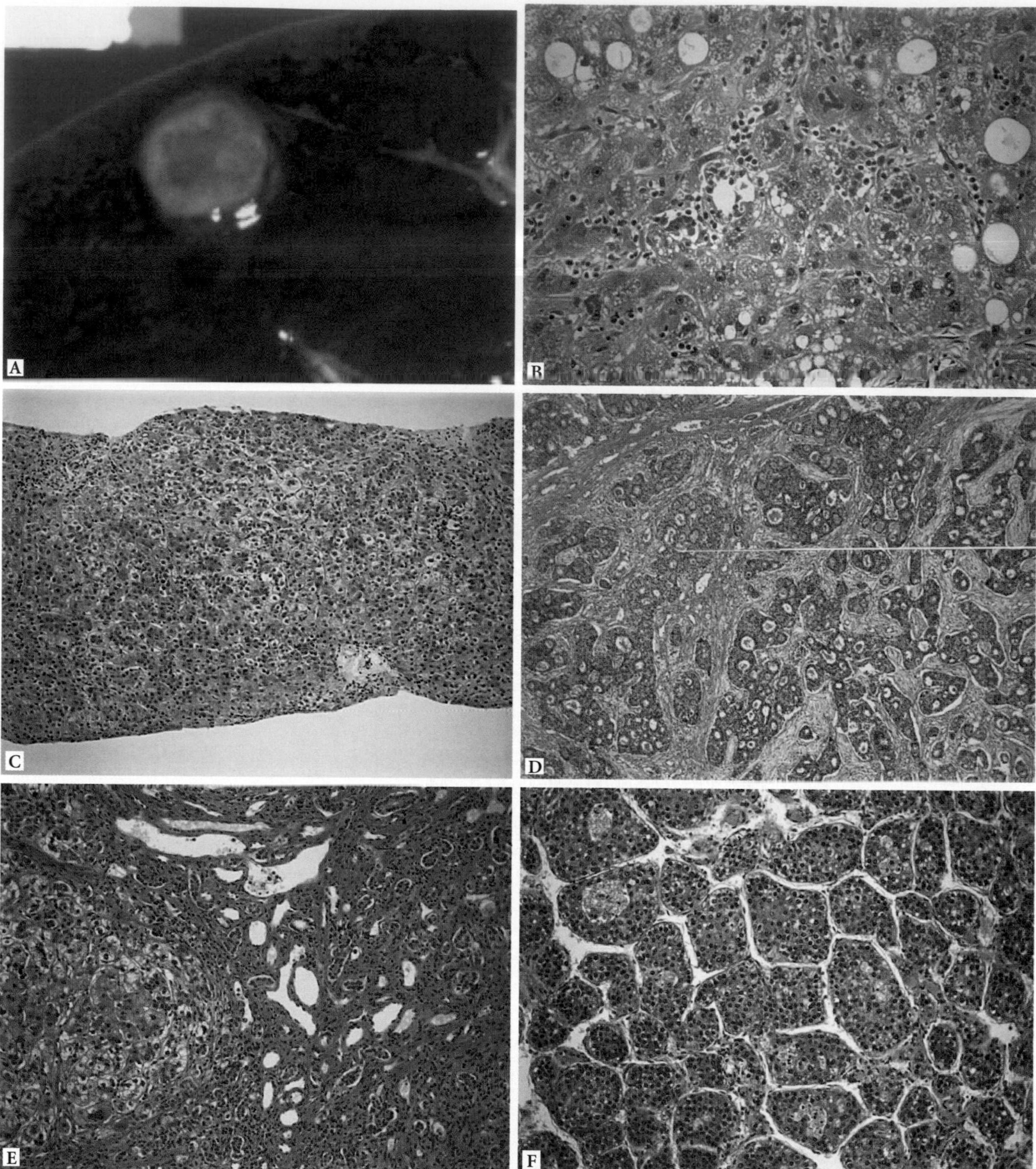

Color Plate 40.2. Metabolic diseases leading to neoplasia. (**A**) Adenoma in autopsy liver of a 12-year-old with glycogen storage disease (GSD), type 1A (glucose 6 phosphatase deficiency). (**B**) Adenoma in GSD 1A has "alcoholic hepatitis"–like histology with fat, Mallory bodies, and inflammation. (**C**) Alagille syndrome. Biopsy at 4 months of age shows bland cholestasis and paucity of the bile ducts. (**D**) Cholangiocarcinoma at age 8 years. (**E**) Biliary cirrhosis at age 29 months, secondary to bile salt excretory protein deficiency (progressive familial intrahepatic cholestasis type 2). (**F**) Hepatocarcinoma found in explant.

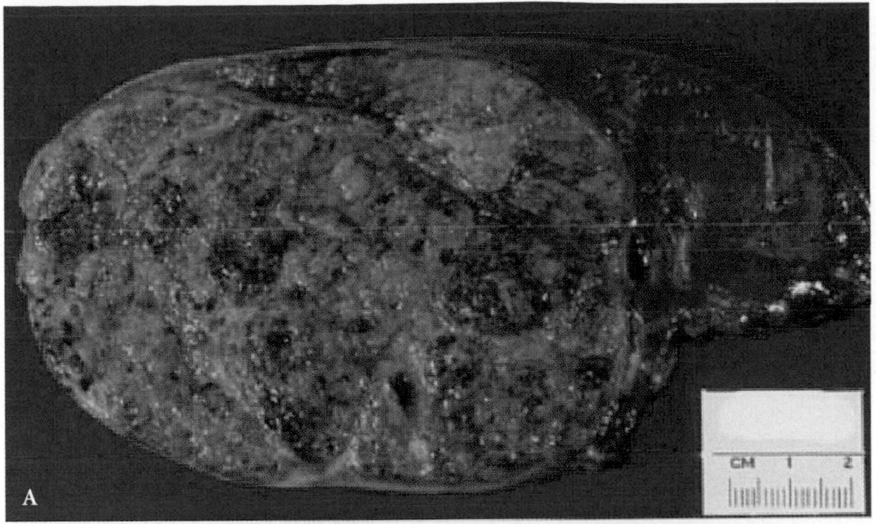

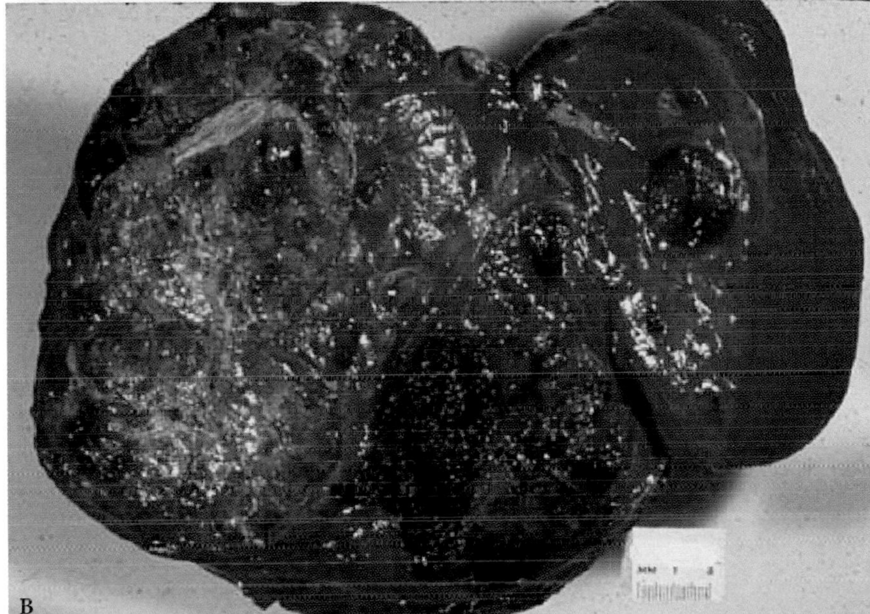

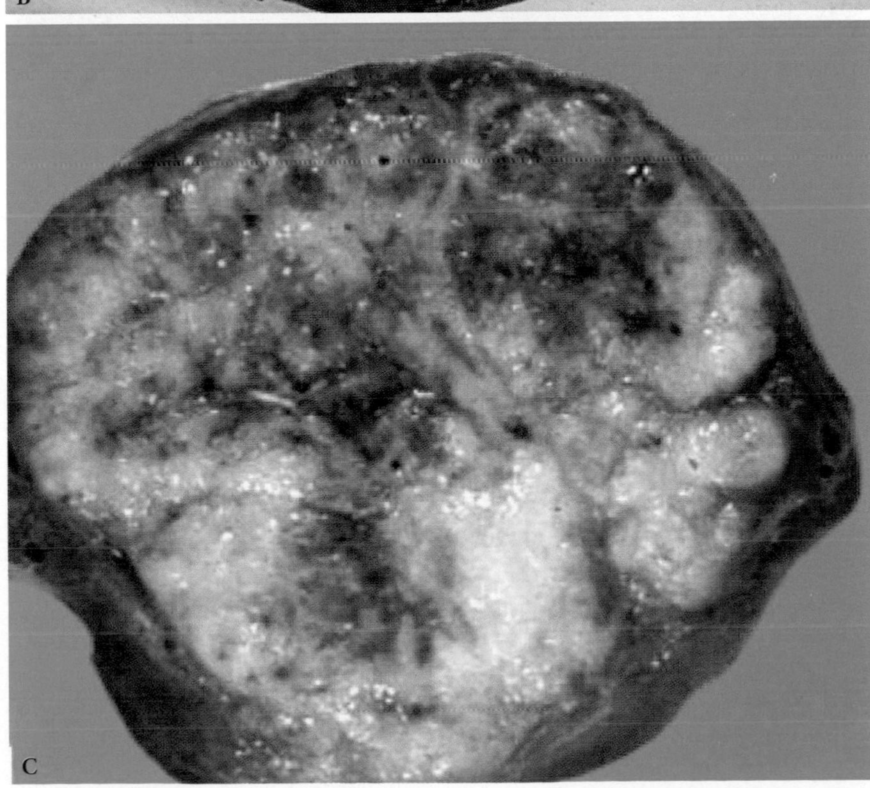

Color Plate 40.6. Gross appearance of hepatoblastoma.
(**A**) Most of this tumor was composed of well-differentiated fetal hepatoblasts.
(**B**) Mixed hepatoblastoma with embryonal, fetal, and mesenchymal tissues. (**C**) Small cell undifferentiated hepatoblastoma is sarcoma like.

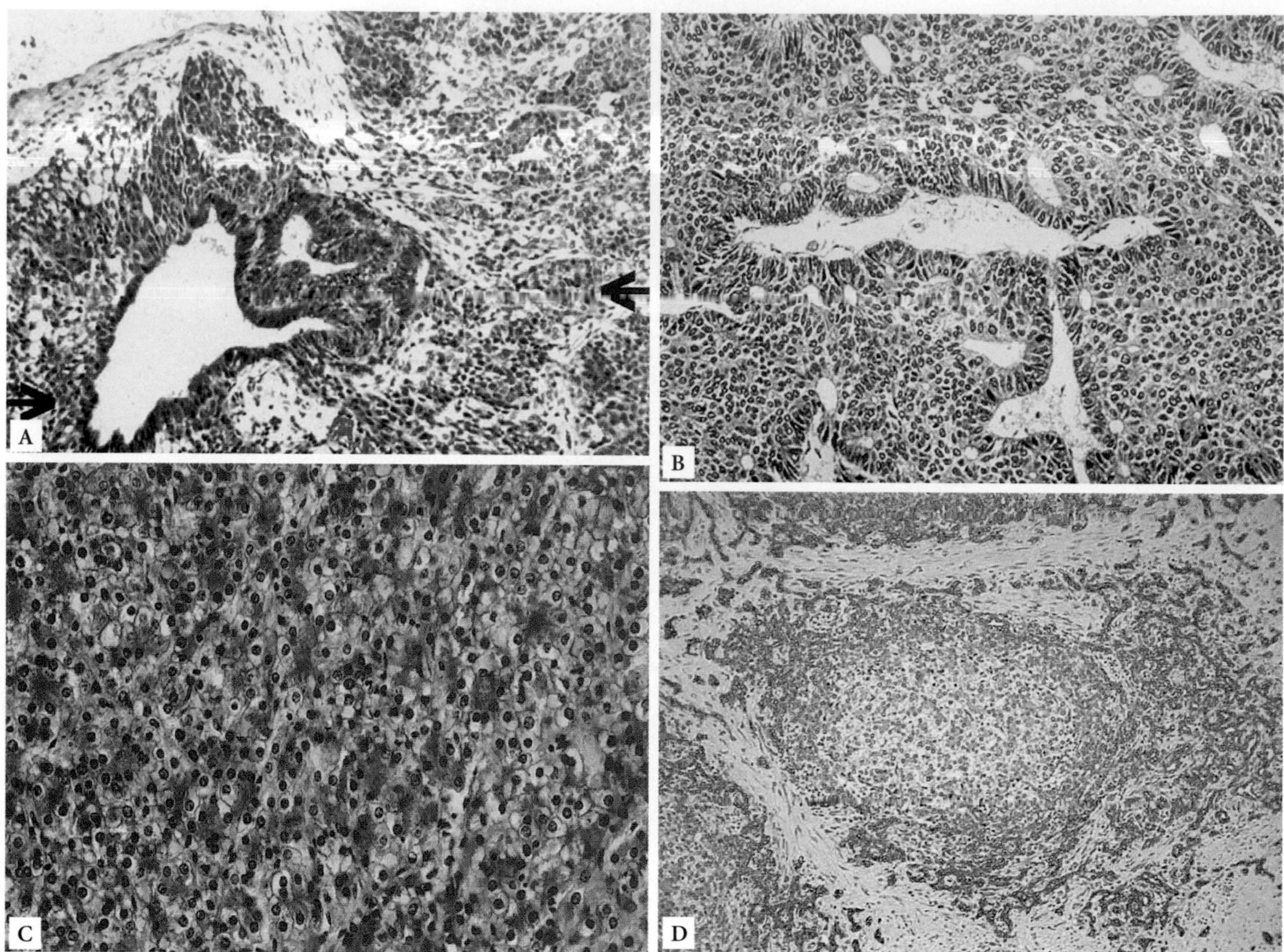

Color Plate 40.7. Histology of hepatoblastomas. (**A**) Histology of the embryo liver at 6–7 weeks postconception. *Arrows* call attention to differentiating hepatoblasts. (**B**) Embryonal hepatoblastoma. Mimicry of the stages of development is the basis for tumor designations. A continuum between tumor types is therefore typical of HB. (**C**) Pure fetal hepatoblastoma. The uniformity of these mature mitotically inactive cells growing in a normal cordlike manner may make them difficult to distinguish from normal hepatocytes in aspirates or small biopsies. The greater nuclear–cytoplasm is helpful. (**D**) Cholangioblastic hepatoblastoma. Cytokeratin 7 decorates the proliferative bile ductular cells, whereas hepatoblasts are unstained.

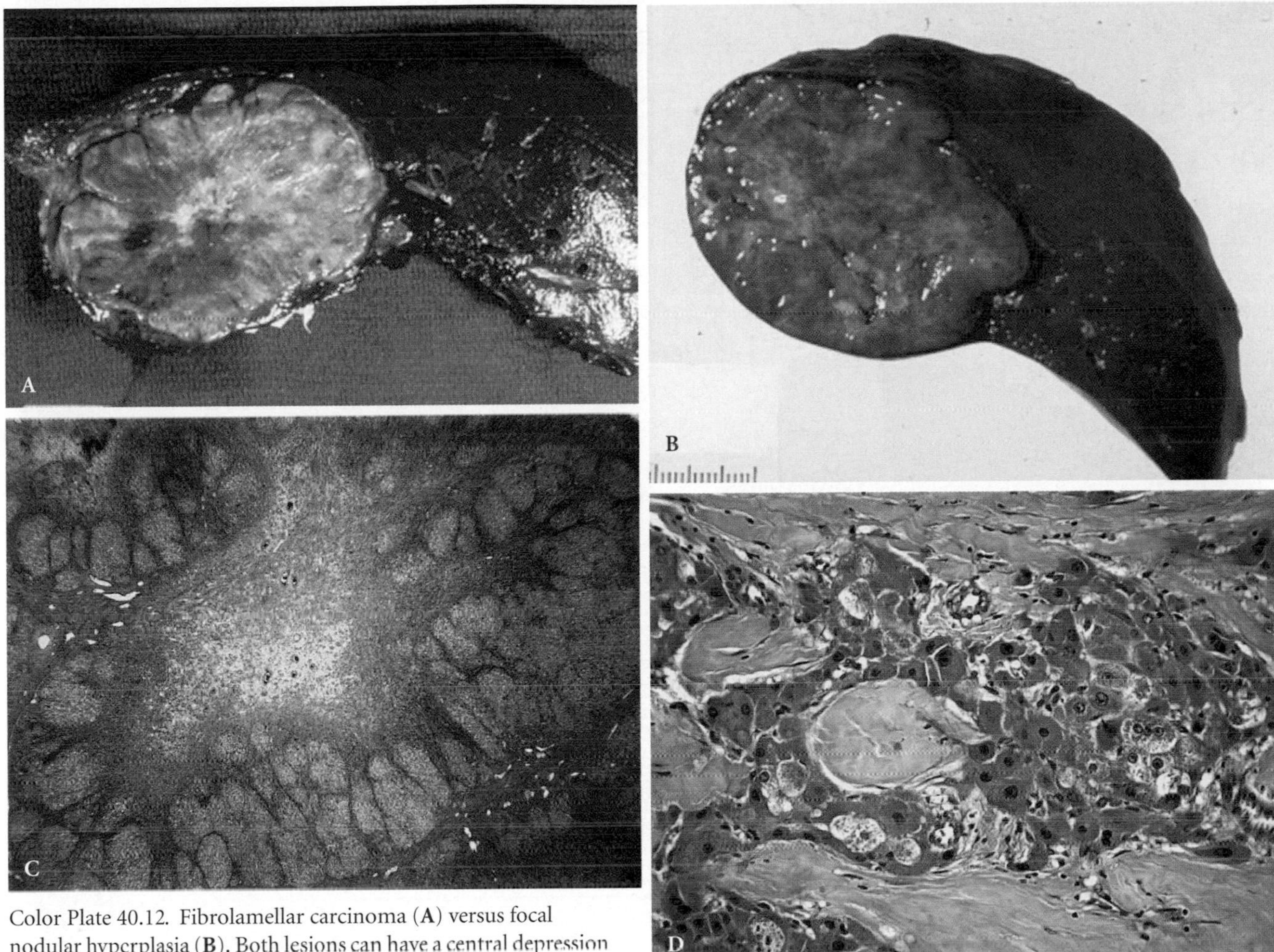

Color Plate 40.12. Fibrolamellar carcinoma (**A**) versus focal nodular hyperplasia (**B**). Both lesions can have a central depression due to scarring and both occur in a noncirrhotic host liver. The hepatocytes surrounding a central scar in focal nodular hyperplasia are normal in appearance (**C**). Histologically there is no difficulty in distinguishing them because large hypereosinophilic hepatocytes in the carcinoma are typically embedded in a dense fibrocollagenous stroma (**D**).

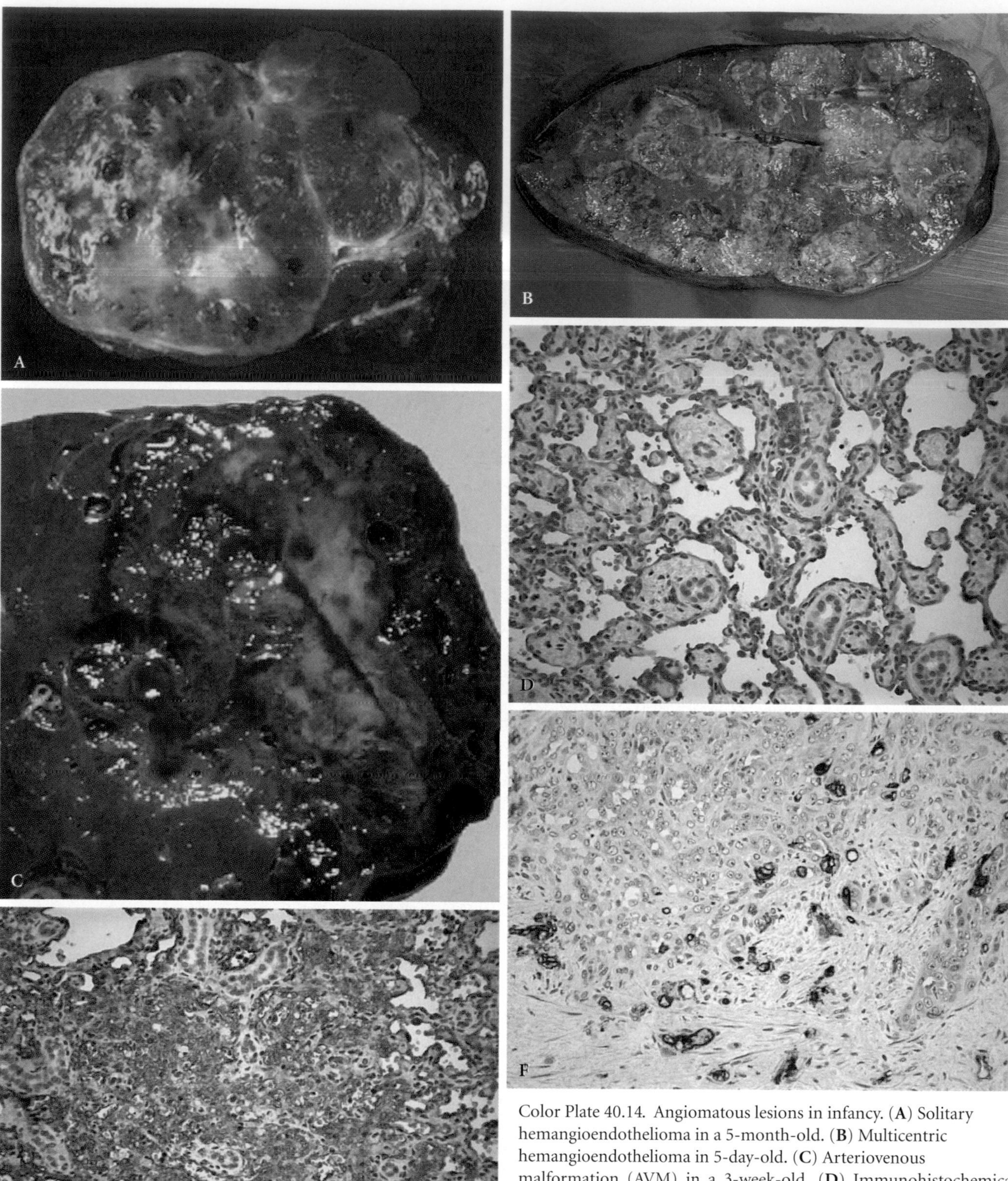

Color Plate 40.14. Angiomatous lesions in infancy. (**A**) Solitary hemangioendothelioma in a 5-month-old. (**B**) Multicentric hemangioendothelioma in 5-day-old. (**C**) Arteriovenous malformation (AVM) in a 3-week-old. (**D**) Immunohistochemical staining for glut 1 is uniformly positive in the endothelium of hemangioendothelioma and negative in the vessels of an AVM. (**E**) The active proliferation and infiltration of vasoformative positive cells as shown with CD 34 correlates with the extensive dissemination of the type 2 hemangioendothelioma. (**F**) Epithelioid hemangioendothelioma in a 15-year-old. Distinguishing this infiltrating pseudoglandular pattern from metastatic carcinoma is not difficult with immunohistochemical stains for endothelium. This is CD 34.

Section III: Hepatitis and Immune Disorders

17

Acute and Chronic Viral Hepatitis

Jay A. Hochman, M.D., and William F. Balistreri, M.D.

Optimal care of children with viral hepatitis necessitates incorporation of recent advances in diagnosis, prevention, and treatment into clinical practice. Though primary viral infection of the liver has been recognized since the time of Hippocrates (460–375 B.C.), only in the past two decades have significant scientific advancements allowed clinicians to alter the outcomes of these infections [1]. Specifically, viral hepatitis can be prevented with vaccines and passive immunization and can be treated with antiviral medications. The availability to detect these infections rapidly and accurately has led to changes in the epidemiology of viral hepatitis.

This chapter details the history, epidemiology, and clinical features as well as the diagnostic, preventative, and therapeutic strategies for the most important group of hepatotropic viruses: hepatitis A (HAV), hepatitis B (HBV), hepatitis C (HCV), hepatitis D (HDV), and hepatitis E (HEV). In 2002, the estimated numbers of new infections in the United States were as follows: 73,000 caused by HAV, 79,000 caused by HBV, and 29,000 caused by HCV/non-A, non-B (NANB) hepatitis [2]. The absolute number of cases of acute hepatitis had been reduced by more than 50% during the preceding 10-year interval (1992–2002). The availability and expansion of vaccination efforts have helped decrease the rates of hepatitis A and hepatitis B. Improvements in the blood supply have dramatically reduced transmission of HCV; the primary means of infection in children is now maternal–infant transmission. Although many other viruses, including cytomegalovirus, herpesvirus, varicella-zoster, Epstein–Barr, adenoviruses, enteroviruses, rubella, and Coxsackie B, can cause hepatitis as part of a generalized illness, they are not the focus of this chapter. To facilitate the discussion of both chronic and acute viral hepatitis, a glossary of the terminology used throughout this chapter is presented in Table 17.1.

HISTORICAL CONTEXT OF VIRAL HEPATITIS

Almost all our knowledge about the hepatitis viruses has been gathered in the past 60 years during a period of scientifically driven preoccupation with this group of diseases (Table 17.2). Before this period, the understanding of these infections was limited. Clinical features of hepatitis, "campaign jaundice," had been observed during wartime in military populations for hundreds of years. However, it was not until the 1940s that there was recognition of the underlying liver cell inflammation and subsequently the confirmation of a viral etiology. In addition, it was observed that infectious hepatitis (hepatitis A) differed from serum hepatitis (hepatitis B); the latter had a longer incubation period [3]. This observation was crystallized by MacCallum [4] who proposed the terminology of *hepatitis A* to differentiate infectious hepatitis from serum hepatitis. Additional work by Krugman et al. [5] documented that one strain of hepatitis, named MS-1, was transmitted predominantly via a fecal–oral route. In an endemic population at the Willowbrook State School, this agent was determined to have an incubation period of about 4 weeks and was highly infectious. This strain was further characterized by the presence in the stool of 27-nm particles on immune electron microscopy in infected persons. It is now recognized that the responsible agent was the HAV.

HEPATITIS A

Viral Characteristics

Hepatitis A is a small spherical, nonenveloped 27- to 32-nm, RNA-containing particle belonging to the hepatovirus group of picornaviruses (Figure 17.1). It is highly infectious and relatively resistant to disinfection, which is likely a result of its stability to heat, cold storage, and acidic conditions. Heating food to greater than 85°C or using disinfectant treatment on surfaces with a 1:100 dilution of sodium hydrochloride (household bleach) in tap water is necessary for inactivation. In the absence of these measures, HAV remains stable in the environment for long periods.

There is only one serotype of HAV. However, there are seven genotypes based on the criterion of 15–20% nucleotide diversity over a 168-base segment at the VP1/2A junction [6]. Genotype 1A predominates in the United States and western Europe [7,8]. The genome for HAV is enclosed in the nucleocapsid, which has been designated HAV antigen. It contains a linear,

Table 17.1: Glossary

Terminology	*Definition*	*Significance*
Hepatitis A virus (HAV)		
Anti-HAV IgM	Antibody (IgM subclass) directed against HAV	Indicates current or recent infection with HAV; detectable for 4–6 mo
Anti-HAV IgG*	Antibody (IgG subclass) directed against HAV	Indicates previous HAV infection and confirms immunity to HAV
Hepatitis B virus (HBV)		
HBsAg	HBV surface antigen; found on the surface of the intact virus and as unattached particles in the serum	Indicates acute or chronic infection
HBcAg	HBV core antigen; found within the core of the intact virus	Detectable in liver tissue but not detectable in serum
HBeAg	Hepatitis B e antigen; soluble antigen produced during cleavage of HBcAg	Indicates active HBV infection and correlates with HBV replication; signifies high infectivity
Anti-HBs*	Antibody to HBsAg	Subclass IgM indicates early response, and IgG indicates immunity to HBV
Anti-HBc	Antibody to HBV core antigen	Subclass IgM indicates early infection; is not a protective antibody. Subclass IgG indicates active acute or chronic infection.
Anti-HBe	Antibody to HBeAg	Seroconversion of HBeAg to anti-HBe indicates resolution of replicative phase in most cases
HBV DNA†	DNA of HBV	Indicates HBV replication
Hepatitis C virus (HCV)		
Anti-HCV	Antibody to HCV	Indicates exposure to HCV; does not indicate protective immunity
HCV RNA	RNA of HCV	Indicates HCV infection
EVR	Early viral clearance rate	Indicates early response to HCV treatment
SVR	Sustained viral clearance rate	Indicates long-term success with HCV treatment
Hepatitis D virus (HDV) (delta)		
HDVAg	δ antigen	Indicates HDV infection
Anti-HDV	Antibody to HCV (IgM and IgG)	Indicates exposure to HDV
HDV RNA	RNA of HDV	Indicates HDV replication
Hepatitis E virus (HEV)		
HEVAg	Antigen associated with HEV	Indicates recent infection when detected in stool
Anti-HEV	Antibody to HEV	Indicates exposure to HEV
HEV RNA	RNA of HEV	Indicates early HEV infection

*Presence may indicate acquisition of antibody through immune globulin administration or protective immunity following infection or vaccination.

†Positive in infection with precore HBV mutants regardless of HBV replicative level.

Table 17.2: Advances in Viral Hepatitis

Advance	*Year*
Hepatitis A recognized	1947
Hepatitis B strains and hepatitis A virus isolated	1967
Fecal excretion of hepatitis A documented	1973
Hepatitis D (delta) identified	1977
Vaccine for hepatitis B licensed	1982
Hepatitis C virus identified	1989
Hepatitis E virus identified	1990
Vaccine for hepatitis A licensed	1996
Ribavirin/interferon treatment for hepatitis C	1996
Pegylated interferon for treatment of hepatitis C	2000
Lamivudine approved for hepatitis B in children	2002

single-stranded molecule of RNA. HAV has been cultured in several cell lines, and the HAV genome has been cloned [9–11].

Humans are thought to be the principal hosts for HAV; however, several nonhuman primates may become infected with HAV. Because there is no known carrier state, HAV infection is maintained in nature by serial transmission from acutely infected individuals to those who are susceptible [9–12]. Because of the large number of individuals with asymptomatic infection and the transmission of the virus usually before the onset of clinical symptoms, HAV continues to be the most common *reported* cause of acute hepatitis in the United States, with 8795 reported cases in 2002 [2]. The total number of acute HAV cases for that year was estimated to be 73,000 [2].

In the infected host, the virus replicates in the liver and is transported through the bile to the stool. Fecal viral excretion begins 1–3 weeks before the onset of illness and continues for a week or more after the onset of clinical symptoms; in children, there is a prolonged period of viral excretion [13]. High concentrations of HAV, up to 10^8 infectious virions per milliliter, are found in the stool. Transmission then occurs through person-to-person spread, primarily via an orofecal route. Viral particles can be identified in the stool by electron microscopy in the early prodromal phase of the illness, during a period of maximal infectivity. The ingested virus replicates in the small bowel and migrates via the portal vein before entering the liver by attachment to a viral receptor on the hepatocyte membrane. The cycle is completed when the replicated mature HAV is then excreted via the bile. The serum and saliva of infected persons have lower concentrations of HAV than the stool, approximately 10^4 and 10^2, respectively. Transmission via saliva has not been reported to occur.

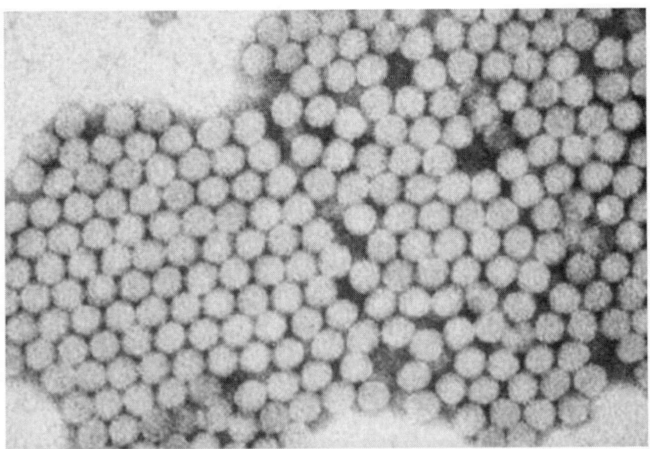

Figure 17.1. Electron micrograph of HAV in stool.

Epidemiology

Hepatitis A is a common illness, with prevalence rates highest in areas with limited hygiene and sanitation practices. High prevalent countries/regions include Mexico, India, the Middle East, and Africa. (A prevalence map is available at www.cdc.gov/ncidod/hepatitis/slideset/hep_a/hep_a.ptt). A direct correlation exists between the prevalence of anti-HAV immunoglobulin G (IgG), the marker of prior HAV exposure, and low socioeconomic status [11,14–16]. In developing countries, where infection is endemic, most people are infected during the first decade of life. As an example, a recent study documented that more than 80% of children in Tamilnadu, India, were anti-HAV positive by 4 years of age and 97%, by 12 years [17].

In developed countries, paradoxically, there is a large population susceptible to periodic outbreaks because of fewer infections in childhood (Table 17.3). In the United States, HAV infection remains a leading vaccine-preventable disease, with an average of more than 200,000 infections annually over the last decade [18,19]. Improved sanitary standards have reduced the likelihood of fecal contamination and subsequent environmental exposure. This, in turn, has resulted in a lower overall incidence of HAV (Figures 17.2 and 17.3). In recent years, the number of infections has been reduced. According to the Centers for Disease Control and Prevention (CDC), the number of *reported* infections in 2003 was 7653, the estimated number of acute clinical cases was 33,000, and the estimated number of all new infections was 61,000 [20]. At the same time, the decreased rates of natural immunity have facilitated the ability of HAV to cause outbreaks owing to an expanding susceptible population and have shifted the burden of HAV to older populations, who are more likely to experience morbidity and mortality from HAV (Table 17.3). Still, HAV infection is common among children. Approximately one third of reported cases of HAV infection occur in children; this is probably an underestimate because children often have minimal manifestations [14,15]. In addition, because of their lack of symptoms and poor hygiene practices, children serve as a frequent transmission source. Therefore, vaccination of children is the key to reducing the incidence of HAV infection further.

Hepatitis A is highly contagious. Factors associated with increased transmission rates include crowding, poor personal

Table 17.3: Global Patterns of Hepatitis A Transmission

Endemicity	*Disease Rate*	*Peak Age of Infection*	*Transmission Patterns*
High	Low to high	Early childhood	Person to person; outbreaks uncommon
Moderate	High	Late childhood/young adults	Person to person; food- and water-borne outbreaks
Low	Low	Young adults	Person to person; food- and water-borne outbreaks
Very low	Very low	Adults	Travelers; outbreaks uncommon

hygiene, improper sanitation, and contamination of food and water; prominent risk factors include close contact with patients with hepatitis A, spending time in child care centers, travel to endemic regions, male homosexual activity, and intravenous drug abuse (Figure 17.4). Transmission by blood transfusion or from mother to newborn (i.e., vertical transmission) is rare. Similarly, transmission from nonhuman primates has rarely been documented.

Surveillance for hepatitis, conducted since 1981 by the CDC in four sentinel counties, has shown that the patterns of hepatitis A epidemiology are heterogeneous. In approximately 50% of patients, the source of the infection could not be identified [12]. Reviewing data from 1990–2000, household or sexual contact with a person with hepatitis A was identified in 14%; a history of injection drug use within the 6 months preceding the onset of illness was the presumed factor in 6% (Figure 17.4) [2]. In this group, it is not clear whether sharing needles was involved in transmission or whether poor hygiene at the time of drug use was the main issue. Attendance or employment in a day care has been identified in 2% of patients, recent male homosexual activity in 10%, and international travel in 5%. These same risk factors are identified in the most recent available data [20]. In 2002, of the 8795 reported cases, 3037 had sufficient information to assign a risk factor. In this group, the proportion of cases due to international travel and injection drug use had increased. Over the previous decade, the proportion attributed to international travel had steadily increased from 1.3% (1992) to 2.8% (1995) to 5.6% (1998) to 9.4% (2002). With regard to illegal drug use, there had been a decline from approximately 10% of cases in 1996 to 3.6% in 2001; this has reversed in the current data to 5.9% (2002). Although hepatitis A has received notoriety from outbreaks related to common source outbreaks (e.g., restaurants), this is actually an infrequent cause of HAV infection [12].

Although food-borne transmission may not cause a large absolute number of infections, these infections illustrate the

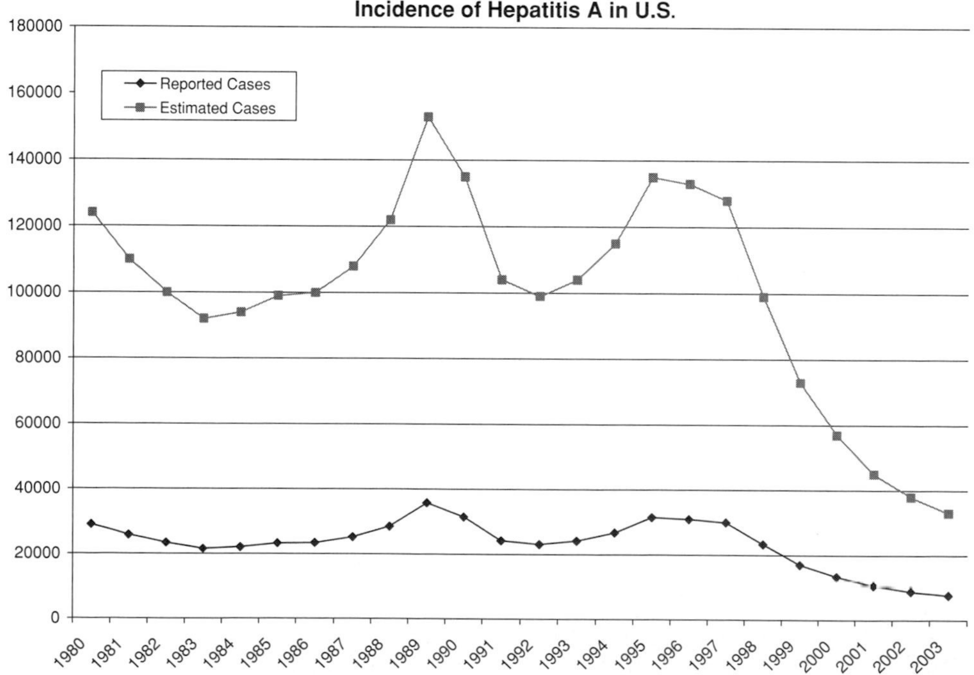

Figure 17.2. The number of reported HAV cases indicates the cases reported to the national notifiable disease surveillance system of the CDC. (From the Centers for Disease Control and Prevention [2].)

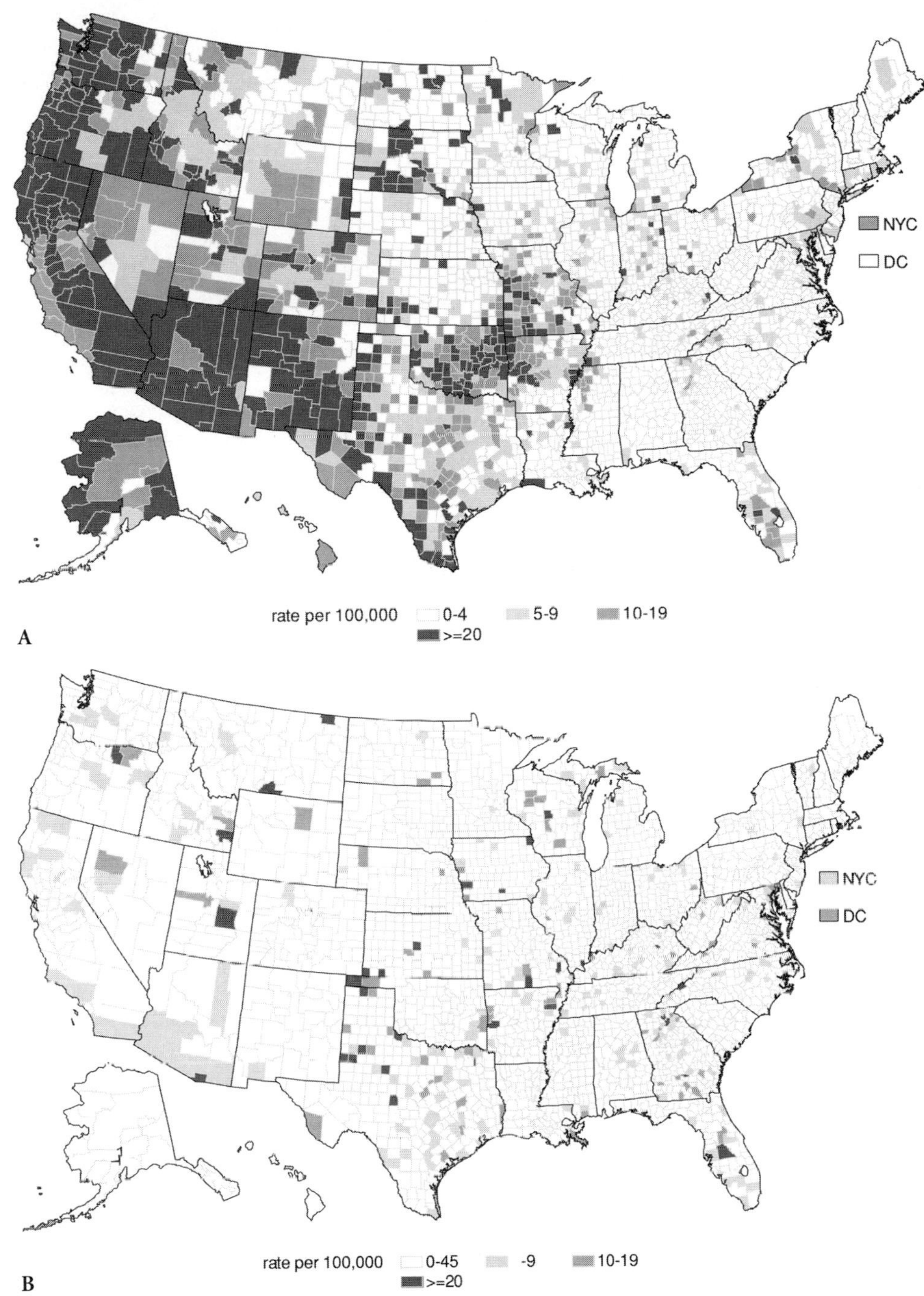

Figure 17.3. The decrease in incidence of HAV over a 5-year period can be seen in this state and county map of the United States. Unlike the baseline period of 1987–1997 (**A**), in 2002 (**B**), there were few counties with more than 20 cases per 100,000. (From the Centers for Disease Control and Prevention [2]; also accessed March 20, 2005, at http://www.cdc.gov/ncidod/diseases/hepatitis/slideset/index.htm.)

difficulty of controlling HAV with the policy of limiting protection to postexposure prophylaxis and to higher-risk individuals. In 2001, the Massachusetts Department of Public Health was notified of an infected worker at a restaurant [21]. Despite apparently high standards of hygiene, including frequent hand washing and use of gloves in food preparation, and lack of gastrointestinal symptoms in this managerial worker, 46 persons became infected. Even though food handlers are not at increased risk for HAV infection, 8% of adults reported with HAV are identified annually as food handlers in the United States [21]. Unlike most HAV cases, which are transmitted to close contacts, food handlers can transmit HAV to many others. A single outbreak of this size can cost approximately $800,000 [22]. The other salient point is that hygiene practices are subjective. In individuals who can be identified within 2 weeks of exposure, postexposure prophylaxis needs to be considered.

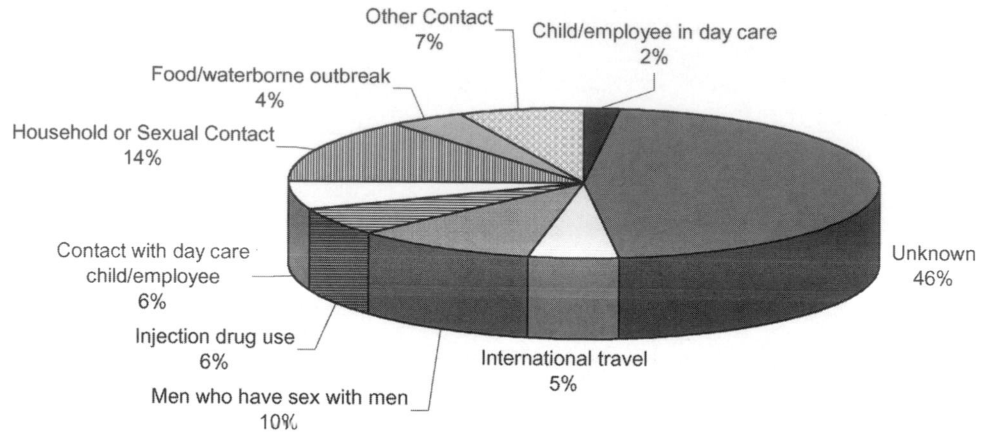

Figure 17.4. This pie chart illustrates the most common sources of HAV infection from 1990 through 2000. Forty-six percent of reported hepatitis A cases could not identify a risk factor for their infection. (Accessed March 20, 2005, at http://www.cdc.gov/ncidod/diseases/hepatitis/slideset/index.htm.)

Multiple steps in the food chain allow dissemination of HAV [22]. An outbreak of 601 persons in Monaca, Pennsylvania, in 2003 resulted from ingestion of green onions imported from Mexico [23,24]. Three people died of liver failure during this outbreak. No ill food service workers could be identified. The green onions were thought to be contaminated before reaching the restaurant; thus, the spread of this infection likely originated during growing, harvesting, packing, or cooling. The fact that this outbreak affected a large number of people may be related to the intermingling of the contaminated food with several uncontaminated foods at the restaurant; previous smaller outbreaks related to green onions have been reported [25].

Many foods have been incriminated as the vehicle for HAV delivery. A multistate food-borne outbreak of hepatitis A illustrates the impact of the disease on children; 213 cases of HAV infection were reported in children attending 23 schools in Michigan and 29 cases from 13 schools in Maine [26]. This outbreak was associated with consumption of frozen strawberries, presumably contaminated during harvesting. The genetic sequences of the infective strains isolated from these cases were linked with strains from patients from Wisconsin and Arizona. The Food and Drug Administration (FDA) has promoted guidelines for control measures to ensure appropriate water quality, use of properly treated manure or biosolids, and provision of sanitary facilities for field workers [27]. The Good Agricultural Practices/Good Manufacturing Practices recommended by the FDA are a worthwhile goal. Nevertheless, there are multiple potential pitfalls. Although the agriculture standards in the United States are high, with a global economy, many foods in the American diet are produced in faraway places. Certain countries that export food to the United States have a high rate of endemic HAV, and contamination of agricultural products is likely to be a frequent occurrence. Once contaminated products are distributed in a population without significant herd immunity, the consequences may prove fatal.

Food-borne infections and travel as sources of HAV are linked. In a recent study, HAV infection among Hispanic children, who are known to have a higher rate of infection (Figure 17.5), was associated with cross-border travel to Mexico and food-borne exposure during travel [28]. Eating foods from a taco stand or street vendor increased the risk of infection more than 17-fold, whereas eating lettuce increased the risk of developing HAV infection more than fivefold. In contrast to previous studies, this study showed an increased risk with higher socioeconomic status. That is, families that could not afford to travel were less likely to be exposed to HAV.

Day care centers serve as a vector for HAV spread throughout local communities [29–32]. Besides viral characteristics that enhance transmission, the high rate of spread is attributable to the crowded conditions, poor hygiene, and mild illness among the infected children. In addition to the attendees and staff, the burden of HAV cases is shared with associated family members. The clinical symptoms in affected children are minimal – almost all are anicteric. This illness may resemble the "flu" or gastroenteritis. It is widely known that many families send their

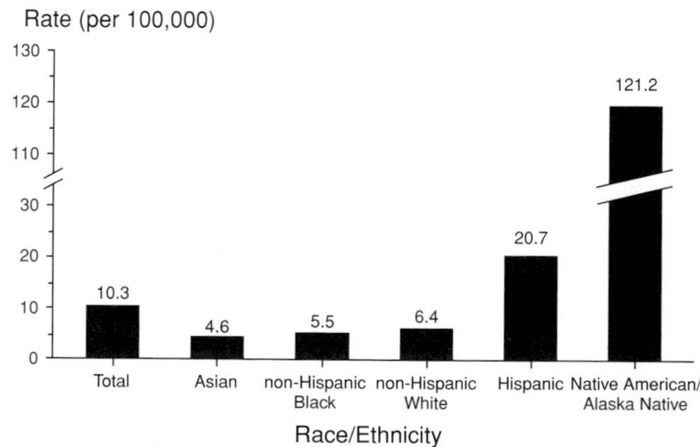

Figure 17.5. Rates of reported hepatitis A by race/ethnicity in the United States, 1994. In 1994, Native Americans had a high incidence of HAV infections. This has changed dramatically, as shown in Figure 17.8. (From the Centers for Disease Control and Prevention [2]; also accessed March 20, 2005, at http://www.cdc.gov/ncidod/diseases/hepatitis/slideset/index.htm.)

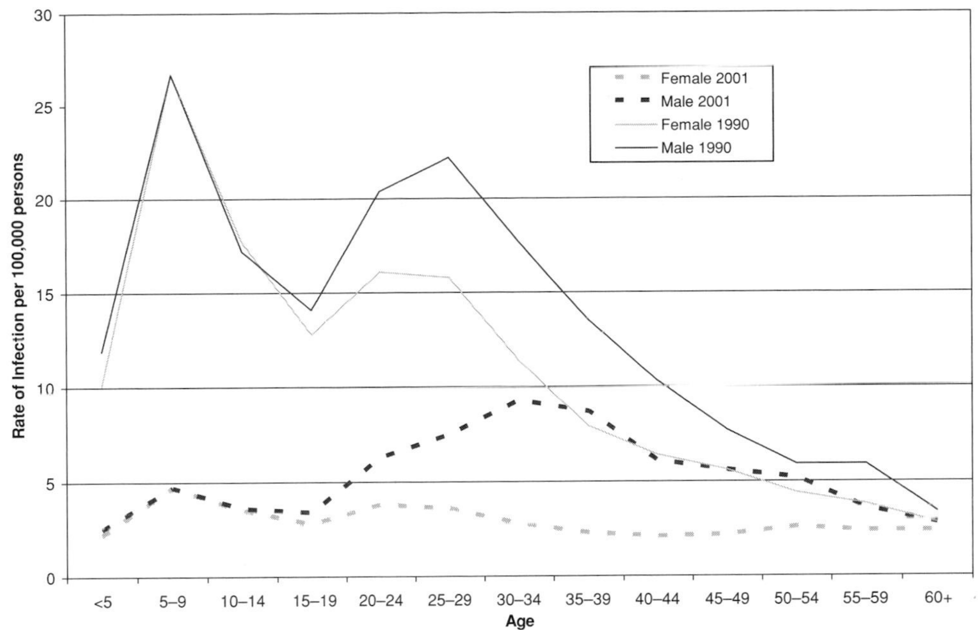

Figure 17.6. With the implementation of vaccination among targeted high-risk groups, the incidence of hepatitis A in 2001 had decreased among all males and females in all age groups. At the same time, a much larger proportion of cases are occurring among older persons and among men. These changes reflect the increased proportion of high-risk groups, including men who have sex with men and users of illicit drugs, which are difficult to target with vaccinations. (From the Centers for Disease Control and Prevention [2].)

children to day care centers with these clinical symptoms. Only diligent hand washing, control of hygiene conditions, and use of prophylactic measures, when indicated, can decrease these infections.

Because HAV infection occurs in so many settings, it is difficult to control. Inside the halls of our hospitals, HAV is a known nosocomial pathogen. It is not surprising that hepatitis A would be transmitted in the setting of diarrheal illnesses [33–36]. Although rarely documented, it can also be transmitted through contaminated transfusions [33–36]. Because HAV infection may represent an occupational hazard, many encourage pediatric health care workers to be vaccinated [18].

In the United States, the incidence of infection is highest in the western states among persons between 5 and 39 years of age (Figure 17.6) [2]. Overall, one third of the U.S. population has serologic evidence of previous HAV infection [12]. The prevalence among 6- to 11-year-olds is 9% and 75% among persons older than 70. Cyclic communitywide outbreaks of hepatitis A occurring every 5–10 years have been noted for decades. Despite these episodic setbacks, there has been a trend of a decreased incidence of HAV infection over the past two decades (Figure 17.6). This decreasing incidence has been most marked among the western states, which now have rates of HAV infection similar to other parts of the country (Figure 17.7, Table 17.4). At-risk groups, such as Native Americans, now have incidence rates below the average U.S. rate (Figure 17.8).

The epidemiology of HAV is changing in the United States (see Figure 17.3). Part of the reason for these epidemiologic changes is immunization. However, even in states where routine HAV vaccination is recommended, in 2003, only 50.9% of children received one or more doses [37]; this compares to a rate of 25% for children in states where vaccination is suggested and 1.4% in states without a vaccination recommendation. Although the overall incidence has declined, there have been areas of increased incidence. In these areas, the increase in HAV is occurring in high-risk groups who are not receiving immunizations, including drug users and men who have sex with men. This is reflected in an increased proportion of cases among men and an increased mean age of infection (see Figure 17.6). The changing epidemiology of HAV infection is of concern because of the higher morbidity and mortality among adults.

Clinical Aspects and Pathogenesis

Hepatitis A virus infection in adults or adolescents is characterized by an abrupt onset of nonspecific features such as fever, headache, anorexia, nausea, dark urine, malaise, right upper quadrant abdominal pain, and jaundice (Table 17.5). Common signs of infection include leukopenia, hepatomegaly, and splenomegaly. Clinical features cannot reliably distinguish hepatitis A from other forms of viral hepatitis and other liver diseases [38]. The illness is usually self-limited, and the severity is age dependent. In infants and preschool-aged children, acute hepatitis A may be clinically inapparent. Only 30% of children in this age range have symptoms; if illness does occur, it is

Table 17.4: States with Highest Incidence of HAV

1987–1997	*Rate**	*2001*	*Rate**
Arizona	48	District of Columbia	14
Alaska	45	Georgia	12
Oregon	40	Arizona	8
New Mexico	40	Rhode Island	7
Utah	33	Connecticut	7
Washington	30	Kansas	7
Oklahoma	24	Maryland	6
South Dakota	24	Massachusetts	6
Idaho	21	Texas	6
Nevada	21	Florida	5
California	20	California	5

*Rate indicates the number of infections per 100,000 persons. During the period between 1987 and 1997, this number reflects an average incidence [2].

not usually accompanied by jaundice [38]. Among older children and adults, symptomatic infection with jaundice occurs in more than 70% [39]. Signs and symptoms typically resolve within 2 months, though 10–15% of symptomatic persons have a relapsing or prolonged course lasting up to 9 months.

The overall case-fatality rate is 0.3%, but it is 1.8% among persons 50 years or older [38]. Persons with underlying chronic liver disease, including HCV infection, have an increased risk of death [38,40]. Other factors that are important in determining a fulminant course may include gender, immune function, and concomitant drug administration. In a recent study from France analyzing these factors, encephalopathy and low factor V level were related to female gender, low serum levels of HAV by polymerase chain reaction (PCR) assay, genotypes other than 1A, and acetaminophen intake [6]. The low viral load was the main factor associated with fulminant hepatic failure in this series of 50 patients. The authors concluded that HAV-induced liver disease is primarily the result of an excessive immunologic response. This conclusion is strengthened by in vitro data showing that most HAV strains have no detectable cytopathic effect in cell culture [41]. Furthermore, in patients with human immunodeficiency virus (HIV)-associated immunodeficiency, HAV-related acute liver failure has not been reported despite increased viral loads and prolonged viremia [42].

The sequence of clinical and serologic events occurring during hepatitis A is shown in Figure 17.9. The incubation period for HAV ranges from 15–40 days (mean, 28 days). With electron microscopy, viral particles can be detected in the stools during the late incubation period. Viremia is detected by qualitative

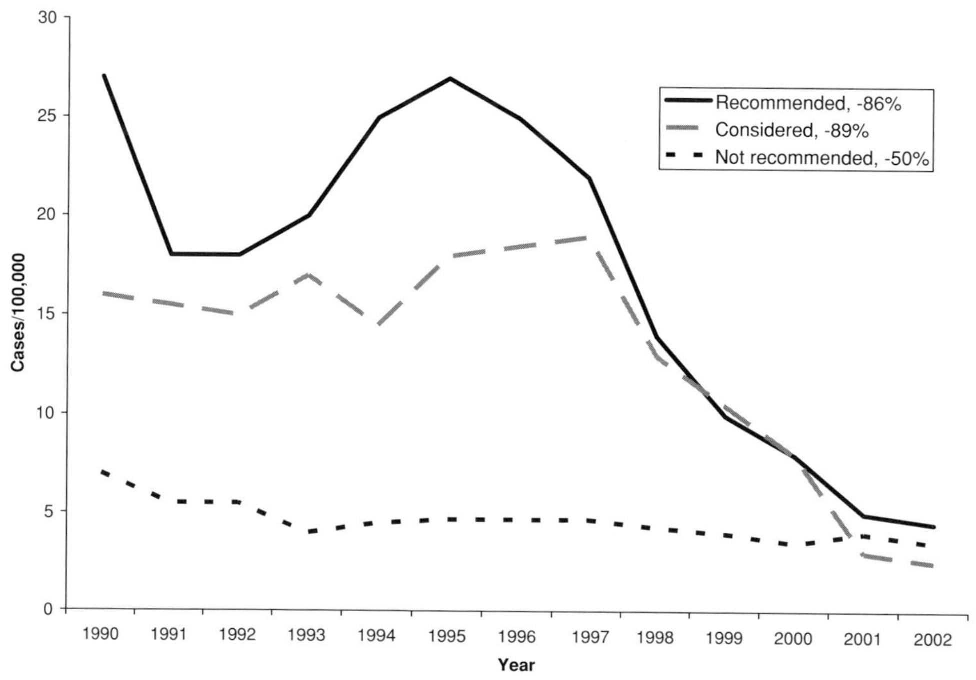

Figure 17.7. Incidence of hepatitis A infection by region, 1990–2002. Coincident with ACIP guidelines in 1996, there has been a reduction in the number of hepatitis A cases, even in regions where routine vaccination was not recommended. In areas with recommended hepatitis A vaccination, the reduction in incidence has been 86%. Rates declined by 89% in states where childhood vaccination is "to be considered." Rates declined by 50% in states where there is no statewide recommendation for routine vaccination of children. (From the Centers for Disease Control and Prevention [2]; http://www.cdc.gov/ncidod/diseases/hepatitis/slideset/index.htm.)

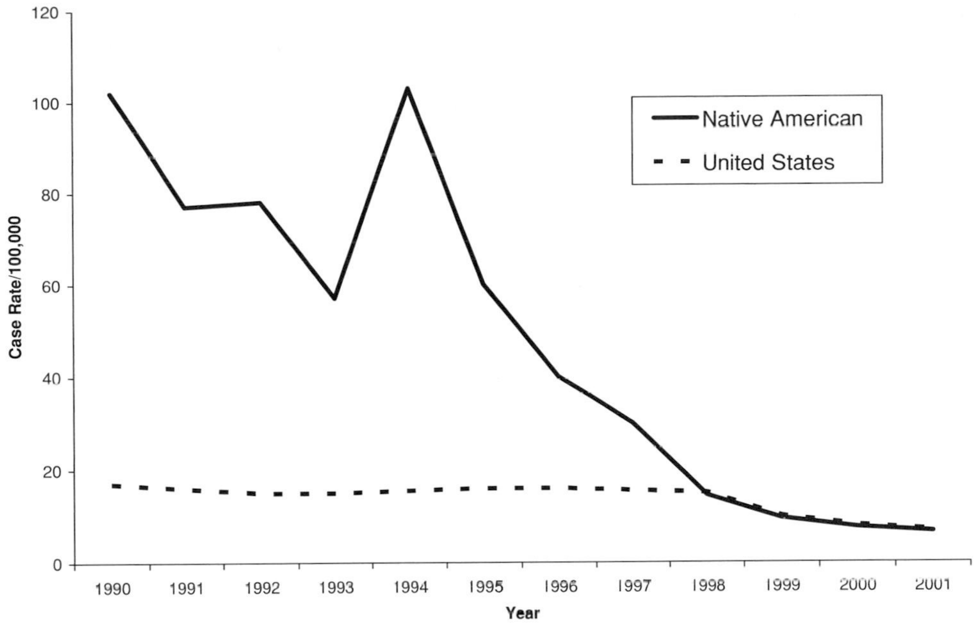

Figure 17.8. Changing incidence of hepatitis A among Native Americans. Before the institution of ACIP guidelines and vaccination, the overall national incidence among Native Americans and Alaska natives was six to ten times higher than the average rate in the United States. Beginning in 1998, the rate among Native Americans and Alaska natives fell below the average U.S. rate. (From the Centers for Disease Control and Prevention [2] and Bialek SR, Thoroughman DA, Hu D, et al. Hepatitis A incidence and hepatitis A vaccination among American Indians and Alaska natives, 1990–2001. Am J Pub Health 2004;94:996–1001; http://www.cdc.gov/ncidod/diseases/hepatitis/slideset/index.htm.)

PCR assay 2 weeks before the aminotransferase peak and for several weeks after symptom onset [43]. Serum aminotransferase levels increase rapidly, peak within 1 week of onset of clinical illness, decrease at a rate of 60–70% per week, and normalize within 1–2 weeks. Bilirubin levels, if elevated, usually peak at the time of maximal aminotransferase levels; subsequently, they decline, albeit slower than the aminotransferase levels. In a small percentage, the course of the illness is prolonged for up to 9 months, with cholestasis characterized by pruritus, fever, and jaundice.

In addition to potentially causing fulminant hepatic failure, HAV can trigger other immunologic problems, resulting in increased morbidity. These complications and associated conditions have included acute disseminated encephalomyelitis [44], autoimmune hepatitis, and Henoch-Schönlein purpura [45].

The burden of HAV infection is twofold. First, in the United States, an estimated 100 people die each year of acute liver failure caused by hepatitis A. Second, 11–22% of people with HAV are hospitalized [38] (Table 17.6). Adults who become ill lose an average of 27 days of work.

Diagnosis

The diagnosis of hepatitis A relies on detection of a specific antibody response to HAV (Table 17.1). The presence of anti-HAV IgM in the serum is indicative of a recent HAV infection. Anti-HAV IgM is present in the serum 5–10 days before the onset of symptoms and may persist for up to 6 months after infection [11].

Alternative means to detect HAV are available but impractical. HAV RNA can be detected in serum and stool during acute infection by nucleic acid amplification. These methods are less readily available and are of little value in clinical practice.

Management

The initial goals in management of patients suspected to be infected with any of the hepatitis viruses are similar: (1) precise, early detection, (2) support and monitoring during acute disease, (3) recognition of the development of fulminant or chronic liver disease, and (4) prevention of disease spread to susceptible persons. This section focuses on management of HAV disease and methods of immunoprophylaxis.

Acute Illness

During the acute phase of viral hepatitis, prescription of bed rest for the child may be appropriate. Specific dietary changes, often advocated, are of no definitive value. Likewise, no demonstrable beneficial role for corticosteroid administration has been found in acute viral hepatitis. Hospitalization is indicated in the presence of coagulopathy, protracted vomiting, or encephalopathy. Because school-aged children rarely transmit the virus to their classmates, they can return to school as soon as they feel well. Infants who may transmit HAV should not return to day care until 2 weeks after the onset of symptoms, when the period of fecal HAV excretion has decreased [46].

Follow-up testing of the patient with HAV should be performed to document biochemical resolution. In addition,

Table 17.5: Clinical Features of Hepatitis A Infection

Clinical Feature	*Characteristics*
Signs and symptoms	Jaundice Fatigue Anorexia Nausea Fever Diarrhea Abdominal pain
Jaundice by age group (% affected)	<6 yr (<10%) 6–14 yr (40–50%) >14 yr (70–80%)
Sources for food-borne infections	Strawberries Blueberries Lettuce Raspberries Green onions Shellfish
Persons at risk of infection	Household contacts of infected persons Sexual contacts of infected persons Persons living in endemic regions Travelers to endemic regions Men who have sex with men Injection and noninjection drug users Day care center attendees and staff
Rare complications	Fulminant hepatitis Cholestatic hepatitis Relapsing hepatitis
Incubation period	Average 30 days (range, 15–50 days)
Chronic sequelae	None

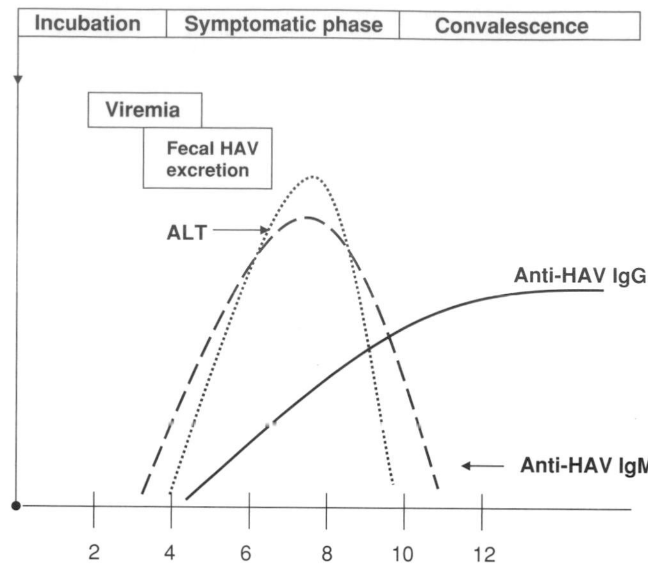

Figure 17.9. Typical course of HAV infection. Following exposure, an average incubation period lasts 4 weeks. During this period, viremia occurs and overlaps the early symptomatic phase. Jaundice, when present, occurs up to 6 weeks following exposure. Other symptoms may include anorexia, malaise, fever, and headache. Immediately before the symptomatic phase, fecal excretion of HAV into the stool is present. Biochemical hepatitis marked by elevation of alanine aminotransferase (ALT) precedes symptomatic infection. The resolution of elevated ALT values typically happens after the normalization of the serum bilirubin and may take 2 months. Early infection with HAV can be detected with anti-HAV IgM antibody, and lasting immunity is indicated by a sustained elevation in anti-HAV IgG. (Balistreri WF. Viral hepatitis. Emerg Clin North Am 1991;9:365–99.)

attention should be given to exclude a coagulopathy suggestive of liver failure. With HAV-induced fulminant hepatic failure, low serum aminotransferase, high serum bilirubin (>15 mg/dL), and low albumin (<2.5 g/dL) levels are associated with a bad outcome [47].

Prevention

The spread of viral infection can theoretically be interrupted by elimination of the virus from the infected population, institution of proper hygiene and isolation procedures, and passive or active immunization [38]. Because transmission of HAV occurs before recognition of clinical infection, hygienic measures alone are often ineffective in preventing infections. Nevertheless, providing information to infected individuals and their contacts regarding the methods of transmission and protection is an important ancillary measure. More effective measures to halt transmission include the use of both passive and active immunization. With these tools, epidemic and endemic spread of HAV can be curtailed.

With regard to hygienic measures, caution should be exercised in handling stool or fomites contaminated with feces to control the spread of HAV. Consistent hand washing and appropriate food-handling techniques are required. If an outbreak of HAV is identified at a day care center, no new admissions should be allowed and transferring children to other centers should be avoided.

Passive Immunization

Immune globulin is an important tool for the prevention of infection and symptomatic disease when administered either before or after exposure to the hepatitis viruses. If contact with a person with acute hepatitis occurs and the exact etiology is unclear, the guidelines listed in Table 17.7 should be followed.

Immune globulin is a preparation of concentrated antibodies from pooled human plasma. The efficacy of immune serum globulin (ISG) in preventing HAV infection has been noted since 1945 [48]. Since then, standard pooled human ISG has been used widely for preexposure and postexposure prophylaxis (Tables 17.8 and 17.9 list specific recommendations). Anti-HAV present in ISG is capable of neutralizing the circulating HAV, preventing viral attack on target cells in the liver and reducing the degree of secondary hepatitis A viremia [49,50]. The efficacy

Table 17.6: Morbidity Associated with Hepatitis A

Measured Outcome	*Washington State, 1989–1990**	*Sentinel Counties, 1991†*
Hospitalization in all ages, %	11	10‡
Mean duration of hospitalization, days (range)	4 (1–10)	2 (1–5)
Outpatient visits per case, average number (range)	4 (0–18)	3 (1–11)
Work loss per case, average days (range)	27 (0–180)	12 (0–40)
Contacts given immunoglobulin per case, avg. number	11	10
Average cost per case in children and adolescents <18 years of age	$433	$1492
Average cost per case in adults	$2459	$1817

*From the Centers for Disease Control and Prevention [38].
†Jefferson County, Alabama; Denver County, Colorado; Pinellas County, Florida; Pierce County, Washington [38].
‡Hospitalization data are for all hepatitis cases identified (n = 287); other data are based on a subset (n = 76) in which no children younger than 18 years were hospitalized.

of ISG, therefore, is presumably the result of the phenomenon of passive/active immunization, whereby the acute disease is modified by administered antibody. At the same time, stimulation of active antibody production occurs because of the low-grade infection. In most cases, the result is an asymptomatic infection followed by long-lasting immunity. By following guidelines for postexposure prophylaxis, HAV disease is prevented in more than 85% of persons [12]. When prophylaxis is administered later in the incubation period, it is less likely to prevent disease but may result in a reduction in the disease severity. Another important caveat is that there is no requirement for testing for antibody against HAV (anti-HAV) before administering immune globulin.

Postexposure prophylaxis with ISG is recommended for all those who have had household contact or intimate exposure to a patient with hepatitis A [46]. Routine use of ISG is not necessary for usual school or work contacts. To be effective, ISG (0.02 mL/kg) must be administered within 2 weeks of exposure. If HAV infection is documented in one day care center employee, child, or parent, ISG should be given to all involved children, employees, and household contacts of the non–toilet-trained attendees. This action has resulted in excellent disease control both within the center and in the community. In a recent study of the effectiveness of ISG in Amsterdam, the authors found that only 12 of 409 susceptible contacts (2.9%) developed symptomatic disease, though 34% had seroconversion despite treatment [51]. ISG is also effective in preventing the spread of HAV in other settings, such as orphanages, institutions for the developmentally disabled, and summer camps. The use of ISG for preexposure prophylaxis against HAV infection has diminished with the availability of an effective HAV vaccine. ISG is recommended for international travelers younger than 1 year, travelers with an imminent departure who need immediate protection, and possibly pregnant travelers [12]. The ISG preparation confers a dose-dependent protection lasting up to 5 months [38].

Even among these populations, some prefer vaccination against hepatitis A over the use of passive immunization [52,53].

Table 17.7: Recommended Immunoprophylaxis after Contact Exposure to Index Case of Acute Viral Hepatitis

Index Case Serology		
Anti-HAV	*HBsAg*	*Recommended Immunotherapy*
Positive, negative, or unknown	Positive	Hepatitis B immune globulin (HBIG), 0.06 mL/kg up to 5.0 mL immediately and at 1 month to regular sexual contacts only*
Positive or unavailable, but disease does not follow blood transfusion	Negative	Immune globulin (Ig), 3–5 mL (0.06 mL/kg) immediately to all contacts†
Negative or unavailable, but disease follows blood transfusion	Negative	Ig (or HBIG), 5 mL immediately to regular sexual contacts only

*HBIG is unnecessary if contact is positive for HBsAg or anti-HBs at time of exposure. HBIG should be administered as soon as possible for maximal effect and must be given within 1 week of exposure.
†With HAV exposure, Ig should be administered as soon as possible for maximal effect and must be given within 2 weeks of exposure.
Data from Balistreri WF. Viral hepatitis. Emerg Clin North Am 1991;9:365–99.

Table 17.8: Recommendations for *Postexposure* Immunoprophylaxis of HAV for Travelers

Age, yr	*Likely Exposure, mo*	*Recommended Prophylaxis*
<1	<3	Ig 0.02 mL/kg*
<1	3–5	Ig 0.06 mL/kg*
<1	Long term	Ig 0.06 mL/kg at departure and every 5 mo thereafter*
≥1	<3†	HAV vaccine‡,§ *or* Ig 0.02 mL/kg*
≥1	3–5†	HAV vaccine‡,§ *or* Ig 0.06 mL/kg*
≥1	Long term	HAV vaccine‡,§

*Immune globulin (Ig) should be administered deep into a large muscle mass. Ordinarily, no more than 5 mL should be administered in one site in an adult or large child; lesser amounts (maximum, 3 mL) should be given to small children and infants.
†Vaccine is preferable, but Ig is an acceptable alternative.
‡To ensure protection in travelers whose departure is imminent, Ig also may be given.
§Dose and schedule of hepatitis A virus (HAV) vaccine as recommended according to age in Table 17.10.
From the American Academy of Pediatrics [81,83].

Table 17.9: Recommendations for *Postexposure* Immunoprophylaxis of Hepatitis A Infection

Time Since Exposure, wk	*Future Exposure Likely*	*Patient Age, yr*	*Recommended Prophylaxis*
≤2	No	All ages	Ig (0.02 mL/kg)*
≤2	Yes	≥1	Ig (0.02 mL/kg)* *and* HAV vaccine†
>2	No	All ages	No prophylaxis
>2	Yes	≥1	HAV vaccine†

*Immune globulin (Ig) should be administered deep into a large muscle mass. Ordinarily, no more than 5 mL should be administered in one site in an adult or large child; lesser amounts (maximum, 3 mL) should be given to small children and infants.
†Dosage and schedule of hepatitis A virus (HAV) vaccine as recommended according to age in Table 17.10.
From the American Academy of Pediatrics [81,83].

The vaccine can elicit a protective response after 2–3 weeks, which is within the incubation period of the disease. Thus it also offers protection against early acquisition of HAV during travel. In addition, it is more widely available than ISG and confers long-lasting immunity.

Active Immunization

There are similarities between the epidemiologies of HAV and poliovirus, suggesting that widespread vaccination of appropriate susceptible populations can substantially lower disease incidence, eliminate virus transmission, and ultimately eradicate HAV [54]. Despite the use of passive immunization, continuing outbreaks of HAV infection, resulting in substantial mortality and morbidity, have emphasized the importance of an aggressive policy for vaccination against HAV [55].

Efficacy of the HAV Vaccine

Because HAV shares structural and biologic features with the polioviruses, the strategy for vaccine development paralleled that used in the development of poliovirus vaccines, namely formalin inactivation and the development of live attenuated vaccine [49,50,54,56–58]. Clinical trials indicated a high degree of efficacy of formalin-inactivated HAV vaccines [50]. Inactivated vaccines limit the intrahepatic replication of the HAV and therefore reduce the amount of virus that is shed in the stool. An HAV vaccine grown in diploid cell cultures, inactivated with formalin, and conjugated to alum was well tolerated and highly immunogenic, inducing an immune response in most people after two doses given 2–4 weeks apart [59]. Viral neutralization tests were used to determine the antibody response after active immunization with an inactivated HAV vaccine [49]. The neutralizing antibody response after two doses of the vaccine (given 1 month apart) was greater than that documented after passive immunization with standard doses of ISG. A third dose, given after 6–12 months, boosted the titer, allowing persistence of the antibody response.

Presently, two inactivated HAV vaccines are licensed by the FDA in the United States: Havrix (GlaxoSmithKline Biologicals) and VAQTA (Merck and Co., Inc.); in addition, a combination vaccine, Twinrix (GlaxoSmithKline Biologicals), is approved for HAV vaccination as well as HBV vaccination in adults (Table 17.10). The HAV portion of the three vaccines is composed of viral antigens purified from HAV-infected human diploid fibroblast cell cultures. Their antigen content is expressed for Havrix and Twinrix as enzyme-linked immunoassay units (EL.U) and for VAQTA as units (U) of HAV antigen. The recommended dosing schedule is a primary intramuscular (deltoid) dose followed by a second dose at 6–18 months for Havrix and VAQTA. Twinrix is dosed analogous to other HBV vaccines; therefore, after the initial dose, additional doses are administered 1 month and 6 months later, respectively. With HAV vaccination, if the second dose is delayed, it can still be given without the need to repeat the primary dose [60]. Also, because of the high rate of seroconversion, testing for antibodies after vaccination is not required.

Similarly, it is not cost-effective to test for *preexisting* immunity (anti-HAV) in the United States and low-HAV–prevalent countries before immunization in children or in *low-risk* adults [38]. High-risk population groups, such as Native Americans, Alaska natives, injection drug users, and

Table 17.10: Recommended Dosages of Hepatitis A Vaccines

Age, yr	*Vaccine*	*Dose*	*Volume, mL*	*No of Doses*	*Schedule, mo*[¶]
1–18	Havrix*	720 EL.U[†]	0.5	2	0, 6–12
>18	Havrix*	1440 EL.U[†]	1.0	2	0, 6
1–17	VAQTA[‡]	25 U[§]	0.5	2	0, 6–18
>17	VAQTA[‡]	50 U[§]	1.0	2	0, 6
≥18	Twinrix[‖]	720 EL.U[†]	1.0	3	0, 1, 6

*Hepatitis A vaccine, inactivated; GlaxoSmithKline Biologicals.
[†]Enzyme-linked immunosorbent assay (ELISA) units.
[‡]Hepatitis A vaccine, inactivated; Merck & Co., Inc.
[§]Units.
[‖]Twinrix is manufactured by GlaxoSmithKline Biologicals; it is a combination of Havrix (720 EL.U) and hepatitis B (Engerix-B 20 μg) vaccines.
[¶]0 months represents timing of the initial dose; subsequent numbers represent months after the initial dose.
From the American Academy of Pediatrics [81] and the Centers for Disease Control and Prevention [92].

immigrants from HAV-endemic countries, may be tested before HAV vaccine administration. Because the seroprevalence for anti-HAV is about 33% in the general population older than 40 years, screening in this group may be cost effective [61]. It is not necessary to test for anti-HAV response after vaccination [38].

The HAV vaccines are highly protective against clinical disease in children. Werzberger et al. [62], in a double-blind, placebo-controlled randomized trial, showed 100% protective efficacy of a prototype HAV vaccine starting 18 days after the first dose in children in a community at high risk for infection. The vaccine was well tolerated and demonstrated complete protective efficacy against clinically apparent hepatitis A. Innis et al. [63], in a randomized study of 40,119 school-aged children in Thailand, demonstrated that 94% of vaccine recipients were positive for anti-HAV at 8 months and 99%, at 17 months. The vaccine was highly effective against clinical disease; 38 clinical cases were noted in the controls versus 2 in the vaccine group, resulting in a clinical efficacy of 94%. With limited data, the vaccine appears to be less immunogenic among patients with chronic liver disease [64,65], immunocompromised persons [66], transplant recipients [67], and the elderly [68]. The seroconversion rates in these groups have been reported to be 93%, 88%, 26%, and 65%, respectively.

Hepatitis A virus vaccines may be capable of interrupting potential secondary or epidemic spread [69–71]. In two villages in Slovakia, a community-wide outbreak ended 2 months after the majority of school-aged children were vaccinated with two doses of vaccine [70]. Limited data indicate excellent immunogenicity in seronegative infants [72]. However, for children less than 1 year of age, ISG is still recommended because residual anti-HAV antibody passively acquired from the mother interferes with the vaccine immunogenicity [73–76].

Long-Term Protection of HAV Vaccine

The long-term protection engendered by the HAV vaccine is still unknown. Estimates of antibody persistence derived from kinetic models indicate that protective levels of anti-HAV will persist for 20 years, without the need for periodic boosters [12,77–79]. Whether other mechanisms (e.g., cellular memory) also contribute to long-term protection remains to be defined.

Adverse Effects

The HAV vaccine has been shown to be very safe. In clinical trials that included more than 26,000 patients, the vaccine was well tolerated. Soreness at the injection site was the most common adverse event, occurring in 18–39%. Headache has been reported in 15% and fever in less than 10% [12,62,63]. No serious adverse events could be attributed to the vaccine in short-term or long-term follow-up [38,80]. The only contraindication to vaccination is a previous allergic reaction to the vaccines or a component of the vaccines. Pregnancy is not considered an absolute contraindication. Although the vaccines have not been studied in pregnant women, given that the HAV vaccines are inactivated, they would most likely be safe. Both Havrix and VAQTA are classified as pregnancy category C.

Recommendation for the Use of HAV Vaccine

The availability of an efficacious HAV vaccine raises questions regarding the rationale for its use and the priority of immunization. The most recent guidelines for use of the HAV vaccine and preexposure prophylaxis issued by the American Academy of Pediatrics (AAP) Committee on Infectious Diseases [81–83] and the Advisory Committee on Immunization Practices (ACIP) of the U.S. Department of Health and Human Services are shown in Table 17.10 [81–83]. Targeted use of HAV vaccine is already in place in several countries. Presently, known risk factors for acquisition and morbidity of HAV hepatitis are occupational exposure, travel to endemic areas, chronic liver disease [84], high risk behaviors, organ transplantation, and receipt of clotting factors. In addition, patients with chronic hepatitis C should be vaccinated against hepatitis A to reduce the risk of fulminant hepatitis [40].

As many affected individuals identify no risk factors, this approach still does not achieve the goal of optimized control and prevention of the disease. Because of their critical role in HAV transmission, children should be a primary target of immunization strategies. Routine ("universal") childhood immunization against HAV is increasingly advocated [12,85,86] and has been adopted by the AAP and ACIP as the best strategy for eliminating HAV infection [83]. Universal vaccination is realistic because there is no animal reservoir of the virus, there is no human carrier state, and there are highly effective vaccines.

Routine vaccination against HAV infection in the states with the highest number of infected people has accelerated the reduction in HAV infections in the United States (see Figures 17.6 and 17.7). In developing countries where HAV is hyperendemic, mass immunization of very young children and improvements in water supplies and sanitary standards are the key to future control of the infection. The major obstacles to achieving those goals include competing health care problems, vaccine cost, and absence of health care infrastructure for vaccine delivery and follow-up. In developed countries, the challenges to globalized HAV vaccination are the cost and the addition of yet another new vaccine to the childhood immunization schedule [11,54,87,88]. Although the universal immunization approach is less costly with combination vaccines, it is feasible even with the current vaccines, as has been demonstrated in routine immunization of young children in areas with high rates of infection [89,90]. Furthermore, this approach has been shown to reduce infections among older persons as well as in the targeted population [91]. Implementation of this new policy will be facilitated by the recent approval of Havrix and VAQTA for children 12 months of age and older [92,93]. Abandoning the selective immunization policy was logical because of the need for frequent reassessment (Table 17.4) and because of its acquiescence of ongoing morbidity and mortality [83,89,90].

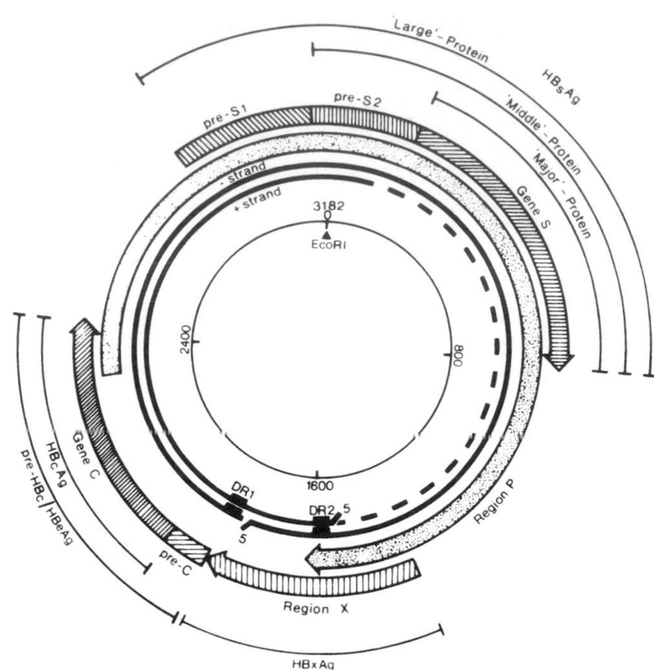

Figure 17.10. Structure of the HBV genome. The circular structure of the HBV genome is sustained by base pairing of 5′ end of (−) and (+) strands of DNA. The long (−) strand of HBV DNA exhibits four long open reading frames, each of which codes for specific proteins: (1) The S gene and the pre-S region encode for surface antigen (HBsAg). (2) The C gene encodes for the major viral nucleocapsid (core) polypeptide (HBcAg) as well as HBeAg. (3) The overlapping P gene encodes for the the DNA polymerase. (4) The X gene encodes for a protein (HBxAg) with transcriptional transactivating function.

HEPATITIS B

Viral Characteristics and Pathogenesis

The hepatitis B virus (HBV) belongs to a family of viruses termed the Hepadnaviridae. The virus contains both double-stranded and single-stranded DNA. The genome consists of approximately 3200 base pairs (Figure 17.10). High levels of HBV DNA are present in the liver of infected individuals; however, HBV DNA is present in smaller quantities in all body fluids, with the exception of stool. DNA sequencing has confirmed the existence of multiple viral genotypes; the prevalence of each genotype is variable in different geographic regions.

The intact virion, called the Dane particle, is spherical and approximately 42 nm in diameter (Figure 17.11); it consists of several identified antigens. The intact virions are double-shelled particles with an outer lipoprotein envelope that contains three related envelope glycoproteins (or surface antigens). Within the envelope is the viral nucleocapsid or core, which contains the partially double-stranded DNA, a DNA polymerase, and hepatitis B e antigen (HBeAg).

The HBV genome has been cloned and sequenced (Figure 17.10) [94]. Hepadnaviruses replicate their DNA genome by reverse transcription of an RNA intermediate [95]. HBV DNA exhibits four overlapping open reading frames, which correspond to four genes. These genes encode the following: (1) envelop proteins (hepatitis B surface antigen [HBsAg]), (2) nucleocapsid (hepatitis B core antigen [HBcAg]), (3) HBV DNA polymerase, and (4) an enhancer–promoter transcription factor (viral X protein [HBV-X]).

The preS-S (presurface–surface) region of the genome encodes the three viral surface antigens by differential initiation of translation at each of three in-frame initiation codons [96]. HBsAg is a 24-kDa protein and is the most abundant protein. HBsAg particles, 20-nm in size, outnumber intact virions by 1000:1 to 10,000:1 [96]. Initiation of translation upstream from the start codon yields the M (or preS2) protein; its function is unknown. Initiation at the most upstream start codon yields the L (or preS1) protein; it is thought to play

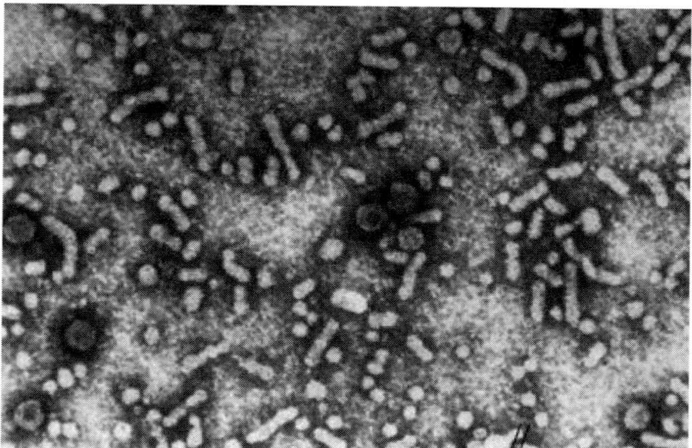

Figure 17.11. Electron micrograph of HBV in serum. The larger spherical objects in this Figure show the intact HBV virion, a 42-nm particle. Outer surface membrane proteins that contain hepatitis B surface antigen also circulate in the blood as smaller (22-nm) spherical and tubular particles. (Accessed May 1, 2005, at http://www.cdc.gov/ncidod/diseases/hepatitis/slideset/index.htm.)

an important role in binding of the virus to the host cell receptor [97]. In addition, the L protein is important in the assembly of the virion and its release from the cell [98].

Hepatitis B core antigen and HBeAg are encoded in the preC-C (precore–core) region. HBcAg functions as the viral capsid. HBeAg plays no role in viral assembly, and its function is not clear. The P coding region is specific for the viral polymerase. This enzyme is essential in DNA synthesis and RNA encapsidation. The X open reading frame encodes for HBV-X; this protein contains an enhancer–promoter complex to direct transcription of host sequences. This protein activity is required for replication and spread of the virus [96,99]. Also, this HBV-X coding gene may play a role in oncogenesis [100].

The replication cycle of HBV begins with the attachment of the virion to the hepatocyte (Figure 17.12) [96]. The virion is internalized into the hepatocyte cytoplasm. Subsequently, viral core particles migrate to the hepatocyte nucleus, where their genomes are repaired to form a covalently closed circular DNA (cccDNA). cccDNA serves as a template for viral messenger RNA (mRNA) transcription. After generation of mRNA, it is transported to the cytoplasm, where the translation of viral mRNA produces HBsAg, HBcAg, HBeAg, HBV DNA polymerase, and HBV-X proteins. This allows for assembly of progeny viral capsids with incorporated viral RNA. Then, this RNA undergoes reverse transcription into viral DNA. After completion of this fully assembled core, some cores will bud into the endoplasmic reticulum to be enveloped and exported from the cell, whereas other cores will undergo a recycling process into the nucleus, with their genomes converted into cccDNA. Most antiviral agents have little or no effect on cccDNA; this accounts for the rapid reappearance of serum HBV DNA after cessation of antiviral therapy [101].

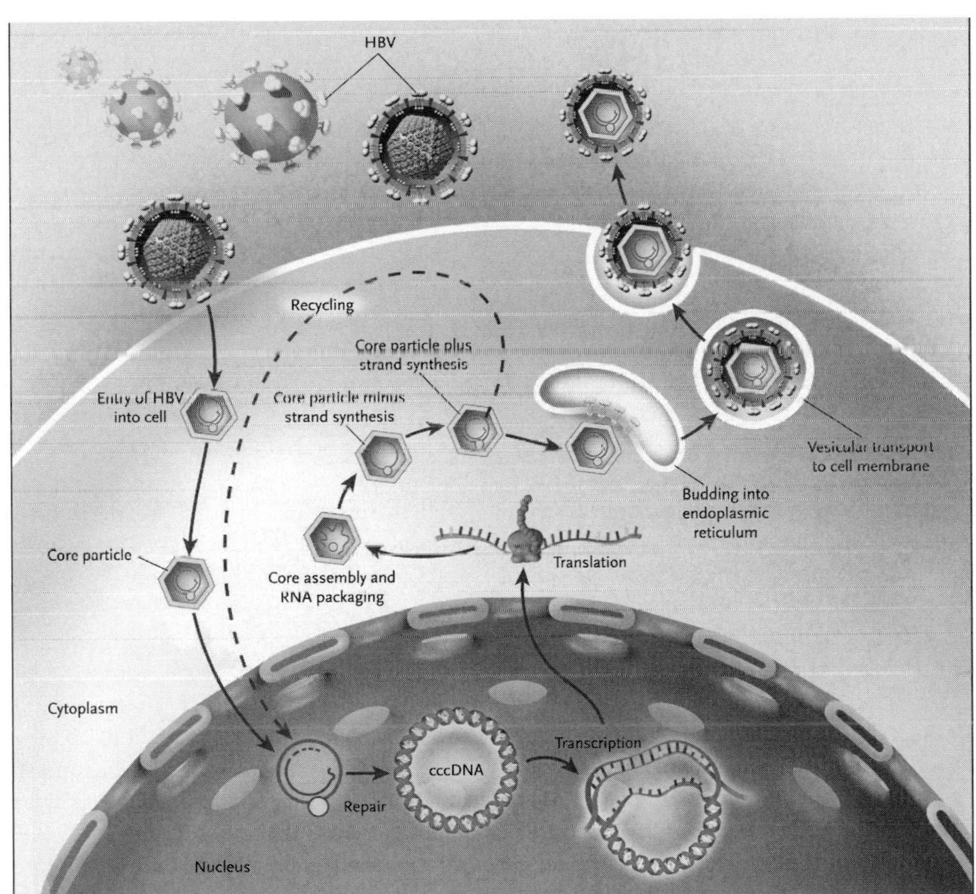

Figure 17.12. Replication cycle of HBV. HBV virions bind to surface receptors and are internalized. Viral core particles migrate to the hepatocyte nucleus, where their genomes are repaired to form a covalently closed circular DNA (cccDNA) that is the template for viral messenger RNA (mRNA) transcription. The viral mRNA that results is translated in the cytoplasm to produce the viral surface, core, polymerase, and X proteins. There, progeny viral capsids assemble, incorporating genomic viral RNA (RNA packaging). This RNA is reverse transcribed into viral DNA. The resulting cores can either bud into the endoplasmic reticulum to be enveloped and exported from the cell or recycle their genomes into the nucleus for conversion to cccDNA. The small sphere inside the core particle is the viral DNA polymerase. (Reprinted with permission from Ganem D, Prince AM. Mechanism of disease: hepatitis B virus infection – natural history and clinical consequences. N Engl J Med 2004;350:1118–29. Copyright © 2004 Massachusetts Medical Society. All rights reserved.)

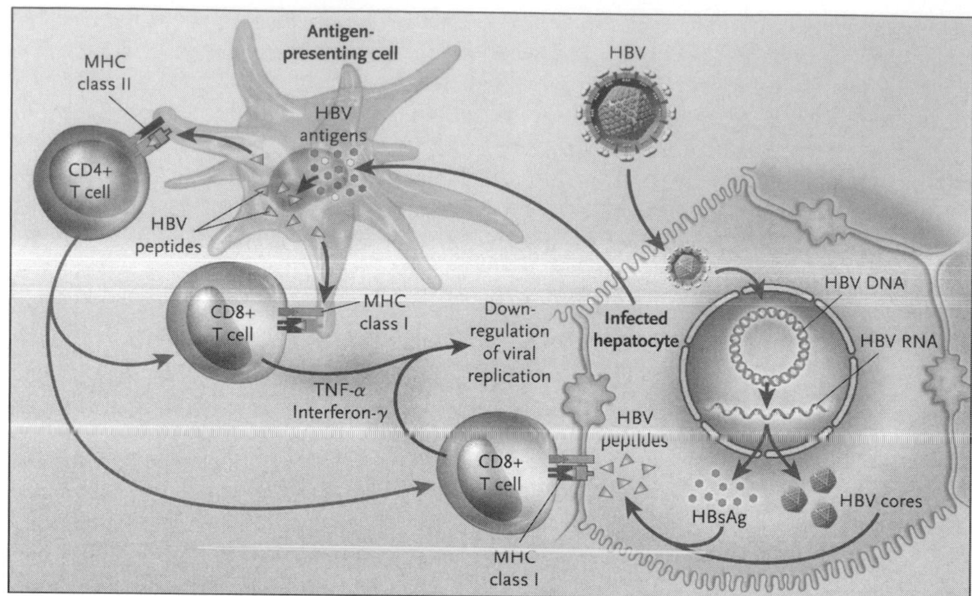

Figure 17.13. Cellular immune responses to HBV. HBV replicates in hepatocytes to produce HBsAg particles and virions. Both types of particles can be taken up by antigen-presenting cells, which degrade the viral proteins to peptides that are then presented on the cell surface bound to major histocompatibility complex (MHC) class I or II molecules. (Antigen-presenting cells can also process and display viral antigens taken up by phagocytosis of killed infected hepatocytes.) These peptide antigens can be recognized by CD8+ or CD4+ T cells, respectively, which are thereby sensitized. Virus-specific CD8+ cytotoxic T cells (with help from CD4+ T cells, *arrow*) can recognize viral antigens presented on MHC class I chains on infected hepatocytes. This recognition reaction can lead to either direct lysis of the infected hepatocyte or the release of interferon gamma and tumor necrosis factor-α (TNF-α), which can down-regulate viral replication in surrounding hepatocytes without direct killing. (Reprinted with permission from Ganem D, Prince AM. Mechanism of disease: hepatitis B virus infection – natural history and clinical consequences. N Engl J Med 2004;350:1118–29.)

HBV Pathogenesis

The immune response to HBV is incompletely understood. It is known that HBV is not directly cytopathic; instead, an immune response to infected hepatocytes is responsible for persistence of hepatic injury or for recovery. Eradication of the virus is thought to occur via lysis by cytotoxic T cells (Figure 17.13). HBV-infected individuals with immune defects often have mild acute liver injury but high rates of chronic carriage [102]. The fact that HBV is not directly cytotoxic allows for many individuals to harbor the infection yet have minimal liver injury and be asymptomatic.

An understanding of the mechanisms of HBV clearance is important when designing therapies. Previously, it had been thought that HBV DNA disappeared from acutely infected individuals as a result of the destruction of virus-infected liver cells. It is now recognized that there are other mechanisms that are important. In addition, low levels of viral DNA may persist after HBV immunity (anti-HBs) has developed [96,103]. The cellular immune response to HBV involves antigen-presenting cells that take up HBV particles and virions. After degrading viral proteins to peptides, these cells present the peptides on the cell surface. In addition, these presenting cells are bound to major histocompatibility complex molecules and to cytotoxic T lymphocytes [96]. This allows sensitization of CD4 helper T cells and CD8 cytotoxic lymphocytes; in turn, virus-specific cytotoxic lymphocytes, with the assistance of CD4 T cells, direct a response against mulitiple epitopes, including surface proteins, polymerase, and HBV core. Viral antigens can be recognized on infected hepatocytes and lead to direct lysis or to the release of interferon (IFN) and tumor necrosis factor, which can down-regulate viral replication without direct hepatocyte killing [104,105]. In a chimpanzee model, 90% of HBV DNA was cleared from the liver without significant destruction of hepatocytes and occurred before maximal infiltration of T cells into the liver [106]. When cytotoxic T lymphocytes are transferred to mice with replicating HBV, viral DNA and RNA disappear from the liver, even from uninjured hepatocytes. This effect can be blocked by antibodies to IFN and tumor necrosis factor [107].

The severity of HBV infection is often correlated with the presence of HBeAg in the serum. HBeAg is a marker for transmissibility and active viral production. Seroconversion to anti-HBe has been equated to a lowered risk of HBV morbidity and mortality; it signifies a decrease in viral replication, a decreased potential for liver injury, and an improved prognosis [108]. Despite the presence of anti-HBe, 70–85% of people will have detectable viral DNA in the circulation by PCR assay. Typically, this is in the range of 10^3–10^5 molecules per milliliter [109]. As

HBV virions have a half-life of approximately 1 day [110], these low levels indicate ongoing viral replication.

With chronic HBV infection, two main serologic patterns have been identified based on the relative frequency of perinatal transmission versus horizontal transmission. The first pattern, notable in Asia, has a predominant transmission via perinatal infections. This serologic pattern involves seroconversion with clearance of HBeAg much later in adulthood. Despite the presence of HBeAg, most individuals have normal alanine aminotransferase (ALT) levels but high HBV DNA levels. The second pattern occurs in areas with frequent person-to-person transmission in childhood or adulthood. Under these circumstances, seroconversion to anti-HBe occurs over a shorter period of time. After spontaneous clearance of HBeAg, 67–80% remain HBeAg negative and anti-HBe positive, with normal ALT and minimal inflammation on liver biopsy [111]. The course of these individuals, often referred to as "inactive carriers," is generally but not always benign; the outcome depends in part on the duration and severity of the preceding chronic hepatitis.

In areas of Asia and the South Pacific Islands, among adults with elevated ALT levels, the rate of HBeAg clearance averages 8–12% per year [111–115]. In the majority of Asian children, most of whom have normal aminotransferase levels, the rate of HBeAg clearance is much lower [116,117].

In other locations, there is also variability in HBeAg clearance rates. In a large study from Alaska, 1536 carrier children and adults were followed for 12 years; spontaneous HBeAg clearance occurred in 45% of carriers in 5 years and in 80% after 10 years [114]. Similar seroconversion rates have been reported in untreated children from Taiwan and Italy [118,119]. Older age and elevated ALT are predictive of HBeAg clearance [115,120].

Similar to HBeAg seronversion, seroconversion of HBsAg also occurs spontaneously but at a slower rate. Approximately 0.5% of HBsAg carriers will clear HBsAg each year in the absence of treatment; most develop anti-HBs [111,114,121,122]. However, even in these individuals, about half have detectable low levels of HBV DNA after disappearance of HBsAg [123].

HBV Genotypes

HBV is currently divided into eight genotypes: A through H; in addition, subtypes have been described [124]. There is growing evidence that these genotypes are each associated with different disease phenotypes. Genotypes B and C are the most common HBV genotypes and predominate in the Far East [125]. Genotypes A and D are predominant in North America and Europe, and genotype F in South America [126]. Recent studies show that adult and pediatric patients with genotype B achieve HBeAg seroconversion a decade earlier than do patients with genotype C [124,127,128]. Therefore, prevalence rates for HBeAg positivity are higher among patients with genotype C than in those with genotype B [126]. It has been suggested that the genotype may be more important than host factors in the outcome of HBV infection; therefore, race-related differences may be secondary to the varied geographic distribution of HBV genotypes as well as to differences in efforts to prevent and eradicate HBV infection.

In a study from Hong Kong, genotype and clinical features were compared among Chinese patients [128]. In this cohort, in which nearly all were infected at birth or in the first 1–2 years of life, persons with genotype B had more severe exacerbations as reflected by higher ALT values and lower albumin values [128]. In addition, these patients had an increased risk for hepatic decompensation and a higher mortality rate.

Besides its relationship to hepatic decompensation, genotype is an important determinant in the development of hepatocellular carcinoma (HCC). HBV genotype C is more prevalent in HCC among patients older than 50 years, whereas genotype B is more prevalent in the development of HCC in patients younger than 50 and in those who have not developed cirrhosis [124].

Not only does the HBV genotype play a role in the outcome of HBV infection, it also is important in predicting response to therapy. In a multicenter study of 307 HBeAg-positive patients, response rates to pegylated IFN varied by HBV genotype. The best response was among those with genotype A (47%), followed by B (44%), then C (28%), and then D (25%) [129].

HBV Mutations

HBV has a mutation rate around ten times that of other DNA viruses [130]. The reverse transcriptase lacks a proofreading function that is common to most other polymerases. This predisposes HBV to mutations either naturally or as the result of selective pressure of antiviral therapy. In many HBeAg-negative infected individuals, much higher levels of HBV DNA are present along with elevated aminotransferase levels; many of these individuals have mutations that prevent the production of HBeAg, and they do not develop anti-HBe. Mutations have been detected in all regions of the HBV genome in patients with HBV infection, but the significance of many of these mutations is unclear.

PRECORE MUTATIONS

Fulminant hepatitis may occur in persons who are HBeAg negative [131,132]. In Asia and parts of southern Europe, 15–20% of HBeAg-negative carriers have elevated ALT levels and viral DNA in the blood [133]. In many such carriers, mutations in the precore (preC region) prevent production of HBeAg. Generally, these patients have more severe liver disease and have been less responsive to IFN therapy [134,135]. The most common mutation, the "precore variant," is characterized by a point mutation (G to A) at nucleotide position 1896 in the precore region of the HBV genome. This single mutation prevents the formation of the precore protein required to make HBeAg by introducing a translational stop codon [131,132]. Because HBeAg is an important target for cell-mediated and antibody-mediated immune responses, the loss of the e antigen production by precore variants may help the virus evade the host immune response. These precore variants have been identified in both adults and infants with fulminant hepatitis B [136–139]. This variant is commonly found in association with HBV genotype D, which is prevalent in the Mediterranean; it is

Table 17.11: Hepatitis B Terminology

Term	*Definition*
Chronic hepatitis B	Chronic inflammation of the liver due to hepatitis B, characterized by the following: Presence of HBsAg >6 mo Serum HBV DNA >10^5 copies/mL Persistent elevated ALT/AST levels Liver biopsy showing chronic hepatitis
Hepatitis B carrier	Persistent HBsAg positivity without significant inflammation of the liver with the following: Presence of HBsAg >6 mo HBeAg negativity, anti-HBe positivity Serum HBV DNA <10^5 copies/mL Normal ALT/AST levels Liver biopsy without significant hepatitis
Resolved hepatitis B infection	Previous hepatitis B infection without evidence of ongoing virologic, biochemical, or histologic disease; features include: HBsAg-negativity Undetectable (or very low) HBV DNA levels Normal ALT levels (if no other liver diseases)
Acute hepatitis B flare	Rise in aminotransferase level to >10 times the upper limit of normal and more than twice the patient's baseline level
HBeAg clearance	Loss of detectable HBeAg in the serum of an individual with previous HBeAg positivity
HBeAg seroconversion	Loss of detectable HBeAg and the appearance of anti-HBe
HBeAg reversion	Reappearance of HBeAg in a person who was previously HBeAg negative

AST, aspartate aminotransferase.
From Lok and McMahon [111].

rarely associated with genotype A, which is the most prevalent genotype in the United States and western Europe [111,140].

SURFACE ANTIGEN MUTATIONS

Surface antigen mutants have been detected in persons who developed HBV despite vaccination. In these individuals, a defect in the major component of antigenicity of HBsAg (the *a*-determinant) is present. Because antibody to the *a* subtype is the protective antibody, patients harboring "escape mutants" develop hepatitis despite adequate levels of anti-HBs. These mutations pose a potential threat to the success of vaccination programs [141]. Also, a small proportion of infants born to HBeAg-positive women become infected despite receiving immunoprophylaxis; these patients may be infected with a variant strain of HBV, which has a point mutation in the S gene [142].

Table 17.12: Global Prevalence of Hepatitis B

Population	*HBsAg, %*	*Any HBV Marker, %*
High endemic regions*	13	70–85
HIV-infected patients	8–11	89–90
Pregnant females (U.S.)	0.4–1.5	—
Men who have sex with men	6	35–80
Injection drug users	7	60–80
Dialysis patients	3–10	20–80
Family/household and sexual contacts	3–6	30–60

*Includes Southeast Asia, Africa, Middle East (except Israel), Dominican Republic, and Haiti.
From Lok and McMahon [111].

Epidemiology

An estimated 350 million people worldwide are chronically infected with HBV [143] (Tables 17.11 and 17.12). High prevalence countries/regions include China, Brazil, Haiti, the Dominican Republic, the Middle East, southeast Asia, and Africa. (A prevalence map can be viewed at www.cdc.gov/ncidod/hepatitis/slideset/101/101_hbv.ptt#440,3,slide_3.) Despite being a "low prevalence" country, the United States has an estimated 1.25 million HBV carriers, defined as persons positive for HBsAg for more than 6 months [46]. Approximately one of four people with chronic hepatitis B will develop serious sequelae during their lifetime [111].

Transmission of HBV typically occurs via the parenteral route through exchange of blood or other secretions. The risk of acquisition of HBV is between 10% and 30% after a single percutaneous exposure; this is much more infectious than either HIV or HCV, which have been estimated at 0.3% and 3% risks, respectively. As HBV has been detected in the saliva, albeit in lower concentrations, transmission may occur through human bites. HBV is not thought to be transmitted via indirect exposure, such as with shared toys. Intimate physical contact of any sort is a common route of infection [46,143–145]. Also, frequent exposure to blood or blood products increases the risk of exposure to infection [146–148]. Transmission of HBV has occurred in the health care setting, even with trivial inattention to hygienic practices [149]. Before widespread

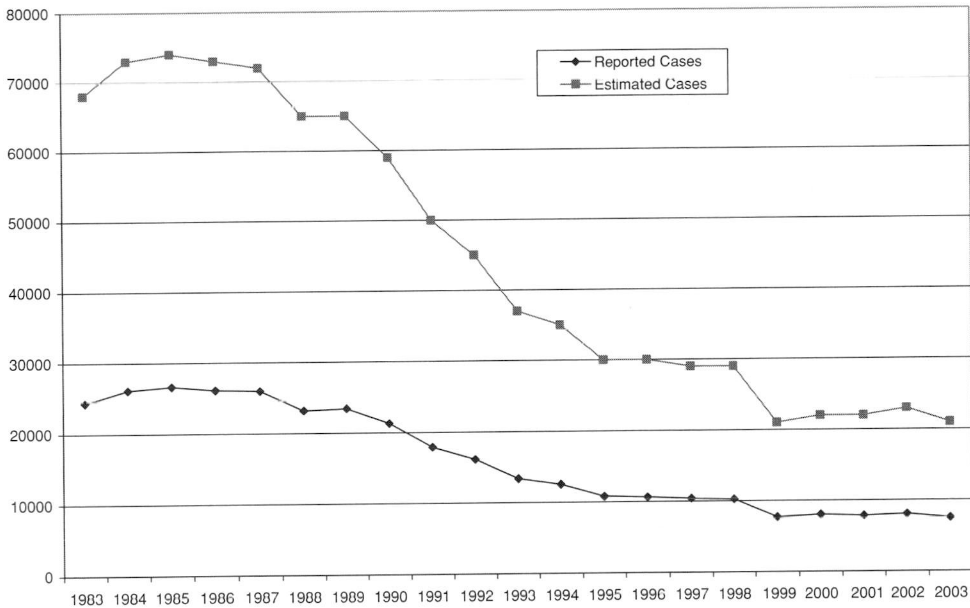

Figure 17.14. The number of reported acute hepatitis B cases indicates the cases reported to the national notifiable disease surveillance system of the CDC (From Centers for Disease Control and Prevention [2].)

vaccination, high-risk groups included individuals with accidental exposure to needles, renal dialysis patients and personnel, clinical laboratory workers, dentists and oral surgeons, emergency department workers, and oncology service health care providers. Transmission from health care providers to patients has been documented as well [46,147,150]. With widespread introduction of vaccination along with blood product screening, the incidence of posttransfusion hepatitis B in the United States is rare but still occurs [151].

Hepatitis B virus remains highly prevalent in Asia, where 75% of HBV-infected persons reside. In the United States and western Europe, there is a low prevalence of chronic HBsAg carriers. The number of chronically infected individuals is likely to further decrease as the number of acute HBV infections has steadily declined over the past two decades (Figure 17.14). Since 1982, when the first vaccine for HBV was introduced, substantial progress has been made toward eliminating HBV in children [152,153] (Figure 17.14). This in turn has reduced complications, including HCC. In Taiwan, the introduction of universal HBV vaccination has resulted in a decline of HCC incidence from 0.54 to 0.20 per 100,000 children from 1981 through 2000 [154]; the children with HCC following the introduction of the immunization policy had either vaccine failure (33–51%) or failure to receive HBV immunoglobulin at birth (42–57%). Almost all children (97%) who did develop HCC were seropositive for HBsAg.

From 1982–2002, in the United States, the rate of HBV infection per 100,000 persons was reduced from 13.8 in 1982, to 6.32 in 1992, to 2.84 in 2002 [153,155]. There are persisting differences in the rate of infection among men and women. In 1990, the incidence of acute hepatitis B was 9.8 per 100,000 for men and 6.3 per 100,000 for women; in 2002, the incidence was 3.7 and 2.2 per 100,000, respectively.

Trends in acute hepatitis B reflect poor immunization coverage among identified high-risk groups (Figure 17.15). During 1994–1998, about half the cases of acute hepatitis B occurred in individuals previously treated for a sexually transmitted disease (STD) or who had been incarcerated [155,156]. Both of these groups are considered high risk and have been targeted for HBV vaccination for more than 20 years. Between 1994 and 1998, the most common reported risk factor for HBV infection was high-risk heterosexual activity (39.8%) followed by male homosexual activity (14.6%) and injection drug use (13.8%).

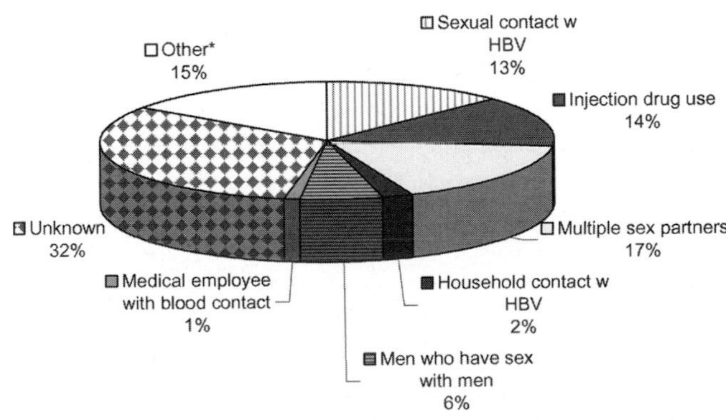

Figure 17.15. This pie chart illustrates frequent risk factors for HBV acquisition. In the 15% of cases in which the cause is listed as "other," transmission factors include surgery, dental procedures, acupuncture, tattoo, or other percutaneous injury. (Accessed May 1, 2005, at http://www.cdc.gov/ncidod/diseases/hepatitis/slideset/index.htm.)

Although targeting high-risk individuals may be difficult, well-identified opportunities have been missed. Recent surveys indicate that only 25% of STD clinics provide HBV vaccine [157]. Furthermore, since 1999, after more than a decade of decline, acute hepatitis B incidence among men older than 19 years and women 40 years and older has increased [153,158]. The incidence of acute hepatitis B has increased 5% among men aged 20–39 and 20% among men 40 years and older. Similarly, in women 40 years and older, the incidence of acute hepatitis B has increased 31%. This increase in acute hepatitis B incidence has been attributed to increases in high-risk sexual behavior among both heterosexual and homosexual individuals [153,158].

Globally, HBV infections cause approximately 620,000 deaths annually; in the United States each year, 5000 deaths are attributable to HBV. Without vaccination, an estimated 1.4 million HBV-related deaths would occur in the 2000 birth cohort over the lifetime of the cohort [156]. Perinatal and early childhood infections account for 21% and 48%, respectively, of subsequent HBV-related deaths worldwide. In 1999, a global initiative was started to make HBV vaccination available for children in the poorest regions of the world. By 2003, HBV immunization was part of more than 151 national immunization programs. However, many countries, mainly in sub-Saharan Africa, have not introduced the vaccine and in many others, the coverage remains low. When these efforts enable the three-dose vaccination to cover more than 90% of children, it is estimated than 84% of global HBV deaths will be prevented [156].

Following the recommendation to vaccinate all infants in the United States for HBV, there has been a steady decline in the incidence of acute hepatitis B. Besides immunizing infants, other factors are important in the reduction in HBV, including a "halo" effect related to the HIV epidemic. Measures important in controlling HIV, such as avoiding contaminated needles and using condoms, are important in decreasing HBV. Nevertheless, the greater than 80% reduction in the rate of acute hepatitis B among children aged 1–9 years is primarily the result of the practice of universal immunization of infants [152].

Immunization has also been effective in health care workers. From 1983–1995, the rate of acute HBV infection among health care workers declined 95% and is now lower than the rate in the general U.S. population [159]. Another example of the changes in the epidemiology has occurred in Alaska. Following vaccination efforts beginning in 1982, the prevalence of *chronic* HBV among Alaska natives younger than 10 years old (i.e., children born after implementation of routine vaccination) declined to zero when assessed in 1994. This compares to a rate of 16% among Alaska natives aged 11–30 years [160].

Despite this progress in eradicating HBV infection in children, HBV remains an important *pediatric* disease in the United States for several reasons. First, even with appropriate immunoprophylaxis at birth, 5–10% of infants born to infected women will develop HBV infection. Second, international adoption and immigration from HBV-endemic regions bring infants and children who were not immunized at birth and have high rates of chronic HBV. Third, adolescents and young adults (born before 1992) remain relatively unprotected and often engage in high-risk behavior.

Table 17.13: Chronology of Hepatitis B Immunization Recommendations from the Advisory Committee on Immunization Practices (ACIP)

Date	*Recommendation*
June 25, 1982	Vaccinate high-risk groups.*
June 1, 1984	Administer hepatitis B immune globulin to all infants with HBsAg-positive mothers, and test high-risk pregnant women.
June 10, 1988	Test all pregnant women for HBsAg during the prenatal period.
November 22, 1991	Immunize all U.S. infants for hepatitis B.
August 4, 1995	Vaccinate all 11- to 12-year-olds.
January 22, 1999	Vaccinate all children 0–18 years who have not been vaccinated previously.
January 18, 2002	Established preference for starting the first vaccine for hepatitis B at birth

*Health care providers, staff of institutions with developmentally disabled people, hemodialysis patients, men who have sex with men, injection drug users, recipients of clotting factors for bleeding disorders, household and sexual contacts of persons with chronic HBV infection, inmates of correctional facilities, and populations with endemic HBV infection (e.g., Alaska natives, Pacific Islanders, immigrants from countries in which HBV is endemic).
From the Centers for Disease Control and Prevention [152].

Adolescents born after 1992 are at low risk for HBV acquisition because of the implementation of the universal infant vaccination policy. This policy occurred following the ACIP recommendation in November 1991 (Table 17.13).

Perinatal Transmission

In areas with a high prevalence of chronic HBV, transmission from asymptomatic carrier mothers to infants is the major route of spread. The offspring of all HBsAg-positive mothers are at risk, but infection is noted most frequently when the mother is HBeAg positive or has acute hepatitis B in the third trimester [161–166]. Specific factors that directly correlate with the development of the HBsAg-positive state in the infant (in the absence of effective prophylaxis) are (1) the maternal HBsAg titer; (2) maternal HBeAg positivity (up to 90% of infants born to HBeAg-positive mothers develop chronic hepatitis B; infants of HBeAg-negative carrier mothers have a 20% risk) [164,166]; (3) HBV DNA in maternal serum [143]; (4) HBsAg-positive cord blood; and (5) HBsAg-positive siblings [166–168]. Infants born to women who have cleared HBeAg and have seroconverted to become anti-HBe positive may retain the potential for the development of HBV infection. Latent HBV residing in maternal mononuclear cells may be responsible for perinatal HBV infection in this setting [168].

Infants who acquire HBV from HBsAg-positive women do not manifest serologic evidence of HBV infection until 1–3 months of age. Therefore, transmission presumably occurs during birth, perhaps following ingestion of maternal blood by the infant during delivery. However, viral transmission may occur in utero via transplacental leakage. HBeAg can cross the human placenta from mother to fetus. Because HBeAg and HBcAg are highly cross-reactive in terms of T helper cell recognition, the exposure to HBeAg in utero may lead to fetal immunotolerance to HBcAg and HBeAg [169].

Although perinatal HBV infection has minimal clinical manifestations, the implications for the neonate of failure to interrupt perinatal HBV infection are significant [170–174]. In approximately 90% of HBsAg-positive infants, chronic hepatitis develops or the chronic carrier state is established; the infected infants therefore may ultimately perpetuate and disseminate HBV. The frequent development of the chronic carrier state following exposure to HBV in the perinatal period has been attributed to the immaturity of the newborn immune system. It has also been postulated that transplacental passage of maternal HBeAg may induce a specific unresponsiveness of helper T cells to HBcAg and HBeAg in the neonates born to HBeAg-positive carrier women [175]. In transgenic mice, in utero exposure to HBeAg through the transplacental route leads to neonatal T-cell tolerance to HBeAg and HbcAg [176]. In rare cases, fatal fulminant hepatitis may follow perinatal transmission; this seems to occur in infants whose mothers are positive for both HBsAg and anti-HBe [177–180]. Infected infants are also at lifelong risk for the development of the known sequelae of chronic HBV infection, cirrhosis, and HCC.

The risk of HBV acquisition does not end in the perinatal period because susceptible infants are at risk for subsequent infection from other family members. Postnatal infection is possible in an environment in which the HBsAg carrier rate is high and vaccination rates are low. Adopted foreign children may spread HBV to susceptible family members [181–188]. In 1989, 46% of cases of HBV infection occurring among U.S.-born children of refugees from a hyperendemic area (Southeast Asia) were not attributable to perinatal transmission but to child-to-child transmission within households [189]. The presumed intrafamilial and interfamilial spread of HBV originating in adoptees has been the basis for the recommendations that directed screening tests be implemented and that the HBV vaccination policy include not only all newborns, but also older siblings of immigrants from areas where HBV infection is endemic.

Clinical Aspects

Acute HBV infection may be either symptomatic or asymptomatic; asymptomatic presentations are more common in young children. In adults, whether symptomatic or not, most acute HBV infections are self-limited, with clearance of virus from blood and liver and the development of long-term immunity to reinfection [96]. In symptomatic individuals, the presentation of acute hepatitis may be indistinguishable from other forms of hepatitis, with predominant symptoms of anorexia, jaundice, fever, abdominal pain, nausea, and fatigue (Table 17.14). The incubation period ranges from 50–180 days before this symptomatic phase, which is followed by a convalescence phase (Figure 17.16).

A prodromal phase precedes the development of jaundice by 2–3 weeks and may include nonhepatic manifestations. In fact, in some infected persons, the presence of certain extrahepatic manifestations may increase the suspicion for HBV infection. For example, a serum sickness–like prodromal phase, also referred to as the "arthritis–dermatitis" prodrome, has been recognized in 10–30% of acute HBV infection [190]. The clinical features of this syndrome include polyarthralgias or arthritis, which may be indistinguishable from acute rheumatoid arthritis until jaundice develops. Most often, the arthritis is symmetric and generalized, involving the small joints of the hands and feet. It is quite painful, out of proportion to the degree of joint swelling; however, the joint lesions are nondestructive and permanent damage does not occur. In some individuals, the arthritis is asymmetric and monoarticular, involving large joints such as the knees, wrists, and ankles. Synovial fluid may contain a variable number of neutrophils [190]; the synovial fluid also contains HBsAg and reduced complement levels [191].

As with the arthritic features, the skin manifestations are variable. In HBV-infected individuals with arthritis, more than 50% have concurrent rashes that range from discrete eruptions to all types of rashes: petechial, urticarial, maculopapular, or purpuric. Unusual dermatologic manifestations have included Henoch-Schönlein–type purpura, erythema multiforme, and lichenoid dermatitis [190]. Biopsies of these skin rashes reveal a cutaneous vasculitis with immunoglobulins, complement, and HBsAg in blood vessel walls [192]. The basis for this serum sickness–like syndrome is thought to be related to circulating immune complexes of HBsAg–anti-HBs [190,191]. Clinical symptoms occur during the period of relative antigen excess and soluble immune complexes. As anti-HBs titers increase, these immune complexes become less soluble and are cleared, with resolution of clinical symptoms. Though these immune complexes of HBsAg are necessary for this syndrome, they alone are not sufficient. A high percentage of infected individuals harbor these complexes [193], yet only a minority develop this serum sickness–like syndrome; this implicates other undetermined host or viral factors that have not been identified.

Many other immunologically mediated manifestations of acute HBV infection have been described. These include various forms of glomerulonephritis and vasculitis [194–197]. These features generally disappear before the onset of the clinical hepatitis illness.

Of the extrahepatic manifestations, papular acrodermatitis of childhood (PAC), also called Gianotti–Crosti syndrome, is frequently cited as an important dermatologic manifestation identified with chronic HBV infection [198]. However, this rash has been described in association with other infections [199,200], and its relationship to HBV infection is unclear [190]. This rash, which is prevalent in the Mediterranean region

Table 17.14: Clinical Features of Hepatitis B Infection

Clinical Feature	Characteristics
Signs and symptoms*	Jaundice Fatigue Anorexia Nausea Fever Diarrhea Abdominal pain Pruritic rash
Extrahepatic manifestations	Polyarteritis nodosa Glomerulonephritis Serum sickness–like prodrome Essential mixed cryoglobulinemia Dermatologic Arthritis Neurologic
Changing incidence	Number of new infections per year has declined from an average of 260,000 in the 1980s to about 78,000 in 2001 in the U.S. Greatest decline among children and adolescents because of vaccination Highest rate of disease occurs in 20- to 49-year-olds
Incubation period	Average ~90 days (range, 50–180 days)
Transmission	Vertical (mother to child) Percutaneous exposure to infected fluids: Unprotected sex Sharing of drugs and needles Occupational exposure
Persons at risk of infection	Sexual contacts of infected persons Infants born to infected mothers International adoptees and immigrants from endemic regions Men who have sex with men Injection drug users Health care and public safety workers Hemodialysis patients† Household contacts of chronically infected persons
Long-term sequelae without vaccination	Chronic infection occurs in: 90% of exposed infants 30% of children between 1–5 years 6% of persons after age 5 years Death from chronic liver disease occurs in 15–25% of chronically infected persons
Fulminant hepatitis	~1% of infants, children, and adults

*About 30% of persons infected with hepatitis B have no signs or symptoms. Signs and symptoms are less common in children than in adults.

†Hemodialysis and blood transfusion were not associated with reported cases of acute hepatitis B in the United States from 1990–2000 [20].

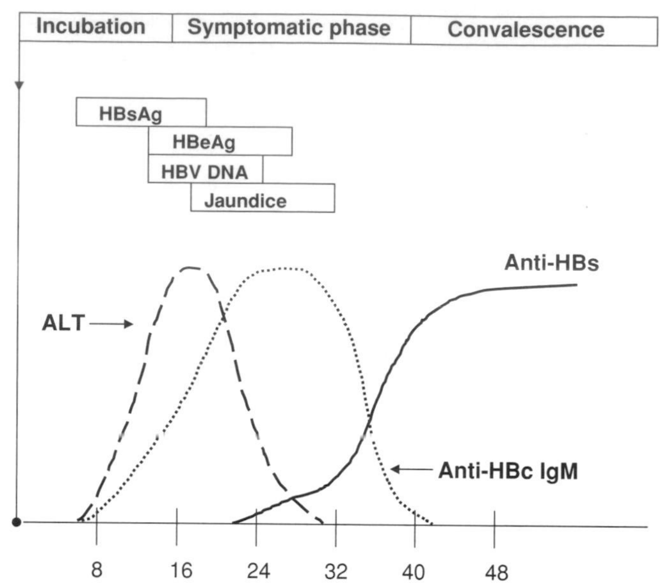

Figure 17.16. Typical course of acute HBV infection. Primary HBV infection has an incubation period of 4–10 weeks. The earliest detectable serum marker of HBV infection is a rise in HBsAg, which may appear between 1 and 10 weeks following exposure. Subsequently, HBeAg and HBV DNA can be identified. HBsAg is present 2–8 weeks before the onset of symptoms, which coincide with a spike in ALT levels, serum bilirubin, and constitutional signs. Clearance of HBsAg with the appearance of anti-HBs typically occurs within 6–8 months following infection. Anti-HBc IgM is present before symptomatic infection and is a marker for acute infection. Anti-HBc does not neutralize HBV infection. (Balistreri WF. Viral hepatitis. Emerg Clin North Am 1991;9:365–99.)

in children usually between 2 and 6 years of age, is characterized by 2- to 3-mm papular erurptions in children, primarily on the face and extremities [198]. PAC typically lasts for 2–3 weeks; in addition, lymphadenopathy is frequent.

Probably the most serious extrahepatic manifestation, albeit rare, is polyarteritis nodosa (PAN). PAN occurs in about 1–5% of chronic HBV patients [190]. However, among individuals identified with PAN, serum HBsAg positivity is observed in 40–50% [190]. This association is found predominantly in North America and Europe. In Asia, PAN associated with HBV has not been observed [190,201], likely because of the predominant perinatal mode of infection acquisition and age-related immunologic responses to HBV infection. Untreated HBV-associated PAN has a poor prognosis, with 30–50% dying as a consequence of the vasculitis [190]. Recently, treatment with a combination of antiviral therapy (IFN-α) and plasma exchange has been effective; newer treatments, including lamivudine and famciclovir, have been promising as well [190]. Seroconversion from HBeAg positive to anti-HBe and loss of detectable HBV DNA have been associated with improvement in PAN and, in many cases, remission of all symptoms.

Diagnosis

The diagnosis of acute and chronic HBV infection relies on serologic markers and molecular testing for hepatitis B DNA

Table 17.15: Interpretation of Serologic Markers of Hepatitis B Virus Infection

HBsAg	*HBeAg*	*Anti-HBe*	*Anti-HBc*	*Anti-HBs*	*HBV DNA*	*Significance*
+	+ or –	–	–	–	+	Early acute hepatitis; persistent carrier
+	+ or –	–	+	–	+	Acute hepatitis (anti-HBc IgM) and persistent carrier or chronic hepatitis (anti-HBc IgG)
+	–	+ or –	+	–	+	Late-phase acute hepatitis; carrier
–	–	–	+	–	+	Recovery phase
–	–	+	+	+	–*	Recovery
–	–	+ or –	+	+	–*	Postinfection
–	–	–	–	+	–*	Immune (no active infection)

*Very low levels of HBV DNA may be detected after the development of anti-HBs antibody.

(Table 17.15). The typical serologic pattern is illustrated in Figure 17.16. HBsAg, which may be detectable in serum as early as 3–6 days after exposure [144,202], is typically not found until approximately 1–3 months after inoculation of the virus, while the patient is still asymptomatic. In most cases, HBsAg becomes nondetectable rapidly after onset of symptoms. If antigenemia persists for longer than 6 months, the patient is considered either a chronic carrier or a chronically infected person. Active hepatic inflammation, as indicated by elevated serum aminotransferase values, may occur 14–60 days after HBsAg is detected in serum. Aminotransferase values commonly remain elevated for 30–60 days.

The initial antibody response detectable in HBV infection is that directed against hepatitis B core antigen (anti-HBc); this is a sensitive indicator of exposure to HBV. Persons acutely infected with HBV exhibit HBsAg and anti-HBc IgM positivity (Figure 17.16); the latter appears shortly after onset of the icteric phase, reaches maximal titers by 5 months, then subsequently declines. Anti-HBc IgG rises later and persists as long as viral replication within the liver cell continues. Anti-HBc IgM may be most helpful in documenting a recent HBV infection in those in whom HBsAg titers have declined to undetectable levels. The presence of HBV DNA in serum, detected by PCR, is a useful marker of viral replication and is usually associated with active liver disease and infectivity [203–206]. HBV DNA is usually present in conjunction with HBeAg; however, as discussed above, HBV mutants that do not secrete HBeAg exist.

During the recovery phase following acute HBV infection, anti-HBc and anti-HBs are detectable in serum (Figure 17.16). In certain people, anti-HBc alone, in the absence of concurrent HBsAg or anti-HBs, may be found. This may represent either the "window phase" between the disappearance of HBsAg and the appearance of anti-HBs (in this case anti-HBc IgM is usually present) or, less commonly, the development of an HBV carrier state, with levels of HBsAg below the limits of detection.

Demonstrable titers of anti-HBs (IgM followed by IgG) may first be noted weeks to months after the aminotransferase elevation and the presence of jaundice. Anti-HBs, a neutralizing antibody, remains detectable for many years after infection, affording antiviral activity. Anti-HBs protects against subsequent infection; successful prophylaxis via active or passive immunization against HBV infection is associated with high serum titers of anti-HBs.

Diagnosis of Chronic HBV Infection

Chronic HBV infection is indicated by detectable HBsAg in serum and liver along with markers of active viral replication, such as HBeAg or HBV DNA in serum or HBcAg in liver [202]. There are two clinical patterns: (1) chronic liver disease, with elevated aminotransferase levels and an abnormal hepatic histology, and (2) the chronic carrier state, defined as persistent viral infection without clinical evidence of hepatic injury (normal aminotransferase values). As noted previously, there may be spontaneous remission of chronic liver disease (loss of HBV DNA and HBeAg from serum, with seroconversion to anti-HBe–positive status) and evolution to the chronic carrier state. HBV DNA detection by PCR may be used to exclude or confirm infection in patients with chronic liver disease who have unusual serologic profiles. HBV DNA has been detected in the serum and liver of patients lacking all markers of HBV infection [207].

Outcome

The outcome of infection with HBV is determined by the interaction between the host immune system and the HBV and is quite variable. The age at the time of HBV acquisition is the major determinant of chronicity [208]. Up to 95% of infected neonates become HBV carriers, whereas fewer than 10% of adults become chronically infected with HBV.

Cirrhosis and HCC occur in nearly one of four persons with chronic hepatitis B. In HBsAg carriers referred to clinical centers, the reported incidence of cirrhosis is as high as 3% per year [111]. Prognostic factors for the development of cirrhosis include HBeAg positivity, older age, and elevated ALT levels. However, even young children with chronic hepatitis B may develop cirrhosis or HCC [209,210]. Although all individuals with HBV may develop these complications, the risk is much less for chronic carriers. In a study from Italy, 296 HBsAg-positive blood donors with ALT less than 1.25 times the upper limit of normal had no difference in survival compared with 157 HBsAg-negative donors [211]. In these individuals, who had a follow-up for a mean of 29 years, there was no difference in death from liver disease or HCC.

For adult patients who develop compensated cirrhosis, the survival rate is 84% at 5 years and 68% at 10 years [111]; after decompensation cirrhosis develops, the 5-year survival rate is only 14%. Clearance of HBeAg, whether spontaneous or with antiviral therapy, reduces the risk of hepatic decompensation and improves survival. Among compensated cirrhotic patients infected with hepatitis B who were HBeAg negative, 5-year survival was 97% in one study [109].

Risk factors for HCC in patients with chronic HBV infection include older age, male gender, family history of HCC, presence of HBeAg, history of reversion from anti-HBe positivity to HBeAg positivity, coinfection with HCV, and perinatal transmission [111,212]. In addition, alcohol use is likely a contributing factor, but studies have been inconclusive. Perinatal transmission has been identified as a risk factor for HCC [212]; the reasons this mode of transmission may increase the risk for HCC include a higher innoculate of HBV DNA, increased immunologic tolerance for HBV infection, and a longer time frame for the development of malignancy. Chronically infected individuals have a risk of HCC that is 100 times that of noncarriers [213]. HCC is much more common among people with cirrhosis, but 30–50% of HCC associated with HBV occurs in the absence of cirrhosis. Clearance of HBeAg and HBsAg lowers, but does not eliminate, the risk of HCC. The prognosis for HCC is poor, with 5-year survival rates of less than 5%.

Of course, the best way to minimize the risk of HCC is primary prevention. In Taiwan, the institution of universal infant vaccination has had a dramatic impact on the incidence of HCC in childhood. The rate of HCC has been followed from 1981 through 2000. Immunization has lowered the rate from 0.54 per 100,000 children in the period before vaccination to 0.20 per 100,000 children in the period after vaccination [154,209].

Throughout this chapter, the outcomes of the hepatotropic viruses have been related to viral factors including HBV genotype and mutations and increased HBV replication. The outcome also is related to so-called "host" factors, including early age of HBV acquisition, gender, and immune status. Besides viral and host factors, the other important contributors to morbidity are external factors including concurrent infection with HCV and HDV as well as hepatotoxins such as alcohol. It has been estimated that 10–15% of HBV patients have HCV coinfection. In patients with HCV and HBV, HCV often becomes the dominant cause of hepatic injury.

Prevention

To limit the spread of HBV, the first task is identification of infected individuals. Once identified, education of carriers and their contacts allows for isolation practices along with passive and/or active immunization of contacts. In addition, treatment in many individuals may decrease the risk of HBV transmission. As HBV can be spread through contaminated blood products, careful screening of blood donors and testing for HBsAg remains an important control measure.

Passive Immunoprophylaxis

Immune globulin is an important tool for the prevention of HBV infection. Initially, when an individual is exposed to a person with acute hepatitis, immune globulin treatment should be given as soon as feasible; hepatitis B immune globulin (HBIG) should be given within 2 weeks of exposure (see Table 17.7). Because of high titers of anti-HBs in commercial ISG lots, ISG may be effective against HBV infection. However, *high-titer* HBIG, prepared from plasma preselected for a high titer of antibody against HBsAg (anti-HBs titer >1:100,000), is more predictably effective for one-time exposures such as accidental needle punctures, pipetting accidents, or other contact of contaminated material with mucous membranes [46,214–217]. To achieve maximum effect, HBIG should be administered as soon as possible after exposure; it should not be given if the delay is greater than 14 days.

Postexposure prophylaxis with HBIG has been recommended for administration following (1) perinatal exposure of an infant born to an HBsAg-positive woman (see Prevention of Perinatal Transmission of Hepatitis B Virus), (2) sexual exposure to an HBsAg-positive person, (3) accidental percutaneous or mucosal exposure to HBsAg-positive products, or (4) household contact (Table 17.16) [218,219].

Active Immunoprophylaxis

The immunization policy for hepatitis B has been modified many times since the initial recommendations from ACIP in June 1982 (see Table 17.13). By 1991, the difficulty of vaccinating high-risk adults along with the significant burden of HBV acquired in childhood prompted ACIP to recommend universal childhood vaccination. In 1995, ACIP recommended the routine vaccination of all adolescents aged 11–12 years who had not been vaccinated previously. The implementation of universal vaccination among these targeted groups along with the previous efforts to identify and immunize high-risk populations has had considerable success in reducing the burden of HBV in the United States. In 1982, there were an estimated 200,000–300,000 persons infected annually with HBV, including 20,000 children [152]. The estimated number of new cases of HBV in 2003 was 73,000; of these new HBV infections, the

Table 17.16: Postexposure Prophylaxis for Individuals Exposed to Hepatitis B Virus

Immune and Vaccine Status of Exposed Person	*Intervention*
Unvaccinated	HBIG,* one dose; initiate hepatitis B vaccine series
Vaccinated	
Known responder	No treatment
Known nonresponder	HBIG, two doses; consider revaccination series
Anti-HBs response unknown	Test for anti-HBs; if inadequate, treat with HBIG × 1 and give vaccine booster

*The dosage of HBIG for perinatal postexposure is 0.5 mL intramuscularly within 12 hours of birth. The dosage for sexual postexposure prophylaxis is 0.06 mL/kg intramuscularly within 14 days of exposure.
From Weinbaum C, Lyerla R, Margolis HS. Centers for Disease Control and Prevention. Prevention and control of infections with hepatitis viruses in correctional settings. MMWR 2003;52:(RR-1): 1–36; and the Centers for Disease Control and Prevention. Recommendations for preventing transmission of human immunodeficiency virus and hepatitis B virus to patients during exposure-prone invasive procedures. MMWR 1991;40(RR-8):1–9.

estimated number of acute clinically symptomatic cases was 21,000 and the actual number of reported cases was 7526 [20].

The greatest challenge for eliminating HBV infection remains the vaccination of high-risk adults. The rates of vaccination for HBV in this population remain low despite two decades of efforts targeting this group. The reasons for this low immunization rate are multifactorial: (1) difficulty in identification of these individuals before they become infected, (2) limited public funding for vaccination of adults, and (3) missed opportunities.

The national health objectives for 2010 call for a reduction of 75–90% in acute hepatitis B cases among high-risk adults [152,220]. To reach this goal, it will be necessary to integrate HBV vaccination into programs that provide services to persons with risk factors for HBV infection. This could include STD clinics, correctional facilities, drug treatment clinics, and HIV clinics. Unless these efforts are undertaken, elimination of HBV as a significant source of morbidity and mortality will have to wait until the cohort of vaccinated infants and adolescents has been expanded by a few more decades.

Prevention of Perinatal Transmission of HBV

Because of the high risk of the development of chronic HBV infection following perinatal exposure, careful attention to immunoprophylaxis in the immediate newborn period remains essential. It is believed that in most cases transmission of HBV from an infected woman to her offspring occurs at the time of delivery. Therefore, immediate treatment of the infant born to an HBsAg-positive mother, using HBIG and HBV vaccine, can abort acquisition and significantly reduce the rate of chronic HBV infection (Tables 17.16 and 17.17). Treatment is predictably effective in modifying the infection and preventing the carrier state if instituted within 48 hours of delivery; therefore, any delay is undesirable. If the maternal HBsAg status is not known, it is *not* necessary to delay treatment until results of the serologic screening document maternal HBsAg positivity and that the cord blood is negative for HBsAg.

When used as the sole prophylactic agent, HBIG has a protective efficacy of approximately 75%, as documented by a significant reduction in the percentage of infants who become chronic HBV carriers following perinatal exposure [221–225]. HBIG has proven efficacy only when given within 12 hours of birth; however, the efficacy of HBIG given at 12–48 hours is presumed but not proved. HBIG *alone* was used for prophylaxis of 14 infants born to HBsAg/HBeAg-positive carrier mothers or to mothers with acute hepatitis B in the third trimester. Four infants became HBsAg-positive carriers, and one infant developed a transient anicteric HBV infection [223]. All HBV infections occurred after the infant reached 9 months of age as HBIG protection diminished, suggesting that adjunctive active immunoprophylaxis with the HBV vaccine is necessary for infants born to HBsAg-positive mothers [179,223,226]. Studies that evaluated this combination regimen serve as the basis for the current recommendations for prevention of perinatal HBV transmission (Table 17.17) [221,227–233]. Concurrent administration of HBIG and HBV vaccine allows both immediate (HBIG) as well as sustained (vaccine) high levels of the protective anti-HBs, thereby reducing the rate of chronic infection to less than 5% [227,230,234–238]. Because an estimated 3–5% of perinatal infections may truly be acquired in utero, further reduction may not be possible. Stevens et al. [239] demonstrated that the administration of HBIG (0.5 mL at birth) with recombinant HBV vaccine (in three doses) protected 94% of infants born to HBsAg/HBeAg-positive mothers from developing the chronic carrier state. The response to HBV vaccine is not impaired by the simultaneous administration of HBIG. HBV vaccine is an inactivated product and therefore does not interfere with other simultaneously administered vaccines. It is presumed that HBIG administered at birth does not interfere with the oral poliovirus or DPT (diphtheria, pertussis, tetanus) vaccination given at 6–8 weeks of age.

Because of the need for concurrent HBIG in infants of HBsAg-positive mothers, the HBV immunoprophylaxis program is dependent on identification of HBV-infected mothers; therefore, prepartum screening is recommended [240–244]. Limitation of antepartum screening to women in high-risk groups will fail to detect many carriers [243,244]. Identifiable risk factors are present in less than 50% of HBsAg-positive pregnant women; therefore, comprehensive routine testing should be carried out in all pregnancies despite a low incidence of HBsAg in the United States [178,243,245,246]. The immediate perinatal period is the only window for intervention against

Table 17.17: Vaccines for Hepatitis B Prevention*

Age	*Recombivax HB*		*Engerix-B*		*Twinrix*	
yr	*μg*	*mL*	*μg*	*mL*	*μg*	*mL*
≤19	5	0.5	10	0.5	—	—
11–15	10†	1.0	—	—	—	—
≥18–20‡	10	1.0	20	1.0	20	1.0
Dialysis patients§	40	1.0‖	40	2.0¶	—	—

*Recombivax HB (Merck & Co, Inc.), Engerix-B (GlaxoSmithKline Biologicals), and Twinrix (GlaxoSmithKline Biologicals) are usually administered in a three-dose schedule. When Recombivax HB or Engerix-B is given at birth, a four-dose schedule may be chosen to complete the series with a combination vaccine (e.g., Pediarix [GlaxoSmithKline Biologicals] or Comvax [Merck & Co., Inc.]) containing hepatitis B. When these vaccines are administered to infants of HBsAg-positive mothers, HBIG (0.5 mL) also is recommended.

†In this age group, a two-dose vaccine schedule is as immunogenic as the three-dose regimen.

‡Recombivax HB and Engerix-B at these doses are administered to adults 20 years or older. Twinrix (GlaxoSmithKline Biologicals) is a combination vaccine of Engerix-B and Havrix licensed for use in persons 18 years or older.

§This high dosage is given to dialysis patients but may be administered to immunocompromised hosts to increase the likelihood of seroprotection.

‖This is a concentrated formulation.

¶Two 1-mL doses are administered at a single site in a four-dose schedule at 0, 1, 2, and 6 months.

From the American Academy of Pediatrics [81] and Weinbaum C, Lyerla R, Margolis HS. Centers for Disease Control and Prevention. Prevention and control of infections with hepatitis viruses in correctional settings. MMWR 2003;52:(RR-1):1–36.

HBV; after infection occurs and the carrier state is established, there is no effective therapy at present.

The HBsAg status of any woman who belongs to a high-risk group and who has not received screening in the perinatal period should be assessed as soon as possible during pregnancy to allow appropriate handling of blood and other secretions and to determine the approach to the neonate. The administration of HBIG depends on the serologic status of the mother [214,247,248]. If a mother is identified as being HBsAg positive more than 1 month after delivery, the infant should be screened for HBsAg and if found to be negative, given HBIG and vaccine.

Each vaccinated infant born to an HBsAg-positive mother should be tested for HBsAg at 6 months of age during routine follow-up evaluation of the infant's health status. If the infant is HBsAg positive, which is unlikely, this indicates failure of immunoprophylaxis, and the third vaccine dose is obviated. On the other hand, the presence of high-titer anti-HBs indicates successful interruption of the spread of HBV, and the third dose of vaccine should be given. Breast-feeding does not pose a risk of transmission of HBV infection for infants who have begun prophylaxis.

Universal Vaccination

The use of HBV vaccination in the targeted programs discussed above, although effective in decreasing the risk for specific groups, such as health care workers, and in preventing perinatal transmission, did not reach the desired goal of a significant decline in the total number of acute hepatitis B cases in the United States. The previously recommended strategy for the control of HBV infection focused on identification and immunization of persons at high risk for acquisition. This strategy was doomed to failure because high-risk behavior is not easily defined or detected and those most likely to be in jeopardy may be the least likely to receive preventive health care [247,249–251]. In more than 30% of cases of acute HBV infection, no risk factor can be identified (see Figure 17.15). Because targeted prophylaxis failed to control HBV infection, *universal vaccination* against HBV infection, regardless of the HBsAg status of the mother, was recommended in 1991 by the ACIP [248] as well as by the Committee on Infectious Diseases of the AAP [247] (Table 17.18). This comprehensive strategy was viewed as cost-effective, even in areas of relatively low endemicity [248,252]. The current program to eliminate transmission of HBV in the United States, which includes incorporation of the HBV vaccine into the schedule of routine immunization for all infants, is aimed at providing protection of all children before the establishment of high-risk behavior [248], thereby reducing the massive human and financial costs of HBV infection [253,254]. The current estimate is that prevention of one case of chronic HBV infection, cirrhosis, or HCC offers significant benefits in health care costs; the cost-effectiveness of HBV vaccination is comparable to other diseases for which vaccination is currently offered [248,255]. The AAP has also recommended adolescent immunization. HBV vaccination requirements for

Table 17.18: Hepatitis B Vaccination: Indications

Recommendation	
Universal	All infants All children and adolescents not previously vaccinated
High-risk groups	Illicit drug users Household contacts* Prisoners Sexual partners of HBV carriers Men having sex with men Those with >1 sexual partner in the previous 6 mo or history of sexually transmitted disease Hemodialysis patients Those with occupational exposure: contact with body fluids Travelers to endemic area >6 mo Recipients of clotting factor concentrates Clients and staff of institutions for the developmentally disabled

*Adoptees from countries where HBV is endemic should be screened for HBsAg at or before the time of adoption. Adoptees found to be HBsAg negative should be immunized. If an adoptee is positive for HBsAg, household contacts should be immunized, preferably before adoption.
From Yu et al. [261].

middle school entry have been implemented in many states and in multiple countries [256–258]. However, where resources are limited, universal immunization of all infants should be given priority [247,249].

Recently, the ACIP has established a preference for the first dose of HBV vaccine to be given at birth for all infants. The second dose may be administered at the first well-baby visit (1–2 months later; Table 17.17) [247,248]. The third dose may be given at a routine visit between 6 and 18 months of age. Alternative schedules for initiation and completion of the vaccine series are possible (e.g., at 0, 12, and 24 months) [250]. Initiation of the HBV vaccine series at birth has the beneficial effect of improving overall immunization rates [251].

Current AAP and ACIP recommendations for HBV immunization in premature infants weighing less than 2 kg at birth born to HBsAg-negative mothers are to delay the initiation of vaccination until such infants reach 1 month of age [259]. In preterm infants weighing less than 2 kg at birth born to HBsAg-positive mothers or to mothers with unknown HBsAg status, HBIG and HBV vaccine should be given within 12 hours of birth; however, the birth vaccine should not be counted toward the completion of the HBV series. Three additional doses should be administered starting at 1 month of age [259].

With the program of universal vaccination established, it is anticipated that rates of HBV infection in the United States will decline when persons immunized as infants reach their period of greatest risk as teenagers and adults. This rationale is further based on the assumption that protection against HBV infection will persist for years or, in those whose anti-HBs titer has declined to low or undetectable levels, a rapid amnestic response to a single booster dose of vaccine will occur because of persistence of immunologic memory [252].

ADOLESCENT IMMUNIZATION

Recent development of a two-dose regimen for adolescents 11–15 years old may facilitate the catch-up efforts in this population (Table 17.17) [258,259]. In immunogenicity studies among this age group, Recombivax HB (Merck & Co., Inc.) at a 1-mL (10-μg) dose conferred seroprotection rates equivalent to the previously established three-dose regimen. All regimens resulted in adequate anti-HBs in 95% or more of vaccines [260]. However, adolescents who have begun vaccination with a 0.5-mL (5-μg) regimen should complete a three-dose schedule.

The goal of completing a vaccination series is important. However, inability to complete either the two-dose regimen or a three-dose regimen does not preclude the initiation of HBV vaccination. In healthy young adults, protective levels of antibody develop in 30–55% following a single conventional (0.5-mL) dose of hepatitis B vaccine and in 75% after two conventional (0.5-mL) doses [152]. Although long-term seroprotection may be diminished, persons with a response to the first dose are expected to have protection for at least 5 years.

GROUPS WITH POOR RESPONSE TO VACCINATION

Several groups have been identified who have low rates of seroconversion with HBV vaccination. Risk factors include increasing age, male gender, obesity, cigarette smoking, immunocompromised status, and dialysis treatment [261]. To improve response in patients with these risk factors, higher doses of HBV vaccines have been given. In a well-controlled trial of double-dose vaccine among hemodialysis patients, 63% developed an adequate antibody response [262]; however, after correction for possible transfer of antibodies by blood transfusion, only 50% had responded. Patients with cirrhosis also have a poor response to immunization. With conventional doses, the seroconversion rate in one study was 28% compared with healthy controls, who had a 97% response [261]; even with double-dosing, the seroconversion rate was 44%. With more effort, the rate can be increased. Among these patients who had a repeat series of vaccination, the rate was 62%, still well below the response rate in healthy adults. Other conditions associated with a poor response to immunization have included HIV infection, chronic cardiopulmonary disease, renal failure, and organ transplantation [261].

Among nonresponders to the initial series of HBV vaccine, half may convert after an additional one to three doses [261]. Hyporesponders are more likely to seroconvert than are nonresponders. Nonresponders to a second series of vaccination are unlikely to develop adequate anti-HBs titers with further vaccine doses [263].

HBV Vaccine Characteristics and Long-Term Protection

The HBsAg particle is the immunogen in both plasma-derived and recombinant HBV vaccines. Plasma-derived vaccines account for more than 80% of all HBV vaccines used worldwide; however, in the United States, HBV immunization relies completely on the recombinant vaccines. The recombinant vaccines became available in 1986 and gained acceptance because of the unfounded concern of blood-borne infectious agents in the plasma-derived vaccine [263]. The recombinant HBV vaccines and combination vaccines are listed in Table 17.17.

Long-term follow-up of current vaccination practices (with recombinant vaccine) is needed to precisely determine the need for booster doses after long intervals [46]. The long-term immunogenicity and protection provided by HBV vaccination have been determined for the initial (plasma-derived) vaccine [261,265]. One follow-up study suggested that anti-HBs levels persisted for at least 7 years but varied inversely with age and directly with the level of anti-HBs attained 1 year after the first dose [265]. This study also indicated that the HBV vaccine provided a high level of protection from adverse HBV events. Two independent long-term follow-up studies of vaccinated children showed persistence of a protective effect up to 15 years following plasma-derived vaccine administration and no added benefit of booster doses [266,267]. To date, there are no data to support the need for booster doses of HBV vaccine in immunocompetent individuals who have responded to a primary course. In a cohort of Yupik Eskimos who had a 94% rate of anti-HBs response to vaccination, 76% had titers greater than or equal to 10 mIU/mL after 10 years of follow-up [265]. None became chronically infected despite exposure to HBV, indicated by the presence of anti-HBc or by the boosting of anti-HBs titers. All adequately vaccinated individuals have shown evidence of immunity in the form of persisting anti-HBs and/or in vitro B-cell stimulation of an anamnestic response to a vaccine challenge [268,269]. Protective antibody levels persist for more than 3 years [270]; however, anti-HBs titers decline and may become undetectable [265]. Despite declining antibody titers, protection against manifest HBV infection seems to be present for more than 10 years [261]. As the titer achieved 1–3 months after the third dose of the basic immunization correlates well with the persistence of long-term protection, measurement of anti-HBs titers in high-risk groups and immunosuppressed patients should be considered. The peak level of anti-HBs that develops after completion of the vaccine series is a good predictor of the duration of antibody persistence [271]. Booster doses of vaccine are not routinely recommended nor is routine serologic testing to assess antibody levels in vaccine recipients necessary for at least 5 years [272–274].

Recommendations for the Use of the HBV Vaccine

Recombinant HBV vaccines are packaged to contain 10–40 μg/mL of HBsAg protein absorbed with aluminum hydroxide (0.5 mg/mL) [46]. Thimerosal was traditionally added as a preservative; however, because of a concern about mercury toxicity in young infants in mid-1999, thimerosal-free preparations became available. The current recommendations for administration include three intramuscular (deltoid) doses of HBV vaccine (Table 17.17). The first two doses of vaccine are given 1 month apart, and a booster dose is typically administered 6 months after the first. This schedule has been shown to provide rapid initial protection in most vaccinees and to induce amplification of memory cells, thereby producing long-term immunity against HBV via an anamnestic recall [46,275,276]. Alternative schedules (0, 1, 2, and 12 months), dosages, and administration modalities (e.g., intradermal) are possible [277–279].

The CDC has recommended that all health care workers exposed to blood in an occupational setting receive HBV vaccine [248,280]. Ideally, this should be accomplished during the period of professional training and before any occupational exposure occurs. The transmission risk for HBV is bidirectional; an estimated total of more than 300 patients, occurring in approximately 20 clusters, have had documented infection with HBV in association with treatment by an HBV-infected health care worker [248]. A combination of risk factors accounts for transmission of HBV in this setting, including HBeAg positivity, major breaks in standard infection control practices, and unintentional injury to the infected health care worker during invasive procedures. Recommendations for the prevention of HBV transmission during invasive procedures that are considered exposure prone have been published [248].

ADVERSE EFFECTS

The recombinant and plasma vaccines are well tolerated [261,263]. The most common adverse effect was transient pain in up to 20% of the vaccine recipients. Low-grade fever occurs in less than 5%. Other effects, such as fatigue, headache, nausea, skin rash, and respiratory distress, affect less than 1%. Because anaphylaxis has been rarely reported, epinephrine should be available. Although rare neurologic events have been reported, no conclusive epidemiologic association has been established. Among 850,000 vaccinees monitored by the CDC and the FDA, 41 neurologic events were reported, including Bell's palsy in 10, Guillain–Barré syndrome in 9, and seizures in 5 [261].

Despite the safety and efficacy of the HBV vaccine, concerns about its safety have resulted in temporary suspension of immunizations. After a mass immunization campaign in France between 1995 and 1997, several cases of multiple sclerosis were reported. In October 1998, the French government halted its school-based HBV vaccination program. This decision was *not* based on any proven association. In fact, at the time, two studies showed a nonsignificant increase in the risk of multiple sclerosis among vaccinated compared with unvaccinated subjects [281]. Further large-scale studies have refuted any connection. Among two cohorts involving 121,700 women and 116,671 women, the relative risk of multiple sclerosis associated with exposure to the HBV vaccine was 0.9 and the relative risk within 2 years of vaccination was 0.7 [281]. Also, in a study involving 260,000 Canadian adolescents, there was no increase in the number of cases of multiple sclerosis after HBV vaccination [282].

In 2002, the Institute of Medicine found that "the epidemiological evidence (i.e., from studies of vaccine-exposed populations and their control groups or of patients with these diseases

Table 17.19: Terminology to Assess Response to Antiviral Therapy

Category	*Definition*
Biologic response (BR)	Decrease in serum ALT level to within normal range
Virologic response (VR)	Decrease in serum HBV DNA to undetectable levels in unamplified assays ($<10^5$ copies/mL) and loss of HBeAg (in patients who were initially HBeAg positive)
Histologic response (HR)	Decrease in histologic activity index by at least 2 points compared with pretreatment liver biopsy
Complete response (CR)	Fulfill criteria of biochemical and virologic response and loss of HBsAg
Sustained response (SR)	Response to therapy that lasts 6 (SR-6) to 12 months (SR-12) after discontinuation of therapy

From Lok and McMahon [111].

and their control groups) favors rejection of a causal relationship between the HBV vaccine in adults and multiple sclerosis. The evidence was inadequate to accept or reject a causal relationship between the HBV vaccine and all other demyelinating conditions" [283].

Another concern raised about HBV vaccination in the United States was related to the preservative thimerosal causing the potential of mercury toxicity. This concern resulted in delaying immunizations [1]; even after thimerosal-free vaccines became available, it was well documented that there were delays in immunization that resulted in HBV acquisition and even in death [1].

Management

When preventive measures fail and an individual has contracted HBV, the focus shifts toward optimizing the outcome using the treatment measures that are available (Tables 17.19, 17.20, and 17.21). The general goals of these therapeutic efforts have been to (1) attempt to eliminate the virus, thereby inducing a remission in liver injury and reducing the risk of transmission; (2) relieve symptoms; and (3) prevent progression to end-stage liver disease. Attainment of these goals has been a formidable task.

A major issue in effective study design and patient management is the determination of whom to treat; this is especially true for pediatric patients. It is known that adults with chronic viral hepatitis are often symptomatic, exhibiting lethargy and fatigue, perhaps associated with nausea, anorexia, abdominal pain, or myalgia. However, these symptoms correlate poorly with the activity or severity of the disease. Physical findings are often absent despite disease activity; however, spider telangiectasias, palmar erythema, hepatomegaly, and splenomegaly may be present. Liver biopsy findings correlate poorly with symptomatology; the biopsy may be useful in assessing prognosis, in planning a therapeutic strategy, and in gauging the response to treatment. In addition, molecular probes applied to liver tissue may be used to confirm active viral replication and to exclude other conditions before initiation of therapy.

Table 17.20: Initial and Follow-Up Evaluation for Chronic Hepatitis B*

Management of Patients with Chronic Hepatitis B
Initial management
History and physical examination
Assess liver disease: complete blood cell count, hepatic panel, prothrombin time, and α-fetoprotein level
Assess HBV replication: HBeAg/anti-HBe, HBV DNA
Assess for concomitant disease: HCV, HDV, alcohol exposure, NAFLD
Screen for hepatitis A and vaccinate if anti-HAV negative
Vaccinate household/sexual contacts
Consider baseline ultrasound
Follow-up management
If ALT $\leq 2 \times$ ULN, observe and do the following:
Follow ALT every 3–12 mo
Consider liver biopsy and/or treatment when ALT levels become elevated
Consider screening for hepatocellular carcinoma with α-fetoprotein levels and ultrasound
If ALT $>2 \times$ ULN† for more than 3 mo, consider treatment (IFN-α, lamivudine, or adefovir) and the following:
Liver biopsy to grade and stage liver disease
Screening for hepatocellular carcinoma with α-fetoprotein levels and ultrasound

*These recommendations have not been validated by clinical trials in children with chronic hepatitis B. Therefore, the approach to each patient needs to be individualized.
†Before instituting treatment, it is important to consider whether ALT values are elevated because of other causes besides HBV, such as nonalcoholic steatohepatitis, medications, or other intrinsic liver diseases.
NAFLD, non-alcoholic fatty liver disease; ULN, upper limit of normal.
From Lok and McMahon [328].

As discussed earlier in this chapter, the patient with chronic liver disease caused by persistent HBV infection must be distinguished from the healthy HBsAg carrier, who harbors infection without active liver disease (see Table 17.11) [111]. The former patient has direct serologic evidence of HBV replication (HBeAg positivity, HBV DNA in serum, or HBcAg in liver). HBeAg-positive patients typically exhibit elevated levels of virus (HBV DNA) in serum, attended by abnormal aminotransferase levels and active liver disease; the latter features are indicative of an active immune response by the host. An important caveat

Table 17.21: Comparison of Treatments for Chronic Hepatitis B

Treatment Parameter	*IFN-α*	*Lamivudine*	*Adefovir*	*Peginterferon*
Indications				
Patient with normal ALT levels	Not indicated	Not indicated	Not indicated	Not indicated
Chronic hepatitis				
HBeAg+	Indicated	Indicated	Indicated	Indicated
HBeAg$^-$	Indicated	Indicated	Indicated	Indicated
Duration of treatment	4–12 mo*	>1 yr	>1 yr	1 yr†
Efficacy, %‡				
Loss of HBeAg	~30	20–30	12–24§	~30
Loss of HBV DNA	37	44	20–50	32–43
ALT normalization	23	40–70	48–72	~60
Route	SC	Oral	Oral	SC
Side effects	Many	Neglible	?Renal toxicity	Many
Drug resistance	None	~15%/yr	~1%/yr	None
Cost/month, $	~1400	260	450	~1400

*Treatment for 12 months has been recommended for HBeAg-negative patients.
†Duration of treatment with peginterferon is based on recent studies from adult patients with HBV.
‡All treatments are 1-year data.
§For adefovir, loss of HBeAg increased to 44% at 72 weeks [130].
SC, subcutaneous.
From Keefe et al. [130] and the Centers for Disease Control and Prevention [248].

when considering elevated ALT values and possible treatment is whether there may be an alternative explanation.

Seroconversion from HBeAg positivity to anti-HBe, indicative of a decrease in viral replication (reduction of HBV DNA levels) and theoretically an improvement in liver disease, may occur spontaneously or in response to antiviral therapy [111]. For this reason, the American Association for the Study of Liver Diseases (AASLD) has published guidelines recommending observation for 3–6 months before instituting treatment in HBeAg-positive patients with increased ALT levels. The ultimate goal of any therapeutic intervention is to induce disappearance of HBsAg, which implies termination of the HBV carrier state. True cure of infection with loss of HBsAg and complete disappearance of viremia, as measured by sensitive PCR assays, is achieved in 1–5% of patients [96].

Multiple forms of anti-inflammatory and antiviral therapy have been studied in patients with chronic hepatitis B. Most agents have proved to be either ineffective or to exert unacceptable toxicity [284–286].

Interferon Therapy

The first effective and clinically useful antiviral agent for chronic viral hepatitis was IFN. The IFNs represent a family of naturally occurring proteins synthesized in response to viral infections. There are three major forms: (1) IFN-α, derived from monocytes and transformed B cells; (2) IFN-β (fibroblasts); and (3) IFN-δ (helper/inducer subset of T lymphocytes) [287]. For treatment purposes, these IFNs have been modulated with the addition of large polyethylene glycol (PEG) moieties to create peginterferons, which have sustained serum levels allowing for once-weekly dosing. The IFNs exert varying degrees of antiviral, immunomodulatory, and antiproliferative effects. They initiate their cellular activity by binding to cell membrane surface receptors and modulating a sequence of intracellular events (induction of enzymes, enhancement of phagocytic activity of macrophages, augmentation of specific cytotoxicity of lymphocytes, and inhibition of virus replication in infected cells). IFNs may act at multiple sites in the viral replication cycle, inhibiting (1) viral entry, (2) uncoating of viral envelope proteins, (3) translation of viral mRNAs, and (4) viral assembly [285,287]. The biologic effects and pharmacokinetics of IFN in patients with chronic hepatitis B have been extensively studied [287,288]. On the basis of clinical studies, IFN-α-2b, made widely available through recombinant DNA technology, has been approved by the FDA for the treatment of chronic hepatitis B. IFN-α-2b is indicated for the treatment of chronic hepatitis B in patients with compensated liver disease and documented HBV replication.

In patients with chronic hepatitis B, serum aminotransferase levels and the intensity of hepatic inflammation are inversely proportional to the degree of HBV replication, which has been interpreted as evidence that liver injury is the result of an immune response to the virus [285,288]. The rationale for using IFN to treat patients with chronic hepatitis B is based

Table 17.22: Laboratory Monitoring with Interferon Therapy

Laboratory Test	*Frequency*
Liver panel, complete blood count, BUN/creatinine	Weeks 0, 1, 2, 4, 8, 12, and 24
HBV DNA, HBeAg, anti-HBe, and HBsAg	Every 3 mo
TSH	Every 3 mo

BUN, blood urea nitrogen; TSH, thyroid-stimulating hormone

on the premise that persistent infection with HBV is the result of a defective immunologic response to the virus. In addition, defective in vitro production of IFN and diminished native IFN-induced cellular activation occur in chronic hepatitis B. Therefore, because patients with chronic hepatitis B not only exhibit active viral replication but appear to have a selective defect in their immune response to HBV, targeted therapy using IFN should theoretically be an ideal therapeutic strategy [285].

A number of factors have been identified that are associated with response to IFN, the most important of which are higher levels of ALT and lower levels of HBV DNA before treatment [111] (Tables 17.22 and 17.23). The usual dose of IFN in immunocompetent patients with chronic hepatitis B is 5 million units (MU) given subcutaneously daily or 10 MU three times weekly for 16 weeks. Attempts to enhance immunologic activity further with corticosteroid "priming" are not recommended because of the risk of fatal hepatic decompensation [111].

Greenberg et al. [289] were the first to successfully use human leukocyte IFN in the treatment of chronic hepatitis B. Subsequent prospective, randomized, controlled clinical trials have indicated that a 3- to 6-month course of IFN induces a long-term remission in approximately 30% of patients with chronic hepatitis B [288,290–298]. In these patients, the IFN-induced remission is indicated by a loss of HBV DNA and HBeAg from serum, a decrease in aminotransferase levels, and an improvement in liver histology [111]. Relapse rates following discontinuation of IFN therapy are low (5–10%) [299]. Long-term follow-up of IFN responders indicates that remission is maintained in the majority, histologic progression of the disease is slowed in responders, and the rate of liver-related deaths is reduced [299–301].

INTERFERON FOR CHILDREN

The efficacy of IFN-α in children is similar to that in adults. Among children with elevated ALT, HBeAg clearance has been reported in 30% of those who received IFN-α compared with 10% of controls [111]. However, among children with normal ALT levels, less than 10% clear HBeAg. One meta-analysis of 240 children found that IFN-α increased HBV DNA clearance (odds ratio, 2.2), HBeAg clearance (odds ratio, 2.2), and ALT normalization (odds ratio, 2.3) compared with untreated controls [302]. Adverse events were similar to those in adults.

In a multinational randomized, controlled trial, Sokal et al. [303] confirmed that in children with chronic hepatitis B (n = 149), INF-α promotes loss of viral replication markers and surface antigen and improves aminotransferase levels and histology [303]. Serum HBeAg became negative in 26% of treated children and 11% of controls; HBsAg became negative in 10% of treated patients and 1% of controls.

These findings were similar to those found in a compilation of the European experience from ten randomized controlled trials spanning 10 years of IFN treatment in pediatric patients with chronic hepatitis B [304]. These studies included 1122 children, 40% of whom were "responders." A consensus was reached about IFN treatment criteria in children: (1) candidates for treatment are children with HBeAg and HBV DNA positivity, with low to intermediate HBV DNA levels and abnormal ALT values, aged 2 years or more; (2) IFN is contraindicated in children with decompensated liver disease, cytopenia, severe renal or cardiac disorders, or autoimmune disease; (3) the standard treatment regimen is 5 MU/m^2 subcutaneously thrice weekly for 6 months; and (4) retreatment in nonresponders is not indicated. This consensus is based on the demonstrated short-term efficacy of IFN; the long-term clinical and virologic effects of the drug, however, remain to be evaluated.

Although clinical trials in adults and children have shown a favorable response, the long-term effect of IFN-α is unclear. Some have suggested that exogenous IFN-α merely expedites seroconversion in predisposed individuals and may not truly change long-term morbidity and mortality. This argument is bolstered by data showing that IFN-α–treated children had no difference in loss of HBeAg compared with untreated children when measured 5 years after randomization [305]. Among this cohort of 107 children in the treatment group (data pooled from two studies) and 59 control patients, 32% of treated children responded with loss of HBeAg during therapy (3–6 months) or during the first year following treatment. High pretreatment ALT levels and a greater histologic activity index were predictors of response. Kaplan-Meier estimates of *cumulative* HBeAg clearance rates at five years were similar between treated patients (60%) and controls (65%). In all patients who cleared HBeAg, there was also loss of detectable HBV DNA using either a quantitative or a semiquantitative dot blot hybridization method; in addition, 94% of these responders had normalization of ALT levels. One significant difference was in the loss of HBsAg; this occurred in four treated patients who responded during treatment but in none of the other treated or untreated patients.

Similar results occurred in a study of 74 children from Belgium [306]. The 7-year cumulative HBeAg and HBsAg clearance rates were similar among the treated group, 47.5% and 8.9%, respectively, compared with a matched control group, 33.5% and 4%, respectively.

PARAMETERS OF RESPONSE TO INTERFERON

Interferon is most likely to be effective in patients in whom the drug is able to fully mediate a two-pronged attack so that IFN

Table 17.23: Comparison of HBV DNA Quantitative Assays

Assay (Manufacturer)	*Sensitivity, pg/mL (Copies/mL)**	*Range, Copies/mL*	*Coefficient of Variation, %*
Branched DNA (Bayer)	2.1 (7×10^5)	7×10^5–5×10^9	6–15
Hybrid capture (Digene)	0.5 (1.4×10^5)	2×10^5–1×10^9	10–15
High volume sample†	0.02 (5×10^3)	5×10^3–3×10^{10}	10–15
Liquid hybridization (Abbott)	1.6 (4.5×10^5)	5×10^5–1×10^{10}	12–22
PCR – Amplicor (Roche)	0.001 (4×10^2)	4×10^2–1×10^7	14–44
Molecular beacons	<50	<50–1×10^5	5–10

*1 pg/mL HBV DNA = 283,000 copies.
†With an increase in sample volume to 1 mL instead of 30 μL, the sensitivity and range of the assay are improved.
From Lok and McMahon [111].

both augments the immune response of the host and inhibits viral replication. A positive indication of an immune response to IFN therapy is a transient increase in serum ALT levels, which typically occurs during the first 90 days of treatment. This is usually associated with a progressive decline in serum HBV DNA levels.

Patients with pretreatment serum ALT levels more than twice the upper limits of normal, low levels of HBV DNA in serum, and HBeAg positivity are most likely to respond. These features presumably indicate a greater inherent immune response to HBV [284,285,307]. The U.S. multicenter study documented that in patients with HBV DNA levels less than 100 pg/mL (1 pg/mL is equivalent to 283,000 copies/mL), a 50% response rate occurred with 5 MU of IFN, whereas only 7% of the patients with HBV DNA levels greater than 200 pg/mL responded [289]. This indicates that patients with high levels of viral replication, often individuals considered immune tolerant of HBV infection, may not be optimal candidates for IFN therapy. Additional factors associated with a positive response to IFN therapy were active hepatitis on liver biopsy, anti-HIV negativity, anti-HDV negativity, female gender, and acquisition of infection later in life compared with exposure at birth [308,309].

In Asian patients, a lower response rate (17%) to IFN therapy has been found [308,310,311]. The low response rate in these patients is postulated to be the result of many factors, including the long average duration of infection; most patients were infected in the perinatal period. Therefore, HBV DNA had become integrated into the host genome, making eradication of the virus difficult.

One of the outcome measures has been whether IFN can reduce the incidence of HCC. Although the exact answer to this question is elusive, the ability to respond to IFN does indicate a lowered risk for this complication. In a recent study of 165 HBeAg patients treated with IFN between 1978 and 2002, over a mean of 8.8 years, it was shown that the relative risk of developing HCC was 0.084 among responders [312]. In addition, responders had improved survival with a relative risk of death of 0.28. However, whether IFN responders are inherently (before treatment) at lower risk than nonresponders is not clear.

ADVERSE EFFECTS

Interferon therapy is expensive and is associated with a high rate of adverse effects. In clinical trials, many patients experienced an adverse effect during the therapeutic course of IFN-α; most of these side effects occurred in a dose-dependent fashion and were rarely serious [287,288]. Most patients experienced a flulike illness shortly after the first dose of IFN, with fever, chills, and myalgia. Premedication with acetaminophen ameliorated these symptoms. A prominent side effect of IFN therapy in adults was fatigue, which became better tolerated as therapy was continued. Other reported side effects were changes in mood such as depression, impaired concentration, and mild alopecia.

Because IFN is myelosuppressive, therapy may be associated with a decrease in peripheral white blood cells (predominantly neutrophils) and platelets, usually within the first month [313]. This may be a significant problem in patients with cirrhosis and hypersplenism and may necessitate dose reduction or withdrawal. In one study, approximately one third of adult patients receiving 5 MU of IFN daily required dose reduction, but less than 5% required discontinuation of therapy [289].

Interferon has the potential to result in the de novo development or exacerbation of autoimmune phenomena. A variety of autoantibodies (e.g., antinuclear antibody, smooth muscle antibody, antibody to thyroid microsomal antigen) may arise during IFN therapy [314]. Thyroid dysfunction (hypothyroidism or, less commonly, hyperthyroidism) has been noted to occur during IFN therapy [315,316], suggesting a need for caution in treating patients with nonhepatic autoimmune disorders. If severe adverse reactions occur, dose modification (reduction) or discontinuation is indicated. Although IFN antibodies may develop in a percentage of treated patients, it is unclear whether these antibodies neutralize the antiviral effects of the drug [284,285,317].

Interferon has been associated with the development and worsening of retinopathy [318]. This often occurs 2 weeks to 3 months after the start of therapy and is more common in individuals with diabetes mellitus and hypertension. Although the cause of the IFN-related retinopathy is unknown, it has been speculated that immune complex deposition may play a role. In most cases, the retinopathy will disappear during therapy or rapidly after stopping treatment. Many clinicians obtain an eye examination before instituting therapy; significant retinopathy is a contraindication for ongoing IFN therapy.

Unique to pediatric patients is the risk of spastic diplegia in children younger than two years [319]. Therefore, IFN should not be administered in this age group.

INTERFERON THERAPY FOR PATIENTS WITH CIRRHOSIS

Initially, patients with decompensated liver disease caused by chronic hepatitis B were excluded from major IFN trials; however, it appears that even in the face of mild to moderate hepatic decompensation, IFN therapy may be beneficial. In one study of patients with cirrhosis, IFN resulted in the sustained disappearance of HBV DNA, in association with marked clinical and biochemical improvement, in 6 of 18 patients [320]. These observations suggest that if viral replication ceases, prolonged survival with improved indices of liver function and good quality of life is possible. However, in view of the low response rate (33%) and the incidence and severity of side effects in this group, therapy with IFN should be initiated with caution. Once complications of end-stage liver disease have developed (ascites, bleeding varices, portosystemic encephalopathy, or HCC), the impact of IFN is limited and is associated with significant adverse events and a real risk of hepatic decompensation.

Consensus guidelines for the use of IFN in children have been published [303]. However, because IFN has limited effectiveness, high costs, and significant adverse risks, even among well-selected individuals without cirrhosis, the search for more effective therapeutic agents continues.

New Treatments for Hepatitis B

At the time of this writing, lamivudine is the only other FDA-approved treatment for chronic hepatitis B in children, though several other agents, including adefovir dipivoxil, famciclovir, tenofovir, entecavir, telbivudine (LdT), emtricitabine (FTC), clevudine, remofovir, and peginterferon, are likely to become accepted treatments in the future.

Several nucleoside (or nucleotide) analogues have been identified that are potent and selective inhibitors of HBV replication: (1) stereoisomers of nucleosides in the "unnatural" L-configuration (e.g., pyrimidine derivatives such as lamivudine), and (2) nucleoside/nucleotides that have modified sugar residues in either cyclic or acyclic configurations (e.g., purine derivatives such as adefovir dipivoxil and famciclovir) [321].

Lamivudine

Lamivudine, an oral nucleoside analogue and reverse-transcriptase inhibitor, has been most widely studied in the treatment of patients with chronic HBV hepatitis [322–324]. Lamivudine given orally once daily (100 mg/d in adults) inhibits reverse-transcriptase activity and inhibits HBV DNA replication with a low incidence of side effects.

Lamivudine has been approved for the treatment of chronic HBV infection despite a high rate of viral mutation under treatment. In a large study from China, lamivudine therapy (25 mg or 100 mg) for 12 months reduced HBV DNA levels by 93–98% and was associated with HBeAg seroconversion in 13–16% of patients and with histologic improvement in 50–56% of patients [322]. Lamivudine-induced normalization of ALT values occurred in 40–50% of patients [322,323]. Dienstag et al. [324] confirmed these results in a U.S. population of previously untreated patients with chronic hepatitis B. After 52 weeks of treatment, lamivudine recipients were more likely than placebo recipients to have a histologic response (52% vs. 23%, $P < 0.001$), loss of HBeAg in serum (32% vs. 11%, $P = 0.003$), sustained suppression of serum HBV DNA to undetectable levels (44% vs. 16%, $P < 0.001$), and sustained normalization of serum ALT levels (41% vs. 7%, $P < 0.001$) [324]. The response rates were increased when treatment was extended for 18 months [325].

During lamivudine treatment and after therapy is withdrawn, ALT elevations are common; these elevations probably reflect a return of liver inflammation associated with unsuppressed HBV replication [326]. These treatment flares tend to be asymptomatic and transient, but they may be associated with clinical deterioration or decompensation in patients with advanced liver disease. After follow-up for 1 year, most patients who have an initial HBeAg response maintain the response [322,325].

Reemergence of HBV DNA during lamivudine therapy (treatment breakthrough) occurred in 14% after 12 months of therapy; these treatment failures among compliant patients are associated with mutations in the YMDD (tyrosine-methionine-aspartate-aspartate) locus of domain C of the polymerase (a nucleotide-binding locus), which lead to decreased sensitivity to lamivudine in vitro [327]. The frequency of YMDD mutations increases with the duration of therapy (as high as 69% after 5 years), but wild-type virus reemerges after cessation of lamivudine therapy. The appearance of these resistant strains has generally not been associated with disease activation in immunocompetent patients [325]. Recent reports suggest that discontinuation of lamivudine in patients with resistant mutations is not associated with increased frequency of hepatitis decompensation compared with those who continue to receive lamivudine [328].

Lamivudine has also been shown to suppress HBV DNA in other patient populations, including those with precore mutations, liver transplant recipients, and those with decompensated liver disease [329]. A recent study of 651 patients has confirmed the effectiveness of lamivudine in patients with advanced fibrosis and cirrhosis [330]. The patients were randomized in a

2:1 ratio to receive either lamivudine (100 mg daily) or placebo. The study was stopped early because of a large difference in disease progression. Over the course of 32 months, there was approximately a 50% reduction in disease progression among the treated group; more specifically, 7.8% of lamivudine-treated patients had clinically significant deterioration versus 17.7% of placebo-treated patients. In this study, disease progression was defined by hepatic decompensation, HCC, spontaneous bacterial peritonitis, bleeding varices, or death related to liver disease.

Lamivudine Use in Children

A large multicenter trial of lamivudine in children was reported in 2002 [331]. The treatment group consisted of 191 children aged 2–17 years at a dosage of 3 mg/kg to a maximum of 100 mg daily; 97 children were randomized to the placebo group. Twenty-three percent of the children in the treatment group cleared HBV DNA and HBeAg compared with 13% in the placebo group. Among children with the higher ALT values and more histologic activity, the response to lamivudine was improved; among children with ALT values greater than five times the upper limit of normal, HBeAg loss occurred in 50% versus 24% in the placebo group. No serious adverse effects were identified; however, 19% of children developed lamivudine-resistant YMDD mutants. Smaller studies of lamivudine treatment in children have confirmed its efficacy in reducing serum HBV DNA and the high mutation rate [332,333]. As in adults, the optimal treatment duration is unclear. Several authors have recommended continuing therapy for at least 6 months after HBeAg seroconversion or until virologic breakthrough occurs [210,328].

Even when virologic breakthrough occurs, other factors besides viral mutants need to be considered. It has been estimated that 30% of breakthrough infection can be attributed to noncompliance, and resumption of lamivudine as directed will result in viral suppression [111].

Lamivudine Adverse Effects and Monitoring

Lamivudine is well-tolerated. However, adverse effects have been reported, though in similar frequency as those in placebo-treated patients. In clinical practice, adverse effects are negligible and the most common issue is the emergence of resistance with increased ALT levels after previous normalization. To monitor for virologic breakthrough and efficacy, it is recommended that HBV DNA levels be followed approximately every 3 months along with serum aminotransferase levels. Additional monitoring may be needed depending on the severity of underlying liver disease and other comorbidities.

Adefovir Dipivoxil

Adefovir dipivoxil is an oral prodrug of adefovir, which is a nucleotide analogue of adenosine monophosphate. The active intracellular metabolite, adefovir disphosphate, inhibits HBV DNA polymerase at levels much lower than those needed to inhibit human DNA polymerases. After preliminary phase 2 studies demonstrated that adefovir was capable of reducing serum HBV DNA by 4 log copies after 12 weeks [334] as well as

Table 17.24: Results of Adefovir Therapy in Adults

	*Adefovir**		
Patient Characteristic	*30 mg, %*	*10 mg, %*	*Placebo, %*
HBeAg positivity			
Loss of HBeAg	12	14	6
Loss of HBV DNA	21	39	0
ALT normalization	48	55	16
Improved histology	53	59	25
HBeAg negativity			
Loss of HBV DNA	—	51	0
ALT normalization	—	72	29
Improved histology	—	64	33

*Percent (%) response at each dose.
From Marcellin et al. [334] and Hadziyannis et al. [335].

being efficacious in lamivudine-resistant HBV infection, large studies of adefovir dipivoxil were undertaken in adults.

In one study of 515 HBeAg-positive adults, one third of the patients were randomized to receive high-dose adefovir dipivoxil (30 mg), one third received 10 mg daily, and one third received placebo [334]. After 48 weeks, histologic improvement was demonstrated among 53%, 59%, and 25%, respectively. Reduction in serum HBV DNA occurred in 21%, 39%, and 0%, respectively. Loss of HBeAg occurred in 12%, and normalization of ALT values occurred in 48%, 55%, and 16%, respectively (Table 17.24). Adefovir was well tolerated. Eight percent of the group receiving adefovir at the 30-mg dosage had a reversible decrease in renal function as measured by serum creatinine levels. Overall, this group of patients had a median increase of serum creatinine of 0.2 mg/dL. In contrast to studies of lamivudine, there were no reports of adefovir-resistant mutants during this 48-week study.

In a study involving 185 research subjects, a 10-mg dose of adefovir dipivoxil was compared with placebo in a 2:1 randomized, double-blind study of HBeAg-negative chronic hepatitis B patients [335]. Again, adefovir dipivoxil administration resulted in improved histology (64% vs. 33%), normalization of ALT values (72% vs. 29%), and loss of HBV DNA to levels less than 400 copies/mL (51% vs. 0%). The adverse effect profile was similar to placebo, and there was no evidence of adefovir-resistant HBV mutations.

Additional studies have confirmed that adefovir dipivoxil is effective in patients with lamivudine-resistant HBV infection [336]. Furthermore, when adefovir dipivoxil monotherapy is compared with combination treatment with lamivudine, the effectiveness of monotherapy is equivalent to combination treatment in patients with YMDD-resistant mutants [337,338].

One disadvantage of adefovir dipivoxil therapy, shared by other orally acting agents, is the need for long-term therapy.

After 48 weeks of therapy, a cohort of 185 patients was assigned to continue adefovir dipivoxil or to placebo in a 2:1 ratio [339]. Only 8% percent of the placebo-treated patients had HBV DNA levels less than 1000 copies/mL at week 144 compared with 79% of patients maintained on adefovir.

ADEFOVIR RESISTANCE

A major advantage of adefovir is the lack of resistance during the first year of therapy; however, drug-resistant mutations do occur. The rtN236T mutation involves an asparagine-to-threonine point mutation downstream of the YMDD motif and confers resistance to adefovir dipivoxil therapy. This has been reported in 2 of 79 patients (2.5%) during the second year of treatment [340]. This mutant remains susceptible to lamivudine and entecavir. Another mutation, rtA181V, also has been described. In a recent long-term study of adefovir dipivoxil, 5.9% of patients developed one of these two resistant mutations after 144 weeks [339].

ADEFOVIR DIPIVOXIL IN CHILDREN

At the time of this writing, a large multicenter trial is ongoing to determine the efficacy and safety of adefovir in children.

ADVERSE EFFECTS OF ADEFOVIR DIPIVOXIL

The main safety concern with adefovir dipivoxil has been nephrotoxicity. Even though the initial trials did not indicate nephrotoxicity with the 10-mg dosage, it has been reported in 2.5% of adult patients with compensated liver disease who received 2 years of treatment, in 12% of transplant recipients, and in 28% of patients with decompensated cirrhosis [328]. Therefore, in patients with renal insufficiency or changes in renal function on therapy, reduction in the 10 mg daily dose is recommended by increasing the dosing interval.

DURATION OF THERAPY

As with lamivudine, the duration of therapy is unclear but likely indefinite in individuals who do not have HBeAg seroconversion. In patients with HBeAg seroconversion, an additional 3–6 months of therapy have been recommended after seroconversion takes place [328]. Anti-HBe positivity should be confirmed on two occasions at least 2 months apart before stopping adefovir.

Novel Hepatitis B Treatments

Numerous treatments for chronic hepatitis B are being investigated. At this time, these treatments have not been studied in children and have only limited data in adults infected with HBV.

Tenofovir

Like adefovir dipivoxil, tenofovir is a nucleotide analogue that inhibits the HBV polymerase.

Several small studies with adult HBV infection have demonstrated that tenofovir improves virologic, serologic, and biochemical parameters in patients with HBV [341–343].

Several studies have involved individuals with HIV and HBV coinfection. A recent study by Van Bommel et al. [342] examined tenofovir and adefovir in patients with lamivudine-resistant infections. By week 48, tenofovir was associated with reduction of HBV DNA levels to less than 10^5 copies/mL in 100% (n = 35), whereas only 44% of the adefovir-treated patients responded in this fashion. In this study, there was no evidence of resistance [342]. Furthermore, tenofovir is unlikely to exert nephrotoxicity [341].

Entecavir

Entecavir has been approved recently by the FDA for chronic HBV infections in adults. Entecavir is a cyclopentyl guanine analogue that is specific for HBV. Unlike many other nucleotide/nucleoside analogues, it has no activity against HIV. Entecavir inhibits several steps in the HBV replication cycle, including the RNA-dependent synthesis of the DNA strand and the DNA-dependent synthesis of the positive-DNA strand. It may affect the priming of the viral polymerase as well by competitively inhibiting the binding of guanosine. Based on several large studies involving more than 1800 patients, entecavir has been shown to have 48-week treatment efficacy exceeding lamivudine in terms of histologic improvement (72% vs. 62%), reduction in HBV DNA levels (67% vs. 36%), seroconversion of HBeAg (21% vs. 18%), and normalization of ALT values (68% vs. 60%) [344,345]. Furthermore, resistance to entecavir was not noted in treatment naïve patients and only occurred in 1% of patients who had preexisting mutations to lamivudine [344].

In one recent phase 2 dosing study of entecavir involving 182 patients who had lamivudine resistance, a dose of 1 mg resulted in undetectable HBV DNA in 79% whereas the 0.5-mg dose resulted in 52% without detectable HBV DNA [346]. Normalization of ALT values similarly was more frequent in those on the 1-mg dose, 68% versus 59%.

Telbivudine

Telbivudine (L-deoxythymidine, or LdT) is an orally bioavailable L-nucleoside (thymidine analogue) that potently inhibits HBV polymerase. Recent data indicated that LdT compared favorably with lamivudine in HBeAg-positive patients (n = 104). At week 52, LdT outperformed lamivudine in HBV DNA clearance 61% versus 32%, normalization of ALT levels 86% versus 63%, and HBeAg seroconversion 31% versus 22% [347]. Virologic breakthrough occurred in 4.5% of LdT patients and 15.8% of lamivudine patients. Furthermore, combination treatment was not more effective than telbivudine monotherapy.

ADDITIONAL NUCLEOTIDE/NUCLEOSIDE ANALOGUES

Small studies have examined the efficacy of famciclovir, remofovir, clevudine, and emtricitabine (FTC) for adults with chronic hepatitis B; in addition, several larger well-controlled studies are under way.

Peginterferon

Although nucleoside/nucleotide analogues have much more favorable safety profiles than IFN, the development of resistance and requirement for indefinite therapy in the majority of patients indicate a need for better treatments. By improving pharmacologic characteristics of IFN, investigators have sought to improve the efficacy, dosing regimen, and safety with the use of peginterferon.

Peginterferon alfa-2a (Pegasys; Hoffmann-La Roche, Nutley, NJ), created by attaching a large branched 40-kDa polyethylene glycol molecule to IFN-α-2a has been studied for HBeAg-negative chronic hepatitis B [348]. In one study, 537 patients were divided into three groups: a peginterferon group, a lamivudine group, and a combination group. After 48 weeks of treatment and an additional 24 weeks of follow-up, loss of HBV DNA below 20,000 copies/mL, normalization of ALT, and loss of HBsAg all occurred more frequently in patients receiving peginterferon. With regard to HBV DNA loss at week 72, this occurred in 43% in the peginterferon group, 44% in the combination treatment group, and 29% in the lamivudine monotherapy group. Sustained loss of HBV DNA to levels below 400 copies/mL occurred in 19%, 20%, and 7%, respectively. Similarly, normalization in ALT levels at week 72 occurred in 59%, 60%, and 44% of patients, respectively. In the peginterferon treatment groups, 12 patients had loss of HBsAg compared with 0 in the lamivudine monotherapy group.

A second study involving 307 HBeAg-positive patients compared peginterferon alfa-2b (Peg-intron, Scherlag-Plough Corporation, Kenilworth, NJ) and lamivudine with peginterferon alfa-2b monotherapy [129]. In this study, combination treatment showed better results after 52 weeks of therapy. However, when measured at 78 weeks, 26 weeks after completing therapy, the results were equivalent. With regard to HBV DNA loss at 78 weeks, this occurred in 35% of the patients in the combination treatment group and 36% in the peginterferon alfa-2b monotherapy group. An HBV DNA response to less than 200,000 copies/mL occurred in 32% and 27%, respectively. HBV DNA levels less than 400 copies/mL occurred in 9% and 7%, respectively, and HBsAg loss occurred in 7% of patients in both groups.

A recent large study of peginterferon involved 814 HBeAg-positive patients [349]. Patients were treated with peginterferon alfa-2a, lamivudine, or combination therapy for 48 weeks and followed for an additional 24 weeks. HBeAg seroconversion occurred in 32% of patients on peginterferon alfa-2a monotherapy, 27% on combination therapy, and 19% on lamivudine monotherapy. A similar response was evident regarding HBV DNA levels, with 32%, 34%, and 22%, respectively, achieving levels less than 100,000 copies/mL. Furthermore, only patients who received peginterferon had loss of HBsAg; this occurred in 16 patients among both groups that received peginterferon. Although more serious adverse events occurred in the peginterferon groups – up to 6% – the only two patients who had liver failure during the course of the study had received lamivudine monotherapy. Both had irreversible liver failure after cessation of treatment, but one recovered following liver transplantation [349].

These studies show that peginterferon may be the most effective of the available agents when used for a 1-year treatment period. More studies of peginterferon in adults and children are needed to further define its role in the treatment of chronic hepatitis B. As with conventional IFN, peginterferon has numerous side effects.

Therapy for Transplant Patients

Liver transplantation in patients with HBV infection is associated with a high rate of recurrence, resulting in severe graft disease [350]. The risk of recurrence is directly proportional to the level of viral replication before transplantation. The pathogenesis of HBV-induced injury in the liver graft is unclear [351]. Initial strategies used to prevent recurrent infection with HBV following liver transplantation, including the administration of HBV vaccine, IFN, and ganciclovir, have proved to be ineffective in patients who are HBV DNA–positive before transplantation [352–356]. In immunocompromised hosts, the massive expression of HBsAg and HBcAg that occurs following liver transplantation presumably transforms the hepatic injury process from an immune-based disorder to one in which the virus exerts a direct cytolytic effect on the hepatocytes with resultant rapid allograft failure [357]. Long-term passive immunoprophylaxis with high-titer immune globulin (HBIG) has reduced the risk of HBV graft infection in those who were HBsAg positive but HBV DNA negative prior to transplantation.

The most effective treatments for immunocompromised hosts are the nucleotide/nucleoside analogues. This observation extends to individuals undergoing chemotherapy for cancer who are at risk for HBV recurrence [328]. Lamivudine has shown promising results in the treatment of hepatitis B post liver transplantation [358]. Of patients treated with lamivudine (100 mg/d for 52 weeks), 60% had undetectable HBV DNA, 31% lost HBeAg, 6% lost HBsAg, 71% had normal ALT, and 50% had an improved histologic activity index. The emergence of YMDD mutants of HBV was detected in 27% of treated patients.

Lamivudine therapy can also reduce the rate of recurrent HBV infection when treatment is started before liver transplantation [356,359]. There is evidence that the response to lamivudine is proportional to the decrease in levels of HBV DNA [360]. A trial evaluated the use of a combination of pre- and posttransplantation lamivudine with intramuscular HBIG (intravenous HBIG has been reserved for HBV DNA–positive patients at transplantation); at a mean 15.6-month follow-up, nine of ten patients maintained protective anti-HBs titers and had no HBV recurrence [361]. This approach seems to hold true for precore mutant HBV infection, with no recurrence in the graft at a mean follow-up of 16 months following a combination of low-dose IFN and lamivudine [362]. Larger numbers of patients need to be studied to confirm these results.

At the time of this writing, the AASLD guidelines recommend the use of lamivudine or adefovir dipivoxil in patients who have recurrent hepatitis B after transplantation [328]. Theoretically, in this vulnerable patient group, adefovir dipivoxil is attractive because of its low resistance rate, as long as the patient's renal function is uncompromised; however,

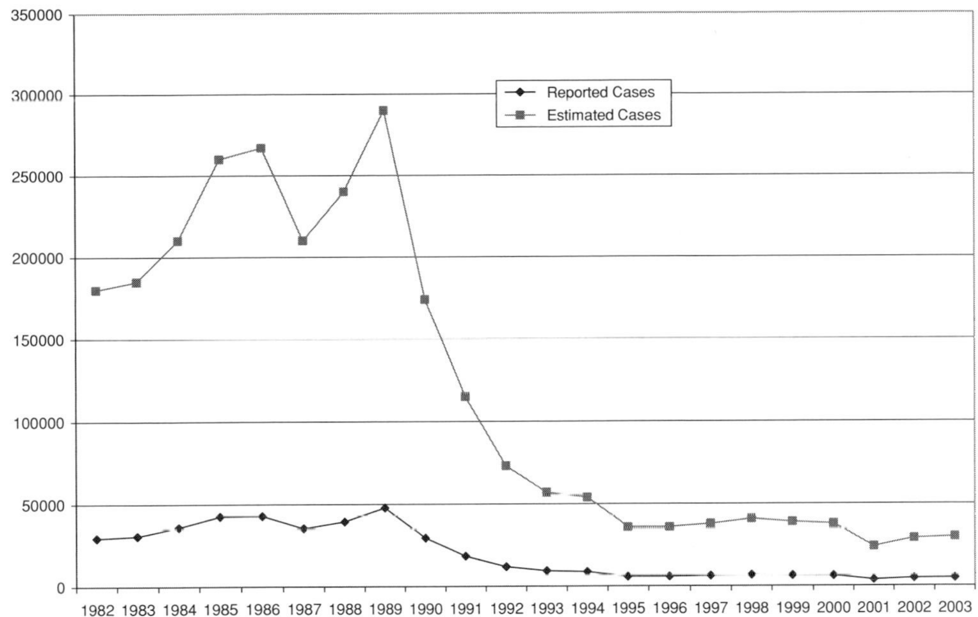

Figure 17.17. The number of reported HCV cases indicates the cases reported to the national notifiable disease surveillance system of the CDC. (From Centers for Disease Control and Prevention [2].)

only limited data are available for adefovir in transplant patient populations [336]. When HBV-infected individuals who have undergone organ transplantation need to be switched from lamivudine to adefovir dipivoxil, it has been recommended to allow a 2- to 3-month overlap period to minimize the risk of graft dysfunction [328].

Treatment of Hepatitis B in the Future

Tailoring therapy for HBV-infected patients based on virologic, histologic, and host factors is the long-term goal. This will require a better understanding of the natural history of the disease and of host and viral responses to emerging therapies. Currently, many patients do not receive treatment because they fall outside the current guidelines for therapy. The availability of drugs with improved potency and tolerability should allow a broader range of patients to benefit from treatment, even those with less extensive liver disease. Although the results to date have not been promising, combination therapies may evolve as an important approach. Novel treatments such as therapeutic vaccines along with nucleoside/nucleotide analogues with or without IFN therapy may help increase the sustained response to HBV. Until that time, assuring that the newest treatments are studied and available for pediatric as well as adult patients is imperative to minimize the burden of HBV disease.

HEPATITIS C

Introduction

Hepatitis C has emerged as the most important cause of viral hepatitis in the United States. It is responsible for more than 10,000 deaths each year [363]. Despite a decline of more than 80% in the incidence of acute hepatitis C (Figure 17.17), the morbidity and mortality of HCV is increasing because of the reservoir of chronically infected individuals [364–366]. Currently, more than 2.7 million individuals have detectable HCV RNA in their blood and about 3.9 million people in the United States have been infected [367]. This is four times the number of individuals infected with HIV. Although these numbers indicate that 1.8% of the U.S. population has detectable anti-HCV, the actual number of infected persons is undoubtedly underestimated as many high-risk populations, such as prisoners, homeless persons, and institutionalized persons, were not included in these prevalence studies. Because of its ability to establish chronic progressive infection, HCV is now the leading indication for liver transplantation. In children, the U.S. prevalence of anti-HCV is lower: 0.2% among 6- to 11-year-olds and 0.4% in 12- to 19-year-olds [367].

Worldwide, HCV is highly prevalent, with an estimated 170 million infected persons, or 3% of the world's population [368,369]. Most populations in Africa, Europe, and Southeast Asia have anti-HCV rates under 2.5%. In western Pacific regions, rates average between 2.5% and 4.9%. The country with the highest prevalence is Egypt, where antibody against HCV is present in 15–20% of the population. The effort to eliminate schistosomal infection with parenteral therapy is a unique risk factor in this country and likely represents the largest iatrogenic transmission of a blood-borne pathogen [370]. As in the United States, worldwide HCV morbidity and mortality are likely to increase over the next two decades.

Historical Context

Phylogenetic analyses indicate that HCV reached the United States around 1910 at the conclusion of the Spanish-American war [371]. However, the discovery of HCV had to wait for the development of molecular cloning techniques in 1989 that indicated that so-called non-A, non-B (NANB) hepatitis was primarily caused by HCV infection [369,372]. This major scientific breakthrough, which led directly to a reduction in the number of acute HCV infections, was achieved after extracting viral nucleic acid from the plasma of an infected chimpanzee. All the extracted genetic material (RNA and DNA) was reverse transcribed to construct a complementary DNA library [372]. Then, the resultant cDNA was inserted into a cloning vector and expressed in *Escherichia coli.* The expressed proteins were screened using an immunoblot assay against serum from a patient with chronic NANB hepatitis, which presumably contained antibodies to the viral proteins. After approximately 1 million clones had been screened, an antigenic protein encoded by HCV was isolated. This allowed expression of the corresponding HCV cDNA in yeast and the development of an immunologic assay to detect the antibody. This innovation was quickly adapted for blood donor screening [373].

Viral Characteristics

Description

The HCV is a small virus, 30–60 nm in diameter, that contains a single-stranded RNA genome that is translated into a single polypeptide, which is cleaved by viral and host enzymes. For taxonomic purposes, it is assigned to the Flaviridae family. Humans are the only known host of HCV, but the virus can be transmitted experimentally to chimpanzees. The virus biology is characterized by the heterogeneity of its genome, resulting from frequent mutations.

Some people infected with HCV experience multiple distinct episodes of acute hepatitis; recurrent episodes of hepatitis have also been observed in chimpanzees. These episodes may represent reinfection or reactivation. During rechallenge experiments carried out in chimpanzees using different HCV strains of proven infectivity, each rechallenge resulted in reappearance of viremia because of infection with the challenge virus [374]. These data indicate that HCV infection does not elicit protective immunity against reinfection with homologous or heterologous strains, raising further concern regarding the development of effective vaccines against HCV [374].

Mechanism of HCV Replication

Hepatitis C virus replicates in infected cells, mainly hepatocytes. Its replication is catalyzed by the viral RdRp, a 68-kDa protein encoded by the NS5B region of the genome located at the 5′ end [375]. The RdRp protein localizes near the perinuclear membranes and then associates with other nonstructural viral proteins and cellular factors to form the replication complex. During replication, RdRp interacts with the 3′ end of the viral RNA. A polymerization reaction proceeds and leads to the synthesis of complementary RNA strands. Positive-strand RNAs are subsequently encapsidated into new virons or used as messenger RNAs, and negative-strand RNAs are used as templates for ongoing replication.

Because of the low fidelity of RNA polymerase, mutations are frequent. On average, one mutation occurs per RNA molecule [375]. Mutations incorporated into negative RNA strands have greater impact because they can be quickly transmitted to a large number of progeny virons containing positive-stranded RNAs.

In the absence of selective pressures, HCV should accumulate nucleotide mutations at random because of the lack of proofreading capabilities of its RNA polymerase. In vivo, however, many regions are hypervariable and others are highly conserved. The regions, like E2, with increased variability, are highly tolerant to changes; in this example, the resultant envelope glycoprotein changes may facilitate the HCV epitopes to avoid host-neutralizing antibody responses, whereas the highly conserved regions do not tolerate amino acid changes in the proteins generated from the translated portions. To conserve the function of proteins like NS5A, NS3 protease, NS3 helicase, and RdRp, mutations in this region have a selective disadvantage [375].

HCV Genotypes

Six distinct genotypes (1–6) of HCV along with about 100 subtypes (designated a, b, c, etc.) have been described. Each genotype differs in its amino acid sequence by 31–34%. Genotypes 1–3 have a worldwide distribution, genotypes 4 and 5 are found prinicipally in Africa, and genotype 6 is primarily in Asia [368]. In the United States, genotype 1 accounts for around 74% (57% 1a, 17% 1b) of HCV infections; genotype 2 for about 15%, genotype 3 for about 7%, genotype 4 for about 1%, and genotype 6 for 3%. Genotypes 1 and 4 are relatively resistant to treatment [367].

In contrast to genotypes, which vary by around 30%, quasi-species may vary by 1–9% of their nucleotide sequence over the entire length of the genome. Mutations in the viral populations likely contribute to drug "resistance" during IFN treatment and to the ineffectiveness of isolate-specific vaccines. However, at the present time, although quasi-species assessment provides important insights into the pathogenesis of disease, this remains a research tool and has no role in the routine clinical management of HCV-infected patients.

Epidemiology

It is estimated that HCV affects 3% of the worldwide population and 1.8% of the U.S. population (Figure 17.18). In the absence of alcohol intake and obesity, HCV is the most common cause of elevated ALT levels in adult American blood donors [376]. Among U.S. children, 240,000 have been infected with HCV, with 68,000–100,000 chronically infected [377].

As noted above, HCV prevalence varies considerably in subpopulations with varied risk factors. Mexican-Americans and non-Hispanic blacks have increased rates of HCV

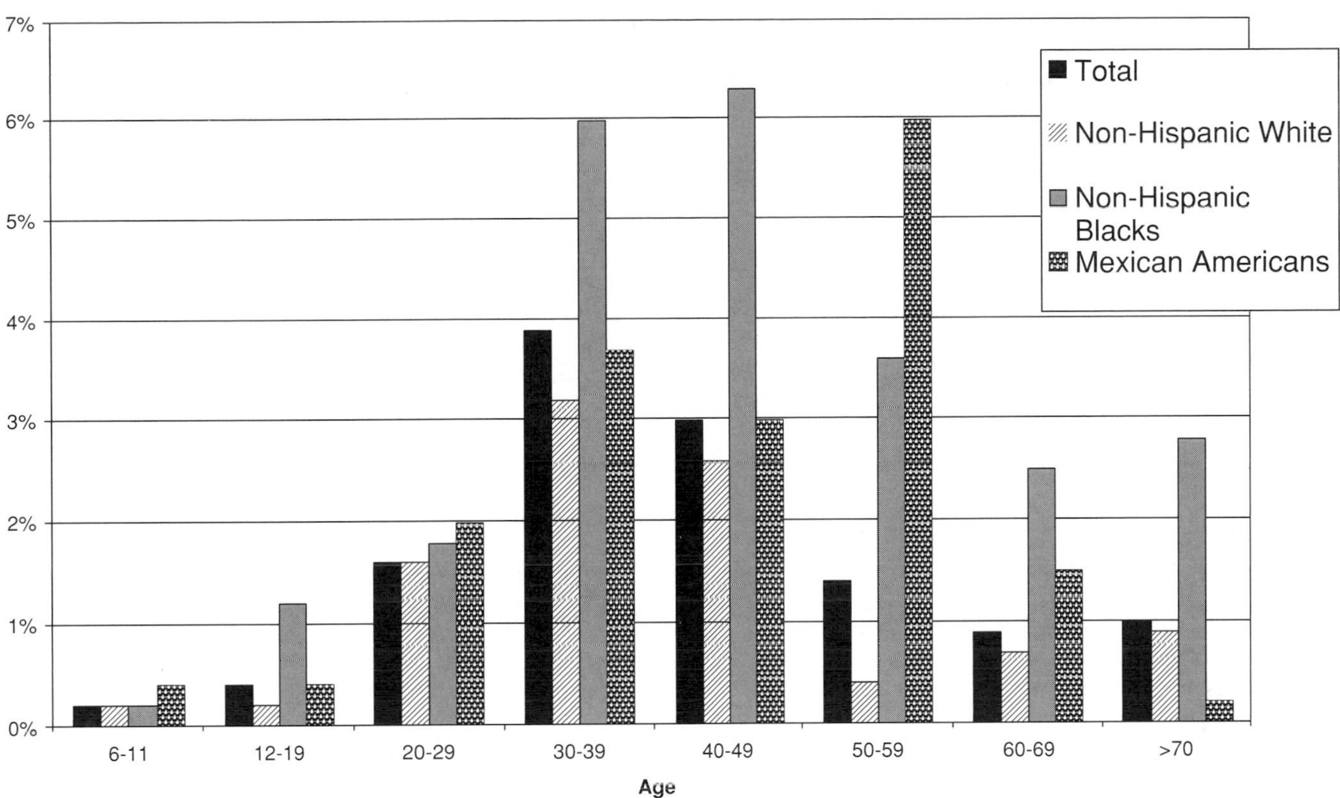

Figure 17.18. Age- and race/ethnic-related prevalence data for HCV antibody. The data are derived from the third National Health and Nutrition Examination Survey (NHANES III), 1988–1994. (From Alter et al. [367].)

seropositivity; the odds ratios for these two populations compared with the general population are 1.6 and 1.4, respectively (Figure 17.18, Table 17.25) [367].

Although HCV is considered a transfusion-related disease, no cases of transfusion-transmitted acute HCV infection have been detected by the CDC's sentinel counties viral hepatitis surveillance system since 1994 [369]. Even when the incidence of infections was much higher, blood transfusions accounted for no greater than about 10% of all infections. Currently, the risk of HCV following a single-unit blood transfusion in the United States is less than 1 in 1 million [378].

The most important risk factor for HCV is injection drug use (Figure 17.19). In fact, up to 90% of illegal intravenous drug users are HCV infected [379]. For reasons that are unclear, there has been a major decline in the incidence of HCV among injection drug users, which has corresponded to the overall decrease in HCV cases. Injection drug use is a risk factor for both HIV and HBV infections; as a result, coinfection with these viruses is common. Some have postulated that the efforts to curtail HIV infection have been responsible for a "halo effect" on the incidence of HCV [380]. Educational programs promoting needle exchange and reducing shared needles have decreased HCV transmission.

Besides injection drug use, other cases of HCV are associated with intranasal cocaine use, high-risk sexual practices, or occupational exposure or are sporadic, community-acquired cases possibly due to nonpercutaneous or covert percutaneous transmission [381]. In the health care setting, HCV infection has been associated with needle-stick injuries, hemodialysis, and organ transplantation [382]. The risk of acquisition of HCV by health care workers following a single needle-stick exposure to blood from an anti-HCV–positive and HCV RNA–positive patient is approximately 2% [363,369]; one study reported that transmission occurred only from hollow-bore needles compared with other sharps [383]. Overall, HCV prevalence is lower among health care workers than the general population. Nevertheless, nosocomial transmission of HCV is possible but has rarely been reported in the United States, other than in chronic hemodialysis settings [369]. One notable exception was an outbreak of HCV following IVIG infusion (Gammagard; Baxter Healthcare Corportation, Glendale, CA) between April 1, 1993, and February 23, 1994 [378]. Currently, all immune globulin products undergo inactivation and are tested for HCV RNA before release.

Transmission of HCV by sexual or close physical contact is possible but uncommon because the virus is inefficiently spread via this manner [369]. Bodily secretions (saliva, seminal fluid, and vaginal secretions) of patients with chronic HCV are rarely contaminated with HCV [369]. Although chimpanzees have been experimentally infected by the injection of saliva from HCV-infected persons [384], casual household contact and contact with saliva of infected persons are very inefficient modes of transmission. Case-control studies have reported an association between exposure to a sex contact with a history

Table 17.25: Prevalence of Antibody to HCV in Relationship to Demographic Characteristics and Potential Risk Factors, 1988–1998

Characteristic	*Prevalence of Anti-HCV, %*	*Adjusted Odds Ratio*
Race/ethnic group		
Non-Hispanic white	1.5	1.0
Non-Hispanic black	3.2	1.6
Mexican American	2.1	1.4
Sex		
Male	2.5	1.2
Female	1.2	1.0
Marital status		
Divorced or separated	5.1	1.7
Married, widowed, or never married	1.8	1.0
Poverty index		
Below poverty level	3.2	2.4
At or above poverty level	1.6	1.0
Education		
≤12 yr	2.8	1.9
>12 yr	1.3	1.0
Area of residence		
City with population ≥1 million	2.2	
City with population <1 million	1.6	
Military service status		
Current or previous	1.7	
No prior military service	2.2	
Born in the U.S.	1.9	
Born outside the U.S.	1.8	
Health-related occupation		
Never	2.0	
Current or previous	1.4	
Lifetime cocaine use		
Never	1.1	1.0
1–10 times	9.3	4.7*
>10 times	17.8	4.7*
Lifetime marijuana use		
Never	0.8	
1–99 times	1.9	
>100 times	9.3	
Age at first sexual intercourse		
≥18 years	0.7	1.0
<18 years	3.2	2.9
No. of lifetime sexual partners		
0–1	0.6	1.0
2–9	1.6	2.54†
10–49	3.3	2.54†
≥50	9.4	5.2
Previous sexually transmitted disease	6	
Injection drug users	79	
Persons with abnormal ALT values	15	
Blood products		
Chronic hemodialysis patients	10	
Hemophiliacs treated with blood products before 1987	87	
Recipients of blood transfusion before 1990	6	
Volunteer blood donors	0.16	
Men who have sex with men	4	
Infants born to infected mothers		
HCV monoinfection	6	
HCV/HIV coinfection	17	

*The adjusted odds ratio for this risk factor is a composite score for any cocaine use compared with the risk never using cocaine.
†The adjusted odds ratio for this risk factor is a composite score for the number of lifetime sexual partners for 2–49 compared with the risk of ≥50 partners and 0–1 partners.
From Alter et al. [367] and the Centers for Disease Control and Prevention [369].

of hepatitis or to multiple sex partners and acquiring hepatitis C; 15–20% of patients with acute hepatitis C have a history of sexual exposure in the absence of other risk factors [369]. In contrast, a low prevalence of HCV infection has been reported by studies of long-term spouses of patients with chronic HCV infection who had no other risk factors for infection. Similar to other blood-borne viruses, sexual transmission of HCV from males to females might be more efficient than from females to males [369].

A definite but low rate of intrafamilial spread has been postulated based on a five- to tenfold higher percentage of anti-HCV positivity in cohabitants than in the general population. The low rate of transmission of HCV in these various settings is presumably related to the low infectivity titer of HCV carriers; however, other undefined factors may be operant.

Many other risk factors have been examined. In the United States, there is no reported association with military service, medical/dental procedures, tattooing, acupuncture, ear piercing, or foreign travel [369]. If transmission occurs in these settings, the frequency may be too low to detect.

Perinatal Transmission

At present, maternal–neonatal transmission of HCV is the most common route of *childhood* infection [385]. Worldwide, one estimate has calculated that 60,000 HCV-infected infants are born yearly [386]. Before the availability of anti-HCV assays, transient or persistent aminotransferase elevations had been

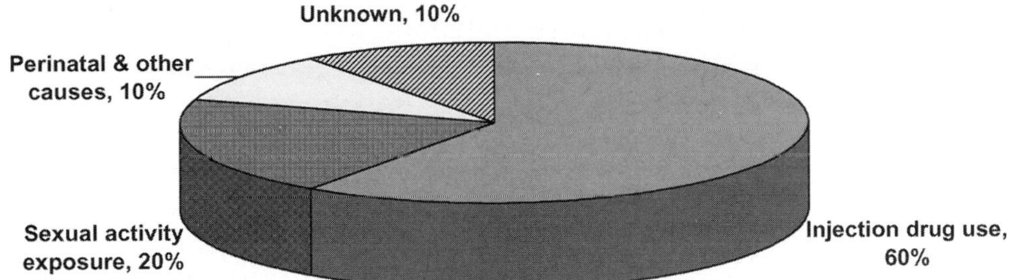

Figure 17.19. This pie chart indicates the current risk factors for HCV transmission. Injection drug use is the most important factor, followed by exposure through sexual activity. In addition to perinatal transmission, other causes include hemodialysis, occupational exposure, and household exposure to contaminated blood. In approximately 10% of cases, the transmission risk factor is unknown. (From the Centers for Disease Control and Prevention [2].)

noted in infants born to women with NANB hepatitis [387]. With the advent of anti-HCV testing, variable rates of maternal-to-infant transmission were reported; however, documentation of infection in early life is difficult because anti-HCV may be passively transferred from mother to child [369,378,388]. Overall, perinatal transmission of HCV is an uncommon event. Of infants born to anti-HCV–positive women, 5–6% (range, 0–25%) acquire HCV. Of infants born to women coinfected with HCV and HIV, the rate of perinatal infection is higher (17%; range, 5–36%). The difference has been speculated to be related to higher titers of HCV RNA in coinfected women [369]; however, recent studies challenge this assumption [389,390]. Conte et al. [389] reported a perinatal transmission rate of 5.1% in a large prospective study (370 pregnancies) performed in Italy [389]. Only mothers with detectable HCV antibody transmitted infection, but the risk of transmission was not related to viral RNA titers. Also in contrast to previous studies, in their cohort, none of the mothers with HIV coinfection (4% of the cohort) transmitted HCV. All these HIV-infected mothers were treated with antiretroviral therapy during their pregnancies. Another recent study of 403 HCV-positive, HIV-negative women reported a 5% transmission rate and no relationship between viral RNA titer and HCV transmission [390].

Most studies have shown no differences in infection rates between infants delivered vaginally and cesarean-delivered infants [369]. However, one study from the United Kingdom involving 441 mother–infant pairs concluded that delivery via elective cesarean section before membrane rupture was associated with a lower risk of transmitting HCV than vaginal delivery or emergency cesarean section [391]. Even if this finding is confirmed, because of the fairly low transmission rate, it would be unclear whether all women should undergo cesarean section. In individuals with coinfection with HIV, cesarean section may be necessary to lower the risk of HIV acquisition. Also, to reduce the risk of HCV infection, the National Institutes of Health has advised caution to avoid the use of fetal scalp monitoring and prolonged rupture of membranes [363].

The variability in reported perinatal transmission rates may be partly ascribed to the noncomparability of the studied populations, which included patients with asymptomatic HCV infection with or without concomitant HIV infection. In addition, the first-generation assays used for anti-HCV detection lacked sensitivity and specificity and therefore underestimated the rate of maternal–infant transmission. Subsequent studies have used the ultrasensitive PCR assay to directly determine the extent and existence of perinatal transmission [392,393]. For example, serum samples were obtained from eight pregnant women who were HIV positive [392]; although none had symptoms of HCV infection, HCV viral sequences were found in five of the mothers and four of the eight children; three of the infants were HCV positive at birth. Viremia was persistent in one infant, coincident with chronic elevation of aminotransferases and persistent anti-HCV positivity. The remaining three infants had intermittent viremia; all were asymptomatic and anti-HCV negative at follow-up. Because viremia was detected at birth in three infants, infection with HCV was presumed to occur in utero or during delivery [392].

The role of breast-feeding in the transmission of HCV has been evaluated in several studies [369,378]. Breast-feeding is not considered to be contraindicated in women who are infected with HCV [363,378]. The AAP recommends that HCV-infected women who wish to breast-feed their infants be counseled that although there appears to be no increased risk of transmission, the data are limited [378].

Neither national nor international adoptees are at increased risk of HCV infection; thus, routine screening is not indicated [378]. The decision to test should be individualized if the child is born to a woman at known risk for HCV infection (e.g., an injection drug user).

Clincial Aspects and Pathogenesis

The majority of people with acute hepatitis C typically are asymptomatic [369]; 20–30% may have jaundice and nonspecific symptoms such as anorexia, malaise, or abdominal pain (Table 17.26). In these patients with clinical features, the illness is similar to other types of viral hepatitis and serologic testing is necessary to determine the etiology. In symptomatic patients, the clinical illness may last for 2–3 weeks. If normalization

Table 17.26: Clinical Features of Hepatitis C Infection

Clinical Feature	*Characteristics*
Signs and symptoms*	Jaundice Fatigue Anorexia Nausea Fever Diarrhea Abdominal pain Pruritic rash
Extrahepatic manifestations	Serum sickness–like disease Essential mixed cryoglobulinemia Keratoconjuncitivits sicca Glomerulonephritis Lichen planus Porphyria cutanea tarda Arthritic presentations Depression
Changing incidence	Number of new infections per year has declined from an average of 230,000 in the 1980s to about 30,000 in 2003 in the U.S. Highest rate of disease occurs in 30- to 49-year-olds
Incubation period	Average ~40–50 days Range 2–26 weeks
Transmission	Vertical (mother to child) Percutaneous exposure to infected fluids Sharing of drugs and needles Unprotected sex (especially if multiple partners) Rarely, occupational exposure
Persons at risk of infection	Injection drug users Sexual contacts of infected persons Infants born to infected mothers Recipients of blood products before 1992 Hemodialysis patients†
Long-term sequelae without vaccination	Chronic infection occurs in 6% of exposed infants 60–80% of persons with acute hepatitis C Death from chronic liver disease occurs in 15–25% of chronically infected persons
Fulminant hepatitis	<1% of adults; not reported in children

*Most persons infected with hepatitits C have minimal clinical signs at presentation.
†After 1992, hemodialysis remains a risk factor because of inadequate infection control practices.

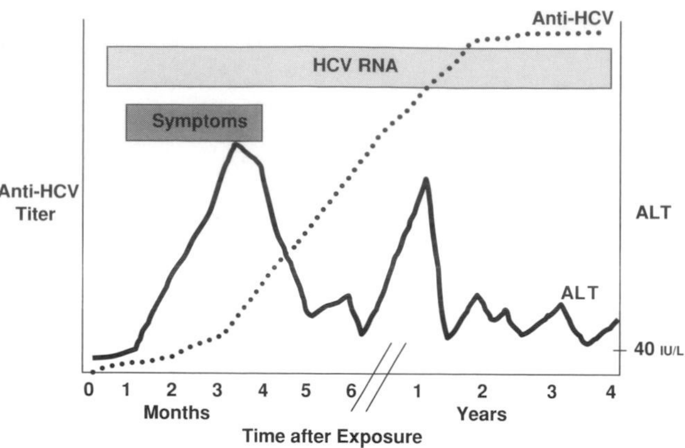

Figure 17.20. Typical sequence of events in HCV infection. Following HCV acquisition at time 0, there is a progressive increase in the ALT level, indicating the onset of clinical hepatitis between 6 and 8 weeks. The appearance of HCV antibody can be detected by radioimmunoassay (RIA), with quantitation of a viral antibody titer. Polymerase chain reaction can indicate infection with HCV within 1–2 weeks of exposure, well before the appearance of detetable anti-HCV, which is typical for 10–12 weeks following exposure. Because anti-HCV does not confer immunity, it can be detected in the majority of patients who progress to chronic infection. In patients who clear HCV infection, ALT values typically normalize and HCV RNA levels become undetectable; over time, anti-HCV decreases when HCV infection resolves. Although not indicated on this figure, quantitative HCV RNA levels do fluctuate through the course of acute and chronic HCV infections [1].

of ALT values occurs, the clinician may think the patient has had a full recovery; however, the fluctuation of ALT values is highly characteristic of HCV infection, and subsequent increases may herald the progression to chronic disease [369]. Fulminant hepatic failure following acute hepatitis C is rare [369] and has not been reported in children [377].

The availability of diagnostic assays has allowed for precise delineation of the sequence of events occurring in a patient with HCV infection; a typical scenario is depicted in Figure 17.20. The serum ALT levels tend to fluctuate [379,378,394]. This polyphasic pattern of serum ALT levels is noted in both acute and chronic HCV. The time interval between exposure to the HCV and the initial detection of anti-HCV is variable; this latency accounts for the long seronegative period of infectivity. HCV RNA can be detected by PCR within 1–2 weeks after exposure.

Outcome in Children

Symptoms of acute viral hepatitis (if any) slowly resolve; however, follow-up studies of patients with posttransfusion HCV as well as sporadic NANB hepatitis ascribed to HCV have documented a high rate of progression to chronic liver disease and cirrhosis. Anti-HCV eventually disappears in those who recover clinically and biochemically. Anti-HCV persists in patients who develop chronic HCV infection.

The natural history of HCV in children is unclear. The outcome of posttransfusion HCV infection has been studied in pediatric patients. In 458 children who underwent cardiac surgery at a mean age of 2.8 years before 1991, when blood donor screening was introduced, 15% became anti-HCV positive versus 1% of control subjects [395]. After more than 17 years following surgery, 55% of the anti-HCV–positive cohort remained HCV positive; the infection had cleared in the other 45%. Only one HCV RNA–positive patient had increased levels of liver enzymes. Among the 17 who had liver biopsies, 2 had significant fibrosis and only 1 had cirrhosis; these 3 patients had additional risk factors for progressive liver disease.

In a study of the natural history of posttransfusion hepatitis, Lai et al. [396] carried out an 8-year prospective study of 135 children newly diagnosed with thalassemia [396]. During the follow-up period, 83 (61%) developed posttransfusion hepatitis and 74 (90%) were anti-HCV positive (ELISA-2). Of the 83 patients, resolution was documented in 17 (20%), recurrent disease in 9 (11%), and chronic hepatitis in 57 (69%). This study documented a high rate of chronicity and severe histologic lesions despite clinically asymptomatic disease.

Another study evaluating the natural history of HCV examined a cohort of children from St. Jude's Children's Research Hospital in Memphis. One child died from liver failure 9 years after the onset of HCV infection, and two others died from HCC after 25 and 27 years [397]. Among 58 survivors with HCV, 35 underwent evaluation with liver biopsy; 8.5% developed cirrhosis [397]. A follow-up investigation involving a larger cohort of St. Jude's patients had 122 of 148 survivors consent to participate [398]. Chronic infection was noted in 81%. Among the 60 who agreed to undergo a liver biopsy, at a median of 12 years following the initial diagnosis of malignancy, 29% had mild fibrosis, 36% had moderate fibrosis, and 14% had cirrhosis. One patient died with decompensated cirrhosis from variceal bleeding. The authors noted an accelerated progression of disease in their cohort thought to be related to either the immunosuppressive or the hepatotoxic effects of chemotherapy [398]. Also, the authors noted that the severity of HCV liver disease in their prospective survivor cohort may be underestimated as a separate retrospective review identified five other HCV-related deaths (three from hepatic failure and two from HCC).

The outcome of perinatal HCV infection has not been well studied; although patients are often asymptomatic despite histologic evidence of chronic hepatitis, recovery is unlikely [399,400]. However, children are more likely to have normal or near-normal ALT values [401]; they tend to have, on average, a slower rate of advancement to end-stage liver disease. Yet a small proportion of perinatally infected children develop advanced liver disease during childhood. According to the Studies of Pediatric Liver Transplantation (SPLIT) Registry, which collects data from 37 North American pediatric liver transplant centers, chronic HCV was the reason for transplantation in 9 of 941 children who underwent liver transplantation between 1995 and 2001 [377]. Besides these children with aggressive infections, the clinical impact of HCV may ultimately be quite significant because the life expectancy at the time of HCV acquisition is much longer.

Outcome in Adults

The natural history of chronic hepatitis C is quite varied in adults. The most remarkable feature of infection with HCV is the high rate of chronic infection, which often leads to chronic liver disease [363,369,401]. Approximately 20% of patients develop progressive signs of liver failure during medical surveillance. Chronic HCV infection, in isolation, is a slowly progressive, insidious disease with a relatively low risk for cirrhosis. Seeff et al. [402] conducted an extended study of the natural history of HCV infection by analyzing archived serum specimens originally collected from military recruits between 1948 and 1954. Of 8568 people, 17 (0.2%) had positive results; during the 45-year follow-up, liver disease occurred in 2 of the 17 HCV-positive people (11.8%) and in 205 of the 8551 HCV-negative people (2.4%). Of persons who were HCV-positive, only one died of liver disease 42 years after the original phlebotomy. In another evaluation of the consequences, 376 women in Ireland were assessed and biopsied 17 years after well-defined iatrogenic HCV infection through receipt of HCV-contaminated anti-D immune globulin [403]. All women who became HCV RNA positive had evidence of hepatic inflammation – 50% had some degree of fibrosis, and only 2% had cirrhosis. These studies suggest that healthy HCV-positive persons may be at a low risk for progressive liver disease. The likelihood of progression to fibrosis appears to be independent of genotype or viral load but increases with alcohol intake, male gender, age over 40 years at infection, iron overload, obesity, and coinfection with HIV or HBV [363–365,369,401,404,405]. Even intake of moderate amounts (>10 g/d) of alcohol in patients with chronic hepatitis C may enhance disease progression [363–365,369]. The issue of coinfections is discussed separately later in this chapter.

The rate of progression to cirrhosis in patients with posttransfusion HCV is estimated to be approximately 20%. The time line from acquisition to this potential consequence is clear; on average, persons developed cirrhosis 20–21 years following infection [363,405–407], whereas on average, HCC developed 28–29 years following HCV acquisition. However, the rate of progression in women and children along with individuals with normal ALT levels may take more than 80 years [363]. In patients who develop cirrhosis, the reported risk for HCC at 5 years is 7% and the risk of decompensation is 18%; the overall probability of survival at 5 years after the first major complication is only 50% [408]. Patients with advanced cirrhosis are at higher risk for decompensation during antiviral treatment and have a higher incidence of side effects [409]. Nevertheless, treatment in selected patients may result in histologic improvement and sustained virologic response (SVR) [409].

Extrahepatic Manifestations

Various nonhepatic manifestations of HCV infection have been described in adults; these include a serum sickness–like illness, autoimmune hepatitis, lymphoma, keratoconjunctivitis sicca, glomerulonephritis, lichen planus, and vasculitis with cryoglobulinemia [369,410]. Many of these HCV-related manifestations, which are rarely seen in children, are immunologically mediated (associated with circulating immune complexes) or a consequence of direct viral injury. Agnello et al. [410] detected HCV RNA in 16 of 19 patients with type II cryoglobulinemia (immune complexes of polyclonal IgG and monoclonal IgM rheumatoid factors) and anti-HCV in 8 [410]. The HCV RNA or anti-HCV was selectively concentrated in the cryoprecipitate, providing evidence of HCV in the pathogenesis of essential mixed cryoglobulinemia. In addition to the disorders listed in Table 17.25, among HCV-infected persons, psychological disorders such as depression are more common as is diabetes mellitus [411].

Occult HCV Infection

As with HBV infection, it is now recognized that occult HCV infections occur and may have important clinical significance. In the context of viral hepatitis, the term *occult* indicates that an infection is present but may remain hidden with all but the most sensitive tests. With HBV infections, it has been shown that infected occult patients may be the source of transmission for posttransfusion hepatitis [412]. Also, these occult HBV-infected patients may have reactivation when undergoing chemotherapy [413]. Recently, the same types of concerns have been voiced with HCV.

Although success with antiviral therapy, usually indicated by an SVR, is associated with histologic and biochemical improvement, it has been recognized that complete elimination of HCV RNA from the body is infrequent. Because an SVR is defined as the elimination of HCV RNA from the blood for at least 6 months after therapy (using an assay with a sensitivity of at least 100 viral copies/mL), this creates an apparent paradox. Although several studies 5–10 years ago supported the notion that only a small percentage (0–14%) of patients had hepatic HCV RNA following an SVR [414–416], recent studies have found HCV RNA in very low levels in the serum, peripheral blood mononuclear cells, and liver [417,418]. In a recent study of 16 HCV patients undergoing SVR, HCV genome was detected up to 5 years after resolution of the infection using a highly sensitive reverse-transcription PCR (RT-PCR)–nucleic acid hybridization assay and real-time PCR. In all 16 patients, investigators found HCV RNA in the sera or peripheral blood mononuclear cells [417]. Another study has confirmed these results in 17 patients who were restudied up to 9 years after treatment [418]. All but 2 had evidence of HCV RNA. In these 17 patients, serum and peripheral blood mononuclear cells were assayed every 3–6 months; in 11 patients, frozen liver tissue samples were available for an average of 64 months after therapy. HCV RNA was detected in the liver of 3 of 11 patients, in the serum of 4 of 11, and in the macrophages of 11.

Also, the role of occult HCV has been investigated as a possible factor in individuals with unexplained persistent elevations in their serum ALT levels [419]. In one study that examined 100 patients with negative serum HCV RNA and negative anti-HCV, the presence of HCV was identified in the liver in 57 patients and in the peripheral blood monocytes in 40 subjects. In those with occult HCV, steatosis, necroinflammatory histology, and fibrosis were more common.

These studies have several implications. First, HCV RNA is present in very low titers in the majority of "successfully treated" patients when highly sensitive assays are used. To detect HCV RNA, multiple assays may be needed and analyzing both hepatic and extrahepatic sites may be necessary. Second, the presence of HCV RNA, even in very low titers, may contribute to the spread of HCV as well as increase the risk of complications such as HCC. Third, HCV may be responsible for many cases of "idiopathic" elevated liver enzymes. Finally, SVR should not be equated with a cure, although it does indicate a significant reduction in the likelihood of progressive liver injury and associated morbidity.

Histology

The histology of *acute* HCV infection is not well defined because biopsies are not commonly obtained. The histology of *chronic* HCV infection has been more clearly illustrated. HCV has characteristic histologic lesions, which are similar in children and adults (Figure 17.21). Typical findings include portal lymphoid aggregates or follicles, sinusoidal lymphocytes, and steatosis [420–423]. In some cases, histology is needed to differentiate HCV from competing etiologies of elevated ALT levels, such as steatohepatitis or autoimmune hepatitis [384,424].

Several studies have assessed the histology of chronic HCV infection in children [421–423,425]; the results are highly variable, which may be related to the mode and age of acquisition of HCV infection. In addition, cofactors that increase or decrease the risk of fibrosis must also be considered. Garcia-Monzon et al. [425] compared the histologic features of chronic posttransfusion HCV in neonates versus adults; at the 11-year follow-up, children uniformly had milder histologic and immunohistochemical forms of chronic hepatitis than did adults. Kage et al. [421] found only grade 1–2 fibrosis in 97% of 109 anti-HCV–positive pediatric patients screened; none of the patients had cirrhosis, but the majority had chronic hepatitis [421]. Guido et al. [422] studied 80 children with biochemical evidence of hepatitis and no underlying chronic disease for a mean duration of 42 months. Inflammatory activity was universal, with high-grade activity in 21%; fibrosis was absent in 28%, mild in 55%, and moderate in 16%; only one patient had cirrhosis. A significant relationship between fibrosis scores and duration of disease was noted, raising the question of disease progression over time. Badizadegan et al. [423], in an evaluation of the hepatic histopathology in 40 children with chronic HCV infection, found portal fibrosis in 75% (bridging fibrosis in 44%) and cirrhosis in 8%. The mode of acquisition of HCV in the above-cited studies was not considerably detailed; therefore, conclusions regarding the factors responsible for the variable outcome are not possible. Overall, the histologic features of HCV in children are often, but not inevitably, mild; because fibrosis is common and may progress with duration of infection, long-term morbidity is possible.

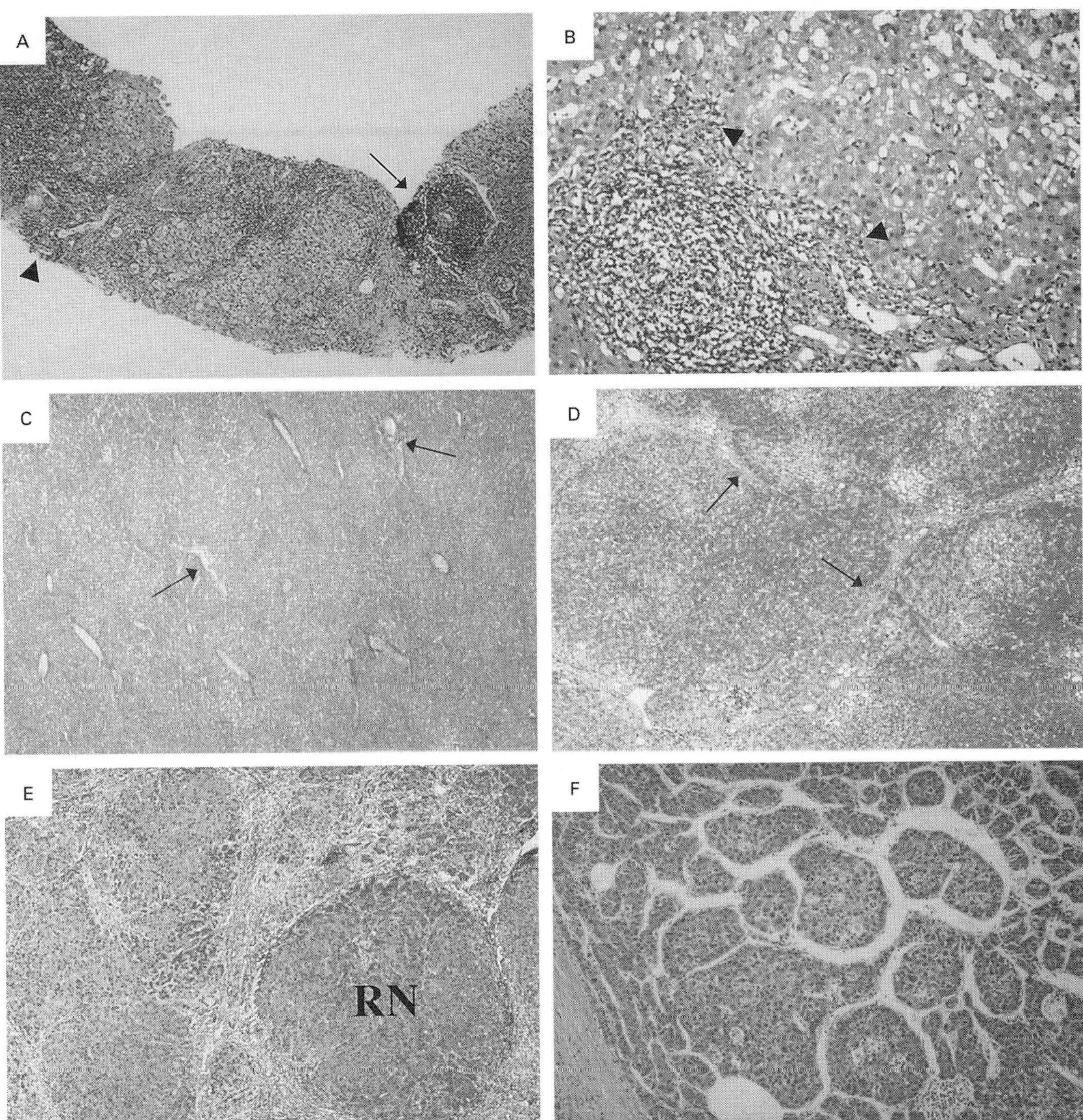

Figure 17.21. Histologic stages of HCV infection. (**A**) A core biopsy specimen from an adult patient chronically infected with HCV shows dense portal lymphocytic infiltrates (*arrow*) and architectural changes (*arrowhead*). (Hematoxylin and eosin [H&E] stain, 10× magnification.) (**B**) The lymphocytes are not limited to the portal tract but extend to the lobules (*arrowheads*). (H&E stain, 100× magnification.) (**C**) Normal liver architecture with scant fibrous tissue (*arrows*) to the portal tracts is evident. (Trichrome stain, 20× magnification.) (**D**) During progressive infections, the fibrotic areas expand and bridging fibrosis develops (*arrows*). (Trichrome stain, 20× magnification.) (**E**) Cirrhosis characterized by marked fibrosis and regenerative nodules (RN) occurs in about 20% of chronically infected persons. (Trichrome stain, 20× magnification.) (**F**) Hepatocellular carcinoma, also a consequence of chronic HCV infection. (H&E stain, 20× magnification.) (Reprinted with permission from Lauer GM, Walker BD. Medical progress: hepatitis C infection. N Engl J Med 2001;345:41–52. Copyright ©2001 Massachusetts Medical Society. All rights reserved.) For color reproduction, see Color Plate 17.21.

Pathogenesis

The HCV genome contains a highly conserved 5′ noncoding region followed by core and envelope structural regions and five nonstructural regions (Figure 17.22) [426]. Structural elements consist of core protein, envelope protein E1, and envelope protein E2, which is a major target of the host immune response. The E2 region contains two hypervariable regions, which may allow HCV to evade the host immune response.

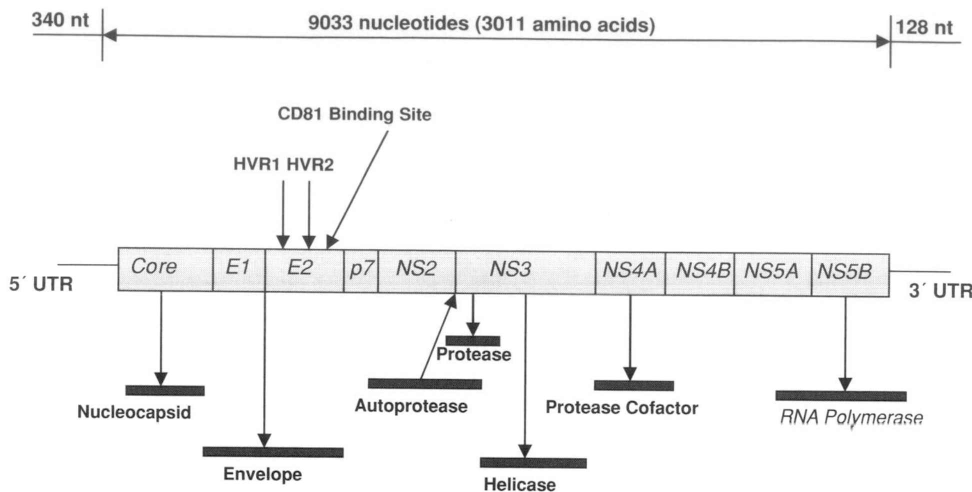

Figure 17.22. HCV genome and expressed proteins. HCV is a single-stranded RNA virus of 9.5 kb that consists of two untranslated regions (UTRs) and a single open reading frame that encodes a 3011 polyprotein. The UTR in the 5′ end contains elements necessary for initiation of viral replication. The polyprotein is cleaved into single proteins by a host peptidase in the structural region, which contains the nucleocapsid core protein and two envelope proteins (E1 and E2). In the nonstructural region, HCV-encoded proteases separate the remaining proteins. The E2 region contains of two hypervariable regions and a binding site for CD81, an HCV receptor. The nonstructural proteins include proteases, a helicase, and an RNA-dependent RNA polymerase. (From Lauer and Walker [384].)

Hepatitis C virus replication is rapid as well as error prone; more than 10 trillion virions are produced each day [427]. The average half-life of an HCV virus is 2.7 hours [427]. Because of the lack of proofreading capabilities of its RNA polymerase, replication errors occur in 1 of 10^4–10^5 nucleotides copied. As a result, viral replication produces quasi-species that are closely related strains of HCV in the same host.

Understanding the pathogenesis of HCV infection has been hindered by the inability to grow HCV in culture. Injection of recombinant transcribed HCV RNA into chimpanzees has resulted in the propagation of virus accompanied by clinical and histologic signs of hepatitis [384]. Recently, cell lines derived from hepatic cells have been used to study HCV replication, viral RNA, and protein synthesis [384]. Furthermore, a rat model has been developed by injecting these cell lines in immunocompetent fetal rats [428]. By inducing tolerance, transplanted HCV-infected human hepatoma cells (Huh 7) can propagate and support HCV gene expression with resultant biochemical and histologic evidence of hepatitis.

In most persons who become infected with HCV, viremia persists and is associated with hepatic inflammation and fibrosis. Studies estimate that 50% or more of hepatocytes harbor the virus in infected persons [429].

The presence of lymphocytes within the hepatic parenchyma suggests an immune-mediated process of inflammation and subsequent fibrosis. The response of the immune system and the T-helper cells in particular are thought to be crucial for the host to clear HCV [384]. Also, the finding that viral diversity is reduced in persons in whom the infection is cleared is consistent with the occurrence of greater immune-mediated control of the virus [430]. In persons in whom chronic HCV develops, the relatively weak response of cytotoxic lymphocytes is insufficient to clear viremia. However, this response is sufficient to cause damage through the elaboration of cytokines in the liver [431]. Studies in humans and chimpanzees support the idea that a vigorous CD4 and CD8 T-cell response against multiple regions of HCV is necessary for elimination of HCV infection. Khakoo et al. [432] have shown that enhanced natural killer function contributes to the spontaneous clearance of HCV. In their study, the authors collected data from 1037 individuals, including 685 with persistent HCV infection and 352 who cleared HCV. The investigators categorized patients based on natural killer (NK) cell receptors and ligands. In individuals without a ligand for inhibiting NK cell activity, there was improved HCV eradication.

Besides host factors that determine the innate ability to ward off HCV infection, the ability of the HCV to suppress IFN signaling and to downgrade the host's immune response are crucial to viral propagation. One mechanism by which HCV accomplishes these tasks is via interference with STAT1, a prinicipal antiviral signal transduction molecule against HCV [433]. It has been shown in human hepatoma cell lines that HCV expression blocks IFN signaling by selectively degrading STAT1. By interfering with IFN signaling, HCV core proteins influence HCV persistence [434]. Other HCV proteins, including NS3A and NS4A, have been shown to interfere with signaling via separate pathways [433]. Decreased expression of anti-inflammatory nuclear receptor peroxisome proliferator–activated receptor-α (PPARα) due to the influence of HCV core proteins is another potential mechanism involved in the pathogenesis of HCV infection; reduced concentrations of PPARα in the liver of untreated HCV-infected patients were noted [434], limiting the ability of the host to mount an effective antiviral response.

Coinfection with HBV

Hepatitis C virus prevalence is about 10–15% in patients with chronic HBV [409], whereas HBV prevalence among HCV-infected patients is approximately 25–30%. Coinfected HCV/HBV patients have an increased risk of fulminant hepatitis, liver fibrosis, and HCC. Chronic HCV patients with HBV superinfection have rates of decompensation of 34%, liver failure of 11%, and mortality of 10% [409]; however, the presence of HBV coinfection does not always change the course of HCV infection, particularly when HBV is present in low levels. Among HCV-infected patients with occult HBV, in which HBV is difficult to detect without the most sensitive techniques, there were no changes in the biochemical or histologic abnormalities in those with or without HBV infection [435,436]. Furthermore, the presence of occult HBV did not affect HCV response to antiviral therapy [437,438]. The presence of occult HBV may be detected in 25–30% of patients with HCV [437,438]. So, the effect of coinfection with HBV and HCV is variable based on host factors and viral virulence. At this juncture, it is prudent to prevent HBV (and HAV) with vaccination in all patients with HCV.

Coinfection with HIV

In the United States, about 10% of HCV-infected persons have HIV infection as well [401]. About 25% of HIV-infected persons in the Western world have chronic HCV [401]. Patients who are coinfected with HCV and HIV-1 are at increased risk for disease progression [363,384,401]. Complications associated with concurrent HCV infection have emerged as one of the most frequent and complex issues in the care of patients with HIV following the introduction of potent antiretroviral therapy for HIV.

Before the advent of highly active antiretroviral therapy (HAART), liver disease mortality was an infrequent cause of death and ranged from 2–13% [409]. Now, mortality from liver disease, chiefly related to HCV, accounts for 7–50% [409]. Even though the effect of HCV on the overall mortality of HIV infection is unclear [439], it is an important clinical problem in the long-term survival of HIV-infected patients. In fact, HCV infection may lessen the severity of untreated HIV infection [439]; however, with improved survival with the administration of HAART, treatment of HCV has assumed much greater significance. Careful consideration about the timing of both HCV and HIV treatment is necessary. In patients with advanced HIV disease, HIV treatment generally is started immediately. In coinfected patients with good immune function and/or advanced liver disease, HCV treatment may be administered first to minimize hepatotoxicity [401]. In coinfected patients who do undergo treatment, side effects from multiple medications need to be carefully monitored and some treatment combinations are contraindicated (e.g., ribavirin and didanosine). Treatment of coinfected patients is similar to that of patients with isolated HCV infection [440,441]; however, a full discussion of the magnitude and management of HCV/HIV-coinfected patients is beyond the scope of this chapter and can be found in recent reviews [401,442].

Table 17.27: Recommended Testing for Hepatitis C Infection

HCV Testing	*Demographic Category*
Recommended	Those with a history of illicit injection drug use
	Those with a history of persistent ALT elevation
	Those who have had a prior transfusion (blood or blood products) or recipients of organs before July 1992
	Persons requiring chronic hemodialysis
	Children born to HCV-positive women
	Persons with HIV infection
	Current sexual partners of HCV-infected persons
	Health care and public safety workers after needle sticks, sharps, or mucosal exposures*
Not recommended	Household (nonsexual) contacts of HCV-positve persons (without additional risk factor)
	Pregnant women
	International adoptees

*Testing of the exposure source would be indicated and subsequent testing of the exposed worker could be undertaken if needed.
From the Centers for Disease Control and Prevention [369] and Strader et al. [401].

Diagnosis

Tests to detect antibody to HCV (anti-HCV) were first licensed by the FDA in 1990. Since that time, improved antibody tests as well as nucleic acid tests for HCV RNA have been developed. No matter which type of test is selected, confirmation of the results is needed. Although false-positive results are rare in at-risk groups (Table 17.27) who have evidence of liver disease, among populations with a low prevalence (<10%) of HCV infection, false-positive results do occur with anti-HCV serology tests [443]. In infants, anti-HCV positivity may indicate placentally transferred maternal antibody for up to 12–18 months rather than HCV infection. Individuals with autoimmune hepatitis are another group with frequent false-positive anti-HCV [444,445]. Finally, anti-HCV positivity may reflect a resolved infection.

There are also circumstances in which HCV may go undetected. Many practitioners order HCV RNA tests because of their widespread availability. An important caveat is that a single HCV RNA test does not exclude HCV infection. Because of the potential for intermittent viremia, repeated HCV RNA testing is needed. In contrast, a negative screening test for anti-HCV is considered reliable.

Serologic Assays

ENZYME IMMUNOASSAY

The initial (first-generation) enzyme immunoassay (EIA), which detected antibody directed against an HCV-related antigen (C100-3 encoded in the NS4 region), was limited because of a lack of sensitivity [446,447]. This was especially problematic early in the course of HCV infection. A negative result in the EIA did not exclude nascent HCV infection because viral RNA could be detected by PCR in serum or liver tissue of patients well in advance of detectable antibody [448]. Equally problematic was the high rate of false positivity of the anti-HCV EIA, a common finding in asymptomatic blood donors and in patients with autoimmune hepatitis [444,445]. In the latter situation, the EIA false positivity was usually attributable to hypergammaglobulinemia because anti-HCV seropositivity, detected in sera tested before immunosuppressive therapy, disappeared during successful therapy [449]. True positivity is also possible; in a certain percentage of anti-LKM (liver-kidney-microsomal) antibody–positive patients with chronic hepatitis, the autoimmune process could be a consequence of HCV infection [450,451]. In children with autoimmune hepatitis, anti-HCV may be falsely positive; before the diagnosis of HCV is accepted in this situation, serum should be negative for autoantibodies and the results of supplementary or confirmatory tests should be determined.

The inherent limitations of the first-generation assay led to the development of second- and third-generation immunoassays that incorporated additional structural and nonstructural antigens encoded by different regions of the HCV genome, including antigens from the viral core (nucleocapsid), a highly conserved portion of the genome. These assays, which detect earlier-appearing antibodies directed against these additional HCV antigens, provide enhanced sensitivity and specificity [452]. Currently available screening serologic assays for HCV (EIA-3) are highly sensitive, but false positive tests still occur, particularly in low-risk populations such as blood donors. Recombinant immunoblot assays (RIBAs) were developed that are able to detect antibody to multiple recombinant HCV antigens. These assays were developed to resolve false-positive EIA results.

NUCLEIC ACID–BASED DETECTION TECHNOLOGY

Amplification of HCV nucleic acid sequences with PCR is a powerful technique for the detection of viremia during acute and chronic HCV infection (Table 17.28) [443]. Most EIA-positive patients with liver disease (>90%) are HCV RNA positive by PCR, suggesting that testing for HCV RNA by PCR may be more appropriate than RIBA to confirm infection. Nucleic acid detection is superior to antibody testing in establishing the diagnosis of HCV infection in patients who lack HCV antibody because of immunosuppression or immunodeficiencies, such as transplant recipients and hemodialysis patients. Detection of HCV RNA is an integral part of assessing response to treatment.

Table 17.28: Interpretation of HCV Test Results

Anti-HCV	*HCV RNA*	*Interpretation*
Negative	Negative	No infection
Positive	Positive	Acute or chronic infection
Negative	Positive	Early infection or chronic infection in an immunosuppressed host
Positive	Negative	Resolved infection or chronic infection or false-positive antibody test

Polymerase chain reaction assays can detect the presence of viremia within a few days after exposure to HCV, weeks before aminotransferase elevation and measurable antibody levels [426]. HCV RNA was detected in the serum of experimentally infected chimpanzees as early as 3 days after inoculation and for an extended period before the appearance of anti-HCV. During this early period of HCV infection (seronegative phase), HCV RNA was the only diagnostic marker of infection [453]. The persistent disappearance of HCV RNA from serum correlates with the resolution of HCV, whereas viremia continues in patients whose disease progresses to chronic hepatitis. A positive HCV RNA is predictive of the presence of liver disease in patients who are anti-HCV positive but have a normal ALT level [454].

Therefore, PCR detection of HCV RNA is applicable in (1) the diagnosis of acute infection before the development of antibodies; (2) confirmation of infection in persons with nonconfirmatory antibody results or those in whom antibody assays are unreliable because of immune compromise; (3) distinguishing resolved from persistent infection; and (4) defining response to treatment.

Qualitative HCV RNA is presently the gold standard to guide treatment and follow-up of patients with chronic hepatitis C. RNA titers fluctuate during the course of chronic disease, and one negative titer in the presence of a positive anti-HCV antibody does not mean resolution of the infection [455]. HCV RNA has been directly detected by in situ hybridization. Other sensitive techniques for HCV detection include immunohistochemistry; with this technique, HCV antigens can be identified in hepatocytes of chimpanzees with acute hepatitis C and patients with chronic hepatitis C [456].

QUANTITATION OF VIRAL GENOMES

A number of different assays are available to measure the amount of virus in specimens. There are two main types of technologies: target amplification and signal amplification [457]. Target amplification tests include PCR and transcription-mediated amplification (TMA), whereas signal amplification refers to branched DNA assays. Because each quantitative assay

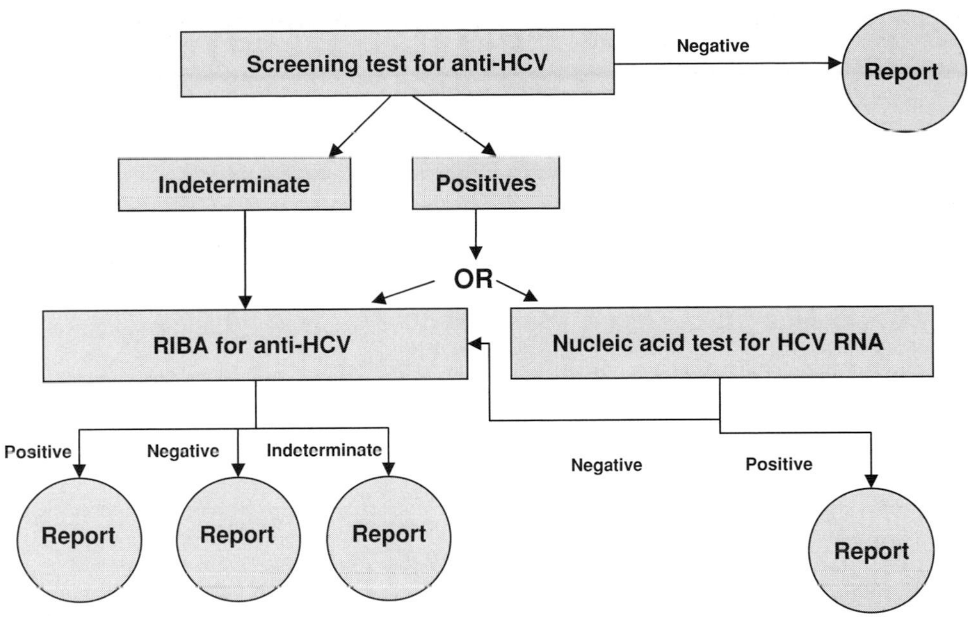

Figure 17.23. Laboratory algorithm for HCV testing. This algorithm depicts screening recommendations from the Centers for Disease Control and Prevention [443]. If anti-HCV (EIA) is negative, no further testing is required. If anti-HCV is positive or indeterminant, confirmatory testing with either a recombinant immunoblot assay (RIBA) or a nucleic acid test for HCV RNA should be performed. The RIBA test is preferred with indeterminant results. When there is a combination of a positive anti-HCV result and a negative nucleic acid test for HCV RNA, RIBA testing should be performed as well [443].

uses a different standard, direct comparisons between the assays may not be meaningful [401]. The range of quantitative assays is between 10 IU/L and 7,700,000 IU/L [401]; however, the conversion of each assay from units to copies per milliliter is variable with each assay. Nevertheless, these assays are useful in following the response to treatment and helpful in deciding the length of treatment. Although quantitative assays can be used to determine the presence of infection, they are less sensitive than qualitative assays; thus a negative result by quantitative assay must be confirmed as negative by qualitative PCR (Figure 17.23).

HCV GENOTYPING

Current indications for HCV genotyping are restricted to patients being considered for treatment, as the duration of therapy is determined by HCV genotype (as discussed subsequently). There are no clear clinical indications for HCV genotyping in other patient subgroups. Genotyping can be performed by direct sequence analysis, by reverse hybridization to genotype-specific oligonucleotide probes, or by use of restriction fragment length polymorphism. These tests, although in clinical use, are not yet FDA approved. Current commercial tests may display mixed genotype results in 1–4% and fail to identify a genotype in less than 3% [458].

Prevention

To reduce the burden of HCV infection and HCV-related disease, primary and secondary prevention activities are necessary. Although the incidence of HCV has declined in the past decade, the absence of an effective vaccine and the lack of an effective passive immunization option indicate that the battle to eliminate and/or reduce the impact of HCV is far from over. Although primary prevention through screening of blood products has resulted in a dramatic reduction in transfusion-associated HCV infection, the major reason for the decline in HCV infection, as alluded to previously, relates to the reduction in the number of HCV infections transmitted among injection drug users [380]. It has been theorized that the decline in the number of HCV infections has been a secondary effect caused by precautions to avoid HIV. As can be seen with the trends of increased HBV among certain demographics, these precautions may be decreasing because the fear of HIV has been reduced subsequent to the introduction of effective therapies.

At the present time, identifying and counseling persons at risk for HCV infection remains the most appropriate medical strategy (Table 17.29). Specifically, efforts at decreasing injection drug use and transmission in this setting, including methadone treatment programs, needle and syringe exchange programs, and education programs, have been effective [363]. As with HBV infection, these efforts can be integrated into existing institutions; important priorities would include correctional facilities and STD clinics.

In household settings, it is prudent to avoid sharing items that may be contaminated with blood, such as razors and toothbrushes. However, there is no evidence that hugging, kissing, coughing, sneezing, or sharing eating utensils or drinking glasses is associated with HCV transmission. HCV infection

Table 17.29: Counseling for Hepatitis C Infection

Clinical Aspect	*Recommendation*
To avoid transmission	HCV-infected persons should avoid sharing toothbrushes and dental/shaving equipment and cover bleeding wounds Stop any illicit drug use. In those who continue, avoid sharing/reusing needles and syringes. HCV-infected persons should avoid donating blood, semen, or body tissues HCV-infected persons should be counseled regarding sexual transmission. Those in long-term relationships are at low risk for HCV transmission*; all others, should use effective barrier methods.
To minimize progressive liver disease:	Assure vaccination against hepatitis A and hepatitis B Avoid alcohol Minimize obesity In selected patients, targeted therapy for HCV will decrease risk for progressive liver disease

*Barrier methods can further lower risk even among individuals in long-term relationships.
From the Centers for Disease Control and Prevention [369] and Strader et al. [401].

Table 17.30: Selecting Patients for Hepatitis C Therapy

Treatment Recommendation	*Characteristics*
Treatment widely accepted	Compensated liver disease in adults* Abnormal liver enzymes† Liver histology showing chronic hepatitis with significant fibrosis High likelihood of compliance
Treatment individualized	Age <18 yr Persistently normal ALT values Acute hepatitis C Coinfection with HIV Chronic renal disease Ongoing use of illicit drugs or alcohol Decompensated cirrhosis Liver transplantation Minimal liver histology changes
Treatment contraindicated	Age <3 yr Severe concurrent disease, such as heart failure, hypertension, diabetes, hyperthyroidism, or pulmonary disease Major depression Autoimmune hepatitis Pregnancy or unwillingness to comply with contraception Renal, heart, or lung transplantation

*Compensated liver disease is characterized by serum bilirubin less than 1.5 g/dL, international normalized ratio less than 1.5, albumin greater than 3.4 g/dL, platelet count greater than 75,000/mm^3, and no evidence of encephalopathy or ascites.
†When liver enzymes are abnormal, other coexisting etiologies, including nonalcoholic fatty liver disease, need to be considered before recommending therapy.
From the Centers for Disease Control and Prevention [369] and Strader et al. [401].

should not preclude school attendance or sports participation. As further improvements in the treatment of HCV are identified, broader screening efforts may be needed to shrink the reservoir of HCV-infected individuals. Ultimately, the development of an effective vaccine, which is not imminent, holds the most promise for eradicating HCV.

Management

The management of chronic hepatitis C in adults has changed significantly over the past 5 years. The ability to increase the eradication rate of HCV with newer therapies has improved the chances of minimizing the progression of HCV-induced liver disease, has decreased the spread of HCV infection to others, and in some cases, has allowed the reversal of cirrhosis [401,459].

Table 17.30 lists guidelines for selecting patients for treatment, and an algorithm for treating adults with chronic hepatitis C is given in Figure 17.24.

Early experience in HCV treatment for adults relied on recombinant IFN, then interferon in combination with ribavirin. These therapies are now mostly of historic interest in adults because of the improved efficacy of pegylated IFN in combination with ribavirin (Figure 17.25). Because damage to the liver in HCV is predominantly immune-mediated, use of IFN as a treatment strategy was logical. An SVR-6, indicated by the disappearance of HCV RNA from the serum for 6 months after the completion of treatment, occurred in approximately 16% of HCV-infected adults with 12 months of IFN monotherapy [317,401,460–462]. The development of pegylated IFN, which decreases renal clearance of the drug (thereby increasing the half-life of IFN) allows weekly dosing. Furthermore, monotherapy with pegylated IFN results in an SVR-6 of 39%, a significant improvement. Currently, there are two licensed products in the United States, the 12-kDa peginterferon alfa-2b (Peg-Intron, Schering-Plough Corporation, Kenilworth, NJ) and the 40-kDa peginterferon alfa-2a (Pegasys; Hoffman-La Roche, Nutley, NJ). The use of ribavirin, which is a synthetic guanosine analogue,

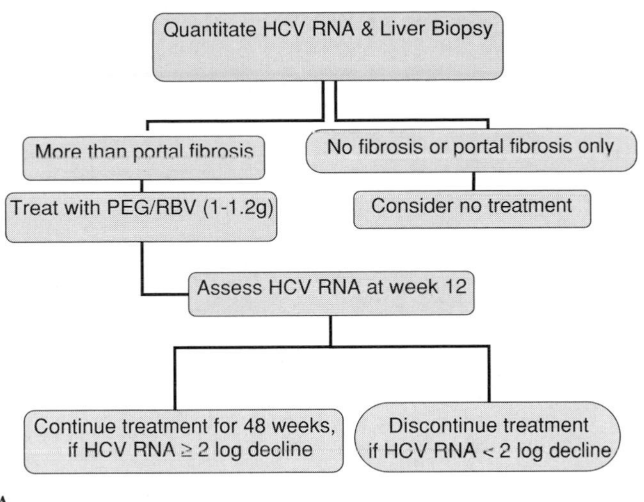

A

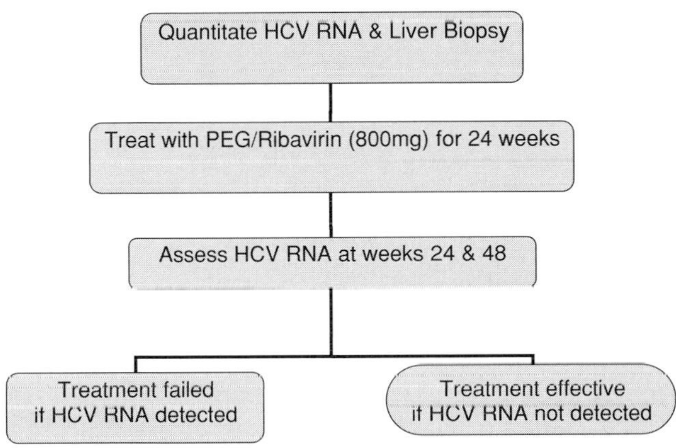

B

Figure 17.24. Suggested algorithms for managing eligible adults with HCV for (**A**) patients with genotype 1 and (**B**) those with genotype 2 or 3 [401]. These algorithms will undoubtedly require modification as new data emerge. For example, recent trials have shown that patients with genotypes 2 and 3 can be treated successfully with shorter treatment courses if HCV RNA is undetectable after 4 weeks of therapy. For pediatric patients, definitive recommendations are not available because of the limited data available. The results of a multicenter study on combination therapy (peginterferon/ribavirin) are awaited and are likely to influence treatment choices in pediatric patients. For now, the only FDA-approved therapy for children older than 3 years is Rebetron (interferon alfa-2b/ribavirin; Schering-Plough Corporation, Kenilworth, NJ).

developed after it was noted to have a partial effect on HCV in pilot trials [463,464]. Combination therapy has been shown to be synergistic: the combination of pegylated IFN with ribavirin achieves SVR-6 in 54–56% of patients [401,465,466].

The toxicities of INF have been discussed previously in the context of hepatitis B in this chapter. Pegylated IFN has essentially the same toxicities as IFN, perhaps at a lower frequency [466]. Ribavirin causes a dose-dependent hemolytic anemia and is teratogenic. In controlled studies, the mean decrease in hemoglobin was 2.5–3 g within the first 4–8 weeks of therapy. Dose reductions, with hemoglobin levels less than 10 g/dL, were required in 6–15% of patients [401,467]. Other side effects of ribavirin include fatigue, itching, rash, sinusitis, and gout. Because of its teratogenic effects, persons who receive ribavirin must use strict contraceptive methods both during treatment and for a period of 6 months after treatment.

Growth factors such as epoetin and granulocyte colony-stimulating factor (G-CSF) have been used to counter the adverse effects of ribavirin and IFN. However, a lack of controlled studies regarding their use precludes specific recommendations for clinical practice.

Combination Therapy: Pegylated Interferon and Ribavirin

The first large published study examining combination therapy involved 1530 patients and compared IFN-α-2b plus ribavirin, and peginterferon alfa-2b plus ribavirin. Overall, the SVR was significantly higher in the high-dose (1.5 μg/kg) peginterferon group compared with the IFN group, 54% versus 47% (Figure 17.26) [465]. These findings were confirmed in a separate study [466] that enrolled 1121 patients and randomly assigned them to one of three treatment groups: peginterferon alfa-2a (180 μg) with ribavirin, peginterferon alfa-2a monotherapy, and IFN-α-2b plus ribavirin [466]. Overall, the SVR was 56% for the combination peginterferon group versus 44% for the combination interferon group and 29% for the peginterferon monotherapy group (Figure 17.27). A third large study that enrolled 1311 patients examined the ribavirin dosage and the optimal duration of peginterferon alfa-2a therapy [467]. The SVR for peginterferon alfa-2a (180 μg) with a weight-based dose of ribavirin (1000 mg or 1200 mg) outperformed that of peginterferon alfa-2a with the "standard" dose (800 mg) of ribavirin among patients with HCV genotype 1 (52% vs. 41%); among patients with genotype 2 or 3, the reduction in ribavirin dosage had no effect on SVR, with an 80% response in individuals receiving the higher dose and a 79% response in those in the lower-dose group (Figure 17.28). The length of therapy, 24 versus 48 weeks, did not improve the SVR in genotypes 2 or 3 but did increase the response from 42% to 52% in HCV-infected individuals with genotype 1 [467]. Also, in patients with genotype 1 – but not those with genotype 2 or 3 – a lower viral load increased the likelihood of response. In the 85 patients with genotype 1, who had a viral load of less than 2×10^6 copies/mL, the SVR was 65% (treated with the higher ribavirin dosage and 48 weeks of peginterferon) [467].

Although SVR rates have improved with combination therapy and longer treatment periods, adverse events are more common with higher doses and longer treatment periods. Among patients treated for 1 year with ribavirin at higher doses, about 15% developed hemoglobin concentrations less than 10 g/dL; only 6% developed this degree of anemia when treated with lower doses of ribavirin [467]. More serious adverse events,

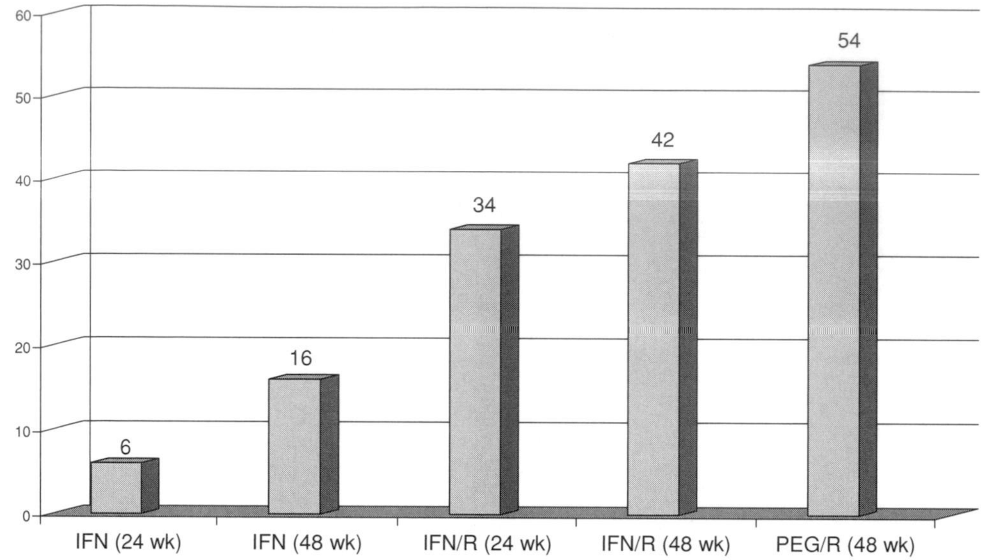

Figure 17.25. Combination treatment with peginterferon/ribavirin (PEG/R) is superior to interferon/ribavirin (IFN/R), which is superior to interferon monotherapy (IFN) with both 24-week and 48-week courses. The additional 6 months of treatment is a benefit only to patients who have HCV genotype 1, which is responsible for approximately 70% of HCV infections in the United States. For patients with genotypes 2 and 3, combination treatment courses of 6 months and 12 months are equally effective. With the PEG/R for 12 months, the average sustained virologic response (for all genotypes) in the United States is 54–56%. (From Hochman and Balistreri [1] and Strader et al. [401].)

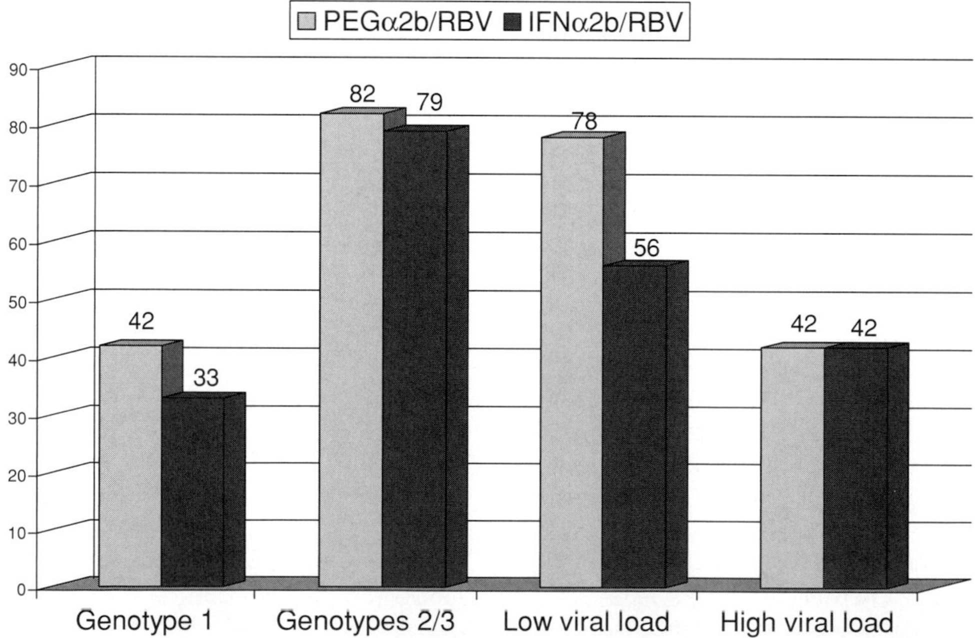

Figure 17.26. Sustained virologic response rates with peginterferon alfa-2b (1.5 μg/kg) combined with ribavirin (800 mg) were greater than those achieved with interferon alfa-2b with ribavirin (800 mg). The difference in SVR was most apparent in HCV-infected persons with genotype 1 and in those with a low viral load, $\leq 2 \times 10^6$/mL (From Manns et al. [465].)

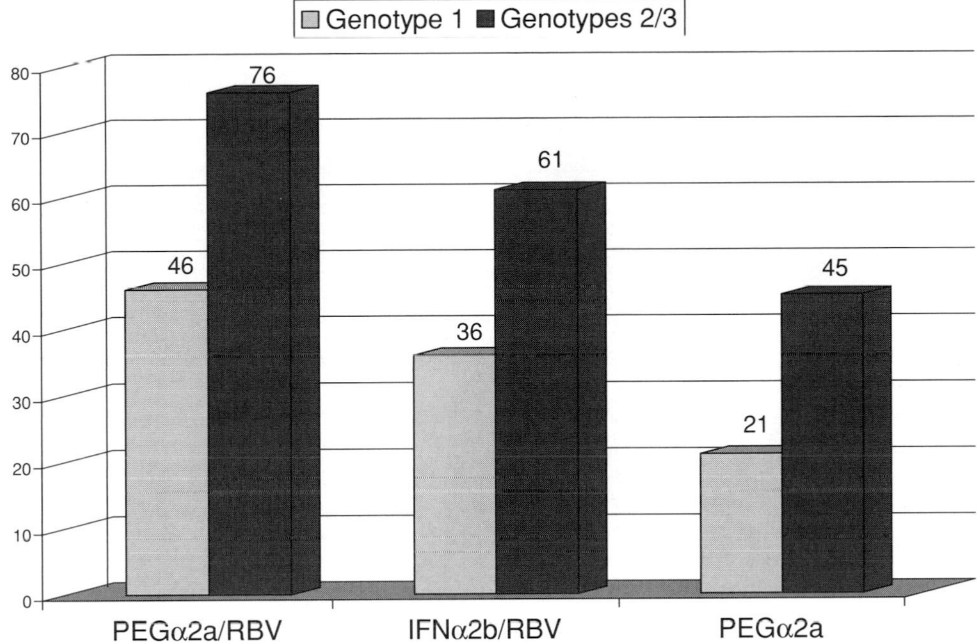

Figure 17.27. Sustained virologic response rates with peginterferon alfa-2a (180 μg) with ribavirin (1.0–1.2 g) were greater than those with combination therapy with interferon alfa-2b with ribavirin and greater than those with peginterferon monotherapy. These differences were present among all genotypes; however, genotypes 2 and 3 had much more favorable responses to all three therapies (From Fried et al. [466].)

including deaths caused by suicide and sepsis, have been reported [401,467].

One way to minimize toxicity is to direct combination therapy toward those most likely to benefit and to stop therapy when it is not effective. Among adults treated with combination therapy, two "stop rules" are useful: (1) therapy should be discontinued in genotype 1 patients who do not achieve undetectable HCV RNA levels or a 2-log (100-fold) drop from baseline at week 12, and (2) treatment should be stopped in genotype 1 patients who have detectable viremia at week 24, even if they had a 2-log reduction at week 12 [401,468]. In these patients, continued therapy is unlikely to yield an SVR.

To minimize the toxicity of therapy, further decreasing the length of treatment in patients with genotypes 2 and 3 has been explored. Mangia et al. [469] explored the efficacy of combination therapy (peginterferon alfa-2b with ribavirin) in 283 patients by randomly assigning the patients to one of two groups; one group received 24 weeks of therapy, and the study group received only 12 weeks of therapy if they had an early viral response (EVR). In this study, patients were considered to have an EVR if the HCV RNA was undetectable after 4 weeks of therapy. Among the study group, 133 patients (62%) had an EVR, allowing a shorter duration of treatment. The SVR among both groups was nearly identical: 76% among the control group and 77% in the variable duration group [469]. This study confirmed the results of an uncontrolled study from Norway in which 89% of patients (n = 95) with genotype 2 or 3 had a response to combination therapy after 14 weeks of therapy [470]. A recent well-controlled randomized study has confirmed the efficacy of shorter treatment periods for HCV-infected patients with genotype 2 or 3 [471]. After identification of patients with an EVR (HCV RNA <600 IU/mL), 142 patients were randomly divided into two groups; both groups received peginterferon alfa-2a (180 μg/wk) along with ribavirin (800–1200 mg/d). The first group was treated for 16 weeks, and the second group was treated for 24 weeks. The SVR-6 rates were 82% and 80%, respectively. Additional analysis noted a suboptimal response among genotype 3 patients with a higher viral load (>800,000 IU/mL).

Caution is necessary in extrapolating these studies to U.S. patients. Although these studies demonstrated that shorter courses of therapy may be effective in genotype 2 and 3 patients, the study subjects had several attributes that may have favored a response to treatment: they had a lower body mass index versus U.S. patients, there were more women, and virtually all were Caucasian. In addition, studies performed in Europe have had higher response rates compared with those from U.S. centers, even after accounting for confounding factors [472].

Because of the improved efficacy of combination treatment, studies have been undertaken to evaluate previous nonresponders; these patients had all been previously treated with IFN with or without ribavirin [473]. In one large study with 604 patients in the Hepatitis C Antiviral Long-Term Treatment against Cirrhosis (HALT-C) trial, 18% achieved SVR with a combination

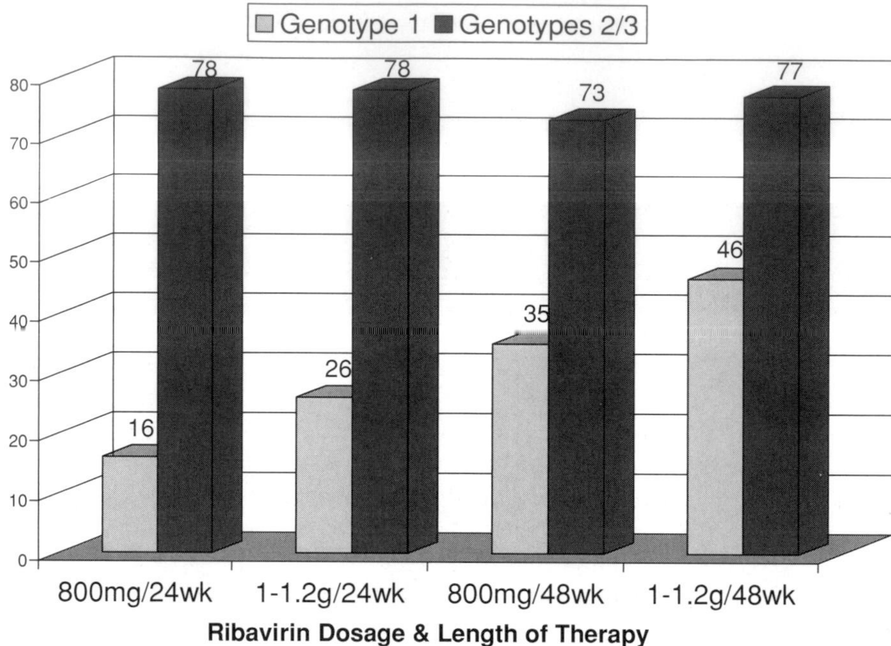

Figure 17.28. Sustained virologic response rates with peginterferon alfa-2a (180 μg) are improved among HCV-infected patients with genotype 1 who receive higher doses of ribavirin and longer treatment periods. Patients with genotypes 2 and 3 respond equally well to shorter treatment periods and with lower ribavirin dosage. Although not shown on this figure, the response of patients with genotype 1 with a low viral load, $\leq 2 \times 10^6$/mL, was better in all treatment groups compared with patients with genotype 1 with a higher viral load; however, even among these patients, there was improvement in treatment response with a longer duration of therapy and higher ribavirin dosage. (From Hadziyannis et al. [467].)

of peginterferon alfa-2a and weight-based ribavirin (1000 mg or 1200 mg). Reduction in the dose of ribavirin to less than 60% of the starting dose lessened the likelihood of response from 21% to 11%.

Ultimately, the ability to clear HCV has important clinical implications. Among patients who respond to therapy, there is usually histologic improvement. Even cirrhosis may be reversed among patients who respond [474]. In one study that pooled data from 3010 patients who received ten different regimens, the impact of treatment on fibrosis was examined by comparing pre- and posttreatment liver biopsy results [474]. Histologic improvement was present in 39% of those who received interferon monotherapy (24 weeks) and 73% of those who received combination peginterferon/ribavirin (48 weeks). Reversal of cirrhosis occurred in 75 of 153 patients (49%) who had baseline cirrhosis. Factors associated with improved histology after treatment included minimal baseline fibrosis/activity, SVR, younger age (<40 years), lower body mass index (<27 kg/m^2), and lower viral load (<3.5 million copies/mL) [474].

Several studies have identified populations that respond less favorably to current HCV therapies. Among African Americans, SVRs for combination peginterferon/ribavirin therapies have ranged from 19–26% [475–477]. The exact reasons for the lower response rate in these patients are unclear. Other patients that have lower response rates include immunocompromised hosts, patients with end-stage renal disease, patients with active substance abuse issues, and patients with cirrhosis [477].

Early Virologic Response

Several studies have shown that an EVR is predictive of an SVR [401,466,468]. An EVR, usually defined by at least a 2-log decline from baseline of the HCV RNA level after 12 weeks of treatment, indicates a 65% probability of subsequently achieving an SVR. Conversely, if an EVR is not present, 97% of patients fail to develop an SVR [468]. As alluded to previously, some studies of patients infected with genotypes 2 and 3 are evaluating an EVR after 4 weeks of therapy to predict patients who may need only 12–16 weeks of therapy [469].

Treatment of Children with Chronic HCV Infection

There have been no published large-scale multicenter prospective placebo-controlled, randomized trials of antiviral therapy for HCV in children. Nevertheless, pooled data from smaller studies have been analyzed and generally demonstrate that HCV-infected children have responses to IFN therapy similar to those of HCV-infected adults [478]. IFN monotherapy has achieved reported SVR rates of 33–45% [377,401,478–484]. An analysis that pooled data from 12 published studies and seven abstracts identified 366 treated and 105 untreated children [478]. The average SVR was 36%; patients with genotype 1 had a 27% response versus 70% for those without genotype 1. In contrast, only 5% of the untreated children had spontaneous resolution of their HCV infections. These data indicate a higher SVR than that reported in adults, but the results may be affected by publication bias or statistical artifact from small uncontrolled studies. The predictors of response have paralleled those identified in adults.

Preliminary experience with combination treatment is limited. A recent review of the literature reviewed the experience of combination treatment in 107 children and adolescents [485]. More than half the published data are from an abstract that reported the results of IFN/ribavirin in 61 children aged 5 to 11 years [486]. Among the cohort in the abstract, the overall SVR was 38% (31% in genotype 1). The ribavirin dose of 15 mg/kg was associated with the highest virologic response rate. In the other studies, the response rate was between 30% and 50% [485,487–490].

Another study of combination therapy examined the effectiveness of peginterferon alfa-2b (1.5 μg/kg) with ribavirin (15 mg/kg/d) in 61 children and adolescents [491]. In this open-label, uncontrolled cohort, 48% of genotype 1 patients (n = 46) achieved an SVR whereas all 13 genotype 2 or 3 patients had an SVR. Side effects were well tolerated; only 3 individuals required dose reduction; 10% developed thyroid autoantibodies and thyroid dysfunction.

Despite limited data, Rebetron (IFN-α-2b/ribavirin; Schering-Plough Corp.) has been approved for use in children and, in fact, is the only current therapy licensed by the FDA for treatment of hepatitis C in children. A large study of peginterferon and ribavirin in children (PEDS-C) is in progress; enrollment began in December 2004 (www.clinicaltrials.gov/show/NCT00100659).

In general, children tolerate IFN-α and ribavirin at least as well as adults. Additional concerns regarding the use of these drugs in children include the potential for side effects involving growth and development. At this time, the practitioner must individualize treatment for children based on the severity of liver disease weighed against the toxicity of therapy. In most children and adolescents, IFN-α-2b along with ribavirin should be selected for initial treatment; however, in older adolescents requiring treatment, the possibility of peginterferon combination therapy should be entertained.

Treatment of Patients with Normal Aminotransferase Levels

As the efficacy of treatments has improved, investigators have started to consider treatment in individuals with milder disease. Most HCV-infected individuals with normal ALT levels have slowly progressive liver disease [363,401]. This group of patients, however, remains controversial for many reasons. First, there are a large number of patients in this category. Up to 60% of patients with HCV infection have normal ALT levels [492–494]. Second, advanced liver disease occurs in 1–10% of patients with normal ALT levels, and at least portal fibrosis occurs in a larger number [454,495–497]. Third, it has been shown that the response rate in this group is similar to the rate in those with abnormal ALT levels [401,498]. Finally, this group of individuals represents a larger reservoir for ongoing spread of HCV. On a personal level, many individuals (e.g., future mothers and surgeons) who are unlikely to develop HCV-related liver disease fear transmission to others.

A confounding issue is determining the optimal upper limit of normal. Each laboratory must establish its normal value; however, ALT values fluctuate based on age, body mass, race, and gender [499]. In addition, alcohol ingestion and comorbid conditions need to be considered in the interpretation of ALT levels. Despite these limitations, currently a normal ALT is defined by two or more determinations identified in the normal range of a licensed laboratory over a minimum of 6 months. Interestingly, when a more stringent definition of a normal ALT value is used, the rate of fibrosis is very slow [500]. Mathurin et al. [500] studied 1353 HCV-infected patients; only 102 patients were considered to have normal ALT values when at least three normal ALT values (mean of six determinations) were obtained during the preceding 6 months. Based on liver histology and progression between liver specimens, the progression to cirrhosis was estimated to be 80 years in those with this more strict definition of normal.

Given these considerations, recent guidelines have recommended an individualized approach to these patients based on the severity of histologic injury, the likelihood of response to therapy, the risk of serious side effects, and the presence of comorbid conditions [401].

Treatment of Acute HCV Infection

Because of the difficulty in recognizing acute HCV infection, only a limited number of studies have been performed. The results are difficult to interpret because in individuals with symptomatic acute hepatitis C, the infection is more likely to resolve spontaneously [501]. Despite these caveats, combinining data from 17 studies using different forms of IFN α monotherapy showed a 62% SVR among treated patients compared with a 12% SVR among untreated patients [401,502]. More impressive results with higher doses of IFN (5–10 MU/d for at least 12 weeks) have been reported. In these uncontrolled studies, eradication rates have been between 83% and 100% [503–505].

Recent data, however, have provided evidence of a high spontaneous resolution in symptomatic acute HCV infection. In one study, 54 of 60 patients were initially observed without treatment [506]. In this group, 37 (68%) spontaneously cleared HCV RNA, with a mean of 8 weeks following diagnosis. However, 13 relapsed, leaving 56% with persistent infection. None of the patients with asymptomatic acute HCV infection spontaneously resolved his or her infection; in contrast, 52% with symptomatic infection had clearance of HCV RNA without treatment. With treatment instituted between 3 and 6 months after the onset of infection, for those who did not spontaneously

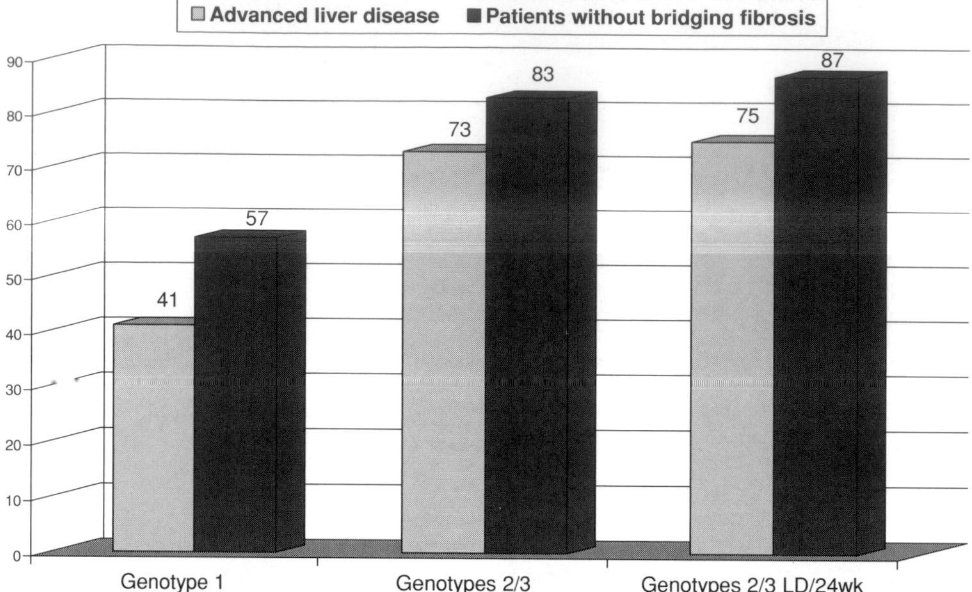

Figure 17.29. Sustained virologic response rates with peginterferon alfa-2a (180 μg)/ribavirin (1.0–1.2 g) are decreased among HCV-infected patients with cirrhosis or bridging fibrosis among all genotypes. The data indicate the response to 48 weeks of combination therapy. As in other patient subpopulations, patients with genotypes 2 and 3 responded more favorably than patients with genotype 1. Furthermore, patients with genotypes 2 and 3, even with advanced liver disease, responded similarly with a lower ribavirin dosage and with a treatment regimen for only 24 weeks; 75% of patients with genotype 2 or 3 with advanced liver disease had an SVR when treated with 24 weeks of therapy using an 800-mg dosage of ribavirin, whereas 87% responded who had no cirrhosis or bridging fibrosis. (From Hadziyannis et al. [467].)

lose HCV, the SVR was 81%. The overall response was 91% among treated and untreated patients [506].

Based on the available data, expert recommendations for acute HCV infection include the following: (1) consider the initiation of therapy 2–4 months after the onset of acute infection, (2) use of peginterferon is preferred because of its ease of administration, and (3) treat for at least 6 months [401]. The addition of ribavirin should be made on a case-by-case basis.

Treatment in Cirrhosis

Overall, the SVR in patients with cirrhosis is about 43–44%, or 10% lower than in patients with minimal fibrosis [401]. In one large study, the investigators examined the relationship between advanced liver disease, genotype, and response to therapy [469]. Across all genotypes, the presence of cirrhosis or bridging fibrosis decreased the SVR rate by 10–15% (Figure 17.29).

In many patients with advanced cirrhosis, liver transplantation may be the only option. However, reinfection with HCV is almost certain and lowers long-term survival to 60–80% [363]. It is unclear whether the benefits of treatment in transplant recipients are greater than the risks associated with treatment, including rejection, anemia, infection, and renal insufficiency.

The pediatric experience with recurrent hepatitis C following liver transplantation is very limited. McDiarmid et al. [507] treated 13 children with de novo hepatitis C post liver transplantation. The mean time to diagnosis was 8.1 years post transplantation. The graft histology showed chronic hepatitis in 11 and cirrhosis in 1 patient. Twelve patients were treated with IFN-α-2. Four patients developed rapidly progressive liver failure requiring urgent retransplantation; 3 of them died within 6 months with evidence of recurrent HCV liver disease. Of the other 8, only 1 became HCV RNA negative.

Future Therapy of Hepatitis C

Despite the significant improvements in HCV therapy witnessed over the previous decade, current treatments are not effective in all patients, are costly, require prolonged treatment periods, and have substantial toxicities. These factors along with a large number of potential patients have led to many new therapies that are in development (Table 17.31) [477]. Newer treatments for HCV are at least 3–5 years away and probably longer for pediatric patients. Therefore, the current treatment goals are to determine conclusively whether combination peginterferon/ribavirin can improve the outlook for pediatric HCV patients and to eliminate other comorbidities for our patients.

DELTA HEPATITIS

Background

Shortly after the discovery of the "delta" antigen in 1977 [508], researchers identified delta hepatitis infection worldwide

Table 17.31: Emerging Hepatitis C Therapies

Drug Category	*Examples*
Interferon alternative	Multiferon Albuferon PEG-alfacon
Ribavirin alternatives	Viramidine Merimepodib (VX-497) Mycophenolic acid
Immune modulators	Civacir (NABI) – HCV immune globulin Hepe-X-C – monoclonal antibodies E1 vaccine – therapeutic vaccine Histamine dihydrochloride – increases interferon's actions on T cells and NK cells Thymosin α_1 – augments T-cell function
Antifibrotics	Enbrel – anti–tumor necrosis factor-α IP-501 – antifibrotic ID-6556 – caspase inhibitor
Viral enzyme inhibitors	BILN 2061 – NS3 inhibitor VX-950 – NS3–4A inhibitor Valopicitabine – RdRp inhibitor ISIS 14803 – antisense oligonucleotide

From Wong and Terrault [477].

[509]. Transmission experiments in susceptible animals confirmed that the delta antigen is a component of a transmissible pathogen whose replication depends on an obligatory association with HBV [508–511]. Subsequently, delta hepatitis virus, or hepatitis D virus (HDV), has been designated as a distinct form of viral hepatitis that has been noted to be more severe than isolated HBV infection.

Viral Characteristics

Hepatitis D virus is found as a concurrent infection in patients with severe acute and chronic HBV-associated hepatitis [512–517]. Although HDV is transmissible as an independent infectious particle and is directly cytopathic, the virus can cause infection and clinical illness only in the presence of active infection with HBV [518]. The δ agent acts as a parasite of HBV, with HDV RNA using structural proteins encoded by the helper virus (HBV). HDV is dissimilar to known families of animal viruses, exhibiting a unique structure and replicative cycle [519]. Elucidation of the structure, sequence, and expression of the HDV genome by Wang et al. [520] clarified the similarities to plant viroids (satellite viruses).

Hepatitis D virus is a viruslike 36–43-nm double-shelled particle that contains a minute RNA, about 1.7 kilobases (kb) in size. The structure of HDV is a hybrid (Figure 17.30). HDV consists of an inner nucleocapsid that contains about 60 copies of the internal δ antigen (HDVAg) in its two forms in addition

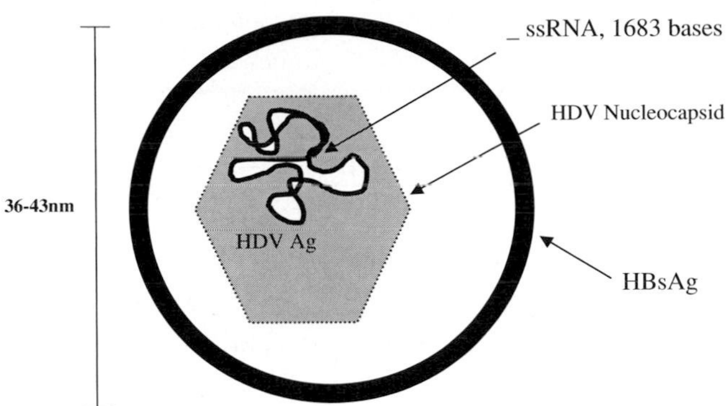

Figure 17.30. The delta hepatitis virus (HDV). Inside the 36–43-nm HBsAg envelope, there is a 19-nm HDV nucleocapsid, which contains about 60 copies of HDAg in its two forms (S and L) and HDV genomic single-stranded, circular RNA (ssRNA). (From the Centers for Disease Control and Prevention. Hepatitis D with notes. [Accessed January 26, 2006, at http://www.cdc.gov/ncidod/diseases/hepatitis/slideset/hep_e/slide_1.htm.])

to the HDV RNA genome enveloped in an external coat of borrowed HBsAg provided by the genome of HBV [521].

The δ antigen, which is a nuclear phosphorylated protein, exists in two forms after posttranscriptional editing, an S-HDAg and an L-HDAg. The S-HDAg, 195 amino acids in length, is necessary for HDV replication, whereas the L-HDAg, 214 amino acids in length, is required for virion assembly. HDAg, in both forms, is the one and only protein expressed by HDV and is present only within the internal nucleocapsid [522]. Although the δ antigen is similar to the HBV capsid, it is antigenically distinct. Inside the HBV capsid, the ds-DNA genome of HBV is nearly twice as long at 3.2 kb.

Hepatitis D virus is the only known animal virus to have a circular RNA genome [522]. Because of a high degree of intramolecular complementarity in the HDV RNA sequence, approximately 70% of the nucleotides are base paired to each other to form an unbranched, double-stranded, rod-shaped structure.

Although about 14 HDV isolates have been identified, based on sequence diversity, HDV is classified into three genotypes. Genotype 1 is the most predominant throughout the world, genotype 2 is more prevalent in Japan and Taiwan, and genotype 3 is associated with outbreaks in Venezuela and Peru [523].

Hepatocyte injury resulting from infection with HDV may be caused by direct virus cytotoxicity, in contrast to immune-mediated injury associated with HBV [522]. HDV replication is limited to the liver, and the pathologic changes in HDV infection are limited to this organ (hepatocellular necrosis and inflammation). The specific features are dependent on the status of the coincidental HBV infection.

Epidemiology

As with the other hepatitis viruses, the incidence of HDV is decreasing [524,525]. Nevertheless, it is estimated that more than 10 million people worldwide have been infected with HDV [524]. The distribution of HDV is uneven throughout the world with parts of South America having the highest incidence. Although HDV requires the presence of HBV to replicate, the distribution of HDV is much different from that of HBV.

In Italy, where HDV was first recognized, anti-HDV antibodies were found in 8.3% of HBsAg-positive patients in 1997, whereas multicenter studies demonstrated anti-HDV positivity rates of 23% in 1987 and 14% in 1992 [524]. When studied in 1997, the highest prevalence rate, 11.7%, was in patients with cirrhosis [524]. Overall, the circulation of HDV decreased by 1.5% per year from 1987–1997. Furthermore, there has been a substantial decrease in the prevalence of HBV in Italy because of universal vaccination. Depriving HDV of its necessary substrate has led to a dramatic reduction in HDV, much more than the reduction in HBV. This indicates that the reduction of HDV incidence is more exponential than colinear when the HBV incidence is decreased [524].

The method of transmission is not entirely understood. Certainly, the mode of transmission has similarities to that of HBV. The strongest risk factors include hemophilia, use of illicit intravenous drugs, and blood product exposure. Conditions with poor hygiene may allow transmission of HDV as well. As with HBV, HDV can be transmitted through sexual contact, but it is less frequently transmitted in this fashion.

Patients immune to HBV, as a result of either previous infection or HBV vaccination, are considered to be immune to HDV [526]. For HBsAg carriers, there are no effective ways of preventing HDV superinfection other than hygienic practices.

Table 17.32: Clinical Features of Delta Hepatitis Infection (HDV)

Clinical Feature	*Characteristics*
Signs and symptoms	Jaundice Fatigue Anorexia Nausea Fever Diarrhea Abdominal pain Pruritic rash
Incubation period	Average ~3–7 wk
Transmission	Percutaneous exposure to infected fluids Sharing of drugs and needles Unprotected sex Vertical transmission rare
Persons at risk of infection	Persons with chronic HBV Injection drug users Sexual contacts of infected persons Infants born to infected mothers Persons with blood product exposure
Long-term sequelae	Chronic infection occurs in 70–80% of exposed superinfected persons 5–20% of exposed coinfected persons Cirrhosis occurs in 5–10 yr in 60–70% of chronically-infected HDV patients Hepatocellular carcinoma Risk is increased more than threefold over isolated HBV infection

Clinical Features

Acute hepatitis D is noted in two disparate forms, *coinfection* and *superinfection.* Coinfection indicates the simultaneous acquisition of HBV and HDV infections, whereas superinfection indicates the appearance of acute HDV infection in a chronic carrier of HBV. Coinfection with the δ agent increases the severity and hastens the progression of HBsAg-associated liver disease [527,528]. Superinfection with the δ agent may be responsible for exacerbation of previously stable disease, a more fulminant course, or a greater tendency to chronicity.

When patients acquire coinfection of HDV with HBV, the incubation period depends on HBV titer but is typically 3–7 weeks (Table 17.32). In the preicteric phase, fatigue, lethargy, anorexia, and nausea occur and may last for 3–7 days. During this phase, ALT levels increase. An icteric phase follows, with increased bilirubin, jaundice, and pale stools. Subsequently, in 80–95% of coinfection cases, a convalescent phase begins, with the resolution of clinical symptoms [529].

Hepatitis D virus infection has a dramatic influence on the clinical course of HBV infection; the alliance of HDV and HBV creates a more ominous situation, both with acute and chronic liver disease. Superinfection of HBV with HDV generally results in a severe acute hepatitis, with chronic HDV persisting in up to 80–97% of cases [530]. Though fulminant hepatitis remains rare, it is about ten times more common with HDV than with other forms of viral hepatitis [531]. The mortality rate for patients with icteric acute HDV ranges from 2–20%, higher than the rate for those with acute HBV, which is less than 1% [526].

Most patients (70–80%) with chronic HDV develop cirrhosis and complications of portal hypertension; this rate is also greater than the 15–30% incidence of end-stage liver disease noted in patients with chronic HBV alone [526]. Chronic HDV is more often a rapidly progressive disease; progression to cirrhosis may occur within 2 years of the onset of infection, though 5–10 years is more typical.

In one long-term study involving 65 HDV patients in institutionalized facilities in Illinois, 11% of residents with HDV died from liver disease 10–35 years after HDV acquisition compared with 0.6% of residents with isolated HBV infection [532]. This study was not able to determine the actual number of deaths caused by HDV before 1986; therefore, the cumulative effect of HDV on the liver was not fully determined. Another long-term study of HDV showed similar results. Bonino et al.

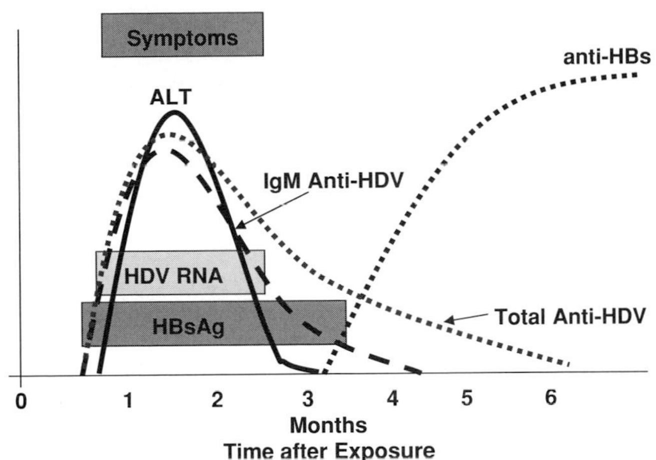

Figure 17.31. Typical serologic pattern with HDV coinfection. Acute HDV–HBV coinfection is characterized by detectable HBsAg followed quickly by detectable HDV RNA. Subsequently, ALT levels increase coincident with clinical symptoms. In some cases, ALT values may fluctuate before improvement. In 80–95% of cases, there is resolution of the infection with disappearance of HBsAg and the development of anti-HBs antibody. When this occurs, HDV replication ceases and biochemical abnormalities resolve [526].

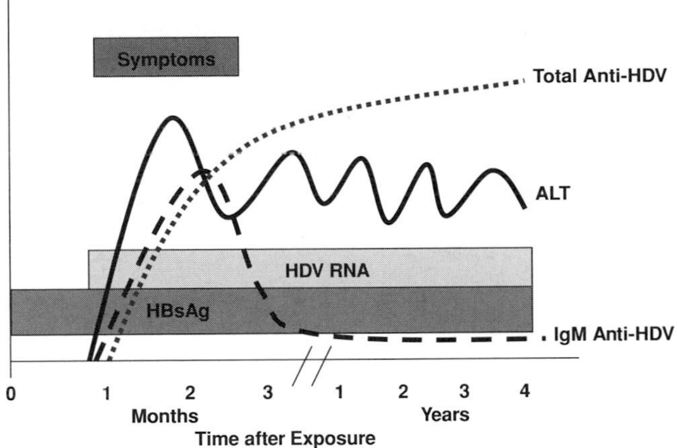

Figure 17.32. Typical serologic pattern with HDV superinfection in a chronic HBV carrier. With HDV superinfection, HBsAg is present before HDV infection. Then, there are marked increases in ALT values and the appearance of HDV RNA, followed by detectable anti-HDV antibody (IgM and total). Unlike in patients with coinfection, chronic progressive liver disease occurs in 70–80% of patients with HDV superinfection. Chronic hepatitis is evident by persistent ALT abnormalities, persistence of HDV RNA replication, and presence of anti-HDV in most cases [526].

[533] followed 176 patients with chronic hepatitis D for 12 years. In this time frame, HDV exerted a 14% mortality rate among this cohort; this rate was three times higher than that of a control group of 149 HBsAg carriers.

In addition to cirrhosis, HDV accelerates the trend toward HCC [534]. The risk of HCC is increased more than threefold [534].

Even among individuals with asymptomatic chronic disease, HDV accelerates liver injury. In a cross-sectional community study in Japan, 210 of 2207 subjects (9.5%) were found to be HBsAg positive. Of this group, 47 (22%) had detectable HDV RNA levels. In these patients, 62% of HDV-infected patients had increased ALT values compared with 9% among isolated HBV-infected patients [535].

The variation in the severity of liver disease noted in different studies has many reasons. Some of the differences are related to study design and patient recruitment variables. Differences in HDV and HBV strains may be related as well.

The typical serologic course of acute HDV and HBV coinfection is shown in Figure 17.31. HBsAg and HDV RNA are detectable before the rise in serum aminotransferase levels and jaundice. The serum ALT levels may rise in a biphasic fashion [526]. There is then clearance of HBsAg, cessation of HDV replication, and resolution of the acute liver disease with the development of antibody to HDV (anti-HDV) and anti-HBs. The anti-HDV titers may be low and appear transiently [526].

The typical serologic profile of acute HDV superinfection of a chronic carrier of HBsAg with normal serum aminotransferase levels, leading to the subsequent development of chronic HDV, is shown in Figure 17.32. This scenario (HDV superinfection) is characterized by a rise in serum ALT levels and the appearance of HDV RNA and, subsequently, anti-HDV in serum. Persistence of HDV replication and consistent abnormalities of liver biochemical tests are present, and HDV RNA remains detectable in serum. Associated with HDV infection acutely is suppression of HBV DNA [532]. Over time, levels of HBV DNA increase with chronic HDV–HBV infection [532].

Hepatitis D in Children

Unusually severe cases of childhood hepatitis, which plagued the Amazon basin and northern Columbia (Santa Marta or Labrea hepatitis), were shown to be caused by HDV superinfection of HBV carriers [536,537]. In a prospective analysis of outbreaks of HBV in alliance with HDV, a high percentage of cases developed fulminant or chronic hepatitis and the case fatality ratio was much higher than expected [517,527,538,539]. Vertical transmission of the δ agent may occur in circumstances that permit perinatal transmission of HBV infection [540,541]. In areas in which HDV infection is endemic, perinatal hepatitis B viremia may allow the coincidental capture of the δ agent.

Diagnosis

Testing for anti-HDV is recommended for any patient with acute or chronic hepatitis who is HBsAg positive. This is especially important when the disease is unusually severe or when the patient emerges from a group at high risk for acquiring hepatitis D (e.g., history of drug abuse, repeated exposures to blood or blood products).

The ability to recognize HDV has been enhanced by more widespread availability of reliable serologic assays (Table 17.33).

Table 17.33: Serologic Differentiation of Acute Hepatitis B Virus, Hepatitis D Virus Coinfection, Hepatitis D Virus Superinfection, and Chronic Hepatitis D Infection

	Anti-HBc (IgM)	*HDVAg*	*Anti-HDV (IgM)*	*HDV RNA*
Acute HBV	+	−	−	−
Acute HDV coinfection	+	+	±	+
Acute HDV superinfection	−	+	+	+
Chronic HDV	−	−	+	+

The diagnostic criteria for chronic hepatitis D are (1) HBsAg positivity and elevated ALT levels for more than 6 months, (2) serum anti-HDV positivity or presence of HDV RNA, and (3) liver biopsy demonstrating HDVAg in hepatocytes attendant to a chronic necroinflammatory disease.

Coinfection with HDV can be distinguished from superinfection through testing for anti-HBc of the IgM subclass, the serologic marker of acute HBV [526,542,543]. Differentiation between acute and chronic HDV infection is based on the presence of anti-HBc IgM, circulating HDV antigen (HDVAg), and anti-HDV IgM [544]. Anti-HBc IgM indicates recent acquisition of HBV (coinfection); HDVAg or anti-HDV IgM indicates acute HDV infection. Superinfected HBV carriers are seronegative for anti-HBc IgM and have circulating HDVAg or anti-HDV IgM [544]. Patients with chronic HDV may be positive for IgA subclass antibodies to the virus (anti-HDV IgA) [544]. The diagnosis of chronic hepatitis D can be confirmed by demonstrating the presence of HDVAg in liver tissue [526].

The most sensitive assay for ongoing HDV infection, both acute and chronic, is RT-PCR. This assay can detect as few as 10 copies of the HDV genome in infected serum [529,531,545]. In individuals with persistently positive RT-PCR results, only about half have a high titer of total anti-HDV [545]. Furthermore, detectable anti-HDV IgM is present in about 60% of patients with chronic disease [545]. This finding is in agreement with previous data that the absence of these anti-HDV antibodies does not rule out active infection in chronic delta hepatitis [546]. Chronic viremia, as indicated by ongoing positivity by PCR, does correlate well with clinical hepatitis; in these subjects, approximately 90% have ALT abnormalities [545].

Treatment

The prognosis of chronic hepatitis D is usually poor. However, several patterns are possible: (1) the disease may be rapidly progressive; (2) insidious disease may be present, which may be relatively asymptomatic but rapidly lead to end-stage liver disease; and (3) in a small percentage of patients, the disease may be nonprogressive [530].

The pattern in an individual patient is not always easy to discern quickly because of the difficulty in monitoring the disease. Analyzing the natural history or response to therapy of patients with chronic HDV infection is problematic. The disappearance of HDV RNA from serum is associated with a decline in ALT levels and improvement in liver histology, but there may be fluctuations in these measurements. Also, HDV RNA reappears with relapse. A decline in the serum anti-HDV titer or disappearance of anti-HDV (IgM) may be useful in monitoring the effects of treatment [526,547]. However, an absence of anti-HDV from serum does not signify complete clearance of virus. Examination of liver tissue for HDV RNA or HDV antigen is a more accurate means of establishing the effect of treatment, though much less pragmatic than serologic tests.

Currently, there is no effective therapy for chronic HDV, and there is a paucity of data regarding antiviral treatments [548–560]. A controlled trial of antiviral therapy of hepatitis D indicated that IFN-α (5 MU/m^2 given three times per week for 4 months followed by 3 MU/m^2 for 8 months) could induce a transient decrease in disease activity and diminish serum HDV RNA levels [549]. Subsequent studies have confirmed that IFN therapy of chronic HDV induces temporary inhibition of HDV replication and lowering of serum ALT levels [548,550–554]. However, relapses are common following discontinuation of therapy. It is possible that either high-dose therapy or long-term maintenance therapy with IFN may be required to control chronic hepatitis D [548]. Besides IFN, several antivirals, including acyclovir, lamivudine, famciclovir, and ribavirin, have not been found to be effective for HDV [556–560].

For those with end-stage liver disease or fulminant failure, liver transplantation should be considered [561,562]. Though graft failure and recurrent HBV–HDV are possible, a multicenter study from Europe reported a 5-year survival rate of 88% among patients with HDV infection who underwent transplantation [561]. To minimize recurrence, anti-HBV prophylaxis is necessary. However, HDV–HBV patients with active HBV replication at the time of transplantation may have an increased risk of HBV recurrence and a poor outcome [562].

Treatment of HDV Infection in Children

Chronic HDV infection usually causes severe liver disease; however, the long-term evolution of HDV infection acquired in childhood is not known. Bortolotti et al. [555] followed 23 children (3–15 years old) with chronic HDV for 5–12 years to determine the outcome. Although 83% of these children had chronic hepatitis when first seen, with cirrhosis in 26%, the clinical and biochemical features remained stable during the observation period. Repeat liver histology, obtained in 14 patients, worsened in 2; 12 were treated with IFN (5 MU three times per week for 12 months), which did not result in any significant change. The clinical and histologic features of these HDV-infected children were more severe than those the authors observed in their series of children with chronic hepatitis B [563–565]. Only 56% of the latter patients had chronic hepatitis, and 3% had cirrhosis [563]; there was also a much higher rate of spontaneous remission [565].

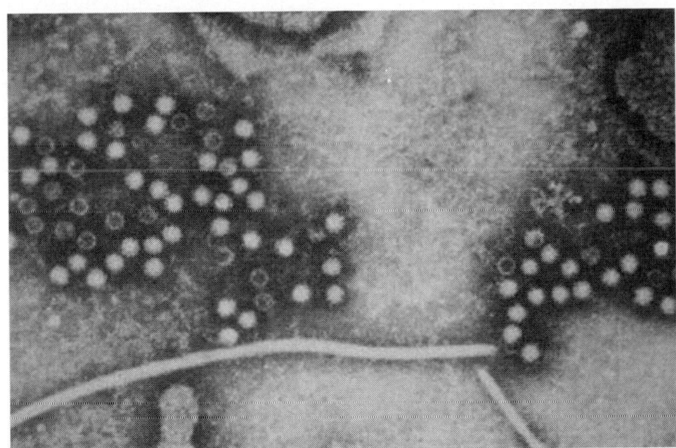

Figure 17.33. Hepatitis E virus in stool on electron microscopy. (From the Centers for Disease Control and Prevention. Hepatitis E virus. [Accessed January 20, 2006, at http:// www.cdc.gov/ncidod/diseases/hepatitis/slideset/hep_e/slide_1.htm.])

HEPATITIS E

Infection by hepatitis E virus (HEV) generally leads to an acute, self-limited, and icteric disease. The first cases of documented HEV occurred in Delhi, India, in 1955 and affected more than 29,000 people [566]. HEV remains highly prevalent, and recent outbreaks in Sudan and Iraq have involved more than 4000 people [567]. HEV infection resembles HAV in many ways [568–576]. HEV has been associated with massive epidemics of hepatitis as well as with sporadic cases in endemic areas.

Viral Characteristics

The hepatitis E virus is a small spherical, nonenveloped, 27- to 32-nm, RNA-containing particle. Its genome is a single-stranded, positive-sense RNA of approximately 7.2 kb with three open reading frames [577].

Hepatitis E, an enterically transmitted virus, has indentations and spikes on its surface and appears similar to calciviruses (Figure 17.33) [569]. On this basis, HEV had been classified in the Calciviridae family from 1988–1998 [566,568]; however, after phylogenetic analysis, differences in the nonstructural regions did not support classification in the Caliciviridae family. At present, HEV is classified in the genus *Hepevirus* of the family Hepeviridae [578].

Hepatitis E virus has been characterized using molecular techniques similar to those successfully applied to the characterization of the HCV [579]. The presumed viral agent was serially transmitted in an animal model (macaque), resulting in typical elevation of aminotransferase values and the detection of characteristic viruslike particles in feces and bile. Bile obtained from the gallbladder of an infected macaque was also shown to be capable of transmitting infection. The bile contained small (32–34-nm) viruslike particles serologically related to HEV, which were used to construct a library of recombinant complementary DNA (cDNAs). Differential hybridization techniques were used to identify putative HEV-cloned sequences. A single-cloned sequence (ET 1.1), absent from uninfected bile, was analyzed by sequence-independent single-primer amplification followed by hybridization probing [579]. ET 1.1 sequences were detected by PCR testing of amplified DNAs isolated from human fecal samples obtained in five geographically disparate areas in which outbreaks of HEV had been documented; these studies suggested that HEV was the primary agent of waterborne hepatitis in these patients.

A specific antigen (HEVAg), expressed in the hepatocytic cytoplasm in the early acute stage of infection, has been shown to induce anti-HEV in infected primates. Anti-HEV is found in acute and convalescent serum samples of patients documented to have enterically transmitted hepatitis (not due to HAV) during outbreaks.

Although only one serotype has been recognized, extensive genomic diversity has been noted among HEV isolates [580]. Currently, HEV isolates have been designated into four genotypes, 1–4 [578,580]. Genotype 1 is most prevalent and accounts for most cases in Asia. In this region, the isolates have 92–99% homology [569]. The second most common genotype, genotype 2, occurs in Mexico and shares only 75% homology with genotype 1. Although HEV is found predominantly in areas with poor sanitation, it has been identified throughout the world, including the United States and Europe [581,582].

Epidemiology

Epidemiologic studies have shown that hepatitis E, like hepatitis A, is predominantly a feces- or water-borne infection noted in developing countries, particularly in areas with inadequate public sanitation or at times of extensive flooding [17,579,583–589]. Outbreaks of enterically transmitted hepatitis (not due to HAV) are often traced to contaminated water supplies. Sporadic cases of HEV have also been described [588]. Even in developed countries, hepatitis E may be identified infrequently. For example, 2.6% of a control population of Japanese children were positive for anti-HEV IgG [590]; however, in this study, HEV was not associated with fulminant hepatitis and was identified in only one case of acute hepatitis.

Hepatitis E virus is the second most common cause of sporadic hepatitis in North Africa and the Middle East [567]. In Hong Kong, HEV was shown to account for one third of the cases of NANB, non-C hepatitis. HEV should therefore be suspected in travelers returning from areas of endemic disease [591].

From epidemiologic studies, it has been postulated that HEV is a zoonosis, with the swine population as a host [567,578,592]. In addition to swine, anti-HEV has been detected in cattle, dogs, rodents, and monkeys [578]. In fact, clusters of HEV in Japan have been traced to the ingestion of undercooked deer meat and pig liver [567].

The development of sensitive assays (most commonly EIAs) for antibody to the HEV (anti-HEV) has confirmed that enterically transmitted HEV is also a major cause of acute sporadic and epidemic hepatitis in children in certain geographic areas [593,594].

There is considerable variability in anti-HEV seroprevalence in endemic regions. In areas such as India, anti-HEV has

Table 17.34: Clinical Features of Hepatitis E Infection

Clinical Feature	*Characteristics*
Signs and symptoms	Jaundice Fatigue Anorexia Nausea Fever Diarrhea Abdominal pain
Incubation period	Average 40 days (range, 15–60 days)
Epidemiology	Highest attack rate among young adults, 15–40 yr Minimal person-to-person transmission Fecal–oral transmission (usually contaminated water) Transmission possible for 14 days after the onset of clinical symptoms Almost all U.S. cases have been related to travel to endemic regions
Persons at risk for more severe infections	Pregnant women Older persons
Complications	Fulminant hepatitis Severe exacerbation of underlying liver disease
Case-fatality rate	~0.2–4% 15–25% among pregnant women
Chronic sequelae	None

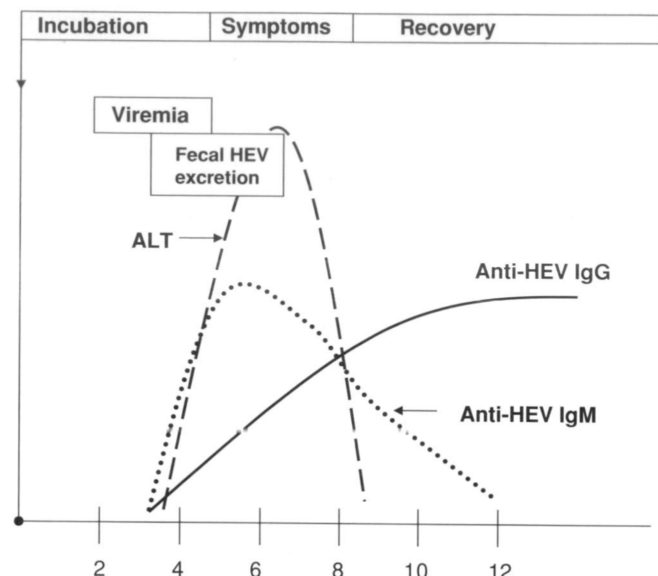

Figure 17.34. Typical course of HEV infection. HEV follows a pattern similar to that of hepatitis A but has a mildly longer incubation period. Following exposure, an average incubation period lasts 5–6 weeks. During this period, viremia and fecal excretion of HEV occur. Biochemical hepatitis marked by elevation of ALT precedes symptomatic infection. Early infection with HEV can be detected with anti-HEV IgM antibody, and lasting immunity is indicated by a sustained elevation in anti-HEV IgG [568].

been detected in as many as 5% of children younger than 10 years; however, in Egypt, antibodies to HEV are found in more than 60% of children by 10 years of age [567]. In India, the seroprevalence rate reaches 30–40% among adults older than 25 years [567,569,595]. In all locations, anti-HEV is less frequent among young children in developing countries than is anti-HAV. This may be the result of its minimal person-to-person transmission along with other variables. Mother-to-child transmission has been documented [596]; in addition, HEV may be transmitted through blood transfusion [597].

Clinical Aspects and Pathogenesis

The clinical manifestations and pathologic features of HEV closely resemble those of HAV; however, there are significant differences (Table 17.34). The incubation period of HEV is somewhat longer, approximately 6 weeks (Figure 17.34). The attack rates for HEV infection are highest in adolescents and young adults (15–40 years), in both epidemic and sporadic forms. HEV infection is predominantly subclinical or anicteric in children [592,598]. Although the overall mortality rate is between 0.2% and 4%, in pregnant women, in whom fulminant disease is highest during the third trimester, the mortality rate is between 15% and 25% [566]. Intrauterine infection with HEV has been observed, contributing significantly to perinatal morbidity and mortality [571]. Apparently, no risk exists for the development of chronic liver disease following acute HEV infection. However, superinfection of HEV in individuals with underlying liver disease may cause severe hepatic decompensation [599–601]. The histology of HEV is somewhat characteristic, with ballooning degeneration, cholestasis, and pseudoglandular changes.

In experimental infections of nonhuman primates, HEV led to variable levels of virus excretion, elevation of ALT levels, and histologic changes in the liver [568]. Although the exact mechanisms for pathogenesis are unknown, ALT elevation typically is coincident with the detection of anti-HEV in the serum and decreasing HEV antigen in hepatocytes. These findings support the role of an immune-mediated response [568]. Additionally, infiltrating lymphocytes in the liver have been found to have a cytotoxic/suppressor immunophenotype [568]. The reasons for more severe liver damage in pregnancy are not known.

Management and Prevention

Currently, passive and active immunizations are not available for hepatitis E. Therefore, the main focus is on prevention. To control infections, it is necessary to provide clean drinking water, assure proper hygiene, and dispose of sewage properly. During an epidemic, improving the water supply can rapidly decrease the number of new cases [602]. Boiling water before consumption appears to reduce the risk of acute HEV infection

[603]. Because of the low person-to-person transmission rate, isolation of affected persons is not indicated.

Administration of immune serum globulin has not been successful in reducing disease in HEV-endemic regions [568,604]. In experimental work, passive transfer of anti-HEV has alleviated HEV infection in monkeys [605]. Similarly, experimental HEV vaccines have shown some promise in experimental models [568,606]. Additional research is needed to further develop effective vaccines and other preventive measures.

CONCLUSION

Because the number of individuals worldwide who have acute and chronic hepatitis is enormous, we must continue to apply proven strategies for eliminating these diseases and discover novel and effective methods of treatment. The rapid pace of viral hepatitis research along with the decrease in the incidence of acute viral hepatitis in the United States indicates that a combination of preventive measures and treatments can limit the morbidity and mortality of these infections. Despite substantial progress, eradicating these viruses remains difficult because of the enormity of the problem, high-risk behaviors, and viral mutations. Furthermore, because of the reservoir of infected individuals, the prevalence of severe chronic liver disease will likely increase despite the decline of acute infections. While awaiting further advances, education of medical care workers and the public about the significant achievements in our understanding of viral hepatitis is essential to realize the benefits of immunoprophylaxis, treatments, and control measures.

REFERENCES

1. Hochman JA, Balistreri WF. Chronic hepatitis: always be current! Pediatr Rev 2003;24:399–409.
2. Centers for Disease Control and Prevention. Hepatitis surveillance report no. 59. Atlanta: U.S. Department of Health and Human Services, Centers for Disease Control and Prevention, 2004:1–60.
3. Havens WP. The etiology of infectious hepatitis. JAMA 1947; 34:653–5.
4. MacCallum FO. Homologous serum jaundice. Lancet 1947;2: 691–2.
5. Krugman S, Giles JP, Hammond DJ. Infectious hepatitis: evidence for two distinctive clinical, epidemiological, and immunologic types of infection. JAMA 1967;200:365–73.
6. Rezende G, Roque-Afonso AM, Samuel D, et al. Viral and clinical factors associated with the fulminant course of hepatitis A infection. Hepatology 2003;38:613–18.
7. Robertson BH, Jansen RW, Khanna B, et al. Genetic relatedness of hepatitis A virus strains recovered from different geographical regions. J Gen Virol 1992;73:1365–77.
8. Fujiwara K, Yokosuka O, Fukai K, et al. Analysis of full-length hepatitis A virus genome in sera from patients with fulminant and self-limited acute type A hepatitis. J Hepatol 2001;35:112–19.
9. Taylor GM, Goldin RD, Karayiannis P, et al. In situ hybridization studies in hepatitis A infection. Hepatology 1992;16:642–8.
10. Ticehurst JR, Racaniello VR, Baroudy BM, et al. Molecular cloning and characterization of hepatitis A virus cDNA. Proc Natl Acad Sci U S A 1983;80:5885–9.
11. Koff RS. Hepatitis A. Lancet 1998;351:1643–9.
12. Craig AS, Schaffner W. Prevention of hepatitis A with the hepatitis A vaccine. N Engl J Med 2004;350:476–81.
13. Rosenblum LS, Villarino M, Nainan OV, et al. Hepatitis A outbreak in a neonatal intensive care unit: risk factors for transmission and evidence of prolonged viral excretion among preterm infants. J Infect Dis 1991;164:476–82.
14. Alter MJ. Nosocomial hepatitis A infection: can we wash our hands of it? Pediatr Infect Dis 1984;3:294–5.
15. Lemon SM. Type A viral hepatitis. N Engl J Med 1985;313:1059–67.
16. Szmuness W, Dienstag JL, Purcell RH, et al. The prevalence of antibody to hepatitis A antigen in various parts of the world. Am J Epidemiol 1977;106:392–8.
17. Mohanavalii B, Dhevahi E, Menon T, et al. Prevalence of antibodies to hepatitis A and hepatitis E virus in urbarn school children in Chennai. Indian Pediatrics 2003;40:328–31.
18. Rosenthal P. Cost-effectiveness of hepatitis A vaccination in children, adolescents, and adults. Hepatology 2003;37:44–51.
19. Centers for Disease Control and Prevention. Hepatitis surveillance report no. 57. Atlanta: U.S. Department of Health and Human Services, Centers for Disease Control and Prevention, 2000.
20. Centers for Disease Control and Prevention. Disease burden from hepatitis A, B, and C in the United States. (Accessed March 20, 2005, at http://www.cdc.gov/nicod/diseases/hepatitis/resource/dz_burden02.htm.)
21. Centers for Disease Control and Prevention. Foodborne transmission of hepatitis A – Massachusetts, 2001. MMWR 2003;52: 565–7.
22. Fiore AE. Hepatitis A transmitted by food. Clin Infect Dis 2004; 38:705–15.
23. Centers for Disease Control and Prevention. Hepatitits A outbreak associated with green onions at a restaurant – Monaca, Pennsylvania, 2003. MMWR 2003;52:1155–7.
24. Wheeler C, Vogt TM, Armstrong GL, et al. An outbreak of hepatitis A associated with green onions. N Engl J Med 2005; 353:890–7.
25. Dentinger CM, Bower WA, Nainan OV, et al. An outbreak of hepatitis A associated with green onions. J Infect Dis 2001;183: 1273–6.
26. Hutin YJF, Pool V, Cramer EH, et al. A multistate, foodborne outbreak of hepatitis A. N Engl J Med 1999;340:595–602.
27. U.S. Food and Drug Administration. Guidance to industry: guide to minimize microbial food safety hazards for fruits and vegetables, 1998. (Accessed at http://www.foodsafety.gov/~dms/prodguid.html.)
28. Weinberg M, Hopkins J, Farrington L, et al. Hepatitis A in Hispanic children who live along the United States-Mexico border: the role of international travel and food-borne exposures. Pediatrics 2004;114:e68–73.
29. Hadler SC, Erben JJ, Francis DP, et al. Risk factors for hepatitis A in day-care centers, J Infect Dis 1982;145:255–61.
30. Benenson MW, Takafuji ET, Bancroft WH, et al. A military community outbreak of hepatitis type A related to transmission in a child care facility. Am J Epidemiol 1980;112:471–81.
31. Vernon AA, Schable C, Francis D. A large outbreak of hepatitis A in a daycare center: association with non-toilet-trained

children and persistence of IgM antibody to hepatitis A virus. Am J Epidemiol 198;115:325–31.

32. Hadler SC, Webster HM, Erber JJ, et al. Hepatitis A in day care centers: a community-wide assessment. N Engl J Med 1980; 302:1222–7.
33. Azimi PH, Roberto RR, Guralnik J, et al. Transfusion acquired hepatitis A in a premature infant with secondary nosocomial spread in an intensive care nursery. Am J Dis Child 1986;140:23–8.
34. Drusin LM, Sohmer M, Groshen SL. Nosocomial hepatitis A infection in a paediatric intensive care unit. Arch Dis Child 1987; 62:690–5.
35. Goodman RA. Nosocomial hepatitis A. Ann Intern Med 1985; 103:452–4.
36. Klein BS, Michaels JA, Rytel MW, et al. Nosocomial hepatitis A: a multi-nursery outbreak in Wisconsin. JAMA 1984;252:2716–21.
37. Amon JJ, Darling N, Fiore AE, et al. Factors associated with hepatitis A vaccination among children 24 to 35 months of age: United States, 2003. Pediatrics 2006;117:30–3.
38. Centers for Disease Control and Prevention. Prevention of hepatitis A through active or passive immunization: recommendations of the Advisory Committee on Immunization Practices (ACIP). MMWR 1999;48(no RR-12):1–39.
39. Lednar WM, Lemon SM, Kirkpatrick JW, et al. Frequency of illness associated with epidemic hepatitis A virus infection in adults. Am J Epidemiol 1985;122:226–33.
40. Vento S, Garofano T, Renzini C, et al. Fulminant hepatitis associated with hepatitis A Virus superinfection in patients with chronic hepatitis C. N Engl J Med 1998;338:286–90.
41. Gauss-Muller V, Deinhardt F. Effect of hepatitis A virus infection on cell metabolism in vitro. Proc Soc Exp Biol Med 1984; 175:10 15.
42. Ida S, Tachikawa N, Nakjima A, et al. Influence of human immunodeficiency virus type I infection on acute hepatitis A virus infection. Clin Infect Dis 2002;34:379–85.
43. Bower WA, Nainan OV, Han X, Margolis HX. Duration of viremia in hepatitis A virus infection. J Infect Dis 2000;182:12–17.
44. Tan H, Kilicaslan B, Onbas O, Buyukavci M. Acute disseminated encephalomyelitis following hepatitis A virus infection. Pediatr Neurol 2004;30:207–9.
45. Islek I, Kalayci AG, Gok F, Muslu A. Henoch-Schonlein purpura associated with hepatitis A infection. Pediatr Int 2003;45:114–16.
46. Centers for Disease Control: Protection against viral hepatitis: recommendations of the Advisory Committee on Immunization Practices (ACIP). MMWR 1990;39(RR-2):1–25.
47. Arora NK, Mathur P, Ahuja A, Oberoi. Acute liver failure. Indian J Pediatr 2003;70:73–9.
48. Stokes J Jr, Neefe JR. The prevention and attenuation of infectious hepatitis by gamma globulin: preliminary note. JAMA 1945;127:144–5.
49. Fujiyama S, Iino S, Odoh K, et al. Time course of hepatitis A virus antibody liter after active and passive immunization. Hepatology 1992;15:983–8.
50. Lemon SM. Inactivated hepatitis A virus vaccines. Hepatology 1992;15:1194–7.
51. Sonder GJB, Van Steenbergen JE, Bovee LPM, et al. Hepatitis A virus immunity and seroconversion among contacts of acute hepatitis A patients in Amsterdam, 1996–2000: an evaluation of current prevention policy. Am J Public Health 2004;94:1620–6.
52. Van Herck K, Van Damme P. Hepatitis A vaccine [letter]. N Engl J Med 2004;350:2211–12.
53. Connor BA, Van Herck K, Van Damme P. Rapid protection and vaccination against hepatitis A for travellers. BioDrugs 2003;17(suppl 1):19–21.
54. Balistreri WF: 'A' new vaccine for an old disease. J Viral Hepat 1996;2:49–59.
55. O'Connor JB, Imperiale TF, Singer ME. Cost-effectiveness analysis of hepatitis a vaccination strategies for adults. Hepatology 1999;30:1077–81.
56. Provost PJ, Banker FS, Giesa PA, et al. Progress toward a live, attenuated human hepatitis A vaccine. Proc Soc Exp Biol Med 1982;170:814.
57. Ellerbeck EF, Lewis JA, Nalin D, et al. Safety profile and immunogenicity of an inactivated vaccine derived from an attenuated strain of hepatitis A. Vaccine 1992;10:668–72.
58. Tilzey AJ, Palmer SJ, Barrow S, et al. Clinical trial with inactivated hepatitis A vaccine and recommendations for its use. Br Med J 1992;304:1272–6.
59. Andre FE, Hepburn A, D'Hondt E: Inactivated candidate vaccines for hepatitis A. Prog Med Virol 1990;37:72–95.
60. Landry P, Tremblay S, Darioli R, Genton B. Inactivated hepatitis A vaccine booster given $\geq$24 months after the primary doses. Vaccine 2000;19:399–402.
61. Das A. An economic analysis of different strategies of immunization against hepatitis A virus in developed countries. Hepatology 1999;29:548–52.
62. Werzberger A, Mensch B, Kuter B, et al. A controlled trial of a formalin-inactivated hepatitis A vaccine in healthy children. N Engl J Med 1992;327:453–7.
63. Innis BL, Snithhan R, Kunasol P, et al. Protection against hepatitis A by an inactivated vaccine. JAMA 1994;271:1328–34.
64. Lee SD, Chan CY, Yu MI, et al. Safety and immunogenicity of inactivated hepatitis A vaccine in patients with chronic liver disease. J Med Virol 1997;52:215–18.
65. Keeffe EB, Iwarson S, McMahon BJ, et al. Safety and immunogenicity of hepatitis A vaccine in patients with chronic liver disease. Hepatology 1998;27:881–6.
66. Neilsen GA, Bodsworth NJ, Watts N. Response to hepatitis A vaccination in human immunodeficiency virus-infected and uninfected homosexual men. J Infect Dis 1997;176:1064–7.
67. Arslan M, Wiesner RH, Poterucha JJ, Zein NN. Safety and efficacy of hepatitis A vaccination in liver transplantation recipients. Transplantation 2001;72:272–6.
68. Wolters B, Junge U, Dziuba S, Roggendorf M. Immunogenicity of combined hepatitis A and B vaccine in elderly persons. Vaccine 2003;21:3623–8.
69. Sagliocca L, Amoroso P, Stroffolini T, et al. Efficacy of hepatitis A vaccine in prevention of secondary hepatitis A infection: a randomised trial. Lancet 1999;353:1136–9.
70. Prikazsky V, Olear V, Cemoch A, et al. Interruption of an outbreak of hepatitis A in two villages by vaccination. J Med Virol 1994;44:457–9.
71. Craig AS, Sockwell DC, Schaffner W, et al. Use of hepatitis A vaccine in a community-wide outbreak of hepatitis A. Clin Infect Dis 1998;27:531–5.
72. Troisi CL, Hollinger FB, Krause DS, et al. Immunization of seronegative infants with hepatitis A vaccine (HAVRIX®;SKB): a comparative study of two dosing schedules. Vaccine 1997;15: 1613–17.

73. Letson GW, Shapiro CN, Kuehn D, et al. Effect of maternal antibody on immunogenicity of hepatitis A vaccine in infants. J Pediatr 2004;144:327–32.
74. Piazza M, Safary A, Vegnente A, et al. Safety and immunogenicity of hepatitis A vaccine in infants: a candidate for inclusion in the childhood vaccination programme. Vaccine 1999;17:585–8.
75. Dagan R, Amir J, Mijalovsky A, et al. Immunization against hepatitis A in the first year of life: priming despite the presence of maternal antibody. Pediatr Infect Dis J 2000;19:1045–52.
76. Fiore AE, Shapiro CN, Sabin K, et al. Hepatitis A vaccination of infants: effecto of maternal antibody status on antibody persistence and response to a booster dose. Pediatr Infect Dis J 2003;22:354–9.
77. Chang CY, Lee SD, Yu MI, et al. Long-term follow-up of hepatitis A vaccination in children. Vaccine 1999;17:369–72.
78. Van Damme P, Banatvala J, Fay O, et al. Hepatitis A booster vaccination: is there a need? Lancet 2003;362:1065–71.
79. Van Herckk, Van Damme P. Inactivated hepatitis A vaccine-induced antibodies: follow-up and estimates of long-term persistence. J Med Virol 2001;63:1–7.
80. Niu MT, Salive M, Krueger C, Ellenberg SS. Two-year review of hepatitis A vaccine safety: data from the Vaccine Adverse Event Reporting System (VAERS). Clin Infect Dis 1998;26:1475–6.
81. American Academy of Pediatrics. Hepatitis A. In: Pickering LK, ed. Red book: 2003 report of the committee on infectious diseases. 26th ed. Elk Grove Village, IL: American Academy of Pediatrics, 2003:309–18.
82. American Academy of Pediatrics, Committee on Infectious Diseases. Recommended childhood and adolescent immunization schedule: United States, 2005. Pediatrics 2005;115:182–6.
83. American Academy of Pediatrics, Committee on Infectious Diseases. Recommended childhood and adolescent immunization schedule – United States, 2006. Pediatrics 2006;117:239–40.
84. Nebbia G, Giacchino R, Soncini R, et al. Hepatitis A vaccination in chronic carriers of hepatitis B. J Pediatr 1999;134:784–5.
85. Koff RS. The case for routine childhood vaccination against hepatitis A. N Engl J Med 1999;340:644–5.
86. Di Giammarino L, Dienstag JL. Hepatitis A – the price of progress [editorial]. N Engl J Med 2005;353:944–6.
87. Bell BP, Shapiro CN, Alter MJ, et al. The diverse patterns of hepatitis A epidemiology in the United States-Implications for vaccination strategies. J Infect Dis 1998;178:1579–84.
88. Centers for Disease Control and Prevention. Combination vaccines for childhood immunization. MMWR 1999;48:1–15.
89. Averhoff F, Shapiro CN, Bell BP, et al. Control of hepatitis A through routine vaccination of children. JAMA 2001;286:2968–73.
90. Werzberger A, Kuter B, Nalin D. Six years' follow-up after hepatitis A vaccination. (Letter to the Editor) N Engl J Med 1998; 338:1160.
91. Armstrong GL, Bell BP. Hepatitis A virus infections in the United States: model-based estimates and implications for childhood immunizations. Pediatrics 2002;109:839–45.
92. Centers for Disease Control and Prevention. Notice to readers: FDA approval of VAQTA®(Hepatititis A vaccine, inactivated) for children aged ≥1 year. MMWR 2005;54:1026.
93. Press release, "CDC's Advisory Committee on Immunization Practices expands Hepatitis A vaccination for children," October 28, 2005. www.havrix.com. Accessed October 30, 2005.
94. Burrell CJ, Mackay P, Greenway DJ, et al. Expression in *Escherichia coli* of hepatitis B virus DNA sequence cloned in plasmid BR-322. Nature 1979;279:43–7.
95. Wang GH, Seeger C. The reverse transcriptase of hepatitis-B virus acts as protein primer for viral DNA synthesis. Cell 1992; 71:663–70.
96. Ganem D, Prince AM. Mechanisms of disease: Hepatitis B virus infection – natural history and clinical consequences. N Engl J Med 2004;350:1118–29.
97. Klingmuller U, Schaller H. Hepadnavirus infection requires interaction between the viral pre-S domain and a specific hepatocellular receptor. J Virol 1993;67:7414–22.
98. Bruss V, Ganem D. The role of envelope proteins in hepatitis B virus assembly. Proc Natl Acad Sci U S A 1991;88:1059–63.
99. Zoulim F, Saputelli J, Seeger C. Woodchuck hepatitis virus X protein is required for viral infection in vivo. J Virol 1994;68: 2026–30.
100. Levrero M, Stemler M, Pasquinelli C, et al. Significance of anti-HBx antibodies in hepatitis B virus infection. Hepatology 1991;13:143–9.
101. Locarnini S, Birch C. Antiviral chemotherapy for chronic hepatitis B infection: lessons learned from treating HIV-infected patients. J Hepatol 1999;30:536–50.
102. Horvath J, Raffanti SP. Clinical aspects of the interactions between human immunodeficiency virus and the hepatotropic viruses. Clin Infect Dis 1994;18:339–47.
103. Prince AM, Lee D-H, Brotman B. Infectivity of blood from PCR-positive, HBsAg-negative, anti-HBs-positive cases of resolved hepatitis B infection. Transfusion 2001;41:329–32.
104. Chisari FV, Ferrari C. Hepatitis B virus immunopathogenesis. Annu Rev Immunol 1995;13:29–60.
105. Chisari FV. Hepatitis B virus transgenic mice: models of viral immunobiology and pathogenesis. Curr Top Mircrobiol Immunol 1996;206:149–73.
106. Guidotti LG, Rochford R, Chung J, et al. Viral clearance without destruction of infected cells during acute HBV infection. Science 1999;284:825–9.
107. Guidotti LG, Ishikawa T, Hobbs MV, et al. Intracellular inactivation of the hepatitis B virus by cytotoxic T lymphocytes. Immunity 1996;4:25–36.
108. DeJongh FE, Janssen HLA, DeMan RA, et al. Survival and prognostic indicators in hepatitis B surface antigen-positive cirrhosis of the liver. Gastroenterology 1992;103:1630–5.
109. Tedder RS, Ijaz S, Gilbert N, et al. Evidence for a dynamic host-parasite relationship in e-negative hepatitis B carriers. J Med Virol 2002;68:505–12.
110. Layden TJ, Laden JE, Ribeiro RM, Perelson AS. Mathematical modeling viral kinetics: a toll to understand and optimize therapy. Clin Liver Dis 2003;7:163–78.
111. Lok AS, McMahon BJ. Chronic hepatitis B (AASLD practice guidelines). Hepatology 2001;34:1225–41.
112. Hoofnagle JH, Dusheiko GM, Seeff LB, et al. Seroconversion from hepatitis B e antigen to antibody in chronic type B hepatitis. Ann Intern Med 1981;94:744–8.
113. Fattovich G, Rugge M, Brollo L, et al. Clinical, virologic and histologic outcome following seroconversion from HBeAg to anti-HBe in chronic hepatitis type B. Hepatology 1986;6:167–72.
114. McMahon BJ, Holck P, Bulkow L, Snowball MM. Serologic and clinical outcomes of 1536 Alaska Natives chronically infected with hepatitis B virus. Ann Int Med 2001;135:759–68.

115. Lok AS, Lai CL, Wu PC, et al. Spontaneous hepatitis e antigen to antibody seroconversion and reversion in Chinese patients with chronic hepatitis B virus infection. Gastroenterology 1987; 92:1839–43.
116. Lok As, Lai CL. A longitudinal follow-up of asymptomatic hepatitis B surface antigen-positive Chinese children. Hepatology 1988;8:1130–3.
117. Chang MH, Hsu HY, Hsu HC, et al. The significance of spontaneous hepatitis e antigen seroconversion in childhood: with special emphasis on the clearance of hepatitis e antigen before 3 years of age. Hepatology 1995;22:1387–92.
118. Lee PI, Chang MH, Lee CY, et al. Changes in serum hepatitis B DNA and aminotransferase levels during the course of chronic hepatitis B virus infection in children. Hepatology 1990;12: 657–60.
119. Bortolotti F, Jara P, Crivellaro C, et al. Outcome of chronic hepatitis B Caucasian children during a 20-year observation period. J Hepatol 1998;29:184–90.
120. Liaw YF, Chu CM, Su IJ, et al. Clinical and histologic events preceding hepatitis B e antigen seroconversion in chronic type B hepatitis. Gastroenterology 1983;84:216–19.
121. Viola LA, Harrison IG, Coleman JC, et al. Natural history of liver disease in chronic hepatitis B surface antigen carriers: survey of 100 patients from Great Britain. Lancet 1981;2:1156–9.
122. Hsu HY, Chang MH, Lee CY, et al. Spontaneous loss of HBsAg in children with chronic hepatitis B virus infection. Hepatology 1992;15:382–6.
123. Gandhi MJ, Yang GG, McMahon B, Vyas G. Hepatitis virions isolated with antibodies to the pre-S1 domain reveal occult viremia in surface antigen negative/antibody-positive carriers by polymerase chain reaction. Transfusion 2000;40:910–16.
124. Yen-Hsuan N, Chang MH, Wang KJ, et al. Clinical relevance of hepatitis B virus genotype in children with chronic infection and hepatocellular carcinoma. Gastroenterology 2004;127: 1733–8.
125. Yuen MF, Sablon E, Wong DKH, et al. Role of hepatitis B virus genotypes in chronic hepatitis B exacerbation. Clin Infect Dis 2003;37:593–7.
126. Furusyo N, Kubo N, Nakashima H, et al. Relationship of genotype rather than race to hepatitis B virus pathogenicity: a study of Japanese and Solomon Islanders. J Trop Med Hyg 2004; 70:571–5.
127. Chu CJ, Hussain M, Lok ASF. Hepatitis B virus genotype B is associated with earlier HBeAg seroconversion compared with hepatitits B virus genotype C. Gastroenterology 2002;122:1756–62.
128. Yuen MF, Sablon E, Yuan HY, et al. Significance of hepatitis B genotype in acute exacerbation, HBeAg serocoversion, cirrhosis-related complications, and hepatocellular carcinoma. Hepatology 2003;37:562–7.
129. Janssen HL, van Zonneveld M, Senturk H, et al. Pegylated interferon alpha-2b alone or in combination with lamivudine for HbeAg-positive chronic hepatitis B: a randomised trial. Lancet 2005;365:123–9.
130. Keefe EB, Dieterich DT, Han SHB, et al. A treatment algorithm for the management of chronic hepatitis B virus infection in the United States. Clin Gastro Hepatol 2004;2:87–106.
131. Stuyver L, Gendt SD, Cadranel JF, et al. Three cases of severe subfulminant hepatitis in heart-transplanted patients after nosocomial transmission of mutant hepatitis B virus. Hepatology 1999;29:1876–83.
132. Bonino F, Brunetto MR, Rizzetto M, et al. Hepatitis B virus unable to secret E antigen. Gastroenterology 1991;100:1138–41.
133. Sung J, Chan HL-Y, Wong ML, et al. Relationship of clinical and virological factors with hepatitis activity in hepatitis B e antigen-negative chronic hepatitis B virus-infected patients. J Viral Hepat 2002;9:229–34.
134. Chan HLY, Leung NWY, Hussain M, et al. Hepatitis B e antigen–negative chronic hepatitis B in Hong Kong. Hepatology 2000;31:763–8.
135. Erhardt A, Reineke U, Blondin D, et al. Mutations of the core promoter and response to interferon treatment in chronic replicative hepatitis B. Hepatology 2000;31:716–25.
136. Liang TJ, Hasegawa K, Rimon N. A hepatitis B virus mutant associated with an epidemic of fulminant hepatitis. N Engl J Med 1991;324:1705–9.
137. Omata M, Ehata T, Yokosuka O, et al. Mutations in the precore region of hepatitis B virus DNA in patients with fulminant and severe hepatitis. N Engl J Med 1991;324:1699–704.
138. Terazawa S, Kojima M, Yamanaka T, et al. Hepatitis B virus mutants with precore-region defects in two babies with fulminant hepatitis and their mothers positive for antibody to hepatitis B antigen. Pediatr Res 1991;29:5–9.
139. Yotsumoto S, Kojima M, Shoji I, et al. Fulminant hepatitis related to transmission of hepatitis B variants with precore mutations between spouses. Hepatology 1992;16:31–5.
140. Magnius LO, Norder H. Subtypes, genotypes and molecular epidemiology of the hepatitis B virus as reflected by sequence variability of the S-gene. Intervirology 1995;38:24–34.
141. Hsu HY, Chang MH, Liaw SH, et al. Changes of hepatitis B surface antigen variants in carrier children before and after universal vaccination in Taiwan. Hepatology 1999;30:1312–17.
142. Okamoto H, Yano K. Nozaki Y, et al. Mutations with the S gene of hepatitis B virus transmitted from mothers to babies immunized with hepatitis B immune globulin and vaccine. Pediatr Res 1992;32:264–8.
143. Lee W. Hepatitis B virus infection. N Engl J Med 1997;337: 1733–45.
144. Alter MJ, Coleman PJ, Alexander WJ, et al. Importance of heterosexual activity in the transmission of hepatitis B and non-A, non-B hepatitis. JAMA 1989;262:1201–9.
145. Rosenblum L, Darrow W, Witte J, et al. Sexual practices in the transmission of hepatitis B virus and prevalence of hepatitis delta virus infection in female prostitutes in the United States. JAMA 1992;267:2477–81.
146. Alter HJ. The evolution, implications, and applications of the hepatitis B vaccine. JAMA 1982;247:2272–5.
147. Kelen GD, Green GB, Purcell RH, et al. Hepatitis B and hepatitis C in emergency department patients. N Engl J Med 1992; 326:1399–404.
148. Nebbia G, Moroni GA, Simoni L, et al. Hepatitis B virus in multitransfused hemophiliacs. Arch Dis Child 1986;61:580–4.
149. Seeff LB, Koff RS. Passive and active immunoprophylaxis of hepatitis B. Gastroenterology 1984;86:958–81.
150. Polish LB, Shapiro CN, Bauer F, et al. Nosocomial transmission of hepatitis B virus associated with the use of spring-loaded finger-stick device. N Engl J Med 1992;326:721–5.
151. Bove JR. Transfusion-associated hepatitis and AIDS: what is the risk? N Engl J Med 1987;317:242–4.
152. Centers for Disease Control and Prevention. Achievements in public health: hepatitis B vaccination – United States, 1982–2002. MMWR 2002;31:549–53, 563.

153. Centers for Disease Control. Summary of notifiable diseases – United States 2002. MMWR 2004;51:1–88.
154. Chang MW, Chen TH-H, Hsu H-M, et al. Prevention of hepatocellular carcinoma by universal vaccination against hepatitis B virus: the effect and problems. Clin Cancer Res 2005;11:7953–7.
155. Goldstein ST, Alter MJ, Williams IT, et al. Incidence and risk factors for acute hepatitis B in the United States, 1982–1998: implications for vaccination programs. J Infect Dis 2002;185:713–19.
156. Weinbaum C, Goldstein S, Subiadur J. Hepatitis B in women: domestically and internationally [conference summary]. Emerg Infect Dis [serial on the internet] 2004. (Accessed March 13, 2005, at http://www.cdc.gov/ncidod/EID/vol10no11/04-0624_02.htm.)
157. Wilson BC, Moyer LA, Schmid G, et al. Hepatitis B vaccination in sexually transmitted disease (STD) clinics: a survey of STD programs. Sex Transm Dis 2001;28:148–52.
158. Centers for Disease Control. Incidence of acute hepatitis B – United States, 1990–2002. MMWR 2004;52:1252–4.
159. Mahoney FJ, Stewart K, Hu H, et al. Progress toward the elimination of hepatitis B virus transmission among health care workers in the United States. Arch Intern Med 1997;157:2601–5.
160. Harpaz R, McMahon BJ, Margolis HS, et al. Elimination of new chronic hepatitis virus infections: results of the Alaska immunization program. J Infect Dis 2000;181:413–18.
161. Tong MJ, Thursby M, Rakela J, et al. Studies on the maternal-infant transmission of the viruses which cause acute hepatitis. Gastroenterology 1981;80:999–1003.
162. Stevens CE, Toy PT, Tong MJ, et al. Perinatal hepatitis B virus transmission in the United States. JAMA 1985;253:1740–5.
163. Woo D, Cummins M, Davies PA, et al. Vertical transmission of hepatitis B surface antigen in carrier mothers in two West London hospitals. Arch Dis Child 1979;54:670–5.
164. Hwang L-Y. Perinatal transmission of hepatitis B virus: role of maternal HBeAg and anti-HBc IgM. J Med Virol 1985;15:265–71.
165. Lee SD, Lo KJ, Wu JC, et al. Prevention of maternal-infant hepatitis B virus transmission by immunization: the role of serum hepatitis B virus DNA. Hepatology 1986;6:369–73.
166. Okada K, Kamiyama I, Inomata M, et al. E antigen and anti-E in the serum of asymptomatic carrier mothers as indicators of positive and negative transmission of hepatitis B virus to their infants. N Engl J Med 1976;294:746–9.
167. Snydman DR. Medical intelligence: current concepts: hepatitis in pregnancy. N Engl J Med 1985;313:1398–404.
168. Shimizu H, Mitsuda T, Fujita S, et al. Perinatal hepatitis B virus infection caused by antihepatitis B e positive maternal mononuclear cells. Arch Dis Child 1991;66:718–21.
169. Wang J, Zhu Q. Infection of the fetus with hepatitis B e antigen via the placenta. Lancet 2000;355:989.
170. Bortolotti P, Cadrobbi P, Armigliato M, et al. Prognosis of chronic hepatitis B transmitted from HBsAg positive mothers. Arch Dis Child 1987;62:201–3.
171. Bortolotti F, Calzia R, Cadrobbi P, et al. Liver cirrhosis associated with chronic hepatitis B infection in childhood. J Pediatr 1986;108:224–7.
172. Chang MH, Hwang LY, Hsu HC, et al. Prospective study of asymptomatic HBsAg carrier children infected in the perinatal period: clinical and liver histologic studies. Hepatology 1988;8:374–7.
173. Schweitzer IL, Dunn AEG, Peters RL. Viral hepatitis B in neonates and infants. Am J Med 1973;55:762–71.
174. Stevens CE, Beasley BP, Tsui J, et al. Vertical transmission of hepatitis B antigen in Taiwan. N Engl J Med 1975;292:771–4.
175. Hsu HY, Chang MH, Hsieh KH, et al. Cellular immune response to HBcAg in mother-to-infant transmission of hepatitis B virus. Hepatology 1992;15:770–6.
176. Milich DR, Jones JE, Hughes JL, et al. Is a function of the secreted hepatitis B antigen to induce immunologic tolerance in utero. Proc Natl Acad Sci U S A 1990;87:6599–603.
177. Beath SV, Boxall EH, Watson RM, et al. Fulminant hepatitis B in infants born to anti-HBe hepatitis B carrier mothers. Br Med J 1992;304:1169–70.
178. Delaplane D, Yogev R, Crussi F, et al. Fatal hepatitis B in early infancy: the importance of identifying HBsAg-positive pregnant women and providing immunoprophylaxis to their newborns. Pediatrics 1983;72:176–80.
179. Sinatra FR, Shah P, Weissman JY, et al. Perinatal transmitted acute icteric hepatitis B in infants born to hepatitis surface antigen-positive and anti-hepatitis B positive carrier mothers. Pediatrics 1982;70:557–9.
180. Chang MH, Lee CY, Chen DS, et al. Fulminant hepatitis in children in Taiwan: the important role of hepatitis B virus. J Pediatr 1987;111:34–9.
181. Hostetter MK, Iverson S, Thomas W, et al. Medical evaluation of internationally adopted children. N Engl J Med 1991;325:479–85.
182. Hershow RC, Hadier SC, Kane MA. Adoption of children from countries with endemic hepatitis B: transmission risks and medical issues. Pediatr Infect Dis J 1987;6:431–7.
183. Hurie MB, Mast EE, Davis JP. Horizontal transmission of hepatitis B virus infection to United States-born children of among refugees. Pediatrics 1992;89:269–73.
184. Christenson B. Epidemiological aspects of the transmission of hepatitis B by HBsAg-positive adopted children. Scand J Infect Dis 1986;18:105–9.
185. Beasley RP, Hwang LY, Lin CC, et al. Hepatitis B immune globulin (HBIG) efficacy in the interpretation of perinatal transmission of hepatitis B virus carrier state. Lancet 1981;ii:388–93.
186. Hsu SC, Chang MH, Ni YH, et al. Horizontal transmission of hepatitis B virus in children. J Pediatr Gastroenterol Nutr 1993;16:66–9.
187. Tsiquaye KN, McCaul TF, Zuckerman AJ, et al. Maternal transmission of duck hepatitis B virus in pedigree Peking ducks. Hepatology 1985;5:622–7.
188. Vegnente A, Iorio R, Guida S, et al. Chronicity rate of hepatitis B virus infection in the families of 60 hepatitis B surface antigen positive chronic carrier children: role of horizontal transmission. Eur J Pediatr 1992;151:188–91.
189. Franks AL, Berg CJ, Kane MA, et al. Hepatitis B virus infection among children born in the United States to Southeast Asian refugees. N Engl J Med 1989;321:1301–5.
190. Han SH B. Extrahepatic manifestations of chronic hepatitis B. Clin Liver Dis 2004;8:403–18.
191. Wands JR, Alpert E, Isselbacher KJ. Arthritis associated with chronic active hepatitis: complement activation and characterization of circulating immune complexes. Gastroenterology 1975;69:1286–91.
192. Popp Jr JW, Harrist TJ, Dienstag JL, et al. Cutaneous vasculitis associated with acute and chronic hepatitis. Arch Intern Med 1981;141:623–9.

193. Alpert E, Isselbacher KJ, Schur PH. The pathogenesis of arthritis associated with viral hepatitis. Complement-component studies. N Engl J Med 1971;285:185–9.
194. Lai KN, Li PKT, Lui SF, et al. Membranous nephropathy related to hepatitis B virus in adults. N Engl J Med 1991;324:1457–63.
195. Southwest Pediatrics Study Group. Hepatitis B surface antigenemia in North American children with membranous glomerulonephropathy. J Pediatr 1985;106:571–8.
196. Duffy J, Lidsky MD, Sharp JT. Polyarthritis, polyarteritis, and hepatitis B. Medicine 1976;55:19–37.
197. McMahon BJ, Alberts SR, Wainwright RB, et al. Hepatitis B-related sequelae: prospective study in 1400 hepatitis B surface antigen-positive Alaska native carriers. Arch Intern Med 1990; 150:1051–4.
198. Gianotti F. Papular acrodermatitis of childhood: an Australian antigen disease. Arch Dis Child 1973;48:794–9.
199. Yoshida, M, Tsuda N, Morihata T, et al. Five patients with localized facial eruptions associated with Gianotti-Crosti syndrome caused by primary Epstein-Barr virus infection. J Pediatr 2004;145:843–4.
200. Draelos ZK, Hansen RC, James WD. Gianotti-Crosti syndrome associated with infections other than hepatitis B. JAMA 1986;256:2386–8.
201. Chan G, Kowdley KV. Extrahepatic manifestations of chronic viral hepatitis. Compr Ther 1995;21:200–5.
202. Hoofnagle JH, DiBisceglie AM. Serologic diagnosis of acute and chronic viral hepatitis. Semin Liver Dis 1991;11:73–83.
203. Malter JS, Gerber MA. The polymerase chain reaction for hepatitis B virus DNA. Hepatology 1991;13:188–90.
204. Shindo M, Okuno T, Arai K, et al. Detection of hepatitis B virus DNA in paraffin-embedded liver tissues in chronic hepatitis B or non A, non B hepatitis using the polymerase chain reaction. Hepatology 1991;13:167–71.
205. Yokosuka O, Omata M, Hosoda K, et al. Detection and direct sequencing of hepatitis B virus genome by DNA amplification method. Gastroenterology 1991;100:175–81.
206. Baker BL, Di Bisceglie AM, Kaneko S, et al. Determination of hepatitis B virus DNA in serum using the polymerase chain reaction: clinical significance and correlation with serological and biochemical markers. Hepatology 1991;13:632–6.
207. Cacciola I, Pollicino T, Squadrito G, et al. Occult hepatitis B virus infection in patients with hepatitis C liver disease. N Engl J Med 1999;341:22–6.
208. Kao JH, Chen PJ, Lai MY, Chen DS. Hepatitis B genotypes correlate with clinical outcomes in patients with chronic hepatitis B. Gastroenterology 2000;118:554–9.
209. Chang MH, Chen CJ, Lai MS, et al. Universal hepatitis B vaccination in Taiwan and the incidence of hepatocellular carcinoma in children. N Engl J Med 1997;336:1855–9.
210. Broderick A, Jonas MM. Management of hepatitis B in children. Clin Liver Dis 2004;8:387–401.
211. Manno M, Camma C, Schepia F, et al. Natural history of chronic HBV carriers in Northern Italy: morbidity and mortallity after 30 years. Gastroeneterology 2004;127:756–63.
212. Chen CH, Chen YY, Chen GH, et al. Hepatitis B virus transmission and hepatocarcinogenesis: a 9 year retrospective cohort of 13,676 relatives with hepatocellular carcinoma. J Hepatol 2004; 40:653–9.
213. Beasley RP. Hepatitis B virus: the major etiology of hepatocellular carcinoma. Cancer 1988;61:1942–56.
214. Committee on Infectious Diseases: Prevention of hepatitis B virus infections. Pediatrics 1985;75:362–4.
215. Dienstag JL. Passive-active immunoprophylaxis after percutaneous exposure to hepatitis B virus [editorial]. Hepatology 1989;10:385–7.
216. Grady GF, Lee VA, Prince AM, et al. Hepatitis B immune globulin for accidental exposures among medical personnel: final report of a multicenter controlled trial. J Infect Dis 1978;138: 625–38.
217. Seeff LB, Wright EC, Zimmerman JH, et al. Type B hepatitis after needlestick exposure: prevention with hepatitis B immunoglobulin: final report of the Veterans Administration Cooperative Study. Ann Intern Med 1978;88:285–93.
218. Mitsui T, Iwano K, Suzuki S, et al. Combined hepatitis B immune globulin and vaccine for postexposure prophylaxis of accidental hepatitis B virus infection in hemodialysis staff members: comparison with immune globulin without vaccine in historical controls. Hepatology 1989;10:324–7.
219. Prince AM, Szmuness W, Mann MK. Hepatitis B immune globulin: final report of a controlled multicenter trial of efficacy in prevention of dialysis-associated hepatitis. J Infect Dis 1978;137:131–44.
220. U.S. Department of Health and Human Services. Healthy people 2010. Conference ed., 2 vols. Washington, D.C.: U.S. Department of Health and Human Services, 2000.
221. Beasley RP, Hwang LY, Lee GCY, et al. Prevention of perinatally transmitted hepatitis B virus infection with hepatitis B immune globulin and hepatitis B vaccine. Lancet 1983;ii:1099–102.
222. Maupas P, Barin F, Chiron JP. Efficacy of hepatitis B vaccine in prevention of early HBsAg carrier state in children: controlled trial in an endemic area (Senegal). Lancet 1981;i:289–95.
223. Nair PV, Weissman JY, Tong MJ, et al. Efficacy of hepatitis B immune globulin in prevention of perinatal transmission of the hepatitis B virus. Gastroenterology 1984;87:293–8.
224. Reesink HW, Reerins-Brongers EE, Lafeber-Schut, et al. Prevention of chronic HBsAg carrier state in infants of HBsAg positive mothers by hepatitis B immunoglobulin. Lancet 1979;ii: 436–8.
225. Tong MJ, Nair PV, Thursby M, et al. Prevention of hepatitis B infection by hepatitis B immune globulin in infants born to mothers with acute hepatitis during pregnancy. Gastroenterology 1985;89:160–7.
226. Zanetti AR, Ferroni P, Magliano EM, et al. Perinatal transmission of the hepatitis B virus and of the HBV-associated delta agent from mothers of offspring in Northern Italy. J Med Virol 1982;9:139–48.
227. Poovorawan Y, Sanpavat S, Pongpunlert W, et al. Protective efficacy of a recombinant DNA hepatitis B vaccine in neonates of HBe antigen-positive mothers. JAMA 1989;261:3278–81.
228. Chung WT, Tong MH, Hwang B, et al. Prevention of perinatal transmission of hepatitis B virus: a comparison between the efficacy of passive and passive-active immunization in Korea. Hepatology 1987;7:46–8.
229. Kanai K, Takehiro A, Noto H, et al. Prevention of perinatal transmission of hepatitis B virus (HBV) to children of E antigen-positive HBV carrier mothers by hepatitis B immune globulin and HBV vaccine. J Infect Dis 1985;151:287–91.
230. Lo KJ, Lee SD, Tsai YT, et al. Long-term immunogenicity and efficacy of hepatitis B vaccine in infants born to HBeAg-positive HBsAg-carrier mothers. Hepatology 1988;8:1647–50.

231. Mazal JA. Passive-active immunization of neonates of HBsAg positive carrier mothers: preliminary observations. Br Med J 1984;288:513–16.
232. Tada H, Yanagida M, Mishini J, et al. Combined passive and active immunization for preventing perinatal transmission of hepatitis virus carrier state. Pediatrics 1982;70:613–19.
233. Wong VCW, Ip HMH, Reesink HW, et al. Prevention of the HBsAg and HBeAg by administration of hepatitis-B vaccine and hepatitis-B immunoglobulin: double blind randomized placebo-controlled study. Lancet 1984;i:921–6.
234. Coursaget P, Yvonnet B, Chotard J, et al. Seven year study of hepatitis B vaccine efficacy in infants from an endemic area (Senegal). Lancet 1986;2:1143–6.
235. Beasley RP, Hwang LY, Stevens CE, et al. Efficacy of hepatitis B immune globulin for prevention of perinatal transmission of the hepatitis B virus carrier state: final report of a randomized double-blind, placebo-controlled trial. Hepatology 1983;3:135–51.
236. Hsu HM, Chen DS, Chuang CH, et al. Efficacy of a mass hepatitis B vaccination program in Taiwan: studies on 3464 infants of hepatitis B surface antigen-carrier mothers. JAMA 1989;260:2231–5.
237. Niu MT, Targonski PV, Stoll BJ, et al. Prevention of perinatal transmission of the hepatitis-B virus- outcome of infants in a community prevention program. Am J Dis Child 1992;146:793 6.
238. Xu ZY, Liu CB, Francis DP, et al. Prevention of perinatal acquisition of hepatitis B virus carriage using vaccine: preliminary report of randomized, double-blind placebo-controlled and comparative trial. Pediatrics 1985;70:713–18.
239. Stevens CE, Taylor PE, Tong MJ, et al. Yeast-recombinant hepatitis B vaccine: efficacy with hepatitis B immune globulin in prevention of perinatal hepatitis B virus transmission. JAMA 1987;257:2612–16.
240. Centers for Disease Control: Prevention of perinatal transmission of hepatitis B virus: prenatal screening of all pregnant women for hepatitis B surface antigen. Recommendations of the Immunization Practices Advisory Committee. MMWR 1988;37:341–5.
241. Kane MA, Hadler SC, Margolis HS, et al. Routine prenatal screening for hepatitis B surface antigen. JAMA 1988;259:408–9.
242. Schalm SW, Mazel HA, de Gast GC, et al. Prevention of hepatitis B infection in newborns through mass screening and delayed vaccination of all infants of mothers with hepatitis B surface antigen. Pediatrics 1989;83:1041–7.
243. Kumar ML, Dawson NL, Heriz R, et al. Hepatitis B risk factors (USPHS) fail to detect HBsAg(+) pregnant women in urban population. Gastroenterology 1987;92:1746–7.
244. McQuillan GM, Townsend TR, Johannes CB, et al. Prevention of perinatal transmission of hepatitis B virus: the sensitivity, specificity, and predictive value of the recommended screening questions to detect high-risk women in an obstetric population. Am J Epidemiol 1987;126:484–91.
245. Summers PR, Biswas MK, Pastorek JG, et al. The pregnant hepatitis B carrier: evidence favoring comprehensive antepartum screening. Obstet Gynecol 1987;69:701–4.
246. Wetzel A. Kirz D. Routine hepatitis screening in adolescent pregnancies: is it cost effective? Am J Obstet Gynecol 1987;156:166–9.
247. Committee on Infectious Diseases. Universal hepatitis B immunization [correction notice appears in Pediatrics 1992;90:715]. Pediatrics 1992;89:795–800.
248. Centers for Disease Control and Prevention. Hepatitis B virus: a comprehensive strategy for limiting transmission in the United States through universal childhood vaccination. Recommendations of the Advisory Committee on Immunization Practices (ACIP). MMWR 1991;40(RR-13):1–25.
249. Hall CB, Halsey NA. Control of hepatitis B: to be or not to be? Pediatrics 1992;90:274–7.
250. Halsey NA, Moulton LH, O'Donovan C, et al. Hepatitis B vaccine administered to children and adolescents at yearly intervals. Pediatrics 1999;103:1243–7.
251. Lauderdale DS, Oram RJ, Goldstein KP, Daum RS. Hepatitis B vaccination among children in inner-city public housing, 1991–1997. JAMA 1999;282:1725–30.
252. Stevens CE, Toy PI, Taylor PE, et al. Prospects for control of hepatitis B virus infection: implications of childhood vaccination and long-term protection. Pediatrics 1992;90:170–3.
253. Chen DS, Hsu NHM, Sung JL, et al. A mass vaccination program in Taiwan against hepatitis B virus infection in infants of hepatitis B surface antigen-carrier mothers. JAMA 1987;257:2597–603.
254. Tabor E. Hepatitis B vaccine: different regimens for different geographic regions. J Pediatr 1985;106:777–8.
255. Krahn M, Guasparini R, Sherman M, Detsky AS. Costs and cost-effectiveness of a universal, school-based hepatitis B vaccination program. Am J Public Health 1998;88:1638–44.
256. Chotard J, Inskip HM, Hall AJ, et al. The Gambia hepatitis intervention study: follow-up of a cohort of children vaccinated against hepatitis-B. J Infect Dis 1992;166:764–8.
257. Salleras L, Bruguera M, Vidal J, et al. Prevalence of hepatitis-B markers in the population of Catalonia (Spain): rationale for universal vaccination of adolescents. Eur J Epidemiol 1992;8:640–4.
258. Klish SW, Wang W, Linton L, et al. Vaccination coverage among adolescents 1 year before the institution of a seventh grade school entry vaccination requirement – San Diego, California, 1998. MMWR 2000;49:101–11.
259. American Academy of Pediatrics. Hepatitis B. In: Pickering LK, ed. Red book: 2003 report of the Committee on Infectious Diseases. 26th ed. Elk Grove Village, IL: American Academy of Pediatrics, 2003:318–36
260. Cassidy WM, Watson B, Ioli VA, et al. A randomized trial of alternative two- and three-dose hepatitis B vaccination regimens in adolescents: antibody responses, safety, and immunologic memory. Pediatrics 2001;107:626–31.
261. Yu AS, Cheung RC, Keeffe EB. Hepatitis B vaccines. Clin Liver Dis 2004;8:283–300.
262. Stevens CE, Alter HJ, Taylor PE, et al. Hepatitis B vaccine in patients receiving hemodialysis. Immunogenicity and efficacy. N Engl J Med 1984;311:496–501.
263. Koff RS. Vaccines and hepatitis B. Clin Liver Dis 1999;3:417–28.
264. Wainwright RB, McMahon BJ, Bulkow LR, et al. Duration of immunogenicity and efficacy of hepatitis B vaccine in a Yupik Eskimo Population. JAMA 1989;261:2362–6.
265. Wainwright RB, McMahon BJ, Bulkow LR, et al. Protection provided by hepatitis B vaccine in a Yupik Eskimo population. Arch Intern Med 1991;151:1634–40.

266. Coursaget P, Leboulleux D, Soumare M, et al. Twelve-year follow-up study of hepatitis B immunization of Senegalese infants. J Hepatol 1994;21:250–4.
267. Liao SS, Li RC, Li H, et al. Long-term efficacy of plasma-derived hepatitis B vaccine: a 15-year follow-up study among Chinese children. Vaccine 1999;17:2661–6.
268. European Consensus Group on Hepatitis B Immunity. Are booster immunisations needed for lifelong hepatitis B immunity? Lancet 2000;355:561–5.
269. Huang LM, Chiang BL, Lee CY, et al. Long-term response to hepatitis B vaccination and response to booster in children born to mothers with hepatitis B e antigen. Hepatology 1999;29:954–9.
270. Szmuness W, Stevens CE, Harley EJ. Hepatitis B vaccine: demonstration of efficacy in a controlled clinical trial in a high-risk population in the United States. N Engl J Med 1980;303:833–41.
271. Hadler SC, Francis DP, Maynard JE, et al. Long-term immunogenicity and efficacy of hepatitis B vaccine in homosexual men. N Engl J Med 1986;315:209–16.
272. Coursaget P, Yvonnet B, Gilks WR, et al. Scheduling of revaccination against hepatitis B virus. Lancet 1991;337:1180–3.
273. Hadler SC. Are booster doses of hepatitis B vaccine necessary? Ann Intern Med 1988;108:457–8.
274. Horowitz MM, Erschler WB, McKinney WP, et al. Duration of immunity after hepatitis B vaccination: efficacy of low-dose booster vaccine. Ann Intern Med 1988;108:185–9.
275. Scolnick EM, McLean AA, West DJ, et al. Clinical evaluation in healthy adults of a hepatitis B vaccine made by recombinant DNA. JAMA 1984;251:2812–15.
276. Zajac BA, West DJ, McAleer WJ, et al. Overview of clinical studies with hepatitis B vaccine made by recombinant DNA. J Infect 1986;13(suppl A):39–43.
277. Bryan JP, Sjogren MH, Perine PL, et al. Low-dose intradermal and intramuscular vaccination against hepatitis B. Clin Infect Dis 1992;14:697–707.
278. Nagafuchi S, Kashiwagi S, Okada K, et al. Reversal of nonresponders and postexposure prophylaxis by intradermal hepatitis B vaccination in Japanese medical personnel. JAMA 1991;265:2679–83.
279. Emini EA, Ellis RW, Miller WJ, et al. Production and immunological analysis of recombinant hepatitis B vaccine. J Infect 1986;13(suppl A):3–9.
280. Murray DL, Goetz A, Yu YL. Protecting tomorrow's health care professionals against hepatitis B virus today. Arch Intern Med 1991;151:1069–70.
281. Ascherio A, Zhang SM, Hernan MA, et al. Hepatitis B vaccination and the risk of multiple sclerosis. N Engl J Med 2001;344:327–32.
282. Sadovnick AD, Scheifele DW. School-based hepatitis B vaccination programme and adolescent multiple sclerosis. Lancet 2000;355:549–50.
283. Institute of Medicine, Stratton K, Almario DA, McCormick MC, eds. Immunization safety review: hepatitis B vaccine and demyelinating neurological disorders. Washington, DC: National Academies Press, 2002.
284. Perrillo RP. Antiviral agents in the treatment of chronic viral hepatitis. In: Boyer JL, Ockner RK, eds. Progress in liver disease. Vol X. Philadelphia: WB Saunders, 1992:283–309.
285. Perrillo RP. Interferon in the management of chronic hepatitis B. Dig Dis Sci 1993;38:577–93.
286. Hoofnagle JH. Current status and future directions in the treatment of chronic viral hepatitis. In: Hollinger FB, Lemon SM, Margolis HS, eds. Viral hepatitis and liver disease. Baltimore: Williams & Wilkins, 1991:632–9.
287. Peters M. Mechanisms of action of interferons. Semin Liver Dis 1989;9:235–9.
288. Peters M, Vierling J, Gershwin ME, et al. Immunology and the liver. Hepatology 1991;13:977–94.
289. Greenberg HBV, Pollard RB, Lutwick LI, et al. Effect of human leukocyte interferon on hepatitis B virus infection in patients with chronic active hepatitis. N Engl J Med 1976;295:517–22.
290. Perrillo RP, Schiff ER, David GL, et al. A randomized, controlled trial of interferon alfa-2b alone and after prednisone withdrawal for the treatment of chronic hepatitis B. N Engl J Med 1990;323:295–301.
291. Alexander GJM, Brahm J, Fagan EA. et al. Loss of HBsAg with interferon therapy in chronic hepatitis B virus infection. Lancet 1987;i:66–8.
292. Hoofnagle GJM, Peters MG, Mullen KD, et al. Randomized controlled trial of a four-month course of recombinant human alpha interferon type B hepatitis. Gastroenterology 1988;95:1318–25.
293. Fevery J, Elewaut A, Michielsen P, et al. Efficacy of interferon alfa-2b with or without prednisone withdrawal in the treatment of chronic viral hepatitis B: a prospective double-blind Belgian-Dutch study. J Hepatol 1990;11:S108–12.
294. Saracco G, Mazzelia G, Rosina F, et al. A controlled trial of human lymphoblastoid interferon in chronic hepatitis B in Italy. Hepatology 1989;10:336–41.
295. Perez V, Tanno H, Vallamil F, et al. Recombinant interferon alfa-2b following prednisone withdrawal in the treatment of chronic type B hepatitis. J Hepatol 1990;11:S113–17.
296. Waked I, Amin M, El Fattah SA, et al. Experience with interferon in chronic hepatitis B in Egypt. J Chemother 1990;2:310–18.
297. Muller R, Baumgarten R, Markus R, et al. Treatment of chronic hepatitis B with interferon alfa-2b. J Hepatol 1990;11:S137–40.
298. Feinman SV, Berris B, Sooknanan R, et al. Effects of interferon-α therapy on serum and liver HBV DNA in patients with chronic hepatitis B. Dig Dis Sci 1992;37:1477–82.
299. Korenman J, Baker B, Waggoner J, et al. Long-term remission of chronic hepatitis B after alpha-interferon in the treatment of chronic type B hepatitis: a randomized, controlled trial. Ann Intern Med 1991;114:629–34.
300. Lin SM, Sheen IS, Chien RN, et al. Long-term beneficial effect of interferon therapy in patients with chronic hepatitis B virus infection. Hepatology 1999;29:971–5.
301. Niederau C, Heintges, T, Lange S, et al. Long-term follow-up of HBeAg-positive patients treated with interferon alfa for chronic hepatitis B. N Engl J Med 1996;334:1422–7.
302. Torre D, Tambini R. Interferon-alpha therapy for chronic hepatitis B in children: a meta-analysis. Clin Infect Dis 1996;23:131–7.
303. Sokal EM, Conjeevaram HS, Roberts EA, et al. Interferon alfa therapy for chronic hepatitis B in children: a multinational randomized controlled trial. Gastroenterology 1998;114:988–95.
304. Jara P, Bortolotti F. Interferon-alpha treatment of chronic hepatitis B in childhood: A consensus advice based on experience in

European children. J Pediatr Gastroenterol Nutr 1999;29:163–70.

305. Bortolotti F, Jara P, Barbera C, et al. Long term effect of alpha interferon in children with chronic hepatitis B. Gut 2000; 46:715–18.
306. Diem HVT, Bourgois A, Bontems P. Chronic hepatitis B infection: long term comparison of children receiving interferon alpha and untreated controls. J Pediatr Gastroenterol Nutr 2005; 40:141–5.
307. Chuang WL, Omata M. Ehata T, et al. Precore mutations and core mutations in chronic hepatitis B virus infection. Gastroenterology 1993;104:263–71.
308. Lok ASF, Lai CL, Su PC. et al. Treatment of chronic hepatitis B with interferon: experience in Asian patients. Semin Liver Dis 1989;9:249–53.
309. Scullard GH, Smith Cl, Merigan TC, et al. Effects of immunosuppressive therapy on viral markers in chronic viral hepatitis B. Gastroenterology 1981;81:987–91.
310. Lok ASF, Wu PC, Lai CL, et al. A controlled trial of interferon with or without prednisone priming for chronic hepatitis B. Gastroenterology 1992;102:2091–7.
311. Ikeda K, Saitoh S, Arase Y, et al. Interferon therapy prevents hepatocellular carcinoma in some patients with chronic HCV: the role of fibrosis. Hepatology 1999;29:1124–30.
312. Van Zonneveld M, Honkoop P, Hansen B, et al. Long-term follow-up of patients with chronic hepatitis B. Hepatology 2004;39:804–10.
313. Renault PF, Hoofnagle JH. Side effects of alpha interferon. Semin Liver Dis 1989;9:273–7.
314. Mayet WJ, Hess G, Gerken G, et al. Treatment of chronic type B hepatitis with recombinant alpha interferon induces autoantibodies not specific for autoimmune chronic hepatitis. Hepatology 1989;10:24–8.
315. Burman P, Karlsson FA, Obert K. Autoimmune thyroid disease in interferon treated patients. Lancet 1985;2:100–1.
316. Fentiman IS, Thomas BS, Balkwill FR, et al. Primary hypothyroidism associated with interferon therapy of breast cancer. Lancet 1985;2:1166.
317. Davis GL, Balari LA, Schiff ER, et al. Treatment of chronic hepatitis C with recombinant interferon alpha: a multicenter randomized, controlled trial. N Engl J Med 1989;321:1501–5.
318. Hayasaka S, Nagaki Y, Matsumoto M, Sato S. Interferon associated retinopathy. Br J Ophthamol 1998;82:323–5.
319. Ballow CF, Priebe CJ, Mulliken JB, et al. Spastic diplegia as a complication of interferon alpha-2a treatment of hemangiomas of infancy. J Pediatr 1998;132:527–30.
320. Hoofnagle JH, Di Bisceglie AM, Waggoner JG, et al. Interferon alfa for patients with clinically apparent cirrhosis due to chronic hepatitis B. Gastroenterology 1993;104:1116–21.
321. Torresi J, Locarnini S. Antiviral chemotherapy for the treatment of hepatitis B virus infections. Gastroenterology 2000;118:S83–103.
322. Lai CL, Chien RN, Leung N, et al. A one-year trial of lamivudine for chronic hepatitis B. N Engl J Med 1998;339:61–8.
323. Dienstag JL, Perrillo RP, Schiff ER, et al. A preliminary trial of lamivudine for chronic hepatitis B infection. N Engl J Med 1995;333:1657–61.
324. Dienstag JL, Schiff ER, Wright TL, et al. Lamivudine as initial treatment for chronic hepatitis B in the United States. N Engl J Med 1999;341:1256–63.
325. Dienstag JL, Schiff ER, Mitchell M, et al. Extended lamivudine retreatment for chronic hepatitis B: maintenance of viral suppression after discontinuation of therapy. Hepatology 1999; 30:1082–7.
326. Boni C, Bertoletti A, Penna A, et al. Lamivudine treatment can restore T cell responsiveness in chronic hepatitis B. J Clin Invest 1998;102:968–75.
327. Allen M, Deslauriers M, Andrews C, et al. Identification and characterization of mutations in hepatitis B virus resistant lamivudine. Hepatology 1998;27:1670–7.
328. Lok ASF, McMahon BJ. Chronic hepatitis B: update of recommendations. Hepatology 2004;39:857–61.
329. Tassopoulos NC, Volpes R, Pastore G, et al. Efficacy of lamivudine in patients with hepatitis B e antigen-negative/hepatitis B virus DNA-positive (precore mutant) chronic hepatitis B. Hepatology 1999;29:889–96.
330. Liaw YF, Sung JJY, Chow WC, et al. Lamivudine for patients with chronic hepatitis B and advanced liver disease. N Engl J Med 2004;1521–31.
331. Jonas MM, Kelley DA, Mizerski J, et al. Clinical trial of lamivudine in children with chronic hepatitis B. N Engl J Med 2002; 346:1706–13.
332. Hagmann S, Chung M, Rochford G, et al. Response to lamivudine in children with chronic hepatitis B virus infection. Clin Infect Dis 2003;37:1434–40.
333. Hartman C, Berkowitz D, Shouval D, et al. Lamivudine treatment for chronic hepatitis B infection in children unresponsive to interferon. Pediatr Infect Dis J 2003;22:224–8.
334. Marcellin P, Chang TT, Lim SG, et al. Adefovir dipivoxil for the treatment of hepatitis B e antigen-positive chronic hepatitis B. N Engl J Med 2003;348:808–16.
335. Hadziyannis SJ, Tassopoulos NC, Heathcote E, et al. Adefovir dipivoxil for the treatment of hepatitis B e antigen-negative chronic hepatitis B. N Engl J Med 2003;348:800–7.
336. Schiff ER, Lai CL, Hadziyannis S, et al. Adefovir dipivoxil therapy for lamivudine-resistant hepatitis B in pre- and post-liver transplantation patients. Hepatology 2003;38:1419–27.
337. Perillo R, Han HW, Mutimer D, et al. Adefovir dipivoxil added to ongoing lamivudine in chronic hepatitis B with YMDD mutant hepatitis B virus. Gastroenterology 2004;126:81–90.
338. Peters MG, Han HW, Martin P, et al. Adefovir dipivoxil alone or in combination with lamivudine in patients with lamivudine-resistant chronic hepatitis B. Gastroenterology 2004;126: 91–101.
339. Hadziyannis S, Tassopoulos NC, Heathcote J, et al. Long-term therapy with adefovir dipivoxil for HBeAg-negative chronic hepatitis B. N Engl J Med 2005;352:2673–81.
340. Angus P, Vaughan R, Xiong S, et al. Resistance to adefovir dipivoxil therapy associated with the selection of a novel mutation in the HBV polymerase. Gastroenterology 2003;125: 292–7.
341. Kuo A, Dienstag JL, Chung RT. Tenofovir disoproxil fumarate for the treatment of lamivudine-resistant hepatitis B. Clin Gastroenterol Hepatol 2004;2:266–72.
342. Van Bommel F, Wunshe T, Mauss S, et al. Comparison of adefovir and tenofovir in the treatment of lamivudine-resisitant hepatitis B virus infection. Hepatology 2004;40:1421–5.
343. Dore GJ, Cooper DA, Pozniak AL, et al. Efficacy of tenofovir disoproxil fumarate in antiretroviral therapy-naive and

–experienced patients coinfected with HIV-1 and hepatitis B virus. J Infect Dis 2004;189:1185–92.
344. Entecavir Review Team. Briefing document for NDA 21–797, entecavir 0.5 and 1mg tablets and NDA 21–798, entecavir oral solution 0.05 mg/mL. February 10, 2005 (memorandum). (Accessed July 7, 2005, at http://www.fda.gov/ohrms/dockets/ac/05/briefing/2005–4094B1_02_FDA-Background-Memo.pdf.)
345. Lok AS. The maze of treatments for Hepatitis B. N Engl J Med 2005;352:2743–6.
346. Chang T-T, Gish RG, Hadziyannis SJ, et al. A dose-ranging study of the efficacy and tolerability of entecavir in lamivudine-refractory chronic hepatitis B patients. Gastroenterology 2005; 129:1198–209.
347. Lai C-L, Leung N, Teo E-K, et al. A 1-year trial of telbivudine, lamivudine, and the combination in patients with hepatitis B e antigen-positive chronic hepatitis B. Gastroenterology 2005; 129:528–36.
348. Marcellin P, Lau GKK, Bonino F, et al. Peginterferon alfa-2a alone, lamivudine alone, and the two in combination in patients with HbeAg-negative chronic hepatitis B. N Engl J Med 2004; 351:1206–17.
349. Lau GKK, Piratvisuth T, Luo KX, et al. Peginterferon alfa-2a, lamivudine, and the combination for HBeAg-positive chronic hepatitis B. N Engl J Med 2005;352:2682–95.
350. Sanchez-Fueyo A, Rimola A, Grande L, et al. Hepatitis B immunoglobulin discontinuation followed by hepatitis B virus vaccination: a new strategy in the prophylaxis of hepatitis B virus recurrence after liver transplantation. Hepatology 2000;31:496–500.
351. Marinos G, Rossol S, Carucci P, et al. Immunopathogenesis of hepatitis B virus recurrence after liver transplantation. Transplantation 2000;69:559–68.
352. Rakela J, Wooten RS, Batts KP, et al. Failure of interferon to prevent recurrent hepatitis B infection in hepatic allograft. Mayo Clin Proc 1989;64:429–32.
353. Chossegros P, Poutiel-Noble C, Samuel D, et al. Ganciclovir is an effective antiviral agent for post-transplantation chronic HBV infection: maintenance therapy may be required in some cases. Gastroenterology 1993;104:A888.
354. Gish RG, Imperial JI, Esquivel CO, et al. Ganciclovir treatment of severe hepatitis B virus (HBV) infection. Gastroenterology 1993;104:A908.
355. Roche B, Samuel D, Gigon M, et al. Long-term ganciclovir therapy for hepatitis B virus infection after liver transplantation. J Hepatol 1999;31:584–92.
356. Marzano A, Debernardi-Vernon W, Smedile A, et al. Recurrence of hepatitis B in liver transplants treated with antiviral therapy. Ital J Gastroenterol Hepatol 1998;30:77–81.
357. Davies SE, Portmann BC, O'Grady JG, et al. Hepatic histological findings after transplantation for chronic hepatitis B virus infection including a unique pattern of fibrosing cholestatic hepatitis. Hepatology 1991;13:150–7.
358. Perrillo R, Rakela J, Dienstag J, et al. Multicenter study of lamivudine therapy for hepatitis B after liver transplantation. Hepatology 1999;29:1581–6.
359. Grellier L, Mutimer D, Ahmed M, et al. Lamivudine prophylaxis against reinfection in liver transplantation for hepatitis B cirrhosis. Lancet 1996;348:1212–15.
360. Gauthier J, Bourne EJ, Lutz MW, et al. Quantitation of hepatitis B viremia and emergence of YMDD variant in patients with chronic hepatitis B treated with lamivudine. J Infect Dis 1999;180:1757–62.
361. Yao FY, Osorio RW, Roberts JP, et al. Intramuscular hepatitis B immune globulin combined with lamivudine for prophylaxis against hepatitis B recurrence after liver transplantation. Liver Transpl Surg 1999;5:491–6.
362. McCaughan GW, Spencer J, Koorey D, et al. Lamivudine therapy in patients undergoing liver transplantation for hepatitis B virus precore mutant associated infection: high resistance rates in treatment of recurrence but universal prevention if used as prophylaxis with very low dose hepatitis B immune globulin. Liver Transpl Surg 1999;5:512–19.
363. National Institutes of Health. National Institutes of Health consensus development conference statement: management of hepatitis C 2002. Hepatology 2002;36:(5 suppl 1):S3–20.
364. Dienstag JL, McHutchison JG. American Gastroenterological Association medical position statement on the management of hepatitis C. Gastroenterology 2006;130:225–30.
365. Dienstag JL, McHutchison JG. American Gastroenterological Association technical review on the management of hepatitis C. Gastroenterology 2006;130:231–64.
366. Wong JB, McQuillan GM, McHutchison JG, Poynard T. Estimating future hepatitis C morbidity, mortality and costs in the United States. Am J Public Health 2000;90:1562–9.
367. Alter MJ, Kruszon-Moran D, Nainan OV, et al. The prevalence of hepatitis C virus infection in the United States, 1988 through 1994. N Engl J Med 1999;341:556–62.
368. Report of World Health Organization. Global surveillance and control of hepatitis C. J Viral Hepatol 1999;6:35–47.
369. Centers for Disease Control and Prevention. Recommendations for prevention and control of hepatitis C virus (HCV) infection and HCV related chronic disease. MMWR 1998;47(no. RR-19): 1–39.
370. Frank C, Mohomed MK, Strickland GT, et al. The role of parenteral antischistosomal therapy in the spread of hepatitis C virus in Egypt. Lancet 2000;355:887–91.
371. Tanaka Y, Hanada K, Mizokami M, et al. A comparison of the molecular clock of hepatitis C virus in the United States and Japan predicts that hepatocellular carcinoma incidence in the United States will increase over the next two decades. Proc Natl Acad Sci U S A 2002;99:15584–9.
372. Choo WL, Koo G, Weiner AJ, et al. Isolation of a cDNA clone derived from a blood-borne non-A, non-B viral hepatitis genome. Science 1989;244:359–62.
373. Koo G, Choo QL, Alter HJ, et al. An assay for circulating antibodies to a major etiologic virus of human non-A, non-B hepatitis. Science 1989;244:362–4.
374. Farci P, Alter HJ, Govindarajan S, et al. Lack of protective immunity against reinfection with hepatitis C virus. Science 1992;259:135–40.
375. Pawlotsky JM. Hepatitis C virus genetic variability: pathogenic and clinical implications. Clin Liver Dis 2003;7:45–66.
376. Katkov WN, Friedman LS, Cody H, et al. Elevated serum alanine aminotransferase levels in blood donors: the contribution of hepatitis C virus. Ann Intern Med 1991;115:882–4.
377. Jonas MM. Children with hepatitis C. Hepatology 2002;36: S173–8.
378. American Academy of Pediatrics. Hepatitis C. In: Pickering LK, ed. Red book: 2003 report of the Committee on Infectious

Diseases. 26th ed. Elk Grove Village, IL: American Academy of Pediatrics, 2003:336–40.
379. Edlin BR. Prevention and treatment of hepatitis C in injection drug users. Hepatology 2002;36:S210–19.
380. McHutchison JG. Understanding hepatitis C. Am J Manag Care 2004;10:S21–9.
381. Alter MJ, Mares A, Hadler SC, et al. The effect of underreporting on the apparent incidence and epidemiology of acute viral hepatitis. Am J Epidemiol 1987;125:133–9.
382. Klein RS, Freeman K, Taylor PE, et al. Occupational risk for hepatitis C virus infection among New York City dentists. Lancet 1991;338:1539–42.
383. Puro V, Petrosillo N, Ippolito G. Risk of hepatitis C seroconversion after occupational exposures in health care workers. Am J Infect Control 1995;23:273–7.
384. Lauer GM, Walker BD. Medical progress: hepatitis C virus infection. N Engl J Med 2001;345:41–52.
385. Bortolotti F, Resti M, Giacchino R, et al. Changing epidemiologic pattern of chronic hepatitis C virus infection in Italian children. J Pediatr 1998;133:378–9.
386. Yeung LTF, King SM, Robert EA. Mother-to-infant transmission of hepatitis C virus. Hepatology 2001;34:223–9.
387. Wejstal R, Norkrans G. Chronic non-A, non-B hepatitis in pregnancy: outcome and possible transmission to the offspring. Scand J Infect Dis 1989;21:485–90.
388. Granovsky MO, Minkoff HL, Tess BH, et al. Hepatitis C virus infection in the mothers and infants Cohort Study. Pediatrics 1998;102:355–9.
389. Conte D, Fraquelli M, Prati D. Prevalence and clinical course of chronic hepatitis C virus infection and rate of HCV vertical transmission in a cohort of 15,250 pregnant women. Hepatology 2000;31:751–5.
390. Resti M, Azzari C, Mannelli F. Mother to child transmission of hepatitis C virus: prospective study of risk factors and timing of infection in children born to women seronegative for HIV-1. Br Med J 1998;317:437–40.
391. Gibb DM, Goodall RL, Dunn DT, et al. Mother-to-child transmission of hepatitis C virus: evidence for preventable peripartum transmission. Lancet 2000;356:904–7.
392. Novati R, Thiers V, Monforte A, et al. Mother-to-child transmission of hepatitis C virus detected by nested polymerase chain reaction. J Infect Dis 1992;165:720–3.
393. Nagata I, Shiraki K, Tanimoto K, et al. Mother-to-infant transmission of hepatitis-C virus. J Pediatr 1992;120:432–4.
394. Alter HJ. Descartes before the horse: I clone, therefore I am: the hepatitis C virus in current perspective. Ann Intern Med 1991;115:644–9.
395. Vogt M, Lang T, Frosner G, et al. Prevalence and clinical outcome of hepatitis C infection in children who underwent cardiac surgery before the implementataion of blood-donor screening. N Engl J Med 2000;341:866–70.
396. Lai ME, De Virgilis S, Argioulu F, et al. Evaluation of antibodies to hepatitis C virus in a long-term prospective study of posttransfusion hepatitis among thalassemic children: comparison between first- and second-generation assay. J Pediatr Gastroenterol Nutr 1993;16:458–63.
397. Strickland DK, Riely CA, Patrick CC, et al. Hepatitis C infection among survivors of childhood cancer. Blood 2000;95:3065–70.
398. Castellino S, Lensing S, Riely C, et al. The epidemiology of chronic hepatitis C infection in survivors of childhood cancer: an update of the St. Jude Children's Research Hospital hepatitis C seropositive cohort. Blood 2004;103:2460–6.
399. Palomba E, Manzini P, Fiammengo P, et al. Natural history of perinatal hepatitis C virus infection. Clin Infect Dis 1996;23:47–50.
400. Tovo PA, Pembrey LJ, Newell ML. Persistence rate and progression of vertically acquired hepatitis C infection. J Infect Dis 2000;181:419–24.
401. Strader DB, Wright T, Thomas DL, Seeff LB. AASLD practice guideline: diagnosis, management, and treatment of hepatitis C. Hepatology 2004;39:1147–71.
402. Seeff LB, Miller RN, Rabkin CS, et al. 45-year follow-up of hepatitis C virus infection in healthy young adults. Ann Intern Med 2000;132:105–11.
403. Kenny-Walsh E. Clinical outcomes after hepatitis C infection from contaminated anti-D immune globulin. N Engl J Med 1999;340:1228–33.
404. Khan MH, Farrell GC, Byth K, et al. Which patients with hepatitis C develop liver complications? Hepatology 2000;31:513–20.
405. Dibisceglie AM. Natural history of hepatitis C: its impact on clinical management. Hepatology 2000;31:1014–18.
406. Kiyosawa K, Sodeyama T, Tanaka E, et al. Interrelationship of blood transfusion, non-A, non-B hepatitis and hepatocellular carcinoma: analysis by detection of antibody to hepatitis C virus. Hepatology 1990;12:671–5.
407. Tong MJ, El-Farra N, Reikes AR, Co RL. Clinical outcomes after transfusion-associated hepatitis C. N Engl J Med 1995;332:1463–6.
408. Fattovich G, Giustina F, Degos F, et al. Morbidity and mortality in compensated cirrhosis type C: a retrospective follow-up study of 384 patients. Gastroenterology 1997;112:463–72.
409. Gish RG, Afdhal NH, Dieterich DT, Reddy KR. Management of hepatitis C virus in special populations: patient and treatment considerations. Clin Gastroenterol Hepatol 2005;3:311–18.
410. Agnello V, Chung RT, Kaplan LM. A role for hepatitis C virus infection in type II cryoglobulinemia. N Engl J Med 1992;327:1490–5.
411. Khalili M, Lim JW, Bass N, et al. New onset diabetes mellitus after liver transplantation: the critical role of hepatitis C infection. Liver Transpl 2004;10:349–55.
412. Hoofnagle JH, Seef LB, Bales ZB, Zimmerman HJ. Type B hepatitis after transfusion with blood containing antibody to hepatitis B core antigen. N Engl J Med 1978;298:1379–83.
413. Hoofnagle JH, Duskeiko GM, Schafer DF, et al. Reactivation of chronic hepatitis B virus infection by cancer chemotherapy. Ann Intern Med 1982;96:447–9.
414. Balart LA, Perillo R, Roddenberry J, et al. Hepatitis C RNA in liver of chronic hepatitis C patients before and after interferon alfa treatment. Gastroenterology 1993;104:1472–7.
415. Shindo M, Arai K, Sokawa Y, Okuno T. Hepatic hepatitis C virus RNA as a predictor of a long-term response to interferon-alpha therapy. Ann Intern Med 1995;122:586–91.
416. Larghi A, Tagger A, Crosignani A, et al. Clinical significance of hepatic HCV RNA in patients with chronic hepatitis C demonstrating long-trm sustained response to interferon-alpha therapy. J Med Virol 1998;55:7–11.
417. Pham TN, MacParland SA, Mulrooney PM, et al. Hepatitis C virus persistence after spontaneous or treatment-induced resolution of hepatitis C. J Virol 2004;78:5867–74.

418. Radkowski M, Gallegos-Orozco JF, Jablonska J, et al. Persistence of hepatitis C virus in patients successfully treated for chronic hepatitis C. Hepatology 2005;41:106–14.
419. Castillo I, Pardo M, Bartolome J, et al. Occult hepatitis C virus infection in patients in whom the etiology of persistently abnormal results of liver-function tests is unknown. J Infect Dis 2004189:7–14.
420. Scheuer PJ, Ashrafzadeh P, Sherlock S, et al. The pathology of hepatitis C. Hepatology 1992;15:567–71.
421. Kage M, Fujisawa T, Shiraki K, et al. Pathology of chronic hepatitis C in children. Hepatology 1997;26:771–5.
422. Guido M, Rugge M, Jara P, et al. Chronic hepatitis C in children: the pathological and clinical spectrum. Gastroenterology 1998; 115:1525–9.
423. Badizadegan K, Jonas MM, Ott MJ, et al. Histopathology of the liver in children with chronic hepatitis C viral infection. Hepatology 1998;28:1416–23.
424. Bach N, Thung SN, Schaffner F. The histological features of chronic hepatitis C and autoimmune chronic hepatitis: a comparative analysis. Hepatology 1992;15:572–7.
425. Garcia-Monzon D, Jara P, Fernandez-Bermejo M, et al. Chronic hepatitis C in children: a clinical and immunohistochemical comparative study with adult patients. Hepatology 1998;28:1696–701.
426. Houghton M, Weiner A, Han J, et al. Molecular biology of the hepatitis C viruses: implications for diagnosis, development and control of viral disease. Hepatology 1991;14:381–8.
427. Neumann AU, Lam NP, Dahari H, et al. Hepatitis C viral dynamics in vivo and the antiviral efficacy of interferon-alpha therapy. Science 1998;282:103–7.
428. Wu GY, Konishi M, Walton C, et al. A novel immunocompetent rat model of HCV infection and hepatitis. Gastroenterology 2005;128:1416 23.
429. Agnello V, Abel G, Knight GB, Muchmore E. Detection of widespread hepatocyte infection in chronic hepatitis. Hepatology 1998;28:573–84.
430. Farci P, Shimoda A, Coiana A, et al. The outcome of acute hepatitis C predicted by the evolution of the viral quasispecies. Science 2000;288:339–44.
431. Koziel MJ, Dudley D, Afdhal N, et al. HLA class I-restricted cytotoxic T lymphocytes specific for hepatitis C virus: identification of multiple epitopes and characterization of pattersn of cytokine release. J Clin Invest 1995;96:2311–21.
432. Khakoo SI, Thoio C, Martin MP, et al. HLA and NK cell inhibitory receptor genes in resolving hepatitis C virus infection. Science 2004;305:872–4.
433. Lin W, Choe WH, Hiasa Y, et al. Hepatitis C virus expression suppresses interferon signaling by degrading STAT1. Gastroenterology 2005;128:1034–41.
434. Dharancy S, Malapel M, Perlemuter G, et al. Impaired expression of the peroxisome proliferator-activated receptor alpha during hepatitis C infection. Gastroenterology 2005;128:334–42.
435. Cacciola I, Pollicino T, Squadrito G, et al. Occult hepatitis B virus infection in patients with chronic hepatitis C liver disease. N Engl J Med 1999;341:22–6.
436. Besisik F, Karaca C, Akyuz F, et al. Occult HBV infection and YMDD variants in hemodialysis patients with chronic HCV infection. J Hepatol 2003;38:506–10.
437. Fabris P, Brown D, Tositti G, et al. Occult hepatitis B virus infection does not affect liver histology or response to therapy with interferon alpha and ribavirin in intravenous drug users with chronic hepatitis C. J Clin Virol 2004;29:160–6.
438. Georgiadou SP, Zachou K, Rigopoulou E, et al. Occult hepatitis B virus infection in Greek patients with chronic hepatitis C and in patients with diverse nonviral hepatic diseases. J Viral Hepat 2004;11:358–65.
439. El-Serag HB, Giordano TP, Kramer J, et al. Survival of hepatitis C and HIV co-infection: a cohort study of hospitalized veterans. Clin Gastroenterol Hepatol 2005;3:175–83.
440. Torriani FJ, Rodriguez-Torres M, Rockstroh JK, et al. Peginterferon alfa-2a plus ribavirin for chronic hepatitis C virus infection in HIV-infected patients. N Engl J Med 2004;351: 438–50.
441. Chung RT, Andersen J, Volberding J, et al. Peginterferon alfa-2a plus ribavirin for chronic hepatitis C in HIV coinfected persons N Engl J Med 2004;351:451–9.
442. Soriano V, Sulkowski M, Bergin C, et al. Care of patients with chronic hepatitis C and HIV co-infection: recommendations from the HIV-HCV international panel. AIDS 2002;16: 813–28.
443. Centers for Disease Control and Prevention. Guidelines for laboratory testing and result reporting of antibody to hepatitis C virus. MMWR 2003;52(no. RR-3):1–15.
444. Maggiore G, Caprai S, Cerino A, et al. Antibody-negative chronic hepatitis C virus infection in immunocompetent children. J Pediatr 1998;132:1048–50.
445. McFarlane IG, Smith HM, Johnson PJ, et al. Hepatitis C virus antibodies in chronic active hepatitis: pathogenetic factor or false-positive result? Lancet 1990;335:754–7.
446. Alter HJ, Purcell RH, Shih JW, et al. Detection of antibody to hepatitis C virus in prospectively followed transfusion recipients with acute and chronic non-A, non-B hepatitis. N Engl J Med 1989;321:1494–500.
447. Larsen J, Skaug K, Maeland A. 2nd-generation anti-HCV tests predict infectivity. Vox Sang 1992;63:39–42.
448. Wang JT, Wang TH, Sheu JC, et al. Post-transfusion hepatitis revisited by hepatitis C antibody assays and polymerase chain reaction. Gastroenterology 1992;103:609–16.
449. Dussaix E, Maggiore G, DeGiacomo C, et al. Autoimmune hepatitis in children and hepatitis C virus testing [letter]. Lancet 1990;335:1160–1.
450. Lunel F, Abuaf N, Frangeul L, et al. Liver/kidney microsome antibody type I and hepatitis C virus infection. Hepatology 1992;16:630–6.
451. Cassani F, Muratori L, Manotti P, et al. Serum autoantibodies and the diagnosis of type-1 autoimmune hepatitis in Italy: a reappraisal in the light of hepatitis-C virus infection. Gut 1992;33:1260–3.
452. Alter HJ. New kit on the block: evaluation of second-generation assays for detection for antibody to the hepatitis C virus. Hepatology 1992;15:350–2.
453. Farci P, Alter JH, Wong D, et al. A long-term study of hepatitis C virus replication in non-A, non-B hepatitis. N Engl J Med 1991;325:98–104.
454. Alberti A, Morsica G, Chemello L, et al. Hepatitis C viraemia and liver disease in symptom-free individuals with anti-HCV. Lancet 1992;340:697–8.
455. Morishima C, Getch DR. Clinical use of hepatitis C virus tests for diagnosis and monitoring during therapy. Clin Liver Dis 1999;3:717–40.
456. Krawczynski K, Beach MJ, Bradley DW, et al. Hepatitis C virus

antigen in hepatocytes: immunomorphologic detection and identification. Gastroenterology 1992;103:622–9.

457. Fang J, Albrecht J, Jacobs S, et al. Quantification of serum hepatitis C virus RNA. Hepatology 1999;29:997–8.
458. Blatt LM, Mutchnick MG, Tong MJ, et al. Assessment of hepatitis C virus RNA and genotype from 6807 patients with chronic hepatitis C in the United States. J Viral Hepat 2000;7:196–202.
459. Polynard T, McHutchison J, Manns M, et al. Impact of pegylated interferon alfa-2b and ribavirin on liver fibrosis in patients with chronic hepatitis C. Gastroenterology 2002;122:1202–313.
460. DiBisceglie AM, Martin P, Kassianides C, et al. Recombinant interferon alpha therapy for chronic hepatitis C: a randomized, doubleblind, placebo-controlled trial. N Engl J Med 1989;321:1506–10.
461. Gerin JL. Antiviral agents for hepatitis B. Hepatology 1991;14: 198–9.
462. Hoofnagle JH, Mullen KD, Jones DB, et al. Treatment of chronic non-A, non-B hepatitis with recombinant human alpha interferon. N Engl J Med 1986;315:1575–8.
463. Reichard O, Andersson J, Schvarcz R, et al. Ribavirin treatment for chronic hepatitis C. Lancet 1991;337:1058–60.
464. DiBisceglie AM, Shindo M. Fong TL, et al. A pilot study of ribavirin therapy for chronic hepatitis C. Hepatology 1992;16:649–54.
465. Manns M, McHutchison JG, Gordon SC, et al. Peginterferon alfa-2b plus ribavirin compared with interferon alfa-2b plus ribavirin for initial treatment of chronic hepatitis C: a randomized trial. Lancet 2001;358:958–65.
466. Fried MW, Shiffman ML, Reddy KR, et al. Peginterferon alfa 2a plus ribavirin for chronic hepatitis C virus infection. N Engl J Med 2002;347:975–82.
467. Hadziyannis SJ, Sette H, Morgan TR, et al. Peginterferon-α2a and ribavirin combination therapy in chronic hepatitis C. Ann Intern Med 2004;140:346–55.
468. Davis GL, Wong JB, McHutchison JG, et al. Early virologic response to treatment with peginterferon alfa 2b plus ribavirin in patients with chronic hepatitis C. Hepatology 2003;38:645–52.
469. Mangia A, Santoro R, Minerva N, et al. Peginterferon alfa-2b and ribavirin for 12 vs. 24 weeks in HCV genotype 2 or 3. N Engl J Med 2005;352:2609–17.
470. Dalgard O, Bjoro K, Hellum KB, et al. Treatment with pegylated interferon and ribavirin in HCV infection with genotype 2 or 3 for 14 weeks: a pilot study. Hepatology 2004;40:1260–5.
471. Von Wagner M, Huber M, Berg T, et al. Peginterferon-alpha-2a (40kd) and ribavirin for 16 or 24 weeks in patients with genotype 2 or 3 chronic hepatitis C. Gastroenterology 2005;129:522–7.
472. Borg BB, Hoofnagle JH. Peginterferon alfa-2b and ribavirin for 12 versus 24 weeks in HCV infection [letter]. N Engl J Med 2005;353:1182–3.
473. Shiffman ML, DiBisceglie AM, Lindsay KL, et al. Peginterferon alfa-2a and ribavirin in patients with chronic hepatitis C who have failed prior treatment. Gastroenterology 2004;126:1015–23.
474. Poynard T, McHutchison J, Manns M, et al. Impact of pegylated interferon alfa-2b and ribavirin on liver fibrosis in patients with chronic hepatitis C. Gastroenterology 2002;122:1303–13.
475. Muir A, Bornstein J, Killenberg P, Atlantic Coast Hepatitis Treatment Group. Peginterferon alfa-2b and ribavirin for the treatment of chronic hepatitis C in blacks and non-Hispnic whites. N Engl J Med 2004;350:2265–71.
476. Jeffers L, Cassidy W, Howell C, et al. Peginterferon alfa-2a (40kd) and ribavirin for black American patients with chronic HCV genotype 1. Hepatology 2004;39:1702–8.
477. Wong W, Terrault N. Update on chronic hepatitis C. Clin Gastroenterol Hepatol 2005;3:507–20.
478. Jacobson KR, Murray K, Zellos A, Schwarz KB. An analysis of published trials of interferon monotherapy in children with chronic hepatitis C. J Pediatr Gastroenterol Nutr 2002;34: 52–8.
479. Ruiz-Moreno M, Rua MJ, Castillo I, et al. Treatment of children with chronic hepatitis C with recombinant interferon-α: a pilot study. Hepatology 1992;16:882–5
480. Bortolotti F, Giacchino R, Vajro P, et al. Recombinant interferon-alpha therapy in children with chronic hepatitis C. Hepatoogyl 1995;22:1623–6.
481. Clemente MG, Congia M, Lai ME, et al. Effect of iron overload on the response to recombinant interferon-alpha treatment in transfusion-dependent patients with thalassemia major and chronic hepatitis C. J Pediatr 1994;125:123–8.
482. Azzari C, Resti M, Bortolotti F, et al. Serum levels of hepatitis C virus RNA in infants and children with chronic hepatitis C. J Pediatr Gastroenterol Nutr 1999;29:314–17.
483. Iorio R, Pensati P, Porzio S, et al. Lymphoblastoid interferon alfa treatment in chronic hepatitis C. Arch Dis Childhood 1996; 74:152–6.
484. Komatsu H, Fujisawa T, Inui A, et al. Efficacy of interferon in treating chronic hepatitis C in children with a history of acute leukemia. Blood 1996;87:4072–5.
485. Puetz J, Thrower M, Kane R, Bouhasin J. Combination therapy with ribavirin and interferon in a cohort of children with hepatitis C and haemophilia followed at a pediatric haemophilia treatment center. Haemophilia 2004;10:87–93.
486. Bunn S, Kelly D, Murray KF, et al. Safety, efficacy and pharmacokinetics of interferon alpha-2b and ribavirin in children with chronic hepatitis C [abstract]. Hepatology 2000;32: 763A.
487. Suoglu O, Elkabes B, Sokucu S, Saner G. Does interferon and ribavirin combination therapy increase the rate of treatment response in children with hepatitis C? J Pediatr Gasto Nutr 2002; 34:199–206.
488. Christensson B, Wiebe T, Akesson A, Widell A. Interferon-alpha and ribavirin treatment of hepatitis C in children with malignancy in remission. Clin Infect Dis 2000;30:585–6.
489. Lackner H, Moser A, Deutsch J, et al. Interferon-alpha and ribavirin in treating children and young adults with chronic hepatitis C after malignancy. Pediatrics 2000;106:353–9.
490. Fried MW, Peter J, Hoots K, et al. Hepatitis C in adults and adolescents with hemophilia and inherited disorders of coagulation: a randomized, controlled, multicenter trial of combination therapy with interferon alfa-2b and ribavirin. Hepatology 2002; 36:967–72.
491. Wirth S, Pieper-Boustani H, Lang T, et al. Peginterferon alfa-2b plus ribavirin treatment in children and adolescents with chronic hepatitits C. Hepatology 2005;41:1013–18.
492. Prieto M, Olaso V, Verdu C, et al. Does the healthy hepatitis C virus carrier state really exist? An analysis using polymerase chain reaction. Hepatology 1995;22:413–17.
493. Estaban JI, Lopez-Talavera JC, Genesca J, et al. High rate of infectivity and liver disease in blood donors with antibodies to hepatitis C virus. Ann Intern Med 1991;115: 443–9.

494. Shakil AO, Conry-Cantilena C, Alter HJ, et al. Volunteer blood donors with antibody to hepatitis C virus: clinical, biochemical, virologic, and histologic features. The Hepatitis C Study Group. Ann Intern Med 1995;123:330–7.
495. Marcellin P, Asselah T, Boyer N. Fibrosis and disease progression in hepatitis C. Hepatology 2002;36(suppl 1):S47–56.
496. Pradat P, Alberti A, Poynard T, et al. Predictive value of ALT levels for histologic findings in chronic hepatitis C: a European collaborative study. Hepatology 2002;36(pt 1):973–7.
497. Hui CK, Belaye T, Montegrande K, Wright TL. A comparison in the progression of liver fibrosis in chronic hepatitis C between persistently normal and elevated transaminases. J Hepatol 2003;38:511–17.
498. Marcellin P, Levy S, Erlinger S. Therapy of hepatitis C: patients with normal aminotransferase levels. Hepatology 1997; 26(suppl 1):S133–6.
499. Dufour DR, Lott JA, Nolte FS, et al. Diagnosis and monitoring of hepatic injury. I. Performance charactersistics of laboratory tests. Clin Chem 2000;46:2027–49.
500. Mathurin P, Moussall J, Cadranel JF, et al. Slow progression rate of fibrosis in hepatitis C virus patients with persistently normal alanine transaminase activity. Hepatology 1998;27:868–72.
501. Villano SA, Vlahov D, Nelson KE, et al. Persistence of viremia and the importance of long-term follow-up after acute hepatitis C infection. Hepatology 1999;29:908–14.
502. Alberti A, Boccato S, Vario A, Benvegnu L. Therapy of acute hepatitis C infection. Hepatology 2002;36(suppl 1):S195–200.
503. Jaeckel E, Cornberg M, Wedemeyer H, et al. Treatment of acute hepatitis C with interferon alfa-2b. N Engl J Med 2001;345: 1452–7.
504. Pimstone NR, Powell JS, Kotfila R, et al. High dose (780MU/52 weeks) interferon monotherapy is highly effective treatment for acute hepatitis C [abstract]. Gastroenterology 2000;118: A960.
505. Vogel W, Graziadei I, Umlauft F, et al. High-dose interferon-alpha-2b treatment prevents chronicicity in acute hepatitis C: a pilot study. Dig Dis Sci 1996;41(suppl):81S–85S.
506. Gerlach JT, Diepolder HM, Zachoval R, et al. Acute hepatitis C: high rate of both spontaneous and treatment-induced viral clearance. Gastroenterology 2003;125:80–8.
507. McDiarmid SV, Conrad A, Ament ME, et al. De novo hepatitis C in children after liver transplantation. Transplantation 1998;66:311–18.
508. Rizzetto M, Canese MG, Arico S, et al. Immunofluorescence detection of a new antigen-antibody system (δ/anti-δ) associated with hepatitis B virus in liver and serum of HBsAg carriers. Gut 1977;18:997–1003.
509. Rizzetto M, Purcell RH, Gerin IL. Epidemiology of HBV-associated delta agent: geographical distribution of anti-delta and prevalence in polytransfused HBsAg carriers. Lancet 1980;i: 1215–18.
510. Rizzetto M, Hoyer B, Canese MG, et al. Delta agent: the association of delta antigen with hepatitis B surface antigen and ribonucleic acid in the serum of delta-infected chimpanzees. Proc Natl Acad Sci U S A 1977;77:6124–8.
511. Rizzetto M, Canese MG, Gerin JL, et al. Transmission of the hepatitis B virus-associated delta antigen to chimpanzees. J Infect Dis 1980;141:590–602.
512. Rizzetto M. The delta agent. Hepatology 1983;3:729–37.
513. Ackerman Z, Valiniuck B, McHutchison JG, et al. Spontaneous exacerbation of disease activity in patients with chronic delta hepatitis infection: the role of hepatitis B, C or D? Hepatology 1992;16:625–9.
514. Farci P, Smedile A, Lavarini C, et al. Delta hepatitis in inapparent carriers of hepatitis B surface antigen: a disease simulating acute hepatitis B progressive to chronicity. Gastroenterology 1983;85:669–73.
515. Rizzetto M, Verme G, Recchia S, et al. Chronic hepatitis in carriers of hepatitis B surface antigen, with intrahepatic expression of the delta antigen: an active and progressive disease unresponsive to immunosuppressive treatment. Ann Intern Med 1983;98:437–41.
516. Rosina F, Saracco G, Rizetto M. Risk of post-transfusion infection with the hepatitis delta virus: a multicenter study. N Engl J Med 1985;312:1488–94.
517. Smedile A, Farci P, Verme G. et al. Influence of delta infection on severity of hepatitis B. Lancet 1982;ii:945–7.
518. Jacobsen IM, Dienstag J. The delta hepatitis agent: viral hepatitis, type D. Gastroenterology 1984;86:1614–16.
519. Taylor JM. The structure and replication of hepatitis delta-virus. Annu Rev Microbiol 1992;46:253–76.
520. Wang KS, Choo QZ, Weiner A, et al. Structure, sequence and expression of the hepatitis delta viral genome. Nature 1986;323: 508–14.
521. Denniston KJ, Hoyer BH, Smedile A, et al. Cloned fragments of the hepatitis delta virus RNA genome: sequence and diagnostic application, Science 1986;232:873–5.
522. Lai MCC. The molecular biology of hepatitis delta virus. Annu Rev Biochem 1995;64:259–86.
523. Casey JL. Molecular biology of HDV: analysis of RNA editing and genotype variations. In: Rizetto M, Purcell RH, Gerin JL, Verme G, eds. Viral hepatitis and liver disease. Turin: Edizioni Minerva Medica, 1997;290–4.
524. Gaeta GB, Stroffolini T, Chiaramonte M, et al. Chronic hepatitis D: a vanishing disease? An Italian multicenter study. Hepatology 2000;32:824–7.
525. Rosina F, Conoscitore P, Cuppone R, et al. Changing pattern of chronic hepatitis D in Southern Europe. Gastroenterology 1999; 117:161–6.
526. Hoofnagle JH. Type D (delta) hepatitis. JAMA 1989;261:1321–5.
527. DeCock KM, Govindarajan S, Chin KP. et al. Delta hepatitis in the Los Angeles area: a report of 126 cases. Ann Intern Med 1986;105:108–14.
528. Kanel GC, Govindarajan S, Peters RJ. Chronic delta infection and liver biopsy changes in chronic active hepatitis B. Ann Intern Med 1984;101:51–4.
529. Hadziyannis SJ. Review: hepatitis delta. J Gastroenterol Hepatol 1997;12:289–98.
530. Wu J-C, Chen T-Z, Huang Y-S, et al. Natural history of hepatitis D viral superinfection: significance of viremia detected by polymerase chain reaction. Gastroenterology 1995;108:796–802.
531. Purcell RH, Gerin JL. Hepatitis Delta virus. In: Fields BN, Knipe DM, Howley PM. eds. Fields virology. 3rd ed. Philadelphia: Lippincott-Raven, 1996:2819–29.
532. Abiad H, Ramani R, Currie JB, et al. The natural history of hepatitis D virus infection in Illinois state facilities for the developmentally disabled. Am J Gastroenterol 2001;96: 534–40.
533. Bonino F, Negro F, Baldi M, et al. The natrual history of chronic delta hepatitis. In: Rizzetto M, Gerin JL, Purcell RH, eds. The

hepatitis delta virus and its infection. New York: Liss, 1987: 145–52.
534. Fattovich G, Giustina G, Pantalena M, et al. Influence of hepatitis delta virus infection on morbidity and mortality in compensated cirrhosis type B. Gut 2000;46:420–6.
535. Sakugawa H, Nakasone H, Kawakami Y, et al. Determination of hepatitis delta virus (HDV) RNA in asymptomatic cases of HDV. Am J Gastroenterol 1997;92:2232–36.
536. Bensabath G, Hadler SC, Pereira Soares MC, et al. Hepatitis delta virus infection and labrea hepatitis. JAMA 1987;258:479–83.
537. Bruitrago B, Hadier SC, Popper H, et al. Epidemiologic aspects of Santa Marta hepatitis over a 40-year period. Hepatology 1986;6:1262–96.
538. Govindarajan S, Chin KP, Redeker AG, et al. Fulminant B viral hepatitis: role of delta antigen. Gastroenterology 1984;86: 1417–20.
539. Hsu HY, Chang MH, Chen DS, et al. Hepatitis D virus infection in children with acute or chronic hepatitis B virus infection in Taiwan. J Pediatr 1988;112:888–992.
540. Farci P, Barbera C, Navone C, et al. Infection with the delta agent in children. Gut 1985;26:4–7.
541. Zanetti AR, Ferroni P, Magliano EM, et al. Perinatal transmission of the hepatitis B virus and of the HBV-associated delta agent from mothers of offspring in Northern Italy. J Med Virol 1982;9:139–48.
542. Aragona M, Macagno S, Caredda F, et al. Serological response to the hepatitis delta virus in hepatitis D. Lancet 1987;i:478–80.
543. DiBisceglie AM, Negro E. Diagnosis of hepatitis delta virus infection. Hepatology 1989;10:1014–16.
544. McFarlane IG, Chaggar K, Davies SL, et al. IgA class antibodies to hepatitis delta virus antigen in acute and chronic hepatitis delta virus infections. Hepatology 1991;14:980–4.
545. Huang Y-H, Wu J C, Sheng W Y, et al. Diagnostic value of anti-hepatitis D virus (HDV) antibodies revisited: a study of total and IgM anti-HDV compared with detection of HDV RNA by polymerase chain reaction. Viral Hepatitis 1998;13:57–61.
546. Govindarajan S, Gupta S, Valinluck B, Redeker AG. Correlation of IgM anti-hepatitis D virus (HDV) to HDV RNA in sera of chronic HDV. Hepatology 1989;10:34–5.
547. Hoofnagle JH. Current status and future directions in the treatment of chronic viral hepatitis. In: Hollinger FB, Lemon SM, Margolis HS, eds. Viral hepatitis and liver disease. Baltimore: Williams & Wilkins, 1991:632–9.
548. Lau DT, Kleiner DE, Park Y, et al. Resolution of chronic delta hepatitis after 12 years of interferon alfa therapy. Gastroneterology 1999;117:1229–33.
549. Rosina F, Rizzetto M. Treatment of chronic type D (delta) hepatitis with alpha interferon. Semin Liver Dis 1989;9:264–6.
550. DiBisceglie AM, Martin P, Lisker-Melman M, et al. Therapy of chronic delta hepatitis with interferon alfa-2b. J Hepatol 1990;11:S151–4.
551. Farci P, Karayiannis P, Brook MG, et al. Treatment of chronic hepatitis delta virus infection with human lymphoblastoid alpha interferon. Q J Med 1989;73:1045–54.
552. Farci P, Mandas A, Lai ME, et al. Treatment of chronic delta hepatitis with high and low doses of interferon alpha-2b: a randomized, controlled trial. Hepatology 1990;12:869–73.
553. Rosina F, Marzano A, Garripoli A, et al. Chronic type D hepatitis: clearance of hepatitis B surface antigen during and after treatment with alfa interferon. Hepatology 1990;12: 883–6.
554. Rosina F, Pintus C, Rizzetto M. Long-term interferon treatment of chronic hepatitis D: a multicentre Italian study. J Hepatol 1990;11:S149–50.
555. Bortolotti F, Di Marco V, Vajro P, et al. Long-term evaluation of chronic delta hepatitis in children. J Pediatr 1993;122: 736–8.
556. Berk L, de Man RA, Housset C, et al. Alpha lymphoblastoid interferon and acyclovir for chronic hepatitis delta. Prog Clin Biol Res 1991;364:411–20.
557. Lau DTY, Doo E, Park Y, et al. Lamivudine for chronic delta hepatitis. Hepatology 1999;30:546–9.
558. Kaymakoglu S, Karac C, Demir K, et al. Alpha interferon and ribavirin combination therapy of chronic hepatitis D. Antimicrob Agents Chemother 2005;49:1135–8.
559. Wolters LM, van Nunen AB, Honkoop P, et al. Lamivudine–high dose interferon combination therapy for chronic hepatitis B patients co-infected with the hepatitis D virus. J Viral Hepatol 2000;7:428–34.
560. Yurdaydin C, Bozkaya H, Gurel S, et al. Famciclovir treatment of chronic delta hepatitis. J Hepatol 2002;37:266–71.
561. Samuel D, Zignego AL, Reynes M, et al. Long-term clinical and virological outcome after liver transplantation for cirrhosis caused by chronic delta hepatitis. Hepatology 1995;21: 333–9.
562. Marsman WA, Wiesner RH, Batts KP, et al. Fulminant hepatitis B virus: recurrence after liver transplantation in two patients also infected with hepatitis delta virus. Hepatology 1997;25: 434–8.
563. Bortolotti F, Calzia R, Cadrobbi P, et al. Liver cirrhosis associated with chronic hepatitis B infection in childhood. J Pediatr 1986;108:224–7.
564. Bortolotti F, Calzia R, Vegnente A, et al. Chronic hepatitis in childhood: the spectrum of the disease. Gut 1988;29:659–64.
565. Bortolotti F, Cadrobbi P, Crivellaro C, et al. Long-term outcome of chronic hepatitis type B in patients who acquire hepatitis B infection in childhood. Gastroenterology 1990;99:805–10.
566. Worm HC, van der Poel WHM, Brandstatter G. Hepatitis E: an overview. Microbes Infect 2002;4:657–66.
567. Emerson SU, Purcell RH. Running like water – the omnipresence of hepatitis E. N Engl J Med 2004;351:2367–8.
568. Aggarwal R, Krawczynski K. Hepatitis E: an overview and recent advances in clinical and laboratory research. J Gastroenterol Hepatol 2000;14:9–20.
569. Krawczynski K, Aggarwal R, Kamili S. Infections of the liver. Infect Dis Clin N Am 2000;14:1–18.
570. Corwin AL, Tien NTK, Bounlu K, et al. The unique riverine ecology of hepatitis E virus transmission in South-East Asia. Trans R Soc Trop Med Hyg 1999;93:255–60.
571. Panda SK, Jameel S. Hepatitis E virus: from epidemiology to molecular biology. Viral Hepat 1997;3:227–51.
572. Bradley DW. Hepatitis-E virus genome: molecular features, expression of immunoreactive proteins and sequence divergence. J Hepatol 1991;13:SI42–54.
573. Koonin EV, Gorbalenya AE, Purdy MA, et al. Computer-assisted assignment of functional domains in the nonstructural polyprotein of hepatitis-E virus delineation of an additional group of positive-strand RNA plant and animal viruses. Proc Natl Acad Sci U S A 1992;89:8259–63.
574. Tsarev SA, Emerson SU, Reyes GR, et al. Characterization of a prototype strain of hepatitis E virus. Proc Natl Acad Sci U S A 1992;89:559–63.

575. Balayan MS. Epidemiology of hepatitis E virus infection. J Viral Hepat 1997;4:155–65.
576. Skidmore SJ. Hepatitis E. BMJ 1995;310:414–15.
577. Ansari IH, Nanda SK, Durgapal H, et al. Cloning sequencing, and expression of the hepatitis E virus (HEV) nonstructural open reading frame 1. J Med Virol 2000;60:275–83.
578. Ahn J-M, Kang S-G, Lee D-Y, et al. Identification of novel human hepatitis E virus (HEV) isolates and determination of the seroprevalence of HEV in Korea. J Clin Microbiol 2005;3042–8.
579. Reyes GR, Purdy MA, Kim JP, et al. Isolation of a cDNA from the virus responsible for enterically transmitted non-A, non-B hepatitis. Science 1990;247:1335–9.
580. Shrestha SM, Srestha S, Tsuda F, et al. Genetic changes in hepatitis E virus of subtype 1a in patients with sporadic acute hepatitis E in Kathmandu, Nepal, from 1997 to 2002. J Gen Virol 2004; 85:97–104.
581. Mansuy JM, Peron JM, Abravanel F, et al. Hepatitis E in the South West of France in individuals who have never visited an endemic area. J Med Virol 2004;74:419–24.
582. Redlinger T, O'Rourke K, Nickey L, Martinez G. Elevated hepatitis A and E seroprevalence rates in a Texas/Mexico border community. Tex Med 1998;94:68–71.
583. Aggarwal R, Naik SR. Faecal excretion of hepatitis-E virus. Lancet 1992;340:787.
584. DeCock KM, Bradley DW, Sandford NL, et al. Epidemic non-A, non-B hepatitis in patients from Pakistan. Ann Intern Med 1987; 106:227–30.
585. Ray R, Aggarwal R, Salunke PN, et al. Hepatitis E virus genome in stools of hepatitis patients during large epidemic in North India, Lancet 1991;338:783–4.
586. Skidmore SJ, Yarbough PO, Gabor KA, et al. Hepatitis E virus: the cause of waterborne hepatitis outbreak. J Med Virol 1992; 37:58–60.
587. Ticehurst J, Popkin TJ, Bryan JP, et al. Association of hepatitis E virus with an outbreak of hepatitis in Pakistan: serologic responses and pattern of virus excretion. J Med Virol 1992; 36:84–92.
588. Chauhan A, Dilawari JB, Jameel S, et al. Common etiological agent for epidemic and sporadic non-A non-B hepatitis. Lancet 1992;339:1509–10.
589. Hau CH, Hien TT, Tien NT, et al. Prevalence of enteric hepatitis A and E viruses in the Mekong delta region of Vietnam. Am J Trop Med Hyg 1998;60:277–80.
590. Goto K, Ito K, Sugiura T, et al. Prevalence of hepatitis E virus infection in Japanese children. J Pediatr Gastroenterol Nutr 2005;42:89–92.
591. Bader TF, Krawczynski K, Polish LB, et al. Hepatitis E in a U.S. traveler to Mexico [letter]. N Engl J Med 1991;325:1659.
592. De Groen PC. Hepatitis E in the United States: a case of "hog fever?" [editorial]. Mayo Clin Proc 1997;72:1197–8.
593. Goldsmith R, Yarbough PO, Reyes GR, et al. Enzyme-linked immunosorbent assay for diagnosis of acute sporadic hepatitis E in Egyptian children. Lancet 1992;339:328–32.
594. Hyams KC, Purdy MA, Kaur M, et al. Acute sporadic hepatitis E in Sudanese children: analysis based on a new Western blot assay. J Infect Dis 1992;165:1001–5.
595. Daniel HDJ, Warier A, Abraham P, Sridharan G. Age-wise exposure rates to hepatitis E virus in a southern Indian patient population without liver disease. Am J Top Med Hyg 2004;71: 675–8.
596. Singh S, Mohanty A, Joshi YK, et al. Mother-to-child transmission of hepatitis E virus infection. Indian J Pediatr 2003;70: 37–9.
597. Khuroo MS, Kamili S, Yattoo GN. Hepatitis E virus infection may be transmitted through blood transfusions in an endemic area. J Gastroenterol Hepatol 2004;19:778–84.
598. Arora NK, Panda SK, Nanda SK, et al. Hepatitis E infection in children: study of an outbreak. J Gastroenterol Hepatol 1999; 14:572–7.
599. Hamid SS, Atiq M, Shehzad F, et al. Hepatitis E virus superinfection in patients with chronic liver disease. Hepatology 2002; 36:474–8.
600. Kumar A, Aggarwal R, Naik SR, et al. Hepatitis E virus is responsible for decompensation of chronic liver disease in an endemic region. Indian J Gastroenterol 2004;23:59–62.
601. Ramachandran J, Eapen CE, Kang G, et al. Hepatitis E superinfection produces severe decompensation in patients with chronic liver disease. J Gastroenterol Hepatol 2004;19: 134–8.
602. Bile K, Isse A, Mohamud O, et al. Contrasting roles of rivers and wells as sources of drinking water on attack and fatality rates in a hepatitis E epidemic in Somalia. Am J Trop Med Hyg 1994; 51:466–74.
603. Corwin AL, Khiem HB, Clayson ET, et al. A waterborne outbreak of hepatitis E virus transmission in southwestern Vietnam. Am J Trop Med Hyg 1996;54:559–62.
604. Khuroo MS, Dar MY. Hepatitis E: Evidence for person-to-person transmission and inability of low dose immune serum globulin from an Indian source to prevent it. Indian J Gastroenterol 1992;3:113–16.
605. Tsarev SA, Tsareva TS, Emerson SU, et al. Successful passive and active immunization of cynomolgus monkeys against hepatitis E. Proc Natl Acad Sci U S A 1994;91:10198–202.
606. Tsarev SA, Tsareva TS, Emerson SU, et al. Recombinant vaccine against hepatitis E: dose response and protection against heterologous challenge. Vaccine 1997;15:1834–8.

18

AUTOIMMUNE HEPATITIS

Giorgina Mieli-Vergani, M.D., Ph.D., and Diego Vergani, M.D., Ph.D.

Autoimmune hepatitis (AIH) is a progressive inflammatory liver disorder preferentially affecting females and characterized serologically by high aminotransferase levels, elevated immunoglobulin G (IgG), and presence of autoantibodies and histologically by interface hepatitis in the absence of a known etiology. AIH is divided into two types according to the autoantibody profile: patients with type 1 are positive for antinuclear antibody (ANA) and/or anti–smooth muscle antibody (ASMA); patients with type 2 are positive for anti–liver-kidney-microsomal antibody type 1 (anti-LKM-1). AIH responds satisfactorily to immunosuppressive treatment.

HISTORY AND EPIDEMIOLOGY

Autoimmune hepatitis is a relatively recently recognized disease, having been first described by Waldenström [1] in 1950. Seropositivity for ANA, the hallmark of systemic lupus erythematosus, led Mackay et al. [2] to call it *lupoid hepatitis,* a term no longer used. Because the disease frequently presents acutely, similarly obsolete is the term *chronic active hepatitis,* which implied that the disease should be chronic, that is, of at least 6 months' duration, before institution of immunosuppression. Before the efficacy of immunosuppression was established, untreated severe AIH had a mortality rate of 50% at 5 years and 90% at 10 years [3,4]. The prevalence of AIH is unknown. Studies in adults have reported rates varying from 1 in 200,000 in the U.S. general population [5] to 20 in 100,000 in females over 14 years of age in Spain [6]; both figures are probably underestimates. At the King's tertiary pediatric hepatology referral center, there has been a sevenfold increase in the incidence of AIH over the last decade, the disease representing approximately 10% of some 400 new referrals per year.

CLINICAL FEATURES

Two types of AIH are recognized according to the presence of ASMA and/or ANA (type 1) or anti-LKM-1 (type 2) antibodies [7–9]. Type 1 AIH represents two thirds of the cases. Severity of disease is similar in the two types [7]. In both, there is a predominance of girls (75–80%). Anti-LKM-1–positive patients are younger and have a higher tendency to present with acute liver failure, but the duration of symptoms before diagnosis and the frequency of hepatosplenomegaly are similar in the two groups. Both have a high frequency of associated autoimmune disorders (about 20%) and a family history of autoimmune disease (40%). Associated autoimmune disorders include thyroiditis, inflammatory bowel disease, vitiligo, insulin-dependent diabetes, and nephrotic syndrome in both types [7]. Type 2 AIH may be associated with autoimmune polyendocrinopathy candidiasis-ectodermal dystrophy (APECED), an autosomal recessive genetic disorder in which liver disease is reportedly present in some 20% of the cases [10].

There are three clinical patterns of disease [7]: (1) In at least 40% of patients, the presentation is indistinguishable from that of an acute viral hepatitis (nonspecific symptoms of malaise, nausea/vomiting, anorexia, and abdominal pain, followed by jaundice, dark urine, and pale stools). Some children, particularly those who are anti-LKM-1 positive, develop acute hepatic failure with grade II–IV hepatic encephalopathy 2–8 weeks from onset of symptoms. (2) In 25–40% of patients, the onset is insidious, with an illness characterized by progressive fatigue, relapsing jaundice, headache, anorexia, and weight loss, lasting from several months and even years before diagnosis. (3) In about 10% of patients, there is no history of jaundice and the diagnosis follows presentation with complications of portal hypertension, such as splenomegaly, hematemesis from esophageal varices, bleeding diathesis, chronic diarrhea, and weight loss. The mode of presentation of AIH in childhood is therefore variable, and the disease should be suspected and excluded in all children presenting with symptoms and signs of prolonged or severe liver disease. The course of disease may be fluctuating, with flares and spontaneous remissions, a pattern that may result in delayed referral and diagnosis. The majority of the children, however, on physical examination have clinical signs of an underlying chronic liver disease, that is, cutaneous stigmata (spider nevi, palmar erythema, leukonychia, and striae), firm liver, and splenomegaly; at ultrasound the liver parenchyma is often nodular and heterogenous.

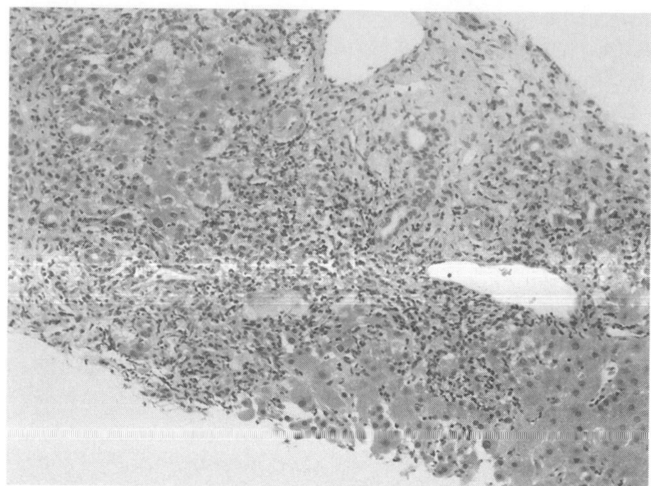

Figure 18.1. Portal and periportal lymphocyte and plasma cell infiltrate extending to and disrupting the parenchymal limiting plate (interface hepatitis). Swollen hepatocytes, pyknotic necroses, and acinar inflammation are present. (Hematoxylin and eosin staining.) (Picture kindly provided by Dr. Alberto Quaglia.) For color reproduction, see Color Plate 18.1.

DIAGNOSIS AND LABORATORY FINDINGS

Diagnosis of AIH is based on a series of positive and negative criteria [11,12]. Liver biopsy is necessary to establish the diagnosis. The typical histologic picture includes a dense mononuclear and plasma cell infiltration of the portal areas, which expands into the liver lobule; destruction of the hepatocytes at the periphery of the lobule, with erosion of the limiting plate ("interface hepatitis"); connective tissue collapse, resulting from hepatocyte death, expanding from the portal area into the lobule ("bridging collapse"); and hepatic regeneration with "rosette" formation (Figure 18.1). In addition to the typical histology, other positive criteria include elevated serum aminotransferase and IgG/γ-globulin levels and presence of ANA, ASMA, or anti-LKM-1. The diagnosis of AIH has been advanced by the criteria developed by the International Autoimmune Hepatitis Group (IAIHG) [11,13], in which negative criteria, such as evidence of infection with hepatitis B or C virus, Wilson's disease, and alcohol, are taken into account in addition to the positive criteria mentioned above. IAIHG has provided a scoring system for the diagnosis of AIH, mainly used for research purposes.

Autoantibodies

A key component of the criteria developed by the IAIHG is detection, by indirect immunofluorescence, of autoantibodies to constituents of the nuclei (ANA), smooth muscle (ASMA), and liver-kidney-microsome type 1 (anti-LKM-1) [11,13,14]. Autoantibody detection not only assists in the diagnosis but also allows differentiation of AIH type 1 and type 2. ANA and ASMA, which characterize type 1 AIH, and anti-LKM-1, which defines type 2 AIH, are mutually exclusive; in those rare instances when they are present simultaneously, the clinical course is similar to that of AIH type 2. Recognition and interpretation of the immunofluorescence patterns are not always straightforward [14]. The operator dependency of the technique and the relative rarity of AIH explain the not-infrequent occurrence of errors in reporting, particularly of less frequent specificities such as anti-LKM-1. Problems do exist between laboratory reporting and clinical interpretation of the results that are partly dependent on (1) insufficient standardization of the tests and (2) the degree of unfamiliarity of some clinicians with the disease spectrum of AIH. In regard to standardization, the lead has been taken by the IAIHG, which has established an internationally representative committee to define guidelines and develop procedures and reference standards for more reliable testing [14]. The basic technique for the routine testing of autoantibodies relevant to AIH is indirect immunofluorescence on a freshly prepared rodent substrate that should include kidney, liver, and stomach to allow the detection of ANA, ASMA, and anti-LKM-1, as well as anti–liver cytosol type 1 (anti-LC-1) and antimitochondrial antibody (AMA), the serologic hallmark of primary biliary cirrhosis. Positive sera should be titrated to extinction, whereas the pattern of nuclear staining for those that are ANA positive may be further characterized by the use of HEp2 cells. Commercially available sections are of variable quality because, to lengthen shelf-life, they are treated with fixatives (acetone, ethanol, or methanol), which results in enhanced background staining that may hinder the recognition of diagnostic autoantibodies, especially when these are present at low titer. Because healthy adults may show reactivity at the conventional starting serum dilution of 1:10, the arbitrary dilution of 1:40 has been considered clinically significant by the IAIHG. In contrast, in healthy children, autoantibody reactivity is infrequent, so titers of 1:20 for ANA and ASMA and 1:10 for anti-LKM-1 are clinically relevant. Hence, the laboratory should report any level of positivity from 1:10 and the attending physician should interpret the result within the clinical context and the age of the patient.

Antinuclear antibody is readily detectable as a nuclear staining in kidney, stomach, and liver. On the latter in particular, the ANA pattern may be detected as homogeneous, or coarsely or finely speckled. In most cases of AIH, but not in all, the pattern is homogeneous. To obtain a much clearer and easier definition of the nuclear pattern, HEp2 cells that have prominent nuclei should be used. HEp2 cells, however, should not be used for screening purposes because nuclear reactivity to these cells is frequent at low serum dilution (1:40) in the healthy population. For ANA, likely molecular targets include nuclear chromatin and histones, akin to lupus, but there are probably several others. The advent of new techniques using recombinant nuclear antigens and immunoassays will enable a better definition of ANA target antigens, an assessment of their specificity for diagnosis, and their possible role in the pathogenesis of AIH type 1.

Smooth muscle antibody is detected on kidney, stomach, and liver, where it stains the walls of the arteries. In the stomach, it also stains the muscularis mucosa and the lamina propria. On the renal substrate, it is possible to visualize the V, G, and

T patterns; V refers to vessels, G to glomeruli, and T to tubules [15]. The V pattern is present also in nonautoimmune inflammatory liver disease, in autoimmune diseases not affecting the liver, and in viral infections, but the VG and VGT patterns are specific for AIH. The VGT pattern corresponds to the so-called F actin or microfilament (MF) pattern observed using cultured fibroblasts as substrate. Neither the VGT nor the anti-MF patterns are, however, entirely specific for the diagnosis of AIH type 1. Although the VGT-MF pattern has been suggested to be the result of a specific antibody uniquely found in AIH type 1, it may just reflect high-titer ASMA. The molecular target of the MF reactivity that is observed in AIH type 1 remains to be identified. Though "anti-actin" reactivity is strongly associated with AIH type 1, some 20% of ASMA-positive AIH type 1 patients do not have the F-actin/VGT pattern. Therefore, the absence, of anti-actin ASMA does not exclude the diagnosis of AIH [16].

Anti-LKM-1 brightly stains the liver cell cytoplasm and the P3 portion of the renal tubules but does not stain gastric parietal cells. Anti-LKM-1 is often confused with AMA because both autoantibodies stain liver and kidney. Compared with LKM-1, AMA stains the liver more faintly and the renal tubules more diffusely, with an accentuation of the small distal ones. In contrast to anti-LKM-1, AMA also stains the gastric parietal cells. In the context of AIH, there can be positivity for AMA in rare cases [17]. The identification of the molecular targets of anti-LKM-1, that is, cytochrome P4502D6 (CYP2D6), and of AMA, that is, enzymes of the 2-oxo-acid dehydrogenase complexes, has led to the establishment of immunoassays based on the use of the recombinant or purified antigens [14]. Commercially available enzyme-linked immunosorbent assays (ELISAs) are accurate for detection of anti-LKM-1, at least in the context of AIH type 2, and reasonably accurate for the detection of AMA. Therefore, if doubt remains after examination by immunofluorescence, this can be resolved by the use of molecular-based immunoassays.

Other autoantibodies less commonly tested but of diagnostic importance include those to liver cytosol type 1 (LC-1), antineutrophil cytoplasm (ANCA), and soluble liver antigen (SLA). Anti-LC-1, which can be present on its own but frequently occurs in association with anti-LKM-1, is an additional marker for AIH type 2 and targets formiminotransferase cyclodeaminase (FTCD) [18]. ANCA may also be positive in pediatric autoimmune liver disease [7]. There are three types of ANCA: cytoplasmic (cANCA), perinuclear (pANCA), and atypical perinuclear, the target of which is a peripheral nuclear and not a cytoplasmic perinuclear antigen (hence, the suggested name of pANNA, i.e., peripheral antinuclear neutrophil antibody). The type found in AIH type 1 is pANNA, which is also found in inflammatory bowel disease and sclerosing cholangitis but is virtually absent in type 2 AIH [7]. Anti-SLA, which was originally described as the hallmark of a third type of AIH [19], is also found in some 50% of patients with type 1 and type 2 AIH, in which it defines a more severe course [20].

After assessment of all the specificities described above, there is a small proportion of patients with AIH without detectable autoantibodies. This condition, which responds to immunosuppression such as the seropositive form, represents seronegative AIH, and its prevalence and clinical characteristics remain to be defined.

Comparison Between Type 1 and Type 2 AIH

Clinical, laboratory, and histologic features of type 1 and 2 AIH are summarized in Table 18.1. Type 1 AIH is associated with the possession of human leukocyte antigen (HLA) DRB1*0301 [7, 21,22], whereas type 2 AIH is associated with DRB1*0701 [23]. Patients with AIH, whether anti-LKM-1 or ANA/ASMA positive, have isolated partial deficiency of the HLA class III complement component C4, which is genetically determined [24].

Anti-LKM-1–positive patients have higher levels of bilirubin and aminotransferases at presentation than those who are ANA/ASMA positive and present significantly more frequently with fulminant hepatic failure [7]. Excluding children with the fulminant presentation, severely impaired hepatic synthetic function, as assessed by the presence of both prolonged prothrombin time and hypoalbuminemia, is more common in ANA/ASMA-positive than in anti-LKM-1–positive patients. The vast majority of patients have increased serum levels of IgG, but some 20% do not, indicating that normal IgG values do not exclude the diagnosis of AIH. Partial IgA deficiency is significantly more common in anti-LKM-1–positive than in ANA/ASMA-positive patients.

The severity of interface hepatitis at diagnosis is similar in both types, but cirrhosis on initial biopsy is more frequent in type 1 than in type 2 AIH, suggesting a more chronic course of disease in the former. Of note is that most patients already cirrhotic at diagnosis present with a clinical picture reminiscent of that of prolonged acute viral hepatitis. Multiacinar or panacinar collapse, which suggests an acute liver injury, is more frequently seen in type 2 AIH. The question as to whether the acute presentation in these patients represents a sudden deterioration of an underlying unrecognized chronic process or genuinely acute liver damage remains open. Progression to cirrhosis during treatment is more frequent in type 1 AIH. As mentioned earlier, in both, a more severe disease and a higher tendency to relapse are associated with the possession of antibodies to SLA, which are present in about half the patients with AIH type 1 or 2 at diagnosis [20].

Differential Diagnosis

Because positive autoimmune serology may be present in conditions other than AIH, particularly autoimmune sclerosing cholangitis [25] (ASC; see below), chronic hepatitis B [26] or C [27], virus infections, and Wilson's disease [28], all these conditions must be considered in the differential diagnosis and excluded. ASC shares the same serologic profile as type 1 AIH but has typical bile duct lesions on cholangiography. Up to 50% of patients with hepatitis B and C are positive for ANA and/or ASMA, usually at low titers, and up to 10% of patients with chronic hepatitis C have anti-LKM-1 antibodies. In these

Table 18.1: Clinical, Laboratory, and Histologic Features at Presentation of Autoimmune Hepatitis Type 1, Autoimmune Hepatitis Type 2, and Autoimmune Sclerosing Cholangitis

	Type 1 AIH	*Type 2 AIH*	*ASC*
Median age, yr	11	7	12
Females, %	75	75	55
Mode of presentation, %			
Acute hepatitis	47	40	37
Acute liver failure	3	25	0
Insidious onset	38	25	37
Complication of chronic liver disease	12	10	26
Associated immune diseases, %	22	20	48
Inflammatory bowel disease, %	20	12	44
Family history of autoimmune disease, %	43	40	37
Abnormal cholangiogram, %	0	0	100
ANA/ASMA, %	100	25	96
Anti–LKM-1, %	0	100	4
pANCA, %	45	11	74
Anti–SLA, %*	58	58	41
Increased IgG level, %	84	75	89
Partial IgA deficiency, %	9	45	5
Low C4 level, %	89	83	70
Increased frequency of HLA DR*0301	Yes	No†	No
Increased frequency of HLA DR*0701	No	Yes	No
Increased frequency of HLA DR*1301	No	No	Yes
Interface hepatitis, %	66	72	35
Biliary features, %	28	6	31
Cirrhosis, %	69	38	15
Remission after immunosuppressive treatment, %	97	87	89

*Measured by radioligand assay.
†But increased in HLA DR*0701-negative patients.
AIH, autoimmune hepatitis; ASC, autoimmune sclerosing cholangitis; ANA, antinuclear antibody; ASMA, anti–smooth muscle antibody; LKM-1, liver-kidney-microsomal type 1 antibody; pANCA, perinuclear antineutrophil cytoplasmic antibody; SLA, soluble liver antigen; IgG, immunoglobulin G; IgA, immunoglobulin A; C4, C4 component of complement; HLA, human leukocyte antigen.
Data from Gregorio et al. [7,25].

patients, the histology may also mimic AIH, though the degree of inflammation is usually milder. Detection of the typical viral markers allows their diagnosis. ANA, and at times ASMA, may be present in Wilson's disease in association with high IgG and an inflammatory liver histology, which can make the differential diagnosis with AIH type 1 difficult. Urinary, serum, and liver tissue copper studies and search for Kayser–Fleischer rings should be performed in all cases.

Autoimmune Polyendocrinopathy-Candidiasis-Ectodermal Dystrophy

Autoimmune polyendocrinopathy-candidiasis-ectodermal dystrophy (APECED) is a monogenic disorder [29,30] with a variable phenotype that includes, in about 20% of the cases, AIH that resembles AIH type 2 [10]. This condition, also known as autoimmune polyendocrine syndrome 1, is an autosomal recessive disorder caused by homozygous mutations in the *AIRE1* gene and characterized by a variety of organ-specific autoimmune diseases, the most common of which are hypoparathyroidism and primary adrenocortical failure, accompanied by chronic mucocutaneous candidiasis.

ETIOLOGY AND PATHOGENESIS

The etiology of AIH is unknown, although both genetic and environmental factors are involved in its expression.

Genetics

Susceptibility to AIH type 1 in children is conferred by the possession of HLA DR3 (DRB1*0301) within the major histocompatibility complex (MHC) in Europe and North America [21,22]. The HLA DRB1*0301 heterodimer contains a lysine residue at position 71 of the DRB1 polypeptide and the hexameric amino acid sequence LLEQKR at positions 67–72, which may be critical for susceptibility to AIH, favoring the binding of autoantigenic peptides, complementary to this hexameric sequence. Interestingly, in South America, possession of the HLA DRB1*1301 allele, which predisposes to pediatric AIH type 1 in that population, is also associated with persistent infection with the endemic hepatitis A virus [31,32], suggesting that these HLA associations may be the molecular footprints of the prevailing environmental triggers that precipitate AIH type 1 in different environments.

The lysine-71 model for AIH type 1 cannot explain the full spectrum of the disease. Thus in Europe and North America, presence of lysine-71 is associated not only with a more severe juvenile form in DRB1*0301-positive patients but also with a milder, late-onset disease in DRB1*0401-positive patients [21,22]. Other genes within and/or without the MHC are therefore likely to be involved in determining the phenotype. Possible candidates are the MHC-encoded complement and tumor necrosis factor-α genes mapping to the class III MCH region and the MHC class I chain-related A and B genes [21,22].

Autoimmune hepatitis type 2 is conferred by the possession of HLA DR7 (DRB1*0701) and, in HLA DRB1*0701-negative patients, to DR3 (DRB1*0301), patients positive for DRB1*0701 having a more aggressive disease and severe prognosis [23].

APECED is the result of mutations of the *AIRE1* gene [29,30]. The *AIRE1* sequence consists of 14 exons containing 45 different mutations, with a 13–base pair deletion at nucleotide 964 in exon 8 accounting for more than 70% of APECED alleles in the United Kingdom [30]. The protein predicted to be encoded by *AIRE1* is a transcription factor. *AIRE1* is highly expressed in medullary epithelial cells and other stromal cells in the thymus involved in clonal deletion of self-reactive T cells. Studies in a murine model indicate that the gene inhibits organ-specific autoimmunity by inducing thymic expression of peripheral antigens in the medulla, leading to central deletion of autoreactive T cells. Interestingly, APECED has a high level of variability in symptoms, especially between populations. Because various gene mutations have the same effect on thymic transcription of ectopic genes in animal models, it is likely that the clinical variability across human populations relates to environmental or genetic modifiers. Of the various genetic modifiers, perhaps the most likely to synergize with *AIRE* mutations are polymorphisms in the HLA region. HLA molecules not only are highly variable and strongly associated with multiple autoimmune diseases but are also able to affect thymic repertoire selection of autoreactive T-cell clones. Carriers of a single *AIRE* mutation do not develop APECED. However, although the inheritance pattern of APECED indicates a strictly recessive disorder, there are anecdotal data of mutations in a single copy of *AIRE* being associated with human autoimmunity of a less severe form than classically defined APECED [29,30]. The role of the *AIRE1* heterozygote state in the development of AIH remains to be established. *AIRE1* mutations have been reported in three children with severe AIH type 2 and extrahepatic autoimmune manifestations [33].

Mechanisms of Liver Autoimmune Attack

The histologic picture of AIH was the first to suggest that autoaggressive cellular immunity might be involved in its pathogenesis. A powerful stimulus must be promoting the formation of the massive inflammatory cell infiltrate present at diagnosis. Whatever the initial trigger, it is most probable that such a high number of activated inflammatory cells cause liver damage. Immunocytochemical studies have shown that T lymphocytes mounting the α/β T-cell receptor predominate and that among the T cells, a majority are positive for the CD4 helper/inducer phenotype and a sizeable minority for the CD8 cytotoxic phenotype [34]. Lymphocytes of non–T-cell lineage are fewer and include (in decreasing order of frequency) natural killer (NK) cells (CD16/CD56 positive), macrophages, and B lymphocytes [34]. The recently described NK T cells (NKT), which express simultaneously markers of both NK (CD56) and T cells (CD3), are involved in liver damage in an animal model of AIH, although there are no studies in humans [35].

The possible pathways that an immune attack can follow to inflict damage on the hepatocyte are summarized in Figure 18.2. Over the past two decades, different aspects of this pathogenic scenario have been investigated.

Defective Immunoregulation

An impairment of immunoregulatory mechanisms has been described in AIH. Both children and young adults with this condition have low levels of T cells expressing the CD8 marker and impaired suppressor cell function [36], which segregates with the possession of the HLA haplotype B8/DR3 and can be corrected by therapeutic doses of corticosteroids [37]. Furthermore, patients with AIH have been reported to have a specific defect in a subpopulation of T cells controlling the immune response to liver-specific membrane antigens [38].

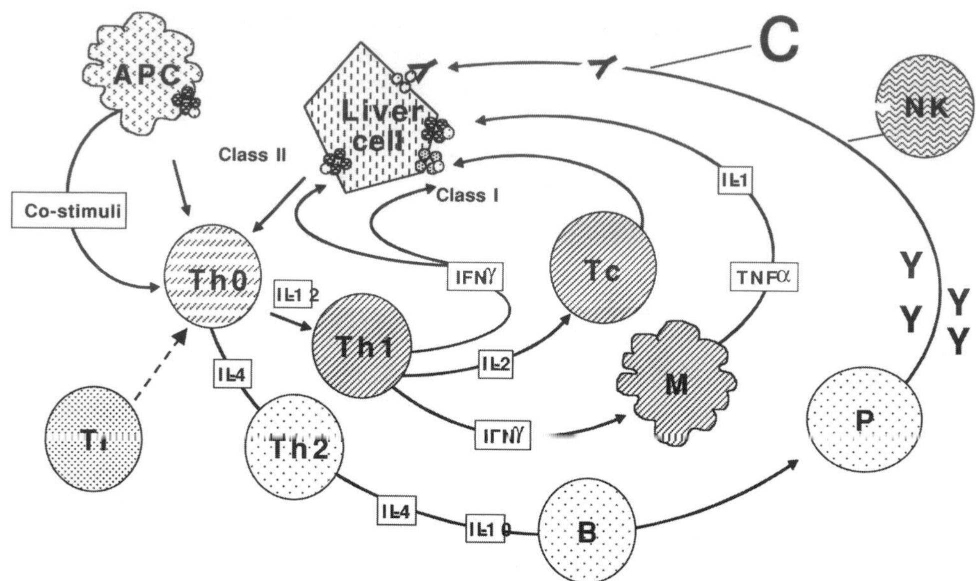

Figure 18.2. Liver damage is believed to be orchestrated by CD4+ T lymphocytes recognizing a self-antigenic peptide. To trigger an autoimmune response, the peptide must be embraced by an HLA class II molecule and presented to uncommitted CD4 T helper 0 (Th0) cells by professional antigen-presenting cells (APCs), with the costimulation of ligand–ligand (CD28 on Th0, CD80 on APC) interaction between the two cells. The Th0 cells become activated, differentiate into functional phenotypes according to the cytokines prevailing in the microenvironment and the nature of the antigen, and initiate a cascade of immune reactions determined by the cytokines they produce. Arising in the presence of the macrophage-produced IL-12, Th1 cells secrete mainly IL-2 and interferon gamma (IFN-γ), which activate macrophages (M), enhance expression of HLA class I (increasing the vulnerability of liver cells to cytotoxic attack), and induce expression of HLA class II molecules on hepatocytes, which then become able to present the autoantigenic peptide to CD4 T helper cells, thus perpetuating the immune recognition cycle. Th2 cells, which differentiate from Th0 if the microenvironment is rich in IL-4, produce mainly IL-4, IL-5, and IL-10, which induce autoantibody production by B lymphocytes and plasma cells (P). Autoantibody-coated hepatocytes may be killed by the action of the complement system (C) or of Fc-bearing lymphocytes such as natural killer cells (NK). Physiologically, Th1 and Th2 cells antagonize each other. The process of autoantigen recognition is strictly controlled by regulatory mechanisms enacted by regulatory T cells, such as CD4$^+$CD25$^+$ T cells (Tr). If these regulatory mechanisms fail, the autoimmune attack is perpetuated.

Further evidence for an impairment of immunoregulatory function in AIH has been obtained in the last few years [39]. Among recently defined T-cell subsets with potential immunosuppression function, CD4$^+$ T cells constitutively expressing the interleukin 2 receptor (IL-2R) α chain (CD25) – regulatory T cells (T-regs) – have emerged as the dominant immunoregulatory population [40]. These cells, which represent 5–10% of the total population of peripheral CD4$^+$ T lymphocytes, control the innate and the adaptive immune response by preventing the proliferation and effector function of autoreactive T cells. Their mechanism of action involves mainly a direct contact with the target cells and, to a lesser extent, the release of immunoregulatory cytokines such as IL-10 and tissue growth factor-β_1. In addition to CD25, which is also present on T cells undergoing activation, T-regs express a number of other markers, such as the forkhead/winged helix transcription factor FOXP3, whose expression has been associated with the acquisition of regulatory properties. In patients with AIH, T-regs are defective in number and their reduction relates to the stage of disease, being more evident at diagnosis than during drug-induced remission [39]. The percentage of T-regs inversely correlates with biomarkers of disease severity, suggesting that a reduction in regulatory T cells favors the serologic manifestations of autoimmune liver disease. If loss of immunoregulation is central to the pathogenesis of autoimmune liver disease, treatment should concentrate on restoring the ability of T-regs to expand, with consequent increases in their number and function. This is at least partially achieved by standard immunosuppression, because T-reg numbers increase during remission [39].

Autoreactive T Cells

Inappropriate expression of HLA class II antigens has been demonstrated on the hepatocytes of patients with AIH [34]. This, in association with impaired immunoregulation, may lead to the presentation of an autoantigenic peptide by the liver cells to helper/inducer cells, leading to their activation. Although no direct evidence exists that an autoantigenic peptide is presented by hepatocytes and recognized by CD4 T helper (Th) cells, activation of these cells has been documented in AIH [34,41].

Investigation of liver antigen–reactive T cells has been based on the generation of T-cell clones from both the peripheral blood and liver parenchyma of patients with AIH [42–44]. Although clones derived from the peripheral blood were mainly $CD4^+$ α/β T cells, a large proportion of those of liver origin were either CD4–CD8 γ/δ or $CD8^+$ α/β T cells. Both α/β and γ/δ T-cell clones demonstrated specific expansion in the presence of liver membrane antigens. Some of the liver membrane–reactive CD4 T-cell clones were found to react with specific membrane antigens, such as liver-specific lipoprotein and/or asialoglycoprotein receptor, and to induce immunoglobulin and autoantibody production by autologous B cells in vitro [42–44].

The most recent advances in the study of T cells have occurred in AIH type 2 since the target of its humoral autoimmune response was identified as cytochrome P4502D6 (CYP2D6). A systematic approach based on the construction of overlapping peptides covering the whole CYP2D6 molecule was recently adopted to define the specificity of ex vivo CYP2D6-reactive T cells in patients with AIH type 2 [23]. This study has shown that T cells from patients positive for the predisposing HLA allele DRB1*0701 recognize, in a proliferation assay, seven regions of CYP2D6, four of which are also partially recognized by T cells of DRB1*0701-negative patients. Whereas distinct peptides induce production of interferon gamma, IL-4, or IL-10, peptides inducing interferon gamma and proliferation overlap. There is also an overlap between sequences inducing T- and B-cell responses. The number of epitopes recognized and the quantity of cytokine produced by T cells are directly correlated to biochemical and histologic markers of disease activity. These results indicate that the T-cell response to CYP2D6 in type 2 AIH is polyclonal, involves multiple effector types targeting different epitopes, and is associated with hepatocyte damage.

Animal Models

Research on the pathogenesis of AIH has been hampered by the lack of animal models faithfully reproducing the human condition. Findings in animal models of AIH have been authoritatively reviewed by Jaeckel [45] and Peters [46]. In early studies aimed at characterizing the nature of the liver antigens responsible for the formation of hepatic mononuclear cell infiltrates in experimental hepatitis, liver cell necrosis and periportal infiltration, reminiscent of the histologic changes seen in human chronic hepatitis, were obtained by multiple immunization of rabbits over a period of several months with allogeneic liver extracts in complete Freund adjuvant. Further studies identified two hepatocyte antigens, one located in the plasma membrane and the other in the cytosolic fraction, targets of autoantibody-containing sera from rabbits with experimental hepatitis, induced by repeated immunizations with human liver antigen over several months. The membrane-associated antigen, which was found to be a lipoprotein, was called liver-specific protein (LSP) and later was also identified in human liver. However, the liver autoantibodies present in serum and on hepatocytes did not correlate with histologic liver damage, questioning their pathogenic relevance and indirectly implying a role for cell-mediated immune damage. Subsequent in vitro studies in the rabbit model did find lymphocyte proliferative responses against liver antigen. In vivo evidence of cell-mediated liver damage was provided in a murine model in which experimental hepatitis could be induced through immunization with syngeneic liver antigen and adoptively transferred to naïve mice with nylon wool–adherent lymphocytes (mainly T cells) [47]. Interestingly, this study showed that the susceptibility to liver damage was strain dependent, implying a genetic influence. Splenocytes from the animals with experimental hepatitis were also able to suppress liver-specific and non–liver-specific immune responses [48]. A balance between effector and regulatory cells may explain the chronic relapsing course of AIH in humans. A widely studied model of experimental hepatitis is that induced by concanavalin A [35]. Though this model does not reflect accurately the pathologic entity of AIH in humans, it has provided evidence that liver damage mainly occurs within a Th1 scenario, with the involvement of activated $CD4^+$ T cells and release of the proinflammatory cytokines interferon gamma and tumor necrosis factor-α against a specific genetic background.

All the models described above, though informative regarding single steps leading to liver inflammation and damage, do not mimic the chronic relapsing course of human AIH. In fact, they demonstrate the difficulty in breaking tolerance toward liver antigens and the involvement of regulatory mechanisms in maintaining it. Researchers have focused on animal models of AIH type 2 because in this condition, the autoantigens are well defined. The model produced by Lapierre et al. [49] is based on immunizing (every 2 weeks for three times) C57BL/6 female mice with a plasmid containing the antigenic region of human CYP2D6, the target of anti-LKM-1, and FTCD, the target of anti-LC-1, together with the murine end terminal region of cytotoxic T lymphocyte antigen 4 (CTLA-4). The latter was added to facilitate antigen uptake by antigen-presenting cells (APCs). In a parallel set of experiments, a plasmid containing the DNA encoding IL-12, a Th1-skewing proinflammatory cytokine, was also used. When autoantigens and IL 12 were used to break tolerance, antigen-specific autoantibodies were produced, a relatively modest elevation of aminotransferase levels at 4 and 7 months was observed, and a portal and periportal inflammatory infiltrate composed of CD4 and CD8 T cells and, to a lesser extent, B cells was demonstrated 8–10 months after the third immunization. When the same immunization protocol was used in different mouse strains, either a mild hepatitis or no inflammatory changes were observed, indicating the importance of a specific genetic background [50]. Another model of AIH type 2 used CYP2D6 transgenic mice aimed at breaking tolerance with an Adenovirus–CYP2D6 vector [51]. Although focal hepatocyte necrosis was seen in both mice treated with the Adenovirus–CYP2D6 vector and control mice treated with Adenovirus alone, only the former developed chronic histologic changes, including fibrosis, reminiscent of AIH. The hepatic lesion was associated with a specific immune response to an immunodominant region of CYP2D6 and a cytotoxic T-cell response to Adenovirus–CYP2D6 vector–infected target cells. Though these two experimental approaches provide useful information on the possible pathogenic mechanisms leading to AIH type 2, a model closely mimicking AIH in humans is still missing.

MANAGEMENT AND PROGNOSIS

Autoimmune hepatitis is exquisitely responsive to immunosuppression. The rapidity and degree of response depend on the disease severity at presentation. All types of presentations, apart from fulminant hepatic failure with encephalopathy, respond to standard treatment with prednisolone with or without azathioprine.

Standard treatment for AIH consists of prednisolone, 2 mg/kg/d (maximum 60 mg/d), which is gradually decreased over a period of 4–8 weeks with progressive normalization of the aminotransferase levels. The patient is then maintained on the minimal dose able to sustain normal aminotransferase levels, usually 5 mg/d [7,52]. During the first 6–8 weeks of treatment, liver tests are checked weekly to allow a frequent fine-tuning, avoiding severe steroid side effects. If progressive normalization of the liver tests is not obtained over this period of time or if too high a dose of prednisolone is required to maintain normal aminotransferase levels, azathioprine is added at a starting dose of 0.5 mg/kg/d. In the absence of signs of toxicity, the dose is increased up to a maximum of 2–2.5 mg/kg/d until biochemical control is achieved. Azathioprine is not recommended as first-line treatment because of its hepatotoxicity in severely jaundiced patients, but 85% of the patients will eventually require azathioprine addition. A preliminary report in a cohort of 30 children with AIH suggests that the measurements of the azathioprine metabolites 6-thioguanine and 6-methylmercaptopurine are useful in identifying drug toxicity or nonadherence and in achieving a level of 6-thioguanine considered therapeutic for inflammatory bowel disease [53]. However, the ideal therapeutic level for AIH has not been determined. Although an 80% decrease of initial aminotransferase levels is obtained within 6 weeks from starting treatment in most patients, complete normalization may take several months. In the King's series, normalization of aminotransferase levels occurred at a median of 6 months in ANA/ASMA-positive children and 9 months in anti-LKM-1–positive children [7]. Relapse while on treatment is common, occurring in about 40% of the patients and requiring a temporary increase of the steroid dose. The risk of relapse is higher if steroids are administered on an alternate-day schedule, often instituted in the belief that it has a less negative effect on the child's growth. Small daily doses are more effective in maintaining disease control and minimize the need for high-dose steroid pulses during relapses (with attendant more severe side effects). Cessation of treatment is considered if a liver biopsy shows minimal or no inflammatory changes after 1 year of normal liver function tests. However, it is advisable not to attempt to withdraw treatment within 2 years from diagnosis or during or immediately before puberty, when relapses are more common. The reasons for this are unclear, though an important role may be played by nonadherence, frequently underestimated in teenagers. In the King's experience, successful long-term withdrawal of treatment was achieved in 20% of patients with AIH type 1 but in none with AIH type 2 [7].

In children, an important role in monitoring the response to treatment is the measurement of autoantibody titers and IgG levels, the fluctuation of which is correlated with disease activity [54].

Despite the efficacy of standard immunosuppressive treatment, severe hepatic decompensation may develop, even after many years of apparently good biochemical control, leading to transplantation 10–15 years after diagnosis in 10% of the patients. Overall, in the King's series, over 97% of the patients treated with standard immunosuppression were alive between 0.3 and 19 years (median, 5 years) after diagnosis, including 8% after liver transplantation. Side effects of steroid treatment were mild, the only serious complication being psychosis during induction of remission in 4%, which resolved after prednisolone withdrawal. All patients developed a transient increase in appetite and mild cushingoid features during the first few weeks of treatment. After 5 years of treatment, 56% of the patients maintained the baseline percentile for height or went up across a percentile line, 38% dropped across one percentile line, and only 6% dropped across two percentile lines [55].

Sustained remission, achieved with prednisolone and azathioprine, has been maintained with azathioprine alone in some patients with AIH type 1, akin to the experience in adults [56], but not in AIH type 2.

Induction of remission has been obtained in 71% of treatment-naïve children with AIH using cyclosporin A alone for 6 months, followed by maintenance with low-dose prednisone and azathioprine [57]. Whether this mode of induction has any advantage over the standard treatment remains to be evaluated in controlled studies in specialized centers.

In patients (up to 10%) in whom standard immunosuppression is unable to induce stable remission or who are intolerant to azathioprine, mycophenolate mofetil at a dose of 20 mg/kg twice daily has been successfully used [55]. In case of persistent no response or of intolerance to mycophenolate mofetil (headache, diarrhea, nausea, dizziness, hair loss, and neutropenia), the use of calcineurin inhibitors (cyclosporin A or tacrolimus) should be considered.

Children who present with acute hepatic failure pose a particularly difficult therapeutic problem. If not encephalopathic, they usually benefit from conventional immunosuppressive therapy, but only one of the six children with acute liver failure and encephalopathy in the King's series responded to immunosuppression and survived without a transplant [7].

AUTOIMMUNE HEPATITIS/SCLEROSING CHOLANGITIS OVERLAP SYNDROME

Autoimmune hepatitis/sclerosing cholangitis overlap syndrome (autoimmune sclerosing cholangitis [ASC]) has the same prevalence as AIH type 1 in childhood [25]. This has been shown in a prospective study conducted over a period of 16 years in which all children with serologic (i.e., autoantibodies, high IgG levels) and histologic (i.e., interface hepatitis) features of autoimmune liver disease underwent a cholangiogram at the time of presentation. Approximately 50% of these patients had alterations of the bile ducts characteristic of sclerosing cholangitis, though generally less advanced than those observed in adult primary sclerosing cholangitis (Figure 18.3). A quarter of the children with ASC, despite abnormal cholangiograms, had no histologic features suggesting bile duct involvement, and the diagnosis of sclerosing cholangitis was possible only because of the cholangiographic studies. Virtually all patients were seropositive for ANA and/or ASMA, 55% were girls, and the mode of presentation was similar to that of typical AIH. Inflammatory bowel disease was present in about 45% of children with ASC compared with about 20% of those with typical AIH, and 90% of children with ASC had greatly increased serum IgG levels. At the time of presentation, standard liver tests did not help in discriminating between AIH and ASC, though the alkaline phosphatase/aspartate aminotransferase ratio was significantly higher in ASC (Table 18.2). pANNA was present in 74% of patients with ASC compared with 45% of patients with AIH type 1 and 11% of those with AIH type 2. Susceptibility to ASC in children is conferred by the possession of HLA DRB1*1301 (Y. May et al., unpublished data). Clinical, laboratory, and histologic features of type 1 and 2 AIH and ASC are compared in Table 18.1.

Children with ASC respond to the same immunosuppressive schedule described earlier for AIH [25], liver test abnormalities resolving within a few months after starting treatment in most patients. Steroids and azathioprine, however, though beneficial in abating the parenchymal inflammatory lesion, appear to be less effective in controlling the bile duct disease. Following favorable reports in adult primary sclerosing cholangitis [58,59], ursodeoxycholic acid is usually added at a dosage of

Table 18.2: Liver Function Tests at Presentation in Children with Autoimmune Hepatitis and Autoimmune Sclerosing Cholangitis

	*AIH (n = 28)**	*ASC (n — 27)**
Bilirubin (nv: <20 μmol/L)	35 (4–306)	20 (4–179)
Albumin (nv: >35 g/L)	35 (25–47)	39 (27–54)
AST (nv: <50 IU/L)	333 (24–4830)	102 (18–1215)
INR (nv: <1.2)	1.2 (0.96–2.5)	1.1 (0.9–1.6)
GGT (nv: <50 IU/L)	76 (29–383)	129 (13–948)
AP (nv: <350 IU/L)	356 (131–878)	303 (104–1710)
AP/AST ratio	1.14 (0.05–14.75)	3.96 (0.20–14.20)

*Results presented as median (range).
AST, aspartate aminotransferase; INR, international normalized (prothrombin) ratio; GGT, γ-glutamyltransferase; AP, alkaline phosphatase; nv, normal value.
Data from Gregorio et al. [7,25].

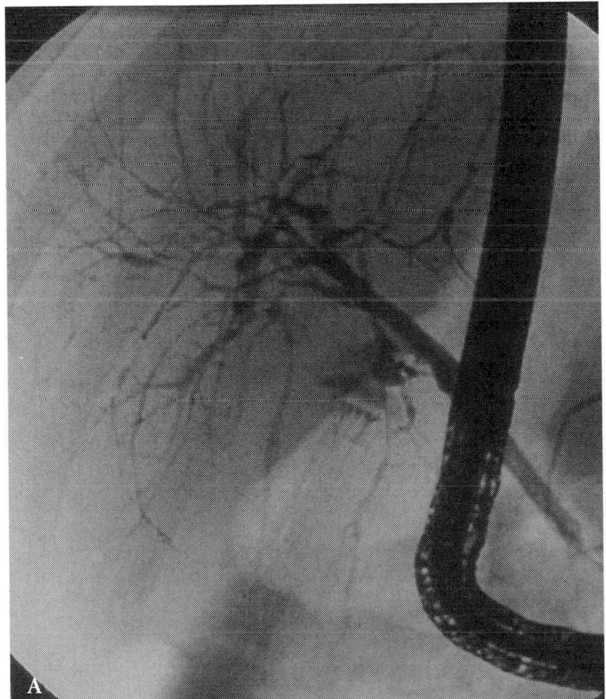

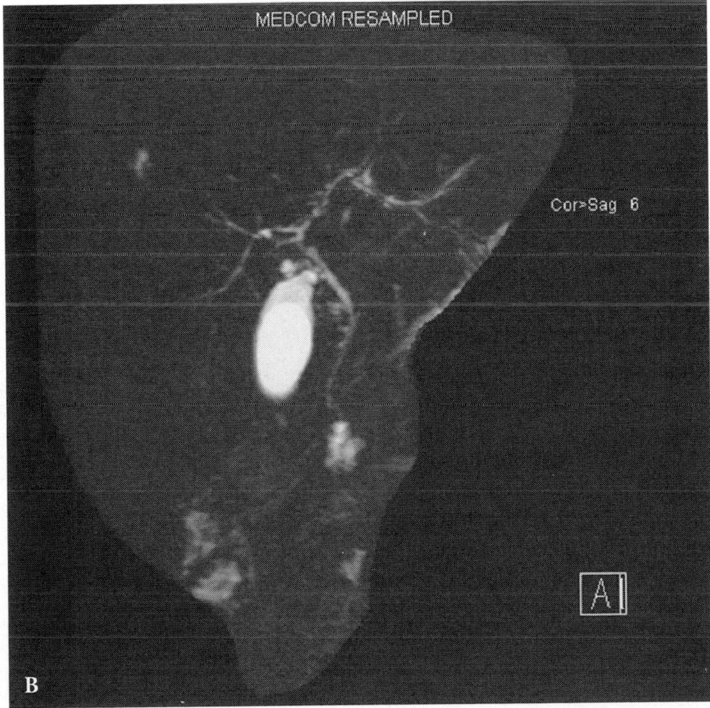

Figure 18.3. Cholangiographic features in two children with autoimmune sclerosing cholangitis. (**A**) Endoscopic cholangiopancreatogram demonstrating cholangiopathy with multiple strictures affecting the intrahepatic bile ducts at all levels. (**B**) Nuclear magnetic resonance cholangiogram demonstrating extensive irregularity of the intra- and extrahepatic bile ducts.

20–30 mg/kg/d, though there is no information as to whether it is helpful in arresting the progression of ASC. Akin to AIH, measurement of autoantibody titers and IgG levels is useful in monitoring disease activity and response to treatment [54]. The medium-term prognosis is good, with a reported 7-year survival of 100%, though 15% of the patients required liver transplantation during this period of follow up [25].

Evolution from AIH to ASC has been documented, suggesting that AIH and ASC are part of the same pathogenic process [25].

RECURRENCE OF AIH AFTER TRANSPLANTATION

Recurrence of AIH after liver transplantation has been shown in several studies [60]. The diagnosis is based on reappearance of clinical symptoms and signs, histologic features of periportal hepatitis, elevation of aminotransferase levels, circulating autoantibodies, and elevated IgG, associated with response to steroids and azathioprine. Possession of the HLA DR3 allele appears to confer predisposition to disease recurrence, as it does to the original AIH, though this has not been universally confirmed. Recurrence has been noted in both adult and pediatric series, and though the rate of this complication increases with the posttransplantation interval, it may appear as early as a month post surgery. Most transplant recipients with recurrent AIH respond to an increase in the dose of corticosteroids and azathioprine, but in a few, recurrence may lead to graft failure and to the need for retransplantation. Caution should be taken in weaning immunosuppression from patients who undergo transplantation for AIH because discontinuation of corticosteroid therapy may increase the risk for recurrent disease.

DE NOVO AIH AFTER TRANSPLANTATION

Tissue autoantibodies after liver transplantation, in particular ANA and ASMA, are also common in patients who have undergone transplantation because of nonautoimmune liver disease [60]. Anti-LKM-1 is the third most frequently reported antibody, but its fluorescence pattern is at times atypical, preferentially staining the renal tubules and sparing the liver. The described prevalence of post–liver transplantation autoantibodies is variable, probably reflecting different techniques used for their detection, the cut-off point above which the autoantibodies are considered positive, the time post transplantation at which they are tested, the nature of the clinical condition leading to transplantation, and the presence or absence of posttransplantation complications. In the late 1990s, it was observed that AIH can arise de novo after liver transplantation in patients who had not received transplants because of autoimmune liver disease [61]. After this original report in children, de novo AIH after liver transplantation has been confirmed by several studies both in adult and pediatric patients [60,62]. Importantly, treatment with prednisolone and azathioprine using the same schedule as that for classic AIH is also effective in de novo AIH, leading to excellent graft and patient survival. It is of interest that these patients do not respond satisfactorily to standard antirejection treatment, making it essential to reach an early diagnosis to avoid graft loss.

Recurrence of AIH post transplantation can be readily explained. The recipient's immune system is sensitized to species-specific antigens and has a pool of memory cells. These are restimulated and reexpanded when the target antigens, "autoantigens," are presented to the recipient's immune system by either the recipient's APCs repopulating the grafted liver or by the donor's APCs sharing histocompatibility antigens with the recipient. In contrast, akin to autoimmune liver disease outside transplantation, the pathogenesis of posttransplantation de novo AIH remains to be defined. There are several non–mutually exclusive explanations: In addition to release of autoantigens from damaged tissue, a possible mechanism is molecular mimicry, whereby exposure to viruses sharing amino acid sequences with autoantigens leads to cross-reactive immunity [63]. Viral infections, which are frequent post transplantation, may lead to autoimmunity also through other mechanisms, including polyclonal stimulation, enhancement and induction of membrane expression of MHC class I and II antigens, interference with immunoregulatory cells and/or with the idiotype anti-idiotype network. Another possible mechanism is suggested by animal experiments showing that the use of calcineurin inhibitors predisposes to autoimmunity and autoimmune disease, possibly by interfering with the maturation of T lymphocytes or with the function of regulatory T cells, with consequent emergence and activation of autoaggressive T-cell clones [62]. Lastly, it has been reported that an antibody directed to glutathione S-transferase T1 is present in patients who develop de novo immune-mediated hepatitis [64]. Because the gene encoding this protein is defective in a fifth of white subjects and the encoded enzyme is absent in some of the reported patients, it is possible to speculate that graft dysfunction results from recognition as foreign of glutathione S-transferase T1 acquired with the graft.

REFERENCES

1. Waldenström J. Leber, Blutproteine und Nahrungseiweiss. Dtsch Z Verdau Staffwechselkr 1950;15:113–19.
2. Mackay IR, Taft LI, Cowling DC. Lupoid hepatitis. Lancet 1956; 271:1323–6.
3. Soloway RD, Summerskill WH, Baggenstoss AH, et al. Clinical, biochemical, and histological remission of severe chronic active liver disease: a controlled study of treatments and early prognosis. Gastroenterology 1972;63:820–33.
4. Cook GC, Mulligan R, Sherlock S. Controlled prospective trial of corticosteroid therapy in active chronic hepatitis. Q J Med 1971; 40:159–85.
5. Manns MP, Luttig B, Obermayer-Straub P. Autoimmune hepatitis. In: Rose NR, Mackay IR, eds. The autoimmune diseases. 3rd ed. San Diego: Academic Press, 1998:511–25.
6. Primo J, Merino C, Fernandez J, et al. Incidence and prevalence of autoimmune hepatitis in the area of the Hospital de Sagunto (Spain). Gastroenterol Hepatol 2004;27:239–43.

7. Gregorio GV, Portmann B, Reid F, et al. Autoimmune hepatitis in childhood: a 20-year experience. Hepatology 1997;25:541–7.
8. Krawitt EL. Autoimmune hepatitis: classification, heterogeneity, and treatment. Am J Med 1994;96:23S–26S.
9. Manns MP, Vogel A. Autoimmune hepatitis, from mechanisms to therapy. Hepatology 2006;43:S132–44.
10. Ahonen P, Myllarniemi S, Sipila I, Perheentupa J. Clinical variation of autoimmune polyendocrinopathy-candidiasis-ectodermal dystrophy (APECED) in a series of 68 patients. N Engl J Med 1990;322:1829–36.
11. Johnson PJ, McFarlane IG. Meeting report: International Autoimmune Hepatitis Group. Hepatology 1993;18:998–1005.
12. Alvarez F, Berg PA, Bianchi FB, et al. International Autoimmune Hepatitis Group Report: review of criteria for diagnosis of autoimmune hepatitis. J Hepatol 1999;31:929–38.
13. Jablonska S, Chorzelski T, Zalewski T, Blaszczyk M. [Autoimmune ("lupoid") hepatitis in the light of immunofluorescence studies]. Dermatol Monatsschr 1972;158:271–7.
14. Vergani D, Alvarez F, Bianchi FB, et al. Liver autoimmune serology: a consensus statement from the committee for autoimmune serology of the International Autoimmune Hepatitis Group. J Hepatol 2004;41:677–83.
15. Bottazzo GF, Florin-Christensen A, Fairfax A, et al. Classification of smooth muscle autoantibodies detected by immunofluorescence. J Clin Pathol 1976;29:403–10.
16. Muratori P, Muratori L, Agostinelli D, et al. Smooth muscle antibodies and type 1 autoimmune hepatitis. Autoimmunity 2002; 35:497–500.
17. Gregorio GV, Portmann B, Mowat AP, et al. A 12-year-old girl with antimitochondrial antibody-positive autoimmune hepatitis. J Hepatol 1997;27:751–4.
18. Lapierre P, Hajoui O, Homberg JC, Alvarez F. Formiminotransferase cyclodeaminase is an organ-specific autoantigen recognized by sera of patients with autoimmune hepatitis. Gastroenterology 1999;116:643–9.
19. Manns M, Gerken G, Kyriatsoulis A, et al. Characterisation of a new subgroup of autoimmune chronic active hepatitis by autoantibodies against a soluble liver antigen. Lancet 1987;1:292–4.
20. Ma Y, Bogdanos BP, Williams R, et al. Anti-SLA antibody is a marker of severity of liver damage in patients with autoimmune liver disease. J Hepatol 2001;34:212.
21. Donaldson PT. Genetics in autoimmune hepatitis. Semin Liver Dis 2002;22:353–64.
22. Donaldson PT. Genetics of autoimmune and viral liver diseases; understanding the issues. J Hepatol 2004;41:327–32.
23. Ma Y, Bogdanos DP, Hussain MJ, et al. Polyclonal T-cell responses to cytochrome P450IID6 are associated with disease activity in autoimmune hepatitis type-2. Gastroenterology 2006; 130:868–82.
24. Vergani D, Wells L, Larcher VF, et al. Genetically determined low C4: a predisposing factor to autoimmune chronic active hepatitis. Lancet 1985;2:294–8.
25. Gregorio GV, Portmann B, Karani J, et al. Autoimmune hepatitis/sclerosing cholangitis overlap syndrome in childhood: a 16-year prospective study. Hepatology 2001;33:544–53.
26. Gregorio GV, Jones H, Choudhuri K, et al. Autoantibody prevalence in chronic hepatitis B virus infection: effect in interferon alfa. Hepatology 1996;24:520–3.
27. Gregorio GV, Pensati P, Iorio R, et al. Autoantibody prevalence in children with liver disease due to chronic hepatitis C virus (HCV) infection. Clin Exp Immunol 1998;112:471–6.
28. Dhawan A, Taylor RM, Cheeseman P, et al. Wilson's disease in children: 37-year experience and revised King's score for liver transplantation. Liver Transpl 2005;11:441–8.
29. Liston A, Lesage S, Gray DH, et al. Genetic lesions in T-cell tolerance and thresholds for autoimmunity. Immunol Rev 2005; 204:87–101.
30. Simmonds MJ, Gough SC. Genetic insights into disease mechanisms of autoimmunity. Br Med Bull 2004;71:93–113.
31. Fainboim L, Canero Velasco MC, et al. Protracted, but not acute, hepatitis A virus infection is strongly associated with HLA-DRB*1301, a marker for pediatric autoimmune hepatitis. Hepatology 2001;33:1512–17.
32. Pando M, Larriba J, Fernandez GC, et al. Pediatric and adult forms of type I autoimmune hepatitis in Argentina: evidence for differential genetic predisposition. Hepatology 1999;30:1374–80.
33. Lankisch TO, Strassburg CP, Debray D, et al. Detection of autoimmune regulator gene mutations in children with type 2 autoimmune hepatitis and extrahepatic immune-mediated diseases. J Pediatr 2005;146:839–42.
34. Senaldi G, Portmann B, Mowat AP, et al. Immunohistochemical features of the portal tract mononuclear cell infiltrate in chronic aggressive hepatitis. Arch Dis Child 1992;67:1447–53.
35. Takeda K, Hayakawa Y, Van Kaer L, et al. Critical contribution of liver natural killer T cells to a murine model of hepatitis. Proc Natl Acad Sci U S A 2000;97:5498–503.
36. Nouri-Aria KT, Lobo-Yeo A, Vergani D, et al. T suppressor cell function and number in children with liver disease. Clin Exp Immunol 1985;61:283–9.
37. Nouri-Aria KT, Hegarty JE, Alexander GJ, et al. Effect of corticosteroids on suppressor-cell activity in "autoimmune" and viral chronic active hepatitis. N Engl J Med 1982;307:1301–4.
38. Vento S, Hegarty JE, Bottazzo G, et al. Antigen specific suppressor cell function in autoimmune chronic active hepatitis. Lancet 1984;1:1200–4.
39. Longhi MS, Ma Y, Bogdanos DP, et al. Impairment of CD4+ CD25+ regulatory T-cells in autoimmune liver disease. J Hepatol 2004;41:31–7.
40. Shevach EM. $CD4^{+}$ $CD25^{+}$ suppressor T cells: more questions than answers. Nat Rev Immunol 2002;2:389–400.
41. Lobo-Yeo A, Alviggi L, Mieli-Vergani G, et al. Preferential activation of helper/inducer T lymphocytes in autoimmune chronic active hepatitis. Clin Exp Immunol 1987;67:95–104.
42. Wen L, Peakman M, Lobo-Yeo A, et al. T-cell-directed hepatocyte damage in autoimmune chronic active hepatitis. Lancet 1990; 336:1527–30.
43. Wen L, Peakman M, Mieli-Vergani G, Vergani D. Elevation of activated gamma delta T cell receptor bearing T lymphocytes in patients with autoimmune chronic liver disease. Clin Exp Immunol 1992;89:78–82.
44. Wen L, Ma Y, Bogdanos DP, et al. Pediatric autoimmune liver diseases: the molecular basis of humoral and cellular immunity. Curr Mol Med 2001;1:379–89.
45. Jaeckel E. Animal models of autoimmune hepatitis. Semin Liver Dis 2002;22:325–38.
46. Peters MG. Animal models of autoimmune liver disease. Immunol Cell Biol 2002;80:113–16.
47. Lohse AW, Meyer zum Buschenfelde KH. Remission of experimental autoimmune hepatitis is associated with antigen-specific and non-specific immunosuppression. Clin Exp Immunol 1993; 94:163–7.

48. Lohse AW, Kogel M, Meyer zum Buschenfelde KH. Evidence for spontaneous immunosuppression in autoimmune hepatitis. Hepatology 1995;22:381–8.
49. Lapierre P, Djilali-Saiah I, Vitozzi S, Alvarez F. A murine model of type 2 autoimmune hepatitis: xenoimmunization with human antigens. Hepatology 2004;39:1066–74.
50. Lapierre P, Beland K, Djilali-Saiah I, Alvarez F. Type 2 autoimmune hepatitis murine model: the influence of genetic background in disease development. J Autoimmun 2006;26:82–9.
51. Christen U, Rhode A, Johnson, E, et al. Development of an animal model for autoimmune hepatitis: breaking of self-tolerance in the CYP2D6 humanized mouse by viral infection. Hepatology; 2003;162A.
52. Mieli-Vergani G, Vergani D. Autoimmune hepatitis in children. Clin Liver Dis 2002;6:623–34.
53. Rumbo C, Emerick KM, Emre S, Shneider BL. Azathioprine metabolite measurements in the treatment of autoimmune hepatitis in pediatric patients: a preliminary report. J Pediatr Gastroenterol Nutr 2002;35:391–8.
54. Gregorio GV, McFarlane B, Bracken P, et al. Organ and non-organ specific autoantibody titres and IgG levels as markers of disease activity: a longitudinal study in childhood autoimmune liver disease. Autoimmunity 2002;35:515–19.
55. Mieli-Vergani G, Bargiota K, Samyn M, Vergani D. Therapeutic aspects of autoimmune liver disease in children. In: Dienes HP, Leuschner U, Lohse AW, Manns MP, eds. Autoimmune liver diseases – Falk Symposium. Dordrecht: Springer, 2005:278–82.
56. Johnson PJ, McFarlane IG, Williams R. Azathioprine for long-term maintenance of remission in autoimmune hepatitis. N Engl J Med 1995;333:958–63.
57. Alvarez F, Ciocca M, Canero-Velasco C, et al. Short-term cyclosporine induces a remission of autoimmune hepatitis in children. J Hepatol 1999;30:222–7.
58. Lindor KD. Ursodiol for primary sclerosing cholangitis. Mayo Primary Sclerosing Cholangitis-Ursodeoxycholic Acid Study Group. N Engl J Med 1997;336:691–5.
59. Mitchell SA, Bansi DS, Hunt N, et al. A preliminary trial of high-dose ursodeoxycholic acid in primary sclerosing cholangitis. Gastroenterology 2001;121:900–7.
60. Vergani D, Mieli-Vergani G. Autoimmunity after liver transplantation. Hepatology 2002;36:271–6.
61. Kerkar N, Hadzic N, Davies ET, et al. De-novo autoimmune hepatitis after liver transplantation. Lancet 1998;351:409–13.
62. Mieli-Vergani G, Vergani D. De novo autoimmune hepatitis after liver transplantation. J Hepatol 2004;40:3–7.
63. Vergani D, Choudhuri K, Bogdanos DP, Mieli-Vergani G. Pathogenesis of autoimmune hepatitis. Clin Liver Dis 2002;6:727–37.
64. Aguilera I, Sousa JM, Gavilan F, et al. Glutathione S-transferase T1 mismatch constitutes a risk factor for de novo immune hepatitis after liver transplantation. Liver Transpl 2004;10:1166–72.

19

Sclerosing Cholangitis

Nissa I. Erickson, M.D., and William F. Balistreri, M.D.

There is a wide spectrum of etiologically obscure inflammatory disorders of the biliary tract, including the obstructive cholangiopathies that occur in infancy (biliary atresia and related entities); primary biliary cirrhosis, which is noted in adults; and primary sclerosing cholangitis (PSC), which may affect patients of all age groups, particularly those with chronic inflammatory bowel disease (IBD). These hepatobiliary disorders differ markedly in clinical expression but display substantial overlap in morphologic features, suggesting that their pathogenesis may be shared [1]. Because the intra- and extrahepatic biliary tree may be assumed to possess a limited repertoire of reactions to injury caused by various inflammatory mechanisms, the association of PSC and IBD may provide insight into other forms of "cholangitis." The frequency of this association also presents an opportunity to trace the evolution of PSC. In this chapter, we focus on idiopathic forms of sclerosing cholangitis (SC) in children, the PSC–IBD complex, and related disorders.

DEFINITION

Sclerosing cholangitis is a chronic hepatobiliary disorder characterized by inflammation of the intrahepatic or extrahepatic ducts (or both), leading to focal dilatation, narrowing, or obliteration accompanied by local periductular fibrosis. Progressive, obliterative fibrosis usually leads to biliary cirrhosis and end-stage liver disease. The structural abnormalities of larger bile ducts are best appreciated by cholangiography, which in most cases is essential in establishing the diagnosis. However, careful delineation of the histology of the hepatic parenchyma and smaller intrahepatic ducts may also suggest the diagnosis [2,3].

Sclerosing cholangitis is the most common form of chronic liver disease seen in patients with IBD, but it also may occur in the absence of IBD and in association with a wide variety of disorders (Table 19.1) [4]. The nosology remains somewhat obscure, with no consensus. By convention, SC is designated as primary regardless of the presence or absence of IBD; in either instance, cholangitis is idiopathic. Cholangitis related to chronic ascending bacterial infection, stones, biliary tract surgery, congenital anomalies of the biliary tract, ischemic injury, neoplasia, or infectious cholangiopathy associated with immunodeficiency are some of the exclusions necessary to justify the use of the term *primary cholangitis* (vs. secondary cholangitis) [5,6]. It is assumed that before the onset of SC, the anatomy of the biliary tree was normal and that the condition has no relationship to disorders such as the congenital hepatic fibrosis–Caroli disease–polycystic kidney disease complex. The term *secondary sclerosing cholangitis* has been used to describe the clinical syndrome resulting from these disorders, as well as from choledocholithiasis, postoperative stricture, or other specific ductal involvement in systemic disease (Table 19.1). Mieli-Vergani and Vergani [7] have suggested that SC be described as *primary* if it occurs (1) outside of the neonatal period, (2) without strong features of autoimmunity and without response to immunosuppression (as seen in so-called autoimmune SC), and (3) in the absence of complicating disorders such as immunodeficiency, Langerhans cell histiocytosis, psoriasis, cystic fibrosis, reticulum cell sarcoma, and sickle cell anemia.

SPECTRUM OF SC

The bulk of the information regarding SC has been generated through studies of adult patients, but in the last 2 decades, an increasing number of reports of pediatric cases has been published, including several large series [8–13]. The wide spectrum of hepatobiliary lesions initially reported to affect a significant proportion of well-studied adults with idiopathic IBD is now being recognized in children with ulcerative colitis (UC) and Crohn's disease, in part because of the increasingly widespread use of cholangiographic techniques in children.

The majority of adult patients with SC have an associated nonhepatic disease, indicating more than a chance occurrence; these disorders include (in addition to IBD) diabetes mellitus, pancreatitis, thyroid diseases, and other autoimmune disorders [2,14]. These comorbidities may precede or develop subsequent to the diagnosis of SC. Similarly in children, SC may be noted in conjunction with IBD, develop in association with a wider variety of disorders, or occur in the absence of any definable associated disease (Table 19.1). For example, SC occurs in

Table 19.1: Spectrum of Sclerosing Cholangitis in Childhood

A. Sclerosing cholangitis
1. Primary sclerosing cholangitis in association with inflammatory bowel disease
   - Ulcerative colitis
   - Crohn's disease
   - Indeterminate colitis
2. SC in association with autoimmune disease
   - Autoimmune hepatitis–sclerosing cholangitis overlap syndrome (autoimmune sclerosing cholangitis)
   - Autoimmune pancreatitis (lymphoplasmocytic sclerosing pancreatitis) [147,148]
   - Celiac disease [149–151]
   - Diabetes mellitus [7,14]
   - Thyroiditis [7,14]
   - Lupus [152,153]
   - Psoriasis [9]
3. SC in association with other inflammatory disorders
   - Inflammatory pseudotumor [154,155]
   - Inflammatory retroperitonitis [156–158]
4. Idiopathic
   - Childhood
   - Neonatal sclerosing cholangitis [9,16–18]
     - Neonatal ichthyosis-sclerosing cholangitis syndrome (NISCH) [22]
     - Kabuki syndrome [19,20]
     - With associated autoimmunity [17]

B. Secondary SC
1. Choledocholithiasis (sludge)
   - Sickle-cell anemia
   - Parenteral nutrition–associated
2. Immunodeficiency (usually associated with infectious cholangitis) [159]
   - AIDS-associated cholangiopathy [160] and Cytomegalovirus, *Cryptosporidium* [161]
   - X-linked hyper-IgM/agammaglobulinemia [162,163] and *Cryptosporidium* [164]
   - Wiskott–Aldrich syndrome [165]
   - Natural killer cell deficiency and *Trichosporon* [166]
   - Agammaglobulinemia, combined variable deficiency, combined immunodeficiency [159,167] and *Cryptosporidium* [168]
   - MHC class II deficiency [169]
   - Undefined immunodeficiency and *Cryptococcus neoformans* [170]
3. Infection
   - Recurrent acute bacterial cholangitis
   - *E. coli 0157:H7* enterocolitis [171]
   - Septic shock [172]
   - *Cryptosporidium* [95]
4. Neoplasm
   - Langerhans cell histiocytosis [15]
   - Hodgkin's disease [173,174]
   - Angioimmunoblastic lymphadenopathy [175]
   - Ductal cancer, gallbladder cancer [162]
   - Reticulum-cell sarcoma [157]
5. Injury
   - Postsurgical stenosis
   - Trauma [176]
   - Caustic injury [177,178]
6. Cystic fibrosis [179,180]

some children with Langerhans cell histiocytosis who have an extensive infiltrate containing the histiocytes around intra- and extrahepatic bile ducts (Figure 19.1); the infiltrates result from uncontrolled proliferation and dissemination of dendritic histiocytes [15]. The clinical, radiographic, and histopathologic features of the hepatobiliary lesions in these various conditions are not yet sufficiently delineated to permit conclusions regarding possible heterogeneity. As we better identify the pathogenesis of secondary SC in systemic disease, we will further our understanding of the pathobiology of biliary diseases in general, and SC in particular.

Information regarding the incidence of conditions associated with sclerosing cholangitis in children was initially provided by Sisto et al. [9], who tabulated 78 cases, including 5 personal cases. In the same year, el-Shabrawi et al. [11] reported 13 cases. Subsequently, Debray et al. [12] described a case series of 56 children with sclerosing cholangitis, and Wilschanski et al. [8] reported on an additional 32 children. More recently, Feldstein et al. [10] published a long-term follow-up

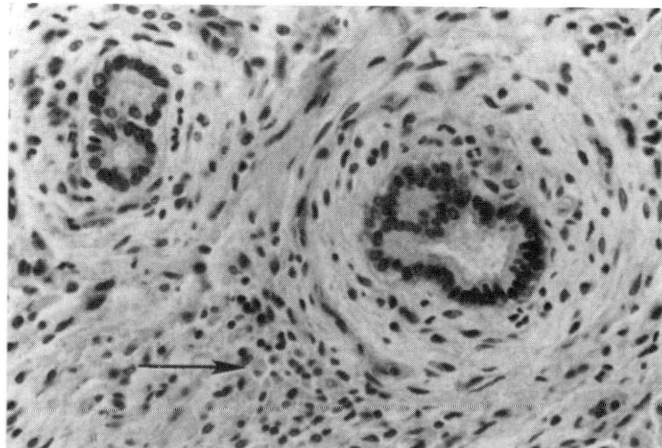

Figure 19.1. Sclerosing cholangitis in a patient with Langerhans cell histiocytosis features periductular mononuclear cells, including scattered histiocytes (*arrow*). (Hematoxylin and eosin [H&E], original magnification ×400.)

Table 19.2: Findings Associated with Sclerosing Cholangitis in Six Large Pediatric Series

	Sisto et al. [9]	*el-Shabrawi et al. [11]*	*Debray et al. [12]*	*Wilschanski et al. [8]*	*Feldstein et al. [10]*	*Batres et al. [13]*	*Totals*
Total cases, n	78	13	56	32	52	20	251
Mean age at diagnosis	6.6 (n = 5)	5.5	7	11	13.8	9.3	8.9
Sex, male, female	3, 2 (n = 5)	5, 8	32, 24	23, 9	34, 18	14, 6	111, 67 (1.7:1)
PSC	49	13	19	30	52	19	182
IBD	37 (76)	9 (69, n = 10)	7 (37)	17 (56)	42 (81)	10 (53)	68%
UC	30 (61)	5 (38, n = 10)	4 (21)	14 (47)	30 (58)	7 (37)	50%
Crohn's disease	2 (4)	0 (n = 10)	3 (16)	3 (10)	8 (15)	3 (16)	11%
Indeterminate colitis	5 (10)	4 (31, n = 10)	0	0	4	(8)	0 7%
AIH	—	5 (38)	2*(11)	5 (17)	4 (35, n = 40)	—	25%
Percent abnormal lab values							
Alk phos	89 (n = 74)	62	88	53	75	—	79% (n = 227)
GGT	—	92	100 (n = 42)	—	94	—	96% (n = 107)
AST	—	92	—	91	92	—	92% (n = 97)
ALT	95 (n = 57)	—	—	—	93	—	94% (n = 109)
Bilirubin	45 (n = 64)	—	—	38	14	—	33% (n = 148)
IgG	—	92	—	53 (n = 31)	70	—	67% (n = 96)
ANA	—	69	—	47 (n = 30)	43	29 (n = 17)	45% (n = 112)
ASMA		69	13 (n = 32)	63 (n = 30)	28	31 (n = 13)	36% (n = 140)
ANCA	—	—	—	42 (n = 24)	72	63 (n = 19)	63% (n = 95)

Several studies included cases of neonatal or secondary sclerosing cholangitis; IBD and AIH percentages reflect patients with PSC only, and laboratory values reflect the percentage abnormal of total cases (unless otherwise indicated). AIH, autoimmune hepatitis; Alk phos, alkaline phosphatase; ALT, alanine aminotransferase; ANA, antinuclear antibody; ANCA, antineutrophil cytoplasmic antibody; ASMA, anti–smooth muscle antibody; AST, aspartate aminotransferase; GGT, γ-glutamyltransferase; IBD, inflammatory bowel disease; IgG, immunoglobulin G; SC, sclerosing cholangitis; UC, ulcerative colitis.
*Described as chronic active hepatitis with positive autoantibodies.

study on a series of 52 children, and Batres et al. [13] reported a histologic study on a cohort of 20 pediatric patients. Some studies included cases of secondary SC and neonatal cases, whereas others restricted their study population to PSC. The composite findings show that 48% of the total cases were associated with IBD (equaling 68% of PSC cases), 27% were associated with another disorder (secondary SC), and 24% occurred in isolation (Table 19.2).

Neonatal SC

The series reported by Debray et al. [12] included 15 patients with the neonatal onset of sclerosing cholangitis. All 15 patients had cholestasis during the first month of life that progressed to cirrhosis. Amedee-Manesme et al. [16] originally described this entity in eight children, initially identified as having neonatal cholestasis, in whom clinical, histologic, and radiologic features compatible with SC developed. Percutaneous cholecystography demonstrated abnormal intrahepatic bile ducts with rarefaction of segmental branches, stenosis, and focal dilation; the extrahepatic ducts were abnormal in six of the eight children. Liver biopsy samples obtained in infancy suggested bile duct obstruction; histologic examination later in life documented ductal proliferation and cirrhosis. Similar cases have been described by Baker et al. [17] and Bar Meir et al. [18]. These reports expand the spectrum of infantile cholangiopathies and beg the question as to whether these cases may represent a forme fruste of biliary atresia or an initial manifestation of progressive familial intrahepatic cholestasis type 3 (MDR3 deficiency) [17]. Recently, neonatal SC has been identified in association with two syndromes: the Kabuki syndrome (involving facial dysmorphisms, mental retardation, growth deficiency, skeletal anomalies, and

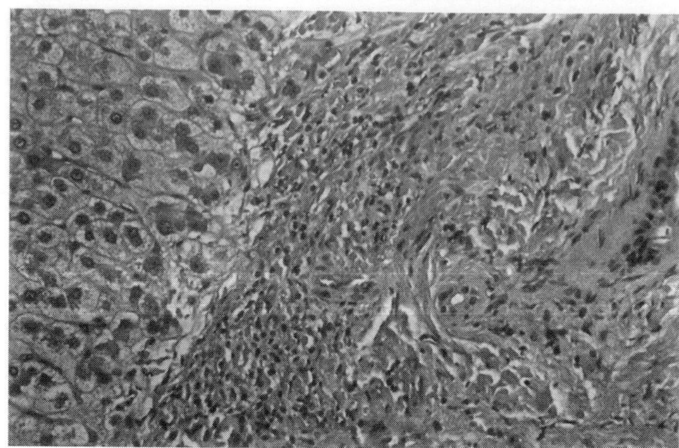

Figure 19.2. Liver biopsy in a patient with AIH and PSC shows periductular stromal edema and inflammation, along with hepatitis along portal margins. (H&E, original magnification ×400.) For color reproduction, see Color Plate 19.2.

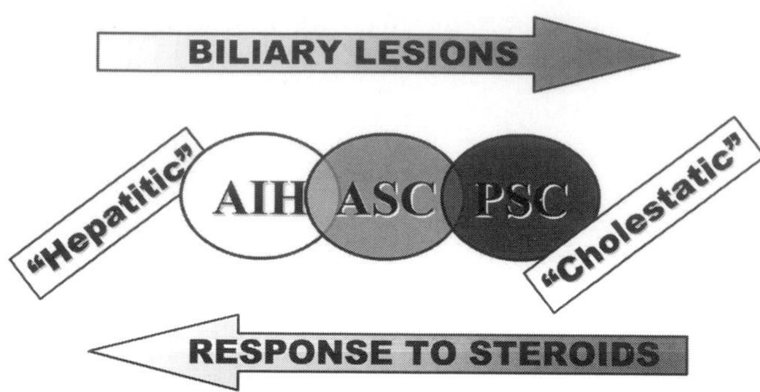

Figure 19.3. Schematic representation of the relationships between AIH and PSC: proposed spectrum of disease.

congenital heart defects), and neonatal ichthyosis-sclerosing cholangitis (NISCH) syndrome, which appears to result from a claudin-1 protein deficiency [19–22]. Early age at onset, rapid progression, and association with congenital disorders suggest that neonatal SC represents a unique form of idiopathic sclerosing cholangitis.

Autoimmune Hepatitis and SC

An overlap syndrome of autoimmune hepatitis (AIH) and SC has received increased attention in recent years, being described in both adults and children [8,10,23–27]. Such patients are defined by elevated serum immunoglobulin levels and positive serum autoantibodies (antinuclear antibody [ANA] or anti–smooth muscle antibody [ASMA]) in addition to histologic and radiologic findings of both autoimmune hepatitis and sclerosing cholangitis (Figure 19.2). As is true for PSC alone, the overlap syndrome often coexists with IBD, and the activity of the hepatitis does not correlate with the activity of the colitis. However, in contrast to isolated PSC, female patients predominate in this overlap syndrome, especially at younger ages of presentation [24,26,27].

In a prospective 16-year study of 55 pediatric patients with AIH, Gregorio et al. [26] found that 50% had radiologic evidence of SC based on screening cholangiograms. Two-thirds had both intra- and extrahepatic findings, whereas in the remaining one-third the cholangiographic abnormalities were intrahepatic only. Eighty-nine percent of patients showed a biochemical and histologic response to immunosuppression in this study; however, no cholangiographic disease regression was noted. Five patients in the series of Wilschanski et al. [8] and five in the series of el-Shabrawi et al. [11] were originally diagnosed to have AIH before cholangiography. Debray et al. [12] gave two patients a diagnosis of both AIH and SC. By contrast, the study by Feldstein et al. [10] found that 35% of patients who had liver biopsies performed were diagnosed with the overlap syndrome. It is interesting to note that there was no difference in the clinical features, aminotransferase levels, or histologic stage of disease in these children compared with those with PSC alone. However, these patients were distinguished by having higher total serum gammaglobulin levels and the presence of ANA or ASMA. The high incidence of overlap syndrome in this study is probably the result of an increased awareness of this condition in children.

The relationship between AIH and PSC is not clear; patients with overlap may simply have concurrence of two disease processes or may be manifesting two features of the same disease, along a spectrum of "hepatitic" to "cholestatic" phenotypes (Figure 19.3). The term *autoimmune sclerosing cholangitis* (ASC) has thus been used interchangeably with AIH–PSC overlap syndrome; there is some suggestion that in these patients, unlike in those without evidence of autoimmunity, the progression of biliary disease might be slowed through the use of immunosuppressive therapy [24,28].

A detailed review of autoimmune liver disease can be found in Chapter 18. It is increasingly clear that, in making the diagnosis of SC, a combination of serum markers, liver histology, and cholangiographic imaging is necessary to distinguish between the classic and autoimmune forms. Conversely, an overlap syndrome should be considered if there is an incomplete response to immunosuppressive medications or development of cholestasis in an individual diagnosed with AIH.

EPIDEMIOLOGY

The overall incidence of sclerosing cholangitis is unknown, and varies widely in geographic regions, with the highest reported cases in Northern Europe [29]. The first population-based estimates in the United States were recently reported: in a study from Olmsted County, Minnesota, a small, predominantly white community, there were 22 new cases of PSC from 1976 to 2000 [30]. The estimated age-adjusted incidence was 1.25 per 100,000 person-years in men, and 0.54 per 100,000 in women. In this study, the prevalence of PSC in 2000 was 20.9 per 100,000 men and 6.3 per 100,000 women; 73% of cases were associated with IBD.

The incidence of PSC in children – even those with IBD – is undefined, but it is likely that the number is largely underestimated; it may be difficult to gain perspective on pediatric PSC because the cholangiographic anatomy of liver diseases prevalent in children is still not well defined. Sclerosing cholangitis occurs at all ages but is most commonly recognized in young adults. In a large Dutch study, for example, the mean age at diagnosis was 40.4 years, whereas in the pediatric reviews, the mean age at diagnosis was 8.9 years (Table 19.2) [8–13,31]. It is consistently more common in male patients, with a ratio approximating 2:1. It also appears that male patients are younger at the time of diagnosis of both PSC and UC [32–34].

Several large independent studies on the natural history of PSC have been published to date, each containing more than 100 adult patients [31,35–38]. Overall, an estimated 70–80% of PSC patients have or will develop UC. An extensive literature review of 572 adult cases of PSC documented that the associated frequency of IBD was 76% (67% for patients with UC and 9% for Crohn's disease) [39].

From 2 to 7.5% of adult patients with UC may simultaneously be affected with PSC [2,33,34,40,41]. Olsson et al. [42] studied 1500 adult patients with UC in Sweden and reported a point prevalence of PSC at 5.5% in patients with substantial colitis but only 0.5% in those with distal colitis. A descriptive report of 36 pediatric cases of PSC–IBD documented similar findings: pancolitis was present on the initial examination in 80%, along with rectal sparing in 26% [43]. Pouchitis also was common after colectomy in this study, occurring in four of five patients after ileal pouch–anal anastomosis.

There is no direct correlation between the activity of PSC and colitis in a given patient at a single time point. In fact, symptomatic PSC may occur during quiescent IBD or after colectomy [31,36,40,44,45]. However, it now appears that chronic, minimally symptomatic pancolitis may predispose to the development of PSC. A recent study evaluating the features of IBD in 71 adult patients with PSC compared with IBD patients without PSC found that, whether diagnosed with UC, Crohn's disease, or indeterminate colitis, patients with PSC–IBD had a high prevalence of pancolitis and rectal sparing, with or without ileitis [40]. This observation, combined with the fact that PSC–IBD patients tend to have mild IBD, led the authors to suggest that PSC might serve as a surrogate marker for chronic, asymptomatic UC.

In the six large pediatric series, an average of 68% of pediatric patients with PSC had IBD (Table 19.2); 50% had UC, and 11% had Crohn's [8–13]. Just as in adults with IBD and PSC, the symptoms and diagnosis of liver disease in children may precede, be coincident with, or follow the diagnosis of IBD. To determine the frequency of PSC in pediatric IBD patients, Hyams et al. [46] screened 555 children with IBD for evidence of liver disease based on an elevated alanine aminotransferase (ALT) level. Primary SC was identified in eight patients with UC (3.5% of all those with UC) and two patients with Crohn's disease (0.6% of those with Crohn's disease). This likely underestimates the incidence because not all patients with PSC will have an elevated ALT.

Primary SC is not as common in patients with Crohn's disease and is seemingly limited to those with extensive colonic involvement (colitis or ileocolitis) [40,47,48]. In the study by Feldstein et al. [10], the proportion of pediatric patients with Crohn's disease was much higher (15%) than the 4–7% reported in adults, yet consistent with other pediatric reports (see Table 19.2) [8,10,11,13,38,43]. The reason for this is unclear but may reflect the degree of colitis in Crohn's disease presenting in childhood [49].

Table 19.3: Clinical Features of Sclerosing Cholangitis in Children

Symptoms	Signs
Abdominal pain	Hepatomegaly
Fatigue	Hepatosplenomegaly
Anorexia	Splenomegaly
Jaundice	Ascites
Fever	Xanthomas
Weight loss	**Other**
Pruritus	Presentation as AIH poorly responsive to therapy
Delayed puberty	
Chronic diarrhea*	
Gastrointestinal hemorrhage	

*Not necessarily associated with IBD.
From references [1,8–13]

CLINICAL FEATURES

In adults, the early clinical course of PSC is similar in patients with or without documented IBD. The early course is insidious, so it may be difficult to determine precisely the onset of the disease; symptoms may be present for months before the diagnosis is made [29,30,37]. Initial symptoms consist of a gradual onset of progressive fatigue, malaise, anorexia, and weight loss. Pruritus followed by fluctuating jaundice may next occur. Clinical evidence of cholangitis, highlighted by recurrent right upper quadrant pain, fever, and hyperbilirubinemia is often noted. The majority of PSC patients are totally asymptomatic when biochemical abnormalities are first detected; this prompts further workup, including cholangiography [10,29,30,37]. Depending on the stage of disease at presentation, patients with PSC may have a normal physical examination or exhibit some abnormality such as hepatomegaly, splenomegaly, or jaundice.

A similar insidious onset has been seen in pediatric patients, with signs and symptoms of liver disease having been present for an average of 3 years before diagnosis in the 56 patients described by Debray et al. [12]. In the study by Wilschanski et al. [8], most of the 32 children presented with relatively nonspecific complaints such as fatigue, anorexia, or pruritus. Twenty-nine percent of patients in the study by Feldstein et al. [10] were asymptomatic at diagnosis. This high number may reflect more frequent laboratory screenings for PSC in pediatric patients with IBD.

The clinical features noted in children with SC are similar to those reported in adults (Table 19.3) [7–14]. Some features are, however, unique to childhood, including poor growth and delayed puberty. The specific clinical features occurring in a relatively large number of pediatric patients have been described in the six large pediatric series [8–13]. In 56 patients reported by Debray et al. [12], the initial signs and symptoms included jaundice in 9, hepatomegaly in 28, splenomegaly in 1, variceal hemorrhage in 1, and abnormal liver function tests in 2 otherwise asymptomatic children. By the time of diagnosis, 25 were cholestatic, almost all had hepatomegaly, three fourths had splenomegaly, and 12 had ascites. Findings by Wilschanski et al. [8] (32 patients) and el-Shabrawi et al. [11] (13 patients) were similar, with jaundice in 11, hepatomegaly in 30 (with coincident splenomegaly in 14), isolated splenomegaly in 1, and pruritus in 7. Of the 52 children reported by Feldstein et al. [10], 13 were asymptomatic, 21 presented with abdominal pain, 14 with fatigue, and 10 with jaundice; hepatomegaly was present in 8, splenomegaly in 10, and weight loss in 9. The differences in the presentations of patients in this recent study may reflect the increasing awareness of PSC and its earlier evaluation and diagnosis.

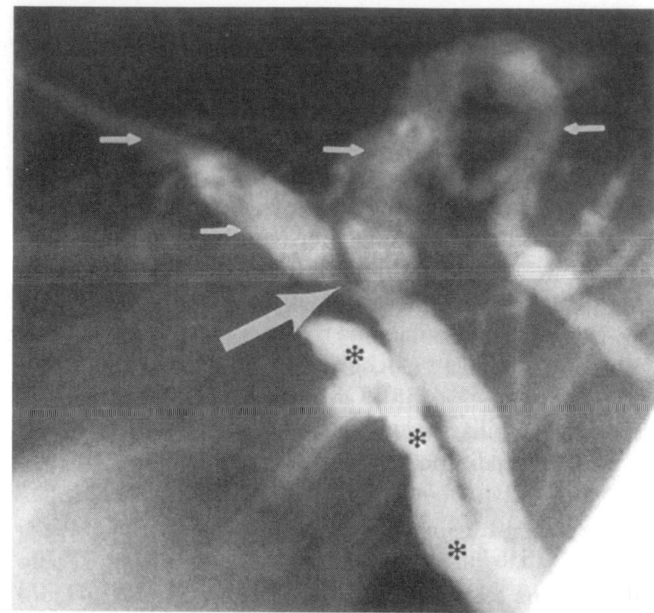

Figure 19.4. Image obtained during ERCP study of an 18-year-old young man with a 7-year history of chronic liver disease and colitis shows typical changes of sclerosing cholangitis. There is overall irregularity of the intrahepatic ducts and areas of distinct stenosis, for example, at the junction of the right and left hepatic ducts (*large arrow*); the distal intrahepatic ducts are relatively spared (*small arrows*). Note the unusually long cystic duct (*asterisks*), which is a normal variant.

Laboratory Findings

There are no specific laboratory findings of PSC. An elevated alkaline phosphatase level is commonly noted in adult patients with PSC, and the vast majority will have mildly increased serum aminotransferase activity [2,4,10,41]. Approximately half have a modest increase in serum bilirubin levels, but wide variations have been noted. Hypoalbuminemia and abnormal prothrombin time are common with advanced disease.

Similarly, most pediatric patients show biochemical evidence of cholestasis. However, although many pediatric patients have an elevated serum alkaline phosphatase level, 15 of 32 had normal levels in the study by Wilschanski et al. [8], and 13 of 52 had normal levels in the study by Feldstein et al. [10]. γ-glutamyltransferase (GGT) levels appear to be more sensitive than alkaline phosphatase levels, with 96% of children with SC having an abnormal GGT level at the time of diagnosis in the large series [8,10,11]. Of those patients tested in the six pediatric series, ALT was increased in 94%, aspartate aminotransferase (AST) in 94%, and the alkaline phosphatase in 79% (Table 19.2) [8–13]. Other laboratory abnormalities noted at diagnosis in these patients included markers of autoimmunity, including elevated immunoglobulin G (IgG) concentrations in 68%, a positive ANA in 45%, and a positive ASMA in 36% of those tested.

DIAGNOSIS

Imaging

The gold standard for the diagnosis of SC is cholangiography, but suspicion of disease rests on a combination of clinical signs and symptoms, laboratory data, and characteristic liver histology. Characteristic findings on endoscopic retrograde cholangiopancreatography (ERCP) are irregular narrowing and stricture of the hepatic and common bile duct caused by fibrosing inflammation with or without involvement of the intrahepatic ducts (Figure 19.4) [31,50–52]. These areas of segmental stenosis can be widespread, diffuse, and multifocal. Strictures may be short (1–2 cm) and annular with intervening segments of apparently normal or minimally dilated ducts that produce the characteristic beaded appearance. Focal minimal dilation or small diverticula may be noted proximal to the stricture [51]. Bandlike strictures are found in approximately 20% of adult patients and diverticular outpouchings in 25%; the latter feature is suggested to be highly specific [53]. The intrahepatic biliary tree may be the site of decreased peripheral arborization, reflecting loss of normal functioning bile ducts, imparting the "pruned tree" appearance [31,50–52].

All of the children described in the six large pediatric series had abnormal cholangiograms as the basis for the diagnosis of sclerosing cholangitis. All patients in the two series by Debray et al. [12] and el-Shabrawi et al. [11] had irregularity of the intrahepatic ducts similar to those shown in adult series; this included duct wall irregularity, filling defects, irregular dilation, pruning of the peripheral branches, absence of opacification of some branches, beading, and confluent strictures. In the study by Feldstein et al. [10], 56% of patients had both intra- and extrahepatic bile duct involvement, 42% had isolated intrahepatic abnormalities, and only 2% had isolated extrahepatic abnormalities.

Recently, magnetic resonance cholangiopancreatography (MRCP) has been used as a noninvasive tool in the diagnosis of abnormalities of the pancreaticobiliary tree. In adults with

PSC, MR imaging has been able to demonstrate abnormalities of both the intra- and extrahepatic biliary tree, including dilation, stenosis, beading, and pruning [54–56]. In a recent study of 150 adult patients comparing ERCP to MRCP for the diagnosis of PSC, the latter showed a sensitivity of 88% and specificity of 99%. More bile duct stenoses and pruning were seen by ERCP, whereas more areas of skip dilatation were visualized by MRCP [56]. MRCP allows for the study of intrahepatic ducts proximal to a site of severe obstruction that would not fill with contrast during ERCP. The major drawback of this technique, however, is that it does not allow for therapeutic interventions such as dilatation of a dominant stricture or brushing for cholangiocarcinoma.

Increasingly MRCP is being used in children as a noninvasive means of diagnosing PSC. In a study by Ferrara et al. [57], ERCPs, MRCPs, and liver biopsies were performed on 21 children with the clinical and laboratory suspicion of PSC; 13 patients (62%) showed duct abnormalities by MRCP, whereas 16 patients (76%) demonstrated abnormal ducts by ERCP [57]. The remaining 5 patients received alternate diagnoses based on liver biopsy results. This study demonstrated a high specificity (100%) and a reasonable sensitivity (81%) of MRCP. The primary advantages of using MRCP – especially in a pediatric population – are that it is noninvasive, requires no radiation or contrast material, and carries a very low complication rate compared with ERCP. In addition, MRCP may visualize the biliary tract in small children in whom ERCP is not feasible and may be useful in following pediatric and adult patients after liver transplantation to evaluate for recurrence of disease [58–60]. In sum, MRCP may be highly suggestive when a strong clinical suspicion of PSC exists. In cases of negative or equivocal studies, traditional cholangiography should be performed.

Computerized tomographic (CT) cholangiography is a new noninvasive technique that has been used to detect biliary tree abnormalities. A recent comparison of MRCP to CT cholangiography for the diagnosis of PSC in 16 adult patients reported a higher sensitivity (94%) in the latter [61]. The projected advantage of CT cholangiography is that it offers information about biliary excretion and more accurate detection of both intra- and extrahepatic bile duct abnormalities in PSC. However, these are preliminary data, and this modality requires substantial further investigation.

Serologic Markers

There are no reliable diagnostic serologic markers for PSC, although circulating non–organ-specific autoantibodies are often present [62]. A study testing autoantibodies in 73 adult patients with PSC found that 97% were positive for at least one in a panel of 20 and that 81% were positive for at least three. The antibodies most frequently identified were ANA in 53%, anticardiolipin antibody in 66%, and antineutrophil cytoplasmic antibody (ANCA) in 84% [63]. Of those tested in the pediatric series, ANCAs were positive in 62% [8,10,13]. Because of the high prevalence of perinuclear ANCA in PSC, this test is useful as a diagnostic marker when combined with other standard diagnostic tests. However, ANCAs are not specific for PSC and often occur in both UC and AIH. They are not helpful for monitoring disease activity, and their role in the pathogenesis of disease is unclear [62,63].

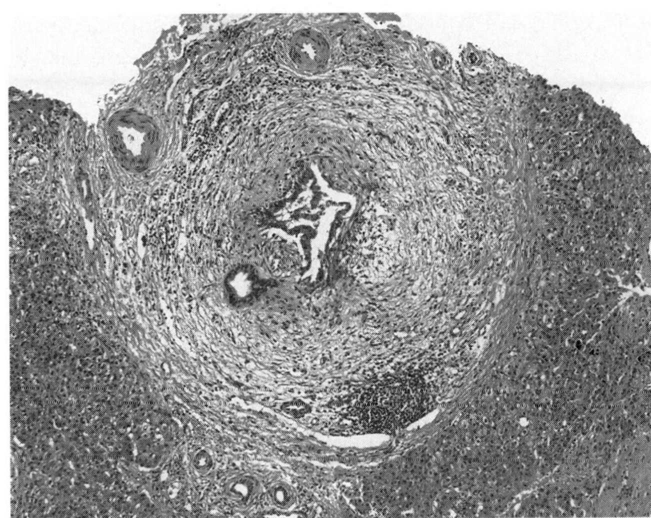

Figure 19.5. Classic "onion-skinning" periductular sclerosis in a patient with primary sclerosing cholangitis. (H&E, original magnification ×400.) For color reproduction, see Color Plate 19.5.

Biopsy

The histologic changes, although characteristic in many cases of PSC, tend to be less dramatic than the cholangiographic changes perhaps because of sampling limitations and the two-dimensional nature of microscopy. The histologic hallmark is progressive ductal lesions. Reported histologic changes range

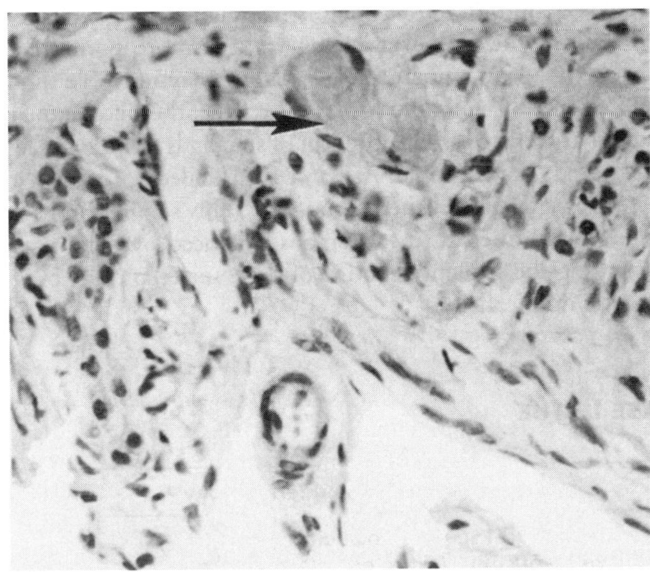

Figure 19.6. Focal fibrous obliteration of a small bile duct (*arrow*) in a patient with inflammatory bowel disease. (H&E, original magnification ×400.)

from nonspecific portal edema and fibrosis and subtle pericholangitis (Figure 19.2: duct changes), to severe pericholangiolar edema and sclerosis (Figure 19.5), to frank obliteration (Figure 19.6). Typically there is portal-to-portal variability. Careful review of serial biopsies, serial sections, or three-dimensional reconstructions of a single biopsy specimen is necessary to appreciate obliteration of ducts with sclerosis or focal duct dilatation. It may be instructive to compare the diameter of the interlobular bile ducts to that of the accompanying artery; these are normally approximately equal.

The most characteristic feature found in liver specimens from patients with PSC is focal concentric edema and fibrosis ("onion-skinning") around interlobular bile ducts [13,64–66]. Synchronous or metachronous histologic changes that have been noted as sequential or concomitant lesions include bile duct proliferation, periductal fibrosis, periductal inflammation, degeneration of bile duct epithelial cells associated with inflammatory infiltration, ductal obliteration, and loss of bile ducts, along with portal edema and fibrosis, portal and periportal hepatitis, and focal parenchymal changes [1]. Pathognomonic histologic change – fibrous-obliterative cholangitis, which occurs in the early stages – may not be present in all biopsy cores or easy to demonstrate. This lesion is succeeded over time by replacement of duct segments by solid cords of connective tissue and extensive loss of interlobular and adjacent septal bile ducts. Ultimately a local condition of bile duct paucity may develop because of substantial reduction in the number of bile duct profiles per portal zone. However, nonobliterated ducts may proliferate, making recognition of the deficit of ducts particularly challenging. With progression, there is an increasing portal fibrosis, bridging, and progression to biliary cirrhosis. At surgery or autopsy, the extrahepatic bile ducts may appear as thickened cords without a change in duct diameter. Cross-sectional examination will reveal the lumen to be narrowed because of concentric fibrous thickening of the wall (up to 10-fold), with the mucosa being unaffected [1,13,64–66].

Liver biopsies from the 56 pediatric patients reported by Debray et al. [12] demonstrated portal fibrosis in 54, neoductular proliferation in 33, ductopenia in 4, and cirrhosis in 23. El-Shabrawi et al. [11] found portal fibrosis and ductular proliferation in all 13 of their patients. In this series, periductal fibrosis, suggestive of sclerosing cholangitis, also was seen in all 13 patients, and 5 had a well-developed periductal onion-skin change around the bile ducts. In contrast, concentric periductular fibrosis or inflammatory infiltrate was found in only 14 of the cases presented by Debray et al. [12]. Of 52 patients in the study by Feldstein et al. [10], 40 had liver biopsy specimens available, each demonstrating features highly suggestive of PSC. Ductular proliferation, ductopenia, and portal edema and fibrosis were the most common features, occurring in 80%, 60%, and 60%, respectively. Periductal fibrosis was seen in 30%. Based on the staging criteria of Ludwig (see following discussion and Table 19.4), nearly half of the patients (46%) had early disease (histologic stage I or II). Wilschanski et al. [8] did not provide details of the histopathology of their patients aside from staging: eight patients were at stage I, 7 at stage II, 6 at stage III, and 11 at the cirrhotic stage (stage IV) [8]. In the recent study by Batres et al. [13], 20 pediatric patients diagnosed with PSC over a 20-year period were retrospectively reviewed, with particular attention to liver histology. Classic periductal concentric fibrosis was found in liver sections of only 5 patients, whereas features of cholangitis and duct or ductular proliferation were present in 11 (55%). Thirteen patients (65%) had advanced disease at presentation: 8 at Ludwig's stage III, and 5 at stage IV.

Table 19.4: Ludwig's Classification of Duct Disease in Primary Sclerosing Cholangitis

Liver Biopsy Features	*Cholangiographic Findings*	*Suggested Terminology*
Typical	Not diagnostic	Small-duct PSC
Not diagnostic	Typical	Large-duct PSC (extra- or intrahepatic)
Typical	Typical	Combined large and small duct PSC (global or classic PSC)

Modified from Ludwig [66], with permission.

Ludwig's Histologic Classification and Small-Duct PSC

Ludwig [66] proposed that the histologic lesions of PSC be divided into four stages (Figure 19.7). The initial stage (I), confined to the portal tract, consists of cholangitis and portal hepatitis; fibrous obliterative cholangitis resulting in eventual loss of interlobular and adjacent septal bile ducts occurs along with lymphocytic infiltration and ductular changes (narrowing, obliteration, or proliferation). In stage II, the inflammatory process has extended beyond the portal tract to involve the periportal region, resulting in periportal fibrosis or hepatitis; the histologic features may resemble autoimmune hepatitis. In stage III (septal stage), fibrosis of the periportal region with portal-to-portal tract bridging occurs; the histologic changes may resemble those noted in PBC in adults. Stage IV reflects the development of biliary cirrhosis. This concept of staging is not universally accepted, and because of the inherent sampling error associated with liver biopsy, it may be unreliable for following the progression of disease [44,67].

Patients who have negative cholangiographic findings, but nevertheless have liver histology and laboratory data consistent with PSC, are considered to have *small-duct PSC* (previously referred to as *pericholangitis*) [68,69]. In a study by Bjornsson et al. [70], the natural history of disease in 33 adult patients with small-duct PSC was compared to that of 260 patients with large-duct PSC. The patients with small-duct PSC had better survival, and none developed cholangiocarcinoma during the 105-month period, compared with 28 patients (11%) with large-duct disease. A cohort of 32 patients with small-duct disease was reported by Broome et al. [45], who found that

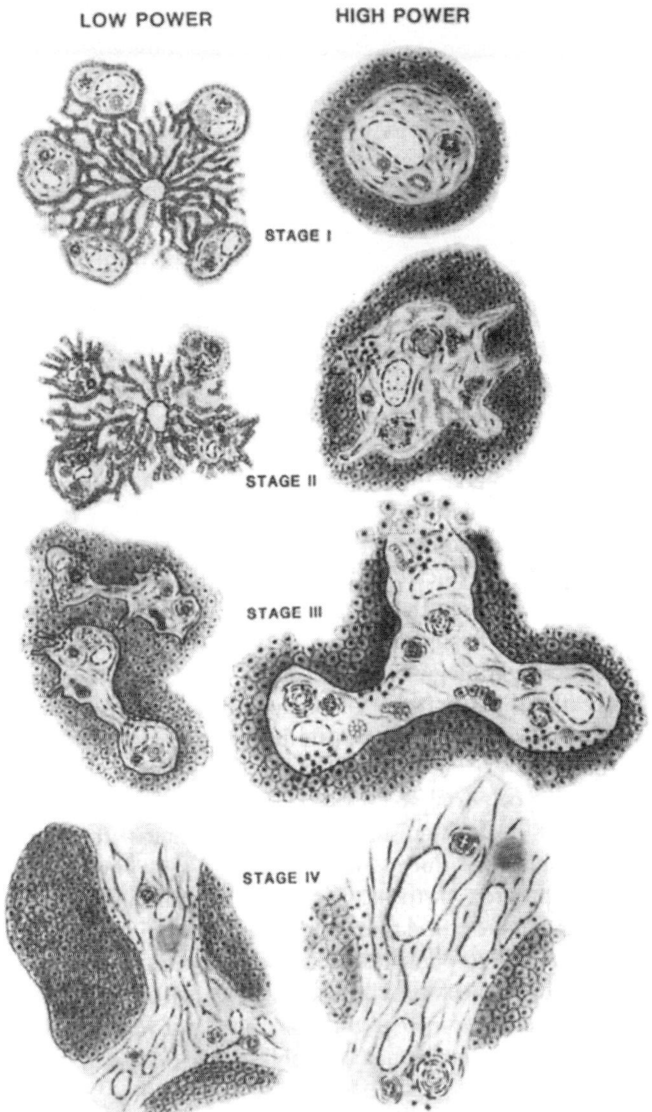

Figure 19.7. Schematic representation of the four stages of liver disease (chronic hepatitis) associated with PSC. In the high-power view of stage II, clusters of hepatocytes are shown within the enlarged portal tract; cholangitis is also depicted. In stage III, portal-to-portal fibrous bridging is present. The low-power view of stage IV shows a garland-shaped regenerative nodule. In stages III and IV, duct obliteration is present; the presence of these duct abnormalities would not be essential for staging. (Reprinted from Ludwig [66], with permission.)

only 4 patients developed large-duct disease in the 63-month follow-up. Although this categorization is still controversial, these results suggest that small-duct PSC may represent a unique, less aggressive, subtype of PSC. The subset of pediatric patients with small-duct PSC has not been closely examined.

PATHOGENESIS

The initiating event and mechanisms responsible for the progressive changes of PSC are unknown, yet they appear to derive from an immune-mediated process. As is the case with many such diseases, the etiology is probably multifactorial: the process may be initiated by various triggers – such as infections, toxins, or ischemic injury – that adversely affect only certain, genetically susceptible, individuals. Three clear abnormalities associated with PSC point to an immune-mediated process: (1) portal tract infiltration with CD3+ T cells, (2) abnormal expression of human leukocyte antigen (HLA) molecules on biliary epithelial cells, and (3) the presence of serum autoantibodies in patients with PSC [3,71,72]. Substantial research is underway to define the role of biliary epithelial cells (BEC) and lymphocytes in PSC, as well as the genetic and autoimmune factors implicated in its pathogenesis.

Biliary Epithelial Cells

To what extent BECs participate in the immune reaction is incompletely understood. They appear to act both as a target of and participant in the immune reaction, expressing cytokines, enzymes, ICAMs, and HLA molecules [73]. The fact that they aberrantly express HLA class II molecules, a classic characteristic of antigen presenting cells, suggests that BECs alone might be capable of initiating an immune response by binding to autoantigens or exogenous antigens [74]. Notably, Xu et al. [75] demonstrated the presence of autoantibodies to surface antigens expressed on BECs in patients with PSC. These cells were found to express the lymphocyte homing receptor (CD44) and to induce IL-6 production, leading to BEC proliferation [76]. It is possible that persistent IL-6 production could account, at least in part, for the bile duct changes of PSC.

Autoimmunity

An autoimmune basis for PSC has long been postulated. This is supported not only by the presence of serum autoantibodies in patients with PSC but also by increased immunoglobulin levels, a strong association with specific HLA types, and the frequent concurrence with other autoimmune diseases [3]. In a study by Saarinen et al. [14], 119 PSC patients with IBD were matched with IBD patients without PSC; 24% of the PSC–IBD patients had one or more autoimmune disorder, compared with only 9% of IBD patients without PSC. In fact, several patients had two or more autoimmune diseases – most frequently, thyroid disease and diabetes mellitus. However, PSC patients do not have a classic autoimmune phenotype because the disease predominantly affects males and shows poor response to immunosuppressive therapies.

Genetics

A genetic predisposition to biliary tract injury initiated by any of the postulated mechanisms must be woven into any etiopathogenetic theory because familial occurrence of PSC has been noted in several reports [77–79]. This genetic predisposition is clearly linked to HLA type. As previously mentioned, healthy BECs express only major histocompatibility complex (MHC) class I antigens, whereas those in PSC aberrantly express the class II molecules, HLA-DR, -DQ, or -DP. Several studies have identified HLA class II haplotypes associated with PSC: DR3,DQ2 and DR6,DQ6 are the most frequently reported [80,81]. In fact, the DR3,DQ2 homozygous haplotype is strongly associated with a susceptibility to PSC, with a relative risk of 16 [80]. By contrast, the DR4,DQ8 haplotype appears to protect against its development [81]. The MICA gene, localized to the class I region, is also associated with susceptibility to PSC: the MICA*008 allele has a strong positive association, and MICA*002 has a strong negative association [82,83]. An illustrative case report described two brothers with PSC who were homozygous for the MICA*008 alleles and for the DR3,DQ2 and DR6,DQ6 HLA haplotypes, whereas their unaffected father and sister carried the protective DR4 allele [78]. The pediatric series reported by Wilschanski et al. [8], which is the only one to include HLA genotyping, found an increased incidence of HLA-B8 and DR2.

Several other gene polymorphisms have been identified in the immunopathogenesis of PSC. Included in this group are TNFα, CTLA-4, ICAM, and metalloproteinases [72]. In addition, one study found an increased prevalence of mild CFTR mutations in patients with PSC; the implication of this is unknown [84]. Several other studies have shown no increased incidence of common CFTR mutations in patients with PSC [85–87].

Lymphocyte Homing

Grant et al. [88] proposed an intriguing new mechanism of disease pathogenesis that might account for how the portal inflammation of PSC can be dyssynchronous from associated colitis. Based on their identification of gut-associated adhesion molecules (such as MAdCAM-1 and VAP-1) on portal endothelium in IBD-associated liver inflammation, they posited that certain lymphocytes activated in the inflamed gut mucosa of IBD patients develop "dual homing," acquiring the ability to bind to both mucosal and hepatic endothelium [89]. These cells can then persist in the liver as memory T cells, and, at some later time point, induce hepatobiliary inflammation in response to a secondary trigger. Furthermore, Eksteen et al. [90,91] reported that the gut-specific chemokine CCL25 is expressed in the livers of patients with PSC, a finding that might help explain how T cells could be recruited to the liver. This new theory not only explains the link between PSC and IBD but also makes teleologic sense because this process of "enterohepatic lymphocyte recirculation" also provides a mechanism for immune surveillance across the liver and gut [88].

Infection

An alternative theory has held that various proinflammatory bacteria-derived products (e.g., peptides or toxic bile acids) play a role in the etiopathogenesis of hepatobiliary disease [72,92,93]. Vierling [92] hypothesized that PSC in patients with IBD is related to repeated episodes of low-grade bacterial infection (or portal bacteremia), suggesting that disruption of the intestinal mucosal barrier allows entry of bacteria into the portal vein. Certainly, bacterial antigens may act through molecular mimicry, whereby microbial molecules containing specific epitopes cross-react with molecules in human antigens, essentially acting as "autoantigens" to set off an inflammatory cascade in a predisposed individual [72].

Several microorganisms have been detected in the livers and biliary tracts of patients with sclerosing cholangitis. For example, explanted livers of patients with SC showed high bacterial positivity, with α-hemolytic *streptococcus* making up 46% of the bacteria found [94]. Moreover, *Cryptosporidiosis* has long been noted in association with SC in immunodeficient patients, but one case report identified the parasite in a patient with SC without documented immunodeficiency [95]. *Helicobacter* species have been identified in human liver samples of patients with SC [96,97], and seropositivity to chlamydial infections has been associated with PSC [98]. The significance of these associations is not clear and requires further study.

A viral etiopathogenesis for PSC, frequently proposed, has largely been abandoned recently. A virus could theoretically infect and alter cholangiocytes, which could then become the target of an autoimmune attack. Serologic evidence for infection by viruses, such as hepatitis B, is seen no more frequently in SC patients than in control subjects [39]. One logical candidate is reovirus 3, which can cause an obliterative cholangitis in weanling mice and perhaps in newborn infants. However, there was no difference in reovirus titers between sera from PSC patients and from control subjects, and cultures and immunohistologic staining for reovirus were also negative [99,100]. These findings do not definitely rule out a pathogenetic role for either virus because a virally initiated immunologic attack could persist long after the viral infection.

Animal Models

Investigation of the pathogenesis of PSC has been bolstered by the development of animal models for hepatobiliary injury. In one such model, lesions reminiscent of PSC (portal inflammation and bile duct proliferation) occur in genetically susceptible rats with experimental small bowel bacterial overgrowth [93, 101]. The hepatobiliary injury noted in this model is not caused by previously postulated factors, such as septicemia or portal bacteremia; instead, the researchers postulated that mucosal absorption of bacterial cell wall polymers occurred and that these bacterial by-products initiated the biliary injury. Targeted disruption of the cell wall polymers prevented hepatobiliary injury [93,101,102]. Koga et al. [103] demonstrated abnormally elevated levels of the bacterial endotoxin lipopolysaccharide in the biliary epithelium of rats with small bowel bacterial overgrowth, linking the pathogenesis of intestinal injury to that of bile duct injury in this model.

A second mouse model may help define the connection between colitis and cholangitis. Numata et al. [104] reported inflammatory cell infiltration and focal necrosis in the livers of mice with dextran sulfate sodium-induced experimental colitis. Cytokine analysis and mononuclear cell isolation from livers of

Table 19.5: Goals of Therapeutic Intervention in the Management of Patients with Sclerosing Cholangitis

I. Provide symptomatic relief:
   A. Decrease pruritus
   B. Improve nutrition
      1. Ameliorate steatorrhea
      2. Prevent fat-soluble vitamin deficiency
   C. Decrease pain (often due to cholangitis)

II. Improve biliary drainage:
   A. Endoscopic balloon dilation (with or without stenting)
   B. Choleretics (ursodeoxycholic acid)

III. Prevent, recognize, and ameliorate complications:
   A. Recurrent cholangitis and bacteremia
   B. Dominant stricture
   C. Cirrhosis (and attendant complications of portal hypertension)
   D. Cholangiocarcinoma; colonic dysplasia/carcinoma

IV. Decrease rate of progression of underlying hepatobiliary disease [retard inflammation]

these mice indicated a Th-1-dominant immune mechanism, similar to that seen in PSC. In a separate study, treatment with α-galactosylceramide reduced the Th-1 dominance in this model, led to improved survival rate and weight gain, and reduced hepatic inflammation [105].

Finally, it has been noted that *Mdr2* knockout mice develop hepatic lesions strongly resembling the onion-skin cholangitis of PSC [106]. Based on their findings of disrupted tight junctions and basement membranes in these mice, Fickert et al. [106,107] suggested that regurgitation of bile acids from leaky bile ducts leads to periductal inflammation and fibrogenesis, and ultimately to cholangitis. In their follow-up study, the *Mdr2* knockout mice demonstrated up regulated fibrogenic genes and down-regulated fibrolytic genes, a finding that may open new avenues for translational and therapeutic research. Although no one animal model accounts for all of the features of PSC, each has helped shed light on elements of its pathogenesis.

TREATMENT

Determination of the efficacy of any specific therapeutic intervention for patients with PSC is bedeviled by the unpredictable natural history. The goals of therapeutic intervention for symptomatic patients with documented PSC, and the treatments that have been tested are listed in Tables 19.5 and 19.6. However, to date, there have been no published reports of large, randomized controlled trials that document an effective form of medical therapy in PSC. Nonspecific management should focus on monitoring for complications and careful assessment and management of nutritional status, including the prevention of fat-soluble vitamin deficiency [108].

Table 19.6: Medical and Surgical Modalities Used to Manage Sclerosing Cholangitis and Attendant Complications

Medical
- Antibiotics [121,181]
- Azathioprine
- Cholestyramine [182]
- Cladribine [183]
- Colchicine [184,185]
- Corticosteroids [28,120,122,186]
- Cyclosporine [187]
- Methotrexate [188,189]
- Mycophenylate mofetil [190]
- Penicillamine [191]
- Pentoxifylline [192]
- Pirfenidone [193]
- Tacrolimus [194]
- Ursodeoxycholic acid [113,115–117,195]
- Combinations (e.g., ursodiol, prednisone, and azathioprine) [122]

Surgical/endoscopic
- Intraductal lavage with steroids [196]
- Strictures
- Balloon dilatation of dominant strictures ($\pm$ stent placement) [124,197,198]
- Resection [199]
- Transplantation [200]

See general discussions of management in PCS reviews [32,41,118, 119,123].

Medications

Ursodeoxycholic acid (UDCA) is the most widely used and studied medication for PSC, despite inconclusive results as to its beneficial effect on the disease. A naturally occurring bile acid that is a potent choleretic, immunomodulatory, and cytoprotective agent, UDCA has been shown to bring about clinical and biochemical improvement in a wide variety of hepatobiliary disorders, via enrichment of the bile acid pool, and displacement of toxic bile acids [109,110]. It also stimulates expression of the cellular transporters MDR3, BSEP, and MRP4 and improves bile acid excretion [111,112]. The Mayo Primary Sclerosing Cholangitis–Ursodeoxycholic Acid Study Group reported their experience in treating 105 patients with either UDCA or placebo: UDCA was associated with improvement in alkaline phosphatase, AST, bilirubin, and albumin levels, but not with an improvement in histology or a delay in time to treatment failure [113]. Similarly, a biochemical response to UDCA has been noted in pediatric patients with PSC. In the series of Debray et al. [12], 3 of 14 patients treated with UDCA had normalization of liver function tests. Of the patients reported by Feldstein et al. [10], there was a significant improvement in alkaline phosphatase, GGT, AST, and ALT levels with UDCA (with or without concurrent immunosuppressive therapy). The proportion of patients with symptoms also decreased after 1 year of treatment. However, these clinical and biochemical improvements have been found to be transient in most patients. A 2002 Cochrane meta-analysis concluded that UDCA improves biochemical profiles of patients with PSC but that there is not enough evidence to support or refute a beneficial effect on the disease process overall [114].

There has been some suggestion that UDCA at 20–25 mg/kg/day may slow the disease process in PSC. In a preliminary study, Mitchell et al. [115] treated 26 adult patients for 2 years and reported improvements in patient biochemistry, liver histology, and cholangiographic findings compared with control subjects. A cohort of 30 patients followed by Harnois et al. [116] for 1 year on high-dose UDCA showed similar improvements. However, the long-term efficacy of high-dose therapy was recently called into question: a large 5-year randomized controlled study concluded that high-dose therapy offered no benefit to low-dose UDCA in either survival or prevention of cholangiocarcinoma [117]. Several points regarding this study warrant discussion: first, although not reaching significance, there did appear to be a trend toward improved survival in the UDCA-treated group. Second, despite it being the largest study to date, following 219 patients, it was still insufficiently powered to detect a dramatic positive effect on survival during the 5-year period. Finally, liver histology was not assessed. Further investigation is required, ideally focusing on treating patients with early disease, before the development of irreversible scarring or stricture. Indeed, initiation of therapy early in disease may well be shown to slow disease progression in the long term. This fact, along with the benign side-effect profile of UDCA, makes high-dose UDCA therapy an attractive treatment for pediatric patients.

Several other medications, including immunosuppressants, antifibrogenics, chelators, and antibiotics, have been used in patients with PSC, with no significant benefit (Table 19.6) [118,119]. Steroids have had nominal effects, with reported benefits only in patients with overlap syndrome or ASC [28,120]. Cox and Cox [121] reported the successful use of oral vancomycin in normalizing ALT levels in three patients with PSC, but this has not been confirmed in larger studies. Still, drug combination regimens may still hold promise. A study of the triple regimen of UDCA plus prednisolone and azathioprine in 15 adult patients resulted in biochemical, histologic, and cholangiographic improvement after 41 months, and only 1 patient developed a dominant stricture [122]. Large follow-up studies are necessary to demonstrate their combined efficacy in the long term.

Surgery

It is now recommended that biliary tract surgery be avoided if possible because it may complicate surgery at the time of transplantation. Endoscopic balloon dilatation, on the other hand, may offer relief for patients with a focal dominant stricture without the disadvantages of a surgical approach [123]. In fact, in selected patients with dominant strictures, endoscopic dilatation and stent placement may significantly improve symptoms and survival free of transplantation [124–126]. For patients with end-stage liver disease, liver transplantation is the only therapeutic option available. Indications for transplant include cirrhosis with impaired liver function, variceal bleeding, intractable ascites, hepatic encephalopathy, and severe recurrent bacterial cholangitis [127,128]. Although PSC is a common reason for adult liver transplantation, it is the reason for only 2.7% of pediatric transplants [129].

PROGNOSIS

There is apparent heterogeneity in the clinical course of PSC, but inexorable progression is the rule. Some series suggest that greater than 80% of patients with PSC will exhibit advancing symptomatology, biochemical features of increasing liver disease, and progression on sequential biopsies [35,36,38,44]. The rate of progression may be slow and insidious or relatively rapid, such that over a 5- to 10-year period, cirrhosis will develop and death will occur without liver transplantation [30,31,37].

Rates of Progression and Survival

Several large adult studies have attempted to clarify the natural history and prognosis of PSC [30,31,35,36,38]. In the series reported by Wiesner et al. [35], which included 174 adults with PSC, 31% died as a result of underlying liver disease and cholangiocarcinoma, and an additional 10% were referred for liver transplantation. The median survival from the time of diagnosis was 11.9 years. Multivariate analysis revealed that age, serum bilirubin and hemoglobin concentrations, the presence of IBD, and histologic stage were independent discriminators of an unfavorable outcome; high-grade strictures and diffuse strictures of the intrahepatic ducts were also indicative of a poor prognosis. Farrant et al. [36] reported on the natural history of 126 adult patients with PSC: liver transplantation was performed in 21%, and an additional 16% died of liver-related disease. The estimated median survival was 12 years. Prognostically significant features included hepatomegaly, splenomegaly, serum alkaline phosphatase, histologic stage, and age. Survival rates have been similar across the largest adult studies, with the exception of a recent study of a Dutch population: median survival was 18 years, and 8% received transplants after a median disease duration of 95 months (range 2–221) [31].

The rate of progression of childhood onset sclerosing cholangitis is still unclear. The pediatric study by Batres et al. [13] reported that 9 of 20 patients required liver transplantation – two who presented with early (stage I or II) disease, and 7 who presented with advanced (stage III or IV) disease. This study compared patient characteristics with liver histology and concluded that the histologic findings at diagnosis are not predictive of disease progression. In the series by Debray et al. [12], which included patients with both primary and secondary sclerosing cholangitis, the mean follow-up was 7 years with a range of 6 months to 19.3 years. Of 56 children in the series, 18 died, and an additional 15 underwent liver transplantation. The estimated median survival in this group was 10 years. In the series by Wilschanski et al. [8], only 1 of 32 children died, with 10 either listed for transplantation or having undergone transplantation. A poor outcome in this group was associated with jaundice, prolongation of prothrombin time, an abnormal bilirubin, and splenomegaly at presentation. In the pediatric cohort reported by Feldstein et al. [10], liver disease was progressive, and 11 of the 52 patients underwent liver transplantation during the 6.6 year (mean) follow-up (range 0.2–16.7 years). The median survival without transplant was 12.7 years; low platelets, splenomegaly, and older age were variables associated with shorter survival.

Posttransplantation Prognosis

Posttransplant survival in adults with PSC is good, with 1-year patient survival rates of 84–97% [130,131]. However, several posttransplantation complications occur more frequently in PSC patients: there is evidence of an increased incidence of acute and chronic rejection, hepatic artery thrombosis, reflux cholangitis, and biliary stricturing in these patients [130,132]. Recurrence of disease is now also well-recognized; the reported incidence averages between 10 and 20% in the largest studies [60,133,134]. However, in a recent study of 152 adult patients followed after transplantation for 14 years, Vera et al. [135] reported a strikingly high recurrence rate of 37%. A late increase in alkaline phosphatase levels almost universally indicated biliary structuring and disease recurrence in the study by Wiesner et al. [35], but multiple studies have identified no consistently significant risk factors. There have been no large posttransplant follow-up studies in pediatrics, but of the 11 transplanted patients in the series by Feldstein et al. [10], three had recurrence of disease. An even higher rate was reported in the series by Batres et al. [13], in which histologic PSC recurrence after transplantation occurred in three of nine patients (1.6, 2.4, and 8.4 yr postoperatively).

Prognostic Factors

There are no reliable prognostic indicators in an individual patient, but multivariate statistical survival models may be of help in identifying individual patients with PSC at low or high risk of dying [35,36,136]. Boberg et al. [136] tested a time-dependent Cox regression model to predict the prognosis of PSC. In this model, bilirubin, albumin, and age at diagnosis were identified as independent prognostic factors. Another prognostic aid may be HLA type: the HLA–DR3,DQ2 heterozygous genotype has been associated with accelerated progression of PSC, and the DR3,DR2 heterozygous genotype has been linked to an increased risk of death after transplantation [137]. The prognostic value of cholangiography has also been assessed: high-grade intrahepatic strictures have been shown to be indicative of a poor prognosis [35,50]. More recently, the Amsterdam cholangiographic classification system was developed, combining intrahepatic and extrahepatic findings with age at first ERCP [31]. Using this system, patient scores were found to correlate inversely with survival. Because this classification reflects disease stage, it has the potential to serve as a predictor of disease progression in patient care. However, more trials are necessary to validate this tool.

The ultimate prognosis may be altered by the fact that PSC is a premalignant condition, complicated by cholangiocarcinoma (CCA) in a certain number of patients, which is often localized to the hepatic hilum (Klatskin tumor) [138–140]. In a prospective study of 161 adult patients with PSC, patients were followed until transplantation, death, or the development of CCA; 7% of patients developed the malignancy over a mean follow-up of 11.5 years [139]. Notably, no association was found between duration of PSC disease and the incidence of CCA, despite the overwhelming majority of cases occurring in adulthood; the youngest reported case of CCA was in a 14-year-old with PSC and longstanding UC [141]. Transplantation may offer hope for long-term survival [142,143].

In addition to being a risk factor for biliary neoplasms, PSC also is a risk factor for colorectal cancer in those with UC [144–146]. In a study of 152 adult patients with PSC after liver transplantation, the incidence of colorectal cancer was 5.3% compared with 0.6% in IBD patients without PSC; pancolitis and duration of colitis greater than 10 years were risk factors [146]. Similarly, in a meta-analysis of eleven studies, Soetikno et al. [145] reported that patients with UC and PSC have a significantly higher risk for the development of colorectal dysplasia and carcinoma than patients with isolated UC, with an odds ratio of 5. In a study of pediatric PSC–IBD, 3 of 43 patients developed colonic dysplasia, with the youngest at 17 years of age [43]. More intensive colonoscopic surveillance should be considered for these patients.

SUMMARY

Primary sclerosing cholangitis is a cholangiopathy that presents as an independent entity and in association with IBD. Idiopathic forms often overlap with AIH, which should be suspected in the setting of elevated aminotransferase and immunoglobulin levels and positive autoantibodies. Secondary forms are associated with immunodeficiencies, malignancies, and infections, among other causes. The clinical presentation of SC is similar to other cholestatic diseases, with fatigue, jaundice, and hepatosplenomegaly predominating. Abnormal laboratory findings include positive ANCAs and elevated ALT, alkaline phosphatase, and GGT levels; particularly in children, an elevated GGT level appears to be a sensitive marker. The diagnosis is based on classic cholangiographic and histologic findings; MRCP is gaining popularity as a noninvasive diagnostic tool. Once a diagnosis is made, patients should be screened for IBD, even if they are asymptomatic. Although there is no current therapy that halts progression of the disease, UDCA may be helpful in inducing biochemical and histologic improvement; further studies are necessary in young patients to determine its potential benefits over the long term. Transplantation is the only option for those with end-stage disease but may be associated with high rates of postoperative complications; the disease recurs in up to one third of patients.

Prospective, controlled collaborative trials performed in clearly defined patient groups should lead to a better understanding of the natural history of SC in children and ideally provide clues to the etiology of the disease, as well as its link to IBD and other disorders.

ACKNOWLEDGMENT

The authors gratefully acknowledge the contributions of Dr. Kevin Bove, who has shared his expertise in reviewing the histologic findings of sclerosing cholangitis, as well as providing images for each edition of this text.

REFERENCES

1. Balistreri WF, Bove KE. Primary sclerosing cholangitis and similar hepatobiliary lesions. In: Balistreri WF, Vanderhoof JA, eds. Pediatric gastroenterology and nutrition. New York: Chapman & Hall, 1990:196–236.
2. Rodriguez HJ, Bass NM. Primary sclerosing cholangitis. Semin Gastrointest Dis 2003;14:189–98.
3. MacFaul GR, Chapman RW. Sclerosing cholangitis. Curr Opin Gastroenterol 2004;20:275–80.
4. Ahmad J, Slivka A. Hepatobiliary disease in inflammatory bowel disease. Gastroenterol Clin North Am 2002;31:329–45.
5. Roberts EA. Primary sclerosing cholangitis in children. J Gastroenterol Hepatol 1999;14:588–93.
6. Gossard AA, Angulo P, Lindor KD. Secondary sclerosing cholangitis: a comparison to primary sclerosing cholangitis. Am J Gastroenterol 2005;100:1330–3.
7. Mieli Vergani G, Vergani D. Sclerosing cholangitis in the paediatric patient. Best Pract Res Clin Gastroenterol 2001;15:681–90.
8. Wilschanski M, Chait P, Wade JA, et al. Primary sclerosing cholangitis in 32 children: clinical, laboratory, and radiographic features, with survival analysis. Hepatology 1995;22:1415–22.
9. Sisto A, Feldman P, Garel L, et al. Primary sclerosing cholangitis in children: study of five cases and review of the literature. Pediatrics 1987;80:918–23.
10. Feldstein AE, Perrault J, El-Youssif M, et al. Primary sclerosing cholangitis in children: a long-term follow-up study. Hepatology 2003;38:210–17.
11. el-Shabrawi M, Wilkinson ML, Portmann B, et al. Primary sclerosing cholangitis in childhood. Gastroenterology 1987;92:1226–35.
12. Debray D, Pariente D, Urvoas E, et al. Sclerosing cholangitis in children. J Pediatr 1994;124:49–56.
13. Batres LA, Russo P, Mathews M, et al. Primary sclerosing cholangitis in children: a histologic follow-up study. Pediatr Dev Pathol 2005;8:568–76.
14. Saarinen S, Olerup O, Broome U. Increased frequency of autoimmune diseases in patients with primary sclerosing cholangitis. Am J Gastroenterol 2000;95:3195–9.
15. Jaffe R. Liver involvement in the histiocytic disorders of childhood. Pediatr Dev Pathol 2004;7:214–25.
16. Amedee-Manesme O, Bernard O, Brunelle F, et al. Sclerosing cholangitis with neonatal onset. J Pediatr 1987;111:225–9.
17. Baker AJ, Portmann B, Westaby D, et al. Neonatal sclerosing cholangitis in two siblings: a category of progressive intrahepatic cholestasis. J Pediatr Gastroenterol Nutr 1993;17:317–22.
18. Bar Meir M, Hadas-Halperin I, Fisher D, et al. Neonatal sclerosing cholangitis associated with autoimmune phenomena. J Pediatr Gastroenterol Nutr 2000;30:332–4.
19. Ewart-Toland A, Enns GM, Cox VA, et al. Severe congenital anomalies requiring transplantation in children with Kabuki syndrome. Am J Med Genet 1998;80:362–7.
20. Nobili V, Marcellini M, Devito R, et al. Hepatic fibrosis in Kabuki syndrome. Am J Med Genet A 2004;124:209–12.
21. Baala L, Hadj-Rabia S, Hamel-Teillac D, et al. Homozygosity mapping of a locus for a novel syndromic ichthyosis to chromosome 3q27-q28. J Invest Dermatol 2002;119:70–6.
22. Hadj Rabia S, Baala L, Vabres P, et al. Claudin-1 gene mutations in neonatal sclerosing cholangitis associated with ichthyosis: a tight junction disease. Gastroenterology 2004;127:1386–90.
23. Beuers U, Rust C. Overlap syndromes. Semin Liver Dis 2005;25:311–20.
24. Floreani A, Rizzotto ER, Ferrara F, et al. Clinical course and outcome of autoimmune hepatitis/primary sclerosing cholangitis overlap syndrome. Am J Gastroenterol 2005;100:1516–22.
25. Hong-Curtis J, Yeh MM, Jain D, Lee JH. Rapid progression of autoimmune hepatitis in the background of primary sclerosing cholangitis. J Clin Gastroenterol 2004;38:906–9.
26. Gregorio GV, Portmann B, Karani J, et al. Autoimmune hepatitis/sclerosing cholangitis overlap syndrome in childhood: a 16–year prospective study. Hepatology 2001;33:544–53.
27. Vergani D, Mieli-Vergani G. Autoimmune hepatitis and sclerosing cholangitis. Autoimmunity 2004;37:329–32.
28. Sekhon JS, Chung RT, Epstein M, Kaplan MM. Steroid-responsive (autoimmune?) sclerosing cholangitis. Dig Dis Sci 2005;50:1839–43.
29. Schrumpf E, Boberg KM. Epidemiology of primary sclerosing cholangitis. Best Pract Res Clin Gastroenterol 2001;15:553–62.
30. Bambha K, Kim WR, Talwalkar J, et al. Incidence, clinical spectrum, and outcomes of primary sclerosing cholangitis in a United States community. Gastroenterology 2003;125:1364–9.
31. Ponsioen CY, Vrouenraets SM, Prawirodirdjo W, et al. Natural history of primary sclerosing cholangitis and prognostic value of cholangiography in a Dutch population. Gut 2002;51:562–6.
32. Talwalkar JA, Lindor KD. Primary sclerosing cholangitis. Inflamm Bowel Dis 2005;11:62–72.
33. Mendes FD, Lindor KD. Primary sclerosing cholangitis. Clin Liver Dis 2004;8:195–211.
34. MacFaul GR, Chapman RW. Sclerosing cholangitis. Curr Opin Gastroenterol 2005;21:348–353.
35. Wiesner RH, Grambsch PM, Dickson ER, et al. Primary sclerosing cholangitis: natural history, prognostic factors and survival analysis. Hepatology 1989;10:430–6.
36. Farrant JM, Hayllar KM, Wilkinson ML, et al. Natural history and prognostic variables in primary sclerosing cholangitis. Gastroenterology 1991;100:1710–17.
37. Okolicsanyi L, Fabris L, Viaggi S, et al. Primary sclerosing cholangitis: clinical presentation, natural history and prognostic variables: an Italian multicentre study. The Italian PSC Study Group. Eur J Gastroenterol Hepatol 1996;8:685–91.
38. Broome U, Olsson R, Loof L, et al. Natural history and prognostic factors in 305 Swedish patients with primary sclerosing cholangitis. Gut 1996;38:610–15.

39. Fausa O, Schrumpf E, Elgjo K. Relationship of inflammatory bowel disease and primary sclerosing cholangitis. Semin Liver Dis 1991;11:31–9.
40. Loftus EV Jr, Harewood GC, Loftus CG, et al. PSC-IBD: a unique form of inflammatory bowel disease associated with primary sclerosing cholangitis. Gut 2005;54:91–6.
41. Portincasa P, Vacca M, Moschetta A, et al. Primary sclerosing cholangitis: updates in diagnosis and therapy. World J Gastroenterol 2005;11:7–16.
42. Olsson R, Danielsson A, Jarnerot G, et al. Prevalence of primary sclerosing cholangitis in patients with ulcerative colitis. Gastroenterology 1991;100:1319–23.
43. Faubion WA Jr, Loftus EV, Sandborn WJ, et al. Pediatric "PSC–IBD": a descriptive report of associated inflammatory bowel disease among pediatric patients with PSC. J Pediatr Gastroenterol Nutr 2001;33:296–300.
44. Aadland E, Schrumpf E, Fausa O, et al. Primary sclerosing cholangitis: a long-term follow-up study. Scand J Gastroenterol 1987;22:655–64.
45. Broome U, Glaumann H, Lindstom E, et al. Natural history and outcome in 32 Swedish patients with small duct primary sclerosing cholangitis (PSC). J Hepatol 2002;36:586–9.
46. Hyams J, Markowitz J, Treem W, et al. Characterization of hepatic abnormalities in children with inflammatory bowel disease. Inflamm Bowel Dis 1995;1:27–33.
47. Juillerat P, Mottet C, Froehlich F, et al. Extraintestinal manifestations of Crohn's disease. Digestion 2005;71:31–6.
48. Raj V, Lichtenstein DR. Hepatobiliary manifestations of inflammatory bowel disease. Gastroenterol Clin North Am 1999;28: 491–513.
49. Kugathasan S, Judd RH, Hoffmann RG, et al. Epidemiologic and clinical characteristics of children with newly diagnosed inflammatory bowel disease in Wisconsin: a statewide population-based study. J Pediatr 2003;143:525–31.
50. Craig DA, MacCarty RL, Wiesner RH, et al. Primary sclerosing cholangitis: value of cholangiography in determining the prognosis. AJR Am J Roentgenol 1991;157:959–64.
51. MacCarty RL, LaRusso NF, Wiesner RH, Ludwig J. Primary sclerosing cholangitis: findings on cholangiography and pancreatography. Radiology 1983;149:39–44.
52. Olsson RG, Asztely MS. Prognostic value of cholangiography in primary sclerosing cholangitis. Eur J Gastroenterol Hepatol 1995;7:251–4.
53. LaRusso NF, Wiesner RH, Ludwig J, MacCarty RL. Current concepts. Primary sclerosing cholangitis. N Engl J Med 1984;310: 899–903.
54. Angulo P, Pearce DH, Johnson CD, et al. Magnetic resonance cholangiography in patients with biliary disease: its role in primary sclerosing cholangitis. J Hepatol 2000;33:520–7.
55. Fulcher AS, Turner MA, Franklin KJ, et al. Primary sclerosing cholangitis: evaluation with MR cholangiography—a case–control study. Radiology 2000;215:71–80.
56. Textor HJ, Flacke S, Pauleit D, et al. Three-dimensional magnetic resonance cholangiopancreatography with respiratory triggering in the diagnosis of primary sclerosing cholangitis: comparison with endoscopic retrograde cholangiography. Endoscopy 2002;34:984–90.
57. Ferrara C, Valeri G, Salvolini L, Giovagnoni A. Magnetic resonance cholangiopancreatography in primary sclerosing cholangitis in children. Pediatr Radiol 2002;32:413–17.
58. Lee WS, Saw CB, Sarji SA. Autoimmune hepatitis/primary sclerosing cholangitis overlap syndrome in a child: diagnostic usefulness of magnetic resonance cholangiopancreatography. J Paediatr Child Health 2005;41:225–7.
59. Norton KI, Lee JS, Kogan D, et al. The role of magnetic resonance cholangiography in the management of children and young adults after liver transplantation. Pediatr Transplant 2001;5: 410–18.
60. Brandsaeter B, Schrumpf E, Bentdal O, et al. Recurrent primary sclerosing cholangitis after liver transplantation: a magnetic resonance cholangiography study with analyses of predictive factors. Liver Transpl 2005;11:1361–9.
61. Macchi V, Floreani A, Marchesi P, et al. Imaging of primary sclerosing cholangitis: preliminary results by two new non-invasive techniques. Dig Liver Dis 2004;36:614–21.
62. Terjung B, Spengler U. Role of auto-antibodies for the diagnosis of chronic cholestatic liver diseases. Clin Rev Allergy Immunol 2005;28:115–33.
63. Angulo P, Peter JB, Gershwin ME, et al. Serum autoantibodies in patients with primary sclerosing cholangitis. J Hepatol 2000;32:182–7.
64. Scheuer PJ. Ludwig Symposium on biliary disorders—part II. Pathologic features and evolution of primary biliary cirrhosis and primary sclerosing cholangitis. Mayo Clin Proc 1998;73: 179–83.
65. Desmet VJ. Histopathology of chronic cholestasis and adult ductopenic syndrome. Clin Liver Dis 1998;2:249–64, viii.
66. Ludwig J. Surgical pathology of the syndrome of primary sclerosing cholangitis. Am J Surg Pathol 1989;13(Suppl 1):43–9.
67. Olsson R, Hagerstrand I, Broome U, et al. Sampling variability of percutaneous liver biopsy in primary sclerosing cholangitis. J Clin Pathol 1995;48:933–5.
68. Ludwig J. Small-duct primary sclerosing cholangitis. Semin Liver Dis 1991;11:11–17.
69. Angulo P, Maor-Kendler Y, Lindor KD. Small-duct primary sclerosing cholangitis: a long-term follow up study. Hepatology 2002;35:1494–500.
70. Bjornsson E, Boberg KM, Cullen S, et al. Patients with small duct primary sclerosing cholangitis have a favourable long term prognosis. Gut 2002;51:731–5.
71. Boberg KM, Lundin KE, Schrumpf E. Etiology and pathogenesis in primary sclerosing cholangitis. Scand J Gastroenterol Suppl 1994;204:47–58.
72. Worthington J, Cullen S, Chapman R. Immunopathogenesis of primary sclerosing cholangitis. Clin Rev Allergy Immunol 2005;28:93–103.
73. Wu CT, Davis PA, Luketic VA, Gershwin ME. A review of the physiological and immunological functions of biliary epithelial cells: targets for primary biliary cirrhosis, primary sclerosing cholangitis and drug-induced ductopenias. Clin Dev Immunol 2004;11:205–13.
74. Broome U, Glaumann H, Hultcrantz R, Forsum U. Distribution of HLA-DR, HLA-DP, HLA-DQ antigens in liver tissue from patients with primary sclerosing cholangitis. Scand J Gastroenterol 1990;25:54–8.
75. Xu B, Broome U, Ericzon BG, Sumitran-Holgersson S. High frequency of autoantibodies in patients with primary sclerosing cholangitis that bind biliary epithelial cells and induce expression of CD44 and production of interleukin 6. Gut 2002;51: 120–7.

76. Cruickshank SM, Southgate J, Wyatt JI, et al. Expression of CD44 on bile ducts in primary sclerosing cholangitis and primary biliary cirrhosis. J Clin Pathol 1999;52:730–4.
77. Quigley EM, LaRusso NF, Ludwig J, et al. Familial occurrence of primary sclerosing cholangitis and ulcerative colitis. Gastroenterology 1983;85:1160–5.
78. Van Steenbergen W, De Goede E, Emonds MP, et al. Primary sclerosing cholangitis in two brothers: report of a family with special emphasis on molecular HLA and MICA genotyping. Eur J Gastroenterol Hepatol 2005;17:767–71.
79. Silber GH, Finegold MJ, Wagner ML, Klish WJ. Sclerosing cholangitis and ulcerative colitis in a mother and her son. J Pediatr Gastroenterol Nutr 1987;6:147–52.
80. Spurkland A, Saarinen S, Boberg KM, et al. HLA class II haplotypes in primary sclerosing cholangitis patients from five European populations. Tissue Antigens 1999;53:459–69.
81. Donaldson PT, Norris S. Evaluation of the role of MHC class II alleles, haplotypes and selected amino acid sequences in primary sclerosing cholangitis. Autoimmunity 2002;35:555–64.
82. Norris S, Kondeatis E, Collins R, et al. Mapping MHC-encoded susceptibility and resistance in primary sclerosing cholangitis: the role of MICA polymorphism. Gastroenterology 2001;120: 1475–82.
83. Wiencke K, Spurkland A, Schrumpf E, Boberg KM. Primary sclerosing cholangitis is associated to an extended B8-DR3 haplotype including particular MICA and MICB alleles. Hepatology 2001;34:625–30.
84. Sheth S, Shea JC, Bishop MD, et al. Increased prevalence of CFTR mutations and variants and decreased chloride secretion in primary sclerosing cholangitis. Hum Genet 2003;113:286–92.
85. Girodon E, Sternberg D, Chazouilleres O, et al. Cystic fibrosis transmembrane conductance regulator (CFTR) gene defects in patients with primary sclerosing cholangitis. J Hepatol 2002; 37:192–7.
86. Gallegos-Orozco JF, E Yurk C, Wang N, et al. Lack of association of common cystic fibrosis transmembrane conductance regulator gene mutations with primary sclerosing cholangitis. Am J Gastroenterol 2005;100:874–8.
87. McGill JM, Williams DM, Hunt CM. Survey of cystic fibrosis transmembrane conductance regulator genotypes in primary sclerosing cholangitis. Dig Dis Sci 1996;41:540–2.
88. Grant AJ, Lalor PF, Salmi M, et al. Homing of mucosal lymphocytes to the liver in the pathogenesis of hepatic complications of inflammatory bowel disease. Lancet 2002;359:150–7.
89. Grant AJ, Lalor PF, Hubscher SG, et al. MAdCAM-1 expressed in chronic inflammatory liver disease supports mucosal lymphocyte adhesion to hepatic endothelium (MAdCAM-1 in chronic inflammatory liver disease). Hepatology 2001;33:1065–72.
90. Eksteen B, Grant AJ, Miles A, et al. Hepatic endothelial CCL25 mediates the recruitment of CCR9+ gut-homing lymphocytes to the liver in primary sclerosing cholangitis. J Exp Med 2004;200:1511–17.
91. Eksteen B, Miles AE, Grant AJ, Adams DH. Lymphocyte homing in the pathogenesis of extra-intestinal manifestations of inflammatory bowel disease. Clin Med 2004;4:173–80.
92. Vierling JM. Hepatobiliary complications of ulcerative colitis and Crohn's disease. In: Zakim D, Boyer TD, eds. Hepatology: a textbook of liver disease. 2nd ed. Philadelphia: WB Saunders, 1990:1126–58.
93. Lichtman SN, Sartor RB, Keku J, Schwab JH. Hepatic inflammation in rats with experimental small intestinal bacterial overgrowth. Gastroenterology 1990;98:414–23.
94. Olsson R, Bjornsson E, Backman L, et al. Bile duct bacterial isolates in primary sclerosing cholangitis: a study of explanted livers. J Hepatol 1998;28:426–32.
95. Goddard EA, Mouton SC, Westwood AT, et al. Cryptosporidiosis of the gastrointestinal tract associated with sclerosing cholangitis in the absence of documented immunodeficiency: cryptosporidium parvum and sclerosing cholangitis in an immunocompetent child. J Pediatr Gastroenterol Nutr 2000;31:317–20.
96. Nilsson HO, Taneera J, Castedal M, et al. Identification of Helicobacter pylori and other Helicobacter species by PCR, hybridization, and partial DNA sequencing in human liver samples from patients with primary sclerosing cholangitis or primary biliary cirrhosis. J Clin Microbiol 2000;38:1072–6.
97. Wadstrom T, Ljungh A, Willen R. Primary biliary cirrhosis and primary sclerosing cholangitis are of infectious origin! Gut 2001;49:454.
98. Ponsioen CY, Defoer J, Ten Kate FJ, et al. A survey of infectious agents as risk factors for primary sclerosing cholangitis: are *Chlamydia* species involved? Eur J Gastroenterol Hepatol 2002; 14:641–8.
99. Minuk GY, Rascanin N, Paul RW, et al. Reovirus type 3 infection in patients with primary biliary cirrhosis and primary sclerosing cholangitis. J Hepatol 1987;5:8–13.
100. Minuk GY, Paul RW, Lee PW. The prevalence of antibodies to reovirus type 3 in adults with idiopathic cholestatic liver disease. J Med Virol 1985;16:55–60.
101. Lichtman SN, Keku J, Clark RL, et al. Biliary tract disease in rats with experimental small bowel bacterial overgrowth. Hepatology 1991;13:766–72.
102. Lichtman SN, Keku J, Schwab JH, Sartor RB. Hepatic injury associated with small bowel bacterial overgrowth in rats is prevented by metronidazole and tetracycline. Gastroenterology 1991;100:513–19.
103. Koga H, Sakisaka S, Yoshitake M, et al. Abnormal accumulation in lipopolysaccharide in biliary epithelial cells of rats with self-filling blind loop. Int J Mol Med 2002;9:621–6.
104. Numata Y, Tazuma S, Nishioka T, et al. Immune response in mouse experimental cholangitis associated with colitis induced by dextran sulfate sodium. J Gastroenterol Hepatol 2004;19: 910–15.
105. Numata Y, Tazuma S, Ueno Y, et al. Therapeutic effect of repeated natural killer T cell stimulation in mouse cholangitis complicated by colitis. Dig Dis Sci 2005;50:1844–51.
106. Fickert P, Fuchsbichler A, Wagner M, et al. Regurgitation of bile acids from leaky bile ducts causes sclerosing cholangitis in Mdr2 (Abcb4) knockout mice. Gastroenterology 2004;127:261–74.
107. Popov Y, Patsenker E, Fickert P, et al. Mdr2 (Abcb4)-/- mice spontaneously develop severe biliary fibrosis via massive dysregulation of pro- and antifibrogenic genes. J Hepatol 2005;43: 1045–54.
108. Ng VL, Balistreri WF. Treatment options for chronic cholestasis in infancy and childhood. Curr Treat Options Gastroenterol 2005;8:419–30.
109. Angulo P. Use of ursodeoxycholic acid in patients with liver disease. Curr Gastroenterol Rep 2002;4:37–44.
110. Balistreri WF. Bile acid therapy in pediatric hepatobiliary disease: the role of ursodeoxycholic acid. J Pediatr Gastroenterol Nutr 1997;24:573–89.

111. Marschall HU, Wagner M, Zollner G, et al. Complementary stimulation of hepatobiliary transport and detoxification systems by rifampicin and ursodeoxycholic acid in humans. Gastroenterology 2005;129:476–85.
112. Trauner M, Graziadei IW. Review article: mechanisms of action and therapeutic applications of ursodeoxycholic acid in chronic liver diseases. Aliment Pharmacol Ther 1999;13:979–96.
113. Lindor KD. Ursodiol for primary sclerosing cholangitis. Mayo Primary Sclerosing Cholangitis-Ursodeoxycholic Acid Study Group. N Engl J Med 1997;336:691–5.
114. Chen W, Gluud C. Bile acids for primary sclerosing cholangitis. Cochrane Database Syst Rev 2003:CD003626.
115. Mitchell SA, Bansi DS, Hunt N, et al. A preliminary trial of high-dose ursodeoxycholic acid in primary sclerosing cholangitis. Gastroenterology 2001;121:900–7.
116. Harnois DM, Angulo P, Jorgensen RA, et al. High-dose ursodeoxycholic acid as a therapy for patients with primary sclerosing cholangitis. Am J Gastroenterol 2001;96:1558–62.
117. Olsson R, Boberg KM, de Muckadell OS, et al. High-dose ursodeoxycholic acid in primary sclerosing cholangitis: a 5-year multicenter, randomized, controlled study. Gastroenterology 2005;129:1464–72.
118. Chapman RW. The management of primary sclerosing cholangitis. Curr Gastroenterol Rep 2003;5:9–17.
119. Rust C, Beuers U. Medical treatment of primary biliary cirrhosis and primary sclerosing cholangitis. Clin Rev Allergy Immunol 2005;28:135–45.
120. Chen W, Gluud C. Glucocorticosteroids for primary sclerosing cholangitis. Cochrane Database Syst Rev 2004:CD004036.
121. Cox KL, Cox KM. Oral vancomycin: treatment of primary sclerosing cholangitis in children with inflammatory bowel disease. J Pediatr Gastroenterol Nutr 1998;27:580–3.
122. Schramm C, Schirmacher P, Helmreich-Becker I, et al. Combined therapy with azathioprine, prednisolone, and ursodiol in patients with primary sclerosing cholangitis. A case series. Ann Intern Med 1999;131:943–6.
123. Stiehl A, Rost D. Endoscopic treatment of dominant stenoses in patients with primary sclerosing cholangitis. Clin Rev Allergy Immunol 2005;28:159–65.
124. Stiehl A, Rudolph G, Kloters-Plachky P, et al. Development of dominant bile duct stenoses in patients with primary sclerosing cholangitis treated with ursodeoxycholic acid: outcome after endoscopic treatment. J Hepatol 2002;36:151–6.
125. Ponsioen CY, Lam K, van Milligen de Wit AW, et al. Four years experience with short term stenting in primary sclerosing cholangitis. Am J Gastroenterol 1999;94:2403–7.
126. van Milligen de Wit AW, Rauws EA, van Bracht J, et al. Lack of complications following short-term stent therapy for extrahepatic bile duct strictures in primary sclerosing cholangitis. Gastrointest Endosc 1997;46:344–7.
127. Angulo P, Larson DR, Therneau TM, et al. Time course of histological progression in primary sclerosing cholangitis. Am J Gastroenterol 1999;94:3310–13.
128. Bjoro K, Schrumpf E. Liver transplantation for primary sclerosing cholangitis. J Hepatol 2004;40:570–7.
129. Annual Report from the Studies of Pediatric Liver Transplantation (SPLIT). (Includes data from the registry as of June 1, 2005.) (Accessed at http:www.splitregistry.com.)
130. Wiesner RH. Liver transplantation for primary sclerosing cholangitis: timing, outcome, impact of inflammatory bowel disease and recurrence of disease. Best Pract Res Clin Gastroenterol 2001;15:667–80.
131. Solano E, Khakhar A, Bloch M, et al. Liver transplantation for primary sclerosing cholangitis. Transplant Proc 2003;35:2431–4.
132. Kugelmas M, Spiegelman P, Osgood MJ, et al. Different immunosuppressive regimens and recurrence of primary sclerosing cholangitis after liver transplantation. Liver Transpl 2003;9:727–32.
133. Abu-Elmagd KM, Balan V. Recurrent primary sclerosing cholangitis: from an academic illusion to a clinical reality. Liver Transpl 2005;11:1326–8.
134. Graziadei IW. Recurrence of primary sclerosing cholangitis after liver transplantation. Liver Transpl 2002;8:575–81.
135. Vera A, Moledina S, Gunson B, et al. Risk factors for recurrence of primary sclerosing cholangitis of liver allograft. Lancet 2002;360:1943–4.
136. Boberg KM, Rocca G, Egeland T, et al. Time-dependent Cox regression model is superior in prediction of prognosis in primary sclerosing cholangitis. Hepatology 2002;35:652–7.
137. Boberg KM, Spurkland A, Rocca G, et al. The HLA-DR3,DQ2 heterozygous genotype is associated with an accelerated progression of primary sclerosing cholangitis. Scand J Gastroenterol 2001;36:886–90.
138. Boberg KM, Schrumpf E. Diagnosis and treatment of cholangiocarcinoma. Curr Gastroenterol Rep 2004;6:52–9.
139. Burak K, Angulo P, Pasha TM, et al. Incidence and risk factors for cholangiocarcinoma in primary sclerosing cholangitis. Am J Gastroenterol 2004;99:523–6.
140. Chalasani N, Baluyut A, Ismail A, et al. Cholangiocarcinoma in patients with primary sclerosing cholangitis: a multicenter case-control study. Hepatology 2000;31:7–11.
141. Ross AMT, Anupindi SA, Balis UJ. Case records of the Massachusetts General Hospital. Weekly clinicopathological exercises. Case 11–2003. A 14-year-old boy with ulcerative colitis, primary sclerosing cholangitis, and partial duodenal obstruction. N Engl J Med 2003;348:1464–76.
142. Belghiti J. Transplantation for liver tumors. Semin Oncol 2005;32:29–32.
143. Brandsaeter B, Isoniemi H, Broome U, et al. Liver transplantation for primary sclerosing cholangitis; predictors and consequences of hepatobiliary malignancy. J Hepatol 2004;40:815–22.
144. Kornfeld D, Ekbom A, Ihre T. Is there an excess risk for colorectal cancer in patients with ulcerative colitis and concomitant primary sclerosing cholangitis? A population based study. Gut 1997;41:522–5.
145. Soetikno RM, Lin OS, Heidenreich PA, et al. Increased risk of colorectal neoplasia in patients with primary sclerosing cholangitis and ulcerative colitis: a meta-analysis. Gastrointest Endosc 2002;56:48–54.
146. Vera A, Gunson BK, Ussatoff V, et al. Colorectal cancer in patients with inflammatory bowel disease after liver transplantation for primary sclerosing cholangitis. Transplantation 2003;75:1983–8.
147. Okazaki K, Uchida K, Matsushita M, Takaoka M. Autoimmune pancreatitis. Intern Med 2005;44:1215–23.
148. Ichimura T, Kondo S, Ambo Y, et al. Primary sclerosing cholangitis associated with autoimmune pancreatitis. Hepatogastroenterology 2002;49:1221–4.
149. Kaukinen K, Halme L, Collin P, et al. Celiac disease in patients with severe liver disease: gluten-free diet may reverse hepatic failure. Gastroenterology 2002;122:881–8.

150. Wurm P, Dixon AD, Rathbone BJ. Ulcerative colitis, primary sclerosing cholangitis and coeliac disease: two cases and review of the literature. Eur J Gastroenterol Hepatol 2003;15:815–17.
151. Al-Osaimi AM, Berg CL. Association of primary sclerosing cholangitis and celiac disease: a case report and review of the literature. Dig Dis Sci 2004;49:438–43.
152. Abraham S, Begum S, Isenberg D. Hepatic manifestations of autoimmune rheumatic diseases. Ann Rheum Dis 2004;63:123–9.
153. Kadokawa Y, Omagari K, Matsuo I, et al. Primary sclerosing cholangitis associated with lupus nephritis: a rare association. Dig Dis Sci 2003;48:911–14.
154. Toda K, Yasuda I, Nishigaki Y, et al. Inflammatory pseudotumor of the liver with primary sclerosing cholangitis. J Gastroenterol 2000;35;304–9.
155. Toosi MN, Heathcote J. Pancreatic pseudotumor with sclerosing pancreato-cholangitis: is this a systemic disease? Am J Gastroenterol 2004;99:377–82.
156. Bartholomew LG, Cain JC, Woolner LB,. Sclerosing cholangitis: its possible association with Riedel's struma and fibrous retroperitonitis. Report of two cases. N Engl J Med 1963;269:8–12.
157. Alpert LI, Jindrak K. Idiopathic retroperitoneal fibrosis and sclerosing cholangitis associated with a reticulum cell sarcoma. Report of a case. Gastroenterology 1972;62:111–17.
158. Kamisawa T, Nakajima H, Egawa N, et al. IgG4-related sclerosing disease incorporating sclerosing pancreatitis, cholangitis, sialadenitis and retroperitoneal fibrosis with lymphadenopathy. Pancreatology 2005;6:132–7.
159. Rodrigues F, Davies EG, Harrison P, et al. Liver disease in children with primary immunodeficiencies. J Pediatr 2004;145: 333–9.
160. Cappell MS. Hepatobiliary manifestations of the acquired immune deficiency syndrome. Am J Gastroenterol 1991;86:1–15.
161. Hashmey R, Smith NH, Cron S, et al. Cryptosporidiosis in Houston, Texas. A report of 95 cases. Medicine (Baltimore) 1997;76:118–39.
162. Rodriguez C, Carrion F, Marinovic MA, et al. [X-linked hyper-IGM syndrome associated to sclerosing cholangitis and gallbladder neoplasm: clinical case]. Rev Med Chil 2003;131:303–8. [Article in Spanish]
163. Lin SC, Shyur SD, Ma YC, et al. Recurrent acalculous cholecystitis and sclerosing cholangitis in a patient with X-linked hyper-immunoglobulin M syndrome. J Formos Med Assoc 2005;104:421–6.
164. Dimicoli S, Bensoussan D, Latger-Cannard V, et al. Complete recovery from Cryptosporidium parvum infection with gastroenteritis and sclerosing cholangitis after successful bone marrow transplantation in two brothers with X-linked hyper-IgM syndrome. Bone Marrow Transplant 2003;32:733–7.
165. Kahn K, Sharp H, Hunter D, et al. Primary sclerosing cholangitis in Wiskott–Aldrich syndrome. J Pediatr Gastroenterol Nutr 2001;32:95–9.
166. Kahana DD, Cass O, Jessurun J, et al. Sclerosing cholangitis associated with trichosporon infection and natural killer cell deficiency in an 8-year-old girl. J Pediatr Gastroenterol Nutr 2003;37:620–3.
167. Misbah SA, Spickett GP, Zeman A, et al. Progressive multifocal leucoencephalopathy, sclerosing cholangitis, bronchiectasis and disseminated warts in a patient with primary combined immune deficiency. J Clin Pathol 1992;45:624–7.
168. Davis JJ, Heyman MB, Ferrell L, et al. Sclerosing cholangitis associated with chronic cryptosporidiosis in a child with a congenital immunodeficiency disorder. Am J Gastroenterol 1987;82:1196–202.
169. Klein C, Lisowska-Grospierre B, LeDeist F, et al. Major histocompatibility complex class II deficiency: clinical manifestations, immunologic features, and outcome. J Pediatr 1993;123: 921–8.
170. Bucuvalas JC, Bove KE, Kaufman RA, et al. Cholangitis associated with Cryptococcus neoformans. Gastroenterology 1985; 88:1055–9.
171. Urushihara N, Ariki N, Oyama T, et al. Secondary sclerosing cholangitis and portal hypertension after O157 enterocolitis: extremely rare complications of hemolytic uremic syndrome. J Pediatr Surg 2001;36:1838–40.
172. Engler S, Elsing C, Flechtenmacher C, et al. Progressive sclerosing cholangitis after septic shock: a new variant of vanishing bile duct disorders. Gut 2003;52:688–93.
173. Gupta A, Roebuck DJ, Michalski AJ. Biliary involvement in Hodgkin's disease. Pediatr Radiol 2002;32:202–4.
174. Man KM, Drejet A, Keeffe EB, et al. Primary sclerosing cholangitis and Hodgkin's disease. Hepatology 1993;18:1127–31.
175. Wegerle W, Garbrecht M, Nerl C, Schmitt W. [Angioimmunoblastic lymphadenopathy with dysproteinemia and sclerosing cholangitis]. Dtsch Med Wochenschr 1994;119:332–7. [Article in German]
176. Benninger J, Grobholz R, Oeztuerk Y, et al. Sclerosing cholangitis following severe trauma: description of a remarkable disease entity with emphasis on possible pathophysiologic mechanisms. World J Gastroenterol 2005;11:4199–205.
177. Castellano G, Moreno-Sanchez D, Gutierrez J, et al. Caustic sclerosing cholangitis. Report of four cases and a cumulative review of the literature. Hepatogastroenterology 1994;41:458–70.
178. Ciftci AO, Karnak I, Senocak ME, et al. Surgical injury of the biliary tract in children. Eur J Pediatr Surg 2000;10:100–5.
179. Strandvik B, Hjelte L, Gabrielsson N, Glaumann H. Sclerosing cholangitis in cystic fibrosis. Scand J Gastroenterol Suppl 1988; 143:121–4.
180. Durieu I, Pellet O, Simonot L, et al. Sclerosing cholangitis in adults with cystic fibrosis: a magnetic resonance cholangiographic prospective study. J Hepatol 1999;30:1052–6.
181. Farkkila M, Karvonen AL, Nurmi H, et al. Metronidazole and ursodeoxycholic acid for primary sclerosing cholangitis: a randomized placebo-controlled trial. Hepatology 2004;40:1379–86.
182. Polter DE, Gruhl V, Eigenbrodt EH, Combes B. Beneficial effect of cholestyramine in sclerosing cholangitis. Gastroenterology 1980;79:326–33.
183. Duchini A, Younossi ZM, Saven A, et al. An open-label pilot trial of cladibrine (2-cholordeoxyadenosine) in patients with primary sclerosing cholangitis. J Clin Gastroenterol 2000;31:292–6.
184. Olsson R, Broome U, Danielsson A, et al. Colchicine treatment of primary sclerosing cholangitis. Gastroenterology 1995;108: 1199–203.
185. Lindor KD, Wiesner RH, Colwell LJ, et al. The combination of prednisone and colchicine in patients with primary sclerosing cholangitis. Am J Gastroenterol 1991;86:57–61.
186. Angulo P, Batts KP, Jorgensen RA, et al. Oral budesonide in the treatment of primary sclerosing cholangitis. Am J Gastroenterol 2000;95:2333–7.

187. Kyokane K, Ichihara T, Horisawa M, et al. Successful treatment of primary sclerosing cholangitis with cyclosporine and corticosteroid. Hepatogastroenterology 1994;41:449–52.
188. Knox TA, Kaplan MM. Treatment of primary sclerosing cholangitis with oral methotrexate. Am J Gastroenterol 1991;86:546–52.
189. Knox TA, Kaplan MM. A double-blind controlled trial of oral-pulse methotrexate therapy in the treatment of primary sclerosing cholangitis. Gastroenterology 1994;106:494–9.
190. Talwalkar JA, Angulo P, Keach JC, et al. Mycophenolate mofetil for the treatment of primary sclerosing cholangitis. Am J Gastroenterol 2005;100:308–12.
191. Klingenberg S, Chen W. D-penicillamine for primary sclerosing cholangitis. Cochrane Database Syst Rev 2006:CD004182.
192. Bharucha AE, Jorgensen R, Lichtman SN, et al. A pilot study of pentoxifylline for the treatment of primary sclerosing cholangitis. Am J Gastroenterol 2000;95:2338–42.
193. Angulo P, MacCarty RL, Sylvestre PB, et al. Pirfenidone in the treatment of primary sclerosing cholangitis. Dig Dis Sci 2002;47:157–61.
194. Van Thiel DH, Carroll P, Abu-Elmagd K, et al. Tacrolimus (FK 506), a treatment for primary sclerosing cholangitis: results of an open-label preliminary trial. Am J Gastroenterol 1995;90:455–9.
195. Gilger MA, Gann ME, Opekun AR, Gleason WA Jr. Efficacy of ursodeoxycholic acid in the treatment of primary sclerosing cholangitis in children. J Pediatr Gastroenterol Nutr 2000;31:136–41.
196. Allison MC, Burroughs AK, Noone P, Summerfield JA. Biliary lavage with corticosteroids in primary sclerosing cholangitis. A clinical, cholangiographic and bacteriological study. J Hepatol 1986;3:118–22.
197. Kaya M, Petersen BT, Angulo P, et al. Balloon dilation compared to stenting of dominant strictures in primary sclerosing cholangitis. Am J Gastroenterol 2001;96:1059–66.
198. Baluyut AR, Sherman S, Lehman GA, et al. Impact of endoscopic therapy on the survival of patients with primary sclerosing cholangitis. Gastrointest Endosc 2001;53:308–12.
199. Hirai I, Ishiyama S, Fuse A, et al. Primary sclerosing cholangitis successfully treated by resection of the confluence of the hepatic duct. J Hepatobiliary Pancreat Surg 2001;8:169–73.
200. Loehe F, Schauer RJ. Surgical treatment of primary biliary cirrhosis and primary sclerosing cholangitis. Clin Rev Allergy Immunol 2005;28:167–74.

20

Drug-Induced Liver Disease

Eve A. Roberts, M.D., F.R.C.P.C.

Drug-induced liver disease is generally regarded as rare in children. Large inpatient [1] and outpatient surveys [2] have generally failed to detect drug hepatotoxicity as a major problem in children, although adverse drug reactions (not necessarily hepatotoxic) are somewhat more frequent in the under-5-year-old group and in children of any age with cancer. A recent study examined deaths from adverse drug reactions in children and found that approximately one sixth of such deaths involved acute liver failure, usually associated with antiepileptic or antineoplastic drugs [3]. Drug hepatotoxicity is now recognized as an important cause of acute liver failure in children as in adults [4]. Why childhood drug hepatotoxicity is otherwise relatively uncommon is not clear. Failure to diagnose and report drug hepatotoxicity in children is a likely explanation. Another important consideration is that most children take relatively few medications, and in particular they rarely take the cardiovascular, antihypertensive, or antidepressant medications commonly associated with hepatotoxicity in adults. Most children have a lean body mass, and most do not use ethanol chronically or smoke cigarettes. Thus, children are usually free of many of the factors predisposing to drug hepatotoxicity in adults. Hepatic drug metabolism in children may be sufficiently different from that in adults to shield against drug hepatotoxicity. Indeed, old age is a risk factor for more severe hepatotoxic reactions, perhaps because the aging liver metabolizes some drugs more slowly. Adult women are somewhat more prone to certain drug hepatotoxicities than men. Changes in drug metabolism possibly associated with puberty may influence the differing incidence of drug hepatotoxicity in childhood and adulthood so that prepubertal children are less likely to develop drug-induced liver disease. However, drug hepatotoxicity definitely occurs in children; adolescents are probably no different from adults in their risk for drug-induced liver disease.

There has been recent interest in modifying terminology for this category of liver disease and referring to drug hepatotoxicity as *drug-induced liver injury* (DILI). Regardless of whether it is called DILI or drug hepatotoxicity, the discussion relating to children must differ from an overview of drug hepatotoxicity in adults. For many of the more frequent DILIs in children, the mechanism of the hepatotoxic process has been hypothesized, investigated, and largely ascertained: this has been important for understanding of drug hepatotoxicity in all ages. The basis for the proposed mechanisms of these toxicities is hepatic drug biotransformation. However, our appreciation of the spectrum of possible drug hepatotoxicity in children is based on the more extensive experience in adults. Readers seeking an all-inclusive discussion of drug hepatotoxicity should consult references drawing on this adult experience [5–7] or adverse drug reaction databases.

HEPATIC DRUG METABOLISM

Drug metabolism, or biotransformation, is one of the most important functions of the liver. These complex biochemical processes can be divided into two broad aspects: activation (Phase I) and detoxification (Phase II). Different families of enzymes perform Phase I and Phase II drug metabolism. With respect to hepatotoxicity, the *balance* between Phase I and Phase II processes is critical. Factors that influence this balance include age or stage of development, state of nutrition (mainly fasting or undernutrition; possibly obesity resulting in hepatic steatosis), coadministered drugs, and immunomodulators resulting from viral infection. Inducers (chemicals that increase the amount of functional enzymes involved in biotransformation) may affect both Phase I and Phase II processes, but not necessarily equally. Coadministered medications may act as inducers or inhibitors of specific drug-metabolizing enzymes. The pharmacokinetics of the drug, especially its absorption from the gastrointestinal tract or other organs and its mode of excretion, also affects hepatic biotransformation. Whether the drug is taken as a single dose or as many doses on a chronic basis may also change its hepatic metabolism. Although not proved conclusively, sporadic recurrent exposure to some drugs may enhance their toxicity. Genetically determined polymorphisms of cytochromes P450 and various Phase II enzymes also influence this balance.

The hemoprotein cytochromes P450 are extremely important in the liver, although they are found in most body tissues [8]. They are associated with Phase I reactions. These diverse reactions include hydroxylation, dealkylation, and dehalogenation, among others. The common feature in all reactions is that one atom of molecular oxygen is inserted into the substrate. Hence these enzymes are *monooxygenases*. Unlike most enzymes, many cytochromes P450 are not absolutely restricted to unique substrates; this characteristic is known as having *overlapping substrate specificity*. Another important characteristic of many hepatic cytochromes P450 is *inducibility*. In hepatocytes various cytochromes P450 are found in the endoplasmic reticulum, mitochondria, and peroxisomes.

The cytochromes P450 were initially classified on the basis of what chemical induced them: basically either phenobarbital or 3-methylcholanthrene, a polycyclic aromatic hydrocarbon. Because they are found in all living organisms, individual cytochromes P450 number in the thousands, and distinct families, which have been now distinguished on the basis of primary amino acid sequence identity, in the hundreds. In addition to detailed information on these genes, the protein structure for some P450s has also been solved. With respect to human hepatic drug metabolism, cytochromes P450 in the 1A, 2B, 2C, 2D, 2E, and 3A subfamilies are particularly important [9,10]. The cytochrome P450 1A subfamily includes two major cytochromes induced by polycyclic aromatic hydrocarbons. Apart from various carcinogens, other common xenobiotics such as caffeine and theophylline are metabolized by these cytochromes. Induction of the cytochrome P450 1A1 (also known as CYP1A1) is regulated through a cytoplasmic protein, the aromatic hydrocarbon (Ah) receptor [11]. The member of this subfamily that is exclusively hepatic is CYP1A2: it is expressed constitutively, and its induction is also regulated by the Ah receptor. The cytochrome P450 2B subfamily includes cytochromes induced by phenobarbital. Some members of the CYP2B subfamily are regulated through a mechanism involving the constitutive androstane receptor (CAR) that dimerizes with the retinoid X receptor (RXR) and then interacts with a regulatory site in the 5′-upstream region of the structural gene. Cytochrome P450 2E1 (CYP2E1) is the ethanol-inducible cytochrome P450, whose regulation is complex and mainly posttranscriptional. The cytochrome P450 3A subfamily includes cytochromes induced by pregnenolone, glucocorticoids, rifampicin, and also phenobarbital. Cytochrome P450 3A4 (CYP3A4) is the most abundant cytochrome P450 in the liver and plays an important role in the biotransformation of many drugs. CYP3A4 is regulated via the pregnane X receptor (PXR) that also interacts with RXR to produce the functional transcriptional regulator. It is increasingly apparent that various members of the nuclear receptor family (CAR, PXR, and others such as hepatocyte nuclear factor-4α) play important roles in the regulation of expression of hepatocellular P450s and also in regulation of expression of these very receptors [12]. Cross-talk between these receptors adds a further level of complexity [13].

Polymorphisms for certain cytochromes P450, relating to differences in the rate of associated enzyme activities, have been identified in humans [14,15]. The first of these polymorphisms for drug oxidations to be identified involves P450 2D6 (CYP2D6). Debrisoquine 4-hydroxylation, an enzyme activity associated with this cytochrome, was found to vary significantly in the Caucasian population: some individuals are "extensive metabolizers" (EM) of debrisoquine and others are "poor metabolizers" (PM) of the drug. Other drugs that are substrates for CYP2D6 show the same pattern: these include antiarrhythmics such as encainide, β-blockers such as metoprolol, various psychoactive agents, and codeine and dextromethorphan [16]. The difference in metabolism between EM and PM appears to be due to changes in the catalytic site of cytochrome CYP2D6 in PM, caused by incapacitating one- or three-base pair deletions or multiple point mutations or complete deletion of the 2D6 gene [17]. Poor metabolizers are at increased risk of toxic drug concentrations, but this polymorphism has not been proven to have a clear relationship to any specific hepatotoxicity. Mephenytoin is subject to polymorphism in its metabolism, which is associated with the P450 2C subfamily. The specific P450 involved is still undetermined, but the most recent candidate is CYP2C18 [18]. The P450 3A subfamily (mainly CYP3A4 and CYP3A5) plays an important role in hepatic drug metabolism of such drugs as nifedipine, erythromycin, cyclosporine, and diltiazem; CYP3A5 is polymorphic and tends to be expressed at a much lower level than CYP3A4. Cytochrome P1A2 has some minor polymorphisms [19]. Polymorphisms affecting the function of the proteins regulating P450 expression may also alter hepatic drug biotransformation.

The outcome of most Phase I biotransformation reactions is to make the substrate a more polar chemical with a substituent poised for further modification via a Phase II reaction. Phase II detoxifying reactions are performed by a variety of enzyme types, including glutathione *S*-transferases, uridine 5′-diphosphate (UDP)-glucuronosyltransferases, epoxide hydrolases, sulfotransferases, *N*-acetyltransferases, and enzymes responsible for glycine conjugation. These reactions complete the transformation of a hydrophobic chemical to a hydrophilic one, which can be excreted easily in urine or bile. Certain Phase II enzymes, such as some glucuronosyl transferases, are inducible. Some are polymorphic. An important example of a Phase II polymorphism involves *N*-acetylation. Arylamine *N*-acetyltransferase 2 (NAT-2) is polymorphic: individuals are either rapid or slow acetylators; a related enzyme, arylamine *N*-acetyltransferase 1, is monomorphic. These enzymes are encoded by two separate genes, and the slow acetylator phenotype of NAT-2 relates to mutations in the gene for NAT-2 causing reduced concentrations of NAT-2 in human liver [20,21]. More recently, the Phase II enzyme involved in metabolism of 6-mercaptopurine, thiopurine methyltransferase, has been shown to be polymorphic [22]. Certain polymorphisms are more or less prevalent in specific ethnic groups; for example, more than 50% of Caucasians are slow acetylators. The UDP-glucuronosyltransferases are diverse and include two large subfamilies that are involved in drug metabolism. Genetic abnormalities in UGT1A1 are associated with Gilbert syndrome, which is highly prevalent and has unconjugated hyperbilirubinemia. In Gilbert syndrome drug metabolism may be affected, but few convincing data exist that this causes drug-induced liver injury except possibly with certain antineoplastic drugs for which UGT1A1-mediated glucuronidation is an important

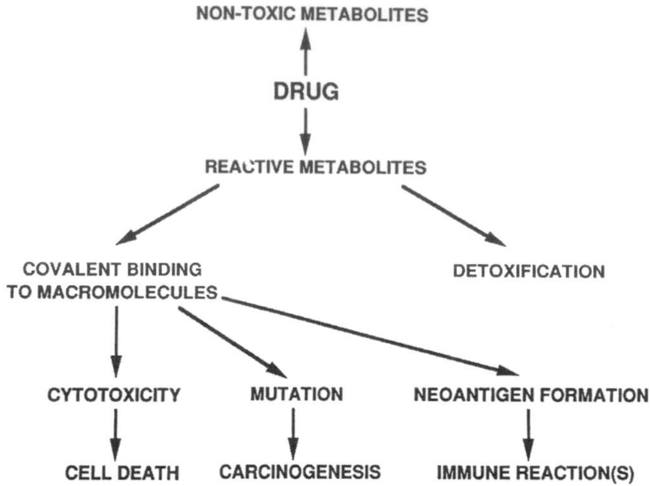

Figure 20.1. The potential fates of a toxic intermediate.

mode of drug disposition [23]. In some metabolic diseases the activity of Phase II enzymes may be abnormal. In hereditary tyrosinemia, for example, glutathione *S*-transferase activity is abnormally low because intermediates in the abnormal tyrosine pathway consume glutathione [24].

The product of a Phase I reaction may be a reactive or "toxic" metabolite. Although this is especially likely when CYP1A cytochromes are involved, as hepatic metabolism of common drugs is studied more extensively, various members of these cytochrome P450 subfamilies are found to be involved. Phase II reactions usually inactivate such chemicals before they damage the hepatocyte. Conjugation with glutathione is particularly important in detoxifying electrophilic toxic metabolites and free radicals [25,26]. It is possible, as in the case of carcinogenic polycyclic aromatic hydrocarbon benzo(*a*)pyrene, for the product of Phase I to be metabolized by the same cytochrome a second time resulting in production of the proximate carcinogen [27]. Whether a reactive metabolite actually damages a cell depends how much reactive metabolite actually binds to cellular components, whether these organelles are critical to cell function, and whether they can be repaired. If the toxic metabolite binds to intracellular proteins or membranes that are vital to cellular integrity, the hepatocyte may die. Damage to proteins within the bile canalicular membrane typically interfere with production of bile and thus cause cholestasis. Changes in the function of P-glycoprotein, the bile salt excretory pump, and other bile canalicular transporters that contribute to excretion of drugs and their metabolites is another mechanism of drug-induced liver injury. If the toxic metabolite binds to cellular DNA, mutagenesis or carcinogenesis may eventually ensue. In fetal tissues, binding of a toxic metabolite can also result in teratogenesis (Figure 20.1).

DEVELOPMENTAL ASPECTS OF DRUG METABOLISM

Hepatic drug metabolism displays complex developmental changes [28]. In addition, developmental expression of hepatic drug-metabolizing enzymes varies from species to species. Inducible Cyp1a1 (murine CYP1A1) was detected in fetal mouse livers at day 15 of gestation [29], whereas CYP1A1 and CYP1A2 were not detected in rat fetuses, although they were detectable after induction in 1-week-old rats [30]. In rabbits, theophylline metabolism was found to increase only gradually over the first 2 months of life [31]. Studies with human fetal tissues indicate that hepatic concentrations of cytochromes P450 are generally undetectable or very low, except for CYP3A7 and possibly CYP1B1. CYP2C9 appears to be absent [32,33]. In other studies, antibodies for CYP2C failed to detect cytochromes in this subfamily in human fetal liver tissue but demonstrated CYP2C cytochromes soon after birth, approaching adult concentrations at 3 weeks of age [34,35]. More recent studies suggest that CYP2C9 and CYP2C19 are not present in the first trimester of fetal development but begin to be expressed in the later fetal period; postnatal expression of CYP2C9 rose faster than that of CYP2C19, consistent with differing regulatory mechanisms, although there was extensive interindividual variation [36]. CYP2D6 and the associated enzyme activity dextromethorphan *O*-demethylation are very low [37], but CYP2D6 expression increases soon after birth. CYP1A2 was not detectable in newborn human livers but increased to approximately 50% of adult levels over the first year of life [34,38]. By contrast, cytochromes in the P450 3A subfamily are detectable in fetal, newborn, and adult human liver tissue [32,34]. CYP3A7 is the main cytochrome P450 in human fetal liver [39–41]. CYP3A4 is absent in fetal liver but increases to approximately 40% of adult levels in the first month of life. Hepatic CYP3A5 is a minor member of the CYP3A subfamily, detected mainly in childhood. Expression of individual cytochromes in CYP3A subfamily appears to correlate with expression of PXR and CAR, although this shows considerable interindividual variation [42]. CYP2E1 is detectable in fetal liver, tends to be low in the first 3 months of life, and then rises fairly rapidly [43].

In the newborn infant, hepatic biotransformation dependent on cytochromes P450 is typically much less active than that in adults. Decreased hepatic drug metabolism is especially severe in premature infants. Metabolism and elimination of caffeine [44,45], theophylline [46], phenobarbital [47], and phenytoin [48] are notably slow. *N*-Demethylation of aminopyrine, measured by an aminopyrine breath test using ^{13}C-labeled aminopyrine, was not detectable in the first days of life in normal infants [49]. Cisapride metabolism was negligible in the neonate but increased with increasing expression of CYP3A4 [50]. All these studies require careful interpretation because of significant interindividual variation in drug-metabolizing enzyme activities at any age, specific stressors of early infancy such as respiratory insufficiency, hypoglycemia, inadequate food intake, or conversely hyperglycemia, and transient physiologic abnormalities such as unconjugated hyperbilirubinemia. In general, however, in early infancy different P450s display different developmental patterns of expression. Some (CYP2A6, CYP2C9, CYP2D6, CYP2E1, and CYP3A4) are expressed and active relatively soon after birth, but others (CYP1A2, CYP2B6, and CYP2C8) take months [51].

In childhood, hepatic drug metabolism, and thus clearance of many drugs, is more rapid than in adults. Prominent examples again include theophylline, phenobarbital, and phenytoin. By puberty, adult patterns of hepatic drug metabolism appear to be well established. Caffeine, which is metabolized in part by CYP1A2, exemplifies these changes. The elimination half-life, which is very long in the newborn period, drops to approximately 3–4 hours around 6 months of age [52]. For the balance of childhood, that is, until puberty, caffeine metabolism remains somewhat more rapid than in adults [53]. In extensive metabolizers, CYP2D6 rises progressively over the first 5 years of life, and this developmental pattern appears to be independent of gestational age [37]. Aminopyrine *N*-demethylase activity reaches adult levels around two years of age [49].

Phase II biotransformation processes also display developmental changes. Among Phase II processes, an important example of late maturation of a detoxifying enzyme is the glu curonosyl transferase for bilirubin conjugation, which is usually deficient for a short time after birth. Sulfation tends to predominate over glucuronidation, for example, in the metabolism of acetaminophen [54]. Hepatic bile acid metabolism also shows maturational changes in the first months of life: in neonates conjugation to taurine is quantitatively more important than conjugation to glycine. Bile acid sulfation is less prominent than in adults. These variations may influence the occurrence and character of hepatotoxicity in children.

Glutathione metabolism is also subject to developmental changes, particularly in the neonatal period. In fetal rat liver, activities of both glutathione peroxidase and glutathione S-transferase are very low compared with adult levels [55]. In guinea pigs, hepatic glutathione concentrations show important differences among preterm neonates, term neonates, and adult animals. Total hepatic glutathione is significantly lower in both neonatal groups, compared with adult animals: with fasting there is no change in the hepatic concentration in preterm neonates but a significant increase in the term neonate. Total hepatic glutathione concentration drops in fasted adult animals [56]. In these animals glutathione peroxidase activity is uniformly lower than in adult animals; γ-glutamyl transpeptidase activity rises from one quarter of adult levels in the preterm neonate to one half of the adult level in the term neonate. In rats the total hepatic concentration of glutathione S-transferase B (ligandin) is approximately one fifth of the adult concentration and rises to adults levels over the first 4 to 5 weeks of life [57]. Other studies in rats have shown that biliary excretion of glutathione and its conjugates rises with age [58]. In the 2-week-old rat hepatobiliary excretion of glutathione appears to be approximately one tenth of that in the adult rat; hepatic γ-glutamyl transpeptidase activity is also low in rat pups [59]. Developmental changes in the relative amounts of various biliary glutathione-derived thiols reflect increasing production of bile over this time, as well as changes in γ-glutamyl transpeptidase activity and other metabolic process related to hepatic bile production.

PATTERNS OF DRUG HEPATOTOXICITY

Because the liver is anatomically and physiologically complex, drug hepatotoxicity presents as a broad spectrum of biochemical, histologic, and clinical abnormalities. Most drug-induced liver disease is cytotoxic, and most often the hepatocyte is the target cell. The exact mechanism of hepatocyte death is not known and probably differs depending on the specific hepatotoxin. Hepatocyte damage may be zonal, reflecting metabolic specialization in the hepatic lobule. Hepatocytes in zone 3 of the Rappaport acinus have the highest concentration of cytochromes P450 and thus the greatest potential for producing toxic intermediates. Zonal hepatocellular necrosis suggests that production of toxic metabolites plays an important role in the pathogenesis of the hepatotoxicity. A toxic metabolite is a short-lived chemically reactive species that usually cannot be detected outside of the cell, that is, in the plasma compartment. The cellular diversity of the liver (nonparenchymal cells as well as hepatocytes) also contributes to the diversity of drug-induced liver disease. Drug-induced injury may involve cells in the liver besides hepatocytes. Cytotoxic damage may predominate in bile duct cells (as with chlorpropamide), hepatic stellate cells (in vitamin A toxicity), or endothelial cells (with pyrrolizadine alkaloid poisoning from certain herbal teas). Damage to bile duct epithelial cells or to larger bile ducts is likely to interfere with bile flow, resulting in cholestasis. However, whenever hepatocellular damage is sufficiently severe, some degree of cholestasis will develop.

Cytotoxicity may have other effects besides cell death. Nonlethal damage to certain subcellular elements may interfere with specific metabolic functions such as protein or lipid synthesis or energy production. Damage to transporters in the bile canalicular membrane can interfere with normal formation of bile. Accumulation of fat or other substances in hepatocytes may then occur. Fatty liver associated with tetracycline hepatotoxicity is an example of such a process. In contrast, cytotoxicity may cause more severe consequences. Extensive damage may lead to fibrosis or cirrhosis. Vascular perfusion of the liver may be altered, as in veno-occlusive disease (VOD). Finally, hepatotoxicity may lead to neoclassic transformation. In some cases, toxic metabolites have been identified that are capable of binding to DNA, thus initiating carcinogenesis.

Drug hepatotoxicity is also classified in terms of the duration of the process. Acute hepatotoxic injuries develop over a relatively short time and cause a lesion without any histologic features of chronicity. Subacute hepatotoxicity refers to lesions that have developed over weeks to months as indicated by areas of fibrosis and possible regeneration. Chronic hepatotoxic lesions include those with fibrosis or cirrhosis, small portal ("interlobular") bile duct paucity, vascular changes, and neoplasia.

A practical and widely used classification of drug-induced hepatotoxicity is based on clinical features. Drug-induced liver disease most often presents as a *hepatitic* process, sometimes accompanied by symptoms associated rather nonspecifically with hepatitis (fatigue, anorexia, nausea, or vomiting). Drug-induced hepatitis is frequently asymptomatic, with isolated elevations in serum aminotransferases. Some drug-induced liver disease, however, is predominantly *cholestatic*. Clinically, there is jaundice, pruritus, prominent elevation of alkaline phosphatase, and mild elevations of aminotransferases. Cholestasis associated with contraceptive steroids is a classic example of this "bland cholestasis." Some drug-induced liver disease presents a *mixed* picture, with elements of both hepatitis and cholestasis. This may be due to injury both to hepatocytes and bile duct epithelial cells. In some cases, the target of the injury may be transport molecules located in the bile canalicular membrane. This *mixed hepatitic–cholestatic* process (sometimes called *hepatocanalicular jaundice*) is characteristic of hepatotoxicity caused by chlorpromazine and erythromycin.

In addition, these three basic clinical types (hepatitic, cholestatic, mixed hepatitic–cholestatic) may be associated with specific systemic syndromes. The "drug hypersensitivity syndrome" includes fever, inflammation of other organ systems (morbilliform rash or Stevens–Johnson syndrome, renal dysfunction, or myocarditis), lymphadenopathy, eosinophilia, and atypical lymphocytosis. These features suggest an immunoallergic component, but they may be found in drug hepatotoxicity associated with production of a toxic metabolite. The other classic systemic syndrome is *chronic active hepatitis*: the features classically associated with autoimmune hepatitis but found in a broad spectrum of viral and metabolic liver disease. Findings include a subacute or chronic course, fatigue, anorexia, variable extrahepatic systemic changes (rash, arthralgias), elevated serum immunoglobulin G, and variable titers of nonspecific autoantibodies such as antinuclear antibody. In some cases, it may be difficult to exclude concurrence of drug administration and underlying autoimmune hepatitis. Drugs that have been associated with chronic active hepatitis include the little-used laxative oxyphenisatin and more common drugs such as methyldopa and nitrofurantoin. In adults, drug-induced hepatotoxicity has been associated with certain anti–liver-kidney-microsomal (anti-LKM) antibodies, similar to those associated with autoimmune hepatitis type 2. These are directed against apoproteins of specific cytochromes P450; recent evidence indicates that some P450 apoproteins can be detected on liver cell membranes [60].

In summary, drug-induced hepatotoxicity can be described in terms of the clinical liver disease (hepatitic, cholestatic, or hepatitic–cholestatic), with or without associated systemic syndromes (drug hypersensitivity, chronic active hepatitis) (Table 20.1), and the time course of the hepatotoxicity (acute, subacute, or chronic). The nature of the process is usually cytotoxic and the target cell is usually the hepatocytes but can be nonparenchymal cells. It may lead to cellular necrosis with eventual scarring, accumulation of specific substances in hepatocytes or nonparenchymal cells, or neoplastic transformation. Clinically, in adults, a hepatitic drug reaction is classically defined as having alanine aminotransferase (ALT) greater than 2 times the upper limit of normal or an ALT:alkaline phosphatase ratio greater than or equal to 5; in contrast, a cholestatic drug reaction has serum alkaline phosphatase greater than 2 times the upper limit of normal or an ALT:alkaline phosphatase ratio less than or equal to 2 [61].

Table 20.1: Clinical Features of Drug-Induced Hepatotoxicity

Hepatic	Symptoms of hepatitis, increased AST/ALT
Mixed = hepatitic–cholestatic	Hepatitis + cholestasis
Cholestatic	Clinical and biochemical cholestasis

+ Systemic syndrome: fever/inflammation of other organ systems (morbilliform or other rash, renal dysfunction, myocarditis)/ atypical lymphocytosis/eosinophilia

+ "Chronic active hepatitis" syndrome: subacute or chronic course + fatigue/anorexia/nonspecific autoantibodies/increased IgG/variable involvement of organ systems (lupoid rash, arthralgias)

AST, aspartate aminotransferase; ALT, alanine aminotransferase.

It has become customary also to characterize hepatotoxicity in terms of *predictability*. This classification attempts to separate chemical poisons from toxicity involving host susceptibility. *Intrinsic hepatotoxicity* is differentiated from *host idiosyncrasy*. In intrinsic hepatotoxicity the agent causes predictable hepatic damage in any person. The toxicity is dose-related, and laboratory animal models can easily be developed that exhibit the same type of hepatotoxicity. Few instances of hepatotoxicity associated with medications fit this description. Instead, most are unpredictable, infrequent, and apparently capricious. The hepatotoxic process is then regarded as idiosyncratic. If such a reaction is accompanied by systemic features such as fever, rash, eosinophilia, atypical lymphocytosis, and possibly other major organ involvement, then classically it has been regarded as an idiosyncratic hypersensitivity reaction, with the connotation of an allergic etiology.

An alternate explanation, put in its most dogmatic form, is that all drug hepatotoxicities have a biochemical basis. Abnormalities in drug biotransformation lead to increased production of toxic metabolites or inadequate provision of appropriate cytoprotective defenses or both. In some cases, these abnormalities are acquired, for example, by drug interaction. In many cases, the abnormality of drug biotransformation is due to an abnormal or defective drug-metabolizing enzyme, inherited as a genetic trait. This pharmacogenetic defect becomes apparent only if elicited by the appropriate drug. The target of the toxic metabolite determines the clinical features of the drug hepatotoxicity. Damage to subcellular organelles may cause cytotoxicity directly. Damage to hepatocellular membranes may also initiate an immune response leading to an immunoallergic reaction similar to a hypersensitivity reaction. According to this view of drug hepatotoxicity, drug hepatotoxicities with mechanisms we understand are predictable even if these toxicities are rare.

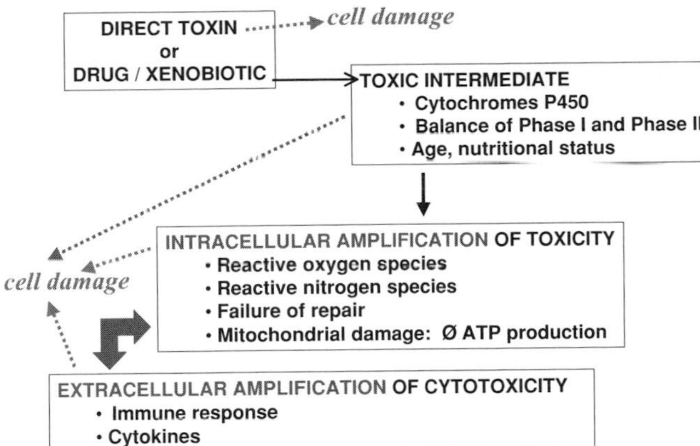

Figure 20.2. A general mechanism of severe drug hepatotoxicity. Most drugs and xenobiotics that cause liver injury elaborate a toxic intermediate within the hepatocytes or nonparenchymal liver cell. The quantity of toxic intermediate is dependent on multiple factors including features of Phase I and Phase II biotransformation and the balance between them. The toxic intermediate can damage the cell itself or initiate various amplifying processes within the cell or external to the cell, such as immune response. Direct toxins typically injure the liver without metabolism, but in principle amplification pathways could also be involved.

Animal models for such hepatotoxicities can be developed but not necessarily in the usual laboratory animals. The importance of the biochemical theory of drug hepatotoxicity is that it provides a basis for research into, and potentially for treatment of, drug hepatotoxicity. In the case of pharmacogenetic disorders of hepatic drug biotransformation, prospective diagnosis (without in vivo drug challenge) may be possible. The importance for pediatric hepatology is that these definable abnormalities in hepatic drug biotransformation are particularly prominent among the drug hepatotoxicities most often found in children.

Biotransformation of drugs may not be the whole story, even though it is critical to generating toxic metabolites that alter cellular proteins. With many drugs, hepatocellular damage seems to be disproportional to the amount of toxic metabolite that might be formed. Both intracellular and extracellular processes may amplify the liver cell damage. This conceptual model is illustrated in Figure 20.2. As an extracellular amplifier, the immune response also plays an important role [62]. For many drugs, whether an individual develops liver injury – as well as its pattern of injury and severity – depends not only on the hepatic processes of drug metabolism but also on that individual's immune reactivity both generally and at the specific point in time of drug exposure, when it might be influenced by transient stimuli such as endotoxinemia. Sometimes the connection between immune-mediated mechanisms and hepatic damage is direct, for example, autoantibodies are expressed against specific components of hepatocytes, usually those involved in drug biotransformation. The targets may be cytochromes P450 or Phase II enzymes such as epoxide hydrolase. The target cytochrome P450 varies with the drug: CYP1A2 for dihydralazine, CYP2E1 for halothane, and CYP2C9 for tienilic acid. Reactive metabolites may alter other hepatocellular

Table 20.2: Classification of Hepatotoxins

Nomenclature Herein	*Previous Usage*
Intrinsic hepatotoxin	Intrinsic toxin
Contingent hepatotoxin (toxic only if biotransformation* is abnormal, whether by genetic or acquired cause)	Metabolic idiosyncrasy
Hepatotoxin eliciting immunoallergic response† (implies some degree of host dependency)	Hypersensitivity

*Generation and/or detoxification of toxic metabolite.
†Fever, eosinophilia, atypical lymphocytosis, or hepatic granulomas or autoantibodies.

proteins to form neoantigens. Immune-mediated damage to hepatocytes may involve either apoptosis or necrosis. Bile acid–associated hepatocyte injury leads to apoptosis via Fas (CD95) activation. When toxic metabolites or reactive oxygen species or cytokines stimulate Kupffer cells, specific mechanisms of cell damage are set into motion involving tumor necrosis factor-α (TNF-α) or nitric oxide produced by Kupffer cells. Nitric oxide elaborated by Kupffer cells and hepatocytes plays a role in acetaminophen hepatotoxicity. Cytokines such as interleukin-8 [63] and other CXC chemokines regulating leukocyte action may become involved. Kupffer cells also elaborate various factors that are cytoprotective to hepatocytes [64]. The vigor of the immune response in general, an individual polygenic trait, most likely determines the extent of immune mechanisms in drug-induced liver injury. For example, genetic polymorphisms affect extent of cytokine production. Such variation may be relevant to diclofenac hepatotoxicity [65]. Thus, in addition to pharmacogenetics, immunogenetics must be considered to explain drug hepatotoxicity.

Classification of chemicals that cause liver injury has to account for these features of simple predictability or for idiosyncrasy, whether mainly a biochemical toxicity or an immune process or some combination of the two (Table 20.2). Hepatotoxic agents can be categorized as follows: *intrinsic hepatotoxin*, *contingent hepatotoxin*, and *hepatotoxin eliciting an immunoallergic response*. The intrinsic hepatotoxin is the true, predictable poison. Environmental xenobiotics usually belong in this category. The contingent hepatotoxin causes hepatotoxicity only when hepatic biotransformation is abnormal so that toxic metabolites are more likely to be generated or detoxification pathways are deficient. Hepatic biotransformation may be abnormal on an acquired or genetic basis. This category encompasses the category denoted as "metabolic idiosyncrasy" by others. A hepatotoxin eliciting an immunoallergic response is identified when hepatotoxicity is accompanied by fever, eosinophilia, and atypical lymphocytosis or is characterized histologically by hepatic granulomatosis; these findings imply some degree of dependency on the host immune response. These mechanisms are poorly understood and have been designated rather imprecisely as "hypersensitivity." Elaboration of autoantibodies, such as anti-LKM antibodies, is another type of immunoallergic reaction. Some chemicals can act as more than one type of hepatotoxin. For example, high-dose acetaminophen acts as an intrinsic hepatotoxin. By contrast, low-dose acetaminophen, normally nontoxic, acts as a contingent hepatotoxin in persons in whom CYP2E1 is induced, as in chronic alcoholics. If the biochemical mechanism of hepatic biotransformation is established for a given chemical, then it is possible to predict circumstances in which that chemical would function as a contingent hepatotoxin. Unfortunately, especially in the case of genetic defects, it is not always possible to identify abnormal hepatic biotransformation until after drug-induced hepatotoxicity has occurred; thus, for the individual, the hepatotoxicity appears to be a chance aberration.

The clinical presentations and liver pathology of drug hepatotoxicity are extremely diverse. There is ample justification for the claim that drug-induced liver injury encompasses the entire spectrum of liver disease. A summary of the broad range of drug hepatotoxicity identified in adults or children is shown in Table 20.3.

Table 20.3: Range of Clinical and Pathologic Findings in Hepatotoxicity from Drugs or Environmental Toxins

Acute hepatitis	a-Methyldopa, isoniazid, halothane
Zonal liver cell necrosis	Acetaminophen
Hepatitis-cholestasis	Erythromycin, chlorpromazine, azathioprine, nitrofurantoin
Cholestasis	Estrogens/oral contraceptive pill, cyclosporine, haloperidol
Steatonecrosis (mimicking alcoholic hepatitis)	Perhexiline, amiodarone
Phospholipidosis	Amiodarone
Microvesicular steatosis	Valproic acid, tetracycline
Macrovesicular fat plus fibrosis	Methotrexate
Granulomatosis	Sulfonamides, phenylbutazone, carbamazepine
Biliary cirrhosis	Practolol, chlorpropamide
Sclerosing cholangitis	Floxuridine (administered via hepatic artery)
Gallstones	Ceftrizxone, dipyridamole
Peliosis	Estrogens, androgens
Hepatic vein thrombosis	Estrogens/oral contraceptive pill
Veno-occlusive disease	Thioguanine, busulfan, pyrrolizidine alkaloids
Noncirrhotic portal hypertension	Vinyl chloride, arsenic, azathioprine
Liver cell adenoma	Estrogens/oral contraceptive pill, anabolic steroids
Malignant tumors	Estrogens/oral contraceptive pill, anabolic steroids, vinyl chloride
Porphyria	2,3,7,8-Tetrachlorodibenzo-p-Dioxin, chloroquine

HEPATOTOXICITY OF SPECIFIC DRUGS

The following drugs are relevant to drug hepatotoxicity in children. Pediatric patients suffering from such drug hepatotoxicities have been diagnosed and treated at the Hospital for Sick Children, Toronto, in the past 20 years. Certain drugs are included because they are frequently used in children and have been associated with major hepatotoxicity in adults.

Acetaminophen

Acetaminophen is an effective antipyretic and analgesic. Taken in a single large dose, however, it is a potent hepatotoxin. The clinical course of this acute acetaminophen toxicity is distinctive. Immediately after the drug is taken, nausea and vomiting occur. These symptoms subside and then there is an asymptomatic interval before liver injury becomes clinically apparent. At that point, jaundice, abnormal serum aminotransferases, and coagulopathy develop. Finally hepatic failure may supervene with progressive coma. Serum aminotransferases may be extremely high in this condition, and the degree of abnormality is not necessarily predictive of outcome. In adults, clinical findings predicting poor outcome (that is, terminal liver failure) are concurrent findings of serum creatinine greater than 300 μmol/L *and* prothrombin time greater than 100 seconds (INR >7) *and* grade 3 or 4 hepatic encephalopathy in patients with a normal pH, or the single finding of arterial pH less than 7.3 in a normovolemic patient [66].

Treatment of acute acetaminophen hepatotoxicity involves the use of what is effectively an antidote, *N*-acetylcysteine. Whether to use *N*-acetylcysteine can be decided on the basis of plotting on a semilogarithmic graph the patient's plasma acetaminophen concentration against time [67]; if it falls in the zone for probable hepatic toxicity, *N*-acetylcysteine should be given. *N*-Acetylcysteine is most effective if given within 10 hours of acetaminophen ingestion, and it may be of little benefit more than 24 hours after ingestion of the acetaminophen. However, even if there is doubt as to its usefulness, it should be given anyway. Late administration of *N*-acetylcysteine has been associated with greater survival in adults with acute acetaminophen intoxication; no adverse side effects of the *N*-acetylcysteine were observed [68–70]. A 72-hour regimen of oral *N*-acetylcysteine appears to be as effective as the 20-hour intravenous regimen; the oral regimen may be more effective if treatment is delayed [67]. Although initial fears that *N*-acetylcysteine administered after 12 hours might increase liver damage appear unfounded, the dose of *N*-acetylcysteine has to be right for body weight because an inappropriately high dose may be toxic, causing respiratory compromise or hypotension. Other measures, such as charcoal, may be effective very early, that is, within 1 hour of ingestion; acetaminophen ingestion itself typically causes vomiting. Hemodialysis must be used early when plasma concentrations of acetaminophen are high or it is not effective. As the metabolism of acetaminophen in adolescents is similar to that of the adult, treatment should be aggressive; younger children also require *N*-acetylcysteine and supportive treatment, even when the timing and total amount of acetaminophen taken are uncertain. Liver transplant may be required for those children in liver failure who show no improvement despite full supportive treatment. Recent experience indicates that the prognosis is good in a child if after 48 hours of treatment with *N*-acetylcysteine the prothrombin time and serum aminotransferases are all normal.

In addition to this acute type of hepatotoxicity, which is encountered in toddlers invading the medicine cabinet or in suicidal teenagers, acetaminophen hepatotoxicity in children can present more subtly, as therapeutic misadventure. This occurs through various sorts of unintentional error: actual dosing error through misunderstanding the dose or using the wrong measuring device, substitution of one formulation for another, failure to appreciate how often acetaminophen turns up in various over-the-counter medications, general belief that acetaminophen is "safe" for children. In typical cases, moderately large doses of acetaminophen (approximately 30–70 mg/kg) are administered at regular intervals (usually every 2–4 hours) for 2 to 3 days, or longer, before hepatotoxicity becomes evident. This is sometimes described as "chronic" overdose, but the actual time frame is comparatively short. The liver disease presents as acute liver failure, and the systemic signs of toxicity and the asymptomatic period do not occur. Alternatively, they are neither distinctive nor noticed. Serum concentrations of acetaminophen are frequently not in a toxic range. Diagnosis is difficult unless a very meticulous drug history is taken to determine exactly what preparation of acetaminophen was used and how often. Getting the actual drug containers, even if they were discarded, may be critically important. The acute liver failure is frequently attributed to another etiology, usually acute viral hepatitis. Numerous cases of this type of acetaminophen hepatotoxicity have now been documented (in addition to those noted previously in this chapter) and reviewed critically [71–74]. The estimate of the lethal per-kilogram dose (140 mg/kg) is based on observations in adults and is probably not accurate for children in this scenario. The threshold for liver injury is highly variable from child to child. A suggested threshold on the order of 90–120 mg/kg/day with more than 1 day of drug administration is highly controversial because it impinges on the dose schedule of 15 mg/kg/day administered every 4 hours around the clock: further data are needed. Fever does not seem to enhance the risk of liver injury [75]. The Rumack nomogram for treatment with *N*-acetylcysteine does not apply in such situations; however, finding a measurable serum concentration of acetaminophen (APAP) 24 hours or more after the last dose should suggest the possibility of APAP hepatotoxicity. The elimination half-life can be estimated from two drug levels obtained at a reasonable interval apart: if it is greater than 4 hours, it suggests hepatotoxicity. Detecting an acetaminophen protein adduct, 3-(cystein-5-yl)-acetaminophen, formed by the binding of the reactive metabolite N-acetyl-*p*-benzoquinoneimine (NAPQI) to glutathione, may be informative [76,77]. In general, it seems reasonable to treat with *N*-acetylcysteine as soon as possible. Anorexia and food avoidance that may have accompanied the underlying illness for which acetaminophen was used may exacerbate the hepatotoxicity by causing acute depletion of glutathione stores. These children tend to present for medical assessment late in the disease course, and this may be an important reason for the poor prognosis.

The primary mechanism for acetaminophen hepatotoxicity involves the formation of a toxic metabolite [78–81]. The important role of drug metabolism in this hepatotoxicity is reflected in the predominance of hepatocellular injury in Rappaport zone 3. Acetaminophen is usually metabolized via sulfation and glucuronidation (Figure 20.3). If a very large amount is taken, these pathways are saturated, and an otherwise minor pathway through cytochromes P450, including CYP1A2, CYP2E1, and CYP3A4 [82], becomes quantitatively important. The product of this pathway is a highly reactive species, NAPQI [83], a potent electrophile. It is conjugated by glutathione, as long as sufficient glutathione is available, to

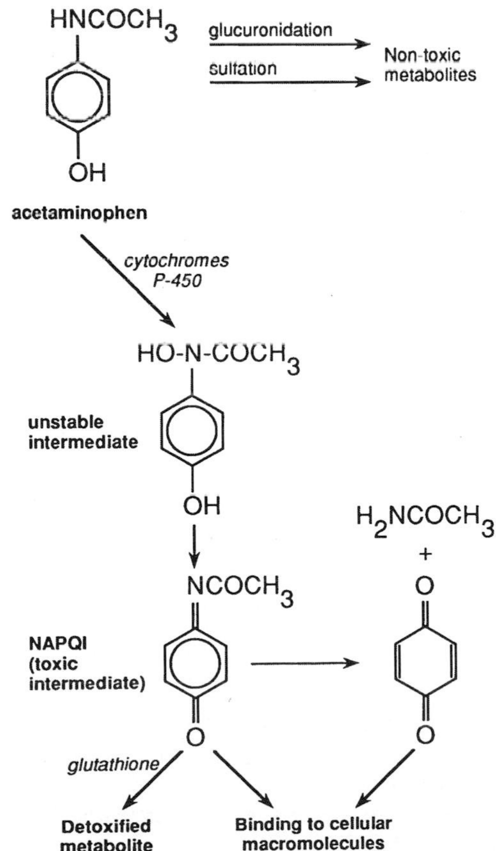

Figure 20.3. Hepatic metabolism of acetaminophen.

form mercapturic acid, which is excreted in the urine. Otherwise NAPQI reacts with cellular proteins, causing cell damage and cell death. Intracellular processes amplifying cellular damage contribute to the liver injury, which may seem to be disproportionate to the amount of toxic intermediate produced. It appears that NAPQI initiates oxidative stress caused by reactive-oxygen and reactive-nitrogen species. This entails mitochondrial damage that itself becomes self-perpetuating and results in failure to produce adenosine triphosphate (ATP) [84]. An intracellular antioxidant response mediated by the nuclear transcription factor NF-E2-related factor (Nrf2) is also activated [85]. As part of an extracellular enhancement mechanism, various cytokines can increase or decrease the liver injury. Polymorphonuclear leukocytes do not appear to enhance the injury. *N*-Acetylcysteine acts by providing substrate for making more glutathione and thus can minimize hepatotoxicity if given early enough. It does not reverse the toxic effects of the toxic intermediate once they have occurred [86]. *N*-acetylcysteine may also promote hepatocellular recovery by enhancing oxygen delivery to the liver tissue [87]. Fasting decreases the amount of glutathione in cells and thus enhances acetaminophen toxicity.

Young children appear to be resistant to acetaminophen hepatotoxicity and tend to recover when it does occur [88,89]. The incidence of hepatotoxicity was 5.5% in a study of 417 children aged 5 years or less, compared with 29% in adolescents and adults at comparable toxic blood levels [90]. Various studies of acetaminophen pharmacokinetics, metabolism, and toxicity in children suggest a biochemical basis for this difference. The elimination half-life is essentially the same in children and adults, although with interindividual variation, it ranges as much as 1–3.5 hours [91]. The elimination half-life is somewhat longer (2.2–5.0 hours) in neonates. The profile of metabolites differs greatly in early childhood from adolescence and adulthood: sulfation predominates over glucuronidation [54]. The switch to the adult pattern seems to occur around 12 years of age. However, even in newborns, urinary metabolites reflecting cytochrome P450-generated intermediates can be found [92,93]; thus, the capacity for producing toxic metabolites seems to be present from an extremely early age. In vitro studies with fetal human hepatocytes have shown that the cytochrome P450–generated intermediates can be formed and conjugated to glutathione as early as at 18 weeks of gestation, but the rate of formation is approximately 10% of that in adult human hepatocytes; sulfation, but not glucuronidation, of acetaminophen also can be detected in the human fetal liver cells [94]. Human infants may also have a greater capacity for synthesis of glutathione than adults and thus can produce enough new glutathione to inactivate toxic metabolites of acetaminophen more effectively.

Despite this relative resistance to this type of hepatotoxicity, young children can develop severe hepatotoxicity from acetaminophen. Some of these reports represent acute poisoning [95–97]. Therapeutic misadventure due to inappropriate dosing is more frequent in this age group: 22 of 47 cases reviewed in the largest published series were children aged 3 years or younger, and 6 of these 22 were infants aged 6 months or younger [71]. Some of this acetaminophen-associated hepatotoxicity might be avoided by clear instructions to parents about dosing and use of conservative dosage guidelines. Hepatotoxicity and extreme prolongation of the elimination half-life of acetaminophen have also been found in infants born after maternal self-poisoning with acetaminophen [92,93].

Initial studies on the mechanism of acetaminophen toxicity showed that toxicity was worse when animals were pretreated with the prototypic polycyclic aromatic hydrocarbon 3-methylcholanthrene, a potent inducer of cytochromes CYP1A1 and CYP1A2. However, in the Cyp1a2 knockout mouse acetaminophen is highly hepatotoxic despite their lacking functional Cyp1a2 [98]; therefore, several different cytochromes P450 are involved. The complement of cytochromes P450 and other factors susceptible to interindividual variation may influence the severity of acetaminophen hepatotoxicity, rendering some individuals unusually prone to toxicity. Chronic alcoholics are more sensitive to acetaminophen than nonalcoholics and can develop subacute acetaminophen hepatotoxicity after taking ordinary therapeutic doses chronically [99]. CYP2E1, which is induced by ethanol is capable of metabolizing acetaminophen [100] and thus induced CYP2E1 enhances its toxicity. Adolescents drinking alcohol regularly may be at risk for this type of acetaminophen hepatotoxicity. Whether exposure to environmental chemicals such as polychlorinated biphenyls or aromatic hydrocarbons increases susceptibility to acetaminophen hepatotoxicity remains unproved. Specifically, the extent to which cigarette smoking, associated with induction of CYP1A1 and CYP1A2, enhances acetaminophen toxicity has not been determined. The potential for the proton pump inhibitor omeprazole to induce CYP1A2 sufficiently to enhance acetaminophen toxicity has not been conclusively demonstrated; individuals with the slow-metabolizer phenotype of the mephenytoin polymorphism would be predicted to be at risk [101]. Phenytoin may induce CYP3A4 and thus enhance acetaminophen hepatotoxicity [102]. Mercury poisoning through exposure to elemental mercury apparently enhanced acetaminophen hepatotoxicity in one child [103]. Some children may have innate defects in acetaminophen detoxification, but this has been difficult to pinpoint mechanistically. Children with 5-oxoprolinuria, who cannot produce glutathione efficiently, are at increased risk of liver injury due to acetaminophen.

The antiviral drug zidovudine has been reported to increase acetaminophen hepatotoxicity, possibly by competing for glucuronidation pathways and forcing a switch-over to the pathways mediated by cytochromes P450 [104]. A similar phenomenon has recently been reported with phenytoin and possibly with phenobarbital [105–107]. Gunn rats, which are deficient in bilirubin UDP-glucuronosyl transferase, are more susceptible to acetaminophen hepatotoxicity than normal rats [108], but whether these data imply that patients with Crigler–Najjar syndromes or Gilbert syndrome are similarly more susceptible is a complex pharmacologic question requiring further investigation [23].

The implications for liver injury of new formulations of acetaminophen, such as sustained-release tablets, are not yet evident. Confusing the sustained-release tablet dosage schedule (every 8 hours) with the conventional dosage schedule (every 4–6 hours) might result in hepatotoxicity. Combining acetaminophen with a potentially habituating analgesic might result in excessive chronic use of acetaminophen. The plethora of over-the-counter medications that contain acetaminophen has been identified as increasing risk of liver injury. Acetaminophen rectal suppositories are used in children, and these pose unique problems of drug absorption and bioavailability depending on the composition of suppository matrix. Severe liver damage in a child was reported attributed to high-dose acetaminophen exposure with rectal suppositories [109]. Although several other potentially hepatotoxic drugs were also administered, this attribution is credible.

Amiodarone

Amiodarone is an iodinated benzofuran derivative used for the treatment of cardiac arrhythmias. Although reserved for more severe disease, it is used from time to time in children. Thyroid dysfunction and pulmonary fibrosis are well-recognized adverse effects of amiodarone. Lamellar inclusion bodies, similar to those found in genetic phospholipid storage diseases, are found in the lungs, lymph nodes, peripheral blood leukocytes, and liver of patients taking amiodarone chronically [110]. Phospholipidosis may be associated with progressive liver damage in some patients [111], but it appears to be independent from pseudo-alcoholic hepatitis due to amiodarone [112,113]. Although iodine accumulation in the liver may produce striking hepatic parenchymal density on computerized tomography (Figure 20.4), it is not in itself a sign of hepatotoxicity.

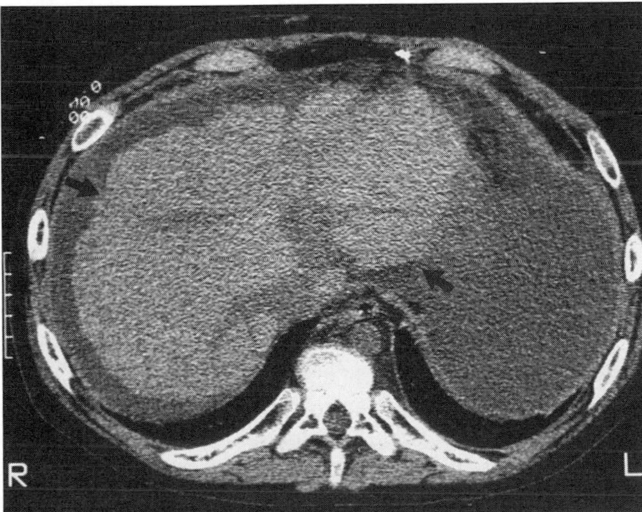

Figure 20.4. Computed tomography of the liver in chronic amiodarone administration. The increased density of the liver (*arrows*) is due to the iodine in the amiodarone accumulated in hepatocytes. (Courtesy of Dr. Paul Babyn, Department of Diagnostic Imaging, the Hospital for Sick Children, Toronto.)

Amiodarone-induced hepatotoxicity, characterized by hepatomegaly and abnormal aminotransferases, may develop within a month of treatment or after 1 year of treatment. Asymptomatic elevations in aminotransferases are frequent, occurring in one quarter to one half of patients treated; these abnormalities may return to normal spontaneously, even if the drug is not discontinued. Alternatively, progressive chronic liver disease occurs in some patients. Cirrhosis may develop, perhaps because excretion of amiodarone is very slow. Hepatotoxic changes mimicking acute alcoholic hepatitis have been described in adults, but not in children [112,114]. Likewise, cholestatic liver injury may occur rarely but has not been described in children [115].

Severe amiodarone hepatotoxicity has been reported in a child [116]. It presented as rapidly progressive hepatic failure beginning after two months of treatment at a relatively high dose of amiodarone (9 mg/kg/day).

The mechanism of amiodarone hepatotoxicity remains undetermined, but it may involve abnormal hepatic biotransformation. Decreased erythrocyte superoxide dismutase activity correlates with pulmonary damage [117]; this might point to a problem with drug or metabolite detoxification, specifically involving generation of free radicals. Amiodarone may also interfere with mitochondrial β-oxidation and oxidative phosphorylation.

Liver injury associated with intravenous administration of amiodarone has recently been described, but it appears that the excipient polysorbate-80 is responsible for the toxicity [118]. This is reminiscent of a similar problem experienced previously with intravenous vitamin E administration in children.

Antineoplastic Drugs

Many drugs used to treat neoplasia in childhood can cause hepatotoxicity [119–122]. However, these drugs are rarely used separately and patients receiving them are usually at risk for multiple types of liver injury. A hepatitic pattern, often asymptomatic with elevation in serum aminotransferases and no other evidence of severe liver toxicity, is common. Antineoplastic drugs, which frequently produce this reaction, include nitrosoureas, 6-mercaptopurine, cytosine arabinoside, cis-platinum, and dacarbazine (DTIC). With cis-platinum the mechanism of liver injury appears to involve oxidative stress [123,124]. For both cis-platinum and DTIC induction of CYP2E1 might enhance the risk of liver damage. Cyclophosphamide may cause a dose-related drug hepatitis [125]. Carmustine and 6-mercaptopurine can also cause severe cholestasis [126]. Adriamycin, dactinomycin, and vinca alkaloids are infrequently associated with hepatotoxicity. However, several patients treated with dactinomycin at the Hospital for Sick Children, Toronto, have developed severe hepatic dysfunction, with extremely elevated serum aminotransferases and coagulopathy, all of which resolved spontaneously when off the drug. Similar experience has been reported in treatment of Wilms' tumor [127,128]. Irradiation may enhance hepatotoxicity of dactinomycin [129,130]. Adriamycin given together with

6-mercaptopurine may increase the hepatotoxic potential of 6-mercaptopurine. Steatosis or portal fibrosis has been found on liver biopsies from children with acute lymphoblastic leukemia, treated with various anticancer drugs [131].

L-asparaginase is associated with severe hepatic injury characterized by severe steatosis, hepatocellular necrosis, and fibrosis, which is usually reversible after the L-asparaginase is stopped [132,133]. The most likely mechanism for this hepatotoxicity is a profound interference with hepatocellular protein metabolism. Thrombocytopenia and acute liver failure were reported in an 18-year-old patient receiving carboplatin [134].

Veno-occlusive disease is an important pattern of hepatotoxicity associated with antineoplastic drugs. It presents acutely with an enlarged tender liver, ascites or unexplained weight gain, and jaundice; serum aminotransferases may be elevated. In surviving patients, the liver disease may progress to cirrhosis with hepatic venular sclerosis and sinusoidal fibrosis. Although 6-thioguanine is a classic cause of VOD, other antineoplastic drugs such as cytosine arabinoside, busulfan, DTIC, carmustine, and dactinomycin have been associated with VOD at conventional or high doses, and drug interactions may enhance their propensity for causing this type of liver injury [135–137]. Currently, VOD most frequently develops after allogeneic bone marrow transplantation [138]; however, it has been reported with other regimens as treatment for childhood solid tumors [139,140]. It has been disputed whether VOD is a consequence of chemotherapeutic conditioning regimens or part of the spectrum of liver injury due to graft-versus-host disease (GVHD) [141,142], and in some individual patients it may in fact be difficult to make this distinction. In some cases cholestasis or cytokines released as part of GVHD might contribute to the development of VOD or increase its severity. Irradiation by itself can lead to VOD [143] possibly because endothelial cells lining hepatic sinusoids are more sensitive to radiation than hepatocytes. The combination of irradiation and chemotherapy in conditioning regimens appears to accelerate development of VOD compared to the effect of a single injurious agent (irradiation or chemical) [144]. Methotrexate plus cyclosporine (used as prophylaxis for GVHD) in patients prepared for bone marrow transplant by a regimen using busulfan and cyclophosphamide led to a higher incidence of jaundice and VOD disease than methylprednisolone and cyclosporine prophylaxis in similarly prepared patients [145,146]. In general, it appears most antineoplastic drugs carry some risk of provoking VOD.

Clinical predictors of likelihood for development of VOD in children have not yet been identified; however, ongoing hepatitis, such as chronic viral hepatitis, before transplant increases susceptibility to hepatic damage [147]. Development of multiorgan failure presages poor survival. Polymorphisms in glutathione *S*-transferases appear to correlate with increased risk [148]; risk associated with other Phase II enzymes is less clear-cut [149]. In many patients, the process resolves, but in a sizable proportion, the process is fatal or leads to chronic liver damage [150,151]. Treatment has generally been aimed at interfering with thrombosis, such as defibrotide [152] or other agents [153], but given the disease mechanism, early treatment with glutathione replacement might be appropriate. Anecdotal evidence suggests its efficacy [154].

The pathogenesis of VOD involves activation of the coagulation cascade in the hepatic sinusoids after injury to endothelial cells [155]. Liver injury progresses from congestion in the sinusoids and hemorrhage into the space of Disse, mainly in zone 3 of the Rappaport acinus, which has been described as sinusoidal obstruction syndrome to damage to the terminal hepatic venules and subsequently to fibrosis [156]. VOD due to DTIC involves damage to sinusoidal endothelial cells by toxic metabolite(s) produced in the endothelial cells; glutathione appears to protect against toxicity [157]. In contrast, with VOD due to cyclophosphamide the toxic metabolites are produced in hepatocytes [158]. In a rat model in which monocrotaline was the toxic chemical, glutathione depletion and decreased hepatic production of nitric oxide contribute to the disease mechanism [159–161]. Among cytokines that may play a role in the disease mechanism, vascular endothelial growth factor has been shown to be elevated in children who develop severe VOD [162].

6-Thioguanine has recently been found to cause nodular regenerative hyperplasia in patients with inflammatory bowel disease, and in one patient sinusoidal obstruction syndrome was also present [163].

Aspirin

Hepatotoxicity has been associated with high-dose aspirin treatment. The hepatotoxicity appears to be dose-dependent, and patients without rheumatoid disease can develop hepatotoxicity. However, most cases are reported in patients with rheumatoid diseases. Approximately 60% of the 300 reported cases have been in patients with juvenile rheumatoid arthritis (not necessarily all children), and a further 10% have occurred in children with acute rheumatic fever [164]. A prospective study of aspirin hepatotoxicity in adult patients with rheumatoid arthritis or osteoarthritis revealed that 5% of those taking aspirin developed asymptomatic elevations of serum aspartate aminotransferase [165]. The preponderance of cases in patients with rheumatologic diseases, however, raises the possibility that these patients have a predisposition to this toxicity. One theory is that chronic inflammation increases generation of oxygen radicals [166]. A single case of apparent hepatotoxicity associated with low-dose aspirin therapy in a young child after liver transplant has been reported; there were essentially asymptomatic elevations of serum aminotransferases, and liver biopsy revealed zonal, but periportal, hepatocellular necrosis [167].

In most cases, salicylate hepatotoxicity has hepatitic features with anorexia, nausea, vomiting, abdominal pain, and elevated serum aminotransferases [168–170]. Hepatomegaly is usually present, and the liver may be tender. Progressive signs of liver damage such as jaundice and coagulopathy are rare. Even in uncomplicated cases, serum aminotransferase levels may be greater than 1000 IU [168]. In some cases encephalopathy (not related to Reye's syndrome) has been present [171,172]. Clinical and laboratory abnormalities resolve when aspirin is stopped. Liver histology typically shows a nonspecific picture with acute, focal hepatocellular necrosis.

Azathioprine

Azathioprine is a potent immunosuppressive drug that consists of 6-mercaptopurine linked to an imidazole side-chain. In effect, it is a prodrug for 6-mercaptopurine. Since its introduction in the 1960s, azathioprine has been associated with hepatotoxicity, including in children, but these early studies are confounded by underdiagnosed concomitant viral liver disease. In adults azathioprine hepatotoxicity has been characterized mainly by cholestasis or a hepatitic-cholestatic picture [173,174]. Liver biopsy in one case showed centrilobular ballooning of hepatocytes and canalicular cholestasis [173]. More recently azathioprine hepatotoxicity has been described in orthotopic liver transplant recipients: endothelial cell damage, as well as hepatocyte damage and cholestasis, was noted [175]. In addition, several cases of nodular regenerative hyperplasia associated with azathioprine have been reported [176,177]. Chronic use has been associated with cirrhosis in some cases.

6-Mercaptopurine has been associated more directly with liver toxicity and causes a mixed hepatitic–cholestatic reaction [178]. Hepatic accumulation of 6-mercaptopurine metabolites was postulated in four children who developed hepatotoxicity from 6-mercaptopurine during treatment for acute lymphoblastic leukemia; one child had severe cholestatic hepatitis [126].

The association of chronic azathioprine therapy with development of malignancy varies with the underlying disease: in inflammatory bowel disease, there seems to be no increased risk [179]. Meta-analysis, however, indicates that azathioprine and 6-mercaptopurine are each associated with increased risk of lymphoma when used chronically in inflammatory bowel disease. Whether azathioprine (or 6-mercaptopurine) predisposes to hepatosplenic T-cell lymphoma in adolescents and young adults with inflammatory bowel disease, either when used alone or in combination with infliximab, is an important new issue because of the severity of this particular lymphoma [180].

Carbamazepine

Carbamazepine is a dibenzazepine derivative, similar structurally to imipramine in that it has fundamentally a tricyclic chemical structure. Hepatotoxicity is uncommon. In adults the predominant type of hepatotoxicity has been granulomatous hepatitis presenting with fever and right upper quadrant pain, suggestive of cholangitis [181,182]. Adults with "vanishing bile duct syndrome" (i.e., small portal bile duct paucity, also known as ductopenia) attributed to chronic toxicity from carbamazepine have been reported [183]. In children the usual clinical picture has been hepatitis, sometimes associated with a drug hypersensitivity syndrome similar to that of phenytoin. Two other children presented with a mononucleosis-like illness consisting of rash, lymphadenopathy, hepatosplenomegaly, and neutropenia [184,185]. A child treated at the Hospital for Sick Children, Toronto, also presented with fever, rash, incipient liver failure, lymphopenia, and eosinophilia. Rechallenge of her lymphocytes in vitro with metabolites of carbamazepine provided evidence of defective detoxification mechanisms. An infant boy also presented to this hospital with only a hepatitic type of toxicity from carbamazepine. Three other children with drug hypersensitivity to carbamazepine (for which hepatitis was not the dominant clinical feature) have been described [186]. However, severe hepatotoxicity has been reported in children. One child died of progressive liver failure when carbamazepine was not stopped [187]. Four children with fatal acute liver failure were taking carbamazepine, phenytoin, and primidone [188]. More recently severe hepatitis was reported in three children taking only carbamazepine: one recovered with corticosteroid treatment but the others died or required liver transplant [189]. Another child developed severe hepatitis with coagulopathy 5 months after beginning treatment with carbamazepine; she survived with prednisone treatment [190].

Like phenytoin and phenobarbital, carbamazepine may be metabolized via arene oxides. These intermediates are ordinarily detoxified by the Phase II enzyme, epoxide hydrolase. Persons with an inherited metabolic idiosyncrasy, possibly involving an abnormal epoxide hydrolase, may be unable to detoxify active metabolite(s) of carbamazepine and thus develop hepatotoxicity. The same metabolic idiosyncrasy which renders them susceptible to carbamazepine hepatotoxicity place them at risk for phenytoin and phenobarbital hepatotoxicity [191]. This may explain the fatal hepatotoxicity reported in children on multiple antiepileptics because primidone contains phenobarbital [188]. Additionally, imipramine can cause cholestasis: the chemical similarity between these two drugs may provide a clue to the mechanism for bile duct injury due to carbamazepine.

Cocaine

Cocaine hepatotoxicity has not yet been reported in children or adolescents. A clinically severe hepatitic reaction has been reported in five young adults: the predominant histologic finding was extensive zonal necrosis of hepatocytes in Rappaport zone 3 with zone 1 steatosis [192,193]. The mechanism of this hepatotoxicity remains undetermined: reactive oxygen species, perhaps generated along with norcaine nitroxide, may lead to lipid peroxidation in a mouse model of cocaine hepatotoxicity [194]. The histologic pattern of hepatic injury in humans is consistent with generation of a toxic metabolite, probably by cytochromes P450. Such a toxic metabolite might be similar to that in the mouse or a potent electrophile. Glutathione appears to protect against cocaine-induced hepatic injury [195]. Cytochromes P450 in the CYP3A subfamily are important in biotransformation of cocaine [196]. Ethanol and phenobarbital-type inducers appear to increase cocaine hepatotoxicity. The interaction of cocaine and ethanol has been studied in vitro in human liver slices: ethanol appears to increase the toxicity of cocaine 10-fold [197]. Studies in primary cultures of human hepatocytes also demonstrate that ethanol potentiates the toxicity of cocaine to hepatocytes, leading depletion of cellular glycogen stores and glutathione [198]. Recent studies in mice also suggest that endotoxin enhances cocaine-induced liver injury [199].

Cyclosporine

The potent immunosuppressive drug cyclosporine has a novel cyclic structure composed of eleven amino acids and is extremely lipophilic. It is metabolized in humans by CYP3A4 [200, 201]. Although at high dosage a mixed hepatitic–cholestatic picture may develop, the more frequent hepatic abnormality is mainly cholestasis: direct hyperbilirubinemia without other evidence of hepatocellular damage [202]. Bland cholestasis after cyclosporine administration has been demonstrated in a rat model [203]. In vitro studies with rat hepatocytes have shown that cyclosporine inhibits taurocholate transport competitively and reversibly [204]. It inhibits the bile salt excretory pump [205], affects gene expression [206], and alters canalicular membrane fluidity [207].

Because cyclosporine is metabolized by cytochromes P450, predictable drug interactions occur. Phenobarbital, phenytoin, and rifampicin all increase clearance of cyclosporine because they are capable of inducing CYP3A4. Cimetidine and ketoconazole, both inhibitors of cytochromes P450, decrease the clearance of cyclosporine. Erythromycin, which is also metabolized by the cytochrome P450 3A subfamily, inhibits cyclosporine metabolism, probably competitively [208]. Verapamil and diltiazem can also inhibit cyclosporine metabolism.

Ecstasy

The synthetic amphetamine 3,4-methylenedioxymetamphetamine (MDMA) is generally known as "Ecstasy" and continues to be a popular "recreational" drug, despite being potentially very hazardous as deaths have occurred with ingestion of only one tablet. It can cause severe hyperthermia with rhabdomyolysis, cardiac damage with arrhythmias, disseminated intravascular coagulation, and acute renal failure. Hepatotoxicity, reported mainly in young adults, led to death or liver transplantation in several [209,210]; more recent reports of severe hepatotoxicity included some adolescents [211–214]. There may be a few days between taking Ecstasy and becoming unwell, or patients may be found "collapsed" within hours of taking it. Some patients have coagulopathy and hypoglycemia without developing full-blown acute liver failure. Liver histology is variable with Ecstasy hepatotoxicity, the spectrum ranging from focal to extensive hepatocellular necrosis, with variable degrees of cholestasis, sometimes microvesicular steatosis. Interindividual variation in susceptibility is a prominent feature of Ecstasy hepatotoxicity; hyperthermia itself, impure drug, or coadministered recreational drugs or ethanol may contribute to the liver damage in some cases. Genetic predisposition involves the CYP2D6 variants with decreased activity; certain drugs (such as paroxetine, fluoxetine, and certain protease inhibitors) inhibit CYP2D6, and indeed Ecstasy may inhibit its own biotransformation by this cytochrome P450 [215,216]. The occurrence of Ecstasy hepatotoxicity with acute liver failure in adolescents depends on emerging trends for teenaged usage; however, fatal multisystem toxicity with hyperthermia and liver failure in a 15-year-old was diagnosed at the Hospital for Sick Children, Toronto. Public education on the risks of using Ecstasy is urgently required.

A second pattern of hepatotoxicity may occur with chronic use and resembles autoimmune hepatitis [210].

Erythromycin

All forms of erythromycin, not just erythromycin estolate, are potentially hepatotoxic [217–222]. The clinical presentation is similar regardless of which erythromycin ester is involved: anorexia, nausea, jaundice, and abdominal pain, predominantly in the right upper quadrant. Pruritus due to cholestasis has been reported in adults. The overall clinical appearance is that of a mixed hepatitic–cholestatic process, although the cholestatic component may be prominent enough to suggest biliary tract obstruction. Hepatomegaly, sometimes with splenomegaly, appears to be common in children [220]. A single report of erythromycin ethylsuccinate hepatotoxicity in a child indicated relatively mild, self-limited disease [219]. Histologic findings include prominent cholestasis and focal necrosis of hepatocytes, both of which tend to be worse in acinar zone 3. Eosinophils are prominent in portal infiltrates and in the sinusoids [217]. The zonality suggests the action of a toxic metabolite.

The mechanism of erythromycin hepatotoxicity remains obscure. Erythromycin and other macrolide antibiotics are metabolized in the liver by the CYP3A subfamily. Hepatocellular damage may be caused by a toxic metabolite, but this is by no means proved. In vitro studies have indicated intrinsic cytotoxicity of erythromycin base and derivatives [223,224]. In a perfused rat liver model, erythromycin estolate caused decreased bile secretion, altered canalicular permeability, and decreased activities of certain ATPases, in contrast to the effect of erythromycin base [225].

Other macrolide antibiotics are also associated with hepatotoxicity. Severe cholestatic liver injury associated with clarithromycin was reported in a 15-year-old girl; it was unresponsive to treatment with ursodiol but subsided with prednisone [226]. Whether nimesulide contributed to this hepatotoxicity is uncertain. Cholestatic liver injury has been reported in adults [227,228]. Telithromycin is a new macrolide antibiotic already proving to be hepatotoxic in adults [229].

An important pharmacologic problem common to erythromycin and related macrolides is that they inhibit CYP3A4 and thus can affect the metabolism of numerous other drugs metabolized by that cytochrome P450, potentially enhancing adverse side effects of those drugs [230]. Recent studies using human liver microsomes and testosterone 6β-hydroxylation as the probe for CYP3A4 function showed erythromycin and clarithromycin to have greater inhibitory effects than azithromycin [231].

Estrogens: Oral Contraceptive Pill

Cholestasis is a well-recognized complication of estrogens administered in oral contraceptives pills [232]. Estrogen-induced changes in bile composition may lead to gallstone formation and diminished gallbladder function.

Hepatic vein thrombosis (Budd–Chiari syndrome) has been associated with use of oral contraceptives [233]. It has been reported in adolescents [234–236]. Other disorders associated with hepatic vein thrombosis, such as paroxysmal nocturnal hemoglobinuria, circulating lupus anticoagulant, and congenital disorders of coagulation proteins, should be excluded. Early diagnosis is important for a good outcome, but the presentation of this disease may be subtle with only gradual increase in abdominal girth due to ascites and nonspecific changes in liver function tests.

Liver cell adenoma is the principal neoplasm associated with prolonged use of oral contraceptives [237]. In some instances hepatocellular carcinoma was found [238], and oral contraceptive-associated adenomas may progress to hepatocellular carcinoma [239]. Uncomplicated liver cell adenomas may regress when the oral contraceptive pill is stopped. Peliosis hepatis, which is focal dilatation of the hepatic sinusoids, is another lesion associated with chronic use of oral contraceptives.

Felbamate

Felbamate is a relatively new anticonvulsant sometimes used for treating seizures in Lennox–Gastaut syndrome and thus available for use in children. It has been associated with serious adverse effects: aplastic anemia and, less commonly, acute liver failure. Severe hepatotoxicity has occurred in young children [240]. The mechanism of this hepatotoxicity is not established but may involve cytochromes P450-generated reactive intermediate(s), which then bind to and modified cellular proteins which then initiate an immune reaction [241,242]. CYP2E1 and CYP3A4 appear to play an important role in hepatic biotransformation of felbamate. One reactive metabolite, 2-phenylpropenal, is detoxified by glutathione but is also capable of inhibiting certain glutathione-*S*-transferases [243]. Felbamate would then be a contingent hepatotoxin capable of causing an immunoallergic reaction, dependant in part on both the pharmacogenetic and immunogenetic complexion of the individual taking the drug.

Felbamate induces CYP3A4 and inhibits CYP2C19 [244]. When combined with other antiepileptic drugs this can alter drugs levels of those dugs and thus affect their efficacy or toxicity.

Haloperidol

Haloperidol may be associated with hepatotoxicity, shown by elevated serum aminotransferases [245]. Cholestasis may dominate the clinical picture, although some degree of hepatocellular damage and eosinophilia may be present. A prolonged severe bland cholestatic reaction, mimicking extrahepatic bile duct obstruction, may develop in children [246]. One such patient, a 9-year-old boy, was diagnosed at the Hospital for Sick Children, Toronto; severe cholestasis resolved when haloperidol was discontinued.

Halothane

Halothane hepatotoxicity is classically hepatitic. It may manifest as asymptomatic hepatitis indicated only by abnormal serum aminotransferases in the first or second week after the anesthetic exposure or as severe hepatitis with extensive hepatocyte necrosis and liver failure. Predictors for developing halothane hepatotoxicity in adults include older age, female sex, obesity, and multiple exposures to halothane. Hepatitis associated with halothane is infrequent in children although halothane is often used in pediatric anesthetic practice. Large retrospective studies in children estimate that the incidence is approximately 1:80,000–1:200,000 [247,248], in contrast to an incidence of 1:4,000–1:30,000 in adults [249]. A more recent study suggests that halothane hepatotoxicity is less common in both adults and children [250]. Certainly there is no longer any doubt that halothane hepatitis occurs in children. Ten cases have been documented in detail in children aged 11 months to 15 years, all of whom had multiple exposures to halothane. Three children died of fulminant liver failure but all others recovered [251,252]. In addition, three cases of halothane hepatitis were found retrospectively [247,248] as well as three additional children who succumbed to fulminant hepatic failure after halothane [253–255]. Other reports of hepatitis or hepatic failure in children after halothane anesthesia are difficult to evaluate because of inadequate data or the presence of complicated, and thus confounding, systemic disease; these may amount to an additional nine cases.

Halothane is metabolized by various cytochromes P450 and toxic metabolites are generated [256–258]. Oxidative or reductive metabolic pathways predominate, depending on the prevailing tissue oxygen tension (Figure 20.5). Reductive metabolism generates a toxic intermediate identified as

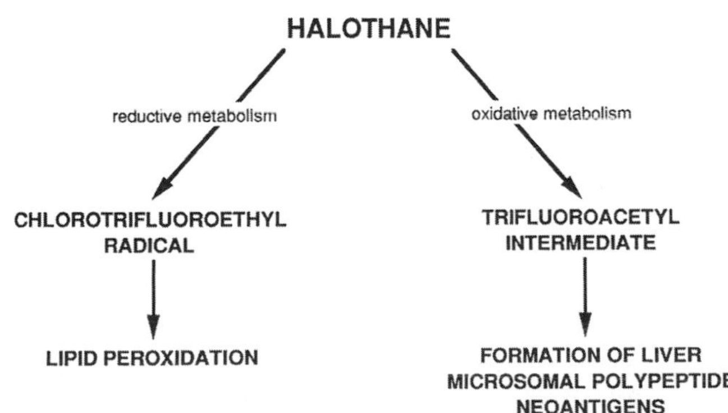

Figure 20.5. Metabolic fates of halothane. Whether reductive or oxidative metabolism predominates depends on the tissue oxygen tension. Formation of neoantigens is associated exclusively with the oxidative pathway.

a chlorotrifluoroethyl radical that leads to lipid peroxidation [256], and oxidative metabolism generates a trifluoroacetyl (TFA) intermediate that can acetylate cellular membranes, thus generating TFA-adducts. The contribution of these complex metabolic systems to human hepatotoxicity remains a matter of some dispute. However, the oxidative pathway is probably predominant in humans. Recent work shows that CYP2A6 and CYP3A4 are associated with the reductive metabolism [259] and CYP2A6 and CYP2E1 (mainly the latter) are associated with the oxidative pathway [260].

Recent studies of the mechanism of halothane hepatotoxicity indicate a connection between cytotoxic damage from reactive intermediates and immunologic phenomena often associated with this hepatotoxicity. The oxidative pathway appears to be associated with hepatocellular membrane damage and immune phenomena typical of the clinical hepatotoxicity syndrome. Patients surviving halothane hepatotoxicity were found to have an antibody to altered hepatocyte membrane constituents [261]. In rabbits, only oxidative metabolism of halothane has been associated with production of this altered hepatocyte membrane antigen, and the effect is greater after pretreatment with the inducer β-naphthaflavone, a polycyclic aromatic hydrocarbon [262]. Other investigators have shown that TFA-adducts can be identified with fluorescent-tagged antibodies in rats, mainly in hepatocytes in Rappaport zone 3 after phenobarbital pretreatment and also on the hepatocyte plasma membrane [263]. Antibodies to these neoantigens have now been identified in sera from patients with halothane hepatitis [264]. Further studies have shown that neoantigens, analogous to these neoantigens derived from halothane-treated animals, are expressed in human liver in individuals exposed to halothane [265]. Only one of these neoantigens has been purified and identified; this particular trifluoroacetylated protein is a microsomal carboxylesterase [266]. Kupffer cells may play a role in the process by which the TFA-adducts initiate an immune response [267]. Other studies in rats suggest that factors such as gender and previous exposure to specific inducers of cytochromes P450 may influence the expression of halothane-associated neoantigens [268].

In summary, severe halothane hepatotoxicity involves several factors. Formation of toxic metabolites varies with tissue oxygenation and possibly with the cytochromes P450 involved. In some instances, halothane may act as a contingent hepatotoxin depending on the adequacy of detoxification of an electrophilic intermediate. In some persons, halothane elicits an immunoallergic response that depends on the adducts formed, as well as the innate immune responsiveness, or immunogenetics, of the host.

Herbal Medications

The hepatotoxic potential of herbal medications is being recognized. The pharmacology of these drugs (active ingredient, metabolism, potential drug interactions) is frequently not well understood. The purity and strength of the actual drug used may not be known; how the herbal preparation is actually manufactured can be important. Patients, including adolescents, may take herbal medications intermittently, and they may not report using herbals to physicians. Use of herbal medications also displays cultural biases. Herbals may be administered to children to promote good health.

Among herbal preparations the toxicity of certain bush teas containing pyrrolizidine alkaloids, which can cause VOD (also known as sinusoidal obstruction syndrome), are best known. Comfrey is also hepatotoxic because it contains pyrrolizidine alkaloids [269,270]. Germander hepatotoxicity [271, 272] appears to be mediated by diterpenoid toxic metabolites formed through biotransformation by CYP3A4 [273,274]. Kava kava, which is used to treat anxiety and promote relaxation, has been removed from the market in some countries because of severe hepatotoxicity [275]. In one instance, a 14-year-old girl required liver transplantation [276]. Some controversy persists as to the real risk of hepatotoxicity, which may depend in part on how the kava is extracted [277]. Kavalactones are capable of inhibiting certain hepatic cytochromes P450 [278]. Other herbals established as hepatotoxic include chaparral leaf [279,280], jin bu huan [281,282], and ma huang (ephedra) [283]. Acute liver failure was reported in a child who received a medication containing various herbs and metals [284]. Fatal VOD associated with herbal medication has also been reported in a child [285]. Echinacea appears to have some hepatotoxic potential.

Isoniazid

Isoniazid (INH) has been associated with a wide spectrum of hepatotoxicity in adults [286]. The most frequent abnormality is asymptomatic elevation of serum aminotransferases. Overt symptoms of hepatitis (fatigue, anorexia, nausea, and vomiting) indicate severe disease; mortality is greater than 10% in patients with jaundice [287]. On histologic examination, INH hepatotoxicity frequently looks exactly like acute viral hepatitis. Submassive hepatic necrosis can occur. Hepatocellular damage sometimes has a zonal pattern, which suggests hepatotoxicity involving drug metabolism.

Isoniazid hepatotoxicity is generally considered to be more common in adults than in children; however, there have been numerous reports of INH hepatotoxicity, including fatal hepatitic necrosis, in children either being treated for tuberculosis or receiving prophylaxis [288–294]. In large studies of children receiving INH alone as prophylaxis against tuberculosis, INH hepatotoxicity (indicated by abnormal serum aminotransferases) had a 7% incidence of a series of 369 children [295] and a 17.1% incidence in 239 patients aged 9–14 years [296]. These findings are nearly equivalent to those in adults, in whom the incidence of transiently elevated serum aminotransferases is estimated at 10–20% [297]. The overall incidence of symptomatic INH hepatitis in children is 0.1–7.1% [298]. Evidence from small studies suggests that hepatic dysfunction occurs in children being treated with INH and rifampicin for tuberculosis. Of 44 patients receiving INH and rifampicin, 36 had some elevation of serum aminotransferases and 15 patients

(42%) of these were jaundiced [299]. In another study, 37% had hepatotoxicity including four of seven children younger than 17 months [300]. These children received conventional doses of INH and rifampicin, as well as brief sequential courses of streptomycin and ethambutal. Other inducers of cytochromes P450 may contribute to INH hepatotoxicity. Severe INH hepatotoxicity has been reported twice in children treated concurrently with INH and carbamazepine [301,302]. As in adults, hepatotoxicity typically develops in the first 2–3 months of treatment; in most children, it resolves with either no change in dose or else a modest dose reduction. Children with more severe tuberculosis seem to be at greater risk for hepatotoxicity, especially if tuberculous meningitis is present [303]. Malnourished children may be at greater risk of hepatotoxicity.

Isoniazid hepatotoxicity appears to be caused by a toxic metabolite. Acetylation via NAT-2 is important in INH metabolism. Acetylisoniazid or its derivatives have been proposed as toxic, and recent studies indicate that acetylhydrazine, derived from acetylisoniazid, undergoes biotransformation by cytochromes P450, principally CYP2E1, to produce these reactive metabolites. Genetically determined activity of CYP2E1 influences whether heptoxicity develops [304]. Likewise, slow acetylators in the NAT-2 polymorphism appear to be a greater risk [305]. Reports in children have failed to show a clear pattern of hepatotoxicity in relation to acetylator status but most were underpowered. Other data suggest that CYP2E1 activity is a more important determinant for hepatotoxicity than acetylator status [306]. Chronic use of alcohol leading to induction of CYP2E1 is known to increase the risk of INH hepatotoxicity. The additive effect of INH and carbamazepine on hepatic cytochromes P450 is complex because INH acts as a potent inhibitor of various cytochromes P450 [307] whereas carbamazepine acts as an inducer.

In summary, INH hepatotoxicity is not uncommon in children. It may be life-threatening. Isoniazid is a contingent hepatotoxin. This is usually contingent on genetic factors relating to the activities of cytochromes P450 and NAT-2. Malnutrition associated with depletion of hepatic glutathione may also play a role. Children with severe tuberculosis and those who receive simultaneous treatment with cytochrome P450 inducers such as rifampicin, phenytoin, or phenobarbital appear to be at greater risk of INH hepatotoxicity. Monitoring with frequent measurement of serum aminotransferases and direct inquiry for hepatitic symptoms is necessary during at least the first 3 months of treatment. If typical hepatitic symptoms develop, INH should be discontinued promptly.

Ketoconazole

In contrast to amphotericin, which is almost never associated with hepatotoxicity, the oral antifungal drug ketoconazole was found to cause significant hepatotoxicity soon after it was introduced for general use. The initial large review of ketoconazole hepatotoxicity in the United States included two children (a 17-year-old boy and a 5-year-old boy, both with chronic mucocutaneous candidiasis) among 54 reported occurrences of which 33 (including both children) were judged as probable or possible cases of ketoconazole-induced hepatotoxicity [308]. Similar series from the United Kingdom and the Netherlands included no children. In these three major series, hepatotoxicity was more frequent in older women. Presenting symptoms included jaundice and hepatitis (anorexia, nausea, vomiting, and malaise) and occurred on average after 6–8 weeks of treatment (range: 5 days–6 months). Peripheral eosinophilia was noted in only one patient in the British series, in 10% of the Dutch patients and in none of the U.S. patients. A patient who developed fulminant hepatitis associated with ketoconazole also had no eosinophilia or rash [309]; other adults with fatal hepatotoxicity have since been reported. In all series, the hepatic lesion was mainly hepatocellular necrosis, often with a centrilobular predominance, or a mixed hepatocellular–cholestatic injury, but some patients had mainly cholestatic features [308,310,311]. In one recent report, protracted jaundice reflecting a predominantly cholestatic lesion was described [309]. Some patients were also noted to have asymptomatic elevations of serum aminotransferases, which returned to normal when the drug was stopped.

The prevailing interpretation of these clinical observations is that ketoconazole-induced hepatotoxicity is due to metabolic idiosyncrasy. A toxic intermediate has been postulated but not defined; no abnormality of drug detoxification has been specifically demonstrated

Itraconazole has been reported to cause a few cases of cholestasis with ductopenia [312].

Lamotrigine

This recently developed anticonvulsant drug can cause the drug hypersensitivity syndrome classically associated with phenytoin [313–316]. Severity of liver damage is variable, but severe acute hepatitis can occur. Lamotrigine can be shown to generate an arene oxide intermediate, which is a candidate for mediating this hepatotoxicity [317]. Children may be more likely to produce this intermediate via cytochromes P450 especially with rapid dose escalation [318]. Ingestion of lamotrigine by a 3-year-old resulted in rash and elevated serum aminotransferases [319].

Methotrexate

Chronic low-dose treatment with methotrexate, as used in psoriasis or certain connective tissue diseases, frequently causes hepatic fibrosis with steatosis [320–322]. The histologic appearance may be similar to that of alcoholic hepatitis with fibrosis. Cirrhosis can develop, and liver transplantation has been performed in some adult patients treated for psoriasis [323]. Self-evidently, these are the characteristics of nonalcoholic steatohepatitis, and the contribution of obesity and fatty liver disease to methotrexate hepatotoxicity in adults is being reexamined [324]. The contribution of specific immune dysregulation in the disease being treated with methotrexate further confounds assessment of methotrexate hepatotoxicity, the features of which may vary in psoriasis or rheumatoid disease or inflammatory bowel disease. In addition to having only relatively small clinical series for examining this problem in adults, a further problem is absence of consensus as to what constitutes mild liver injury.

Hepatic fibrosis has occasionally been found in children with juvenile rheumatoid arthritis (JRA). It is difficult to screen for liver damage by biochemical testing. Serum aminotransferases may not reflect ongoing liver damage, and in fact they may be normal even after the development of cirrhosis or fibrosis [325]. Using an aggregate of aminotransferase determinations (% abnormal over 6 or 12 months) may compensate for the relative insensitivity of these measurements [326,327]. Risk factors for the likely development of liver disease proposed for adults (advanced age, chronic ethanol use, obesity, diabetes mellitus, and renal insufficiency) [328] have limited utility for children, except obesity. Although daily administration of methotrexate appears more prone to cause hepatotoxicity, weekly pulse doses are also associated with the development of hepatic fibrosis [329]. Higher cumulative doses are more likely to be associated with hepatotoxicity, but liver damage has sometimes been found at low cumulative doses. The cumulative dose at which hepatotoxicity becomes likely in children has not been determined.

Because of the difficulty in predicting the likelihood of methotrexate-induced liver damage and in detecting it biochemically, regular histologic examination of the liver by liver biopsy has been customary. Liver biopsy before treatment and at regular, often yearly, intervals during prolonged treatment has been advised, but this may involve a considerable number of invasive procedures for a child. The need for such stringent surveillance has been questioned, especially for children with JRA. The risk of methotrexate hepatotoxicity in JRA appears to be comparatively low. No child in a cross-sectional study of 14 children with JRA who had received a methotrexate cumulative dose greater than 3000 mg or greater than 4000 mg/1.73 m^2 body surface area had significant fibrosis and only one had moderate-to-severe hepatocellular, fatty, inflammatory, or necrotic changes on liver biopsy [330]. In a larger study of 37 liver biopsies from 25 patients with JRA, most were normal or near-normal, 4 had moderate-to-severe fatty or inflammatory changes, and 2 had mild portal fibrosis. Weak but significant correlations were found between abnormal histology and percent of aminotransferase elevations and body mass index [331]. In similar previous studies normal or near-normal liver histology was found [332,333]. Two patients with JRA treated with methotrexate have been reported as developing some degree of liver fibrosis [334].

The surveillance strategy should be individualized for each patient. Children with JRA on methotrexate should have serum aminotransferases checked frequently (monthly or bimonthly). Those with elevated aspartate aminotransferase or alanine aminotransferase on 40% or more tests in 1 year should be considered for liver biopsy. Those with other risk factors such as obesity or diabetes mellitus should also be considered for liver biopsy surveillance. Performing a liver biopsy after a large cumulative dose of methotrexate has been taken may still be judicious, especially if continued treatment is anticipated. The merits of a pretreatment liver biopsy should not be disregarded because several studies indicate that hepatic abnormalities may be present before treatment, which would otherwise be (wrongly) attributed to methotrexate hepatotoxicity. This is especially important if the child is overweight or obese. Children with other indications for methotrexate, such as psoriasis, may require closer surveillance, because it is not evident that the guidelines for JRA can be generalized to other diseases. Observations in adults suggest that methotrexate is relatively free of hepatotoxicity in inflammatory bowel disease, but again the relevance of these data to children with inflammatory bowel disease is not certain [335].

Considerable interest is emerging in the application of noninvasive methods for assessing liver fibrosis to how methotrexate hepatotoxicity is monitored. These may prove to be advantageous, but their applicability to methotrexate hepatotoxicity in children will require separate and detailed investigation.

Methotrexate is also associated with acute hepatitis. High-dose methotrexate treatment used in some antineoplastic treatment regimens may produce acute hepatitis as shown by a sudden rise in aminotransferases [336,337]. After chronic treatment for malignancy, usually at comparatively low doses, hepatic damage may be relatively mild, with some steatosis and fibrosis [338]. However, severe liver disease with ascites, hepatosplenomegaly, and transient jaundice has been reported. In a small study of liver histology after maintenance high-dose methotrexate for 1–2 years, portal fibrosis was found in more than half of the patients, but this was neither severe nor accompanied by clinical liver disease [339].

The mechanism of methotrexate toxicity remains undetermined although a toxic metabolite has been postulated. The poorly soluble metabolite 7-hydroxymethotrexate has been detected after treatment with high-dose regimens and may be associated with renal toxicity from methotrexate. Studies in rats suggest that methotrexate can damage the bile canalicular transporter MRP2, and this may contribute to hepatotoxicity [340]. The mechanism of chronic hepatotoxicity may differ from that of acute toxicity.

Minocycline

Although tetracycline is well known to cause microvesicular steatosis when administered intravenously, this is currently rare. A tetracycline derivative, minocycline, is often used to treat acne in adolescents. Minocycline appears to have a greater potential for causing liver damage than generally appreciated. Specifically, minocycline hepatotoxicity may mimic autoimmune hepatitis. Several cases of hepatotoxicity in teenagers have been reported: hepatic symptoms, jaundice, elevated serum aminotransferases, and positive antinuclear antibodies were common [341–343]. Another typical presentation was polyarthritis with biochemical hepatitis; jaundice was present when hepatitis was severe. Histologic features of chronic active hepatitis may be found on biopsy. In many patients, liver damage resolved when the drug was discontinued. Two cases of acute liver failure in adolescents have been reported [344,345]: one died before transplant, and the other underwent liver transplant. Careful monitoring of liver function is indicated whenever minocycline is used chronically. The mechanism of hepatotoxicity is undetermined but includes immunoallergic features.

Nonsteroidal Anti-Inflammatory Drugs (NSAIDs)

Many NSAIDs have little or no risk of hepatic toxicity. Two widely used NSAIDs, ibuprofen and naproxen, have been associated with hepatotoxicity in only a very few reported instances [287,346]. A study of adverse effects associated with NSAIDs in children revealed a variety of adverse side effects, but liver injury was not prominent [347].

Sulindac can cause important hepatotoxicity as a hepatitic–cholestatic reaction, which may be accompanied by systemic involvement including fever and rash [287,348]. Diclofenac causes elevated serum aminotransferases in 10–15%, but it also causes severe liver injury in rare patients, usually at least 1–3 months into chronic treatment. This is typically a mixed hepatitic–cholestatic injury. Serum aminotransferases are greatly elevated, and in some cases features of the drug hypersensitivity syndrome or a "chronic active hepatitis" pattern is present. Diclofenac appears to a contingent hepatotoxin that can sometimes elicit immunoallergic features. Biotransformation via CYP3A4 and CYP2C9 can produce two quinoneimine toxic metabolites, or an arene oxide can be produced. Glucuronidated metabolites excreted into bile via MRP2 can damage the bile canalicular excretory apparatus; because it is a weak acid, it can act as an uncoupler of mitochondrial ATP production. Environmental factors that may enhance hepatotoxicity may include concurrent medication with other CYP3A4 substrates and systemic inflammatory disease [349].

Nimesulide is a recently developed selective cyclooxygenase (COX)-2 inhibitor, highly efficacious, and less likely than some NSAIDs to cause renal or gastrointestinal damage. It is related to sulfonamides. It appears to be somewhat more hepatotoxic than most other NSAIDs [350], with greater severity of liver injury. Thus far children have not been affected except an adolescent simultaneously treated with clarithromycin. Oxidative injury to mitochondria may play a role in the mechanism of hepatotoxicity [351], and genetically determined differences in hepatocellular defenses could contribute to susceptibility.

Pemoline

Pemoline, used for the treatment of attention-deficit disorders, has been associated with hepatotoxicity ranging from asymptomatic elevation of serum aminotransferases to acute liver failure [352–356]. Other cases of acute liver failure have been reported to regulatory agencies, and several children have now required liver transplantation. The drug has largely been withdrawn from the market. If pemoline is used, serum aminotransferases and other liver function tests must be followed at least monthly throughout the first year of treatment and frequently thereafter because onset of hepatotoxicity may be late in the course of treatment, possibly because it inhibits its own biotransformation. An autoimmune basis for hepatotoxicity seems unlikely. When pemoline is associated with elevated aminotransferases, it must be discontinued promptly. The usual alternative drug, methylphenidate, has also been associated with some hepatotoxicity [357].

Penicillins

Semisynthetic derivatives of penicillin have been associated with liver injury. Oxacillin has been associated with hepatitis [358]; oxacillin, cloxacillin, and flucloxacillin have all caused severe cholestasis [358–362]. Amoxicillin–clavulanic acid may pose the greatest risk of hepatotoxicity among antibiotics [363]. It has been associated with cholestasis [364] or a mixed hepatitic–cholestatic reaction [365]. Cholestatic hepatitis has been reported in one child [366]. Acute liver failure due to amoxicillin–clavulanic acid has been reported in a few adults [367]. Susceptibility may relate to human leukocyte antigen class II markers [368]. With prolonged cholestasis, the development of small portal bile duct paucity (ductopenia) has been observed [361,369]. Notably, ductopenia with severe cholestasis has been reported in a 3-year-old boy treated briefly with amoxicillin–clavulanic acid; severe progressive disease mandated liver transplantation [370].

Phenobarbital

In view of how widely phenobarbital is used, hepatitis is rare. When it occurs, it is usually associated with a multisystemic drug hypersensitivity syndrome, but liver involvement may dominate the clinical picture [371]. Of 13 patients reported in the world literature, 7 were children. Three additional children, a girl aged 3 years and boys aged 10 months and 18 months, have been treated at the Hospital for Sick Children, Toronto; all had severe hepatic dysfunction with coagulopathy or ascites but ultimately survived [372]. In most cases with clinically significant hepatotoxicity, jaundice began within 8 weeks of starting phenobarbital, along with generalized rash and fever. Eosinophilia and other systemic involvement may occur. Usually the liver disease was moderately severe but self-limited; however, two children died of fulminant hepatic failure [373]. One child developed chronic liver disease.

The mechanism of phenobarbital-induced hepatotoxicity remains unclear. Results from in vitro rechallenge of lymphocytes indicate an inherited defect in detoxification of an active metabolite. Phenobarbital may also be metabolized via arene oxide intermediates, which are typically detoxified via epoxide hydrolase. In in vitro rechallenge, if lymphocyte epoxide hydrolase is inhibited, the extent of cytotoxicity of metabolites generated from phenobarbital, as from phenytoin, increases [374]. These observations raise the possibility that defective epoxide hydrolase function may contribute to the development of phenobarbital hepatotoxicity.

Persons who develop hepatotoxicity from phenobarbital typically develop adverse reactions from other barbiturates.

Sedation for a diagnostic procedure in a child is an important opportunity for such a drug exposure. It is also important to note that persons who develop hepatitis from phenobarbital may also be likely to develop hepatitis from carbamazepine or phenytoin. It is possible that such individuals cannot detoxify the toxic metabolite(s) of phenobarbital, carbamazepine, or phenytoin [186]. Thus, substituting either of these latter anticonvulsants may worsen the hepatitis.

Phenytoin

Diphenylhydantoin has been associated with a broad range of adverse effects. Phenytoin-induced hepatitis is not infrequent in children; the incidence is estimated at 2–4 per 100,000 exposures. It was the only drug-induced hepatitis mentioned specifically among adverse drug reactions in a large prospective study of adverse drug reactions in children [1]. There are numerous cases of phenytoin hepatotoxicity reported in the literature [375,376], and an additional nine cases in children in whom hepatic dysfunction was incidental to other organ system involvement [186].

Phenytoin hepatotoxicity presents as a hepatitic process associated with a drug hypersensitivity syndrome. Aminotransferases are elevated, and the patient may be moderately jaundiced. In severe cases, clinical features of hepatic failure (coagulopathy, ascites, altered level of consciousness) are also present. The drug hypersensitivity syndrome typically includes fever, rash (such as morbilliform rash, Stevens–Johnson syndrome, or toxic epidermal necrolysis), lymphadenopathy, leukocytosis, eosinophilia, and atypical lymphocytosis. Histopathologic examination of the liver shows spotty necrosis of hepatocytes, along with features reminiscent of mononucleosis in some case or of viral hepatitis in others; cholestasis may complicate more severe hepatocellular injury; granulomas are sometimes found [377]. Reports of a diphenylhydantoin-induced cholestatic hepatitis are unconvincing. In severe cases treatment with high-dose corticosteroids has appeared effective in some patients, although this has not been tested in a controlled trial and anecdotal reports do not consistently show a clear benefit.

A toxic metabolite may be the cause of phenytoin hepatotoxicity. Phenytoin is metabolized via an arene oxide intermediate, which is ordinarily metabolized and detoxified by epoxide hydrolase [374]. This hypothesis has been investigated in vitro with lymphocytes, which are easy to isolate and retain most Phase II biotransformation pathways. When lymphocytes from persons who have developed the drug hypersensitivity syndrome to phenytoin are incubated in vitro with phenytoin and a murine microsomal system to generate the intermediate metabolites of phenytoin, these lymphocytes are killed to a greater extent than lymphocytes from normal control subjects [378]. If lymphocytes from normal individuals are pretreated with chemicals that inhibit cellular epoxide hydrolase, these lymphocytes become similar to those from affected individuals [374]. Studies of parents indicate an intermediate sensitivity to the toxic metabolite(s), consistent with an inherited defect in drug detoxification. Instead of only causing cell death, the toxic metabolite may bind to certain cellular proteins and thus create haptens for initiating an immune response. This may account for the features of a drug hypersensitivity syndrome clinically and for positive immune challenges noted by others [379]. The finding of hepatic granulomas in some patients with phenytoin hepatotoxicity corroborates the importance of immune mechanisms in this adverse reaction. Phenytoin thus appears to be a contingent hepatotoxin that is capable of eliciting an immunoallergic response.

Three of four children reported with fatal diphenylhydantoin hepatotoxicity were taking phenobarbital at the same time. The same problem has been reported when phenytoin and carbamazepine are used concurrently [191]. The potential for this cross susceptibility was established years ago by in vitro studies indicating that some patients who cannot detoxify toxic intermediates of phenytoin are similarly sensitive to phenobarbital, carbamazepine, or both. One other patient was switched from phenytoin to phenobarbital and then relapsed; he improved when high-dose corticosteroids were given along with the phenobarbital [375]. The prevalence of this cross-sensitivity is approximately 40–50% in those with intolerance for one of these antiepileptics. In general, patients experiencing hepatotoxicity from phenytoin should not be treated with phenobarbital or carbamazepine.

Phenytoin may enhance certain types of drug hepatotoxicity by interfering with glucuronidation. This problem may be most relevant to acetaminophen hepatotoxicity, but its relevance to children is still unclear [105–107].

Propylthiouracil

Hepatitis is a rare, but potentially dangerous, complication of propylthiouracil (PTU) treatment for hyperthyroidism. Several cases have been reported in children and additional children with PTU hepatotoxicity have been treated at the Hospital for Sick Children, Toronto; one child underwent liver transplantation [380–383]. PTU hepatotoxicity appears to be more frequent in girls, and overall females predominate 8:1 [383]. The clinical presentation includes nonspecific symptoms of hepatitis such as anorexia, nausea, vomiting, and jaundice. Serum aminotransferases are moderately elevated. Symptoms typically begin within 2–3 months of starting treatment, but in one child treated at the Hospital for Sick Children, Toronto, liver disease began at least 9 months after starting treatment and in two reported cases liver disease was not apparent until at least 15 months after beginning PTU [384,385]. Because asymptomatic elevation of aminotransferases may be the earliest sign of hepatotoxicity, these should be checked regularly throughout treatment. A mixture of hepatitic and cholestatic features has been reported in some adults with PTU hepatotoxicity. Liver histology shows mild to severe hepatocellular necrosis, characterized as submassive in three cases. Acute liver failure has increasingly been reported.

Several cases of PTU-associated liver disease were called "chronic active hepatitis" [386], and PTU is classified as a drug capable of causing liver injury indistinguishable from autoimmune hepatitis. Until recently, this was reported only in adults. Liver biopsy was interpreted as showing the histologic hallmark of chronic active hepatitis, piecemeal necrosis. Although the IgG and complement C3 and C4 concentrations were not reported, some patients had nonspecific autoantibodies. Thyroiditis may be an accompanying feature of autoimmune hepatitis. Given the available data, it is difficult to confirm these as true cases of drug-induced chronic active hepatitis, and the association of PTU hepatotoxicity with the chronic active hepatitis pattern in reported adult cases remains problematic. In contrast, a more convincing case of PTU hepatotoxicity associated with this chronic active hepatitis picture has been reported in one child who developed urticaria during treatment with methimazole and nonicteric hepatomegaly with elevated aminotransferases after more than 1 year of treatment with PTU [384]. Liver biopsy revealed portal inflammation and moderate piecemeal necrosis; treatment with corticosteroids and stopping the PTU led to prompt clinical improvement in the liver disease. Because neither anti–smooth muscle antibodies nor anti-LKM antibodies were positive, a drug-induced liver injury may be more likely. Because thyroid disease is more likely to accompany type 2 autoimmune hepatitis [387], the presence of anti-LKM antibodies should be sought in any child in whom PTU-induced chronic active hepatitis is suspected.

A single case of neonatal hepatitis attributed to lymphocyte sensitization during gestation while the mother was taking PTU during pregnancy has been reported [388].

Retinoids

Vitamin A taken chronically in excess is a well known cause of hepatotoxicity, with changes in hepatic stellate (Ito) cells, steatosis, and fibrosis [389]. The retinoids currently in clinical use are isotretinoin and etretinate. Severe teratogenicity has been the major adverse side effect. Hepatotoxicity associated with these compounds has been variable, generally with a hepatitic pattern, as evidenced by asymptomatic elevations in serum aminotransferases [390]. Of the two, etretinate shows greater potential for liver toxicity [391], possibly because it is more lipophilic than isotretinoin and accumulates in the liver with chronic administration. On liver biopsy, there has been variable degrees of hepatocellular necrosis; rare patients have developed cirrhosis.

Sulfonamides

Any sulfonamide can cause hepatotoxicity. Children are most commonly treated with these drugs for otitis media, upper respiratory infections, or inflammatory bowel disease. Sulfanilamide, trimethoprim-sulfamethoxazole, and pyrimethamine-sulfadoxine have all been reported as causing significant hepatotoxicity [392,393]. Sulfasalazine has been associated with severe liver disease in adolescents and young adults [394–397]. In some cases, acute, sometimes fatal, liver failure occurred [398]. The spectrum of sulfa-associated liver toxicity also includes asymptomatic elevation of serum aminotransferases [399] and granulomatous hepatitis. A bland cholestatic pattern has sometimes been reported [400]. In general, sulfa hepatotoxicity is associated with a systemic drug hypersensitivity reaction. Fever, significant rash, periorbital edema, atypical lymphocytosis, lymphadenopathy, and renal dysfunction with proteinuria all may occur. The incidence of hepatotoxicity associated with erythromycin and sulfisoxazole is not clear. Dapsone resulting in acute liver failure with typical features of the sulfa drug hypersensitivity syndrome in a child has been reported [401].

Sulfonamide hepatotoxicity is due to elaboration of an electrophilic toxic metabolite in the liver. The toxic metabolite appears to be a reactive species, possibly the nitroso, derived from the hydroxylamine metabolite of the particular sulfonamide [402,403]. Simple administration of nitroso sulfamethoxazole in a susceptible animal model does not reproduce clinical syndrome found in humans. The hydroxylamine metabolite of sulfamethoxazole has been identified in humans, and microsomes prepared from human liver specimens generate this metabolite in the presence of nicotinamide adenosine dinucleotide phosphate [404]. Some patients who developed sulfa hepatotoxicity have been shown to be slow acetylators (in the rapid/slow polymorphism for NAT-2) as well as being unable to detoxify this reactive metabolite. Upon in vitro rechallenge of their lymphocytes with sulfonamide and a metabolite-generating system, the patient's lymphocytes show significantly more cytotoxicity than control lymphocytes [392]. Glutathione appears to be important for detoxifying the toxic intermediate [405,406].

In summary, sulfonamides appear to be contingent hepatotoxins that are capable of eliciting an immunoallergic response. The pattern of hepatotoxicity is usually hepatitis or mixed hepatitic–cholestatic. The hypersensitivity features involving multiple organ systems are probably subsequent to metabolic events, in that the reactive metabolite apparently acts as a hapten to initiate the immune mechanisms. Extrahepatic metabolism may contribute to the development of the immunoallergic response [407].

Valproic Acid

Valproic acid is an eight-carbon, branched fatty acid. Its systemic and hepatic toxicity remain an important problem [408]. It causes a hepatitic reaction that takes two main forms. A certain proportion of patients, estimated at 11% [409] to 30% [318], develop abnormal serum aminotransferases usually within a short time of starting treatment. This is a dose-responsive biochemical abnormality that resolves when the dose of valproic acid is decreased. Much more rarely, patients develop progressive liver failure that may resemble Reye's syndrome clinically [410,411]. This severe form of hepatotoxicity usually does not improve when the drug is withdrawn and is frequently fatal in children [409,412–415]. It cannot be predicted by regular monitoring of serum aminotransferases and other liver function tests [416]. The time from initiating treatment with valproic acid and onset of liver disease is usually less than 4 months, but longer duration of treatment does not preclude hepatotoxicity. Severe valproic acid hepatotoxicity occurs more often in children than in adults. Specific risk factors in children include age under 2 years, multiple anticonvulsant treatment along with valproic acid, coexistent medical problems such as mental retardation, developmental delay, or congenital abnormalities. In such children the risk of fatal hepatotoxicity is 1:600 [417]. Hyperammonemia, not associated with liver failure, is another metabolic adverse effect of valproic acid and is rarely associated with encephalopathy [418,419].

The severe hepatotoxicity typically presents with a hepatitis-like prodrome, mainly malaise, anorexia, nausea, and vomiting. A noteworthy feature is that seizure control may deteriorate over the same time period. A febrile illness may appear to trigger the onset of liver failure. Coagulopathy is often present early; jaundice typically develops later, along with other signs of progressive hepatic insufficiency such as ascites and hypoglycemia. Hypoglycemia indicates a poor prognosis. Death due to liver failure, complicated by renal failure or infection, is frequent. A child with valproic acid–induced acute liver failure along with an unusual skin eruption (lichenoid dermatitis) has been reported [420]. Liver histology reviewed in one large series [412] showed hepatocellular necrosis, which may be zonal, with outright loss of hepatocytes and moribund hepatocytes remaining. Acidophilic bodies, ballooned hepatocytes, and small duct reaction may be present. Microvesicular steatosis is the most common finding overall and is often present in addition to features of cell necrosis. Hepatocellular mitochondria may be sufficiently prominent on light microscopy to make hepatocytes look granular and excessively eosinophilic. In cases presenting clinically like Reye's syndrome, fever, coagulopathy, progressive loss of consciousness, severe acidosis, and variably abnormal aminotransferases are present, but the patient is not jaundiced. Hepatocellular necrosis, as well as microvesicular fat, is found on histologic examination of the liver, unlike the characteristic histologic findings of Reye's syndrome. The succinate dehydrogenase stain, reflecting mitochondrial function, is negative in Reye's syndrome but positive in drug-induced Reye-like hepatotoxicity (Figure 20.6). On electron microscopic examination,

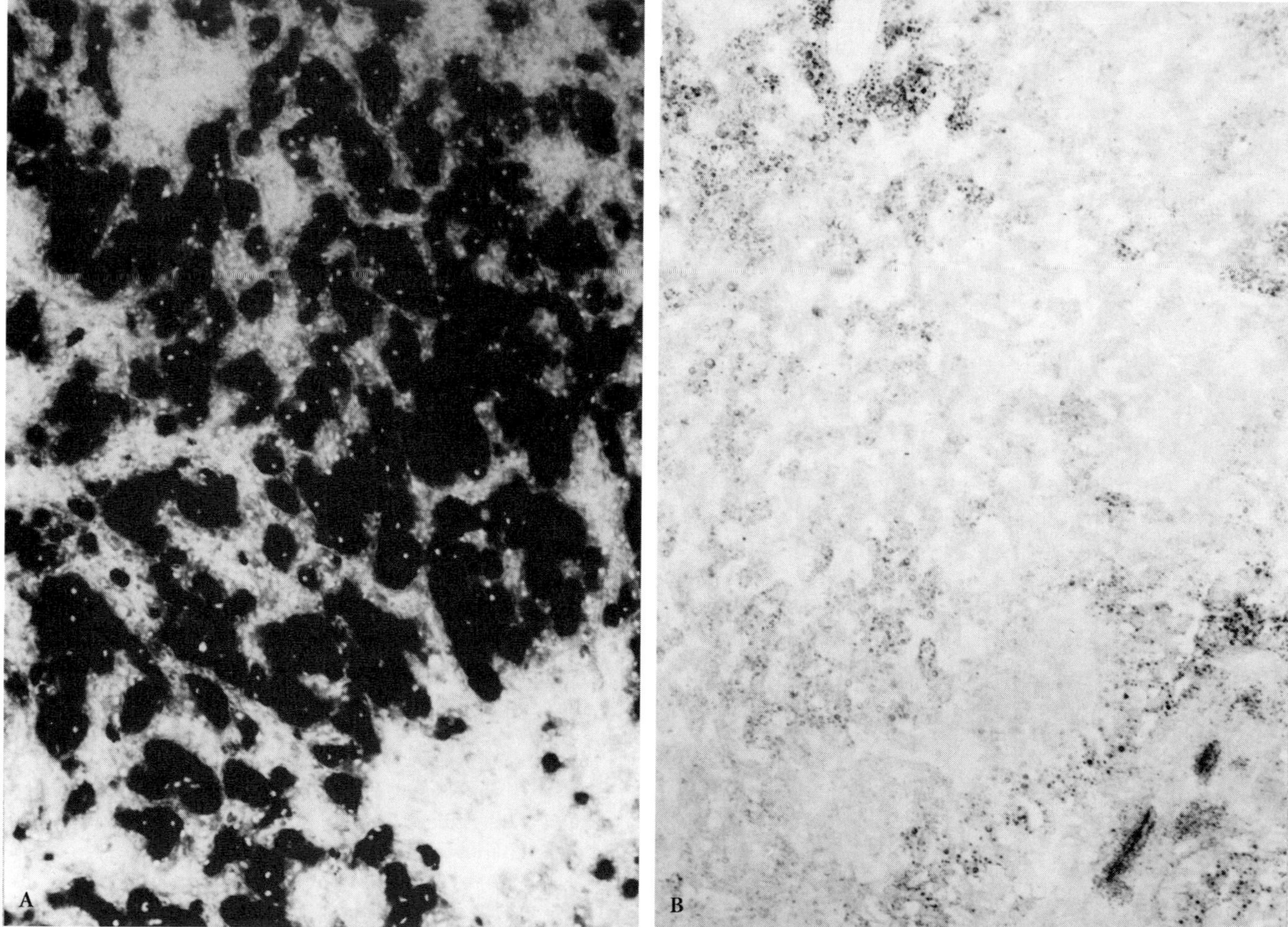

Figure 20.6. Comparison of liver biopsies processed histochemically for the mitochondrial enzyme succinic acid dehydrogenase in Reye-like hepatotoxicity due to valproic acid and in Reye's syndrome. (**A**) Liver lobule from a patient with valproic acid toxicity: note positive cytoplasmic staining indicative of normal succinic acid dehydrogenase activity (×250). (**B**) Liver lobule from a patient with Reye's syndrome: note virtual absence of staining for succinic acid dehydrogenase in that only a few hepatocytes in zones 1 and 3 show weak staining (×250). (Courtesy of Dr. M. James Phillips, Department of Pathology, the Hospital for Sick Children, Toronto.)

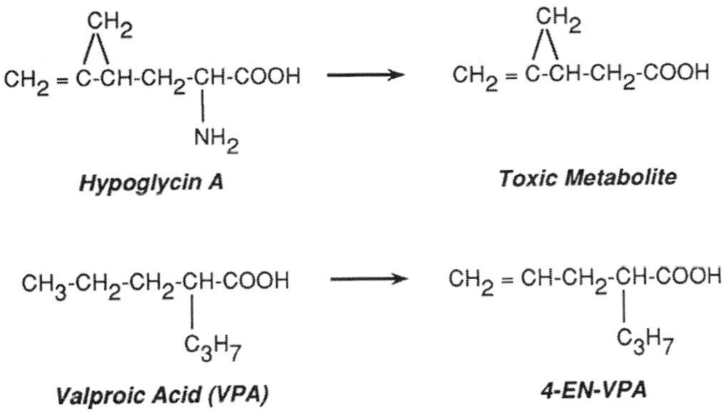

$CH_2 = C(CH_2)\text{-}CH\text{-}CH_2\text{-}CH(NH_2)\text{-}COOH$ ⟶ $CH_2 = C(CH_2)\text{-}CH\text{-}CH_2\text{-}COOH$

Hypoglycin A ⟶ ***Toxic Metabolite***

$CH_3\text{-}CH_2\text{-}CH_2\text{-}CH(C_3H_7)\text{-}COOH$ ⟶ $CH_2 = CH\text{-}CH_2\text{-}CH(C_3H_7)\text{-}COOH$

Valproic Acid (VPA) ⟶ ***4-EN-VPA***

Figure 20.7. Similarity in the chemical structures of the toxic metabolite of hypoglycin A and the metabolite of valproic acid, 4-en-valproic acid.

the mitochondrial changes associated with valproic acid hepatotoxicity differ from those of Reye's syndrome [421].

Valproic acid is extensively metabolized in the liver [422], mainly by glucuronidation. Because it is a fatty acid, valproic acid also can undergo mitochondrial or peroxisomal β-oxidation. Mitochondrial metabolism is the more important. Valproic acid passes through the mitochondrial membrane spontaneously and is converted to its coenzyme A (CoA) thioester in the mitochondrial matrix; the major product of mitochondrial metabolism, 2-propylpentanoyl-CoA, can be hydrolyzed to form valproic acid again or conjugated to carnitine and excreted [423]. Two other pathways, ω- and ω_1-hydroxylation, are via cytochromes P450.

The mechanism of severe valproic acid hepatotoxicity appears to involve generation of toxic metabolite(s) plus some type of metabolic idiosyncrasy. Metabolic idiosyncrasy is probable not only because severe hepatotoxicity is rare but because toxic ingestions do not necessarily lead to liver necrosis. Valproic acid and more specifically its partially unsaturated metabolite 4-en-valproic acid (4-en-VPA) are related structurally to two known hepatotoxins which both cause microvesicular steatosis: *hypoglycin*, responsible for Jamaican vomiting sickness, a Reye-like hepatopathy with, and *4-pentenoic acid*, which inhibits β-oxidation (Figure 20.7). Valproic acid itself is capable of inhibiting mitochondrial β-oxidation; some of its metabolites also have this effect. 4-en-VPA, which is produced by ω-oxidation, has been demonstrated in a primate model [424] and in patients with liver failure developing on valproic acid treatment [425]. Administration of 4-en-VPA to rats caused accumulation of microvesicular fat in hepatocytes, changes in hepatocyte organelles and inhibition of β-oxidation [426,427]. Both VPA and 4-en-VPA inhibit β-oxidative metabolism of the fatty acid decanoic acid whereas 4-pentenoic acid is only a weak inhibitor in this system [428]. In preliminary studies 4-en-VPA has been shown to be toxic to human cells in in vitro testing. Thus valproic acid and its metabolite(s) are capable of causing adverse changes in liver cell metabolism that may lead to observed features of this hepatotoxicity. Similarities and differences in these metabolic toxicities compared with hypoglycin and 4-pentenoic acid merely reflect the complexity of this metabolic system. Furthermore, the β-oxidation metabolite of 4-en-VPA, (*E*)-2,4-dien-VPA, may also act as a toxic intermediate. Urinary levels of thiol conjugates of 4-en-VPA and (*E*)-2,4-dien-VPA were elevated in children less than 7.5 years old receiving valproic acid monotherapy and also in older children if they were receiving treatment with an antiepileptic drug capable of inducing cytochromes P450 along with the valproic acid [429]. Concentrations of the thiol conjugates of (*E*)-2,4-dien-VPA were higher than those of 4-en-VPA.

Investigations of valproic acid metabolism in patients with severe hepatotoxicity indicate that β-oxidation is inhibited in these patients [425,430,431]; however, biochemical abnormalities consistent with inhibition of β-oxidation have also been found in children on valproic acid treatment at low risk for hepatotoxicity [432]. There is interindividual variation in the exact step in β-oxidation blocked [431]. Increased amounts of 4-en-VPA have been measured in some cases [425,433,434]. In one case, increased propylglutaric acid, the product of a cytochrome P450-associated pathway, was found, as was evidence of decreased β-oxidation [431]. These observations suggest a combination of inhibited β-oxidation and use of alternative pathways such as those associated with cytochromes P450 to produce toxic metabolites. Recent experimental evidence suggests that oxidative stress plays a secondary role [435,436].

It is likely that some people have anomalous mitochondrial β-oxidation that renders them more susceptible to adverse metabolic effects of valproic acid. An intercurrent problem, such as a viral illness, might additionally inhibit β-oxidation. If such a person were also taking drugs that strongly induce cytochromes P450 (such as phenytoin, phenobarbital, or carbamazepine), the effect of inhibiting mitochondrial β-oxidation and shunting into cytochrome P450-associated pathways would be magnified. An individual who develops severe valproic acid hepatotoxicity may not be able to make metabolic adjustments to detoxify these metabolites or subsequent toxic intermediates before significant mitochondrial damage occurs. The metabolic idiosyncrasy might thus be a functional defect in the mitochondrion itself. Experimental data in the ornithine transcarbamylase–deficient mouse support the hypothesis of an intrinsic metabolic defect in the mitochondrion. The ornithine transcarbamylase–deficient mouse develops hepatocellular necrosis and microvesicular steatosis at doses of valproic acid that do not affect the normal control adversely [437]. Ornithine transcarbamylase deficiency may be one such definable abnormality and has been suspected in some patients [438,439]. Cytochrome c oxidase deficiency appeared to predispose to valproic acid hepatotoxicity in another study [440], and valproic acid hepatotoxicity has been reported in an adult with Friedreich's ataxia [441]. The apparently high incidence of valproic acid hepatotoxicity in children with Alpers syndrome, known to be associated with abnormalities in the mitochondrial DNA polymerase, also supports the hypothesis that genetically determined mitochondrial dysfunction contributes to susceptibility to valproic acid hepatotoxicity [442–445].

In summary, valproic acid hepatotoxicity has a hepatitic pattern. The major target organelle is the hepatocellular mitochondrion. Valproic acid appears to be a contingent hepatotoxin. In the severe form of hepatotoxicity, an important pathway of biotransformation, mitochondrial β-oxidation, is inhibited, and pathways capable of producing toxic products may assume more importance quantitatively. Interindividual variation in mitochondrial function may determine susceptibility to inhibition of β-oxidation. Intrinsic metabolic defects in mitochondria may contribute to the mechanism of liver injury. Screening young patients for mitochondrial and other metabolic disorders before starting valproic acid may identify some patients with a risk of severe hepatotoxicity. Although inhibition of β-oxidation has important adverse consequences in itself, it does not appear to be sufficient to explain all the features of valproic acid hepatotoxicity. The most toxic metabolite, 4-en-VPA, inhibits β-oxidation further and probably plays an important role in causing direct cellular damage. However, the exact mechanism of valproic acid hepatotoxicity remains uncertain, and other unidentified primary and secondary metabolites may also play key roles in the cytotoxicity.

Decreased serum carnitine has been found in valproic acid hepatotoxicity [430,446]. Serum carnitine is also low in patients treated chronically, without any clinical evidence of hepatotoxicity [446–448]. Conjugation to carnitine is a minor metabolic pathway for valproic acid [449]. It is not known whether this pathway is important for the development of hepatotoxicity. Equally, the value of carnitine repletion as treatment for severe hepatotoxicity remains somewhat controversial [450]. A recent retrospective study indicated efficacy if carnitine is started very early in the course of severe hepatotoxicity [451].

Valproic acid can also cause pancreatitis in children, but it is not known whether the mechanism is the same as with liver injury [452]. It is also teratogenic.

PRINCIPLES OF TREATMENT

Once the drug responsible is stopped, most drug-induced liver disease resolves spontaneously. Severe chronic changes may not regress. However, bridging necrosis on liver biopsy does not indicate aggressive chronic liver damage in drug-induced liver disease [453]. Specific antidotes are available for some hepatotoxins, such as *N*-acetylcysteine in acetaminophen hepatotoxicity. The use of steroids in drug-induced liver disease is controversial. Steroid treatment has merit when severe acute hepatitis dominates a multisystem hypersensitivity reaction as with phenytoin, phenobarbital, or carbamazepine. The use of steroids in these circumstances may reduce mortality. The treatment of fulminant hepatic failure due to drug hepatotoxicity is otherwise essentially the same as in viral hepatitis. Liver transplantation may be necessary.

The most important question is how to diagnose drug-induced liver disease. A high index of suspicion is important. The history of the illness must be comprehensive, with detailed attention to all drugs taken, including over-the-counter and herbal preparations. Potential exposure to environmental or industrial toxins must be sought by direct questioning. The possibility of a child taking a parent's or grandparent's medication must be considered. In children, it is important to ensure that the appropriate dosage was actually given. With acetaminophen, for example, this may involve examining the actual medication bottle used and determining how the caregiver understood the dosing regimen. Liver biopsy is often informative and sometimes definitive. Electron microscopy may reveal features highly suggestive of drug hepatotoxicity. Algorithms for determining the likelihood of an adverse drug reaction [454–457] may be helpful. In vitro rechallenge of the patient's lymphocytes with generated toxic metabolites may provide important corroborative evidence [458], but this investigation remains primarily a research tool. In vitro rechallenge assays using immunologic endpoints have proved less informative.

A preemptive approach to hepatotoxicity may be possible in the near future. Methods are being developed for cell-based screening of prospective drugs. Genomic and bioinformatics technologies may also permit novel methods to identify potential hepatotoxicity early in drug development. Methods to describe an individual's pharmacogenetic profile are being considered to permit a truly individualized approach to drug therapy; avoiding drug-induced liver injury would be one goal.

SUMMARY

Drug-induced hepatotoxicity presents a wide spectrum of clinical disease. Cytotoxic processes, presenting as hepatitis, are most common, but virtually every major type of hepatic pathology can occur. Acute liver failure is an important problem with drug-induced liver injury. Hepatic drug metabolism plays an important role in hepatotoxicity in children. With many hepatotoxic drugs, an imbalance between generation of a toxic metabolite and detoxification processes can be identified. Focal defects in detoxification, frequently leading to this imbalance, may be inherited. Developmental changes in drug disposition and biotransformation add to the complexity of drug hepatotoxicity in children. Making the diagnosis of drug hepatotoxicity in children depends largely on including it in the differential diagnosis. In particular, drug-induced or environmental xenobiotic–induced hepatotoxicity should be considered when other etiologies of childhood liver disease are excluded. Children taking medications known to be hepatotoxic need close monitoring.

REFERENCES

1. Mitchell AA, Lacouture PG, Sheehan JE, et al. Adverse drug reactions in children leading to hospital admission. Pediatrics 1988;82:24–9.
2. Woods CG, Rylance ME, Cullen RE, et al. Adverse reactions to drugs in children. Br Med J 1987;294:689–90.
3. Clarkson A, Choonara I. Surveillance for fatal suspected adverse drug reactions in the UK. Arch Dis Child 2002;87:462–7.

4. Squires RH, Jr., Shneider BL, Bucuvalas J, et al. Acute liver failure in children: the first 348 patients in the pediatric acute liver failure study group. J Pediatr 2006;148:652–8.
5. Zimmerman HJ. Hepatotoxicity: the adverse effects of drugs and other chemicals on the liver. 1st ed. New York: Appleton-Century-Crofts, 1978.
6. Farrell GC. Drug induced liver disease. New York: Churchill Livingstone, 1994.
7. Kaplowitz N, DeLeve L. Drug hepatotoxicity. New York: Marcel Dekker, 2002.
8. Ingelman-Sundberg M. Human drug metabolising cytochrome P450 enzymes: properties and polymorphisms. Naunyn Schmiedebergs Arch Pharmacol 2004;369:89–104.
9. Guengerich FP. Characterization of human microsomal cytochrome P-450 enzymes. Annu Rev Pharmacol Toxicol 1989; 29:241–64.
10. Wrighton SA, Stevens JC. The human hepatic cytochromes P450 involved in drug metabolism. Crit Rev Toxicol 1992;22:1–21.
11. Whitlock JPJ. Induction of cytochrome P4501A1. Annu Rev Pharmacol Toxicol 1999;39:103–25.
12. Tirona RG, Kim RB. Nuclear receptors and drug disposition gene regulation. J Pharm Sci 2005;94:1169–86.
13. Chen Y, Kissling G, Negishi M, et al. The nuclear receptors constitutive androstane receptor and pregnane X receptor cross-talk with hepatic nuclear factor 4alpha to synergistically activate the human CYP2C9 promoter. J Pharmacol Exp Ther 2005;314:1125–33.
14. Weinshilboum R. Inheritance and drug response. N Engl J Med 2003;348:529–37.
15. Cascorbi I. Genetic basis of toxic reactions to drugs and chemicals. Toxicol Lett 2006;162:16–28.
16. Lennard MS. Genetic polymorphism of sparteine/debrisoquine oxidation: a reappraisal. Pharmacol Toxicol 1990;67:273–83.
17. Cholerton S, Daly AK, Idle JR. The role of individual human cytochromes P450 in drug metabolism and clinical response. Trends Pharmacol Sci 1992;13:434–9.
18. Murray M. P450 enzymes. Inhibition mechanisms, genetic regulation and effects of liver disease. Clin Pharmacokinet 1992; 23:132–46.
19. Butler MA, Lang NP, Young JF, et al. Determination of CYP1A2 and NAT2 phenotypes in human populations by analysis of caffeine urinary metabolites. Pharmacogenetics 1992;2:116–27.
20. Grant DM, Moerike K, Eichelbaum M, et al. Acetylation pharmacogenetics. The slow acetylator phenotype is caused by decreased or absent arylamine *N*-acetyltransferase in human liver. J Clin Invest 1990;85:968–72.
21. Blum M, Grant DM, McBride W, et al. Human *N*-acetyltransferase genes: Isolation, chromosomal localization, and functional expression. DNA Cell Biol 1990;9:193–203.
22. Glauser TA, Kerremans AL, Weinshilboum RM. Human hepatic microsomal thiol methyltransferase. Assay conditions, biochemical properties, and correlation studies. Drug Metab Dispos 1992;20:247–55.
23. Burchell B, Soars M, Monaghan G, et al. Drug-mediated toxicity caused by genetic deficiency of UDP-glucuronosyltransferases. Toxicol Lett 2000;112–113:333–40.
24. Stoner E, Starkman H, Wellner D, et al. Biochemical studies of a patient with hereditary hepatorenal tyrosinemia: evidence of a glutathione deficiency. Pediatr Res 1984;18:1332–6.
25. Moldeus P, Quanguan J. Importance of the glutathione cycle in drug metabolism. Pharmacol Ther 1987;33:37–40.
26. Reed DJ. Glutathione: Toxicological implications. Annu Rev Pharmacol Toxicol 1990;30:603–31.
27. Oesch F. Significance of various enzymes in the control of reactive metabolites. Arch Toxicol 1987;60:174–8.
28. Hines RN, McCarver DG. The ontogeny of human drug-metabolizing enzymes: phase I oxidative enzymes. J Pharmacol Exp Ther 2002;300:355–60.
29. Ikeda T, Altieri M, Chen Y-T, et al. Characterization of cytochrome P_2-450 (20S) mRNA: association with the P_1-450 genomca gene and differential response to the inducers 3-methylcholanthrene and isosafrole. Eur J Biochem 1983;134:13–18.
30. Giachelli CM, Omiecinski CJ. Developmental regulation of cytochrome P-450 genes in the rat. Mol Pharmacol 1987;31:477–84.
31. Corada M, Bortolottie A, Barzago MM, et al. Pharmacokinetic profile of theophylline in isolated perfused liver of rabbits at different ages. Development of drug-metabolizing activity during ontogenesis. Drug Metab Dispos 1992;20:826–31.
32. Cresteil T, Beaune PH, Kremers P, et al. Immunoquantitation of epoxide hydrolase and cytochrome P-450 isozynes in fetal and adult human liver microsomes. Eur J Biochem 1985;151:345–50.
33. Shimada T, Misono KS, Gungerich FP. Human liver microsomal cytochrome P-450 mephenytoin 4-hydroxylase, a probable genetic polymorphism in oxidative drug metabolism. Purification and characterization of two similar forms involved in the reaction. J Biol Chem 1986;261:909–21.
34. Ratanasavanh D, Beaune P, Morel F, et al. Intralobular distribution and quantitation of cytochrome P-450 enzymes in human liver as a function of age. Hepatology 1991;13:1142–51.
35. Treluyer JM, Gueret G, Cheron G, et al. Developmental expression of CYP2C and CYP2C-dependent activities in the human liver: in-vivo/in-vitro correlation and inducibility. Pharmacogenetics 1997;7:441–52.
36. Koukouritaki SB, Manro JR, Marsh SA, et al. Developmental expression of human hepatic CYP2C9 and CYP2C19. J Pharmacol Exp Ther 2004;308:965–74.
37. Treluyer J-M, Jacqz-Aigran E, Alvarez F, et al. Expression of CYP2D6 in developing human liver. Eur J Biochem 1991;202: 583–8.
38. Sonnier M, Cresteil T. Delayed ontogenesis of CYP1A2 in the human liver. Eur J Biochem 1998;251:893–8.
39. Wrighton SA, Molowa DT, Guzelian PS. Identification of a cytochrome P-450 in human fetal liver related to glucocorticoid inducible cytochrome P-450HLp in the adult. Biochem Pharmacol 1988;37:3053–5.
40. Wrighton SA, VandenBranden M. Isolation and characterization of human fetal liver cytochrome P450HLp2: a third member of the P450III gene family. Arch Biochem Biophys 1989;268: 144–51.
41. Lacroix D, Sonnier M, Moncion A, et al. Expression of CYP3A in the human liver – evidence that the shift between CYP3A7 and CYP3A4 occurs immediately after birth. Eur J Biochem 1997;247:625–34.
42. Vyhlidal CA, Gaedigk R, Leeder JS. Nuclear receptor expression in fetal and pediatric liver: correlation with CYP3A expression. Drug Metab Dispos 2006;34:131–7.
43. Johnsrud EK, Koukouritaki SB, Divakaran K, et al. Human hepatic CYP2E1 expression during development. J Pharmacol Exp Ther 2003;307:402–7.
44. Aldridge A, Aranda JV, Neims AH. Caffeine metabolism in the newborn. Clin Pharmacol Ther 1979;25:447–53.

45. Pons G, Carrier O, Richard M-O, et al. Developmental changes of caffeine elimination in infancy. Dev Pharamcol Ther 1988;11: 258–64.
46. Aranda JV, Sitar DS, Parsons WD, et al. Pharmacokinetic aspects of theophylline in premature newborns. N Engl J Med 1976;295:413–16.
47. Painter MJ, Pippinger C, MacDonald H, et al. Phenobarbital and diphenylhydantoin levels in neonates with seizures. J Pediatr 1978;92:315–19.
48. Loughnan PM, Greenwald A, Purton WW, et al. Pharmacokinetic observations of phenytoin disposition in the newborn and young infant. Arch Dis Child 1977;52:302–9.
49. Jaeger-Roman E, Rating D, Platzek T, et al. Development of N-demethylase activity measured with the ^{13}C-aminopyrine breath test. Eur J Pediatr 1982;139:129–31.
50. Treluyer JM, Rey E, Sonnier M, et al. Evidence of impaired cisapride metabolism in neonates. Br J Clin Pharmacol 2001;52: 419–25.
51. Tateishi T, Nakura H, Asoh M, et al. A comparison of hepatic cytochrome P450 protein expression between infancy and postinfancy. Life Sci 1997;61:2567–74.
52. Aranda JV, Collinge JM, Zinman R, et al. Maturation of caffeine elimination in infancy. Arch Dis Child 1979;54:946–9.
53. Lambert GH, Schoeller DA, Kotake AN, et al. The effect of age, gender, and sexual maturationon the caffeine breath test. Dev Pharmacol Ther 1986;9:375–88.
54. Miller RP, Roberts RJ, Fischer LF. Acetaminophen elimination kinetics in neonates, children and adults. Clin Pharmacol Ther 1976;19:284–94.
55. Di Ilio C, Del Boccio G, Casalone E, et al. Activities of enzymes associated with the metabolism of glutathione in fetal rat liver and placenta. Biol Neonate 1986;49:96–101.
56. Langley SC, Kelly FJ. Differing response of the glutathione system to fasting in neonatal and adult guinea pigs. Biochem Pharmacol 1992;44:1489–94.
57. Hales BF, Neims AH. Developmental aspects of glutathione S-transferase B (ligandin) in rat liver. Biochem J 1976;160:231–6.
58. Ballatori N, CLarkson TW. Developmental changes in the biliary excretion of methylmercury and glutathione. Science 1982; 216:61–2.
59. Zoltan G, Stein AF, Klaassen CD. Age-dependent biliary excretion of glutathione-related thiols in rats: role of gamma-glutamyltranspeptidase. Am J Physiol 1987;16:G86–92.
60. Loeper J, Descatoire V, Maurice M, et al. Cytochromes P-450 in human hepatocyte plasma membrane: Recognition by several autoantibodies. Gastroenterology 1993;104:203–16.
61. Benichou C. Criteria of drug induced liver disorders: report of an international consensus meeting. J Hepatol 1990;11:272–6.
62. Jaeschke H, Gores GJ, Cederbaum AI, et al. Mechanisms of hepatotoxicity. Toxicol Sci 2002;65:166–76.
63. James LP, Farrar HC, Darville TL, et al. Elevation of serum interleukin 8 levels in acetaminophen overdose in children and adolescents. Clin Pharmacol Ther 2001;70:280–6.
64. Ju C, Reilly TP, Bourdi M, et al. Protective role of Kupffer cells in acetaminophen-induced hepatic injury in mice. Chem Res Toxicol 2002;15:1504–13.
65. Aithal GP, Ramsay L, Daly AK, et al. Hepatic adducts, circulating antibodies, and cytokine polymorphisms in patients with diclofenac hepatotoxicity. Hepatology 2004;39:1430–40.
66. Makin AJ, Wendon J, Williams R. A 7-year experience of severe acetaminophen-induced hepatotoxicity (1987–1993). Gastroenterology 1995;109:1907–16.
67. Smilkstein MJ, Knapp GL, Kulig KW, et al. Efficacy of oral N-acetylcysteine in the treatment of acetaminophen overdose. N Engl J Med 1988;319:1557–62.
68. Harrison PM, Keays R, Bray GP, et al. Improved outcome of paracetamol-induced fulminant hepatic failure by late administration of acetylcysteine. Lancet 1990;335:1572–3.
69. Keays R, Harrison PM, Wendon JA, et al. Intravenous acetylcysteine in paracetamol induced fulminant hepatic failure: a prospective controlled trial. BMJ 1991;303:1026–9.
70. Mutimer DJ, Ayres RCS, Neuberger JM, et al. Serious paracetamol poisoning and the results of liver transplantation. Gut 1994;35:809–14.
71. Heubi JE, Barbacci MB, Zimmerman HJ. Therapeutic misadventures with acetaminophen: hepatoxicity after multiple doses in children. J Pediatr 1998;132:22–7.
72. Rivera-Penera T, Gugig R, Davis J, et al. Outcome of acetaminophen overdose in pediatric patients and factors contributing to hepatotoxicity. J Pediatr 1997;130:300–4.
73. Anderson BD, Shepherd JG, Klein-Schwartz W. Outcome of acetaminophen overdose. J Pediatr 1998;132:1080.
74. Pershad J, Nichols M, King W. "The silent killer": chronic acetaminophen toxicity in a toddler. Pediatr Emerg Care 1999;15: 43–6.
75. Shaoul R, Novikov J, Maor I, et al. Silent acetaminophen-induced hepatotoxicity in febrile children: does this entity exist? Acta Paediatr 2004;93:618–22.
76. Roberts DW, Bucci TJ, Benson RW, et al. Immunohistochemical localization and quantification of the 3-(cystein-S-yl)-acetaminophen protein adduct in acetaminophen hepatotoxicity. Am J Pathol 1991;138:359–71
77. Webster PA, Roberts DW, Benson RW, et al. Acetaminophen toxicity in children: diagnostic confirmation using a specific antigenic biomarker. J Clin Pharmacol 1996;36:397–402.
78. Mitchell JR, Jollow DJ, Potter WZ, et al. Acetaminophen-induced hepatic necrosis. I. Role of drug metabolism. J Pharmacol Exp Ther 1973;187:185–94.
79. Jollow DJ, Mitchell JR, Potter WZ, et al. Acetaminophen-induced hepatic necrosis. II. Role of covalent binding in vivo. J Pharmacol Exp Ther 1973;187:195–202.
80. Potter WZ, Davis DC, Mitchell JR, et al. Acetaminophen-induced hepatic necrosis. III. Cytochrome P-450-mediated covalent binding *in vitro*. J Pharmacol Exp Ther 1973;187:203–10.
81. Mitchell JR, Jollow DJ, Potter WZ, et al. Acetaminophen-induced hepatic necrosis. IV. Protective role of glutathione. J Pharmacol Exp Ther 1973;187:211–17.
82. Thummel KE, Lee CA, Kunze KL, et al. Oxidation of acetaminophen to N-acetyl-p-aminobenzoquinone imine by human CYP3A4. Biochem Pharmacol 1993;45:1563–9.
83. Miner DJ, Kissinger PT. Evidence for the involvement of *N*-acetyl-*p*-quinoneimine in acetaminophen metabolism. Biochem Pharmacol 1979;28:3285–90.
84. Jaeschke H, Knight TR, Bajt ML. The role of oxidant stress and reactive nitrogen species in acetaminophen hepatotoxicity. Toxicol Lett 2003;144:279–88.
85. Goldring CE, Kitteringham NR, Elsby R, et al. Activation of hepatic Nrf2 in vivo by acetaminophen in CD-1 mice. Hepatology 2004;39:1267–76.

86. Corcoran GB, Racz WJ, Smith CV, et al. Effects of N-acetylcysteine on acetaminophen covalent binding and hepatic necrosis in mice. J Pharmacol Exp Ther 1985;232:864–72.
87. Harrison PM, Wendon JA, Gimson AES, et al. Improvement by acetylcysteine of hemodynamics and oxygen transport in fulminant hepatic failure. New Engl J Med 1991;324:1852–7.
88. Peterson RG, Rumack BH. Age as a variable in acetaminophen overdose. Arch Intern Med 1981;141:390–3.
89. Meredith TJ, Newman B, Goulding R. Paracetamol poisoning in children. Br Med J 1978;2:478–9.
90. Rumack BH. Acetaminophen overdose in young children. Treatment and effects of alcohol and other additional ingestants in 417 cases. Am J Dis Child 1984;138:428–33.
91. Peterson RG, Rumack BH. Pharmacokinetics of acetaminophen in children. Pediatrics 1978;62:877–9.
92. Lederman S, Fysh WJ, Tredger M, et al. Neonatal paracetamol poisoning: treatment by exchange transfusion. Arch Dis Child 1983;58:631–3.
93. Roberts I, Robinson MJ, Mughal MZ, et al. Paracetamol metabolites in the neonate following maternal overdose. Br J Clin Pharmacol 1984;18:201–6.
94. Rollins DE, Von Bahr C, Glaumann H, et al. Acetaminophen: Potentially toxic metabolites formed by human fetal and adult liver microsomes and isolated fetal liver cells. Science 1979; 205:1414–16.
95. Arena JM, Rourk MH, Jr., Sibrack CD. Acetaminophen: Report of an unusual poisoning. Pediatrics 1978;61:68–72.
96. Lieh-Lai MW, Sarnaik AP, Newton JF, et al. Metabolism and pharmacokinetics of acetaminophen in a severely poisoned young child. J Pediatr 1984;105:125–8.
97. Hickson GB, Altemeier WA, Martin ED, et al. Parental administration of chemical agents: a cause of apparent life threatening events. J Pediatr 1989;83:772–6.
98. Tonge RP, Kelly EJ, Bruschi SA, et al. Role of CYP1A2 in the hepatotoxicity of acetaminophen: investigations using Cyp1a2 null mice. Toxicol Appl Pharmacol 1998;153:102–8.
99. Seeff LB, Cuccherini BA, Zimmerman HJ, et al. Acetaminophen hepatotoxicity in alcoholics. A therapeutic misadventure. Ann Intern Med 1986;104:399–404.
100. Raucy JL, Lasker JM, Lieber CS, et al. Acetaminophen activation by human liver cytochromes P450IIE1 and P4501A2. Arch Biochem Biophys 1989,271:270–83.
101. Sarich T, Kalhorn T, Magee S, et al. The effect of omeprazole pretreatment on acetaminophen metabolism in rapid and slow metabolizers of S-mephenytoin. Clin Pharmacol Ther 1997;62: 21–8.
102. Brackett CC, Bloch JD. Phenytoin as a possible cause of acetaminophen hepatotoxicity: case report and review of the literature. Pharmacotherapy 2000;20:229–33.
103. Zwiener RJ, Kurt TL, Day LC, et al. Potentiation of acetaminophen hepatotoxicity in a child with mercury poisoning. J Pediatr Gastroenterol Nutr 1994;19:242–5.
104. Shriner K, Goetz MB. Severe hepatotoxicity in a patient receiving both acetaminophen and zidovudine. Am J Med 1992;93: 94–6.
105. Suchin SM, Wolf DC, Lee Y, et al. Potentiation of acetaminophen hepatotoxicity by phenytoin, leading to liver transplantation. Dig Dis Sci 2005;50:1836–8.
106. Kostrubsky SE, Sinclair JF, Strom SC, et al. Phenobarbital and phenytoin increased acetaminophen hepatotoxicity due to inhibition of UDP-glucuronosyltransferases in cultured human hepatocytes. Toxicol Sci 2005;87:146–55.
107. Mutlib AE, Goosen TC, Bauman JN, et al. Kinetics of acetaminophen glucuronidation by UDP-glucuronosyltransferases 1A1, 1A6, 1A9 and 2B15. Potential implications in acetaminophen-induced hepatotoxicity. Chem Res Toxicol 2006;19:701–9.
108. De Morais SMF, Wells PG. Deficiency in bilirubin UDP-glucuronyl transferase as a genetic determinant of acetaminophen toxicity. J Pharmacol Exp Ther 1988;247:323–31.
109. Bruun LS, Elkjaer S, Bitsch-Larsen D, et al. Hepatic failure in a child after acetaminophen and sevoflurane exposure. Anesth Analg 2001;92:1446–8.
110. Poucell S, Ireton J, Valencia-Mayoral P, et al. Amiodarone-associated phospholipidosis of the liver. Light, immunohistochemical and electron microscopic studies. Gastroenterology 1984;86:926–36.
111. Shepherd NA, Dawson AM, Crocker PR, et al. Granular cells as a marker of early amiodarone hepatotoxicity: a pathological and analytical study. J Clin Pathol 1987;40:418–23.
112. Lewis JH, Ranard RC, Caruso A, et al. Amiodarone hepatotoxicity: prevalence and clinicopatholic correlations among 104 patients. Hepatology 1989;9:679–85.
113. Somani P, Bandyopadhyay S, Klaunig JE, et al. Amiodarone- and desethylamiodarone-induced myelinoid inclusion bodies and toxicity in cultured rat hepatocytes. Hepatology 1990;11:81–92.
114. Geneve J, Zafrani ES, Dhumeaux D. Amiodarone induced liver disease. J Hepatol 1989;9:130–3.
115. Chang CC, Petrelli M, Tomashefski JF, Jr., et al. Severe intrahepatic cholestasis caused by amiodarone toxicity after withdrawal of the drug: a case report and review of the literature. Arch Pathol Lab Med 1999;123:251–6.
116. Yagupsky P, Gazala E, Sofer S. Fatal hepatic failure and encephalopathy associated with amiodarone therapy. J Pediatr 1985;107:967–70.
117. Pollak PT, Sharma AD, Carruthers SG. Relation of amiodarone hepatic and pulmonary toxicity to serum drug concentrations and superoxide dismutase activity. Am J Cardiol 1990;65:1185–91.
118. Bravo AE, Drewe J, Schlienger RG, et al. Hepatotoxicity during rapid intravenous loading with amiodarone: description of three cases and review of the literature. Crit Care Med 2005; 33:128–34; discussion 245–6.
119. Menard DB, Gisselbrecht C, Marty H, et al. Antineoplastic agents and the liver. Gastroenterology 1980;78:142–64.
120. Perry MC. Hepatotoxicity of chemotherapeutic agents. Sem Oncol 1982;9:65–74.
121. Sznol M, Ohnuma T, Holland JF. Hepatic toxicity of drugs used for hematologic neoplasia. Sem Liver Dis 1987;7:237–56.
122. Shanholtz C. Acute life-threatening toxicity of cancer treatment. Crit Care Clin 2001;17:483–502.
123. Pratibha R, Sameer R, Rataboli PV, et al. Enzymatic studies of cisplatin induced oxidative stress in hepatic tissue of rats. Eur J Pharmacol 2006;532:290–3.
124. Lu Y, Cederbaum AI. Cisplatin-induced hepatotoxicity is enhanced by elevated expression of cytochrome P450 2E1. Toxicol Sci 2006;89:515–23.
125. Honjo I, Suou T, Hirayama C. Hepatotoxicity of cyclophosphamide in man: pharmacokinetic analysis. Res Commun Chem Pathol Pharmacol 1988;61:149–65.

126. Berkovitch M, Matsui D, Zipursky A, et al. Hepatotoxicity of 6-mercaptopurine in childhood acute lymphocytic leukemia: pharmacokinetic characteristics. Med Pediatr Oncol 1996;26: 85–9.
127. Hazar V, Kutluk T, Akyuz C, et al. Veno-occlusive disease-like hepatotoxicity in two children receiving chemotherapy for Wilms' tumor and clear cell sarcoma of kidney. Pediatr Hematol Oncol 1998;15:85–9.
128. Ludwig R, Weirich A, Abel U, et al. Hepatotoxicity in patients treated according to the nephroblastoma trial and study SIOP-9/GPOH. Med Pediatr Oncol 1999;33:462–9.
129. Flentje M, Weirich A, Potter R, et al. Hepatotoxicity in irradiated nephroblastoma patients during postoperative treatment according to SIOP9/GPOH. Radiother Oncol 1994;31:222–8.
130. Bisogno G, de Kraker J, Weirich A, et al. Veno-occlusive disease of the liver in children treated for Wilms tumor. Med Pediatr Oncol 1997;29:245–51.
131. Topley J, Benson J, Squier MV, et al. Hepatotoxicity in the treatment of acute lymphoblastic leukemia. Med Pediatr Oncol 1979;7:393–9.
132. Pratt CB, Johnson WW. Duration and severity of fatty metamorphosis of the liver following L-asparaginase therapy. Cancer 1971;28:361–4.
133. Sahoo S, Hart J. Histopathological features of L-asparaginase-induced liver disease. Semin Liver Dis 2003;23:295–9.
134. Hruban RH, Sternberg SS, Meyers P, et al. Fatal thrombocytopenia and liver failure associated with carboplatin therapy. Cancer Invest 1991;9:263–8.
135. Penta JS, Van Hoff DD, Muggia FM. Hepatotoxicity of combination chemotherapy for acute myelocytic leukemia. Ann Intern Med 1977;87:247–8.
136. Rollins BJ. Hepatic veno-occlusive disease. Am J Med 1986;81: 297–306.
137. D'Antiga L, Baker A, Pritchard J, et al. Veno-occlusive disease with multi-organ involvement following actinomycin-D. Eur J Cancer 2001;37:1141–8.
138. Barker CC, Anderson RA, Sauve RS, et al. GI complications in pediatric patients post-BMT. Bone Marrow Transplant 2005;36:51–8.
139. Sulis ML, Bessmertny O, Granowetter L, et al. Veno-occlusive disease in pediatric patients receiving actinomycin D and vincristine only for the treatment of rhabdomyosarcoma. J Pediatr Hematol Oncol 2004;26:843–6.
140. Elli M, Pinarli FG, Dagdemir A, et al. Veno-occlusive disease of the liver in a child after chemotherapy for brain tumor. Pediatr Blood Cancer 2006;46:521–3.
141. Berk PD, Popper H, Krueger GF, et al. Veno-occlusive disease of the liver after allogeneic bone marrow transplantation. Possible association with graft-versus-host disease. Ann Intern Med 1979;90:158–64.
142. Beschorner WE, Pino J, Boitnott JK, et al. Pathology of the liver with bone marrow transplantation. Effects of busulfan, carmustine, acute graft-versus-host disease, and cytomegalovirus infection. Am J Pathol 1980;99:369–86.
143. Fajardo LF, Colby TV. Pathogenesis of veno-occlusive disease after radiation. Arch Pathol Lab Med 1980;104:584–8.
144. McDonald GB, Sharma P, Matthews DE, et al. The clinical course of 53 patients with veno-occlusive disease of the liver after marrow transplantation. Transplantation 1985;39:603–8.
145. Essell JH, Thompson JM, Harman GS, et al. Marked increase in veno-occlusive disease of the liver associated with methotrexate use for graft-versus-host disease prophylaxis in patients receiving busulfan/cyclophosphamide. Blood 1992;79:2784–8.
146. McDonald GB, Slattery JT, Bouvier ME, et al. Cyclophosphamide metabolism, liver toxicity, and mortality following hematopoietic stem cell transplantation. Blood 2003;101:2043–8.
147. El-Sayed MH, El-Haddad A, Fahmy OA, et al. Liver disease is a major cause of mortality following allogeneic bone-marrow transplantation. Eur J Gastroenterol Hepatol 2004;16:1347–54.
148. Srivastava A, Poonkuzhali B, Shaji RV, et al. Glutathione S-transferase M1 polymorphism: a risk factor for hepatic venoocclusive disease in bone marrow transplantation. Blood 2004;104:1574–7.
149. Stoneham S, Lennard L, Coen P, et al. Veno-occlusive disease in patients receiving thiopurines during maintenance therapy for childhood acute lymphoblastic leukaemia. Br J Haematol 2003;123:100–2.
150. Reiss U, Cowan M, McMillan A, et al. Hepatic venoocclusive disease in blood and bone marrow transplantation in children and young adults: incidence, risk factors, and outcome in a cohort of 241 patients. J Pediatr Hematol Oncol 2002;24:746–50.
151. Ravikumara M, Hill FG, Wilson DC, et al. 6-Thioguanine-related chronic hepatotoxicity and variceal haemorrhage in children treated for acute lymphoblastic leukaemia-a dual-centre experience. J Pediatr Gastroenterol Nutr 2006;42:535–8.
152. Corbacioglu S, Greil J, Peters C, et al. Defibrotide in the treatment of children with veno-occlusive disease (VOD): a retrospective multicentre study demonstrates therapeutic efficacy upon early intervention. Bone Marrow Transplant 2004;33:189–95.
153. Shin-Nakai N, Ishida H, Yoshihara T, et al. Control of hepatic veno-occlusive disease with an antithrombin-III concentrate-based therapy. Pediatr Int 2006;48:85–7.
154. Ringden O, Remberger M, Lehmann S, et al. N-acetylcysteine for hepatic veno-occlusive disease after allogeneic stem cell transplantation. Bone Marrow Transplant 2000;25:993–6.
155. Shulman HM, Gown AM, Nugent DJ. Hepatic veno-occlusive disease after bone marrow transplantation. Immunohistochemical identification of the material within occluded central venules. Am J Pathol 1987;127:549–58.
156. Shulman HM, Fisher LB, Schoch HG, et al. Veno-occlusive disease pf the liver after marrow transplantation: histological correlates of clinical signs and symptoms. Hepatology 1994;19:1171–81.
157. DeLeve LD. Dacarbazine toxicity in murine liver cells: a model of hepatic endothelial injury and glutathione defense. J Pharmacol Exp Ther 1994;268:1261–70.
158. DeLeve LD. Cellular target of cyclophosphamide toxicity in the murine liver: role of glutathione and site of metabolic activation. Hepatology 1996;24:830–7.
159. DeLeve LD, McCuskey RS, Wang X, et al. Characterization of a reproducible rat model of hepatic veno-occlusive disease. Hepatology 1999;29:1779–91.
160. Wang X, Kanel GC, DeLeve LD. Support of sinusoidal endothelial cell glutathione prevents hepatic veno-occlusive disease in the rat. Hepatology 2000;31:428–34.
161. DeLeve LD, Wang X, Kanel GC, et al. Decreased hepatic nitric oxide production contributes to the development of rat sinusoidal obstruction syndrome. Hepatology 2003;38:900–8.
162. Iguchi A, Kobayashi R, Yoshida M, et al. Vascular endothelial growth factor (VEGF) is one of the cytokines causative and predictive of hepatic veno-occlusive disease (VOD) in stem cell transplantation. Bone Marrow Transplant 2001;27:1173–80.

163. Geller SA, Dubinsky MC, Poordad FF, et al. Early hepatic nodular hyperplasia and submicroscopic fibrosis associated with 6-thioguanine therapy in inflammatory bowel disease. Am J Surg Pathol 2004;28:1204–11.
164. Benson GD. Hepatotoxicity following the therapeutic use of antipyretic analgesics. Am J Med 1983;75:85–93.
165. Freeland GR, Northington RS, Hedrich DA, et al. Hepatic safety of two analgesics used over the counter: ibuprofen and aspirin. Clin Pharmacol Ther 1988;43:473–9.
166. Parke DV. Activation mechanisms to chemical toxicity. Arch Toxicol 1987;60:5–15.
167. Chen TC, Ng KF, Jeng LB, et al. Aspirin-related hepatotoxicity in a child after liver transplant. Dig Dis Sci 2001;46:486–8.
168. Doughty R, Giesecke L, Athreya B. Salicylate therapy in juvenile rheumatoid arthritis. Am J Dis Child 1980;134:461–3.
169. Barron KS, Person DA, Brewer EJ. The toxicity of non-steroidal anti-inflammatory drugs in juvenile rheumatoid arthritis. J Rheumatol 1982;9:149–55.
170. Hamdan JA, Manasra K, Ahmed M. Salicylate-induced hepatitis in rheumatic fever. Am J Dis Child 1985;139:453–5.
171. Ulshen MH, Grand RJ, Crain JD, et al. Hepatotoxicity with encephalopathy associated with aspirin therapy in rheumatoid arthritis. J Pediatr 1978;93:1034–7.
172. Petty BG, Zahka KG, Bernstein MT. Aspirin hepatitis associated with encephalopathy. J Pediatr 1978;93:881–2.
173. DePinho RA, Goldberg CS, Lefkowitch JH. Azathioprine and the liver. Evidence favoring idiosyncratic, mixed cholestatic-hepatocellular injury in humans. Gastroenterology 1984;86: 162–5.
174. Jeurissen ME, Boerbooms AM, van de Putte LB, et al. Azathioprine induced fever, chills, rash, and hepatotoxicity in rheumatoid arthritis. Ann Rheum Dis 1990;49:25–7.
175. Sterneck M, Wiesner R, Ascher N, et al. Azathioprine hepatotoxicity after liver transplantation. Hepatology 1991;14:806–10.
176. Duvoux C, Kracht M, Lang P, et al. Hyperplasie nodulaire régénérative du foie associée à la prise d'azathioprine. Gastroenterol Clin Biol 1991;15:968–73.
177. Seiderer J, Zech CJ, Diebold J, et al. Nodular regenerative hyperplasia: a reversible entity associated with azathioprine therapy. Eur J Gastroenterol Hepatol 2006;18:553–5.
178. Lennard L. The clinical pharmacology of 6-mercaptopurine. Eur J Clin Pharmacol 1992;43:329–39.
179. Fraser AG, Orchard TR, Robinson EM, et al. Long-term risk of malignancy after treatment of inflammatory bowel disease with azathioprine. Aliment Pharmacol Ther 2002;16:1225–32.
180. Navarro JT, Ribera JM, Mate JL, et al. Hepatosplenic T-gamma-delta lymphoma in a patient with Crohn's disease treated with azathioprine. Leuk Lymphoma 2003;44:531–3.
181. Mitchell MC, Boitnott JK, Arregui A, et al. Granulomatous hepatitis associated with carbamazepine therapy. Am J Med 1981;71:733–5.
182. Williams SJ, Ruppin DC, Grierson JM, et al. Carbamazepine hepatitis: the clinicopathological spectrum. J Gastroenterol Hepatol 1986;1:159–68.
183. Ramos AM, Gayotto LC, Clemente CM, et al. Reversible vanishing bile duct syndrome induced by carbamazepine. Eur J Gastroenterol Hepatol 2002;14:1019–22.
184. Lewis IJ, Rosenbloom L. Glandular fever-like syndrome, pulmonary eosinophilia and asthma associated with carbamazepine. Postgrad Med J 1982;58:100–1.
185. Brain C, MacArdle B, Levin S. Idiosyncratic reactions to carbamazepine mimicking viral infection in children. Br Med J 1984;289:354.
186. Shear NH, Spielberg SP. Anticonvulsant hypersensitivity syndrome. In vitro assessment of risk. J Clin Invest 1988;82:1826–32.
187. Zucker P, Daum F, Cohen MI. Fatal carbamazepine hepatitis. J Pediatr 1977;91:667–8.
188. Smith DW, Cullity GJ, Silberstein EP. Fatal hepatic necrosis associated with multiple anticonvulsant therapy. Aust N Z J Med 1988;18:575–81.
189. Hadzic N, Portmann B, Davies ET, et al. Acute liver failure induced by carbamazepine. Arch Dis Child 1990;65:315–17.
190. Morales-Diaz M, Pinilla-Roa E, Ruiz I. Suspected carbamazepine-induced hepatotoxicity. Pharmacotherapy 1999;19:252–5.
191. Sierra NM, Garcia B, Marco J, et al. Cross hypersensitivity syndrome between phenytoin and carbamazepine. Pharm World Sci 2005;27:170–4.
192. Perino LE, Warren GH, Levine JS. Cocaine-induced hepatotoxicity in humans. Gastroenterology 1987;93:176–80.
193. Wanless IR, Dore S, Gopinath G, et al. Histopathology of cocaine hepatotoxicity. Report of four cases. Gastroenterology 1990;98:497–501.
194. Gottfried MR, Kloss MW, Graham D, et al. Ultrastructure of experimental cocaine hepatotoxicity. Hepatology 1986;6:299–304.
195. Boelsterli UA, Goldlin C. Biomechanisms of cocaine-induced hepatocyte injury mediated by the formation of reactive metabolites. Arch Toxicol 1991;65:351–60.
196. Pellinen P, Honkakoshi P, Stenback F, et al. Cocaine N-demethylation and the metabolism-related hepatotoxicity can be prevented by cytochrome P450 3A inhibitors. Eur J Pharmacol 1994;270:35–43.
197. Jover R, Ponsoda X, Gomez-Lechon MJ, et al. Potentiation of cocaine hepatotoxicity by ethanol in human hepatocytes. Toxicol Appl Pharmacol 1991;107:526–34.
198. Ponsoda X, Jover R, Castell JV, et al. Potentiation of cocaine hepatotoxicity in human hepatocytes by ethanol. Toxicol In Vitro 1992;6:155–8.
199. Labib R, Turkall R, Abdel-Rahman MS. Endotoxin potentiates cocaine-mediated hepatotoxicity by nitric oxide and reactive oxygen species. Int J Toxicol 2003;22:305–16.
200. Kronbach T, Fischer V, Meyer UA. Cyclosporine metabolism in human liver: Identification of a cytochrome P-450 III gene family as the major cyclosporine-metabolizing enzyme explains interaction of cyclosporine with other drugs. Clin Pharmacol Ther 1988;43:630–5.
201. Combalbert J, Fabre I, Fabre G, et al. Metbolism of cyclosporin A IV. Purification and identification of the rifampin-inducible human liver cytochrome P-450 (cyclosporin A oxidase) as a product of the P450IIIA gene subfamily. Drug Metab Dispos 1989;17:197–207.
202. Kassianides C, Nussenblatt R, Palestine AG, et al. Liver injury from cyclosporine A. Dig Dis Sci 1990;35:693–7.
203. Stone BG, Udani M, Sanghvi A, et al. Cyclosporin A-induced cholestasis. The mechanism in a rat model. Gastroenterology 1987;93:344–51.
204. Kuhongviriyapan V, Stacey NH. Inhibition of taurocholate transport by cyclosporin A in cultured rat hepatocytes. J Pharmacol Exp Ther 1988;247:685–9.
205. Stieger B, Fattinger K, Madon J, et al. Drug- and estrogen-induced cholestasis through inhibition of the hepatocellular bile

salt export pump (Bsep) of rat liver. Gastroenterology 2000;118: 422–30.

206. Bramow S, Ott P, Thomsen Nielsen F, et al. Cholestasis and regulation of genes related to drug metabolism and biliary transport in rat liver following treatment with cyclosporine A and sirolimus (Rapamycin). Pharmacol Toxicol 2001;89: 133–9.
207. Yasumiba S, Tazuma S, Ochi H, et al. Cyclosporin A reduces canalicular membrane fluidity and regulates transporter function in rats. Biochem J 2001;354:591–6.
208. Freeman DJ, Martele R, Carruthers SG, et al. Cyclosporin-erythromycin interaction in normal subjects. Br J Clin Pharmacol 1987;23:776–8.
209. Henry JA, Jeffreys KJ, Dawling S. Toxicity and deaths from 3,4-methylenedioxymethamphetamine ("ecstasy"). Lancet 1992; 340:384–7.
210. Ellis AJ, Wendon JA, Portmann B, et al. Acute liver damage and ecstasy ingestion. Gut 1996;38:454–8.
211. Brauer RB, Heidecke CD, Nathrath W, et al. Liver transplantation for the treatment of fulminant hepatic failure induced by the ingestion of ecstasy. Transpl Int 1997;10:229–33.
212. Andreu V, Mas A, Bruguera M, et al. Ecstasy: a common cause of severe acute hepatotoxicity. J Hepatol 1998;29:394–7.
213. Greene SL, Dargan PI, O'Connor N, et al. Multiple toxicity from 3,4-methylenedioxymethamphetamine ("ecstasy"). Am J Emerg Med 2003;21:121–4.
214. Smith ID, Simpson KJ, Garden OJ, et al. Non-paracetamol drug-induced fulminant hepatic failure among adults in Scotland. Eur J Gastroenterol Hepatol 2005;17:161–7.
215. Ramamoorthy Y, Yu A-M, Suh N, et al. Reduced +/–3,4-methylenedioxymethampetamine ("Ecstasy") metabolism with cytochrome P450 2D6 inhibitors and pharmacogenetic variants *in vitro*. Biochem Pharmacol 2002;63:2111–19.
216. Heydari A, Yeo KR, Lennard MS, et al. Mechanism-based inactivation of CYP2D6 by methylenedioxymethamphetamine. Drug Metab Dispos 2004;32:1213–17.
217. Zafrani ES, Ishak KG, Rudzki C. Cholestatic and hepatocellular injury associated with erythromycin esters. Report of nine cases. Dig Dis Sci 1979;24:385–96.
218. Keeffe EB, Reis TC, Berland JE. Hepatotoxicity to both erythromycin estolate and erythromycin ethylsuccinate. Dig Dis Sci 1982;27:701–4.
219. Phillips KG. Hepatotoxicity of erythromycin ethylsuccinate in a child. Can Med Assoc J 1983;129:411–12.
220. Funck-Brentano C, Pessayre D, Benhamou JP. Hépatites dues a divers dérives de l'érythromycine. Clin Biol (Paris) 1983;7:362–9.
221. Diehl AM, Latham P, Boitnott JK, et al. Cholestatic hepatitis from erythromycin ethylsuccinate. Am J Med 1984;76:931–4.
222. Principi N, Esposito S. Comparative tolerability of erythromycin and newer macrolide antibacterials in paediatric patients. Drug Saf 1999;20:25–41.
223. Villa P, Begue JM, Guillouzo A. Erythromycin toxicity in primary cultures of rat hepatocytes. Xenobiotica 1985;15:767–73.
224. Sorensen EMB, Acosta A. Erythromycin toxicity in primary cultures of rat hepatocytes. Toxicol Lett 1985;27:73–82.
225. Gaeta GB, Utili R, Adinolfi LE, et al. Characterization of the effects of erythromycin estolate and erythromycin base on the excretory function of the isolated rat liver. Toxicol Appl Pharmacol 1985;80:185–92.
226. Giannattasio A, D'Ambrosi M, Volpicelli M, et al. Steroid therapy for a case of severe drug-induced cholestasis. Ann Pharmacother 2006;40:1196–9.
227. Brown BA, Wallace RJ Jr, Griffith DE, et al. Clarithromycin-induced hepatotoxicity. Clin Infect Dis 1995;20:1073–4.
228. Fox JC, Szyjkowski RS, Sanderson SO, et al. Progressive cholestatic liver disease associated with clarithromycin treatment. J Clin Pharmacol 2002;42:676–80.
229. Clay KD, Hanson JS, Pope SD, et al. Brief communication: severe hepatotoxicity of telithromycin: three case reports and literature review. Ann Intern Med 2006;144:415–20.
230. Pai MP, Graci DM, Amsden GW. Macrolide drug interactions: an update. Ann Pharmacother 2000;34:495–513.
231. Polasek TM, Miners JO. Quantitative prediction of macrolide drug-drug interaction potential from in vitro studies using testosterone as the human cytochrome P4503A substrate. Eur J Clin Pharmacol 2006;62:203–8.
232. Schreiber AJ, Simon FR. Estrogen-induced cholestasis: clues to pathogenesis and treatment. Hepatology 1983;3:607–13.
233. Lewis JH, Tice HL, Zimmerman HJ. Budd-Chiari syndrome associated with oral contraceptive steroids. Review of treatment of 47 cases. Dig Dis Sci 1983;28:673–83.
234. Lockhat D, Katz SS, Lisbona R, et al. Oral contraceptives and liver disease. Can Med Assoc J 1981;124:993–9.
235. Valla D, Le MG, Poynard T, et al. Risk of hepatic vein thrombosis in relation to recent use of oral contraceptives. A case control study. Gastroenterology 1986;90:807–11.
236. Barnet B, Joffe A. Hepatic vein thrombosis in a teenager: a case report. J Adolesc Health 1991;12:60–2.
237. Edmonson HA, Henderson B, Benton B. Liver cell adenomas associated with the use of oral contraceptives. N Engl J Med 1976;294:470–2.
238. Neuberger J, Nunnerley HB, Davis M, et al. Oral-contraceptive-associated liver tumours: Occurrence of malignancy and difficulties in diagnosis. Lancet 1980;i:273–6.
239. Tesluk H, Lawrie H. Hepatocellular adenoma. Its transformation to carcinoma in a user of oral contraceptives. Arch Pathol Lab Med 1981;105:296–9.
240. Pellock JM. Felbamate. Epilepsia 1999;40 Suppl 5:S57–62.
241. Kapetanovic IM, Torchin CD, Thompson CD, et al. Potentially reactive cyclic carbamate metabolite of the antiepileptic drug felbamate produced by human liver tissue in vitro. Drug Metab Dispos 1998;26:1089–95.
242. Popovic M, Nierkens S, Pieters R, et al. Investigating the role of 2-phenylpropenal in felbamate-induced idiosyncratic drug reactions. Chem Res Toxicol 2004;17:1568–76.
243. Dieckhaus CM, Roller SG, Santos WL, et al. Role of glutathione S-transferases A1-1, M1-1, and P1-1 in the detoxification of 2-phenylpropenal, a reactive felbamate metabolite. Chem Res Toxicol 2001;14:511–16.
244. Hachad H, Ragueneau-Majlessi I, Levy RH. New antiepileptic drugs: review on drug interactions. Ther Drug Monit 2002;24: 91–103.
245. Gaertner I, Altendorf K, Batra A, et al. Relevance of liver enzyme elevations with four different neuroleptics: a retrospective review of 7,263 treatment courses. J Clin Psychopharmacol 2001;21:215–22.
246. Dincsoy HP, Saelinger DA. Haloperidol-induced chronic cholestatic liver disease. Gastroenterology 1982;83:694–700.
247. Wark HJ. Postoperative jaundice in children. Anaesthesia 1983; 38:237–42.

248. Warner LO, Beach TP, Gariss JP, et al. Halothane and children: The first quarter century. Anesth Analg 1984;63:838–40.
249. Farrell G, Prendergast D, Murray M. Halothane hepatitis: detection of a constitutional susceptibility factor. N Engl J Med 1985;313:1310–14.
250. Lo SK, Wendon J, Mieli-Vergani G, et al. Halothane-induced acute liver failure: continuing occurrence and use of liver transplantation. Eur J Gastroenterol Hepatol 1998;10:635–9.
251. Kenna JG, Neuberger J, Mieli-Vergani G, et al. Halothane hepatitis in children. Br Med J 1987;294:1209–11.
252. Hassall E, Israel DM, Gunasekaran T, et al. Halothane hepatitis in children. J Pediatr Gastroenterol Nutr 1990;11:553–7.
253. Psacharopoulos HJ, Mowat AP, Davies M, et al. Fulminant hepatic failure in childhood: An analysis of 31 cases. Arch Dis Child 1980;55:252–8.
254. Inman WHV, Mushin WW. Jaundice after repeated exposure to halothane: A further analysis of reports to the Committee of Safety of Medicines. Br Med J 1978;2:1455–6.
255. Campbell RL, Small EW, Lesesne HR, et al. Fatal hepatic necrosis after halothane anesthesia in a boy with juvenile rheumatoid arthritis: a case report. Anesth Analg 1977;56:589–93.
256. DeGroot H, Noll T. Halothane hepatotoxicity: Relation between metabolic activation, pyrexia, covalent binding, lipid peroxidation and liver cell damage. Hepatology 1983;3:601–6.
257. Farrell GC. Mechanism of halothane-induced liver injury: is it immune or metabolic idiosyncrasy? J Gastroenterol Hepatol 1988;3:465–82.
258. Pohl LR, Satoh H, Christ DD, et al. The immunologic and metabolic basis of drug hypersensitivities. Annu Rev Pharmacol Toxicol 1988;28:367–87.
259. Spracklin DK, Thummel KE, Kharasch ED. Human reductive halothane metabolism in vitro is catalyzed by cytochrome P450 2A6 and 3A4. Drug Metab Dispos 1996 1996;24:976–83.
260. Spracklin DK, Hankins DC, Fisher JM, et al. Cytochrome P450 2E1 is the principal catalyst of human oxidative halothane metabolism in vitro. J Pharmacol Exp Ther 1997;281:400–11.
261. Vergani D, Mieli-Vergani G, Alberti A, et al. Antibodies to the surface of halothane-altered rabbit hepatocytes in patients with severe halothane-associated hepatitis. N Engl J Med 1980;303: 66–71.
262. Neuberger J, Mieli-Vergani G, Tredger JM, et al. Oxidative metabolism of halothane in the production of altered hepatocyte membrane antigens in acute halothane-induced hepatic necrosis. Gut 1981;22:669–72.
263. Satoh H, Fukada Y, Anderson DK, et al. Immunological studies on the mechanism of halothane-induced hepatotoxicity: immunohistochemical evidence of trifluoroacetylated hepatocytes. J Pharmacol Exp Ther 1985;233:857–62.
264. Kenna JG, Satoh H, Christ DD, et al. Metabolic basis for a drug hypersensitivity: antibodies in sera from patients with halothane hepatitis recognize liver neoantigens that contain the trifluoroacetyl group derived from halothane. J Pharmacol Exp Ther 1988;245:1103–9.
265. Kenna JG, Neuberger J, Williams R. Evidence for expression in human liver of halothane-induced neoantigens recognized by antibodies in sera from patients with halothane hepatitis. Hepatology 1988;8:1635–41.
266. Satoh H, Martin BM, Schulick AH, et al. Human enti-endoplasmic reticulum antibodies in sera of patients with halothane-induced hepatitis are directed against a trifluoroacetylated carboxylesterase. Proc Natl Acad Sci U S A 1989;86:322–6.
267. Christen U, Buergin M, Gut J. Halothane metabolism: Kupffer cells carry and partially process triflouroacetylated protein adducts. Biochem Biophys Res Commun 1991;175:256–62.
268. Kenna JG, Martin JL, Satoh H, et al. Factors affecting the expression of trifluoracteylated liver microsomal protein neoantigens in rats treated with halothane. Drug Metab Dispos 1990;18:788–93.
269. Yeong ML, Swinburn B, Kennedy M, et al. Hepatic veno-occlusive disease associated with comfrey ingestion. J Gastroenterol Hepatol 1990;5:211–14.
270. Rode D. Comfrey toxicity revisited. Trends Pharmacol Sci 2002; 23:497–9.
271. Laliberte L, Villeneuve JP. Hepatitis after the use of germander, a herbal remedy. CMAJ 1996;154:1689–92.
272. Larrey D, Vial T, Pauwels A, et al. Hepatitis after germander (Teucrium chamaedrys) administration: another instance of herbal medicine hepatotoxicity. Ann Intern Med 1992;117:129–32.
273. Lekehal M, Pessayre D, Lereau JM, et al. Hepatotoxicity of the herbal medicine germander: metabolic activation of its furano diterpenoids by cytochrome P450 3A Depletes cytoskeleton-associated protein thiols and forms plasma membrane blebs in rat hepatocytes. Hepatology 1996;24:212–18.
274. Fau D, Lekehal M, Farrell G, et al. Diterpenoids from germander, an herbal medicine, induce apoptosis in isolated rat hepatocytes. Gastroenterology 1997;113:1334–46.
275. Clouatre DL. Kava kava: examining new reports of toxicity. Toxicol Lett 2004;150:85–96.
276. Campo JV, McNabb J, Perel JM, et al. Kava-induced fulminant hepatic failure. J Am Acad Child Adolesc Psychiatry 2002;41: 631–2.
277. Whitton PA, Lau A, Salisbury A, et al. Kava lactones and the kava kava controversy. Phytochemistry 2003;64:673–9.
278. Anke J, Ramzan I. Pharmacokinetic and pharmacodynamic drug interactions with Kava (*Piper methysticum Forst. f.*). J Ethnopharmacol 2004;93:153–60.
279. Batchelor WB, Heathcote J, Wanless IR. Chaparral-induced hepatic injury. Am J Gastroenterol 1995;90:831–3.
280. Sheikh NM, Philen RM, Love LA. Chaparral-associated hepatotoxicity. Arch Intern Med 1997;157:913–19.
281. Woolf GM, Petrovic LM, Rojter SE, et al. Acute hepatitis associated with the Chinese herbal product jin bu huan. Ann Intern Med 1994;121:729–35.
282. Horowitz RS, Feldhaus K, Dart RC, et al. The clinical spectrum of Jin Bu Huan toxicity. Arch Intern Med 1996;156:899–903.
283. Skoulidis F, Alexander GJ, Davies SE. Ma huang associated acute liver failure requiring liver transplantation. Eur J Gastroenterol Hepatol 2005;17:581–4.
284. Webb N, Hardikar W, Cranswick NE, et al. Probable herbal medication induced fulminant hepatic failure. J Paediatr Child Health 2005;41:530–1.
285. Zuckerman M, Steenkamp V, Stewart MJ. Hepatic veno-occlusive disease as a result of a traditional remedy: confirmation of toxic pyrrolizidine alkaloids as the cause, using an in vitro technique. J Clin Pathol 2002;55:676–9.
286. Maddrey WC, Boitnott JK. Isoniazid hepatitis. Ann Intern Med 1973;79:1–12.
287. Zimmerman HJ. Update of hepatotoxicity due to classes of drugs in common clinical use: non-steroidal drugs, anti-inflammatory drugs, antibiotics, antihypertensives, and cardiac and psychotropic drugs. Sem Liver Dis 1990;10:322–38.

288. Rudoy R, Stuemky J, Poley R. Isoniazid administration and liver injury. Am J Dis Child 1973;125:733–6.
289. Casteels-Van Daele M, Igodt-Ameye L, Corbell L, et al. Hepatotoxicity of rifampicin and isoniazid in children. J Pediatr 1975;86:739–41.
290. Vanderhoof JA, Ament ME. Fatal hepatic necrosis due to isoniazid chemoprophylaxis in a 15 year-old girl. J Pediatr 1976;88:867–8.
291. Litt IF, Cohen MI, McNamara H. Isoniazid hepatitis in adolescents. J Pediatr 1976;89:133–5.
292. Walker SH, Park-Hah JO. Possible isoniazid-induced hepatotoxicity in a two-year-old child. J Pediatr 1977;91:344–5.
293. Pessayre D, Bentata M, Degott C, et al. Isoniazid-rifampin fulminant hepatitis. A possible consequence of the enhancement of isoniazid hepatotoxicity by enzyme induction. Gastroenterology 1977;72:284–9.
294. Gal AA, Klatt EC. Fatal isoniazid hepatitis in a child. Pediatr Infec Dis 1986;5:490–1.
295. Beaudry P, Brickman H, Wise M, et al. Liver enzyme disturbances during isoniazid chemoprophylaxis in children. Am Rev Resp Dis 1974;110:581–4.
296. Spyridis P, Sinantios C, Papadea I, et al. Isoniazid liver injury during chemoprophylaxis in children. Arch Dis Child 1979; 54:65–7.
297. Mitchell J, Zimmerman H, Ishak K, et al. Isoniazid liver injury: clinical spectrum, pathology and probable pathogenesis. Ann Intern Med 1976;84:181–96.
298. Palusci VJ, O'Hare D, Lawrence RM. Hepatotoxicity and transaminase measurement during isoniazid chemoprophylaxis in children. Pediatr Infect Dis J 1995;14:144–8.
299. Tsagaropoulou-Stinga H, Mataki-Emmanouilidou T, Karadi-Kavalioti S, et al. Hepatotoxic reactions in children with severe tuberculosis treated with isoniazid-rifampin. Pediatr Infect Dis 1985;4:270–3.
300. Martinez-Roig A, Cami J, Llorens-Teroi J, et al. Acetylation phenotype and hepatotoxicity in the treatment of tuberculosis of children. Pediatrics 1986;77:912–15.
301. Berkowitz FE, Henderson SL, Fajman N, et al. Acute liver failure caused by isoniazid in a child receiving carbamazepine. Int J Tuberc Lung Dis 1998;2:603–6.
302. Campos-Franco J, Gonzalez-Quintela A, Alende-Sixto MR. Isoniazid-induced hyperacute liver failure in a young patient receiving carbamazepine. Eur J Intern Med 2004;15:396–7.
303. O'Brien RJ, Long MW, Cross FS, et al. Hepatotoxicity from isoniazid and rifampin among children treated for tuberculosis. Pediatrics 1983;72:491–9.
304. Huang YS, Chern HD, Su WJ, et al. Cytochrome P450 2E1 genotype and the susceptibility to antituberculosis drug-induced hepatitis. Hepatology 2003;37:924–30.
305. Huang YS, Chern HD, Su WJ, et al. Polymorphism of the N-acetyltransferase 2 gene as a susceptibility risk factor for antituberculosis drug-induced hepatitis. Hepatology 2002;35: 883–9.
306. Vuilleumier N, Rossier MF, Chiappe A, et al. CYP2E1 genotype and isoniazid-induced hepatotoxicity in patients treated for latent tuberculosis. Eur J Clin Pharmacol 2006;62:423–9.
307. Desta Z, Soukhova NV, Flockhart DA. Inhibition of cytochrome P450 (CYP450) isoforms by isoniazid: potent inhibition of CYP2C19 and CYP3A. Antimicrob Agents Chemother 2001;45: 382–92.
308. Lewis JH, Zimmerman HJ, Benson GD, et al. Hepatic injury associated with ketoconazole therapy. Analysis of 33 cases. Gastroenterology 1984;86:503–13.
309. Bercoff E, Bernuau J, Degott C, et al. Ketoconazole-induced fulminant hepatitis. Gut 1985;26:636–8.
310. Stricker BHC, Blok APR, Bronkhurst FB, et al. Ketoconazole-associated hepatic injury. A clinicopathological study of 55 cases. J Hepatol 1986;3:399–406.
311. Lake-Bakaar G, Scheuer PJ, Sherlock S. Hepatic reactions associated with ketoconazole in the United Kingdom. Br Med J 1987; 294:419–22.
312. Adriaenssens B, Roskams T, Steger P, et al. Hepatotoxicity related to itraconazole: report of three cases. Acta Clin Belg 2001; 56:364–9.
313. Schlienger R, Knowles S, Shear N. Lamotrogine-associated anticonvulsant hypersensitivty syndrome. Neurology 1998;51: 1172–5.
314. Brown TS, Appel JE, Kasteler JS, et al. Hypersensitivity reaction in a child due to lamotrigine. Pediatr Dermatol 1999;16:46–9.
315. Fayad M, Choueiri R, Mikati M. Potential hepatotoxicity of lamotrigine. Pediatr Neurol 2000;22:49–52.
316. Overstreet K, Costanza C, Behling C, et al. Fatal progressive hepatic necrosis associated with lamotrigine treatment: a case report and literature review. Dig Dis Sci 2002;47:1921–5.
317. Maggs JL, Naisbitt DJ, Tettey JN, et al. Metabolism of lamotrigine to a reactive arene oxide intermediate. Chem Res Toxicol 2000;13:1075–81.
318. Anderson GD. Children versus adults: pharmacokinetic and adverse-effect differences. Epilepsia 2002;43 Suppl 3:53–9.
319. Zidd AG, Hack JB. Pediatric ingestion of lamotrigine. Pediatr Neurol 2004;31:71–2.
320. Tolman KG, Clegg DO, Lee RG, et al. Methotrexate and the liver. J Rheumatol 1985;12 Suppl 12:29–34.
321. Van de Kerkhof PCM, Hoegnagels WHL, Van Haelst UJGM, et al. Methotrexate maintenance therapy and liver damage in psoriasis. Clin Exp Dermatol 1985;10:194–200.
322. Kremer JM, Lee RG, Tolman KG. Liver histology in rheumatoid arthritis patients receiving long-term methotrexate therapy. A prospective study with baseline and sequential biopsy samples. Arthritis Rheum 1989;32:121–7.
323. Gilbert SC, Klintmalm G, Mentor A, et al. Methotrexate-induced cirrhosis requiring liver transplantation in three patients with psoriasis: a word of caution in light of the expanding use of this "steroid sparing" agent. Arch Intern Med 1990; 150:889–91.
324. Langman G, Hall PM, Todd G. Role of non-alcoholic steatohepatitis in methotrexate-induced liver injury. J Gastroenterol Hepatol 2001;16:1395–401.
325. Newman M, Auerbach R, Feiner H, et al. The role of liver biopsies in psoriatic patients receiving long-term methotrexate treatment. Arch Dermatol 1989;125:1218–24.
326. Kremer JM, Alarcón GS, Lightfoot RWJ, et al. Methotrexate for rheumatoid arthritis. Suggested guidelines for monitoring liver toxicity. Arthritis Rheum 1994;37:316–28.
327. Kremer JM, Furst DE, Weinblatt ME, et al. Significant changes in serum AST across hepatic histological grades: prospective analysis of 3 cohorts receiving methotrxate therapy for rheumatoid arthritis. J Rheumatol 1996;23:489–61.
328. Zachariae H, Kragbulle K, Sugaard H. Methotrexate induced liver cirrhosis. Br J Dermatol 1980;102:407–12.

329. Shergy WJ, Polisson RP, Caldwell DS, et al. Methotrexate-associated hepatotoxicity: Retrospective analysis of 210 patients with rheumatoid arthritis. Am J Med 1988;85:771–4.
330. Hashkes PJ, Balistreri WF, Bove KE, et al. The long-term effect of methotrexate therapy on the liver in patients with juvenile rheumatoid arthritis. Arthritis Rheum 1997;40:2226–34.
331. Hashkes PJ, Balistreri WF, Bove KE, et al. The relationship of hepatotoxic risk factors and liver histology in methotrexate therapy for juvenile rheumatoid arthritis. J Pediatr 1999;134:47–52.
332. Graham LD, Myones BL, Rivas-Chacon RF, et al. Morbidity associated with long-term methotrexate therapy in juvenile rheumatoid arthritis. J Pediatr 1992;120:468–73.
333. Kugathasam S, Newman AJ, Dahms BB, et al. Liver biopsy findings in patients with juvenile rheumatoid arthritis receiving long-term, weekly methotrexate therapy. J Pediatr 1996;128: 149–51.
334. Keim D, Ragsdale C, Heidelberger K, et al. Hepatic fibrosis with the use of methotrexate for juvenile rheumatoid arthritis. J Rheumatol 1990;17:846–8.
335. Te HS, Schiano TD, Kuan SF, et al. Hepatic effects of long-term methotrexate use in the treatment of inflammatory bowel disease. Am J Gastroenterol 2000;95:3150–6.
336. Perez C, Sutow WW, Wang YM, et al. Evaluation of overall toxicity of high-dosage methotrexate reigmens. Med Pediatr Oncol 1979;6:219–28.
337. Locasciulli A, Mura R, Fraschini D, et al. High-dose methotrexate administration and acute liver damage in children treated for acute lymphoblastic leukemia. A prospective study. Haematologica 1992;77:49–53.
338. Harb JM, Werlin SL, Camitta BM, et al. Hepatic ultrastructure in leukemic children treated with methotrexate and 6-mercaptopurine. Am J Pediatr Hematol Oncol 1983;5:323–31.
339. McIntosh S, Davidson DL, O'Brien RT, et al. Methotrexate hepatotoxicity in children with leukemia. J Pediatr 1977;90:1019–21.
340. Ng C, Xiao YD, Lum BL, et al. Quantitative structure-activity relationships of methotrexate and methotrexate analogues transported by the rat multispecific resistance-associated protein 2 (rMrp2). Eur J Pharm Sci 2005;26:405–13.
341. Malcolm A, Heap TR, Eckstein RP, et al. Minocycline-induced liver injury. Am J Gastroenterol 1996;91:1641–3.
342. Gough A, Chapman S, Wagstaff K, et al. Minocycline induced autoimmune hepatitis and systemic lupus erythematosus-like syndrome. BMJ 1996;312:169–72.
343. Bhat G, Jordan J Jr, Sokalski S, et al. Minocycline-induced hepatitis with autoimmune features and neutropenia. J Clin Gastroenterol 1998;27:74–5.
344. Davies MG, Kersey PJW. Acute hepatitis and exfoliative dermatitis associated with minocycline. BMJ 1989;298:1523–4.
345. Boudreaux JP, Hayes DH, Mizrahi S, et al. Fulminant hepatic failure, hepatorenal syndrome, and necrotizing pancreatitis after minocycline hepatotoxicity. Transplant Proc 1993;25:1873.
346. Traversa G, Bianchi C, Da Cas R, et al. Cohort study of hepatotoxicity associated with nimesulide and other non-steroidal anti-inflammatory drugs. BMJ 2003;327:18–22.
347. Titchen T, Cranswick N, Beggs S. Adverse drug reactions to nonsteroidal anti-inflammatory drugs, COX-2 inhibitors and paracetamol in a paediatric hospital. Br J Clin Pharmacol 2005; 59:718–23.
348. Whittaker SJ, Amar JN, Wanless IR, et al. Sulindac hepatotoxicity. Gut 1982;23:875–7.
349. Boelsterli UA. Diclofenac-induced liver injury: a paradigm of idiosyncratic drug toxicity. Toxicol Appl Pharmacol 2003;192: 307–22.
350. Merlani G, Fox M, Oehen HP, et al. Fatal hepatoxicity secondary to nimesulide. Eur J Clin Pharmacol 2001;57:321–6.
351. Ong MM, Wang AS, Leow KY, et al. Nimesulide-induced hepatic mitochondrial injury in heterozygous Sod2(+/−) mice. Free Radic Biol Med 2006;40:420–9.
352. Pratt DS, Dubois RS. Hepatotoxicity due to pemoline (Cylert). A report of two cases. J Pediatr Gastroenterol Nutr 1990;10:239–41.
353. Elitsur Y. Pemoline (Cylert)-induced hepatotoxicity. J Pediatr Gastroenterol Nutr 1990;11:143–4.
354. Adcock KG, MacElroy DE, Wolford ET, et al. Pemoline therapy resulting in liver transplantation. Ann Pharmacother 1998;32: 422–5.
355. Marotta PJ, Roberts EA. Pemoline hepatotoxicity in children. J Pediatr 1998;132:894–7.
356. Rosh JR, Dellert SF, Narkewicz M, et al. Four cases of severe hepatotoxicity associated with pemoline: possible autoimmune pathogenesis. Pediatrics 1998;101:921–3.
357. Mehta H, Murray B, Iolodice TA. Hepatic dysfunction due to intravenous abuse of methylphenidate hydrichloride. J Clin Gastroenterol 1984;6:149–51.
358. Bruckstein AH, Attia AA. Oxacillin hepatitis. Am J Med 1978; 64:519–22.
359. Tauris P, Jorgensen NF, Petersen CM, et al. Prolonged severe cholestasis induced by oxacillin derivatives. A report on two cases. Acta Med Scand 1985;217:567–9.
360. Kleinman MS, Presberg JE. Cholestatic hepatitis after dicloxacillin-sodium therapy. J Clin Gastroenterol 1986;8:77–8.
361. Turner IB, Eckstein RP, Riley JW, et al. Prolonged hepatic cholestasis after flucloxacillin therapy. Med J Aust 1989;151: 701–5.
362. Miros M, Kerlin P, Walker N, et al. Flucloxacillin induced delayed cholestatic hepatitis. Aust N Z J Med 1990;20:251–3.
363. Gresser U. Amoxicillin-clavulanic acid therapy may be associated with severe side effects – review of the literature. Eur J Med Res 2001;6:139–49.
364. Reddy KR, Brillant P, Schiff ER. Amoxicillin-clavulinate potassium-associated cholestasis. Gastroenterology 1989;96:1135–41.
365. Larrey D, Vial T, Babany G, et al. Hepatitis associated with amoxycillin-clavulanic acid combination report of 15 cases. Gut 1992;33:368–71.
366. Stricker BH, Van den Broek JW, Keuning J, et al. Cholestatic hepatitis due to antibacterial combination of amoxicillin and clavulanic acid (augmentin). Dig Dis Sci 1989;34:1576–80.
367. Fontana RJ, Shakil AO, Greenson JK, et al. Acute liver failure due to amoxicillin and amoxicillin/clavulanate. Dig Dis Sci 2005;50:1785–90.
368. O'Donohue J, Oien KA, Donaldson P, et al. Co-amoxiclav jaundice: clinical and histological features and HLA class II association. Gut 2000;47:717–20.
369. Degott C, Feldmann G, Larrey D, et al. Drug-induced prolonged cholestasis in adults: a histological semiquantitative study demonstrating progressive ductopenia. Hepatology 1992;15: 244–51.
370. Chawla A, Kahn E, Yunis EJ, et al. Rapidly progressive cholstasis: an unusual reaction to amoxicillin/clavulinic acid in a child. J Pediatr 2000;136:121–3.

371. Shapiro PA, Antonioli DA, Peppercorn MA. Barbiturate-induced submassive hepatic necrosis. Am J Gastroenterol 1980; 74:270–3.
372. Roberts EA, Spielberg SP, Goldbach M, et al. Phenobarbital hepatotoxicity in an 8-month-old infant. J Hepatol 1990;10:235–9.
373. Li AM, Nelson EA, Hon EK, et al. Hepatic failure in a child with anti-epileptic hypersensitivity syndrome. J Paediatr Child Health 2005;41:218–20.
374. Spielberg SP, Gordon GB, Blake DA, et al. Anticonvulsant toxicity in vitro: possible role of arene oxides. J Pharmacol Exp Ther 1981;217:386–9.
375. Powers NG, Carson SH. Idiosyncratic reactions to phenytoin. Clin Pediatr 1987;26:120–4.
376. Bessmertny O, Hatton RC, Gonzalez-Peralta RP. Antiepileptic hypersensitivity syndrome in children. Ann Pharmacother 2001;35:533–8.
377. Mullick FG, Ishak KG. Hepatic injury associated with diphenylhydantoin therapy. Am J Clin Pathol 1980;74:442–52.
378. Spielberg SP, Gordon GB, Blake DA, et al. Predisposition to phenytoin hepatotoxicity assessed in vitro. N Engl J Med 1981;305:722–7.
379. Kahn HD, Faguet GB, Agee JF, et al. Drug-induced liver injury. In vitro demonstration of hypersensitivity to both phenytoin and phenobarbital. Arch Intern Med 1984;144:1677–9.
380. Jonas MM, Edison MS. Propylthiouracil hepatotoxicity: Two pediatric cases and review of the literature. J Pediatr Gastroenterol Nutr 1988;7:776–9.
381. Kirkland JL. Propylthiouracil-induced hepatic failure and encephalopathy in a child. Ann Pharmacother 1990;24:470–1.
382. Levy M. Propylthiouracil hepatotoxicity. A review and case presentation. Clin Pediatr 1993;32:25–9.
383. Williams KV, Nayak S, Becker D, et al. Fifty years of experience with propylthiouracil-associated hepatotoxicity: what have we learned? J Clin Endocrinol Metab 1997;82:1721–33.
384. Maggiore G, Larizza D, Lorini R, et al. PTU hepatotoxicity mimicking autoimmune chronic active hepatitis in a girl. J Pediatr Gastroenterol Nutr 1989;8:547–8.
385. Aydemir S, Ustundag Y, Bayraktaroglu T, et al. Fulminant hepatic failure associated with propylthiouracil: a case report with treatment emphasis on the use of plasmapheresis. J Clin Apher 2005;20:235–8.
386. Safani MM, Tatro DS, Rudd P. Fatal propylthiouracil-induced hepatitis. Arch Intern Med 1982;142:838–9.
387. Homberg J-C, Abuaf N, Bernard O, et al. Chronic active hepatitis associated with antiliver/kidney microsome antibody type 1: A second type of "autoimmune" hepatitis. Hepatology 1987; 7:1333–9.
388. Hayashida CY, Duarte AJ, Sato AE, et al. Neonatal hepatitis and lymphocyte sensitization by placental transfer of propylthiouracil. J Endocrinol Invest 1990;13:937–41.
389. Jacques EA, Buschmann RJ, Layden TJ. The histopathologic progression of vitamin A-induced hepatic injury. Gastroenterology 1979;76:599–602.
390. Roenigk HH Jr. Liver toxicity of retinoid therapy. J Am Acad Dermatol 1988;19:199–208.
391. Fallon MB, Boyer JL. Hepatic toxicity of vitamin A and synthetic retinoids. J Gastroenterol Hepatol 1990;5:334–42.
392. Shear NH, Spielberg SP, Grant DM, et al. Differences in metabolism of sulfonamides predisposing to idiosyncratic toxicity. Ann Intern Med 1986;105:179–84.
393. Zitelli BJ, Alexander J, Taylor S, et al. Fatal hepatic necrosis due to pyrimethamine-sulfadoxine (Fansidar). Ann Intern Med 1987;106:393–5.
394. Sotolongo RP, Neefe LI, Rudzki C, et al. Hypersensitivity reaction to sulfasalazine with severe hepatotoxicity. Gastroenterology 1978;75:95–9.
395. Losek JH, Werlin SL. Sulfasalazine hepatotoxicity. Am J Dis Child 1981;135:1070–2.
396. Ribe J, Benkov KJ, Thung SN, et al. Fatal massive hepatic necrosis: a probable hypersensitivity reaction to sulfasalazine. Am J Gastroenterol 1986;81:205–8.
397. Gremse DA, Bancroft J, Moyer SA. Sulfasalazine hypersensitivity with hepatotoxicity, thrombocytopenia, and erythroid hypoplasia. J Pediatr Gastroenterol Nutr 1989;9:261–3.
398. Besnard M, Debray D, Durand P, et al. [Fulminant hepatitis in two chilldren treated with sulfasalazine for Crohn disease]. Arch Pediatr 1999;6:643–6. [Article in French.]
399. Karpman E, Kurzrock EA. Adverse reactions of nitrofurantoin, trimethoprim and sulfamethoxazole in children. J Urol 2004;172:448–53.
400. Ghishan FK. Trimethoprim-sulfamethoxazole-induced intrahepatic cholestasis. Clin Pediatr 1983;22:212–14.
401. Bucaretchi F, Vicente DC, Pereira RM, et al. Dapsone hypersensitivity syndrome in an adolescent during treatment during of leprosy. Rev Inst Med Trop Sao Paulo 2004;46:331–4.
402. Rieder MJ, Uetrecht J, Shear NH, et al. Diagnosis of sulfonamide hypersensitivity reactions by in-vitro "rechallenge" with hydroxylamine metabolites. Ann Intern Med 1989;110: 286–9.
403. Cribb AE, Spielberg SP. Hepatic microsomal metabolism of sulfamethoxazole to the hydroxylamine. Drug Metab Dispos 1990;18:784–7.
404. Cribb AE, Spielberg SP. Sulfamethoxazole is metabolized to the hydroxylamine in humans. Clin Pharmacol Ther 1992;51:522–6.
405. Shear NH, Spielberg SP. In vitro evaluation of a toxic metabolite of sulfadiazine. Can J Physiol Pharmacol 1985;63:1370–2.
406. Rieder MJ, Uetrecht J, Shear NH, et al. Synthesis and in vitro toxicity of hydroxylamine metqbolites of sulfonamides. J Pharmacol Exp Ther 1988;244:724–8.
407. Cribb AE, Miller M, Tesoro A, et al. Peroxidase-dependent oxidation of sulfonamides by monocytes and neutrophils from humans and dogs. Mol Pharmacol 1990;38:744–51.
408. Sztajnkrycer MD. Valproic acid toxicity: overview and management. J Toxiocl Clin Toxicol 2002;40:789–801.
409. Powell-Jackson PR, Tredger JM, Williams R. Hepatotoxicity to sodium valproate: a review. Gut 1984;25:673–81.
410. Suchy FJ, Balistreri WF, Buchino J, et al. Acute hepatic failure associated with the use of sodium valproate. Report of two fatal cases. N Engl J Med 1979;300:962–6.
411. Gerber N, Dickinson RG, Harland RC, et al. Reye-like syndrome associated with valproic acid therapy. J Pediatr 1979;95:142–4.
412. Zimmerman HJ, Ishak KG. Valproate-induced hepatic injury: Analysis of 23 fatal cases. Hepatology 1982;2:591–7.
413. Dreifuss FE, Santilli N, Langer DH, et al. Valproic acid hepatic fatalities. Neurology 1987;37:379–85.
414. Scheffner D, Konig ST, Rauterberg-Ruland I, et al. Fatal liver failure in 16 children with valproate therapy. Epilepsia 1988;29: 530–42.
415. Koenig SA, Siemes H, Blaker F, et al. Severe hepatotoxicity during valproate therapy: an update and report of eight new fatalities. Epilepsia 1994;35:1005–15.

416. Green SH. Sodium valproate and routine liver function tests. Arch Dis Child 1984;59:813–14.
417. Bryant AE 3rd, Dreifuss FE. Valproic acid hepatic fatalities. III. U.S. experience since 1986. Neurology 1996;46:465–9.
418. McCall M, Bourgeois JA. Valproic acid-induced hyperammonemia: a case report. J Clin Psychopharmacol 2004;24:521–6.
419. Gerstner T, Buesing D, Longin E, et al. Valproic acid induced encephalopathy – 19 new cases in Germany from 1994 to 2003 – a side effect associated to VPA-therapy not only in young children. Seizure 2006;15:443–8.
420. Huang YL, Hong HS, Wang ZW, et al. Fatal sodium valproate-induced hypersensitivity syndrome with lichenoid dermatitis and fulminant hepatitis. J Am Acad Dermatol 2003;49: 316–19.
421. Partin JS, Suchy FJ, Bates SR. An ultrastructural analysis of sodium valproate associated hepatopathy. Gastroenterology 1983;84:1389.
422. Eadie MJ, Hooper WD, Dickinson RG. Valproate-associated hepatotoxicity and its biochemical mechanisms. Med Toxicol Adverse Drug Exper 1988;3:85–106.
423. Li X, Norwood DL, Mao L-F, et al. Mitochondrial metabolism of valproic acid. Biochemistry 1991;30:388–94.
424. Rettenmeier AW, Gordon WP, Prickett KS, et al. Metabolic fate of valproic acid in the rhesus monkey. Formation of a toxic metabolite, 2-*n*-propyl-4-pentenoic acid. Drug Metab Dispos 1986; 14:443–53.
425. Kochen W, Schneider A, Ritz A. Abnormal metabolism of valproic acid in fatal hepatic failure. Eur J Pediatr 1983;14: 30–5.
426. Kesterson JW, Granneman GR, Machinist JM. The hepatotoxicity of valproate in rats. I. Toxicologic, biochemical and histopathologic studies. Hepatology 1984;4:1143–52.
427. Granneman GR, Wang SI, Kesterson JW, et al. The hepatotoxicity of valproic acid and its metabolites in rats. II. Intermediary and valproic acid metabolism. Hepatology 1984;4:1153–8.
428. Bjorge SM, Baillie TA. Inhibition of medium-chain fatty acid beta-oxidation in vitro by valproic acid and its unsaturated metabolite, 2-*n*-propyl-4-pentenoic acid. Biochem Biophys Res Commun 1985;132:245–52.
429. Gopaul S, Farrell K, Abbott F. Effects of age and polytherapy, risk factors of valproic acid (VPA) hepatotoxicity, on the excretion of thiol conjugates of (E)-2,4-diene VPA in people with epilepsy taking VPA. Epilepsia 2003;44:322–8.
430. Böhles H, Richter K, Wagner-Thiessen E, et al. Decreased serum carnitine in valproate induced Reye syndrome. Eur J Pediatr 1982;139:185–6.
431. Eadie MJ, McKinnon GE, Dunstan PR, et al. Valproate metabolism during hepatotoxicity associated with the drug. Quart J Med 1990;77:1229–40.
432. Kossak BD, Schmidt-Sommerfeld E, Schoeller DA, et al. Impaired fatty acid oxidation in children on valproic acid and the effect of L-carnitine. Neurology 1993;43:2362–8.
433. Keulen FP, Kochen W. Hepatotoxität unter Valproinsaure Behandlung. Klin Pädiatrie 1985;197:431–6.
434. Dickinson RG, Bassett ML, Searle J, et al. Valproate hepatotoxicity: a review and report of two instances in adults. Clin Exp Neurol 1985;21:79–91.
435. Tong V, Teng XW, Chang TK, et al. Valproic acid I: time course of lipid peroxidation biomarkers, liver toxicity, and valproic acid metabolite levels in rats. Toxicol Sci 2005;86:427–35.
436. Tong V, Teng XW, Chang TK, et al. Valproic acid II: effects on oxidative stress, mitochondrial membrane potential, and cytotoxicity in glutathione-depleted rat hepatocytes. Toxicol Sci 2005;86:436–43.
437. Qureshi IA, Letarte J, Tuchweber B, et al. Heptotoxicology of sodium valproate in ornithine transcarbamylase-deficient mice. Toxicol Lett 1985;25:297–306.
438. Hjelm M, De Silva LVK, Seakins IWT, et al. Evidence of inherited urea cycle defect in a case of fatal valproate toxicity. Br Med J 1986;292:23–4.
439. Kay JDS, Hilton-Jones D, Hyman N. Valproate toxicity and ornithine carbamoyltransferase deficiency. Lancet 1986;2: 1283–4.
440. Chabrol B, Mancini J, Chretien D, et al. Valproate-induced hepatic failure in a case of cytochrome c oxidase deficiency. Eur J Pediatr 1994;153:133–5.
441. Konig SA, Schenk M, Sick C, et al. Fatal liver failure associated with valproate therapy in a patient with Friedreich's disease: review of valproate hepatotoxicity in adults. Epilepsia 1999; 40:1036–40.
442. Schwabe MJ, Dobyns WB, Burke B, et al. Valproate-induced liver failure in one of two siblings with Alpers disease. Pediatr Neurol 1997;16:337–43.
443. Delarue A, Paut O, Guys JM, et al. Inappropriate liver transplantation in a child with Alpers-Huttenlocher syndrome misdiagnosed as valproate-induced acute liver failure. Pediatr Transplant 2000;4:67–71.
444. Kayihan N, Nennesmo I, Ericzon BG, et al. Fatal deterioration of neurological disease after orthotopic liver transplantation for valproic acid-induced liver damage. Pediatr Transplant 2000;4:211–14.
445. Rasmussen M, Sanengen T, Skullerud K, et al. Evidence that Alpers-Huttenlocher syndrome could be a mitochondrial disease. J Child Neurol 2000;15:473–7.
446. Murphy JV, Maquardt KM, Shug AL. Valproic acid associated abnormalities of carnitine metabolism. Lancet 1985;1: 820–1.
447. Matsuda I, Ohtani Y, Ninomiya N. Renal handling of carnitine in children with carnitine deficiency and hyperammonemia associated with valproate therapy. J Pediatr 1986;109:131–4.
448. Beghi E, Bizzi A, Codegoni AM, et al. Valproate, carnitine metabolism, and biochemical indicators of liver function. Epilepsia 1990;31:346–52.
449. Millington DS, Bohan TP, Roe CR, et al. Valproylcarnitine: a novel drug metabolite identified by fast atom bombardment and thermospray liquid chromatography-mass spectroscopy. Clin Chim Acta 1985;145:69–76.
450. Lheureux PE, Penaloza A, Zahir S, et al. Science review: carnitine in the treatment of valproic acid-induced toxicity – what is the evidence? Crit Care 2005;9:431–40.
451. Bohan TP, Helton E, McDonald I, et al. Effect of L-carnitine treatment for valproate-induced hepatotoxicity. Neurology 2001;56:1405–9.
452. Grauso-Eby NL, Goldfarb O, Feldman-Winter LB, et al. Acute pancreatitis in children from Valproic acid: case series and review. Pediatr Neurol 2003;28:145–8.
453. Spitz RD, Keren DF, Boitnott JR, et al. Bridging hepatic necrosis: etiology and prognosis. Am J Dig Dis 1978;23:1076–8.
454. Naranjo CA, Busto U, Sellers EM, et al. A method for estimating the probability of adverse drug reactions. Clin Pharmacol Ther 1981;30:239–45.

455. Begaud B, Evreux JC, Jongland W, et al. Imputabilite des effets inattendus ou toxiques des medicaments. Therapie 1985;40: 111–18.
456. Danan G, Benichou C. Causality assessment of adverse reactions to drugs – I. A novel method based on the conclusions of international consensus meetings: application to drug-induced liver injuries. J Clin Epidemiol 1993;46:1323–30.
457. Benichou C, Danan G, Flahault A. Causality assessment of adverse reactions to drugs – II. An original model for validation of drug causality assessment methods: case reports with positive rechallenge. J Clin Epidemiol 1993;46:1331–6.
458. Spielberg SP. In vitro assessment of pharmacogenetic susceptibility to toxic drug metabolites in humans. Fed Proc 1984;43: 2308–13.

21

Liver Disease in Immunodeficiencies

Nedim Hadžić, M.D.

Man and microbes are committed to a perennial evolutionary conflict in which the human immune system represents a powerful tool of protection against invasion. The liver plays an important role in the immune defense because of its central position adjacent to the gastrointestinal tract, representing the first line of defense against ingested pathogens and various antigens from food.

There are two types of immune response *innate* and *adaptive*. Innate immunity represents the first line of immune defense in which cells such as phagocytes, natural killer (NK) cells, and NK T cells recognize highly conserved antigens from the invading microorganisms and provide a prompt nonspecific inflammatory response. The principal intrahepatic defenders are Kupffer cells – resident macrophages, strongly supported by the action of NK cells, previously also known as Pit cells, which represent approximately 50% of the lymphocyte pool in a healthy liver. In contrast, the adaptive immune system is more phylogenetically advanced and includes more highly specialized cells such as T and B lymphocytes, produced and differentiated in the lymphoid organs. On stimulation, these cells undergo sophisticated processes of immune diversification enabling them to mount specific immune responses to different invading antigens from the environment. These events are much slower and involve mechanisms such as cell-to-cell interaction, proliferation of B cells, production of antibodies and cytokines, and activation of effector cytotoxic cells.

Historically, the adaptive immune response has been divided into the following categories: (1) the humoral arm, mediated by B cells capable of producing antibodies and responsible for mounting defense against bacterial and fungal infections, and (2) the cellular arm, predominantly controlling viral, protozoan, mycobacterial, and other intracellular pathogens. In reality, this distinction is relatively artificial because the immune system, to control the infection, must have both of the components activated. This is achieved through a network of complex feedback mechanisms affecting both arms, orchestrated by CD4-positive T cells via various costimuli on the lymphocyte surface and serine mediators such as acute phase proteins, cytokines, and complement components.

ROLE OF THE LIVER IN IMMUNE DEFENSES

The main immunologic functions of the liver include participation in acute inflammatory response, production of acute phase proteins, induction of tolerance to various antigens, tumor surveillance, and elimination of activated lymphocytes [1]. These are achieved through a complex interaction between macrophages, antigen presenting cells, hepatocytes and effector cells of the innate and adaptive immune system trafficking through the liver. The portal vein is a principal supplier of the liver with massive amount of lymphocytes and antigens from the intestine, which come into close contact with the endothelial cells through an extensive sinusoid network. Kupffer cells control the influx of microorganisms and toxins from the gastrointestinal tract by ensuring that the majority of the pathogens are eliminated via phagocytosis before even entering the systemic circulation. The hepatocytes are a major production site for compounds of systemic inflammatory response, such as C-reactive protein, fibrinogen, α-1-antitrypsin, α-1-antichymotrypsin, mannose-binding lectin, amyloid, and ceruloplasmin [1]. These acute phase reactants assist in infection control and clearance of the pathogens. Finally, most of the activated lymphocytes, after fulfilling their immunologic duties, are destroyed by the hepatic elements of the reticulo–endothelial system or via apoptosis. Thus, the term "immunologic graveyard" has been recently coined for the liver [2].

An intriguing physiologic function inherent to the liver, encompassing elements from both innate and adaptive immunity, is immunologic tolerance. To distinguish between self- and foreign antigens, the immune system undergoes perpetual sophisticated mechanisms of T-cell clonal selection in the thymus and at the periphery. The key players in maintaining mechanisms of "central" and "peripheral" tolerance are T regulatory (T-reg) cells. In addition, the intrahepatic antigen-presenting cells, including Kupffer cells, dendritic cells, sinusoidal endothelial cells, and stellate cells, are heavily involved in the processes of induction and maintenance of immunologic tolerance [1–3]. This critical role of the liver may help in understanding its relatively immune-privileged position and the lesser degree of tissue compatibility required for successful liver transplantation.

A variety of immunologic disturbances have been observed as a consequence of both acute liver failure [4] and chronic liver disease [5]. These include up-regulation of various cytokines, such as interleukin 1 (IL-1), interleukin 6 (IL-6), tumor necrosis factor alpha (TNF-α), and interferon-gamma, abnormal synthesis of acute phase reactants and complement components [6]. It is noteworthy that despite the frequent overexpression of immunologic components, the overall immune function remains impaired, suggesting a lack of immunologic coordination. This immune paresis often adds to the infection-related mortality in liver disorders, particularly in acute liver failure [4]. Conversely, inborn defects of the immune function per se can also contribute to both acute and chronic liver disorders, a fact particularly relevant from the pediatric perspective because these conditions tend to present in childhood.

Defects in the defense mechanisms can be divided in *primary* immunodeficiencies in which there is a genetic cause of the impaired immunity, and *secondary* immunodeficiencies in which the presence of viruses, such as human immunodeficiency virus (HIV), or some major medical intervention, such as chemotherapy or immunosuppressive medications, render the immune responses abnormal. Much of our current understanding of the physiology of the immune reactions originates from recognition of clinical patterns of immune dysfunction in immunodeficient patients and the identification of specific types of microorganisms isolated from them.

PRIMARY IMMUNODEFICIENCIES

Primary immunodeficiencies (PIDs) are rare but potentially fatal disorders of the innate and adaptive immune systems. More than 100 PIDs have been identified at clinical and genetic levels, with an estimated incidence of approximately 1 in 10,000 live births [7,8].

Broadly speaking, PIDs can be divided into disorders of innate and adaptive immunity. Over the last 20 years, the diagnosis and management of PIDs have been dramatically improved because of advances in immunogenetics, better anti-infectious strategies, and the increased use of hematopoietic stem cell transplantation (HSCT) [9].

Secondary immunodeficiencies, related to HIV infection, chemotherapy, post–organ transplantation immunosuppression, or immune ablation, are also better controlled because of the use of modern anti-infectious strategies. In particular, progression of HIV infection has been significantly reduced by the advent of combination antiviral treatment [10].

Primary immunodeficiencies are inherited in either an autosomal recessive or an X-linked manner. Thus, boys are more likely to be affected by PIDs. A simplified classification of PIDs is presented at Table 21.1. A majority of children with significant PIDs present early in infancy, when passive protection from transplacentally and lactation-acquired immunoglobulins starts to wane. Life-threatening chest infections, often caused by *Pneumocystis carinii,* are a typical clinical presentation for children with severe combined immune deficiency (SCID) or hyper-IgM syndrome. Milder forms of PIDs could be diagnosed following investigation into chronic diarrhea; recurrent chest, skin, or ear infections; or failure to thrive. Many children are found to come from consanguineous families. Some have a positive family history of unexplained neonatal and infantile deaths in siblings or maternal relatives because of the X-linked pattern of inheritance in some PIDs [9].

The main clinical problems in the management of immunodeficiencies are recurrent and opportunistic infections. In addition, these patients have an increased lifelong risk of developing malignancies and autoimmune disorders [9]. Frequently, the type of infection broadly indicates whether the problem affects the humoral (e.g., recurrent pyogenic pathogens – bacteria, protozoa) or the cellular (e.g., opportunistic pathogens – viruses, fungi, atypical bacteria) arm of the immune system. For example, isolation of protozoan *P. carinii* from the bronchial aspirate suggests a significant problem in cellular immunity, and identification of *Staphylococcus aureus* from a liver abscess points to neutrophil dysfunction. However, in most immune deficiencies, both cellular and humoral pathways are affected to some degree. For example, the X-linked form of hyper-IgM syndrome – CD40 ligand deficiency, an inborn immunoglobulin defect in class-switch recombination that renders the patients unable to produce other than IgM forms of immunoglobulin, is caused by abnormal interaction between activated lymphocytes and B cells [11]. Consequently, early antibiotic prophylaxis and intravenous or subcutaneous immunoglobulin replacement therapy is indicated for the majority of PIDs. This therapeutic approach, by reducing the incidence of infections, has greatly improved the quality of life of children with PIDs, although there are no data regarding their impact on the longer term incidence of complications.

LIVER COMPLICATIONS IN CHILDREN WITH IMMUNE DEFICIENCIES

Hepatic complications in children with immune deficiencies can be related to chronic infections unaffected by antimicrobial prophylaxis, drugs used to control the infections, or complications before or after HSCT. Approximately 25% of children with PIDs are estimated to have some form of liver involvement [12]. By far the most common hepatic complication of the PIDs is sclerosing cholangitis (SC) (SC is discussed in detail in Chapter 19) [12]. Typically, immunodeficient children with SC do not present with classical symptoms of cholangiopathy such as jaundice, fatigue, or pruritus. Elevation of liver enzymes (aspartate aminotransferase, γ-glutamyltransferase, or alkaline phosphatase) may be trivial or absent. Expert ultrasonography could indicate mild dilatation of the extrahepatic or, less frequently, intrahepatic bile ducts and splenomegaly. In the presence of biochemical or ultrasound changes, further evaluation with liver biopsy and cholangiography is indicated.

Table 21.1: Common Primary Immunodeficiencies

X-Linked Immunodeficiencies

Condition	*Chromosome*	*Gene*	*Function*
X-linked SCID	Xq13	Common γ chain	T- and NK-cell development, T- and B-cell function
X-linked agammaglobulinemia (Bruton)	Xq22	Bruton's tyrosine kinase (Btk)	Pre–B-cell maturation
X-linked hyper-IgM syndrome (CD40 ligand deficiency)	Xq26	CD40 ligand (CD154)	Isotype switching, T-cell function
Wiskott–Aldrich syndrome	Xp11	WASP	Cytoskeletal defect affecting HSC derivatives
X-linked chronic granulomatous disease (CGD)	Xp21	gp91*phox*	Component of NADPH oxidase-phagocytic burst
X-linked lymphoproliferative disease (Duncan's syndrome)	Xq25	SAP	T-cell response to EBV
Properdin deficiency	Xp21	Properdin	Component of complement cascade

Autosomal Recessive Immunodeficiencies

Condition	*Chromosome*	*Gene*	*Function*
SCID type			
Adenosine deaminase (ADA) deficiency	20q12-13	Adenosine deaminase	Removal of toxic metabolites from purine salvage pathway
Purine nucleoside phosphorylase (PNP) deficiency	14q11	Purine nucleoside phosphorylase	Removal of toxic metabolites from purine salvage pathway
Recombinase activating gene (RAG 1 and 2) deficiency	11p13	RAG1 and RAG2	Defective DNA recombination
JAK3 deficiency (T-B+NK SCID)	19p13	JAK3	Abnormal T- and NK-cell development
Zap70 deficiency	2q12	ZAP70	Abnormal intrathymic T-cell selection
Non-SCID type			
Leukocyte adhesion deficiency (LAD) type 1	21q22	CD11/CD18	Defective leukocyte adhesion and migration
Chronic granulomatous disease (CGD)	7q11 1q25 16p24	p47*phox* p67*phox* p22 *phox*	Defective respiratory burst and phagocytic intracellular killing
Chediak–Higashi syndrome	1q42	LYST	Abnormalities in lysosomal protein trafficking
MHC class I deficiency	6p21	TAP1 & TAP2	Abnormal presentation of HLA class I molecules
MHC class II deficiency	16p13 19p12 1q21 13q13	CIITA (MHC2TA) RFXANK RFX5 RFXAP	Defective regulation of MHC II molecule expression
Autoimmune lymphoproliferative syndrome (ALPS)	10q24	APT1 (Fas)	Defective apoptosis
Ataxia telangiectasia	11q22	ATM	Cell cycle control and DNA repair responses

SCID, severe combined immunodefiency
Modified from Jones and Gaspar [8].

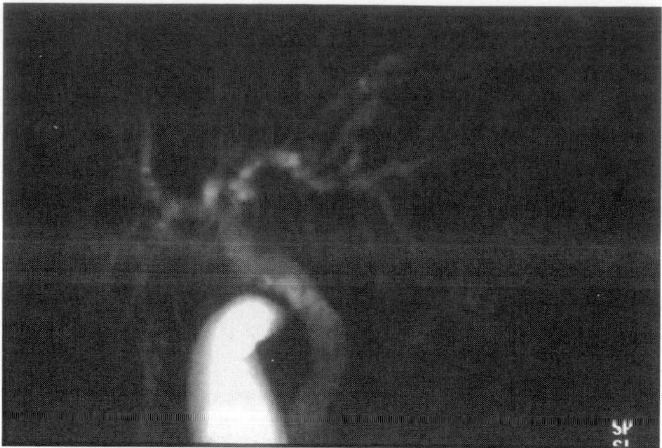

Figure 21.1. Magnetic resonance cholangio-pancreatography (MRCP) demonstrating advanced intrahepatic and extrahepatic cholangiopathy in a patient with combined immunodeficiency (CID).

The increased sensitivity of magnetic resonance cholangiopancreatography (MRCP) has reduced the requirement for the more aggressive direct cholangiographic techniques, such as endoscopic retrograde cholangiopancreatography (ERCP) and percutaneous transhepatic cholangiography (PTC). One study has reported a good concordance between MRCP and ERCP in diagnosing cholangiopathy when the disease is advanced [12] (Figure 21.1). However, subtler radiologic changes may be missed on MRCP. The same study indicated a good correlation, but a slightly increased sensitivity of radiologic compared with histologic methods for diagnosing PIDs-related SC in children [12].

ROLE OF OPPORTUNISTIC INFECTIONS IN THE DEVELOPMENT OF SCLEROSING CHOLANGITIS

Sclerosing cholangitis has been described in a number of immunodeficiencies, predominantly of the combined cellular and humoral type (Table 21.2) [13–16], the most common association being with hyper-IgM syndrome [17]. In a significant proportion of these patients *Cryptosporidium* (CS) is identified, in particular with the use of more sensitive detection approaches, such as polymerase chain reaction–based assays [18]. Standard microscopy, following a modified acid-fast stain, can often overlook the focal presence of CS oocysts in the gastrointestinal tract, where the microbe usually resides in the intestinal and biliary epithelium. Rarely, CS can be identified in liver biopsy specimens at the surface of the biliary epithelium by light microscopy (Figure 21.2). There are 10 CS species, with CS parvum (CSP) representing the most common human pathogen. Two distinct genotypes of CSP relevant to humans – human type 1 and bovine type 2 – have been identified. In immunocompetent individuals, this ubiquitous organism can cause small waterborne outbreaks of diarrhea, but it has not been associated with cholangiopathy [19]. The pathogenic role

Table 21.2: Primary Immunodeficiencies Reported with Sclerosing Cholangitis

Hyper IgM syndrome
Combined immunodeficiency
Common variable deficiency
Wiskott–Aldrich syndrome
MHC class II deficiency
Interferon-gamma deficiency
DiGeorge syndrome
Immunoglobulin subclass deficiency

of CSP in immune deficiency has not been fully elucidated, but animal models of CS-related cholangiopathy have been described [20,21]. Interferon-gamma knockout mice appear to be particularly susceptible to CS infection, suggesting that this cytokine plays a critical role in the immune defense against this pathogen [21]. Biliary damage in humans appears to be caused by a direct cytopathic effects of CSP via apoptotic mechanisms [22]. In addition, CSP can induce cholangiopathy in HIV infection [23–26] and after organ transplant [27,28]. Other intracellular parasites such as *Microsporidium, Mycobacterium avium intracellulare*, and cytomegalovirus [CMV] have also been reported in association with cholangiopathy in adult patients infected with HIV [25]. It is possible that the particularly fast evolution of CSP cholangiopathy in patients with HIV is due to the synergistic effect of multiple biliary infections [24].

Children with chronic cholangiopathy have been reported to have an increased number of gastrointestinal malignancies, including cholangiocarcinoma, lymphoma, and hepatocellular carcinoma. One multicenter study has reported that

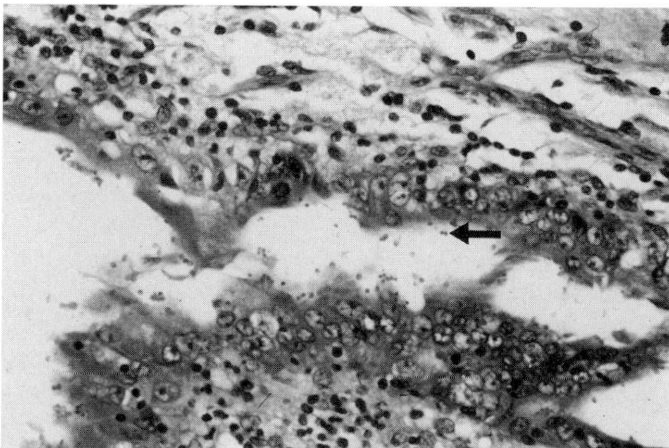

Figure 21.2. Cryptosporidium oocysts (*arrow*) in the section of the liver biopsy of the patient with hyper IgM syndrome and sclerosing cholangitis. (Hematoxylin and eosin, ×150.)

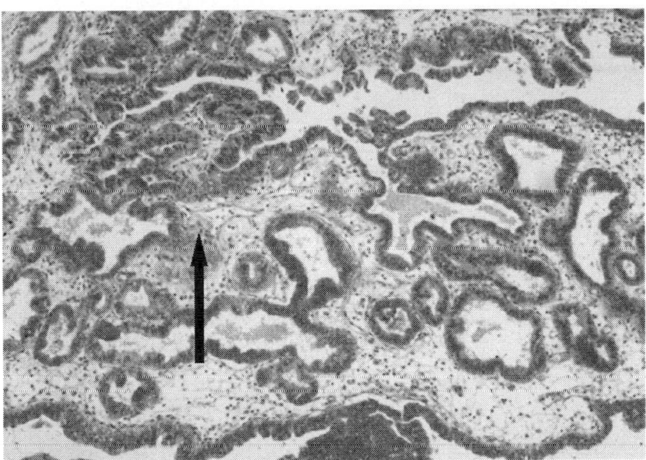

Figure 21.3. Dysplastic changes (*arrow*) in the biliary epithelium of the explanted liver of the patient with CD40 ligand deficiency and end-stage chronic liver disease. (Hematoxylin and eosin, ×400.)

55% of hyper-IgM patients with sclerosing cholangitis had cryptosporidiosis [17]. One 18-year-old patient with hyper-IgM syndrome, undergoing curative sequential liver and stem cell transplantation, was found to have dysplastic biliary changes in the explanted liver (Figure 21.3) [29]. Similar histologic appearances have been noted in patients with HIV infection [25]. Thus, it is conceivable that the failure of antimicrobials to clear CSP or other protozoans from the biliary tract could lead to chronic cholangiopathy, dysplastic changes, and, ultimately, biliary malignancies. The mechanisms for other described immunodeficiency associated malignancies, such as lymphoma and hepatocellular carcinoma, however, remain less than clear, although it can be speculated that inability to mount an effective immune surveillance against potentially neoplastic antigens or clones may play a role.

HYPER-IgM SYNDROME

This condition is a paradigm for immune deficiency–associated SC, which, if not corrected, progresses to chronic biliary disease and cirrhosis in the majority of the patients. In addition, children with hyper-IgM suffer from neutropenia, opportunistic infections, chronic mouth ulcers, chronic diarrhea, failure to thrive, and poorly defined chronic encephalopathy [30]. The estimated incidence is between 1 in 500,000–1,000,000 live births [11,30]. One study reported only 20% survival at 20 years of age in this condition, with life-threatening opportunistic infections and progressive hepatobiliary complications being the main cause of death [17]. Hyper-IgM syndrome is caused by absence of CD40 ligand on activated lymphocytes and lack of interaction with CD40 molecules from B cells in the X-linked form (CD40 ligand deficiency), or defective expression of activation-induced cytidine deaminase (AID) on B cells in the autosomal recessive form of the disease [11]. Therefore, in both forms, B cells are unable to direct physiologic IgM class switching to other immunoglobulin types.

In the past, the majority of children with hyper-IgM syndrome presented to the hepatologist with well-established signs of advanced liver disease, such as biochemical abnormalities and portal hypertension. An increased awareness of the hepatic involvement in PIDs among immunologists in recent years has led to earlier referrals and preventative measures with a consequent reduction of severe liver involvement. Many children with hyper-IgM syndrome may remain surprisingly clinically asymptomatic well into the second decade of life, when progression of the liver disease typically occurs. Thus, pediatricians and parents alike have felt uneasy about considering mortality-associated transplantation options in children with hyper-IgM syndrome, who often have a practically normal quality of life on immunoglobulin replacement and anti-infectious prophylaxis.

Liver transplantation has been attempted for end-stage biliary disease in hyper-IgM syndrome, but fatal cholangiopathy recurs within months after the operation [31,32]. The recurrence may well be accelerated by the effect of post–transplant immunosuppression on quiescent infections of the gastrointestinal tract. It has become clear that correction of the immune defect is essential for patient and graft survival. Hematopoietic stem cell transplantation is able to correct the immune deficiency [33,34], but associated hepatic complications such as sinusoidal obstruction syndrome (also known as veno-occlusive disease), drug hepatotoxicity, and graft-versus-host-disease, significantly reduce survival [35]. Therefore, a reduced intensity conditioning approach that avoids irradiation and uses less hepatotoxic chemotherapeutics, for example, melphalan, and a smaller amount of infused cells, has been introduced for HSCT in the presence of significant pre-existing organ (lungs, liver, or heart) damage. This modified gentler approach has been termed nonmyeloablative or "mini" HSCT [36,37]. A sequential approach with combined liver and "mini" HSCT 1 month later has proved successful in a teenager with decompensated biliary cirrhosis secondary to hyper-IgM syndrome [29]. Some children with less advanced liver disease can survive isolated nonmyeloablative HSCT, but generally patients with hyper-IgM should be identified and screened for a matched donor for HSCT early, while the liver involvement is absent or minimal. In future, the use of umbilical cord grafts will expand the availability of donors for the correction of this and other immune defects.

MANAGEMENT OF CRYPTOSPORIDIOSIS AND SCLEROSING CHOLANGITIS IN IMMUNODEFICIENT PATIENTS

Cryptosporidiosis represents a frequent problem in patients with PIDs [18,19,23] but has also been described after solid organ transplantation [27,28]. Infected patients often have vague abdominal symptoms with watery diarrhea and fever but may also be completely asymptomatic [18,28]. One seven-year old child who was HIV-positive developed acute CSP-associated hydrops of the gallbladder, requiring urgent cholecystectomy [38]. Jejunal biopsy can increase the diagnostic yield in suspected CSP infection, showing nonspecific features such as mild to moderate villous atrophy, submucosal inflammatory infiltrate, and crypt hyperplasia [27]. Some studies have observed a disproportionate elevation of alkaline phosphatase in HIV patients with CSP-associated cholangiopathy [39].

Although most commonly seen in hyper-IgM syndrome and its variant CD40 ligand deficiency, SC, often in conjunction with cryptosporidiosis, has also been described in patients with other PIDs (Table 21.1) [12,13,15,40]. Therefore, this condition needs to be considered in all immunodeficient patients with abnormal hepatic biochemical markers, regardless of their primary diagnosis.

The medical management of cryptosporidiosis is not satisfactory. Clearly, the critical therapeutic maneuver is to increase the immune competence of the host whenever possible. Despite availability of several anti-CS drugs, their efficacy is uncertain, particularly in the setting of chronic immunosuppression. Paromomycin, azithromycin, letrazuril, and recombinant interleukin-2 have been investigated in HIV-positive patients, but without convincing evidence about their benefits [41–44]. Intravenous paromomycin poses considerable risks for inducing conductive deafness, even when the serum levels are kept within the therapeutic range. Nitazoxanide is a novel drug with a proven activity in cryptosporidial diarrhea of immunocompetent patients [45], but no information is available yet in the immunodeficiency setting.

It is prudent to initiate anti-CSP prophylaxis with oral medications, effective in the intestinal lumen, and the boiling of drinking water in all children with hyper-IgM syndrome. The standard choice is paromomycin 250–500 mg twice daily. Once CSP has penetrated the hepatic barriers, any treatment short of reestablishing the immunity is likely to be futile. We also recommend starting choleretic treatment with ursodeoxycholic acid (20 mg/kg/d) [46] in the hope that it will reduce the likelihood of CSP ascending from the gut into the biliary tract.

Children with PIDs who have evidence of persistent hepatic biochemical derangement, even only of a mild degree, should be promptly considered for HSCT because these changes are likely to progress. In the presence of more advanced liver involvement, clinically documented by dilated ducts on ultrasound, splenomegaly, or mild jaundice, each patient should be evaluated individually to assess the relative risks for HSCT. Availability of a well-matched donor, lack of evidence for CSP colonization, satisfactory renal and lung function, and absence of neutropenia increase the chances of a successful outcome. Finally, if the patient with PID presents with end-stage chronic liver disease (coagulopathy, hypoalbuminemia, or ascites) the only viable option is sequential liver and HSCT. The reverse order for these procedures is unlikely to succeed because the decompensated liver would probably not tolerate the effects of pre-HSCT conditioning. Furthermore, the risks of early post-HSCT complications such as sinusoidal obstruction syndrome, acute graft-versus-host disease, or reactivation of quiescent pathogens are much higher with end-stage liver damage [33,35]. The same concerns would apply to a theoretically possible simultaneous living-related liver and HSCT.

MISCELLANEOUS IMMUNODEFICIENCIES AND LIVER DISEASE

Several rare metabolic liver-based conditions have been associated with immune deficiency, such as adenosine deaminase (ADA) deficiency [47], lysinuric protein intolerance [48,49], and propionic acidemia [50,51]. Their immune phenotype may vary from severe combined immune deficiency in ADA deficiency to increased frequency of infections in propionic acidemia. The hepatic damage is thought to be inflicted by accumulation of toxic metabolites and appears to improve on pegylated-ADA supplements in ADA deficiency [48]. Another rare association is severe combined immunodeficiency and multiple intestinal atresia (MIA) with ensuing parental nutrition-induced liver damage [52,53]. In this otherwise fatal condition a recent report suggested amelioration of the immune phenotype following a liver–small bowel transplant, possibly related to the transfer of the peripheral stem cells into the heavily immunosuppressed host during the operation [54].

CHRONIC VIRAL HEPATITIS IN IMMUNODEFICIENCIES

Immunodeficient patients often have abnormal responses to viral pathogens. Given their common long-term requirements for blood products, they may have been exposed to hepatotropic viruses despite the much improved safety of such products. Moreover, these patients are less likely to mount an adequate immune response to vaccines, when they are available, as is the case for hepatitis B (HBV). Longer term, chronic viral infections in immunodeficient patients could have a more aggressive clinical course, particularly in the setting of coinfection. One study from Italy found evidence of HBV, hepatitis C (HCV), and hepatitis G virus (HGV) in 6 of 11 children with PIDs and liver disease, with a 5-year survival of 60% [55].

HIV INFECTION

Liver Disease in HIV Infection

It was estimated that 38 million adults and 2.3 million children worldwide were infected with HIV at the end of 2005 (http://www.unaids.org). The majority of children acquire the infection vertically from their HIV-infected mothers. The advent of highly active antiretroviral therapy (HAART) in 1996 has considerably modified the natural history of this infection in geographic regions where the treatment is affordable [10]. Compared with adults with HIV infection, the survival time in children is significantly shorter even with the use of long-term

HAART. Unfortunately, this treatment has also created a frustrating dual scenario; in the developed world, HIV infection has become a potentially controllable chronic disease with yet-unknown medium-term morbidity, whereas it remains a major killer in the developing countries where HAART is unavailable [56]. An 81% decrease in mortality of children who are HIV-positive diagnosed in the United States between 1987 and 1999 has been reported, albeit with no significant change in morbidity [57]. The median age at death of children infected with HIV was 5 years, with hepatic causes contributing in only around 4% of cases [57].

The gastrointestinal tract is a common port of entry for HIV. The term *HIV-enteropathy* has been coined to describe characteristic histologic changes including monocytic mucosal inflammation and an increased number of intraepithelial lymphocytes caused by invasion of the lamina propria and intestinal macrophages by HIV. As the CD4 count declines, further histologic changes follow, such as crypt hyperplasia and villous atrophy. Activated lymphocytes release a variety of cytokines, such as interferon-gamma and TNF-α, causing further disturbances in the life cycle and function of the enterocytes [58]. Diverse ultrastructural changes including irregular, broadened, and short microvilli, mitochondrial swelling, and deposition of intracytoplasmic inclusion bodies in the various cellular organelles have been described [59]. Inevitably, these chronic morphologic changes in the intestinal tract give rise to clinical symptoms of chronic diarrhea, malnutrition, and weight loss [58]. Breast-feeding may play a role in reducing the rate of progression in countries where HAART is not available [56]. As HIV infection progresses further, the virus spreads to Kupffer cells in the liver, where it can be detected in a characteristically scattered appearance [60]. More advanced disease, reflected in an increased viral load and lower CD4 counts, overwhelms the macrophage scavenger control in the lungs and in the liver, frequently leading to opportunistic infections in the respiratory and gastrointestinal tract, including the liver.

The hepatic pathology in HIV infection in children shares some similarities with the findings in adults, such as nonspecific portal inflammation, Kupffer cell hyperplasia, and high incidence of opportunistic infections, including CMV, *Mycobacterium avium* complex [MAC], *Cryptococcus*, and *Cryptosporidium* [61,62]. However, some intriguing differences such as decreased incidence of granulomas and fatty change, more prominent giant cell transformation of the hepatocytes [63], cholestasis [63], and occasional presence of diffuse lymphoplasmocytic infiltrate associated with lymphoid interstitial pneumonitis have been reported [61,64,65]. Moreover, children from the developing world appear to have more prominent inflammatory features and increased incidence of opportunistic infections contributing to earlier deaths than those observed in their peers from the developed world [65]. Because most of the pediatric studies have been based on autopsy material [61,62,64,65], the role of liver biopsy in the clinical management of HIV-positive patients with minor biochemical abnormalities is uncertain [66]. Less invasive tests for the diagnosis of opportunistic infections, which are the most common reason for the liver involvement, are available.

OPPORTUNISTIC INFECTIONS AND HIV CHOLANGIOPATHY

During the pre-HAART era, HIV-related cholangiopathy associated with *Cryptosporidia, Microsporidia,* and CMV, was frequently reported from both adults and children [67]. This condition, clinically and radiologically very similar to SC in primary immunodeficiencies, is still the most common hepatic feature of HIV infection [68], although it is less frequent with a better preserved immunocompetence of the HIV-infected patients through HAART [10]. Clinical symptoms include abdominal pain, scleral jaundice, hepatomegaly, and diarrhea. Mild to moderate elevation of alkaline phosphatase, γ-glutamyl-transferase, aspartate-aminotransferase, and bilirubin levels is common. Abdominal ultrasonography often demonstrates a mild dilatation of the bile ducts, enlarged gallbladder, and abnormal echo pattern of the liver with minimal splenomegaly [69]. Although MRCP may be useful in documenting suspected HIV cholangiopathy, ERCP is preferred because of the additional possibility of bile sampling to identify the pathogens and of therapeutic biliary stenting or papillotomy in the presence of distal biliary stricture or papilary stenosis, respectively [68,70].

Management of HIV-related hepatic involvement in children is limited. A range of liver disorders has been described in association with HIV infection (Table 21.3). Often, presence of the liver complications simply reflects the general clinical condition of the patient. Therefore, it is hoped that the wider use of effective antiretroviral treatment will arrest their development. By analogy to prevention of cholangiopathy in primary immunodeficiencies, where protozoans such as *Cryptosporidium parvum* or *Microsporidium* are also frequently implicated, it is prudent to initiate antiprotozoal prophylaxis with azythromycin or paromomycin as soon as a decline in peripheral CD4 count is observed. At present, however, there are no controlled data to endorse this suggestion. Choleretic treatment with ursodeoxycholic acid (20 mg/kg/day) may be of benefit when evidence of cholangiopathy is present [46].

Some research indicates that HAART treatment per se may be hepatotoxic [71–74]. In addition to liver involvement, affected patients may have profound lactic acidosis, myopathy, hypercapnia, organic aciduria, anemia, and a range of neurologic symptoms. The underlying mechanism for these symptoms appears to be mitochondrial injury resulting in mtDNA depletion in the liver and muscle. On withdrawal of nucleoside analogues, the clinical symptoms have been reported to revert, with normalization of mtDNA content in the muscle [74,75].

Following the success of HAART, HIV infection has ceased to be a contraindication for liver transplantation. Short-term transplant results in adults are comparable to other indications, although the longer term outcome is likely to be affected by

Table 21.3: Hepato–Biliary Conditions Described with HIV Infection

Viral hepatitis
Chronic hepatitis B
Chronic hepatitis C
Adenovirus
CMV
Epstein–Barr virus
Cholangiopathy
Cryptosporidium parvum
Microsporidium
CMV
Opportunistic infections
Mycobacterium intracellulare
Histoplasma capsulatum
Cryptococcus neoformans
Pneumocystis Carinii
Malignancies
Non–Hodgkin B-cell lymphoma
Kaposi's sarcoma
Hepatoblastoma
Acute B-cell lymphoblastic leukemia
Burkitt lymphoma
Secondary to antiretroviral treatment
Mitochondrial injury
mtDNA depletion syndrome
Pancreatitis
Miscellaneous
Peliosis hepatis
Acalculous cholecystitis

progression of associated pathologies, such as recurrent HCV infection [76,77].

COINFECTION WITH HIV AND OTHER HEPATOTROPIC VIRUSES

Evolution of chronic liver disease caused by hepatotropic viruses (HBV and HCV) in the presence of HIV infection appears to be accentuated [78–80]. The prolonged survival of the coinfected children requires tailored therapeutic strategies. It has been suggested that children with HIV and HCV coinfection need to be treated early, while immune competence of the host is preserved [80,81]. However, this is less clear for children coinfected with HIV and HBV. It is conceivable that impaired cytotoxic, HBV-specific, T-cell function may result in a lesser degree of hepatocyte damage despite ongoing HBV replication. Whether HIV infection–related decline in immune competence is associated with reduced liver injury is possible but uncertain. There is an increased risk of HBV-related acute liver failure observed in adults coinfected with HIV [79]. Of note, the nucleoside analogue lamivudine and the nucleotide inhibitor adefovir, which have proven suppressive activity against HBV, are frequent components of the combined antiretroviral regimens together with some other novel antivirals, such as tenofovir and emtricitabine, that are currently under investigation for potential anti-HBV activity. Studies in adults coinfected with HIV and HCV show that combination therapy with pegylated interferon and ribavirin is safe but that the response is less good than in patients infected with HCV alone [81].

HEPATITIS B VIRUS AND PRIMARY IMMUNODEFICIENCY

Chronic hepatitis B is rarely diagnosed in children with PIDs. There are two primary reasons for this: (1) the countries where PIDs are predominantly diagnosed have a lower incidence of HBV and (2) to inflict hepatocellular injury to HBV-infected hepatocytes, cytotoxic T lymphocytes, sensitized against cells expressing HBV-related peptides, need to be fully operational, which is often not the case in children with PIDs. Thus, their HBV DNA titers and amount of HBe antigen could be high but the liver damage remains minimal because of the lack of host immune response required to cause injury to the hepatocytes.

No published data on the long-term outcome of HBV-positive patients with PIDs are available, but some analogy can be drawn from HBV/HIV coinfected adult patients who, despite the earlier postulate, appear to have an accelerated course of HBV. In a study of adults coinfected with HBV and HIV dating from a pre-HAART era, the histologic features of hepatitis were less advanced as HIV infection progressed [79]. More recent studies indicate reduced rates of anti-HBe and anti-HBs seroconversion with a higher incidence of decompensated end-stage cirrhosis [82]. Antiretroviral treatment can trigger spontaneous anti-HBe and anti-HBs seroconversion and enhance immune control of HBV replication by restoring T-cell integrity but may also induce hepatitic flares. Current recommendations suggest the use of interferon, adefovir, or entecavir in HBV/HIV coinfected naïve patients who do not require antiretroviral treatment. Combination of tenofovir with the nucleoside analogues lamivudine or emtricitabine has been proposed as treatment potentially effective for both viruses [83].

If the immunity is restored, for example, after successful HSCT, there is a danger of overwhelming hepatitis B. Therefore, the use of lamivudine or adefovir is recommended for the HBV-positive patients undergoing HSCT. Recently, it has been reported that using anti-HBc-positive donors may lead to a transfer of adoptive HBV immunity after HSCT [84]. This approach should minimize the likelihood of post-HSCT acute hepatitis B.

HEPATITIS C VIRUS AND PRIMARY IMMUNODEFICIENCY

Evidence of HCV infection in patients with PIDs should be sought by measuring serum HCV RNA because of their frequently assumed deficiency in producing antibodies. Nevertheless, one study suggested that 8 of 18 adult patients with various primary impairments of antibody production, such as common variable immunodeficiency (CVI), hyper-IgM syndrome, and IgG subclass deficiency, were able to produce anti-HCV antibodies [85].

Chronic hepatitis C has an accelerated course in individuals with immune deficiencies [86,87]. One 15-year-old girl with CVI developed fatal end-stage liver disease only 5 years after contracting the virus [87]. When compared with immunocompetent individuals, immunodeficient patients have significantly higher HCV RNA titers during acute hepatitis [88]. Before 1990, there were several well-documented outbreaks of HCV infection in patients with immune deficiencies due to contaminated immunoglobulins, leading to progressive liver disease often requiring liver transplantation [55,89,90]. The results of transplantation were largely disappointing with prompt recurrence and fatal infectious complications [91]. It is likely that posttransplant immunosuppression played a significant contributory role in these adverse outcomes. However, an adult patient with CVI has been reported to have cleared the virus after liver transplantation, but aggressive recurrence with severe cholestatic hepatitis and liver failure prompted withdrawal of immunosuppression. Five years posttransplant, he remained well on low-dose immunosuppression, subsequently reintroduced [92].

There are no data on whether immunodeficient patients should be treated early with the emerging more efficient anti-HCV strategies. Early treatment would appear logical, although it is unlikely that there will ever be a sufficient number of immunodeficient patients to endorse this speculation through a formal trial. The same would apply to children perinatally coinfected by HIV and HCV in view of the highly effective antiretroviral therapy now available.

HEMOPHAGOCYTIC LYMPHOHISTIOCYTOSIS

Hemophagocytic lymphohistiocytosis (HLH) is a hyperinflammatory syndrome characterized by high fever, pancytopenia, hypercytokinemia, and coagulopathy [93]. Cardinal clinical features are hepatosplenomegaly, ascites, respiratory failure, skin infiltrates, and central nervous system involvement. Frequent laboratory findings are hypofibrinogenemia, hyperferritinemia, hypertriglyceridemia, and elevated serum lactate dehydrogenase. Hallmark of the disease is the presence of hemophagocytosis in activated macrophages in the bone marrow, ascitic, or cerebrospinal fluid (Figure 21.4). This diagnostic feature may not be seen at presentation and cytologic examination of the bone marrow or ascitic fluid may need to be repeated if clinically indicated. At postmortem, the hemophagocytic infiltrates can be found in the liver, lungs, skin, kidneys, and brain. This systemic disease is often triggered by infection and may progress to hepatic and renal failure. The microorganisms reported in association with HLH include viruses (Epstein–Barr

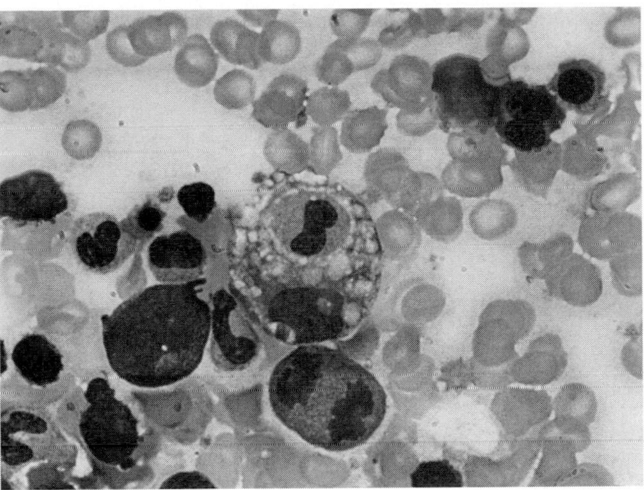

Figure 21.4. Phenomenon of hemophagocytosis demonstrated by a large histiocyte (*center*) engulfing two smaller cells in the bone marrow aspirate.

virus [EBV], herpes simplex and zoster, CMV), bacteria, and fungi, but often no organism is identified [93]. Children with HLH who present with liver involvement and multiorgan failure have a very high mortality [94]. Clinical diagnostic criteria are presented in the (Table 21.4).

Despite its recognition more than 50 years ago [95] and recent progress in understanding its pathogenesis [96], HLH remains underdiagnosed, probably because of its nonspecific clinical features and often fulminant progression. Its incidence is estimated to be approximately 1 in 50,000 live births [97].

Most patients with HLH will have abnormal NK cell function, with evidence of impaired granule-dependent cytotoxic pathways. Perforin is a 60 kDa polypeptide, secreted by cytoplasmic granules of NK cells and cytotoxic lymphocytes. Its physiologic role, on stimulation, is to form "pores" or perforations in the membrane of the target cells, allowing other mediators of cell death (i.e., granzyme) to enter the cell and facilitate osmotic cell lysis [96,98]. The ongoing yet inefficient stimulation of the immune system via various complex pathogenic mechanisms results in overexpression of proinflammatory cytokines, such as TNF-α, interleukin-6, interleukin-8, interleukin-12, interleukin-18, interferon-gamma, and macrophage inhibitory protein 1-α, but also of a number of hemopoietic growth factors released by the overstimulated lymphocytes and macrophages [93,96].

Approximately 70–80% of the HLH patients, predominantly presenting in infancy, have an autosomal recessive primary immune defect (primary or familial form of HLH), often unmasked by an acute infection [98]. Only 20–30% of these children have documented perforin mutations [96], and it is speculated that other modifiers or yet unrecognized defects of immune function could play a role in the remaining patients. In older HLH patients, the "overstimulation" of the immune system may also be triggered by a microbial stimulus, but in the absence of documented underlying immunodeficiency or consanguinity (secondary form). This sporadic form of HLH

Table 21.4: Diagnostic Criteria for Hemophagocytic Lymphohistiocytosis*

1. A molecular diagnosis consistent with HLH

or

2. Diagnostic criteria for HLH fulfilled (5 of the 8 criteria that follow)

A) Initial diagnostic criteria (*to be evaluated in all patients with HLH*)

Clinical criteria

- Fever
- Splenomegaly

Laboratory criteria

- Cytopenias (affecting ≥2 of 3 lineages in the peripheral blood):
  - Hemoglobin (<90 g/L) (In infants <4 weeks: Hb <100 g/L)
  - Platelets (<100 × 10^9/L)
  - Neutrophils (<1.0 × 10^9/L)
- Hypertriglyceridemia and/or hypofibrinogenemia (fasting triglycerides ≥3.0 mmol/L (i.e., ≥265 mg/dL, fibrinogen ≤1.5 g/L)

Histopathologic criteria

- Hemophagocytosis in bone marrow, ascitic fluid, liver, spleen, or lymph nodes. No evidence of malignancy.

B) New diagnostic criteria

- Low or absent NK-cell activity (according to local laboratory reference)
- Ferritin ≥500 μg/L
- Soluble CD25 (i.e., soluble IL-2 receptor) ≥2400 U/mL

*Modified from Henter JI. Hemophagocytic lymphohistiocytosis (HLH). (Accessed February 10, 2006, at http://histio.org/society.)

can also be seen in association with malignancy, autoimmune disorders, or after organ transplant [99]. *Macrophage activation syndrome* is an alternative term sometimes used in rheumatology to describe a phenomenon similar to HLH.

Familial HLH is a heterogeneous group with possibly different degrees of clinical severity. There are now at least four variants of familial HLH for which a number of mutations in the genes involved in the intracellular perforin- and granzyme-related intracellular killing homeostasis have been identified in children from various ethnic groups (Table 21.5) [100–104]. The best documented are the defects in perforin synthesis (FHL2) in which absence of perforin-1 in the cytotoxic granules of NK cells can also be demonstrated immunohistochemically [105]. Expression of perforin in peripheral lymphocytes using a fluorescence activated cell sorter (FACS) technique can be used as a simple and rapid screening test for confirmation of perforin deficiency in a child with clinically suspected HLH [105].

Griscelli syndrome is another autosomal recessive form of HLH associated with variable pigment distribution, ranging from hair hypopigmentation and albinism to hyperpigmentation of sun-exposed areas. The underlying genetic defect is mutation in RAB27A, located at chromosome 15q21, encoding several Rab proteins involved in melanin synthesis by melanosomes in the skin melanocytes and intracellular killing in the lymphocytes [98].

A milder clinical phenotype of HLH has recently been described in patients with lysinuric protein intolerance [48,49]. Hyperammonemia and aminoaciduria may be suggestive of this metabolic condition, but in children presenting with acute liver failure, these findings could be of limited help.

TREATMENT OF HEMOPHAGOCYTIC LYMPHOHISTIOCYTOSIS

The clinical manifestations of acute HLH are invariably associated with infection [96,106]. However, the majority of symptoms are related to the effects of the over-stimulated immune system and antimicrobial treatment may have a limited role [93]. Thus, the main aim of treatment is to neutralize the effects of the ongoing overwhelming, yet inefficient inflammatory response. Paradoxically, the initial treatment of these patients, including those who could have a primary immune defect, is with immunosuppressive agents such as epidophyllotoxin etoposide (VP-16), corticosteroids and cyclosporine A, in conjunction with a high dose intravenous immunoglobulin [93,97,107].

The recently modified HLH-94 treatment protocol recommends 8 weeks of initial therapy with VP-16 (150 mg/m^2 twice weekly for 2 weeks and then weekly), with daily oral cyclosporin A, aiming at trough levels of 200 μg/L, and dexamethasone (initially 10 mg/m^2 for 2 weeks followed by 5 mg/m^2 for 2 weeks, 2.5 mg/m^2 for 2 weeks, 1.25 mg/m^2 for 1 week, and 1 week of tapering). From week 9 onward, the maintenance therapy includes dexamethasone pulses (10 mg/m^2 for 3 days every second week) and VP-16 infusions (150 mg/m^2) on alternate weeks. Full details of the treatment protocol are available elsewhere [97, http://histio.org/society/protocols]. Some children with milder forms may respond to this treatment, but severe and primary forms may lead to consideration for anti–thymocyte globulin with intrathecal methotrexate, if deemed safe on clinical grounds [107].

Children who present with liver involvement and HLH are often critically ill and need intensive supportive management [94]. Aggressive broad-spectrum antibiotic, antiviral, and antifungal treatment is given while awaiting culture results. Liposomal amphotericin B is the antifungal of choice because it is also effective against Leishmania, a common trigger for HLH in some geographic areas. Assisted ventilation is required early because of lung involvement and development of central nervous system complications. Renal support with hemofiltration or dialysis is often indicated because of impending renal failure.

Table 21.5: Genetic Variants of Familial Hemophagocytic Lymphohistiocytosis

	Locus	*Gene*	*Function*	*Group*
FHL1	9q21.3–22	Unknown		Ohadi et al. [100]
FHL2	10q21–22	Perforin 1 (*PRF1*)	Perforin synthesis	Dufourcq Lagelouse et al. [101]
FHL3	17q25	*UNC13D*	hMunc 13–4 synthesis, granule priming	Feldmann et al. [102]
FHL4	6q24	Syntaxin 11 (*STX11*)	Vesicle trafficking, membrane fusion	zur Stadt et al. [103]

In parallel with the intensive medical management children with HLH need to be worked up for urgent diagnosis of primary immunodeficiency and consideration for HSCT [108–110]. Familial HLH is universally relapsing and search for a familial or an unrelated donor must start immediately after diagnosis. Secondary HLH usually responds to medical treatment and does not require HSCT [110]. Of note, asymptomatic relatives of children with primary HLH secondary to perforin deficiency (FHL2) have reduced perforin expression in their lymphocytes [105]. There is a possibility that some of these prospective donor siblings may be in a preclinical phase of the same disease, which could then be accelerated by post-HSCT immunosuppression. Thus, unrelated donors are preferable, particularly in the absence of convincingly better results of HSCT from the familial donors [109,111]. Overall, 1- to 3-year survival post-HSCT is approximately 30–75% [93,110], but one recent single center study reports 100% survival in 12 children with more than 2-year follow-up [109]. Another series also reports no fatalities in 12 children, including 3 with mild liver involvement, after nonmyeloablative HSCT [111].

Liver transplantation has traditionally been considered to be contraindicated in the acute phase of HLH because of the hyperactivated immune system, multiorgan failure, and the critical condition of the patient. The assumption was that the abnormality of the immune system would recur and promptly affect the liver graft. A recent case report by Matthes-Martin et al. [112] has broadened the discussion about familial HLH. A 4-month-old girl presenting with HLH-related acute liver failure initially received a living-related liver transplant from her mother, followed by myeloablation and haploidentical stem-cell grafting from the same donor 70 days later. Two months later, a complete donor chimerism was obtained after a further maternal T-cell infusion, which led to a complete withdrawal of immunosuppression. The child is alive and well 5 years later (Dr. Helmut Gadner, personal communication).

X-LINKED LYMPHOPROLIFERATIVE DISEASE

X-linked lymphoproliferative (XLP) disease is a rare familial condition; affected males present with fulminant, often fatal, infectious mononucleosis, B-cell lymphomas or progressive dysgammaglobulinaemia. The condition was described more than 30 years ago in a large U.S. family, the Duncan kindred, in which six of the boys but none of the girls were affected, which led to the initial name (Duncan's disease) [113]. In the majority, but not in all patients, the disease becomes symptomatic on acquiring EBV infection [114,115].

Clinically, children usually present with fever; liver involvement including hepatitis, hepatosplenomegaly, or frank liver failure; and lymphadenopathy. Female carriers can have a milder involvement. Less frequently, XLP disease can present with lymphomas and autoimmune disorders such as colitis, vasculitis, psoriasis, or Wegener granulomatosis in children younger than 5 years [116]. Histologically, the affected organs exhibit a polyclonal infiltration by EBV-infected cells but also reactive CD4+ and CD8+ T cells and sometimes hemophagocytosis [117]. Thus, XLP disease should also be considered in the differential diagnosis of HLH.

X-linked lymphoproliferative disease is caused by mutations in the Src homology 2 (SH2) domain-containing gene 1A (*SH2D1A*), encoding a cytoplasmic adapter called signalling lymphocytic activation molecule (SLAM)-associated protein (SAP) [117, 118]. Cytoplasmic adapters are intracellular molecules modulating intracellular signalling processes. Aberrant reactivity within the SAP pathway induces a severe disruption of cytotoxic T-cell function, which, when triggered by EBV, leads to uncontrolled B-cell proliferation [115,117,119]. By positional cloning, XLP disease has been mapped to a single locus at chromosome Xq24–25 [120].

X-linked lymphoproliferative disease may not always been triggered by EBV infection. Measles virus and Neisseria meningitidis have also been implicated [117]. The immune response against EBV is controlled by primary and memory CD8+ cytotoxic T lymphocyte (CTL) reaction toward major histocompatibility complex (MHC)-peptide complexes produced by EBV latent proteins: EBNA-3A, -3B, and -3C. The CTL function is genetically determined via various mechanisms, including the SAP-dependent pathway, possibly explaining the variable individual clinical response against infectious mononucleosis in immunocompetent individuals. In XLP patients, the failure of CTLs to control ongoing EBV-driven B-cell proliferation may ultimately give rise to lymphoid malignancies [121].

The treatment options for XLP disease are very limited. Characterization of the immune defect in an acutely unwell child usually takes longer than the fulminant course of the disease. In families with a previous positive history, it is possible to perform elective HSCT before the affected boys are exposed to EBV [122]. Novel treatments with anti–B-cell monoclonal antibodies or adoptive transfer of immunity by infusions of EBV-sensitized, HLA-matched CTLs, both of potential theoretical benefit in XLP disease, have not yet been reported.

A better understanding of the interaction between invading pathogens, SLAM and SAP proteins, and activation of cytotoxic T cells will help not only in the understanding of the pathogenesis of XLP disease but potentially also of posttransplant lymphoproliferative disorder, for which EBV also represents a common trigger [121].

CHRONIC GRANULOMATOUS DISEASE

Chronic granulomatous disease (CGD) is a primary neutrophil disorder caused by a defect in the production of the respiratory oxidative burst leading to ineffective phagocytosis. About two thirds of affected patients are boys with a mutation at chromosome Xp21, and the remaining children have a less severe, autosomal recessive form of the disease with mutations at 7q11, 1q25, or 16p25 [9,123].

The patients with CGD are particularly susceptible to infections caused by catalase-producing bacteria and fungi. The failure to clear these infections effectively leads to granuloma formation in the skin, liver, bone, brain, or gut. Approximately 25% of children with CGD will present with hepatic abscesses [123]. One series from the United Kingdom reported a 33% incidence of newly diagnosed CGD among children with pyogenic liver abscesses [124]. The diagnosis is made via a simple nitroblue-tetrazolium (NBT) test in which a failure of intracytoplasmic granules to change color suggests abnormal neutrophil function. Carriers, including mothers of the X-linked cases, will often have a history of recurrent mouth ulcers or prolonged infections and mildly abnormal NBT tests. Following the diagnosis in a proband, the whole family should undertake screening with NBT test because the disease could be initially asymptomatic. It is strongly recommended to rule out CGD in any child presenting with a liver abscess even in the absence of a history of pyogenic skin lesions or recurrent infections [124].

Hepatic abscesses require aspiration both for diagnostic and therapeutic purposes. The most common isolated microorganism in children is *Staphylococcus aureus* [124]. Intravenous antibiotics often need to be given for several months until ultrasonographic resolution is evident and until fever and inflammatory markers, such as leukocytosis and C-reactive protein, normalize. Resistant infections may be considered for interferon-gamma treatment and infusions of purified white cells. Indefinite antimicrobial prophylaxis with itraconazole and septrin is mandatory, sometimes in association with subcutaneous interferon-gamma [125]. If this strategy fails, HSCT is increasingly being performed with satisfactory results [126].

REFERENCES

1. Mackay IR. Hepatoimmunology: a perspective. Immunol Cell Biol 2002;80:36–44.
2. Crispe IN, Dao T, Klugewitz K, et al. The liver as a site of T-cell apoptosis: graveyard, or killing field? Immunol Rev 2000;174:47–62.
3. Weiler-Normann C, Rehermann B. The liver as an immunological organ. J Gastroenterol Hepatol 2004;19:S279–83.
4. Rolando N, Wade J, Davalos M, et al. The systemic inflammatory response syndrome in acute liver failure. Hepatology 2000; 32:734–9.
5. Tilg H, Wilmer A, Vogel W, et al. Serum levels of cytokines in chronic liver diseases. Gastroenterology 1992;103:264–74.
6. Izumi S, Hughes RD, Langley PG, et al. Extent of the acute phase response in fulminant hepatic failure. Gut 1994;35:982–6.
7. Notarangelo L, Casanova JL, Fischer A, et al. Primary immunodeficiency diseases: an update. J Allergy Clin Immunol 2004;114: 677–87.
8. Jones AM, Gaspar HB. Immunogenetics: changing the face of immunodeficiency. J Clin Pathol 2000;53:60–5.
9. Rosen FS, Cooper MD, Wedgwood RJP. The primary immunodeficiencies. N Engl J Med 1995;333:431–40.
10. Hammer SM. Management of newly diagnosed HIV infection. N Engl J Med 2005;353:1702–10.
11. Durandy A, Honjo T. Human genetic defects in class-switch recombination (hyper-IgM syndromes). Curr Opin Immunol 2001;13:543–8.
12. Rodrigues F, Davies ED, Harrison P, et al. Liver disease in primary immunodeficiencies. J Pediatr 2004;145:333–9.
13. Record CO, Shilkin KB, Eddleston ALWF, Williams R. Intrahepatic sclerosing cholangitis associated with a familial immunodeficiency syndrome. Lancet 1973;ii:18–20.
14. Thomas IT, Ochs HD, Wedgwood RJ. Liver disease and immunodeficiency syndromes [letter]. Lancet 1974;ii:311.
15. Naveh Y, Mendelsohn H, Spira G, et al. Primary sclerosing cholangitis associated with immunodeficiency. Am J Dis Child 1983;137:114–17.
16. Davis JJ, Heyman MB, Ferrell L, et al. Sclerosing cholangitis associated with chronic cryptosporidiosis in a child with a congenital immunodeficiency disorder. Am J Gastroenterol 1987; 82:1196–202.
17. Hayward AR, Levy J, Facchetti F, et al. Cholangiopathy and tumours of the pancreas, liver and biliary tree in boys with X-linked immunodeficiency with hyper-IgM. J Immunol 1997; 158:977–83.
18. McLauchlin J, Amar CFL, Pedraza-Diaz S, et al. Polymerase chain reaction-based diagnosis of infection with Cryptosporidium in children with primary immunodeficiencies. Pediatr Inf Dis J 2003;22:329–34.
19. Chen XM, Keithly JS, Paya CV, LaRusso NF. Cryptosporidiosis. N Engl J Med 2002;346:1723–31.
20. Mead JR, Arrowood MJ, Sidwell RW, Healey MC. Chronic *Cryptosporidium parvum* infections in congenitally immunodeficient SCID and nude mice. J Infect Dis 1991;163:1297–304.
21. Stephens J, Cosyns M, Jones M, Hayward A. Liver and bile duct pathology following *Cryptosporidium parvum* infection of the immunodeficient mice. Hepatology 1999;30:27–35.
22. Chen XM, Levine SA, Tietz P, et al. *Cryptosporidium parvum* is cytopathic for cultured human biliary epithelia via an apoptotic mechanism. Hepatology 1998;28:906–13.

23. Petersen J. Cryptosporidiosis in patients infected with human immunodeficiency virus. Clin Infect Dis 1992;152:2497–9.
24. Chen XM, LaRusso NF. Cryptosporidiosis and the pathogenesis of AIDS cholangiopathy. Semin Liver Dis 2002;22: 277–89.
25. Kline TJ, De Las Morenas T, O'Brien M, et al. Squamous metaplasia of extrahepatic biliary system in an AIDS patient with cryptosporidia and cholangitis. Dig Dis Sci 1993;38:960–2.
26. Cello JP. Acquired immunodeficiency syndrome cholangiopathy: spectrum of disease. Am J Med 1989;86:539–46.
27. Gerber DA, Green M, Jaffe R, Greenberg D, et al. Cryptosporidial infections after solid organ transplantation in children. Pediatr Transplant 2000;4:50–5.
28. Campos M, Jouzdani E, Sempoux C, et al. Sclerosing cholangitis associated to cryptosporidiosis in liver-transplanted children. Eur J Pediatr 2000;159:113–15.
29. Hadzic N, Pagliuca A, Rela M, et al. Correction of the hyper IgM-syndrome after liver and bone marrow transplantation. N Engl J Med 2000;342:320–4.
30. Winkelstein JA, Marino MC, Ochs H, et al. The X-linked hyper-IgM syndrome. Clinical and immunological features of 79 patients. Medicine 2003;82:373–84.
31. Martinez Ibanez V, Espanol T, Matamoros N, et al. Relapse of sclerosing cholangitis after liver transplantation in patients with hyper-IgM syndrome. Transplant Proc 1997;29:432–3.
32. Hadzic N, Heaton ND, Davies G, et al. Liver transplantation in children with primary immunodeficiencies [abstract]. Hepatology 1999;30:182A.
33. Horwitz ME. Stem-cell transplantation for inherited immunodeficiency disorders. Pediatr Clin North Am 2000;47:1371–87.
34. Thomas C, De Saint BG, Le Deist F, et al. Brief report: correction of X-linked hyper-IgM syndrome by allogeneic bone marrow transplantation. N Engl J Med 1995;333:426–9.
35. Khawaja K, Gennery AR, Flood TJ, et al. Bone marrow transplantation for CD40 ligand deficiency: a single centre experience. Arch Dis Child 2001;84:508–11.
36. Amrolia P, Gaspar HB, Hassan A, et al. Nonmyeloablative stem cell transplantation for congenital immunodeficiencies. Blood 2000;96:1239–46.
37. Jacobsohn DA, Emerick KM, Scholl P, et al. Nonmyeloablative hematopoietic stem cell transplant for X-linked hyper-immunoglobulin M syndrome with cholangiopathy. Pediatrics 2004;113:122–7.
38. Boige N, Bellaiche M, Cornet D, et al. Hydrops-like cholecystitis due to cryptosporidiosis in an HIV-infected child. J Pediatr Gastroenterol Nutr 1998;26:219–21.
39. Ramratnam B, Flanigan TP. Cryptosporidiosis in persons with HIV infection. Postgrad Med J 1997;73:713–16.
40. Kahn K, Sharp H, Hunter D, Kerzner B, et al. Primary sclerosing cholangitis in Wiskott–Aldrich syndrome. J Pediatr Gastroenterol Nutr 2001;32:95–9.
41. Hicks P, Zwiener RJ, Squires J, Savell V. Azithromycin therapy for Cryptosporidium parvum infection in four children infected with human immunodeficiency virus. J Pediatr 1997;130: 1009–10.
42. Armitage K, Flanigan T, Carey J, et al. Treatment of cryptosporidiosis with paromomycin. A report of 5 cases. Arch Intern Med 1992;152: 2497–9.
43. Blanshard C, Shanson DC, Gazzard BG. Pilot studies of azithromycin, letrazuril and paromomycin in the treatment of Cryptosporidiosis. Int J Std AIDS 1997;8:124–9.
44. Nachbaur D, Kropshofer G, Feichtinger H, et al. Cryptosporidiosis after CD34-selected autologous peripheral blood stem cell transplantation (PBSCT). Treatment with paromomycin, azithromycin and recombinant human interleukin-2. Bone Marrow Transplant 1997;19:1261–3.
45. Rosignol JF, Ayoub A, Ayers MS. Treatment of diarrhea caused by Cryptoporidium parvum: a prospective randomized, double-blind, placebo-controlled study of nitazoxanide. J Infect Dis 2001;184:103–6.
46. Gilger MA, Gann ME, Opekun AR, Gleason WA Jr. Efficacy of ursodeoxycholic acid in the treatment of primary sclerosing cholangitis in children. J Pediatr Gastroenterol Nutr 2000;31: 136–41.
47. Bollinger ME, Arredongo-Vega FX, Santisteban I, et al. Brief report: hepatic dysfunction as a complication of adenosine deaminase deficiency. N Engl J Med 1996;334:1367–71.
48. Duval M, Fenneteau O, Doireau V, et al. Intermittent hemophagocytic lymphohistiocytosis is a regular feature of lysinuric protein intolerance. J Pediatr 1999;134:236–9.
49. Bader-Meunier B, Parez N, Muller S. Treatment of hemophagocytic lymphohistiocytosis with cyclosporin A and steroids in a boy with lysinuric protein intolerance. J Pediatr 2000;136:134.
50. Raby RB, Ward RB, Herrod HG. Propionic academia and immunodeficiency. J Inher Metab Dis 1994;17:250–1.
51. Al Essa M, Rahbeeni Z, Jumaah S, et al. Infectious complications of propionic academia in Saudi Arabia. Clin Genet 1998;54: 90–4.
52. Moreno LA, Gottrand F, Turck D, et al. Severe combined immunodeficiency syndrome associated with autosomal recessive familial multiple gastrointestinal atresias: study of a family. Am J Med Genet 1990;37:143–6.
53. Walker MW, Lovell MA, Kelly TE, et al. Multiple areas of intestinal atresia associated with immunodeficiency and posttransfusion graft-versus-host disease. J Pediatr 1993;123:93–5.
54. Gilroy RK, Coccia PF, Talmadge JE, et al. Donor immune reconstitution after liver-small bowel transplantation for multiple intestinal atresia with immunodeficiency. Blood 2004;103: 1171–4.
55. Fiore M, Ammendola R, Gaetaniello L, et al. Chronic unexplained liver disease in children with primary immunodeficiency syndromes. J Clin Gastroenterol 1998;26:187–92.
56. Wittenberg D, Benítez CV, Canani RB, et al. HIV infection: working group report of the Second World Congress of Pediatric Gastroenterology, Hepatology, and Nutrition. J Pediatr Gastroenterol Nutr 2004;39 Suppl 2:S640–6.
57. Selik RM, Lindegren ML. Changes in deaths reported with human immunodeficiency virus infection among United States children less than thirteen years old, 1987 through 1999. Pediatr Infect Dis J 2003;22:635–41.
58. Guarino A, Bruzzese E, De Marco G, Buccigrossi V. Management of gastrointestinal disorders in children with HIV infection. Pediatr Drugs 2004;6:347–62.
59. Fontana M, Boldorini R, Zuin G, et al. Ultrastructural changes in duodenal mucosa of HIV-infected children. J Pediatr Gastroenterol Nutr 1993;17:255–9.
60. Duffy LF, Daum F, Kahn E, et al. Hepatitis in children with acquired immune deficiency syndrome: histopathologic and immunocytologic features. Gastroenterology 1986;90:173–81.
61. Jonas MM, Roldan EO, Lyons HJ, et al. Histopathologic features of the liver in pediatric acquired immune deficiency syndrome. J Pediatr Gastroenterol Nutr 1989;9:73–81.

62. Viriyavejakul P, Rojanasunan P, Viriyavejakul A, et al. Opportunistic infections in the liver of HIV-infected patients in Thailand: a necropsy study. Southeast Asian J Trop Med Public Health 2000;31:663–7.
63. Gaur S, Rosenthal S, Dadhania J, et al. Cholestatic giant cell hepatitis associated with ultrastructural evidence of intrahepatic retroviral infection in a human immunodeficiency virus-seropositive infant. J Pediatr Gastroenterol Nutr 1993;16:199–202.
64. Kahn E, Greco MA, Daum F, et al. Hepatic pathology in pediatric acquired immunodeficiency syndrome. Hum Pathol 1991;22:1111–19.
65. Morotti RA, Tata M, Drut R, et al. Liver pathology in children with AIDS: a comparison between the South American and North American population. Pediatr Pathol Mol Med. 2001;20:537–45.
66. Lacaille F, Fournet JC, Blanche S. Clinical utility of liver biopsy in children with acquired immunodeficiency syndrome. Pediatr Infect Dis J 1999;18:143–7.
67. Bouche H, Housset C, Dumont JL, et al. AIDS-related cholangitis: diagnostic features and course in 15 patients. J Hepatol 1993;17:34–9.
68. Yabut B, Werlin SL, Havens P, et al. Endoscopic retrograde cholangiopancreatography in children with HIV infection. J Pediatr Gastroenterol Nutr 1996;23:624–7.
69. Chung CJ, Sivit CJ, Rakusan TA, et al. Hepatobiliary abnormalities on sonography in children with HIV infection. J Ultrasound Med 1994;13:205–10.
70. Cello JP. Human immunodeficiency virus-associated biliary tract disease. Semin Liver Dis 1992;12:213–18.
71. Lacaille F, Ortigao MB, Debre M, et al. Hepatic toxicity associated with 2′-3′dideoxy-inosine in children with AIDS. J Pediatr Gastroenterol Nutr 1995;20:287–90.
72. Clark SJ, Creighton S, Portmann B, et al. Acute liver failure associated with antiretroviral treatment for HIV: a report of six cases. J Hepatol 2002;36:295–301.
73. Scherpbier HJ, Hilhorst MI, Kuijpers TW. Liver failure in a child receiving highly active antiretroviral therapy and voriconazole. Clin Infect Dis 2003;37:828–30.
74. Church JA, Mitchell WG, Gonzales-Gomes I, et al. Mitochondrial DNA depletion, near-fatal metabolic acidosis, and liver failure in an HIV-infected child treated with combination antiretroviral therapy. J Pediatr 2001;138:748–51.
75. De la Asuncion JG, del Olmo ML, Sastre J, Pallardo FV, Vina J. Zidovudine (AZT) causes an oxidation of mitochondrial DNA in mouse liver. Hepatology 1999;29:985–7.
76. Prachalias AA, Pozniak A, Taylor C, et al. Liver transplantation in adults coinfected with HIV. Transplantation 2001;72:1684–8.
77. Neff GW. Bonham A, Tzakis AG, et al. Orthotopic liver transplantation in patients with human immunodeficiency virus and end-stage liver disease. Liver Transplant 2003;9:239–47.
78. Martin P, DiBisceglie AM, Kassianides C, et al. Rapidly progressive non–A non–B hepatitis in patients with human immunodeficiency virus infection. Gastroenterology 1989;97:1559–61.
79. Housset C, Pol S, Carnot F, et al. Interactions between human immunodeficiency virus-1, hepatitis delta virus and hepatitis B virus infections in 260 chronic carriers of hepatitis B virus. Hepatology 1992;15:578–83.
80. Resti M, Azzari C, Bortolotti F. Hepatitis C virus infection in children coinfected with HIV: epidemiology and management. Pediatr Drugs 2002;4:571–80.
81. Strader DB, Wright T, Thomas TL, Seeff LB. Diagnosis, management, and treatment of hepatitis C. Hepatology 2004;39:1147–71.
82. Puoti M, Torti C, Bruno R, et al. Natural history of chronic hepatitis B in co-infected patients. J Hepatol 2006;44:S65–70.
83. Benhamou Y. Treatment algorithm for chronic hepatitis B in HIV-infected patients. J Hepatol 2006;44:S90–4.
84. Lau G, Suri D, Liang R, et al. Resolution of chronic hepatitis B and anti-HBs seroconversion in humans by adoptive transfer of immunity to hepatitis B core antigen. Gastroenterology 2002;122:614–24.
85. Quinti I, Pandolfi F, Paganelli R, et al. HCV infection in patients with primary defects of immunoglobulin production. Clin Exp Immunol 1995;102:11–16.
86. Christie JM, Healey CJ, Watson J, et al. Clinical outcome of hypogammaglobulinaemic patients following outbreak of acute hepatitis C: 2 year follow up. Clin Exp Immunol 1997;110:4–8.
87. Sumazaki R, Matsubara T, Aoki T, et al. Rapidly progressive hepatitis C in a patient with common variable immunodeficiency. Eur J Pediatr 1996;155:532–4.
88. Watson JP, Bewitt DJ, Spickett GP, et al. Hepatitis C virus density heterogeneity and viral titre in acute and chronic infection: a comparison of immunodeficient and immunocompetent patients. J Hepatol 1996;25:599–607.
89. Bjoro K, Froland SS, Yun Z, et al. Hepatitis C infection in patients with primary hypogammaglobulinemia after treatment with contaminated immune globulin. N Engl J Med 1994;331:1607–11.
90. Yap PL, McOmish F, Webster ADB, et al. Hepatitis C virus transmission by intravenous immunoglobulin. J Hepatol 1994;21:455–60.
91. Smith MSH, Webster DB, Dhillon AP, et al. Orthotopic liver transplantation for chronic hepatitis in two patients with common variable immunodeficiency. Gastroenterology 1995;108:879–84.
92. Gow PJ, Mutimer D. Successful outcome of liver transplantation in a patient with hepatitis C and common variable immune deficiency. Transplant Int 2002;15:380–3.
93. Janka GE, Schneider EM. Modern management of children with haemophagocytic lymphohistiocytosis. Br J Hematol 2004;124:4–14.
94. Hirst WJ, Layton DM, Singh S, et al. Haemophagocytic lymphohistiocytosis: experience at two U.K. centres. Br J Hematol 1994;88:731–9.
95. Farquhar JW, Claireaux AE. Familial haemophagocytic reticulosis. Arch Dis Child 1952;27:519–25.
96. Arico M, Danesino C, Pende D, Moretta L. Pathogenesis of haemophagocytic lymphohistiocytosis. Br J Hematol 2001;114:761–9.
97. Henter JI, Samuelsson-Horne, Arico M, et al. Treatment of hemophagocytic lymphohistiocytosis with HLH-94 immunochemotherapy and bone marrow transplantation. Blood 2002;100:2367–73.
98. Menasche G, Feldmann J, Fischer A, de Saint Basile G. Primary hemophagocytic syndromes point to a direct link between lymphocyte cytotoxicity and homeostasis. Immunol Rev 2005;203:165–79.
99. Chisuwa H, Hashikura Y, Nakazawa Y, et al. Fatal hemophagocytic syndrome after living-related liver transplantation: a report of two cases. Transplantation 2001;72:1843–6.

100. Ohadi M, Lalloz MR, Sham P, et al. Localization of a gene for familial hemophagocytic lymphohistiocytosis at chromosome 9q21.3–22 by homozygosity mapping. Am J Hum Genet 1999;64:165–71.
101. Dufourcq-Lagelouse R, Jabado N, Le Deist F, et al. Linkage of familial hemophagocytic lymphohistiocytosis to 10q21–22 and evidence for heterogeneity. Am J Hum Genet 1999;64:172–9.
102. Feldmann J, Callebaut I, Raposo G, et al. Munc13–4 is essential for cytolytic granules fusion and is mutated in a form of familial hemophagocytic lymphohistiocytosis (FHL3). Cell 2003;115:461–73.
103. zur Stadt U, Schmidt S, Kasper B, et al. Linkage of familial hemophagocytic lymphohistiocytosis (FHL) type-4 to chromosome 6q24 and identification of mutations in syntaxin 11. Hum Mol Gen 2005;14:827–34.
104. Stepp SE, Dufourcq-Lagelouse R, Le Deist F, et al. Perforin gene defects in familial hemophagocytic lymphohistiocytosis. Science 1999;286:1957–9.
105. Kogawa K, Lee SM, Villanueva J, et al. Perforin expression in cytotoxic lymphocytes from patients with hemophagocytic lymphohistiocytosis and their family members. Blood 2002; 99:61–6.
106. McClain K, Gehrz R, Grierson H, et al. Virus-associated histiocytic proliferations in children. Frequent association with Epstein-Barr virus and congenital or acquired immunodeficiencies. Am J Pediatr Hematol Oncol 1988;10:196–205.
107. Stephan JL, Donadieu J, Ledeist F, et al. Treatment of familial hemophagocytic lymphohistiocytosis with antithymocyte globulins, steroids, and cyclosporin A. Blood 1993;82:2319–23.
108. Fischer A, Cerf Bensussan N, Blanche S, et al. Allogeneic bone marrow transplantation for erythrophagocytic lymphohistiocytosis. J Pediatr 1986;108:267–70.
109. Durken M, Horstmann M, Bieling P, et al. Improved outcome in haemophagocytic lymphohistiocytosis after bone marrow transplantation from related and unrelated donors: a single-centre experience of 12 patients. Br J Hematol 1999;106:1052–8.
110. Horne A, Janka G, Maarten Egeler R, et al. Haematopoietic stem cell transplantation in haemophagocytic lymphohistiocytosis. Br J Hematol 2005;129:622–30.
111. Cooper N, Rao K, Gilmour K, et al. Stem cell transplantation with reduced intensity conditioning for haemophagocytic lymphohistiocytosis. Blood 2006;107:1233–6.
112. Matthes-Martin S, Peters C, Koningsrainer A, et al. Successful stem cell transplantation following liver transplantation from the same haploidentical family donor in a girl with hemophagocytic lymphohistiocytosis. Blood 2000;96:3997–9.
113. Purtilo DT, Cassel CK, Yang JPS, et al. X-linked recessive progressive combined variable immunodeficiency (Duncan's disease). Lancet 1975;i:935–41.
114. Bar RS. DeLor CJ, Clausen KP, et al. Fatal infectious mononucleosis in a family. N Engl J Med 1974;290:363–7.
115. Howie D, Sayos J, Terhorst C, Morra M. The gene defective in X-linked lymphoproliferative disease controls T cell dependent immune surveillance against Epstein-Barr virus. Curr Opin Immunol 2000;12:474 8.
116. Sullivan JL, Byron KS, Brewster FE, et al. X-linked lymphoproliferative syndrome: natural history of the immunodeficiency. J Clin Invest 1983;71:1765–8.
117. Nichols KE, Ma CS, Cannons JL, et al. Molecular and cellular pathogenesis of X-linked lymphoproliferative disease. Immunol Rev 2005;203:180–99.
118. Sayos J, Wu C, Morra M, et al. The X linked lymphoproliferative–disease gene product SAP regulates signals induced through the co-receptor SLAM. Nature 1998;395:462–9.
119. Sharifi R, Sinclair JC, Gilmour KC, et al. SAP mediates specific cytotoxic T-cell functions in X-linked lymphoproliferative disease. Blood 2004;103:3821–7.
120. Skare JC, Sullivan JL, Milunsky A. Mapping the mutation causing the X-linked lymphoproliferative syndrome in relation to restriction fragment length polymorphisms on Xq. Hum Genet 1989;82:349–53.
121. Pinkerton CR, Hann I, Weston CL, et al. Immunodeficiency-related lymphoproliferative disorders: prospective data from the United Kingdom Children's Cancer Study Group Registry. Br J Hematol 2002;118:456–61.
122. Gross TG, Filipovich AH, Conley ME, et al. Cure of X-linked lymphoproliferative disease (XLP) with allogeneic hematopoietic stem cell transplantation (HSCT): report from the XLP registry. Bone Marrow Transplant 1996;17:741–4.
123. Finn A, Hadzic, Morgan G, Strobel S, Levinsky RJ. Prognosis of chronic granulomatous disease. Arch Dis Child 1990;65: 942–5.
124. Muorah M, Hinds R, Verma A, et al. Liver abscesses in children in the developed world: a single centre experience. J Pediatr Gastroenterol Nutr 2006;42:201–6.
125. Bylund J, Goldblatt D, Speert DP. Chronic granulomatous disease: from genetic defect to clinical presentation. Adv Exp Med Biol 2005;568:67–87.
126. Gungor T, Halter J, Klink A, et al. Successful low toxicity hematopoietic stem cell transplantation for high-risk adult chronic granulomatous disease patients. Transplantation 2005; 79:1596–606.

SECTION IV: METABOLIC LIVER DISEASE

22

Laboratory Diagnosis of Inborn Errors of Metabolism

Devin Oglesbee, Ph.D., and Piero Rinaldo, M.D., Ph.D

Inborn errors of metabolism are recognized with increasing frequency as a cause of disease manifestations in every organ and at every life interval from the fetus to the geriatric patient [1]. Yet their collective incidence is often underestimated, and diagnostic errors often occur, leading to devastating consequences for patients and their families [2]. Among an increasing number of single-gene disorders that are currently recognized, inborn errors of the intermediate metabolism of amino acids, carbohydrates, and fatty acids deserve special attention. The majority of these diseases have been identified within the past 30 years, primarily through the detection of endogenous metabolites abnormally accumulating in biologic fluids [3]. This chapter focuses predominantly on the laboratory diagnosis of three major groups of metabolic diseases: organic acidurias, congenital lactic acidemias, and disorders of fatty acid transport and oxidation. Aspects of urea cycle defects and amino acid disorders are covered to a lesser extent.

The inborn errors listed in Table 22.1 share a common natural history, which is the occurrence of either acute life-threatening illness in early infancy or unexplained developmental delay with intercurrent episodes of metabolic decompensation in later childhood. Unfortunately, the clinical presentations of these diseases are often attributed to a variety of other causes (Table 22.2). Indeed, once a patient is properly diagnosed with a metabolic condition, it is not uncommon to find retrospectively that a sibling within the same family presented with similar symptoms but had passed away without a precise diagnosis.

Two major misconceptions stand behind the frequent failure of correctly diagnosing a metabolic disorder: (1) a high degree of specialization is needed to suspect and initially manage acutely ill patients with inborn errors of metabolism and (2) very expensive analytic instruments are required to undertake a diagnostic challenge of this apparent magnitude. Even today, in what has been called the Genomic Era, specific training in metabolic genetic diseases receives minimal coverage in the curriculum of medical students and pediatric residents at many academic institutions. This situation is disconcerting because newborns and infants with life-threatening illnesses of the type covered here are initially placed under the responsibility of either a general practitioner or a pediatric subspecialist [4] and rarely immediately into the hands of a metabolic specialist.

The aim of this review is to emphasize that a methodic use of routine laboratory tests supplemented by one or two specialized investigations should allow a prompt biochemical diagnosis of patients affected with one of these metabolic diseases, preventing serious sequelae or almost inevitable fatality. Although effective treatment for many metabolic disorders remains unavailable or unreachable in terms of financial requirements, ample evidence has demonstrated that a growing number of these diseases can be treated effectively and efficiently [5,6]. Therefore, high morbidity and mortality should not be systematically assumed in reference to these inborn errors of intermediate metabolism.

Recognition of Signs and Symptoms

The clinical aspects of metabolic disorders with primary hepatic disease are specifically addressed in Chapters 22 and 31–35 of this book and elsewhere [5–7]. For a better understanding of the diagnostic process generally pertinent to these and other conditions, a brief recapitulation of the cardinal clinical findings of these disorders is necessary to put the laboratory analyses to be described in a practical perspective.

Although the final diagnosis of a specific inborn error of metabolism is a laboratory process, several clinical elements should effectively raise the level of suspicion in that diagnostic direction. Saudubray et al. [8–11] delineated up to five basic patterns of clinical presentation, the recognition of which may provide valuable diagnostic signs. It is their observation that a clinical picture in a newborn or infant that is dominated by severe neurologic deterioration is more informative than one may assume from the notion that limited, stereotyped responses are evoked by several causes (sepsis, encephalitis, ingestion, Reye's syndrome, and others). In the neonatal period, a patient who becomes rapidly comatose after a variable (hours to days) symptom-free period could be clinically categorized as being in an intoxication-type of neurologic distress. On the other hand, the absence of a symptom-free period associated with a delayed

Table 22.1: Most Common Inborn Errors of Metabolism Associated with Acute Life-Threatening Illness

Organic acidurias
Congenital lactic acidemias
Pyruvate oxidation defects
Gluconeogenesis defects
Krebs cycle defects
Respiratory chain defects
Disorders of fatty acid transport and oxidation
Defects of membrane-bound enzymes and transporters
Defects of mitochondrial matrix enzymes
Urea cycle disorders
Amino acid disorders
Maple syrup urine disease
Nonketotic hyperglycinemia

Table 22.2: Possible Misdiagnoses of Inborn Errors of Metabolism

Accidental ingestion
Acute liver failure
Cerebral palsy
Child abuse (including Munchausen-by-proxy syndrome)
Cyclic vomiting syndrome
Developmental delay
Intraventricular brain hemorrhage
Reye's syndrome
Seizure disorder
Sepsis
Sudden infant death syndrome
Sudden unexpected death in early life (attributed to infections)

evolution of coma is rather indicative of an energy-deficit type of neurologic distress. In both cases, a failure to respond to symptomatic therapy, followed by rapid deterioration of an infant's general status is a typical manifestation of certain types of metabolic disease [10]. Many organic acidemias, urea cycle disorders, and selected disorders of amino acid metabolism belong to the former category, and primary lactic acidemias, mitochondrial fatty acid β-oxidation disorders pertain to the latter one. Additional stratification of clinical symptoms can also be beneficial. For instance, the predominant occurrence of generalized seizures is indicative of two treatable disorders of vitamin metabolism, such as folinic acid–responsive and vitamin B_6–responsive seizures [8]. The presence of cardiac failure and other functional heart disorders are characteristic for fatty acid oxidation disorders and mitochondrial diseases [8]. Lastly, if persistent hypoglycemia and liver dysfunction are the most prominent features observed for a patient, these findings would suggest a possible disorder of carbohydrate metabolism, such as glycogenosis type I or III, fructose intolerance, or galactosemia [7]. These disorders are discussed in Chapter 25.

ROUTINE LABORATORY INVESTIGATIONS

Table 22.3 lists the basic laboratory investigations that are recommended when a clinical picture compatible with an inborn error of metabolism has been recognized. Recognition of a diagnostic pattern, potentially within hours from the time of admission, may allow the implementation of adequate therapeutic measures pending confirmation of the preliminary diagnosis by specialized laboratory investigations [12,13]. Although blood gases, electrolytes, and glucose are routinely part of the evaluation of any acutely ill pediatric patient, ammonia, lactate, and pyruvate are not consistently requested at admission. In urine, the qualitative determination of 3-keto acids by a commercial dip strip (e.g., Chemstrip, Roche Diagnostics, Basel, Switzerland) and 2-keto acids by the dinitrophenylhydrazine (DNPH) test are particularly important in the early stage of evaluation of an acutely ill patient and can be performed at bedside. A guideline for diagnostic orientation by routine laboratory investigations is shown in Table 22.4 and discussed in the context of each specific group of disorders. Obviously, partial deviations from a model pattern are always possible, in light of the variable nature of a particular metabolic block and the role that environmental factors play in individual cases.

Other simple manual tests that could aid the differential diagnosis of other disorders in acutely ill patients include the detection in urine of reducing substances and sulfites. A positive reducing substances test (Clinitest, Bayer AG, Leverkusen, Germany) may be indicative for galactosemia or hereditary fructose intolerance. Gross galactosuria, however, also may occur in cases with severe liver disease of any origin [7], and false-negative reactions for reducing substances have been observed in symptomatic newborns with galactosemia [14]. Qualitative detection of sulfites in fresh urine (Baker Testrips for Sulfite, J.T. Baker, Phillipsburg, New Jersey) of a patient presenting with severe neurologic distress, lactic acidosis, and hypouricemia is indicative of a diagnosis of molybdenum cofactor deficiency [15].

SPECIALIZED LABORATORY INVESTIGATIONS

On admission, special consideration should be given to the immediate collection and proper storage of urine and blood samples from patients in severe decompensation. These samples may not be available postmortem, or material collected even after a partial recovery may not show certain diagnostic abnormalities otherwise detectable, or more easily detectable,

Table 22.3: Routine Laboratory Investigations in the Initial Evaluation of Patients with Inborn Errors of Metabolism

Serum
- Blood gases, electrolytes
- Glucose, ammonia, uric acid
- Lactic acid, pyruvic acid (L:P ratio)
- Ketone bodies (3OHB:AcAc ratio)

Urine
- Ketone bodies (3-keto acids)
- 2-keto acids (DNPH)
- Reducing substances
- Sulfites
- pH

DNPH, dinitrophenylhydrazine

under acute conditions. Any volume of urine (stored at –20°C with no preservatives, or even a wet diaper obtained at the emergency room) and plasma and serum (≤0.5 mL, stored at –20°C) should be considered adequate for testing. Alternatively, a blood spot on filter paper could provide enough material for one or more of the specialized laboratory investigations described later in this chapter. In case of death, collection of body fluids and tissues should be secured according to available protocols [16].

Quantitative profiling of amino acids, carnitine, acylcarnitines, and free fatty acids in plasma, as well as urine organic acids and acylglycines are the analyses of choice to reach a biochemical diagnosis for the vast majority of these disorders. There are, of course, indications, advantages, and limitations to these tests in the differential diagnosis of each group of inborn errors of metabolism. Furthermore, the provision of a detailed interpretation is essential [17], because a biochemical genetics service differs from a conventional clinical chemistry laboratory in the expectation to provide an overview of abnormal and relative negative results (i.e., ketotic vs. nonketotic dicarboxylic aciduria, methylmalonic aciduria with or without homocystinuria), to quantify pertinent abnormal compounds whenever possible, correlate available clinical information, explain the elements of the differential diagnosis, provide recommendations for additional biochemical testing and in vitro confirmatory studies (enzyme assay, molecular analysis), give the name and phone number of key contacts who may provide these studies, and provide a phone number for the laboratory director in case a referring physician has additional questions.

Group I: Organic Acidurias

Organic acids are water-soluble compounds containing one or more carboxyl groups as well as other functional groups (-keto, -hydroxy), which are intermediate metabolites of all major groups of organic cellular components: amino acids, lipids, carbohydrates, nucleic acids, and steroids. Organic acidurias are a biochemically heterogeneous group of inborn errors of metabolism biochemically characterized by the accumulation of metabolites that are not present under physiologic conditions, from the activation of alternative pathways in response to the loss of function of a specific gene product, or pathologic amounts of normal metabolites [18–22]. These disorders share a common natural history, which is the occurrence of either acute life-threatening illness in early infancy or unexplained developmental delay with intercurrent episodes of metabolic decompensation in later childhood. The incidence of individual inborn errors of organic acid metabolism varies from 1 in 10,000 to more than 1 in 1,000,000 live births. However, their collective incidence approximates 1 in 3000 live births. This estimation does not include other inborn errors of metabolism (i.e., amino acid disorders, urea cycle disorders, congenital lactic acidemias), for which diagnosis and monitoring also require organic acid analysis. All possible disease entities included, the incidence of conditions in which informative organic acid profiles could be detected in urine is likely to approach 1 in 1000 live births.

A situation of severe and persistent metabolic acidosis of unexplained origin, elevated anion gap, and severe neurologic manifestations should always be considered as a strong diagnostic indicator for one of these diseases, findings that warrant immediate verification and should not be postponed, as occurs frequently, when more common causes have been ruled out. The presence of ketonuria, occasionally massive, provides an important clue toward the recognition of disorders such as methylmalonic aciduria, propionic aciduria, and isovaleric aciduria, especially in the neonatal period [23]. Hyperammonemia, hypoglycemia, and hyperlactacidemia are frequently associated findings, especially during acute episodes of metabolic decompensation. Plasma amino acid analysis may provide only limited and generally nonspecific information for enzyme deficiencies affecting distal steps of amino acid catabolism [23]. Thus, the biochemical diagnosis of individual organic acidemias ultimately relies on urine organic acid analysis by gas chromatography/mass spectrometry (GC/MS) [18,19]. Detection, positive identification, and eventually quantitation of pathognomonic organic acids by GC/MS could be available in a matter of hours if the analysis is performed at a local laboratory. Otherwise, results from a referral laboratory should be available within 24 hours for an urgent case.

A large proportion of organic acidurias known to date affect the intermediate metabolism of the essential branched-chain amino acids isoleucine, leucine, and valine [24]. The diagnostic specificity of organic acid analysis under acute and asymptomatic conditions is outlined for individual defects in Table 22.5. Informative profiles may not always be detected in disorders where the excretion of diagnostic metabolites depends on the residual activity of the defective enzyme, the dietary load of precursors, and the anabolic status of a patient. In some cases, methods with higher specificity and sensitivity, such as acylcarnitine determination by electrospray-tandem mass spectrometry [25,26] and acylglycine determination by GC/MS stable isotope dilution analysis [27,28] can overcome the limitations of standard organic acid analysis to assess patients who are not

Table 22.4: Interpretation of Routine Laboratory Investigations for the Diagnosis of Inborn Errors of Metabolism

		Primary Lactic Acidemias						*Amino Acid Disorders*	
	Organic Acidurias	*Pyruvate Oxidation*	*Gluco-neogenesis*	*Pyruvate Carboxylase*	*Respiratory Chain*	*Fatty Acid Oxidation Disorders*	*Urea Cycle Disorders*	*MSUD*	*NKHG*
Approximate number of IEMs	>50	7	3	3	>100	23	8	4	1
Neurologic distress	I	ED	ED	ED	ED	ED	I	I	I
Metabolic acidosis	+++	+++	+++	+++	+++	+	−	−	−
3-Keto aciduria (KB)	+++	−	+	++	++	−	−	+	−
2-Keto aciduria (DNPH-positive)	−	+++	−	+	−	−	−	+++	−
Hyperammonemia	+	+	+	+++	+	+	+++	−	−
Hypoglycemia	+	−	+++	+	+	+++	−	−	−
Lactic acidemia	+	+++	+++	+++	+++	+	−	−	−
		Permanent	Intermittent (fasting)	Permanent	Permanent (fed)				
L:P ratio		<15	>20	>30	>50				
3OHB:AcAc ratio		>2	>2	<1	>3				

DNPH, dinitrophenylhydrazine; IEM, inborn error of metabolism; KB, ketone bodies; MSUD, maple syrup urine disease; I, intoxication type; ED, energy deficiency type of neurologic distress; +, possibly present; +++, typically present with high diagnostic significance; −, not typically present.

acutely ill. However, these tests are rarely needed to diagnose the most frequent and acute organic acidurias.

Group II: Congenital Lactic Acidemias

A classification of enzyme defects leading to a primary lactic acidemia is shown in Table 22.6. In addition to a clinical picture of energy deficiency neurologic distress [10,29], a marked elevation in blood or cerebrospinal fluid (CSF) of lactate concentrations warrant special attention. This should not be assumed to indicate a phenomenon secondary to sepsis, peripheral hypoxia, or merely suboptimal sampling of a patient under severely compromised conditions. Any unexplained occurrence of hyperlactacidemia should be systematically investigated by evaluation of the parameters shown in Table 22.3, particularly the simultaneous determination of serum lactate and pyruvate [30].

Obtaining a plasma lactate:pyruvate (L:P) ratio (normal values in fed state, <15) [31] may be highly informative in acutely ill patients. However, a reliable measurement demands accurate specimen sampling for both lactate and pyruvate obtained at the same time as well as fastidious processing of collected specimens. Lactic acidemia with a normal L:P ratio is indicative of disorders of the pyruvate dehydrogenase (PDH) complex [32]; lactic acidemia with a high L:P ratio is indicative of either pyruvate carboxylase deficiency, one of four known gluconeogenesis defects [33], or a mitochondrial respiratory chain defect [29,34]. In the latter case, the L:P ratio could be markedly elevated. A possible diagnosis of pyruvate carboxylase deficiency may be corroborated by documenting a decreased 3–hydroxy butyrate: acetoacetate ratio (normal values in fed state, 1.0–1.5), which occurs from the consequence of forced accumulation of reducing equivalents (NADH) in the cytosolic compartment via malate–aspartate shuttling. The oxidized status of the mitochondrial matrix halts the reduction of acetoacetate to 3-hydroxy butyrate, a functional block reflected by a decrease of their relative ratio in blood. In respiratory chain disorders affecting the liver, the ratio of 3OHB:AcAc is typically elevated [31].

Ketonuria is more commonly observed in a primary rather than secondary lactic acidemia, and hyperammonemia can be a key element in the recognition of the cross-reacting material–negative form of pyruvate carboxylase deficiency [33], a defect of gluconeogenesis with typical diagnostic features also at the amino acid level, as described subsequently. Other gluconeogenesis defects present with hypoglycemia as the dominant sign in association with lactic acidemia, hepatomegaly, and liver disease [7,10,33]. The more pronounced and apparent are symptoms such as hypoglycemia and hepatomegaly, the more distal a defect is to pyruvate carboxylase in the gluconeogenic pathway.

Beyond the varied clinical signs and symptoms, some of that bear high diagnostic specificity [10], amino acid and organic acid analyses may provide precise laboratory information for

Table 22.5: Organic Acidurias: Diagnostic Significance of Organic Acid, Acylcarnitine, and Acylglycine Analyses

		Organic Acids			
Common Name	*Enzyme Deficiency*	*Acute*	*Asymptomatic*	*Acylcarnitines*	*Acylglycines*[a]
Branched-chain amino acid metabolism					
Isovaleric aciduria	Isovaleryl-CoA dehydrogenase	+	+	+	|
3-Methyl crotonylglycinuria	3-Methyl crotonyl-CoA carboxylase	+	–	+	+[b]
3-Methyl glutaconic aciduria	3-Methyl glutaconyl-CoA hydratase	+	+	+	0
3-Hydroxy 3-methyl glutaric aciduria	3-Hydroxy 3-methyl glutaryl-CoA lyase	+	+	+	0
2-Methyl acetoacetic aciduria	2-Methyl acetoacetyl-CoA thiolase	+	–	+	+
3-Hydroxy isobutyric aciduria	3-Hydroxy isobutyryl-CoA dehydrogenase	+	+	0	0
	Methylmalonyl/malonyl semialdehyde dehydrogenase	+	–	0	0
Propionic aciduria	Propionyl-CoA carboxylase	+	+	+	+
Methylmalonic aciduria	Methylmalonyl-CoA mutase	+	+	+	+[c]
Methylmalonic aciduria	Cobalamin metabolism (multiple defects)	+	+	+	+[c]
	Succinyl-CoA transferase	+	+	0	0
Malonic aciduria	Malonyl-CoA decarboxylase	+	–	+	0
Miscellaneous					
Ethylmalonic encephalopathy	ETHE1 (unknown function)	+	+	+	+
Glutaric aciduria type I	Glutaryl-CoA dehydrogenase	+	+	+	+
D-2-hydroxy glutaric aciduria	Unknown	+	–	0	0
L-2-hydroxy glutaric aciduria	Unknown	+	–	0	0
2-Ketoadipic aciduria	2-Keto adipic dehydrogenase	+	–	0	0
4-Hydroxy butyric aciduria	Succinic semialdehyde dehydrogenase	+	–	0	0
Hyperoxaluria type I	Alanine:glyoxylate aminotransferase	+	+	0	0
Hyperoxaluria type II	D-glyceric dehydrogenase	+	+	0	0
Glyceroluria	Glycerol kinase	+	+	0	0
Pyroglutamic aciduria	Glutathione synthetase	+	+[d]	0	0
Alcaptonuria	Homogentisic acid oxidase	+	+	0	0
Mevalonic aciduria	Mevalonic synthetase	+	+	0	0

Acute, analysis of a urine sample collected during an episode of metabolic decompensation; asymptomatic, analysis of a urine sample collected in clinical remission; +, diagnostic profile; –, possible occurrence of an uninformative urinary organic acid profile in asymptomatic patients, depending on the clinical status and effectiveness of therapy; 0, test not informative.

[a] Stable isotope dilution analysis of the metabolites (acylglycines and organic acids) listed in Table 22.8.

[b] 3-Methylcrotonylglycine independently measured by gas chromatography/mass spectrometry (GC/MS) stable isotope dilution analysis.

[c] Propionylglycine independently measured by GC/MS stable isotope dilution analysis.

[d] If applicable, rule out transient pyroglutamic aciduria in response to acetaminophen intake (see Pitt JJ, Hauser S. Transient 5-oxoprolinuria and high anion gap metabolic acidosis: clinical and biochemical findings in eleven subjects. Clin Chem 1998;44:1497–503).

Table 22.6: Congenital Lactic Acidemias: Diagnostic Significance of Clinical Information and Specialized Laboratory Investigations

	Clinical Findings	*Urine Organic Acids*	*Plasma Amino Acids*
Disorders of gluconeogenesis			
Glucose-6-phosphatase deficiency	+	–	–
Fructose 1,6-diphosphatase deficiency	–	–	–
Phosphoenolpyruvate carboxykinase deficiency	–	–	–
Pyruvate carboxylase deficiency			
Apoenzyme deficiency			
CRM-positive	–	+	–
CRM-negative	–	+	|
Coenzyme deficiency			
Holocarboxylase deficiency	+	+	–
Biotinidase deficiency	+	+	–
Disorders of pyruvate metabolism (PDH complex)			
Pyruvate decarboxylase (E_1) deficiency			
α-subunit deficiency (X-linked)	+	+	–
β-subunit deficiency	+	+	–
E_1 phosphatase deficiency	–	–	–
Dihydrolipoyl transacetylase (E_2) deficiency	–	–	–
Dihydrolipoyl dehydrogenase (E_3) deficiency	–	+	+
Krebs cycle's disorders			
α-ketoglutarate dehydrogenase deficiency	–	+	+
Fumarase deficiency	–	+	–
Aconitase deficiency	–	+	–
Respiratory chain defects			
NADH-CoQ reductase (complex I)			
Myopathy	|	+	–
Encephalomyopathy	+	+	–
MELAS	+	+	–
Succinate dehydrogenase (complex II)	–	+	–
CoQ–cytochrome *c* reductase (complex III)			
Myopathy	+	–	–
Encephalopathy	+	–	–
Cytochrome *c* oxidase (complex IV)			
Myopathy			
Fatal infantile myopathy	+	–	+[a]
Benign infantile myopathy	+	–	–
Encephalopathy			
Leigh's syndrome			
Kearns–Sayre syndrome	+	–	–
MERRF	+	–	–
ATP synthase (complex V)	+	+	–

ATP, adenosine triphosphate; CoQ, coenzyme Q; CRM, cross-reacting material; MELAS, mitochondrial encephalopathy lactic acidosis strokelike episodes; MERRF, myoclonus epilepsy with ragged red fibers; NADH, nicotinamide adenine dinucleotide (reduced); PDH, pyruvate dehydrogenase; +, typical clinical findings or informative profiles by either urine organic acid or plasma amino acid analysis; –, not informative beyond a possible elevated plasma alanine level.

[a]Generalized amino aciduria (Fanconi's syndrome).

the diagnosis of the lactic acidemias (Table 22.6). The presence of an elevated plasma alanine concentration is a common feature of these defects and could actually corroborate a potential diagnosis of primary lactic acidemia in early diagnostic stages [35]. The cross-reacting material–negative form of pyruvate carboxylase deficiency presents with elevated plasma concentration of citrulline and lysine [36]. A defect of the E_3 subunit of the PDH complex also compromises the catalytic function of 2-keto glutarate and branched-chain amino acid dehydrogenase complexes as well, with the accumulation of valine, isoleucine, leucine, and alloisoleucine to an extent that this disorder was once thought to be a variant of maple syrup urine disease (MSUD) [37]. Additionally, elevated plasma glutamic acid concentrations have been reported in isolated 2-ketoglutarate dehydrogenase deficiency [38], although incorrect sample handling is a much more frequent cause of the same finding [39]. Moreover, generalized amino aciduria concurrent with lactic acidemia is an important element in the recognition of cytochrome *c* oxidase deficiency with renal involvement and Fanconi's syndrome [40].

Significant lactic acidemia is typically accompanied by an increased excretion of 2-hydroxy butyric acid, observable by an organic acid analysis, and is a signature finding much like an observed elevation of plasma alanine [41,42]. Marked elevations of Krebs cycle intermediates (succinate, fumarate, and malate) have been quantitatively reported in patients with pyruvate carboxylase deficiency [43]. Although these findings have been found in additional cases with pyruvate carboxylase deficiency confirmed by enzyme assays [44], an increased excretion of Krebs cycle intermediates is often overlooked, possibly because of the broad reference values for these organic acids among different age groups [44]. Patients with multiple carboxylase deficiencies give a typical urine organic acid profile characterized by the presence of 3-hydroxy isovaleric acid, 3-methylcrotonylglycine, propionylglycine, 3-hydroxy propionic acid, and methylcitric acid [45]. As discussed earlier, PDH complex defects show a characteristic elevation of both lactate and pyruvate, 2-ketoglutaric acid, and the 2-keto/2-hydroxy organic acids that originate from branched-chain amino acid metabolism are present in urine from patients with an E_3 defect of the PDH complex [37,43]. Organic acid analysis is obviously the method of choice for the recognition of fumarase deficiency and 2-keto glutarate dehydrogenase deficiency, two disorders primarily affecting the Krebs cycle, the key compounds of which fumarate and 2 keto glutarate, respectively, are found in massive levels in urine [34]. Moreover, an elevated excretion of succinic acid could be an indication of succinate dehydrogenase deficiency [46]. However, this compound is also elevated in urine because of diet, medication, and even bacterial contamination, and these artifacts must be ruled out. Abnormal excretions of 3-hydroxy isobutyric acid, 2-ethyl hydracrylic acid, 2-methyl 3-hydroxy butyric acid, and tiglylglycine have been reported in a handful of patients with NADH-CoQ reductase (complex I) deficiency [47]. However, they are general abnormalities associated with an increase in the NADH:NAD ratio and are the consequence of the inhibition of NAD-requiring dehydrogenases found in the mitochondria.

Group III: Disorders of Fatty Acid Transport and Oxidation

Fatty acid oxidation (FAO) plays a major role in energy production during periods of fasting. At the cellular level, long-chain fatty acids are oxidized to acetyl-coenzyme A (CoA) in mitochondria following transport through the cell membrane and carnitine-mediated mitochondrial import [48]. Under fasting conditions, acetyl-CoA fuels the hepatic synthesis of ketone bodies [49], which are used by extrahepatic tissues as alternative substrates for energy production.

Inherited FAO disorders represent a more widely recognized class of metabolic diseases [50,51]. Symptoms may appear at any age, from birth [52,53] to adult life [54,55], frequently leading to life-threatening episodes of metabolic decompensation after a period of inadequate caloric intake or intercurrent illness. Typical manifestations include hypoketotic hypoglycemia, liver disease, or cardiomyopathy, each of which can be so severe as to warrant organ transplantation [56], as well as sudden and unexpected death [57].

During an acute episode of metabolic decompensation, routine laboratory tests may reveal nonketotic hypoglycemia, a characteristic feature of many FAO disorders. However, there have been several reports of patients unexpectedly presenting with ketonuria [58, personal observations], and hyperketonuria is actually a characteristic features of short-chain 3-hydroxy acyl-CoA dehydrogenase deficiency [59]. Liver function tests, ammonia, and creatine phosphokinase may be markedly abnormal [50,60]. Serum lactate is often increased under acute conditions, especially in cases with long-chain FAO disorders. Once suspicion of an FAO disorder has been raised, it is necessary to rely on specialized biochemical investigations to formulate a more specific diagnosis. For this purpose, the collection of plasma and urine specimens at the earliest possible stage of an acute episode is strongly recommended.

Table 22.7 summarizes the characteristic biochemical findings in plasma and urine of patients with individual disorders [61]. The correct identification of FAO disorders is an increasingly complex process that can hardly be achieved by a single test but requires the performance of multiple analyses and their integrated interpretation. Moreover, uninformative metabolite profiles occur frequently in affected patients on the basis of their clinical and nutritional status and therefore should not be taken as sufficient evidence to rule out the possibility of an underlying FAO disorder in a patient with clinical evidence of fasting intolerance.

In urine, analyses of organic acids and acylglycines, performed by GC/MS methods, are recommended [60,61]. Organic acid profiles may vary significantly from one defect to another and are dependant on the clinical status of the patient. A signature pattern of hypoketotic medium-chain dicarboxylic acidemia ($C_6 > C_8 > C_{10}$) with multiple unsaturated species ($C_{8:1} < C_8$, $C_{10:1} > C_{10}$) is seen in patients with the three most common FAO disorders: medium-chain acyl-CoA dehydrogenase (MCAD) deficiency, very-long-chain acyl-CoA dehydrogenase (VLCAD) deficiency, and long-chain 3-hydroxy acyl-CoA dehydrogenase (LCHAD) deficiency. In the latter, C_6 to C_{14} 3-hydroxy dicarboxylic acidemia is often a dominant feature. However, supportive therapy may alleviate the need for fatty acid oxidation as an energy source and this rapidly diminishes the excretion of characteristic organic acids. The systemic form of short-chain 3-hydroxy acyl-CoA dehydrogenase deficiency presents with organic acid patterns similar to LCHAD

Table 22.7: Disorders of Fatty Acid Transport and Oxidation: Diagnostic Significance of Specialized Investigations

	Carnitine					
	FC	*AC/FC*	*Acylcarnitines*	*Free Fatty Acids*	*Organic Acids*	*Acylglycines*[a]
Disorders of membrane-bound enzymes						
Long-chain fatty acid transport defect	N to low	–	–	+ (acute)	–	–
Carnitine transport defect	Very low	–	–	–	–	–
CPT-I deficiency (liver)	High	–	–	?	–	–
Carnitine acylcarnitine translocase deficiency	N to low	High	+	?	–	–
CPT-II deficiency						
Neonatal onset (liver, heart, kidney)	N to low	High	+	?	–	–
Late onset (skeletal muscle)	N to low	High	+	?	–	–
VLCAD deficiency	N to low	High	+	+	+ (acute)	–
ETF-ubiquinone oxidoreductase deficiency	N to low	High	+	+	+	+
Trifunctional protein (TFP) deficiency						
LCHAD deficiency	N to low	High	+ (acute)	+	+ (acute)	–
α-TFP deficiency	N to low	High	+ (acute)	+	+ (acute)	–
β-TFP deficiency	N to low	High	+	+	+ (acute)	–
Defects of mitochondrial matrix enzymes						
MCAD deficiency	N to low	High	+	+	+ (acute)	+
M/SCHAD deficiency	N to low	High	+	+	+ [acute]	–
MCKAT deficiency	N to low	High	?	?	+ [acute]	+
SCAD deficiency	N to low	High	+	–	+ [acute]	+
SCHAD deficiency						
Myopathic form	N to low	High	+	?	–	–
Systemic form	N to low	High	+	?	+ (acute)	–
Hepatic form	N to low	High	?	+	+ (acute)	–
Glutaric acidemia type II						
α-ETF deficiency	N to low	High	+	+	+	+
β-ETF deficiency	N to low	High	+	+	+	+
Riboflavin responsive form	N to low	High	+	+	+ (acute)	+
2,4-Dienoyl-CoA reductase deficiency	N to low	High	+	?	–	–

AC, esterified fraction (acylcarnitines); FC, free carnitine; CPT, carnitine palmitoyltransferase; ETF, electron transport flavoprotein; ETF-QO, ETF ubiquinone-oxidoreductase; LCHAD, long chain 3-hydroxy acyl-CoA dehydrogenase; MCAD, medium-chain acyl-CoA dehydrogenase; SCAD, short-chain acyl-CoA dehydrogenase; M/SCHAD, medium and short-chain 3-hydroxy acyl-CoA dehydrogenase; VLCAD, very long chain acyl-CoA dehydrogenase; +, diagnostic profile; + (acute), possible occurrence of an uninformative profile of urinary organic acids in asymptomatic patients, depending on clinical status and effectiveness of therapy; –, test not informative; N, normal; ?, insufficient information available to establish diagnostic significance.

[a] Stable isotope dilution analysis of the metabolites (acylglycines and organic acids) listed in Table 22.8.

Modified from Rinaldo P et al. Fatty acid oxidation disorders: clinical and biochemical features. Curr Opin Pediatr 1998;10:615–21; with permission.

deficiency, with the notable addition of marked ketoaciduria [59].

Figure 22.1 presents two profiles obtained from asymptomatic patients affected with electron transfer flavoprotein subunit β deficiency and MCAD deficiency, respectively. In both cases, the organic acid profiles were essentially normal. Profiles such as these underscore the fact that a diagnosis of FAO disorders could be missed if a standard organic acid analysis is the only biochemical test performed, especially when a patient is free of clinical symptoms or even shortly after recovery from an acute episode of metabolic decompensation. One test indicated for the recognition of patients with mild or intermittent biochemical phenotypes, which may be missed by organic acid analysis, is the quantitative analysis of acylglycines by stable isotope dilution methods (Table 22.7). Table 22.8 summarizes the patterns of excretion of acylglycine compounds in eight disorders and three common circumstances related to dietary or pharmacologic treatment. The acylglycine profile is particularly effective for the differential diagnosis of ethylmalonic acidemia, a biochemical phenotype that could be linked to multiple disorders [62–67].

In plasma, carnitine (total and free), acylcarnitines, and free fatty acids are necessary components of the laboratory workup of a patient suspected of having an FAO disorder. Despite the

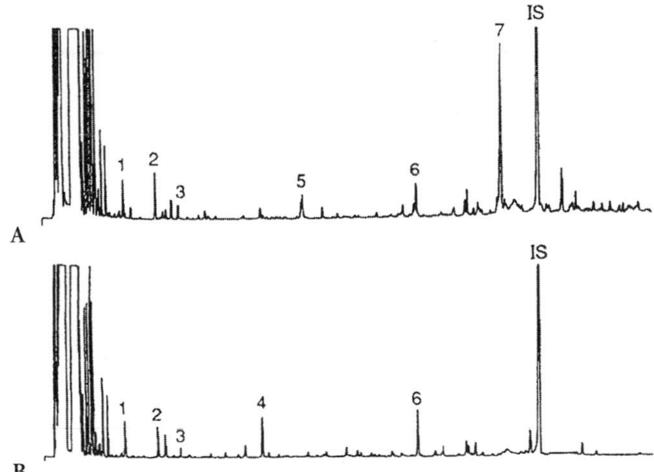

Figure 22.1. Urine organic acid profiles in asymptomatic patients with fatty acid β-oxidation disorders. Capillary gas chromatographic profiles of organic acid trimethylsilyl derivatives. (**A**) A 7-year-old boy with MCAD deficiency (diagnosed by acylglycine determination and confirmed by molecular analysis performed in the laboratory of Dr. Kay Tanaka, Yale University). (**B**) A 3-day-old boy with electron transfer flavoprotein subunit β deficiency (diagnosed prenatally by immunoblot analysis, pulse-labeling experiments, and metabolite analysis in amniotic fluid). Peak legend: 1, lactic acid; 2, oxalic acid; 3, 3-hydroxy isobutyric acid; 4, 4-deoxythreonic acid; 5, adipic acid; 6, 4-hydroxy phenylacetic acid; 7, hippuric acid; IS, internal standard (pentadecanoic acid). All peak identifications were confirmed by GC/MS analysis.

higher significance of acylcarnitine profiling, plasma carnitine determination cannot be overlooked because it offers the only method to biochemically recognize patients affected with a carnitine uptake deficiency without performing a tissue biopsy [68]. Indeed, it may also offer an important clue in the differential diagnosis of disorders such as carnitine palmitoyltransferase type 1 deficiency, which lacks a characteristic metabolite pattern in plasma acylcarnitines or organic acids [61]. The biochemical workup of plasma specimens should also include the analysis of free fatty acids and 3-hydroxy fatty acids in plasma [69,70]. In particular, quantitatively modest ($<5\ \mu$mmol/mL) but nevertheless significant amounts of C_{14}-C_{18} 3-hydroxy fatty acids are consistently found in plasma of patients with LCHAD deficiency, even when they are asymptomatic or treated with a low-fat diet [70].

The analysis of acylcarnitines is best performed by tandem mass spectrometry (MS/MS) [71] with or without electrospray ionization (ESI) [72] because these methods are more sensitive and superior to conventional high performance liquid chromatography and GC/MS systems. The commercial availability of relatively affordable bench-top triple quadrupole mass spectrometers and the reliability of liquid chromatography MS interface based on ESI have made the application of these techniques a cornerstone of the clinical biochemical genetics laboratory. Indeed, the analyses of amino acids, acylcarnitines, and a growing number of other metabolites are now routinely performed by MS/MS to evaluate patients suspected of having an inborn error of metabolism [25,26,73]. Accordingly, MS/MS is at the forefront of technology revolutionizing state and national newborn screening programs aimed at identifying inborn errors of metabolism [74,75].

Fatty acid oxidation disorders frequently manifest with sudden and unexpected death [16,57]. Figure 22.2 summarizes a diagnostic protocol that allows detection of multiple disorders, based on the evaluation of independent diagnostic criteria. If parental permission to perform an autopsy is not granted, an immediate effort should be made to retrieve specimens that may still be available: if death occurred in a nursery or hospital setting, the laboratory should be immediately contacted and asked to hold any unused portions of blood or urine specimens previously collected for routine tests. If available, these specimens should be subjected to a complete metabolic workup as described previously. If death occurs at home after discharge, retrieval of any unused portion of the patient's blood spot card, collected for newborn screening, could be easily arranged via a request submitted by a physician to the state laboratory. Blood spots may be sent for acylcarnitine analysis by electrospray MS/MS [25,26,75] or for DNA isolation for mutation analysis. Assays of biochemical markers are preferable to direct DNA tests, which may be too limited in scope, focused around relatively common mutations, and have the disadvantage of precluding the ability to screen effectively for multiple conditions, not to mention the tangible risk of missing patients carrying less common mutations [76]. If the acylcarnitine profile is not informative, testing of parental plasma carnitine levels for biochemical markers of heterozygosity may also be indicated, especially if the aim of testing is to rule out the possibility that the patient passed away from a carnitine uptake defect [52].

When the procedures listed here are negative or not available, a biochemical workup of all sibs should be considered. Although this approach must take into consideration the variable biochemical phenotype of different FAO disorders, it has proven to be effective in the specific case of MCAD deficiency [16].

Group IV: Urea Cycle Disorders

As with the inborn errors described earlier, the clinical presentations of almost all urea cycle disorders are similar to each other. Given this fact, it is of special concern that the diagnostic possibility of a urea cycle defect is often neglected in favor of more common diseases or those thought to be more common [77]. In neonatal cases, it has been estimated that the median delay is 16 months between the onset of major symptoms before a correct diagnosis is made [78]. A delay of this magnitude is often too late to prevent severe and irreversible neurologic damage to the patient [79].

In urea cycle disorders, routine laboratory investigations (Table 22.4) are often dominated by the presence of hyperammonemia and respiratory alkalosis. However, in some cases, such as argininemia, blood ammonia may be within normal

Table 22.8: Diagnostic Specificity of Acylglycine and Organic Acid Determination by Stable Isotope Dilution Analysis for the Differential Diagnosis of Acyl-Coa Dehydrogenase Deficiencies, Physiologic Ketosis, and Iatrogenic Conditions

Metabolite	*SCAD*	*EMA Encephalo-pathy*	*ETF/ ETF-QO*	*MCAD*	*MCKAT*	*GDH*	*IVDH*	*2MBCAD*	*KET*	*MCT*	*VALP*
Ethylmalonic acid	+++	+++	+++	–	–	–	–	–	+	–	–
Methylsuccinic acid	+	+	+	–	–	–	–	–	–	–	–
Glutaric acid	–	–	+++	–	–	+++	–	–	+	–	–
Isobutyrylglycine	–	+++	+	–	–	–	–	–	+	–	–
Butyrylglycine	+	+	+	–	–	–	–	–	+	+	+
2-Methylbutyryl-glycine	–	+++	+	–	–	–	–	+++	–	–	+
Isovalerylglycine	–	+	+++	–	–	–	+++	–	–	–	–
Hexanoylglycine	+	–	+++	+++	+	–	–	–	–	–	+
Octanoylglycine	–	–	+	+	–	–	–	–	–	+	–
Phenylpropionyl-glycine	–	–	–	+++	–	–	–	–	–	–	–
Suberylglycine	–	–	+	+++	–	–	–	–	+	+	–
Dodecanedioic acid	–	–	+	–	+++	–	–	–	+	–	–
Tetradecanedioic acid	–	–	+	–	+++	–	–	–	–	–	–
Hexadecanedioic acid	–	–	+	–	+++	–	–	–	–	–	–

2MBCAD, 2-methyl branched-chain acyl-CoA dehydrogenase deficiency; EMA, ethylmalonic acid; ETF, electron transport flavoprotein deficiency; ETF-QO, ETF ubiquinone-oxidoreductase deficiency; GDH, glutaryl-CoA dehydrogenase deficiency; IVDH, isovaleryl-CoA dehydrogenase deficiency; MCAD, medium-chain acyl-CoA dehydrogenase deficiency; MCKAT, medium-chain 3-keto acyl-CoA thiolase deficiency; SCAD, short-chain acyl-CoA dehydrogenase deficiency; KET, physiologic ketosis; MCT, medium chain triglycerides (diet supplemented with); VALP, valproic acid therapy; +++, high diagnostic significance; +, possibly present; –, not typically present.

range, and there have been conflicting reports about significance of respiratory alkalosis [79]. Indeed, it has been reported that patients presenting with urea cycle disorders may be either acidotic or alkalotic during acute episodes of metabolic decompensation [80]. Therefore, an organic acid analysis could be of benefit to definitively rule out whether hyperammonemia in a patient is secondary to an underlying organic aciduria.

Plasma amino acids and urine orotic acid are required for a differential diagnosis that can be effectively achieved according to established protocols [81]. High glutamine and alanine concentrations are typical but not diagnostic for these disorders, reflecting a nonspecific consequence of cellular nitrogen accumulation. A low or absent citrulline concentration is consistent with either ornithine transcarbamylase (OTC) or carbamylphosphate synthetase (CPS) deficiencies. Indeed, these two disorders can be differentiated by testing orotic acid in urine, which is only elevated in OTC deficiency. Therefore, the diagnosis of CPS deficiency is made biochemically by the step-by-step exclusion of other disorders. Although a more than 20-fold increase of citrulline concentration (normal values <50 μmmol/mL) indicates a defect of argininosuccinic synthetase, a condition commonly known as citrullinemia, a two- to five-fold elevation of plasma citrulline in the presence of argininosuccinic acid in urine is indicative of argininosuccinase deficiency. Clinical and more detailed diagnostic aspects of urea cycle defects are discussed in Chapter 35.

Group V: Amino Acid Disorders

Two disorders are briefly considered in this last section: MSUD and nonketotic hyperglycinemia (NKHG), which should always be contemplated in the context of a differential diagnosis among those inborn errors listed in Tables 22.1 and 22.4.

Maple syrup urine disease is caused by a defect of one of the three components of the branched-chain 2-keto acid dehydrogenase complex [82]. In untreated or decompensated patients,

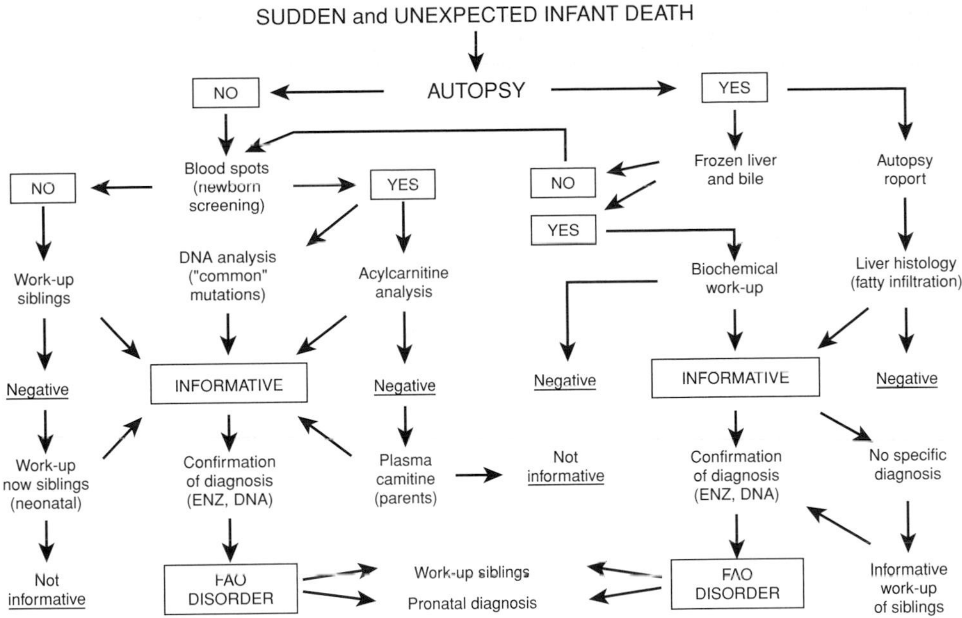

Figure 22.2. Protocol for the postmortem screening of fatty acid oxidation disorders. DNA, molecular analysis; ENZ, enzymatic assay; FAO, fatty acid oxidation. (Reprinted from Rinaldo P, Yoon HR, Yu C, et al. Sudden and unexpected neonatal death: a protocol for the postmortem diagnosis of fatty acid oxidation disorders. Semin Perinatol 1999;23:204–10; with permission.)

a diagnosis of MSUD could be suspected by a positive dinitrophenylhydrazine test or simply by the presence of a characteristically sweet smell in urine or earwax, the latter in older patients [82]. A diagnosis is more reliably substantiated by either plasma amino acid or urine organic acid analysis. Through the keto-enol tautomerization of (2*S*) 2-keto 3-methyl valeric acid to its (2*R*) enantiomer (mirror image), L alloisoleucine is formed in vivo [83]. The detection of L-alloisoleucine in plasma is a pathognomonic finding of MSUD, along with a high concentration of the three branched-chain amino acids (especially leucine). Their accumulation is due to the freely reversible transamination of 2-keto acids (2-ketoisocaproic acid, 2-keto 3-methylvaleric acid, and 2-keto isovaleric acid) to the corresponding amino acid. 2-Hydroxy isovaleric acid may also be present in large amounts. When organic acids are analyzed by GC/MS [18,19], the 2-keto acids should first be stabilized by oximation with hydroxylamine hydrochloride or other equivalent reagents.

Nonketotic hyperglycinemia is a severe condition caused by a defect of the mitochondrial glycine cleavage system [84]. The key element that raises the suspicion of NKHG is the sum of all uninformative results by routine laboratory investigations in a child with progressive neurologic symptoms (Table 22.4) and the observation that plasma and CSF amino acid analysis reveal high concentrations of glycine (plasma, frequently >1,000 μmmol/mL, normal values <500 μmmol/mL in newborns, <300 μmmol/mL in older infants; CSF, >30 μmmol/mL, normal values <10 μmmol/mL*M*). The calculation of a CSF:plasma glycine concentration ratio (NKHG, >0.09, normal <0.04) is critical in the differential diagnosis of this condition [85]. Of course, the reliability of this parameter hinges on the fact that both the plasma and CSF specimens must be collected simultaneously. No other abnormalities are detectable by amino acid or organic acid analysis for this disorder.

There exist many more in vivo provocative tests, in vitro enzyme assays, and molecular investigations available for the diagnosis of inborn errors of metabolism. These procedures have not been considered here for the sole reason that they have no significant impact on the way physicians confront the occurrence of a life-threatening episode of metabolic decompensation at the bedside. In the very critical initial hours, the diagnosis of an inborn error of metabolism must rely on the kind of routine and specialized biochemical laboratory investigations described within this chapter.

REFERENCES

1. Scriver CR. Foreword. In: Blau N, Duran M, Blaskovics ME, et al., eds. Physician's guide to the laboratory diagnosis of metabolic diseases. 2nd ed. Berlin: Springer-Verlag, 2003:v–xii.
2. Hoffman M. Scientific sleuths solve a murder mystery. Science 1991;254:931.
3. Beaudet AL, Scriver CR, Beaudet AL, et al. Genetics and biochemistry of variant human phenotypes. In: Scriver CR, Beaudet AL, Sly WS, et al., eds. The metabolic and molecular bases of inherited disease. 8th ed. New York: McGraw-Hill, 2001:3–45.
4. Hostetler MA, Arnold GL, Mooney R, et al. Hypoketotic hypoglycemic coma in a 21 month old. Ann Emerg Med 1999;34:394–8.
5. Fernandes J, Saudubray JM, van den Berghe G, eds. Inborn metabolic diseases. Diagnosis and treatment. 3rd ed. Berlin: Springer-Verlag, 2000.

6. Blau N, Hoffman GF, Leonard J, et al., eds. Physician's guide to the treatment and follow-up of metabolic diseases. Berlin: Springer-Verlag, 2006.
7. Odievre M. Clinical presentation of metabolic liver disease. J Inherit Metab Dis 1991;14:526–37.
8. Saudubray JM, Nassogne MC, de Lonlay P, et al. Clinical approach to inherited metabolic disorders in neonates: an overview. Semin Neonatol 2002;7:3–15.
9. Saudubray JM, Ogier de Baulny H, Charpentier C. Clinical approach to inherited metabolic disorders. In: Fernandes J, Saudubray JM, van den Berghe G, eds. Inborn metabolic diseases. Diagnosis and treatment. 3rd ed. Berlin: Springer-Verlag, 2000:3–41.
10. Saudubray JM, Charpentier C. Clinical phenotypes: diagnosis algorithms. In: Scriver CR, Beaudet AL, Sly WS, et al., eds. The metabolic and molecular bases of inherited disease. 8th ed. New York: McGraw-Hill, 2001:1327–403.
11. Saudubray JM, Martin D, Poggi-Travert F, et al. Clinical presentations of inherited mitochondrial fatty acid oxidation disorders: an update. Int Pediatr 1997;12:34–40.
12. Hommes F, ed. Techniques in diagnostic human biochemical genetics – a laboratory manual. New York: Wiley-Liss, 1991.
13. Blau N, Duran M, Blaskovics ME, et al., eds. Physician's guide to the laboratory diagnosis of metabolic diseases. 2nd ed. Berlin: Springer-Verlag, 2003.
14. Wraith JE. Diagnosis and management of inborn errors of metabolism. Arch Dis Child 1989;64:1410–15.
15. Johnson JL, Wadman SK. Molybdenum cofactor deficiency and isolated sulfite oxidase deficiency. In: Scriver CR, Beaudet AL, Sly WS, et al., eds. The metabolic and molecular bases of inherited disease. 8th ed. New York: McGraw-Hill, 2001:3163–77.
16. Rinaldo P, Yoon HR, Yu C, et al. Sudden and unexpected neonatal death: a protocol for the postmortem diagnosis of fatty acid oxidation disorders. Semin Perinatol 1999;23:204–10.
17. ACMG Laboratory Practice Committee. Standards and guidelines for clinical genetics laboratories. 2006 ed. Bethesda, Md.: American College of Medical Genetics, 2006:F.7.7.3.7.
18. Goodman SI, Markey SP. Diagnosis of organic acidemias by gas chromatography–mass spectrometry. New York: Alan R Liss, 1981.
19. Chalmers RA, Lawson AM. Organic acids in man. Analytical chemistry, biochemistry and diagnosis of the organic acidurias. London: Chapman & Hall, 1982.
20. Sweetman L. Organic acid analysis. In: Hommes F, ed. Techniques in diagnostic human biochemical genetics – a laboratory manual. New York: Wiley-Liss, 1991:143–76.
21. Lehotay DC, Clarke JTR. Organic acidurias and related abnormalities. Crit Rev Clin Lab Sci 1995;32:377–429.
22. Hoffman GF, Feyh P. Organic acid analysis. In: Blau N, Duran M, Blaskovics ME, et al. eds. Physician's guide to the laboratory diagnosis of metabolic diseases. 2nd ed. Berlin: Springer-Verlag, 2003:27–44.
23. Burlina AB, Bonafé L, Zacchello F. Clinical and biochemical approach to the neonate with a suspected inborn error of amino acid and organic acid metabolism. Semin Perinatol 1999;23:162–73.
24. Sweetman L, Williams JC. Branched chain organic acidurias. In: Scriver CR, Beaudet AL, Sly WS, et al., eds. The metabolic and molecular bases of inherited disease. 8th ed. New York: McGraw-Hill, 2001:2125–63.
25. Millington DS, Chace DH, Hillman SL, et al. Diagnosis of metabolic disease. In: Matsuo T, Caprioli RM, Gross ML, et al., eds. Biological mass spectrometry: present and future. New York: Wiley, 1994:559–79.
26. Rashed MS, Bucknall MP, Little D, et al. Screening blood spots for inborn errors of metabolism by electrospray tandem mass spectrometry with a microplate batch process and a computer algorithm for automated flagging of abnormal results. Clin Chem 1997;43:1129–41.
27. Rinaldo P, O'Shea JJ, Coates PM, et al. Medium chain acyl-CoA dehydrogenase deficiency: diagnosis by stable isotope dilution analysis of urinary n-hexanoylglycine and 3-phenylpropionylglycine. N Engl J Med 1988;319:1308–13.
28. Yamaguchi S, Shimuzu N, Orii T, et al. Prenatal diagnosis of Glutaric aciduria type II due to electron transfer flavoprotein (β-subunit) deficiency and the time course of metabolite excretion after birth. Pediatr Res 1991;30:439–43.
29. Sue CM, Hirano M, DiMauro S, et al. Neonatal presentations of mitochondrial metabolic disorders. Semin Perinatol 1999; 32:113–24.
30. Vassault A, Bonnefont JP, Specola N, et al. Lactate, pyruvate, and ketone bodies. In: Hommes F, ed. Techniques in diagnostic human biochemical genetics – a laboratory manual. New York: Wiley-Liss, 1991:285–308.
31. Smeitink J, van den Heuvel B, Trijbels F, et al. Mitochondrial energy metabolism. In: Blau N, Duran M, Blaskovics ME, et al., eds. Physician's guide to the laboratory diagnosis of metabolic diseases. 2nd ed. Berlin: Springer-Verlag, 2003:519–36.
32. Robinson BH, MacMillan H, Petrova-Benedict R, et al. Variable clinical presentation in patients with defective E1 component of the pyruvate dehydrogenase complex. J Pediatr 1987;111: 525–33.
33. Robinson BH. Lactic academia: disorders of pyruvate carboxylase and pyruvate dehydrogenase complex. In: Scriver CR, Beaudet AL, Sly WS, et al., eds. The metabolic and molecular bases of inherited disease. 8th ed. New York: McGraw-Hill, 2001:2275–95.
34. Leonard JV, Schapira AHV. Mitochondrial respiratory chain disorders. I: mitochondrial DNA defects. Lancet 2000;355:299–304.
35. Robinson BH, Taylor J, Sherwood WG. The genetic heterogeneity of lactic acidosis: occurrence of recognizable inborn errors of metabolism in a pediatric population with lactic acidosis. Pediatr Res 1980;14:956–62.
36. Coude FX, Ogier H, Marsac C, et al. Secondary citrullinemia with hyperammonemia in four neonatal cases of pyruvate carboxylase deficiency. Pediatrics 1981;68:914.
37. Munnich A, Saudubray J-M, Taylor J, et al. Congenital lactic acidosis, α-ketoglutaric aciduria and variant form of maple syrup urine disease due to a single enzyme defect: dihydrolipoyldehydrogenase deficiency. Acta Paediatr Scand 1982;71:167–71.
38. Bonnefont JP, Chretien D, Rustin P, et al. Alpha-ketoglutarate dehydrogenase deficiency presenting as congenital lactic acidosis. J Pediatr 1992;121:255–8.
39. Shih VE. Amino acid analysis. In: Blau N, Duran M, Blaskovics ME, et al., eds. Physician's guide to the laboratory diagnosis of metabolic diseases. 2nd ed. Berlin: Springer-Verlag, 2003:11–26.
40. Tein I. Neonatal metabolic myopathies. Semin Perinatol 1999;23: 125–51.
41. Pettersen JE, Landaas S, Eldjarn L. The occurrence of 2-hydroxy butyric acid in urine from patients with lactic acidosis. Clin Chim Acta 1973;48:213–19.

42. Landaas S, Pettersen JE. Clinical conditions associated with urinary excretion of 2-hydroxy butyric acid. Scand J Clin Lab Invest 1975;35:259–66.
43. Chalmers RA. Organic acids in urine of patients with congenital lactic acidosis: an aid to differential diagnosis. J Inherit Metab Dis 1984;7 Suppl 1:79–89.
44. Rinaldo P, Marcon M, Dussini N, et al. Urinary organic acids in inherited disorders of mitochondrial metabolism: presumptive differential diagnosis of lactic acidoses by gas chromatography-mass spectrometry. Perspect Inherit Metab Dis 1985;6:53–63.
45. Wolf B. Disorders of biotin metabolism. In: Scriver CR, Beaudet AL, Sly WS, et al., eds. The metabolic and molecular bases of inherited disease. 8th ed. New York: McGraw-Hill, 2001:3935–62.
46. Bourgeron T, Rustin P, Chretien D, et al. Mutation of a nuclear succinate dehydrogenase gene results in mitochondrial respiratory chain deficiency. Nat Genet 1995;11:144–9.
47. Bennett MJ, Sherwood WG, Gibson KM, et al. Secondary inhibition of multiple NAD-requiring dehydrogenases in respiratory chain complex I deficiency: possible metabolic markers for the primary defect. J Inherit Metab Dis 1993;16:560–2.
48. Eaton S, Bartlett K, Pourfarzam M. Mammalian mitochondrial β-oxidation. Biochem J 1996;320:345–57.
49. McGarry JD, Foster DW. Regulation of hepatic fatty acid oxidation and ketone body production. Ann Rev Biochem 1980;49:395–420.
50. Bennett MJ, Rinaldo P, Strauss AW. Inborn errors of mitochondrial fatty acid oxidation. Crit Rev Clin Lab Sci 2000;37:1–44.
51. Nyhan WL, Barshop BA, Ozand PT. Disorders of fatty acid oxidation. In: Nyhan WL, Barshop BA, Ozand PT, eds. Atlas of metabolic diseases. London: Hodder Arnold, 2005:239–99.
52. Rinaldo P, Stanley CA, Sanchez LA, et al. Sudden neonatal death in carnitine transporter deficiency. J Pediatr 1997;131:304–5.
53. Chalmers RA, Stanley CA, English N, et al. Mitochondrial carnitine-acylcarnitine translocase deficiency presenting as sudden neonatal death. J Pediatr 1997;131:220–5.
54. Smelt AHM, Poorthuis BJHM, Onkenhout W, et al. Very long chain acyl-coenzyme A dehydrogenase deficiency with adult onset. Ann Neurol 1998;43:540–4.
55. Raymond K, Bale AE, Barnes CA, et al. Medium-chain acyl-CoA dehydrogenase deficiency: sudden and unexpected death of a 45 year old woman. Genet Med 1999;1:293–4.
56. Al Odaib A, Shneider BL, Bennett MJ, et al. A defect in the transport of long-chain fatty acids associated with acute liver failure. N Engl J Med 1998;339:1752–7.
57. Boles RG, Buck EA, Blitzer MG, et al. Retrospective biochemical screening of fatty acid oxidation disorders in postmortem liver of 418 cases of sudden unexpected death in the first year of life. J Pediatr 1998;132:924–33.
58. Patel JS, Leonard JV. Ketonuria and medium-chain acyl-CoA dehydrogenase deficiency. J Inherit Metab Dis 1995;18:98–9.
59. Bennett MJ, Weinberger MJ, Kobori JA, et al. Mitochondrial short-chain L-3-hydroxybutyryl-CoA dehydrogenase deficiency: a new defect of fatty acid oxidation. Pediatr Res 1996;39:185–8.
60. Duran M. Disorders of mitochondrial fatty acid oxidation and ketone body handling. In: Blau N, Duran M, Blaskovics ME, et al., eds. Physician's guide to the laboratory diagnosis of metabolic diseases. 2nd ed. Berlin: Springer-Verlag, 2003:309–34.
61. Rinaldo P, Raymond K, Al Odaib A, et al. Fatty acid oxidation disorders: clinical and biochemical features. Curr Opin Pediatr 1998;10:615–21.
62. Lehnert W, Ruitenbeek W. Ethylmalonic aciduria associated with progressive neurological disease and partial cytochrome C oxidase deficiency. J Inherit Metab Dis 1993;16:557–9.
63. Christensen E, Brandt NJ, Schmalbruch H, et al. Muscle cytochrome C oxidase deficiency accompanied by a urinary organic acid pattern mimicking multiple acyl-CoA dehydrogenase deficiency. J Inherit Metab Dis 1993;16:553–6.
64. Burlina AB, Dionisi-Vici C, Bennett MJ, et al. A new encephalopathy with ethylmalonic aciduria and normal fatty acid oxidation in fibroblasts. J Pediatr 1994;124:79–86.
65. Bhala A, Willi SM, Rinaldo P, et al. The emerging clinical and biochemical picture of short-chain acyl-CoA dehydrogenase deficiency. J Pediatr 1995;126:910–15.
66. Corydon MJ, Gregersen N, Lehnert W, et al. Ethylmalonic aciduria is associated with an amino acid variant (G209S) of short-chain acyl-coenzyme A dehydrogenase (SCAD). Pediatr Res 1996;39:1059–66.
67. Gregersen N, Winter V, Corydon MJ, et al. Identification of four new mutations in the short-chain acyl-CoA dehydrogenase (SCAD) gene in two patients: one of the variant alleles, 511CT, is present at an unexpectedly high frequency in the general population, as was the case for 625GA, together conferring susceptibility to ethylmalonic aciduria. Hum Mol Genet 1998;7:619–27.
68. Stanley CA, DeLeeuw S, Coates PM, et al. Chronic cardiomyopathy and weakness or acute coma in children with a defect in carnitine uptake. Ann Neurol 1991;30:709–16.
69. Costa CG, Dorland L, Holwerda U, et al. Simultaneous analysis of plasma free fatty acids and their 3-hydroxy analogs in fatty acid β-oxidation disorders. Clin Chem 1998;44:463–71.
70. Jones PM, Quinn R, Fennessey P, et al. An improved method for measuring serum or plasma free 3-hydroxy-fatty acids using stable isotope dilution gas chromatography-mass spectrometry and its utility for the study of disorders of mitochondrial fatty acid β-oxidation. Clin Chem 2000;46:149–55.
71. McLafferty FW. Tandem mass spectrometry. Science 1981;214:280–7.
72. Fenn JB, Mann M, Meng CK, et al. Electrospray ionization for mass spectrometry of large molecules. Science 1989;246:64–71.
73. Magera MJ, Lacey JM, Casetta B, et al. A method for the determination of total homocysteine in plasma and urine by stable isotope dilution and electrospray tandem mass spectrometry. Clin Chem 1999;45:1517–22.
74. Levy HL. Newborn screening by tandem mass spectrometry: a new era [Editorial]. Clin Chem 1998;44:2401–2.
75. Chace DH, DiPerna JC, Naylor EW. Laboratory integration and utilization of tandem mass spectrometry in neonatal screening: a model for clinical mass spectrometry in the next millennium. Acta Pediatr 1999;88:45–7.
76. Andresen BS, Bross P, Udvari S, et al. The molecular basis of medium-chain acyl-CoA dehydrogenase (MCAD) deficiency in compound heterozygous patients: is there correlation between genotype and phenotype? Hum Mol Genet 1997;6:695–707.
77. Brusilow SW, Horwich AL. Urea cycle enzymes. In: Scriver CR, Beaudet AL, Sly WS, et al., eds. The metabolic and molecular bases of inherited disease. 8th ed. New York: McGraw-Hill, 2001:1909–63.
78. Rowe PC, Newman SL, Brusilow SW. Natural history of symptomatic partial ornithine transcarbamylase deficiency. N Engl J Med 1986;314:541–7.
79. Leonard JV. Disorders of the urea cycle. In: Fernandes J,

Saudubray JM, van den Berghe G, eds. Inborn metabolic diseases. Diagnosis and treatment. 3rd ed. Berlin: Springer-Verlag, 2000:213–22.

80. Bachmann C, Colombo JP. Acid-base status and plasma glutamine in patients with hereditary urea cycle disorders. In: Soeters PB, Wilson JHP, Meijer AJ, et al., eds. Advances in ammonia metabolism and hepatic encephalopathy. Amsterdam: Elsevier, 1988:72–8.
81. Bachmann C. Satellite meeting on advances in inherited urea cycle disorders. Recent results – new questions. J Inherit Metab Dis 1998;21 Suppl 1:1–5.
82. Chuang DT, Shih VE. Maple syrup urine disease (branched-chain ketoaciduria). In: Scriver CR, Beaudet AL, Sly WS, et al., eds. The metabolic and molecular bases of inherited disease. 8th ed. New York: McGraw-Hill, 2001:1971–2006.
83. Matthews DE, Ben-Galim E, Haymond MW, et al. Alloisoleucine formation in maple syrup urine disease: isotopic evidence for the mechanism. Pediatr Res 1980;14:854–7.
84. Hamosh A, Johnston MV. Nonketotic hyperglycinemia. In: Scriver CR, Beaudet AL, Sly WS, et al., eds. The metabolic and molecular bases of inherited disease. 8th ed. New York: McGraw-Hill, 2001:2065–78.
85. Tada K, Narisawa K. Non-ketotic hyperglycinemia: clinical and biochemical aspects. Eur J Pediatr 1987;146:221–7.

23

α_1-Antitrypsin Deficiency

David H. Perlmutter, M.D.

Homozygous PIZZ α_1-antitrypsin (α_1-AT) deficiency is a relatively common genetic disorder, affecting 1 in 1600 to 1 in 2000 live births [1,2]. It is an autosomal codominant disorder associated with 85–90% reduction in serum concentrations of α_1-AT. A single amino acid substitution results in an abnormally folded protein that is unable to traverse the secretory pathway. The mutant α_1-ATZ protein is retained in the endoplasmic reticulum (ER) rather than secreted into the blood and body fluids.

α_1-Antitrypsin is an approximately 55-kDa secretory glycoprotein that inhibits destructive neutrophil proteases, elastase, cathepsin G, and proteinase 3. Plasma α_1-AT is derived predominantly from the liver and increases three- to fivefold during the host response to tissue injury or inflammation. It is the archetype of a family of structurally related circulating serine protease inhibitors called *serpins.*

Nationwide prospective screening studies done by Sveger [1,3] in Sweden have shown that only 8–10% of the PIZZ population develops clinically significant liver disease over the first 20 years of life. Nevertheless, this deficiency is the most frequent genetic cause of liver disease in children and the most frequent genetic disease for which children undergo orthotropic liver transplantation. It also has been associated with chronic hepatitis, cirrhosis, and hepatocellular carcinoma in adults [4].

Although the condition does not affect children, many α_1-AT-deficient individuals develop destructive lung disease and emphysema. Most of the data in the literature indicate that emphysema results from a loss-of-function mechanism whereby decreased number of α_1-AT molecules within the lower respiratory tract allow unregulated elastolytic attack on the connective tissue matrix of the lung [5,6]. Oxidative inactivation of residual α_1-AT as a result of smoking accelerates lung injury [7]. Moreover, the elastase–antielastase theory for the pathogenesis of emphysema is based on the concept that oxidative inactivation of α_1-AT as a result of cigarette smoking plays a key role in the emphysema of α_1-AT-sufficient individuals, the vast majority of patients with emphysema [5,8].

It has been more difficult to explain the pathogenesis of liver injury in this deficiency. Results of transgenic animal experiments have provided further evidence that the liver disease does not result from a deficiency in antielastase activity [9,10]. Most of the data in the literature corroborate the concept that liver injury in α_1-AT deficiency results from a gain-of-toxic function mechanism whereby retention of the mutant α_1-ATZ molecule in the ER of liver cells eventually exacts hepatotoxic effects.

The diagnosis of α_1-AT deficiency is based on the altered migration of the abnormal α_1-ATZ molecule in serum specimens subjected to isoelectric focusing gel analysis. Treatment of α_1-AT deficiency–associated liver disease is mostly supportive. Liver transplantation has been used successfully for severe liver injury. Although the clinical efficacy has not been demonstrated, many patients with emphysema caused by α_1-AT deficiency are being treated by intravenous and intratracheal aerosol administration of purified plasma α_1-AT. An increasing number of patients with severe emphysema has been undergoing lung transplantation. Several new pharmacologic and genetic strategies for prophylaxis of both liver and lung disease are under development for clinical application.

LIVER DISEASE: CLINICAL MANIFESTATIONS

Liver involvement is often noticed first at 1–2 months of age, because of persistent jaundice (Table 23.1). Conjugated bilirubin levels in the blood and serum aminotransferase levels are mildly to moderately elevated. Blood levels of alkaline phosphatase and γ-glutamyl transpeptidase also may be elevated. The liver may be enlarged. There is a tendency for some affected infants to be small for gestational age. Because these clinical and laboratory characteristics are similar to other causes of liver injury in the newborn period, these infants may initially be given the diagnosis of neonatal hepatitis syndrome and subjected to a diagnostic evaluation for various disorders including α1-AT deficiency [11]. Infants also may be evaluated initially for α_1-AT deficiency because of an episode of gastrointestinal bleeding, bleeding from the umbilical stump, or bruising [12]. A small number of affected infants, approximately 10% of the deficient population, have hepatosplenomegaly, ascites, and liver synthetic dysfunction in early infancy. An even smaller

Table 23.1: Liver Disease Associated with α_1-Antitrypsin Deficiency

Clinical features
- Prolonged jaundice in infants
- Neonatal hepatitis syndrome
- Mild elevation of aminotransferases in toddler
- Portal hypertension in child/adolescent
- Severe liver dysfunction in child/adolescent
- Chronic hepatitis in adult
- Cryptogenic cirrhosis in adult
- Hepatocellular carcinoma in adult

Diagnostic features
- Diminished serum levels of α_1-antitrypsin
- Abnormal mobility of α_1-antitrypsin in isoelectric focusing
- Periodic acid–Schiff positive, diastase-resistant globules in liver cells

number have severe fulminant liver failure in infancy [13]. A few infants are recognized initially because of a cholestatic clinical syndrome characterized by pruritus and hypercholesterolemia. The clinical picture in these patients resembles extrahepatic biliary atresia, but histologic examination shows paucity of intrahepatic bile ducts.

Liver disease associated with α_1-AT deficiency may also be discovered first in late childhood or early adolescence, when the affected individual develops abdominal distention from hepatosplenomegaly or ascites, has splenomegaly, or has upper intestinal bleeding caused by esophageal variceal hemorrhage. In some of these patients, there is a history of unexplained prolonged obstructive jaundice during the neonatal period. In others, there is no evidence of any previous liver injury, even if the neonatal history is carefully reviewed (Table 23.1).

α_1-Antitrypsin deficiency should be considered in the differential diagnosis of any adult who presents with chronic hepatitis, cirrhosis, portal hypertension, or hepatocellular carcinoma of unknown origin. An autopsy study in Sweden showed a higher risk of cirrhosis in adults with α_1-AT deficiency than was previously suspected and that α_1-AT deficiency has a strong association with primary liver cancer [4]. Moreover, the risk of liver cancer was greater than could be accounted for by the known increase associated with cirrhosis alone [4]. Interestingly, cirrhosis and liver cancer may be initially diagnosed in a patient with little in the way of clinical manifestations of liver disease, perhaps only asymptomatic hepatomegaly or elevated transaminases or bilirubin levels. Primary liver cancer is also observed in the absence of cirrhosis in some patients with α1-AT deficiency [14]. The histology of the hepatic cancer can be characteristic of hepatocellular carcinoma, cholangiocarcinoma or have features of both [14]. Although it has been said that heterozygotes are at increased risk of primary liver cancer [15], it has not been possible to prove that the cancers in these patients are caused by the allelic variant itself.

The only prospective data on the natural history of α_1-AT deficiency–associated liver injury is the Swedish nationwide screening study done by Sveger [1]. In this study, 200,000 newborn infants were screened, and 127 PIZZ individuals were identified. Of these 127 infants, 14 had prolonged obstructive jaundice, and 9 of the 14 had severe liver disease, as indicated by clinical and laboratory criteria. Another 8 of the 127 PIZZ infants had mild abnormalities of serum bilirubin or serum aminotransferase levels or hepatomegaly. Approximately 50% of the remainder of the 127 had only abnormal aminotransferase levels [1]. Published follow-up studies of the original cohort of 127 PIZZ children at 18 years of age showed that more than 85% had persistently normal serum transaminase levels with no evidence of liver dysfunction [3]. Issues not addressed by the Sveger study include whether 18-year-olds with α_1-AT deficiency have persistent subclinical histologic abnormalities, despite lack of clinical or biochemical evidence of liver injury, and whether liver disease eventually becomes clinically evident during adulthood.

It still is not clear what clinical manifestations or abnormal laboratory test results can be used to predict a poor prognosis for individuals with α_1-AT deficiency–associated liver disease. One study suggested that persistence of hyperbilirubinemia, hard hepatomegaly, early development of splenomegaly, and progressive prolongation of prothrombin time are indicators of poor prognosis [16]. In another study, elevated aminotransferase levels, prolonged prothrombin time, and a lower trypsin inhibitor capacity correlated with worse prognosis [17]. In my experience, however, some children with α_1-AT deficiency–associated liver disease can lead relatively normal lives for years after the development of hepatosplenomegaly and mild prolongation of prothrombin time. In a review of 44 patients with α_1-AT deficiency seen at St. Louis Children's Hospital from 1984 to 2000, 17 had cirrhosis or portal hypertension [18]. Nine of these have had a prolonged, relatively uneventful course for at least 4 years after the diagnosis of cirrhosis or portal hypertension. Two of these patients eventually underwent liver transplantation, but seven have led relatively healthy lives for up to 22 years after diagnosis. These nine patients could be distinguished from the remaining eight only by overall functioning and not by any single clinical or biochemical characteristic. Starzl et al. [19] reported three children with severe liver disease as a result of α_1-AT deficiency who underwent portocaval or splenorenal shunt and had survived 10 to 15 years at the time of the report. Hence, predictions of poor prognosis for α_1-AT deficiency–associated liver disease and for timing of liver transplantation depend more on the overall functioning of the affected child than on the liver histologic analysis or laboratory data.

There is no evidence that the heterozygous α_1-AT (MZ) phenotype by itself causes liver disease during childhood. Moreover, it is not clear whether the heterozygous MZ phenotype predisposes to liver disease in adults. An early study of a liver biopsy collection suggested that there was a relation between heterozygosity and the development of liver disease [20]. A retrospective study of liver transplant recipients at the Mayo Clinic showed a higher prevalence for heterozygosity for α_1-ATZ than in the general population, including a group of patients without another explanation for liver disease [21]. However, both of these studies are biased in ascertainment and do not include concurrent prospective controls. A cross-sectional study of patients with α_1-AT deficiency in a referral-based Austrian university hospital who were reexamined with the most sophisticated and sensitive assays available suggests that liver disease in heterozygotes can be accounted for, to a great extent, by infections with hepatitis B or C virus or autoimmune disease [22]. Thus the literature does not provide convincing evidence that liver injury can be explained by the α_1-AT MZ heterozygous state alone, but clinical experience with MZ individuals that have severe liver disease and no other explanation for it gives the impression that this is due to the difficulties in study design more than anything else.

Liver disease has been described for several other allelic variants of α_1-AT. Children with compound heterozygosity type PISZ are affected by liver injury in a manner similar to PIZZ children [1,3]. There are several reports of liver disease in the α_1-AT deficiency variant PIM_{malton} [23,24]. These are particularly interesting associations because the mutant PIM_{malton} and PISZ α_1-AT molecules has been shown to undergo polymerization and retention within the ER [25–27]. Liver disease has been detected in single patients with several other α_1-AT allelic variants – such as PIM_{Duarte} [28], PI_W [29], and PI_{FZ} [30] – but it is not clear whether other causes of liver injury for which we have more sophisticated diagnostic assays, such as infection with hepatitis C and autoimmune hepatitis, have been excluded completely in these cases.

LUNG DISEASE: CLINICAL MANIFESTATIONS

The incidence and prevalence of emphysema in α_1-AT deficiency have not been studied prospectively. Autopsy studies suggest that 60–65% of persons with homozygous PIZZ α_1-AT deficiency develop clinically significant lung injury [31]. There are PIZZ smokers, however, who do not have any symptoms of lung disease or evidence of pulmonary function abnormalities until the seventh or eighth decade of life [32].

The typical person with lung disease is a man and a cigarette smoker. Onset of dyspnea is insidious in the third to fourth decade of life. About 50% of affected persons develop cough and recurrent lung infections. The disease progresses to a severe limitation of airflow. A reduction in the forced expiratory volume, an increase in total lung capacity, and a reduction in diffusing capacity occur. Chest radiographs demonstrate hyperinflation with marked lucency at the lung bases [33]. Histopathologic studies demonstrate panacinar emphysema, more prominent in the lower lung [33,34].

It is rare for emphysema to affect an α_1-AT-deficient patient during childhood. A number of patients have been described in the literature, but for each of these, an alternative explanation can be offered. In the most convincing case, emphysema developed several years after a portocaval shunt procedure was done [35]. In three early cases, there are problems with the phenotypic diagnosis of α_1-AT deficiency [36–38]. In a more recent report, two patients had pulmonary abnormalities that could have been attributed to severe systemic illness associated with end-stage liver disease [39]. A number of infants with α_1-AT deficiency have had pulmonary function testing suggesting a subtle degree of hyperinflation [40]. Another study, however, did not detect any significant difference between the pulmonary function of PIZZ children between the ages of 13 and 17 and that of an age-matched control group [41]. These data indicate that it is extremely rare for α_1-AT deficiency to cause emphysema in individuals aged younger than 25 years.

The destructive effect of cigarette smoking on the outcome of lung disease in α_1-AT deficiency has been demonstrated in many studies. Actuarial studies suggest that cigarette smoking reduces median survival by more than 20 years in deficient persons [42]. The rate of decline in forced expiratory volume is 4 times greater in smoking than in nonsmoking persons with α_1-AT deficiency [43].

There is still limited information about the incidence of liver disease in α_1-AT-deficient individuals with emphysema. In one recent study of 22 PIZZ patients with emphysema, there was an elevated aminotransferase level in 10 patients, and cholestasis was present in one patient [44]. Liver biopsies were not done in this study; they may be necessary to determine accurately the extent of liver injury in these patients.

PATHOPHYSIOLOGY

Structure of α_1-Antitrypsin

α_1-Antitrypsin is a single-chain, approximately 52- to 55-kDa polypeptide with 394 amino acids and three asparagine-linked complex carbohydrate side chains [45]. There are two major isoforms in serum, depending on the presence of a biantennary or triantennary configuration for the carbohydrate side chains [46]. It has a globular shape and a highly ordered internal domain composed of two central β sheets surrounded by a small β sheet and nine α helices [45]. The dominant structure is the five-stranded β-pleated sheet termed the *A sheet*.

α_1-Antitrypsin is the archetype of the serpins (or *serine protease inhibitors*), including antithrombin III, α_1-antichymotrypsin, C1 inhibitor, α_2-antiplasmin, protein C inhibitor, heparin cofactor II, plasminogen activator inhibitors I and II, protease nexin I, ovalbumin, angiotensinogen, corticosteroid-binding globulin, and thyroid-binding globulin, among others [47]. These proteins share about 25–40% primary structural homology, with higher degrees of regional homology in functional domains. Most serpins function as suicide inhibitors by forming equimolar complexes with a specific target protease. Other serpins are not inhibitory. For instance, corticosteroid and thyroid hormone–binding globulins, which are thought to represent carriers for corticosteroid and thyroid hormone, respectively, form complexes but do not inactivate their hormone ligands.

A comparison of α_1-AT with other members of the serpin supergene family has generated several important concepts

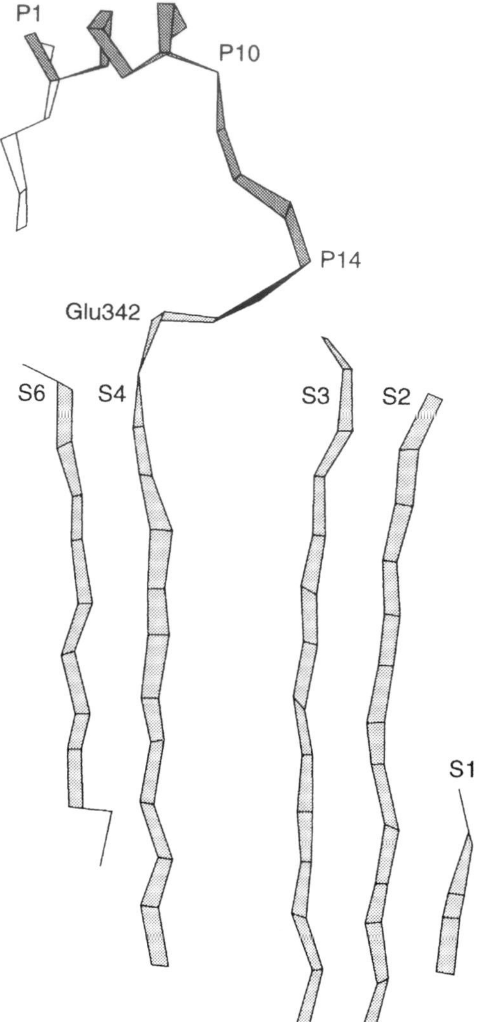

Figure 23.1. Ribbon diagram of the A sheet and reactive centre loop of native α_1-AT. Because native α_1-AT has not been crystallized, this ribbon diagram is generated by computer models based on the crystal structures of cleaved α_1-AT and native ovalbumin. The reactive center loop is shown in black. Residues P10 and P14 are numbered from the reactive-site methionine P1. The carboxyl terminal fragment is shown as white ribbons. β-helices of the A sheet are shown as gray ribbons and referred to as S_1, S_2, S_3, S_5, and S_6. The Glu 342 residue, which is replaced by Lys in α_1-ATZ PIZ α_1-AT, is designated. (Adapted from Carrell RW, Evans DL, Steen DE. Mobile reactive centre of serpins and the control of thrombosis. Nature 1991;353:376; with permission.)

about the structure and function of α_1-AT. For instance, the reactive site, P1 residue, of α_1-AT is localized to a canonic loop that rises above the gap in the center of the A sheet [48,49] (Figure 23.1). This loop may provide a certain degree of flexibility to the functional activity of the inhibitor. The reactive loop conformation of serpins is also thought to make them susceptible to proteolytic cleavage by thiolenzymes and metalloenzymes. The P1 residue itself is the most important determinant of functional specificity for each serpin molecule. This concept was confirmed dramatically by the discovery of α_1-AT Pittsburgh, a variant in which the P1 residue of α_1-AT, Met 358, is replaced by Arg. In this variant, α_1-AT functions as a thrombin inhibitor, and severe bleeding diathesis results [50].

The carboxyl-terminal fragment of α_1-AT and the other serpins also bears important structural and functional characteristics. There is a much higher degree of sequence homology among serpins in the carboxyl terminus. A small fragment at this terminus is cleaved during formation of the inhibitory complex with serine protease. This carboxyl-terminal fragment possesses chemotactic activity [51,52]. Moreover, this fragment bears the receptor-binding domain for cell surface binding, internalization of α_1-AT elastase and other serpin-enzyme complexes, and activation of a signal-transduction pathway for upregulation of α_1-AT gene expression [53,54].

α_1-Antitrypsin is encoded by a 12.2-kilobase (kb) gene (Figure 23.2) located on human chromosome 14q31–32.2 [55–58]. The first two exons and a short 5′ segment of the third exon code for 5′ untranslated regions of the α_1-AT messenger RNA (mRNA). Most of the fourth exon and the remaining three exons encode the protein sequence of α_1-AT. A 72-base sequence constitutes the 24–amino acid amino-terminal signal sequence. The three sites for asparagine-linked carbohydrate attachment are at residues 46, 83, and 247. The active site, the so-called P1 residue, Met 358, is encoded in the seventh exon. It is not yet known whether the two exons, also called *short open-reading frames*, in the upstream untranslated region of the α_1-AT gene are involved in translational regulation of its expression [59]. There is a "sequence-related gene" about 12 kb downstream from the α_1-AT gene [56,60–62]. Because no evidence exists that the sequence-related gene is expressed, it is considered a pseudogene. The genes for two other serpins, α_1-antichymotrypsin and corticosteroid-binding globulin, also are linked closely on chromosome 14 [58,63]. The α_1-AT mRNA expressed in liver is 1.4 kb long [55]. In macrophages, the α_1-AT mRNA is slightly longer [59]. In fact, there are three forms of α_1-AT mRNA in macrophages, depending on transcription initiation sites in two upstream exonic structures (exons IA and IB) [59,64].

Structural variants of α_1-AT in humans are classified according to the protease inhibitor phenotype system as defined by agarose electrophoresis or isoelectric focusing of plasma [65]. The PI classification assigns a letter to variants according to position of migration of α_1-AT in these gel systems, using alphabetic order from low to high isoelectric point. For example, the most common normal variant migrates to an intermediate isoelectric point, designated *M*. Persons with the most common severe deficiency have an α_1-AT allelic variant that migrates to a high isoelectric point, designated *Z*.

More than 100 allelic variants of α1-AT have been reported [66]. Structural variants of α_1-AT not associated with changes in serum concentration or functional activity from the normal range are termed *normal allelic variants* and include the M1 [67], M2, M3 [68–70], M1 (Ala 213) [67], X [71], Christchurch [72], and $P_{\text{Saint Alban's}}$ alleles [73]. In each case examined, a single relatively conservative substitution is present. α_1-AT variants in which α_1-AT is not detectable in serum are called *null*

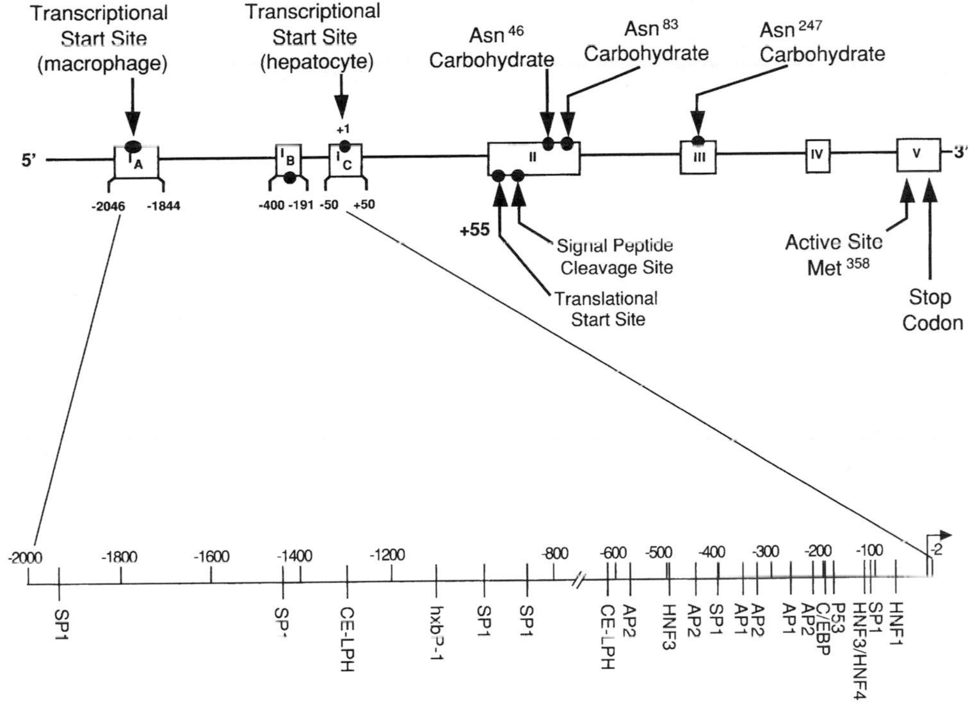

Figure 23.2. Schematic representation of the structure of the α_1-antitrypsin gene (not to scale) and map of potential regulatory elements based on its sequence.

allelic variants (Table 23.2) and, if inherited with another null variant or deficiency variant, are associated with premature development of emphysema [74]. Several types of defects, including insertions and deletions, appear to be responsible for these variants (Table 23.2). In two instances, α_1-AT Null$_{\text{isola di procida}}$ and α_1-AT Null$_{\text{Reidenburg}}$, there is deletion of all α_1-AT coding regions [75,76]. In two other cases, α_1-AT Null$_{\text{Bellingham}}$ and α_1-AT Null$_{\text{Granite Falls}}$, α_1-AT mRNA is undetectable [77–80]. Three other null alleles result in truncated proteins that are degraded in the ER – Null$_{\text{Mattawa}}$, Null$_{\text{hong kong}}$, and Null$_{\text{Clayton}}$ [81–84].

Several variants of α_1-AT associated with a reduction in serum concentrations of α_1-AT have been described and are called *deficiency variants* (Table 23.3). Some of these variants are not associated with clinical disease, such as the S variant [55,85,86]. Other deficiency variants are associated with emphysema such as M$_{\text{Heerlen}}$ [87], M$_{\text{Procida}}$ [88], M$_{\text{Malton}}$ [22,89], M$_{\text{Duarte}}$ [24], M$_{\text{Mineral Springs}}$ [90], P$_{\text{Lowell}}$ [73], and W$_{\text{Bethesda}}$ [91]. In two persons with M$_{\text{Malton}}$ and one with M$_{\text{Duarte}}$, hepatocyte α_1-AT inclusions and liver disease have been reported [21,22,24]. In one person with the deficiency variant S$_{\text{iiyama}}$, emphysema and hepatocyte inclusions were reported, but this person did not have liver disease [92]. Dysfunctional variants of α_1-AT include α_1-AT Pittsburgh [50]. There also is a decrease in serum concentration and functional activity for α_1-AT M$_{\text{Mineral Spring}}$ [90]. For several variants that have been identified in compound heterozygotes such as α_1-AT F [93], α_1-AT Null$_{\text{Newport}}$, and α_1-AT Z$_{\text{Wrexham}}$ [94], it is not clear whether the variants result in normal, null, deficient, or dysfunctional changes.

Function of α_1-Antitrypsin

α_1-Antitrypsin is an inhibitor of serine proteases in general, but its most important targets are neutrophil elastase, cathepsin G, and proteinase 3, proteases released by activated neutrophils. Several lines of evidence suggest that inhibition of these neutrophil proteases is the major physiologic function of α_1-AT. First, individuals with α_1-AT deficiency are susceptible to premature development of emphysema, a lesion that can be induced in experimental animals by instillation of excessive amounts of neutrophil elastase [95]. These observations have led to the concept that destructive lung disease may result from perturbations of the net balance of elastase and α_1-AT within the local environment of the lung [5]. Second, the kinetics of association for α_1-AT and neutrophil elastase are more favorable, by several orders of magnitude, than those for α_1-AT and any other serine protease [96]. Third, α_1-AT constitutes more than 90% of the neutrophil elastase inhibitory activity in the one body fluid that has been examined, pulmonary alveolar lavage fluid [5].

α_1-Antitrypsin acts competitively by allowing its target enzymes to bind directly to a substrate-like region within its reactive center loop [96]. The reaction between enzyme and inhibitor is essentially second order, and the resulting complex contains one molecule of each of the reactants. A reactive-site peptide bond within the inhibitor is hydrolyzed during formation of the enzyme–inhibitor complex. Hydrolysis of this bond, however, does not proceed to completion. An equilibrium, near unity, is established between complexes in which the

Table 23.2: Null Variants of α_1-Antitrypsin

	Defect		*Clinical Disease*		*Cellular Defect*
			Liver	*Lung*	
$Null_{Granite Falls}$	Single base deletion	Tyr 160	−	+	No detectable RNA
$Null_{Bellingham}$	Single base deletion	Lys 217	−	+	No detectable RNA
$Null_{Mattawa}$	Single base insertion	Phe 353	−	+	IC degradation?
$Null_{Hong Kong}$	Dinucleotide deletion	Leu 318	−	+	IC accumulation
$Null_{Ludwigshafen}$	Single base substitution	Isoleu 92-Asp	−	+	Dysfunctional protein (EC degradation?)
$Null_{Clayton}$	Single base insertion	Glu 363	−	+	IC degradation?
$Null_{Bolton}$	Single base deletion	Glu 363	−	+	IC degradation?
$Null_{Isola di Procida}$	Deletion	Exons II–V	−	+	Unknown
$Null_{Riedenburg}$	Deletion	Exons II–V	−	+	Unknown
$Null_{Newport}$	Single base substitution	Gly 115-Ser	−	+	Unknown
$Null_{bonny blue}$	Intron deletion		−	+	Unknown
$Null_{new hope}$	Two base substitutions	Gly 320-Glu	−	+	Unknown
		Glu 342-Lys	−		
$Null_{Trastavere}$	Single base substitution	Trp 194-stop	−	+	Unknown
$Null_{Kowloon}$	Single base substitution	Tyr 38-stop	−	+	Unknown
$Null_{Saarbruecken}$	Single base insertion	Pro 362-stop	−	+	Unknown
$Null_{Lisbon}$	Single base substitution	Thr 68-Ile	−	+	Unknown
$Null_{West}$	Intron deletion		−	+	Unknown

IC, intracellular; EC, extracellular.

reactive-site peptide bond of α_1-AT is intact (native inhibitor) and those in which this peptide bond is cleaved (modified inhibitor). The complex of α_1-AT and serine protease is a covalently stabilized structure that is resistant to dissociation by denaturing compounds, including sodium dodecyl sulfate and urea. The interaction between α_1-AT and serine protease is suicidal in that the modified inhibitor is no longer able to bind with or inactivate the enzyme.

The net functional activity of α_1-AT in complex biologic fluids may be modified by several factors. First, the reactive-site methionine may be oxidized and thereby rendered inactive as an elastase inhibitor [97]. In vitro, α_1-AT is oxidatively inactivated by activated neutrophils [98] and by oxidants released by alveolar macrophages of cigarette smokers [99]. Second, the functional activity of α_1-AT may be modified by proteolytic inactivation. Several members of the metalloprotease family – including collagenase and *Pseudomonas* elastase – and of the thiol protease family can cleave and inactivate α_1-AT [100].

Although α_1-AT from the plasma or liver of individuals with PIZZ α_1-AT deficiency is functionally active [101], there may be a decrease in its specific elastase inhibitory capacity. Ogushi et al. [102] have shown that the kinetics of association with neutrophil elastase and the stability of complexes with neutrophil elastase were decreased significantly for α_1-AT isolated from PIZZ plasma. There was no decrease in the functional activity of α_1-AT from PiSS individuals.

α_1-AT has also been shown to protect experimental animals from the lethal effects of tumor necrosis factor (TNF) [103,104]. Most of the evidence from these studies indicates that this protective effect results from inhibition of the synthesis and release of platelet-activating factor from neutrophils [104,105], presumably through the inhibition of neutrophil-derived proteases.

Several studies indicate that α_1-AT has functional activities other than inhibition of serine protease. The carboxyl-terminal fragment of α_1-AT, which can be generated during the formation of a complex with serine protease or during proteolytic inactivation by thiol- or metalloproteases, is a potent neutrophil chemoattractant [51,52,106].

Although effects on lymphocyte activities and immune function have been attributed to α_1-AT [107,108], there are inherent conflicts in some of the reports, and the data have not been duplicated. There is no evidence that the immune response is altered systemically in α_1-AT-deficient individuals.

Table 23.3: Deficiency Variants of α_1-Antitrypsin

	Defect		*Clinical Disease* *Liver*	*Lung*	*Cellular Defect*
Z	Single base substitution M_1 (Ala 213)	Glu 342-Lys	+	+	IC accumulation
S	Single base substitution	Glu 264-Val	–	–	IC accumulation
$M_{Heerlen}$	Single base substitution	Pro 369-Leu	–	+	IC accumulation
$M_{Procida}$	Single base substitution	Leu 41-Pro	–	+	IC accumulation
M_{Malton}	Single base deletion	Phe 52	?	+	IC accumulation
M_{Duarte}	Unknown	Unknown	+?	+	Unknown
$M_{Mineral\ Springs}$	Single base substitution	Gly 57-Glu	–	+	No function; EC degradation?
S_{iiyama}	Single base substitution	Ser 53-Phe	–	+	IC accumulation
P_{Duarte}	Two base substitution	Arg 101 His	+?	+	Unknown
		Asp 256-Val			
P_{Lowell}	Single base substitution	Asp 256-Val	–	+	IC accumulation; reduced function
	Single base substitution				
$W_{Bethesda}$	Single base substitution	Ala 336-Thre	–	+	EC degradation?
$Z_{Wrexham}$		Ser19-Leu	?	?	Unknown
F	Single base substitution	Arg 223-Cys	–	–	Unknown
T	Single base substitution	Glu 264-Val	–	–	Unknown
I	Single base substitution	Arg 39-Cys		–	IC accumulation; reduced function
$M_{palermo}$	Single base deletion	Phe 51	–	–	Unknown
$M_{nichinan}$	Single base deletion and single base substitution	Phe 52	–	–	Unknown
		Gly 148-Arg			
Zausburg	Single base substitution	Glu 342-Lys	–	–	Unknown

IC, intracellular; EC, extracellular.

Biosynthesis of α_1-Antitrypsin

The predominant site of synthesis of plasma α_1-AT is the liver. This is most clearly shown by conversion of plasma α_1-AT to the donor phenotype after orthotopic liver transplantation [109]. It is synthesized in human hepatoma cells as a 52-kDa precursor; undergoes posttranslational, dolichol phosphate-linked glycosylation at three asparagine residues [110]; and undergoes tyrosine sulfation [111]. It is secreted as a 55-kDa native single-chain glycoprotein with a half-time for secretion of 35 to 40 minutes.

Tissue-specific expression of α_1-AT in human hepatoma cells is directed by structural elements within a 750-nucleotide region upstream of the hepatocyte transcriptional start site in exon Ic. Within these regions are structural elements that are recognized by hepatocyte nuclear transcription factors (HNFs), including HNF1α, HNFβ, C/EBP, HNF4, and HNF3 [112]. HNF1α and HNF4 appear to be particularly important for expression of the human α_1-AT gene. Two distinct regions within the proximal element bind these two transcription factors. In fact, substitution of five nucleotides within the region of nucleotides -77 through -72 disrupts binding of HNF1α and dramatically reduces expression of the human α_1-AT gene in the liver of transgenic mice [113]. Substitution of four nucleotides at positions -118 through -115 disrupts the binding of HNF4 but does not alter expression of the human α_1-AT gene in the liver of adult transgenic mice. The latter mutation does result in a reduction in the expression of human α_1-AT in the liver during embryonic development. HNF1α and HNF4 have a synergistic effect on expression of the α_1-AT gene in hepatocytes and enterocytes [114].

Plasma concentrations of α_1-AT increase three- to fivefold during the host response to inflammation or tissue injury [115]. Because the source of this additional α_1-AT has been thought to be the liver, α_1-AT is known as a positive hepatic acute phase reactant. Synthesis of α_1-AT in human hepatoma cells (HepG2, Hep3B) is up-regulated by interleukin-6 but not by interleukin-1 or TNF [116]. Plasma concentrations of α_1-AT also increase during oral contraceptive therapy and pregnancy [117].

α_1-Antitrypsin is also synthesized and secreted in primary cultures of human blood monocytes and bronchoalveolar and breast milk macrophages [118]. Expression of α_1-AT in monocytes and macrophages is influenced by products generated during inflammation, such as bacterial lipopolysaccharide [119] and interleukin-6 [116].

Expression of α_1-AT is also regulated by a feed-forward mechanism in which elastase – α_1-AT complexes mediate an increase in synthesis of α_1-AT through the interaction of a pentapeptide domain in the carboxylterminal tail of α_1-AT with a novel cell surface receptor [53,54,106,120,121]. This class of receptor molecules is now referred to as *serpin–enzyme complex (SEC) receptors* because they recognize the highly conserved domains of other SECs, such as antithrombin III–thrombin, α_1-antichymotrypsin–cathepsin G, and, to a lesser extent, C1 inhibitor–C1s and tissue plasminogen activator – plasminogen activator inhibitor I complexes, as well as that of elastase – α_1-AT complexes [53,122]. Substance P, several other tachykinins, bombesin, and the amyloid-β peptide bind to the SEC receptor through a similar pentapeptide sequence [123]. Recent studies indicate that the SEC receptor can mediate endocytosis of soluble amyloid-β peptide, but it does not recognize the aggregated form of amyloid-β peptide, which is toxic to neurons and other cell types [124]. The SEC receptor may play a role in preventing amyloid-β peptide from accumulating in the amyloid deposits associated with Alzheimer's disease.

Because its ligand specificity is similar to that required for in vivo clearance of SECs [125], the SEC receptor also may be involved in the clearance and catabolism of elastase – α_1-AT and other serpin–enzyme complexes [54]. The low-density lipoprotein receptor–related protein can also mediate clearance and catabolism of elastsase–α_1-AT complexes [126,127].

α_1-Antitrypsin mRNA has been isolated from multiple tissues in transgenic mice [128–130], but in many cases it has not been possible to distinguish whether this mRNA is in ubiquitous tissue macrophages or other cell types. α_1-AT is synthesized in enterocytes and paneth cells, as indicated by studies in intestinal epithelial cell lines, ribonuclease protection assays of human intestinal RNA, and in situ hybridization analyses in cryostat sections of human intestinal mucosa [131]. Expression of α_1-AT in enterocytes increases during differentiation from crypt to villus, in response to interleukin-6 and during inflammation in vivo. α_1-AT is also synthesized by pulmonary epithelial cells [132,133]. Interestingly, synthesis of α_1-AT in pulmonary epithelial cells is less responsive to regulation by interleukin-6 than by a related cytokine, oncostatin M [133].

Clearance and Distribution

The half-life of α_1-AT in plasma is approximately 5 days [134]. It is estimated that the daily production rate of α_1-AT is 34 mg/kg body weight, with 33% of the intravascular pool of α_1-AT degraded daily. There is a slight increase in the rate of clearance of radiolabeled α_1-ATZ compared with that of wild-type α_1-AT if infused into PIMM individuals, but this difference does not account for the decrease in serum levels of α_1-AT in deficient individuals [135].

α_1-Antitrypsin diffuses into most tissues and is found in most body fluids [5]. Its concentration in lavage fluid from the lower respiratory tract is approximately equivalent to that in serum. α_1-AT also is found in feces, and increased fecal concentrations of α_1-AT correlate with the presence of inflammatory lesions of the bowel [136]. In each case, it has been assumed that α_1-AT was derived from serum. Local sites of synthesis, however, such as macrophages and epithelial cells, also may make important contributions to the α_1-AT pool in these tissues and body fluids. It has been reported that the rate of fecal α_1-AT clearance is higher in patients with homozygous PIZZ α_1-AT deficiency than in normal persons [137]. Because the former have only 10–15% of the normal serum concentrations of α_1-AT, a local intestinal source for fecal α_1-AT is implicated. One possible explanation is that the bulk of α_1-AT in feces is derived from sloughed enterocytes. Increased fecal α_1-AT in those with homozygous PIZZ α_1-AT deficiency would result from intracellular accumulation of the abnormal α_1-AT molecule in enterocytes that are being sloughed at the usual rate. Increased fecal α_1-AT in normal PIMM persons with inflammatory-related, protein-losing enteropathy would result from increased sloughing of enterocytes alone.

Mechanism for Deficiency of α_1-AT in PIZZ Individuals

The mutant α_1-ATZ molecule is characterized by a single nucleotide substitution, which results in an amino acid substitution, Lys for Glu 342 [138–140]. There is a selective decrease in the secretion of α_1-AT, with the mutant protein accumulating in the ER [141,142]. The defect is not specific for liver cells; it also affects extrahepatic sites of α_1-AT synthesis, such as macrophages [141] and transfected cell lines [142–144]. Site-directed mutagenesis studies have shown that this single amino acid substitution is sufficient to produce the cellular defect [145]. Once translocated into the lumen of the ER, the mutant α_1-AT protein is unable to traverse the remainder of the secretory pathway because it is folded abnormally.

Several studies have recently provided evidence that the substitution for Glu 342 of Lys in the α_1-ATZ variant reduces the stability of the molecule in its monomeric form and increases the likelihood that it will form polymers by means of a so-called loop-sheet insertion mechanism [146]. In this mechanism, the reactive center loop of one α_1-AT molecule inserts into a gap in the β-pleated A sheet of another α_1-AT molecule (Figure 23.1). Lomas et al. [146] were the first to notice that the site of the amino acid substitution in the α_1-ATZ variant was at the base of the reactive center loop, adjacent to the gap in the A sheet. These investigators predicted that a change in the charge at this residue, as occurs with the substitution of Lys for Glu, prevents the insertion of the reactive-site loop into the gap in the A sheet and renders mutant α_1-ATZ susceptible to the insertion of the reactive center loop of adjacent molecules into the gap in I sheet. This in turn causes the mutant α_1-ATZ to be more susceptible to polymerization than the wild-type α_1-AT. These experiments showed that α_1-ATZ undergoes this form of polymerization to a certain extent spontaneously and to a greater extent during relatively minor perturbations, such as a rise in temperature. Presumably, an increase in body temperature during systemic inflammation would exacerbate this tendency in vivo. Polymers also could be detected by electron microscopy in the ER of hepatocytes in a liver biopsy specimen from a PIZZ individual [146]. Similar polymers have been found in the plasma of patients with the S_{iiyama} α_1-AT variant and the M_{malton} α_1-AT variant [23,147]. The mutation in α_1-ATS_{iiyama} (Ser 53 to Phe) [92], and in α_1-ATM_{malton} (Phe 52 deletion) [22] affect residues that provide a ridge for the sliding movement that opens the A sheet. Those mutations would be expected to interfere with the insertion of the reactive center loop into the gap in the A sheet and, therefore, leave the gap in the A sheet available for spontaneous loop-sheet polymerization. It is notable that hepatocytic α_1 AT globules have been observed in a few patients with these two variants. Recent observations suggest that the α_1-ATS variant also undergoes loop-sheet polymerization [148] and that this may account for its retention in the ER, albeit a milder degree of retention than that for α_1-ATZ [26]. Moreover, α_1-ATS apparently can form heteropolymers with α_1-ATZ [27], providing a potential explanation for liver disease in patients with the SZ phenotype.

Two series of studies have suggested that polymerization of α_1-ATZ is the cause of its retention in the ER, including, most notably, studies in which its secretion is partially corrected by introduction of a second mutation that suppresses loop-sheet polymerization [149,150]. However, these studies have not excluded the possibility that retention is caused by a distinct abnormality in folding that is partially corrected by the second, experimentally introduced mutation. Indeed, several recent observations militate against the idea that polymerization is the cause of ER retention. First, naturally occurring variants of α_1-AT in which the carboxyl terminal tail of α_1-AT is truncated, including a double mutant with the substitution that characterizes the Z allele and the substitution that results in carboxyl terminal truncation, are retained in the ER even though they do not polymerize [151]. Second, only approximately 18% of the intracellular pool of α_1-ATZ at steady state is in the form of polymers in model cell lines characterized by marked ER retention [151,152]. A greater degree of polymerization is thought to be prevented by the activity of ER chaperones. Most of the cellular pool of α_1-ATZ in the ER in vivo is in heterogeneous soluble complexes with multiple ER chaperones (Figure 23.3) [152], a state that cannot be modeled by studies of purified α_1-ATZ in vitro. These observations suggest the possibility that polymerization of α_1-ATZ in the ER is an effect, rather than a cause, of the retention. This possibility does not preclude a specific role of polymers in the pathogenesis of tissue injury. In fact, three new lines of evidence argue for the specific role of polymers in injury to the liver. The first of these is the discovery that an inherited form of progressive dementia is associated with mutations in neuroserpin that have effects on the structure of that molecule that are almost identical to the effects of the Z mutation on α_1-AT [153]. Second, there is now evidence suggesting that polymers that accumulate in the ER are degraded by a mechanism distinct from that of polymers, autophagic as distinct from proteosomal degradation [154,155]. Third, recent studies indicate that accumulation of the polymerogenic mutant α_1-ATZ activates cellular signaling pathways that are distinct from those activated by nonpolymerogenic α_1-AT mutants [156].

CELLULAR ADAPTIVE RESPONSES TO MUTANT α1-ATZ RETAINED IN THE ER

We now know that cells have elaborate mechanisms for degrading mutant proteins that are retained in the ER. The pathway, or pathways, by which retained α_1-ATZ is degraded is also a candidate for genetic variations that predispose some homozygotes or protect other homozygotes from liver injury by the gain-of-toxic function mechanism. One study has provided a substantiation of this concept by showing that there is a lag in ER degradation of α_1-ATZ after gene transfer into cell lines derived from *susceptible hosts*, homozygotes with liver disease, when compared with cell lines from *protected hosts*, homozygotes completely free of liver disease [157].

Several pathways appear to be involved in the ER degradation of α_1-ATZ. The proteosomal system was implicated first and has since been demonstrated in a number of model systems [158–162]. Both the classical ubiquitin-dependent and the ubiquitin-independent proteosomal pathways play a role [160]. However, it is still not entirely clear how the α_1-ATZ on the luminal side of the ER membrane reaches the proteosome in the cytoplasm. Some luminal substrates have been shown to traverse the ER membrane to reach the cytoplasm by a retrograde translocation mechanism. The only evidence that this mechanism is a part of the ER degradation pathway for α_1-ATZ comes from the studies of Werner et al. [158] in which α_1-ATZ could be detected in the cytosolic fraction of yeast when the proteosome was inhibited, but only a minor fraction of the α_1-ATZ was undergoing degradation. A mechanism in which the proteosome directly mediates extraction of substrates from the ER membrane that has been described for model ER degradation substrates [163] represents one possible alternative.

There are at least nonproteosomal pathways that contribute to ER degradation of α_1-ATZ as well [160]. Cabral et al. [164] have provided evidence for a nonproteosomal pathway that is sensitive to tyrosine phosphatase inhibitors. We have shown that macroautophagy contributes to the disposal of α_1-ATZ that is retained in the ER, using chemical inhibitors of autophagy

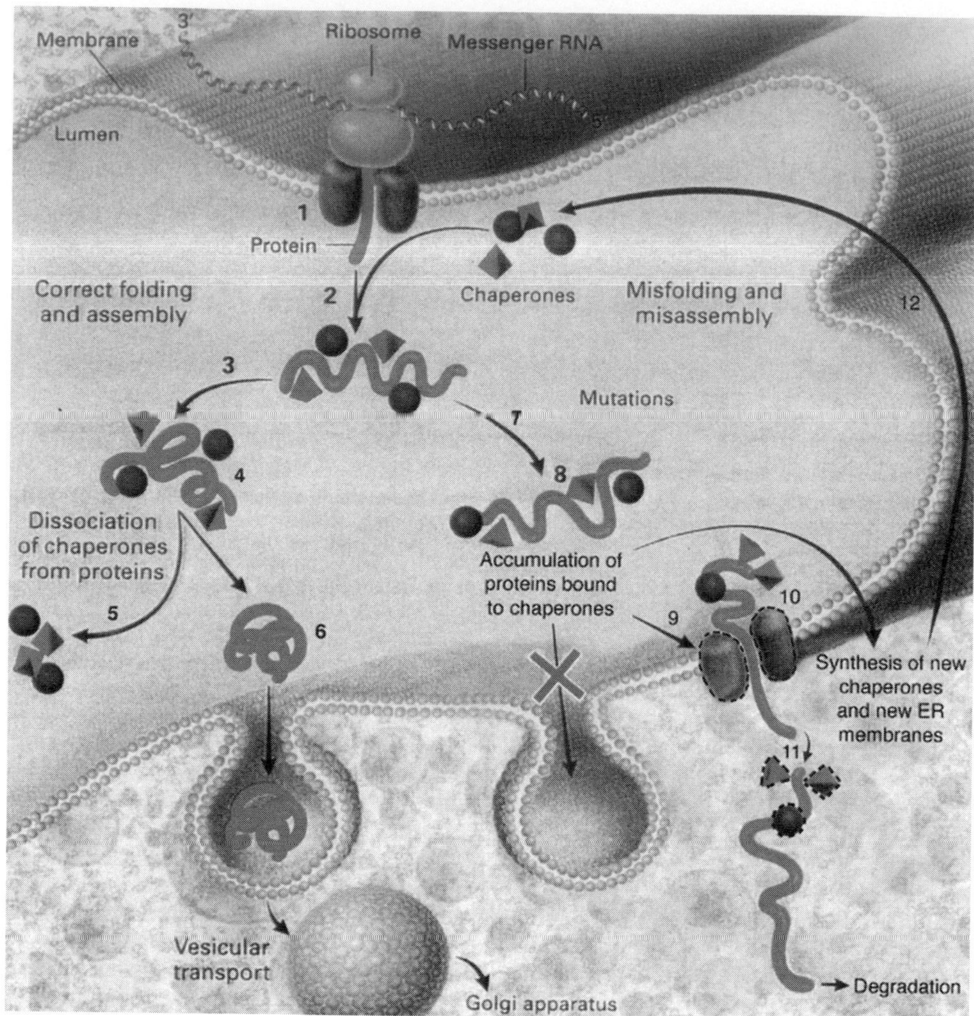

Figure 23.3. The fate of polypeptides in the ER. Secretory and membrane proteins are cotranslationally translocated into the lumen of the ER through the import channel associated with Sec61p (1). These polypeptides transiently interact with several chaperones (2) to facilitate folding (3). Once folding is completed (4), there is dissociation of chaperones (5) and vesicular transport out of the ER (6). In the cases of mutant proteins (7) that remain misfolded even after interaction with chaperones (8), there is accumulation of misfolded proteins bound to their chaperones. The quality control apparatus of the ER mediates transport of these misfolded proteins, free or bound to chaperones, to the ER membrane (9) or through a channel, perhaps even through the import channel associated with Sec61p (10), into the cytoplasm (11) for degradation. The accumulation of misfolded proteins induces the synthesis of new chaperones and new ER membrane to accommodate the increased load of misfolded proteins and thereby protect the cells (12). (Adapted from Kuznetsov G, Nigam SK. Folding of secretory and membrane proteins. N Engl J Med 1998;339:1688–95; with permission.)

[165] as well as cell lines that are genetically engineered for deficient autophagy [154]. Macroautophagy is a general stress-activated degradative mechanism whereby cytosol and intracellular organelles are first enveloped by distinct, newly forming vesicles and then delivered to the lysosome for degradation. This process, which has been highly conserved in evolution, is activated by starvation and bacterial invasion and plays a role in differentiation, morphogenesis, and senescence. Recent studies in autophagy-deficient mammalian cell lines [154] and autophagy-deficient yeast [155] suggest that the autophagic response is particularly important for insoluble polymers and aggregates of α_1-ATZ when there are high levels of expression.

In addition to degradation mechanisms, cells appear to have a number of other mechanisms by which they attempt to adapt to, or protect themselves, from proteins that are retained in the ER. Because differences in an adaptive response could theoretically explain variation in the liver disease phenotype, we have recently begun a series of studies designed to characterize how cells respond to ER retention of α_1-ATZ using cell line and transgenic mouse model systems with tetracycline-inducible expression of the mutant gene. These models permit us to see the earliest responses and to separate them from compensatory adaptations that arise later. Because the relative expression of the mutant gene can be regulated in this kind of model system, it is also possible to determine the effect of expressing the mutant gene product at specific concentrations, at specific stages of development and for specific intervals.

First, we found that accumulation of α_1-ATZ in the ER elicits mitochondrial dysfunction [166]. It has long been known that mitochondria are closely apposed to the ER, and recent studies have shown that there are elaborate mechanisms by which the ER and mitochondrion communicate with each other [167,168]. This mitochondrial injury was demonstrated functionally and by detailed ultrastructural studies in the liver of affected patients as well as in the model cell lines and transgenic mice. It is not yet clear whether this is directly mediated by the ER accumulation or results indirectly from an overexuberant autophagic response. Antagonism of mitochondrial dysfunction by administration of cyclosporine A is associated with reduction in mitochondrial ultrastructural change, caspase-3 activation, and liver disease morbidity in the PiZ transgenic mouse [166]. These data raise the interesting possibility that the adaptive response actually contributes to liver injury by the release of active oxygen intermediates that accompanies mitochondrial dysfunction.

Second, we have found that accumulation of α_1-ATZ in the ER is sufficient to activate the autophagic response. This was demonstrated by mating two types of transgenic mice: the Z mouse with liver-specific inducible expression of α_1-ATZ in which α_1-ATZ accumulates in the ER of hepatocytes only when doxycycline is removed from the drinking water [156], and the GFP-LC3 mouse in which autophagosomes have green fluorescence because LC3 is an autophagosomal membrane–specific protein [169]. Although green fluorescent autophagosomes are only seen in the liver of the GFP-LC3 mouse when it is starved, they are seen in the liver of the Z × GFP-LC3 mouse simply by removing doxycycline from the drinking water and inducing the accumulation of mutant α_1-ATZ in the ER of hepatocytes [165]. This is a particularly important observation because it represents the first evidence that a single protein can activate the autophagic response.

To our great surprise, accumulation of α_1-ATZ in the ER does not activate the unfolded protein response (UPR). The UPR is a signaling pathway activating a number of genes in response to accumulation of unfolded proteins in the ER [170]. In addition to new synthesis of ER chaperones, such as BiP, and enzymes that facilitate disulfide bond formation, bolstering the protein-folding capacity of the ER, and lipids for synthesis of new ER membrane required to handle the increased protein load, an increase in synthesis of proteins that participate in degradative and other cellular translocation mechanisms occurs. There is also a decrease in initiation of translation in such a way that only specific mRNAs can be translated and thereby prevent the de novo synthesis of proteins that will further accumulate in the ER [171]. Although we do not detect activation of the UPR when α_1-ATZ accumulates in the ER, we do detect it when truncated nonpolymerogenic α_1-AT mutants do so, suggesting that it is the formation of polymers in the ER by α_1-ATZ that suppresses the UPR [156].

In contrast, the ER overload pathway and its signature target nuclear transcription factor kappa B (NFκB) is activated when α_1-ATZ accumulates in the ER [156]. The ER overload pathway was first described as activation of the transcription factor NFκB in response to the type of "ER stress" that is generated by treatment of cells with brefeldin A or by experimental accumulation of adenovirus E3 protein in the ER [172]. The fact that ER accumulation of α_1-ATZ activates NFκB but not the UPR provides strong corroborating evidence for the previously held contention that the ER overload pathway was distinct from the UPR [172]. Activation of NFκB has potentially important implications for target organ injury in α_1-AT deficiency. First, through NFκB, accumulation of α_1-ATZ in liver cells and respiratory epithelial cells [173] could mediate inflammation in the liver and the lung, particularly neutrophil infiltration in response to the NFκB target interleukin-8. Second, activation of NFκB has been shown to play a key role in inflammation-associated carcinogenesis [174–176] and therein could be involved in the pathogenesis of hepatocellular carcinoma in α_1-AT deficiency.

We also examined two other signal transduction pathways that have been associated with ER stress. For one, we found that ER accumulation of α_1-ATZ led to cleavage and activation of the ER caspases – caspase-12 in mouse cells and caspase-4 in human cells [156]. These results indicate that both the mitochondrial and ER caspase pathways are activated in α_1-AT deficiency. For another, we found that accumulation of α_1-ATZ in the ER specifically mediated cleavage and activation of BAP31 [156], an integral membrane protein of the ER that is involved in the ER retention of several proteins [177] and appears to mediate proapoptotic signals from the ER to mitochondria [178]. This last result may provide a mechanistic basis for the mitochondrial dysfunction that was recently found in cell line and transgenic mouse models as well as in the liver of deficient patients [166].

PATHOGENESIS OF LIVER INJURY IN α_1-ANTITRYPSIN DEFICIENCY

There are several theories for the pathogenesis of liver injury in α_1-AT deficiency. According to the *immune theory*, liver damage results from an abnormal immune response to liver antigens [179]. This theory is based on the observation that peripheral blood lymphocytes from PIZZ infants are cytotoxic for isolated hepatocytes; however, this is probably a nonspecific effect of liver injury, in that peripheral blood lymphocytes from PIMM infants with a similar degree of liver injury caused by idiopathic neonatal hepatitis syndrome are also cytotoxic for isolated hepatocytes. More recent studies have indicated an increase in the HLA DR3-DW25 haplotype in α_1-AT-deficient individuals with liver disease [180]. There is no difference, however, in the expression of class II major histocompatibility complex (MHC) antigen in the livers of these individuals compared with normal control subjects [181]. Moreover, an increase in the prevalence of a particular HLA DR haplotype in the affected population does not by itself imply altered immune function. Because of the linkage disequilibrium displayed by genes within the MHC, it is possible that increased susceptibility is caused by the products of unrelated but linked genes. For instance, the MHC contains genes for several heat shock/stress proteins [182,183], proteins that play an important role in the biogenesis and transport of other proteins through the secretory pathway.

The *accumulation theory*, in which liver damage is thought to be caused by accumulation of mutant α_1-AT molecules in the ER of liver cells, is the most widely accepted. Experimental results in transgenic mice are most consistent with this theory and completely exclude the possibility that liver damage is caused by "proteolytic attack" as a consequence of diminished serum of α_1-AT concentrations. Transgenic mice carrying the mutant Z allele of the human α_1-AT gene develop periodic acid–Schiff–positive, diastase-resistant intrahepatic globules and liver injury early in life [9,10]. Because there are normal levels of α_1-AT and presumably other antielastases in these animals, as directed by endogenous murine genes, the liver injury cannot be attributed to proteolytic attack.

Some have argued that the histologic characteristics of the liver in the transgenic mouse model are not identical to those in humans. Detailed histologic characterization of the liver in one transgenic mouse model by Geller et al. [184] has shown that there are focal areas of liver cell necrosis, microabcesses with an accumulation of neutrophils and regenerative activity in the form of multicellular liver plates, and focal nodule formation during the neonatal period. Nodular clusters of altered hepatocytes that lack α_1-AT-immunoreactivity are also seen during the neonatal period. With aging, there is a decrease in the number of hepatocytes containing α_1-ATZ globules; there is also an increase in the number of nodular aggregates of α_1-AT-negative hepatocytes and development of periosinusoidal fibrosis [185]. Within 6 weeks, there are dysplastic changes in these aggregates. Adenomas occur within 1 year, and invasive hepatocellular carcinoma is seen between 1 and 2 years of age [185]. The relationship between the α_1-ATZ globules and inflammation or dysplasia, however, is not yet apparent from these animal studies. It is still unclear why the liver injury in this transgenic mouse model is somewhat milder and less fibrogenic than that seen in children with α_1-AT deficiency–associated liver disease. It is possible that there are strain-specific factors that condition the response to injury in the mouse. There are certainly host-specific factors that determine the amount of liver injury in α_1-AT deficiency [157], and we find that the amount of inflammation and fibrosis varies widely among our patients with liver disease from α_1-AT deficiency.

Data from individuals who have null alleles of α_1-AT, and therefore negligible serum levels of α_1-AT, have also been used as evidence against the proteolytic attack theory. These individuals do not develop liver injury – at least not sufficiently to result in clinical detection. However, only a few individuals with null alleles have been reported, and each has a different allele. Based on data in PiZZ individuals showing that only 10–15% of these individuals develop clinically significant liver injury, it might be necessary to evaluate seven to eight individuals with each null allele before detecting one with liver injury.

The recognition that several other naturally occurring variant alleles of α_1-AT associated with deficiency can undergo polymerization has provided some support for the accumulation theory. The most important of these is the compound heterozygous α_1-ATSZ phenotype. Recent work by Mahadeva et al. [26] has shown that α_1-ATS and α_1-ATZ may form heteropolymers. We know from the nationwide study of α_1-AT deficiency in Sweden that the incidence of liver disease among individuals with the PISZ phenotype is similar to that of individuals with the PIZZ phenotype [1,3]. We also know that the $\text{PiM}_{\text{malton}}$ allele undergoes polymerization, and several of the $\text{PiM}_{\text{malton}}$ patients have been reported to have α_1-AT globules in their liver and liver injury [21–23]. However, there is a report of an individual with $\text{PIS}_{\text{iiyama}}$ allele having hepatocyte α_1-AT globules but no liver injury [92,145]. Moreover, a report by Ray and Brown has indicated that the $\text{PIM}_{\text{heerlen}}$ and $\text{PIM}_{\text{procidia}}$ undergo aggregation and that the $\text{PIM}_{\text{mineral springs}}$ and $\text{PI-Null}_{\text{Ludwigshafen}}$ may undergo aggregation, but there are no reports of liver disease in individuals carrying these alleles (J. Brown, personal communication). There are only a few patients, however, with M_{malton}, S_{iiyama}, $\text{M}_{\text{heerlen}}$, $\text{M}_{\text{procida}}$, $\text{M}_{\text{mineral springs}}$, and $\text{Null}_{\text{Ludwigshafen}}$ who have been identified. It is also not clear how many of these patients have been thoroughly examined for liver disease, infection with hepatitis C virus, or evidence for autoimmune or alcoholic hepatitis. Again, on the basis of what we know about the PIZZ and PISZ phenotype, at least seven to eight individuals with each of these alleles would need to be examined to detect one with liver injury.

It has been difficult to reconcile the accumulation theory with the observations of Sveger [1,3], which show that only a subset of PIZZ α_1-AT-deficient individuals develop significant liver damage. We have made the prediction that a subset of the PIZZ population is more susceptible to liver injury by virtue of one or more additional inherited traits or environmental factors that exaggerate the intracellular accumulation of the mutant Z α_1-AT protein or exaggerate the cellular pathophysiologic consequence of mutant α_1-AT accumulation. To address this prediction experimentally, we transduced skin fibroblasts from α_1-AT PIZZ individuals, with or without liver disease, with amphotropic recombinant retroviral particles designed for constitutive expression of the mutant α_1-ATZ gene [157]. Human skin fibroblasts do not express the endogenous α_1-AT gene but, presumably, express other genes involved in the postsynthetic processing of secretory proteins. The results show that expression of the human α_1-AT gene was conferred on each fibroblast cell line. Compared with the same cell line transduced with the wild-type α_1-ATM gene, there was selective intracellular retention of the mutant α_1-ATZ protein in each case. However, there was a marked delay in degradation of the mutant α_1-ATZ protein, after it accumulated in the fibroblasts from PIZZ individuals with liver disease (susceptible hosts) compared with those without liver disease (protected hosts; Figure 23.4). These data provide evidence that other factors affecting the fate of the

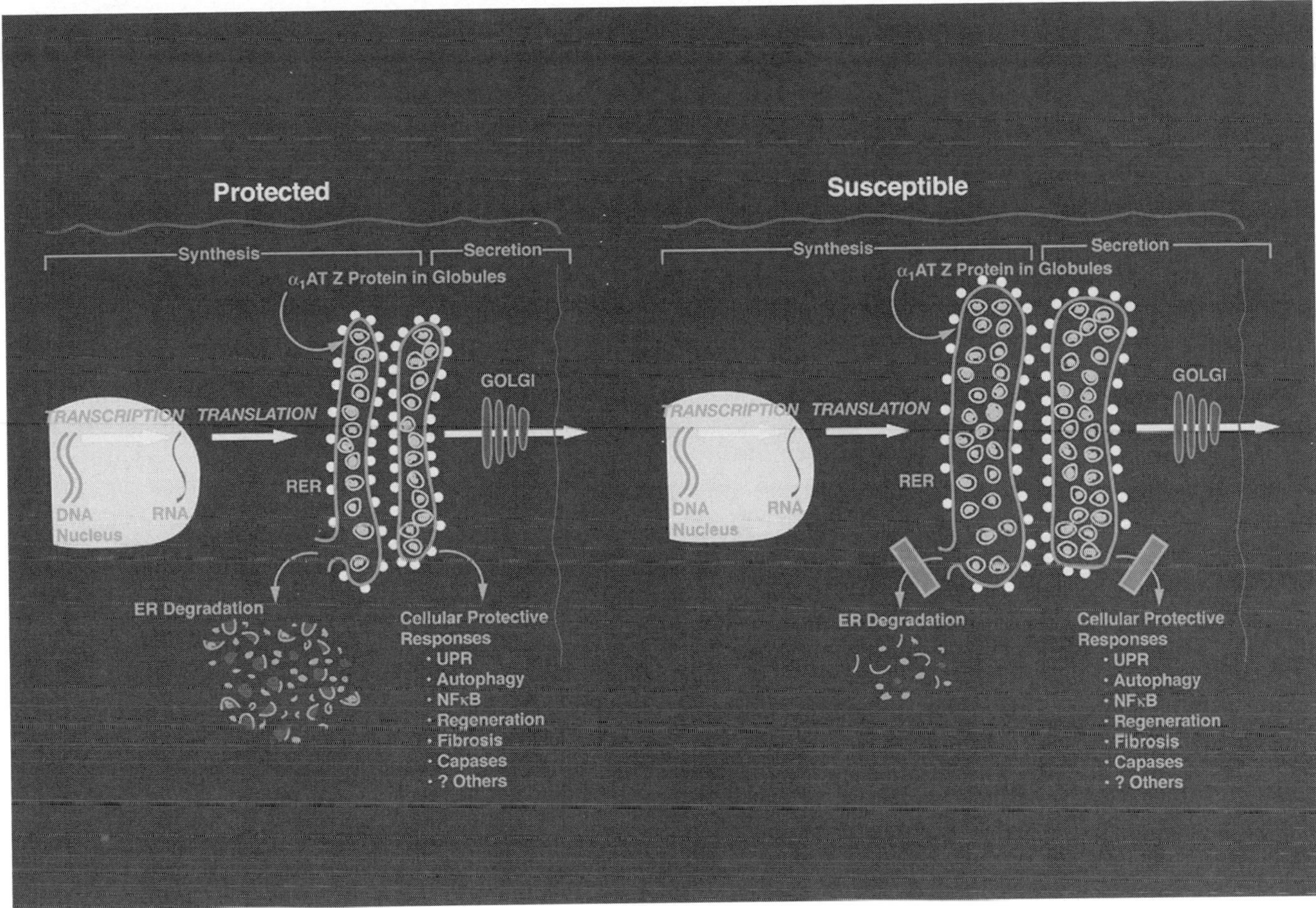

Figure 23.4. Difference in endoplasmic reticulum degradation of α_1-ATZ in protected and susceptible hosts. The block in degradation in susceptible hosts is represented by a small dark bar. (Adapted from Teckman JH, Perlmutter DH. Conceptual advances in the pathogenesis and treatment of childhood metabolic liver disease. Gastroenterology 1995;108:1263–79; with permission.)

mutant α_1-ATZ molecule, such as a lag in ER degradation, at least in part determine susceptibility to liver disease.

The lag in ER degradation of α_1-ATZ in susceptible hosts may involve several distinct mechanisms. In one susceptible host, the retained α_1-ATZ interacts poorly with calnexin [157]. In the liver cells of this host, there is likely to be only a very little polyubiquitinated calnexin-α_1-ATZ complex that can be recognized for proteolysis by the proteasome. In several other susceptible hosts, the retained α_1-ATZ interacts well with calnexin but is degraded slowly (J. Teckman, D. Qu, D. H. Perlmutter, unpublished observations). These hosts may have a defect in calnexin that prevents its ubiquitination or a defect in the ubiquitin system of the proteasome. Hosts with the latter defect also would be more likely to respond to a pharmacologic agent such as interferon-gamma [186] that enhances the activity of the ubiquitin-dependent proteasomal system. Recent studies involving yeast that have identified at least 30 putative recessive mutants and seven complementation groups of strains defective in ER degradation of α_1-ATZ [155] are likely to lead to recognition of other mechanisms for excessive ER retention of α_1-ATZ.

There is still relatively limited information about the mechanism through which ER retention of α_1-ATZ leads to liver cell injury. In the transgenic mice that express the human α_1-ATZ, mild inflammation and necrosis, formation of adenomas, and ultimately carcinoma occur. Relatively little information is also lacking regarding the short- and long-term effects of ER retention of α_1-ATZ in cell culture systems. In one report, the accumulation of α_1-ATZ in *Xenopus* oocytes was associated with the release of lysosomal enzymes [187]. Several studies in model systems have provided interesting and, perhaps, relevant information. Raposo et al. [188] used a novel approach to establish cell lines with marked retention of MHC class I molecules in the ER. This led to a marked alteration in the structure of the ER into an expanded network of tubular and fenestrated membranes. Marker studies suggest that this altered network is derived from the ER and ER–Golgi intermediate compartment. Electron-dense compartments resembling lysosomes appear to bud off from this altered network. Because ubiquitin and ubiquitin-activating enzymes were associated with the cytosolic aspect of the electron-dense bodies, the bodies were thought to represent compartments in which ER degradation takes place. The electron-dense bodies also resemble autophagic vacuoles. Autophagic vacuoles are now known to be derived in part from subdomains of the rough ER [189]. The autophagic response is thought to be a general mechanism by which intracellular organelles are first sequestered away from the cytosol and then degraded within lysosomes. It occurs in many cell types, especially during stress states –such as nutrient deprivation – and during the cellular remodeling that accompanies differentiation, metamorphosis, and aging. Recent studies have shown that the ubiquitin system, or at least molecules and mechanisms that are almost identical to those of the ubiquitin system, are essential for autophagy in yeast [190,191]. Work in several labs has shown that a novel structure called the *aggresome* is formed in cells if expression of misfolded membrane proteins such as CFTRΔF508, other mutant membrane proteins, and mutant viral proteins exceeds the capacity of the proteasome to degrade them [192,193]. The aggresome is a pericentriolar membrane-free cytoplasmic inclusion containing misfolded, ubiquitinated protein ensheathed in a case of vimentin and perhaps other intermediate filaments. Our studies indicate that retention of α_1-ATZ induces expansion, and alteration in the structure, of the ER and formation of autophagic vesicles but does not cause aggresome formation [165].

Recently, we examined the autophagic response to ER retention of α_1-ATZ in vivo by testing the effect of fasting on the liver of the PiZ mouse model of α_1-AT deficiency [194]. Starvation is a well-defined physiologic stimulus of autophagy, as well as a known environmental stressor of liver disease in children. The results show that there is a marked increase in fat accumulation and in α_1-AT containing, ER-derived globules in the liver of the PiZ mouse, induced by fasting. These changes were particularly exaggerated at 3–6 months of age. Three-month-old PiZ mice had a significantly decreased tolerance for fasting compared with nontransgenic C57 Black mice. Although fasting induced a marked autophagic response in wild-type mice, the autophagic response was already activated in PiZ mice to levels that were more than 50% higher than those in the liver of fasted wild-type mice, and they did not increase further during fasting. These results indicate that autophagy is constitutively activated in α_1-AT deficiency and that the liver is unable to mount an increased autophagic response to physiologic stressors. Based on our search of the literature, the only other condition in which there is accumulation of autophagic vacuoles under homeostatic conditions is Danon disease [39]. In contrast to α_1-AT deficiency, however, autophagosomes accumulate in Danon disease because of a genetic defect in the terminal phases of autophagy, that is, the fusion of autophagic vacuoles with lysosomes and subsequent degradation within autolysosomes [195,196].

In the course of our ultrastructural studies of the liver of the PiZ mouse and of patients with α_1-AT deficiency, we have been struck by the degree of mitochondrial autophagy that is induced [166]. A comparison of the liver from four α_1-AT-deficient patients with livers from eight patients with other liver diseases and four normal livers showed a marked specific increase in mitochondrial autophagy associated with α_1-AT deficiency. Even more interesting is the observation that many mitochondria that are not surrounded by autophagic vacuolar membranes are nevertheless damaged or in various phases of degeneration in liver cells from α_1-AT-deficient hosts. This damage is characterized by the formation of multilamellar structures within the limiting membrane, condensation of the cristae and matrix, and, in some cases, dissolution of the internal structures, often leaving only electron-dense debris compressed into a thin rim at the periphery of the mitochondrion.

Mitochondrial autophagy and injury are also marked in the liver of the PiZ transgenic mouse model of α_1-AT deficiency. Immunofluorescence analysis shows the presence of activated caspase-3 in the PiZ mouse liver [166]. Because cyclosporine A (CsA) has been shown to reduce mitochondrial injury and inhibit starvation-induced autophagy [197], we examined the effect of CsA on PiZ mice. We found that it significantly reduces hepatic mitochondrial injury, increases activation of caspase-3 and improves the animals' tolerance of starvation. These results provide evidence for the novel concept that mitochondrial damage and caspase activation play a role in the mechanism of liver cell injury in α_1-AT deficiency. Although this analysis suggests that there is mitochondrial injury that is separate from the autophagic process, the possibility that autophagy plays some role in mitochondrial damage cannot be completely excluded. One model of mitochondrial damage in this deficiency holds that accumulation of α_1-ATZ in the ER is in itself responsible for mitochondrial dysfunction, and indeed, there is now ample evidence in the literature for functional interactions between mitochondrial and closely apposed ER cisternae [198,199]. Recent studies show that specific signals are transmitted between these two intracellular compartments [200,201] and that mitochondrial dysfunction, including release of cytochrome c and caspase-3 activation, is associated with the ER dilatation and stress induced by brefeldin A, tunicamycin, or thapsigargin [202,203]. It is not yet known, however, whether mitochondrial dysfunction in the latter cases is due to ER dilatation or ER stress (or both) or to independent effects on mitochondria by these experimental drugs. A second possible explanation, not necessarily incompatible with the first, envisages mitochondrial dysfunction as a result of the autophagic response to ER retention of α_1-ATZ. In this scenario, mitochondria are recognized nonspecifically by the autophagic response, which is constitutively activated to somehow remove and degrade areas of the ER that are distended by aggregated mutant protein. Although our data indicate that CsA inhibits hepatic mitochondrial injury in vivo, this benefit could reflect the drug's known effects on the mitochondrial permeability transition, on autophagy, or both [197].

The CsA findings are also noteworthy for their therapeutic implications. They indicate that CsA can prevent mitochondrial damage even under circumstances in which α_1-ATZ continues to accumulate in the ER. Thus, they provide a proof-in-principle for mechanism-based therapeutic approaches to liver disease in α_1-AT deficiency – pharmacologic intervention directed as distal steps in the pathobiologic pathway that leads to liver injury (the mitochondrial step, for instance), rather than at the primary defect or the early events in the pathway.

HEPATIC REGENERATION AND CARCINOGENESIS IN α1-AT DEFICIENCY

To begin to understand how the liver is injured and how it regenerates in AT deficiency, Rudnick et al. [204] used the PiZ mouse model of AT deficiency and measured the degree of injury by bromodeoxyuridine (BrdU) labeling to quantify hepatocellular proliferation. These studies showed that there was increased hepatocellular proliferation in the liver of the PiZ mouse at baseline. Although the increase was five- to ten-fold above the control mice and highly statistically significant, there was still a relatively low number of BrdU+ hepatocytes at one time (2–3% detected over 72 hours of continuous labeling). These data indicate that liver injury in the mouse model is relatively mild and appropriately corresponds to the smoldering and slowly progressing liver disease that is seen in most AT-deficient patients. The increase in hepatocellular proliferation was entirely accounted for by male mice and correlated with an increased number of hepatocytes that had periodic acid–Schiff (PAS)-positive, diastase-resistant globules as well as increased steady-state levels of AT mRNA and protein. Systemic administration of testosterone to female PiZ mice led to an increase in number of globule-containing hepatocytes, steady-state levels of AT mRNA and protein, and an increase in BrdU labeling that was comparable to that in male PiZ mice. These results were consistent with previous studies showing that androgens had a positive regulatory effect on the human AT gene; in this mouse, this would represent a positive regulatory effect on the human transgene. More important, however, these results indicated that the increase in hepatocellular proliferation in the PiZ mouse liver was proportional to the number of globule-containing cells, the level of ATZ accumulation within these cells, or both.

Next, double labeling for PAS staining and BrdU staining was used to determine whether the globule-containing or the globule-devoid cells were proliferating. The results showed that almost all of the BrdU-positive cells in the PiZ mouse liver were globule-devoid and, conversely, very few of the globule-containing cells were BrdU-positive. These results provided evidence that the globule-devoid hepatocytes had a selective proliferative advantage in the PiZ liver.

To further characterize this selective proliferative advantage, the hepatocellular proliferative response to partial hepatectomy in the PiZ mice was determined. Although partial hepatectomy resulted in increased mortality among PiZ mice compared with their C57/BL6 nontransgenic littermates, those PiZ mice that survived had a similar proliferative response to the C57 littermates. In particular, there was a comparable increase in BrdU labeling of globule-containing and globule-devoid hepatocytes. These data indicate that the block in proliferation of globule-containing cells is relative – that is, when the stimulus is as powerful as the one that follows partial hepatectomy, those cells are able to replicate.

Finally, these studies showed that there was increased caspase-9 and caspase-3 activation in the PiZ mouse liver. Together with the observation that the liver-to-body-weight ratio in PiZ mice was identical to that observed in wild-type mice, these data suggest that hepatocytes undergo programmed cell death at a rate equivalent to the rate of increased cellular proliferation. However, increased apoptosis was not detected either histologically or by terminal deoxynucleotidyl transferase mediated dUTP nick end labeling (TUNEL) staining in the livers of these animals. Thus the increase in cell death that must be occurring in the PiZ mouse liver is at a rate that is lower than the limits for detection of apoptosis using currently available in situ methods. This is, again, consistent with the slowly progressing nature of the disease. Most informative, however, is the lack of apoptosis histologically and by TUNEL staining of cells that obviously have globules. If we take this together with our data on how cells respond to accumulation of ATZ, we suggest that the globule-containing cells are "sick but not dead" – they have activated ER- and mitochondrial-caspases, NFκB, and autophagy with a relative block in proliferation, but they are not apoptotic.

These data have led to a hypothetical paradigm in which the accumulation of α_1-ATZ in the ER activates ER and mitochondrial caspases, NFκB, and autophagy, but the caspase pathway is blocked at terminal steps, so that the globule-containing hepatocytes are "sick but not dead." An "injury–regeneration" signal is generated by these cells in proportion to the amount of α_1-ATZ accumulation per cell or the number of cells with α_1-ATZ accumulation. Hepatocytes with lesser amounts of α_1-ATZ, globule-devoid hepatocytes are therein chronically stimulated "in trans" to divide. The cancer-prone state is then engendered by having cells that are unable to die at the appropriate time and cells that are chronically dividing in an inflamed milieu. The paradigm anticipates that some of the globule-containing hepatocytes eventually die, but, because the block in their proliferation is relative, they can be replenished, at least to the extent that there are always some of these cells present in the affected liver. The mechanism by which globule-devoid hepatocytes arise in unknown, but one possibility is that they are progenitors or relatively young cells for which there has not been enough time to accumulate as much α_1-ATZ. Furthermore, because of the proliferative advantage, it would presumably only take one or a few of these to lead ultimately to many more.

This model is consistent with the observations of Geller et al. [184], using the Z#2 transgenic mouse model of AT deficiency. These authors found that increasing areas of the liver were negative for AT immunostaining as the mice aged so that by age 12 months, more than 90% of the liver was AT-negative, corresponding to the globule-devoid hepatocytes. Moreover, by 6 months, adenomas began developing in the AT-negative areas and by 18 months more than 80% of these mice had hepatocellular carcinoma arising from the AT-negative areas [184,185].

Why adenomas and carcinomas arise rather specifically from the AT-negative regions is not clear. There are many possible explanations. Certainly, this is where the most rapid cell proliferation is occurring. The mechanism by which the caspase pathway is blocked in globule-containing hepatocytes is not known, but one possibility is the antiapoptotic effect of heat shock proteins [205]. We have shown that accumulation of α_1-ATZ leads to an increase in expression of several heat shock proteins [206].

A similar model may be involved in the mechanism of hepatocarcinogenesis in the fumarylacetoacetate hydrolase–deficient (FAH) mouse model of tyrosinemia [207]. In these studies, the liver of the FAH mouse was found to contain hepatocytes that were damaged but not dead. In fact, these cells were found to be resistant to cell death and, therein, prone to carcinogenesis. By the paradigm that we are proposing here, these hepatocytes would be considered equivalent to the globule-containing hepatocytes in the PiZ mouse liver. They are damaged by an entirely different mechanism than the globule-containing hepatocytes, and the damage is much more severe and rapidly progressing. However, they share the property of being TUNEL-negative, and upregulation of antiapoptotic heat shock proteins has also been implicated in the block in their cell death [207]. There is also evidence in the FAH mouse for chronic stimulation in "trans" of hepatocytes that are not damaged and have a selective proliferative advantage. According to the paradigm we are proposing here, these hepatocytes correspond to the globule-devoid hepatocytes in the PiZ mouse liver. The mechanism by which some undamaged hepatocytes arise in the FAH mouse as well as in tyrosinemic patients is known and appears to involve mutation reversion [208], whereas the origin and mechanism of globule-devoid hepatocytes in the PiZ mouse and AT-deficient patient is still unknown. Evidence for a "trans" effect in the FAH mouse comes from studies with transplanted normal hepatocytes that are capable of undergoing multiple rounds of replication in the FAH liver, but only if disease is present. Once the mouse is given the drug 2-(2-nitro-4-fluoromethylbenzoyl)-1,3-cyclohexanedione (NTBC), which prevents the accumulation of toxic intermediates in the damaged cells, transplanted hepatocytes will no longer replicate in the FAH mouse liver [209]. However, at least one part of this paradigm does not fit with what has been found in humans with hereditary tyrosinemia – this is, that dysplasia and carcinoma have only been found to arise from the damaged cell compartment [210]. It is possible that this difference relates to the net balance of carcinogenic and anticarcinogenic factors in each compartment in the two diseases. For instance, activation of NFκB and of autophagy is present in the damaged cell compartment in the AT deficiency models but not in the tyrosinemia model.

A similar situation has been described for hepatocarcinogenesis in hepatitis B surface antigen (HBsAg) transgenic mice [211]. In this model of hepatitis B–associated liver injury, as in the PiZ model, the degree of hepatocellular proliferation correlated with the presence of injury and carcinomas and with the cellular load of HBsAg, but the proliferating cells, adenomas, and carcinomas had significantly lesser amounts of retained HBsAg. However, because this transgenic model only expresses HBsAg and not complete hepatitis B virus, it is not clear whether the model truly reflects hepatocarcinogenesis in chronic hepatitis B virus infection. It is of some interest that HBsAg is known to be selectively retained in the ER of hepatocytes, and this process is thought to be responsible for the so-called ground glass hepatocyte [212]. Prolonged ER retention has also been observed for several proteins encoded by hepatitis C virus in infected hepatocytes [213], raising the possibility that a similar paradigm applies to cancer predisposition in hepatitis C infection. Several studies have shown an increase in the proliferation of hepatocytes with lesser loads of fat accumulation in mouse models of obesity-related hepatic steatosis [214]. Moreover, these cells have some of the staining characteristics of a type of progenitor cell known as the oval cell [215]. Thus, the paradigm in which hepatocarcinogenesis involves cross-talk between inappropriately surviving, damaged cells and younger cells with a selective proliferative advantage may be applicable to chronic liver disease due to viral infections or associated with obesity in addition to genetic liver disease.

DIAGNOSIS

Diagnosis is established by a serum α_1-AT phenotype determination in isoelectric focusing or by agarose electrophoresis at acid pH. The phenotype should be determined in cases of neonatal hepatitis or unexplained chronic liver disease in older children, adolescents, and adults. It is particularly important in the neonatal period because it may be very difficult to distinguish patients with α_1-AT deficiency from those with biliary atresia. Moreover, it is not uncommon for neonates with a PIZZ phenotype to have no biliary excretion on scintographic studies [216]. There is one report of α_1-AT deficiency and biliary atresia in a single patient [217]. We have had several patients with homozygous PIZZ α_1-AT deficiency and cholestasis and no biliary excretion of technetium-labeled mebrofenin, but in each of these cases, with more prolonged observation, cholestasis remitted, and it was obvious that the patient did not also have biliary atresia.

Serum concentrations of α_1-AT may be helpful, if used with phenotype, to distinguish individuals who are homozygous for the Z allele from SZ compound heterozygotes, both of whom may develop liver disease. In some cases, phenotype determinations of parents or other relatives are also necessary to ensure the distinction between ZZ and SZ allotypes, a distinction that is important for genetic counseling. Serum concentrations of α_1-AT occasionally are misleading. For instance, serum α_1-AT concentrations may increase during the host response to inflammation, even in homozygous PIZZ individuals, giving a falsely reassuring impression.

PATHOLOGY

The distinctive histologic feature of homozygous PIZZ α_1-AT deficiency, periodic acid–Schiff–positive, diastase-resistant

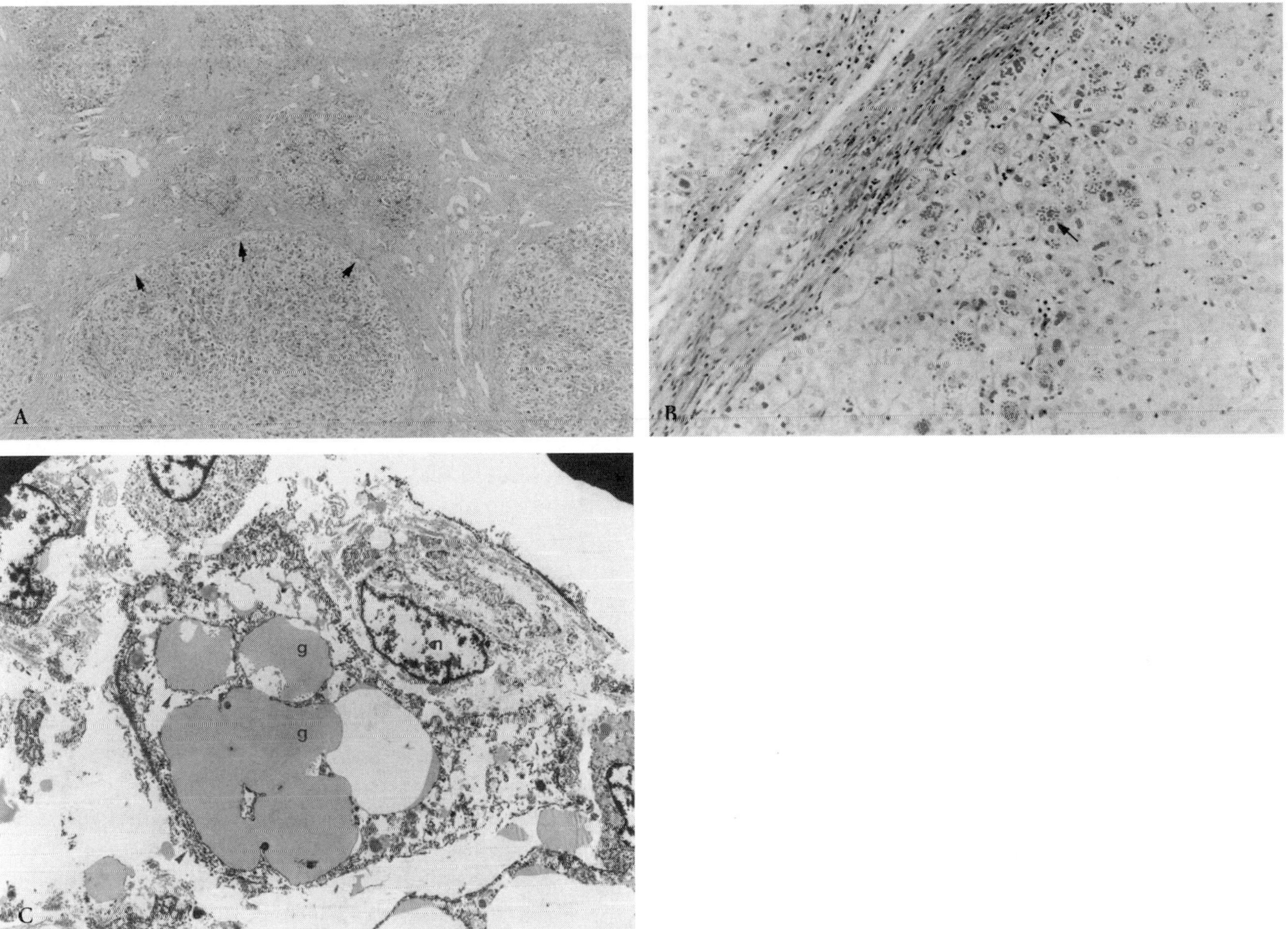

Figure 23.5. Hepatic histology in homozygous PiZZ α-AT deficiency. (**A**) Micrograph of liver biopsy specimen in α_1-AT deficiency demonstrating increased fibrous tissue deposition *(arrowheads)* and nodular transformation. (PAS–diastase staining, 4× magnification.) (**B**) Micrograph of liver biopsy in α_1-AT deficiency demonstrating the PAS-positive, diastase-resistant globules. (Two of the hepatocytes with globules are indicated by *arrows.*) (PAS–diastase staining, 40× magnification.) (**C**) Electron micrograph of same biopsy specimen demonstrating globules in endoplasmic reticulum. N, nucleus; g, globules; arrowheads, ribosomes. For color reproduction of (**A**) and (**B**), see Color Plate 23.5.

globules in the ER of hepatocytes substantiates the diagnosis (Figure 23.5). According to some observers, these globules are not as easy to detect in the first few months of life [218,219]. The presence of these inclusions should not be interpreted as diagnostic of α_1-AT deficiency. Similar structures occasionally are observed in PIMM individuals with other liver disease [220]. The inclusions are eosinophilic, round to oval, and 1–40 μm in diameter. They are most prominent in periportal hepatocytes but also may be seen in Kupffer cells and cells of biliary ductular lineage [221]. There may be evidence of variable degrees of hepatocellular necrosis, inflammatory cell infiltration, periportal fibrosis, or cirrhosis. There is often evidence of bile duct epithelial cell destruction, and occasionally there is a paucity of intrahepatic bile ducts. Our recent study has shown that there also may be an intense autophagic reaction detected by electron microscopic examination of liver biopsy specimens, with a full array of nascent and degradative-type autophagic vacuoles [165].

TREATMENT

The most important principle in the treatment of α_1-AT deficiency is avoidance of cigarette smoking. Cigarette smoking markedly accelerates the destructive lung disease that is associated with α_1-AT deficiency, reduces the quality of life, and significantly shortens longevity of these individuals [38,39,222].

There is no specific therapy for α_1-AT deficiency–associated liver disease. Clinical care largely involves supportive management of symptoms resulting from liver dysfunction and the prevention of complications (Chapter 10). Although ursodeoxycholic acid and colchicine have been mentioned in the literature, there is no evidence for biochemical or clinical efficacy for either drug. Udall et al. [223] reported that breast-fed α_1-AT-deficient infants had less severe liver disease than their bottle-fed counterparts and suggested that the α_1-AT present in breast milk provides the protective effect. Presumably, breast milk α_1-AT formed complexes with serine proteases in the gut that prevented these proteases from being transported to the liver because of enhanced intestinal permeability of the neonatal gut to macromolecules [224]. However, the study was retrospective, and interpretation limited by bias in ascertainment of patients. There is no evidence that breast milk α_1-AT is present or functionally active in the intestinal lumen or that there are increased levels of α_1-AT-protease complexes in the intestinal fluid or portal circulation of breast-fed compared with bottle-fed infants. Finally, there is no evidence for more liver disease or more severe liver disease in bottle-fed PIZZ infants identified prospectively in the Swedish nationwide screening study [3].

Orthotopic Liver Transplantation

Progressive liver dysfunction and liver failure in children has been treated by orthotopic liver transplantation, with survival rates approaching 90% at 1 year and 80% at 5 years [225]. Nevertheless, a number of PIZZ individuals with severe liver disease, even cirrhosis or portal hypertension, may have relatively low rates of disease progression and lead relatively normal lives for extended periods of time. With the availability of living related donor transplantation techniques, it may be possible to manage these patients expectantly for some time. Children with α_1-AT deficiency and mild liver dysfunction (elevated transaminase levels or hepatomegaly) without functional impairment may never need liver transplantation.

Shunt Surgery

Most α_1-AT-deficient children with liver disease are not candidates for alternative surgical interventions. There are rare specific clinical situations in which a portocaval or splenorenal shunt might be considered (such as a child with only mild liver synthetic dysfunction and mild parenchymal liver injury but severe portal hypertension). Several children with severe liver disease and α_1-AT deficiency have survived 10–15 years after shunt surgery before requiring orthotropic liver transplantation [17].

Pharmacologic Therapy

Trials of pharmacologic therapy for α_1-AT deficiency have been conducted. Patients have been given synthetic androgens danazol or stanozolol because of the dramatic effects of these agents in those with hereditary angioedema [226], which is a deficiency of the homologous serine proteinase inhibitor C1 inhibitor, and because danazol initially was found to increase serum levels of α_1-AT in PIZZ individuals [227]. Further evaluation, however, has demonstrated that danazol increases serum levels of α_1-AT in only 50% of deficient persons, and the magnitude of the effect is small [228]. Moreover, it was not clear from any of the studies whether the effect of androgens occurred at the level of synthesis and might therefore also be associated with increased accumulation of α_1-ATZ in the ER with potential hepatotoxic consequences.

Several studies have shown that chemical chaperones can reverse the cellular mislocalization or misfolding of mutant plasma membrane, lysosomal, nuclear, and cytoplasmic proteins including CFTRΔF508, prion proteins, mutant aquaporin molecules associated with nephrogenic diabetes insipidus, and mutant galactosidase A associated with Fabry disease [229–233]. These compounds include glycerol, trimethylamine oxide, deuterated water, and 4-phenylbutyric acid (PBA). We recently found that glycerol and PBA mediated an increase in secretion of α_1-ATZ in a model cell culture system [234]. Oral administration of PBA was well tolerated by PiZ mice (transgenic for the human α_1-ATZ gene) and consistently mediated an increase in blood levels of human α_1-AT reaching 20–50% of the levels present in PiM mice and normal humans. PBA did not affect the synthesis or intracellular degradation of α_1-ATZ. The α_1-ATZ secreted in the presence of PBA was functionally active, in that it could form an inhibitory complex with neutrophil elastase. Because PBA has been used safely for years in children with urea cycle disorders as an ammonia scavenger and because clinical studies have suggested that only partial correction of the deficiency state is needed for prevention of both liver and lung injury in α_1-AT deficiency, PBA constitutes an excellent candidate for chemoprophylaxis of target organ injury in α_1-AT deficiency.

Several iminosugar compounds may be useful for chemoprophylaxis of liver and lung disease in α_1-ATZ deficiency. These compounds are designed to interfere with oligosaccharide side chain trimming of glycoproteins and are now being examined as potential therapeutic agents for viral hepatitis and other types of infections [235,236]. We have examined several of these compounds initially to determine the effect of inhibiting glucose or mannose trimming from the carbohydrate side chain of α_1-ATZ on its fate in the ER. To our surprise, we found that a glucosidase inhibitor, castanospermine (CST), and two α-mannosidase I inhibitors, kifunensine (KIF) and deoxymannojiromicin (DMJ), mediate increased secretion of α_1-ATZ and that the secreted molecules are functionally active [237]. KIF and DMJ are not as attractive as CST as a basis for chemoprophylaxis because these compounds also mediate a decrease in intracellular degradation of α_1-ATZ. The mechanism of action of CST on α_1-ATZ is unknown. An interesting hypothesis for the action of KIF and DMJ has mutant α_1-ATZ interacting with ERGIC-53 for transport from ER to Golgi when mannose trimming is inhibited.

Treatment of Emphysema or Destructive Lung Disease

Patients with α_1-AT deficiency and emphysema have undergone replacement therapy with purified and recombinant plasma α_1-AT, either by intravenous or intratracheal aerosol administration [8]. This therapy is associated with improvement in serum concentrations of α_1-AT and in α_1-AT and neutrophil elastase inhibitory capacity in bronchoalveolar lavage fluid, without significant side effects. Although initial studies have suggested that there is a slower decline in forced expiratory volume in patients on replacement therapy, this only occurred in a subgroup of patients, and the study was not randomized [238].

Protein replacement therapy is designed only for individuals with established and progressive emphysema. It is not being considered for individuals with liver disease because there is no information to support the notion that deficient serum levels of α_1-AT are related mechanistically to liver injury.

A number of patients with severe emphysema from α_1-AT deficiency have undergone lung transplantation in the past 10 years. The latest data from the St. Louis International Lung Transplant Registry show that 91 patients with emphysema and α_1-AT deficiency had undergone single or bilateral lung transplantation by 1993. Actuarial survival for patients in this category who underwent transplantation between 1987 and 1994 is approximately 50% for 5 years. Lung function and exercise tolerance is significantly improved [239].

Gene Replacement Therapy

Replacement of α_1-AT by somatic gene therapy has also been discussed in the literature [8]. This strategy is potentially less expensive than replacement therapy with purified protein and would alleviate the need for intravenous or inhalation therapy. Again, this form of therapy would be useful only in ameliorating emphysema because liver disease associated with α_1-AT deficiency is not caused by deficient levels of α_1-AT in the serum or tissue. Of course, it would be helpful to know that replacement therapy with purified α_1-AT, as it is currently applied, is effective in ameliorating emphysema in this deficiency before embarking on clinical trials involving gene therapy. There also are still major issues that need to be addressed before gene therapy becomes a realistic alternative [240]. Several novel types of gene therapy, such as repair of mRNA by transsplicing ribozymes [241,242] and chimeric RNA/DNA oligonucleotides [243–245], triplex-forming oligonucleotides [246], small fragment homologous replacement [247], or RNA silencing [248,249] are theoretically attractive alternative strategies for liver disease in α_1-AT deficiency because they would prevent the synthesis of mutant α_1-ATZ protein and ER retention. In fact, a chimeric RNA-DNA oligonucleotide based on the sequence of coagulation factor IV in complex with lactose so that it could be taken up by asialoglycoprotein receptor–mediated endocytosis was delivered to hepatocytes with surprisingly high efficiency after intravenous administration [243].

Other Strategies

Recent studies have shown that transplanted hepatocytes can repopulate the diseased liver in several mouse models [209,250], including a mouse model of a childhood metabolic liver disease termed *hereditary tyrosinemia*. Replication of the transplanted hepatocytes occurs only if there is injury or regeneration in the liver. The results provide evidence that it may be possible to use hepatocyte transplantation techniques to treat hereditary tyrosinemia and, perhaps, other metabolic liver diseases in which the defect is cell-autonomous. For instance, α_1-AT deficiency involves a cell-autonomous defect and would be an excellent candidate for this strategy.

Alternative strategies for at least partial correction of α_1-AT deficiency may result from a more detailed understanding of the fate of the α_1-ATZ molecule in the ER. For instance, delivery of synthetic peptides to the ER to insert into the gap in the A sheet or into a particular hydrophobic pocket of the α_1-AT molecule [47] and prevent polymerization of α_1-AT might result in release of the mutant α_1-ATZ molecules into the extracellular fluid and prevent its accumulation in the ER. Although it is not yet entirely clear, some evidence from studies on the assembly of MHC class I molecules suggests that synthetic peptides may be delivered to the ER from the extracellular medium of cultured cells [251]. There is also evidence that certain molecules may be transported retrograde to the ER by receptor-mediated endocytosis [252,253]. Second, elucidation of the biochemical mechanism by which abnormally folded α_1-AT undergoes intracellular degradation might allow pharmacologic manipulation of this degradative system, such as enhancing proteasomal activity with interferon-gamma in the subpopulation of PIZZ individuals predisposed to liver injury. Third, a competitive antagonist of binding or signal transduction by α_1-AT-proteinase complexes at the SEC receptor might prevent increases in intracellular accumulation of α_1-AT during augmentation of α_1-AT levels with protein replacement or gene replacement therapies.

PREVENTION

Restriction fragment length polymorphisms detected with synthetic oligonucleotide probes [254,255] and family studies [256] allow prenatal diagnosis of α_1-AT deficiency. Nevertheless, it is not clear how prenatal diagnosis for this deficiency should be used and how families should be counseled regarding the diagnosis. Data indicate that 80–85% of persons with α_1-AT deficiency do not have evidence of liver disease at age 18 years and that PIZZ persons may not develop emphysema or even pulmonary function abnormalities until age 60–70 years. These data could support a counseling strategy in which amniocentesis and abortion are discouraged. The only other data on this subject suggest a 78% chance that a second PIZZ child will have serious liver disease if the older sibling had serious liver disease [257]. This study, however, is retrospective and heavily influenced by bias in ascertainment of patients. The issue will not be resolved until studied prospectively, as, for example, in the Swedish population [1,3].

Several recent studies have suggested that population screening for α_1-AT deficiency would be efficacious. First, there is now evidence that knowledge of and counseling regarding the consequences of α_1-AT deficiency is associated with a reduced rate of smoking among affected adolescents [258,259]. Second, although there was some evidence for adverse psychologic effects from knowledge of the deficiency by affected families [260], more recent studies have indicated that there were no significant negative psychosocial consequences in early adulthood from neonatal screening for α_1-AT deficiency in Sweden [261]. These data should give new momentum to reconsideration of screening programs for α_1-AT deficiency.

REFERENCES

1. Sveger T. Liver disease in α_1-antitrypsin deficiency detected by screening of 200,000 infants. N Engl J Med 1976;294:1216–21.
2. Silverman EK, Miletich JP, Pierce JA, et al. Alpha-1-antitrypsin deficiency: prevalence estimation from direct population screening. Am Rev Respir Dis 1989;140:961–6.
3. Sveger T. The natural history of liver disease in alpha-1-antitrypsin deficient children. Acta Paediatr Scand 1995;77: 847–51.
4. Eriksson S, Carlson J, Velez R. Risk of cirrhosis and primary liver cancer in alpha-1-antitrypsin deficiency. N Engl J Med 1986; 314:736–9.
5. Gadek JE, Fells GA, Zimmerman RL, et al. Antielastases of the human alveolar structure: implications for the protease–antiprotease theory of emphysema. J Clin Invest 1981;68:889–98.
6. Perlmutter DH, Pierce JA. The alpha-1-antitrypsin gene and emphysema. Am J Physiol 1989;257:L147–62.
7. Janoff A. Elastases and emphysema: current assessment of the protease–antiprotease hypothesis. Am Rev Respir Dis 1985;132: 417–33.
8. Crystal RG. Alpha-1-antitrypsin deficiency, emphysema and liver disease: genetic basis and strategies for therapy. J Clin Invest 1990;95:1343–52.
9. Carlson JA, Rogers BB, Sifers RN, et al. Accumulation of PiZ antitrypsin causes liver damage in transgenic mice. J Clin Invest 1988;83:1183–90.
10. Dyaico JM, Grant SGN, Felts K, et al. Neonatal hepatitis induced by alpha-1-antitrypsin: a transgenic mouse model. Science 1988;242:1409–12.
11. Sharp HL, Bridges RA, Krivit W. Cirrhosis associated with alpha-1-antitrypsin deficiency: a previously unrecognized inherited disorder. J Lab Clin Med 1969;73:934–9.
12. Hope PL, Hall MA, Millward-Sadler GH, et al. Alpha-1-antitrypsin deficiency presenting as a bleeding diathesis in the newborn. Arch Dis Child 1982;57:68–70.
13. Ghishan FR, Gray GF, Greene HL. α_1-antitrypsin deficiency presenting with ascites and cirrhosis in the neonatal period. Gastroenterology 1983;85:435–8.
14. Zhou H, Fischer H-P. Liver carcinoma in PiZ alpha-1-antitrypsin deficiency. Am J Surg Pathol 1998;22:742–8.
15. Zhou H, Ortiz-Pallardo ME, Ko Y, Fischer H-P. Is heterozygous alpha-1-antitrypsin deficiency type PiZ a risk factor for primary liver carcinoma? Cancer 2000;88:2668–76.
16. Nebbia G, Hadchouel M, Odievre M, et al. Early assessment of evolution of liver disease associated with α_1-antitrypsin deficiency in childhood. J Pediatr 1983;102:661–5.
17. Ibarguen E, Gross CR, Savik SK, Sharp HL. Liver disease in α_1-antitrypsin deficiency: prognostic indicators. J Pediatr 1990;117:864–70.
18. Volpert D, Molleston JP, Perlmutter DH. Alpha1-antitrypsin deficiency-associated liver disease progresses slowly in some children. J Pediatr Gastro Nutr 2000;31:258–63.
19. Starzl TE, Porter KA, Busuttil RW, et al. Liver disease in alpha-1-antitrypsin deficiency: prognostic indicators. J Pediatr 1990;117:864–70.
20. Hodges JR, Millward Sadler GH, Barbatis C, et al. Heterozygous MZ α_1-antitrypsin deficiency in adults with chronic active hepatitis and cryptogenic cirrhosis. N Engl J Med 1981;304:357–60.
21. Graziadei IW, Joseph JJ, Wiesner RH, et al. Increased risk of chronic liver failure in adults with heterozygous α_1-antitrypsin deficiency. Hepatology 1998;28:1058–63.
22. Propst T, Propst A, Dietze O, et al. High prevalence of viral infections in adults with homozygous and heterozygous α_1-antitrypsin deficiency and chronic liver disease. Ann Intern Med 1992;117:641–5.
23. Reid CL, Wiener GJ, Cox DW, et al. Diffuse hepatocellular dysplasia and carcinoma associated with the M_{malton} variant of α_1-antitrypsin. Gastroenterology 1987;93:181–7.
24. Curiel DT, Holmes MD, Okayama H, et al. Molecular basis of the liver and lung disease associated with α_1-antitrypsin deficiency allele M_{malton}. J Biol Chem 1989;264:13938–45.
25. Lomas DA, Elliott PR, Sidhar SK, et al. α_1-antitrypsin M_{malton} [$Phe^{52\ deleted}$] forms loop-sheet polymers in vivo: evidence for the C-sheet mechanism of polymerization. J Biol Chem 1995;270:16864–74.
26. Mahadeva R, Chang W-SW, Dafforn TR, et al. Heteropolymerization of S, I, and Z α_1-antitrypsin and liver cirrhosis. J Clin Invest 1999;103:999–1006.
27. Teckman JH, Perlmutter DH. The endoplasmic reticulum degradation pathway for mutant secretory proteins α_1-antitrypsin Z and S is distinct from that for an unassembled membrane protein. J Biol Chem 1996;271:13215–20.
28. Crowley JJ, Sharp HL, Freier E, et al. Fatal liver disease associated with α_1-antitrypsin deficiency PIM/PIM_{duarte}. Gastroenterology 1987;93:242–4.
29. Clark P, Chong AYH. Rare alpha-1-antitrypsin allele PI_W and a history of infant liver disease. Am J Med Genet 1992;45: 674–6.
30. Kelly CP, Tyrrell DNM, McDonald GSA, et al. Heterozygous FZ α_1-antitrypsin deficiency associated with severe emphysema and hepatic disease: case report and family study. Thorax 1989; 44:758–9.
31. Eriksson S. Alpha-1-antitrypsin deficiency and liver cirrhosis in adults. Acta Med Scand 1987;221:461–7.
32. Silverman EK, Province MA, Rao DC, et al. A family study of the variability of pulmonary function in alpha-1-antitrypsin deficiency. Am Rev Respir Dis 1990;142:1015–21.
33. Guenter CA, Welch MH, Russell TR, et al. The pattern of lung disease associated with alpha-1-antitrypsin deficiency. Arch Intern Med 1968;122:254–9.
34. Thurlbeck WM, Henderson JA, Fraser RG, et al. Chronic obstructive disease: a comparison between clinical, roentgenologic, functional and morphologic criteria in chronic bronchitis, emphysema, asthma and bronchiectasis. Medicine 1970; 49:81–98.
35. Glasgow JFT, Lynch MJ, Hercz A, et al. $Alpha_1$ antitrypsin deficiency in association with both cirrhosis and chronic obstructive lung disease in two sibs. Am J Med 1973;54:181–94.
36. Talamo RC, Levison H, Lynch MJ, et al. Symptomatic pulmonary emphysema in childhood associated with hereditary alpha-1-antitrypsin and elastase inhibitor deficiency. J Pediatr 1971;79:20–6.

37. Houstek J, Copova M, Zapletal A, et al. Alpha1-antitrypsin deficiency in a child with chronic lung disease. Chest 1973;64:773–6.
38. Dunand P, Cropp GA, Middleton E Jr. Severe obstructive lung disease in a 14-year-old girl with alpha-1 antitrypsin deficiency. J Allergy Clin Immunol 1975;57:615–22.
39. Wagener JS, Sobonya RE, Taussig LM, et al. Unusual abnormalities in adolescent siblings with α_1-antitrypsin deficiency. Chest 1983;83:464–8.
40. Hird MF, Greenough A, Mieli-Vergani G, et al. Hyperinflation in children with liver disease due to α_1-antitrypsin deficiency. Pediatr Pulmonol 1991;11:212–16.
41. Wiebicke W, Niggermann B, Fischer A. Pulmonary function in children with homozygous alpha-1-protease inhibitory deficiency. Eur J Pediatr 1996;155:603–7.
42. Larsson C. Natural history and life expectancy in severe alpha-1-antitryspin deficiency, PiZ. Acta Med Scand 1978;204:345–51.
43. Janus ED, Phillips NT, Carrell RW. Smoking, lung function and alpha-1-antitrypsin deficiency. Lancet 1985;I:152–4.
44. Schonfeld JV, Brewer N, Zotz, R, et al. Liver function in patients with pulmonary emphysema due to severe alpha-1-antitrypsin deficiency (PIZZ). Digestion 1996;57:165–9.
45. Huber R, Carrell RW. Implications of the three-dimensional structure of alpha-1-antitrypsin for structure and function of serpins. Biochemistry 1990;28:8951–66.
46. Vaughan L, Lorier MA, Carrell RW. Alpha-1-antitrypsin microheterogeneity: isolation and physiological significance of isoforms. Biochim Biophys Acta 1982;701:339–45.
47. Silverman GA, Bird PI, Carrell RW, et al. The serpins are an expanding superfamily of structurally similar but functionally diverse proteins. Evolution, mechanism of inhibition, novel functions and a revised nomenclature. J Biol Chem 2000; 276:33293–6.
48. Elliott PR, Lomas DA, Carrell RW, et al. Inhibitory conformation of the reactive loop of α_1-antitrypsin. Nat Struct Biol 1996;3:676–81.
49. Elliott PR, Abrahams J-P, Lomas DA. Wild-type α_1-antitrypsin is in the cannonical inhibitory conformation. J Mol Biol 1998; 275:419–25.
50. Owen MC, Brennan SO, Lewis JH, et al. Mutation of antitrypsin to antithrombin: alpha-1-antitrypsin Pittsburgh (358 Met-Arg), a fatal bleeding disorder. N Engl J Med 1983;309: 694–8.
51. Banda MJ, Rice AG, Griffin GL, et al. Alpha-1-proteinase inhibitor is a neutrophil chemoattractant after proteolytic inactivation by macrophage elastase. J Biol Chem 1988;263:4481–4.
52. Banda MJ, Rice AG, Griffin GL, et al. The inhibitory complex of human alpha-1-proteinase inhibitor and human leukocyte elastase is a neutrophil chemoattractant. J Exp Med 1988;167:1608–15.
53. Perlmutter DH, Glover GI, Rivetna M, et al. Identification of a serpin-enzyme complex (SEC) receptor on human hepatoma cells and human monocytes. Proc Natl Acad Sci U S A 1990;87:3753–7.
54. Perlmutter DH, Joslin G, Nelson P, et al. Endocytosis and degradation of alpha-1-antitrypsin-proteinase complexes is mediated by the SEC receptor. J Biol Chem 1990;265:16713–16.
55. Long GL, Chandra T, Woo SLC, et al. Complete nucleotide sequence of the cDNA for human alpha-1-antitrypsin and the gene for the S variant. Biochemistry 1984;23:4828–37.
56. Lai EC, Kao F-F, Law ML, et al. Assignment of the alpha-1-antitrypsin gene and sequence-related gene to human chromosome 14 by molecular hybridization. Am J Hum Genet 1983; 35:385–92.
57. Pearson SJ, Tetri P, George DL, et al. Activation of human alpha-1-antitrypsin gene in rat hepatoma x human fetal liver cell hybrids depends on presence of human chromosome 14. Somat Cell Mol Genet 1983;9:567–92.
58. Rabin M, Watson M, Kidd V, et al. Activation of human alpha-1-antichymotrypsin and alpha-1-antitrypsin genes on human chromosome 14. Somat Cell Mol Genet 1986;12:209–14.
59. Perlino E, Cortese R, Ciliberto G. The human alpha-1-antitrypsin gene is transcribed from two different promoters in macrophages and hepatocytes. EMBO J 1987;6:2767–71.
60. Hofker MH, Nelen M, Klasen EC, et al. Cloning and characterization of an alpha-1-antitrypsin-like gene 12 kb downstream of the genuine alpha-1-antitrypsin gene. Biochem Biophys Res Comm 1988;155:634–42.
61. Kelsey GD, Parker M, Povey S. The human alpha-1-antitrypsin-related sequence gene: isolation and investigation of its sequence. Ann Hum Genet 1988:52:151–60.
62. Sefton L, Kelsey G, Kearney P, et al. A physical map of human PI and AACT genes. Genomics 1990;7:382–8.
63. Seralini G-E, Berube D, Gagne R, et al. The human corticosteroid binding globulin gene is located on chromosome 14q31-q32.1 near two other serine protease inhibitor genes. Hum Genet 1990;80:75–8.
64. Hafeez W, Ciliberto G, Perlmutter DH. Constitutive and mod ulated expression of the human alpha-1-antitrypsin gene: different transcriptional initiation sites used in three different cell types. J Clin Invest 1992;89:1214–22.
65. Pierce JA, Erdio BG. Improved identification of antitrypsin phenotypes through isoelectric focusing with dithioerythritol. J Lab Clin Med 1979;94:826–31.
66. Barker A, Brantly M, Campbell E, et al. α_1-antitrypsin deficiency: memorandum from a WHO meeting. Bull World Health Organ 1997;75:397–415.
67. Nukiwa T, Brantly ML, Ogushi F, et al. Characterization of the M1 (ala 213) type of alpha-1-antitrypsin haplotype. Biochemistry 1987;26:5259–67.
68. Dykes D, Miller S, Polesky H. Distribution of alpha-1-antitrypsin variants in a U.S. white population. Hum Hered 1984;34:308–10.
69. Kueppers F, Christopherson MJ. Alpha-1-antitrypsin: further genetic heterogeneity revealed by isoelectric focusing. Am J Hum Genet 1978;85:381–2.
70. Graham A, Hayes K, Weidinger S, et al. Characterization of alpha-1-antitrypsin M3 gene, a normal variant. Hum Genet 1990;85:381–2.
71. Jeppsson J-O, Laurell C-B. The amino acid substitutions of human alpha-1-antitrypsin M3, X and Z. FEBS Lett 1988;231: 327–30.
72. Brennan SO, Carrell RW. Alpha-1-antitrypsin Christchurch, 363Glu-Lys: mutation at the P′5 position does not affect inhibitory activity. Biochim Biophys Acta 1986;573:13–19.
73. Holmes MD, Brantly ML, Crystal RG. Molecular analysis of the heterogeneity among the P-family of alpha-1-antitrypsin alleles. Am Rev Respir Dis 1990;142:1185–92.
74. Talamo RC, Langley CE, Reed CE, et al. Alpha-1-antitrypsin deficiency: a variant with no detectable alpha-1-antitrypsin. Science 1973;181:70–1.
75. Takahashi H, Crystal RG. Alpha-1-antitrypsin null isola di procida: alpha-1-antitrypsin deficiency allele caused by deletion

of all alpha-1-antitrypsin coding exons. Am J Hum Genet 1990;47:403–13.
76. Poller W, Faber J-P, Neidinger S, et al. DNA polymorphisms associated with a new alpha-1-antitrypsin PIQO variant (PIQO reidenberg). Hum Genet 1991;86:522–4.
77. Garver RI, Mornex J-P, Nukiwa T, et al. Alpha-1-antitrypsin deficiency and emphysema caused by homozygous inheritance of on-expressing alpha-1-antitrypsin genes. N Engl J Med 1986;314:762–6.
78. Satoh K, Nukiwa T, Brantly M, et al. Emphysema associated with complete absence of alpha-1-antitrypsin in serum and the homozygous inheritance of stop codon in an alpha-1-antitrypsin coding exon. Am J Hum Genet 1988;42:77–83.
79. Holmes M, Curiel D, Brantly M, et al. Characterization of the intracellular mechanism causing the alpha-1-antitrypsin $\text{Null}_{\text{granite falls}}$ deficiency state. Am Rev Respir Dis 1989;140: 1662–7.
80. Nukiwa T, Takahashi H, Brantly M, et al. Alpha-1-antitrypsin $\text{Null}_{\text{granite Falls}}$: a nonexpressing alpha-1-antitrypsin gene associated with a frameshift stop mutation in a coding exon. J Biol Chem 1987;262:11999–2004.
81. Curiel D, Brantly M, Curiel E, et al. Alpha-1-antitrypsin deficiency caused by the alpha-1-antitryspin null mattawa gene: an insertion mutation rendering the alpha-1-antitrypsin gene incapable of producing alpha-1-antitrypsin. J Clin Invest 1989;83:1144–52.
82. Muensch H, Gaidulis L, Kueppers F, et al. Complete absence of serum alpha-1-antitrypsin in conjunction with an apparently normal gene structure. Am J Hum Genet 1986;38:898–907.
83. Sifers RN, Brashears-Macatee S, Kidd VJ, et al. A frameshift mutation results in a truncated alpha-1-antitrypsin that is retained within the rough endoplasmic reticulum. J Biol Chem 1988;263:7330–5.
84. Brantly M, Lee JH, Hildeshiem J, et al. α_1-antitrypsin gene mutation hot spot associated with the formation of a retained and degraded null variant. Am J Respir Cell Mol Biol 1997; 16:224–31.
85. Carrell RW. Alpha-1-antitrypsin molecular pathology, leukocytes and tissue damage. J Clin Invest 1986;77:1427–31.
86. Curiel D, Chytil A, Courtney M, et al. Serum alpha-1-antitrypsin deficiency associated with the common S-type (Glu^{364}-Val) mutation results in intracellular degradation of alpha-1-antitrypsin prior to secretion. J Biol Chem 1989;264: 10477–86.
87. Hofker MH, Nukiwa T, Van Paassen HMB, et al. A Pro-Leu substitution in codon 369 in the alpha-1-antitrypsin deficiency variant $\text{PiM}_{\text{heerlen}}$. Am J Hum Genet 1987;41:A220[abstract].
88. Takahashi H, Nukiwa T, Satoh K, et al. Characterization of the gene and protein of the alpha-1-antitrypsin "deficiency" allele M procida. J Biol Chem 1988;263:15528–34.
89. Sproule BJ, Cox SW, Hsu K, et al. Pulmonary function associated with the M malton deficient variant of alpha-1-antitrypsin. Am Rev Respir Dis 1983;127:237–40.
90. Curiel DT, Vogelmeier C, Hubbard RC, et al. Molecular basis of alpha-1-antitrypsin deficiency and emphysema associated with alpha-1-antitrypsin M mineral springs allele. Mol Cell Biol 1990;10:47–56.
91. Holmes MD, Brantley ML, Fells GA, et al. Alpha-1-antitrypsin $\text{W}_{\text{Bethesda}}$: molecular basis of an unusual alpha-1-antitrypsin deficiency variant. Biochem Biophys Res Comm 1990;170:1013–22.
92. Seyama K, Nukiwa T, Takabe K, et al. S_{iiyama} serine 53 [TCC] to phenylalanine 53 (TTC): a new alpha-1-antitrypsin deficient variant with mutation on a predicted conserved residue of the serpin backbone. J Biol Chem 1991;266:12627–32.
93. Okayama H, Brantly M, Holmes M, et al. Characterization of the molecular basis of the alpha-1-antitrypsin F allele. Am J Hum Genet 1991;47:1154–8.
94. Graham A, Kalsheker NA, Bamforth FJ, et al. Molecular characterization of two alpha-1-antitrypsin deficiency variants: proteinase inhibitor (Pi) Null newport (Gly165-Ser) and (Pi) Z Wrexham (Ser-19-Leu). Hum Genet 1990;85:537–40.
95. Senior RM, Tegner H, Kuhn C, et al. The induction of pulmonary emphysema with human leukocyte elastase. Am Rev Respir Dis 1977;116:469–75.
96. Travis J, Salvesen GS. Human plasma proteinase inhibitors. Annu Rev Biochem 1983;52:655–709.
97. Carp H, Janoff A. Possible mechanisms of emphysema in smokers: in vitro suppression of serum elastase inhibitory capacity by fresh cigarette smoke and its prevention by antioxidants. Am Rev Respir Dis 1978;118:617–21.
98. Ossanna PJ, Test S, Matheson NR, et al. Oxidative regulation and neutrophil elastase-alpha-1-proteinase inhibitor interactions. J Clin Invest 1986;72:1939–51.
99. Hubbard RC, Ogushi F, Fells GA, et al. Oxidants spontaneously released by alveolar macrophages of cigarette smokers can inactivate the active site of α_1-antitrypsin, rendering it ineffective as an inhibitor of neutrophil elastase. J Clin Invest 1987;80: 1289–95.
100. Mast AE, Enghild J, Nagase H, et al. Kinetics and physiologic relevance of the inactivation of α_1-proteinase inhibitor, α_1-antichymotrypsin, and antithrombin III by matrix metalloproteinases-1 (tissue collagenase), -1 (72-kDa gelatinase/ type IV collagenase), and -3 (stromelysin). J Biol Chem 1991; 266:15810–16.
101. Bathurst IC, Travis J, George PM, et al. Structural and functional characterization of the abnormal $Z\alpha_1$-antitrypsin isolated from human liver. FEBS Lett 1984;177:179–83.
102. Ogushi F, Fells GA, Hubbard RC, et al. Z-type α_1-antitrypsin is less competent than M1-type α_1-antitrypsin as an inhibitor of neutrophil elastase. J Clin Invest 1987;89:1366–74.
103. Libert C, Van Molle W, Brouckaert P, et al. α_1-antitrypsin inhibits the lethal response to TNF in mice. J Immunol 1996; 157:5126–9.
104. Van Molle W, Libert C, Fiers W, et al. α_1-acid glycoprotein and α_1-antitrypsin inhibit TNF-induced, but not anti-Fas-induced apoptosis of hepatocytes in mice. J Immunol 1997;159: 3555–64.
105. Camussi G, Tetta C, Bussolino F, et al. Synthesis and release of platelet-activating factor is inhibited by plasma α_1-proteinase inhibitor or α_1-antichymotrypsin and is stimulated by proteinases. J Exp Med 1988;168:1293–306.
106. Joslin G, Griffin GLI, August AM, et al. The serpin-enzyme complex [SEC] receptor mediate the neutrophil chemotactic effect of α_1-antitrypsin-elastse complexes and amyloid-β peptide. J Clin Invest 1992;90:1150–4.
107. Wilson-Cox D. Alpha-1-antitrypsin deficiency. In: Scriber CB, Beaudet AL, Aly QA, eds. The metabolic basis of inherited disease. New York: McGraw-Hill, 1989:2409–37.
108. Breit SN, Wakefield D, Robinson JP, et al. The role of alpha-1-antitrypsin deficiency in the pathogenesis of immune disorders. Clin Immun Immunopathol 1985;35:363–80.

109. Hood JM, Koep LJ, Peters RL, et al. Liver transplantation for advanced liver disease with α_1-antitrypsin deficiency. *N Engl J Med* 1980;302:272–6.
110. Lodish HF, Kong N. Glucose removal from N-linked oligosaccharides is required for efficient maturation of certain secretory glycoproteins from the rough endoplasmic reticulum to the Golgi complex. J Cell Biol 1987;104:221–30.
111. Liu M-C, Yu S, Sy J, et al. Tyrosine sulfation of proteins from human hepatoma cell line HepG2. Proc Natl Acad Sci U S A 1985;82:7160–4.
112. DeSimone V, Cortese R. Transcription factors and liver-specific genes. J Biol Biophys Acta 1992;1132:119–26.
113. Tripodi M, Abbott C, Vivian M, et al. Disruption of the LF-A1 and LF-B1, binding sites in the human alpha-1-antitrypsin gene, has a differential effect during development in transgenic mice. EMBO J 1991;10:3177–82.
114. Hu C, Perlmutter DH. Regulation of α_1-antitrypsin gene expression in human intestinal epithelial cell line Caco2 by HNF1α and HNF4. Am J Physiol 1999;276:G1181–94.
115. Dickson I, Alper CA. Changes in serum proteinase inhibitor levels following bone surgery. Clin Chim Acta 1974;54:381–5.
116. Perlmutter DH, May LT, Sehgal PB. Interferon $\beta_2$interleukin-6 modulates synthesis of α_1-antitrypsin in human mononuclear phagocytes and in human hepatoma cells. J Clin Invest 1989;264:9485–90.
117. Laurell C-B, Rannevik G. A comparison of plasma protein changes induced by danazol, pregnancy and estrogens. J Clin Endocrinol Metab 1979;49:719–25.
118. Perlmutter DH, Cole FS, Kilbridge P, et al. Expression of the α_1-proteinase inhibitor gene in human monocytes and macrophages. Proc Natl Acad Sci U S A 1985;82:795–9.
119. Barbey-Morel C, Pierce JA, Campbell EJ, et al. Lipopolysaccharide modulates the expression of α_1-proteinase inhibitor and other serine proteinase inhibitors in human monocytes and macrophages. J Exp Med 1987;166:1041–54.
120. Perlmutter DH, Travis J, Punsal PI. Elastase regulates the synthesis of its inhibitors, α_1-proteinase inhibitor, and exaggerates the defect in homozygous PIZZ α_1-proteinase inhibitor deficiency. J Clin Invest 1988;81:1774–8.
121. Joslin G, Fallon RJ, Bullock J, et al. The SEC receptor recognizes a pentapeptide neo-domain of α_1-antitrypsin protease complexes. J Biol Chem 1991;266:11281–8.
122. Joslin G, Wittwer A, Adams S, et al. Cross-competition for binding of α_1-antitrypsin (α-1-AT)-elastase complexes to the serpin-enzyme complex receptor by other serpin-enzyme complexes and by proteolytically modified α-1-AT. J Biol Chem 1993;268:1886–93.
123. Joslin G, Krause JE, Hershey ED, et al. Amyloid-β peptide, substance P and bombesin bind to the serpin-enzyme complex receptor. J Biol Chem 1991;266:21897–902.
124. Boland K, Behrens M, Choi D, et al. The serpin-enzyme complex receptor recognizes soluble, nontoxic amyloid-β peptide but not aggregated, cytotoxic amyloid-β peptide. J Biol Chem 1996;271:18032–44.
125. Mast AE, Enghild JJ, Pizzo SV, et al. Analysis of plasma elimination kinetics and conformation stabilities of native, proteinase-complexed and reactive site cleaved serpins: comparison of α_1-proteinase inhibitor, α_1-antichymotrypsin, antithrombin III, α_2-antiplasmin, angiotensinogen, and ovalbumin. Biochemistry 1991;30:1723–30.
126. Poller W, Willnow TE, Hilpert J, et al. Differential recognition of α_1-antitrypsin-elastase and α_1-antichymotrypsin-cathespin G complexes by the low density lipoprotein receptor-related protein. J Biol Chem 1995;270:2841–5.
127. Kounnas MZ, Church FC, Argraves WS, et al. Cellular internalization and degradation of antithrombin-III-thrombin, heparin cofactor II-thrombin, and α_1-antitrypsin-trypsin complexes is mediated by the low density lipoprotein receptor-related protein. J Biol Chem 1996;271:6523–9.
128. Kelsey GD, Povey S, Bygrave AE, et al. Species-and tissue-specific expression of human alpha-1-antitrypsin in transgenic mice. Genes Dev 1987;1:161–70.
129. Koopman P, Povey S, Lovel-Badge RH. Widespread expression of human alpha-1-antitrypsin in transgenic mice revealed by in situ hybridization. Genes Dev 1989;3:16–25.
130. Carlson JA, Rogers BB, Sifers RN, et al. Multiple tissues express alpha-1-antitrypsin in transgenic mice and man. J Clin Invest 1988;82:26–36.
131. Molmenti EP, Perlmutter DH, Rubin DC. Cell-specific expression of α_1-antitrypsin in human intestinal epithelium. J Clin Invest 1993;92:2022–34.
132. Venembre P, Boutten A, Seta N, et al. Secretion of α_1-antitryupsin by alveolar epithelial cells. FEBS Lett 1994;346:171–4.
133. Cichy J, Potempa J, Travis J. Biosynthesis of α_1 proteinase inhibitor by human lung-derived epithelial cells. J Biol Chem 1997;272:8250–5.
134. Makino S, Reed CE. Distribution and elimination of exogenous alpha-1-antitrypsin. J Lab Clin Med 1977;52:457–61.
135. Laurell C B, Nosslin B, Jeppsson J O. Catabolic rate of α_1 antitrypsin of P1 type M and Z in man. Clin Sci Mol Med 1977;52:457–61.
136. Thomas DW, Sinatra FR, Merritt RJ. Random fecal alpha-1-antitrypsin concentration in children with gastrointestinal disease. Gastroenterology 1981;80:776–82.
137. Grill B, Tinghitella T, Hillemeier C, et al. Increased intestinal clearance of alpha-1-antitrypsin in patient with alpha-1-antitrypsin deficiency. J Pediatr Gastroenterol Nutr 1983;2:95–8.
138. Kidd VJ, Walker RB, Itakura K, et al. α_1-antitryupsin deficiency detection by direct analysis of the mutation of the gene. Nature (London) 1983;304:230–4.
139. Jeppsson J-O. Amino acid substitution Glu-Lys in α_1-antitrypsin PiZ. FEBS Lett 1976;65:195–7.
140. Owen MC, Carrell RW. α_1-antitrypsin: sequence of the Z variant tryptic peptide. FEBS Lett 1976;79:247–9.
141. Perlmutter DH, Kay RM, Cole FS, et al. The cellular defect in α_1-proteinase inhibitor deficiency is expressed in human monocytes and xenopus oocytes injected with human liver mRNA. Proc Natl Acad Sci U S A 1985;82:6918–21.
142. Foreman RC, Judah JD, Colman A. Xenopus oocytes can synthesize but do not secrete the Z variant of human α_1-antitrypsin. FEBS Lett 1984;169:84–8.
143. McCracken AA, Kruse KB, Brown JL. Molecular basis for defective secretion of variants having altered potential for salt bridge formation between amino acids 240 and 242. Mol Cell Biol 1989;9:1408–14,
144. Sifers RN, Hardick CP, Woo SLC. Disruption of the 240–342 salt bridge is not responsible for the defect of the PIZ α_1-antitrypsin variant. J Biol Chem 1989;264:2997–3001.

145. Wu Y, Foreman RC. The effect of amino acid substitutions at position 342 on the secretion of human α_1-antitrypsin from xenopus oocytes. FEBS Lett 1990;268:21–3.
146. Lomas DA, Evans DL, Finch JJ, et al. The mechanism of Z α_1-antitrypsin accumulation in the liver. Nature 1992;357: 605–7.
147. Lomas DA, Finch JT, Seyama K, et al. α_1-antitrypsin S_{iiyama} (SER53→Phe): further evidence for intracellular loop-sheet polymerization. J Biol Chem 1993;268:15333–5.
148. Elliott PR, Stein PE, Bilton D, et al. Structural explanation for the deficiency of S α_1-antitrypsin. Nature Struct Biol 1996;3: 910–11.
149. Sidhar SK, Lomas DA, Carrell RW, et al. Mutations which impede loop-sheet polymerization enhance the secretion of human α_1-antitrypsin deficiency variants. J Biol Chem 1995; 270:8393–6.
150. Kang HA, Lee KN, Yu M-H. Folding and stability of the Z and S_{iiyama} genetic variants of human α_1-antitrypsin. J Biol Chem 1997;272:510–16.
151. Lin L, Schmidt B, Teckman J, Perlmutter DH. A naturally occurring non-polymerogenic mutant of α_1-antitrypsin characterized by prolonged retention in the endoplasmic reticulum. J Biol Chem 2001;276:33893–8.
152. Schmidt BZ, Perlmutter DH. GRP78, GRP94 and GRP170 interact with α1 AT mutants that are retained in the endoplasmic reticulum. Am J Physiol Gastrointest Liver Physiol 2005;289:G444–55.
153. Davis RL, Shrimpton AE, Holohan PD, et al. Familial dementia caused by polymerization of mutant neuroserpin. Nature 1999; 401:376–9.
154. Kamimoto T, Shoji S, Mizushima N, et al. Intracellular inclusions containing mutant α1 ATZ are propagated in the absence of autophagy. J Biol Chem 2006;281:4467–76
155. Kruse KB, Brodsky JL, McCracken AA. Characterization of an ERAD gene as VPS30/ATG6 reveals two alternative and functionally distinct protein quality control pathways: one for soluble α1 PiZ and another for aggregates of α1 PiZ. Mol Biol Cell 2006;17:203–12. Epub 2005 Nov 2.
156. Hidvegi T, Schmidt BZ, Hale P, Perlmutter DH. Accumulation of mutant α_1-antitrypsin Z in the ER activates caspases-4 and -12, NFκB and BAP31 but not the unfolded protein response. J Biol Chem 2005;280:39002–15. Epub 2005 Sep 23.
157. Wu Y, Whitman I, Molmenti E, et al. A lag in intracellular degradation of mutant α_1-antitrypsin correlates with the liver disease phenotype in homozygous PiZZ α_1-antitrypsin deficiency. Proc Natl Acad Sci U S A 1994;91:9014–18.
158. Werner ED, Brodsky JL, McCracken AA. Proteasome-dependent endoplasmic reticulum-associated protein degradation: an unconventional route to a familiar fate. Proc Natl Acad Sci U S A 1996;93:13797–801.
159. Qu D, Teckman JH, Omura S, Perlmutter DH. Degradation of mutant secretory protein, α_1-antitrypsin Z, in the endoplasmic reticulum requires proteasome activity. J Biol Chem 1996;271:22791–5.
160. Teckman JH, Gilmore R, Perlmutter DH. Role of ubiquitin in proteasomal degradation of mutant α_1-antitrypsin Z in the endoplasmic reticulum. Am J Physiol 2000;278:G39–48.
161. Teckman JH, Burrows J, Hidvegi T, et al. The proteasome participants in degradation of mutant α_1-antitrypsin Z in the endoplasmic reticulum of hepatoma-derived hepatocytes. J Biol Chem 2001;276:44865–72.
162. Cabral CM, Liu Y, Moremen KW, Sifers RN. Organizational diversity among distinct glycoprotein endoplasmic reticulum-associated degradation programs. Mol Biol Cell 2002;13: 2639–50.
163. Mayer T, Braun T, Jentsch S. Role of the proteasome in membrane extraction of a short-lived ER-transmembrane protein. EMBO J 1998;17:3251–7.
164. Cabral CM, Choudhury P, Liu Y, Sifers RN. Processing by endoplasmic reticulum mannosidases partitions a secretion-impaired glycoprotein into distinct disposal pathways. J Biol Chem 2000;275:25015–22.
165. Teckman JH, Perlmutter DH. Retention of mutant α_1-antitrypsin Z in endoplasmic reticulum is associated with an autophagic response. Am J Physiol 2000;279:G961–74.
166. Teckman JH, An JK, Blomenkamp K, et al. Mitochondrial autophagy and injury in the liver in α_1-antitrypsin deficiency. Am J Physiol 2004;286:G851–62.
167. Perkins G, Renken C, Martone ME, et al. Electron tomography of neuronal mitochondria: three-dimensional structure and organization of cristae and membrane contacts. J Struct Biol 1997;119:260–72.
168. Achleitner G, Gaigg B, Krasser A, et al. Association between the endoplasmic reticulum and mitochondria of yeast facilitates intraorganelle transport of phospholipids through membrane contact. Eur J Biochem 1999;264:545–53.
169. Mizushima N, Yamamoto A, Matsui M, et al. In vivo analysis of autophagy in response to nutrient starvation using transgenic mice expressing a fluorescent autophagosome marker. Mol Biol Cell 2004;15:1101–11.
170. Zhang K, Kaufman RJ. Signaling the unfolded protein response from the endoplasmic reticulum. J Biol Chem 2004;279: 25935–8.
171. Ron D. Translational control in the endoplasmic reticulum stress response. J Clin Invest 2002;110:1383–8.
172. Pahl HL, Sester M, Burgert HG, Baeuerle PA. Activation of transcription factor NFκB by the adenovirus E3/19K protein requires its ER retention. J Cell Biol 1996;132:511–22.
173. Hu C, Perlmutter DH. Cell-specific involvement of HNF-1β in α_1-antitrypsin gene expression in human respiratory epithelial cells. Am J Physiol 2002;282:L757–65.
174. Pikarsky E, Porat RM, Stein I, et al. NFκB functions as a tumor promoter in inflammation-associated cancer. Nature 2004;431:461–6.
175. Greten FR, Eckman L, Greten TF, et al. IKKβ links inflammation and tumorigenesis in a mouse model of colitis-associated cancer. Cell 2004;118:285–96.
176. Maeda S, Kamata H, Luo J-L, et al. IKKβ couples hepatocyte death to cytokine-driven compensatory proliferation that promotes chemical hepatocarcinogenesis. Cell 2005;121:977–90.
177. Schamel WW, Kuppig S, Becker B, et al. A high-molecular-weight complex of membrane proteins BAP29/BAP31 is involved in the retention of membrane-bound IgD in the endoplasmic reticulum. Proc Natl Acad Sci U S A 2003;100:9861–6.
178. Breckenridge DG, Stojanovic M, Marcellus RC, Shore GC. Caspase cleavage product of BAP31 induces mitochondrial fission through endoplasmic reticulum calcium signals, enhancing cytochrome c release to the cytosol. J Cell Biol 2003;160:1115–27.
179. Povey S. Genetics of α_1-antitrypsin deficiency in relation to neonatal liver disease. Mol Biol Med 1990;7:161–2.

180. Dougherty DG, Donaldson PT, Whitehouse DB, et al. HLA phenotype and gene polymorphism in juvenile liver disease associated with α_1-antitrypsin deficiency. Hepatology 1990;12:218–23.
181. Lobo-Yeo A, Senaldi G, Portmann R, et al. Class I and class II major histocompatibility complex antigen expression on hepatocytes: a study in children with liver disease. Hepatology 1990;12:224–32.
182. Sargent CA, Dunham I, Trowsdale J, et al. Human major histocompatibility complex contains genes for the major heat shock protein HSP 70. Proc Natl Acad Sci U S A 1989;1968–77.
183. Albertella MR, Jones H, Thomson W, et al. Localisation of eight additional genes in the human major histocompatibility complex, including the gene encoding the casein kinase II beta subunit, and DNA sequence analysis of the class III region. DNA Sequence 1996;7:9–12.
184. Geller SA, Nichols WS, Dycacio MJ, et al. Histopathology of α_1-antitrypsin liver disease in a transgenic mouse model. Hepatology 1990;12:40–7.
185. Geller SA, Nichols WS, Kim SS, et al. Hepatocarcinogenesis is the sequel to hepatitis in Z#2 α_1-antitrypsin transgenic mice: histopathological and DNA ploidy studies. Hepatology 1994;19:389–97.
186. Gaczynska M, Rock KL, Goldber AL. Gamma-interferon and expression of MHC genes regulate peptide hydrolysis by proteasomes. Nature 1993;365:264–7.
187. Bathurst IC, Errington DM, Foreman RC, et al. Human Z alpha-1-antitrypsin accumulates intracellularly and stimulates lysosomal activity when synthesized in the xenopus oocyte. FEBS Lett 1985;183:304–8.
188. Raposo G, van Santen HM, Liejendekker R, et al. Misfolded major histocompatibility complex class I molecules accumulate in an expanded ER-Golgi intermediate compartment. J Cell Biol 1995;131:1403–19.
189. Dunn WA. Studies on the mechanism of autophagy: formation of autophagic vacuole. J Cell Biol 1991;110:1923–33.
190. Mizushima N, Noda T, Yoshimori T, et al. A protein conjugation system essential for autophagy. Nature 1998;195:395–8.
191. Klionsky DJ. Autophagy. Curr Biol 2005;15:R282–3.
192. Johnston JA, Ward CL, Kopito RR. Aggresomes: a cellular response to misfolded proteins. J Cell Biol 1998;143:1883–98.
193. Anton LC, Schubert U, Bacik I, et al. Intracellular localization of proteasomal degradation of a viral antigen. J Cell Biol 1999;146:113–24.
194. Teckman JH, An J-K, Loethen S, Perlmutter DH. Effect of fasting on liver in a mouse model of α_1-antitrypsin deficiency: constitutive activation of the autophagic response. Am J Phys iol 2002;283:61117–24.
195. Tanka Y, Guhde G, Suter A, et al. Accumulation of autophagic vacuoles and cardiomyopathy in LAMP-2-deficient mice. Nature 2000;406:902–6.
196. Nishino I, Fu J, Tanji K, et al. Primary LAMP-2 deficiency causes X-linked vacuolar cardiomyopathy and myopathy (Danon disease). Nature 2000;406:906–10.
197. Elmore SP, Qian T, Grissom DF, Lemasters JJ. The mitochondrial permeability transition initiates autophagy in rat hepatocytes. FASEB J 2001;15:2286–7.
198. Perkins G, Renken C, Martone ME, et al. Electron tomography of neuronal mitochondria: three-dimensional structure and organization of cristae and membrane contacts. J Struct Biol 1997;119:260–72.
199. Achleitner G, Gaigg B, Krasser A, et al. Association between the endoplasmic reticulum and mitochondria of yeast facilitates interorganelle transport of phospholipids through membrane contact. Eur J Biochem 1999;264:545–53.
200. Wang H-J, Guay G, Pogan L, et al. Calcium regulates the association between mitochondria and a smooth subdomain of the endoplasmic reticulum. J Cell Biol 2000;150:1489–97.
201. Arnaudeau S, Kelley WL, Walsh JV, Demaurex N. Mitochondria recycle Ca2+ to the endoplasmic reticulum and prevent the depletion of neighboring endoplasmic reticulum regions. J Biol Chem 2001;276:29430–9.
202. Hacki J, Egger L, Monney L, et al. Apoptotic crosstalk between the endoplasmic reticulum and mitochondria controlled by Bcl-2. Oncogene 2000;19:2286–95.
203. Wei MC, Zong WX, Cheng EH, et al. Proapoptotic BAX and BAK; a requisite gateway to mitochondrial dysfunction and death. Science 2001;292:727–30.
204. Rudnick DA, Liao Y, An JK, et al. Analyses of hepatocellular proliferation in a mouse model of α1-antitrypsin deficiency. Hepatology 2004;39:1048–55.
205. Bruey JM, Ducasse C, Bonniaud P, et al. Hsp27 negatively regulates cell death by interacting with cytochrome c. Nat Cell Biol 2000;2:645–52.
206. Perlmutter DH, Schlesinger MJ, Pierce JA, et al. Synthesis of stress proteins is increased in individuals with homozygous PiZZ α1-antitrypsin deficiency and liver disease. J Clin Invest 1989;84:1555–61.
207. Vogel A, van Den Berg IE, Al-Dhalimy M, et al. Chronic liver disease in murine hereditary tyrosinemia type 1 induces resistance to cell death. *Hepatology* 2004;39:433–43.
208. Kvittingen EA, Rootwelt H, Berger R, Brandtzaeg P. Self-induced correction of the genetic defect in tyrosinemia type I. J Clin Invest 1994;94:1657–61.
209. Overturf K, Al-Dhalimy M, Tanguay R, et al. Hepatocytes corrected by gene therapy are selected in vivo in a murine model of hereditary tyrosinaemia type I. Nat Genet 1996;12:266–73.
210. Demers SI, Russo P, Lettre F, Tanguay RM. Frequent mutation reversion inversely correlates with clinical severity in a genetic liver disease, hereditary tyrosinemia. Hum Pathol 2003;34:1313–20.
211. McLachlan A, Milich DR, Raney AK, et al. Expression of hepatitis B virus surface and core antigens: influences of pre-S and precore sequences. J Virol 1987;61:683–92.
212. Wang HC, Wu HC, Chen CF, et al. Different types of ground glass hepatocytes in chronic hepatitis B virus infection contain specific pre-S mutants that may induce endoplasmic reticulum stress. Am J Pathol 2003;163:2441–9.
213. Dubuisson J. Folding, assembly and subcellular localization of hepatitis C virus glycoproteins. Curr Top Microbiol Immunol 2000;242:135–48.
214. Yang SQ, Lin HZ, Hwang J, et al. Hepatic hyperplasia in noncirrhotic fatty livers: is obesity-related hepatic steatosis a premalignant condition? Cancer Res 2001;61:5016–23.
215. Roskams T, Yang SQ, Koteish A, et al. Oxidative stress and oval cell accumulation in mice and humans with alcoholic and nonalcoholic fatty liver disease. Am J Pathol 2003;163:1301–11.
216. Johnson K, Alton HM, Chapman S. Evaluation of mebrofenin hepatoscintigraphy in neonatal-onset jaundice. Pediatr Radiol 1998;28:937–41.

217. Nord KS, Saad S, Joshi VV, et al. Concurrence of α_1-antitrypsin deficiency and biliary atresia. J Pediatr 1987;111:416–18.
218. Ghishan FK, Greene HL. Inborn errors of metabolism that lead to permanent liver injury. In: Zakim D, Boyer TD, eds. Hepatology: a textbook of liver disease. Philadelphia: WB Saunders, 1982:1351.
219. Mowat AP. Hepatitis and cholestasis in infancy: intrahepatic disorders. In: Mowat AP, ed. Liver disorders in childhood. London: Butterworth, 1982:50.
220. Qizibash A, Yong-Pong O. Alpha-1-antitrypsin liver disease: differential diagnosis of PAS-positive diastase-resistant globules in liver cells. Am J Clin Pathol 1983;79:697–702.
221. Yunis EJ, Agostini RM, Glew RH. Fine structural observations of the liver in α_1-antitryspin deficiency. Am J Clin Pathol 1976;82:265–86.
222. Tobin MJ, Cook PJL, Hutchison DCS. Alpha-1-antitrypsin deficiency: the clinical and physiological features of pulmonary emphysema in subjects homozygous for Pi type Z. Br J Dis Chest 1983;77:14–27.
223. Udall JN, Dixon M, Newman AP, et al. Liver disease in α_1-antitrypsin deficiency: a retrospective analysis of the influence of early breast- vs bottle-feeding. *JAMA* 1985;253:2679–82.
224. Udall JN, Bloch KJ, Walker WA. Transport of proteases across neonatal intestine and development of liver disease in infants with α_1-antitrypsin deficiency. Lancet 1982;ii:1441–3.
225. Kayler LK, Merion RM, Lee S, et al. Long-term survival after liver transplantation in children with metabolic disorders. Pediatr Transplant 2002;6:295–300.
226. Gelfand JA, Sherins RJ, Alling DW, et al. Treatment of hereditary angiodema with danazol: reversal of clinical and biochemical abnormalities. N Engl J Med 1976;195:1444–8.
227. Gadek JE, Fulmer JD, Gelfand JA, et al. Danazol-induced augmentation of serum alpha-1-antitrypsin levels in individuals with marked deficiency of this anti-protease. J Clin Invest 1980;66:82–7.
228. Wewers MD, Gadek JE, Loegh BA, et al. Evaluation of danazol therapy for patients with PiZZ alpha-1-antitrypsin deficiency. Am Rev Respir Dis 1986;134:476–80.
229. Sato S, Ward CL, Krouse ME, et al. Glycerol reverses the misfolding phenotype of the most common cystic fibrosis mutation. J Biol Chem 1996;271:635–8.
230. Tatzelt J, Prusiner SB, Welch WJ. Chemical chaperones interfere with the formation of scrapie prion protein. EMBO J 1996;15:6363–73.
231. Tamarappoo B, Verkman AS. Defective aquaporin-2 trafficking in nephrogenic diabetes insipidus and correction by chemical chaperones. J Clin Invest 1998;101:2257–67.
232. Brown CR, Hong-Brown LQ, Welch WJ. Correcting temperature-sensitive protein folding defects. J Clin Invest 1997; 99:1432–44.
233. Fan J-Q, Ishii S, Asano N, et al. Accelerated transport and maturation of lysosomal alpha-galactosidase A in Fabry lymphoblasts by an enzyme inhibitor. Nat Med 1999;5:112–15.
234. Burrows JAJ, Willis LK, Perlmutter DH. Chemical chaperones mediate increased secretion of mutant α_1-antitrypsin (α_1-AT) Z: a potential pharmacological strategy for prevention of liver injury and emphysema in α_1-AT deficiency. Proc Natl Acad Sci U S A 2000;97:1796–801.
235. Jacob GS. Glycosylation inhibitors in biology and medicine. Curr Opin Struct Biol 1995;5:605–11.
236. Zitzmann N, Mehta AS, Carrouee S, et al. Imino sugars inhibit the formation and secretion of bovine viral diarrhea virus, a pestivirus model of hepatitis C virus: implications for the development of broad-spectrum anti-hepatitis virus agents. Proc Natl Acad Sci U S A 1999;96:11878–82.
237. Marcus NY, Perlmutter DH. Glucosidase and mannosidase inhibitors mediate increased secretion of mutant α1-antitrypsin Z. J Biol Chem 2000;275:1987–92.
238. Abboud RT, Ford GT, Chapman KR. Emphysema in alpha1antitrypsin deficiency: Does replacement therapy affect outcome? Treat Respir Med 2005;4:1–8.
239. Cassivi SD, Meyers BF, Battafarano RJ, et al. Thirteen year experience in lung transplantation for emphysema. Ann Thorac Surg 2002;74:1663–9.
240. Anderson WF. The current status of clinical gene therapy. Hum Gene Ther 2002;13:1261–2.
241. Long MB, Jones JP, Sullenger BA, Byun J. Ribozyme-mediated revision of RNA and DNA. J Clin Invest 2003;112:312–18.
242. Garcia-Blanco MA. Messenger RNA reprogramming by spliceosome-mediated RNA trans-splicing. J Clin Invest 2003; 112:474–80.
243. Kren BT, Bandyopadhyay P, Steer CJ. In vivo site-directed mutagenesis of the *factor IX* gene by chimeric RNA/DNA oligonucleotides. Nat Med 1998;4:285–90.
244. Metz R, Dicola M, Kurihara T, et al. Mode of action of RNA/DNA oligonucleotides. Chest 2002;121:915–25.
245. Kmiec EB. Targeted gene repair – in the arena. J Clin Invest 2003; 112:632–6.
246. Seidman MM, Glazier PM. The potential for gene repair via triple helix formation. J Clin Invest 2003;114:487–94.
247. Gruenert DC, Bruscia E, Novelli G, et al. Sequence-specific modification of genomic DNA by small DNA fragments. J Clin Invest 2003;112:637–41.
248. Davidson BL. Hepatic diseases – hitting the target with inhibitory RNAs. N Engl J Med 2003;349:2357–9.
249. Rubinson DA, Dillon CP, Kwiatkowski AV, et al. A lentivirus-based system to functionally silence genes in primary mammalian cells, stem cells and transgenic mice by RNA interference. Nat Gen 2003;33:401–6.
250. Rhim JA, Sandgen EP, Degen JL, et al. Replacement of disease mouse liver by hepatic cell transplantation. Science 1994; 263:1149–52.
251. Day PM, Yewdell JW, Porgador A, et al. Direct delivery of exogenous MHC class I molecule-binding oligopeptides to the endoplasmic reticulum of viable cells. Proc Natl Acad Sci U S A 1997; 94:8064–9.
252. Johannes L, Goud B. Surfing on a retrograde wave: how does Shiga toxin reach the endoplasmic reticulum? Trends Cell Biol 1998;8:158–62.
253. Lord, JM, Roberts LM. Toxin entry: retrograde transport through the secretory pathway. J Cell Biol 1998;140:733–6.
254. Kidd VJ, Golbus MS, Wallace RB, et al. Prenatal diagnosis of alpha-1-antitrypsin deficiency by direct analysis of the mutation site in the gene. N Engl J Med 1984;310:639–42.
255. Cox DW, Mansfield T. Prenatal diagnosis of alpha-1-antitrypsin deficiency and estimates of fetal risk for disease. J Med Genet 1987;24:52–9.

256. Nukiwa T, Brantly M, Garver R, et al. Evaluation of "at risk" alpha-1-antitrypsin genotype SZ with synthetic oligonucleotide gene probes. J Clin Invest 1986;77:528–37.
257. Psacharopoulos HT, Mowat AP, Cook PJL, et al. Outcome of liver disease associated with alpha-1-antitrypsin deficiency (PiZ). Arch Dis Child 1983;58:882–7.
258. Thelin T, Sveger T, McNeil TF. Primary prevention in a high-risk group: smoking habits in adolescents with homozygous alpha-1-antitrypsin deficiency. Acta Paediatr 1996;85:1207–12.
259. Wall M, Moe E, Eisenberg J, et al. Long-term follow-up of a cohort of children with alpha-1-antitrypsin deficiency. J Pediatr 1990;116:248–51.
260. McNeil TF, Sveger T, Thelin T. Psychosocial effects of screening for somatic risk: the Swedish α_1-antitrypsin experience. Thorax 1988;43:505–7.
261. Sveger T, Thelin T, McNeil TF. Young adults with α_1-antitrypsin deficiency identified neonatally: their health, knowledge about and adaptation to the high-risk condition. Acta Paediatr 1997; 86:37–40.

24

Cystic Fibrosis Liver Disease

Andrew P. Feranchak, M.D.

Cystic fibrosis (CF) is a genetic disorder characterized by epithelial electrolyte transport abnormalities, elevated sweat Cl^- concentrations, pancreatic insufficiency, and chronic lung disease in most patients. It is the most common potentially fatal genetic disorder in the Caucasian population, affecting 1 in 2400–3500 live births [1,2]. It is an autosomal recessive disorder caused by a mutation in the gene for the cystic fibrosis transmembrane conductance regulator (CFTR), a membrane channel protein. The clinical significance of hepatobiliary disease in CF has not been well characterized primarily because of two factors: (1) pulmonary involvement leads to early mortality in a majority of patients, and (2) the clinical identification of CF-associated liver disease has been difficult because, although it is progressive, liver involvement is often asymptomatic until the appearance of end-stage complications. Recently, with improved pulmonary treatments, median life expectancy now exceeds 30 years [3] and CF-associated hepatobiliary disease is recognized and characterized more comprehensively. Liver disease is now the second major cause of death in CF [4]. In recent years, advances in our understanding of the function of CFTR in bile duct epithelia have provided a stronger scientific basis for the pathogenesis of the disease, leading to insights concerning potentially novel therapeutic approaches.

The earliest reports of CF, probably date to the Middle Ages with reports of malnourished and "sickly" children that tasted "salty" when kissed [5]. In 1905, Landsteiner [6] published the first description of an abnormal pancreas and meconium ileus in CF, although it was Anderson's [7] description in 1938 that gave us a more modern description of "cystic fibrosis of the pancreas." This initial description was revised in 1945 by Farber [8], who used the term "mucoviscidosis" to described the multiple organs affected by thickened mucus. This term is still used in many areas to describe the "duct organs" containing viscid, mucus secretions. In 1953, di Sant'Agnese et al. [9], from astute observations following the high incidence of CF patients with heat prostration during the New York City heat wave of 1948, described the abnormal sweat electrolyte concentrations. The diagnostic sweat test was subsequently developed by Gibson and Cooke [10] and has served as the basis of the diagnosis until the recent availability of genetic analysis. On a cellular level, meticulous studies of the sweat duct led Quinton [11] to describe the Cl^- transport defect. Finally, it was the discovery the CF gene in 1989 by Riordan et al. [12] that permitted critical breakthroughs in the understanding of CF pathogenesis. It was hoped that the gene discovery would herald a quick and forthcoming cure for CF, and although this dream has not been realized to date, the intense study of the role of CFTR in cell and organ function has advanced our knowledge of basic cellular physiology enormously. For a review of the remarkable history of the scientific discovery related to this disease see reviews by Quinton [13] and Doershuk [14].

CFTR: A CHANNEL

The CF gene is located on the long arm of chromosome 7. Containing 250,000 base pairs with 27 exons, it encodes a polypeptide product of 1480 amino acids known as the CF transmembrane conductance regulator (CFTR). The protein belongs to a family of transmembrane proteins known as adenosine triphosphate (ATP)-binding cassette (ABC) proteins, which all contain transmembrane sequences and hydrolize ATP for activation. CFTR contains two domains, capable of spanning the membrane six times, separated by regulatory cytoplasmic domains consisting of two consensus nucleotide binding domains (NBD) and an intervening regulatory domain (Figure 24.1). It is now well established that CFTR functions as a cyclic adenosine monophosphate (cAMP)-dependent Cl^- channel in the apical membrane of secretory epithelia. CFTR-associated Cl^- channels have a small unitary conductance of approximately 8 picosiemens and a linear current-voltage relation [15,16]. Under normal conditions, cAMP-dependent protein kinase A (PKA) phosphorylates CFTR, causing channel opening and transport of Cl^- ions.

In addition to Cl^-, evidence suggests that CFTR may also directly transport HCO_3^- [17–19]. In CF epithelia with some retained Cl^- secretion (associated with minor CFTR mutations), HCO_3^- transport is still significantly impaired,

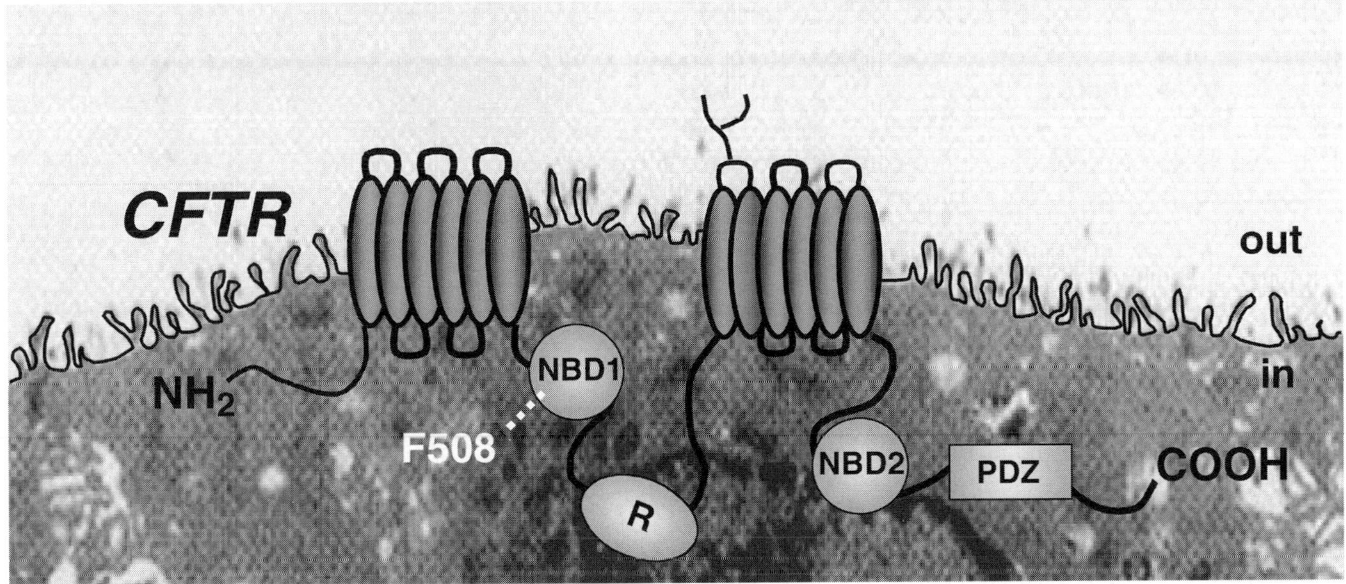

Figure 24.1. Putative monomeric structure for the cystic fibrosis transmembrane conductance regulator (CFTR). The 1480 amino acids of CFTR are arranged into 12 membrane-spanning domains. The first six transmembrane domains are followed by an intracellular regulatory domain, or R-domain, containing phosphorylation sites for protein kinase A (PKA). Transmembrane segments 6 and 12 are followed by sequences containing ATP-binding domains or nucleotide binding domains (NBD). The most common CF-associated mutation (ΔF508) results from a base pair deletion in exon 10, causing a deletion of phenylalanine at position 508 in the first NBD region. The C-terminal end of the protein contains PDZ-domains that may facilitate protein–protein interactions.

suggesting that HCO_3^- transport may be a primary problem related to abnormal CFTR and not necessarily secondary to abnormal Cl^- efflux [20]. Additionally, it has been proposed that CFTR may transport glutathione [21] or ATP [22,23], both constituents of bile, in a conductive manner. Whether CFTR directly transports these molecules or regulates another transport protein is unknown. Further studies to determine the pore and conductive properties of CFTR in mediating these transport events are ongoing.

CFTR: A REGULATOR

There is increasing evidence to suggest that, in addition to its role as a Cl^- channel, CFTR, as the name implies, also functions as a *regulator* of other membrane proteins and channels [24]. This was first suggested by the observation that, in addition to abnormal Cl^- and HCO_3^- transport, CF tissues display other transport abnormalities such as defective regulation of outwardly rectified Cl^- channels and increased Na^+ absorption through epithelial Na^+ channels (ENaC) [25–27]. Expression of wild-type CFTR not only corrects the cAMP-dependent Cl^- conductance but leads to normalization of outwardly rectified Cl^- channel regulation and ENaC channel activity [23,28,29]. It also appears that CFTR regulates inwardly rectifying K^+ channels such as the renal outer medullary K^+ channel [30]. These observations suggest that CFTR is multifunctional, serving as both an ion channel and as a protein that regulates other ion channels.

In other secretory epithelia, CFTR has been shown to regulate glutathione transport [31,32], mucin secretion [33], water transport through aquaporins [34–36], and ATP permeability [37]. In addition to its effect on membrane transport activity, CFTR appears to play a role in vesicular transport as evidenced by the abnormal cAMP-dependent exocytosis and abnormal acidification of intracellular organelles observed in CF cells [38,39]. How CFTR regulates these membrane proteins and transport activities is currently unknown. The finding that CFTR contains specific sequences that bind integral membrane proteins and cytoskeletal elements raises the possibility of *membrane regulatory complexes* in the apical domain of epithelial cells. Recent studies demonstrate that the intracellular portion of CFTR binds to protein modules referred to as PSD-95/Discs-large/ZO-1 (PDZ) domains that promote protein–protein interactions. Several PDZ-domain-containing proteins have been shown to bind to CFTR including EBP50 and E3KARP [40], which are both expressed in cholangiocytes and may be important regulators of ductular bile formation [41]. In fact, overexpression of the PDZ-1 domain of EBP50 decreases endogenous cAMP Cl^- channel activity in a cholangiocyte cell line, suggesting that this protein–protein interaction has direct regulatory effects on Cl^- secretion [41]. Overall, CFTR, through PDZ domain interactions, forms macromolecular signaling complexes and engages in interactions with a wide variety of transporters and signaling molecules to regulate cellular events. Understanding the nature of these interactions is an area for future investigation and may serve as the basis for novel therapies for CF.

ROLE OF CFTR IN LIVER FUNCTION

In human liver, CFTR is expressed on the apical membrane of bile duct cells (cholangiocytes) and gallbladder epithelia but is not expressed in hepatocytes or other cells of the liver [42]. Its location on the apical (luminal) membrane of cholangiocytes as well as the large increase in cAMP-stimulated CFTR activity observed with secretory agonists, suggests it plays a role in bile formation.

The formation of bile by the liver depends on complementary interactions between hepatic parenchymal cells, or hepatocytes, and intrahepatic bile duct cells, or cholangiocytes. Both of these cell types work in a complementary manner to initiate and modify bile flow. Although bile formation is initiated at the hepatocyte canalicular membrane through the transport of bile acids, organic and inorganic solutes, electrolytes, and water, the cholangiocyte contribution to bile formation is significant and may account for approximately 40% of bile flow in humans. This is even more remarkable in that cholangiocytes only constitute 3–5% of the nuclear mass of the liver, suggesting that these cells have a prodigious capacity for secretion.

Studies in isolated cholangiocytes, biliary epithelial monolayers, and isolated bile duct segments have recently helped to elucidate the basic mechanisms of constitutive and stimulated secretion in biliary epithelium. One of the current working models is shown in Figure 24.2. Intracellular Cl^- accumulation occurs via uptake of Cl^- at the basolateral membrane by a bumetadine-sensitive $Na^+/K^+/2Cl^-$ cotransporter. Whereas the intracellular accumulation of Cl^- ions leads to values above the electrochemical equilibrium, the Cl^- permeability of the apical membrane under basal conditions is low. However, exposure to agonists, such as secretin, which increase intracellular cAMP levels, leads to a rapid series of events including 1) opening of Cl^- channels in the apical membrane and efflux of Cl^- ions into the duct lumen, 2) an increase in Cl^-/HCO_3^- exchange activity with a resultant increase in ductal HCO_3^- concentration, and 3) movement of water out of the cell through water channels or aquaporins. The findings that CFTR is localized to the apical membrane of cholangiocytes and secretin-stimulated Cl^- channels have properties analogous to CFTR, support a working model that postulates a role for CFTR in the regulation of ductular secretion. According to this model, the secretin-stimulated increase in Cl^- and HCO_3^- permeability is through PKA-dependent activation of CFTR. The generation of a lumen-negative potential favors movement of Na^+ into the bile duct through a paracellular pathway and water through aquaporins. Additionally, a small conductance, K^+ channel (SK2) has been identified in the basolateral membrane of cholangiocytes and plays an important role in maintaining the membrane potential difference necessary for continued transepithelial secretion [43]. Thus, CFTR appears to contribute to normal bile formation and alkalinization through the

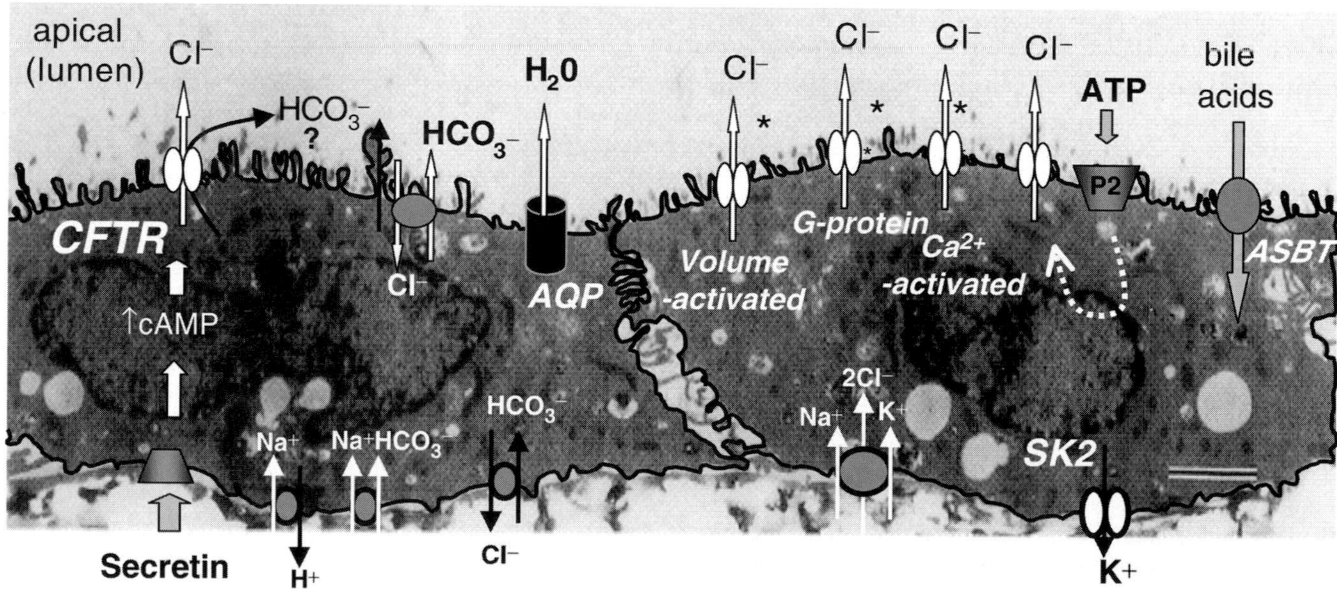

Figure 24.2. Model of cholangiocyte bile formation highlighting channels involved in secretion. Stimulation of basolateral receptors by secretin results in increases in cAMP and PKA-dependent stimulation of Cl^- efflux through CFTR. The transmembrane Cl^- gradient drives Cl^-/HCO_3^- exchange. Alternatively, HCO_3^- may enter bile through a conductive manner or through CFTR. Water is transported via aquaporin proteins. The increase in HCO_3^- and water secretion leads to alkalinization and dilution of bile. Other Cl^- channels, including volume-sensitive, P2 receptor linked, G-protein stimulated, and Ca^{2+}-activated, have been identified. Lumenal ATP and bile acids may also stimulate Cl^- efflux though the mechanisms are not defined. An apical transporter for bile acids has been identified (ASBT). On the basolateral membrane, Na^+/H^+ exchange, Na^+-dependent Cl^-/HCO_3^- exchange, and Na^+/HCO_3^- symport help to maintain intracellular pH and HCO_3^- concentrations. Cl^- uptake is mediated by an $Na^+/K^+/2Cl^-$ cotransporter. A small conductance Ca^{2+}-activated K^+ channel (SK2) has been identified in the basolateral membrane and may work in parallel with apical Cl^- channels to hyperpolarize the membrane and provide the driving force for continued secretion. See text for details. P2, purinergic receptor; ∗, location (apical vs. basolateral) not definitively established.

regulation of Cl^-, HCO_3^-, and water transport (Figure 24.1). Although this model implies a prominent role for CFTR in normal bile formation, it fails to explain why only a minority of patients with CF develop liver disease despite the fact that they all have abnormal or absent CFTR in bile duct epithelia. This observation suggests that CFTR may not be the predominant pathway for Cl^- secretion in cholangiocytes.

ALTERNATE CHANNELS AND CHOLANGIOCYTE SECRETION

In addition to CFTR, cholangiocytes express several other Cl^- channels, including a G-protein activated Cl^- channel [44], a Ca^{2+}-activated Cl^- channel [45,46], a purinergic receptor-linked Cl^- channel [47,48], and a volume-stimulated Cl^- channel [49] (Figure 24.2). However, their regulation and overall contribution to biliary secretion is largely unknown at present. It is attractive to speculate, however, that these alternate Cl^- conductances may partly compensate for the CF secretory defect in the liver and may serve to suggest alternate strategies to bypass the Cl^- secretory defect associated with CF. In other organs, the expression of alternate Cl^- channels may modulate the expression of disease. In fact, in the *cftr −/−* mouse model, increased expression of Ca^{2+}-activated Cl^- channels in tracheal epithelial cells is associated with mild pulmonary disease [50]. Exploring the pathways involved in the regulation of these alternate Cl^- channels has therefore become an exciting area of investigation.

It is interesting to note that these alternate channels are regulated independently of CFTR. Although CFTR is regulated in part through secretin acting on basolateral receptors to increase intracellular cAMP concentrations, these alternate channels may be stimulated by other agonists, including those acting from the luminal or apical membrane. In fact, constituents of bile, such as bile acids and ATP, have been shown to modulate cholangiocyte secretion in isolated cells in culture [47,51,52]. This exciting finding suggests that factors released by hepatocytes into bile may serve as signals coordinating the separate hepatic and biliary components of secretion, a process termed *hepatobiliary coupling.*

Cholangiocytes express transporters for bile acids on the apical membrane (Figure 24.2) [53]. Recent evidence in the rat cholangiocytes demonstrates the presence of an apical Na^+-dependent bile acid transporter (ASBT) similar to the ileal bile acid transporter and capable of transporting conjugated bile acids [53]. Additionally, bile acid uptake stimulates cholangiocyte secretion in isolated cells [52], suggesting a mechanism by which lumenal bile acids may modulate ductular secretion. This provides further evidence for the cholehepatic shunt hypothesis proposed by Hofmann et al. [54,55] and may help to explain the hypercholeresis, out of proportion to bile salt pool enrichment alone, observed with bile acid therapy [56]. In fact, in rats taurocholate feeding results in cholangiocyte proliferation and increases in secretion [57].

Another constituent of bile and shown to regulate cholangiocyte secretion is ATP. Recently, extracellular ATP has been identified as an important signaling molecule that regulates diverse cellular processes by binding to one or more *purinergic receptors* in the plasma membrane of target cells. Purinergic signaling may provide a means of regulating biliary secretion through hepatobiliary coupling [58]. ATP, in fact, is released by primary human hepatocytes [59] and model liver and biliary cell lines [48,60]; it is present in mammalian bile in concentrations (>100 nmol/mL) sufficient to activate purinergic receptors [61]. Cholangiocytes express a variety of nucleotide/nucleoside receptors, including both P2X and P2Y subtypes [62–64], and P2 receptor binding results in large increases in Cl^- secretion [47,51]. Although both hepatocytes and cholangiocytes are capable of the regulated release of ATP, the molecular identity of the ATP channel–transporter is currently unknown. There has been evidence both for [22] and against [65] CFTR as an ATP permeable channel. Recent studies suggest that CFTR may in fact regulate, but is distinct from, an ATP permeable pathway [37,66]. In fact, in *CFTR −/−* cells, extracellular ATP has been shown to elicit large increases in Cl^- secretion, suggesting that purinergic signaling activates non-CFTR Cl^- channels and may be a potential site for stimulation of secretion to bypass the Cl^- secretory defect associated with CF [63,67–69]. These findings have led to recent therapeutic trials of extracellular nucleotides in patients with CF. Aerosolized UTP, for instance, has been shown to increase mucociliary clearance in the lungs of patients with CF [70].

In summary, CFTR is a cAMP-dependent Cl^- channel expressed on the apical membrane of cholangiocytes that contributes to ductular secretion. However, the possible role of other membrane Cl^- channels is yet to be determined. Intriguing studies have established that CFTR, in addition to its role as a Cl^- channel, is in fact a "transmembrane regulator" modulating other membrane permeability pathways. Further study of CFTR function and regulation may help to elucidate the mechanisms of cholangiocyte function and bile formation. The remainder of this chapter focuses on the hepatobiliary effects of abnormal CFTR function, namely, CF-associated liver disease.

CFTR MUTATIONS

There are now more than 1400 recognized mutations in the CFTR gene (CFTR Mutation Data Base: http://www.genet.sickkids.on.ca/cftr). Worldwide, the ΔF508 mutation accounts for 66% of the described mutations while G542X and G551D, the next two most common mutations, account for 2.4% and 1.6%, respectively (CFTR Mutation Data Base) [71]. The incidence of CF in the Caucasian population corresponds to a carrier frequency of approximately 5%. This high carrier frequency in a lethal genetic disease suggests the possibility of a survival advantage for heterozygotes. In fact, it has been suggested that the absent or unresponsive Cl^- channel associated with CFTR mutations may have protected infants during epidemics of cholera, which causes secretory diarrhea through toxin-mediated, cAMP-dependent activation of Cl^- channels. The *cftr −/−* mouse has been shown to be resistant to the effects

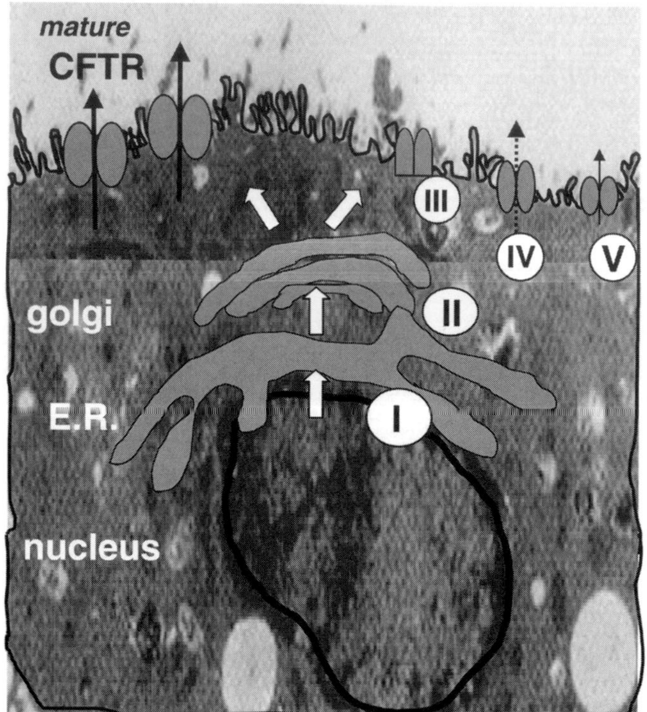

Figure 24.3. Classification of CFTR mutations. Class I mutations (nonsense and frameshift) result in abnormal mRNA production and no CFTR protein. Class II mutations (amino acid deletion, missense) result in abnormal CFTR protein trafficking with subsequent degradation. Class III mutations (missense) result in a mature CFTR protein that is refractory to normal activation. Class IV mutations (missense) result in a CFTR protein that localizes normally, but with a reduction in single-channel conductance. Class V mutations (alternative splicing, missense) result in a decreased full length mRNA and a decrease in the number of functional CFTR channels at the apical membrane. E.R., endoplasmic reticulum.

of cholera infection, providing some evidence for this theory [72].

The mutations are classified into five classes according to their effect on CFTR protein function [73] (Figure 24.3). Class I mutations (such as G542X and R553X) cause impairment of CFTR messenger RNA production. Class II mutations result in defective processing or trafficking of CFTR protein to the apical membrane. The most common mutation, ΔF508, is of this class and results in a base pair deletion in exon 10 with a consequent deletion of phenylalanine at position F508 in the first NBD region of the protein [12]. The ΔF508-CFTR protein does not fold correctly and is subsequently diverted from normal trafficking to the apical membrane and degraded by the ubiquitin–proteosome pathway. Class III mutations (G551D and others) are associated with defective regulation of CFTR, which locates correctly to the apical membrane but does not respond to cAMP agonists. Class IV mutations (R117H and others) demonstrate some residual Cl^- conductance but at a significantly decreased amplitude. Class V mutations (A455E, P574H, and others) lead to abnormal splicing of CFTR with partial reduction in the number of functioning Cl^- channels. Mutations of classes I, II, and III are considered severe because they result in an absence of functioning CFTR at the plasma membrane, whereas class IV and V are "mild" mutations with some residual CFTR activity demonstrated.

The report from the CFF registry, which records data from the United States CF centers, reveals that ΔF508/ΔF508 homozygotes account for 50.6% and ΔF508/other heterozygotes account for 37.9% of the mutations reported in the United States (CFF Registry) [3]. This is similar to data provided by the European Epidemiologic Registry of Cystic Fibrosis (ERCF) [74]. In this population, class II mutation homozygotes accounted for 56% of all mutations and comprised the largest group. The other classes of mutations, class I, class III, and class IV homozygotes represented 0.8%, 0.2%, and 0.05%, respectively. There were no class V homozygotes. Class II/III mutation compound heterozygotes comprised 2.9% of the genotypes, and class IV/any (mild mutations) accounted for 2% of the mutations. Interestingly, abnormal elevation of serum liver enzymes (1.5× normal) was much less frequent in class IV/any heterozygotes than in any other group. Patients heterozygous for a class IV mutation had milder disease in general, and it is suggested that class IV mutations may offer some protection from pancreatic insufficiency and diabetes.

Overall, although specific gene mutations have been associated with the severity of pancreatic involvement, there is no correlation between specific genotype and clinically detectable liver disease in patients with CF [75–77]. However, there appears to be a lower frequency of liver disease in pancreatic-sufficient patients who generally have milder mutations [78]. Because all patients with CF have abnormal CFTR in the biliary tree, it is unclear why significant liver disease does not develop in all patients. Because patients with CF and identical CFTR mutations exhibit variable onset and severity of liver disease, it is postulated that there are other modifying genetic or environmental factors that determine whether clinically significant hepatobiliary involvement will occur.

PATHOGENESIS OF LIVER INJURY

The pathophysiology underlying the development of CF-associated liver disease is still only speculative. Definitive studies directly assessing the effects of abnormal CFTR in the liver are lacking. Several proposed pathways in the pathogenesis of CF liver disease are shown in Figure 24.4. One leading hypothesis is that impaired secretory function of cholangiocytes results in a decrease in bile flow (cholestasis) and thickened, inspissated secretions in the bile ductules. The subsequent bile duct obstruction leads to liver cell injury and the development of fibrosis and cirrhosis. The histologic finding of inspissated eosinophilic material in bile ducts, a pathognomonic lesion in CF, provides some morphologic evidence for this "bile duct plugging" theory [79]. Theoretically, abnormal viscosity of bile could result from several factors including defective transport of Cl^-, HCO_3^-, and mucins, Na^+ reabsorption, altered composition of the bile acid pool, or a combination of these. Bile duct

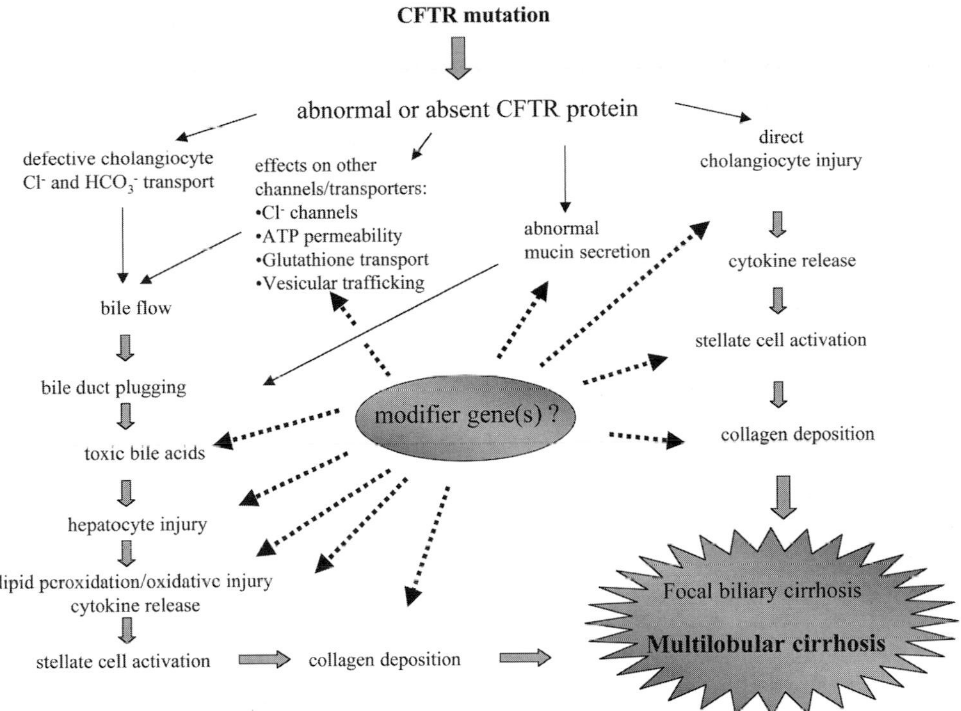

Figure 24.4. A proposed model of the pathogenesis of CF liver disease.

plugging would be anticipated to initiate a series of secondary steps including cholangiocyte injury, release of inflammatory mediators, and stellate cell activation with subsequent deposition of collagen, ultimately leading to fibrosis and cirrhosis.

Alternatively, the initiating step may be direct cholangiocyte injury due to an abnormal CFTR protein. As mentioned earlier, the most common mutation ΔF508 results in protein misfolding and subsequent degradation by the ubiquitin proteosome pathway. The misfolded protein can potentially form aggresomes, which may lead to cellular injury as seen in many neurodegenerative diseases [80]. This suggests a possible role of chaperone proteins, which are responsible for quality control mechanisms in the cell by targeting and degrading abnormal or misfolded proteins in the disease pathogenesis [81]. In fact, diseases associated with abnormal protein degradation (such as CF or alpha-1-antitrypsin deficiency) are receiving more interest and suggest that mechanisms that target chaperone proteins and the degradation pathway may provide therapeutic strategies for these diseases in the future.

Although the initiating event in the development of liver disease is unknown, it appears that a progressive fibrogenic process ultimately leads to cirrhosis in a subset of patients. It is felt that this continuum from cholestasis to focal biliary obstruction and ultimately to cirrhosis may progress over many years. Genetic and environmental factors may modify any and all components of the pathway and may explain the heterogeneity in the liver response to abnormal CFTR function. Several potential factors that have been proposed to contribute to, or modify, the liver injury in CF include altered mucin secretion, accumulation of toxic bile acids, abnormal oxidant–antioxidant balance, stellate cell activation, and fat accumulation (steatosis).

Mucins

Hypersecretion of mucus is a major contributor to the lung pathology in CF. If similar factors are operable in the bile duct, then one potential etiology of increased bile viscosity would be altered mucin secretion. The viscous properties of mucus are determined in large part by mucin glycoproteins. The role of mucins in the bile duct is not defined, and there is conflicting evidence linking CFTR and mucin secretion [33,82]. Although secretion of chondroitin sulfate was shown to be markedly elevated in CF biliary epithelium in vitro [83]. Assessing the presence of altered viscosity and the role of mucin secretion in the development of CF liver disease awaits further evaluation.

Toxic Bile Acids

Patients with CF may have an altered bile acid pool, with an increase in hydrophobic and a decrease in hydrophilic bile acids. In fact, a recent study examining bile acid profiles in CF patients found a higher level of endogenous biliary ursodeoxycholic acid (UDCA) in CF patients without liver disease compared with those with CF-associated liver disease [84]. The authors suggested that the elevated UDCA in CF patients without liver disease may play a possible protective role. In addition to a decrease in hyprophilic bile acids, retaining hydrophobic bile acids may be responsible for subsequent hepatocyte injury, as seen in other cholestatic disorders. Hydrophobic bile acids have been associated with altered mitochondrial respiration and stimulation of the mitochondrial membrane permeability transition, a key process involved in cellular apoptosis and necrosis [85].

The increase in hydrophobic bile acids may provide a possible explanation of how the biliary plugging and cholangiocyte injury translates into subsequent hepatocyte injury.

Antioxidants

Several studies have suggested that there is an imbalance between oxidant injury and antioxidant defenses in cystic fibrosis [86]. This imbalance may be due to the malabsorption of dietary antioxidants such as vitamin E, tocopherols, beta-carotene, and other carotenoids or through direct effects of CFTR on the transport of antioxidants such as glutathione. In fact, recent evidence suggests that glutathione transport is an intrinsic property of CFTR [21]. Potentially, CFTR-mediated glutathione transport may decrease mucus viscosity by disruption of bond formation in mucin proteins or may exert effects through modulation of redox reactions at the epithelial surface. In the liver, a decrease in lipid-soluble antioxidant activity may potentially result in increased free radical production and oxidative hepatic injury [87]. Antioxidants may counteract these effects on the mitochondrial membrane and suggest other potential novel therapies for CF associated liver disease [88–90].

Stellate Cells

Hepatic stellate cells have been implicated in the pathogenesis of cystic fibrosis and may play a role in the progressive fibrosis characteristic of this disorder [91]. Potentially, activation of stellate cells could occur through direct cholangiocyte or indirect hepatocyte injury with subsequent release of proinflammatory cytokines. In liver biopsy specimens of CF patients, stellate cells have been found located in the periportal regions of the liver and, their activation has been correlated with areas of collagen deposition and fibrosis [91]. One of the earliest effects of stellate cell activation is an increase in the production of extracellular matrix proteins, including types II, III, and IV collagen [92,93]. Elucidation of the role of stellate cells in the progressive fibrosis associated with liver disease, may suggest novel therapies targeting these cells.

Steatosis

Hepatic steatosis is a common finding in CF, although it is unclear whether it is due to abnormal CFTR and the cholangiocyte transport defect or represents a separate, secondary entity. Several factors may contribute to hepatic steatosis in CF including malnutrition, essential fatty acid deficiency, ethanol ingestion, and elevated circulating levels of cytokines [94–96]. How increased levels of intracellular fat cause liver disease is an ongoing area of investigation. It may be that the hepatic steatosis as observed in CF provides an increased substrate for lipid peroxidation and oxidative injury. It is unclear whether hepatic steatosis progresses to fibrosis or multilobular cirrhosis; however, the progressive nature of other disorders associated with fat accumulation (nonalcoholic fatty liver disease) suggests that steatosis may not be as benign a condition in CF as once thought.

Further studies into the pathogenesis of CF liver disease are clearly needed. It is hoped that the use of novel models of biliary epithelium and animal models will help to further our knowledge. Recently, a mouse model has been developed that develops liver disease similar to that observed in humans and may provide important insight into the factors responsible for the development and progression of CF liver disease [97].

POTENTIAL GENETIC MODIFIERS

Family studies suggest that factors independent of CFTR contribute to the development of liver disease. Studies of families with multiple members with CF and at least one with liver disease revealed a concordance rate of CF liver disease of 20% [77]. Another study of sets of CF siblings discordant for liver disease could not identify any overt environmental factor contributing to the development of liver disease [98]. These observations have led to the intense scrutiny of the role of modifier genes in the pathogenesis of CF liver disease. Several associations or risk factors for the development of liver disease in CF have been described, including male sex, history of meconium ileus, human leukocyte antigen (HLA) type, and heterozygosity for mutations of other ion channel or liver diseases.

Male Sex

A preponderance of male patients has been described in all age groups of patients with CF and liver disease [4,99,100]. Given the reported survival advantage for males with CF [101], it is unclear whether male sex is indeed an independent risk factor or represents an overrepresentation in the study population. Although it is becoming clear that sex hormones may influence hepatic transporter expression as well as other liver functions [102], providing a possible cellular rationale for this potential correlation.

Meconium Ileus

Several studies have suggested that a history of meconium ileus as an infant is a risk factor for the subsequent development of liver disease. Maurage et al. [103] reported this risk factor to be present in 50% of patients with CF-associated cirrhosis and 14% of those without. Colombo et al. [75,104] have described a history of meconium ileus in 35% of patients with liver disease but in only 12% of patients without liver disease, and these authors suggested that there may be an overall sixfold increase in the development of liver disease in those infants with a history of meconium ileus. However, other studies have failed to find such an association [105]. A gene locus, termed CF Modifier gene 1 (CFM1), on chromosome 19q13 was initially identified as a modifier of meconium ileus expression [106]. Although the actual gene and protein product are unknown, a candidate gene in the region codes for KCCN, a K^+ channel. More recent studies using high-performance single nucleotide polymorphisms and complex linkage analysis have not confirmed a linkage in this region, and further studies are ongoing [107].

Immune System and Antioxidant Status

Several studies have shown an association between certain histocompatibility antigens (HLA) and susceptibility for liver disease in CF. A higher frequency of HLA-DQw6 has been reported in British CF patients with liver disease compared with those without liver disease [108,109]. Duthie et al. [110] found HLA haplotype DQ6 in 66% of patients with liver disease but in only 33% without it. Two other antigens, DR15 and B7, with linkage disequilibrium with this locus, were also significant risk factors. It is interesting to note that the association was greater in male than in female subjects, and only in male subjects when the phenotype was restricted to portal hypertension (representing more severe disease). These findings suggest a possible immune contribution to the pathogenesis of hepatobiliary injury or, alternatively, another susceptibility gene linked with specific haplotypes lies at or near the HLA-DQ locus. Other studies have shown an association between the development of liver disease and polymorphisms for the genes for TGF-β [111] and angiotensin converting enzyme [112], an enzyme involved in TGF-β activation. Mannose-binding lectin (MBL), a component of innate immunity involved in complement activation in response to infection, is encoded by the MBL2 gene, and in one study homozygous and compound heterozygotes for MBL variants were found in significant excess among CF patients with cirrhotic liver disease [113]. Lastly, one study has shown an association between polymorphisms in the gene for glutathione S-transferase, a hepatic detoxifying enzyme, and the development of CF liver disease [114]. This is interesting in light of the association between CFTR and glutathione transport, suggesting that patients with altered CFTR function may have a primary imbalance in antioxidant defenses. The role of modifier genes in the immune and antioxidant defense systems may provide important insight into the pathogenesis of disease, as well as suggest new therapeutic options.

Other Ion Channels

It has been proposed that other Cl^- channels may modify phenotypic expression of CF. Several mouse models of CF have demonstrated the importance of other Cl^- channels in modulating organ-level disease expression. Clarke et al. [50] demonstrated that expression of Ca^{2+}-activated Cl^- channels in the lung of cftr –/– mice may explain the mild pulmonary disease in these animals. Rozmahel et al. [115] described modulation of the severity of the gastrointestinal disease by a locus that may code for ion channel proteins [115], and Ritzka et al. [116] described the CLCA gene locus, encoding for a Ca^{2+}-activated Cl^- channel as a modulator of the gastrointestinal disease in humans. The role of other ion channels and transporters in normal bile formation as well as the pathogenesis of CF liver disease remains to be established.

Other Liver Diseases

Recent studies have sought to determine whether patients with CF liver disease are heterozygote carriers of another genetic mutation for common liver diseases that render the liver more susceptible to injury in the presence of abnormal CFTR function. Although hemochromatosis is one of the most common genetic liver diseases in the Caucasian population, no increased frequency of heterozygote carriers for this genetic disease was found in patients with CF liver disease or meconium ileus [117]. Another commonly inherited genetic disease with known liver involvement is α-1 antitrypsin deficiency. Preliminary data suggest an increase in frequency of heterozygote carriers for the α-1 antitrypsin mutation allele among CF patients with liver disease compared with those without [118,119]. This association was greatest for female subjects, although larger confirmatory studies are required for validation of this interesting observation. Over the last several years, the genetic basis of many cholestatic liver disorders have been identified and have shed light on the basic mechanisms of bile formation. The contribution of these genes and corresponding proteins (e.g., BSEP, MDR3, FIC-1, or cMOAT) to the development of CF liver disease should be evaluated.

PREVALENCE

Determining the true prevalence of CF liver disease has been difficult because 1) no universally accepted definition has been established, 2) many patients with significant liver disease are compensated and remain asymptomatic, and 3) there are no sensitive and specific markers for the diagnosis of CF liver disease.

The most recent data (from 2003) from the CF foundation national CF registry [3] reported elevated liver enzymes in 4.3% of patients older than 18 years of age and in 3.2% of those 18 years or older, whereas liver cirrhosis was reported in 1.4% of patients seen in U.S. CF centers. It should be noted that these numbers rely on self-reporting and therefore appear to underestimate significantly the true prevalence of liver disease. Although retrospective analyses have reported prevalence figures between 4.2 and 24% with a slight predominance in males and a peak in adolescence [99,100,120], autopsy data indicate a progressive increase in prevalence with age from 10% in infants to 72% in adults [79,121].

Four large prospective studies from different countries have been performed and may help to provide more accurate estimates of the true prevalence of clinically significant CF-associated liver disease. A prospective study of 153 CF patients in Australia by Gaskin et al. [122] revealed the presence of hepatomegaly in 30% of patients, whereas 13% had multilobular cirrhosis defined by biochemical, clinical, and imaging criteria [122]. A prospective study from Sweden by Lindblad et al. [123] in 124 patients with CF, followed over a 15-year period, revealed abnormal biochemical markers of liver disease in 25% of children and the development of cirrhosis in 10% as confirmed by liver biopsy [123]. In this study, severe liver disease occurred predominantly by preadolescence or adolescence. Additionally, no risk factors for the development of liver disease were identified. However, deficiency of essential fatty acids was associated with steatosis. A prospective study from Italy by Colombo et al. [124] followed 177 CF patients up to a median of 14 years [124]. Significant liver disease (defined by persistent hepatomegaly, elevated liver enzymes on two consecutive visits, and ultrasound abnormalities) developed in 47 patients (26.5%) with an incidence rate of 1.8 cases per 100 patient years. Cirrhosis was present in 5 (10%) and developed in 12 other patients, giving an incidence rate of 4.5 per 100 liver disease patient years. In this study, meconium ileus, male sex, and severe CFTR mutations were associated with the development of liver disease. Lastly, a study from Canada by Lamireau et al. [125] reported a prevalence of 18% at 2 years, 29% at 5 years, and 41% at 12 years.. Cirrhosis developed in 7.8% of patients at a median of 10 years, and the development of liver disease was independently associated with a history of meconium ileus and pancreatic insufficiency. The high prevalence rates in this study may reflect the more lenient definition of liver disease used (the findings on more than one occasion of either abnormal liver enzymes or abnormal ultrasound imaging). Together, based on these prospective studies, the best current estimate for clinically significant liver disease in children with CF is approximately 10–26% with cirrhosis occurring in approximately 7–13%. Additionally, in contrast to the autopsy data, which suggest that there is an increase in the development of liver disease over time, most prospective studies revealed that liver disease developed before or during adolescence, suggesting that most patients who will develop clinically significant liver disease will do so at an early age.

CLINICAL MANIFESTATIONS

The two most common clinical presentations of liver disease in CF are 1) an abnormal liver on physical examination (hepatomegaly or a small hard liver) or 2) elevated serum liver enzymes on routine screening. A small, hard liver on exam or signs of portal hypertension suggest cirrhosis. It should be noted that patients with CF can present with end-stage liver disease and even cirrhosis with few, if any, outward signs to suggest chronic liver disease. Hepatomegaly suggests steatosis or focal biliary cirrhosis but may also suggest congestive hepatopathy associated with cor pulmonale and right heart failure. These distinct clinical manifestations including hepatic steatosis, neonatal cholestasis, focal biliary cirrhosis, and multilobular cirrhosis have been described based on clinical or histologic criteria and have variable prevalence rates (Table 24.1 [75,79,100, 120–123,126–134]).

Congestive Hepatopathy

Although hepatic congestion is not a direct result of defective CFTR protein in bile duct epithelial cells, it nonetheless should be considered a clinically significant cause of hepatomegaly in CF. Chronically elevated right-sided heart pressures or cor pulmonale may lead to congestive hepatopathy through increased hepatic vein and sinusoidal pressures. The elevated sinusoidal pressure is thought to cause hepatocyte injury and necrosis. Eventually this can progress to "cardiac cirrhosis" with the development of bands of fibrosis extending between centrilobular areas with intervening normal portal areas. Other signs of elevated right-sided pressures, such as jugular venous distention, are often present. The diagnosis should be considered in those CF patients with chronic lung disease, clinical signs of cor pulmonale, a large liver (and sometimes tender) on exam, and dilated hepatic veins on ultrasound examination. Ultrasonography with Doppler and echocardiography are therefore the main modalities that aid in the diagnosis. Additionally, Doppler ultrasonography or angiography can be helpful to exclude other vascular complications such as thrombosis of hepatic veins or inferior vena cava. Biochemical analysis usually reveals aminotransferase levels that are only mildly elevated (<2–3 times normal), and a prothrombin time that is normal or only slightly prolonged (<5 seconds prolonged) [135]. If aminotransferases are greater than 3 times normal, consideration should be given to the co-occurrence of other liver disorders. It is important to exclude hepatic congestion as a cause of hepatomegaly before any consideration of a percutaneous liver biopsy because the dilated hepatic veins associated with this condition increase the risk of bleeding, and therefore, a transjugular or surgical approach should be considered in that circumstance. Treatment of this disorder relies on improving the underlying cardiac or lung disease. Correcting any existing nutritional and antioxidant deficiencies may be of theoretical benefit in reducing oxidant injury associated with ischemia-reperfusion injury.

Table 24.1: Hepatobiliary Manifestations of Cystic Fibrosis

Condition	*% Affected*	*Reference*
Asymptomatic elevation of liver enzymes	10–46	[75,126]
Liver		
Hepatomegaly	30	[75,122,123]
Hepatic steatosis	20–60	[127]
Neonatal cholestasis	2–38	[128–130]
Focal biliary cirrhosis	10–72	[79,121]
Multilobular cirrhosis	7–20	[75,100,121,122]
Hepatocellular carcinoma	Very rare	[131]
Biliary Tract		
Microgallbladder	20–30	[129,132]
Cholelithiasis	1–10	[100,133]
Common bile duct stenosis	<2	[120]
Sclerosing cholangitis	<1	[120]
Cholangiocarcinoma	Very rare	[134]

Neonatal Cholestasis

Prolonged neonatal cholestasis may be quite common in newborns with CF. In one CF report, 35% of infants with CF had evidence of hepatomegaly or cholestasis within the first few months of life [129], and autopsy data has revealed histologic evidence of obstructive cholestasis in 38% of patients aged less than 3 years with CF [79]. Other series of patients have not reported such a high incidence of prolonged neonatal cholestasis [130,136], and most patients with CF do not have an early history of jaundice. Infants with CF and cholestasis should be evaluated thoroughly to exclude other cholestatic liver diseases, such as biliary atresia. On exam, hepatomegaly may be present and biochemical evaluation reveals elevation of serum direct bilirubin and GGT concentrations. Stools may be acholic as in other cholestatic disorders, such as biliary atresia. The etiology of this disorder is unknown but may be multifactorial. Coexistent factors such as abdominal surgery, parenteral nutrition, or infection may contribute to prolonged cholestasis. Some studies have suggested an association between meconium ileus and neonatal cholestasis, occurring together in up to 50% of cases [103,130]; however, others have not confirmed such an association [99]. The natural history of this disorder is unknown and may resolve without any long-term sequela. There does not appear to be an increased risk for the long-term development of cirrhosis with an early history of neonatal cholestasis [122]. It is important, however, to consider the diagnosis of CF in infants who present with cholestasis. A sweat test or genotype testing should therefore be performed as part of the evaluation of neonatal cholestasis.

Steatosis

Hepatic steatosis is characterized by a large but soft liver on palpation (Figure 24.5A). Other signs of chronic liver disease or portal hypertension are usually not present. Histologic examination reveals hepatic parenchymal cells filled with micro- and macrovesicular fat (Figure 24.5B). Ultrasound has been used to aid in the diagnosis; however, the true sensitivity or specificity of this modality to determine the presence of steatosis and exclude other causes is still unknown. Other imaging

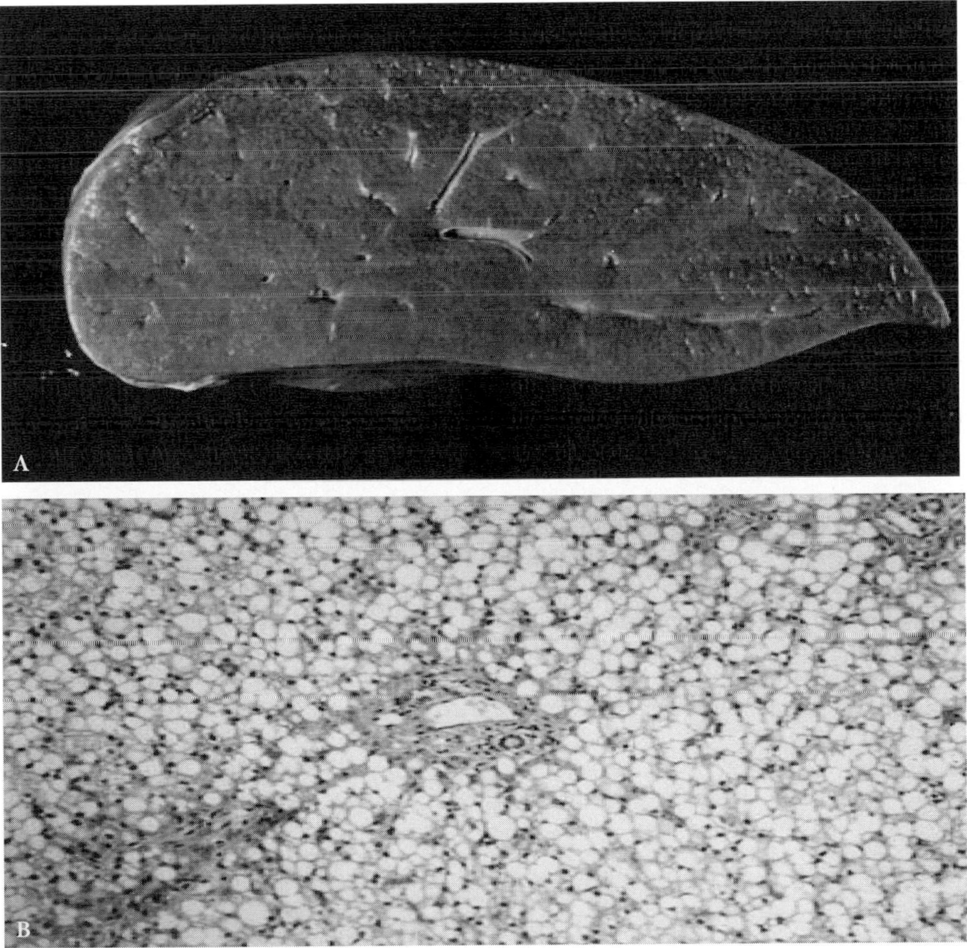

Figure 24.5. Steatosis in cystic fibrosis. (**A**) Cut section of the liver revealing extensive fatty infiltration. The liver is large and soft. (**B**) Photomicrograph of a histologic section from the liver above. Histology reveals extensive micro- and macrovesicular fat. (Hematoxylin and eosin staining.) (Courtesy of Dr. Arthur Weinberg, University of Texas Southwestern Medical Center, Dallas, Texas.)

studies such as computed tomography (CT) or magnetic resonance imaging (MRI) have also been used to reveal fat density of the liver, although once again the sensitivity of these modalities to diagnosis steatosis in CF is unknown. This lesion is relatively common in CF, occurring in 20–60% of affected patients depending on the study [127]. The etiology is unknown; however, it has been suggested that steatosis may result from the effect of circulating cytokines on hepatic fatty acid oxidation [89]. It is unclear whether this is a result of abnormal CFTR function in cholangiocytes or reflects a secondary effect due to malnutrition or deficiency of trace element or minerals. Hepatic steatosis has been associated with deficiencies in trace elements, essential fatty acids, and carnitine, as well as diabetes and ethanol use [137–139]. In fact, steatosis may resolve with improved nutritional status and correction of trace mineral, vitamin, or fatty acid deficiencies. Although this lesion is felt to be benign and nonprogressive, the recent interest in nonalcoholic steatohepatitis (NASH) as a cause of cirrhosis in adults may lead to a reappraisal of this belief [138].

Focal Biliary Cirrhosis and Multilobular Cirrhosis

Focal biliary cirrhosis is characterized histologically by focal areas of portal inflammation and fibrosis, bile duct obstruction and proliferation, and the inclusion of eosinophilic material in bile ductules (Figure 24.6). This lesion is considered pathonogmonic of CF liver disease. The focal areas of fibrosis may give the liver a furrowed appearance (Figure 24.6A). The pink-staining eosinophilic material seen in the bile ductules, as well as the focal nature of the lesion, provides more evidence for the "bile duct plugging" hypothesis as contributing to the pathogenesis of this disease. The clinical diagnosis of focal biliary cirrhosis is difficult as both the physical exam and biochemical evaluation may be normal. Additionally, ultrasound examination has

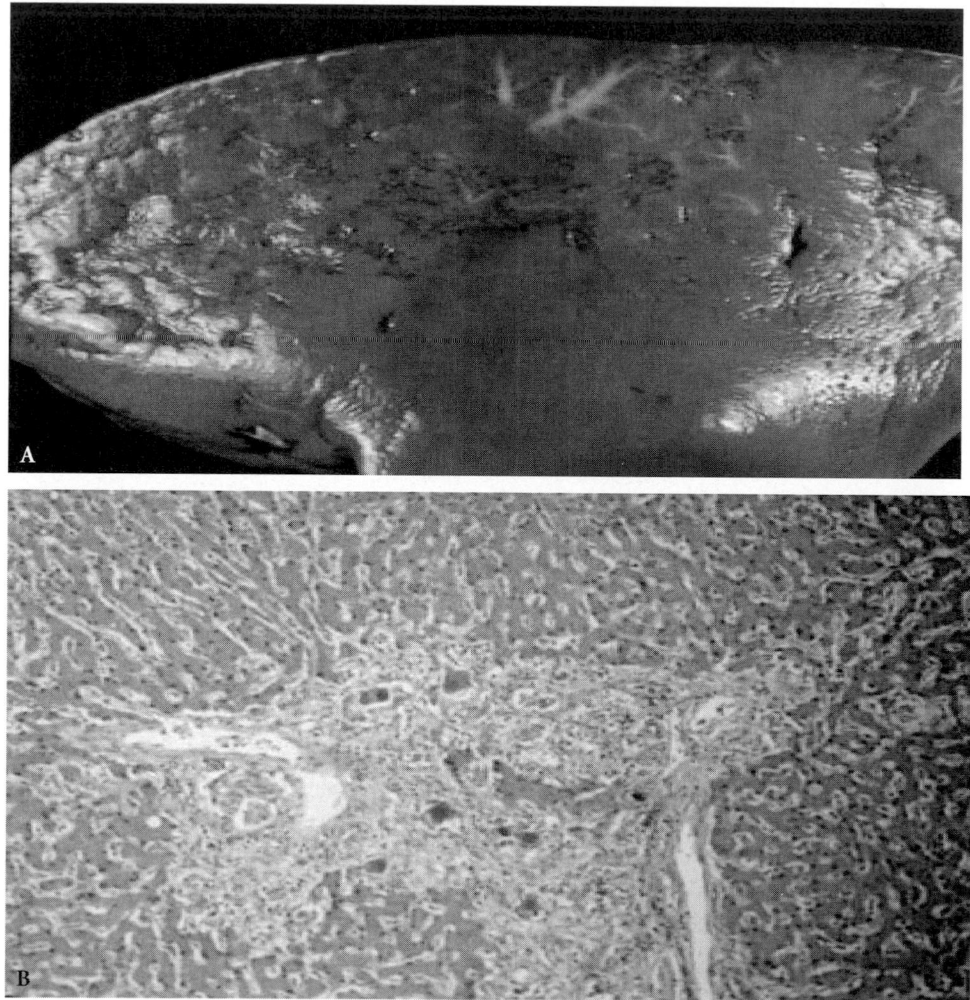

Figure 24.6. Focal biliary cirrhosis in cystic fibrosis. (**A**) The surface of the liver displays focal areas of scarring and furrowing. Large areas of normal preserved hepatic architecture are present. (**B**) Photomicrograph of a histologic section from liver above. The portal tract is expanded with bile duct proliferation and plugging of ducts with "eosinophilic material." Cholestasis and significant bands of fibrosis are present. (Hematoxylin and eosin staining.) (Courtesy of Dr. Arthur Weinberg, University of Texas Southwestern Medical Center, Dallas, Texas.) For color reproduction of (**A**), see Color Plate 24.6.

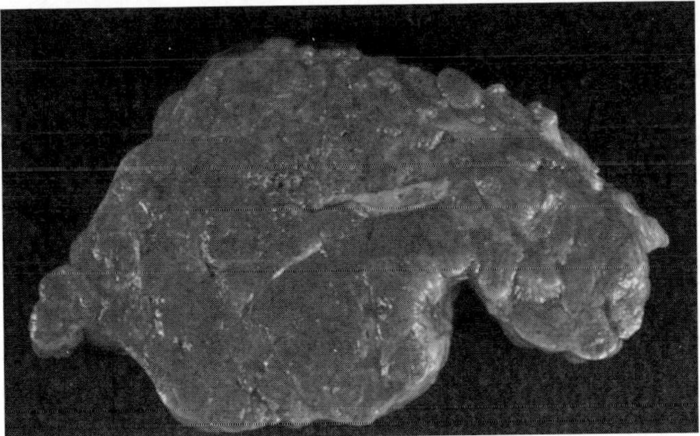

Figure 24.7. Multilobular cirrhosis in cystic fibrosis. Cut section of the liver revealing significant lobulation, fibrosis, scarring, and cirrhosis. (Courtesy of Dr. Arthur Weinberg, University of Texas Southwestern Medical Center, Dallas, Texas.) For color reproduction, see Color Plate 24.7.

not proved to detect this lesion reliably. Given the silent nature of this lesion, the prevalence of focal biliary cirrhosis can only be estimated from autopsy series. Autopsy studies indicate an increasing incidence of this lesion with increasing age, and focal biliary cirrhosis may progress into the more severe multilobular cirrhosis with portal hypertension or liver failure [140]. The disease was identified after death in 10% of infants dying in the first 3 months of life, in 27% dying after 1 year [79], and in 72% of adults [121]. It is unknown why a subset of patients with focal biliary cirrhosis will progress to more severe liver disease and eventually multilobular cirrhosis.

Multilobular cirrhosis is characterized histologically by extensive, broad bands of fibrosis extending between portal areas (Figure 24.7). The liver is extensively lobulated, and within the individual lobules, both focal areas of scarring, as well as intervening areas of normal hepatocyte parenchyma, are present. Physical examination reveals a multilobulated and firm liver; in fact, the extensive lobulation is characteristic of this lesion. Signs of chronic liver disease such as clubbing, spider angiomata, and palmar erythema may be present. The identification of splenomegaly or ascites may herald the development of portal hypertension. Prospective studies have suggested prevalence rates of multilobular cirrhosis as high as 17%, and the majority of patients identified were less than 14 years of age [75,100,122]. This is consistent with an adult autopsy study demonstrating cirrhosis in 20% [121]. Recent studies from Colombo et al. [124] have confirmed that the majority of patients with significant CF liver disease develop it by early adolescence. Patients with multilobular cirrhosis are at risk from complications of end-stage liver disease and portal hypertension, including esophageal varices, ascites, encephalopathy, fatigue, splenomegaly, hypersplenism, and coagulopathy. In fact, complications from portal hypertension cause the majority of morbidity with this liver lesion. Impaired bile flow may lead to fat malabsorption and fat-soluble vitamin deficiencies. Treatment is based on correction of these deficiencies, optimizing nutritional status, and therapy with UDCA, as described in more detail later.

Biliary Tract Disease

Biliary abnormalities are common in CF, although it is unclear how a defective or absent CFTR protein results in the biliary manifestations such as gallbladder atrophy or bile duct stenosis. These findings may suggest even another potential role of CFTR, namely, as a developmental regulator of the biliary tree and gallbladder. A small or microgallbladder is present in 20–30% of patients with CF, and although it appears to be a benign condition without clinical sequela [129], the finding in an infant should at least raise the suspicion of biliary atresia, which has been described in CF patients.

Cholelithiasis is found in 1–10% of patients, however clinical symptoms of cholecystitis have been reported to occur in less than 4% of cases, usually in older children [141]. The main component of gallstones in CF is calcium bilirubinate, which is resistant to dissolution by UDCA therapy [142]. Cholecystectomy is therefore the treatment of choice for gallbladder stones in symptomatic patients. The approach is not as clearly defined in the asymptomatic patient, in whom stones are identified with routine ultrasound, although consideration should be given to elective cholecystectomy, if pulmonary function is stable, because these stones increase the risk of cholecystitis and future complications.

Common bile duct stenosis is a rare complication of CF, occurring in less than 1% of patients. Although sclerosing cholangitis has been described in association with CF, the true incidence is unknown as the characteristic endoscopic retrograde cholangiography (ERCP) findings may be misleading in the face of inspissated biliary secretions. An increased prevalence of CFTR mutations has been reported in patients with primary sclerosing cholangitis, suggesting that patients with inflammatory bowel disease who are heterozygote carriers of CF gene mutations may be at an increased risk for the development of sclerosing cholangitis [143].

DIAGNOSIS AND SCREENING

It is important to note that at present there are no established diagnostic criteria universally accepted to establish the presence of CF liver disease. The diagnosis is usually established by a constellation of findings, including (1) an abnormal physical exam (hepatomegaly; or a small, hard liver; splenomegaly; signs of portal hypertension; or other signs of chronic liver disease), (2) persistently elevated liver enzymes (greater than 3 times normal on two or more sequential occasions), (3) abnormal imaging studies (abnormal ultrasound or other imaging modality demonstrating multilobular cirrhosis), or 4) abnormal liver histology.

Physical Examination

A meticulous clinical examination is the fundamental means for detecting and following the progression of liver disease in CF. A careful liver examination should be performed at every clinic visit and at least yearly. An abnormal examination suggests underlying pathology and warrants further evaluation. Hepatomegaly is the most important finding to suggest the presence of liver disease. However, simply noting the degree that the liver edge is below the rib margin may be misleading due to the lung hyperinflation often present in CF. Therefore, the entire span should be carefully measured and recorded. Hepatomegaly should be defined as a liver size above the upper limit of normal for age. If hepatomegaly is confirmed, then consideration should be given to the predominant lesion present (steatosis, focal biliary cirrhosis, or congestive hepatopathy secondary to chronic pulmonary or cardiac disease). Conversely, the presence of a small, hard liver or a multilobulated liver edge suggests cirrhosis. In this setting, portal hypertension is suggested by splenomegaly and dilated abdominal wall vasculature. Examination for other signs of chronic liver disease (palmar erythema, clubbing, or spider nevi) should always be conducted. A complete nutritional assessment should be performed in conjunction with a dietician including an evaluation for any clinical signs of fat-soluble deficiency (a detailed description of the manifestations and evaluation of fat-soluble vitamin deficiencies can be found in Chapter 10).

Biochemical Evaluation

Serum liver enzyme analysis should be performed on a yearly basis as recommended by the CF Foundation Hepatobiliary Disease Consensus guidelines [144]. These should include aspartate aminotransferase, alanine aminotransferase, bilirubin (total and direct), alkaline phosphatase, and glutamyltransferase. It should be noted that none of the biochemical measures have been shown to correlate with the degree of hepatic fibrosis in CF. In fact, patients may have completely normal liver enzymes in the presence of cirrhosis. Conversely, elevations in serum liver enzymes are common in CF, occurring in 10–46% of patients and may not represent true liver disease [126,133]. Therefore the diagnosis of CF liver disease cannot rely solely on elevated liver enzymes at one point in time. Based on these uncertainties in the evaluation of serum liver enzymes, the CFF hepatobiliary consensus group has proposed a strategy for the interpretation of these tests (Figure 24.8). If a value is greater than 1.5 times the upper limit of normal for age, it is recommended that that value should be repeated in 3–6 months. If the level remains elevated for more than 6 months, without another explanation, it is indicative of possibly clinically significant liver involvement. At any time, if a value is greater than 3 times normal, tests of liver synthetic function, including prothrombin time, total protein, albumin, blood ammonia, cholesterol, and glucose should be performed and further evaluation into the etiology performed. Exclusion of other causes of aminotransferase elevation, such as drugs, toxins, infectious hepatitis, biliary atresia, α-1-antitrypsin deficiency, autoimmune hepatitis, or other metabolic liver diseases, should be done when appropriate. It should be noted that in large series of patients with suspected CF liver disease, other liver diseases, such as biliary atresia and α-1-antitrypsin deficiency, have been reported.

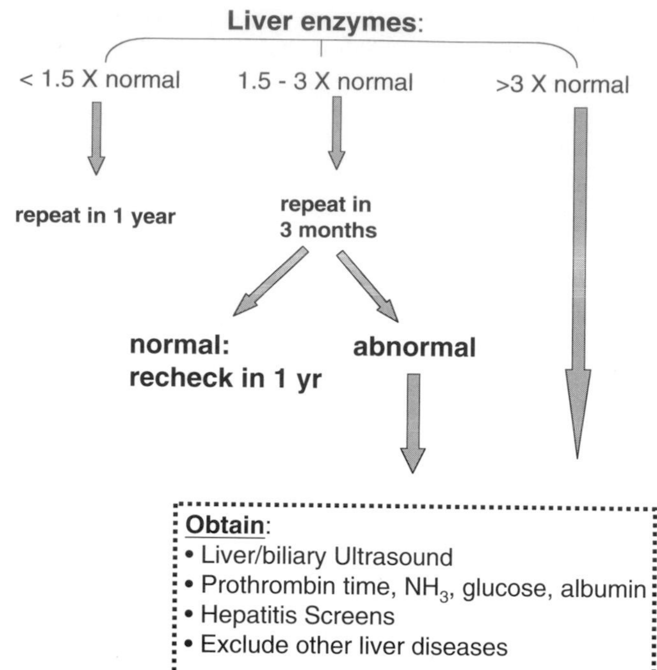

Figure 24.8. Serum liver enzyme screening protocol for the detection of CF liver disease. Based on the CF Foundation Hepatobiliary Disease Consensus Guidelines. Assumes physical exam is normal and patient has no clinical evidence of liver disease. Serum liver enzymes should be obtained annually. If levels are persistently greater than 1.5 times normal (on at least two consecutive occasions) or greater than 3 times normal, then further evaluation is indicated. See text for further description.

Ultrasonography

One of the most helpful imaging studies is ultrasonography (US) of the liver and biliary tract. The CF Hepatobiliary Consensus Group has recommended obtaining an U/S in all patients with CF in whom liver disease is suspected [144]. US is presently the modality of choice to screen for biliary tract abnormalities in CF (biliary obstruction or stricture, gallstones, gallbladder abnormalities). Additionally, combined with Doppler, US is helpful in evaluating the vasculature. Reversal of flow (hepatofugal) in the portal vein usually indicates portal hypertension. Likewise, dilated hepatic veins suggest cor pulmonale or right heart failure. However, in one study Doppler US was found to be inaccurate for the diagnosis of portal hypertension in CF [145]. Some recent studies suggest that US may be useful in the initial screening to determine the predominant lesion present as well as following the progression of liver disease. In fact, a US scoring system has been proposed and may correlate with markers of hepatic disease, specifically signs of portal hypertension [146]. In a large study by Patriquin et al. [147] of 195 patients with CF, a correlation between US findings of cirrhosis and abnormal liver enzymes was found [147]. In a follow-up study of this original cohort, the authors repeated US exam in the 106 patients originally without findings of liver disease [148] and found that after 10 years 19 of the 106 [18%] patients had developed abnormal US changes with 8 having signs of portal hypertension. The earliest abnormality identified was a "heterogenous parenchyma" and almost two thirds of the children with a heterogenous or nodular parenchyma (or both) and half of those with portal hypertension had no evidence of abnormal liver enzymes at the time when US changes were first noted. Another long-term study of 168 CF patients in whom annual US were routinely performed revealed persistently abnormal US exams in 23% and cirrhosis in 4%. Overall, the majority of these studies revealed a disparity between US findings and serum liver enzyme levels. Nonetheless, observations from these long-term studies suggest that routine US may be a valuable marker of early liver disease; however, findings may be subjective and operator-dependent, and the true sensitivity and specificity of this test to detect clinically significant liver disease has not been determined. Clearly larger studies are needed to determine the accuracy of US to predict the degree of liver involvement, track changes over time, and monitor treatment response.

CT and MRI

Other imaging studies that have been evaluated in small numbers of CF patients include abdominal CT and MRI. Computed tomography is very effective at identifying cirrhosis from any cause including multilobular cirrhosis associated with CF [149]. Additionally, CT may be of benefit in identifying fat density of the liver associated with hepatic steatosis. The accuracy of CT in detecting early liver changes associated with CF is unknown, and the radiation exposure makes CT unsuitable for screening purposes. However, CT is the modality of choice for identifying mass lesions and hepatic tumors. Like CT, MRI is effective in detecting findings associated with cirrhosis and portal hypertension, although its sensitivity in the detection of early changes is unknown [150]. Magnetic resonance cholangiopancreatography (MRCP) has become a valuable modality for the imaging of the biliary tree and has been described in CF [150].

ERCP

Endoscopic retrograde cholangiography is a useful modality for diagnosis of distal stenosis of the common bile duct, sclerosing cholangitis, and choledocholithiasis. However, it is an invasive procedure with considerable potential for complications and should not used for routine diagnostic or screening purposes in patients with CF.

Hepatobiliary Scintigraphy (Iminodiacetic Acid Derivatives)

Hepatobiliary scintigraphy (iminodiacetic acid [IDA] derivatives) involves the detection, by a scintillation camera, of radioisotopes after uptake and then excretion from the liver. This test is most useful for the detection of biliary obstruction as well as in the evaluation of cholecystitis, by demonstrating absence of gallbladder filling, characteristic of this condition [151]. In CF, several abnormalities have been described including dilated bile ducts and delayed excretion of radioisotope [120,151,152]. Additionally, it has been suggested that scintigraphy may be of value in the initiation and monitoring of the therapeutic response to UDCA [152,153]; however, this has not been validated in controlled clinical trials.

Liver Biopsy

The role of liver biopsy in the evaluation of suspected liver disease in the CF patient is controversial. Arguments in favor of performing a liver biopsy include: (1) it is the most accurate means to define the predominant lesion present (steatosis or focal biliary cirrhosis), (2) it may help to quickly exclude other causes, and (3) it will help to determine the degree of fibrosis present. Arguments against performing a liver biopsy include: (1) the recognized risk of sampling error due to the heterogenous distribution of liver lesions, (2) that patients may be at a higher risk for complications (pneumothorax due to lung hyperexpansion and bleeding due to the dilated hepatic veins secondary to cor pulmonale), and (3) that no definitive treatment exists, and therefore there is no reason to make an accurate diagnosis. At this time, the decision to perform a liver biopsy must be an individual determination based on the clinical scenario. If a percutaneous liver biopsy is felt to be indicated, US should always be performed immediately before the procedure to exclude dilated hepatic veins and ascites and to locate an appropriate spot with special care to avoid the lower lobe of the lung. If dilated hepatic veins or ascites are present, a percutaneous liver biopsy should not be performed and consideration should be given to a surgical or transjugular biopsy if indicated. Given the elusive nature of the diagnosis of CF liver disease, it is strongly advised to obtain a surgical liver biopsy, if it can be done without difficulty or additional significant risk, during abdominal surgery for any reason in the patient with CF.

Biomarkers

Given the difficulty in identifying the presence and severity of liver disease in CF, serum biomarkers of early disease have been sought, including bile acid profiles, inflammatory markers, matrix remodeling proteins, and functional tests of hepatic reserve.

In one recent study comparing CF patients with and without liver disease, significant correlations were seen among serum cholic acid levels, or the ratio of serum cholic acid: chenodeoxycholic acid; and hepatic fibrosis score, the degree of inflammation; and limiting plate disruption [84]. The use of serum bile acid profiles in the early detection of CF liver disease warrants further study.

Several markers of hepatic injury and inflammation, including Glutathione S-transferase B1 activity [154], high molecular mass alkaline phosphatase [155], and serum hyaluronic acid [156], have been shown to be elevated in subsets of CF patients with liver disease. Additionally, serum markers to detect liver fibrosis have been evaluated in CF. Both collagen VI [157] and serum prolyl hydroxylase [158] have been shown to be increased in a small number of CF patients with compared with those without liver disease. A study by Pereira et al. [159] analyzed the serum of 36 patients with CF-associated liver disease, 30 CF patients without liver disease, and 39 control patients for several markers of hepatic fibrosis, including tissue inhibitor of matrix metalloproteinase (TIMP-1), collagen type IV, matrix metalloproteinase type II (MMP-2), hyaluronic acid, and prolyl hydroxylase. TIMP-1, prolyl hydroxylase, and collagen-IV were increased in CF patients with liver disease compared with those without (or control subjects), and the TIMP-1 and prolyl hydroxylase levels correlated negatively with fibrosis score. In this study, collagen-IV and TIMP-1 differentiated CF patients with from those without liver disease. Although studies of serum markers of fibrosis and matrix remodeling appear promising in the detection of liver disease, one concern is that these markers may be affected by growth as well as the airway epithelial cell remodeling associated with chronic lung disease. The use of these serum markers of liver injury, inflammation, and fibrosis therefore require further study to determine the usefulness in screening programs.

Tests of hepatic clearance, as a measure of liver function, have been studied in small groups of patients with cholestatic liver diseases. Studies of caffeine clearance have not shown it to be useful in the detection of liver disease in CF patients [160]. Galactose clearance, an indirect measure of hepatic blood flow and hepatic functional mass, has been shown to correlate with the presence of hepatic fibrosis in a small number of patients with intrahepatic cholestasis [161], although the role of this test in the detection of CF liver disease is unknown. The technical difficulties in performing these studies, as well as the equivocal results, make these tests unsuitable for screening purposes at the present time.

TREATMENT

Once the presence of liver disease has been identified, the predominant lesion defined, and other diseases excluded, consideration should be given to treatment. A multidisciplinary approach is recommended for the management of liver disease in CF involving all members of the CF care team, including a hepatologist, surgeon, and radiologist.

Hepatic Congestion

The treatment of hepatic congestion or congestive hepatopathy involves optimizing pulmonary and cardiac function and should be coordinated by an appropriate team of pulmonology and cardiology specialists. Correcting any oxidant–antioxidant imbalance that may be present in CF may be of theoretical benefit in congestive hepatopathy. Antioxidant therapy, including vitamin E, may be beneficial in reducing injury to the liver by ischemia and reperfusion injury. The role of antioxidant therapy in cystic fibrosis is still undergoing evaluation.

Hepatic Steatosis

The fundamental treatment of hepatic steatosis is nutritional rehabilitation, normalizing biochemical parameters of micronutrients, and maximizing growth. Optimizing intake of protein, fat, energy, and pancreatic enzyme replacement therapy, as well as identifying and correcting any trace element, mineral, or vitamin deficiencies, is essential. Biochemical evaluation of essential fatty acids and fat-soluble vitamins should be assessed and replaced if found to be inadequate. It is important to exclude contributing factors such as ethanol, hepatotoxic medications, and other drugs or toxins. Lastly, given the recent interest of insulin resistance in the development of hepatic steatosis, consideration should be given to evaluation of diabetes by glucose tolerance testing.

Focal Biliary Cirrhosis and Multilobular Cirrhosis

Ursodeoxycholic acid, a hydrophilic bile acid normally produced in small quantities by the human liver, has been shown to improve bile flow and biochemical parameters of liver injury in CF. However, no treatment, including UDCA, has yet been shown to alter the progression of liver disease or the development of cirrhosis in CF. Ursodeoxycholic acid may have several mechanisms of action, including enrichment of the hydrophilic bile acid pool [162], stimulation of Cl^- and HCO_3^- transport [162,163], and direct cytoprotective [164] and immunomodulatory effects [165]. Prospective clinical trials of UDCA, at doses of 10–20 mg/kg/day for 6–12 months, have shown significant improvements in serum liver enzyme levels in pediatric patients with CF liver disease [166,167]. It should be noted that higher doses of UDCA (20 mg/kg/day) may be necessary in the treatment of CF liver disease compared with other forms of cholestasis [167,168]. In a 2-year, uncontrolled study, UDCA therapy improved the liver histology, with less inflammation and bile duct proliferation, in 7 of 10 patients with CF-related liver disease [169]. A 10-year prospective study in 70 patients with CF liver disease suggested that UDCA (20 mg/kg/day) may improve the ultrasound appearance of the liver [170]. Lastly, UDCA may improve the nutritional status of patients with CF-related liver disease including rises in serum essential fatty acid and fat-soluble vitamin levels [171]. Despite these findings, there is still no long-term data to prove that UDCA alters the natural course of liver disease in CF patients. However, given the improved biochemical parameters, ultrasound findings, and, perhaps, histologic data, the Cystic Fibrosis Foundation Hepatobiliary Disease Consensus Group has recommended it is "prudent to treat patients with CF who have cholestasis-fibrosis-cirrhosis with 20 mg/kg/day UDCA divided into two doses" [144].

After initiating therapy, serum liver enzymes should be obtained in 1 month and then at least every 6–12 months, as recommended by the Consensus Group [144]. A repeat liver biopsy is not recommended in the routine monitoring of UDCA therapy because the "patchy" distribution of the liver lesion may make the assessment of change over time in the individual patient difficult. Long-term clinical trials to determine the ultimate effect of UDCA on morbidity and mortality are needed. Therefore, ideally patients receiving UDCA therapy should be enrolled in clinical trials. It will be important to determine whether early treatment will alter the natural progression of the disease and decrease the occurrence of cirrhosis and the complications associated with portal hypertension. At present, there are no studies to promote the routine, prophylactic use of UDCA in all patients with CF. Clearly, this would result in overtreatment in a significant portion of patients. Once again, this highlights the need for research into the basic pathogenesis of the disease to identify risk factors and markers for screening. Patients in whom liver disease is identified should receive counseling and education concerning the promotion of "liver health" including the avoidance of alcohol, liver-toxic medications, herbal therapies, and obesity. Additionally, patients should receive vaccines against hepatitis A and B.

NUTRITIONAL MANAGEMENT

An important component of the management of liver disease in CF is maintenance of a normal nutritional state. Patients with CF may require energy intake that exceeds recommendations by 20–40% because of the continued fat malabsorption, increased caloric expenditure from chronic lung disease, and the increased oxygen consumption associated with cholestasis [172]. Protein intake should not be restricted in children with CF unless decompensated hepatic failure with encephalopathy and hyperammonemia are present. Infants with significant cholestasis may require formulas containing medium-chain triglyceride (MCT) to promote intestinal absorption of dietary lipid. Attention should be given to the optimization of pancreatic enzyme replacement therapy (PERT) in those patients with pancreatic insufficiency. Dosing of PERT should ideally be based on dietary composition with a goal to minimize fat malabsorption and steatorrhea while maximizing growth and weight gain. High doses (>3000 U lipase/kg/meal) should be avoided because these have been associated with the development of fibrosing colonapathy [173,174]. The CFF consensus committee on PERT has recommended dosage ranges of 1000–2500 U of lipase/kg/meal for ages 4 and younger and 500–2500 U of lipase/kg/meal for ages 4 and older in patients with CF and pancreatic insufficiency [174]. Monitoring fat-soluble vitamin status is even more important in the presence of liver disease [87] than in the patient with CF who has pancreatic insufficiency alone [175]. A multidisciplinary approach including physicians, nurses, dieticians, nutritionists, and pharmacists is essential to the successful management of the complex nutritional issues facing the patient with CF liver disease. A more detailed description of the nutritional management of cholestatic liver disease, including fat-soluble vitamin monitoring and dosing, is found in Chapter 10 of this text.

PORTAL HYPERTENSION AND LIVER TRANSPLANTATION

Cystic fibrosis–associated liver disease rarely causes acute liver failure; rather it leads to the complications of end-stage liver disease, namely, those associated with portal hypertension. At this point, UDCA is not effective, and treatment relies on the management of the complications of portal hypertension. In a recent long-term study of 40 patients with CF liver disease, Efrati et al. [176] reported the development of portal hypertension in 10 (25%), all of whom had variceal hemorrhage [176]. Prevention of recurrent variceal hemorrhage with the use of β-blocking agents may be contraindicated in patients with CF because of adverse effects on bronchial reactivity. Surgical portosystemic shunt and transjugular portosystemic shunt (TIPS) may be indicated for the management of portal hypertension in these patients allowing for prolonged survival, a bridge to liver transplant, or both. Partial splenectomy was used in the past management of hypersplenism in CF patients with liver disease; however, this procedure has been abandoned in favor of other approaches. Partial splenic embolization has been used to treat hypersplenism and extreme splenomegaly with success in other conditions [177], and using smaller volume embolization reduces the morbidity associated with this procedure [178].

Liver transplantation should be offered to those patients with life-threatening complications of portal hypertension or severe functional impairment and who have adequate pulmonary function, good compliance with care, and no other contraindications. Some controversy has existed regarding the possible adverse role of pulmonary infections in CF patients before liver transplant. However, two reports suggest that both graft and patient survival is similar in pediatric patients with CF as for those children undergoing liver transplantation for other indications [179,180]. Fridell et al. [179] reported 16 liver transplants in 12 patients with a 1-year patient survival of 92% and a 5-year survival of 75% [179]. Molmenti et al. [180] reported a series of 10 children who underwent liver transplantation for CF, with an average 1-year survival of approximately 90% and a 5-year survival of approximately 70% [180]. In both studies, there was no statistically significant difference between preoperative pulmonary colonization between survivors versus nonsurvivors. Patients in both studies had mild to moderate pulmonary disease before transplant that remained stable without deterioration following transplantation. In fact, the majority of patients had improved pulmonary function following liver transplant thought to be due to decreased airway inflammation from immunosuppressive treatment or to decreased abdominal pressure (after correction of portal hypertension and ascites) allowing for better lung expansion. Experience with combined lung–liver transplantation or small bowel–liver transplantation is limited but has been performed in CF patients [181,182]. Selection of the most appropriate intervention (repeated sclerotherapy or banding, portosystemic shunt, partial splenectomy, or liver transplantation) for the management of end-stage CF liver disease and portal hypertension must be individualized in as much as there is insufficient data to support a best practices approach.

FUTURE THERAPIES

Based on our growing knowledge of CFTR function in cellular physiology, potentially new and exciting therapies may be developed in the future for the treatment and prevention of CF. Strategies to correct the basic biliary defect, target and correct the abnormal CFTR trafficking, activate other Cl^- channels or transport pathways, and treat the progressive fibrosis through antioxidants or antifibrotic therapies are all being evaluated.

Gene Therapy

One fundamental goal of treatment strategies has been to correct the basic gene defect through the use of somatic gene transfer. Successful insertion of normal CFTR into normal and CF bile duct cell lines in culture has been achieved [183] and has been performed experimentally by retrograde infusion into the biliary tree of the rat [184]. It is doubtful that this approach will be successful in humans because of the invasive nature of ERCP. Strategies for clinically feasible approaches for gene transfer to the biliary tree (e.g., appropriate vector development) will need to be developed and validated before clinical application of this novel approach becomes feasible.

Correctors and Potentiators of CFTR

New pharmacologic treatments are being studied that target specific CFTR mutant proteins to correct protein structure, folding, or trafficking. For example, class I mutations, associated with a premature stop signal and therefore no functional CFTR protein, can be corrected in vitro by certain aminogylcoside antibiotics, which cause the aberrant stop signal to be skipped [185,186]. Class II mutations (e.g., ΔF508) result in an unstable protein that does not traffic to the apical membrane correctly. The protein can potentially be restored to a normal pathway by manipulation of chaperone protein/CFTR interactions. This has been accomplished in vitro by the use of chemical chaperones or drugs, such as butyrate or adenosine receptor antagonists, that affect modulation of protein folding [187,188]. Curcumin, a component of the spice turmeric, is a known inhibitor of ER Ca^{2+}-ATPase pumps and therefore may theoretically prevent the degradation of the misfolded CFTR protein. In one study, curcumin appeared to improve nasal epithelial potential difference (PD) measurements and prevent death by intestinal obstruction in ΔF508 homozygous mice [189]; others have not been able to reproduce these findings [190,191], however. The factors responsible for the discrepancies between these studies is not known, but the effects of curcumin may depend on high doses as well as other genetic modifiers, and therefore it may not be a reliable treatment option. Class III mutations result in CFTR with reduced Cl^- secretory capacity, which can be augmented by the drug genistein, a flavonoid compound [192,193], and milrinone, a phosphodiesterase inhibitor, can partially restore the decreased Cl^- conductance associated with the class IV mutations [194,195]. At present, all of these approaches require significant further development, and their potential application to the treatment of liver disease is unknown. Although further studies are warranted, given the suggestion that "non–CFTR factors" may determine the development of liver disease, these strategies to correct an abnormal CFTR protein may be of limited benefit in the treatment of CF liver disease.

Alternate Channels

Understanding the basic mechanisms involved in cholangiocyte transport and secretion may suggest other areas of intervention to modulate bile flow. Indeed, the apical membrane of cholangiocytes contains several other Cl^- channels, which at least in single cell or epithelial monolayer studies, have a larger unitary conductance than CFTR itself [43–45,48,49]. Both Ca^{2+}-activated Cl^- channels and Ca^{2+}-activated K^+ channels have been described in cholangiocytes and appear to contribute importantly to secretion [43,46]. The presence of alternate channels may modify organ-level disease expression in CF. For instance, the mild lung disease in the CF mouse may be explained by the high expression of Ca^{2+}-activated Cl^- channels in the epithelial airway cells of these animals [50]. In other CF epithelial models, overexpression of CLC-2 channels improves Cl^- transport in vitro [196]. Understanding the regulation of these alternate channels may provide strategies to bypass the secretory defect associated with CF.

Choleretic Agents

Currently, although UDCA is the only choleretic agent that may be beneficial in CF liver disease, other bile acids or analogues are being developed. One such synthetic bile acid is 24-norursodeoxycholic acid, a side chain shortened C23 homologue of UDCA. This agent has recently been studied in Multidrug resistance-2 gene (ABCB4) knockout mice (MDR2 –/–), a model of primary sclerosing cholangitis (PSC) [197]. After a 4-week diet of chow supplemented with 24-norursodeoxycholic acid, MDR2 –/– mice had lower aminotransferases, less hepatic fibrosis, and improved biliary HCO_3^- secretion and bile flow compared with control animals fed only chow. Although this is a very preliminary report, it suggests that modification of UDCA may increase the hydrophilicity of bile acids and increase HCO_3^--rich bile flow, and further studies in other cholestatic conditions, including CF, are warranted. Another novel approach for the treatment of cholestatic liver disorders is to increase expression of bile acid transporters by the use of nuclear receptor agonists [198–200]. Although the use of these agents is potentially an exciting therapeutic modality, studies are clearly needed to determine the safety and efficacy of nuclear receptor agonists in cholestatic liver conditions such as CF.

Antioxidants

Given a possible imbalance in oxidants versus antioxidants in CF, there may be a rationale for exploring the use of antioxidants as a therapeutic strategy. In early clinical trials, aerosolized glutathione has been delivered to the lung in patients with CF and was shown to increase airway glutathione levels but only had a modest effect on markers of oxidant injury [201]. Although *N*-acetylcysteine, a substrate for glutathione production, has been used in an acetaminophen-induced liver injury, its role in the treatment of CF liver disease is unknown. Current results of antioxidant treatment in experimental models of oxidative liver injury appear promising [202,203]; however, there is no direct clinical evidence to support this therapy for CF liver disease at this time.

Antifibrotic Agents

Understanding the role of the hepatic stellate cell in the progressive fibrosis associated with CF may lead to new treatment strategies to prevent ongoing cellular injury and interrupt fibrogenesis [204,205]. Although a number of antifibrogenic agents that target stellate cells are in the development phase and may prove to be beneficial in the future [206–208], the role of antifibrotic agents in the treatment of CF liver disease warrants further study.

CONCLUSION

The pathogenesis of CF liver disease continues to be a mystery. However, our knowledge of CFTR structure, function, and regulation in novel models of biliary epithelium continues to increase at a rapid rate. In the future, it is anticipated that this knowledge will translate into therapeutic strategies for the successful treatment and prevention of CF liver disease.

ACKNOWLEDGMENTS

Research supported by the Cystic Fibrosis Foundation and the National Institute of Diabetes, Digestive and Kidney Diseases of the National Institutes of Health (grant DK KO8 61480).

REFERENCES

1. Dodge JA, Morison S, Lewis PA, et al. Incidence, population, and survival of cystic fibrosis in the UK, 1968–95. UK Cystic Fibrosis Survey Management Committee. Arch Dis Child 1997;77: 493–6.
2. Kosorok MR, Wei WH, Farrell PM. The incidence of cystic fibrosis. Stat Med 1996;15:449–62.
3. Cystic Fibrosis Foundation Patient Registry 2003 Annual Data Report. Bethesda, Md.: 2004 Cystic Fibrosis Foundation, 2004.
4. Fitzsimmons SC. Cystic Fibrosis Foundation Patient Registry, 1996. 1997.
5. Busch R. On the history of cystic fibrosis. Acta Univ Carol 1990;36:13–15.
6. Landsteiner K. Darmverschluss durch eingedicktes meconium pankreatitis. Centr Allg Pathol 1905;16:903–7.
7. Anderson DH. Cystic fibrosis of the pancreas and its relation to celiac disease. 56th ed. 1938. 344–99.
8. Farber S. Some organic digestive disturbances in early life. J Mich State Med Soc 1945;44:587–94.
9. Di Sant'Agnese PA, Darling R, Perera G, Shea E. Abnormal electrolyte composition of sweat in cystic fibrosis of the pancreas. 12th ed. 1953. 549–63.
10. Gibson LE, Cooke RE. A test for concentration of electrolytes in sweat in cystic fibrosis of the pancreas utilizing pilocarpine by iontophoresis. Pediatrics 1959;23:545–9.
11. Quinton PM. Chloride impermeability in cystic fibrosis. Nature 1983;301:421–2.
12. Riordan JR, Rommens JM, Kerem B-S, et al. Identification of the cystic fibrosis gene: cloning and characterization of complementary DNA. Science 1989;245:1066–73.
13. Quinton PM. Physiological basis of cystic fibrosis: a historical perspective. Physiol Rev 1999;79 Suppl 1:S3–22.
14. Doershuk CF. Cystic Fibrosis in the 20th century. People, events, and progress. Cleveland, Ohio: AM Publishing, 2001.
15. Anderson MP, Gregory RJ, Thompson S, et al. Demonstration that CFTR is a chloride channel by alteration of its anion selectivity. Science 1991;253:202–5.
16. Fuller CM, Benos DJ. CFTR! Am J Physiol 1992;263:C267–86.
17. Smith JJ, Welsh MJ. cAMP stimulates bicarbonate secretion across normal but not cystic fibrosis airway epithelia. J Clin Invest 1992;89:1148–53.
18. Poulsen JH, Fischer H, Illek B, Machen TE. Bicarbonate conductance and pH regulatory capability of cystic fibrosis transmembrane conductance regulator. Proc Natl Acad Sci U S A 1994;91:5340–4.
19. Reddy MM, Quinton PM. Control of dynamic CFTR selectivity by glutamate and ATP in epithelial cells. Nature 2003;423: 756–60.
20. Choi JY, Muallem D, Kiselyov K, et al. Aberrant CFTR-dependent HCO3- transport in mutations associated with cystic fibrosis. Nature 2001;410:94–7.
21. Kogan I, Ramjeesingh M, Li C, et al. CFTR directly mediates nucleotide-regulated glutathione flux. EMBO J 2003;22: 1981–9.
22. Reisin IL, Prat AG, Abraham EH, et al. The cystic fibrosis transmembrane conductance regulator is a dual ATP and chloride channel. J Biol Chem 1994;269:20584–91.
23. Schwiebert EM, Egan ME, Hwang T-H, et al. CFTR regulates outwardly rectifying chloride channels through an autocrine mechanism involving ATP. Cell 1995;81:1063–73.
24. Schwiebert EM, Benos DJ, Egan ME, et al. CFTR is a conductance regulator as well as a chloride channel. Physiol Rev 1999;79 Suppl 1:S145–66.
25. Chinet TC, Fullton JM, Yankaskas JR, et al. Mechanism of sodium hyperabsorption in cultured cystic fibrosis nasal epithelium: a patch-clamp study. Am J Physiol 1994;266:C1061–8.
26. Gabriel S, Clarke LL, Boucher RC, Stutts MJ. CFTR and outward rectifying chloride channels are distinct proteins with a regulatory relationship. Nature 1993;363:263–6.
27. Grubb BR, Vick RN, Boucher RC. Hyperabsorption of Na+ and raised Ca(2+)-mediated Cl– secretion in nasal epithelia of CF mice. Am J Physiol 1994;266:C1478–83.

28. Egan M, Flotte T, Afione S, et al. Defective regulation of outwardly rectifying Cl$^-$ channels by protein kinase A corrected by insertion of CFTR. Nature 1992;358:581–4.
29. Hyde SC, Gill DR, Higgins CF, Trezise AE, et al. Correction of the ion transport defect in cystic fibrosis transgenic mice by gene therapy. Nature 1993;362:250–5.
30. McNicholas CM, Guggino WB, Schwiebert EM, et al. Sensitivity of a renal K+ channel (ROMK2) to the inhibitory sulfonylurea compound glibenclamide is enhanced by coexpression with the ATP-binding cassette transporter cystic fibrosis transmembrane regulator. Proc Natl Acad Sci U S A 1996;93:8083–8.
31. Gao L, Kim KJ, Yankaskas JR, Forman HJ. Abnormal glutathione transport in cystic fibrosis airway epithelia. Am J Physiol 1999;277:L113–18.
32. Linsdell P, Hanrahan JW. Glutathione permeability of CFTR. Am J Physiol 1998;275:C323–6.
33. Kuver R, Ramesh N, Lau S, et al. Constitutive mucin secretion linked to CFTR expression. Biochem Biophys Res Commun 1994;203:1457–62.
34. Roberts SK, Yano M, Ueno Y, et al. Cholangiocytes express the aquaporin CHIP and transport water via a channel-mediated mechanism. Proc Nat Acad Sci U S A 1994;91:13009–13.
35. Schreiber R, Nitschke R, Greger R, Kunzelmann K. The cystic fibrosis transmembrane conductance regulator activates aquaporin 3 in airway epithelial cells. J Biol Chem 1999;274:11811–16.
36. Schreiber R, Pavenstadt H, Greger R, Kunzelmann K. Aquaporin 3 cloned from Xenopus laevis is regulated by the cystic fibrosis transmembrane conductance regulator. FEBS Lett 2000;475:291–5.
37. Braunstein GM, Roman RM, Clancy JP, et al. Cystic fibrosis transmembrane conductance regulator facilitates ATP release by stimulating a separate ATP release channel for autocrine control of cell volume regulation. J Biol Chem 2001;276:6621–30.
38. Bradbury NA, Lilling T, Berta G,. Regulation of plasma membrane recycling by CFTR. Science 1992;256:530–2.
39. Barasch J, Kiss B, Prince A, et al. Defective acidification of intracellular organelles in cystic fibrosis. Nature 1991;352:70–3.
40. Guggino WB. The cystic fibrosis transmembrane regulator forms macromolecular complexes with PDZ domain scaffold proteins. Proc Am Thorac Soc 2004;1:28–32.
41. Fouassier L, Duan CY, Feranchak AP, et al. Ezrin-radixin-moesin-binding phosphoprotein 50 is expressed at the apical membrane of rat liver epithelia. Hepatology 2001;33:166–76.
42. Cohn JA, Strong TA, Picciotto MA, et al. Localization of CFTR in human bile duct epithelial cells. Gastroenterology 1993;105:1857–64.
43. Feranchak AP, Doctor RB, Troetsch M, et al. Calcium-dependent regulation of secretion in biliary epithelial cells: the role of apamin-sensitive SK channels. Gastroenterology 2004;127:903–13.
44. McGill J, Gettys TW, Basavappa S, Fitz JG. GTP-binding proteins regulate high conductance anion channels in rat bile duct epithelial cells. J Membr Biol 1993;133:253–61.
45. Fitz JG, Basavappa S, McGill J, Melhus O, Cohn JA. Regulation of membrane chloride currents in rat bile duct epithelial cells. J Clin Invest 1993;91:319–28.
46. Schlenker T, Fitz JG. Calcium-activated chloride channels in a human biliary cell line: Regulation by calcium/calmodulin-dependent protein kinase. Am J Physiol 1996;271:G304–10.
47. Roman RM, Feranchak AP, Salter KD, et al. Endogenous ATP regulates Cl$^-$ secretion in cultured human and rat biliary epithelial cells. Am J Physiol 1999;276:G1391–400.
48. Feranchak AP, Roman RM, Doctor RB, et al. The lipid products of phosphoinositide 3-kinase contribute to regulation of cholangiocyte ATP and chloride transport. J Biol Chem 1999;274:30979–86.
49. Roman RM, Wang Y, Fitz JG. Regulation of cell volume in a human biliary cell line: Calcium-dependent activation of K+ and Cl- currents. Am J Physiol 1996;271:G239–48.
50. Clarke LL, Grubb BR, Yankaskas J, et al. Relationship of a non-cystic fibrosis transmembrane conductance regulator-mediated chloride conductance to organ-level disease in cftr(-/-) mice. Proc Nat Acad Sci U S A 1994;91:479–83.
51. McGill J, Basavappa S, Shimokura GH, et al. Adenosine triphosphate activates ion permeabilities in biliary epithelial cells. Gastroenterology 1994;107:236–43.
52. Alpini G, Glaser S, Robertson W, et al. Bile acids stimulate proliferative and secretory events in large but not small cholangiocytes. Am J Physiol 1997;273:G518–29.
53. Lazaridis KN, Pham L, Tietz PS, et al. Rat cholangiocytes absorb bile acids at their apical domain via the ileal sodium-dependent bile acid transporter. J Clin Invest 1997;100:2714–21.
54. Hofmann AF. Bile acids. In: Arias IM, ed. The liver: biology and pathobiology. 3th ed. New York: Raven Press, 1994. 677–718.
55. Yoon YB, Hagey LR, Hofmann AF, et al. Effect of side chain shortening on the physiologic properties of bile acids: hepatic transport and effect on biliary secretion of 23-Nor-ursodeoxycholate in rodents. Gastroenterology 1986;90:837–52.
56. Palmer R, Gurantz D, Hofmann AF, et al. Hypercholeresis induced by norchenodeoxycholate in biliary fistula rodent. Am J Physiol 1987;252:G219–28.
57. Alpini G, Glaser SS, Ueno Y, et al. Bile acid feeding induces cholangiocyte proliferation and secretion: evidence for bile acid-regulated ductal secretion. Gastroenterology 1999;116:179–86.
58. Feranchak AP, Fitz JG. Adenosine triphosphate release and purinergic regulation of cholangiocyte transport. Semin Liver Dis 2002;22:251–62.
59. Feranchak AP, Fitz JG, Roman RM. Volume-sensitive purinergic signaling in human hepatocytes. J Hepatol 2000;33:174–82.
60. Roman RM, Wang Y, Lidofsky SD, et al. Hepatocellular ATP-binding cassette protein expression enhances ATP release and autocrine regulation of cell volume. J Biol Chem 1997;272:21970–6.
61. Chari RS, Schutz SM, Haebig JA, et al. Adenosine nucleotides in bile. Am J Physiol 1996;270:G246–52.
62. Schlenker T, Romac JMJ, Sharara A, et al. Regulation of biliary secretion through apical purinergic receptors in cultured rat cholangiocytes. Am J Physiol 1997;273:G1108–17.
63. Taylor AL, Schwiebert LM, Smith JJ, et al. Epithelial P2x purinergic receptor channel expression and function. J Clin Invest 1999;104:875–84.
64. Doctor RB, Matzakos T, McWilliams R, et al. Purinergic regulation of cholangiocyte secretion: identification of a novel role for P2X receptors. Am J Physiol Gastrointest Liver Physiol 2005;288:G779–86.
65. Al-Awqati Q. Regulation of ion channels by ABC transporters that secrete ATP. Science 1995;269:805–6.

66. Pasyk EA, Foskett JK. Cystic fibrosis transmembrane consuctance regulator-associated ATP and adenosine 3′-phosphate 5′-phosphosulfate channels in endoplasmic reticulum and plasma membranes. J Biol Chem 1997;272:7746–51.
67. Knowles MR, Clarke LL, Boucher RC. Activation by extracellular nucleotides of chloride secretion in the airway epithelia of patients with cystic fibrosis. N Engl J Med 1991;325:533–8.
68. Parr CE, Sullivan DM, Paradiso AM, et al. Cloning and expression of a human P2u nucleotide receptor, a target for cystic fibrosis pharmacotherapy. Proc Nat Acad Sci U S A 1994;91:3275–9.
69. Chan HC, Cheung WT, Leung P, et al. Purinergic regulation of anion secretion by cystic fibrosis pancreatic duct cells. Am J Physiol 1996;271:C469–77.
70. Bennett WD, Olivier KN, Zeman KL, et al. Effect of uridine 5′-triphosphate plus amiloride on mucociliary clearance in adult cystic fibrosis. Am J Respir Crit Care Med 1996;153:1796–801.
71. Zielenski J, Tsui LC. Cystic fibrosis: genotypic and phenotypic variations. Annu Rev Genet 1995;29:777–807.
72. Gabriel SE, Brigman KN, Koller BH, et al. Cystic fibrosis heterozygote resistance to cholera toxin in the cystic fibrosis mouse model. Science 1994;266:107–9.
73. Wilschanski M, Zielenski J, Markiewicz D, et al. Correlation of sweat chloride concentration with classes of the cystic fibrosis transmembrane conductance regulator gene mutations. J Pediatr 1995;127:705–10.
74. Koch C, Cuppens H, Rainisio M, et al. European Epidemiologic Registry of Cystic Fibrosis (ERCF): comparison of major disease manifestations between patients with different classes of mutations. Pediatr Pulmonol 2001;31:1–12.
75. Colombo C, Apostolo MG, Ferrari M, et al. Analysis of risk factors for the development of liver disease associated with cystic fibrosis. J Pediatr 1994;124:393–9.
76. De Arce M, O'Brien S, Hegarty J, et al. Deletion delta F508 and clinical expression of cystic fibrosis-related liver disease. Clin Genet 1992;42:271–2.
77. Duthie A, Doherty DG, Williams C, et al. Genotype analysis for delta F508, G551D and R553X mutations in children and young adults with cystic fibrosis with and without chronic liver disease. Hepatology 1992;15:660–4.
78. Augarten A, Kerem BS, Yahav Y, et al. Mild cystic fibrosis and normal or borderline sweat test in patients with the 3849 + 10 kb C –> T mutation. Lancet 1993;342:25–6.
79. Oppenheimer EH, Esterly JR. Hepatic changes in young infants with cystic fibrosis: possible relation to focal biliary cirrhosis. J Pediatr 1975;86:683–9.
80. Burnett BG, Pittman RN. The polyglutamine neurodegenerative protein ataxin 3 regulates aggresome formation. Proc Natl Acad Sci U S A 2005;102:4330–5.
81. Welch WJ. Role of quality control pathways in human diseases involving protein misfolding. Semin Cell Dev Biol 2004;15:31–8.
82. Peters RH, French PJ, van Doorninck JH, et al. CFTR expression and mucin secretion in cultured mouse gallbladder epithelial cells. Am J Physiol 1996;271:G1074–83.
83. Bhaskar KR, Turner BS, Grubman SA, et al. Dysregulation of proteoglycan production by intrahepatic biliary epithelial cells bearing defective (delta-f508) cystic fibrosis transmembrane conductance regulator. Hepatology 1998;27:7–14.
84. Smith JL, Lewindon PJ, Hoskins AC, Pereira TN, Setchell KD, O'Connell NC, et al. Endogenous ursodeoxycholic acid and cholic acid in liver disease due to cystic fibrosis. Hepatology 2004 Jun;39[6]:1673–82.
85. Sokol RJ, Straka MS, Dahl R, et al. Role of oxidant stress in the permeability transition induced in rat hepatic mitochondria by hydrophobic bile acids. Pediatr Res 2001;49:519–31.
86. Hudson VM. New insights into the pathogenesis of cystic fibrosis: pivotal role of glutathione system dysfunction and implications for therapy. Treat Respir Med 2004;3:353–63.
87. Sokol RJ. Fat-soluble vitamins and their importance in patients with cholestatic liver diseases. Gastroenterol Clin North Am 1994;23:673–705.
88. Yerushalmi B, Dahl R, Devereaux MW, et al. Bile acid-induced rat hepatocyte apoptosis is inhibited by antioxidants and blockers of the mitochondrial permeability transition. Hepatology 2001;33:616–26.
89. Pessayre D, Berson A, Fromenty B, Mansouri A. Mitochondria in steatohepatitis. Semin Liver Dis 2001;21:57–69.
90. Cantin AM. Potential for antioxidant therapy of cystic fibrosis. Curr Opin Pulm Med 2004;10:531–6.
91. Lewindon PJ, Pereira TN, Hoskins AC, et al. The role of hepatic stellate cells and transforming growth factor-beta(1) in cystic fibrosis liver disease. Am J Pathol 2002;160:1705–15.
92. Friedman SL, Roll FJ, Boyles J, Bissell DM. Hepatic lipocytes: the principal collagen-producing cells of normal rat liver. Proc Natl Acad Sci U S A 1985;82:8681–5.
93. Maher JJ, McGuire RF. Extracellular matrix gene expression increases preferentially in rat lipocytes and sinusoidal endothelial cells during hepatic fibrosis in vivo. J Clin Invest 1990;86:1641–8.
94. Wilroy RS Jr, Crawford SE, Johnson WW. Cystic fibrosis with extensive fat replacement of the liver. J Pediatr 1966;68:67–73.
95. Strandvik B, Hultcrantz R. Liver function and morphology during long-term fatty acid supplementation in cystic fibrosis. Liver 1994;14[1]:32–6.
96. Feingold KR, Serio MK, Adi S, et al. Tumor necrosis factor stimulates hepatic lipid synthesis and secretion. Endo 1989; 124:2336–42.
97. Durie PR, Kent G, Phillips MJ, Ackerley CA. Characteristic multiorgan pathology of cystic fibrosis in a long-living cystic fibrosis transmembrane regulator knockout murine model. Am J Pathol 2004;164:1481–93.
98. Castaldo G, Fuccio A, Salvatore D, Raia V, et al. Liver expression in cystic fibrosis could be modulated by genetic factors different from the cystic fibrosis transmembrane regulator genotype. Am J Med Genet 2001;98:294–7.
99. Scott-Jupp R, Lama M, Tanner MS. Prevalence of liver disease in cystic fibrosis. Arch Dis Child 1991;66:698–701.
100. Feigelson J, Anagnostopoulos C, Poquet M, et al. Liver cirrhosis in cystic fibrosis – therapeutic implications and long term follow up. Arch Dis Child 1993;68:653–7.
101. Davis PB. The gender gap in cystic fibrosis survival. J Gend Specif Med 1999;2:47–51.
102. Simon FR, Fortune J, Iwahashi M, et al. Multihormonal regulation of hepatic sinusoidal Ntcp gene expression. Am J Physiol Gastrointest Liver Physiol 2004;287:G782–94.
103. Maurage C, Lenaerts C, Weber A, et al. Meconium ileus and its equivalent as a risk factor for the development of cirrhosis: an autopsy study in cystic fibrosis. J Pediatr Gastroenterol Nutr 1989;9:17–20.

104. Colombo C, Battezzati PM, Strazzabosco M, Podda M. Liver and biliary problems in cystic fibrosis. Semin Liver Dis 1998;18: 227–35.
105. Lindblad A, Strandvik B, Hjelte L. Incidence of liver disease in patients with cystic fibrosis and meconium ileus. J Pediatr 1995;126:155–6.
106. Zielenski J, Corey M, Rozmahel R, et al. Detection of a cystic fibrosis modifier locus for meconium ileus on human chromosome 19q13. Nat Genet 1999;22:128–9.
107. Blackman SM, Deering RS, Naughton K, et al. Modifier genes are responsible for meconium ileus in cystic fibrosis patients, but a major modifier gene is not located on chromosome 19q13. [abstract]. Pediatr Pulm 2005;Suppl 28:247.
108. Tanner MS, Taylor CJ. Liver disease in cystic fibrosis. Arch Dis Child 1995;72:281–4.
109. Williams SG, Westaby D, Tanner MS, Mowat AP. Liver and biliary problems in cystic fibrosis. Br Med Bull 1992;48:877–92.
110. Duthie A, Doherty DG, Donaldson PT, et al. The major histocompatibility complex influences the development of chronic liver disease in male children and young adults with cystic fibrosis. J Hepatol 1995;23:532–7.
111. Arkwright PD, Laurie S, Super M, et al. TGF-beta(1) genotype and accelerated decline in lung function of patients with cystic fibrosis. Thorax 2000;55:459–62.
112. Arkwright PD, Pravica V, Geraghty PJ, et al. End-organ dysfunction in cystic fibrosis: association with angiotensin I converting enzyme and cytokine gene polymorphisms. Am J Respir Crit Care Med 2003 Feb 1;167:384–9.
113. Buranawuti K, Cheng S, Merlo C, et al. Variants in the mannose binding lectin gene modify survival of cystic fibrosis patients [abstract]. Pediatr Pulm 2003;Suppl 25:215.
114. Henrion-Caude A, Flamant C, Roussey M, et al. Liver disease in pediatric patients with cystic fibrosis is associated with glutathione S-transferase P1 polymorphism. Hepatology 2002; 36:913–17.
115. Rozmahel R, Wilschanski M, Matin A, et al. Modulation of disease severity in cystic fibrosis transmembrane conductance regulator deficient mice by a secondary genetic factor. Nat Genet 1996;12:280–7.
116. Ritzka M, Stanke F, Jansen S, et al. The CLCA gene locus as a modulator of the gastrointestinal basic defect in cystic fibrosis. Hum Genet 2004;115:483–91.
117. Rohlfs EM, Shaheen NJ, Silverman LM. Is the hemochromatosis gene a modifier locus for cystic fibrosis? Genet Test 1998;2:85–8.
118. Friedman K, Ling S, Macek M, et al. Complex multigenic inheritence influences the development of severe liver disease in CF [A]. Proceedings of the 15th North American Cystic Fibrosis Conference, Orlando, Florida, 2001.
119. Friedman KJ, Ling SC, Lange EM, et al. Genetic modifiers of severe liver disease in cystic fibrosis [abstract]. Pediatr Pulm 2005;Suppl 28:247.
120. Nagel RA, Westaby D, Javaid A, et al. Liver disease and bile duct abnormalities in adults with cystic fibrosis. Lancet 1989;2: 1422–5.
121. Vawter GF, Shwachman H. Cystic fibrosis in adults: an autopsy study. Pathol Annu 1979;14:357–82.
122. Gaskin KJ, Waters DLM, Howman-Giles R, et al. Liver disease and common bile duct stenosis in cystic fibrosis. N Engl J Med 1988;318:340–6.
123. Lindblad A, Glaumann H, Strandvik B. Natural history of liver disease in cystic fibrosis. Hepatology 1999;30:1151–8.
124. Colombo C, Battezzati PM, Crosignani A, et al. Liver disease in cystic fibrosis: A prospective study on incidence, risk factors, and outcome. Hepatology 2002;36:1374–82.
125. Lamireau T, Monnereau S, Martin S, et al. Epidemiology of liver disease in cystic fibrosis: a longitudinal study. J Hepatol 2004;41:920–5.
126. Sokol RJ, Carroll NM, Narkewicz MR, et al. Liver blood tests during the first decade of life in children with cystic fibrosis identified by newborn screening. Pediatr Pulm 1994;10:275.
127. Craig JM. The pathological changes in the liver in cystic fibrosis of the pancreas. 93rd ed. 1957. 357–69.
128. Vlaman HB, France NE, Wallis PG. Prolonged neonatal jaundice in cystic fibrosis. 46th ed. 1971. 805–9.
129. Roy CC, Weber AM, Morin CL, et al. Hepatobiliary disease in cystic fibrosis: a survey of current issues and concepts. J Pediatr Gastroenterol Nutr 1982;1:469–78.
130. Lykavieris P, Bernard O, Hadchouel M. Neonatal cholestasis as the presenting feature in cystic fibrosis. Arch Dis Child 1996;75:67–70.
131. McKeon D, Day A, Parmar J, et al. Hepatocellular carcinoma in association with cirrhosis in a patient with cystic fibrosis. J Cyst Fibros 2004;3:193–5.
132. Willi UV, Reddish JM, Teele RL. Cystic fibrosis: its characteristic appearance on abdominal sonography. AJR Am J Roentgenol 1980;134:1005–10.
133. Kovesi T, Corey M, Tsui L-C, et al.The association between liver disease and mutations of the cystic fibrosis gene. Pediatr Pulm 1992;8:244.
134. Neglia JP, Fitzsimmons SC, Maisonneuve P, et al. The risk of cancer among patients with cystic fibrosis. Cystic Fibrosis and Cancer Study Group. N Engl J Med 1995;332:494–9.
135. Narkewicz MR, Sondheimer HM, Ziegler JW, et al. Hepatic dysfunction following the Fontan procedure. J Pediatr Gastroenterol Nutr 2003;36:352–7.
136. Forstner GG, Durie PR. Cystic Fibrosis. In: Walker WA, Durie PR, Hamilton JR, eds. Pediatric Gastroinetstinal disease. 2nd ed. Toronto: BC Decker, 1996, 1466–87.
137. Videla LA, Rodrigo R, Araya J, Poniachik J. Oxidative stress and depletion of hepatic long-chain polyunsaturated fatty acids may contribute to nonalcoholic fatty liver disease. Free Radic Biol Med 2004;37:1499–507.
138. Browning JD, Horton JD. Molecular mediators of hepatic steatosis and liver injury. J Clin Invest 2004;114:147–52.
139. Treem WR, Stanley CA. Massive hepatomegaly, steatosis, and secondary plasma carnitine deficiency in an infant with cystic fibrosis. Pediatrics 1989;83:993–7.
140. di Sant'Agnese PA, Blanc WA. A distinctive type of biliary cirrhosis of the liver associated with cystic fibrosis of the pancreas. Pediatrics 1956;18:387–409.
141. Stern RC, Rothstein FC, Doershuk CF. Treatment and prognosis of symptomatic gallbladder disease in patients with cystic fibrosis. J Pediatr Gastroenterol Nutr 1986;5:35–40.
142. Colombo C, Bertolini E, Assaisso ML, et al. Failure of ursodeoxycholic acid to dissolve radiolucent gallstones in patients with cystic fibrosis. Acta Paediatr 1993;82:562–5.
143. Sheth S, Shea JC, Bishop MD, et al. Increased prevalence of CFTR mutations and variants and decreased chloride secretion in primary sclerosing cholangitis. Hum Genet 2003;113:286–92.

144. Sokol RJ, Durie PR. Recommendations for management of liver and biliary tract disease in cystic fibrosis. Cystic Fibrosis Foundation Hepatobiliary Disease Consensus Group. J Pediatr Gastroenterol Nutr 1999;28 Suppl 1:S1–13.
145. Valletta EA, Loreti S, Cipolli M, Cazzola G, Zanolla L. Portal hypertension and esophageal varices in cystic fibrosis. Unreliability of echo-Doppler flowmetry. Scand J Gastroenterol 1993; 28:1042–6.
146. Williams SG, Evanson JE, Barrett N, Hodson ME, Boultbee JE, Westaby D. An ultrasound scoring system for the diagnosis of liver disease in cystic fibrosis. J Hepatol 1995;22: 513–21.
147. Patriquin H, Lenaerts C, Smith L, Perreault G, Grignon A, Filiatrault D, et al. Liver disease in children with cystic fibrosis: US-biochemical comparison in 195 patients. Radiology 1999; 211:229–32.
148. Lenaerts C, Lapierre C, Patriquin H, et al. Surveillance for cystic fibrosis-associated hepatobiliary disease: early ultrasound changes and predisposing factors. J Pediatr 2003;143:343–50.
149. Dodd GD III, Baron RL, Oliver JH III, Federle MP. Spectrum of imaging findings of the liver in end-stage cirrhosis: part I, gross morphology and diffuse abnormalities. AJR Am J Roentgenol 1999;173:1031–6.
150. King LJ, Scurr ED, Murugan N, et al. Hepatobiliary and pancreatic manifestations of cystic fibrosis: MR imaging appearances. Radiographics 2000;20:767–77.
151. Dogan AS, Conway JJ, Lloyd-Still JD. Hepatobiliary scintigraphy in children with cystic fibrosis and liver disease. J Nucl Med 1994;35:432–5.
152. Colombo C, Castellani MR, Balistreri WF, et al. Scintigraphic documentation of an improvement in hepatobiliary excretory function after treatment with ursodeoxycholic acid in patients with cystic fibrosis and associated liver disease. Hepatology 1992;15:677–84.
153. O'Connor PJ, Southern KW, Bowler IM, et al. The role of hepatobiliary scintigraphy in cystic fibrosis. Hepatology 1996; 23:281–7.
154. Rattenbury JM, Taylor CJ, Heath PK, et al. Serum glutathione S-transferase B1 activity as an index of liver function in cystic fibrosis. J Clin Pathol 1995;48:771–4.
155. Schoenau E, Boeswald W, Wanner R, et al. High-molecular-mass ("biliary") isoenzyme of alkaline phosphatase and the diagnosis of liver dysfunction in cystic fibrosis. Clin Chem 1989; 35:1888–90.
156. Wyatt HA, Dhawan A, Cheeseman P, et al. Serum hyaluronic acid concentrations are increased in cystic fibrosis patients with liver disease. Arch Dis Child 2002;86:190–3.
157. Gerling B, Becker M, Staab D, Schuppan D. Prediction of liver fibrosis according to serum collagen VI level in children with cystic fibrosis. N Engl J Med 1997;336:1611–12.
158. Leonardi S, Giambusso F, Sciuto C, et al. Are serum type III procollagen and prolyl hydroxylase useful as noninvasive markers of liver disease in patients with cystic fibrosis? J Pediatr Gastroenterol Nutr 1998;27:603–5.
159. Pereira TN, Lewindon PJ, Smith JL, et al. Serum markers of hepatic fibrogenesis in cystic fibrosis liver disease. J Hepatol 2004; 41:576–83.
160. Bianchetti MG, Kraemer R, Passweg J, et al. Use of salivary levels to predict clearance of caffeine in patients with cystic fibrosis. J Pediatr Gastroenterol Nutr 1988;7:688–93.
161. Narkewicz MR, Smith D, Gregory C, et al. Effect of ursodeoxycholic acid therapy on hepatic function in children with intrahepatic cholestatic liver disease. J Pediatr Gastroenterol Nutr 1998;26:49–55.
162. Heuman DM. Hepatoprotective properties of ursodeoxycholic acid. Gastroenterology 1993;104:1865–70.
163. Shimokura GH, McGill J, Schlenker T, Fitz JG. Ursodeoxycholate increases cytosolic calcium concentration and activates Cl^- currents in a biliary cell line. Gastroenterology 1995;109: 965–72.
164. Botla R, Spivey JR, Aguilar H, et al. Ursodeoxycholate (UDCA) inhibits the mitochondrial membrane permeability transition induced by glycochenodeoxycholate: a mechanism of UDCA cytoprotection. J Pharmacol Exp Ther 1995;272:930–8.
165. Calmus Y, Gane P, Rouger P, Poupon R. Hepatic expression of class I and class II major histocompatibility complex molecules in primary biliary cirrhosis: effect of ursodeoxycholic acid. Hepatology 1990;11:12–15.
166. Colombo C, Battezzati PM, Podda M, et al. Ursodeoxycholic acid for liver disease associated with cystic fibrosis: A double-blind multicenter trial. Hepatology 1996;23:1484–90.
167. Colombo C, Setchell KD, Podda M, et al. Effects of ursodeoxycholic acid therapy for liver disease associated with cystic fibrosis. J Pediatr 1990;117:482–9.
168. van de Meeberg PC, Houwen RH, Sinaasappel M,. Low dose versus high-dose ursodeoxycholic acid in cystic fibrosis-related cholestatic liver disease. Results of a randomized study with 1-year follow-up. Scand J Gastroenterol 1997;32:369–73.
169. Lindblad A, Glaumann H, Strandvik B. A two-year prospective study of the effect of ursodeoxycholic acid on urinary bile acid excretion and liver morphology in cystic fibrosis-associated liver disease. Hepatology 1998;27:166–74.
170. Nousia-Arvanitakis S, Fotoulaki M, Economou H, et al. Long-term prospective study of the effect of ursodeoxycholic acid on cystic fibrosis-related liver disease. J Clin Gastroenterol 2001;32: 324–8.
171. Lepage G, Paradis K, Lacaille F, et al. Ursodeoxycholic acid improves the hepatic metabolism of essential fatty acids and retinol in children with cystic fibrosis. J Pediatr 1997;130: 52–8.
172. Pierro A, Koletzko B, Carnielli V, et al. Resting energy expenditure is increased in infants and children with extrahepatic biliary atresia. J Pediatr Surg 1989;24:534–8.
173. Fitzsimmons SC, Burkhart GA, Borowitz D, et al. High-dose pancreatic-enzyme supplements and fibrosing colonopathy in children with cystic fibrosis. N Engl J Med 1997;336:1283–9.
174. Borowitz DS, Grand RJ, Durie PR. Use of pancreatic enzyme supplements for patients with cystic fibrosis in the context of fibrosing colonopathy. Consensus Committee. J Pediatr 1995; 127:681–4.
175. Ramsey BW, Farrell PM, Pencharz P. Nutritional assessment and management in cystic fibrosis: a consensus report. The Consensus Committee. Am J Clin Nutr 1992;55:108–16.
176. Efrati O, Barak A, Modan-Moses D, et al. Liver cirrhosis and portal hypertension in cystic fibrosis. Eur J Gastroenterol Hepatol 2003;15:1073–8.
177. Nio M, Hayashi Y, Sano N, et al. Long-term efficacy of partial splenic embolization in children. J Pediatr Surg 2003;38:1760–2.
178. Harned RK, Thompson HR, Kumpe DA, et al. Partial splenic embolization in five children with hypersplenism: effects of

reduced-volume embolization on efficacy and morbidity. Radiology 1998;209[3]:803–6.
179. Fridell JA, Bond GJ, Mazariegos GV, et al. Liver transplantation in children with cystic fibrosis: a long-term longitudinal review of a single center's experience. J Pediatr Surg 2003;38:1152–6.
180. Molmenti EP, Squires RH, Nagata D, et al. Liver transplantation for cholestasis associated with cystic fibrosis in the pediatric population. Pediatr Transplant 2003;7:93–7.
181. Couetil JP, Houssin DP, Soubrane O, et al. Combined lung and liver transplantation in patients with cystic fibrosis. A 4 1/2-year experience. J Thorac Cardiovasc Surg 1995;110[5]:1415–22.
182. Fridell JA, Mazariegos GV, Orenstein D, et al. Liver and intestinal transplantation in a child with cystic fibrosis: a case report. Pediatr Transplant 2003;7:240–2.
183. Grubman SA, Fang SL, Mulberg AE, et al. Correction of the cystic fibrosis defect by gene complementation in human intrahepatic biliary cell lines. Gastroenterology 1995;108:584–92.
184. Yang Y, Raper SE, Cohn JA, et al. An approach for treating the hepatobiliary disease of cystic fibrosis by somatic gene transfer. Proc Nat Acad Sci U S A 1993;90:4601–5.
185. Palmer E, Wilhelm JM, Sherman F. Phenotypic suppression of nonsense mutants in yeast by aminoglycoside antibiotics. Nature 1979;277:148–50.
186. Bedwell DM, Kaenjak A, Benos DJ, et al. Suppression of a CFTR premature stop mutation in a bronchial epithelial cell line. Nat Med 1997;3:1280–4.
187. Rubenstein RC, Egan ME, Zeitlin PL. In vitro pharmacologic restoration of CFTR-mediated chloride transport with sodium 4-phenylbutyrate in cystic fibrosis epithelial cells containing delta F508-CFTR. J Clin Invest 1997;100:2457–65.
188. Eidelman O, Guay-Broder C, van Galen PJ, et al. A1 adenosine-receptor antagonists activate chloride efflux from cystic fibrosis cells. Proc Natl Acad Sci U S A 1992;89:5562–6.
189. Egan ME, Pearson M, Weiner SA, et al. Curcumin, a major constituent of turmeric, corrects cystic fibrosis defects. Science 2004;304:600–2.
190. Song Y, Sonawane ND, Salinas D, et al. Evidence against the rescue of defective DeltaF508-CFTR cellular processing by curcumin in cell culture and mouse models. J Biol Chem 2004; 279:40629–33.
191. Dragomir A, Bjorstad J, Hjelte L, Roomans GM. Curcumin does not stimulate cAMP-mediated chloride transport in cystic fibrosis airway epithelial cells. Biochem Biophys Res Commun 2004;322:447–51.
192. Illek B, Yankaskas J, Machen TE. cAMPand genistein stimulate HCO3- conductance through CFTR in human airway epithelia. Am J Physiol 1997;272:L752–61.
193. Illek B, Zhang L, Lewis NC, et al. Defective function of the cystic fibrosis-causing missense mutation G551D is recovered by genistein. Am J Physiol 1999;277:C833–9.
194. Kelley TJ, Al Nakkash L, Cotton CU, Drumm ML. Activation of endogenous deltaF508 cystic fibrosis transmembrane conductance regulator by phosphodiesterase inhibition. J Clin Invest 1996;98:513–20.
195. Kelley TJ, Thomas K, Milgram LJ, Drumm ML. In vivo activation of the cystic fibrosis transmembrane conductance regulator mutant deltaF508 in murine nasal epithelium. Proc Natl Acad Sci U S A 1997;94:2604–8.
196. Schwiebert EM, Cid-Soto LP, Stafford D, et al. Analysis of ClC-2 channels as an alternative pathway for chloride conduction in cystic fibrosis airway cells. Proc Nat Acad Sci U S A 1998;95:3879–84.
197. Fickert P, Wagner M, Fuchsbichler A, et al. 24-Norursodeoxycholic acid as novel therapeutic approach to sclerosing cholangitis in MDR2 (ABCB4) knockout mice. Hepatology 2005;42 Suppl 1:274A.
198. Wagner M, Trauner M. Transcriptional regulation of hepatobiliary transport systems in health and disease: implications for a rationale approach to the treatment of intrahepatic cholestasis. Ann Hepatol 2005;4:77–99.
199. Liu Y, Binz J, Numerick MJ, et al. Hepatoprotection by the farnesoid X receptor agonist GW4064 in rat models of intra- and extrahepatic cholestasis. J Clin Invest 2003;112:1678–87.
200. Fiorucci S, Clerici C, Antonelli E, et al. Protective effects of 6-ethyl chenodeoxycholic acid, a farnesoid X receptor ligand, in estrogen-induced cholestasis. J Pharmacol Exp Ther 2005;313: 604–12.
201. Griese M, Ramakers J, Krasselt A, et al. Improvement of alveolar glutathione and lung function but not oxidative state in cystic fibrosis. Am J Respir Crit Care Med 2004;169:822–8.
202. Britton RS, Bacon BR. Role of free radicals in liver diseases and hepatic fibrosis. Hepatogastroenterology 1994;41:343–8.
203. Zhang M, Song G, Minuk GY. Effects of hepatic stimulator substance, herbal medicine, selenium/vitamin E, and ciprofloxacin on cirrhosis in the rat. Gastroenterology 1996;110:1150–5.
204. Friedman SL. Molecular mechanisms of hepatic fibrosis and principles of therapy. J Gastroenterol 1997;32:424–30.
205. Friedman SL. Molecular regulation of hepatic fibrosis, an integrated cellular response to tissue injury. J Biol Chem 2000;275: 2247–50.
206. Yata Y, Gotwals P, Koteliansky V, Rockey DC. Dose-dependent inhibition of hepatic fibrosis in mice by a TGF-beta soluble receptor: implications for antifibrotic therapy. Hepatology 2002; 35:1022–30.
207. Jonsson JR, Clouston AD, Ando Y, et al. Angiotensin-converting enzyme inhibition attenuates the progression of rat hepatic fibrosis. Gastroenterology 2001;121:148–55.
208. Di SA, Bendia E, Svegliati BG, et al. Effect of pirfenidone on rat hepatic stellate cell proliferation and collagen production. J Hepatol 2002;37:584–91.

25

Inborn Errors of Carbohydrate Metabolism

Fayez K. Ghishan, M.D., and Mona Zawaideh, M.D.

This chapter deals with three inborn errors of carbohydrate metabolism that lead to hepatic dysfunction: galactosemia, hereditary fructose intolerance (HFI), and glycogen storage disease (GSD) types I, III, and IV. The clinical presentation of such patients includes varying degrees of hypoglycemia, acidosis, growth failure, and hepatic dysfunction. Appropriate steps in obtaining clinical history, physical examination, and laboratory evaluation support a definitive diagnosis. Advances in biochemistry and molecular biology, which have made significant contributions toward better understanding of the molecular defects underlying these disorders, are anticipated to result eventually in the development of newer treatment strategies. The newer information is highlighted in this chapter.

GALACTOSEMIA

The first detailed characterization of a galactose-intolerant individual was provided by Mason and Turner in 1935 [1]. Since then, three distinct disorders of galactose metabolism and several variant forms of the disease have been identified. These disorders are transmitted by autosomal recessive inheritance and are expressed as a cellular deficiency of one of three enzymes in the metabolic pathway through which galactose is converted to glucose: galactose-1-phosphate uridyl transferase, galactokinase, and uridine diphosphate (UDP) galactose-4-epimerase. The terms *transferase deficiency galactosemia*, *galactokinase deficiency galactosemia*, and *epimerase deficiency galactosemia* traditionally have been used to distinguish between the various forms of the disease. Until recently, the genetic basis of galactosemia was discerned primarily through quantification of red cell activity of these enzymes. Recent advances in molecular biology, however, have led to the identification of more than 150 genetic mutations, which soon may be used to characterize this metabolic disorder [2,3]. Each enzymatic defect associated with galactosemia results in a distinctive clinical presentation. Clinical manifestations of toxicity in transferase-deficiency galactosemia, the classic form of the disease, include malnutrition, growth failure, cataract formation, progressive liver disease, mental retardation, and ovarian failure [4,5]. Galactokinase deficiency, originally described by Gitzelmann in 1967 [6], results primarily in cataract formation. In most cases of UDP galactose-4-epimerase deficiency, the defect is limited to erythrocytes and leukocytes; therefore, affected individuals display no clinical or laboratory manifestations of galactosemia [7,8]. In a variant form of epimerase deficiency galactosemia identified by Holton and colleagues in 1981 [9], however, the defect is more generalized and results in a severe clinical presentation resembling the classic form of the disease [9–12].

Treatment of galactosemia has remained essentially unchanged since the disorder first was described more than 60 years ago. Confidence in dietary strategies that effectively minimize galactose intake in affected individuals, however, has declined significantly in the past decade. This coincides with recognition that long-term complications such as learning difficulties, speech disorders, ovarian failure, and ataxia syndromes commonly occur in well-treated patients. It is now clear that development of new treatment strategies is necessary to have a positive impact on the outcome of this disorder. To this end, future research efforts should be focused on developing a complete understanding of the molecular and biochemical basis of galactosemia, particularly as they relate to the pathogenesis of these long-term complications [13].

Physiology and Biochemistry of Galactose Metabolism

Galactose is a monosaccharide that is derived from the hydrolysis of lactose, the sugar in dairy products. Lactose is hydrolyzed into glucose and galactose by the disaccharidase, lactase, in the brush border membranes of the enterocytes. Galactose is transported across the brush border membrane of the enterocyte through the Na^+-dependent glucose–galactose transporter [14]. Galactose is metabolized to glucose in a series of reactions as depicted in Figure 25.1. The first step in galactose metabolism involves phosphorylation of galactose by adenosine triphosphate (ATP) utilizing the enzyme galactokinase. This enzyme is present in bacteria [15], yeast [16], and mammalian tissues [17]. Galactokinase in the human liver shows developmental changes, with progressive increase from the seventh week until term [18]. The level of activity in the red blood cells is higher

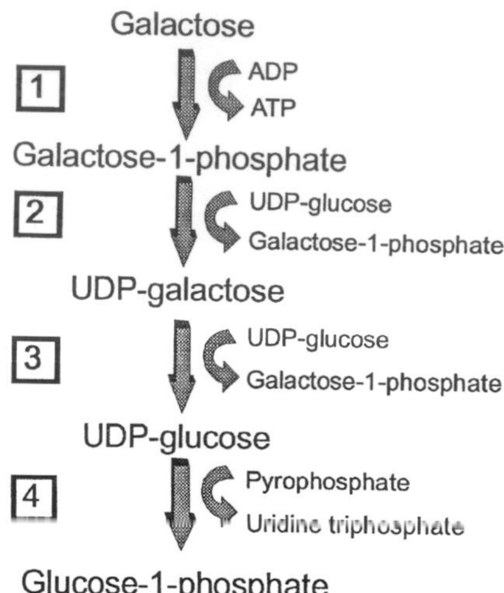

Figure 25.1. Galactose metabolism. 1, Galactokinase; 2, galactose-1-phosphate uridyl; 3, uridine diphosphate galactose-4-epimerase; 4, uridine diphosphate glucose pyrophosphorylase.

in the newborn than in the adult. The enyzme, however, is not regulated by galactose.

The second step in galactose metabolism involves the reaction of galactose-1-phosphate with UDP glucose, which is catalyzed by the enzyme galactose-1-phosphate uridyl transferase. The enzyme is present in most mammalian tissues including the liver [19]. This reaction results in the formation of UDP galactose and glucose-1-phosphate. The complementary DNA (cDNA) encoding for the human transferase enzyme is 1295 bases in length and encodes a 43,000-dalton protein [20].

The third step in galactose metabolism involves the interconversion of UDP galactose to UDP glucose through the catalysis of the enzyme UDP galactose-4-epimerase [21]. The fourth step in galactose metabolism involves the generation of glucose-1-phosphate from UDP glucose by the enzyme UDP glucose pyrophosphorylase. This enzyme has been crystallized from the mammalian liver [22], and it appears to play a role in the synthesis of UDP glucose from UDP and glucose.

Alternative pathways of galactose metabolism involve reduction to galactitol through two enzymes, namely, aldose reductase and L-hexonate dehydrogenase [23]. The existence of this alternative pathway explains the presence of galactitol in the urine of patients with both transferase and galactokinase deficiencies [24,25]. The other pathway involves oxidation of galactose to galactonate. Patients with transferase deficiency excrete galactonate in their urine [26].

Humans are able to metabolize large amounts of galactose as evidenced by rapid clearance of galactose from blood. Fifty percent of injected radiolabeled galactose is found in glucose pools within 30 minutes [27]. The removal mechanism of galactose from the blood is saturated at 50 mg/dL secondary to the limited ability of galactokinase to phosphorylate the sugar [28]. During the infancy period, 40% of calories is derived from the hydrolysis of lactose to galactose and glucose. Therefore, the conversion of galactose to glucose is of importance to maintain euglycemia.

Consequently, transferase deficiency typically results in more severe symptoms compared with the other defects in galactokinase and UDP galactose-4-epimerase deficiency.

Molecular Basis of Galactosemia

Galactosemia is an inborn error of metabolism resulting from a deficiency of the human galactose-1-phosphate uridyl transferase enzyme. The sequences of the homologous proteins from *Escherichia coli* [29], *Saccharomyces cerevisiae* [30], and humans [20] have been reported. The overall amino acid sequence identity of the enzymes in bacteria, yeast, and humans is approximately 35%. The cDNA that encodes the human transferase enzyme is 1295 bases in length and encodes a 43,000-dalton molecular weight protein. The gene has been mapped to chromosome 9p18. The gene has eleven exons and spans 4 kilobases (kb). Southern, Northern, and Western blot experiments suggested that the majority of the patients with galactosemia have missense mutations [31]. These mutations result in low or undetectable enzymatic activity. More than 180 mutations have been identified [3]. The most common galactosemia mutation characterized so far involves glutamine 188 substitution by arginine Q188R, which has a prevalence of 60–70% in galactosemic Caucasians and results in no enzymatic activity [32]. The mutated glutamine is a highly conserved residue in evolution and is two amino acid residues downstream from the active site histidine–proline–histidine triad [33]. Several other mutations have been described and suggest that galactosemia results from a multiplicity of mutations at the molecular level. These mutations involve evolutionary conserved amino residues. Mutation S135L, involving leucine substitution by serine, occurs mainly in African Americans and results in residual enzyme activity. The N314D mutation occurs in Caucasians, Asians, and African Americans. The basis of the Durate variant involves an asparagine to aspartate change, which is benign because it expresses diminished enzyme activity [34]. Polymorphisms occurring in nonconserved domains result in normal enzymatic function [35]. The molecular heterogeneity is thought to be responsible for the variability in clinical outcome.

Transferase-Deficiency Galactosemia

The first described metabolic defect resulting in galactosemia occurs at the second step in galactose metabolism (Figure 25.1). Transferase-deficiency galactosemia is inherited through autosomal recessive transmission and occurs in approximately 1 in 50,000 live births [36].

Clinical Presentation

Several reports of large groups of patients with galactosemia followed over the course of years have been published. In 1961, Hsia and Walker [37] reported the variable clinical presentations of 45 patients. Donnell et al. [38] described growth patterns of 24 children with galactosemia and more recently reported follow-up on findings from a series of 39 patients [39]. Observations of 55 galactosemic individuals were reported by Nadler et al. in 1969 [40]. In 1980, Fishler et al. [41] updated long-term follow-up data from 47 families in the Los Angeles area. Komrower and Lee [42,43] in 1982 updated previously published findings in the 60 known patients of galactosemia in Great Britain. Finally, Waggoner et al. [44] reported findings from a survey of 350 patients related to long-term prognosis of galactosemia in 1990. These reports, coupled with numerous case descriptions published since 1935, have established clearly the clinical entity of this disease.

The clinical presentation of transferase-deficiency galactosemia varies in severity from an acute fulminant illness characterized by abdominal distention, vomiting, diarrhea, anorexia, and hypoglycemia after the first milk feeding to a subacute illness beginning within the first few days of life. Most certainly, the great variation in clinical characteristics among patients with this complex disorder ultimately will be elucidated through correlation of genotypic and phenotypic features [2,34]. Failure to thrive is the most common presenting symptom and occurs in almost all patients. Vomiting or diarrhea may occur in 95% of patients [40]. Jaundice and hepatomegaly develop almost as frequently after the first week of life. Severe hemolysis and erythroblastosis may occur in some patients and may accentuate jaundice caused by intrinsic liver disease. Prolonged conjugated hyperbilirubinemia is a common presenting symptom in infants with this form of galactosemia. Urine tests for reducing sugars should be performed in all infants presenting with this symptom. Ascites may develop within 2–5 weeks after birth with continued galactose ingestion and is present in most infants who succumb to the disease.

Cataracts may develop early within the postnatal period, or they may be present at birth if the mother ingested generous amounts of dairy products late in pregnancy. These punctate lesions in the nucleus of the lens may be so small that slit-lamp examination is required for visualization. Signs of increased intracranial pressure and cerebral edema also have been observed as a presenting feature [45]. Mental retardation may become apparent after several months.

In 1977, Levy et al. [46] identified a direct correlation between galactosemia and neonatal *E. coli* sepsis. In their review of more than 700,000 infants screened during a 12-year period, four of eight infants were diagnosed with septicemia and transferase-deficiency galactosemia during the second week of life; three of the four died. Thirty-five more patients with classic galactosemia were identified through further review of data from routine screening of over 2.5 million infants from eight other states. *E. coli* sepsis was documented in 10 of the 35 patients, and 9 of 10 died despite antibiotic therapy. Systemic infection seems to develop at approximately 7–14 days of age and appears to be directly associated with continued galactose ingestion secondary to inhibition of leukocyte bactericidal activity by the sugar [47]. As a result of these important clinical observations, neonates diagnosed with galactosemia or *E. coli* sepsis should undergo further evaluation to rule out the alternate condition.

Mild symptoms of vomiting or diarrhea following milk ingestion may be the only presenting symptoms in mild forms of the disease. A few individuals have been found to be entirely asymptomatic on milk feedings. These patients, who are usually black, are homozygous for the disease and may have the ability to metabolize moderate amounts of galactose [48].

Lactose-free formulas have become increasingly accessible, and feeding trials with these products are employed in infants who experience recurrent vomiting and growth failure early in life. Because these are the most common presenting symptoms of galactosemia, a child with the disorder may display improvement in symptoms without recognition of the underlying defect. In such patients, galactosemia may remain undetected through the first several months of life until motor retardation, hepatomegaly, or cataracts develop [49]. Still others may be diagnosed after several years of life. These individuals usually suffer from mental retardation and visual disturbances caused by cataracts and frequently have a history of vomiting after milk intake managed by reduced intake or use of milk substitutes [50].

Biochemical Features and the Pathogenesis of Galactose Toxicity

Aberrant laboratory findings in galactosemia vary but may include elevations in blood and urinary galactose levels, hyperchloremic acidosis, hypoglycemia (occasionally severe and prolonged in nature), abnormal liver function tests, albuminuria, and aminoaciduria [51–54]. Galactosuria occurs only intermittently during periods of substantial food intake and completely resolves within 3–4 days of intravenous feeding. Diagnosis of the disease may be overlooked if a urine test for reducing sugar is timed inappropriately. In contrast, the presence of urinary reducing sugar does not confirm the diagnosis, because other conditions that impair blood galactose clearance such as severe liver disease, fructosuria, and lactosuria resulting from intestinal lactase deficiency may produce this finding [49]. Further tests to establish the diagnosis should be done if urinary reducing substances do not react with the glucose oxidase test.

Pathologic changes that accompany galactosemia affect the liver, lens of the eye, brain, and kidney. Toxicity seems to result primarily from accumulation of two by-products of galactose metabolism, galactose-1-phosphate and galactitol (Figure 25.1). Although the mechanisms resulting in pathologic changes of all organs are not clearly understood, defective galactosylation of complex molecules may play a role in the pathogenesis of galactosemia.

Liver

Hepatic changes associated with transferase-deficiency galactosemia result entirely from abnormal galactose metabolism. In affected individuals, galactose ingestion results in elevated levels of both galactose-1-phosphate and galactitol in the liver. Other findings, however, suggest that one or more additional metabolites act alone or together to produce the liver damage seen in this form of the disease. For example, liver damage does not occur in normal laboratory animals fed diets rich in galactose, despite hepatic galactitol accumulation in chicks [55] and hepatic accumulation of galactose-1-phosphate in rats [56]. Furthermore, humans with galactokinase deficiency accumulate large amounts of galactitol but develop no liver damage. The amount of galactosamine, which is known to stimulate hepatocellular changes in animals, was found to be increased in one patient with galactosemia [57].

Kidney

Individuals with transferase-deficiency galactosemia develop renal tubular dysfunction following galactose ingestion; over time, levels of galactose-1-phosphate and galactitol accumulate in the kidneys [57,58]. Alteration in kidney function appears to result primarily from increased galactose-1-phosphate levels, because patients with galactokinase deficiency who characteristically excrete large amounts of galactitol develop renal impairment. Galactose-1-phosphate accumulation also may produce the aminoaciduria seen in this disorder through secondary inhibition of amino acid accumulation by the tubules [59]. The inhibition is noncompetitive and similar to that seen in human intestine [60]. Large amounts of galactose can induce aminoaciduria in normal man and rats [61,62].

Lenticular Changes

The specific mechanisms for cellular changes in the eye are more clearly understood than in other organs. Changes in the lens seem to result primarily from galactitol accumulation, which initially was reported by van Heyningen in 1959 [63]. Later, Kinoshita et al. [64,65] demonstrated that a concomitant increase in water content occurred with galactitol buildup caused by oncotic pressure exerted by the alcohol. Poor diffusion of galactitol from these tissues leads to further damage and cataract formation. Application of an osmotically balanced incubation medium prevents opacification [64].

Nutrient supplementation has been shown to alter the rate of cataract formation in animals [66]. Biochemical changes induced by galactose feeding include decreases in several enzymatic reactions, amino acid transport, protein synthesis, and alterations in ion fluxes. These occur simultaneously as cataract formation takes place [64,65,67–71]. As little as 2 days of galactose ingestion can reduce glycolysis and lenticular respiration by approximately 30%, and this reduction is sustained until cataracts are formed. Nutrient imbalances and changes in lenticular water content resulting from galactitol accumulation are principal initiators of lenticular opacification.

Brain

Galactitol accumulates in higher concentrations in brain tissue of humans and rats fed galactose than in any other tissue except the lens [56,72]. Therefore, galactitol appears to be a factor in the development of brain function abnormalities seen in transferase-deficiency galactosemia. On the other hand, damage from galactitol accumulation in patients with galactokinase deficiency seems to be limited to the lens.

Pathologic alterations in brain tissue of individuals with transferase-deficiency galactosemia may not be completely reversible through dietary galactose restriction. Considerable attention has been paid to defining the specific mechanism for galactose-induced brain damage. In laboratory studies, galactose administration resulted in diminished levels of ATP, reduced brain glucose and glycolytic intermediate concentrations, altered the usual distribution of hexokinase, heightened fragility of neural lysosomes, and impaired fast axoplasmic transport [73–77]. These changes seem to be associated with other conditions, namely, hyperosmolality [77], alteration in energy metabolism [74], abnormal serotonin levels [78], and interference with active uptake of glucose into neurons. Glucose administration temporarily reversed the changes [79]. In more recent studies by Tsakiris et al. [80], in vitro galactosemia involving suckling and adult rat brains showed inhibition of (Na^+,K^+)- ATPase and activation of Mg^{2+}ATPase in classical and galactokinase deficiency galactosemia. This effect was reversed by the addition of antioxidants to the mix.

Intestine

Many infants with transferase-deficiency galactosemia experience vomiting and diarrhea after galactose ingestion. It has been shown that transferase activity in the intestinal epithelium is deficient in this form of the disease [60]; however, intestinal transport of galactose appears to remain normal. This supports the hypothesis that gastrointestinal symptoms of the disease are secondary to effects on the central nervous system rather than a direct effect on the intestine.

Gonads

The majority of galactosemic females have ovarian failure, as characterized by hypergonadotropic hypogonadism [81,82]. Because of the observation that a 5-day-old child with galactosemia had normal follicles, it is thought that the ovarian failure occurs postnatally [83]. The mechanism underlying ovarian failure in galactosemic women is not known, although galactose toxicity has been implicated. Despite the documented ovarian failure in most of the affected patients, successful pregnancies have been reported [84]. Affected male patients do not appear to have gonadal atrophy.

Cellular Mechanisms for Cell Toxicity by Galactose

Red blood cells from patients with transferase deficiency exhibit impaired oxygen uptake if incubated with galactose [85]. Similarly, fibroblast cultures from such patients show no growth if incubated with galactose [86]. Because mutant *E. coli* organisms deficient in transferase enzyme have an impaired growth in galactose media but galactokinase mutants do not, it has been suggested that cell toxicity is related to accumulation of galactose-1-phosphate [87,88].

Diagnosis

The presence of urinary reducing sugar that does not react with glucose oxidase reagents in an infant with vomiting and growth failure on milk feedings supports a presumptive diagnosis of galactosemia. During the first 2 weeks of life, some normal premature and term infants excrete up to 60 mg/dL galactose in urine. Furthermore, lactose, fructose, and pentose can produce the same urine test result, and the specific sugar may be identified only by paper or gas–liquid chromatography. More recently, screening for galactosuria has been simplified by the availability of paper impregnated with galactose oxidase. Regardless, galactose restriction should be instituted promptly if no other dietary carbohydrate is identified. Confirmation of the diagnosis should be made through direct measurement of transferase activity. Recently, Xu et al. [89] developed a highly sensitive radiochemical assay that can detect galactose-1-phosphate uridyl transferase (GalT) activity as low as 0.1% of normal in erythrocytes and leukocytes. Galactose tolerance tests should never be employed for this purpose, because it has been suggested that a single exposure to a large quantity of galactose may produce brain injury resulting from prolonged severe hypoglycemia [49,90].

During the past 15 years, measurement of red cell UDP glucose consumption has been employed extensively as a diagnostic test for galactosemia [49,91,92]. It is based on quantitation of UDP glucose before and after incubation of galactose-1-phosphate, using added red cell hemolysate as the enzyme source. Results are obtained through spectrophotometric measurement of nicotinamide adenine dinucleotide (NAD), which is formed from hepatic NAD through the conversion of UDP glucose to UDP glucuronic acid by UDP glucose dehydrogenase. Homozygous patients exhibit complete absence of red cell transferase activity. Heterozygous carriers typically display intermediate levels of enzyme activity. Multiple variants of galactosemia have been identified and are more prevalent than classic transferase-deficiency galactosemia. Infants with 50% of normal enzyme activity should undergo further tests to identify the presence of a specific variant of the disease [93].

More recently, cloning of the cDNA encoding for the transferase enzyme, as well as the observation that the majority of galactosemic patients have a missense mutation, allowed introduction of rapid molecular techniques for analysis of common mutations such as Q188R [31–33,35].

Genetic Screening for Galactosemia

Multiple variants of galactosemia have become apparent since the advent of genetic screening for the disease [94–99]. Three homozygotic types exist: (1) “Classic” galactosemia is autosomal recessive, and transferase activity is absent in red cells, fibroblasts, the liver, and presumably all other tissues. Asymptomatic, heterozygotic carriers, on the other hand, exhibit 50% enzyme activity. The prevalence of classic galactosemia in the United States has been estimated to be 1 in 63,000. (2) The most frequently detected abnormality in neonatal screening is the compound heterozygous state, consisting of allelic genes for classic galactosemia and the Duarte variant; it is the most common form of the disease, affecting up to 10–15% of the population. Some infants with this form of the disease exhibit characteristic symptoms and metabolic manifestations of galactosemia. Others, however, are asymptomatic at birth and remain so throughout infancy. Diagnosis of the disease requires enzyme screening. On starch gel electrophoresis, red cells of patients with the Duarte variant produce two distinct bands rather than a normal single band. Red cells of a parent of a homozygous Duarte variant patients have three bands for the variant enzyme, and its mobility is increased on starch gel electrophoresis. (3) Erythrocyte transferase activity is absent in the negro variant; the liver and intestine exhibit 10% of normal activity. Clinical manifestations of the Duarte and negro variants range from asymptomatic to a galactose toxicity syndrome occurring in the postnatal period.

Several heterozygotic forms of galactosemia also have been identified: the Indiana variant, characterized by erythrocyte transferase activity at approximately 35% of normal with delayed enzyme migration; the Rennes variant, also characterized by delayed enzyme migration on starch gel electrophoresis; the Los Angeles variant, distinguished by rapid electrophoretic mobility like that of the Duarte variant and erythrocyte transferase activity at 140% of normal; and Chicago and West German variants.

Treatment

Ongoing efforts to incorporate expanding molecular data in increasing knowledge regarding the full panorama of normal and pathologic aspects of galactose metabolism is anticipated to lead to new therapeutic strategies in treatment of galactosemia. To date, two possible new treatment strategies have emerged. The first, involving administration of uridine to patients, has been hypothesized to correct problems related to reduced galactosylation [100] by increasing the level of sugar nucleotides (including UDP galactose) in red cells. Unfortunately, clinical trials of this strategy have produced no convincing evidence of its therapeutic value [100,101]. Second, animal studies have indicated that the use of aldose reductase inhibitors may be effective in restoring the balance of tissue polyols by blocking production of galactitol from galatose; this strategy has not undergone trials in human subjects [12,102].

Elimination of dietary galactose is currently the only available approach to treatment of transferase-deficiency galactosemia. Early diagnosis and nutritional intervention consistently results in survival, reversal of acute symptoms and biochemical manifestations, normal growth, and complete normalization of liver function in many patients. Nevertheless, long-term follow-up data have shown great variability among those equally well treated by conventional management [41,42, 44,45,48–50,90]. Mental retardation, neurologic disorders, ovarian failure, and growth inhibition continue to occur among survivors of this metabolic disorder. Other factors that may contribute to suboptimal therapeutic impact have been identified. For years, there has been concern that the diet of patients with galactosemia is not sufficiently restrictive, and endogenous production of galactose in galactosemic patients is viewed as a potential significant cause of ongoing galactose toxicity in seemingly well-treated patients [2].

Traditionally, patient management has focused on the elimination of milk and dairy products. Several studies since the 1950s, however, have raised concerns that ongoing galactose toxicity may result from the presence of galactose in grains [103], fruits [104,105], and vegetables [106–111]. Gross and Acosta [112] determined that various fruits and vegetables contain significant amounts of soluble galactose, as delineated in Table 25.1, and it has been recommended that appropriate consideration be given to this information in designing therapeutic nutritional regimens. These foodstuffs contain B-1,4-linked galactosyl residues in cell wall structures, primarily in the form of pectin-associated B-1,4-galactan. Galactose is hydrolyzed from the nonreducing end of the galactan molecule by B-galactosidase present in the human gut, rendering it available for absorption [112,113]. Realization of the actual impact of this dietary constituent in galactosemia requires further clinical investigation, although the newer information related to substantial endogenous production of galactose has minimized this concern [111].

In 1969 [114] and again in 1974 [115], Gitzelmann and Hansen postulated that galactose could be formed from UDP galactose breakdown in individuals with galactosemia, resulting in chronic self-intoxication. Undertaken in an effort to explain the development of long-term complications of galactosemia despite meticulous dietary galactose restriction, studies by Berry et al. [116] have shed new light on this phenomenon. Using ^{13}C galactose, these researchers have shown that galactose and glucose-1-phosphate are synthesized endogenously from glucose-1-phosphate at a rate of more than 1 g/d, corresponding to estimates made from urinary galactitol excretion reported earlier [117]. Endogenous production far exceeds exogenous galactose intake, which typically amounts to 20–40 mg/d on an appropriately restricted diet.

Commercial infant formulas appropriate for use in the management of transferase-deficiency galactosemia include soy formulas, Enfamil LactoFree (Mead-Johnson, Evansville, Indiana), and Similac Lactose Free (Ross-Abbott Laboratories, Chicago, Illinois). The use of soy preparations has been questioned in the past, because of the presence of galactose in oligosaccharides such as raffinose and stachyose. Gitzelmann and Auricchio [113] have demonstrated, however, that these α-linked galactosyl residues are not hydrolyzed by human digestive enzymes. A clinical investigation of the use of soy products in the management of several patients by Donnell et al. [39] concluded that galactose absorption does not occur from these products. Pregestimil (Mead Johnson Nutritionals) and Alimentum (Ross Laboratories, Columbus, Ohio), casein-based protein hydrolysate formulas that contain medium-chain triacylglycerol (MCT) oil, should be used until liver dysfunction associated with the acute galactose toxicity has resolved [111].

Careful attention to elimination of galactose should be given throughout the progression to solid foods, because of the frequent use of dairy products in food preparation. Complete elimination is the desired goal, but this may be difficult to accomplish. Some have advocated that diets be restricted to

Table 25.1: Soluble Galactose Content (mg/100 g Fresh Weight ± SE) of Various Fruits and Vegetables

Fruit/Vegetable	*Content*
Persimmon, American	35.4 ± 2.5
Papaya	28.6 ± 1.9
Tomato	23.0 ± 2.0
Watermelon	14.7 ± 2.0
Date	11.5 ± 0.6
Pepper, bell	10.2 ± 0.4
Pumpkin	9.9 ± 2.5
Kiwi	9.8 ± 0.4
Pepper, cayenne	9.7 ± 4.0
Banana	9.2 ± 0.8
Brussels sprouts	9.2 ± 0.7
Apple	8.3 ± 0.7
Potato, sweet	7.7 ± 0.7
Pear	7.3 ± 1.4
Broccoli	6.8 ± 0.7
Carrot	6.2 ± 0.4
Onion, bunching	6.1 ± 0.3
Onion, yellow	5.1 ± 0.3
Pea, sweet	4.9 ± 0.8
Turnip	4.9 ± 0.6
Eggplant (aubergine)	4.7 ± 0.2
Bean sprouts, green	4.3 ± 0.2
Cantaloupe melon	4.3 ± 0.2
Cauliflower	4.3 ± 0.3
Orange, sweet	4.3 ± 0.4
Grapefruit	4.1 ± 0.1
Cucumber	4.0 ± 0.3
Corn, sweet	3.7 ± 0.3
Cabbage, common	3.3 ± 0.2
Zucchini squash	3.3 ± 0.1
Lettuce, garden	3.1 ± 0.3
Grape, green	2.9 ± 0.1
Celery	2.4 ± 0.1
Kale	2.3 ± 0.2
Asparagus	1.2 ± 0.6
Apricot	1.1 ± 0.6
Potato, white	1.2 ± 0.3
Beet, red	0.8 ± 0.2
Radish, red	0.5 ± 0.3
Avocado	<0.5
Spinach	<0.5
Artichoke	Not detectable
Mushroom, common	Not detectable
Olive, green	Not detectable
Peanut	Not detectable

Adapted from Gross and Acosta [112], with permission.

less than 125 mg galactose daily [118]. Regardless, successful dietary management is dependent entirely on thorough education of caregivers.

Within 72 hours of initiation of a galactose-free diet, all acute symptoms associated with transferase-deficiency galactosemia show marked improvement, and hepatic dysfunction begins to normalize by the end of 1 week. Ingestion of small amounts of galactose may reinduce symptoms during childhood. On the other hand, most patients experience an improved tolerance to galactose around puberty. Segal and Cuatrecasas [119] postulated the development of an alternative metabolic pathway for oxidation of galactose to explain this phenomenon. As illustrated in Figure 25.1, the formation of UDP galactose from the interaction of galactose-1-phosphate and uridine triphosphate bypasses the deficient transferase reaction. This would result in normal concentrations of galactose-1-phosphate in liver and brain, protecting against further effects of the enzyme defect. This hypothesis sets forth a plausible explanation for the increased galactose tolerance later in life. Isotope studies have not demonstrated an increased rate of galactose metabolism, however, and do not support this theory [48,49,90]. A third pathway without significance in normal humans, involving formation of xylulose, may increase the duration of survival in some patients with the disease who continue to consume galactose. In older patients, liberalization of the diet to include limited quantities of foods containing milk and dairy products should be considered to minimize the psychologic effect of lifelong stringent dietary restrictions [50]. Milk restriction, however, should be maintained.

Dietary galactose restriction is warranted during subsequent pregnancies in asymptomatic heterozygotic mothers who have given birth to children with galactosemia. These women may have elevated serum galactose levels with liberal milk and dairy product ingestion. Consequently, their infants may exhibit symptoms of galactosemia at birth [48,49,90]. Donnell et al. [39] employed this strategy in 11 pregnancies resulting in transferase-deficient infants; in only one were cataracts detectable at birth.

Subsequent Course

All acute manifestations of the galactose toxicity syndrome show marked improvement by the end of 1 week of treatment. Cataracts regress substantially with elimination of galactose from the diet. Findings from the long-term follow-up studies in the United States provide the basis for current knowledge regarding the subsequent course of transferase-deficiency galactosemia and substantiate the value of early diagnosis and intervention in minimizing the overall impact of this disease. In the U.S. series, normal growth and development have resulted from effective diet therapy [39,41]. In general, this conflicts with findings of British observers, who have reported that most patients remain below the 50th percentile in height despite rigid dietary control [42].

Mental retardation is the most significant result of galactose toxicity. Very low IQ values, however, are seen infrequently in transferase-deficiency galactosemia, even if diet therapy is initiated late in the first year of life. In the U.S. experience, eventual intelligence level appears highly correlated with adequate dietary control and may even be influenced by intrauterine exposure. In the series of 41 patients followed by Donnell and colleagues [39], 29 (71%) had IQs greater than 85, 7 (17%) had IQs between 70 and 84, and only 3 (7%) were determined to be severely retarded. Furthermore, normal IQ values were found among those whose mothers were on galactose-free diets during pregnancy and were treated from birth. One other individual who was treated initially at age 14 months also had a normal IQ. Nadler et al. [40] reported IQs between 71 and 89 in 10 (23%) of 44 patients and IQs below 70 in 8 (18%) patients. These researchers found that the average IQ of individuals in the normal range was lower than the average IQ of their siblings. Once again, reports from the British experience have not been as favorable. Komrower and Lee [42] reported an average IQ of 84 in 34 patients on appropriately restricted diets; another 22 patients with histories of moderate to poor dietary treatment had an average IQ of 77.

Functional deficits in a high percentage of individuals with galactosemia has been noted, even in those with normal IQs. Consequently, the association of adequate treatment and functional impairment is less clear. Learning disabilities involving spatial relationships and mathematics, behavioral problems resulting from short attention spans, and psychologic problems manifested by inadequate drive, shyness, and social withdrawal occur often in these patients. Many are behind by one or more grades in school [40,42]. Waisbren et al. [120] have documented speech and language deficits in children treated from an early age.

Four reports of neurologic sequelae in older children and adults with galactosemia have appeared in the literature [121–124]. Symptoms have included cerebellar ataxia, tremor, choreoathetosis, and encephalopathy. In two instances, these findings could have resulted from severe jaundice and kernicterus [121,122]. Ataxia and tremor, however, have been described in adequately treated patients [123,124]. As a result of these reports, a neurologic syndrome encompassing mental retardation, tremor, and cerebellar dysfunction has been proposed to occur in a subgroup of individuals with transferase-deficiency galactosemia. These clinical manifestations are associated with cerebral atrophy and lack of normal myelination on magnetic resonance imaging of the brain [50].

A high incidence of ovarian failure with hypergonadotrophic hypogonadism in female patients has been documented [5,81,82,125,126]. It has been proposed that this phenomenon occurs despite adequate dietary control; other findings, however, suggest that ovarian failure develops as a result of ongoing galactose exposure. Levy et al. [83] found abundant oocytes and evidence of normal folliculogenesis in a 5-day-old galactosemic infant who died of sepsis. Far fewer but normal follicles were identified by Robinson et al. [126] through ovarian biopsy in a 16-year-old. Kaufman et al. [125] reported the incidence of ovarian dysfunction in galactosemia at 92% and documented that it occurs as early as 1 year of age by gonadotropin release stimulation tests. Ovarian failure was shown to develop over a 4-year period in a group of patients with normal ovarian function, and successful pregnancies in women with galactosemia have taken place [84,127]. Related findings include primary and secondary amenorrhea, which may develop even after pregnancy, and diminished or absent ovarian tissue on pelvic ultrasound. In 1987, Fraser et al. [128] reported findings from a study of women with premature ovarian failure; none were heterozygous for uridyl transferase deficiency. Male gonadal function appears to be resistant to the effects of the disease.

Osteoporosis is a frequent finding among female patients with galactosemia. It is assumed that this condition results from low calcium intake, lack of sex hormones associated with ovarian failure, and an independent defect in collagen synthesis resulting from disturbances in bone mineralization [129]. Renner et al. [130] recently reported onset of menarche and increased bone density in two 28-year-old galactosemic twins who underwent extended hormone replacement therapy and vitamin D therapy (cholecalciferol 1000 U/d) beginning at age 25 years for delayed pubertal development and decreased bone density, as demonstrated through dual-energy radiographic absorptiometry of the lumbar spine. Lactose-free nutrient supplements should be prescribed to address this consequence of galactosemia.

GALACTOKINASE-DEFICIENCY GALACTOSEMIA

The incidence of galactokinase-deficiency galactosemia is less than that of the classic form of the disease, approximately 1 in 10,000 [51]. It is appropriate to compare this disorder with the transferase-deficiency variety, because it affects both the first reaction (kinase) and the second reaction (transferase) in galactose metabolism (Figure 25.1). Studies involving comparison of these conditions with that involving the third reaction (epimerase) in galactose metabolism have elucidated the mechanisms of toxicity affecting several organs. Unlike transferase-deficiency galactosemia, galactokinase deficiency does not result in mental retardation or progressive liver disease, but galactose exposure may lead to cataract formation [6,131,132]. Development of cataracts results from formation of galactitol in the lens and osmotic disruption of lens fiber architecture. Treatment involves lifelong galactose elimination because of the ongoing potential for cataract formation. Fetal cataract formation even may result from maternal galactokinase deficiency [49].

URIDINE DIPHOSPHATE GALACTOSE-4-EPIMERASE DEFICIENCY GALACTOSEMIA

Uridine diphosphate galactose-4-epimerase catalyzes the third reaction in galactose metabolism (Figure 25.1). Epimerase deficiency apparently is caused by diminished stability of the enzyme leading to an inadequate reserve in cells such as erythrocytes, in which turnover is slow or absent [133]. Incidence of epimerase deficiency has been reported to be 1 in 46,000 in Switzerland [7]. Affected individuals have elevated galactose-1-phosphate activity despite normal erythrocyte transferase activity. This form of galactosemia was discovered incidentally through screening for galactosemia.

Initially, epimerase-deficiency galactosemia was considered a benign condition, because of the lack of symptoms in affected individuals and limitation of the deficiency to erythrocytes and leukocytes. Recently, however, patients with generalized epimerase deficiency have been reported [11,13] who exhibit symptoms identical to the classic form of the disease. One individual was unable to synthesize UDP glucose from UDP galactose, the galactose precursor required for synthesis of glycolipids and glycoproteins. These compounds contribute to normal growth and development by enhancing cell membrane integrity, particularly in the central nervous system. In contrast to transferase-deficiency galactosemia, treatment of epimerase deficiency may mandate inclusion of small quantities of dietary galactose. Frequent monitoring of erythrocyte galactose-1-phosphate is required to determine the optimal level of dietary restriction.

Disorders of Fructose Metabolism

The three recognized disorders of fructose metabolism include essential fructosuria, hereditary fructose intolerance (HFI), and fructose-1,6-diphosphatase deficiency. A fourth potential defect characterized by incomplete fructose absorption in one of three healthy adults and two of three children recently has been reported [134–136], but the underlying defect remains to be described.

Essential fructosuria, a benign disorder first described in 1876, was renamed *hepatic fructokinase deficiency* after identification of the specific enzyme defect. This condition is characterized by alimentary hyperfructosemia and fructosuria and usually is diagnosed after detection of urinary reducing substances in a seemingly healthy individual. Fructosuria unrelated to feeding also has been observed in one child [137].

Fructose-1,6-diphosphatase deficiency is a severe disorder of gluconeogenesis characterized by both fructose- and fasting-induced hypoglycemia, lactic acidosis, and hepatomegaly. In this condition, symptoms appear within the first 1–4 days of life in approximately half of affected individuals and can be life threatening in this age group. A mild variant of this condition has been described in which patients are resistant to the development of lactic acidosis, presumably because of partial enzyme activity [138]. Microscopic examination of liver tissue usually reveals fatty infiltration without fibrosis or altered hepatic architecture; hepatomegaly in this condition is reversible with appropriate treatment.

Hereditary fructose intolerance results from a deficiency of fructose-1-phosphate aldolase in the liver, renal cortex, and small intestine. Accumulation of fructose-1-phosphate in the liver leads to the major clinical manifestations of the disorder including permanent liver injury. A detailed discussion of this condition is included here.

Physiology and Biochemistry of Fructose Metabolism

Fructose is a monosaccharide that belongs to the ketose group and is a widely distributed compound in nature. Free fructose is found in fruits and in honey. A major source of fructose is the disaccharide, sucrose, which is hydrolyzed into fructose and glucose by the disaccharidase, sucrase, at the brush border membrane of enterocytes. Fructose is transported across the intestinal and liver plasma membranes via a carrier protein called *GLUT5*, a sodium-independent transporter [139,140]. Once absorbed, fructose is used mainly by the liver, kidney, and small intestine. Approximately 75% of fructose is taken up by the liver; the kidney and small intestine take up the remaining 25%. These tissues possess specialized enzymes involved in fructose metabolism. These enzymes are fructokinase aldolase type B and triokinase (Figure 25.2).

The first step in fructose metabolism involves the enzyme fructokinase, which catalyzes the phosphorylation of fructose to fructose-1-phosphate. The next step involves the enzyme fructoaldolase. Three aldolase isoenzymes have been identified. Aldolase B is present in the liver, kidney, and small intestine and acts on fructose-1-phosphate to produce D-glyceraldehyde and dihydroxyacetone phosphate. The two other aldolases are aldolase A, found in the muscle, and aldolase C, found in the brain. Both aldolase A and C have much greater activity against fructose-1,6-diphosphate than aldolase B. The presence of these two enzymes allows gluconeogenesis and glycolysis to continue even in the absence of aldolase B enzyme. The cDNA encoding for human and rat aldolase B has been cloned [141–143]. The aldolase B gene is localized to chromosome 9q22.3 [144]. The resulting D-glyceraldehyde is converted into D-glyceraldehyde-3-phosphate, as catalyzed by the enzyme triokinase.

Other enzymes involved in fructose metabolism include fructose-1,6-diphosphatase, which catalyzes the splitting of fructose-1,6-diphosphate to fructose-6-phosphate and phosphate. This process is irreversible; however, the opposite conversion also occurs through the enzyme phosphofructokinase. Alternative pathways of fructose metabolism involve the conversion of fructose directly to fructose-6-phosphate by the enzymes hexokinase and glucokinase. The affinity of these two enzymes to fructose, however, is several-fold lower compared with glucose.

Hereditary Fructose Intolerance

Hereditary fructose intolerance first was described by Chambers and Pratt in 1956 [145]. This case report involved a young woman who complained of vomiting after ingestion of fruit or sugar. Testing with glucose failed to produce the same effect, but she reported an aversion to its taste. According to the history obtained, symptoms first appeared after weaning at age 10 months. The authors recognized the variation in symptoms from those of essential fructosuria and

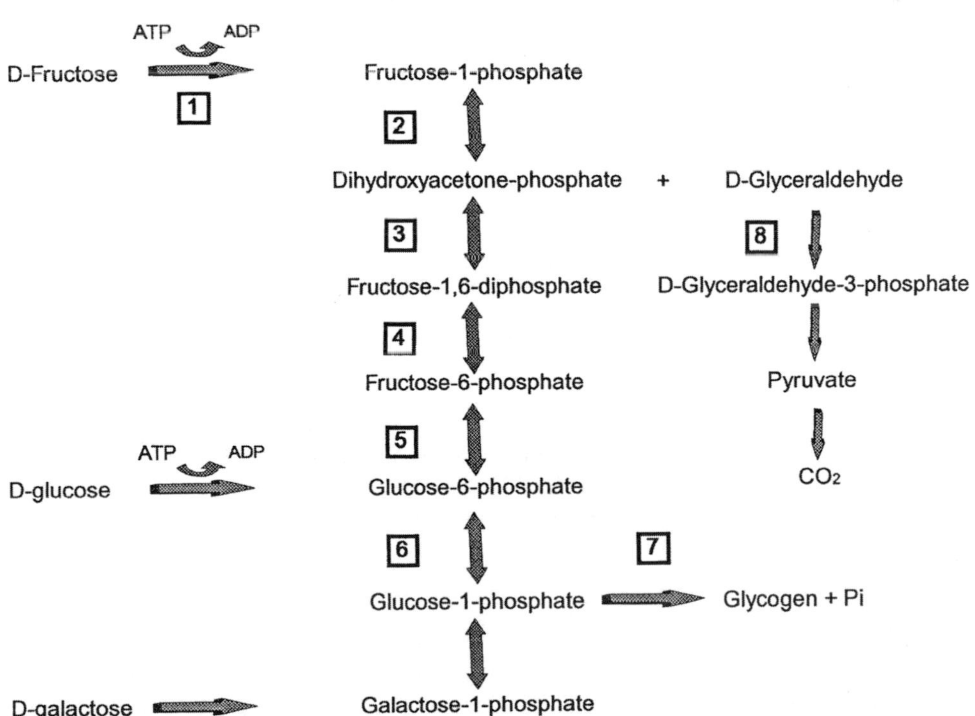

Figure 25.2. Fructose metabolism. 1, Fructokinase; 2, fructoaldolase; 3, fructose-1,6-diphosphate aldolase; 4, fructose-1,6-biphosphatase; 5, phosphohexose; 6, phosphoglucomutase; 7, glycogen phosphorylase; 8, triokinase.

speculated that the illness resulted from accumulation of a toxic intermediate. In 1957, Froesch et al. [146] described the syndrome in two siblings and two relatives and proposed that aldolase deficiency was the causative factor, based on the results of two liver biopsies. Hers and Joassin [147] later characterized the defect as an inability of the aldolase enzyme to split fructose-1-phosphate.

Molecular Basis of Hereditary Fructose Intolerance

Hereditary fructose intolerance is inherited as an autosomal recessive trait, with an estimated frequency of 1 in 20,000 individuals. The disorder is caused by catalytic deficiency of aldolase B in the liver, kidney, and small intestine. The enzymatic activities of aldolase A and C are normal [148]. The activity of tissue aldolase B is reduced to less than 15% of normal values.

The aldolase B gene has been sequenced and mapped to human chromosome 9q22.3 [144]. The gene consists of nine exons; the first is untranslated. The cognate messenger RNA encodes 364 amino acids [149,150]. The first demonstration of a common missense mutation was by Cross et al. [151]. A single base pair change was found by cloning and sequencing a genomic library, which was constructed from leukocyte DNA prepared from a patient with HFI. The single base change [G → C] was found at codon 149. The mutation causes a proline residue to be substituted for an alanine at this position; hence, it is designated *A149P*. The alanine at position 149 is a conserved amino acid, because it is present in the aldolase B gene of humans, rats, and chicken [151]. The A149P mutation creates a new recognition site for the restriction enzyme AhaII. The insertion of a protein residue, an imido acid in which peptide bond formation involves the rigid pyrollidine ring, is known to alter protein secondary structure. Mutation resulting in the change of alanine to proline is likely to disrupt the spatial configuration of juxtaposed residues in aldolase B and adversely affect its catalytic activities. The mutation A149P was found in 67% of 50 patients studied by Cross et al. [152]. This mutation was more common in patients from northern Europe than in those from southern Europe. Two other mutations involving A174D [C → A] and ala174 → asp were found in subjects from Italy, Switzerland, and Yugoslavia but not in those from the United Kingdom, France, or the United States. Testing for these mutations in amplified DNA by the polymerase chain reaction with a limited panel of allele specific oligonucleotides identifies more than 95% of patients with HFI. Twenty-two genetic mutations have been identified [153]. Tolan and Brooks [154] characterized the molecular defects in the aldolase B gene in 31 North Americans with HFI. Fifty-five percent of mutant North American alleles were A149P, the most common mutation in the European population. The other two alleles, A174D (ala174 → asp) and N334K (asn334 → lys), represent 11% and 2% of North American alleles, respectively. Nine subjects representing 32% of independent alleles studied had HFI alleles that were not of this common missense mutation. The two most common mutations (A149P and A174D), which cause more than 70% of HFI worldwide, lie within exon 5 of the aldolase B gene and can be detected by a reverse dot blot screening method [155].

Table 25.2: Symptoms and Signs of Hereditary Fructose Intolerance

Acute
Nausea, vomiting
Tremor
Dizziness
Lethargy, coma
Chronic
Failure to thrive
Jaundice, cirrhosis
Vomiting and diarrhea
Feeding difficulties

Clinical Presentation

Once considered a rare metabolic disorder, HFI is sufficiently common to have enabled several centers to compile observations from dozens of patients [156–158]. Clinical presentation of the disease depends entirely on exposure to fructose and sucrose. Severity of symptoms depends on age at exposure and fructose load; that is, the younger the child and the higher the load, the more severe the reaction. During breast-feeding or feeding with sucrose free formulas, infants are asymptomatic and appear healthy. Initial symptoms usually appear with introduction of fruits, juices, vegetables, or sucrose to the diet.

Symptoms associated with HFI may be categorized as resulting from acute and chronic exposure to the sugar, as shown in Table 25.2. All symptoms result directly from accumulation of fructose-1-phosphate in tissues in which aldolase B is normally present – the liver, small intestine, and kidney – and can be related to chemical characteristics of the compound [159]. Fructose-1-phosphate is osmotically active, producing abdominal distention, pain, colic, vomiting, and diarrhea. Hypophosphatemia, hypoglycemia, hyperlacticacidemia, and hyperuricemia result from its ability to sequester phosphate. Tissue toxicity results in hepatic enlargement, hepatic failure, and renal dysfunction.

Biochemical Features and the Pathogenesis of Fructose Toxicity

The metabolic consequences of the catalytic deficiency of aldolase B enzyme are the accumulation of fructose-1-phosphate in liver, kidney, and small intestine after the ingestion of physiologic amounts of fructose [160]. The inability to metabolize fructose-1-phosphate leads to sequestration of large amounts of phosphate and depletion of ATP and phosphate. Patients with aldolase B deficiency have high levels of fructose-1-phosphate, which inhibit both gluconeogenesis and

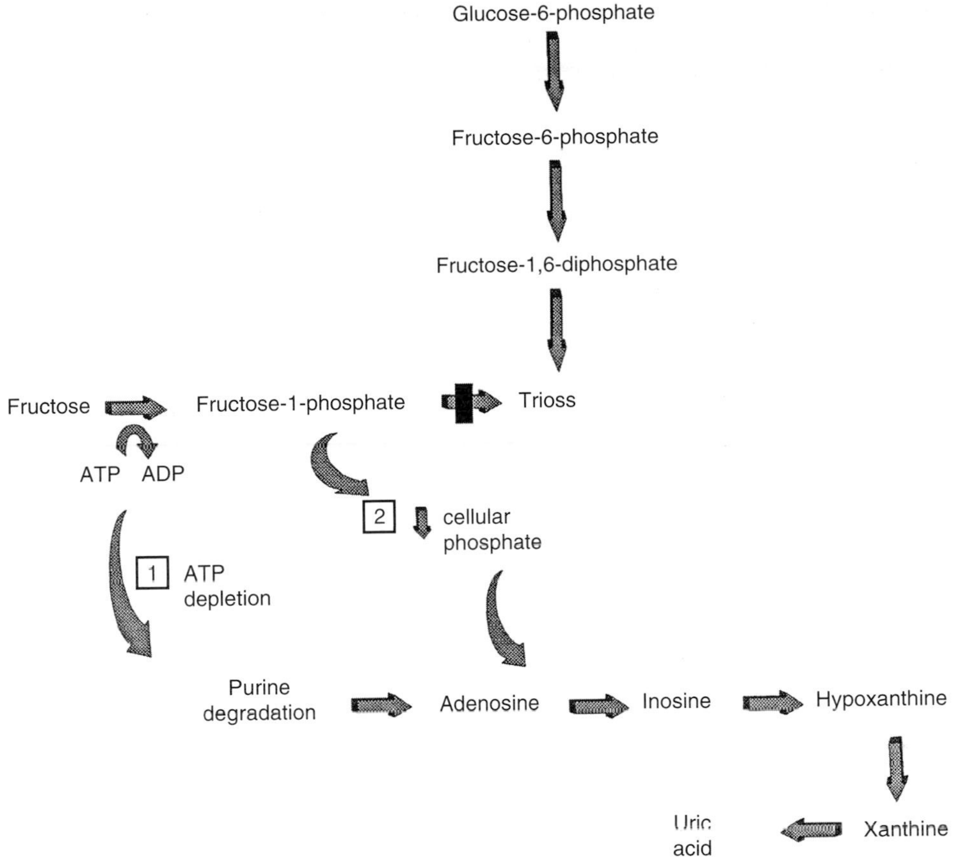

Figure 25.3. Mechanism of hyperuricemia and hypophosphatemia in aldolase B deficiency. Because of aldolase B defect, ATP is consumed in the fructokinase reaction, leading to ATP depletion. Fructose-1-phosphate accumulation inhibits ATP generation from anaerobic glycolysis. Phosphate is trapped in fructose-1-phosphate leading to depletion of intracellular phosphate. Both depletions favor degradation of purines to uric acid.

glycogenolysis [161–164]. The inhibition occurs at the level of fructose-1,6-diphosphate aldolase enzyme. Inhibition at this site is supported by the observation that patients with aldolase B deficiency do not form glucose from ^{14}C glycerol if fructose is present, whereas oxidation of ^{14}C glycerol is apparently unaffected by fructose. Moreover, fructose-induced hypoglycemia is not prevented by simultaneous infusions of gluconeogenic substrates such as dihydroxyacetone or glycerol. The inhibition of glycogenolysis occurs above the level of phosphoglucomutase. In support of this observation is the demonstration that administration of galactose together with fructose results in less pronounced hypoglycemia; therefore, a defect in the phosphorylation of glycogen to glucose-1-phosphate has been incriminated.

Other major metabolic consequences of HFI besides hypoglycemia are hyperuricemia [165–167] and lactic acidosis [168]. The hyperuricemic effect of fructose is secondary to degradation of adenine nucleotides [169,170]. Fructose infusion in rats and humans results in a decrease in hepatic ATP to 40% of its normal value without an equivalent increase in adenosine diphosphate or monophosphate [171]. Moreover, inorganic phosphate (P_i) concentration falls before the noted decrease in ATP. The decrease in ATP is secondary to its utilization in the fructokinase reaction. P_i depletion is secondary to rephosphorylation of adenosine diphosphate within the mitochondria. These findings have been confirmed by ^{31}P nuclear magnetic resonance spectroscopy [172]. In patients with aldolase B deficiency, there is marked exaggeration of the hyperuricemia secondary to sequestration of P_i within fructose-1-phosphate, because this compound cannot be metabolized further; ATP is utilized continually in the fructokinase reaction. The decreases in ATP and P_i increase the rate of purine degradation to uric acid (Figure 25.3). Serum magnesium levels increase in patients with aldolase B deficiency secondary to release of cellular magnesium from the loss of chelating effects of ATP [161]. Adenosine triphosphate is a well-known strong magnesium chelator. The loss of hepatic ATP, by its effect on protein synthesis, may explain the hyperaminoacidemia and the decrease in clotting factors seen in HFI. Renal tubular dysfunction is likely to be secondary to degradation of ATP in the kidney tubules [158,173,174]. Table 25.3 summarizes the metabolic derangement following acute and chronic exposure to fructose in affected patients.

Table 25.3: Biochemical Abnormalities of Hereditary Fructose Intolerance

Renal tubular dysfunction: increased urine losses of fructose, glucose, amino acids, proteins, urate, HCO_3, phosphate
Blood
Hematologic: anemia, thrombocytopenia
Liver: conjugated hyperpotassium bilirubinemia, prolonged prothrombin time
Metabolic: Hypoglycemia, hypophosphatemia, hypomagnesmia, lactic acidosis, hyperuricemia

Diagnosis

In the largest series of patients reported [158], 5 of 55 patients with HFI were diagnosed as a result of having a sibling with the disorder. The remaining 50 became symptomatic following ingestion of fructose. Fourteen of these individuals received fructose in their first feeding through a sucrose-containing, soy-based formula. Thirty-two (64%) of the 50 patients were diagnosed at younger than 6 months of age, 12 (24%) between 6 and 12 months of age, and 6 (12%) during the second year of life.

Because the clinical presentation of HFI is highly variable and many of its characteristic features commonly occur with other disorders, the differential diagnosis may include hepatitis, intrauterine infection, septicemia, hemolytic uremic syndrome, galactosemia, tyrosinosis, Wilson's disease, and other storage disorders. A detailed nutritional history correlating onset of symptoms with intake of fructose-containing foods is often a key component in the diagnostic process. Most often, young infants with HFI present for workup of vomiting, hepatomegaly, poor feeding, and failure to thrive [157,158]. Older infants and children usually present with similar symptoms, or occasionally for evaluation for a storage disorder or anomalous behavior [175]. Suspicion is fostered by the presence of reducing substances in urine. Amino acid profiles show increased urinary amino acids and elevations in serum methionine and tyrosine levels. On suspicion of the diagnosis, all food and pharmaceutical sources of fructose, sucrose, and sorbitol are eliminated from the diet. Resolution of symptoms may be observed within days to weeks and further supports the diagnosis.

Traditionally, direct measure of fructose-1-phosphate aldolase in hepatic or small intestine tissue samples has been employed in the diagnosis of HFI. The liver is the preferred source for biopsy specimens because an assessment of tissue damage as indicated by the presence of limited and scattered necrosis of hepatocytes, intralobular and periportal fibrosis, and diffuse fatty vacuolization resulting from fructose-1-phosphate accumulation can be made simultaneously [158,176]. Assay of enzyme activity in serum and blood cells shows only slightly reduced levels and is of little diagnostic value. Likewise, cultured skin fibroblasts and placental tissue appear to express predominantly aldolase A [177–180]. Currently, more than 95% of patients with HFI can be diagnosed through amplification of DNA with a limited number of allele-specific oligonucleotides, circumventing the need for tissue biopsy [152].

Treatment

Prompt and permanent removal of fructose and sucrose from the diet is the only effective therapy for HFI. Sorbitol also must be eliminated, because of its conversion to fructose in the human body. Complete elimination of the offending sugars is rarely a therapeutic goal, however, because of the wide distribution and high concentration of fructose in foods (primarily honey, fruits, and vegetables) and liberal use of sucrose and sorbitol as sweetening agents in countless commercial food products and pharmaceuticals [159]. A trend toward increased use of fructose as a sweetening agent also has been recorded [181]. This has been attributed to the intense sweetening power of the monosaccharide – 1.5–1.7 times that of sucrose at isocaloric concentrations – and the development of technologies for its commercial production.

In Western societies, per capita intake of fructose as sucrose or the free monosaccharide currently is estimated at 100 g/d [181] or more [182]. Optimal levels of restriction in individuals with HFI have not been established. Some are able to achieve sufficiently low intake to normalize hepatic and renal function [183]. Still others suffer chronic, nonspecific symptoms despite treatment [183]. Unfortunately, no biochemical method exists for monitoring the adequacy of fructose restriction. Dietary indiscretion, however, has been detected in an adult patient through the use of ^{31}P magnetic resonance spectroscopy [172].

Gitzelmann et al. [183] stressed that dietary restriction should be rigid during infancy. This can be achieved in early infancy through exclusive use of breast milk or sucrose-free infant formulas. A delay in the introduction of solid foods is not advisable; however, care must be taken to avoid introduction of fructose-containing foods until age 2–3 years, at which time some degree of liberalization seems to be tolerable [183,184]. The lack of more specific guidelines stems from the fact that food composition tables detailing the sugar content of foods, which traditionally have been used to design diets for individuals with HFI, contain significant discrepancies as well as incomplete data [185–187]. Recently, investigators have conducted an examination of current practices among centers managing HFI, and updated recommendations for dietary treatment of this condition have been published [159].

Subsequent Course

Small infants recover more slowly from fructose exposure than older infants and children. They may die secondary to organ failure several days after fructose removal, because recovery of renal and hepatic function may require days. Exchange transfusions or fresh frozen plasma may be necessary to alleviate clotting disorders and complement deficiency resulting from

Table 25.4: Glycogen Storage Diseases

Disease	*Enzyme*	*Clinical Manifestations*
Type 1a	Glucose-6-phosphatase	Hepatomegaly, hypoglycemia, acidosis
Type 1b	Glucose-6-phosphatase transporter	Hepatomegaly, hypoglycemia, infection
Type II	Lysosomal acid α-glucosidase	Muscle hypotonia
Type III	Debrancher	Hepatomegaly
Type IV	Brancher	Liver cirrhosis
Type V	Muscle phosphorylase	Muscle cramps
Type VI	Liver phosphorylase	Hepatomegaly
Phosphorylase kinase deficiency	Liver α subunit	Hepatomegaly
Phosphorylase kinase deficiency	Muscle α subunit	Muscle cramps
Phosphorylase kinase deficiency	β subunit	Hepatomegaly
Phosphorylase kinase deficiency	Muscle γ subunit	Muscle cramps
Phosphorylase kinase deficiency	Liver γ subunit	Hypoglycemia, liver fibrosis
Fanconi–Bickel syndrome	GLUT2	Hepatomegaly, renal Fanconi syndrome
Glycogen synthase deficiency	Liver glycogen synthase 2	Ketotic hypoglycemia

Adapted from Elpeles ON. The molecular background of glycogen metabolism disorders. J Pediatr Endocrinol Metab 1999;12:263–379, with permission.

fructose ingestion [188]. If a child survives the severe reaction and appropriate dietary restriction is implemented and maintained, the future course is usually uneventful, and normal growth and intellectual development proceed. In children, hepatomegaly, which may persist for months or years despite seemingly adequate therapy, may be caused by a high degree of intolerance during childhood [163] or ongoing intake of hidden sources of fructose, sucrose, and sorbitol [158]. Self-imposed dietary restriction is sufficient to prevent gastrointestinal discomfort; however, it cannot be relied on to prevent hepatomegaly and growth retardation, particularly in children [183].

Adults with HFI usually remain asymptomatic and appear healthy. The oldest known patient died at age 83 years of an unrelated cause [189]. Premature deaths resulting from routine postoperative infusions of solutions containing fructose, sorbitol, or invert sugar have been reported [190]. Therefore, individuals should report the diagnosis to appropriate personnel on hospitalization or when undergoing medical procedures.

GLYCOGEN STORAGE DISEASE

Glycogen, a polysaccharide, is the primary carbohydrate storage compound in animals. It is present in virtually all animal cells and is particularly abundant in liver and muscle tissue. It undergoes depolymerization through phosphorolysis and hydrolysis to release free glucose as needed to sustain cellular processes and to maintain normal blood glucose concentrations during fasting. The formation and degradation of glycogen are highly regulated processes involving at least eight enzymes. Deficiencies of each enzyme have been identified in humans and result in the 12 recognized forms of GSD. The discussion here is limited to types I, III, and IV, because their clinical expressions primarily involve the liver; however, the clinical features of all GSDs are provided in Table 25.4.

Physiology and Biochemistry of Glycogen Metabolism

Glycogen is a polymer of glucose units linked between the C_1 of one D-glucopyranosyl residue and the hydroxyl at C_4 of the adjacent residue (1,4 linkage). Short chains of glucose residues linked through the hydroxyl groups at C_6 of some of the residues (α-1,6 linkage) represent 7–8% of the glycogen, which allows a highly branched structure. Glycogen is present in most animal cells but is particularly abundant in liver and muscle. The role of glycogen in the liver is to provide glucose to the blood for various organs [191]. At times of stress or if blood glucose levels fall, the liver rapidly releases glucose into the blood stream, which carries it to organs such as the brain that cannot make glucose. Glycogen in the muscle serves as a reserve of glycolytic fuel to be used locally if oxygen or glucose availability declines.

Figure 25.4 illustrates the pathways involved in glycogen metabolism. Glycogen is synthesized from and degraded to

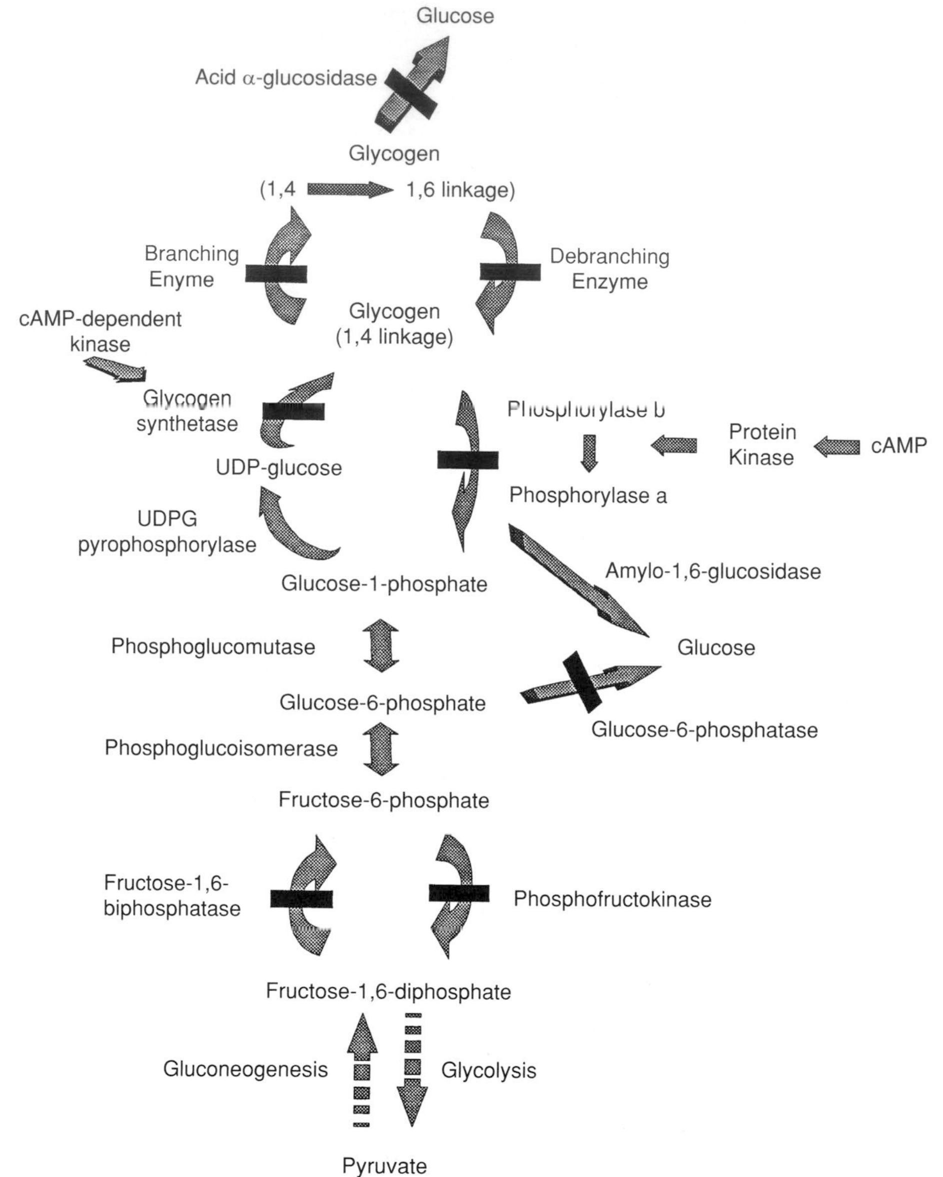

Figure 25.4. Pathways of glycogen metabolism. ▬ indicates site of a block in enzymatic activity. Phosphorylase a, active form; Phosphorylase b, inactive form.

glucose. Glycogen synthesis occurs through the action of glycogen synthase and branching enzymes. Hydrolysis occurs through phosphorylase and amylo-1,6-glucosidase. Glycogen synthase catalyzes the synthesis of glycogen from UDP glucose. Several protein kinases can phosphorylate glycogen synthase. Branching of glycogen is carried out by the transfer of α-1, 4-linked glucosyl units from the outer chains of glycogen into a 1,6 position. Glycogen phosphorylase is an interconvertible enzyme, with the α and β forms representing the active and inactive forms, respectively. The phosphorylase enzyme catalyzes the transfer of a glucose unit at the nonreducing end of α-1,4 glucosyl chain glycogen to liberate glucose-1-phosphate. Activation of this enzyme by epinephrine and glucagon plays a major role in controlling glycogenolysis. After extensive phosphorylase action on glycogen, the molecule contains four glucose residues in α-1,4 glucosidic bonds attached by an α-1,6 link. This unit is termed *phosphorylase limit dextrin.* The enzyme oligo (1,4 $\rightarrow$ 1,4) glucan transferase removes three of the four glucose residues, exposing the 1,6 linkages to be acted on by the amylo-1,6-glucosidase enzyme to yield free glucose. Both enzymes represent the catalytic activity of the debrancher enzyme.

Because glycogen contains 8% branch points (1,6 links), glycogen degradation by phosphorylase and debrancher enzymes yields about 8% free glucose. The major end product of glycogen hydrolysis by phosphorylase is glucose-1-phosphate, which is acted on by the enzyme phosphoglucomutase to yield glucose-6-phosphate. There is no known deficiency of the enzyme phosphoglucomutase. Glucose-6-phosphatase is responsible for the formation of the majority of glucose

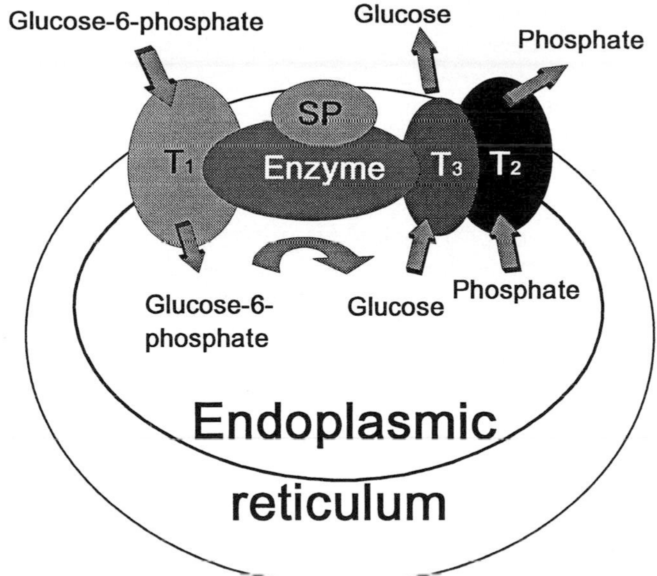

Figure 25.5. Schematic model of hepatic microsomal glucose-6-phosphatase. Glucose-6-phosphate entry into the endoplasmic reticulum is through a transport protein (T_1). Hydrolysis occurs by the catalytic subunit of the glucose-6-phosphatase. Phosphate is returned to the cytosol through another transport protein (T_2). Glucose is returned through T_3. SP, stabilizing protein.

from gluconeogenesis and glycogenolysis; it is a microsomal enzyme that catalyzes the hydrolysis of glucose-6-phosphate into glucose and phosphate. Glucose-6-phosphatase is present in the liver and kidney and in intestinal mucosa. Glucose-6-phosphatase is located with its active site inside the lumen of the endoplasmic reticulum. Arion et al. [192] and later Burchell [193] proposed that glucose-6-phosphatase was a multicomponent system consisting of three transport proteins, T_1, T_2, and T_3, which transport glucose-6-phosphate, phosphate and pyrophosphate, and glucose, respectively, across the endoplasmic membrane. The other two units of this system include the catalytic subunit of the enzyme and a regulatory calcium stabilizing protein and are shown in Figure 25.5. An alternative model predicts tight linkage of hydrolytic and transport activities by various domains of a single protein [194].

Glycogen Metabolism in Liver

The control of glycogen metabolism is mediated by several factors that control glycogen synthesis and degradation by the enzymes glycogen synthetase and phosphorylase, respectively. Control of these enzymes occurs through several factors, including hormonally mediated changes in the concentrations of glucose and glycogen [195]. As illustrated in Figure 25.4, glycogen synthetase and phosphorylase occur in active form and in an inactive form. During feeding, high glucose concentration in the sinusoids allows glucose to bind to the phosphorylase enzyme and causes conversion of active phosphorylase into inactive phosphorylase, resulting in a halt in glycogenolysis. Because active phosphorylase is an inhibitor of synthetase enzyme, its inactivation allows glycogen synthesis to proceed. During fasting, a hormonally mediated (glucagon) increase in cyclic adenosine monophosphate allows activation of protein kinase, which converts inactive to active phosphorylase, initiating glycogenolysis. High glycogen content also favors glycogenolysis by inhibiting glycogen synthetase.

Type I Glycogen Storage Disease (Glucose-6-Phosphatase Deficiency)

In 1929, von Gierke [196] published detailed reports of autopsies of two young children in whom the most remarkable findings were excessive glycogen accumulation in hepatic and renal tissues, resulting in respective threefold and twofold increases in organ size. Although sparse, their clinical records included reports of frequent nosebleeds. In the 1950s, further investigation by Cori and Cori [197] led to recognition of the biochemical heterogeneity of hepatic glycogenosis. In their study of six patients, enzyme activity ranging from normal to near complete deficiency was identified. In 1954, von Gierke's disease was classified as type I GSD [198]. It is the most commonly diagnosed form of hepatic glycogenosis, representing approximately 25% of all cases.

Classification

Patients with type Ia GSD have complete absence of glucose-6-phosphatase activity. Biochemical purification of the catalytic subunit by Burchell [193] suggests that a double polypeptide of 36.5 kDa is the active unit of the glucose-6-phosphatase enzyme. Type Ia stabilizing protein subtype describes patients with clinically classic type Ia GSD with normal activity of the enzyme but lacking a 21-kDa stabilizing polypeptide protein. Type Ib has a clinical picture like that of type Ia; however, in these patients, the activity of glucose-6-phosphatase in fully disrupted microsomes is completely normal, but the activity in intact microsomes and in vivo is abnormal. These patients have a defect in the transport protein T_1 (glucose-6-phosphatase transporter) and classically have neutropenia. Type Ic is characterized by a deficiency of T_2, the microsomal phosphate and pyrophosphate transport protein [199–201]. These patients may have impaired insulin release [202], because T_2 is present in liver, kidney, and pancreatic cells [203]. For practical purposes, there are only two types: type Ia and Ib. Types Ic and Id are exceedingly rare [204].

Molecular Basis

Glycogen storage disease type Ia is caused by the deficiency of D-glucose-6-phosphatase, which is a key enzyme in glucose homeostasis. The gene has been localized to chromosome 17q21. The gene spans 12.5 kb, is composed of five exons, and encodes a 357–amino acid protein [205–207]. So far more than 30 mutations have been described in the gene encoding the glucose-6-phosphate enzyme. These mutations alter amino acid residues within the transmembrane helices or in the luminal side of the endoplasmic reticulum [208]. The two most common mutations occur in R83C and Q347X, which account for about 70% of mutations in Caucasian populations [209].

Glycogen storage disease type Ib is caused by mutation in the gene encoding microsomal glucose-6-phosphate transporter [210]. The gene is localized to 11q23.3 [211] and is composed of nine exons spanning a genomic region of 4 kb. The gene is expressed in the liver, kidney, and leukocytes [212]. Several mutations have been described in the gene, resulting in functional deficiency of glucose-6-phosphate transporter, which explains the neutropenia and neutrophil–monocyte dysfunction characteristic of GSD type Ib [210].

Clinical Presentation

The expression of clinical and biochemical symptoms of type I GSD varies considerably among patients, even in the absence of differences in age, measurable enzyme activity, or treatment. Some individuals require frequent hospitalizations as a result of marked metabolic abnormalities. Others may experience only mild symptoms and slightly delayed growth. Still others may succumb to the disease during infancy or early childhood.

Children with type I GSD are generally of short stature and prone to adiposity but without disproportionate head circumference or limb or trunk lengths. Bone films may reveal delayed bone age and osteoporosis [213]. On physical examination, increased fat deposition is most notable on cheeks, breasts, buttocks, and the backs of arms and thighs. A protuberant abdomen and lumbar lordosis result from hepatomegaly, which may be detected as early as 2 months. The spleen is usually normal in size. Xanthomas, which usually appear around puberty, may be present on elbows, knees, and buttocks; their presence on the nasal septum may contribute to frequent nosebleeds in patients with type I GSD. Profound hypoglycemia after relatively short periods of fasting and severe hepatomegaly are the most striking features of the disorder. Except in severe cases, hypoglycemia may not become apparent during the first several weeks of life, in which the infant feeds every 2–3 hours; however, septicemia may lead to earlier recognition of this symptom, particularly in patients with type Ib GSD. Metabolic acidosis resulting from hypoglycemia may cause weakness, malaise, headache, increased respiratory rate, and fruity breath; a few patients experience recurrent fevers with these symptoms [214]. Hypoglycemic convulsions and severe metabolic acidosis may result in death. In other patients, severe hypoglycemia may occur without clinical symptoms. This phenomenon is presumably caused by concomitantly high blood lactate levels, which provide an alternative source of energy for the brain [215].

Liver abnormalities usually include only slight elevations in serum transaminase levels, which improve quickly with stabilization of the blood glucose concentration between 70 and 110 mg/dL. Type I GSD does not lead to hepatic cirrhosis or liver failure. On the other hand, by age 15 years, most patients develop hepatic adenomas, and these have been documented by ultrasound as early as 3 years. Solitary hepatocellular carcinomas within individual nodules also have been found in a number of patients [216–218]. The kidneys show no abnormalities beyond substantial enlargement caused by excessive glycogen accumulation and the inability to release free glucose. Individuals who survive puberty, however, may develop

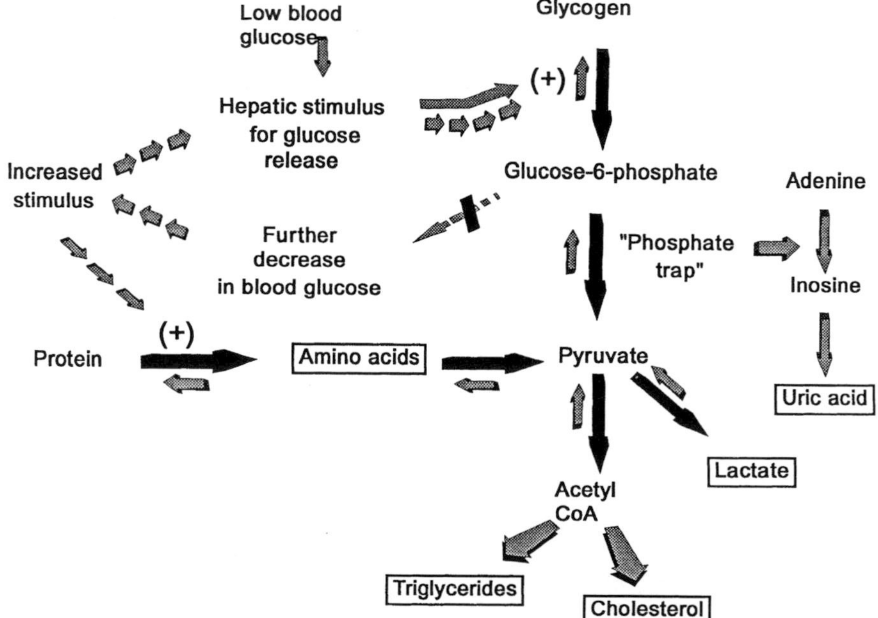

Figure 25.6. Biochemical basis for the primary laboratory finding in patients with glucose-6-phosphate deficiency (*solid rectangle*). The increased production of glucose-6-phosphate that results from continuous stimulation of glycogen breakdown apparently increases glycolysis, which in turn results in a net increase (*dark arrows*) in the production of lactate, triglycerides, cholesterol, and uric acid. Both glycogenolysis and gluconeogenesis are involved in the overproduction of substrate. (From Zakim D, Boyer T, eds. Textbook of liver diseases, 3rd ed. Philadelphia: WB Saunders, 1996, 1589, with permission.)

progressive nephropathy [219] and gouty complications secondary to persistent hyperuricemia.

Metabolic Consequences

Figure 25.6 depicts the biochemical consequences of a block in glucose-6-phosphatase. These abnormalities include those described in the following sections.

Hypoglycemia

Blood glucose levels are normally maintained by exogenous sources of the sugar and endogenous sources by glycogenolysis and gluconeogenesis. In patients with type I GSD, degradation of glycogen and gluconeogenesis proceed normally until formation glucose-6-phosphate, which cannot be converted to glucose, leads to the development of hypoglycemia. During hypoglycemia, insulin levels are appropriately low; glucagon levels are high [220].

Lactic Acidosis

Under normal circumstances, lactic acid generated from anaerobic glycolytic processes in muscle and from red blood cell metabolism is removed and metabolized by the liver by pyruvate in the tricarboxylic acid cycle into fatty acid or enters the gluconeogenic pathway. In patients with type I GSD, much of the lactate generated from hepatic glycolysis is not converted to glucose resulting in lactic acidemia [221]. Blood lactate levels in these patients are, in general, 4–8 times normal values.

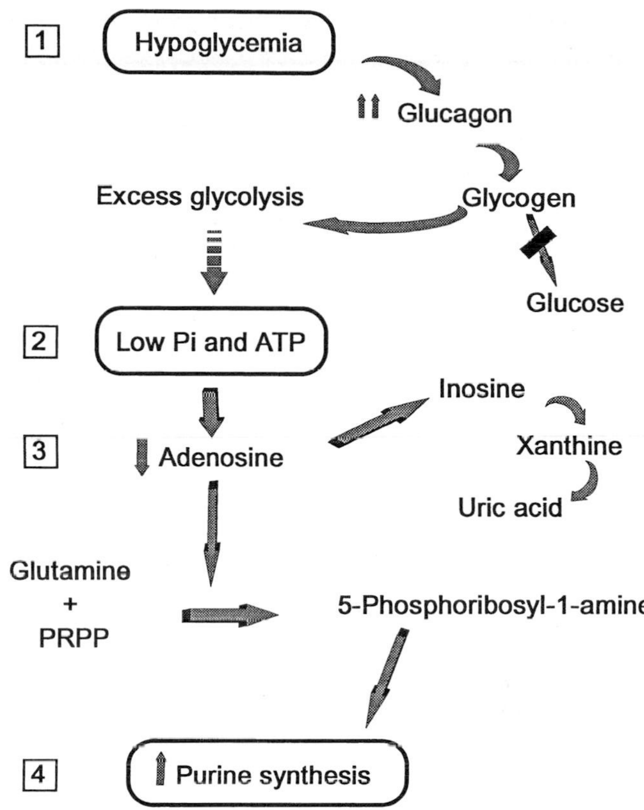

Figure 25.8. Mechanism of increased purine synthesis secondary to low inorganic phosphate (P_i) and adenosine triphosphate.

Hyperuricemia

Hyperuricemia, gouty arthritis, and nephropathy are well-known manifestations of type I GSD [222,223]. Hyperuricemia appears to be related to an increased rate of purine synthesis de novo. Two mechanisms have been suggested to explain this observation. The first implicates an increase in substrate availability, that is, in phosphoribosyl pyrophosphate and glutamine levels, which represents the first committed reaction in purine synthesis (Figure 25.7). In addition, increased levels of glucose-6-phosphate produced during glycogenolysis result in an increase in the level of ribose-5-phosphate, another important substrate [224,225].

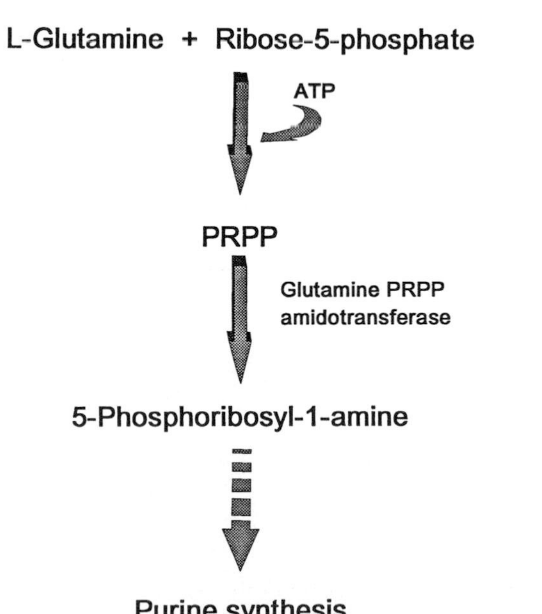

Figure 25.7. Mechanism of increased purine synthesis secondary to increased concentration of precursors.

The second mechanism relates to decreased intracellular ATP and phosphate levels [226], which favor the rapid degradation of adenyl- or guanylribonucleotides to xanthine and uric acid, as depicted in Figure 25.8. A decrease in adenosine level favors increased purine synthesis.

Hypophosphatemia

Low serum phosphate levels are generally seen during hypoglycemic episodes. Glucagon injection in patients with type I GSD is followed by a decrease in serum phosphate level. Because glucose-6-phosphate cannot be converted to glucose, phosphate is trapped within the compound, resulting in intracellular depletion of phosphate and a compensatory shift of extracellular phosphate into the cell. A similar phenomenon has been well documented in patients with HFI [163].

Hyperlipidemia

Hyperlipidemia is a well-recognized abnormality in patients with type I GSD. Serum levels of triglyceride may rise to 4000 to 6000 mg/dL, and elevation of cholesterol levels to 400–600 mg/dL is common. The mechanisms underlying hyperlipidemia relate to the increased products of glycolytic pathways, such as in hepatic NAD, NAD phosphate, glycerol-3-phosphate, and acetyl coenzyme A. These compounds are essential for fatty acid and cholesterol synthesis. They are synthesized abundantly in patients with type I GSD, as a result of the block in the glycolytic and gluconeogenic pathways [221]. Moreover, carnitine palmityl transferase enzyme is inhibited by malonyl coenzyme A, which is produced by acetyl coenzyme A, preventing the transfer of fatty acids to the mitochondria. Furthermore, there is elevation of free fatty acid levels in the serum secondary to hypoglycemia.

Platelet Dysfunction

Abnormalities in platelet aggregation and adhesiveness have been described in patients with type I GSD [227]. These abnormalities were thought to be the result of impairment in the ability of the platelet membranes to release adenosine diphosphate secondary to changes in membrane fluidity. This hypothesis, however, has not been proven. Platelet dysfunction may also occur secondary to depletion of nucleotide pools, which also result from hypoglycemia [228].

Neutropenia

Neutropenia has been documented in most patients with type Ib GSD. The degree of neutropenia is varied among such patients, especially during periods of infection. The functional impairment may be related to impaired carbohydrate metabolism caused by a phosphorylation defect after glucose uptake across the neutrophil membranes [229]. Treatment of patients with granulocyte colony–stimulating factor corrects neutropenia and defects in phagocytic cell function [230].

Pathogenesis of Growth Impairment and Hepatocellular Changes

One of the major clinical manifestations of type I GSD is growth failure. Glucose-6-phosphatase deficiency results in a surprising nutritional status. Whereas the liver has an excess supply of metabolic intermediates and it is in the fed state, the periphery remains in the fasted state because of the marked decrease in endogenous glucose production. Hypoglycemia results and leads to lactic acidosis, as glucose-6-phosphate is diverted through the glycolytic pathway. Correction of hypoglycemia and metabolic acidosis results in improved growth and development.

The hepatocellular changes seen in type I GSD relate mainly to the development of hepatic adenomas. The cause of the hepatic adenomas is not known, but they are believed to be secondary to chronic stimulation of the liver by hepatotrophic agents (such as glucagon). Our own experience with two patients who had adenomas prior to nocturnal feeding showed resolution of these adenomas after 3 years of treatment [231]. This finding supports the hypothesis that hypoglycemia-induced hyperglucagonemia may play a role in the pathogenesis of hepatic adenomas. Hepatocellular carcinoma has been documented in patients who had adenomas [232]. The mechanism for this malignant transformation is not known.

Diagnosis

Accurate diagnosis of type I GSD has become crucial for the development of an effective approach to treatment. Direct assay of hepatic enzyme activity, that is, glucose-6-phosphatase hydrolysis, in a fresh liver biopsy specimen is advocated. The use of the percutaneous needle biopsy technique avoids exposure to potential complications of surgery and general anesthesia [233]. To provide some selectivity in the application of this procedure, determination of serial blood glucose and lactate levels during a 4- to 6-hour fast as well as maximum blood glucose response to glucagon is recommended. A deficiency of phosphorylase kinase, which is not routinely measured in liver tissue samples, should be suspected if blood glucose rises more than 30 mg/dL [214].

Traditionally, glucagon, galactose, fructose, and glucose tolerance tests were used to diagnose GSD [234,235]. Glucagon administration typically fails to produce an increase in blood glucose in these patients. Within 20 minutes after administration, however, patients may experience a substantial decrease in blood glucose, followed by development of severe metabolic acidosis. Patients with type I GSD are unable to convert galactose and fructose to free glucose. Administration of either of these sugars results in a flat blood glucose curve. Oral galactose administration results in an increase in blood lactate [234]. On the contrary, a decrease in blood lactate and hypoinsulinism can be observed after glucose administration [235]. The use of these tests provides the advantage of avoiding risks associated with more invasive diagnostic techniques; however, a substantial blood volume is required for completion, and results frequently fail to yield a definitive diagnosis. Liver biopsy specimens have hepatocytes filled with glycogen. Figure 25.9A shows a significant amount of glycogen in the hepatocyte, as evident by strong periodic acid–Schiff (PAS) staining, which disappears after diastase treatment (Figure 25.9B).

Treatment

The pioneering work of Folkman et al. [236] led to the development of current treatment strategies for type I GSD. Through the use of total parenteral nutrition, these researchers were able to effect dramatic improvement in most biochemical abnormalities associated with the disease. Similar results had been demonstrated in a group of patients after portocaval shunting [237,238], although lack of response to this form of treatment also had been reported [239]. Thus, it appeared that delivery of nutrients primarily into the systemic circulation minimizing hepatic exposure to nutrients diverted a major stimulus in the pathogenesis of the disease. Later, the

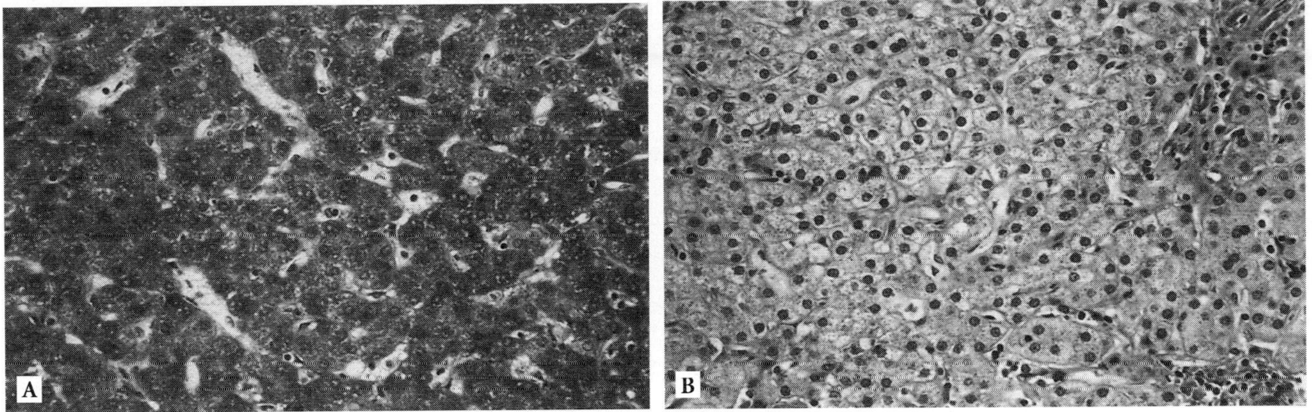

Figure 25.9. Type 1 glycogen storage disease. Hepatocytes are filled with glycogen, demonstrated with periodic acid–Schiff stain (**A**) and removed with diastase treatment (**B**).

strength of this hypothesis was diminished when Greene et al. [240] demonstrated equally positive results with continuous nasogastric infusion of nutrients and formulated a new hypothesis relating to the pathogenesis type I GSD: if blood glucose levels fall below a critical level (70–90 mg/dL), compensatory mechanisms result in the breakdown of glycogen to glucose-6-phosphate. Deficiency of glucose-6-phosphatase inhibits the conversion of glucose-6-phosphate to glucose, resulting in formation of metabolic intermediates through pathways previously described. Any treatment that maintains blood glucose above the critical level reduces the stimulus for glycogenolysis. Parenteral and enteral nutrition produce the desired effect by providing a continuous source of glucose. A glucose infusion rate of 8–9 mg/kg/min has been recommended [241]. Portocaval shunting is presumed to reduce the hormonal stimulus by diluting hepatotropic agents in the systemic circulation and should be effective in reversing most biochemical manifestations of type I GSD with the exception of hypoglycemia. The surgical approach therefore is not recommended for small children in whom shunts are more likely to undergo spontaneous closure or in those anticipated to experience frequent episodes of very low blood sugar concentration [214].

Continuous infusions of either parenteral or enteral nutrients are impractical for long-term use. A more feasible approach employing frequent daytime feedings of a high-starch diet (which provides a "time release" source of glucose) in combination with a continuous nocturnal nutrient infusion has been devised. This form of treatment has been employed in numerous patients and has proved effective in maintaining blood glucose concentrations within a range that prevents stimulation of excess glycogenolysis and glycolysis [214].

Chen et al. [242] modified the dietary treatment regimen for type I GSD by incorporating raw cornstarch, which undergoes slow degradation to glucose by α-amylase, into the diet. Given in doses of 2 g/kg every 6 hours, it provides a suitable alternative to nasogastric nutrient infusions in some patients. Blood glucose and lactate levels, however, may not be maintained as effectively in young infants if cornstarch is used in place of continuous feedings, because of the low level of α-amylase in these patients. Consequently, optimal growth rates may not be achieved [214]. It has been suggested that, to achieve maximum growth potential, many children require an intensive feeding regimen consisting of high-starch meals given at 2- to 3-hour intervals during waking hours, coupled with a continuous nocturnal infusion of a nutritionally complete, high-glucose, low-fat (less than 5% of calories) formula. As growth ceases and glucose requirements concomitantly decrease, many of these patients are able to maintain adequate metabolic control on the cornstarch regimen [214]. Detailed recommendations for nutritional management of GSD have been published elsewhere [241,243–245].

More drastic approaches have been employed in the treatment of type I GSD. Renal transplantation was performed in one patient with type I GSD but failed to correct hypoglycemia [246]. To date hepatic transplantation been reported in 17 patients with GSD Ia and in two patients with GSD Ib [247,248]. In most cases, the transplantation was performed because of multiple malignant hepatic adenomas. In terms of short-term follow-up, all reports show correction of the hepatic enzyme defect, providing an improvement in both metabolic disturbances and quality of life [249,250]. However, only a few reports describe long-term follow-up. More recently, simultaneous liver–kidney transplantation has been successfully reported in a 25-year-old patient with history of hepatic adenomatosis and kidney failure [251]. On the contrary, hepatic transplantation proved to be effective therapy in another patient [252]. It is recommended that surgical treatment be reserved for those patients who experience life-threatening complications of the disease, such as bleeding adenomas or malignant degeneration, despite aggressive nutritional therapy.

Recommendations for treatment of type Ib GSD are identical to those for type Ia, and similar results may be expected with one exception: Treatment does not correct the neutropenia that accompanies this form of the disease. Prophylactic antibiotics may reduce the incidence of infections in these patients [253–257]. Some investigators have documented improvement in neutrophil function with this therapy [255,256], but the relationship between hepatic enzyme deficiency and leukocyte dysfunction is poorly understood.

Subsequent Course

Current treatment strategies have altered the clinical course significantly and dramatically improved the prognosis in type I GSD, and life expectancy now extends beyond the third decade. Before the mid-1970s, patients required frequent hospitalizations for hypoglycemia, fever, and acidosis. A high rate of mortality and permanent neurologic impairment secondary to recurrent or prolonged hypoglycemia were associated with the disease, and survivors often suffered from both physical and intellectual developmental delay.

Current treatment has been used successfully in a group of patients who have experienced near normal growth and have remained relatively symptom-free for more than 10 years [258]. Furthermore, the tendency to develop hypoglycemia seems to mitigate as patients reach adulthood [259]. In fact, reports of successful pregnancies in more than one patient with type I GSD have appeared in the literature [260,261]. Complete resolution of hepatic adenomas has been documented as a result of this therapy [231]. One case report of a child who remained unresponsive to aggressive nutritional therapy has appeared in the literature [262].

Suboptimal treatment continues to result in the consequences of poor metabolic control. Persistent hyperuricemia, which has been managed successfully with allopurinol in some patients, often leads to the development of gouty complications in the second and third decades of life. Compared with a normal population, higher rates of cardiovascular disease and pancreatitis resulting from hyperlipidemia have been reported in these patients [263–267]. Hepatic adenomas may progress to malignant hepatomas. Progressive renal disease has recently been documented in these patients. Of 20 patients older than 13 years of age with type I GSD, 14 had disturbed renal function manifested by altered creatinine clearance. Progressive renal insufficiency developed in 6 of these 14 patients, leading to three deaths from renal failure [219].

Type III Glycogen Storage Disease (Amylo-1,6-Glucosidase Deficiency)

This form of GSD first was recognized in 1952, when examination of liver and muscle tissue from a patient followed by Forbes [268] revealed atypical structure of glycogen molecules present in excess in both tissues. Illingworth and Cori [269] noted the presence of short outer chains as in phosphorylase limit dextrin and proposed a deficiency of the debranching enzyme, amylo-1,6-glucosidase. This was confirmed in 1956 [270]. Debranching enzyme contains two catalytic activities on a single polypeptide chain. The two activities are oligo-1,4–1, 4-glucantransferase and amylo-1,6-glucosidase [271,272]. The debrancher enzyme has been purified and has a 160-kDa molecular weight [273]. In 1967, van Hoof and Hers [274] measured debranching enzyme activity by four methods in hepatic and muscle tissue samples from 45 patients known to have the disease. Thirty-four patients exhibited complete absence of enzyme activity in both tissues regardless of the method of measurement; these cases were designated type IIIa. In the remaining patients, residual enzyme activity was apparent in either muscle (type IIIb) or hepatic tissue through at least one method of measurement. Ding et al. [275] have confirmed these findings by immunoblot analysis of glycogen debranching enzyme in 41 patients with type III GSD. Three patients had isolated oligo-1,4–1,4-glucantransferase deficiency, with retention of glucosidase activity (type IIId). Thirty-one patients had disease involving both liver and muscle (type IIIa), four patients had disease involving the liver only (type IIIb), and three had disease of unknown status.

Type III glycogenosis also is known as *limit dextrinosis* or *Forbes disease*. Transmission of the disease is autosomal recessive, and it may be diagnosed prenatally [275,276]. A higher incidence of type III GSD (1 in 5400 births) occurs in non-Ashkenazi Jewish communities of North African descent [244].

Molecular Basis

The human gene encoding for glycogen debranching enzyme is 85 kb in length and is composed of 35 exons [277]. The gene has been localized to chromosome 1p21 [278]. Translation begins in exon 3, and the predicated protein contains 1532 amino acids. Six messenger RNA isoforms have been identified [279]. Isoform 1 is expressed mainly in the liver; isoforms 2, 3, and 4 are muscle-specific. Isoforms 5 and 6 are minor isoforms. Mutations in the glycogen debranching gene have been described in patients with types IIIa and IIIb GSD. These mutations include nonsense, splicing, missense, and deletion–insertion lesions [280]. Certain mutations in exon 3, such as 17delAG and Q6X are seen only in type IIIb, indicating that specific mutations in exon 3 are associated only with type IIIb [281].

Clinical Presentation

The clinical manifestations of type III GSD result directly from its effects on hepatic and muscle tissue, although amylo-1,6-glucosidase deficiency is generalized to all types of cells. Individuals with type III GSD generally tolerate longer periods of fasting without hypoglycemia; therefore, the clinical course of the disease is usually much milder than that of type I GSD.

Symptoms and their severity vary from patient to patient and with age. In infancy and childhood, type III and type I GSD are not readily distinguishable by physical examination alone, primarily because hepatic manifestations predominate in this age group. Growth failure and hepatomegaly may be striking early in life. Hepatic fibrosis may lead to the development of splenomegaly in some children by age 4–6 years [282]. A decrease in liver size, however, has been noted to occur in some patients around puberty [283–286], and in some adult patients, normal physical examination results have been documented. Nevertheless, hepatic fibrosis has progressed to cirrhosis and liver failure in a few patients with type III GSD [238,263,286]. Additional deficiencies of phosphorylase and phosphorylase kinase have been identified in these unfortunate individuals [263].

The onset of muscular symptoms usually occurs in adulthood and is manifested primarily as progressive muscle weakness, which may be intensified by brisk walking or climbing, and muscle wasting [285]. Accumulation of glycogen in peripheral nerve axons has been demonstrated in one adult patient with unsteady gait [287].

Renal enlargement is not seen in type III GSD. Glycogen accumulation in the heart may produce cardiomegaly and nonspecific electrocardiographic changes [282]. Congestive heart failure and arrhythmias have not been reported; however, sudden death as a result of cardiac failure has occurred even in infancy [288,289].

Metabolic Consequences

Laboratory aberrations seen in type III GSD are similar to but less severe than those in type I. The onset of fasting-induced hypoglycemia occurs more slowly in most patients with type III GSD. Elevations in lipid levels appear to correlate directly with the tendency toward hypoglycemia; that is, moderately high lipid levels are seen in those patients who develop lower blood glucose levels after 6- to 8-hour fasts [286]. Moderate elevations in serum transaminase levels (300–600 IU) are seen consistently [290], with the exception of an occasional patient with more severe enzyme elevations. Lactic acid and uric acid levels are usually normal, although a rare patient has levels slightly above normal.

Patients with type III GSD exhibit characteristic responses to the administration of various hormones and nutrients. Galactose and fructose are transformed freely to glucose in these patients, and protein and amino acids cause small but protracted increases in blood glucose levels [220,286]. Similarly, glucagon and epinephrine administration between 1.5 and 3 hours after a meal raise blood glucose levels. Failure of these hormones to produce increases in blood glucose levels after a prolonged fast seems to provide evidence of available 1,4 glucosyl linkages that can undergo phosphorolysis shortly after a meal [291]. After a prolonged fast, access to 1,4 linkages would be blocked by terminal 1,6 glycosyl linkages, preventing an increase in blood glucose. This has been called the *double glucagon tolerance test;* however, patient response has been inconsistent, possibly because of glucose formation through this pathway. Such testing is therefore of little diagnostic value.

Biochemical and Pathologic Characteristics

Patients with type III GSD have abnormally high hepatic glycogen content; levels of 17.4% have been reported [284]. Structurally, hepatic glycogen has been found to have abnormally short outer branch points. These patients also may exhibit alterations in the activity of other enzymes involved in glycogen degradation. For example, Hug [263] demonstrated defects in phosphorylase and phosphorylase kinase activity in patients with type III GSD who had developed cirrhosis. Depression of glucose-6-phosphatase activity has also been identified in numerous patients [214].

The appearance of the liver in type III GSD varies from that in type I in two ways: the presence of fibrous septa, and the paucity of fat. Likewise, the ultrastructural appearance of the liver in type III GSD is characterized by small and frequent lipid vacuoles [274]. The progression of fibrosis to frank cirrhosis in type III GSD has been reported only recently. Figure 25.10A shows glycogen deposition in hepatocytes as stained by PAS stain, and removal of glycogen after diastase treatment (Figure 25.10B).

Diagnosis

There are several distinguishing laboratory and clinical features of type III glycogenosis, and patients with this disorder exhibit characteristic responses to various stimulation or challenge tests. No one test or feature, however, provides information that will differentiate this form of the disease from all others. Therefore, direct measurement of amylo-1,6-glucosidase activity in liver and muscle tissue samples and concomitant examination for abnormal glycogen structure should be relied on to yield a definitive diagnosis. The presence of excess glycogen in muscle and excess plasma creatine kinase also strongly support the diagnosis.

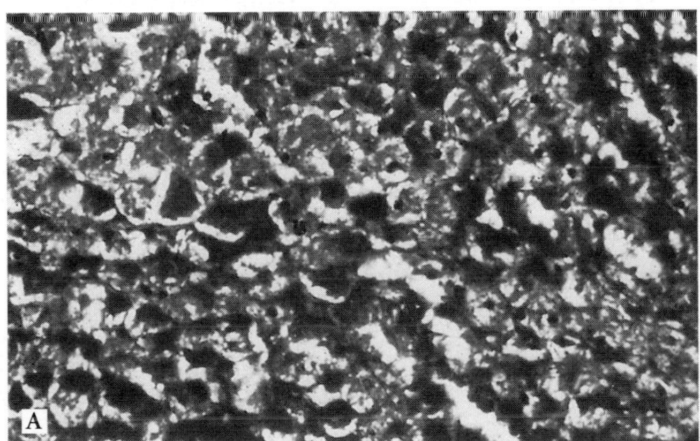

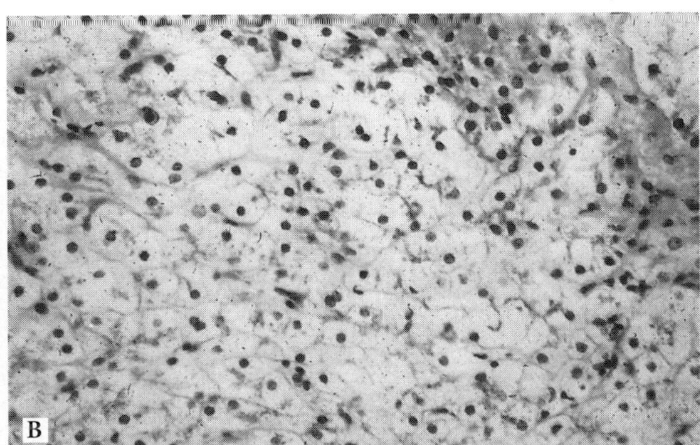

Figure 25.10. Type III glycogen storage disease. Glycogen accumulates with hepatocytes, demonstrated with periodic acid–Schiff stain (**A**), which is removed easily with diastase treatment (**B**).

Treatment

Traditionally, dietary regimens similar to but less stringent than those for type I GSD have been employed in the management of debranching enzyme deficiency. Borowitz and Greene [292] demonstrated improvement in liver transaminase levels with a high-starch diet containing only the recommended dietary allowances for protein. Slonim et al. [293] demonstrated improved growth and increased muscle strength in one patient with type III GSD in response to a high-protein diet and continuous nocturnal nutrient infusion of a high-protein formula.

Liver transplantation has been reported in three adult patients with type III GSD one with cirrhosis and hepatocellular carcinoma, and two with liver failure [250]. For the most part, treatment of type III GSD remains investigative and should be reserved for patients with progressive muscle involvement, hepatic fibrosis, or both.

Type IV Glycogen Storage Disease (-1,4 Glucan-6-Glycosyl Transferase Deficiency)

This form of GSD initially was described by Andersen in 1956 [294]. An infant, who died of cirrhosis at 17 months of age, had been noted to have hepatomegaly and an abnormal glycemic response to epinephrine. Recognizing the abnormally long inner and outer chains of glucose units, Illingworth and Cori [198,269] proposed a deficiency of branching enzyme, because of the similarity between amylopectin and the glycogen contained in tissue samples from this patient at autopsy. Brown and Brown [295] were credited with actual demonstration of the enzyme deficiency in 1966.

Type IV GSD also is known as *amylopectinosis* and as *Andersen's disease.* The disorder is most likely inherited through autosomal recessive transmission [294,296]; the possibility of X-linked transmission has not been eliminated because of the preponderance of males among reported patients [214].

Molecular Basis

The human gene encoding for the branching enzyme has been localized to chromosome 3p12 [297]. The human cDNA is 3 kb in length, encoding a 702–amino acid protein [297]. There appears to be a phenotype–genotype correlation, which may explain the clinical variability of the patients [298]. Mutations R515C, F257L, and R524X result in infantile cirrhosis; mutations 873del210 and 873del210 result in infantile myopathy and cardiomyopathy. Mutation Y3295/L224P results in nonprogressive liver disease [298]; prenatal diagnosis can be made using polymerase chain reaction–based DNA mutation analysis [299].

Clinical Presentation

Clinically, GSD type IV is a heterogeneous disorder with variability that may have congenital [300], infantile, childhood, or adulthood presentation. The most common form is the classic progressive liver cirrhosis, with onset of symptoms between ages 3 and 15 months. These children usually present with failure to thrive, abdominal distention, hepatosplenomegaly, and other vague gastrointestinal complaints. Later, symptoms associated with progressive liver dysfunction and cirrhosis usually dominate the clinical picture.

Approximately 50% of patients with type IV glycogenosis also experience abnormal neuromuscular development, with abnormal polysaccharide deposition in skeletal muscle [301–304]. A neuromuscular form of the disease has been described with the usual manifestations of hypotonia, muscular atrophy, and decreased or absent tendon reflexes, and evidence that all levels of the neuromuscular axis, that is, skeletal muscles and the peripheral and central nervous systems, may be affected [302]. A few patients have developed cardiac failure, presumably resulting from myofibrillar damage caused by amylopectin deposition within myocardial cells [214]. In exceptional patients, cardiac and neuromuscular symptoms predominate [305–307]. A few patients with features suggestive of GSD type IV with amylopectinosis have been reported to have severe progressive cardiomyopathy with and without skeletal myopathy but normal or near-normal GBE activity in liver, muscle, and cultured skin fibroblasts [308,309]. Adults with diffuse central and peripheral nervous systems dysfunction accompanied by accumulation of polyglucosan bodies have been described (adult polyglucosan body disease) [310,311].

Finally, four case reports involving adult patients with amylopectin-like storage myopathy have appeared in the literature. One, a 59-year-old man, reported symptoms of progressive, asymmetric limb–girdle weakness. Skeletal muscle branching enzyme deficiency was present, and vacuoles were noted to contain glycogen partially resistant to diastase [305]. Two of the other three patients ultimately developed heart and brain involvement [306,307]. None of these patients exhibited any symptoms of hepatic involvement.

Metabolic Consequences

Biochemical abnormalities associated with branching enzyme deficiency vary considerably from those seen in other forms of hepatic glycogenosis. Hypoglycemia is an uncommon manifestation of type IV GSD; it has been documented in only one instance in the literature [312]. The response to glucagon and epinephrine administration varies from normal to subnormal to flat in these patients [296,313–315] with maximum response occurring approximately 30 minutes after injection and 2 hours after a meal [314]. Both hormones allow detection of urinary ketone bodies. These patients exhibit a normal glycemic response if challenged with glucose, fructose, and galactose, however. Serum cholesterol levels usually are slightly elevated. Moderate elevations (3–6× normal) in serum transaminase and alkaline phosphatase levels are characteristic of the disease. Serum lactate and pyruvate levels are normal in most patients [314]; however, chronic and severe acidosis as well as abnormal electrolyte concentrations may result from renal tubular defects [296,316,317]. As liver failure ensues, these patients exhibit the characteristic laboratory abnormalities associated with this clinical condition including hypoglycemia and hypocholesterolemia.

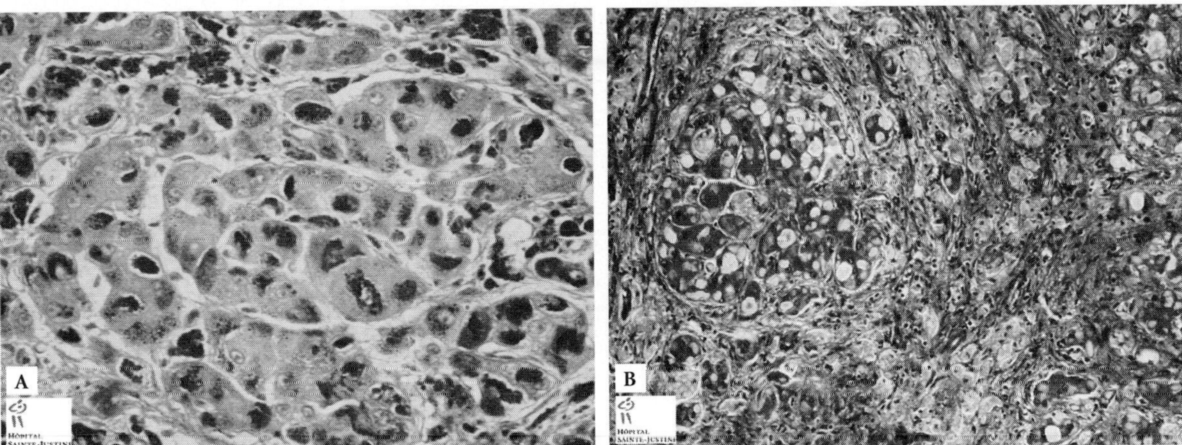

Figure 25.11. Glycogen storage disease type IV. (**A**) Periodic acid–Schiff stain positive inclusions in cytoplasm and (**B**) micronodular cirrhosis with hepatocytes containing cytoplasmic inclusions. (Masson trichrome stain.) (Image courtesy of humpath.com.) For color reproduction, see Color Plate 25.11.

Biochemical and Pathologic Features

Individuals with type IV GSD characteristically have hepatic glycogen contents of 3.5–5.0%, compared with approximately 6% of wet weight in normal subjects. In one patient, hepatic glycogen content measured 10.7% [296]. The chemical properties of the polysaccharide also differ from those of normal glycogen, because of the abnormal structure of the compound. In type IV GSD, more than 40% of the glucose units are highly susceptible to phosphorylase-induced hydrolysis (normal: ~36%); this could be attributed to its longer outer chain lengths (normal: 8–12 glycosyl U) and fewer branch points (~6%) compared with normal mammalian glycogen (~8%). The polysaccharide is highly chromogenic, with a maximal KI:I2 absorption band at approximately 525 nm (nL: 460 nm) [296]. Leukocytic glycogen also is abnormal, presumably because of the deficiency of branching enzyme in these cells. Skeletal muscle glycogen appears normal. Liver and myocardial glycosyl deposits appear similar histochemically; both are resistant to digestion by α-amylase.

Macroscopically, the liver shows micronodular cirrhosis. Microscopically, the hepatocytes contain cytoplasmic PAS stain–positive deposits. The nuclei of the hepatocytes is displaced by inclusions, which characteristically are limited to the periphery of the lobule (Figure 25.11A). Ultrastructural studies show three types of cytoplasmic deposits including glycogen particles, fibrils, and finely granular material. The abnormal glycogen can be detected ultrastructurally or histochemically. Similarly, changes in cytoplasmic deposits are seen in the myocardium, central nervous system, and skeletal muscles. Histochemically, the liver deposits represent an abnormal glycogen with fewer branch points [301,302,313,314,316,317]. Figure 25.11A shows characteristic cytoplasmic inclusion–like artifacts. Fibrosis is demonstrated by Masson trichone stain (Figure 25.11B).

Diagnosis

Identification of the characteristic abnormal structure of glycogen and ramification of branching enzyme deficiency in muscle, leukocytes, cultured fibroblasts, and amniotic cells [295,296,304,305,307] are critical steps in the diagnosis of type IV GSD.

Treatment

Liver transplantation is the only available option for patients with type IV GSD who progress to liver cirrhosis.

Subsequent Course

In most patients, hepatosplenomegaly quickly progresses to cirrhosis, and the terminal course of the disease usually is highlighted by complications of chronic liver failure. Most patients have succumbed within 3 years after diagnosis, although a few case reports documenting survival considerably beyond this time period can be found in the literature [312,315,318]. These include two patients managed at our center, both of whom were determined to have branching enzyme deficiency in skin fibroblasts as well as the liver. Of those, one patient developed cirrhosis and liver failure by 18 months of age [312]. Six months later, he underwent liver transplantation. He has subsequently been managed with standard immunosuppressive therapy. Follow-up evaluations over the subsequent 7 years posttransplantation showed no evidence of liver, muscle, nerve, or cardiac dysfunction. A second child was initially evaluated at age 3 years for hepatomegaly and chronically elevated serum transaminases. Liver biopsy results showed moderate, generalized micronodular fibrosis. Present in approximately 25% of hepatocytes were PAS-positive, diastase-resistant deposits.

Drochman fibril accumulation was demonstrated through electron microscopy but was not present in all cells [319]. Over the next 3 years, this patient experienced normal growth and development and spontaneous normalization of liver enzymes. Repeat liver biopsy at age 6 showed equally remarkable changes including minimal periportal fibrosis and complete absence of PAS-positive, diastase-resistant deposits. Electron microscopy revealed normal glycogen structure. Branching enzyme activity remained undetectable in hepatocytes and skin fibroblasts.

The reports of patients with amylopectin-like storage myopathy that have appeared in the literature demonstrate that in the absence of hepatic involvement, survival into adulthood is possible with type IV GSD [305–307].

ACKNOWLEDGMENT

We acknowledge Jean F. Simpson, M.D., associate professor of pathology and director of anatomic pathology, Vanderbilt University Medical Center, for providing the photomicrographs.

REFERENCES

1. Mason HH, Turner ME. Chronic galactosemia. Am J Dis Child 1935;50:359–74.
2. Segal S. Galactosaemia today: the enigma and the challenge. J Inherit Metab Dis 1998;21:455–71.
3. GALTdB (the Galactose-1-Phosphate Uridyl Transferase Mutation Analysis Database Home Page). (Accessed November 2, 2006 at http://www.ich.bris.ac.uk/galtdb/.)
4. Isselbacher KJ, Anderson EP, Kurahashi K, et al. Congenital galactosemia, a single enzymatic block in galactose metabolism. Science 1956;123:635–6.
5. Steinmann B, Gitzelmann R, Zachmann M. Hypogonadism and galactosaemia. N Engl J Med 1981;305:464–5.
6. Gitzelmann R. Hereditary galactokinase deficiency, a newly recognized cause of juvenile cataracts. Pediatr Res 1967;1:14–23.
7. Gitzelmann R. Deficiency of uridine diphosphate galactose-4-epimerase in blood cells of an apparently healthy infant. Helv Paediatr Acta 1972;27:125–30.
8. Gitzelmann R, Steinmann B, Mitchell B, et al. Uridine diphosphate galactose-4-epimerase deficiency. IV. Report of eight cases in three families. Helv Paediatr Acta 1977;31:441–52.
9. Holton JB, Gillett MG, MacFaul R, et al. Galactosemia: a new severe variant due to uridine diphosphate galactose-4-epimerase deficiency. Arch Dis Child 1981;56:885–7.
10. Henderson MJ, Holton JB, MacFaul R. Further observations in a case of uridine diphosphate galactose-4-epimerase deficiency with a severe clinical presentation. J Inherited Metab Dis 1983;6:17–20.
11. Garibaldi LR, Canine S, Superti-Furga A, et al. Galactosemia caused by generalized uridine diphosphate galactose-4-epimerase deficiency. J Pediatr 1983;103:927–30.
12. Bowling FG, Fraser DK, Clague AE, et al. A case of uridine diphosphate galactose-4-epimerase deficiency detected by neonatal screening for galactosemia. Med J Aust 1986;144: 150–1.
13. Holten, JB. Galactosaemia: pathogenesis and treatment. J Inherit Metab Dis 1996;19:3–7.
14. Hopfer U. Membrane transport mechanisms for hexoses and amino acids in the small intestine. In: Johnson LR, Christensen J, Jackson MJ, eds. Physiology of the gastrointestinal tract. 2nd ed. New York: Raven Press, 1987:1499–526.
15. Sherman JR, Adler J. Galactokinase from *E. coli*. J Biol Chem 1963;238:873–8.
16. Heinrich MR. The purification and properties of yeast galactokinase. J Biol Chem 1964;239:50–3.
17. Cardini CE, Leloir LF. Enzymatic phosphorylation of galactosamine and galactose. Arch Biochem Biophys 1953;45:55–64.
18. Shin-Buehring YS, Beier T, Tan A, et al. Galactokinase and galactose-1-phosphate uridyltransferase (transferase) and galactokinase in human fetal organs [abstract]. Pediatr Res 1977;11:1012.
19. Tedesco TA. Human galactose-1-phosphate uridyl transferase: purification, antibody production, and comparison of the wild type, Duarte variant, and galactosemic gene products. J Biol Chem 1972;247:6631–6.
20. Flach JE, Reichardt TKV, Elsas LJ. Sequence of a cDNA encoding human galactose-1-phosphate uridyl transferase. Mol Biol Med 1990;7:365–9.
21. Bergren WR, Ng WG, Donnell GN. Uridine diphosphate galactose-4-epimerase in human and other mammalian hemolysates. Biochim Biophys Acta 1973;315:464–72.
22. Knop J, Hansen R. Uridine diphosphate glucose pyrophosphorylase: IV. Crystallization and properties of the enzyme from human liver. J Biol Chem 1970;245:2499–504.
23. Clements R, Weaver J, Winegrad A. The distribution of polyol: NADP oxidoreductase in mammalian tissues. Biochem Biophys Res Commun 1969;37:347–53.
24. Wells W, Pittman T, Egan T. The isolation and identification of galactitol from urine of patients with galactosemia. J Biol Chem 1964;239:3192–5.
25. Gitzelmann R, Curtius HC, Muller M. Galactitol excretion in the urine of a galactokinase deficient man. Biochem Biophys Res Commun 1966;22:437–41.
26. Bergren WR, NG WG, Donnell GN. Galactonic acid in galactosemia: identification in the urine. Science 1972;176:683–4.
27. Segal S, Blair A. Some observations on the metabolism of D-galactose in normal man. J Clin Invest 1961;40:2016–25.
28. Tygstrup N. Determination of the hepatic elimination capacity (LM) of galactose by single injection. Scand J Clin Lab Invest 1966;92 Suppl 18:118–25.
29. Lemaire HG, Mueller-Hill B. Nucleotide sequences of the galE gene and the galT gene of *E. coli*. Nucleic Acid Res 1986;14:7705–11.
30. Tajima J, Nogi Y, Fukasawa T. Primary structure of the *Saccharomyces cerevisiae* GAL7 gene. Yeast 1985;1:67–77.
31. Reichardt JKV, Woo SLC. Molecular basis of galactosemia: mutations and polymorphisms in the gene encoding human galactose-1-phosphate uridyl transferase. Proc Natl Acad Sci U S A 1991;88:2633–7.
32. Reichardt JKV, Packman S, Woo SLC. Molecular characterization of two galactosemic mutations: correlation of mutations with highly conserved domains in galactose-1-phosphate uridyl transferase. Am J Hum Genet 1991;49:860–7.
33. Field TL, Reznikoff WS, Frey PA. Galactose-1-phosphate uridyl transferase: identification of histidine-164 and histidine-166 as critical residues by site directed mutagenesis. Biochemistry 1989;28:2094–9.
34. Wang B, Xu Y, Ng WG, et al. Molecular and biochemical basis of galactosemia. Mole Geneti Metab 1998;63:263–9.
35. Reichardt JK, Levy HL, Woo SL. Molecular characterizations of two galactosemic mutations and one polymorphorism: implications for structure-function analysis of human galactose-1-phosphate uridyl transferase. Biochemistry 1992;311:5430–3.
36. Williams JC, Howell RR. Nutrition in inborn errors of carbohydrate metabolism. In: Grand RJ, Sutphen JL, Dietz WH, eds.

Pediatric nutrition: theory and practice. Boston: Butterworths. 1987:665–70.

37. Hsia DYY, Walker FA. Variability in the clinical manifestations of galactosemia. J Pediatr 1961;59:872–83.
38. Donnell GN, Collado M, Koch R. Growth and development of children with galactosemia. J Pediatr 1961;58:836–44.
39. Donnell GN, Koch R, Bergren WR. Observations on results of management of galactosemic patients. In: Hsia DYY, ed. Galactosemia. Springfield, IL: Charles C Thomas, 1969:247–68.
40. Nadler HL, Inouye T, Hsia DYY. Clinical galactosemia: a study of fifty-five cases. In: Hsia DYY, ed. Galactosemia. Springfield, IL: Charles C. Thomas, 1969:127.
41. Fishler K, Koch R, Donnell GN, et al. Developmental aspects of galactosemia from infancy to childhood. Clin Pediatr 1980, 19:38–44.
42. Komrower GM, Lee DH. Long-term follow-up of galactosemia. Arch Dis Child 1970;45:367–73.
43. Komrower GM. Galactosaemia: thirty years on the experience of a generation. J Inherit Metab Dis 1982;5:96.
44. Waggoner DD, Buist NRM, Donnell GH. Long-term prognosis in galactosaemia: results of a survey of 350 cases. J Inherit Metab Dis 1990;13:802–18.
45. Belman AL, Moshe SL, Zimmerman RD. Computered tomographic demonstration of cerebral edema in a child with galactosemia. Pediatrics 1986;78:606–9.
46. Levy HL, Sepe SJ, Shih VE, et al. Sepsis due to *Escherichia coli* in neonates with galactosemia. N Engl J Med 1977;297:823–5.
47. Litchfield WJ, Wells WW. Effects of galactose on free radical reactions of polymorphonuclear leukocytes. Arch Biochem Biophys 1978;188:26–30.
48. Segal S, Blair A, Roth H. The metabolism of galactose by patients with congenital galactosemia. Am J Med 1965;38:62–70.
49. Segal S. Disorders of galactose metabolism. In: Stanbury JB, Wyngaarden JB, Frederickson DS, eds. The metabolic basis of inherited disease. 4th ed. New York: McGraw-Hill, 1978:160–81.
50. Segal S. Disorders of galactose metabolism. In: Stanbury JB, Wyngaarden JB, Frederickson DS, eds. The metabolic basis of inherited disease. 6th ed. New York: McGraw-Hill, 1989:453–80.
51. Komrower GM, Schwarz V, Holzel A, et al. A clinical and biochemical study of galactosemia. Arch Dis Child 1956;31:254–64.
52. Holzel A, Komrower GM, Schwarz V. Galactosemia. Am J Med 1957;22:703–11.
53. Holzel A, Komrower GM, Wilson VK. Amino-aciduria in galatosemia. Br Med J 1952;1:194–5.
54. Cusworth DC, Dent CE, Flynn FV. The amino-aciduria in galactosemia. Arch Dis Child 1955;30:150–4.
55. Keppler D, Decker K. Studies on the mechanisms of galactosamine hepatitis: accumulation of galactosamine-1-phosphate and its inhibition of UDP-glucose pyrophosphorylase. Eur J Biochem 1969;10:219–25.
56. Quan-Ma R, Wells W. The distribution of galactitol in tissues of rats fed galactose. Biochem Biophys Res Commun 1965;20:486–90.
57. Schwarz V. The value of galactose phosphate determinations in the treatment of galactosemia. Arch Dis Child 1960;35:428–32.
58. Quan-Ma R, Wells H, Wells W, et al. Galactitol in the tissues of a galactosemic child. Am J Dis Child 1966;112:477–8.
59. Thier S, Fox M, Rosenberg L, et al. Hexose inhibition of amino acid uptake in the rat kidney cortex slice. Biochim Biophys Acta 1964;93:106–15.
60. Saunders S, Isselbacher KJ. Inhibition of intestinal amino acid transport by hexoses. Biochim Biophys Acta 1965;102:397–409.
61. Fox M, Thier S, Rosenberg L, et al. Impaired renal tubular function induced by sugar infusion in man. J Clin Endocrinol 1964;24:1318–27.
62. Rosenberg L, Weinberg A, Segal S. The effect of high galactose diets on urinary excretion of amino acids in the rat. Biochim Biophys Acta 1961;48:500–5.
63. van Heyningen R. Formation of polyols by the lens of the rat with "sugar" cataract. Nature 1959;184:194–5.
64. Kinoshita JH, Dvornik D, Krami M, et al. The effect of aldose reductase inhibitor on the galactose-exposed rabbit lens. Biochim Biophys Acta 1968;158:472–5.
65. Kinoshita JH, Barber GW, Merola LO, et al. Changes in levels of free amino acids and myo-inositol in the galactose-exposed lens. Invest Ophthalmol 1969;8:625–32.
66. Heffley JD, Williams RJ. The nutritional teamwork approach: prevention and regression of cataracts in rats. Proc Natl Acad Sci U S A 1974;71:4164–8.
67. Dische Z, Zelmenis G, Youlous J. Studies on protein and protein synthesis during the development of galactose cataract. Am J Ophthalmol 1957;44:332–40.
68. Sippel TO. Enzymes of carbohydrate metabolism in developing galactose cataracts of rats. Invest Ophthalmol 1967;6:59–63.
69. Korc I. Biochemical studies on cataracts in galactose-fed rats. Arch Biochem 1961;94:196–200.
70. Sipple TO. Energy metabolism in the lens during development of galactose cataract in rats. Invest Ophthalmol 1966;5:576–82.
71. Kinoshita JH, Merola LO, Tung B. Changes in cation permeability in the galactose-exposed rabbit lens. Exp Eye Res 1968;7:80–90.
72. Wells W, Pittman T, Wells H, et al. The isolation and identification of galactitol from the brains of galactosemia patients. J Biol Chem 1965;240:1002–4.
73. Wells HJ, Gordon M, Segal S. Galactose toxicity in the chick: oxidation of radioactive galactose. Biochim Biophys Acta 1970;222:327–32.
74. Granett SE, Kozak LP, McIntyre JP, et al. Studies on cerebral energy metabolism during the course of galactose neurotoxicity in chicks. J Neurochem 1972;19:1659–70.
75. Knull HR, Lobert PF, Wells WW. Galactose neurotoxicity in chicks: effects on fast axoplasmic transport. Brain Res 1974;79:524–7.
76. Malone J, Wells H, Segal S. Decreased uptake of glucose by brain of the galactose toxic chick. Brain Res 1972;43:700–4.
77. Malone JI, Wells HJ, Segal S. Galactose toxicity in the chick: hyperosmolality. Science 1971;174:952–4.
78. Woolley DW, Gommi BW. Serotonin receptors, IV: specific deficiency of receptors in galactose poisoning and its possible relationship to the idiocy of galactosemia. Proc Natl Acad Sci U S A 1964;52:14–19.
79. Knull HR, Wells WW. Recovery from galactose-induced neurotoxicity in the chick by the administration of glucose. J Neurochem 1973;20:415–22.
80. Tsakiris S, Karagiorgiou H, Schulpis KH. The protective effect of L-Cystine and Glutathione on the adult and aged rat brain (Na+,K+)-ATPase and Mg2+-ATPase activities in galactosemia in vitro. Metab Brain Dis 2005;20:87–95.
81. Kaufman FR, Kogut MD, Donnell GN, et al. Hypergonadotropic hypogonadism in female patients with galactosemia. N Engl J Med 1981;304:994–8.

82. Fraser IS, Russell P, Greco S, et al. Resistant ovary syndrome and premature ovarian failure in young women with galactosemia. Clin Reprod Fertil 1986;4:133–8.
83. Levy HL, Driscoll SG, Porensky RS, et al. Ovarian failure in galactosemia. N Engl J Med 1984;310:50.
84. Roe TF, Hallat JG, Donnell GN, et al. Childbearing by a galactosemic woman. J Pediatr 1971;78:1026–30.
85. Schwarz V, Goldberg L, Komrower GM, et al. Some disturbances of erythrocyte metabolism in galactosemia. Biochem J 1956;62:34–40.
86. Miller LR, Gordon GB, Bensch KG. Cytologic alterations in hereditary metabolic disorders: I. The effects of galactose on galactosemia fibroblasts in vitro. Lab Invest 1968;19:428–36.
87. Kurahashi K, Wahba AJ. Interference with growth of certain *E. coli* mutants by galactose. Biochim Biophys Acta 1958;30:298–302.
88. Yarmolinsky MB, Wiesmeyer H, Kalckar HM, et al. Hereditary defects in galactose metabolism in *E. coli* mutants: II. Galactose-induced sensitivity. Proc Natl Acad Sci U S A 1959;45:1786–91.
89. Xu YK, Kaufman FR, Donnell GN, et al. Radiochemical assay of minute quantities of galactose-1-phosphage uridyl transferase activity in erythrocytes and leukocytes of galactosemia patients. Clin Chim Acta 1995;235:125–36.
90. Koch R, Donnell GN, Fishler K, et al. Galactosemia. In: Kelley VC, ed. Practice of pediatrics. Hagerstown, MD: Harper and Row, 1979:1–14.
91. Brandt MJ. Frequency of heterozygotes for hereditary galactosemia in a normal population. Acta Genet (Basel) 1967;17:289–98.
92. Tedesco TA, Miller KL, Rawnsley BE, et al. Human erythrocyte galactokinase and galactose-1-phosphate uridylyltransferase: a population survey. Am J Hum Genet 1975;27:737–47.
93. Kliegman RM, Sparks JW. Perinatal galactose metabolism. J Pediatr 1985;107:831–41.
94. Scriver CR. Population screening: report of a workshop. Prog Clin Biol Res 1985;163B:89–152.
95. Robbins SL, Cotran RS. Diseases of infancy and childhood. In: Robbins SL, Cotran RS, eds. Pathologic basis of disease. 2nd ed. Philadelphia: WB Saunders, 1979:561–92.
96. Smetana HF, Olen E. Hereditary galactose disease. Am J Clin Pathol 1962;38:3–25.
97. Walker FA, Hsia DYY, Slatis HM, et al. Galactosemia: a study of 27 kindreds in North America. Ann Hum Genet 1962;25:287–311.
98. Kirkman HN, Bynum E. Enzymic evidence of a galactosemic trait in parents of galactosemic children. Ann Hum Genet 1959; 23:117–26.
99. Mellman WJ, Tedesco TA, Feigl P. Estimation of the gene frequency of the Duarte variant of galactose-1-phosphate uridyl transferase. Ann Hum Genet 1968;32:1–8.
100. Ng WG, Xu YK, Kaufman FR, et al. Deficit of uridine diphosphate galactose in galactosaemia. J Inherit Metab Dis 1989;12: 257–66.
101. Manis FR, Cohn LB, McBride-Chang C, et al. A longitudinal study of cognitive functioning in patients with classical galactosaemia, including a cohort treated with oral uridine. J Inherit Metab Dis 1997;20:549–55.
102. Berry GT. The role of polyols in the pathophysiology of galactosemia. Eur J Pediatr 1995;154 Suppl 2:40–4.
103. Pomeranz Y. Interaction between glycolipids and wheat flour macromolecules in bread making. Adv Food Res 1973;20:153–88.
104. Gross KC, Sams CE. Changes in cell wall neutral sugar composition during fruit ripening: a species survey. Phytochemistry 1984;23:2457–61.
105. Jermyn MA, Isherwood FA. Changes in the cell wall of the pear during ripening. Biochem J 1956;64:123–32.
106. Shallenberger RS, Moyer JC. Relationship between changes in glucose, fructose, galactose, sucrose and stachyose and the formation of starch in peas. Agri Food Chem 1961;8:137–40.
107. Weier TE, Benson AA. The molecular organization of chloroplast membranes. Am J Bot 1967;54:389–402.
108. Wood PJ, Siddiqui IR. Isolation and structural studies of a water-soluble galactan from potato (solanum tuberosum) tubers. Carbohydr Res 1972;22:212–20.
109. Fry SC. Phenolic components of the primary cell wall: feruloylated disaccharides of D-galactose and L-arabinose from spinach polysaccharide. Biochem J 1982;203:493–504.
110. Gross KC. Changes in free galactose, myo-inositol and other monosaccharides in normal and non-ripening mutant tomatoes. Phytochemistry 1983;22:1137–9.
111. Walter JH, Collins JE, Leonard JV. Recommendations for the management of galactosaemia: UK Galactosaemia Steering Group. Arch Dis Child 1999;80:93–6.
112. Gross KC, Acosta PB. Fruits and vegetables are a source of galactose: implications in planning the diets of patients with galactosemia. J Inherit Metab Dis 1991;14:253–8.
113. Gitzelmann R, Auricchio S. The handling of soya alpha-galactosides by a normal and a galactosemic child. Pediatrics 1965;36:231–5.
114. Gitzelmann R. Formation of galactose-1-phosphate from uridine diphosphate galactose in erythrocytes from patients and galactosemics. Pediatr Res 1969;3:279–86.
115. Gitzelmann R, Hansen RG. Galactose biogenesis and disposal in galactosemics. Biochim Biophys Acta 1974;372:374–8.
116. Berry GT, Nissim I, Lin Z, et al. Endogenous synthesis of galactose in normal man and patients with hereditary galactosaemia. Lancet 1995;346:1073–4.
117. Berry GT, Palmieri MJ, Gross KC, et al. The effects of dietary fruits and vegetables on urinary galactitol excretion in galactose-1-phosphate uridyltransferase deficiency. J Inherit Metab Dis 1993;16:91–100.
118. Bower BD, Smallpiece V. Lactose-free diet in galactosemia. Lancet 1955;ii:873.
119. Segal S, Cuatrecasas P. The oxidation of 14C galactose by patients with congenital galactosemia: evidence for a direct oxidative pathway. Am J Med 1968;44:340–7.
120. Waisbren SE, Norman RT, Schnell RR, et al. Speech and language deficits in early treated children with galactosemia. J Pediatr 1983;102:75–7.
121. Haberland C, Perou M, Brunngraber EG, et al. The neuropathology of galactosemia: a histopathological and biochemical study. J Neuropathol Exp Neurol 1971;30:431–47.
122. Crome L. A case of galactosemia with the pathological and neuropathological findings. Arch Dis Child 1962;37:415–21.
123. Jan JE, Wilson RA. Unusual late neurological sequelae in galactosemia. Dev Med Child Neurol 1973;15:72–4.
124. Lo W, Packman S, Nash S, et al. Curious neurologic sequelae in galactosemia. Pediatrics 1984;73:309–12.

125. Kaufman FR, Donnell GN, Roe TF, et al. Gonadal function in patients with galactosaemia. J Inherited Metab Dis 1986;9: 140–6.
126. Robinson ACR, Dockeray CJ, Cullen MJ, et al. Hypergonadotrophic hypogonadism in classical galactosemia: evidence for defective oogenesis. Br J Obstet Gynaecol 1984;91: 199–200.
127. Tedesco TA, Morrow G, Mellman WJ. Normal pregnancy and childbirth in a galactosemic woman. J Pediatr 1972;81:1159–61.
128. Fraser IS, Shearman RP, Wilcken B, et al. Failure to identify heterozygotes for galactosaemia in women with premature ovarian failure. Lancet 1987;ii:566.
129. Kaufman FR, Loro ML, Azen C, et al. Effect of hypogonadism and deficient calcium intake on bone density in patients with galactosemia. J Pediatr 1993;123:365–70.
130. Renner C, Razeghi S, Uberall MA, et al. Hormone replacement therapy in galactosaemic twins with ovarian failure and severe osteoporosis. J Inherit Metab Dis 1999;22:194–5.
131. Chacko CM, McCrone L, Nadler HL. A study of galactokinase and glucose-4-epimerase from normal and galactosemic skin fibroblasts. Biochim Biophys Acta 1972;284:552–5.
132. Dahlqvist A, Gamstorp I, Madsen H. A patient with hereditary galactokinase deficiency. Acta Pediatr Scand 1970;59:669–75.
133. Gitzelmann R, Haigis E. Appearance of active UPD-galactose-4-epimerase in cells cultured from epimerase-deficient persons. J Inherit Metab Dis 1978;i:41.
134. Ravich WJ, Bayless TM, Thomas M. Fructose: incomplete intestinal absorption in humans. Gastroenterology 1983;84: 26–9.
135. Steinmann B. Personal communication.
136. Kneepkens CMF, Vonk RJ, Fernandes J. Incomplete intestinal absorption of fructose. Arch Dis Child 1984;59:735–8.
137. Khachadurian AK. Nonalimentary fructosuria. Pediatrics 1963; 32:455–7.
138. Taunton OD, Greene HL, Stifel FB, et al. Fructose-1,6-diphosphatase deficiency, hypoglycemia, and response to folate therapy in a mother and her daughter. Biochem Med 1978;19: 260–76.
139. Sigrist Nelson K, Hopfer U. A distinct D-fructose transport system in isolated brush border membrane. Biochim Biophys Acta 1974;367:247–54.
140. Thorens B. Glucose transporters in the regulation of intestinal, renal, and liver glucose fluxes. Am J Physiol 1996;270:G541–53.
141. Tsutsumi K, Tsunehiro M, Hidaka S, et al. Rat aldolase isozyme gene: cloning and characterization of cDNA for aldolase B messenger RNA. J Biol Chem 1983;258:6537–42.
142. Besmond C, Dreyfus J-C, Gregori C, et al. Nucleotide sequence of a cDNA clone for human aldolase B. Biochem Biophys Res Commun 1983;117:601–9.
143. Rottmann WH, Tolan DR, Penhoet EE. Complete amino acid sequence for human aldolase B derived from cDNA and genomic clones. Proc Natl Acad Sci U S A 1984;81:2738–42.
144. Lench NJ, Telford EA, Andersen SE, et al. An EST and STS-based YAC contig map of human chromosome 9q22.3. Genomics 1996;38:199–205.
145. Chambers RA, Pratt RTC. Idiosyncrasy to fructose. Lancet 1956;ii:340.
146. Froesch VER, Prader A, Labhart A, et al. Die hereditare Fructoseintoleranz, eine bisher nicht bekannte kongenitale Stoffwechselstorung. Schweiz Med Wochenschr 1957;87:1168–71.
147. Hers HG, Joassin G. Anomaly of hepatic adolase in intolerance to fructose. Enzymol Biol Clin 1961;1:4–14.
148. Penhoet EE, Kochman M, Rutter WJ. Isolation of fructose diphosphate aldolases A, B and C. Biochemistry 1969;8: 4391–5.
149. Mukai T, Yatsuki H, Arai Y, et al. Human aldolase B gene: characterization of the genomic aldolase B gene and analysis of sequences required for multiple polyadenylations. J Biochem 1987;102:1043–51.
150. Tolan DR, Penhoet EE. Characterization of the human aldolase B gene. Mol Biol Med 1986;3:245–64.
151. Cross NCP, Tolan DR, Cox TM. Catalytic deficiency of human aldolase B in hereditary fructose intolerance caused by a common missense mutation. Cell 1988;53:881–5.
152. Cross NCP, Franchis RD, Sebastio G, et al. Molecular analysis of aldolase B genes in hereditary fructose intolerance. Lancet 1990;335:306–9.
153. Ali M, Rellos P, Cox TM. Hereditary fructose intolerance. J Med Genet 1998;35:353–65.
154. Tolan DR, Brooks CC. Molecular analysis of common aldolase B alleles for hereditary fructose intolerance in North Americans. Biochem Med Metabol Biol 1992;48:19–25.
155. Lau J, Tolan DR. Screening for hereditary fructose intolerance mutations by reverse dot-blot. Mol Cell Probes 1999;13:35–40.
156. Steinmann B, Gitzelmann R. The diagnosis of hereditary fructose intolerance. Helv Paediatr Acta 1981;36:297–316.
157. Baerlocher K, Gitzelmann R, Steinmann B, et al. Hereditary fructose intolerance in early childhood: a major diagnostic challenge. Survey of 20 symptomatic cases. Helv Paediatr Acta 1978;33:465–87.
158. Odievre M, Gentil C, Gautier M, et al. Hereditary fructose intolerance in childhood. Am J Dis Child 1978;132:605–8.
159. Bell L, Sherwood WG. Current practices and improved recommendations for treating hereditary fructose intolerance. J Am Diet Assoc 1987;87:721–30.
160. Baker L, Winegrad AI. Fasting hypoglycaemia and metabolic acidosis associated with deficiency of hepatic fructose-1,6-diphosphatase activity. Lancet 1970;ii:13–16.
161. Levin B, Snodgrass GJAI, Oberholzer VG, et al. Fructosaemia. Observations on seven cases. Am J Med 1968;45:826–38.
162. Cornblath M, Rosenthal IM, Reisner SH, et al. Hereditary fructose intolerance. N Engl J Med 1963;269:1271–8.
163. Froesch ER, Wolf HP, Baitsch H, et al. Hereditary fructose intolerance: an inborn defect of hepatic fructose-1-phosphate splitting aldolase. Am J Med 1963;34:151–67.
164. Perheentupa J, Raivio KO, Nikkila EA. Hereditary fructose intolerance. Acta Med Scand 1972;542 Suppl:65–75.
165. Fox IH, Kelley WN. Studies on the mechanism of fructose-induced hyperuricemia in man. Metabolism 1972;21:713–21.
166. Narins RG, Weisberg JS, Myers AR. Effects of carbohydrates on uric acid metabolism. Metabolism 1974;23:455–65.
167. Heuckenkamp P-U, Zollner N. Fructose-induced hyperuricaemia. Lancet 1971;ii:808–9.
168. Sahebjami H, Scalettar R. Effects of fructose infusion on lactate and uric acid metabolism. Lancet 1971;i:366–9.
169. van den Berghe G, Bronfman M, Vanneste R, et al. The mechanism of adenosine triphosphate depletion in the liver after a load of fructose: a kinetic study of liver adenylate deaminase. Biochem J 1977;162:601–9.

170. Bode JC, Zelder O, Rumpelt HJ, et al. Depletion of liver adenosine phosphate and metabolic effects of intravenous infusion of fructose or sorbitol in man and in the rat. Eur J Clin Invest 1973;3:436–41.
171. Maenpaa PH, Raivio KO, Kekomaki MP. Liver adenine nucleotides: fructose-induced depletion and its effect on protein synthesis. Science 1968;161:1253–4.
172. Oberhaensli RD, Rajagopalan B, Taylor DJ, et al. Study of hereditary fructose intolerance by use of ^{31}P magnetic resonance spectroscopy. Lancet 1987;ii:931–7.
173. Morris RC. Fructose induced disruption of renal acidification in patients with hereditary fructose intolerance. J Clin Invest 1965;44:1076–7.
174. Morris RC. Evidence for an acidification defect of the proximal renal tubule in experimental and clinical renal disease. J Clin Invest 1966;45:1048–52.
175. Swales JD, Smith ADM. Adult fructose intolerance. Q J Med 1966;35:455–73.
176. Black JA, Simpson K. Fructose intolerance. Br Med J 1967; 4:138–41.
177. Burton BK, Chacko CM, Nadler HL. Aldolase in cultivated human fibroblasts. Proc Soc Exp Biol Med 1974;146:605–7.
178. Izzo P, Costanzo P, Lupo A, et al. A new human species of aldolase A mRNA from fibroblasts. Eur J Biochem 1987;164:9–13.
179. Gliksman R, Ghosh NR, Cox RP. Comparison of aldolase Iisozymes in placenta, HeLa cells, and human fibroblast cultures. Enzyme 1977;22:416–19.
180. Shin YS, Rimbock H, Endres W. Fructose-1-phosphate aldolase activity in human fetal and adult tissues as well as leukocytes and cultured fibroblasts in hereditary fructose intolerance. J Inherit Metab Dis 1982;5 Suppl:45.
181. Anderson TA. Recent trends in carbohydrate consumption. Annu Rev Nutr 1982;2:113–32.
182. Yudkin J. Sugar and health. Lancet 1987;i:918.
183. Gitzelmann R, Steinmann B, Van den Berghe G. Disorders of fructose metabolism. In: Stanbury JB, Wyngaarden JB, Fredrickson DS, eds. The metabolic basis of inherited disease. 6th ed. New York: McGraw-Hill, 1989:399–424.
184. Mock DM, Perman JA, Thaler MM, et al. Chronic fructose intoxication after infancy in children with hereditary fructose intolerance: a cause of growth retardation. N Engl J Med 1983;309:764–70.
185. Shallenberger RS. Occurrence of various sugars in foods. In: Sipple HL, McNutt KW, eds. Sugars in nutrition. New York: Academic Press, 1974:67–80.
186. Hardinge MG, Swarner JB, Crooks H. Carbohydrates in foods. J Am Diet Assoc 1965;46:197–204.
187. Somogyi JC, Trautner K. Der Glukose-, Fructose- und Saccharosegehalt verschiedener Gemusearten. Schweiz Med Wochenschr 1974;104:177–82.
188. Wyke RJ, Rajkovic IA, Eddleston AL, et al. Defective opsonization and complement deficiency in serum from patients with fulminant hepatic failure. Gut 1980;21:643–9.
189. Brauman J, Kentos P, Frisque P, et al. Intolerance hereditaire au fructose chez une femme de 83 ans. Acta Clin Belg 1971;26: 65–77.
190. Gitzelmann R, Steinmann B, Muller-Wiefel DE, et al. Infusionslosungen. Dtsch Med Wochenschr 1983;108:1656.
191. Nordlie RC. Fine tuning of blood glucose concentrations. Trends Biochem Sci 1985;10:70–5.
192. Arion WJ, Lange AJ, Walls HE, et al. Evidence for the participation of independent translocation for phosphate and glucose-6-phosphate in the microsomal glucose-6-phosphatase system: interactions of the system with orthophosphate, inorganic pyrophosphate, and carbonyl phosphate. J Biol Chem 1980;255:10396–406.
193. Burchell A. Molecular pathology of glucose-6-phosphatase. FASEB J 1990;4:2978–88.
194. Schulze HU, Nolte B, Kannler R. Evidence for changes in the conformational status of rat liver microsomal glucose-6-phosphate: phosphohydrolase during detergent-dependent membrane modification. Effect of p-mercuribenzoate and organomercurial agarose gel on glucose-6-phosphatase of native and detergent-modified microsomes. J Biol Chem 1986; 261:16571–8.
195. Hers HG. The control of glycogen metabolism in the liver. Ann Rev Biochem 1976;45:167–89.
196. von Gierke E. Hepato-nephromegalia glykogenica (Glykogenspeicherkrankheit der Leber und Nieren). Beitr Pathol Anat 1929;82:497–513.
197. Cori GT, Cori CF. Glucose-6-phosphatase of the liver in glycogen storage disease. J Biol Chem 1952;199:661–7.
198. Cori GT. Glycogen structure and enzyme deficiencies in glycogen storage disease. Harvey Lect 1953;48:145–71.
199. Burchell A, Jung RT, Lang CC, et al. Diagnosis of type Ia and Ic glycogen storage diseases in adults. Lancet 1987;i:1059–62.
200. Waddell ID, Lindsay JD, Burchell A. The identification of T_2: the phosphate/pyrophosphate transport protein of the hepatic microsomal glucose-6-phosphatase system. FEBS Lett 1988;229:179–82.
201. Burchell A, Waddell ID, Stewart L, et al. Perinatal diagnosis of Type Ic glycogen storage disease. J Inherit Metab Dis 1989;12:315–17.
202. Nordlie RC, Sukalski K, Munoz JM, et al. Type Ic, a novel glycogenosis. J Biol Chem 1983;258:9139–744.
203. Waddell ID, Burchell A. The microsomal glucose-6-phosphatase enzyme of pancreatic islets. Biochem J 1988;255: 471–6.
204. Veiga-da-Cunha M, Gerin I, Chen YT, et al. The putative glucose 6-phosphate translocase gene is mutated in essentially all cases of glycogen storage disease type I non-a. Eur J Hum Genet 1999;7:717–23.
205. Brody LC, Abel KJ, Castilla LH, et al. Construction of a transcription map surrounding the BRCA1 locus of human chromosome 17. Genomics 1995;25:238–47.
206. Lei KJ, Shelly LL, Pan CJ, et al. Mutations in the glucose-6-phosphatase gene that cause glycogen storage disease type 1a. Science 1993;262:580–3.
207. Lei KJ, Pan CJ, Shelly LL, et al. Identification of mutations in the gene for glucose-6-phosphatase, the enzyme deficient in glycogen storage disease type 1a. J Clin Invest 1994;93:1994–9.
208. Pan CF, Lei KJ, Annabi B, et al. Transmembrane topology of glucose-6-phosphatase. J Biol Chem 1998;273:6144–8.
209. Stroppiano M, Regis S, DiRocco M, et al. Mutations in the glucose-6-phosphatase gene of 53 Italian patients with glycogen storage disease type Ia. J Inherit Metab Dis 1999;22: 43–9.
210. Hiraiwa H, Pan CJ, Lin B, et al. Inactivation of the glucose 6-phosphate transporter causes glycogen storage disease type 1b. J Biol Chem 1999;274:5532–6.

211. Hershkovitz E, Mandel H, Fryman M, et al. The gene for glycogen-storage disease type 1b maps to chromosome 11q23. Am J Hum Genet 1998;62:400–5.
212. Gerin I, Veiga-de-Cunha M, Achouri Y, et al. Sequence of a putative glucose 6-phosphate translocase, mutated in glycogen storage disease type 1b. FEBS Lett 1997;419:235–8.
213. Hers H, Van Hoof F, de Barsy T. glycogen storage disease. In: Stanbury JB, Wyngaarden JB, Frederickson DS, eds. The metabolic basis of inherited disease. 6th ed. New York: McGraw-Hill, 1989:425–52.
214. Ghishan FK, Greene HL. Inborn errors of metabolism that cause permanent injury to the liver. In: Zakim D, Boyer T, eds. Hepatology: a textbook of liver disease. 2nd ed. Philadelphia: WB Saunders, 1990:49:1300–48.
215. Fernandes J, Berger R, Smit GPA. Lactate as a cerebral metabolic fuel for glucose-6-phosphatase deficient children. Pediatr Res 1984;18:335–9.
216. Howell RR, Stevenson RE, Ben-Menachen Y, et al. Hepatic adenomata with type I glycogen storage disease. JAMA 1976;236: 1481–4.
217. Coire CI, Qizilbash AH, Castelli MF. Hepatic adenomata in type Ia glycogen storage disease. Arch Pathol Lab Med 1987;111:166–9.
218. Levine G, Mierau G, Favara BE. Hepatic glycogenosis, renal glomerular cysts and hepatocarcinoma. Am J Pathol 1976;82: PPC 37.
219. Chen Y-T, Coleman RA, Sheinman JI, et al. Renal disease in type I glycogen storage disease. N Engl J Med 1988;318: 7–11.
220. Slonim AE, Lacy WW, Terry AB, et al. Nocturnal intragastric therapy in type I glycogen storage disease: effect on hormonal and amino acid metabolism. Metabolism 1979;28:707–2.
221. Sadeghi-Nejad A, Presente E, Binkiewicz A, et al. Studies in Type I glycogenosis of the liver: the genesis and deposition of lactate. J Pediatr 1974;85:49–55.
222. Fine RN, Strauss J, Connel GN. Hyperuricemia in glycogen storage disease, type I. Am J Dis Child 1966;1125:572–5.
223. Howell RR. The interrelationship of glycogen storage disease and gout. Arthritis Rheum 1965;8:780–4.
224. Howell RR, Ashton DM, Wyngaarden JB. Glucose-6-phosphatase deficiency glycogen storage disease: studies on the interrelationships of carbohydrates, lipid and purine abnormalities. Pediatrics 1962;29:553–9.
225. Howell RR. Hyperuricemia in childhood. Fed Proc 1968; 27:1078–84.
226. Greene HL, Wilson FA, Hefferan S, et al. ATP depletion, a possible role in the pathogenesis of hyperuricemia in glycogen storage disease, type I. J Clin Invest 1978;62:321–8.
227. Corby DG, Putnam CW, Greene HL. Impaired platelet function in glucose-6-phosphate deficiency. J Pediatr 1974;85: 71–6.
228. Hutton RA, Macnab AJ, Rivers PA. Defects of platelet function associated with chronic hypoglycemia. Arch Dis Child 1976;51:49–55.
229. Bashan N, Hagai R, Potashnik R, et al. Impaired carbohydrate metabolism of polymorphonuclear leukocytes in glycogen storage disease, Ib. J Clin Invest 1988;81:1317–22.
230. McCawley LJ, Korchak HM, Douglas SD, et al. In vitro and in vivo effects of granulocyte colony-stimulating factor on neutrophils in glycogen storage disease type 1B: granulocyte colony-stimulating factor therapy corrects the neutropenia and the defects in respiratory burst activity and $Ca2^{+}$ mobilization. Pediatr Res 1994;35:84–90.
231. Parker PH, Burr I, Slonim AE, et al. Regression of hepatic adenomas in type Ia glycogen storage disease with dietary therapy. Gastroenterology 1987;81:534–6.
232. Limmer J, Feig WE, Leupold D, et al. Hepatocellular carcinoma in type I glycogen storage disease. Hepatology 1988;8:531–7.
233. Edelstein G, Hirschman CA. Hyperthermia and ketoacidosis during anesthesia in a child with glycogen storage disease. Anesthesiology 1980;52:90–2.
234. Schwartz R, Ashmore J, Renold AE. Galactose tolerance in glycogen storage disease. Pediatrics 1957;19:585–94.
235. Fernandes J, Huijing F, Van de Kamer JH. A screening method for liver glycogen diseases. Arch Dis Child 1969;44:311–17.
236. Folkman J, Philippart A, Tze WJ, et al. Portacaval shunt for glycogen storage disease: value of prolonged intravenous hyperalimentation before surgery. Surgery 1972;72:306–14.
237. Boley SJ, Cohen MI, Gliedman ML. Surgical therapy of glycogen storage disease. Pediatrics 1970;46:929–32.
238. Starzl TE, Putnam CW, Porter KA, et al. Portal diversion for the treatment of glycogen storage disease in humans. Ann Surg 1973;178:525–39.
239. Borowitz SM, Greene HL, Gay JC, et al. Case report: Comparison of dietary therapy and portacaval shunt in the management of a patient with type Ib glycogen storage disease. J Pediatr Gastroenterol Nutr 1987;6:635–9.
240. Greene HL, Slonim AE, O'Neil Jr JA, et al. Continuous nocturnal intragastric feeding for management of type I glycogen-storage disease. N Engl J Med 1976;294:423–5.
241. Schwenk WF, Haymond MW. Optimal rate of enteral glucose administration in children with glycogen storage disease type I. N Engl J Med 1986;314:682–5.
242. Chen Y-T, Cornblath M, Sidbury JB. Cornstarch therapy in type I glycogen storage disease. N Engl J Med 1984;310:171–5.
243. Moses SW. Pathophysiology and dietary treatment of the glycogen storage diseases. J Pediatr Gastroenterol Nutr 1990;11: 155–74.
244. Folk CC, Greene HL. Dietary management of type Ia glycogen storage disease. J Am Diet Assoc 1984;84:293–301.
245. Fernandes J, Leonard JV, Moses SW, et al. glycogen storage disease: recommendations for treatment. Eur J Pediatr 1988; 147:226–8.
246. Emmett M, Narins RG. Renal transplantation in type I glycogenosis: failure to improve glucose metabolism. JAMA 1978;239:1642–6.
247. Matern D, Seydewitz HH, Bali D, et al. Glycogen storage disease type I: diagnosis and phenotype/genotype correlation. Eur J Pediatr 2002;161 Suppl 1:S10–19.
248. Rake JP, Visser G, Labrune P, et al. Glycogen storage disease type I: diagnosis, management, clinical course and outcome. Results of the European Study on Glycogen Storage Disease Type I (ESGSD I). Eur J Pediatr 2002;161 Suppl 1: S20–34.
249. Faivre L, Houssin D, Valayer J, et al. Long-term outcome of liver transplantation in patients with glycogen storage disease type Ia. J Inherit Metab Dis 1999;22:723–32.
250. Matern D, Starzl TE, Arnaout W, et al. Liver transplantation for glycogen storage disease types I, III, and IV. Eur J Pediatr 1999;158 Suppl 2:S43–8.
251. Panaro F, Andorno E, Basile G, et al. Simultaneous liver-kidney transplantation for glycogen storage disease type IA (von Gierke's disease). Transplant Proc 2004;36:1483–4.

252. Malatack JJ, Finegold DN, Iwatsuki S, et al. Liver transplantation in type I glycogen storage disease. Lancet 1983;i:1073–4.
253. Anderson DC, Mace ML, Brinkley BR, et al. Recurrent infection in glycogenosis Type IB: abnormal neutrophil motility related to impaired redistribution of adhesion sites. J Infect Dis 1981;143:447–59.
254. Beaudet AL, Anderson DC, Michels VV, et al. Neutropenia and impaired neutrophil migration in type IB glycogen storage disease. J Pediatr 1980;97:906–10.
255. Seger R, Steinmann B, Tiefenauer L, et al. Glycogenosis Ib: neutrophil microbicidal defects due to impaired hexose monophosphate shunt. Pediatr Res 1984;18:297–9.
256. Arion WJ, Wallin BK, Lange AJ. On the involvement of a glucose-6-phosphate transport system in the function of microsomal glucose-6-phosphatase. Mol Cell Biochem 1975;6:75–83.
257. Ambruso DR, McCabe ERB, Anderson D, et al. Infectious and bleeding complications in patients with glycogenosis Ib. Am J Dis Child 1985;139:691–7.
258. Greene HL, Slonim AE, Burr IM. Type I glycogen storage disease: a metabolic basis for advances in treatment. Adv Pediatr 1979;26:63–92.
259. Kalhan SC, Gilfillan C, Tserng KY, et al. Glucose production in type I glycogen storage disease. J Pediatr 1982;101:159–60.
260. Sidbury JB. The genetics of the glycogen storage diseases. Prog Med Genet 1965;4:32–58.
261. Farber M, Knuppel RA, Binkiewicz A, et al. Pregnancy and von Gierke's disease. Obstet Gynecol 1976;47:226–8.
262. Michels VV, Beaudet AL. Hemorrhagic pancreatitis in a patient with glycogen storage disease type I. Clin Genet 1980;17:220–2.
263. Hug G. Glycogen storage diseases. Birth Defects 1976;12:145–75.
264. Howell RR. The glycogen storage diseases. In: Stanbury JB, Wyngaarden JB, Fredrickson DS, eds. The metabolic basis of inherited disease. 4th ed. New York: McGraw-Hill, 1978:137–59.
265. Senior B, Sadeghi-Nejad A. The glycogenoses and other inherited disorders of carbohydrate metabolism. Clin Perinatol 1976;3:79–98.
266. Coleman JE. Metabolic interrelationships between carbohydrates, lipids, and proteins. In: Bondy PK, Rosenberg LE, eds. Diseases of metabolism. 7th ed. Philadelphia: WB Saunders, 1974:107–220.
267. Greene HL, Slonim AE, Burr IM, et al. Type I glycogen storage disease: five years of management with nocturnal intragastric feeding. J Pediatr 1980;96:590–5.
268. Forbes GB. Glycogen storage disease: report of a case with abnormal glycogen structure in liver and skeletal muscle. J Pediatr 1953;42:645–53.
269. Illingworth B, Cori GT. Structure of glycogens and amylopectins: III. Normal and abnormal human glycogen. J Biol Chem 1952;199:653–60.
270. Illingworth B, Cori GT, Cori CF. Amylo-1,6-glucosidase in muscle tissue in generalized glycogen storage disease. J Biol Chem 1956;218:123–9.
271. Bates EJ, Heaton GM, Taylor C, et al. Debranching enzyme from rabbit skeletal muscle: evidence for the location of two active centres on a single polypeptide chain. FEBS Lett 1975;58:181–5.
272. Gillard BK, Nelson TE. Amylo-1,6-glucosidase/4-β-glucanotransferase: use of reversible substrate model inhibitors to study the binding and active sites of rabbit muscle debranching enzyme. Biochemistry 1977;16:3978–87.
273. Chen Y-T, He J-K, Ding J-H, et al. Glycogen debranching enzyme: purification, antibody characterization, and immunoblot analyses of type III glycogen storage disease. Am J Hum Genet 1987;41:1002–15.
274. van Hoof F, Hers HG. The subgroups of type III glycogenosis. Eur J Biochem 1967;2:265–70.
275. Ding J-H, de Barsy T, Brown BI, et al. Immunoblot analyses of glycogen debranching enzyme in different subtypes of glycogen storage disease type III. J Pediatr 1990;116:95–100.
276. Brown BI. Diagnosis of glycogen storage disease. In: Wanir RA, ed. Congenital metabolic diseases. Basel: Dekker, 1985:227–50.
277. Bao Y, Dawson TL Jr, Chen YT. Human glycogen debranching enzyme gene (AGL): complete structural organization and characterization of the 5' flanking region. Genomics 1996;38:155–65.
278. Yang-Feng TL, Zheng K, Yu J, et al. Assignment of the human glycogen debrancher gene to chromosome 1p21. Genomics 1992;13:931–4.
279. Bao Y, Yang BZ, Dawson TL, et al. Isolation and nucleotide sequence of human liver glycogen debranching enzyme mRNA: identification of multiple tissue-specific isoforms. Gene 1997;197:389–98.
280. Okubo M, Kanda F, Horinishi A, et al. Glycogen storage disease type IIIa: first report of a causative missense mutation (G1448R) of the glycogen debranching enzyme gene found in a homozygous patient. Hum Mutat 1999;14:542–3.
281. Shen J, Bao Y, Liu HM, et al. Mutations in exon 3 of the glycogen debranching enzyme gene are associated with glycogen storage disease type III that is differentially expressed in liver and muscle. J Clin Invest 1996;98:352–7.
282. Levin S, Moses Sw, Chayoth R, et al. Glycogen storage disease in Israel: a clinical, biochemical and genetic study. Isr J Med Sci 1967;3:397–410.
283. Brandt IK, DeLuca VA Jr. Type III glycogenosis: a family with an unusual tissue distribution of the enzyme lesion. Am J Med 1966;40:779–84.
284. Brown B, Brown DH. The glycogen storage diseases: types I, III, IV, V, VII, and unclassified glycogenoses. In: Dickens F, Randle PJ, Whelan WJ, ed. Carbohydrate metabolism and its disorders. New York: Academic Press, 1968:123–50.
285. Murase T, Ikeda H, Muro T, et al. Myopathy associated with Type III glycogenosis. J Neurol Sci 1973;20:287–95.
286. van Creveld S, Huijing F. Glycogen storage disease: biochemical and clinical data in sixteen cases. Am J Med 1965;38:554–61.
287. Ugawa Y, Inoue K, Takemura T, et al. Accumulation of glycogen in peripheral nerve axons in adult-onset type III glycogenosis. Ann Neurol 1986;19:294–7.
288. Miller CG, Alleyne GA, Brooks SEH. Case report: gross cardiac involvement in glycogen storage disease type III. Br Heart J 1972;34:862–4.
289. Bost M. La myocardiopathie de la glycogenose type III. Arch Fr Pediatr 1979;36:303–9.
290. Alagille D, Odievre M. Inborn errors of metabolism. In: Alagille D, Odievre M, eds. Liver and biliary tract disease in children. New York: John Wiley, 1979:196–242.
291. Hug G, Krill CE Jr, Perrin EV, et al. Cori's disease (amylo-1,6-glucosidase deficiency): report of a case in a Negro child. N Engl J Med 1963;268:113–20.
292. Borowitz SM, Greene HL. Case report: cornstarch therapy in a patient with type III glycogen storage disease. J Pediatr Gastroenterol Nutr 1987;6:631–4.

293. Slonim AE, Terry AB, Moran R, et al. Differing food consumption for nocturnal intragastric therapy in Types I and III glycogen storage disease. Pediatr Res 1978;12:512.
294. Andersen DH. Familial cirrhosis of the liver with storage of abnormal glycogen. Lab Invest 1956;5:11–20.
295. Brown BI, Brown DH. Lack of an α-1,4-glucan: α-1,4-glucan 6-glycosyl transferase in a case of type IV glycogenosis. Proc Natl Acad Sci U S A 1966;56:725–9.
296. Fernandes J, Huijing F. Branching enzyme-deficiency glycogenosis: studies in therapy. Arch Dis Child 1968;43:347–52.
297. Thon VJ, Khalil M, Cannon JF. Isolation of human glycogen branching enzyme cDNAs by screening complementation in yeast. J Biol Chem 1993;268:7509–13.
298. Bao Y, Kishnani P, Wu J-Y, et al. Hepatic and neuromuscular forms of glycogen storage disease type IV caused by mutations in the same glycogen-branching enzyme gene. J Clin Invest 1996;97:941–8.
299. Shen J, Liu HM, McConkie-Rosell A, et al. Prenatal diagnosis of glycogen storage disease type IV using PCR-based DNA mutation analysis. Prenat Diagn 1999;9:837–9.
300. Maruyama K, Suzuki T, Koizumi T, et al. Congenital form of glycogen storage disease type IV: a case report and a review of the literature. Pediatr Int 2004;46:474–7.
301. Ishihara T, Uchino F, Adachi H. Type IV glycogenosis: a study of two cases. Acta Pathol Jpn 1975;25:613–33.
302. McMaster KR, Powers JM, Hennigar GR Jr, et al. Nervous system involvement in type IV glycogenosis. Arch Pathol Lab Med 1979;103:105–11.
303. Schochet SS, McCormick WF, Zellweger H. Type IV glycogenosis (amylopectinosis): light and electron microscopic observations. Arch Pathol 1970;90:354–63.
304. Howell RR, Kaback MM, Brown BI. Type IV glycogen storage disease: branching enzyme deficiency in skin fibroblasts and possible heterozygote detection. J Pediatr 1971;78:638–42.
305. Ferguson IT, Mahon M, Cumming WJK. An adult case of Andersen's disease: type IV glycogenosis. J Neurol Sci 1983;60:337–51.
306. Holmes JM, Houghton CR, Woolf AL. A myopathy presenting in adult life with features suggestive of glycogen storage disease. J Neurol Neurosurg Psychiatr 1960;23:302–11.
307. Torvik A, Dietrichson P, Svaar H, et al. Myopathy with tremor and dementia: a metabolic disorder? Case report with post mortem study. J Neurol Sci 1974;21:181–90.
308. de La Blanchardiere A, Vayssier C, Duboc D, et al. Severe cardiomyopathy revealing amylopectinosis. Two cases in adolescents from the same family. Presse Med 1994;23:1124–7.
309. Das BB, Narkevicz MR, Sokol RJ, et al. Amylopectinosis disease isolated to the heart with normal glycogen branching enzyme activity and gene sequence. Pediatr Transplant 2005;9:261–5.
310. Lossos A, Barash V, Soffer Z, et al. Hereditary branching enzyme dysfunction in adult polyglucosan body disease: a possible metabolic cause in two patients. Ann Neurol 1991;30:655–62.
311. Bruno C, Servidei S, Shanske G, et al. Glycogen branching enzyme deficiency in adult polyglucosan body disease. Ann Neurol 1993;33:88–93.
312. Greene HL, Ghishan FK, Brown B, et al. Hypoglycemia in type IV glycogenosis: hepatic improvement in two patients with nutritional management. J Pediatr 1988;112:55–8.
313. Reed GB Jr, Dixon JFP, Neustein HB, et al. Type IV glycogenosis: patient with absence of a branching enzyme α-1,4-glucan: α-1,4-glucan 6-glycosyl transferase. Lab Invest 1968;19:546–57.
314. Levin B, Burgess EA, Mortimer PE. Glycogen storage disease type IV, amylopectinosis. Arch Dis Child 1968;43:548–55.
315. Holleman LWJ, van der Haar JA, de Vann GAM. Type IV glycogenosis. Lab Invest 1966;15:357–67.
316. Motoi M, Sonobe H, Ogawa K. Two autopsy cases of glycogen storage disease: cirrhotic type. Acta Pathol Jpn 1973;23:211–23.
317. Brass K. Zur histologischen Diagnose der glykogenose Type IV (Amylopektinose). Z Kinderheilkd 1974;117:187–203.
318. Servidei S, Riepe RE, Langston C, et al. Severe cardiopathy in branching enzyme deficiency. J Pediatr 1987;111:51–6.
319. Greene HL, Brown BI, McClenathan DT, et al. A new variant of type IV glycogenosis: deficiency of branching enzyme activity without apparent progressive liver disease. Hepatology 1988;8:302–6.

26

Copper Metabolism and Copper Storage Disorders

Judith A. O'Connor, M.D., and Ronald J. Sokol, M.D.

The accumulation of excess copper in the liver is toxic in humans and other mammals and may lead to hepatitis, fulminant hepatic failure, cirrhosis, and death. Of the several human copper storage diseases that have been described, the molecular basis of only Wilson's disease is understood, with the discovery of the Wilson's disease gene (*ATP7B*) in 1993. The therapeutic success using oral copper chelating agents and zinc therapy makes Wilson's disease one of the few treatable metabolic liver diseases. In cases with a fulminant presentation or advanced disease at diagnosis, copper chelation is ineffective and liver transplantation is lifesaving. Indian childhood cirrhosis (ICC) has been defined as a copper storage disorder affecting children primarily of Indian descent and evolving to cirrhosis and death before age 3–4 years without treatment. Children from North America, Asia, Austria, Germany, and other countries have been described with a similar condition, which has been termed *idiopathic copper toxicosis* (ICT). In this chapter, copper physiology and mechanisms of copper hepatotoxicity are reviewed, followed by descriptions of the major copper storage diseases of childhood.

COPPER ABSORPTION AND METABOLISM

The normal adult Western diet contains 2–5 mg/d of copper. The efficiency of copper absorption in adults ranges from 55–75% [1], with higher absorption at lower intakes [1,2] (Figure 26.1). Foods containing high amounts of copper include unprocessed wheat, dried beans, peas, shellfish (particularly oysters), chocolate, liver, and kidney. The estimated daily copper requirement for adults is approximately 1.3–1.7 mg [3]. Dietary and chemical factors may impair copper absorption. For example, excess intake of zinc [4], cadmium [4], and ascorbic acid [5] can interfere with copper bioavailability because of the formation of insoluble copper salts at an alkaline pH [6]. A vegetarian diet, as well as ingested raw meat, has been associated with decreased copper absorption [7–9]. Gastrointestinal secretions (e.g., saliva, gastric juice, duodenal secretions) form low molecular weight soluble complexes that aid in the absorption of copper by preventing the precipitation of copper salts [5,6], and certain digestive products (e.g., L-amino acids) facilitate copper absorption [7,8]. It is the balance between these exogenous and endogenous factors that regulate intestinal absorption of copper. Because dietary intake and absorption generally exceed metabolic needs, a large amount of ingested copper is eventually excreted in bile (see below).

Within the small intestine epithelial cells, absorbed copper is either bound to the protein metallothionein or complexed to amino acids and transported into the portal venous circulation. Although enterocyte metallothionein also binds zinc and cadmium, copper is bound most avidly. Because zinc stimulates metallothionein synthesis, it has been postulated that increased dietary zinc may impair copper absorption by causing retention of copper in the enterocyte, which is then excreted in the feces following desquamation of the enterocyte. This proposed mechanism forms the basis for trials of oral zinc therapy in Wilson's disease (see below).

Once absorbed into the portal venous blood, copper is complexed to albumin and amino acids in equilibrium with a very small fraction of free ionic copper. Copper is then transported into hepatocytes by a specific membrane transport system for albumin-bound copper by hCTR (human copper transporter) [10–17] (Figure 26.2). Among the amino acids present in blood, the binding affinities for copper in decreasing order are histidine, threonine, glutamine, and asparagine [9]. This amino acid–bound copper is most likely the form in which copper is transported to various tissues other than the liver [10,11]. Within 3 hours of absorption, 60–90% of copper has been transported to and taken up by hepatocytes [18–20], where copper initially interacts with low molecular weight ligands, such as cytosolic metallothionein, glutathione, and HAH1 [15]. The function of these proteins is to store copper for subsequent metabolic needs of the hepatocyte, to bind and detoxify excess copper, and to provide copper to chaperones that assist in incorporating it into essential proteins that are secreted (as in ceruloplasmin) or assist in copper excretion in bile (*ATP7B*). Important hepatic copper metalloenzymes include superoxide dismutase (molecular weight [MW], 32,000 daltons), mitochondrial monoamine oxidase (MW, 195,000 daltons), cytochrome C oxidase (MW,

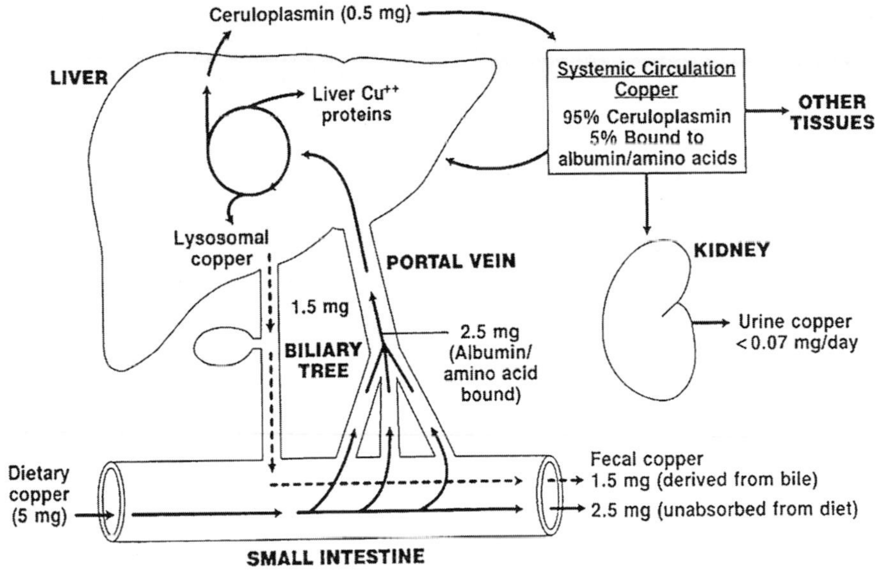

Figure 26.1. Copper balance in humans. Relative amounts of copper arising from 5 mg of daily dietary intake in an adult. (Adapted from Sokol RJ. Copper storage diseases. In: Kaplowitz N, ed. Liver and biliary diseases. Baltimore: Williams & Wilkins, 1992:322–33.)

290,000 daltons), and ceruloplasmin. In other tissues, copper is incorporated into tyrosinase and lysyl oxidase.

The *ATP7B* gene (80 kilobases [kb]) is located on chromosome 13, contains 21 exons, and is highly expressed in liver and kidney, with lower levels of expression in lung, placenta, and other tissues. Splicing variants of the gene may be present in brain. The encoded protein, ATP7B, is a P-type cation-transporting adenosine triphosphatase (ATPase), homologous to the Menkes' disease gene product and the copper transporting ATPase (copA) in copper-resistant *enterococcus hirae.* The protein structure (Figure 26.3) includes domains for copper binding (six sites), adenosine triphosphate (ATP)-binding, a phosphorylation region, a transmembrane cation channel, and a transduction domain. Within one membrane-spanning domain is a sequence of amino acids (cysteine-proline-cysteine) that is characteristic of all metal-transporting ATPases. *ATP7B* is located in the trans-Golgi complex of the hepatocyte and appears necessary for transport of copper into vesicles bound for lysosomes and eventual excretion into the bile canaliculus (Figure 26.2). *ATP7B* also makes copper available for the synthesis of ceruloplasmin, possibly within the Golgi apparatus as

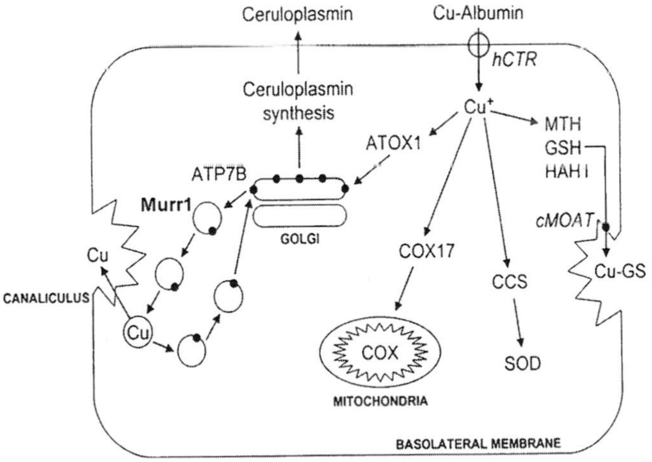

Figure 26.2. Copper metabolism in the hepatocyte. MTH, metallothionein; SOD, superoxide dismutase; COX, cytochrome *c* oxidase; GSH, glutathione; cMOAT, canalicular multiple organic anion transporter (MRP2). (Adapted from Bacon BR, Schilsky ML. New knowledge of genetic pathogenesis of hemochromatosis and Wilson's disease. Adv Intern Med 1999;44:91–116.)

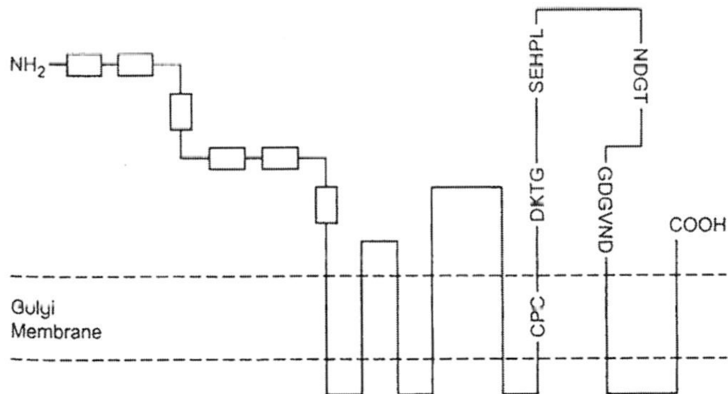

Figure 26.3. Structural features of *ATP7B*, the Wilson's disease gene, include six cysteine-rich metal-binding regions (*open boxes*) near the amino terminus in the cytosol of the cell; eight transmembrane domains, one of which includes the cysteine–proline–cysteine (CPC) sequence common to other metal transporters; the DKTG phosphatase and phosphorylation domain; the TGDN ATP-binding domain; and the hinge region (GDGVND). (Adapted from Bacon BR, Schilsky ML. New knowledge of genetic pathogenesis of hemochromatosis and Wilson's disease. Adv Intern Med 1999;44:91–116; and Petrukhin K, Lutsenko S, Chernov I, et al. Characterization of the Wilson disease gene encoding a P-type copper transporting ATPase: genomic organization, alternative splicing, and structure/function predictions. Hum Mol Genet 1994;3:1647–56.)

well. When *ATP7B* is mutated in Wilson's disease, both copper secretion into bile and copper incorporation into ceruloplasmin are impaired, resulting in copper accumulation within the hepatocyte.

It is now clear that metallochaperones play an essential role in copper homeostasis in mammalian (and yeast) cells. These proteins control delivery of copper to specific intracellular targets, in which copper is incorporated into synthesis of critical enzymes and proteins [21]. Three mammalian copper chaperones (Figure 26.2) have been well characterized, including human CCS (homologous to yeast Lys7p), which delivers copper to copper/zinc superoxide dismutase (SOD) in cytosol [22–24]; human COX17 (homologous to yeast Cox17p), which delivers copper to cytochrome *c* oxidase in mitochondria [25]; and human ATOX1/HAH1 (homologous to yeast Atx1p), which delivers copper to the secretory pathway for incorporation into the copper transport protein *ATP7B* (homologous to yeast Ccc2p) in the Golgi compartment [26]. Atx1p has also been found to function as an antioxidant.

Ceruloplasmin, a blue-colored copper-containing α_2-globulin (MW, 134,000 daltons) is secreted from the liver into the systemic circulation [27,28]. One of the major roles of ceruloplasmin is to promote iron mobilization from tissues by oxidizing ferrous iron for transfer into transferrin. Patients homozygous for mutations in the ceruloplasmin gene develop iron overload in the liver, pancreas, and brain [29,30]. Ceruloplasmin may also transport copper to other tissues [30] as an oxidase toward aromatic amines (e.g., epinephrine, 5-hydroxytryptamine, and dopamine) [31], phenols, cystine, ferrous ion [30], and ascorbic acid, or as an antioxidant [32,33]. The normal plasma concentration of ceruloplasmin in older children and adults, measured by the oxidase enzymatic assay, is between 20 and 45 mg/dL, and the normal plasma concentration of copper is between 70 and 150 μg/dL. In the human newborn, ceruloplasmin levels are 1.8–13.1 mg/dL and copper levels vary between 12 and 26 μg/dL [34], increasing to adult levels by age 2 years. This is in contrast to the parturient mother, whose levels are 40–89 mg/dL and 118–302 μg/dL, respectively [34]. Non–ceruloplasmin-bound copper does not differ between newborn and mother and ranges between 5 and 15 μg/dL [32]. It should be noted that the classic assays for ceruloplasmin were based on its oxidase activity in vitro, hence they depended on the presence of copper in the molecule [30,35]. More recent immunoassays detect apoceruloplasmin (which does not contain copper) as well as holoceruloplasmin (which contains copper), and may thus give higher serum values of ceruloplasmin in Wilson's disease patients than does the oxidase method, which only detects holoceruloplasmin [35]. This may affect the predictive value of ceruloplasmin levels in diagnosing Wilson's disease.

More than 80% of absorbed copper is excreted in bile (Figure 26.1), totaling approximately 1.2–1.7 mg/d [36,37]. Exocytosis of lysosomal copper across the canalicular membrane is the major source of biliary copper, which is then complexed to large proteins (e.g., metallothionein) that prevent reabsorption by the small intestine. Recent identification of a new gene in the Bedlington terrier [38] suggests that the gene product, MURR1, is required for vesicular copper (*ATP7B*) movement and excretion (Figure 26.2). The human *MURR1* has been mapped to chromosome region 2p13-16 [39]. Human *MURR1* has been excluded as the gene causing non–Wilson's disease hepatic copper toxicosis syndromes [39]. This protein has recently been shown to interact with the copper-binding N-terminus of *ATP7B*, providing biochemical evidence in support of the proposed role of the MURR1 gene product in hepatic copper toxicosis [40]. An initial report identified polymorphisms in *MURR1* in 19 of 63 Wilson's disease patients [41]. Fifteen patients with early-onset Wilson's had the same base pair change at Asn 164, suggesting that the timing of disease onset could potentially be influenced by polymorphisms in this gene [41]. These provocative findings suggest that genetic modifiers may be important in the phenotypic expression of Wilson's disease.

Metallothionein-bound copper does not account for all of biliary copper. An additional pathway for copper secretion into bile may involve glutathione-conjugated copper secreted into the canaliculus by cMOAT (MRP2), the canalicular multiorganic ion transporter (Figure 26.2). There is minimal enterohepatic circulation of copper. Urine, sweat, and menstrual blood are minor pathways for copper excretion. Urine copper (<100 μg/d) is neither indicative of dietary intake nor is it important in copper homeostasis under normal circumstances. Pathologic processes that interfere with biliary excretion of copper, such as intrahepatic and extrahepatic hepatobiliary cholestatic disorders, produce copper retention in the liver, generally in the lysosomal fraction of hepatocytes, and are associated with elevated plasma copper and ceruloplasmin levels. In fact, hepatic concentrations of copper in intrahepatic cholestatic disorders of childhood [42] and primary biliary cirrhosis in adults [43] may exceed levels found in Wilson's disease. Whether or not excess hepatic copper in cholestasis is hepatotoxic is under debate.

The organ distribution of the 80–100 mg of copper in an adult includes 15% in the liver, with brain, heart, and kidneys storing copper in decreasing order [44]. Fifty percent of the body's copper is stored in muscle and bone; however, the concentration is low in these tissues. In fetal liver, copper concentration is several-fold higher than that present in older children and adults [45], most of which is bound to metallothionein in hepatocyte lysosomes [46,47]. During fetal life, the amount of copper present in the liver declines from over 90% of total body copper during early development to approximately 50–60% at birth. After birth, hepatic copper content falls rapidly, reaching adult levels by 3 months of age. Because of delayed maturation of ceruloplasmin synthesis in the infant's liver, plasma levels of both ceruloplasmin and copper remain low during the first 6–12 months of life. Increased blood levels of thyroxine, estrogens, and testosterone [46,47] can increase plasma ceruloplasmin and copper and can make laboratory values difficult to interpret. Insufficiency of corticosteroids decreases biliary copper excretion, resulting in elevated plasma copper and ceruloplasmin levels.

MECHANISMS OF COPPER TOXICITY

High levels of orally or parenterally administered copper accumulate in the liver in most mammalian species. Excess hepatic copper has been shown to cause liver injury in rodents, chickens, ruminants, sheep, Bedlington terriers, and humans [46,47]. Endogenous copper detoxification mechanisms, such as sequestration with metallothionein, export via copper-translocating ATPases, and biliary secretion [48], have allowed certain animal species (e.g., the normal dog [49], Dominican toad [46], and mute swan [46]) to tolerate higher hepatic copper content. The newborn human has the capacity to tolerate 5–100-fold the hepatic copper content of normal adults [50,51]. Hepatic lysosomal sequestration of excess copper is also an effective mechanism to render nontoxic enormous concentrations of intracellular copper [52]. However, in some species, natural accumulation of dietary copper leads to severe liver injury and death, as observed in sheep [53] and the Bedlington terriers [54,55].

The precise intracellular target for the toxic action of copper is uncertain. Many cytosolic enzymes that contain sulfhydryl groups may be inhibited in vitro by copper [46]. Copper inhibits polymerization of tubulin, the chief protein of microtubules, possibly perturbing intracellular trafficking of proteins and mitotic spindle formation [56]. Copper also functions as a pro-oxidant, catalyzing the transformation of hydrogen peroxide to the hydroxyl free radical, which, in turn, may react with and damage polyunsaturated fatty acid residues of cell membranes, thiol-rich proteins, and nucleic acids [57], and may activate intrinsic apoptotic cell death pathways. These effects may lead to disturbances in plasma membrane function, mitochondrial oxidative phosphorylation, nuclear control of cell processes, protein synthesis by endoplasmic reticulum, and leakage of lysosomal enzymes into the cytosol. In addition, by-products of lipid peroxidation, such as malondialdehyde and 4-hydroxynonenal, have been shown to stimulate collagen gene expression in hepatic stellate cells and promote fibrogenesis [58] as well as stimulate nuclear factor κB (NFκB) and cytokine gene expression [59].

There is considerable evidence that oxidative injury is a key factor in copper toxicity. Lipid peroxidation has been documented in both hepatic lysosomes [60] and mitochondria [61] isolated from copper-loaded rats. Moreover, hepatic mitochondria isolated from copper-overloaded rats have abnormal respiration and diminished mitochondrial activity of cytochrome *c* oxidase in conjunction with increased lipid peroxidation [62]. Elevated hepatic mitochondrial copper concentrations in patients with Wilson's disease and copper-overloaded Bedlington terriers have been associated with excessive lipid peroxidation of these organelles [63] and in Wilson's disease patients, with oxidative modification of mitochondrial DNA [64]. Furthermore, the ultrastructurally abnormal mitochondria in hepatocytes of Wilson's disease [65] and ICC [66] patients support the hepatic mitochondrion being one of the target organelles in copper toxicity. Metallothionein has been shown to function as an antioxidant [67], thus it may not only chelate excess copper but may play a role in reducing oxidative stress stimulated by copper. Several studies suggest that hepatocyte apoptosis may be the primary mode of cell death in copper toxicity [68,69], possibly explaining the characteristic mild elevation of serum aminotransferases associated with Wilson's disease. In addition, oxidative modification of mitochondria DNA may result in impaired oxidative phosphorylation and amplification of oxidative stress.

WILSON'S DISEASE (HEPATOLENTICULAR DEGENERATION)

History

In 1912, Kinnear Wilson, an American neurologist, described the degenerative disease of the central nervous system associated with cirrhosis that now bears his name [70]. He proposed the term *progressive lenticular degeneration* for this rare, familial, invariably fatal disease of young people that was characterized by softening of the lenticular nuclei and hepatic cirrhosis. In 1921, Hall [71] further characterized hepatic involvement and introduced the term *hepatolenticular degeneration.* It was not until 1948 that Cumings [72] proposed that copper toxicity caused the tissue injury and suggested the novel use of 2,3-dimercaptopropanol (British antilewisite [BAL]) to increase urinary copper excretion and thus treat the disorder. In 1952, Scheinberg and Gitlin [73] discovered that low circulating ceruloplasmin levels were a practical diagnostic test for the disorder. In 1956, Walshe [74] reported the successful use of the oral copper chelator penicillamine for treatment of this condition, and in 1968, Sternlieb and Scheinberg [75] showed that penicillamine could prevent neurologic and hepatic injury in asymptomatic affected siblings.

Walshe showed in 1982 [76] that triethylene tetramine (trientine) was effective, with less toxicity than penicillamine The role of liver transplantation as a treatment option under certain circumstances has been defined [77]. In the 1990s, the search for the Wilson's disease gene localized the gene to within 13q14-q21 [78,79] on chromosome 13 [80,81]. Using positional cloning techniques in 1993, three groups independently reported the identification of the gene responsible for Wilson's disease, designated *ATP7B* [82–84]. Since this discovery, there has been a burst of activity characterizing not only the Wilson's gene [85] but gene mutations and intracellular copper trafficking [86–89].

Epidemiology

It has long been known that Wilson's disease is transmitted by autosomal recessive inheritance, thus consanguinity is relatively common in affected families. Wilson's disease is ubiquitous, with a worldwide prevalence of approximately 1 in 30,000 and the heterozygote carrier state in approximately 1 in 90 persons [90]. There are certain isolated communities in Japan, Sardinia, and Israel with a higher prevalence [90]. Patients present with a variety of clinical manifestations, including hepatic

Table 26.1: Clinical Presentation in 802 Patients of All Ages with Wilson's Disease

Series	*Patients, No.*	*Hepatic, No. (%)*	*Neuropsychiatric, No. (%)*	*Hematologic, No. (%)*	*Endocrine, No. (%)*	*Asymptomatic, No. (%)*
Walshe [93]	217	101 (47)	90 (42)			28 (13)
Scheinberg and Sternlieb [90]	151	68 (45)	85 (56)	19 (13)	4 (3)	
Saito [158]	140	82 (59)	58 (41)			
Giagheddu et al. [370]	68	30 (40)	23 (34)			15 (22)
Dobyns et al. [371]	53	25 (47)	28 (53)			
Stremmel et al. [111]	51	34 (67)	31 (61)	5 (10)		
Aksoy and Erdem [372]	49	14 (29)	31 (63)			4 (8)
Oder et al. [112]	45	27 (60)	12 (27)			6 (13)
Park et al. [161]	28	12 (43)	10 (36)			6 (21)
Total	802	393 (49)	368 (46)	24 (3)	4 (<1)	59 (7)

presentations common in childhood and a later-onset, predominately neurologic form. Although there are often similarities in the age of onset and clinical findings of Wilson's disease in affected siblings, there may be marked differences in organ system involvement and biochemical findings, suggesting that polygenic or environmental factors may play a role in expression of the disease [90]. The disease has been described as late as the eighth decade of life [91]. Rarely are clinical symptoms present before age 3–4 years, although a 3-year-old with severe liver involvement has been described [92]. Forty to 60% of patients will present with a primary hepatic presentation in the second decade of life [90,93]. The remainder of patients come to clinical attention during the third and fourth decades with a primarily neurologic (34%) or psychiatric (10%) presentation [90,92] (Table 26.1). Other presenting features include hematologic and endocrine abnormalities (e.g., amenorrhea) in 12% and renal symptoms in 1% of patients [90]. All patients have liver involvement, although it may be asymptomatic and well compensated. Although symptoms attributable to Wilson's disease may start in childhood, the diagnosis may not be made for several years or even decades because of a low index of suspicion by the clinician. Not infrequently this delay results in advanced hepatic or neurologic manifestations at the time of diagnosis that could have been prevented.

Genetics

Genetic linkage of Wilson's disease to the locus of the red blood cell esterase D gene indicated that the Wilson's disease gene is on the long arm of chromosome 13 [67,81]. The chromosomal location of the gene was further mapped to a smaller region, 13q14-13q21 [78,79]. The identification of the Menkes' disease gene prompted the search for the Wilson's disease gene. Menkes' disease is a rare autosomal recessive–inherited copper deficiency disorder caused by impaired copper absorption at the intestinal level. Because the Menkes' disease gene, *ATP7A* [94], is a putative cation-transporting P-type ATPase involved in copper transport, the search began for a homologous gene located in the Wilson's disease locus of chromosome 13. In 1993, three groups reported isolation and identification of the gene for Wilson's disease [82–84], designated *ATP7B* (Figure 26.3), with mutations unique to patients with Wilson's disease [83,85]. The database maintained by the University of Alberta lists over 250 distinct mutations identified from patients with Wilson's disease (http://www.medicalgenetics.med.ualberta.ca/wilson/index.php). Most of these are small deletions or missense mutations, the latter requiring confirmation that they are not merely polymorphisms. Missense mutations are associated with a predominance of neurologic symptoms and a later clinical presentation. Deletions and other mutations causing premature stop codons are associated with an earlier clinical presentation predominated by symptoms of liver disease [95]. Specific mutations appear to be more common among certain ethnic groups [95,96]. The most common mutation in descendents from northern Europe, H1069Q, may be present in as many as 40% of cases, whereas in Asian populations, an A778L mutation occurs in 30% of affected individuals. However, over half of all mutations occur rarely in any population. This degree of heterogeneity suggests most affected individuals are compound heterozygotes. Because of the wide variety of mutations, genetic techniques to establish the diagnosis of Wilson's disease have significant limitations. A battery of mutations common to a given ethnic group can be screened; however, the absence of one of these mutations does not exclude the diagnosis. Haplotype analysis (microsatellite markers) may be particularly helpful in evaluating relatives of a known case, in which microsatellite markers are informative [97].

Pathogenesis

Mutations in *ATP7B* cause impaired biliary copper excretion that leads to progressive accumulation of copper in the liver followed by subsequent deposition in other organs, causing the varied clinicopathologic features of Wilson's disease. The initial accumulation of copper in the liver begins in the first few years of life and may be substantial. It has been proposed that there is also failure to clear the high hepatic copper burden that is usually well tolerated in the neonate. By the end of the first or into the second decade of life, the hepatic burden of copper is exceeded, causing release of free copper into the circulation that penetrates other tissues [90]. During this time, hepatic copper may actually decrease in concentration, whereas brain, kidney, and ocular copper increase [90].

The cause of the copper accumulation in the liver and other organs has been intensely studied. Although initial studies suggested increased intestinal absorption of copper [98,99], using more sophisticated methodology, other investigators proved that intestinal absorption of copper was not increased [100,101]. It is clear that mutations in *ATP7B* cause decreased biliary excretion of copper [36,102,103] and defective hepatocyte incorporation of copper into ceruloplasmin. Serum ceruloplasmin levels are low in Wilson's disease because of decreased synthesis of holoceruloplasmin [90] and rapid clearance of apoceruloplasmin; however, the structure of apoceruloplasmin and its saturation with copper are normal. Studies have shown that the rate of transcription of the ceruloplasmin gene is reduced in Wilson's disease [104] with the possibility of a translational or posttranslational defect [105]. However, the ceruloplasmin gene on chromosome 3 is normal in patients with Wilson's disease [106]. Aceruloplasminemia, a congenital deficiency of ceruloplasmin caused by lack of synthesis of apoceruloplasmin due to homozygous mutations in its gene [106], causes iron deposition (not copper) in liver, brain, and spleen; retinal degeneration; diabetes; and dementia [107]. Ceruloplasmin is essential for cellular iron efflux [108], with little apparent role in copper homeostasis. Heterozygotes for Wilson's disease may have low ceruloplasmin levels yet no pathologic accumulation of copper in tissues [90,109]. Conversely, approximately 5–25% of Wilson's disease patients [110] have normal plasma ceruloplasmin levels yet they manifest elevated tissue copper levels and toxicity [90,93,111,112]. The normal ceruloplasmin level results from ceruloplasmin being an acute phase reactant. In addition, circulating apoceruloplasmin may be detected by newer immunologic assays for ceruloplasmin. Intravenous purified ceruloplasmin infusions do not normalize copper metabolism in Wilson's disease patients [113]. Thus, although a useful biomarker for this disease, the impairment in ceruloplasmin synthesis appears to be a result of, rather than the cause of, the disturbance of copper metabolism in Wilson's disease and does not in itself appear related to any of the manifestations of Wilson's disease.

Studies in animal models of Wilson's disease have revealed that mutations in Wilson's disease impair the passage of copper from the hepatocyte into bile. The Long–Evans cinnamon (LEC) rat is an inbred strain of rat with a recessive disorder of copper transport causing hepatotoxicity. Deletions in the rat homolog (*ATP7B*) to the Wilson's disease gene have been described [114]. Studies in the LEC rat show that transport of copper into the vesicular pathway from the Golgi to the canaliculus [115] is abnormal, not delivery of lysosomal copper to bile as previously thought [103]. *ATP7B* is localized in hepatocytes to the trans-Golgi part of the late secretory pathway. With increasing intracellular copper concentrations, the ATPase traffics to a cytoplasmic vesicular compartment that distributes near the canaliculus, where it participates in copper excretion into bile. Once the *ATP7B* sequestration of copper in vesicles reduces the cytoplasmic copper content, *ATP7B* is recycled back to the trans-Golgi network [116] (Figure 26.2).

The role of *ATP7B* in the incorporation of copper into ceruloplasmin has been investigated in yeast. The *ATP7B* orthologue Ccc2 transports copper to Fet3, which is analogous to apoceruloplasmin in mammalian tissues. In yeast lacking Ccc2, *ATP7B* replaced this activity whereas mutant *ATP7B* did not [117]. Mutations in the metal-binding sites closest to the transmembrane domain 1 are more important for this copper transporting activity than are sites closer to the N-terminus [118]. These studies illustrate the dependence of copper incorporation into ceruloplasmin on the copper transport function of *ATP7B*. Mutations in *ATP7B* result in failure to incorporate copper in ceruloplasmin and in the secretion of apoceruloplasmin, which is rapidly removed from circulation.

Clinical Features of Wilson's Disease

Wilson's disease is one of the great masqueraders and can present at almost any age. Although the failure to excrete biliary copper is present from birth, clinical manifestations of Wilson's disease are rarely apparent before age 5 years [90]. Clinical symptoms develop sequentially based on the pathophysiologic disturbance of copper metabolism in Wilson's disease. Copper silently accumulates in the liver during childhood. After the liver storage capacity for copper becomes saturated, circulating non–ceruloplasmin-bound "free copper" levels rise and copper is then redistributed systemically, accumulating in the nervous system, cornea, kidneys, and other organs and tissues. This change in organ distribution of copper over time is paralleled by the clinical presentations of Wilson's disease. Based on data from the combined patient series of Walshe [93] and Scheinberg and Sternlieb [90], before age 10 years, 83% of patients presented with hepatic symptoms and 17% with neuropsychiatric manifestations; between 10 and 18 years, 52% presented with hepatic and 48% with neuropsychiatric symptoms; and after age 18 years, 24% presented with hepatic and 74% with neuropsychiatric symptoms (Figure 26.4). Considering patients of all ages using data derived from nine combined series, approximately 49% of patients present with hepatic and 46% with neuropsychiatric symptoms (Table 26.1). The median delay in establishing the diagnosis of Wilson's disease in those with neuropsychiatric symptoms is 18 months, which is

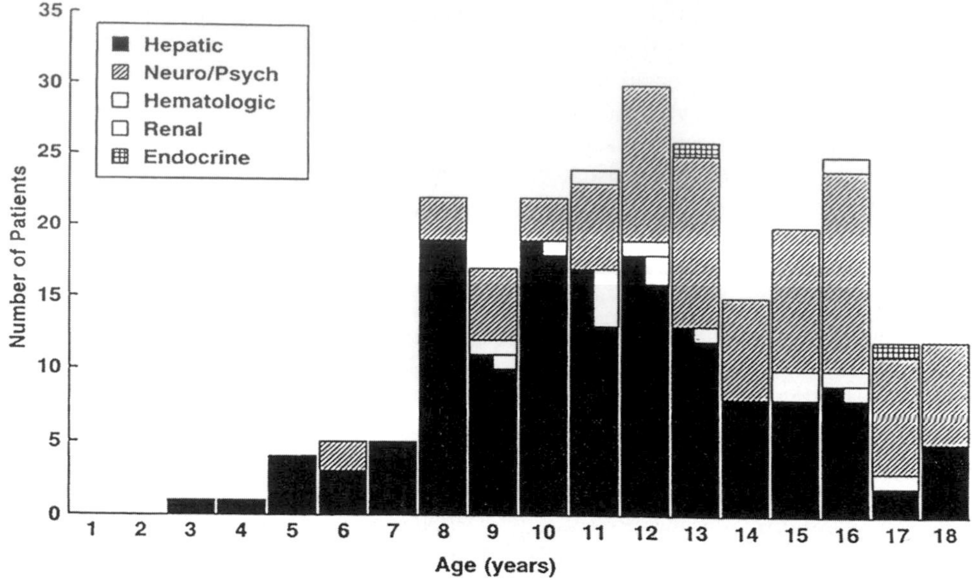

Figure 26.4. Histogram of age distribution of initial mode of clinical presentation in children and adolescents with Wilson's disease. *Split vertical bars* represent combined clinical presentation. (Based on combined data from Scheinberg and Sternlieb [90] and Walshe [93].)

considerably longer than for those with hepatic presentation (median, 6 months) [112]. During the phase of copper redistribution, other organ systems become involved, with renal, endocrine, and hematologic manifestations appearing after age 10 years (Figure 26.4). A combination of liver dysfunction and other organ system involvement, at any age, should suggest Wilson's disease.

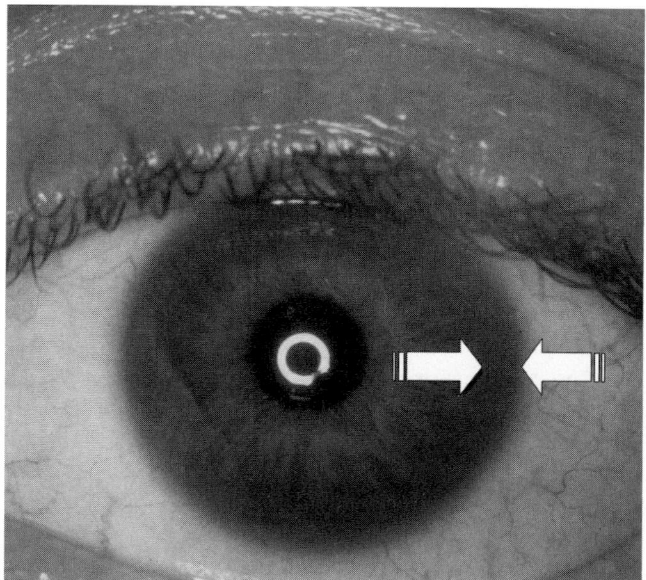

Figure 26.5. Kayser–Fleischer ring (noted by *arrows*) in a 30-year-old man with Wilson's disease. (Used by permission from Sokol RJ. Copper storage diseases. In: Kaplowitz N, ed. Liver and biliary diseases. Baltimore: Williams & Wilkins, 1992:322–33.) For color reproduction, see Color Plate 26.5.

After hepatic saturation, copper accumulating in the ocular cornea may cause the characteristic Kayser–Fleischer (K-F) ring (Figure 26.5), a greenish brown ring at the periphery of the cornea on its posterior surface in Descemet's membrane [119]. This is best detected by slit-lamp examination by an ophthalmologist, although a prominent K-F ring can be seen easily, particularly if the iris has light pigmentation. The color of the ring is the result of scattering and reflection of light by layers of copper granules. The K-F ring initially appears at the superior poles of the cornea only, with subsequent involvement of inferior poles followed by circumferential involvement [120]. Treatment with copper chelators results in gradual resolution of the rings over 3–5 years in reverse order of area of appearance, occasionally leading to complete disappearance [119,120]. This pattern of copper deposition has been said to be the result of a relative stagnation of solvent flow in the superior poles of the cornea, allowing the precipitation of copper to occur [121]. Using atomic absorbance spectroscopy, it was shown that the central region of the cornea in Wilson's disease actually contains as much copper as the periphery [120]. However, by analysis of x-ray energy spectroscopy, the K-F ring at the periphery of the cornea consisted of granules that were rich not only in copper, but also in sulfur [120]. This suggested that metallothionein-bound copper in Descemet's membrane is essential for the visual appearance characteristic of K-F rings. The K-F ring does not interfere with visual function. The K-F ring is virtually always present at the time when neurologic or psychiatric symptoms develop, although there are rare exceptions (5% of patients with neurologic symptoms) [122]. Importantly, the K-F ring is frequently absent in children without neurologic involvement who present with hepatic symptoms. The K-F ring is not pathognomonic for Wilson's disease but may also be seen in patients with prolonged cholestatic liver disease, such as chronic hepatitis, chronic intrahepatic and neonatal cholestasis, cryptogenic cirrhosis, and primary biliary cirrhosis [123–128]. This is a result of diminished biliary excretion and secondary copper overload. It is of particular interest that five of ten infants found to have pigmented corneal rings were preterm infants who received standard intravenous copper supplementation as part of parenteral nutrition in the face of significant parenteral nutrition–associated cholestasis [128]. Thus, during cholestasis in the neonate, failure to transport copper by the low plasma levels of ceruloplasmin may predispose to extrahepatic deposition of "free copper." For this reason, intravenous copper supplementation should be reduced in the cholestatic infant, with appropriate monitoring of copper status to prevent deficiency.

Another characteristic, but less common, ophthalmologic feature of Wilson's disease is the grayish brown "sunflower cataract" that may develop because of deposits of copper in the anterior and posterior lens capsule [121]. Visualizing these cataracts requires an ophthalmoscopic examination; they rarely interfere with vision and resolve with therapy [121,129]. The other circumstance in which these cataracts may develop is from a copper-containing foreign body lodged intraocularly (chalcosis) [130]. Because of these characteristic ocular findings, all patients in whom Wilson's disease is suspect should undergo a thorough ophthalmologic examination.

Hepatic Presentation

The liver is both the site of the biochemical defect in Wilson's disease and the initial target of copper toxicity. Although symptoms and signs of liver disease were initially considered "minimal and subservient to the central nervous system features" [131], reports of Chalmers et al. [132] and Silverberg and Gellis [131] brought attention to the important manifestations of liver dysfunction in childhood Wilson's disease. Clinical symptoms of liver disease virtually never occur before age 3–5 years (Figure 26.4); however, asymptomatic mild elevation of serum aminotransferase levels has been reported and a rare patient developed fulminant liver failure before age 5 years [92]. Thereafter, symptoms of acute or chronic liver disease may interrupt a presymptomatic period at any time in the first two decades of life. Hepatic presentations include acute hepatitis, fulminant hepatic failure, chronic active hepatitis, and cirrhosis (Table 26.2). Elevated aminotransferase levels may be detected in completely asymptomatic patients for whom a chemistry panel is drawn for unrelated reasons, such as seizure medication monitoring. Exclusion of more common causes of abnormal liver blood tests should lead to consideration of Wilson's disease if the tests do not normalize. It is essential that the clinician maintain a high level of suspicion and thoroughly investigate the child with persisting asymptomatic elevation of aminotransferase levels to facilitate diagnosis and initiate treatment early in the course of Wilson's disease.

Acute hepatitis is the mode of presentation in approximately 25% of patients [90]. Clinical signs of jaundice, anorexia, nausea, malaise, pale stools, and dark urine mimic infectious hepatitis. Laboratory investigation reveals a conjugated hyperbilirubinemia associated with elevated aminotransferases but normal serum albumin and prothrombin time. Although serologic testing for viral hepatitis types A, B, and C and Epstein–Barr virus is negative, this presentation may be confused with acute viral hepatitis, particularly if the patient makes a complete, although temporary, recovery.

Table 26.2: Hepatic Presentations of Wilson's Disease

Acute hepatitis
Fulminant hepatic failure
Chronic hepatitis
Portal hypertension
Cirrhosis
Asymptomatic elevation of serum aminotransferases
Gallstones

Fulminant hepatic failure, an infrequent but devastating presentation of Wilson's disease, usually occurs in adolescence as an acute icteric hepatitis that rapidly evolves over a few days to several weeks. Symptoms progress to fatigue, hepatic insufficiency, extreme jaundice (because of the accompanying hemolysis), severe coagulopathy, ascites, hepatic coma, renal failure, and death if liver transplantation is not performed [133–141]. This presentation may appear identical to that encountered in acute fulminant viral hepatitis or following ingestion of a hepatotoxin.

A similar, and unfortunate, fulminant presentation has been described in patients who had been successfully treated for up to 20 years with copper chelators but who discontinued therapy or became noncompliant for as little as 8 months' time [142,143]. The mean survival of eight such patients who died after discontinuing penicillamine was 2.6 years after an average of 10.5 years of treatment [142]. This rapid development of fatal hepatic disease suggests that the therapeutic action of penicillamine may be the result of formation of nontoxic copper–penicillamine or copper–protein complexes (e.g., copper–metallothionein) rather than the generally accepted action of penicillamine in removing excess copper from the patient. The abrupt discontinuation of penicillamine may expose the liver to a large load of free toxic copper released by dissociation of this complex [142]. Similar presentations have occurred after the discontinuation of zinc therapy. Whatever the mechanism of fulminant liver injury, Wilson's disease patients must be repeatedly and frequently reminded that copper chelation, or zinc maintenance therapy, is lifelong and discontinuation could be fatal.

Chronic hepatitis is a more common presentation in 10–30% of Wilson's disease patients during adolescence or young adulthood. Frequently, cirrhosis is already present at the time of diagnosis [90,144–147]. Malaise, anorexia, fatigue, abdominal pain, and nausea may precede the onset of jaundice and hepatic dysfunction [90,146]. Amenorrhea, delayed puberty, polyarthralgias, edema, gynecomastia, ascites, clubbing, or spider angiomata, when present, indicate the chronic nature and likelihood of hepatic fibrosis or cirrhosis. Tender hepatomegaly and splenomegaly are typically found on examination. K-F rings may be absent in up to 50% [147]. Obviously, neurologic dysfunction, psychiatric symptoms, or a family history of Wilson's disease should raise suspicion. Laboratory tests reveal raised serum aminotransferases, low albumin, elevated γ-globulin, and a variably abnormal prothrombin time. Except for lower aminotransferase levels, wilsonian chronic hepatitis patients appear clinically no different than other patients [146], except that liver biopsies may reveal steatohepatitis. Unless appropriate diagnostic studies are performed, the patient will carry a diagnosis of autoimmune, viral, alcoholic, or nonalcoholic steatohepatitis or idiopathic chronic hepatitis until neurologic symptoms develop or the liver is examined at transplantation or autopsy. Thus, it is imperative that biochemical screening for Wilson's disease be undertaken in all patients with chronic hepatitis without a defined diagnosis. The response to copper chelation therapy is generally excellent, even if cirrhosis is present [146,148]. In a series of 20 chronic hepatitis patients, Schilsky et al. [146] described long-term survival in 90% of cirrhotic patients who were compliant with copper chelation therapy. This compares favorably with survival rates of 55–80% in patients with chronic hepatitis and cirrhosis caused by hepatitis B virus, autoimmune hepatitis, or other causes [149,150].

The cirrhotic presentation of Wilson's disease may be insidious, with cutaneous signs of chronic liver disease or splenomegaly being the only clues. Alternatively, anorexia, fatigue, abdominal pain, weight loss, jaundice, ascites, gastrointestinal hemorrhage, hypersplenism, coagulopathy, spontaneous bacterial peritonitis, encephalopathy, poor school function, or hepatorenal syndrome may signal the onset [131,132, 151–154]. Indeed, none of these features is specific to wilsonian cirrhosis, so, sadly, patients may be misdiagnosed as having postnecrotic steatohepatitis, cryptogenic cirrhosis, or, in adult patients, alcoholic cirrhosis. Although cirrhosis and its complications are relatively common presenting features of Wilson's disease in childhood, the disease may remain silent and asymptomatic well into adulthood, when patients present with neurologic, psychiatric, endocrine, or other symptoms.

Cholelithiasis is relatively common in adolescents with Wilson's disease and results from ongoing hemolysis in the presence of cirrhosis [153,154]. Abdominal pain in a patient with Wilson's disease should prompt ultrasonographic evaluation for gallstones. Analysis of gallstones showed twice the level of cholesterol as found in gallstones from children with hemolytic disease, but less than 30% of that measured in typical cholesterol gallstones [153]. Interestingly, the copper content of gallstones removed from Wilson's disease patients (5.2–85.4 μg/g) was significantly lower than that in pigment gallstones found in nonwilsonian patients (571.7–1951.8 μg/g) [93], a consequence of impaired biliary excretion of copper.

Despite the frequent finding of nuclear atypia and pleomorphism on hepatic histology [90], hepatocellular carcinoma has been thought to be unusually rare in cirrhotic patients with Wilson's disease compared with other causes of cirrhosis [90,93]. Perhaps this is because long-term survival in Wilson's disease is unusual without chelation therapy, which may have a protective effect. In contrast, a recent retrospective evaluation of 363 Wilson's disease patients in the United Kingdom and Sweden demonstrated intra-abdominal malignancies (primarily hepatomas, cholangiocarcinomas, and poorly differentiated adenocarcinomas) in 4.2–5.3% of patients followed for 10–29 years and in 15% of those followed for 30–39 years [155]. No case of hepatocellular carcinoma has been reported in an affected child or adolescent.

Neuropsychiatric Presentation

In 40–45% of Wilson's disease patients, neurologic or psychiatric signs are the first indication of illness (Table 26.1). Neurologic onset has been recorded in children as young as 6 years [90] and in adults as old as 72 years [91]. Neurologic symptomatology is generally limited to motor manifestations of extrapyramidal or cerebellar dysfunction [111,112,156–158]. Psychiatric symptomatology can take many forms (Table 26.3). Neurologic symptoms most commonly present during the second and third decades of life with the insidious appearance of a single symptom, followed by gradual worsening of the symptom with development of other motor abnormalities. Recently, neurologic features have been broken down into three subsets by correlating neuropsychiatric symptoms to magnetic resonance imaging (MRI) of the brain [159]. The first subgroup, termed *pseudoparkinsonian*, describes patients with bradykinesia, cognitive impairment, cogwheel rigidity, and an organic mood syndrome. This presentation correlates with dilation of the third ventricle on brain MRI scanning. The second subgroup, termed *pseudosclerosis*, is manifested by ataxia, tremor, and reduced functional capacity and is characterized by focal thalamic lesions. Tremors may be of the resting, intention, or postural forms and may become incapacitating. The third subgroup, termed *dyskinesia*, includes patients who exhibit dyskinesia, dysarthria, and organic personality syndrome and correlates with MRI findings of focal lesions in the putamen and globus pallidus. Extrapyramidal symptoms include facial grimaces, stereotypic gestures, drooling, a fixed grin, dysphagia, and finally, contractures of the jaw or extremities. Titubation, dysmetria, scanning speech, illegible handwriting, and rarely, choreiform and athetoid movements also occur. The nature of these abnormalities frequently leads to misdiagnoses such as multiple sclerosis, Parkinson's disease, and Friedreich's ataxia [160,161]. Because intelligence is unaffected, the patient generally becomes frustrated and depressed.

The neurologic basis for these motor abnormalities is dysfunction of the basal ganglia and cerebellum [90,93]. The corticospinal and corticobulbar pathways are also affected to some extent. Walshe and Gibbs [162] reported that patients with neurologic symptoms had brain copper content above 40 μg/g wet weight, whereas those with normal neurologic function had

Table 26.3: Neurologic and Psychiatric Symptoms Associated with Wilson's Disease

Neurologic	*Psychiatric*
Tremor (resting, intention)	Organic dementia
Drooling, hypersalivation Dysarthria	Neuroses: Anxiety, depression, Obsessive/compulsive disorder
Coordination defects, clumsiness	Schizophrenia
Dystonia	Bipolar disorder
Writing difficulties	Antisocial behavior
Choreiform movements	Alcoholism
Ataxic gait	
Fixed grin	
Headache	
Seizures	

brain copper below this level. Thus, there appears to be a critical threshold of brain copper deposition above which neurologic injury and symptomatology ensue.

Sensory function and intelligence in Wilson's disease patients remain normal; however, there may be mild memory impairment [163]. Lower scores reported on various intelligence tests are most likely the result of impaired ability to perform motor tasks [163]. Other symptoms that may develop include migraine headaches; grand mal, focal motor, or partial complex seizures; and various gait disturbances caused by both the tremor and dystonia. Dening et al. [164] found 13 of 200 Wilson's disease patients had seizures at some time, yielding a prevalence rate of seizures of 6.2% at one point in time. Both these figures exceed the frequency of epilepsy in the general population by tenfold. Seizures were rarely present initially but developed not infrequently within weeks or months of starting copper chelation therapy. It has thus been proposed that sudden mobilization of large quantities of copper by chelating agents may be responsible for these seizures; pyridoxine deficiency was not contributory [164]. Neurologic presentations of Wilson's disease are summarized in Table 26.2.

At some time during the course of their life, many patients will suffer from organic dementia, neurotic behavior, bipolar or schizophrenic psychosis, or behavioral abnormalities that may be antisocial in nature [165–167]. Aggressive behavioral outbursts, deterioration in school performance, or a major change in affect or personality may be the initial symptoms in an adolescent or college student. Sometimes it is difficult to be certain that a psychiatric disturbance is present rather than severe neurologic dysfunction, leading to the impression of mental illness. In addition, the frustration of a progressive, undiagnosed neurologic illness has been said to contribute to the development of psychoemotional distress and symptomatology [90]. Therefore, psychiatric evaluation and ongoing psychotherapy in addition to chelation therapy are important elements in the total care of these patients.

In approximately 10–25% of Wilson's disease patients, a psychiatric disturbance is the initial clinical presentation, even before the appearance of any movement disorder. If the diagnosis of Wilson's disease is not made, the development of a movement disorder during therapy with drugs for the psychiatric disorder may be attributed to a medication side effect rather than to the possibility of undiagnosed Wilson's disease [90]. Psychiatrists must therefore maintain a high index of suspicion of Wilson's disease and should measure plasma ceruloplasmin and obtain a slit-lamp examination in patients with psychiatric disorders (even if chronic in nature). This is of particular importance if there is a history of liver disease or a family history of a psychiatric disorder or Wilson's disease, if the patient is under age 50 years, or if the patient is not responding satisfactorily to conventional psychiatric treatment [90].

Other Presentations

Renal disturbances may occur in patients with Wilson's disease [90,168–170]; however, renal disease as a presenting symptom is extremely rare. Copper has been shown to accumulate in the kidneys of Wilson's disease patients, with up to 100 times the normal concentration being observed [90]. Proximal renal tubular dysfunction, decreased glomerular filtration rate, and decreased renal plasma flow characterize the resulting renal dysfunction [168–170]. The renal tubular dysfunction is manifested by proteinuria, glucosuria, phosphaturia, uricosuria, generalized aminoaciduria, and microscopic hematuria [168–170]. Distal renal tubular acidosis is reflected by the inability to acidify urine to a pH of less than 5.2 in response to an ammonium chloride load [171–173] and contributes to an increased tendency for formation of renal stones. In one series [172], 16% of 45 patients developed renal stones. Patients with the fulminant presentation of Wilson's disease and those with end-stage liver disease may develop severe renal insufficiency requiring temporary dialysis. Finally, isosthenuria has been reported. Many of the renal abnormalities improve during copper chelation therapy [170,174]; however, severe proteinuria and the nephrotic syndrome [90,175] or a Goodpasture-like syndrome [176] are more likely to occur as a consequence of penicillamine administration rather than of copper toxicity.

A variety of hematologic manifestations have been reported in Wilson's disease. Intravascular hemolysis is frequent and may be the presenting abnormality in approximately 15% [177–179]. Hemolysis may be transient and occur when there are no associated neurologic or hepatic clinical manifestations. Therefore, Wilson's disease should be considered in all children and adolescents with Coombs-negative hemolytic anemia. When associated with the acute fulminant hepatic presentation, hemolysis is a poor prognostic factor, contributing to renal failure by excess hemoglobinuria [133–138]. Hemolysis is considered secondary to sudden release of copper from the liver, initiating an oxidant stress capable of peroxidizing red cell membrane lipids [179,180]. If hepatic involvement is advanced, circulating hepatic-derived coagulation factor levels may be low, platelets may have impaired function [181], and portal hypertension may cause splenomegaly and resultant thrombocytopenia and leukopenia [182].

Cardiac involvement has been recognized in Wilson's disease. Electrocardiographic abnormalities were present in 34% of 53 patients with a mean age of 21 years [183,184], including left ventricular hypertrophy, ST wave depression, and T wave inversion. Arrhythmias were present in 13% of patients, and 19% had orthostatic hypotension (although asymptomatic), indicating autonomic dysfunction. Histologic findings at autopsy have included cardiac hypertrophy, interstitial fibrosis, intramyocardial small vessel sclerosis, and focal inflammation [183]. Factor et al. [183] postulated that sudden death may be caused by arrhythmias in Wilson's disease patients.

Skeletal manifestations of Wilson's disease are not uncommon and may even be the first clinical symptoms of the disease [185]. Bone demineralization is the most common feature [157], possibly caused by the hypercalciuria and hyperphosphaturia resulting from renal tubular dysfunction [90]. Other radiologic changes include rickets and osteomalacia, osteoporosis, spontaneous fractures, bone fragmentation near joints, osteochondritis dessicans, chondromalacia patellae, premature osteoarthrosis, and premature degenerative arthritis of the knees and wrists [186–190]. Stiffness of larger joints is a complaint of many patients [188].

Skin pigmentation may be increased, particularly on the anterior aspect of the lower legs, because of deposition of melanin [191], and acanthosis nigricans may be present. Blue lunulae of the fingernails have also been reported [192]. Other associated dermatologic findings may be caused by cirrhosis and portal hypertension. Hormonal imbalance secondary to chronic liver disease has been thought to lead to amenorrhea in women and gynecomastia in boys [90,193]. However, more recent studies suggest that primary ovarian dysfunction may be present [193] and that increased androgen levels and abnormalities in the hypothalamic–pituitary–testicular axis in males is probably not a result of liver dysfunction [194]. Additional infrequent associations with Wilson's disease include diabetes mellitus [195,196], exocrine pancreatic insufficiency [197], and hypoparathyroidism [198].

Laboratory Findings

Patients with Wilson's disease may present with almost any combination of abnormalities in liver blood tests, or even no abnormality at all. Serum aminotransferase levels are characteristically only mildly to moderately elevated, with aspartate aminotransferase (AST) higher than alanine aminotransferase (ALT) [90,199–202], even in patients with the fulminant hepatic failure presentation. Serum alkaline phosphatase is usually in the low range [200–202], particularly when fulminant hepatic failure is present. Serum copper is usually low; however, during the fulminant presentation, serum copper is actually elevated because of massive copper release from the necrosing liver and may be helpful in establishing this diagnosis [199]. This released copper also contributes to the hemolytic anemia, hemoglobinuria, and renal failure that are common during this presentation [90].

Serum phosphate and uric acid may be low because of renal tubular losses [90]. Recent studies suggest that uric acid may

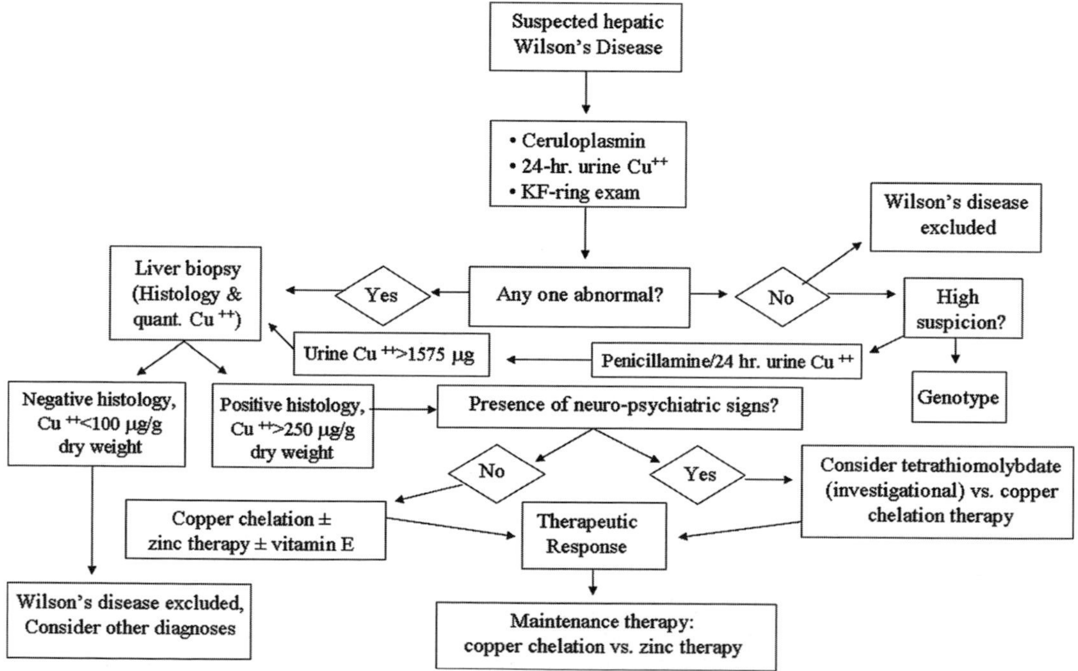

Figure 26.6. Approach to the evaluation and treatment of a pediatric patient with suspected Wilson's disease because of presentation with liver disease.

Table 26.4: Diagnostic Studies Used in Evaluation for Wilson's Disease

Diagnostic Test	*Diagnostic Values*	*Causes of False Positive*	*Causes of False Negative*
Serum ceruloplasmin	$<$20 mg/dL	Kwashiorkor, nutritional copper deficiency, protein-losing state, fulminant hepatitis, hepatic failure, hereditary hypoceruloplasminemia or aceruloplasminemia, Wilson's disease heterozygote, Menkes' syndrome, normal neonate	Acute inflammation (hepatitis), malignancy, pregnancy or estrogen therapy in Wilson's disease (5% of patients), immunoassays of apoceruloplasmin
Hepatic copper concentration	$>$250 μg/g dry wt.	Primary biliary cirrhosis, Indian childhood cirrhosis, chronic cholestatic liver disease, primary sclerosing cholangitis, Alagille syndrome, liver tumors, newborn liver	Copper chelation therapy in Wilson's disease
24-Hour urine copper excretion	$>$100 μg/24 hr	Copper chelation therapy, chronic active hepatitis, chronic cholestatic liver diseases, primary sclerosing cholangitis, hepatic failure, nephrotic syndrome	Copper chelation therapy in Wilson's disease
Presence of Kayser–Fleischer rings	Present	Chronic cholestatic liver diseases, primary biliary cirrhosis, neonatal cholestasis	Early Wilson's disease
Incorporation of ^{64}Cu into ceruloplasmin	Low	Ceruloplasmin $<$20 mg/dL, Wilson's disease heterozygote	Pregnancy, estrogens, inflammation or malignancy in Wilson's disease
Genotyping	Identification of two disease-causing mutations in *ATP7B*	Laboratory error	Mutation not identified but present
Haplotype analysis (microsatellite markers)	Presence of informative markers on both chromosomes	Laboratory error	Absence of informative microsatellite markers in family

Adapted from Scheinberg and Sternlieb [90].

also be oxidized as a result of oxidative stress [203]. A complete Fanconi's syndrome, including aminoaciduria and glycosuria, may be evident upon appropriate urine testing [168–170]. Changes on radiologic evaluation of the skeleton may include osteoporosis, rickets, osteomalacia, localized demineralization, osteoarthritis, and other lesions [185–188].

Diagnosis of Wilson's Disease

Establishing the diagnosis of Wilson's disease may be problematic (Figure 26.6) but is essential if copper chelation therapy is to be instituted as early as possible in the course of the disease (Table 26.4). For instance, if the patient has oliguric renal failure, it is not possible to quantify urinary copper excretion. Alternatively, plasma ceruloplasmin values in Wilson's disease may be elevated into the low normal range during acute hepatitis or estrogen therapy, or may be low in patients with other causes of hepatic failure [96]. Severe coagulopathy may prevent percutaneous liver biopsy. Therefore, the specific criteria used to establish the diagnosis of Wilson's disease must be tailored to the patient's clinical presentation. No single laboratory test result can establish this diagnosis without confirmatory clinical and laboratory data, with the possible exception of genetic testing under certain circumstances. A recent international group has attempted to develop a scoring system to assist with the diagnosis of Wilson's disease [204]. The following sections discuss diagnostic criteria in classic and problematic clinical presentations.

Hepatic Presentations

In a patient with liver dysfunction, the finding of a plasma or serum ceruloplasmin level less than 20 mg/dL suggests the diagnosis of Wilson's disease; however, confirmatory studies are necessary because a number of disease states may also yield low ceruloplasmin values. For example, low serum ceruloplasmin levels may also occur in patients with massive protein loss, kwashiorkor, severe copper deficiency, severe hepatic insufficiency [90], hereditary hypoceruloplasminemia [205] or aceruloplasminemia [106], or fulminant hepatitis; in the normal neonate; in those with Menkes' syndrome; and in 10% of heterozygotes for Wilson's disease (Table 26.4). Thus, the diagnosis of Wilson's disease must be confirmed by an elevated urine 24-hour copper excretion above 100 μg/24 hr (normal, <40 μg/24 hr), an elevated urine copper during a penicillamine challenge (see below), the presence of a K-F ring (and the absence of other cholestatic liver disorders), or elevated hepatic copper content (>250 μg/g dry weight) with consistent liver histology.

Urine must be collected in copper-free containers to avoid contamination. Additionally, determining if the collection was a full 24-hour collection should be confirmed by measuring total urinary creatinine excretion (normal, 10–20 mg/kg/24 hr). False-positive results of a 24-hour urine copper excretion (i.e., >100 μg/24 hr) may be seen if the patient is receiving any type of copper chelation therapy, if the collection is contaminated by exogenous copper, or if the patient has chronic active hepatitis, cholestatic cirrhosis, or nephrotic syndrome. Perman et al. [145], DaCosta et al. [206], and Frommer [207] showed that although Wilson's disease patients as a group had higher mean values in 24-hour urine copper excretion than did children and young adults with autoimmune chronic active hepatitis, acute hepatitis, primary sclerosing cholangitis, acute liver failure, and primary biliary cirrhosis, there was a significant overlap in values. Recent studies indicate that basal 24-hour urinary copper excretion may be even less than 100 μg at presentation in 16–23% of patients [110,208], leading some to recommend a threshold of 40 μg for diagnosis [209]. Using this threshold would certainly increase the number of false-positive urinary coppers in patients with other liver diseases. Thus, to improve the diagnostic accuracy of urine copper, the King's College Hospital group [206,210] demonstrated virtually complete discrimination between Wilson's disease and other liver disorders when 24-hour urine copper excretion was measured *after* a penicillamine challenge (500 mg given orally immediately before and repeated 12 hours into the urine collection); values above 25 μmol/24 hr (1575 μg) indicated Wilson's disease. Gregorio and Mieli-Vergani [211] subsequently reported similar postpenicillamine copper excretion in three children with acute persistent hepatitis A virus infection, cautioning against the use of this test as the sole criterion for diagnosing Wilson's disease.

If the serum ceruloplasmin concentration is greater than 20 but less than 30 mg/dL, the diagnosis of Wilson's disease is not excluded if clinical circumstances are suggestive, because 5–17% of patients will have serum ceruloplasmin in this low-normal range [90,206,212]. Recently, Steindl et al. [110] reported that 40% of 25 patients presenting with liver disease had ceruloplasmin values in the normal range, with several exceeding 30 mg/dL. In this study, ceruloplasmin was measured by radial immunodiffusion, an immunologic technique that recognizes both the oxidase-active holoprotein that contains six copper atoms per molecule and the enzymatically inactive apoceruloplasmin [213]. Thus, immunologic techniques may yield higher values than those obtained by the "gold standard" oxidase reaction, confusing the diagnosis. Unfortunately, many commercial laboratories have adopted the more convenient immunoassay, making low ceruloplasmin concentration less valuable as a diagnostic pillar for Wilson's disease. If ceruloplasmin is normal but there is a high index of suspicion, then a 24-hour urine copper excretion (best after penicillamine challenge), slit-lamp examination, and liver biopsy should be performed to confirm or exclude the diagnosis. If a sibling has Wilson's disease, then haplotype analysis can potentially be performed.

A percutaneous liver biopsy should be obtained for light microscopy, electron microscopy, and quantitative copper analysis if coagulation studies allow it to be performed safely. Transjugular liver biopsy may be performed if a significant coagulopathy is present. Characteristic histologic findings of Wilson's disease (fatty change, periportal glycogenated nuclei) or of other liver disorders (e.g., primary biliary cirrhosis) aid in the diagnosis. Ultrastructural mitochondrial changes of Wilson's disease are also valuable. Measuring a quantitative hepatic copper concentration is absolutely essential. Normal hepatic copper content is less than 50 μg/g dry weight of liver [214]. Assuming an adequate sample has been obtained, it is virtually always above 250 μg/g dry weight in Wilson's disease and may reach 3000 μg/g in liver tissue [90]. In affected asymptomatic siblings of Wilson's disease patients, liver copper content may be borderline elevated [215]. Although a normal hepatic copper content excludes the diagnosis of Wilson's disease, a false-positive result may occur in the proper clinical setting. Other conditions associated with elevated hepatic copper values must be excluded by specific diagnostic studies as the clinical circumstances dictate (Table 26.4). The disorders that arise most commonly are autoimmune and infectious chronic hepatitis. The presence of autoimmune markers, serum ceruloplasmin above 30 mg/dL, and 24-hour urine copper excretion (with or without penicillamine challenge) below the threshold will generally exclude Wilson's disease.

If the diagnosis remains uncertain despite the testing already described, or if liver biopsy is contraindicated, the rate of incorporation of radiolabeled copper into ceruloplasmin can also be determined as a diagnostic study [90,216]. A dose of 2 mg of cupric acetate containing 0.3–0.5 mCi copper Cu 64 (^{64}Cu) is administered orally in 100–150 mL of fruit juice following an 8-hour fast. The concentration of ^{64}Cu in serum is determined serially (at +1, 2, 4, 24, and 48 hours) over 48 hours. Normally, the radio-labeled copper rises at 1 and 2 hours and falls thereafter, with a secondary rise over the ensuing 24 or 48 hours representing incorporation of the radio-labeled copper into newly synthesized ceruloplasmin. In Wilson's disease, the secondary rise in serum copper that normally occurs after 4 hours is absent. The pattern is intermediate in Wilson's disease heterozygotes [217]. Although this test has been performed in the past on occasion, it is now rarely used because of the difficulty in obtaining the isotope.

Molecular genetic testing has been available in recent years and is most helpful if the diagnosis remains in doubt despite the testing already discussed. DNA haplotype testing may establish the diagnosis if another family member (proband) has Wilson's disease. Evaluation of DNA haplotype markers (microsatellite markers) that flank *ATP7B* on chromosome 13 is available in a number of commercial laboratories [96]. Prenatal diagnosis is also possible using this approach [218], although this has limited application because early diagnosis allows appropriate timing for treatment. Alternatively, direct genotyping of ATPb can be attempted. Because of a multitude of mutations of *ATP7B*, genetic mutation analysis generally employs a panel of likely mutations for a given ethnic population [95,219]. Some specific ethnic groups that have a single predominant mutation and for whom genotyping may be useful include populations in Sardinia, Iceland, Korea, Japan, and the Canary Islands [209]. Most genotyping is still being performed in research laboratories, hence this testing is not readily available. Although genotyping might prove to be very helpful in individual cases, it still will not yield complete diagnostic accuracy [220]. Genotype–phenotype correlations are hampered by the high prevalence of compound heterozygotes in *ATP7B*.

Tests that appear to be of no value in establishing the diagnosis of Wilson's disease include computed tomography (CT) scanning and MRI of the liver, because liver copper content cannot currently be detected or quantitated by these modalities [221–223]. Although advocated by some experts as useful, the nonceruloplasmin serum copper fraction "free copper" may be elevated in a variety of liver diseases as well as in Wilson's disease [224], so its value in establishing the diagnosis is questionable. It is of more value in monitoring treatment.

Figure 26.6 illustrates a suggested approach to diagnosing Wilson's disease in patients with a hepatic presentation. Serum ceruloplasmin, a 24-hour urine collection for copper analysis, and an ophthalmology examination for a K-F ring should be obtained. A liver biopsy should be obtained if any of these are abnormal or if there is a high suspicion for Wilson's disease and the ceruloplasmin is 20–30 μg/dL or it was measured by an immunologic method and is in the normal range. In addition to routine histology, electron microscopy and quantitative copper analysis should be obtained. If quantitative hepatic copper exceeds 250 μg/g dry weight and other diagnoses are excluded by histology and other appropriate laboratory tests, then the diagnosis of Wilson's disease is established. Alternatively, DNA mutation analysis can be performed for a defined *ATP7B* mutation, common mutations in the appropriate ethnic population, or haplotype (microsatellite) marker analysis if a first-degree relative has Wilson's disease.

HISTOPATHOLOGY OF THE LIVER

Although the diagnosis of Wilson's disease may not be evident from a single liver biopsy, the sequential changes observed over several years are characteristic. Therefore, a high index of suspicion and an understanding of the characteristic pathology are required to suggest the diagnosis on a single liver biopsy. Earliest histologic findings, that may be present in asymptomatic children [75,90], include periportal glycogen-filled, swollen nuclei [225,226] and hepatic steatosis, initially microvesicular that evolves into macrovesicular fat [65,227] (Figure 27.7). Soon mononuclear cell infiltrates of portal tracts become evident with increasing periportal fibrosis, hyperplasia of Kupffer cells, and pericentral venular fibrosis [90,226]. In adolescents and adults, the macrovesicular steatosis might mistakenly suggest alcohol-induced liver disease or nonalcoholic steatohepatitis. During the acute hepatitis phase of Wilson's disease, hepatocyte swelling and individual hepatocyte necrosis, mild cholestasis, and lymphocytic infiltration are present [90]. The chronic hepatitis lesion exhibits ballooning of hepatocytes, focal hepatocyte necrosis with interface hepatitis, glycogenated nuclei, erosion of the periportal limiting plate, lymphocytic and plasma cell inflammatory infiltrates in portal tracts, periportal fibrosis, and, when advanced, combined micronodular and macronodular cirrhosis (Figures 27.8 and 27.9) [144,147,228]. This appearance may be indistinguishable from that of autoimmune or chronic infectious hepatitis. The fulminant hepatitis lesion is characterized by microvesicular fat, coagulative cell necrosis,

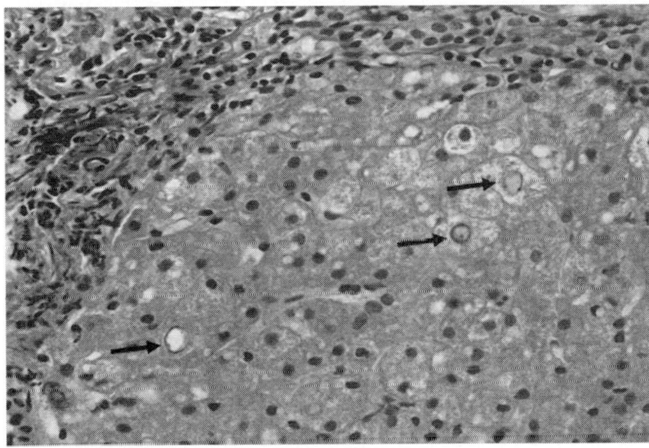

Figure 26.7. Liver histology of Wilson's disease in a 3-year-old asymptomatic boy diagnosed because his sister presented with fulminant liver failure caused by Wilson's disease. Portal tract mononuclear infiltrate and prominent periportal glycogenated hepatocyte nuclei (*arrows*) are present. Early evidence of portal fibrosis is also present. (Hematoxylin and eosin [H&E] stain, 400× magnification.) For color reproduction, see Color Plate 26.7.

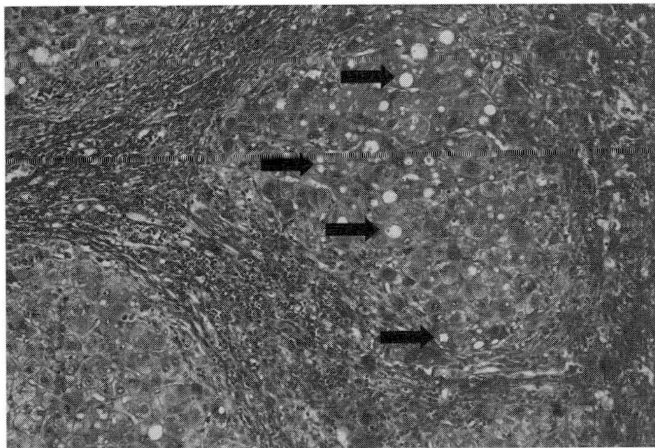

Figure 26.8. Liver histology of Wilson's disease in a 16-year-old girl presenting with fulminant liver failure. Macrovesicular steatosis (*arrows*), mononuclear cell portal tract inflammatory infiltrate, bridging fibrosis, and micronodular cirrhosis are present. (Masson trichrome stain, 200× magnification.) For color reproduction, see Color Plate 26.8.

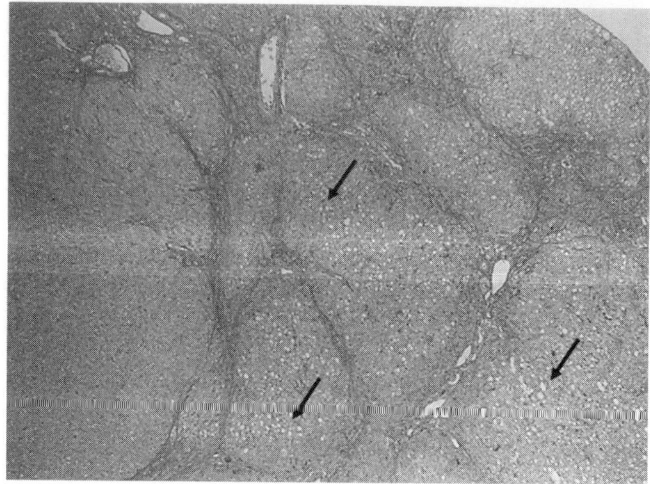

Figure 26.9. Liver histology of Wilson's disease in a 13-year-old girl. Bridging fibrosis and both mild micro- and macrovesicular hepatocytic steatosis (*arrows*) are present, with less inflammatory infiltrate than that seen in Figure 26.8. (H&E stain, 100× magnification.) For color reproduction, see Color Plate 26.9.

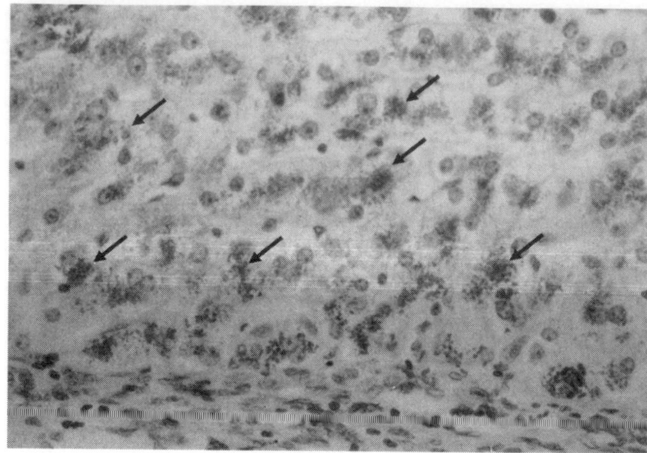

Figure 26.10. Copper staining of liver removed at the time of liver transplantation from a 16-year-old girl with fulminant hepatic failure caused by Wilson's disease (see Figure 26.8). Staining of copper-associated proteins in multiple hepatocytes (*arrows*) by rhodanine histochemical stain is strongly positive. (1000× magnification.) For color reproduction, see Color Plate 26.10.

pigment-laden Kupffer cells, collapse of stoma with drop out of hepatocytes, Mallory's hyaline present in cytoplasm, and occasional multi-nucleated giant cells and bile duct proliferation in a background of cirrhosis [90].

Cirrhosis develops invariably in untreated patients and is characterized by fibrous bands separating regenerative nodules of either a macronodular or mixed micro/macronodular pattern (Figure 26.8) [90,229,230]. Pericentral venular fibrosis and a pseudo-acinar pattern may be observed. Periportal steatosis and glycogenated nuclei may still be present and are characteristic [90]. Mallory's hyaline may be present in hepatocytes at the periphery of regenerative nodules, leading to confusion with Laënnec's cirrhosis [226,230]. Dark pigment representing lipofuscin, copper-associated protein, or occasionally iron may also be observed in individual hepatocytes. Hepatocellular carcinoma is rarely found in cirrhotic livers from Wilson's disease patients [231–233], possibly because copper may be protective against hepatocellular carcinoma [234].

Histochemical stains for copper or copper-associated proteins, such as rhodamine, rubeanic acid, orcein, or Timms silver sulfide, provide qualitative evidence of increased liver copper. However, despite elevated hepatic copper content, these stains are frequently negative in Wilson's disease patients [90,147] and may be very misleading. Although a positive stain for copper is helpful (Figure 26.10), a negative histochemical stain for copper on a liver biopsy never rules out the diagnosis of Wilson's disease. These stains are invariably positive in other conditions causing elevated hepatic copper levels, such as cholestatic liver disorders and ICC [235–239]; however, in Wilson's disease, there is no correlation between histochemical staining of copper and quantitative copper measurements on biopsy samples. There are several possible reasons for the absence of stainable copper in Wilson's disease: copper is not present in hepatocytes of regenerating nodules that have had insufficient time to accumulate copper, copper has been released because of cell injury [230], or cytosolic copper is more difficult to identify by histochemistry than the granular appearance of lysosomal copper present in other conditions [90,240]. For these reasons, quantitative measurement of copper in liver biopsies is mandatory. Liver biopsies must be performed with steel biopsy needles and at least 5 mg, if not 10–15 mg, used for determination of quantitative copper by a reputable laboratory.

Electron microscopy may be helpful in establishing the diagnosis because Wilson's disease is one of the few liver diseases with characteristic ultrastructural lesions [65,241]. In the early stages of Wilson's disease, hepatocellular mitochondria are pleomorphic and abnormally large and show widened intracristal spaces, increased matrix density, large granules, and sometimes crystalline, vacuolated, or dense inclusions in the mitochondrial matrix (Figure 26.11) [65,241]. This

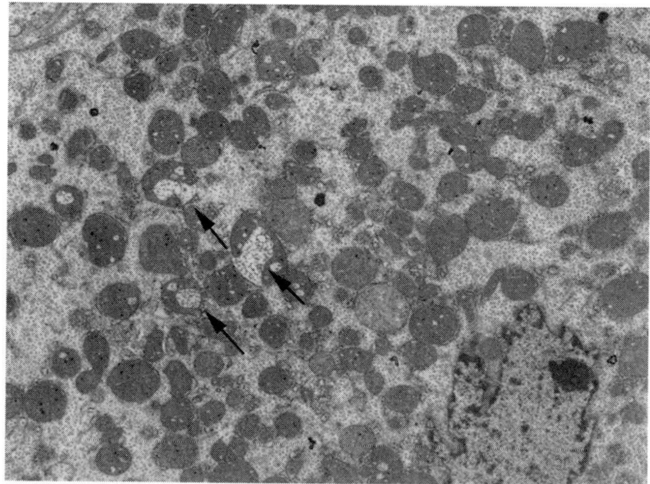

Figure 26.11. Electron microscopy of liver from a 10-year-old boy with Wilson's disease and liver failure. Pleomorphic mitochondria with dilated and cystic cristae are abundant (*arrows*). (14,000× magnification.)

constellation of mitochondrial changes in a liver with fatty changes is characteristic Wilson's disease [90]; however, similar changes may be observed in nonalcoholic steatohepatitis. During penicillamine therapy, these mitochondrial changes regress or disappear [242]. These mitochondrial changes also disappear during progression of the lesion toward cirrhosis [65]. Peroxisomes may become enlarged and granular or flocculent. In the later stages of cirrhosis, these ultrastructural lesions are absent; however, excess copper-rich lipofuscin granules are present [65,243].

In the central nervous system, lesions include degeneration of the putamen and globus pallidus and atrophy of the caudate. Degeneration of the cerebral cortex, cerebellum, and white matter in the region of the dentate nucleus has also been described [90].

Neuropsychiatric Presentation

If a patient presents with neurologic or psychiatric symptomatology, the absence of a K-F ring makes the diagnosis of Wilson's disease unlikely, although in a recent series, 2 of 20 patients presenting with neurologic symptoms did not have K-F rings [110]. Thorough examination for a K-F ring must be carried out by an experienced ophthalmologist using a slit lamp. However, copper might also be deposited in the cornea in chronic cholestatic liver disease, such as primary biliary cirrhosis or familial cholestatic syndromes [123–127], and even in neonates with cholestasis [128]. Consequently, hepatic histology and other blood tests are necessary to exclude other forms of liver disease. Thus, it can be seen that no single test can be used to diagnose Wilson's disease in all circumstances; it is the constellation of clinical history, family history, physical examination, and key laboratory tests that establish the diagnosis.

Computed tomography of the head shows that cerebral injury is not limited to the lenticular nuclei in Wilson's disease. Williams and Walshe [244] evaluated 60 patients and found a surprisingly high frequency of CT abnormalities: 73% with ventricular dilation, 63% cortical atrophy, 55% brainstem atrophy, 45% hypodense areas in basal ganglia, and 10% posterior fossa atrophy. This combination of findings appeared specific for Wilson's disease, although the findings alone are observed in a variety of clinical conditions. Only 2 of 40 patients with neurologic symptoms had normal CT scans. Interestingly, 75% of those with hepatic presentation and 50% of presymptomatic patients had abnormal scans. Penicillamine therapy resulted in improvement in basal ganglia hypodensities in 10 of 14 patients as well as clinical improvement [244]. Despite striking abnormalities on brain CT scans, patients may still respond well to chelation treatment [244]. Therefore, CT examination may be valuable in diagnosis and management of patients with neurologic involvement; however, it is of little prognostic value. In fact, patients have been reported who clinically improved on chelation therapy despite progression of abnormalities on CT scan [245].

Magnetic resonance imaging has been used to better characterize and follow central nervous system lesions during copper chelation therapy [160,223,246,247]. The most common abnormalities noted by MRI are lesions in the basal ganglia, ventricular dilatation, and generalized atrophy. MRI has identified abnormalities in patients with normal CT scans [223]. Prolongation of T1, or darker areas on T1 images, corresponds to necrosis, cystic change or edema, whereas a shortened T1, which produces a lighter image, represents increased copper content [223,246]. On MRI, 46% of 22 patients had lesions in the caudate, 41% had lesions in the putamen, 36% had brain atrophy, 27% had midbrain lesions, 23% had subcortical white matter lesions, 23% had pons lesions, and less than 10% had lesions in the thalamus, vermis, dentate, or globus pallidus [160]. Dystonia and bradykinesia correlated with putamen lesions and dysarthria with both putamen and caudate lesions [160]. Using a more sensitive ultra-low-field MRI technique with computerized image processing, Linne et al. [247] were able to demonstrate gradual return toward normality in brain lesions of a 13-year-old boy with Wilson's disease concomitant with clinical improvement during copper chelation therapy. More recently, positron emission tomography (PET) has been used to evaluate brain lesions in Wilson's disease [248]. Glucose consumption was reduced in the cerebellum, striatum, cortex, and thalamus in Wilson's disease patients [249]. In addition, there was a significant reduction in dopa-decarboxylase, which indicates impaired function of the striatal dopaminergic pathway [250].

A variety of electrophysiologic and imaging techniques have been used to evaluate Wilson's disease patients and the response to chelation therapy. Auditory evoked potentials showed increased wave latencies in patients with central nervous system involvement [251–254], were normal in neurologic symptom-free Wilson's disease patients [253,254], and improved during copper chelation therapy [253]. Visual evoked potentials revealed abnormally prolonged latency in three of eight symptomatic patients tested [254]. Likewise, somatosensory evoked potentials showed central conduction delay in symptomatic patients [254], were normal in symptom-free patients, and improved during therapy [253,254]. These findings suggest involvement of sensory pathways as they course through the brainstem [251–254], although hearing, vision, and sensory function are unimpaired.

Specific Clinical Circumstances

ACUTE HEPATITIS

This presentation is most often confused with acute viral hepatitis, particularly if the patient makes a complete recovery. Serologic markers for viral hepatitis types A, B, and C as well as Epstein–Barr virus, cytomegalovirus, and other hepatotrophic viruses are negative. Additionally, markers for toxin-induced hepatitis are negative. Some key findings that should alert the clinician to the diagnosis of Wilson's disease include a mild hemolytic anemia or a depressed serum uric acid level due to renal tubular losses. In the absence of positive serologies, patients with acute nonspecific hepatitis should be screened for evidence of subclinical chronic liver disease, such as Wilson's disease and autoimmune hepatitis.

FULMINANT HEPATIC FAILURE

Establishing the diagnosis of Wilson's disease in the patient with fulminant hepatic failure may be particularly difficult. Liver biopsy may not be possible because of coagulopathy, renal failure may preclude collection of urine, and K-F rings are often absent because of the young age of the patients. However, if these can be examined, the diagnostic criteria are similar to those described above. This presentation may appear similar to acute fulminant viral, autoimmune, or toxin-induced hepatitis, although several clues should suggest Wilson's disease. A Coombs-negative hemolytic anemia with elevated reticulocyte count caused by rapid release of massive amounts of copper from the necrosing liver is characteristic of Wilson's disease and makes this the most likely diagnosis [90]. Occasionally, hepatitis A virus triggers hemolysis in patients with glucose-6-phosphate dehydrogenase deficiency or thalassemia trait; however, hepatitis A virus infection can quickly be excluded serologically [255]. Other findings that should suggest Wilson's disease include relatively low serum aminotransferase levels for fulminant hepatic failure of two to ten times the upper limit of normal [90,199,200] and an abnormally low serum alkaline phosphatase level for patient age [200–202]. This latter finding is not caused by interference of copper or bilirubin with the alkaline phosphatase assay [201,202], nor is it the result of abnormalities in zinc metabolism [202]. In addition, the serum AST is significantly more elevated than the ALT [200,202]. In one study of patients in this clinical setting, a ratio of alkaline phosphatase (IU/L) to total serum bilirubin (mg/dL) less than 2 in association with an AST–ALT ratio greater than 4 appeared to be diagnostic of Wilson's disease [200]. However, others have not been able to verify these findings [256]. In this presentation, serum copper levels are actually quite elevated, rather than depressed, because of the hepatocyte copper release with hepatic necrosis [199]. McCullough et al. [141] suggested that elevated serum copper could differentiate wilsonian patients; however, subsequent studies [200,256] failed to confirm this finding. Berman et al. [200] proposed that the ratio of serum alkaline phosphatase (IU/L) to total bilirubin (mg/dL) of less than 2 was 100% specific and sensitive for Wilson's disease. However, Sallie et al. [256] studied 21 cases of fulminant Wilson's disease and showed that this ratio may be helpful in suggesting Wilson's disease; however, values greater than 2 did not exclude the diagnosis. Thus, it was not possible to reliably differentiate Wilson's disease from other causes by this ratio alone. K-F rings, if present on slit-lamp examination, will confirm the diagnosis of Wilson's disease, although K-F rings are commonly absent in the typical adolescent Wilson's disease patient with fulminant hepatic failure in whom neuropsychiatric symptoms have not yet developed [90].

Transjugular liver biopsy now allows for obtaining tissue even if a significant coagulopathy is present. Characteristic histologic findings of Wilson's disease, such as fatty change, periportal glycogenated nuclei, and an elevated hepatic copper content, aid in the diagnosis. Ultrastructural mitochondrial changes of Wilson's disease are also valuable. If Wilson's disease cannot be diagnosed or excluded based on the histology, electron microscopy, and quantitative copper content of the removed recipient liver, then DNA mutation analysis should be performed. If a mutation cannot be found, then ceruloplasmin levels can be determined for the patient's parents, if available; if the levels in both parents are near the lower limit of normal, this supports the heterozygote state in each parent and the possibility that the patient may be homozygous.

If the diagnosis of Wilson's disease escapes detection, all patients with this presentation will die of hepatic or renal failure. Even when appropriately diagnosed, these patients virtually never recover despite copper chelation therapy [133,137,138, 140], plasmapheresis [133,257], or postdilution hemofiltration [258]. In many patients, it will be obvious that liver transplantation will be required regardless of the underlying diagnosis. Prompt referral to a liver transplantation center is essential and may be lifesaving [133,258–260].

CHRONIC HEPATITIS AND CIRRHOSIS

Other than finding a mild hemolytic anemia, there is little to distinguish this cause of cirrhosis from others. A high degree of suspicion is necessary to pursue slit-lamp examination for a K-F ring, investigate for a positive family history, or recognize neuropsychiatric symptoms. For this reason, all children age 3–4 years or older with cirrhosis should undergo evaluation for Wilson's disease as described. Referral for a liver transplantation evaluation should be considered if at diagnosis there is an irreversible coagulopathy, encephalopathy, or renal insufficiency, or if hepatic decompensation develops despite the initiation of copper chelation therapy [89].

CHRONICALLY ELEVATED AMINOTRANSFERASES

All children and adults who have unexplained chronically elevated serum aminotransferase levels require a serum ceruloplasmin, slit-lamp examination, 24-hour urine copper excretion, and most likely, a liver biopsy to establish the underlying diagnosis. Attributing elevated aminotransferases as being caused by nonalcoholic fatty liver disease in obese or overweight patients has the potential of overlooking Wilson's disease in a significant number of patients. Institution of copper chelation at this stage of Wilson's disease assuredly will prevent serious hepatic or neurologic sequelae if cirrhosis has not yet developed.

ASYMPTOMATIC PATIENTS WITH KAYSER–FLEISCHER RINGS

In an asymptomatic patient in whom a K-F ring is found on routine ophthalmologic examination, a serum ceruloplasmin level should be performed. If it is low or there is high suspicion and it is normal, a 24-hour urine copper excretion should be performed and consideration given to a liver biopsy. Elevated urine copper excretion, a low ceruloplasmin, and a K-F ring establish the diagnosis. However, if the liver or spleen is enlarged or liver blood tests are abnormal, a liver biopsy should be performed.

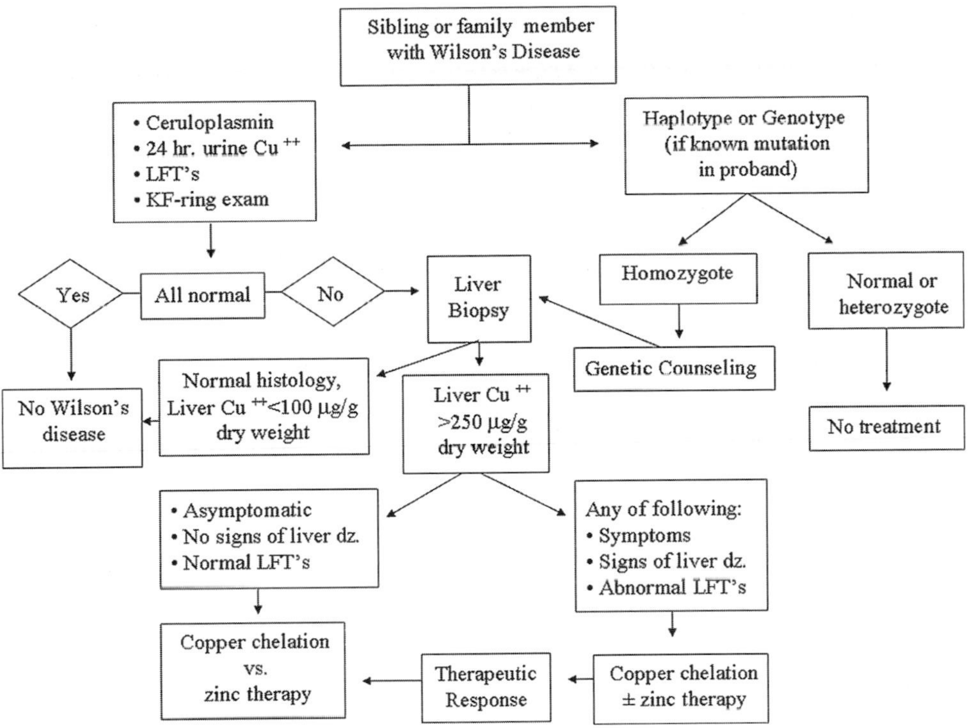

Figure 26.12. Approach to evaluation and treatment of asymptomatic siblings (or other first-degree relatives) of a patient with Wilson's disease. Illustrated are both a "phenotype" and a "genotype" approach to evaluation. LFTs, liver function tests.

ASYMPTOMATIC SIBLINGS OF WILSON'S DISEASE PATIENTS

Asymptomatic siblings and other first-degree relatives of a Wilson's disease patient should be screened for the disease after age 3 or 4 years unless hepatomegaly or abnormal aminotransferase levels are found earlier. A thorough history and physical examination, slit-lamp examination, and laboratory analysis should be performed (Figure 26.12). If all tests are normal, it is very unlikely that the relative has Wilson's disease. However, if any of those tests are abnormal, a liver biopsy should be performed for histology, electron microscopy, and quantitative copper analysis. An alternative, less invasive approach is to evaluate the known patient, the sibling, and the parents for DNA haplotype (microsatellite markers) to determine if the sibling in question has inherited the Wilson's disease gene. Haplotype analysis is informative in over 90–95% of cases. Another approach is to genotype the affected relative and if *ATP7B* mutations are identified, to test the sibling in question for these mutations. Finding two mutations or informative microsatellite markers will establish the diagnosis of Wilson's disease and preclude the need for liver biopsy unless there are signs or symptoms of chronic liver disease.

Treatment

Without treatment, Wilson's disease is uniformly fatal. The hallmark of medical management in Wilson's disease is reducing or chelating the stored copper and preventing copper from reaccumulating. This is accomplished by instituting therapy with one of several copper chelating agents, a low-copper diet, oral zinc, and possibly antioxidants (Table 26.5). Stringent dietary restriction of copper-containing foods is impractical, although it is recommended that patients avoid foods with very high copper content, such as chocolate, nuts, legumes, mushrooms, shellfish, and liver. Domestic water softeners should *not* be used because they may increase copper concentrations in drinking water substantially [261].

Copper Chelation Therapy

Until the 1950s, little effective therapy was available for Wilson's disease. BAL was then introduced and shown to effectively chelate copper [74]; however, daily intramuscular injections limited its usefulness. There are currently three commercially available anticopper agents and a fourth agent that is being used under an Investigational New Drug (IND) application to the U.S. Food and Drug Administration (FDA). These include D-penicillamine, trientine, zinc, and the investigational drug ammonium tetrathiomolybdate. There is only one recently published randomized trial comparing two of these therapies [262]. Published data include primarily single-center experience and combined-center reviews. D-penicillamine has the most published experience because it was the first orally effective drug developed for the treatment of Wilson's disease.

Table 26.5: Medications Used in Treatment of Wilson's Disease

Medication	*Action*	*Dosage*	*Comments*
D-penicillamine	Copper chelator	*Initial*: 20 mg/kg/d (up to 1.5–2.0 g/d), 3 doses per day between meals *Maintenance*: 10–20 mg/kg/d (up to 0.75–1.0 g/d) *Oral pyridoxine*: 25–50 mg/d	Initial and maintenance therapy
Trientine	Copper chelator	Same dose as penicillamine	Same as above
Zinc acetate	Inhibits copper absorption Stimulates hepatic metallothionein	25–50 mg 3 times daily between meals	Slower action than copper chelators Useful for maintenance and during pregnancy
Ammonium tetrathiomolybdate	Inhibits copper absorption Copper chelator	120–200 mg/d	Investigational drug used for limited (6–8 wk) periods of time
Vitamin E	Antioxidant	400–1200 IU/d (2–3 doses per day with meals)	Adjunctive therapy

D-PENICILLAMINE

The paramount work of Walshe [74] clearly demonstrated the benefits of D-penicillamine in Wilson's disease. D-Penicillamine (β-β-dimethylcysteine) is a sulfhydryl-containing metabolite of penicillin that is absorbed well from the gastrointestinal tract, effectively chelates copper, and is then excreted in the urine. The actual mechanism on how this drug works is not known. The major action of penicillamine was originally thought to be a "decoppering effect," although there are conflicting data as to whether D-penicillamine actually reduces total copper content of the liver and other organs. Alternatively, a "detoxification" effect has been proposed [263] in which copper is directly complexed to the drug and induction of metallothionein synthesis occurs [264]. Thus, unbound or "toxic" copper will not be available to injure the liver and central nervous system.

It is recommended to begin the penicillamine therapy with one fourth to half of the desired dose and increase the dose slowly over 1–2 weeks. The dosage for older children and adults is 1 g of penicillamine orally per day in four divided doses given ideally at least 30 minutes before or 2 or more hours after meals [90]. If an overtly ill patient fails to show clinical improvement, the dosage can be increased to 1.5–2.0 g/d. In young children, a dosage of 20 mg/kg/d rounded to the nearest multiple of 250 mg is given ideally in three divided doses. After stabilization, the dose may be divided into two or three daily doses not to be given with meals. D-penicillamine may have an antipyridoxine effect, thus all treated patients should also receive 25–50 mg of pyridoxine daily [90].

During the first month of penicillamine therapy, the patient should be monitored weekly for fever or rash. A complete blood count and platelet count, urinalysis, and renal and liver blood tests should be obtained every 1–2 weeks. If the patient responds appropriately with resolution of symptoms and normalization of liver blood tests, monitoring is performed every 1–3 months for the first year and every 6–12 months thereafter. Abnormalities in liver blood tests may persist for at least a year of treatment; however, the trend should be toward improvement. An annual 24-hour urinary copper excretion is helpful in monitoring chronic penicillamine therapy. Initially, several grams of copper may be excreted in 24 hours; however, after months to years of chelation, as little as 200–500 μg of copper should be excreted per day [90,209]. If urinary copper excretion is less than 200 μg/24 hr, poor compliance with chelation therapy should be suspected. If copper excretion increases suddenly, this suggests a lapse in compliance followed by resumption of penicillamine a few days before the urine collection. Sternlieb and Scheinberg [90] recommend assessing free serum copper as a means of monitoring compliance. To calculate free serum copper, one multiplies the ceruloplasmin concentration (in milligrams per deciliter) by 3, and then subtracts it from the total measured serum copper level (in micrograms per deciliter). Values should be between 5 and 15 μg/dL during effective therapy. Noncompliance is suspected if during chronic therapy the free copper is above 20 μg/dL [96]. Values less than 5 μg/dL should be repeated and, if confirmed, indicate copper deficiency; the dose of penicillamine should be gradually reduced by 25% and the patient monitored closely. For patients in whom K-F rings had been initially detected, serial ophthalmologic examination is helpful in documenting disappearance or significant reduction of these lesions with adequate copper chelation [90]. Serial ophthalmologic examination may also be useful in patients without K-F rings, as the development of rings would also indicate poor compliance. For patients who require higher doses of penicillamine, the dosage may be reduced to 0.75–1.0 g/d once clinical symptoms have resolved [90,93]. If he or she is compliant, penicillamine therapy will maintain the asymptomatic patient in good health [75,90]. Uninterrupted lifelong therapy is mandatory. A yearly discussion with the patient and family should reinforce the importance of compliance. Patients should be reminded of the essential need to take the penicillamine without fail and the possible fatal consequences of discontinuing this therapy suddenly. In one series, 8 of 11 patients who discontinued therapy died of fulminant liver failure within 2.6 years [142].

In 10–50% of patients, neurologic symptoms worsened shortly after penicillamine therapy was started [160,265]. Continued or altered penicillamine therapy generally resulted in reversal of this worsening [90,266], although irreversible neurologic abnormalities have been reported [265]. Thus, it is recommended that the penicillamine dosage be reduced to 250 mg/d if neurologic symptoms worsen and gradually increased every 4–7 days by 250 mg/d until urinary copper excretion exceeds 2000 μg/d [267]. The cause of this neurologic worsening is unknown. Some propose that there is a transient brain exposure to increased blood copper as the penicillamine mobilizes hepatic copper stores [265,268] or that penicillamine may form a complex with intracellular copper that is more toxic [268]. Although this type of neurologic exacerbation is more common with penicillamine, it does not appear to be specific to this agent. Worsening neurologic function has also been reported following initiation of treatment with trientine [269], thiomolybdates [270], and zinc [271], but in lower frequency. A seriously neurologically handicapped patient may respond poorly to penicillamine therapy alone and require combined therapy with BAL [90]. Alternatively, recent data suggest that the investigational drug ammonium tetrathiomolybdate may be a better alternative in patients with neurologic symptoms [262].

The effect of penicillamine therapy on psychiatric disturbances is difficult to predict, although improved school performance is commonly observed in treated children [90]. Liver dysfunction generally improves rapidly (by 2–6 months) with penicillamine therapy; however, if overt fibrosis and cirrhosis are present, the signs of portal hypertension show little response, although histology may gradually improve [242,272–274]. Hepatic copper content generally decreases but may remain quite elevated despite years of therapy and clinical improvement [242,273,274]. Patients with psychiatric disturbances require not only copper chelation therapy but also psychotherapy and appropriate psychotropic medications.

Penicillamine may produce both allergic and toxic side effects in up to 30% of patients. Early side effects of penicillamine include a hypersensitivity reaction manifested as fever, skin rash, lymphadenopathy, and pancytopenia [274]. After the first year of therapy, late toxic reactions include proteinuria, nephrotic syndrome [175], drug-associated systemic lupus erythematosus [275], Goodpasture's syndrome [176], optic neuritis, agranulocytosis, thrombocytopenia, myasthenia gravis, low serum IgA levels, loss of taste, and anaphylactic reactions [90]. The most common late reactions caused by penicillamine are observed in the skin because of the interference with cross-linking of collagen and elastin [276,277]. These include a dermatopathy (cutis laxa) associated with weakening of subcutaneous tissue [276], elastosis perforans serpiginosa [277], lichen planus, aphthous stomatitis, systemic sclerosis-like lesions [278], and pemphigoid lesions in the mouth, vagina, and skin [279]. Rarely, hepatotoxicity [280], hair loss, and dysgeusia have been reported. For treatment of these reactions, penicillamine should be temporarily discontinued until the lesions resolve, and 2 or 3 days before restarting therapy, 0.5 mg/kg/d of prednisone should be started. Penicillamine is then reintroduced at a lower dosage and increased gradually, with weaning of prednisone when the final dose is reached and tolerated [90]. Alternatively, nowadays trientine therapy should be substituted for penicillamine for any significant toxic reaction. If bone marrow toxicity is observed, penicillamine should be immediately withdrawn and trientine substituted. Overall, trientine appears to be associated with a lower frequency of side effects and is recommended by some authorities as a safer initial chelator for Wilson's disease.

Penicillamine therapy is ineffective in patients with fulminant Wilson's disease, in patients who develop hepatic failure after penicillamine therapy has been discontinued, and in those with advanced cirrhosis [90]. These patients rarely will survive unless liver transplantation is performed. As in other patients with fulminant hepatic failure, survival is dependent on intensive care therapy and a rapid evaluation for liver transplantation.

TRIETHYLENE TETRAMINE DIHYDROCHLORIDE (TRIENTINE)

In 1985, trientine was approved by the FDA for patients who are intolerant of penicillamine [76,281]. It does not contain sulfhydryl groups; rather it chelates copper by forming a stable complex with copper through its four nitrogen atoms in a planar ring. It is very effective and some advocate it as an alternative initial copper-chelating drug [209,281,282] primarily because of its better safety profile. The initial dosage for adolescents and adults is 750–1500 mg daily in two to three divided doses before meals. Maintenance therapy is typically 750 or 1000 mg/d. In children, the dose generally used is 20 mg/kg/d rounded off to the nearest 250 mg. The drug appears to be less toxic than penicillamine [209]. The toxicity includes bone marrow suppression (a sideroblastic anemia), nephrotoxicity, and skin and mucosal lesions [76]. Female patients may become iron deficient and require iron supplementation [76]. Initiation of therapy requires a clinical and laboratory assessment and adjustment of doses similar to that for D-penicillamine. Patients are monitored with 24-hour urinary coppers and other laboratory tests as they are for penicillamine. There appears to be no cross-reactivity in toxicity in patients who have toxic reactions to penicillamine.

AMMONIUM TETRATHIOMOLYBDATE

Brewer et al. [283] have proposed an alternative approach to the treatment of Wilson's disease that is based on whether the patient presents with neurologic or hepatic symptoms. Because up to 50% of patients in an earlier series [270] who had neurologic disease showed worsening of their symptoms with penicillamine therapy, Brewer's group proposed using an alternative drug, ammonium tetrathiomolybdate, for initial therapy in neurologically affected patients [283]. This investigational compound acts by forming a stable three-way complex between protein, copper, and itself [282,284–288]. Given with food, it complexes with dietary copper, preventing its absorption, and when taken between meals, it is absorbed and complexes with copper and albumin in blood, preventing cellular uptake and resulting in decreased intracellular copper stores [282]. This drug may exhibit a higher affinity for copper than metallothionein in vitro, providing a rationale for its proposed ability to remove copper from cells [282]. An initial study of 33 neurologically affected patients treated for 8 weeks as initial therapy reported that there was no worsening of neurologic symptoms [282]. After 8 weeks, the drug was stopped and patients were maintained on oral zinc acetate, 50 mg three times a day [282]. Brewer [282] estimated that this drug is extremely fast acting, with copper toxicity essentially halted within 2 weeks of treatment. In a follow-up study with 22 additional patients, the incidence of side effects was slightly higher. Of the 22 patients, 3 dropped out of the study, 2 developed neurologic deterioration, and 5 had bone marrow suppression [289]. Indeed, Walshe [270] pointed out concerns over possible bone marrow suppression and other toxicities of this drug, although he has treated a patient successfully with this drug for 9 years [266].

Recently, a randomized comparison of tetrathiomolybdate and trientine as initial treatment in 48 Wilson's disease patients presenting with neurologic symptoms was conducted. Six in the trientine arm and one in the tetrathiomolybdate arm showed neurologic progression during therapy ($P < 0.05$). Seven receiving tetrathiomolybdate had an adverse event (none of the events was serious; four patients had elevations of aminotransferases), whereas only one patient receiving trientine had an adverse event. These data suggest a possible benefit of tetrathiomolybdate short term for neurologically affected patients. Continued ongoing prospective evaluation of this potential treatment will hopefully yield useful guidelines for its use and more information about possible side effects.

ZINC THERAPY

Zinc has been proposed as maintenance or adjunctive therapy for Wilson's disease [290]. Zinc inhibits intestinal absorption of copper and, possibly, increases metallothionein binding of copper in the liver [291–296]. The dosage of zinc acetate, given between meals, that currently is advocated is 50 mg of elemental zinc three times daily [276] or zinc sulfate, 150–220 mg three times daily [293,295,296]. Common side effects include headache and gastrointestinal upset, which are perhaps less common with zinc acetate. Because of its slower onset of action, zinc therapy is generally not used as initial therapy for symptomatic patients. It is not known whether zinc therapy is beneficial for patients receiving a copper chelator, so it is not recommended as combined therapy. Because chelators bind zinc, giving them together to a patient may interfere with the action of both. Zinc therapy may play a role in presymptomatic patients or siblings. Some authorities suggest that because these children have normal liver blood tests, normal or mildly increased urinary copper excretion, and mild to moderate elevations of hepatic copper, they should not be exposed to the possible side effects of copper chelators [297]. Because these children have not yet accumulated a toxic burden of copper, it is proposed that sole treatment with zinc (1 mg/kg/dose of elemental zinc three times a day between meals) is effective and less toxic. Prospective long-term follow-up of such children under various forms of treatment is needed to establish the safest and most effective manner of treating this enlarging group of patients. Although there are a number of reports of successful maintenance therapy with zinc, it should be used cautiously as a sole agent and patients should be monitored very closely. It should also be stressed that patients have deteriorated and developed fulminant liver failure after the discontinuation of zinc therapy.

Antioxidant Therapy

The role of antioxidants as adjunctive therapy in Wilson's disease has not been thoroughly explored. The basis for this type of therapy is the demonstrated oxidative damage to the hepatocyte in rats with copper overload [61], Bedlington terriers, and patients with Wilson's disease [63]. In addition, Sokol et al. [298] have shown that α-tocopherol (vitamin E) protects isolated rat hepatocytes from the toxicity of in vivo copper loading [298]. Furthermore, hepatic concentrations of antioxidants, such as glutathione and vitamin E [63], are depressed and circulating vitamin E levels are lower in Wilson's disease patients compared with controls. There are several anecdotal reports of patients with liver failure being "rescued" by adjuvant vitamin E therapy in addition to aggressive copper chelation therapy [299]. Vitamin E, 400–1200 IU/d, may be given orally in divided doses with meals safely. Because high-dose vitamin E may interfere with vitamin K–dependent clotting factor synthesis, the prothrombin time should be monitored and vitamin K supplementation used if necessary. Other antioxidants are not currently recommended until further testing is performed.

Liver Transplantation

Orthotopic liver transplantation is well established as a lifesaving therapy in Wilson's disease patients with acute fulminant hepatic failure, those with fulminant hepatic failure after inadvisably discontinuing copper chelation therapy, and those with decompensated cirrhosis unresponsive to medical therapy. A recent survey of 57 patients who received transplants showed a survival rate of 77% at a mean of 2.7 years after transplantation, a poorer outcome in patients with neurologic disease, and disappearance of K-F rings in 18 of 20 patients examined [300]. Neurologic symptoms improved in survivors [301]. In another series of 45 patients who received liver transplants, survival at 5 years was 73%, with a poorer outcome for those with fulminant hepatic failure [302]. Living-related transplantation from heterozygote parent donors has also been shown to be successful [303]. Liver engraftment appears to cure the underlying biochemical defect, making further copper chelation therapy unnecessary.

To better determine the criteria for referral for liver transplantation, Nazer et al. [304] developed a prognostic index based on grading from 1–4 points the serum bilirubin concentration, serum AST, and prolongation of prothrombin time (Table 26.6). Patients with 7 or more of a possible 12 points at presentation had fatal courses or required transplantation,

Table 26.6: Prognostic Index in Fulminant Wilson's Disease

	Score*				
Test	*0*	*1*	*2*	*3*	*4*
Serum bilirubin, μmol/L (mg/dL)†	<100 (<5.9)	100–150 (5.9–8.8)	151–200 (8.9–11.8)	201–300 (11.9–17.5)	>300 (>17.5)
Serum AST, IU/L‡	<100	100–150	151–200	201–300	>300
Prolongation of prothrombin time, sec	<4	4–8	9–12	13–20	>20

*A prognostic total score of 7 or more indicates the need for liver transplantation.
†Normal: 3–20 μmol/L (0.2–1.2 mg/dL).
‡Normal: 7–20 IU/L.
Adapted from Nazer et al. [304], with permission of BMJ Publishing Group.

and those with 6 or fewer points survived with medical therapy alone. Dhawan et al. [305] recently evaluated the validity of this scoring system for pediatric patients by retrospectively reviewing the data from 74 patients who either died or survived on medical management. Using 7 as the cut-off number for death without transplantation, 5 children with a score greater than 7 survived on chelation therapy. Importantly, 4 children who had a score less than 7 died on medical management. This translates into a sensitivity of 87% and a specificity of 90%. The authors developed a new index based on serum bilirubin, INR (international normalized ratio), AST, albumin, and WCC (white cell count) at presentation. A score greater than 11 of a possible 20 was predictive for death, with a 93% sensitivity, 98% specificity, and 88% positive predictive value [305]. The new index was then prospectively evaluated in 14 patients. Four patients were predicted to need transplantation, whereas no patient with a score less than 11 died on medical management [305]. One patient with a score of 11 survived on medical management. This index appears to be more sensitive and specific in predicting mortality without transplantation. If further prospective evaluation of this index proves its validity, it may help to facilitate selection of patients for potential liver transplantation. Currently, there does not appear to be a role for gene transfer therapy in Wilson's disease because of the availability of other effective treatments and the uncertainties of gene therapy.

Special Circumstances

PREGNANCY

During pregnancy, it is advisable to continue penicillamine therapy at a dosage of 750–1000 mg/d, although one authority advises discontinuation during the first 12 weeks of gestation if possible [93]. Several patients who have discontinued therapy for longer periods during pregnancy have had episodes of acute hemolysis or worsening of liver disease [96], including fulminant hepatic failure. Penicillamine has been administered to more than 150 pregnant Wilson's disease patients [305–307], and there have been two cases of neonatal transient cutis laxa [308,309]. However, one infant developed a connective tissue defect [309] although the mother was being treated with penicillamine for cystinuria. The overall risk of miscarriage and fetal abnormalities in infants whose mothers were maintained on D-penicillamine during pregnancy (750–1000 mg/d for the first two trimesters and 500 mg/d for the last trimester) appear to be the same (144 normal neonates in 153 pregnancies) [306] as for those whose mothers received trientine therapy (19 normal neonates in 22 pregnancies) [307] and as for those whose mothers received zinc therapy (24 normal neonates in 26 pregnancies) [310]. Therefore, trientine [307,311] and zinc therapy [306,312] are probably equivalent to penicillamine therapy as far as safety during pregnancy [306]. All children fathered by patients with Wilson's disease have been normal [96]. Although infants may be at a small risk for a connective tissue or skin abnormality during penicillamine therapy, the risk to mother and infant of discontinuing copper chelation therapy appears to be greater [96,313]. If cesarean section is anticipated, some authorities recommend reducing the dose of penicillamine to 250 mg/d 6 weeks before delivery to reduce the risk for impaired wound healing [314].

SURGERY

Penicillamine has inhibitory effects on collagen cross-linking [315]. Therefore, to prevent interference with wound healing, it is recommended that when patients with Wilson's disease undergo surgery, the dose of penicillamine be reduced, but not stopped, for 10–14 days postoperatively.

INDIAN CHILDHOOD CIRRHOSIS AND IDIOPATHIC COPPER TOXICOSIS

There are several additional disorders of hepatic copper toxicosis in childhood. ICC has been a significant cause of mortality in the preschool-aged child in India and neighboring countries. The cause of this toxicosis has been attributed to excess copper exposure from ingestion of contaminated milk or water sources. Liver biopsies of these patients show extraordinarily high levels of hepatic copper, suggesting that copper may be involved in the pathogenesis of this condition [316,317]. Clusters of children living in the Austrian province of Tyrol and in northern Germany and isolated cases from North America and other countries have been described in which the clinical course, hepatic histology, and hepatic copper levels are similar to those in the classic cases from India. These entities have been called endemic Tyrolean infantile cirrhosis and idiopathic copper toxicosis, respectively. They may represent several distinct diseases or the same disease in different populations. Although dietary copper restriction has markedly reduced the number of cases, it is unclear whether excessive intake of copper alone is enough to cause disease. This suggests that there is a second factor contributing to these disorders. Two mechanisms have been suggested for the etiologic role of copper in the development of childhood hepatic toxicosis: (1) copper may act in synergy with a hepatoxin or (2) patients may have a genetic predisposition to copper-associated liver damage (a so-called ecogenetic disease) [318]. Treatment with copper chelation is promising; without treatment, these diseases are invariably fatal. Both ICC and ICT of childhood are discussed.

Indian Childhood Cirrhosis

Epidemiology and Genetics

Indian childhood cirrhosis classically occurs in children 1–3 years of age, but it has occurred up to age 10 years [319]. There is a positive family history in 30% of the cases; however, the genetics have not been well established. ICC has been one of the leading causes of cirrhosis in children in India and was said to be the fourth most common cause of death in pediatric centers in that country [319] before changes in feeding practices that were associated with excessive copper intake. Boys outnumber girls three to one, without discrimination by social class [320]. A striking epidemiologic association discovered in the 1980s was the observation that boiled animal milk stored in brass utensils, which was the common practice in India, has a very high copper concentration and that this copper is bound to casein [321]. Compared with control infants who did not develop ICC, children with ICC who lived in small rural communities were less likely to be exclusively breast-fed, received animal milk earlier, and stopped breast-feeding at a younger age [322,323]. Patients with ICC seemed to have an earlier and larger exposure to milk contaminated with copper leached from brass utensils. However, several other studies dispute these findings. In one study, brass utensils were not used in 46% of 120 cases of ICC [324], although it is possible that water transported in copper utensils may have been a source of contamination [317]. Asymptomatic siblings have also been found to have mild to moderate accumulation of copper but no evidence of liver dysfunction. Thus, it has been proposed that there might be a genetic predisposition to the liver injury in ICC that requires excessive copper intake to lead to disease expression [325,326]. Indeed, family data from a series of cases from Pune, India, showed that 26% of cases were from consanguineous parents, higher than the 13% in children with other liver disorders. The *ATP7B* gene causing Wilson's disease has been excluded in nonwilsonian syndromes [317,327]. A defect in metallothionein synthesis was shown in an American child with an ICC-like illness [328]; however, this defect was not found in three ICC patients or two other ICT patients [329]. Additionally, the *MURR1* gene, responsible for the Bedlington terrier copper toxicosis, has been recently identified [38] and has been excluded as the gene causing nonwilsonian syndromes [39]. Studies to determine the possible genetic linkage for ICC are in progress.

Clinical Features

The clinical presentation of ICC has been divided into three clinical stages [317,320]. In the early stage, anorexia, irritability, and low-grade fever develop and abdominal distention due to an enlarged, smooth liver with a sharp, firm edge is found. During the intermediate stage, jaundice and signs of portal hypertension such as splenomegaly and ascites appear, associated with an increased susceptibility to infection. Progression to cirrhosis takes from 1–8 months in patients. The late stage is characterized by decompensated cirrhosis with jaundice, a shrinking liver, gastrointestinal bleeding, repeated infections, edema, and, finally, hepatic encephalopathy and death.

Serum aminotransferase levels, serum bilirubin, albumin, and coagulation studies follow the expected changes for the various stages of ICC. Renal tubular dysfunction reveals a generalized amino aciduria and the presence of reducing substances. Other characteristic findings include elevated serum immunoglobulin levels, positive smooth muscle antibodies in up to 45% of cases, elevated serum α-fetoprotein level, and low complement levels [317,319,320]. Serum ceruloplasmin and copper levels are normal to elevated [330], distinguishing this disease from Wilson's disease.

The course of decompensation from cirrhosis in untreated patients is rapid. The mortality rate is 45% within 4 weeks of presentation and 86% within 6 months [331]. Occasional children survive longer untreated; however, it is possible that these children suffer from a separate entity. Copper chelation therapy has dramatically changed the natural course of ICC, and changes in storage of milk in India have led to a welcome reduction in the number of cases.

Histopathology

The hepatic histology in ICC shows several distinguishing characteristics [66]: (1) hepatocellular necrosis with prominent Mallory's hyaline, (2) marked pericellular fibrosis throughout the hepatic lobule (*micro*-micronodular cirrhosis), (3) a lack of regenerative nodules, and (4) coarse brown aggregates of copper-associated protein in the hepatocytes (Figures 26.13 through 26.15). The early histologic lesion consists of ballooned hepatocytes reflecting hepatocellular injury, with focal inflammatory cell infiltrates near necrotic hepatocytes [66,320]. For the most part, portal tracts remain uninflamed. Mallory's hyaline affects approximately 15% of the hepatocytes; however, it may be more prominent in rapidly progressive and fatal cases. Hepatic steatosis is characteristically absent. Creeping

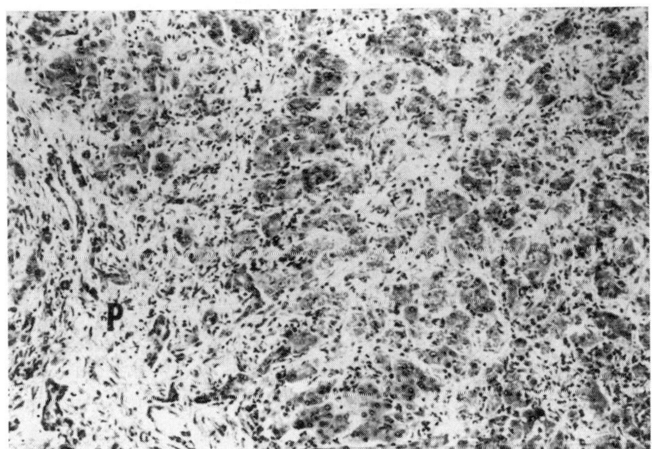

Figure 26.13. Histology of liver in Indian childhood cirrhosis. Low-power view of liver from an American child with features of ICC showing extensive fibrosis throughout the hepatic lobules, entrapment of clusters of hepatocytes, and parenchymal inflammation that includes neutrophils and lymphocytes. P, portal tract. (H&E stain, 150× magnification.) (Used by permission from Sokol RJ. Copper storage diseases. In: Kaplowitz N, ed. Liver and biliary diseases. Baltimore: Williams & Wilkins, 1992:322–33.)

intercellular fibrosis creates the characteristic micro-micronodular cirrhosis that eventually develops as small islands of hepatocytes that are segregated from the rest of the hepatic lobule by fibrosis. Hepatocyte regenerative changes and regenerative nodules are conspicuously absent. Inflammatory infiltrates in the parenchyma and portal tracts are composed mostly of mononuclear cells and some neutrophils around degenerating hepatocytes. Bile ductular proliferation is a constant feature, with variable degrees of hepatocellular and canalicular cholestasis [320].

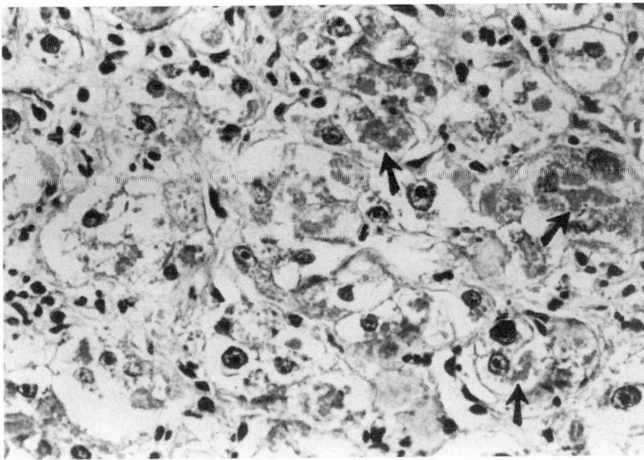

Figure 26.14. Histology of liver in ICC. Hepatocytes are diffusely ballooned, and many contain Mallory bodies (*arrows*). Note the infiltrate of neutrophils and lymphocytes surrounding the hepatocytes. (H&E stain, 600× magnification.) (Used by permission from Sokol RJ. Copper storage diseases. In: Kaplowitz N, ed. Liver and biliary diseases. Baltimore: Williams & Wilkins, 1992:322–33.)

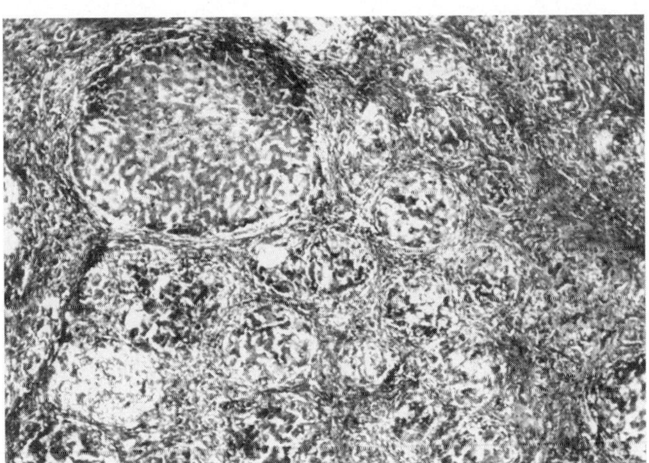

Figure 26.15. Histology of liver in ICC. Low-power micrograph demonstrating the "micro-micronodular" nature of ICC. The majority of nodules are much smaller than normal hepatic lobules. (Masson trichrome stain, 60× magnification.) (Used by permission from Sokol RJ. Copper storage diseases. In: Kaplowitz N, ed. Liver and biliary diseases. Baltimore: Williams & Wilkins, 1992:322–33.)

Increased amounts of hepatocellular copper and copper-associated protein are indicated by appropriate histochemical staining, such as the rhodamine and orcein stains, respectively [66,332]. Glycogen depletion and multinucleated giant cells are characteristic of the advanced cirrhotic lesion. Kupffer cells contain iron and lipofuscin.

Electron microscopy reveals Mallory's hyaline, indistinct mitochondria, and dilated rough endoplasmic reticulum [319, 320,333]. Lysosomal copper is also evident.

Pathogenesis

Many factors have been considered in the pathogenesis of ICC. Although many etiologic agents may lead to liver failure in children in India [334,335], infectious agents have only rarely been associated with ICC [335]. The hepatitis viruses do not play a role in ICC [335]. Aflatoxin, a hepatotoxin produced by the fungus *Aspergillus flavus*, has been implicated because this fungus commonly contaminates grain, nuts, and animal feed in India and appears in cows' milk [336]. In addition, cirrhosis in children has been linked to ingestion of peanuts contaminated by aflatoxin [337]. It has been proposed that in addition to copper in milk, ingestion of a second contaminant, such as aflatoxin, might compound the copper toxicity, leading to cirrhosis [338]; however, there are little data to support its role.

It has also been proposed that synergistic toxicity of pyrrolizidine alkaloids secreted in milk of lactating cows or buffalo may produce liver injury in human infants if the milk is subsequently contaminated with copper [338]. Such a synergy has been demonstrated in sheep [339] and suckling rats [340], with severe liver damage caused by the combination of agents. Although these alkaloids have been more commonly associated with veno-occlusive disease of the liver in the West Indies [341], when administered with excess copper, they increase copper accumulation and toxicity in animals [339]. Although this is an interesting hypothesis, currently, little human data support a role of pyrrolizidine alkaloids in ICC.

A nutritional etiology has not been supported because the liver in ICC lacks steatosis, which is common in nutritional liver disease. The immunologic abnormalities of hypergammaglobulinemia, reduced complement levels, depressed delayed-type hypersensitivity, and reduced T-cell numbers [66] present in ICC probably reflect hepatocellular damage and malnutrition rather than an autoimmune component. The role of chronic ingestion of copper in this disorder is supported by both the high incidence and earlier introduction of animal milk feedings from brass utensils used to heat and store milk, compared with unaffected children [321–323], and the documented increase of milk copper concentration from 11.5–625 μg/dL when milk is heated and stored in this fashion [321].

The liver in ICC has the highest copper levels of any human condition. The average hepatic copper content is approximately 1400 μg/g dry weight of liver, with values reported up to 4788 μg/g liver [316,332]. Furthermore, the intracellular distribution of copper includes diffuse hepatocyte cytoplasmic staining for copper and copper-laden hepatocytes show evidence of severe damage, suggesting that this copper is toxic and involved in the pathogenesis of liver injury [332]. It has been proposed that the excessive copper interferes with the assembly of microtubes, leading to the accumulation of intermediate filaments that constitute the Mallory's hyaline characteristic of ICC and interfering with intracellular transport of secretory proteins, causing ballooning of hepatocytes [332].

Compelling evidence that copper is the cause of liver injury in ICC is derived from studies of both treatment and prevention of ICC. Treatment with D-penicillamine early in the course of the disease reduces mortality [342], improves liver histology [343], reverses cirrhosis [344], and leads to long-term survival [317,345]. In fact, D-penicillamine therapy has been discontinued in a number of children after a mean of 3–5 years of therapy, without recurrence of disease or relapse [345]. Moreover, the recurrence rate of ICC in children born subsequently to families with an index case was significantly reduced in families who received dietary advice to avoid boiling and storing animal milk in brass utensils compared with those not receiving such advice [317,346]. Thus, most experts believe copper is the primary factor in the pathogenesis of liver injury in ICC; however, a genetic defect in copper metabolism or excretion has not been excluded as being a predisposing factor [66].

Diagnosis and Treatment

The diagnosis of ICC is established based on the age of the patient, rapid onset and progression of severe liver disease, absence of other common causes of liver disease, negative serologies for hepatitis viruses, histologic findings on liver biopsy, normal serum ceruloplasmin, and markedly elevated hepatic copper concentration. In a well-conducted controlled trial [342], copper chelation therapy with D-penicillamine in 15 patients with advanced cirrhosis showed no benefit when compared with untreated cases. In 20 children with less advanced disease, that is, no ascites or jaundice, treatment with 20 mg/kg/d of D-penicillamine reduced mortality from 93% to 53% during a treatment period of 1.5 years. Copper concentration in hepatic biopsies decreased dramatically during therapy. Addition of prednisolone therapy did not seem to improve survival beyond D-penicillamine therapy alone. Inasmuch as penicillamine may have other effects besides copper chelation, it is not certain that the copper chelation was the precise means by which the hepatic disease was stabilized or improved, but this seems to be very likely. In another trial of penicillamine, histologic evidence of disease regressed and correlated with clinical recovery [343]. Long-term survival after D-penicillamine therapy (>5 years) was associated with normal growth and development, absence of neurologic abnormalities, reduction of hepatosplenomegaly, and normalization of liver function tests [345]. Liver histology continued to improve and normalized in a number of treated patients [345]. These data support the role of copper in the pathogenesis of ICC and indicate that penicillamine chelation therapy should be instituted in cases in the preicteric phase, before end-stage liver disease is present. In patients with decompensated cirrhosis or those unresponsive to penicillamine, hepatic transplantation should be considered [347]. The use of trientine or other copper chelators or zinc therapy in ICC has not been reported to date. Because copper initiates generation of oxygen free radicals, it is possible that adjuvant antioxidant therapy might be of benefit during copper chelation therapy, although this has not been investigated in ICC.

An important study has validated that prevention of ICC may be possible by the institution of public health measures designed to reduce copper ingestion by infants and young children in India [317]. In this study, decreased use of brass utensils for storage of milk in the Pune district of India as a result of a public health interventional program resulted in a dramatic drop of ICC recurrences in families (1 of 86) compared with older siblings (12 of 125) when no dietary advice was given. In an adjacent district without the public education campaign, the prevalence of ICC was unchanged during the study period. Based on these data, it is clear that children in India and nearby countries should not be fed milk that is boiled or stored in copper-containing vessels, such as those made of brass, particularly if there is a family history of ICC. In non-Indian children with hepatic lesions that resemble ICC, copper metabolism should be investigated, drinking water tested for copper contamination, and therapy instituted with copper chelation therapy. If unresponsive end-stage liver disease ensues, liver transplantation should be performed.

Idiopathic Copper Toxicosis

A growing number of cases of an ICC-like illness have been described in non-Indian infants and young children in Europe, North America, Asia, and the Middle East [348–365]. The clinical course, liver histology, and hepatic copper content of these children most closely resemble those of ICC and are clearly different from those of Wilson's disease. This disorder, or group of disorders, has variably been labeled as idiopathic copper toxicosis [366], copper-associated childhood cirrhosis [358], copper-associated liver disease [359], and non-Indian childhood cirrhosis [351] and may be identical to endemic Tyrolean infantile cirrhosis [364]. Overall, approximately 30 cases have been reported from a variety of countries, a cluster of 138 cases from the Tyrol area of western Austria [364], and a recent cluster of 8 cases from the Emsland area of northern Germany [367,368]. In general, these patients demonstrate an onset of clinical liver disease in the first 2 years of life with a relatively rapidly progressive course to cirrhosis and liver failure. The liver histology is similar to that of ICC, with cytoplasmic Mallory's hyaline and a markedly elevated hepatic copper content greater than 400 μg/g dry weight. In addition, these patients have a normal or elevated serum ceruloplasmin concentration [367].

Clinical Features

The age of onset of reported cases of ICT ranges from 2 months to 10 years. Most cases have an onset in the first 2 years of life; however, several patients have not been identified until age 5 years, with one patient presenting at age 10 years [352]. Clinical features include a distended abdomen and hepatosplenomegaly. Occasionally, patients have fever, lethargy, anemia, malaise, and ascites. Jaundice is rare as an initial symptom. Within several weeks to 1 year, complications of cirrhosis and portal hypertension progress rather rapidly to death, suggesting the presence of compensated cirrhosis before clinical presentation. Patients with ICT come to clinical recognition at an earlier age range than do patients with Wilson's disease. ICT may be confused with other metabolic liver diseases that present at this age with cirrhosis, such as α_1-antitrypsin deficiency and hereditary tyrosinemia.

Diagnostic Testing

The diagnosis of ICT requires a high index of suspicion. A family history of infantile liver disease, use of brass utensils to store milk, and the use of well water or water supplied through old copper plumbing might be clinical clues to this diagnosis; however, these factors are frequently not present. Liver function blood tests are abnormal, consistent with the extent of liver injury and hepatic failure. Serum ceruloplasmin must be normal. Urinary copper excretion is raised [352,358]. Other causes of cholestatic liver disease that may also lead to copper accumulation must be excluded. These include α_1-antitrypsin deficiency, paucity of intralobular bile ducts, progressive familial intrahepatic cholestasis, and autoimmune hepatitis. In some older cases, it may be necessary to perform DNA mutation analysis of *ATP7B* to exclude common mutations for Wilson's disease. Finally, copper incorporation into ceruloplasmin using ^{65}Cu was normal, unlike that found in Wilson's disease, in a patient studied by Horslen et al. [358] and is not useful in establishing the diagnosis of ICT.

Histopathology

Careful examination of the liver reveals the characteristic lesion of ICC. There is micro-micronodular cirrhosis, Mallory's hyaline, pericellular fibrosis, a mixed inflammatory infiltrate, and on histochemical stain, granular copper or copper-associated protein. Early in the clinical course, the liver lesion may be less florid and Mallory's hyaline may be absent. Most importantly, the tissue must be preserved appropriately at the time of biopsy for quantitative copper analysis by an experienced laboratory. Hepatic copper content has usually been greater than 1000 μg/g dry weight but is occasionally in the 400–1000 μg/g range [365,366].

Etiopathogenesis

There is evidence for both a genetic and an environmental component in the etiology of ICT. Cases in Tyrolia [364] and northern Germany [368] had both familial clustering and consanguinity, suggesting an autosomal recessive inheritance. However, expression of ICT in the Tyrolean patients was linked closely to the early introduction of copper-contaminated milk from copper or brass vessels [364], analogous to the suspected etiology of true ICC. Importantly, the Tyrolean endemic cirrhosis disappeared after 1974, when traditional copper cooking utensils were replaced by stainless steel, thus eliminating the excessive copper exposure to infants [364]. Two ICT patients have also been treated successfully with D-penicillamine [358]. These data, coupled with the extraordinarily high hepatic copper levels, leave little doubt that copper toxicity is the major factor causing the liver injury and cirrhosis in ICT. The burning question is whether this is merely an environmental exposure or a genetic predisposition requiring an additional environmental exposure, a so-called ecogenetic disease [364]. As with ICC, both mutations in *ATP7B*, the Wilson's gene, and *MURR1*, the Bedlington terrier gene, have been eliminated as causes of ICT [39,327]. Müller et al. [366] reviewed a number of ICT cases that have been associated with excess copper intake from a domestic water supply suggesting copper toxicity as the sole etiologic factor. However, Scheinberg and Sternlieb [369] evaluated the incidence of deaths from liver disease in children under 6 years of age in three Massachusetts towns with elevated drinking water copper concentrations of 8.5–8.8 mg/L. Representing 64,124 child years, no deaths from liver disease were reported over a 23-year period. In contrast, in six published cases of ICT, the excess copper intake was attributed to the ingestion of drinking water containing up to 6.8 mg/L. Scheinberg and Sternlieb [369] concluded that chronic excess copper intake alone was unlikely the etiology of ICT. The Tyrolean and northern Germany cases, as well as other reported cases with a suggested hereditary influence, strongly suggest a genetic defect exacerbated by a high copper intake during infancy as the etiology of ICT. The candidate gene for ICT has yet to be identified; however, the continued discovery of new proteins involved in cellular copper homeostasis and new genetic techniques, such as homozygosity mapping, should lead to identification of a genetic etiology for ICT.

Treatment

Current treatment of ICT involves establishing an early diagnosis, eliminating excess copper intake, and instituting copper chelation therapy. Evaluation for liver transplantation is indicated if standard criteria for transplantation are met. The water supply of patients should be evaluated for copper content or substituted by bottled distilled drinking water. Brass and copper utensils should not be used to store or administer infant formula, milk, or water. Some advocate for dietary elimination of foods high in copper, such as liver, chocolate, nuts, mushrooms, and shellfish. Consideration should be given to therapy with vitamin E to reduce ongoing oxidant damage until hepatic copper levels are reduced by chelation therapy. Siblings should be screened by liver blood tests, physical examination, and possibly, urinary copper excretion. To assist with identification of the genetic defect in this rare illness, caretakers of newly identified patients should contact current investigators in this field.

ACKNOWLEDGMENTS

This work is supported in part by grants R01-DK38446, U01-DK062453–01, U54 -DK 078377, and M01-R00069 from the National Institutes of Health and the Abbey Bennett Liver Research Fund.

The authors thank Dr. Jay Lefkowitch and Dr. Bruce Beckwith for providing the photomicrographs and Cynthia Wyman for typing this manuscript.

REFERENCES

1. Klevay LM, Sandstead H, Munoz J, et al. The copper requirement of healthy men. Am J Clin Nutr 1978;31:711.
2. Linder MC, Hazegh-Azam M. Copper biochemistry and molecular biology. Am J Clin Nutr 1996;96(suppl):797–811.
3. Weber PM, O'Reilly S, Pollycove M, et al. Gastrointestinal absorption of copper: studies with ^{64}Cu, ^{95}Zr, a whole body counter and the scintillation camera. J Nucl Med 1969;10:591–6.
4. Van Campen DR, Scaife PU. Zinc interference with copper absorption in rats. J Nutr 1967;91:473–6.
5. Gollan JL, Davis PS, Deller DJ. A radiometric assay of copper binding in biological fluids and its application to alimentary secretions in normal subjects and Wilson's disease. Clin Chim Acta 1971;31:197–204.
6. Gollan JL. Studies on the nature of complexes formed by copper with human alimentary secretions and their influence on copper absorption in the rat. Clin Sci Mol Med 1975;49:237.
7. Kirchgessner M, Grassman E. The dynamics of copper absorption. In: Mills CF, ed. Trace element metabolism in animals. Edinburgh: Churchill Livingstone, 1970:277.
8. Chou T-P, Adolph WH. Copper metabolism in man. Biochem J 1935;29:476–9.
9. Moore T, Constable BJ, Day KC, et al. Copper deficiency in rats fed upon raw meat. Br J Nutr 1964;18:135–46.
10. Schmitt RC, Darwish HM, Cheney JC, et al. Copper transport kinetics by isolated rat hepatocytes. Am J Physiol 1983;244: 1–83.
11. Ettinger MJ, Darwish HM, Schmitt RD. Mechanism of copper transport from plasma to hepatocytes. Fed Proc 1986;45: 2800–4.
12. Zhou B, Gitscher J. hCTRI: a human gene for copper uptake identified by complementation in yeast. Proc Natl Acad Sci U S A 1997;94:7481–6.
13. Lee J, Pena M, Nose Y, Thiele D. Biochemical characterization of the human Copper transporter Ctr1. J Biol Chem 2002; 277:4380–7.
14. Harris DIM, Sass-Kortsak A. The influence of amino acids on copper uptake by rat liver slices. J Clin Invest 1967;46:659–67.
15. Klomp LW, Liu SJ, Yuan DS, et al. Identification and functional expression of HAH1, a novel human gene involved in copper homeostasis. J Biol Chem 1997;272:9221–6.
16. Klomp AE, Juijin JA, Vand Der Gun LT, et al. The N-terminus of the human copper transporter 1 (hCTR1) is localized extracellularly, and interacts with itself. Biochem J 2003;370:881–9.
17. Petris MJ, Smith K, Lee J Thiele DJ. Copper-stimulated endocytosis and degradation of the human copper transporter, hCtr1. J Biol Chem 2003;278:9639–46.
18. Cartwright GE, Hodges RE, Gubler CJ, et al. Studies on copper metabolism. XIII. Hepatolenticular degeneration. J Clin Invest 1954;33:1487–501.
19. Canelas HM, De Jorge FG, Tognola WA. Metabolic balances of copper in patients with hepatolenticular degeneration submitted to vegetarian and mixed diets. J Neurol Neurosurg Psychiatry 1967;30:371–3.
20. Turnlung JR, Keyes WR, Anderson HL, et al. Copper absorption and retention in young men at three levels of dietary copper using the stable isotope, ^{65}Cu. Am J Clin Nutr 1989;49:870–8.
21. Harrison MD, Jones CE, Dameron CT. Copper chaperones: function, structure and copper-binding properties. J Biol Inorg Chem 1999;4:145–53.
22. Rae TD, Torres AS, Pufahl RA, O'Halloran TV. Mechanism of Cu;Zn-superoxide dismutase activation by the human metallochaperone hCCS. J Biol Chem 2001;276:5166–76.
23. O'Halloran TV, Culotta VC. Metallochaperones, an intracellular shuttle service for metal ions. J Biol Chem 2000;275:25057–60.
24. Culotta VC, Klomp LW, Strain J, et al. The copper chaperone for superoxide dismutase. J Biol Chem 1997;272:23469–72.
25. Amaravadi R, Glerum DM, Tzagoloff A. Isolation of a cDNA encoding the human homolog of COX17, a yeast gene essential for mitochondrial copper recruitment. Hum Genet 1997;99: 329–33.
26. Portnoy ME, Rosenzweig AC, Roe T, et al. Structure-function analyses of the ATX1 metallochaperone. J Biol Chem 1999;274:15041–5.
27. Sternlieb I, Morell AG, Tucker WD, et al. The incorporation of copper into ceruloplasmin *in vivo*: studies with copper 64 and copper 67. J Clin Invest 1961;40:1834–40.
28. Neifakh SA, Monakhov NK, Shaponshnikov AM, et al. Localization of ceruloplasmin synthesis in human and monkey liver cells and its copper regulation. Experientia 1969;25:337–44.
29. Harris ZL, Klomp LWJ, Gitlin JD. Aceruloplasminemia: an inherited neurodegenerative disease with impairment of iron homeostasis. Am J Clin Nutr 1998;67(suppl):972–7.
30. Frieden E, Hsieh HS. The biological role of ceruloplasmin and its oxidase activity. Adv Exp Med Biol 1976;74:505–29.
31. Barass BC, Coult DB, Pinder RM, et al. Substrate specificity of ceruloplasmin indoles and indole isosteres. Biochem Pharmacol 1973;22:2891.
32. Dormandy TL. Free-radical oxidation and antioxidants. Lancet 1978;1:647–50.
33. Cranfield LM, Gollan JL, White AG, et al. Serum antioxidant activity in normal and abnormal subjects. Ann Clin Biochem 1979;16:299–306.

34. Scheinberg IH, Cook CD, Murphy JA. The concentration of copper and ceruloplasmin in maternal and infant plasma at delivery. J Clin Invest 1954;33:963.
35. Schilsky ML, Sternlieb I. Overcoming obstacles to the diagnosis of Wilson's disease. Gastroenterology 1997;113:350–3.
36. Frommer DJ. Defective biliary excretion of copper in Wilson's disease. Gut 1974;15:125–9.
37. Van Berge Henegouwen GP, Tangedahl TN, Hofmann AF, et al. Biliary secretion of copper in healthy man. Quantitation by an intestinal perfusion technique. Gastroenterology 1977;72: 1228–31.
38. Van De Sluis B, Rothuizen J, Pearson PL, et al. Identification of a new copper metabolism gene by positional cloning in a purebred dog population Hum Mol Genet 2002;11:165–73.
39. Mueller T, Van de Sluis B, Zhernakova A, et al. The canine copper toxicosis gene MURR1 does not cause non-Wilsonian hepatic copper toxicosis. J Hepatol 2003;38:164–8.
40. Tao TY, Liu F, Klomp L, et al. The copper toxicosis gene product Murr1 directly interacts with the Wilson disease protein. J Biol Chem 2003;278:41593–6.
41. Stuehler B, Reichert J, Stemmel W, Schaefer M. Analysis of the human homologue of the canine copper toxicosis gene MURR1 in Wilson disease patients. J Mol Med 2004;82:629–6.
42. Evans J, Newman S, Sherlock S. Liver copper levels in intrahepatic cholestasis of childhood. Gastroenterology 1978;75:875–8.
43. Fleming CR, Dickson ER, Baggenstoss AH, et al. Copper and primary biliary cirrhosis. Gastroenterology 1974;67:1182–7.
44. Evans GW. Copper homeostasis in the mammalian system. Physiol Rev 1973;53:535–70.
45. Ryden L, Deutsch HF. Preparation and properties of the major copper-binding component in human fetal liver. J Biol Chem 1978;253:519–24.
46. Sternlieb I. Copper and the liver. Gastroenterology 1980;78: 1615–28.
47. Sass-Kortsak A. Copper metabolism. Adv Clin Chem 1965;8: 1–67.
48. Dameron CT, Harrison MD. Mechanisms for protection against copper toxicity. Am J Clin Nutr 1998;67(suppl):1091–7.
49. Twedt DC, Sternlieb I, Gilbertson SR. Clinical morphologic, and chemical studies on copper toxicosis of Bedlington terriers. J Am Vet Med Assoc 1979;175:269–75.
50. Porter H. Copper proteins in brain and liver in normal subjects and in cases of Wilson's disease. In: Bergsma D, Scheinberg IH, Sternlieb I, eds. Wilson's disease. Birth defects original article series. Vol. 4. New York: National Foundation–March of Dimes, 1968:23.
51. Reed GB, Butt EM, Landing BH. Copper in childhood liver disease. A histologic, histochemical and chemical survey. Arch Pathol 1972;93:249–55.
52. Walshe JM. Copper: its role in the pathogenesis of liver disease. Semin Liver Dis 1984;4:252–63.
53. Ishmael J, Gopinath C, Howell JM. Experimental chronic copper toxicity in sheep. Histological and histochemical changes during the development of lesions in the liver. Res Vet Sci 1971;12:358.
54. Sternlieb I, Twedt DC, Johnson GF, et al. Inherited copper toxicity of the liver in Bedlington terriers. Proc R Soc Med 1977;70(suppl 3):8–9.
55. Su L-C, Owen CA, Zollman PE, et al. A defect of biliary excretion of copper in copper-laden Bedlington terriers. Am J Physiol 1982;243:G231–6.
56. Wallin M, Larsson H, Edstrom A. Tubulin sulfhydryl groups and polymerization *in vitro*. Effects of di- and trivalent cations. Exp Cell Res 1977;107:219–25.
57. Aust SD, Morehouse LA, Thomas CE. Role of metals in oxygen radical reactions. Free Rad Biol Med 1985;1:3–25.
58. Parola M, Robino G, Marra F, et al. HNE interacts directly with JNK isoforms in human hepatic stellate cells. J Clin Invest 1998;102:1942–50.
59. Lee KS, Buck M, Houglum K, et al. Activation of hepatic stellate cells by TGF alpha and collagen type I is mediated by oxidative stress through c-myb expression. J Clin Invest 1995;96:2461–8.
60. Meyers BM, Kuntz SM, LaRusso NF. Alterations in the structure and physical properties of hepatic lysosomes in experimental metal overload [abstract]. Hepatology 1987;7:1045.
61. Sokol RJ, Devereaux M, Mierau GW, et al. Oxidant injury to hepatic mitochondrial lipids in rats with dietary copper overload. Modification by vitamin E deficiency. Gastroenterology 1990;99:1061–71.
62. Sokol RJ. Abnormal hepatic mitochondrial respiration and cytochrome C oxidase activity in rats with copper overload. Gastroenterology 1993;105:178–87.
63. Sokol RJ, Twedt D, McKim JM Jr, et al. Oxidant injury to hepatic mitochondria in patients with Wilson's disease and Bedlington terriers with copper toxicosis. Gastroenterology 1994;107:1788–98.
64. Mansouri A, Gaou I, Fromenty B, et al. Premature oxidative aging of hepatic mitochondrial DNA in Wilson's disease. Gastroenterology 1997;113:599–605.
65. Sternlieb I. Mitochondrial and fatty changes in hepatocytes of patients with Wilson's disease. Gastroenterology 1968;55:354–67.
66. Joshi VV. Indian childhood cirrhosis. Perspect Pediatr Pathol 1987;11:175–92.
67. Coppen DE, Richardson DE, Cousins RJ. Zinc suppression of free radicals in cultures of rat hepatocytes by iron, t-butyl hydroperoxide, and 3-methylindole. Proc Soc Exp Biol Med 1988;189:100–9.
68. Strand S, Hofmann WJ, Grambihler A, et al. Hepatic failure and liver cell damage in acute Wilson's disease involve CD95 (APO-1/Fas) mediated apoptosis. Nat Med 1998;4:588–93.
69. Yamate J, Kumagai D, Tsujino K, et al. Macrophage populations and apoptotic cells in the liver before spontaneous hepatitis in Long-Evans Cinnamon (LEC) rats. J Comp Pathol 1999;120:333–46.
70. Wilson AK. Progressive lenticular degeneration: a familial nervous disease associated with cirrhosis of the liver. Brain 1912;34:295.
71. Hall HC. La degenerescence hepato-lenticulaire: maladie de Wilson pseudo-sclerose. Paris: Masson, 1921:190.
72. Cumings JN. The copper and iron content of brain and liver in the normal and in hepatolenticular degeneration. Brain 1948;71:410–15.
73. Scheinberg IH, Gitlin D. Deficiency of ceruloplasmin in patients with hepatolenticular degeneration (Wilson's disease). Science 1952;116:484–5.
74. Walshe JM. Penicillamine, a new oral therapy for Wilson's disease. Am J Med 1956;21:487–95.
75. Sternlieb I, Scheinberg IH. Prevention of Wilson's disease in asymptomatic patients. N Engl J Med 1968;278:352–4.
76. Walshe JM. Treatment of Wilson's disease with trientine (triethylene tetramine) dihydrochloride. Lancet 1982;1:643–7.

77. Sternlieb I. Wilson's disease: indications for liver transplantation. Hepatology 1984;4(suppl):15–17.
78. Bowcock AM, Farrer LA, Hebert JM, et al. Eight closely linked loci place the Wilson's disease locus within 13q14-q21. Am J Hum Genet 1988;43:664–74.
79. Honwen RHJ, Roberts EA, Thomas GR, et al. DNA markers for the diagnosis of Wilson's disease. J Hepatol 1993;17:269–76.
80. Frydman M, Bonn-Tamir B, Farrer LA, et al. Assignment of the gene for Wilson's disease to chromosome 13: linkage to the esterase D locus. Proc Natl Acad Sci U S A 1985;82:1819–21.
81. Bowcock AM, Farrer LA, Cavalli-Sforza LL, et al. Mapping the Wilson disease locus to a cluster of linked polymorphic markers on chromosome 13. Am J Hum Genet 1987;14:27–35.
82. Petrukhin K, Fischer SG, Pirastu M, et al. Mapping, cloning and genetic characterization of the region containing the Wilson disease gene. Nat Genet 1993;5:338–43.
83. Bull PC, Thomas GR, Rommens JM, et al. The Wilson's disease gene is a putative copper transporting P-type ATPase similar to the Menkes' gene. Nat Genet 1993;5:327–37.
84. Yamaguchi Y, Heiny ME, Gitlin JD. Isolation and characterization of a human liver cDNA as a candidate gene for Wilson's disease. Biochem Biophys Res Commun 1993;197:271–7.
85. Tanzi RE, Petrukhin K, Chernov I, et al. The Wilson's disease gene is a copper transporting ATPase with homology to the Menkes' disease gene. Nat Genet 1993;5:344–50.
86. Vandarwarf SM, Cooper MLJ, Stetsenko IV, et al. Copper specifically regulates intracellular phosphorylation of the Wilson's disease protein, a human copper-transporting ATPase. J Biol Chem 2001;276:36289–94.
87. Schaefer M, Gitlin JD. Genetic disorders of membrane transport. IV. Wilson's disease and Menkes disease. Am J Physiol 1999;276:G311–14.
88. Lutsenko S, Petris MJ. Function and regulation of the mammalian copper-transporting ATPases: insights from biochemical and cell biological approaches. J Membr Biol 2003;191: 1–12.
89. Cater MA, Forges J, LaFontaine S et al. Intracellular trafficking of the human Wilson protein: the role of the six N-terminal metal-binding sites. Biochem J 2004;380:805–13.
90. Scheinberg IH, Sternlieb I, eds. Wilson's disease. Philadelphia: WB Saunders, 1984.
91. Ala A, Borjigin J, Rochwarger A, Schilsky M. Wilson disease in septuagenarian siblings: Raising the bar for diagnosis. Hepatology 2005;41:668–70.
92. Wilson DC, Phillips MJ, Cox DW, Roberts EA. Severe hepatic Wilson's disease in preschool-aged children. J Pediatr 2000;137:719–22.
93. Walshe JM. The liver in Wilson's disease (hepatolenticular degeneration). In: Schiff L, Schiff ER, eds. Diseases of the liver. Philadelphia: JB Lippincott, 1982:1037–50.
94. Tumer Z, Moller LB, Horn N. Mutation spectrum of ATP7A, the gene defective in Menkes' disease. Adv Exp Med Biol 1999; 448:83–95.
95. Shah AB, Chernov I, Zhang HT, et al. Wilson's disease gene (ATP7B): population frequencies, genotype-phenotype correlation, and functional analysis. Am J Hum Genet 1997;61:317–28.
96. Maier-Dobersberger T, Mannhalter C, Rack S, et al. Diagnosis of Wilson's disease in an asymptomatic sibling by DNA linkage analysis. Gastroenterology 1995;109:2015–18.
97. Maier-Dobersberger T, Ferenci P, Polli C, et al. Detection of the His1069G/n mutations in Wilson's disease by rapid polymerase chain reaction. Ann Intern Med 1997;127:21–6.
98. Matthews WB. The absorption and excretion of radiocopper in hepatolenticular degeneration (Wilson's disease). J Neurol Neurosurg Psychiatry 1954;17:242–6.
99. Beam AG, Kunkel HG. Metabolic studies in Wilson's disease using Cu. J Lab Clin Med 1955;45:623.
100. Sternlieb I, Scheinberg IH. Radiocopper in diagnosing liver disease. Semin Nucl Med 1972;2:176–88.
101. Strickland GT, Beckner WM, Leu M-L. Absorption of copper in homozygotes and heterozygotes for Wilson's disease and controls: isotope tracer studies with ^{61}Cu and ^{64}Cu. Clin Sci 1972;43:617–25.
102. Gibbs K, Walshe JM. Biliary excretion of copper in Wilson's disease. Lancet 1980;2:538–9.
103. Sternlieb I, Van den Hamer CJ, Morell AG, et al. Lysosomal defect of hepatic copper excretion in Wilson's disease (hepatolenticular degeneration). Gastroenterology 1973;64:99–105.
104. Koschinsky ML, Funk WD, Vanoost BA, et al. Complete cDNA sequence of human preceruloplasmin. Proc Natl Acad Sci U S A 1986;83:5086–90.
105. Czaja MJ, Weiner FR, Schwarzenberg SJ, et al. Molecular studies of ceruloplasmin deficiency in Wilson's disease. J Clin Invest 1987;80:1200–4.
106. Gitlin JD. Aceruloplasminemia. Pediatr Res 1998;44:271–6.
107. Logan JI, Harveyson KB, Wisdom GB, et al. Hereditary ceruloplasmin deficiency, dementia, and diabetes mellitus. Q J Med 1994;87:663–70.
108. Harris ZL, Durley AP, Man TK, et al. Targeted gene disruption reveals an essential role for ceruloplasmin in cellular iron efflux. Proc Natl Acad Sci U S A 1999;96:10812–17.
109. Gibbs K, Walshe JM. A study of the ceruloplasmin concentrations found in 75 patients with Wilson's disease. Their kinships and various control groups. Q J Med 1979;48:447–63.
110. Steindl P, Ferenci P, Dienes HP, et al. Wilson's disease in patients presenting with liver disease: a diagnostic challenge. Gastroenterology 1997;113:212–18.
111. Stremmel W, Meyerrose K-W, Niederau C, et al. Wilson's disease: clinical presentation, treatment, and survival. Ann Intern Med 1991;115:720–6.
112. Oder W, Grimm G, Kollegger H, et al. Neurological and neuropsychiatric spectrum of Wilson's disease: a prospective study of 45 cases. J Neurol 1991;238:281–7.
113. Scheinberg IH, Sternlieb I. The long-term management of hepatolenticular degeneration. Am J Med 1960;29:316–33.
114. Wu J, Forbes JR, Shiene Chen H, et al. The LEC rat has a deletion in the copper transporting ATPase gene homologous to the Wilson's disease gene. Nat Genet 1994;7:541–5.
115. Schilsky ML, Stockert RJ, Sternlieb I. Pleiotropic effect of the LEC mutation: a rodent model of Wilson's disease. Am J Physiol 1994;266:G907–13.
116. Tao YT, Gitlin JD. Hepatic copper metabolism: insights from genetic disease. Hepatology 2003;37:1241–7.
117. Nagano K, Nakamura K, Urakami KI, et al. Intracellular distribution of the Wilson's disease gene product (ATPase 7B) after *in vitro* and *in vivo* exogenous expression in hepatocytes from the LEC rat, an animal model of Wilson's disease. Hepatology 1998;27:799–807.

118. Forbes JR, His G, Cox DW. Role of the copper-binding domain in the copper transport function of ATP7B proteins. Hum Mol Genet 2000;9:127–35.
119. Harry J, Tripathi R. Kayser-Fleischer ring: a pathologic study. Br J Ophthalmol 1980;54:794–800.
120. Johnson RE, Campbell RJ. Wilson's disease. Electron microscopic, x-ray energy spectroscopic, and atomic absorption spectroscopic studies of corneal copper deposition and distribution. Lab Invest 1982;46:564–9.
121. Wiebers DO, Hollenhorst RW, Goldstein NP. The ophthalmologic manifestations of Wilson's disease. Mayo Clin Proc 1977;52:409–16.
122. Demirkiran M, Jankovic J, Lewis RA, Cox DW. Neurologic presentation of Wilson Disease without Kayser-Fleischer rings. Neurology 1996;46:1040–3.
123. Fleming CR, Dickson ER, Hollenhorst RW, et al. Pigmented corneal rings in a patient with primary biliary cirrhosis. Gastroenterology 1975;69:220–5.
124. Fleming CR, Dickson ER, Walmer HW, et al. Pigmented corneal rings in non-Wilsonian liver disease. Ann Intern Med 1977;86:285–8.
125. Jones EA, Rabin L, Buckley CH, et al. Progressive intrahepatic cholestasis of infancy and childhood. A clinicopathological study of a patient surviving to the age of 18 years. Gastroenterology 1976;71:675–82.
126. Rimola A, Bruguera M, Rodes J. Kayser-Fleischer–like rings in cryptogenic cirrhosis. Arch Intern Med 1978;138:1857–8.
127. Kaplinsky C, Sternlieb I, Javitt N, et al. Familial cholestatic cirrhosis associated with Kayser-Fleischer rings. Pediatrics 1980; 65:782–8.
128. Dunn LL, Annable WL, Kliegman RM. Pigmented corneal rings in neonates with liver disease. J Pediatr 1987;110:771–6.
129. Cairns JE, Williams BP, Walshe JM. "Sunflower cataract" in Wilson's disease. BMJ 1969;3:95–6.
130. Rosenthal AR, Marmor MF, Levenberger PL. Chalcosis: a study of natural history. Ophthalmology 1979;86:1956–72.
131. Silverberg M, Gellis SS. The liver in juvenile Wilson's disease. Pediatrics 1962;30:402–13.
132. Chalmers TC, Iber FL, Uzman LL. Hepatolenticular degeneration (Wilson's disease) as a form of idiopathic cirrhosis. N Engl J Med 1957;256:235–42.
133. Sokol RJ, Francis PO, Gold SH, et al. Orthotopic liver transplantation for acute fulminant Wilson's disease. J Pediatr 1985; 107:549–52.
134. Forbes JR, Cox DW. Functional characterization of missense mutations in ATP7B: Wilson's disease mutation or normal variant? Am J Hum Genet 1998;63:1663–74.
135. Kraut JR, Yogev R. Fatal fulminant hepatitis with hemolysis in Wilson's disease. Clin Pediatr 1984;23:637–40.
136. Adler R, Mahnovski V, Heuser ET, et al. Fulminant hepatitis: a presentation of Wilson's disease. Am J Dis Child 1977;131:870–2.
137. Roche-Sicot J, Benhamou J-P. Acute intravascular hemolysis and acute liver failure associated as a first manifestation of Wilson's disease. Ann Intern Med 1977;86:301–3.
138. Harnlyn AN, Gollan JL, Douglas AP, et al. Fulminant Wilson's disease with haemolysis and renal failure: copper studies and assessment of dialysis regimens. BMJ 1977;2:660–3.
139. Vielhauer W, Eckadt V, Holtertnuller KH, et al. D-penicillamine in Wilson's disease presenting as acute liver failure and hemolysis. Dig Dis Sci 1982;27:1126–9.
140. Doering EJ, Savage RA, Dittmer TE. Hemolysis, coagulation defects, and fulminant hepatic failures: a presentation of Wilson's disease. Am J Dis Child 1979;133:440–1.
141. McCullough AJ, Wiesner RH, Fleming CR, et al. Antemortem diagnosis and short-term survival of a patient with Wilson's disease presenting as fulminant hepatic failure. Dig Dis Sci 1984;9:862–4.
142. Scheinberg IH, Jaffe ME, Sternlieb I. The use of trientine in preventing the effects of interrupting penicillamine therapy in Wilson's disease. N Engl J Med 1987;317:209–13.
143. Walshe JM, Dixon AK. Dangers of non-compliance in Wilson's disease. Lancet 1986;1:845–7.
144. Sternlieb I, Scheinberg IH. Chronic hepatitis as a first manifestation of Wilson's disease. Ann Intern Med 1972;76:59–64.
145. Perman JA, Werlin SL, Grand RJ, et al. Laboratory measures of copper metabolism in the differentiation of chronic active hepatitis and Wilson's disease in children. J Pediatr 1979;94:564–8.
146. Schilsky ML, Scheinberg IH, Sternlieb I. Prognosis of Wilsonian chronic active hepatitis. Gastroenterology 1991;100:762–7.
147. Scott J, Gollan JL, Samourian S, et al. Wilson's disease presenting as chronic active hepatitis. Gastroenterology 1978;74:645–51.
148. Santus-Silva EE, Sarles J, Buts JP, et al. Successful medical treatment of severely decompensated Wilson's disease. J Pediatr 1996;128:285–7.
149. Czaja AJ. Natural history, clinical features, and treatment of autoimmune hepatitis. Semin Liver Dis 1984;4:1–12.
150. Lashner BA, Jones RB, Tang HS, et al. Chronic hepatitis: disease factors at diagnosis predictive of mortality. Am J Med 1988;85:609–14.
151. Taylor WJ, Jackson EC, Jensen WN. Wilson's disease, portal hypertension and extrahepatic vascular obstruction. N Engl J Med 1959;260:1160–4.
152. Strickland GT, Chang NK, Beckner WM. Hypersplenism in Wilson's disease. Gut 1972;13:220–4.
153. Sternlieb I, Scheinberg IH, Walshe JM. Bleeding esophageal varices in patients with Wilson's disease. Lancet 1970;1:638–41.
154. Rosenfield N, Grand RJ, Watkins JB, et al. Cholelithiasis and Wilson's disease. J Pediatr 1978;92:210–13.
155. Walshe JM, Waldenstrom E, Sams V, et al. Abdominal malignancies in patients with Wilson's disease. Q J Med 2003;96:657–62.
156. Lau JYN, Lai CL, Wu PC, et al. Wilson's disease: 35 years' experience. Q J Med 1990;75:597–605.
157. Strickland GT, Frommer D, Leu M-L, et al. Wilson's disease in the United Kingdom and Taiwan. I. General characteristics of 142 cases and prognosis. II. A genetic analysis of 88 cases. Q J Med 1973;42:619–38.
158. Saito T. Presenting symptoms and natural history of Wilson's disease. Eur J Pediatr 1987;146:261–5.
159. Oder W, Prayer L, Grimm G, et al. Wilson's disease: evidence of subgroups derived from clinical findings and brain lesions. Nature 1993;43:120–4.
160. Starosta-Rubinstein S, Young A, Kluin K, et al. Clinical assessment of 31 patients with Wilson's disease. Correlations with structural changes on magnetic resonance imaging. Arch Neurol 1987;44:365–70.
161. Park RHR, McCabe P, Fell GS, et al. Wilson's disease in Scotland. Gut 1991;32:1541–5.
162. Walshe JM, Gibbs KR. Brain copper in Wilson's disease. Lancet 1987;2:1030.

163. Medalia A, Isaacs-Glaberman K, Scheinberg IH. Neuropsychological impairment in Wilson's disease. Arch Neurol 1988; 45:502–4.
164. Dening TR, Berrios GE, Walshe JM. Wilson's disease and epilepsy. Brain 1988;111:1139–55.
165. Goldstein NP, Ewert JC, Randall RV, et al. Psychiatric aspects of Wilson's disease (hepatolenticular degeneration): results of psychometric tests during long term therapy. Am J Psychiatry 1968;124:1555–61.
166. Scheinberg IH, Sternlieb I, Richman J. Psychiatric manifestations in patients with Wilson's disease. Birth Defects (Original Article Series) 1968;4:85.
167. Dening TR, Berrios GE. Wilson's disease: clinical groups in 400 cases. Acta Neurol Scand 1989;80:527–34.
168. Uzman LL, Denny-Brown D. Amino-aciduria in hepatolenticular degeneration (Wilson's disease). Am J Med Sci 1948;215:599.
169. Beam AG, Tu TF, Gutman AB. Renal function in Wilson's disease. J Clin Invest 1957;36:1107.
170. Leu M-L, Strickland GT, Gutman RA. Renal function in Wilson's disease: response to penicillamine therapy. Am J Med Sci 1970;260:381–98.
171. Fulop M, Sternlieb I, Scheinberg IH. Defective urinary acidification in Wilson's disease. Ann Intern Med 1968;68: 770–7.
172. Wiebers DO, Wilson DM, McLeod RA, et al. Renal stones in Wilson's disease. Am J Med 1979;67:249–54.
173. Wilson DM, Goldstein NP. Bicarbonate excretion in Wilson's disease (hepatolenticular degeneration). Mayo Clin Proc 1974; 49:394–400.
174. Walshe JM. Effect of penicillamine on failure of renal acidification in Wilson's disease. Lancet 1968;1:775–8.
175. Adams DA, Goldman R, Maxwell MH, et al. Nephrotic syndrome associated with penicillamine therapy of Wilson's disease. Am J Med 1964;36:330–6.
176. Sternlieb I, Bennett B, Scheinberg IH. D-penicillamine induced Goodpasture's syndrome in Wilson's disease. Ann Intern Med 1975;82:673–6.
177. McIntyre N, Clink HM, Levi AG, et al. Hemolytic anemia in Wilson's disease. N Engl J Med 1967;276:439.
178. Iser JH, Stevens BJ, Stening GF, et al. Hemolytic anemia of Wilson's disease. Gastroenterology 1974;67:290–3.
179. Deiss A, Lee GR, Cartwright GE. Hemolytic anemia in Wilson's disease. Ann Intern Med 1970;73:413–18.
180. Forman SJ, Kumar KS, Redeker AG, et al. Hemolytic anemia in Wilson's disease: clinical findings and biochemical mechanisms. Am J Hematol 1980;9:269–75.
181. Owen CA Jr, Goldstein NP, Bowie EJ. Platelet function and coagulation in patients with Wilson's disease. Arch Intern Med 1976;136:148–52.
182. Hoagland HC, Goldstein NP. Hematologic (cytopenic) manifestations of Wilson's disease (hepatolenticular degeneration). Mayo Clin Proc 1978;53:498.
183. Factor SM, Cho S, Sternlieb I, et al. The cardiomyopathy of Wilson's disease. Myocardial alterations in nine cases. Virchows Arch [A] 1982;397:301–11.
184. Kuan P. Cardiac Wilson's disease. Chest 1987;91:579–83.
185. Walshe JM. Wilson's disease. The presenting symptoms. Arch Dis Child 1962;37:253–6.
186. Mindelzun R, Elkin M, Scheinberg IH, et al. Skeletal changes in Wilson's disease: a radiological study. Radiology 1970;94:127–32.
187. Feller ER, Schumacher BR. Osteoarticular changes in Wilson's disease. Arthritis Rheum 1972;15:259–66.
188. Golding DN, Walshe JM. Arthropathy of Wilson's disease. Study of clinical and radiological features in 32 patients. Ann Rheum Dis 1977;36:99–111.
189. Menerey KA, Eider W, Brewer GJ, et al. The arthropathy of Wilson's disease: clinical and pathologic features. J Rheumatol 1988;15:331–7.
190. Yu-Zhang X, Xue-Zhe Z, Xian-Hao X, et al. Radiologic study of 42 cases of Wilson's disease. Skel Radiol 1985;13:114–19.
191. Leu ML, Strickland T, Wang CC, et al. Skin pigmentation in Wilson's disease. JAMA 1970;211:1542–3.
192. Bearn AG, McKusick VA. Azure lunale. An unusual change in the fingernails in two patients with hepatolenticular degeneration (Wilson's disease). JAMA 1958;166:904–6.
193. Kaushansky A, Frydman M, Kaufman H, et al. Endocrine studies of the ovulatory disturbances in Wilson's disease (hepatolenticular degeneration). Fertil Steril 1987;47:270–3.
194. Frydman M, Kauschansky A, Bonne-Tamir B, et al. Assessment of the hypothalamic-pituitary-testicular function in male patients with Wilson's disease. J Androl 1991;12:180–4.
195. Johansen K, Gregersen G. Glucose intolerance in Wilson's disease. Normalization after treatment with penicillamine. Arch Intern Med 1972;129:587–90.
196. Sulochana G, Viswanathan J. Wilson's disease with associated diabetes mellitus presenting as renal tubular acidosis. J Assoc Phys India 1982;30:405–7.
197. Lankisch G, Kaboth U, Koop H. Involvement of the exocrine pancreas in Wilson's disease? Klin Wochenschr 1978;56:969.
198. Carpenter TO, Cames DL, Anast CS. Hypoparathyroidism in Wilson's disease. N Engl J Med 1983;309:873–7.
199. McCullough AJ, Fleming CR, Thistle JL, et al. Diagnosis of Wilson's disease presenting as fulminant hepatic failure. Gastroenterology 1983;84:161–7.
200. Berman DH, Leventhal RI, Gavaler JS, et al. Clinical differentiation of fulminant Wilsonian hepatitis from other causes of hepatic failure. Gastroenterology 1991;100:1129–34.
201. Shaver WA, Bhatt H, Combes B. Low serum alkaline phosphatase activity in Wilson's disease. Hepatology 1986;6:859–63.
202. Willson RA, Clayson KJ, Leon S. Unmeasurable serum alkaline phosphatase activity in Wilson's disease associated with fulminant hepatic failure and hemolysis. Hepatology 1987;7:613–18.
203. Ogihara H, Ogihara T, Miki M, et al. Plasma copper and antioxidant status in Wilson's disease. Pediatr Res 1995;37:219–26.
204. Ferenci P, Caca K, Loudianos G, et al. Diagnosis and phenotypic classification of Wilson disease. Liver Int 2003;23:139–42.
205. Edwards CQ, Williams DM, Cartwright GE. Hereditary hypoceruloplasminemia. Clin Genet 1979;15:311–16.
206. DaCosta CM, Baldwin D, Portmann B, et al. Value of urinary copper excretion after penicillamine challenge in the diagnosis of Wilson's disease. Hepatology 1992;15:609–15.
207. Frommer DJ. Urinary copper excretion and hepatic copper concentrations in liver disease. Digestion 1981;21:169–78.
208. Sanchez-Albisua I, Garde T, Hierro L, et al. A high index of suspicion: the key to an early diagnosis of Wilson's disease in childrenood. J Pediatr Gastroenterol Nutr 1999;28:186–90.
209. Roberts EA, Schilsky ML. A practice guideline on Wilson disease. Hepatology 2003;37:1475–92.
210. Martins da Costa C, Baldwin D, Protmann B, et al. Value of urinary copper excretion afrter penicillamine challenge in the diagnosis of Wilson's disease. Hepatology 1991;15:609–15.

211. Gregorio GV, Mieli-Vergani G. Urinary copper excretion after penicillamine challenge in children with prolonged hepatitis A infection. Hepatology 1993;18:706–7.
212. Sternlieb I. Diagnosis of Wilson's disease. Gastroenterology 1978;74:787–9.
213. Matsuda I, Pearson T, Holtzman NA. Determination of apoceruloplasmin by radioimmunoassay in nutritional copper deficiency, Menkes' kinky hair syndromes, Wilson's disease and umbilical cord blood. Pediatr Res 1976;8:821–4.
214. Smallwood RA, Williams HA, Rosenoer VM et al. Liver copper levels in liver disease: studies using neutron activation analysis. Lancet 1968;2:1310–13.
215. Ferenci P, Steindl-Munda P, Vogel W, et al. Diagnostic value of quantitative hepatic copper determination in patients with Wilson's disease. Clin Gastroenterol Hepatol. 2005;3:811–18.
216. Sternlieb I, Scheinberg IH. The role of radiocopper in the diagnosis of Wilson's disease. Gastroenterology 1979;77:138–42.
217. Sternlieb I, Morell AG, Bauer CD, et al. Detection of the heterozygous carrier of the Wilson's disease gene. J Clin Invest 1961;40:707–15.
218. Cossu P, Pirastu M, Nucaro A, et al. Prenatal diagnosis of Wilson's disease by analysis of DNA polymorphisms. N Engl J Med 1992;327:57.
219. Sternlieb I. The outlook for the diagnosis of Wilson's disease. J Hepatol 1993;17:263–4.
220. Gollan JL, Gollan TJ. Wilson disease in 1998: genetic, diagnostic and therapeutic aspects. J Hepatol 1998;28:28–36.
221. Dixon AK, Walshe JM. Computed tomography of the liver in Wilson's disease. J Comput Assist Tomogr 1984;8:46–9.
222. Smevik B, Ritland S, Nilsen T, et al. Liver attenuation values at computed tomography related to liver copper content. Scand J Gastroenterol 1982;17:461–3.
223. Lawler GA, Pennock JM, Steiner RE, et al. Nuclear magnetic resonance (NMR) imaging in Wilson's disease. J Comput Assist Tomogr 1983;7:1–8.
224. Frommer DJ. Direct measurement of serum non-ceruloplasmin copper in liver disease. Clin Chim Acta 1976;68:303–7.
225. Schaffner F, Sternlieb I, Barka T, et al. Hepatocellular changes in Wilson's disease. Histochemical and electron microscopic studies. Am J Pathol 1962;41:315–28.
226. Anderson PJ, Popper H. Changes in hepatic structure in Wilson's disease. Am J Pathol 1960;36:483–97.
227. Scheinberg IH, Sternlieb I. The liver in Wilson's disease. Gastroenterology 1959;37:550–64.
228. Johnson RC, De Ford JW, Gebhart RJ. Chronic active hepatitis and cirrhosis in Wilson's disease. South Med J 1977;70:753–4.
229. Sternlieb I. The development of cirrhosis in Wilson's disease. Clin Gastroenterol 1975;4:367–79.
230. Stromeyer FW, Ishak HG. Histology of the liver in Wilson's disease. A study of 34 cases. Am J Clin Pathol 1980;73:12–24.
231. Kamakura K, Kimura S, Igarashi S, et al. A case of Wilson's disease with hepatoma. J Jpn Soc Intern Med 1975;64:232–8.
232. Buffet C, Servent L, Pelletier G, et al. Hepatocellular carcinoma in Wilson's disease. Gastroenterol Clin Biol 1984;8:681–2.
233. Guan R, Oon Cj, Wong PK, et al. Primary hepatocellular carcinoma associated with Wilson's disease in a young woman. Postgrad Med J 1985;61:357–9.
234. Wilkinson ML, Portmann B, Williams R. Wilson's disease and hepatocellular carcinoma: possible protective role of copper. Gut 1983;24:767–71.
235. Salaspuro M, Sipponen P. Demonstration of an intracellular copper-binding protein by orcein staining in long-standing cholestatic liver diseases. Gut 1976;17:787–90.
236. Evans J, Newman SP, Sherlock S. Observations on copper-associated protein in childhood liver disease. Gut 1980;21: 970–6.
237. Jain S, Scheuer PJ, Archer B, et al. Histological demonstration of copper and copper-associated protein in chronic liver disease. J Clin Pathol 1978;31:784–90.
238. Goldfischer S, Popper H, Sternlieb I. The significance of variations in the distribution of copper in liver disease. Am J Pathol 1980;99:715–30.
239. Guarascio P, Yentis F, Cevikbas U. Value of copper-associated protein in diagnostic assessment of liver biopsy. J Clin Pathol 1983;36:18–23.
240. Nartey NO, Frei JV, Cherian MG. Hepatic copper and metallothionein distribution in Wilson's disease (hepatolenticular degeneration). Lab Invest 1987;57:397–401.
241. Sternlieb I. Characterization of the ultrastructural. Changes of hepatocytes in Wilson's disease. Birth Defects (Original Article Series) 1968;4:92.
242. Sternlieb I, Feldmann G. Effects of anticopper therapy on hepatocellular mitochondria in patients with Wilson's disease. An ultrastructural and stereological study. Gastroenterology 1976;71:457–61.
243. Goldfischer S, Sternlieb I. Changes in the distribution of hepatic copper in relation to the progression of Wilson's disease (hepatolenticular degeneration). Am J Pathol 1968;53: 883–901.
244. Williams FJB, Walshe JM. Wilson's disease. An analysis of the cranial computerized tomographic appearances found in 60 patients and the changes in response to treatment with chelating agents. Brain 1981;104:735–52.
245. Harik SI, Donovan Post MJ. Computed tomography in Wilson's disease. Neurology 1981;31:107–10.
246. Aisen AM, Martel W, Gabrielsen TO, et al. Wilson disease of the brain: MR imaging. Radiology 1985;157:137–41.
247. Linne T, Agartz I, Saaf J, et al. Cerebral abnormalities in Wilson's disease as evaluated by ultra-low-field magnetic resonance imaging and computerized image processing. Magn Reson Imaging 1990;8:819–24.
248. Schwarz J, Antonini A, Kraft E, et al. Treatment with D-penicillamine improves dopamine D_2-receptor binding and T_2-signal intensity in de novo Wilson's disease. Neurology 1994;44: 1079–82.
249. Kuwert T, Hefter H, Scholz D, et al. Regional cerebral glucose consumption measured by positron emission tomography in patients with Wilson's disease. Eur J Nucl Med 1992;19:96–101.
250. Snow BJ, Bhatt M, Martin WRW, et al. The nigrostriatal dopaminergic pathway in Wilson's disease with positron emission tomography. J Neurol Neurosurg Psychiatry 1991;54:12–17.
251. Fujita M, Hosoki M, Miyazaki M. Brainstem auditory evoked responses in spinocerebellar degeneration and Wilson's disease. Ann Neurol 1981;9:42–7.
252. Roach ES, Ford CS, Spudis EV, et al. Wilson's disease: evoked potentials and computed tomography. J Neurol 1985;232:20–3.
253. Grimm G, Oder W, Prayer L, et al. Evoked potentials in assessment and follow-up of patients with Wilson's disease. Lancet 1990;336:963–4.
254. Chu NS. Sensory evoked potentials in Wilson's disease. Brain 1986;109:491–507.

255. Kattamis CA, Tjortjatou F. The hemolytic process of viral hepatitis in children with normal or deficient glucose-6-phosphate dehydrogenase activity. J Pediatr 1970;77:422–30.
256. Sallie R, Katsiyiannakis L, Baldwin D, et al. Failure of simple biochemical indices to reliably differentiate fulminant Wilson's disease from other causes of fulminant hepatic failure. Hepatology 1992;16:1206–11.
257. Bennan DH, Leventhal RI, Kiss J, et al. Plasmapheresis in the management of fulminant Wilson's disease. Gastroenterology 1989;96:A577.
258. Rakela J, Kurtz SB, McCarthy JT, et al. Fulminant Wilson's disease treated with post-dilution hemofiltration and orthotopic liver transplantation. Gastroenterology 1986;90:2004–7.
259. Emre S, Atillasoy EQ, Ozdemir S, et al. Orthotopic liver transplantation for Wilsons disease: a single-center experience. Transplantation 2001;72:1232–6.
260. Schilsky ML. Diagnosis and treatment of Wilson's disease. Pediatr Transplant 2002;6:15–19.
261. Underwood EJ. Trace elements in human and animal nutrition. New York: Academic, 1971:57.
262. Brewer GJ, Askari F, Lorincz MT, et al. Treatment of Wilson disease with ammonium tetrathiomolybdate: IV. Comparison of tetrathiomolybdate and trientine in a double-blind study of treatment of the neurologic presentation of Wilson disease. Arch Neurol 2006;63:521–7.
263. Scheinberg IH, Sternlieb I, Schilsky M, et al. Penicillamine may detoxify copper in Wilson's disease. Lancet 1987;2:95.
264. Heilmaicr HE, Jiang JL, Griem H, et al. D-penicillamine induces rat hepatic metallothionein. Toxicology 1986;42:23–31.
265. Brewer GJ, Terry CA, Aisen AM, Hill GM. Worsening of neurologic syndrome in patients with Wilson's disease with initial penicillamine therapy. Arch Neurol 1987;44:490–3.
266. Walshe JM, Yealland M. Chelation treatment of neurological Wilson's disease. Q J Med 1993;86:197–204.
267. Marsden CD. Wilson's disease. Q J Med 1987;65:959–66.
268. Pall HS, Williams AC, Blake DR. Deterioration of Wilson's disease following the start of penicillamine therapy [letter]. Arch Neurol 1989;46:359–61.
269. Saito H, Watanabe K, Sahara M, et al. Triethylene-tetramine (Trien) therapy for Wilson's disease. Tohoku J Exp Med 1991; 164:29.
270. Walshe JM. Thiomolybdates in the treatment of Wilson's disease. Arch Neurol 1992;49:132–3.
271. Lang CJG, Rabas-Kolominsky P, Engelhart A, et al. Fatal deterioration of Wilson's disease after institution of oral zinc therapy. Arch Neurol 1993;50:1007.
272. Grand RJ, Vawter GF. Juvenile Wilson's disease: histologic and functional studies during penicillamine therapy. J Pediatr 1975;87:1161–70.
273. Marecek Z, Heyrovsky A, Volek V. The effect of long term treatment with penicillamine on the copper content in the liver in patients with Wilson's disease. Acta Hepatol Gastroenterol 1975;22:292–6.
274. Sternlieb I, Scheinberg IH. Penicillamine therapy in hepatolenticular degeneration. JAMA 1964;189:748–54.
275. Walshe JM. Penicillamine and the SLE syndrome. J Rheumatol 1981;8(suppl 7):155–60.
276. Sternlieb I, Fischer M, Scheinberg IH. Penicillamine-induced skin lesions. J Rheumatol 1981;8(suppl 7):149–54.
277. Pass F, Goldfischer S, Sternlieb I, et al. Elastosis perforans serpiginosa during penicillamine therapy for Wilson's disease. Arch Dermatol 1973;108:713–15.
278. Miyagawa S, Yoshioka A, Hatoko M, et al. Systemic sclerosis-like lesions during long-term penicillamine therapy for Wilson's disease. Br J Dermatol 1987;116:95–100.
279. Eisenberg E, Ballow M, Wolfe SH, et al. Pemphigus-like mucosal lesions: a side effect of penicillamine therapy. Oral Surg Oral Med Oral Pathol 1981;51:409–14.
280. Menara M, Aancan L. Penicillamine hepatotoxicity in the treatment of Wilson's disease. J Pediatr Gastroenterol Nutr 1992;14: 353.
281. Dubois RS, Rodgerson DO, Hambidge KM. Treatment of Wilson's disease with triethylene tetramine hydrochloride (Trientine). J Pediatr Gastroenterol Nutr 1990;10:77–81.
282. Brewer GJ. Recognition, diagnosis, and management of Wilson's disease. Proc Soc Exp Biol Med. 2000;223:30–46.
283. Brewer GJ, Johnson V, Dick RD, et al. Treatment of Wilson's disease with ammonium tetrathiomolybdate. II. Initial therapy in 33 neurologically affected patients and follow up with zinc therapy. Arch Neurol 1996;53:1017–25.
284. Mason J. The biochemical pathogenesis of molybdenum-induced copper deficiency syndromes in ruminants: towards the final chapter. Ir Vet J 1990;43:18–21.
285. Mills CF, El-Gallad TT, Bremmer I. Effects of molybdate, sulphide and tetrathiomolybdate on copper metabolism in rats. J Inorg Biochem 1981;14:189–207.
286. Bremner I Mills CF, Young BW. Copper metabolism in rats given di or trithiomolybdates. J Inorg Biochem 182;16:109–19.
287. Mills CF, ElGallad TT, Bremner I Weham G. Copper and molybdenum absorption by rats given ammonium tetrahiomolybdate. J Inorg Biochem 1981;14:163–75.
288. Gooneratne SR, Howell JM, Gawthorne JM. An investigation of the effects of intravenous administration of thiomolybdate on copper metabolism in chronic Cu-poisoned sheep. Br J Nutr 181;46:469–80.
289. Brewer GJ, Hedera P, Kluin KJ, et al. Treatment of Wilson disease with ammoniumtetrathiomolybdate. III. Initial therapy in a total of 55 neurologically affected patients and follow-up with zinc therapy. Arch Neurol 2003;60:379–85.
290. Lipsky MA, Gollan JL. Treatment of Wilson's disease: in D-penicillamine we trust – what about zinc? Hepatology 1987; 7:593–5.
291. Hoogenraad TU, Koevoet R, de Ruyter Korvr EG. Oral zinc sulphate as long-term treatment in Wilson's disease (hepatolenticular degeneration). Eur Neurol 1979;18:205–11.
292. Brewer GJ, Hill GM, Prasad AS, et al. Oral zinc therapy for Wilson's disease. Ann Intern Med 1983;99:314–19.
293. Van Caillie-Bertrand M, Degenhart HJ, Visser HKA, et al. Oral zinc sulphate for Wilson's disease. Arch Dis Child 1985;60: 656–9.
294. Hill GM, Brewer GJ, Prasad AS, et al. Treatment of Wilson's disease with zinc: 1. Oral zinc therapy regimens. Hepatology 1987;7:522–8.
295. Hoogenraad TU, Van Hattum J, Van den Hamer CJA. Management of Wilson's disease with zinc sulphate. Experience in a series of 27 patients. J Neurol Sci 1987;77:137–46.
296. Rossaro L, Sturniolo GC, Giacon G, et al. Zinc therapy in Wilson's disease: observations in five patients. Am J Gastroenterol 1990;85:665–8.

297. Roberts EA, Cox DW. Wilson's disease. Baillieres Clin Gastroenterol 1998;12:237–356.
298. Sokol RJ, McKim JM Jr, Devereaux MW. Alpha-tocopherol ameliorates oxidant injury in isolated copper overload rat hepatocytes. Pediatr Res 1996;39:259–63.
299. Zeid I, Perrault J, Cox D, et al. Vitamin E in the treatment of Wilson's disease. J Pediatr Gastroenterol Nutr 1996;26:345.
300. Schilsky ML, Scheinberg IH, Sternlieb I. Liver transplantation for Wilson's disease: indications and outcome. Hepatology 1994;19:583–7.
301. Mason AL, Marsh W, Alpers DH. Intractable neurologic Wilson's disease treatment with orthotopic liver transplantation. Dig Dis Sci 1993;38:1746.
302. Eghtesad B, Nezakatgoo N, Geraci LC, et al. Liver transplantation for Wilson's disease: a single-center experience. Liver Transpl Surg 1999;5:467–74.
303. Asonuma K, Inomata Y, Kasahara M, et al. Living related liver transplantation from heterozygote genetic carriers to children with Wilson's disease. Pediatr Transplant 1999;3:201–5.
304. Nazer H, Ede RJ, Mowat AP, et al. Wilson's disease: clinical presentation and use of prognostic index. Gut 1986;27:1377–81.
305. Dhawan A, Taylor RM, Cheeseman P, et al. Wilson's disease in children: 37-year experience and revised King's score for liver transplantation. Liver Transpl 2005;11:441–8.
306. Cossack ZT. The efficacy of oral zinc therapy as an alternative to penicillamine for Wilson's disease [letter]. N Engl J Med 1988;318:322–3.
307. Chin RKH. Pregnancy and Wilson's disease [letter]. Am J Obstet Gynecol 1991;165:488.
308. Sternlieb I. Wilson's disease and pregnancy. Hepatology 2000;31:531–2.
309. Linares A, Zarranz JJ, Rodriguez-Alacron J, et al. Reversible cutis laxa due to maternal penicillamine treatment. Lancet 1979;2:43.
310. Yarze JC, Martin P, Munoz SJ, et al. Wilson's disease: current status. Am J Med 1992;92:643–54.
311. Mjolnerod IK, Rasmussen K, Dormnerud SA, et al. Congenital connective tissue defect probably due to d-penicillamine treatment in pregnancy. Lancet 1971;1:673–6.
312. Brewer GJ, Johnson VD, Dick RD, et al. Treatment of Wilson's disease with zinc XVII: treatment during pregnancy. Hepatology 2000;31:364–70.
313. Walshe JM. The management of pregnancies in Wilson's disease. Q J Med 1986;58:81–7.
314. Scheinberg IH, Sternlieb I. Pregnancy in penicillamine-treated patients with Wilson's disease. N Engl J Med 1975;293:1300–2.
315. Morris JJ, Seifter E, Rettura G, et al. Effect of penicillamine upon wound healing. J Surg Res 1969;9:142–9.
316. Tanner MS, Portmann B, Mowat AP, et al. Increased hepatic copper concentration in Indian childhood cirrhosis. Lancet 1979;1:1203–5.
317. Tanner MS. Role of copper in Indian childhood cirrhosis. Am J Clin Nutr 1998;67(suppl):1074–81.
318. Müller T, Feichtinger H, Berger H, et al. Endemic Tyrolean infantile cirrhosis: an ecogenetic disorder. Lancet 1996;347:877–80.
319. Mowat AT. Liver disorders in childhood. London: Butterworths, 1987:294–7.
320. Nayak NC, Ramalingaswammi V. Indian childhood cirrhosis. Clin Gastroenterol 1975;4:333–49.
321. O'Neill NC, Tanner MS. Uptake of copper from brass vessels by bovine milk and its relevance to Indian childhood cirrhosis. J Pediatr Gastroenterol Nutr 1989;9:167–72.
322. Bhave SA, Pandit AN, Tanner MS. Comparison of feeding history of children with Indian childhood cirrhosis and paired controls. J Pediatr Gastroenterol Nutr 1987;6:562–7.
323. Tanner MS, Kantarjian AH, Bhave SA, et al. Early introduction of copper-contaminated animal milk feeds as a possible cause of Indian childhood cirrhosis. Lancet 1983;2:992–5.
324. Sethi S, Grover S, Khodaskar MB. Role of copper in Indian childhood cirrhosis. Ann Trop Paediatr 1993;13:3–5.
325. Adelson JW. Indian childhood cirrhosis is a result of copper hepatotoxicity – in all likelihood. J Pediatr Gastroenterol Nutr 1987;6:491–2.
326. Kalra V. Dietary copper and Indian childhood cirrhosis. Ind Pediatr 1986;23:399–401.
327. Wijmenga C, Muller T, Murli IS, et al. Endemic Tyrolean infantile cirrhosis is not an allelic variant of Wilson's disease. Eur J Hum Genet 1998;6:624–8.
328. Hahn SH, Brantly ML, Oliver C, et al. Metallothionein synthesis and degradation in Indian childhood cirrhosis fibroblasts. Pediatr Res 1994;35:197–204.
329. Hahn SH, Tanner MS, Danks DM, et al. Normal metallothionein synthesis in fibroblasts obtained from children with Indian childhood cirrhosis or copper-associated childhood cirrhosis. Biochem Mol Med 1995;54:142–5.
330. Kapoor SK, Singh M, Ghai OP. Study of serum copper and copper oxidase in patients with Indian childhood cirrhosis. Ind J Med Res 1971;59:115–21.
331. Bhave SA, Pandit AN, Pradhan AM, et al. Liver disease in India. Arch Dis Child 1982;57:922.
332. Popper H, Goldfischer S, Sternlieb I, et al. Cytoplasmic copper and its toxic effects. Studies in Indian childhood cirrhosis. Lancet 1979;1:1205–8.
333. Roy S, Ramalingaswami V, Nayak NC. An ultrastructural study of the liver in Indian childhood cirrhosis with particular reference to the structure of cytoplasmic hyaline. Gut 1971;12:693–701.
334. Bhagwat AG, Walia BNS, Koshy A, et al. Will the real Indian childhood cirrhosis please stand up? Cleve Clin Q 1983;50:323–37.
335. Arora NK, Nanda SK, Gulati S, et al. Acute viral hepatitis types E, A and B singly and in combination in acute liver failure in children in North India. J Med Virol 1996;48:215–21.
336. Suryanarayan Rao K, Madhavan TV, Tulpule PG. Incidence of toxigenic strains of Aspergillus flavus affecting ground nut crop in certain coastal districts of India. Ind J Med Res 1965;53:1196–201.
337. Amla I, Kamala C, Gopalakrishna GS, et al. Cirrhosis in children from peanut meal contaminated by alfatoxin. Am J Clin Nutr 1971;24:609–14.
338. Tanner MS, Mattocks AR. Hypothesis: plant and fungal biocides, copper and Indian childhood cirrhosis. Ann Trop Paediatr 1987;7:264–9.
339. Howell JM, Deol HS, Thomas JB, et al. Experimental copper and heliotrope intoxication in sheep: morphological changes. J Comp Pathol 1991;105:49–74.
340. Aston NS, Morris PA, Tanner MS. Retrorsine exacerbates liver damage from copper ingestion in neonatal rats [abstract]. Z Gastroenterol 1995;33:473.

341. Bras G, Jelliffe DB, Stuart KL. Veno-occlusive disease of the liver with non-portal type of cirrhosis occurring in Jamaica. Arch Pathol 1954;57:285–300.
342. Tanner MS, Bhave SA, Pradham AM, et al. Clinical trials of penicillamine in Indian childhood cirrhosis. Arch Dis Child 1987;62:1118–24.
343. Bhusnurmath SR, Walia BN, Singh S, et al. Sequential histopathologic alterations in Indian childhood cirrhosis treated with d-penicillamine. Hum Pathol 1991;22:653–8.
344. Pradhan AM, Bhave AM, Joshi VV, et al. Reversal of Indian childhood cirrhosis by d-penicillamine. J Pediatr Gastroenterol Nutr 1995;20:28–35.
345. Bavdekar AR, Bhave SA, Pradhan AM, et al. Long term survival in Indian childhood cirrhosis treated with d-penicillamine. Arch Dis Child 1996;74:32–5.
346. Bhave SA, Pandit AN, Singh S, et al. The prevention of Indian childhood cirrhosis. Ann Trop Paediatr 1992;12:23–30.
347. Superina RA, Pearl RH, Roberts EA, et al. Liver transplantation in children: the initial Toronto experience. J Pediatr Surg 1989;24:1013–19.
348. Müller-Höcker J, Weiss M, Meyer U, et al. Fatal copper storage disease of the liver in a German infant resembling Indian childhood cirrhosis. Virchows Arch 1987;411:379–85.
349. Walker-Smith JA, Blomfield J. Wilson's disease or chronic copper poisoning? Arch Dis Child 1973;48:476–9.
350. Lefkowitch J, Honig CL, King M, et al. Hepatic copper overload and features of Indian childhood cirrhosis in an American sibship. N Engl J Med 1982;307:271–7.
351. Müller-Höcker J, Meyer U, Wiebecke B, et al. Copper storage disease of the liver and chronic dietary copper intoxication in two further German infants mimicking Indian childhood cirrhosis. Pathol Res Pract 1988;183:39–45.
352. Maggiore G, De Giacomo C, Sessa F, et al. Idiopathic hepatic copper toxicosis in a child. J Pediatr Gastroenterol Nutr 1987;6:980–3.
353. Bartok I, Szabo L, Horvath E, et al. Juvenile Zirrhose mit hochgradiger kupferspeicherung in der Leber. Acta Hepatosplenol 1971;18:119–28.
354. Weiss M, Müller-Höcker J, Wiebecke B, et al. First description of "Indian childhood cirrhosis" in a non-Indian infant in Europe. Acta Paediatr Scand 1989;78:152–6.
355. Adamson M, Reiner B, Olson JL, et al. Indian childhood cirrhosis in an American child. Gastroenterology 1992;102:1771–7.
356. Dubois RS, Giles G, Rodgerson DO, et al. Orthotopic liver transplantation for Wilson's disease. Lancet 1991;1:505–8.
357. Aljajeh IA, Mughal S, Al-Tahou B, et al. Indian childhood cirrhosis-like liver disease in an Arab child. A brief report. Virchows Arch 1994;424:225–7.
358. Horslen SP, Tanner MS, Lyon TDB, et al. Copper associated childhood cirrhosis. Gut 1994;35:1497–500.
359. Baker A, Gormally S, Saxena R, et al. Copper-associated liver disease in childhood. J Hepatol 1995;23:538–43.
360. Ludwig J, Farr GH, Freese DK, et al. Chronic hepatitis and hepatic failure in a 14-year-old girl. Hepatology 1996;22: 1874–9.
361. Lim CT, Choo KE. Wilson's disease in a 2 year old child. J Singapore Paediatr Soc 1979;21:99–102.
362. Bent S, Bohm K. Copper-induced liver cirrhosis in a 13-month-old boy. Gesundheitswesen 1995;57:667–9.
363. Valencia MP, Gamboa MJ, Mediana J. Copper overload and cirrhosis in four Mexican children [abstract]. Lab Invest 1993; 68:10P.
364. Müller T, Feichtinger H, Berger H, et al. Endemic Tyrolean infantile cirrhosis: an ecogenetic disorder. Lancet 1996;347:877–80.
365. Scheinberg IH, Sternlieb I. Wilson's disease and idiopathic copper toxicosis. Am J Clin Nutr 1996;63(suppl):842–5.
366. Müller T, Müller W, Feichtinger H. Idiopathic copper toxicosis. Am J Clin Nutr 1998;67(suppl):1082–6.
367. Müllendahl KE, Lange H. Copper and childhood cirrhosis. Lancet 1994;344:1515–16.
368. Müller T, Schöfer H, Rodeck B, et al. Familial clustering of infantile cirrhosis in Northern Germany: a clue to the etiology of idiopathic copper toxicosis. J Pediatr 1999;135:189–96.
369. Scheinberg IH, Sternlieb I. Is non-Indian childhood cirrhosis caused by excess dietary copper. Lancet 1994;344:1002–4.
370. Giagheddu A, Demelia L, Puggioni G, et al. Epidemiologic study of hepatolenticular degeneration (Wilson's disease) in Sardinia (1902–1983). Acta Neurol Scand 1985;72:43–55.
371. Dobyns WB, Goldstein NP, Gordon H. Clinical spectrum of Wilson's disease (hepatolenticular degeneration). Mayo Clin Proc 1979;54:35–42.
372. Aksoy M, Erdem S. Wilson's disease in Turkey, a review of 49 cases in 41 families. New Istanbul Contrib Clin Sci 1975;11: 92–7.

27

Iron Storage Disorders

Alex S. Knisely, M.D., and Michael R. Narkewicz, M.D.

IRON OVERLOAD DISORDERS

Hereditary Hemochromatosis (OMIM 235200)

Iron overload states can be classified as primary or secondary. There are many disorders that can lead to iron overload (Table 27.1). This chapter focuses on hereditary hemochromatosis (HHC), juvenile hemochromatosis (JHC), and secondary iron overload (primarily transfusion associated) in the pediatric patient and on neonatal hemochromatosis. For a discussion of the rarer entities, the reader is referred to several recent reviews [1,2].

Physiology and Pathophysiology of Iron Overload

Iron is one of the more tightly regulated nutrients in the body. Humans have no significant excretory pathway for iron. Thus, body iron stores are normally controlled at the level of absorption, matching absorption to physiologic requirements. Under normal circumstances, only about 1 mg of elemental iron is absorbed per day (Figure 27.1), in balance with gastrointestinal losses. Intestinal iron absorption is increased by low body iron stores (storage regulation) [3], increased erythropoiesis (erythropoietic regulation) [3], anemias associated with ineffective erythropoiesis (thalassemias, congenital dyserythropoietic anemias, and sideroblastic anemia), and acute hypoxia. Both dietary iron intake (dietary regulation) and systemic inflammation can temporarily decrease iron absorption and availability, even in the presence of iron deficiency [4–6].

Duodenal crypt cells sense body iron status and are programmed for iron absorption as they mature. Duodenal and proximal jejunal enterocytes are responsible for iron absorption. Low gastric pH helps dissolve iron, which is then enzymatically reduced to the ferrous form by ferrireductase [7]. Divalent metal transporter 1 (DMT-1) transfers iron to the enterocyte, where it is either stored as ferritin or moved across the basolateral membrane to reach the plasma, where it is rapidly oxidized to the ferric form by hephaestin and bound to transferrin. DMT-1 levels are altered in response to body iron stores [8].

The recent discoveries of hepcidin and ferroportin have shed new light on the regulation of iron in humans. Hepcidin is produced in the liver, and its expression and secretion in iron sufficiency is elevated. Hepcidin acts to down-regulate the cell-surface expression of ferroportin [9], a transmembrane iron transporter that acts to transfer iron out of intestinal epithelial cells and macrophages [10,11]. During times of low iron status, hepcidin is low and ferroportin expression on the basolateral membrane of the enterocyte is maintained. As a consequence, intestinal epithelial cells transport more dietary iron across their basolateral membranes leading to increased iron absorption. Mutations in both the hepcidin (juvenile hemochromatosis) [12,13] and ferroportin [14] (autosomal dominant hemochromatosis) genes have been described. Hepcidin expression is regulated by the HFE protein (mutated in HHC type 1), transferrin receptor 2 (TfR2; see below), and hemojuvelin (mutated in juvenile hemochromatosis). This regulation provides a probable link for the mechanism of iron overload in the various forms of hemochromatosis (Figure 27.2). In animal models and in humans with hemochromatosis, the normal increase in hepcidin expression with iron loading is lost, leading to lower hepcidin levels and continued iron absorption in the face of iron overload [15–19].

In humans, iron in the circulation is tightly bound to transferrin [20]. Transferrin can bind up to two molecules of ferric iron, with about 30% of the binding sites on transferrin normally occupied by ferric iron. Diferric transferrin binds to the transferrin receptor on the cellular plasma membrane. This complex is then endocytosed into the cell, where iron is released by the acid environment of the endocytic vesicle. The iron is then transported across the endosomal membrane to the cytoplasm. Thus, in the setting of a highly saturated transferrin (e.g., HHC), more of the transferrin is in the diferric state, or the more readily absorbable state. The uptake of iron is primarily regulated by the expression of the transferrin receptor on the cell surface. In iron deficiency, iron regulatory proteins are increased and bind to the transferrin receptor iron-responsive elements in the 3′-untranslated region of the transferrin receptor messenger RNA (mRNA). This stabilizes the transferrin receptor transcript, leading to increased transferrin receptor expression on the cell surface, increasing iron uptake. Simultaneously, these same iron regulatory proteins bind to the 5′-untranslated region of ferritin (the iron storage

Table 27.1: Classification of Iron Overload States

Primary forms of iron overload

Hereditary hemochromatosis, *HFE*-associated
- C282Y homozygotes
- C282Y/H63D compound heterozygotes

Hereditary hemochromatosis, non–*HFE*-associated
- Hereditary hemochromatosis, *TFR2*-associated
- Juvenile hemochromatosis (hemojuvelin-associated, hepcidin-associated)
- Ferroportin-associated hemochromatosis (autosomal dominant)

Heavy–chain ferritin disease

Neonatal hemochromatosis

Autosomal dominant hemochromatosis (Solomon Islands)

Aceruloplasminemia

Atransferrinemia

Secondary iron overload

Iatrogenic (transfusional iron overload)

Anemias (sideroblastic anemia, hereditary spherocytosis, β-thalassemia)

Dietary or medicinal iron overload

Long-term hemodialysis

Chronic liver disease (hepatitis B and C, alcoholic liver disease, NASH, post portocaval shunt)

Porphyria cutanea tarda

Cystic fibrosis

Tyrosinemia

Zellweger syndrome

Adapted from Pietrangelo [2].

and intracellular sequestration molecule), decreasing its synthesis [21]. In states of iron repletion or excess, there is a reduced level of iron-binding proteins, leading to less transferrin receptor production and an increase in ferritin and hepcidin synthesis [21]. In the intestine and at other sites, iron is also transported by at least one transporter that is independent of transferrin and the transferrin receptor. An active transporter for divalent cations, including iron, called the divalent cation transporter 1 (DCT-1) has been reported [8,22]. This mRNA is strongly expressed in the enterocytes at the villous tips and is increased in states of iron deficiency [8,21].

A second transferrin receptor (TfR2) [23] binds holotransferrin/diferric transferrin and mediates the uptake of transerrin-bound iron. This protein is predominately expressed in the liver, where, in contrast to TfR, it is not down-regulated by dietary iron overload or in the mouse model for HHC [24]. Hepatic TfR2 provides an explanation for the continued hepatic iron uptake in HHC despite the down-regulation of TfR. TfR2 also regulates hepcidin synthesis in the liver [17].

In HHC and JHC, net iron absorption is increased above endogenous losses [25,26]. In addition, in both disorders, there is loss of the normal down-regulation of iron absorption as iron accumulates in the body. Recent evidence suggests that this is directly related to dysregulation of hepatic hepcidin expression [5,16–18,27]. The result is a net gradual increase in total body iron. In HHC, the net increase in total body iron has been estimated at 4–7 mg/d. The increased iron absorption in HHC is the result of inappropriate transfer of iron at the basolateral surface of the enterocyte due to suppression of hepatic hepcidin secretion [18]. In JHC, iron accumulates more rapidly than in HHC, perhaps related to a more significant rôle of hemojuvelin in the regulation of hepcidin [28]. Excessive iron intake in the diet can accelerate the accumulation of iron in both HHC and JHC. In a similar manner, increased iron losses (most commonly in menstruating females) can retard the accumulation of iron. In secondary iron overload due to hemoglobinopathies, iron overload is related to both the anemia and increased iron absorption and excess iron provided by transfusions. In contrast, in aplastic anemias, iron overload is primarily related to transfusion.

Genetics of Hereditary Hemochromatosis

Hereditary hemochromatosis has long been recognized as an autosomal recessive disorder. In 1976, HHC was linked to the human leukocyte antigen (HLA) region of the short arm of chromosome 6 [29]. In 1996, using positional cloning in a defined cohort of patients with HHC, the candidate gene for HHC, called *HFE*, was discovered [30]. The *HFE* gene encodes a novel major histocompatibility (MHC) class 1–like molecule [30]. Two principal missense mutations of *HFE* have been identified. One results in a change from a cysteine to tyrosine at position 282 (C282Y) [30]. A second mutation results in a change from a histidine to aspartate at position 63 (H63D) [30]. Upward of 85–90% of patients with classic HHC are homozygous for C282Y, and another 5% are compound heterozygotes (C282Y/H63D) [21]. The H63D mutation is quite common (15–20% heterozygote state in the general population), but H63D homozygotes generally do not have significant iron loading [31,32]. It is also important to note that in the majority of studies, 10–15% of patients with a clinical syndrome of typical HHC do not have either the C282Y or H63D mutation [33]. However, in a recent study from Shaheen et al. [34], 55% of patients initially felt to have HHC who carried neither mutation were found to have previously unrecognized causes for secondary iron overload. There still remains a subgroup of mutation-negative iron-overloaded patients with typical HHC. This one study suggested that these patients may have more severe iron overloading compared with C282Y homozygotes [34]. Recently, several new mutations in *HFE* have been described in patients with iron overload, suggesting that other *HFE* mutations may be found in "wild-type" HHC [35–37].

The formation of a heterodimer between *HFE* and β_2-microglobulin (β_2m) is essential for correct intracellular trafficking

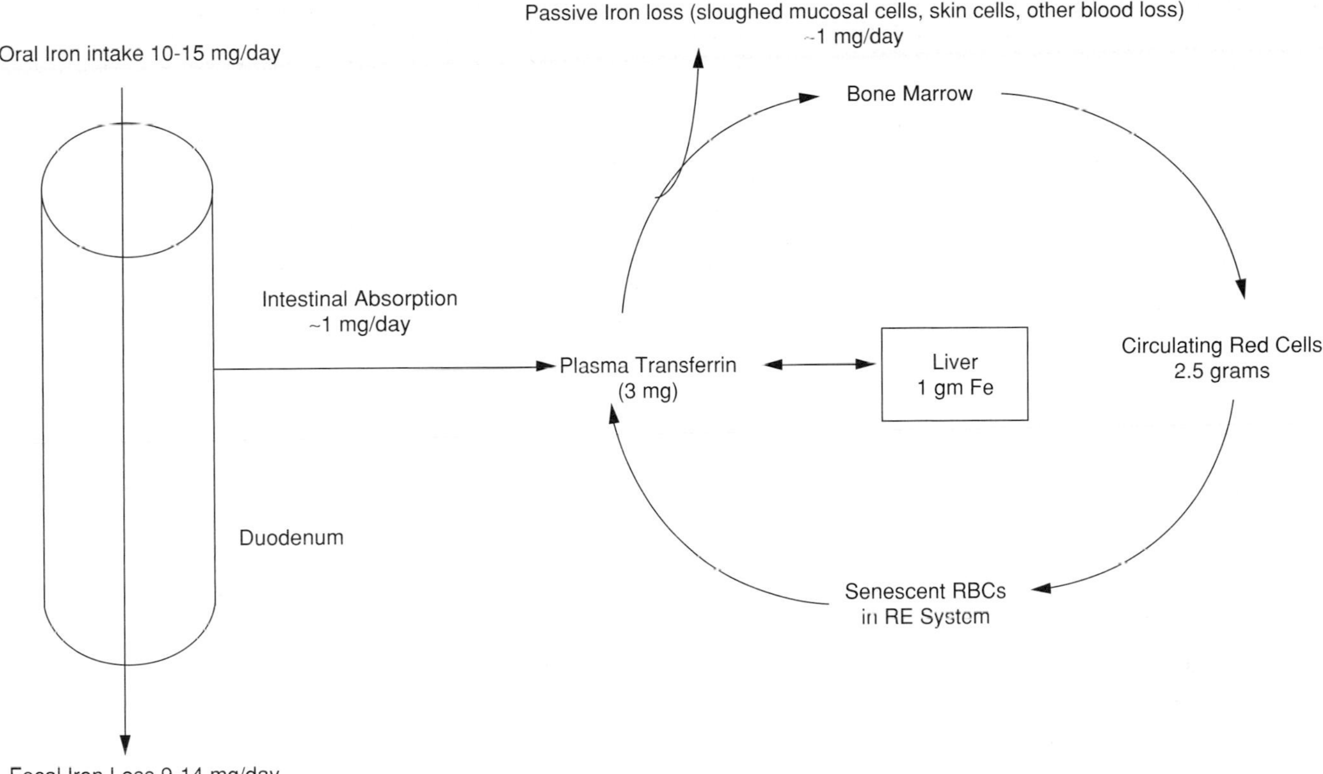

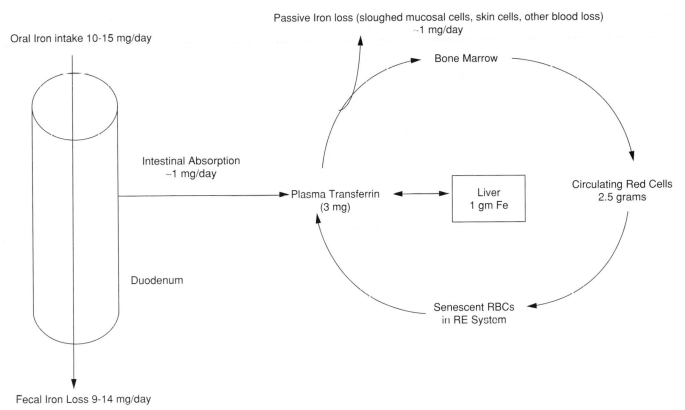

Figure 27.1. Physiology of normal iron metabolism in humans. RE, reticuloendothelial; RBCs, red blood cells; Fe, iron.

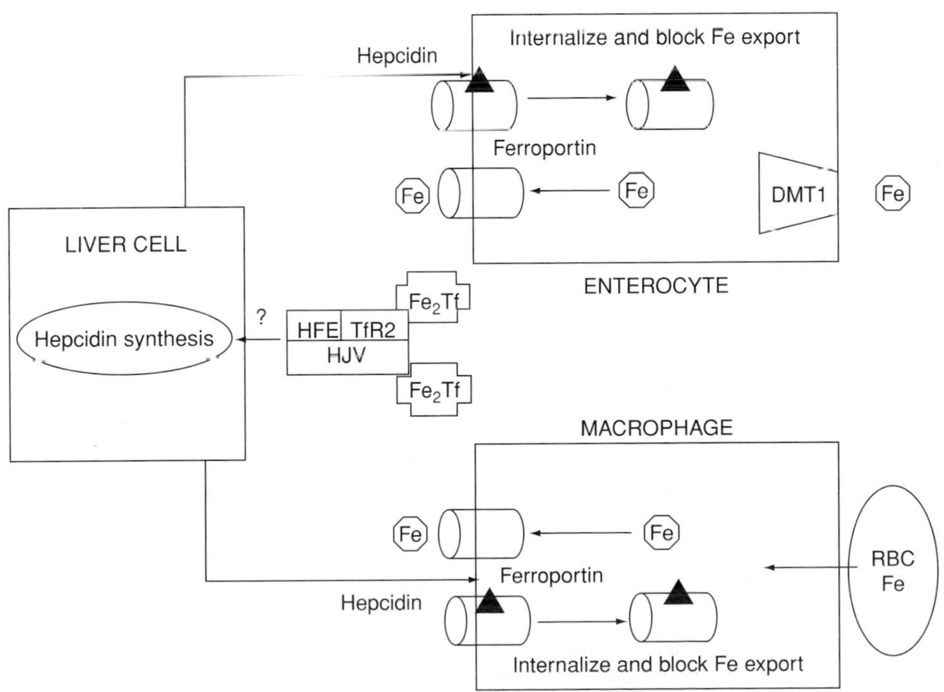

Figure 27.2. Proposed roles of hepcidin, *HFE*, TfR2, and ferroportin in iron absorption. In states of high iron stores and inflammation, hepatic hepcidin synthesis is increased with signaling from *HFE*, TfR2, and hemojuvelin (HJV). Hepcidin results in internalization of ferroportin in both enterocytes and macrophages, reducing transport of iron. (Adapted from Vaulont et al. [11].)

and transport of *HFE* to the plasma membrane and cell surface expression of an *HFE*–β_2m complex [38]. The C282Y mutant gene product does not associate with β_2m, resulting in a reduction in cell surface expression of the *HFE*–β_2m complex in transfected cells [38]. The C282Y mutant *HFE* fails to undergo late Golgi processing and is retained in the endoplasmic reticulum, undergoing accelerated degradation [39]. In contrast, the H63D mutation has no effect on the binding of β_2m or cell surface expression of *HFE* [21]. Further work has demonstrated that *HFE* associates with the transferrin receptor on the cell surface, decreasing the affinity of the transferrin receptor for diferric transferrin [40]. The C282Y *HFE* mutant does not arrive at the cell surface; thus, it does not associate with the transferrin receptor. The H63D mutant does associate with the transferrin receptor. The affinity of the transferrin receptor for diferric transferrin decreases less with binding to the H63D mutant than with binding to wild-type *HFE* [40].

HFE is widely expressed throughout the body; the highest levels are found in the liver and small intestine [30]. *HFE* is prominently expressed in the deep crypt cells of the duodenum [30]. A proposed mechanism by which mutant *HFE* would contribute to abnormal iron uptake has been put forward [21]. Normally, high serum iron would increase transferrin receptor and *HFE*-mediated uptake of iron into the crypt cells and would provide a signal for high iron stores and a reduction in the production of DMT-1, leading to a reduction in villous tip iron absorption. In the setting of a mutant *HFE*, transferrin receptor–mediated iron uptake would be reduced and would send a false signal for iron depletion, resulting in overproduction of DMT-1. Preliminary studies have suggested that DMT-1 is up-regulated in the *HFE* knockout mouse [21]. It has been proposed that the unifying mechanism for this observation is that *HFE* is involved in an as yet unknown complex regulation of hepcidin secretion, with subsequent lack of hepcidin mRNA expression and hepcidin secretion in the face of excessive total body iron stores [16–18,41].

Further evidence for the role of *HFE* in iron metabolism comes from two recently developed animal models. Studies in the β_2m knockout mouse have shown that these mice accumulate iron in a pattern similar to that of HHC [42,43]. The murine *HFE* homologue has been disrupted. The phenotype of this mouse is very similar to HHC, with an elevated transferrin saturation and iron accumulation in the parenchymal cells of the liver [44]. Although most studies in this model suggest that the key factor in iron overload is the dysregulation of hepcidin, one study suggests that the ferric reductase duodenal cytochrome *b* (Dcytb) may act as a possible mediator of iron overload in *HFE* deficiency [45].

Epidemiology

Hereditary hemochromatosis is one of the most common genetic diseases in the white population, with a prevalence of the C282Y homozygous state of 1 in 200 to 1 in 400 [46]. The disease is most common in individuals of northern European descent. The frequency of the C282Y mutation is highest in subjects from northwest Europe (10–20%), less frequent in southern and eastern European populations (2–4%), and rare in natives of Africa, Central or South America, Eastern Asia, and the Pacific Islands [47]. The H63D mutation has a distribution similar to that of C282Y, but it is more common in European groups (15–40%). In a large population-based study of 3011 unrelated white adults in Brusselton, Australia, 14.1% were heterozygous for the C282Y mutation and 0.5% were homozygous [47]. It is very unusual to find HHC in African American or Asian patients [46]. Indeed, no instances of C282Y/C282Y have been found in African patients with iron overload [48]. There also have been reports of non-C282Y/C282Y iron overload in Italian patients [49].

Overall estimates are that about 6.8% of the U.S. white population are heterozygotes for the C282Y mutation and 0.5% are homozygous. This is fairly similar to the estimates of 1 in 200 incidence of iron overload in the worldwide white population [50,51]. HHC and the C282Y mutation are uncommon in African Americans or Asian Americans [47], the prevalence of clinically diagnosed HHC in African Americans being about 1 in 1000 [46].

Thus, although HHC is a disease with worldwide distribution, it remains predominately a disease of individuals of northern European descent. The distribution of genotypes in this population is shown in Figure 27.3. Although mutation analysis has assisted in defining the prevalence of the disease in this population, it has not proved useful in other selected populations. Nevertheless, HHC remains one of the more common, if not the most common, inherited disorder in humans.

Clinical Features

In adults, HHC may present with the clinical syndrome of diabetes, cirrhosis, and increased skin pigmentation as initially described in 1865 [52]. Although the genetic defect is present at birth, years of increased iron absorption and tissue accumulation (usually >5 g of excess total body iron) are required for the development of clinical symptoms (Figure 27.4). As such,

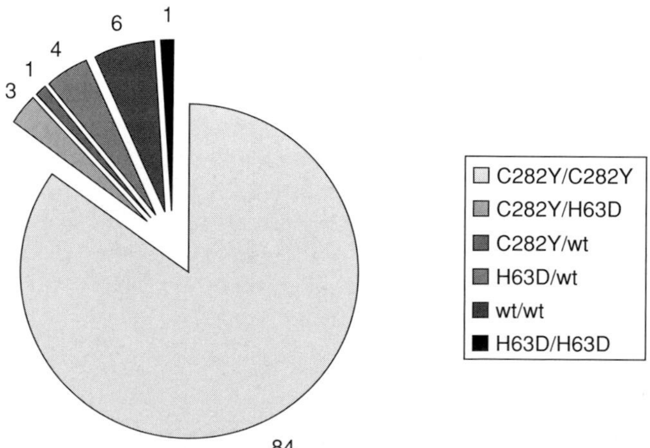

Figure 27.3. Distribution of genotypes in patients with hemochromatosis. Combination of 19 studies encompassing 1618 patients. wt, wildtype. (Adapted from Ramrakhiani and Bacon [33], with permission.)

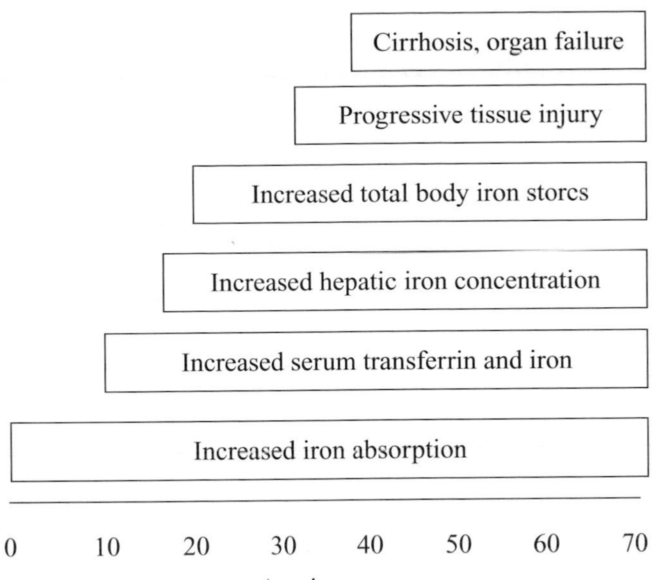

Figure 27.4. Typical progression of iron accumulation and pathology in hereditary hemochromatosis.

clinical symptoms are rare before adulthood [53]. Before the discovery of the gene for HHC, most adults were diagnosed with clinical symptoms that included liver disease (fibrosis or cirrhosis), diabetes, skin pigmentation, heart failure, arthritis, and endocrinologic disturbances. Screening of asymptomatic adults was restricted to first-degree relatives of affected adults. Thus, the true prevalence of symptoms was uncertain. Since the discovery of the *HFE* gene, it is recognized that many adults who are homozygous for the C282Y mutation are asymptomatic [47]. HHC can be classified into four stages: (1) a genetic predisposition with no abnormality other than possibly a raised serum transferrin saturation, (2) iron overload (2–5 g) without symptoms, (3) iron overload with early symptoms (lethargy, arthralgia), and (4) iron overload with organ damage [54,55]. For further data on the clinical manifestations in adults, the reader is referred to recent reviews [56,57].

As iron accumulates in the tissues, there is progressive fibrosis and injury. As organ failure results, the classic clinical consequences of hemochromatosis are recognized. The organs involved and pathologic findings are listed in Table 27.2.

Disease expression is dependent not only on the mutation but on other genetic and environmental factors, such as sex, age, dietary iron, and other factors affecting iron balance. For example, males with HHC typically present earlier than females, presumably because of the ongoing iron losses in menstruating females. In addition, recent population studies have found that the penetrance of the mutations is quite variable and less common than previously thought [58,59].

Most children and adolescents with HHC are asymptomatic. Indeed, although most will have abnormal transferrin saturation, a normal ferritin is the rule. Reports of elevated ferritin and death from congestive heart failure in pediatric

Table 27.2: Organ Involvement in Hereditary Hemochromatosis

Organ	*Histology*
Liver	Periportal iron deposition, fibrosis, cirrhosis
Pancreas	Fibrosis with normal exocrine and β-cell function. Abnormal β-cell function.
Skin	Bronzing secondary to increased melanin
Heart	Dilated and restrictive cardiomyopathy
Joints	Hip, shoulder, knee, metacarpophalangeal joint involvement, and chondrocalcinosis
Pituitary	Fibrosis leading to hypogonadotropic hypogonadism

patients have not been confirmed by genotype analysis and may represent JHC, a truly distinct disorder [60,61]. A recent study screening the children of 179 homozygotes found that even at a mean age of 37 years, most affected children of parents with HHC were asymptomatic [62].

Several studies in heterozygotes have shown that unless another illness is present, heterozygotes do not have clinically important iron overload. Heterozygotes do have slightly higher transferrin saturations than those in normal individuals (men 38% vs. 30%; women 32% vs. 29%) [63–65]. This suggests that the heterozygote state may be protective for iron deficiency in women [63,66].

Diagnosis and Screening

Prior to the discovery of *HFE*, the diagnosis of HHC required the documentation of iron overload or HLA linkage to an affected individual. Criteria for iron overload consistent with HHC include (a) grade 3 or 4 stainable iron on liver biopsy; (b) hepatic iron concentration greater than 4500 μg (80 μmol)/g dry weight; (c) a hepatic iron index (iron concentration in micromoles per gram of dry weight divided by age in years) of more than 1.9; or (d) evidence of iron overload of more than 5 g [21]. These criteria are rarely encountered in children because in the absence of confounding factors (high dietary intake, hepatitis C viral infection, etc.), children typically have not developed this degree of iron overload. Indeed, these criteria are probably not acceptable for individuals identified by family screening, who may be early in the course of iron overload. Some investigators have suggested that any individual with an abnormal hepatic iron concentration (>30 μmol/g or 1500 μg/g dry weight) who has no other reason for iron overload should be suspected of having HHC [21]. A variety of disorders can lead to hepatic iron overload, including chronic liver diseases such as alcoholic liver disease, nonalcoholic steatohepatitis (NASH), chronic viral hepatitis, cystic fibrosis, and porphyria cutanea tarda. There is no association with an increased prevalence of the *HFE* mutations in either alcoholic liver disease or viral hepatitis [67]. However, in both NASH and porphyria cutanea tarda, a higher frequency of the C282Y mutation has been observed [68–70].

In adults, the transferrin saturation is used to screen individuals, with the threshold for further investigation being 45% in men and 42% in premenopausal women. Abnormal transferrin saturation has been reported in children as young as 2 years [71]. However, fasting transferrin saturation and ferritin level in affected children can be normal, even in known homozygous subjects [72–74]. Indeed, as many as 30% of women with HHC who are under 30 years of age have normal transferrin saturation [72,73]. Thus, transferrin saturation appears to be helpful in children when it is abnormal but does not exclude HHC when normal. In contrast, ferritin may be elevated in many inflammatory liver diseases such as chronic viral hepatitis and NASH in the absence of HHC.

Liver biopsy has been primarily studied in adults. Increased hepatic iron can be demonstrated by Prussian blue staining. Hepatic iron quantitation with the determination of the hepatic iron index (micromoles of iron per gram of dry weight divided by age in years) has been considered one of the more sensitive and specific tests for HHC. Several studies have demonstrated that a hepatic iron index of greater than 1.9 in the absence of secondary iron overload is indicative of HHC. However, 10–15% of HHC patients identified by genetic testing will have a hepatic iron index of less than 1.9, calling into question the use of this test for diagnosis in children [72,73]. In children with HHC, an abnormal hepatic iron index has been reported in those as young as 7 years [75]. The role of magnetic resonance imaging (MRI) quantitation of hepatic iron content is under study [76–78].

Genetic testing is available on a commercial basis. The distribution of genotypes in patients with hemochromatosis is shown in Figure 27.3. In 150 family members of 61 white American probands, 34 family members had an HHC phenotype. Among the family members, 92% of the C282Y homozygotes and 34% of the C282Y/H63D compound heterozygotes had the HHC phenotype [79]. None of the H63D homozygotes had an HHC phenotype. A few individuals were heterozygous for one mutation and had iron overload. Thus, testing for HFE mutations should include both the C282Y and the H63D mutation. Heterozygosity may contribute to iron overload with an associated condition, but it should not be considered the sole cause of iron overload. Only C282Y/C282Y and compound heterozygosity (C282Y/H63D) should be considered indicative of HHC. However, not all compound heterozygotes will develop HHC. In most cases, these individuals will not require liver biopsy for confirmation of the diagnosis. However, C282Y homozygotes with evidence of liver disease (elevated aminotransferases or hepatomegaly) or with serum ferritin levels greater than 1000 μg/L should undergo a liver biopsy to assess the degree of liver injury and the possible contribution of other liver disorders to the clinical picture. Liver biopsy is also recommended in suspected iron overload in non-C282Y homozygotes (C282Y heterozygotes, C282Y/H63D, or no mutations).

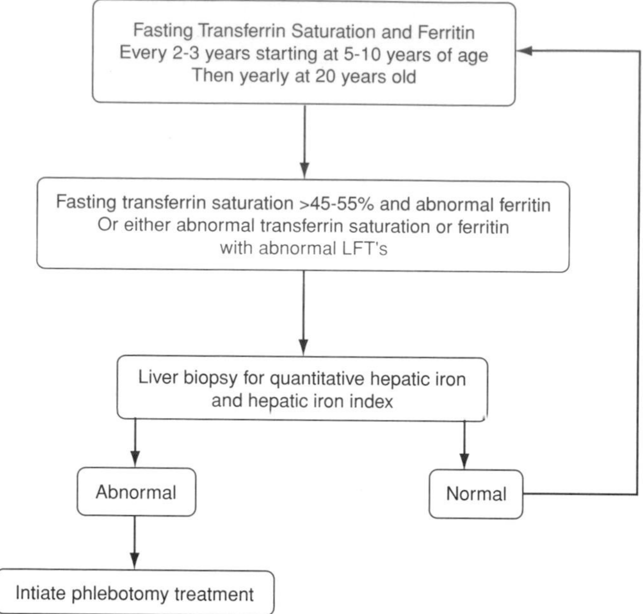

Figure 27.5. Phenotypic strategy for screening for iron overload in a child with a parent with hemochromatosis when the affected parent has no detectable mutation in *HFE*. LFTs, liver function tests.

Approach to the Child with a Parent with Hereditary Hemochromatosis

The preferred clinical assessment of a child whose parent has HHC is open to debate. Because symptomatic end-stage organ disease from HHC is easily preventable with early therapy, screening of potentially affected children has been advocated. However, the majority of patients present with clinical disease after the age of 20 years. Biochemical screening (phenotypic strategy, Figure 27.5) may require sequential transferrin saturation and ferritin determinations and even liver biopsy. With the advent of genetic mutation testing, Adams et al. [62] have shown that it is cost-effective to screen the spouse of the affected parent with mutation analysis (genetic strategy, Figure 27.6). If the unaffected parent is either heterozygous or homozygous for C282Y, the potentially affected children are then screened with mutation analysis following appropriate counseling and consent [62]. Subsequently, at-risk children are followed with fasting transferrin saturation, ferritin, and liver blood tests. This strategy was found to be more cost-effective when compared with the phenotypic strategy [80]. When the ferritin is greater than 200 μg/L or aminotransferases increase, phlebotomy therapy is then initiated.

Iron Overload in Children with Liver Dysfunction

In pediatric patients, iron overload should be considered in the differential diagnosis of liver disease. Testing for transferrin saturation and ferritin should be considered in the evaluation of hepatic dysfunction in children (Figure 27.7). If liver biopsy is performed as part of the evaluation, staining for iron should be done and quantitative hepatic iron determination should be considered. There are older reports of children presenting as young as 5 years with iron overload and presumed HHC that

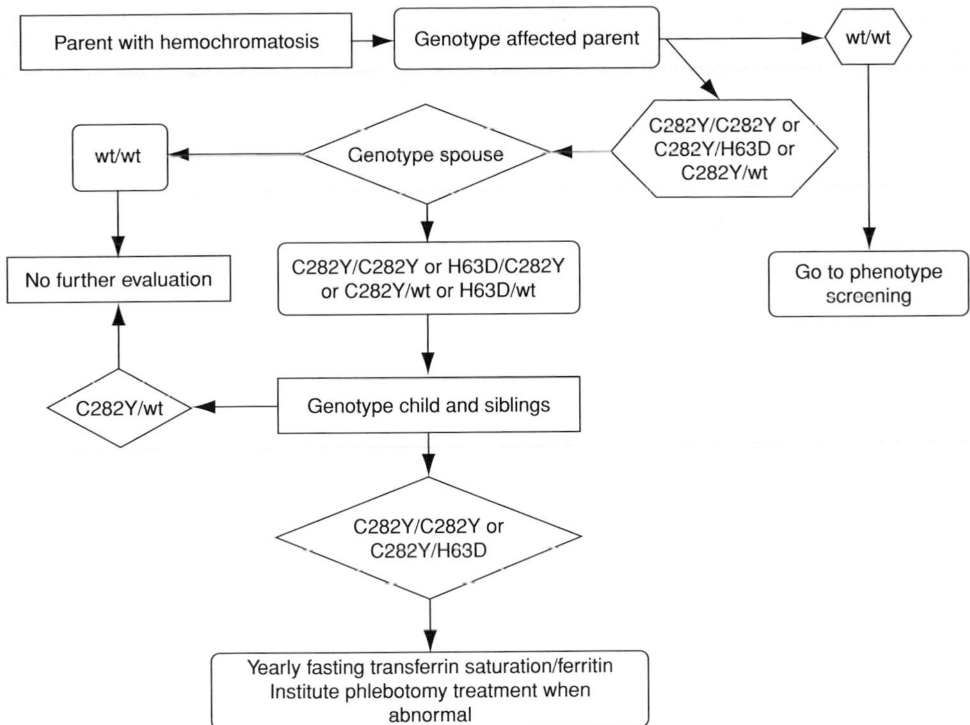

Figure 27.6. Genotypic strategy for screening for hereditary hemochromatosis in a child with a parent with hemochromatosis.

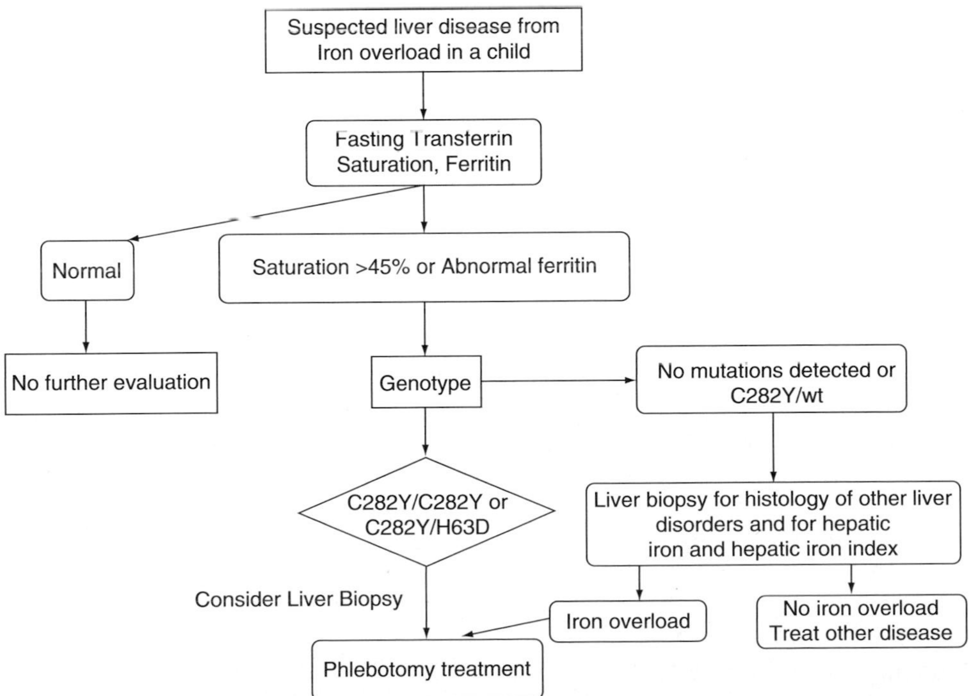

Figure 27.7. Phenotypic strategy for screening for iron overload in a child with liver disease and suspected iron overload.

may have been JHC, as these reports predate *HFE* testing [71]. White children with evidence of iron overload (elevated transferrin saturation of >50%, elevated ferritin, increased stainable iron or hepatic iron concentration) would be candidates for possible *HFE* mutation analysis. The yield of *HFE* analysis in African American and Asian American children would be expected to be quite low. *HFE* mutation analysis also may be helpful in patients with other diseases that can lead to iron overload (NASH, porphyria cutanea tarda).

The role of liver biopsy has not been studied in children. Data from one large adult study has shown that 50% of HHC patients with a ferritin level greater than 1000 μg/L, abnormal aspartate aminotransferase (AST), or hepatomegaly had significant fibrosis on liver biopsy [81]. In contrast, none of the HHC patients without those factors had significant fibrosis [81]. Even before genotyping was available, Niederau et al. [82] demonstrated that patients diagnosed in the precirrhotic stage who were treated with venisection had a normal life expectancy. Thus, in patients homozygous for the C282Y mutation, these noninvasive measures may be used to avoid liver biopsy.

Because HHC is a common genetic disorder whose effects can be prevented by presymptomatic intervention, screening of the general population has been considered. Until the cost of the testing is reduced and the implications for insurability and management are clarified, newborn testing has not been recommended [83,84]. In adults, screening strategies have been suggested using a combination of transferrin saturation and confirmation with *HFE* testing [21].

Treatment

The goals of treatment are to reduce total body iron overload and prevent reaccumulation of iron. When instituted before end organ injury, successful treatment would ideally prevent the development of cirrhosis and other end organ disease and reduce the incidence of hepatocellular carcinoma. A standard adult treatment schedule is shown in Table 27.3. Current recommendations are that venisection is indicated if serum ferritin is greater than 300 μg/L in males or 200 μg/L in females [85]. The goals of therapy are to maintain a ferritin level less than 50 μg/L [85]. There are little published data on phlebotomy therapy in children. Initial therapy in symptomatic children should include weekly or every-other-week phlebotomy of 5–8 mL/kg until the ferritin has decreased to <300 μg/L. Thereafter, two to four sessions per year will probably be required [75]. In our experience, therapeutic phlebotomy may need to be less frequent in children with HHC who have asymptomatic iron overload, probably because of their lower total body iron load. Careful attention to the development of iron deficiency is required when treating children. Once identified, children with HHC should be counseled to maintain a low-iron diet and avoid ascorbic acid and vitamin supplements containing iron.

Table 27.3: Standard Adult Treatment Schedule

1. Remove excess iron
   - Phlebotomy: 1–2 times/wk, 500 mL (250 mg iron/500 mL blood) = 12–35 g iron removed in 1 yr
   - Check hemoglobin every week
   - Serum iron, transferrin saturation, and ferritin every 2 mo
   - Serum ferritin more frequently when <100 mg/dL
   - Document iron depletion by liver biopsy or MRI
2. Prevent reaccumulation of iron
   - Phlebotomy every 2–3 mo
   - Serum iron, transferrin saturation, and ferritin every year
   - Screen for hepatocellular carcinoma if cirrhosis is present

Adapted from Niederau C, Erhardt A, Haussinger D, et al. Haemochromatosis and the liver. J Hepatology 1999;30:6–11; with permission.

Juvenile Hemochromatosis (OMIM 602390)

Juvenile hemochromatosis, or hemochromatosis type 2, is a rare iron-loading disorder that leads to severe iron loading and organ failure, typically before 30 years of age [60]. JHC is characterized by autosomal recessive inheritance and a pattern of iron distribution and tissue injury similar to that of HHC. However, JHC is not associated with mutations in *HFE* and does not show linkage to chromosome 6p [30,86]. In contrast to HHC, males and females are equally affected, and hypogonadism and cardiac dysfunction are the most common symptoms at presentation [61,87]. The disorder has been reported in several ethnic groups [87–89]. Most patients present in the second and third decades of life, which may be partly the result of a higher rate of iron accumulation in JHC as compared with HHC. Indeed, the phlebotomy requirements to maintain normal iron balance are significantly higher in JHC as compared with HHC [90]. The JHC locus was initially localized to chromosome 1q [86]. Further study demonstrated that the gene *HJV* at this site encodes hemojuvelin, a key regulatory protein for hepcidin [41], and accounts for about 90% of the cases reported to date [91–93]. The most frequent mutation is G320V, which was reported to account for 60% of the mutations in the original description [93] and all individuals identified in a French Canadian study [92]. *HAMP*, which encodes hepcidin and is located on chromosome 19, accounts for only 10% of the reported cases [12,91]. A recent report suggests that combined mutations in *HFE* and *TFR2* may also present with a phenotype of JHC without mutations in either *HJV* or *HAMP* [94].

As a consequence, this disorder should be considered when children and adolescents present with clinically significant liver disease and iron overload. A family history of iron overload and hypogonadism in the absence of *HFE* mutations should raise the clinical suspicion for JHC. It is possible that some of the earlier reports of children with clinically apparent liver disease and iron overload [71] dealt with this disorder and not the classic HHC. With the identification of candidate genes involved in JHC, genetic diagnosis is available for *HJV*, *HAMP*, and the *HFE/TFR2* combination. These offer the opportunity for presymptomatic diagnosis in children from affected families. However, the overall incidence of this disorder must be small in comparison with classic HHC, as in the Australian population study, only 0.5% of the adults with the wild-type/wild-type hemochromatosis genotype had an elevated (>45%) fasting transferrin saturation.

Secondary Iron Overload

Secondary iron overload is a common problem for children with transfusion-dependent diseases such as the thalassemias, sickle cell disease, and aplastic anemias. This disorder has been referred to as hemosiderosis, primarily because of the accumulation of iron in the reticuloendothelial cells in the liver. The pathophysiology of secondary iron overload is related to the provision of parenteral iron that bypasses the normal intestinal regulation of iron absorption. In addition, the anemias of ineffective erythropoiesis (thalassemias, congenital dyserythropoietic anemias, and sideroblastic anemias) stimulate iron absorption [95], resulting in an additional 2–5 g of iron absorbed from the diet per year [96,97]. With inadequate chelation therapy, clinical symptoms of iron overload typically are not manifest until the second decade of life. However, tissue iron overloading of parenchymal cells is apparent after only 1 year of transfusion therapy [98]. In patients who are receiving transfusions without chelation therapy, symptomatic heart disease has been reported within 10 years [99]. Iron-induced liver disease is a common cause of death in older patients, often aggravated by hepatitis C infection [100]. Fibrosis is present as early as 2 years after starting transfusions, with cirrhosis reported in the first decade of life [101,102]. With improved survival with iron chelation, iron loading of the anterior pituitary and associated disturbed sexual maturation are quite common [103].

Although the amount of excess iron that has been provided in the form of transfused iron can be calculated from the volume of red blood cells administered, the biochemical markers of iron overload may be unreliable. Some researchers advocate following ferritin levels for signs of iron overload [104,105]. Under normal conditions, 1 μg/L of ferritin is equivalent to 8–10 mg of storage iron. Thus, a ferritin of 1000 μg/L is equal to about 10,000 mg of storage iron. However, above 4000 μg/L ferritin, there is no longer a correlation between ferritin and iron stores. In addition, ferritin may be increased with hepatic inflammation that may be related to other factors, such as hepatitis C infection. This has led others to suggest that ferritin concentrations are not an accurate reflection of tissue iron accumulation [106]. More accurate estimations of tissue iron burden are obtained by liver or cardiac biopsy [105,106] and by recent techniques for iron quantitation by MRI [107–110] or by investigative SQUID (superconducting quantum interference device) biomagnetometry, which may be better at assessing high tissue iron concentrations [111].

Treatment

Standard treatment of transfusional iron overload centers on chelation therapy. Deferoxamine is generally given by continuous subcutaneous administration and is capable of inducing negative iron balance [112]. In general, ferritin should begin to decrease by the end of 1 year of treatment. Generally, the goal is to maintain a ferritin level of less than 1000 μg/L on treatment. Deferoxamine prevents early cardiac death, arrests the progression to cirrhosis, and stabilizes or reduces total body iron load [113]. The major risks of deferoxamine are growth failure, hearing impairment, and bone abnormalities. These are more common in patients with low iron loads [114]. Direct dose-related toxicities involve the kidneys, lungs, and visual loss. Iron chelation is generally successful at reducing liver and early cardiac toxicity. Indeed, the early use of deferoxamine in an amount proportional to the transfusional iron overload reduces iron burden and the risk of the development of diabetes mellitus, cardiac disease, and early death in patients with thalassemia major [113]. However, alternative strategies have been applied for serious iron overload. When possible, such as in some cases of sickle cell disease, exchange transfusion can reduce the iron burden from transfusions [115]. Other strategies include intravenous deferoxamine, which can rapidly reduce tissue iron burden in situations of severe iron overload (Figure 27.8). A newer oral chelation agent, deferiprone, has been used in Europe and was recently approved for use in the United States [116–119]. Preliminary data suggest that deferiprone may be more effective at removal of cardiac iron load than deferoxamine [120] and similar in efficacy or slightly less effective for hepatic iron reduction. However, the efficacy of deferiprone was an area of controversy [121–123] regarding a recent study that shows no evidence of the development of an increase in hepatic fibrosis with deferiprone therapy [124]. The major side effects of deferiprone are bone marrow suppression, arthropathy, gastrointestinal symptoms, and zinc deficiency. Combination treatment with deferoxamine and deferiprone or other oral chelators, such as deferasirox, are now under study.

Some researchers have recommended serial liver biopsy to follow iron overload in transfusion-dependent patients. If performed, multiple liver biopsies may be required to adequately assess the degree of injury and iron overload [102]. We have found that liver biopsy is helpful in determining the contribution from hepatitis C and iron overload and in guiding the use of more aggressive therapies, such as intravenous deferoxamine. Recent work suggests that MRI may be reliable in quantitating hepatic iron overload and may be preferable for serial determinations [107–109,111]. Liver biopsy could then be reserved for assessment of hepatic injury and fibrosis and for the assessment of the relative contribution of non–iron-related disorders to the process.

NEONATAL HEMOCHROMATOSIS (OMIM 321100)

Several disorders of infancy reportedly are associated with tissue iron overload. The term infant liver is normally iron replete; siderosis of hepatocytes, however, generally cannot be observed in biopsy materials after the third postnatal month. This reflects

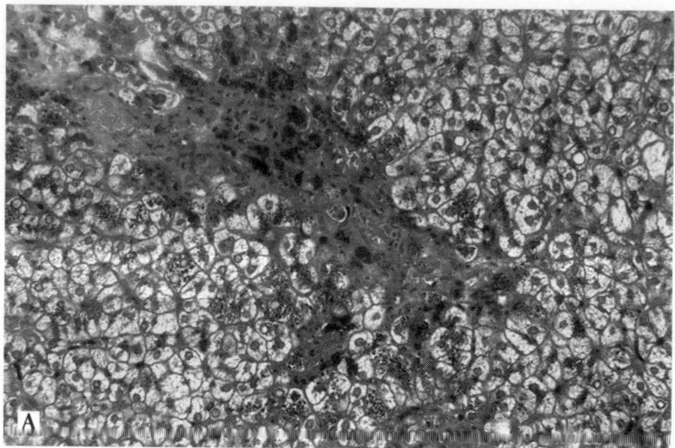

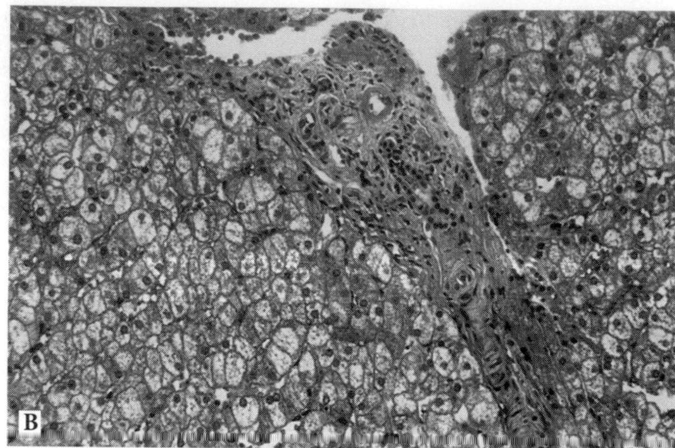

Figure 27.8. Effects of intravenous deferoxamine treatment. (**A**) Liver biopsy from a 16-year-old girl with β-thalassemia. Increased stainable iron shown on Prussian blue stain. Quantitative hepatic iron of 15,483 μg/g dry weight. (**B**) Repeat liver biopsy with Prussian blue stain in the same patient following 1 year of daily intravenous deferoxamine (hepatic iron, 669 μg/g dry weight). Note the dramatic reduction in stainable iron. For color reproduction, see Color Plate 27.8.

the mobilization, and depletion, of hepatic iron stores in support of growth [125]. Illness can slow this process. (Perhaps claims several decades ago that infants with tyrosinemia or Zellweger syndrome were iron overloaded reflected not simply a judgment of infant livers by adult standards but also these infants' failure to thrive.) Prominent iron stores, found only in the liver, have been thought to characterize the mitochondriopathy of one form of *BCS1L* mutation [126] (*g*rowth *r*etardation, *a*minoaciduria, *c*holestasis, *i*ron overload, *l*actic acidosis, *e*arly death [GRACILE] syndrome), but this feature of the disorder may be adventitious. Two of the four infants to date identified with the tricho-hepato-enteric syndrome [127] had both extrahepatic and hepatic siderosis on death at 6 months; this entity awaits further study. The last to be considered is likely not a disorder but a syndrome and is called fetal, congenital, or neonatal hemochromatosis.

Neonatal hemochromatosis (NH; also called neonatal iron storage disease) appears to be a misnomer. Fifty years ago, a Swiss hematologist encountered two infants born with end-stage liver disease and siderosis of extrahepatic tissues. The pattern of iron deposition, involving pancreas, myocardium, and epithelia of mucosal and ductless glands, recalled that of adult hemochromatosis. The findings in the livers, with hepatocellular loss, scarring, and nodular regeneration, also were reminiscent of adult hemochromatosis. This case report of a disease picture resembling hemochromatosis in two newborn infants [128] defined NH as a form of cholestatic liver disease of infancy and set implicit guidelines for further work.

Although isolated case reports followed every several years, only in the 1980s had understanding of adult hemochromatosis and its inheritance, as well as of the biology and biochemistry of iron handling, made it possible to assemble and to test hypotheses on the origins of the clinicopathologic entity of NH. There were two hypotheses on the cause of NH. In one, disordered fetoplacental metabolism of iron was held to lead to liver disease. In the other, fetal liver disease was considered primary, with disordered iron handling a sequela [129,130]. (Attempts to assess the role of iron, if any, in liver disease of fetal onset have been hampered by failure to recognize that the term conceptus is physiologically iron replete to a degree that would constitute iron overload in adult life.)

Work summarized elsewhere [131] has failed to demonstrate, among other things, that NH is an unusual manifestation of adult hemochromatosis and that cultured fibroblasts from NH patients respond abnormally to iron loading or withdrawal. In addition, none of the recently described species that serve as intermediates in iron handling (see above) has yet been implicated as primarily defective in NH [132]. Observation of several kindreds into which children with NH were born has made clear that occurrence risks within a sibship do not fit usual patterns for heritable metabolic disorders, with several instances of maternal half-siblings affected by NH [131]. Attention in NH accordingly has turned to evaluation of maternally harbored, transplacentally transmissible agents that damage the fetal liver, with promising initial yield (see below). Even without primary lesions of iron handling being implicated in NH, however, the appellation NH seems likely to persist. Severe liver disease of intrauterine onset, with extrahepatic hemochromatotic siderosis, is not catchy enough to prevail.

Clinical Manifestations

The clinical picture in NH is that of acute liver failure superimposed on chronic liver disease. In some instances, illness is manifest well before birth and can be identified as intrauterine growth retardation or fetal or placental edema; general collapse supervenes in the delivery suite. In others, the picture is that of a well-grown infant who suffers hypoglycemia, hypocoagulability, and circulatory collapse within a few hours after birth.

Once sepsis is excluded (including echovirus in particular [133,134]) and generalized hepatocellular synthetic insufficiency is recognized, few diagnostic candidates other than NH remain. Features that may point to acute liver failure include not only hypoalbuminemia but also nonspecifically low serum concentrations of a variety of proteins [135]. Abnormal bile acid species in urine, coupled with a failure of serum concentrations of γ-glutamyltransferase activity to rise despite conjugated hyperbilirubinemia, may suggest a disorder of bile acid synthesis [136] but likely reflect hepatocellular failure [137,138]. As seen in infants with hemophagocytic syndrome, hyperferritinemia in the setting of liver failure is not specific for NH [139]; hypotransferrinemia, with hypersaturation of available transferrin, is a better marker. Particularly in infants with Down's syndrome, a megakaryocyte-predominant transient myeloproliferative disorder should be considered [140]. Commonly, aminotransferase activity is disproportionately low for the degree of liver dysfunction [141] and α-fetoprotein is high.

Magnetic resonance imaging studies may identify siderosis at extrahepatic sites (pancreas, myocardium), which supports the diagnosis of NH [142]. Iron-intense signaling from the liver alone does not support a diagnosis of NH. Demonstration of siderosis in glands of oropharyngeal mucosa obtained at biopsy also supports the diagnosis of NH (Figure 27.9) [143]. Some infants with NH have dysmature proximal tubular epithelium in later-formed nephrons, likely a sequela of severe liver disease during nephrogenesis. Whether findings at renal biopsy have prognostic implications is unclear [144].

The liver is not frequently biopsied in NH because of the profound coagulopathy. In necropsy or hepatectomy specimens, various patterns of injury are found. These range from a liver almost devoid of hepatocytes (*le foie vide* [145]) to a liver, also almost devoid of hepatocytes, in which diffuse perisinusoidal fibrosis accompanies neocholangiolar metaplasia of parenchymal elements. Centrilobular vaso-obliterative fibrosis often is encountered. Varying degrees of hepatocellular loss, stromal collapse, and nodular regeneration of hepatocytic parenchyma may be seen. Giant cell change of hepatocytes, with intracellular and canalicular cholestasis, is sometimes observed, particularly in regenerated regions.

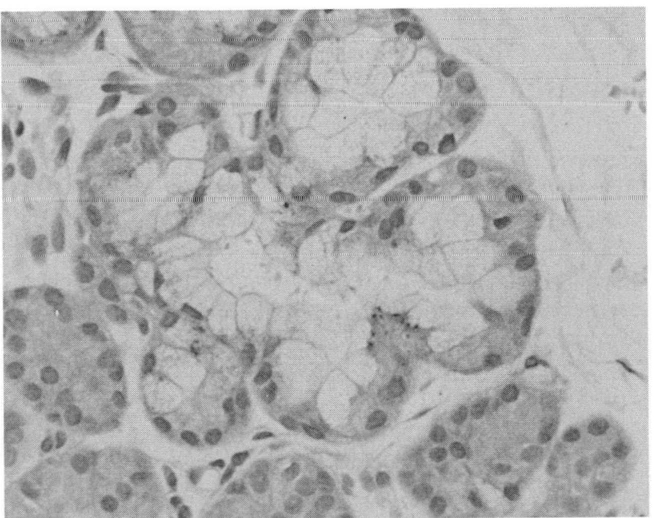

Figure 27.9. Buccal biopsy from a patient with neonatal hemochromatosis. Finely granular stainable iron is seen, particularly within mucus cells, in epithelium of a minor salivary gland from the inner aspect of the lower lip. (Prussian blue/nuclear fast red, original magnification 400×.) For color reproduction, see Color Plate 27.9.

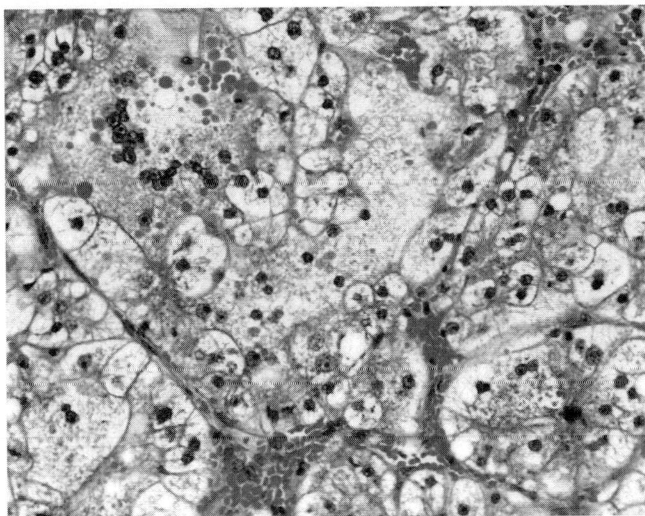

Figure 27.10. Liver biopsy from a patient with neonatal hemochromatosis. Edema, pigment accumulation (both bile and hemosiderin), and giant cell change with rosetting are seen in severely injured liver. (Hematoxylin and eosin stain, original magnification 200×.) For color reproduction, see Color Plate 27.10.

All these features, with two exceptions, may be found in necropsy or hepatectomy specimens from adults with acute or subacute liver failure. The exceptions are giant cell change of hepatocytes (Figure 27.10) and centrilobular vaso-obliterative fibrosis. The adult liver generally does not respond to injury with giant cell change. The adult liver also lacks the pop-off valve of the ductus venosus, which, in the presence of fetal lobular injury, may facilitate blood shunting away from parenchyma, with accentuation of centrilobular hypoxic–ischemic injury and scarring [146].

Treatment

Care in NH is supportive, with the option of liver transplantation as a backstop. Some infants with presumed NH recover [147,148]. In others, liver scarring may resolve incompletely, with portal hypertension. An antioxidant/chelation cocktail (Table 27.4) is controversial but appears to be useful principally in infants with less severe liver disease [148,149] and must be employed with caution; the component deferoxamine, in particular, may potentiate bacterial or fungal sepsis [148]. Disordered iron handling in childhood or early adulthood has not been reported in patients who recovered from NH or in patients who have received allografts.

Although the experience with liver transplantation is limited, survival is approximately 50% at 1 year in limited case

Table 27.4: Antioxidant/Chelation Treatment Proposed for Neonatal Hemochromatosis

Vitamin E (α-tocopheryl–polyethylene succinate)	25 IU/kg/d orally
N-acetylcysteine	100 mg/kg/d IV
Prostaglandin-E_1	0.4 μg/kg/hr IV (max. 2 wk)
Selenium	3 μg/kg/d IV
Deferoxamine	30 mg/kg/d IV until ferritin <500 ng/mL

IV, intravenously.

series [141,148–150]. Although iron does not usually accumulate in the new liver, there is one report of hepatic iron overload in the transplanted liver [151]. The authors speculated that this was the result of redistribution of iron. The major impediment to liver transplantation in this disorder is survival of the infant until transplantation [148]. This may be the area where chelation therapy may play a role.

Whitington and Hibbard [152] hypothesized that the recurrence risk of NH within a sibship suggests a disorder of maternofetal alloimmunization and demonstrated that administration of immunoglobulin to pregnant mothers with previously affected children reduced, but did not eliminate, liver injury in the fetus. Comparison with historical controls suggests that immunoglobulin therapy during pregnancy converts an often fatal disorder into a survivable or even minor one.

Although sera from NH mothers react with an antigen present in fetal but not in adult human or mouse liver, and sera from non-NH mothers do not react with this antigen [153], the identity of this antigen and the mechanisms by which maternal immunization against it may lead to fetal disease remain to be defined. In addition, intravenous immunoglobulin therapy might nonspecifically palliate different types of insult leading to NH: It might ablate a maternal immune response, mask target antigens, or even suppress recrudescence of a dormant maternal infection with a hepatotropic agent that can be transplacentally transmitted. Serologic studies in NH may define subsets of liver disease of fetal onset as well as subsets of response to the immunoglobulin therapy. Elucidation of mechanisms of fetal liver injury may, in turn, lead to an understanding of how such injury produces extrahepatic siderosis in a hemochromatotic distribution.

ACKNOWLEDGMENTS

Michael Narkewicz thanks Dr. Sarah Mengshol for providing the photomicrographs. This work was supported in part by grant M01 R00069 from the General Clinical Research Centers Program of the National Center for Research Resources, National Institutes of Health and the Hewit-Andrews Endowed Chair in Pediatric Liver Disease.

REFERENCES

1. Wallace DF, Summerville L, Lusby PE, Subramaniam VN. First phenotypic description of transferrin receptor 2 knockout mouse, and the role of hepcidin. Gut 2005;54:980–6.
2. Pietrangelo A. Non-HFE hemochromatosis. Semin Liver Dis 2005;25:450–60.
3. Finch C. Regulators of iron balance in humans. Blood 1994;84:1697–702.
4. Sturrock A, Alexander J, Lamb J, et al. Characterization of a transferrin-independent uptake system for iron in HeLa cells. J Biol Chem 1990;265:3139–45.
5. Ganz T, Nemeth E. Iron imports. IV. Hepcidin and regulation of body iron metabolism. Am J Physiol Gastrointest Liver Physiol 2006;290:G199–203.
6. Nicolas G, Chauvet C, Viatte L, et al. The gene encoding the iron regulatory peptide hepcidin is regulated by anemia, hypoxia, and inflammation. J Clin Invest 2002;110:1037–44.
7. Riedel HD, Remus AJ, Fitscher BA, Stremmel W. Characterization and partial purification of a ferrireductase from human duodenal microvillus membranes. Biochem J 1995;309 (pt 3):745–8.
8. Gunshin H, Mackenzie B, Berger UV, et al. Cloning and characterization of a mammalian proton-coupled metal-ion transporter. Nature 1997;388:482–8.
9. Nemeth E, Tuttle MS, Powelson J, et al. Hepcidin regulates cellular iron efflux by binding to ferroportin and inducing its internalization. Science 2004;306:2090–3.
10. Donovan A, Lima CA, Pinkus JL, et al. The iron exporter ferroportin/Slc40a1 is essential for iron homeostasis. Cell Metab 2005;1:191–200.
11. Vaulont S, Lou DQ, Viatte L, Kahn A. Of mice and men: the iron age. J Clin Invest 2005;115:2079–82.
12. Roetto A, Papanikolaou G, Politou M, et al. Mutant antimicrobial peptide hepcidin is associated with severe juvenile hemochromatosis. Nat Genet 2003;33:21–2.
13. Nicolas G, Bennoun M, Devaux I, et al. Lack of hepcidin gene expression and severe tissue iron overload in upstream stimulatory factor 2 (USF2) knockout mice. Proc Natl Acad Sci U S A 2001;98:8780–5.
14. Njajou OT, Vaessen N, Joosse M, et al. A mutation in SLC11A3 is associated with autosomal dominant hemochromatosis. Nat Genet 2001;28:213–14.
15. Ahmad KA, Ahmann JR, Migas MC, et al. Decreased liver hepcidin expression in the Hfe knockout mouse. Blood Cells Mol Dis 2002;29:361–6.
16. Gehrke SG, Kulaksiz H, Herrmann T, et al. Expression of hepcidin in hereditary hemochromatosis: evidence for a regulation in response to the serum transferrin saturation and to non-transferrin-bound iron. Blood 2003;102:371–6.
17. Nemeth E, Roetto A, Garozzo G, et al. Hepcidin is decreased in TFR2 hemochromatosis. Blood 2005;105:1803–6.
18. Bridle KR, Frazer DM, Wilkins SJ, et al. Disrupted hepcidin regulation in HFE-associated haemochromatosis and the liver as a regulator of body iron homoeostasis. Lancet 2003;361:669–73.
19. Papanikolaou G, Tzilianos M, Christakis JI, et al. Hepcidin in iron overload disorders. Blood 2005;105:4103–5.
20. Rouault T, Klausner R. Regulation of iron metabolism in eukaryotes. Curr Top Cell Regul 1997;35:1–19.

21. Bacon BR, Powell LW, Adams PC, et al. Molecular medicine and hemochromatosis: at the crossroads. Gastroenterology 1999;116:193–207.
22. Fleming MD, Trenor CC 3rd, Su MA, et al. Microcytic anaemia mice have a mutation in Nramp2, a candidate iron transporter gene. Nat Genet 1997;16:383–6.
23. Kawabata H, Yang R, Hirama T, et al. Molecular cloning of transferrin receptor 2. A new member of the transferrin receptor-like family. J Biol Chem 1999;274:20826–32.
24. Fleming RE, Migas MC, Holden CC, et al. Transferrin receptor 2: continued expression in mouse liver in the face of iron overload and in hereditary hemochromatosis. Proc Natl Acad Sci U S A 2000;97:2214–19.
25. Cox TM, Peters TJ. Uptake of iron by duodenal biopsy specimens from patients with iron-deficiency anaemia and primary haemochromatosis. Lancet 1978;1:123–4.
26. Cox TM, Peters TJ. In vitro studies of duodenal iron uptake in patients with primary and secondary iron storage disease. Q J Med 1980;49:249–57.
27. Niederkofler V, Salie R, Arber S. Hemojuvelin is essential for dietary iron sensing, and its mutation leads to severe iron overload. J Clin Invest 2005;115:2180–6.
28. Huang FW, Pinkus JL, Pinkus GS, et al. A mouse model of juvenile hemochromatosis. J Clin Invest 2005;115:2187–91.
29. Simon M, Bourel M, Fauchet R, Genetet B. Association of HLA-A3 and HLA-B14 antigens with idiopathic haemochromatosis. Gut 1976;17:332–4.
30. Feder JN, Gnirke A, Thomas W, et al. A novel MHC class I-like gene is mutated in patients with hereditary haemochromatosis. Nat Genet 1996;13:399–408.
31. Beutler E. Genetic irony beyond haemochromatosis: clinical effects of HLA-H mutations. Lancet 1997;349:296–7.
32. Sham RL, Ou CY, Cappuccio J, et al. Correlation between genotype and phenotype in hereditary hemochromatosis: analysis of 61 cases. Blood Cells Mol Dis 1997;23:314–20.
33. Ramrakhiani S, Bacon BR. Hemochromatosis: advances in molecular genetics and clinical diagnosis. J Clin Gastroenterol 1998;27:41–6.
34. Shaheen NJ, Bacon BR, Grimm IS. Clinical characteristics of hereditary hemochromatosis patients who lack the C282Y mutation. Hepatology 1998;28:526–9.
35. Barton JC, Sawada-Hirai R, Rothenberg BE, Acton RT. Two novel missense mutations of the HFE gene (I105T and G93R) and identification of the S65C mutation in Alabama hemochromatosis probands. Blood Cells Mol Dis 1999;25:147–55.
36. Mura C, Raguenes O, Ferec C. HFE mutations analysis in 711 hemochromatosis probands: evidence for S65C implication in mild form of hemochromatosis. Blood 1999;93:2502–5.
37. Wallace DF, Dooley JS, Walker AP. A novel mutation of HFE explains the classical phenotype of genetic hemochromatosis in a C282Y heterozygote. Gastroenterology 1999;116:1409–12.
38. Feder JN, Tsuchihashi Z, Irrinki A, et al. The hemochromatosis founder mutation in HLA-H disrupts beta2-microglobulin interaction and cell surface expression. J Biol Chem 1997;272:14025–8.
39. Waheed A, Parkkila S, Zhou XY, et al. Hereditary hemochromatosis: effects of C282Y and H63D mutations on association with beta2-microglobulin, intracellular processing, and cell surface expression of the HFE protein in COS-7 cells. Proc Natl Acad Sci U S A 1997;94:12384–9.
40. Feder JN, Penny DM, Irrinki A, et al. The hemochromatosis gene product complexes with the transferrin receptor and lowers its affinity for ligand binding. Proc Natl Acad Sci U S A 1998;95:1472–7.
41. Lin L, Goldberg YP, Ganz T. Competitive regulation of hepcidin mRNA by soluble and cell-associated hemojuvelin. Blood 2005;106:2884–9.
42. de Sousa M, Reimao R, Lacerda R, et al. Iron overload in beta 2-microglobulin-deficient mice. Immunol Lett 1994;39:105–11.
43. Rothenberg BE, Voland JR. Beta2 knockout mice develop parenchymal iron overload: a putative role for class I genes of the major histocompatibility complex in iron metabolism. Proc Natl Acad Sci U S A 1996;93:1529–34.
44. Zhou XY, Tomatsu S, Fleming RE, et al. HFE gene knockout produces mouse model of hereditary hemochromatosis. Proc Natl Acad Sci U S A 1998;95:2492–7.
45. Herrmann T, Muckenthaler M, van der Hoeven F, et al. Iron overload in adult Hfe-deficient mice independent of changes in the steady-state expression of the duodenal iron transporters DMT1 and Ireg1/ferroportin. J Mol Med 2004;82:39–48.
46. Phatak PD, Sham RL, Raubertas RF, et al. Prevalence of hereditary hemochromatosis in 16031 primary care patients. Ann Intern Med 1998;129:954–61.
47. Olynyk JK, Cullen DJ, Aquilia S, et al. A population-based study of the clinical expression of the hemochromatosis gene. N Engl J Med 1999;341:718–24.
48. Monaghan KG, Rybicki BA, Shurafa M, Feldman GL. Mutation analysis of the HFE gene associated with hereditary hemochromatosis in African Americans. Am J Hematol 1998;58:213–17.
49. Pietrangelo A, Montosi G, Totaro A, et al. Hereditary hemochromatosis in adults without pathogenic mutations in the hemochromatosis gene. N Engl J Med 1999;341:725–32.
50. Baer DM, Simons JL, Staples RL, et al. Hemochromatosis screening in asymptomatic ambulatory men 30 years of age and older. Am J Med 1995;98:464–8.
51. Edwards CQ, Griffen LM, Goldgar D, et al. Prevalence of hemochromatosis among 11,065 presumably healthy blood donors. N Engl J Med 1988;318:1355–62.
52. Trousseau A. Glycosurie, diabete, sucre. In: Clinique medicale de l'Hôtel-Dieu de Paris. Paris: Balliere, 1865:663.
53. Adams PC, Deugnier Y, Moirand R, Brissot P. The relationship between iron overload, clinical symptoms, and age in 410 patients with genetic hemochromatosis. Hepatology 1997;25:162–6.
54. Powell LW, Dixon JL, Hewett DG. Role of early case detection by screening relatives of patients with HFE-associated hereditary haemochromatosis. Best Pract Res Clin Haematol 2005;18:221–34.
55. Tavill AS. Diagnosis and management of hemochromatosis. Hepatology 2001;33:1321–8.
56. O'Neil J, Powell L. Clinical aspects of hemochromatosis. Semin Liver Dis 2005;25:381–91.
57. Franchini M, Veneri D. Hereditary hemochromatosis. Hematology 2005;10:145–9.
58. Waalen J, Felitti V, Gelbart T, et al. Prevalence of hemochromatosis-related symptoms among individuals with mutations in the HFE gene. Mayo Clin Proc 2002;77:522–30.
59. Waalen J, Nordestgaard BG, Beutler E. The penetrance of hereditary hemochromatosis. Best Pract Res Clin Haematol 2005;18:203–20.

60. Camaschella C. Juvenile haemochromatosis. Baillieres Clin Gastroenterol 1998;12:227–35.
61. Camaschella C, Roetto A, Cicilano M, et al. Juvenile and adult hemochromatosis are distinct genetic disorders. Eur J Hum Genet 1997;5:371–5.
62. Adams PC, Kertesz AE, Valberg LS. Screening for hemochromatosis in children of homozygotes: prevalence and cost-effectiveness. Hepatology 1995;22:1720–7.
63. Datz C, Haas T, Rinner H, et al. Heterozygosity for the C282Y mutation in the hemochromatosis gene is associated with increased serum iron, transferrin saturation, and hemoglobin in young women: a protective role against iron deficiency? Clin Chem 1998;44:2429–32.
64. Distante S, Berg JP, Lande K, et al. High prevalence of the hemochromatosis-associated Cys282Tyr HFE gene mutation in a healthy Norwegian population in the city of Oslo, and its phenotypic expression. Scand J Gastroenterol 1999;34:529–34.
65. McLaren CE, McLachlan GJ, Halliday JW, et al. Distribution of transferrin saturation in an Australian population: relevance to the early diagnosis of hemochromatosis. Gastroenterology 1998;114:543–9.
66. Rossi E, Olynyk JK, Cullen DJ, et al. Compound heterozygous hemochromatosis genotype predicts increased iron and erythrocyte indices in women. Clin Chem 2000;46:162–6.
67. Grove J, Daly AK, Burt AD, et al. Heterozygotes for HFE mutations have no increased risk of advanced alcoholic liver disease. Gut 1998;43:262–6.
68. Bonkovsky HL, Jawaid Q, Tortorelli K, et al. Non-alcoholic steatohepatitis and iron: increased prevalence of mutations of the HFE gene in non-alcoholic steatohepatitis. J Hepatol 1999;31:421–9.
69. Bonkovsky HL, Poh-Fitzpatrick M, Pimstone N, et al. Porphyria cutanea tarda, hepatitis C, and HFE gene mutations in North America. Hepatology 1998;27:1661–9.
70. Roberts AG, Whatley SD, Morgan RR, et al. Increased frequency of the haemochromatosis Cys282Tyr mutation in sporadic porphyria cutanea tarda. Lancet 1997;349:321–3.
71. Kaikov Y, Wadsworth LD, Hassall E, et al. Primary hemochromatosis in children: report of three newly diagnosed cases and review of the pediatric literature. Pediatrics 1992;90(1 pt 1):37–42.
72. Adams PC, Chakrabarti S. Genotypic/phenotypic correlations in genetic hemochromatosis: evolution of diagnostic criteria. Gastroenterology 1998;114:319–23.
73. Kowdley KV, Trainer TD, Saltzman JR, et al. Utility of hepatic iron index in American patients with hereditary hemochromatosis: a multicenter study. Gastroenterology 1997;113:1270–7.
74. Powell LW, Summers KM, Board PG, et al. Expression of hemochromatosis in homozygous subjects. Implications for early diagnosis and prevention. Gastroenterology 1990;98:1625–32.
75. Escobar GJ, Heyman MB, Smith WB, Thaler MM. Primary hemochromatosis in childhood. Pediatrics 1987;80:549–54.
76. Brittenham GM, Badman DG. Noninvasive measurement of iron: report of an NIDDK workshop. Blood 2003;101:15–19.
77. Martin DR, Semelka RC. Magnetic resonance imaging of the liver: review of techniques and approach to common diseases. Semin Ultrasound CT MR 2005;26:116–31.
78. Pomerantz S, Siegelman ES. MR imaging of iron depositional disease. Magn Reson Imaging Clin N Am 2002;10:105–20, vi.
79. Barton JC, Rothenberg BE, Bertoli LF, Acton RT. Diagnosis of hemochromatosis in family members of probands: a comparison of phenotyping and HFE genotyping. Genet Med 1999;1:89–93.
80. Adams PC. Implications of genotyping of spouses to limit investigation of children in genetic hemochromatosis. Clin Genet 1998;53:176–8.
81. Guyader D, Jacquelinet C, Moirand R, et al. Noninvasive prediction of fibrosis in C282Y homozygous hemochromatosis. Gastroenterology 1998;115:929–36.
82. Niederau C, Fischer R, Sonnenberg A, et al. Survival and causes of death in cirrhotic and in noncirrhotic patients with primary hemochromatosis. N Engl J Med 1985;313:1256–62.
83. Burke W, Thomson E, Khoury MJ, et al. Hereditary hemochromatosis: gene discovery and its implications for population based screening. JAMA 1998;280:172–8.
84. Qaseem A, Aronson M, Fitterman N, et al. Screening for hereditary hemochromatosis: a clinical practice guideline from the American College of Physicians. Ann Intern Med 2005;143:517–21.
85. Barton JC, McDonnell SM, Adams PC, et al. Management of hemochromatosis. Hemochromatosis Management Working Group. Ann Intern Med 1998;129:932–9.
86. Roetto A, Totaro A, Cazzola M, et al. Juvenile hemochromatosis locus maps to chromosome 1q. Am J Hum Genet 1999;64:1388–93.
87. Cazzola M, Ascari E, Barosi G, et al. Juvenile idiopathic haemochromatosis: a life-threatening disorder presenting as hypogonadotropic hypogonadism. Hum Genet 1983;65:149–54.
88. Kelly AL, Rhodes DA, Roland JM, et al. Hereditary juvenile haemochromatosis: a genetically heterogeneous life-threatening iron-storage disease. Q J Med 1998;91:607–18.
89. Lamon JM, Marynick SP, Roseblatt R, Donnelly S. Idiopathic hemochromatosis in a young female. A case study and review of the syndrome in young people. Gastroenterology 1979;76:178–83.
90. Cazzola M, Cerani P, Rovati A, et al. Juvenile genetic hemochromatosis is clinically and genetically distinct from the classical HLA-related disorder. Blood 1998;92:2979–81.
91. Gehrke SG, Pietrangelo A, Kascak M, et al. HJV gene mutations in European patients with juvenile hemochromatosis. Clin Genet 2005;67:425–8.
92. Lanzara C, Roetto A, Daraio F, et al. Spectrum of hemojuvelin gene mutations in 1q-linked juvenile hemochromatosis. Blood 2004;103:4317–21.
93. Papanikolaou G, Samuels ME, Ludwig EH, et al. Mutations in HFE2 cause iron overload in chromosome 1q-linked juvenile hemochromatosis. Nat Genet 2004;36:77–82.
94. Pietrangelo A, Caleffi A, Henrion J, et al. Juvenile hemochromatosis associated with pathogenic mutations of adult hemochromatosis genes. Gastroenterology 2005;128:470–9.
95. Andrews NC. Disorders of iron metabolism. N Engl J Med 1999;341:1986–95.
96. Pippard MJ, Callender ST, Warner GT, Weatherall DJ. Iron absorption and loading in beta-thalassaemia intermedia. Lancet 1979;2:819–21.
97. Pootrakul P, Kitcharoen K, Yansukon P, et al. The effect of erythroid hyperplasia on iron balance. Blood 1988;71:1124–9.
98. Risdon RA, Flynn DM, Barry M. The relation between liver iron concentration and liver damage in transfusional iron

overload in thalassaemia and the effect of chelation therapy. Gut 1973;14:421.
99. Wolfe L, Olivieri N, Sallan D, et al. Prevention of cardiac disease by subcutaneous deferoxamine in patients with thalassemia major. N Engl J Med 1985;312:1600–3.
100. Zurlo MG, De Stefano P, Borgna-Pignatti C, et al. Survival and causes of death in thalassaemia major. Lancet 1989;2:27–30.
101. Jean G, Terzoli S, Mauri R, et al. Cirrhosis associated with multiple transfusions in thalassaemia. Arch Dis Child 1984;59:67–70.
102. Thakerngpol K, Fucharoen S, Boonyaphipat P, et al. Liver injury due to iron overload in thalassemia: histopathologic and ultrastructural studies. Biometals 1996;9:177–83.
103. Low LC. Growth, puberty and endocrine function in beta-thalassaemia major. J Pediatr Endocrinol Metab 1997;10:175–84.
104. Lombardo T, Ferro G, Frontini V, Percolla S. High-dose intravenous desferrioxamine (DFO) delivery in four thalassemic patients allergic to subcutaneous DFO administration. Am J Hematol 1996;51:90–2.
105. Lombardo T, Tamburino C, Bartoloni G, et al. Cardiac iron overload in thalassemic patients: an endomyocardial biopsy study. Ann Hematol 1995;71:135–41.
106. Nielsen P, Fischer R, Engelhardt R, et al. Liver iron stores in patients with secondary haemosiderosis under iron chelation therapy with deferoxamine or deferiprone. Br J Haematol 1995;91:827–33.
107. Alexopoulou E, Stripeli F, Baras P, et al. R2 relaxometry with MRI for the quantification of tissue iron overload in beta-thalassemic patients. J Magn Reson Imaging 2006;23:163–70.
108. Carneiro AA, Fernandes JP, de Araujo DB, et al. Liver iron concentration evaluated by two magnetic methods: magnetic resonance imaging and magnetic susceptometry. Magn Reson Med 2005;54:122–8.
109. Wood JC, Enriquez C, Ghugre N, et al. MRI R2 and R2* mapping accurately estimates hepatic iron concentration in transfusion-dependent thalassemia and sickle cell disease patients. Blood 2005;106:1460–5.
110. St Pierre TG, Clark PR, Chua-anusorn W, et al. Noninvasive measurement and imaging of liver iron concentrations using proton magnetic resonance. Blood 2005;105:855–61.
111. Carneiro AA, Vilela GR, Fernandes JB, et al. In vivo tissue characterization using magnetic techniques. Neurol Clin Neurophysiol 2004;2004:85.
112. Olivieri NF, Brittenham GM. Iron-chelating therapy and the treatment of thalassemia. Blood 1997;89:739–61.
113. Brittenham GM, Griffith PM, Nienhuis AW, et al. Efficacy of deferoxamine in preventing complications of iron overload in patients with thalassemia major. N Engl J Med 1994;331:567–73.
114. Gabutti V, Borgna-Pignatti C. Clinical manifestations and therapy of transfusional haemosiderosis. Baillieres Clin Haematol 1994;7:919–40.
115. Cabibbo S, Fidone C, Garozzo G, et al. Chronic red blood cell exchange to prevent clinical complications in sickle cell disease. Transfus Apher Sci 2005;32:315–21.
116. Barman Balfour JA, Foster RH. Deferiprone: a review of its clinical potential in iron overload in beta-thalassaemia major and other transfusion-dependent diseases. Drugs 1999;58:553–78.
117. Piga A, Roggero S, Vinciguerra T, et al. Deferiprone: new insight. Ann N Y Acad Sci 2005;1054:169–74.
118. Kontoghiorghes GJ, Eracleous E, Economides C, Kolnagou A. Advances in iron overload therapies. prospects for effective use of deferiprone (L1), deferoxamine, the new experimental chelators ICL670, GT56–252, L1NA11 and their combinations. Curr Med Chem 2005;12:2663–81.
119. Taher A, Sheikh-Taha M, Sharara A, et al. Safety and effectiveness of 100 mg/kg/day deferiprone in patients with thalassemia major: a two-year study. Acta Haematol 2005;114:146–9.
120. Victor Hoffbrand A. Deferiprone therapy for transfusional iron overload. Best Pract Res Clin Haematol 2005;18:299–317.
121. Olivieri NF, Brittenham GM, Matsui D, et al. Iron-chelation therapy with oral deferipronein patients with thalassemia major. N Engl J Med 1995;332:918–22.
122. Olivieri NF, Brittenham GM, McLaren CE, et al. Long-term safety and effectiveness of iron-chelation therapy with deferiprone for thalassemia major. N Engl J Med 1998;339:417–23.
123. Tondury P, Zimmermann A, Nielsen P, Hirt A. Liver iron and fibrosis during long-term treatment with deferiprone in Swiss thalassaemic patients. Br J Haematol 1998;101:413–15.
124. Wanless IR, Sweeney G, Dhillon AP, et al. Lack of progressive hepatic fibrosis during long-term therapy with deferiprone in subjects with transfusion-dependent beta-thalassemia. Blood 2002;100:1566–9.
125. Dallman PR, Siimes MA, Stekel A. Iron deficiency in infancy and childhood. Am J Clin Nutr 1980;33:86–118.
126. Visapaa I, Fellman V, Vesa J, et al. GRACILE syndrome, a lethal metabolic disorder with iron overload, is caused by a point mutation in BCS1L. Am J Hum Genet 2002;71:863–76.
127. Verloes A, Lombet J, Lambert Y, et al. Tricho-hepato-enteric syndrome: further delineation of a distinct syndrome with neonatal hemochromatosis phenotype, intractable diarrhea, and hair anomalies. Am J Med Genet 1997;68:391–5.
128. Cottier H. [A hemochromatosis similar disease in newborn.] Schweiz Med Wochenschr 1957;87:39–43.
129. Thaler MM. Fatal neonatal cirrhosis: entity or end result? A comparative study of 24 cases. Pediatrics 1964;33:721–34.
130. Witzleben CL, Uri A. Perinatal hemochromatosis: entity or end result? Hum Pathol 1989;20:335–40.
131. Knisely AS, Mieli-Vergani G, Whitington PF. Neonatal hemochromatosis. Gastroenterol Clin North Am 2003;32:877–89, vi–vii.
132. Whitington PF. Fetal and infantile hemochromatosis. Hepatology 2006;43:654–60.
133. Mostoufizadeh M, Lack EE, Gang DL, et al. Postmortem manifestations of echovirus 11 sepsis in five newborn infants. Hum Pathol 1983;14:818–23.
134. Ventura KC, Hawkins H, Smith MB, Walker DH. Fatal neonatal echovirus 6 infection: autopsy case report and review of the literature. Mod Pathol 2001;14:85–90.
135. Silver MM, Beverley DW, Valberg LS, et al. Perinatal hemochromatosis. Clinical, morphologic, and quantitative iron studies. Am J Pathol 1987;128:538–54.
136. Shneider BL, Setchell KD, Whitington PF, et al. Delta 4-3-oxosteroid 5 beta-reductase deficiency causing neonatal liver failure and hemochromatosis. J Pediatr 1994;124:234–8.
137. Clayton PT. Delta 4-3-oxosteroid 5 beta-reductase deficiency and neonatal hemochromatosis. J Pediatr 1994;125(5 pt 1): 845–6.

138. Siafakas CG, Jonas MM, Perez-Atayde AR. Abnormal bile acid metabolism and neonatal hemochromatosis: a subset with poor prognosis. J Pediatr Gastroenterol Nutr 1997;25:321–6.
139. Parizhskaya M, Reyes J, Jaffe R. Hemophagocytic syndrome presenting as acute hepatic failure in two infants: clinical overlap with neonatal hemochromatosis. Pediatr Dev Pathol 1999;2:360–6.
140. Ruchelli ED, Uri A, Dimmick JE, et al. Severe perinatal liver disease and Down syndrome: an apparent relationship. Hum Pathol 1991;22:1274–80.
141. Rand EB, McClenathan DT, Whitington PF. Neonatal hemochromatosis: report of successful orthotopic liver transplantation. J Pediatr Gastroenterol Nutr 1992;15:325–9.
142. Hayes AM, Jaramillo D, Levy HL, Knisely AS. Neonatal hemochromatosis: diagnosis with MR imaging. AJR Am J Roentgenol 1992;159:623–5.
143. Smith SR, Shneider BL, Magid M, et al. Minor salivary gland biopsy in neonatal hemochromatosis. Arch Otolaryngol Head Neck Surg 2004;130:760–3.
144. Morris S, Akima S, Dahlstrom JE, et al. Renal tubular dysgenesis and neonatal hemochromatosis without pulmonary hypoplasia. Pediatr Nephrol 2004;19:341–4.
145. Gilmour SM, Hughes-Benzie R, Silver MM, Roberts EA. Le foie vide: a unique case of neonatal liver failure. J Pediatr Gastroenterol Nutr 1996;23:618–23.
146. Bowen A 3rd, Sane SS, Knisely AS. Patent ductus venosus in neonatal hemochromatosis: US and pathologic findings. Pediatr Radiol 2001;31:B21.
147. Colletti RB, Clemmons JJ. Familial neonatal hemochromatosis with survival. J Pediatr Gastroenterol Nutr 1988;7:39–45.
148. Rodrigues F, Kallas M, Nash R, et al. Neonatal hemochromatosis–medical treatment vs. transplantation: the king's experience. Liver Transpl 2005;11:1417–24.
149. Sigurdsson L, Reyes J, Kocoshis SA, et al. Neonatal hemochromatosis: outcomes of pharmacologic and surgical therapies. J Pediatr Gastroenterol Nutr 1998;26:85–9.
150. Flynn DM, Mohan N, McKiernan P, et al. Progress in treatment and outcome for children with neonatal hemochromatosis. Arch Dis Child Fetal Neonatal Ed 2003;88:F124–7.
151. Egawa H, Berquist W, Garcia-Kennedy R, et al. Rapid development of hepatocellular siderosis after liver transplantation for neonatal hemochromatosis. Transplantation 1996;62:1511–13.
152. Whitington PF, Hibbard JU. High-dose immunoglobulin during pregnancy for recurrent neonatal haemochromatosis. Lancet 2004;364:1690–8.
153. Whitington PF, Malladi P. Neonatal hemochromatosis: is it an alloimmune disease? J Pediatr Gastroenterol Nutr 2005;40:544–9.

28

Heme Biosynthesis and the Porphyrias

Robert J. Desnick, M.D., Ph.D., Kenneth H. Astrin, Ph.D., and
Karl E. Anderson, M.D.

The porphyrias are metabolic disorders, each resulting from the deficiency of a specific enzyme in the heme biosynthetic pathway (Figure 28.1; Table 28.1). These enzyme deficiencies are inherited as autosomal dominant or recessive traits, with the exception of porphyria cutanea tarda (PCT), which usually is sporadic. The porphyrias are classified as either *hepatic* or *erythropoietic* depending on the primary site of overproduction and accumulation of porphyrin precursors or porphyrins (Table 28.2) although some have overlapping features. The hepatic porphyrias are characterized by overproduction and initial accumulation of porphyrin precursors and/or porphyrins primarily in the liver, whereas in the erythropoietic porphyrias, overproduction and initial accumulation of the pathway intermediates occur primarily in bone marrow erythroid cells.

The major manifestations of the acute hepatic porphyrias, which typically present after puberty, are neurologic, including neuropathic abdominal pain, neuropathy, and mental disturbances. The neurologic involvement appears to be the result of hepatic production of a neurotoxic substance, as liver transplantation prevented further occurrences in a patient who had frequent attacks of acute intermittent porphyria (AIP) [1]. Steroid hormones, drugs, and nutrition influence the hepatic production of porphyrin precursors and porphyrins, thereby precipitating or increasing the severity of some hepatic porphyrias. Rare homozygous variants of the autosomal dominant hepatic porphyrias have been identified and usually manifest clinically before puberty. The symptoms in these patients are usually more severe and occur earlier than those of patients with the respective autosomal dominant porphyria (see below) [2].

The erythropoietic porphyrias usually present with cutaneous photosensitivity at birth or in early childhood, or in the case of congenital erythropoietic porphyria (CEP), even in utero as nonimmune hydrops fetalis [3,4]. Cutaneous sensitivity to sunlight results from excitation of excess porphyrins in the skin by long-wave ultraviolet light, leading to cell damage, scarring, and deformation. Thus, the porphyrias are metabolic disorders in which environmental, physiologic, and genetic factors interact to cause disease.

Because many symptoms of the porphyrias are nonspecific, diagnosis is often delayed [5]. First-line diagnostic testing involves the determination of the porphyrin precursors and/or porphyrins in urine, plasma, or erythrocytes (see below). A definitive diagnosis is based on demonstration of the specific enzyme deficiency and/or gene mutation(s). The isolation and characterization of the genes encoding the heme biosynthetic enzymes have permitted identification of the mutations causing each porphyria. Molecular genetic analyses now make it possible to provide precise heterozygote or homozygote identification and prenatal diagnoses in families with known mutations.

Recent reviews of the porphyrias are available [3,6–8]. Informative and up-to-date websites are sponsored by the American Porphyria Foundation (www.porphyriafoundation.com) and the European Porphyria Initiative (www.porphyria-europe.org). An extensive list of unsafe and safe drugs for individuals with porphyria is given at the Drug Database for Acute Porphyrias (www.drugs-porphyria.com).

HEME BIOSYNTHESIS

Heme biosynthesis involves eight enzymatic steps in the conversion of glycine and succinyl–coenzyme A (CoA) to heme (Figure 28.1 and Table 28.1) [3]. These eight enzymes are encoded by nine genes, as the first enzyme in the pathway, 5′-aminolevulinate synthase (ALA-synthase), has two genes that encode unique housekeeping and erythroid-specific isozymes. The first and last three enzymes in the pathway are located in the mitochondrion, whereas the other four are in the cytosol. Heme is required for a variety of hemoproteins, such as hemoglobin, myoglobin, respiratory cytochromes, and the cytochrome P450 enzymes (CYPs). Hemoglobin synthesis in erythroid precursor cells accounts for approximately 85% of daily heme synthesis in humans. Hepatocytes account for most of the rest, primarily for synthesis of CYPs, which are especially abundant in the liver endoplasmic reticulum, and turn over more rapidly than many other hemoproteins, such as the mitochondrial respiratory cytochromes. As shown in Figure 28.1, pathway intermediates are the porphyrin precursors, 5′-ALA and porphobilinogen

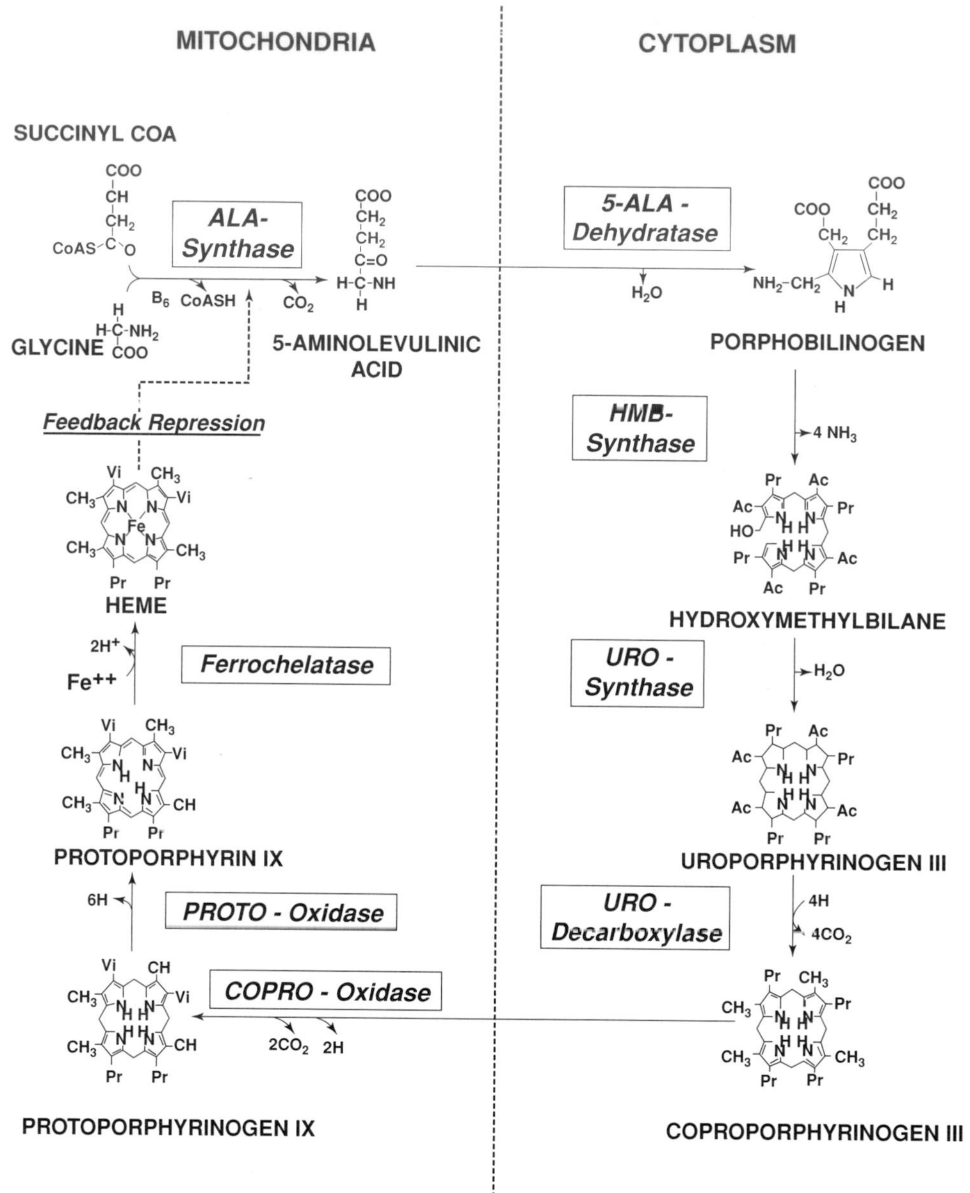

Figure 28.1. The human heme biosynthetic pathway.

(PBG), and porphyrins (mostly in their reduced forms, known as porphyrinogens). At least in humans, these intermediates do not accumulate in significant amounts under normal conditions or have important physiologic functions.

The first enzyme, ALA-synthase, catalyzes the condensation of glycine, activated by pyridoxal phosphate and succinyl-CoA, to form ALA. In the liver, this rate-limiting enzyme can be induced by a variety of drugs, steroids, and other chemicals. The distinct nonerythroid (i.e., housekeeping) and erythroid-specific forms of ALA-synthase are encoded by separate genes located on chromosomes 3p21.1 (ALA-synthase 1 [*ALAS1*]) and Xp11.2 (ALA-synthase 2 [*ALAS2*]), respectively. Defects in the erythroid gene *ALAS2* cause X-linked sideroblastic anemia [3].

The second enzyme, 5′-aminolevulinate dehydratase (ALA-dehydratase), catalyzes the condensation of two molecules of ALA to form PBG. Four molecules of PBG condense to form the tetrapyrrole uroporphyrinogen (URO) III by a two-step process catalyzed by hydroxymethylbilane (HMB)-synthase (also known as PBG-deaminase) and uroporphyrinogen III synthase (URO-synthase). HMB-synthase catalyzes the head-to-tail condensation of four PBG molecules by a series of deaminations to form the linear tetrapyrrole HMB. URO-synthase catalyzes the rearrangement and rapid cyclization of HMB to form URO III, the asymmetric, physiologic, URO isomer required for heme synthesis.

The fifth enzyme in the pathway, uroporphyrinogen decarboxylase (URO-decarboxylase), catalyzes the sequential removal of the four carboxyl groups from the acetic acid side chains of URO III to form coproporphyrinogen (COPRO) III, a tetracarboxylate porphyrinogen. COPRO III then enters the mitochondrion, where COPRO-oxidase, the sixth enzyme,

Table 28.1: Human Heme Biosynthetic Enzymes and Genes

Enzyme	*Gene Symbol*	*Chromosomal Location*	*cDNA, bp*	*Gene*		*Protein, aa*	*Subcellular Location*	*Known Mutations†*	*3D Structure‡*
				Size, kb	*Exons**				
ALA-synthase									
Housekeeping	*ALAS1*	3p21.1	2199	17	11	640	M	—	
Erythroid-specific	*ALAS2*	Xp11.2	1937	22	11	587	M	26	—
ALA-dehydratase									
Housekeeping	*ALAD*	9q32	1149	15.9	12 (1A + 2–12)	330	C	9	Y
Erythroid-specific	*ALAD*	9q32	1154	15.9	12 (1B + 2–12)	330	C	—	
HMB-synthase									
Housekeeping	*HMBS*	11q23.3	1086	11	15 (1 + 3–15)	361	C	246	E
Erythroid-specific	*HMBS*	11q23.3	1035	11	15 (2–15)	344	C	—	
URO-synthase									
Housekeeping	*UROS*	10q26.2	1296	34	10 (1 + 2B–10)	265	C	32	H
Erythroid-specific	*UROS*	10q26.2	1216	34	10 (2A+ 2B–10)	265	C	4	
URO-decarboxylase	*UROD*	1p34.1	1104	3	10	367	C	65	H
COPRO-oxidase	*CPOX*	3q12.1	1062	14	7	354	M	37	H
PROTO-oxidase	*PPOX*	1q23.3	1431	5.5	13	477	M	129	—
Ferrochelatase	*FECH*	18q21.31	1269	45	11	423	M	88	B

*Number of exons and those encoding separate housekeeping and erythroid-specific forms indicated in parentheses.
†Number of known mutations from the Human Gene Mutation Database (www.hgmd.org) as of January 1, 2007.
‡Crystallized from human (H), murine (M), *Escherichia coli* (E), *Bacillus subtilis* (B), or yeast (Y) purified enzyme; references in Protein Data Bank (www.rcsb.org).
3D, three-dimensional; aa, amino acid; bp, base pairs; C, cytoplasm; kb, kilobases; M, mitochondria.
From Anderson et al. [3].

catalyzes the decarboxylation of two of the four propionic acid groups to form the two vinyl groups of protoporphyrinogen (PROTO) IX, a dicarboxylate porphyrinogen. Next, PROTO-oxidase oxidizes PROTO IX to protoporphyrin IX by the removal of six hydrogen atoms. The product of the reaction is a porphyrin (oxidized form), in contrast to the preceding tetrapyrrole intermediates, which are porphyrinogens (reduced forms). Finally, ferrous iron is inserted into protoporphyrin IX to form heme, a reaction catalyzed by the eighth enzyme in the pathway, ferrochelatase (FECH; also known as heme synthetase or protoheme ferrolyase).

REGULATION OF HEME BIOSYNTHESIS

Regulation of heme synthesis differs in the two major heme-forming tissues, the liver and erythron. In the liver, "free" heme regulates the synthesis and mitochondrial translocation of the housekeeping form of ALAS1 [9]. Heme represses the synthesis of the ALAS1 mRNA and interferes with the transport of the enzyme from the cytosol into mitochondria. Hepatic ALAS1 is increased by many of the same chemicals that induce CYPs in the endoplasmic reticulum of the liver. Because most of the heme in the liver is used for the synthesis of CYPs, hepatic ALAS1 and CYPs are regulated in a coordinated fashion, and many drugs that induce hepatic ALAS1 also induce CYPs. The other hepatic heme biosynthetic enzymes are presumably expressed at constant levels, although their relative activities and kinetic properties differ. For example, normal individuals have much higher activities of ALA-dehydratase compared with HMB-synthase, the latter being the second rate-limiting step in the pathway [5].

In the erythron, novel regulatory mechanisms allow for the production of the very large amounts of heme needed for hemoglobin synthesis. The response to stimuli for hemoglobin synthesis occurs during cell differentiation, leading to an increase in cell number. The erythroid-specific ALAS2 is expressed at higher levels than the hepatic enzyme, and an erythroid-specific control mechanism regulates iron transport into erythroid cells. During erythroid differentiation, the activities of other heme biosynthetic enzymes may be increased. Separate erythroid-specific and nonerythroid or "housekeeping" transcripts are known for the first four enzymes in the pathway. As noted above, ALAS1 and ALAS2 are encoded by genes on different chromosomes, but for each of the next three genes in the pathway, both erythroid and nonerythroid transcripts are transcribed by alternative promoters from their single respective genes [10–12].

Table 28.2: Human Porphyrias: Major Clinical and Laboratory Features

Porphyria	*Deficient Enzyme*	*Inheritance*	*Principal Symptoms, NV or CP*	*Enzyme Activity, % of Normal*	*Increased Porphyrin Precursors and/or Porphyrins**		
					Erythrocytes	*Urine*	*Stool*
Hepatic							
5-ALA dehydratase–deficient porphyria	ALA-dehydratase	AR	NV	~5	Zn-protoporphyrin	ALA, Coproporphyrin III	—
Acute Intermittent porphyria	HMB-synthase	AD	NV	~50	—	ALA, PBG, Uroporphyrin	—
Porphyria cutanea tarda	URO-decarboxylase	AD	CP	~20	—	Uroporphyrin, 7-carboxylate porphyrin	Isocoproporphyrin
Hereditary coproporphyria	COPRO-oxidase	AD	NV & CP	~50	—	ALA, PBG, coproporphyrin III	Coproporphyrin III
Variegate porphyria	PROTO-oxidase	AD	NV & CP	~50	—	ALA, PBG, coproporphyrin III	Coproporphyrin III, protoporphyrin
Erythropoietic							
Congenital erythropoietic porphyria	URO-synthase	AR	CP	1–5	Uroporphyrin I, coproporphyrin I	Uroporphyrin I, coproporphyrin I	Coproporphyrin I
Erythropoietic protoporphyria	Ferrochelatase	AD†	CP	~20–30	Protoporphyrin	—	Protoporphyrin

*Increases that may be important for diagnosis.
†A polymorphism in intron 3 of the wild-type allele affects the level of enzyme activity and clinical expression.
AR, autosomal recessive; AD, autosomal dominant; NV, neurovisceral; CP, cutaneous photosensitivity.

CLASSIFICATION OF THE PORPHYRIAS

As mentioned above, the porphyrias can be classified as either *hepatic* or *erythropoietic*, depending on whether the heme biosynthetic intermediates that accumulate arise initially from the liver or developing erythrocytes, or as *acute* or *cutaneous*, based on their clinical manifestations. Table 28.2 lists the porphyrias, their principal symptoms and major biochemical abnormalities. Of the five hepatic porphyrias, AIP, hereditary coproporphyria (HCP), variegate porphyria (VP), and ALA-dehydratase deficient porphyria (ADP), present with acute attacks of neurologic manifestations and elevated levels of one or both of the porphyrin precursors, ALA and PBG, and are thus classified as acute porphyrias. Symptoms of neuropathic abdominal pain, peripheral neuropathy, and mental disturbances typically develop during adult life [3,5,8]. The fifth hepatic porphyria, PCT, usually presents in adults with blistering skin lesions and not acute attacks. HCP and VP may cause cutaneous manifestations similar to those of PCT in addition to acute neurologic symptoms.

The erythropoietic porphyrias, CEP, and erythropoietic protoporphyria (EPP), are characterized by elevations of porphyrins in bone marrow and erythrocytes and usually present in infancy with cutaneous photosensitivity. The skin lesions in CEP resemble those of PCT but are usually much more severe, whereas EPP causes a more immediate, painful, and nonblistering type of photosensitivity. EPP is the porphyria that most commonly causes symptoms before puberty. Around 20% of EPP patients develop minor abnormalities of liver function, and up to 5% develop more severe hepatic complications that may be life threatening.

DIAGNOSIS OF PORPHYRIAS

A few specific and sensitive first-line laboratory tests should be used whenever symptoms or signs suggest the diagnosis of porphyria [5]. If a first-line test is significantly abnormal, more comprehensive testing should follow to establish the type of porphyria.

Acute Porphyrias

An acute porphyria should be suspected in patients with neurovisceral symptoms after puberty, such as abdominal pain, when the initial clinical evaluation does not suggest another cause, and the urinary porphyrin precursors (ALA and PBG) should be measured. Urinary PBG is virtually always increased during acute attacks of AIP, HCP, and VP, and is not substantially increased in any other medical condition. Therefore, this measurement is both sensitive and specific. A method for rapid, in-house testing for urinary PBG, such as the Trace PBG kit (Trace America/Trace Diagnostics, Louisville, CO), should be available. Results from spot (single-void) urine specimens are highly informative because very substantial increases in PBG are expected during acute attacks of porphyria. A 24-hour collection may unnecessarily delay diagnosis. The same spot urine specimen should be saved for quantitative determination of ALA and PBG to confirm the qualitative PBG result and also to detect elevations of ALA in rare patients with ADP. Urinary porphyrins may remain increased longer than porphyrin precursors in HCP and VP. Therefore, it is useful to measure total urinary porphyrins in the same sample, keeping in mind that urinary porphyrin increases are often nonspecific. Measurement of urinary porphyrins alone should be avoided for screening, because these may be increased in disorders other than porphyrias, such as chronic liver disease, and misdiagnoses of porphyria may result from minimal increases in urinary porphyrins that have no diagnostic significance. Measurement of erythrocyte HMB-synthase is not useful as a first-line test in the acute setting because it does not differentiate latent from active AIP. Moreover, the enzyme activity is not decreased in all AIP patients and is never deficient in other acute porphyrias.

Cutaneous Porphyrias

Blistering skin lesions caused by porphyria are virtually always accompanied by increases in total plasma porphyrins. A fluorometric method is preferred because the porphyrins in plasma in VP are mostly covalently linked to plasma proteins and may be less readily detected by high-performance liquid chromatography. The normal range for plasma porphyrins is somewhat increased in patients with end-stage renal disease. Although a total plasma porphyrin determination will usually detect EPP, which has symptoms of nonblistering photosensitivity, an erythrocyte protoporphyrin determination is more sensitive. However, because increases in erythrocyte protoporphyrin occur in many other conditions, the diagnosis of EPP must be confirmed by showing a predominant increase in free protoporphyrin rather than zinc protoporphyrin.

More extensive testing is justified when an initial test is positive [5]. A substantial increase in PBG may be caused by AIP, HCP, or VP. These acute porphyrias can be distinguished by measuring erythrocyte HMB-synthase, urinary porphyrins (using the same spot urine sample), fecal porphyrins, and plasma porphyrins. Enzymatic assays for COPRO-oxidase and PROTO-oxidase are not widely available. The various porphyrias that cause blistering skin lesions are differentiated by measuring porphyrins in urine, feces, and plasma. Confirmation at the DNA level by the demonstration of the causative mutation(s) is important after the diagnosis is established by biochemical testing and also permits family studies. Further details are provided in the following sections on each type of porphyria.

Testing for Subclinical Porphyria

It is often difficult to diagnose or "rule out" porphyria in patients who had suggestive symptoms months or years in the past, and in relatives of patients with acute porphyrias, because porphyrin precursors and porphyrins may be normal. More extensive testing and consultation with a specialist laboratory and physician may be needed. Before evaluating relatives, the diagnosis of porphyria should be firmly established in an index case and the laboratory results reviewed to guide the choice of tests for the family members. The index case or another family member with confirmed porphyria should be retested if necessary. Identification of a disease-causing mutation in an index case greatly facilitates detection of additional gene carriers.

THE HEPATIC PORPHYRIAS

The major manifestations of the hepatic porphyrias, which typically present after puberty, are neurologic, although some also have cutaneous symptoms.

ALA-Dehydratase Deficient Porphyria

ALA-dehydratase deficient porphyria is a rare autosomal recessive acute hepatic porphyria caused by the severe deficiency of ALA-dehydratase activity [3,5]. To date, there are only six documented cases, five in children or adolescents, in which specific gene mutations have been identified [3,13–15]. These affected homozygotes had less than 10% of normal ALA-dehydratase activity in erythrocytes, but their clinically asymptomatic parents and heterozygous relatives had about half-normal levels of activity and did not excrete increased levels of ALA. The frequency of ADP is unknown, but the frequency of heterozygous individuals with less than 50% normal ALA-dehydratase activity was approximately 2% in a population screening study in Sweden. Because there are multiple causes for deficient ALA-dehydratase activity, it is important to confirm the diagnosis of ADP by mutation analysis.

Clinical Features

The clinical presentation is variable, presumably depending on the amount of residual ALA-dehydratase activity. All patients had significantly elevated levels of plasma and urinary ALA and markedly decreased ALA-dehydratase activity. Four of the reported patients were male adolescents with symptoms resembling those of AIP, including abdominal pain and neuropathy [13–15]. One patient was an infant with more severe disease, including failure to thrive beginning at birth. Earlier onset and more severe manifestations in this patient reflected a more significant deficiency of ALA-dehydratase activity [16]. Another patient was essentially normal until age 63, when he developed an acute motor polyneuropathy that was associated with a myeloproliferative disorder. This patient was heterozygous for an ALA-dehydratase mutation that presumably was present in erythroblasts that underwent clonal expansion because of the bone marrow malignancy [17].

Diagnosis

Patients have increased urinary levels of ALA and COPRO III. Urinary PBG is normal or slightly increased. ALA-dehydratase activity in erythrocytes is less than 10% of normal. Hereditary tyrosinemia type 1 (fumarylacetoacetase deficiency) and lead intoxication should be considered in the differential diagnosis because either succinylacetone (which accumulates in hereditary tyrosinemia type 1 and is structurally similar to ALA) or lead can inhibit ALA-dehydratase, increase urinary excretion of ALA, and cause manifestations that resemble those of the acute porphyrias. Heterozygotes are clinically asymptomatic and do not excrete increased levels of ALA but can be detected by demonstration of intermediate levels of erythrocyte ALA-dehydratase activity or a specific mutation in the ALA-dehydratase gene. To date, molecular studies of ADP patients have identified eight point mutations, two splice-site mutations, and a two-base deletion in the ALA-dehydratase gene (Human Gene Mutation Database, www.hgmd.org) [14,15,18,19]. The parents in each case were not consanguineous, and the index cases had inherited a different ALA-dehydratase mutation from each parent. Prenatal diagnosis of this disorder should be possible by determination of the ALA-dehydratase activity and/or gene mutation in cultured chorionic villi or amniocytes. Of note, a common polymorphism (K59N) has been identified that alters zinc binding but retains normal activity [20].

Treatment

The treatment of acute attacks in the four males who developed symptoms during adolescence was similar to that of AIP (see below) and included decreased symptoms from intravenous hemin treatment. The severely affected patient who did not survive infancy was supported by hyperalimentation and periodic blood transfusions but did not respond biochemically or clinically to hemin or liver transplantation.

Acute Intermittent Porphyria

This hepatic porphyria is an autosomal dominant condition resulting from the half-normal level of HMB-synthase activity. The disease is widespread but may be more common in Scandinavia and Great Britain. In most heterozygous individuals, clinical expression is highly variable. Activation of the disease is often related to environmental or hormonal factors, such as drugs, diet, and steroid hormones. Attacks can often be prevented by avoiding known precipitating factors. Rare homozygous dominant AIP also has been described in children (see below).

Clinical Features

Induction of the rate-limiting hepatic enzyme ALAS1 is thought to underlie acute attacks in AIP and the other acute porphyrias. AIP remains latent (or asymptomatic) in the great majority of heterozygous carriers of HMB-synthase mutations, and this is almost always the case before puberty. In patients with no history of acute symptoms, porphyrin precursor excretion is usually normal, suggesting that half-normal hepatic HMB-synthase activity is sufficient for normal hepatic heme synthesis and ALAS1 activity is not increased. When heme synthesis is increased in the liver, half-normal HMB-synthase activity may become limiting and ALA, PBG, and other heme pathway intermediates may accumulate. Common precipitating factors include endogenous and exogenous gonadal steroids, porphyrinogenic drugs, alcohol ingestion, and low-calorie diets, usually instituted for weight loss.

The fact that AIP is almost always latent before puberty suggests that adult levels of steroid hormones are important for clinical expression. Symptoms are more common in women, which suggests a role for female hormones. Premenstrual attacks are probably the result of endogenous progesterone. Acute porphyrias are sometimes exacerbated by exogenous steroids, including oral contraceptive preparations containing progestins. Surprisingly, pregnancy is usually well tolerated, suggesting that beneficial metabolic changes may ameliorate the effects of high levels of progesterone. Table 28.3 is a partial list of the major drugs that are harmful in AIP (and also in HCP, VP, and probably ADP). An extensive list of unsafe and safe drugs for individuals with porphyria is given at the Drug Database for Acute Porphyrias (www.drugs-porphyria.com). Reduced intake of calories and carbohydrates, as may occur with illness or attempts to lose weight, may also increase porphyrin precursor excretion and induce attacks of porphyria. Increased carbohydrates may ameliorate attacks. Recent findings indicate that hepatic ALAS1 is regulated by the peroxisome proliferator-activated receptor γ coactivator 1α (PGC-1α), which may represent an important link between nutritional status and the acute porphyrias [21]. Attacks also may be provoked by infections, surgery, and ethanol. Some patients have repeated attacks without identifiable precipitants.

Because the neurovisceral symptoms are often nonspecific, a high index of suspicion is required to make the diagnosis. The disease is rarely fatal if diagnosed promptly. Abdominal pain, the most common symptom, is usually steady and poorly localized but may be cramping. Constipation, abdominal distention, and decreased bowel sounds are common. Increased bowel sounds and diarrhea are less common. Because inflammation is absent, abdominal tenderness, fever, and leukocytosis are usually not prominent. Additional common manifestations include nausea; vomiting; tachycardia; hypertension; mental symptoms; extremity, neck, or chest pain; headache; muscle weakness; sensory loss; tremors; sweating; dysuria; and bladder distention.

The peripheral neuropathy is the result of axonal degeneration (rather than demyelinization) and primarily affects motor neurons. Findings such as tachycardia, hypertension,

Table 28.3: Some Major Drugs Considered Unsafe and Safe in Acute Porphyrias*

Unsafe	*Safe*
Alcohol	Acetaminophen
Barbiturates†	Aspirin
Carbamazepine†	Atropine
Carisoprodol†	Bromides
Clonazepam (high doses)	Cimetidine
Danazol†	Erythropoietin†‡
Diclofenac and possibly other	Gabapentin
NSAIDs†	Glucocorticoids
Ergots	Insulin
Estrogens‡§	Narcotic analgesics
Ethchlorvynol‡	Penicillin and derivatives
Glutethimide†	Phenothiazines
Griseofulvin†	Ranitidine†‡
Mephenytoin	Streptomycin
Meprobamate† (also mebutamate,† tybutamate†)	
Methyprylon	
Metoclopramide†	
Phenytoin†	
Primidone†	
Progesterone and synthetic progestins†	
Pyrazinamide†	
Pyrazolones (aminopyrine, antipyrine)	
Rifampin†	
Succinimides (ethosuximide, methsuximide)	
Sulfonamide antibiotics†	
Valproic acid†	

*A more extensive list of drugs and their status is available in Anderson et al. [3] and at the following websites:
www.porphyriafoundation.com
www.porphyria-europe.com
www.drugs-porphyria.com

†Porphyria is listed as a contraindication, warning, precaution, or adverse effect in U.S. labeling for these drugs. For drugs listed as unsafe, absence of such cautionary statements in U.S. labeling does not imply lower risk.

‡Although porphyria is listed as a precaution in U.S. labeling, these drugs are regarded as safe by other sources.

§Estrogens have been regarded as harmful, mostly from experience with estrogen–progestin combinations and because they can exacerbate porphyria cutanea tarda. Although evidence that they exacerbate acute porphyrias is weak, they should be used with caution. Low doses of estrogen (e.g., transdermal) have been used safely to prevent side effects of gonadotropin-releasing hormone analogues in women with cyclic attacks. NSAIDs, nonsteroidal anti-inflammatory drugs.

sweating, and tremors may be the result of sympathetic overactivity. Motor neuropathy affects the proximal muscles initially, more often in the shoulders and arms. Muscle weakness may progress to respiratory and bulbar paralysis and death, especially when diagnosis and treatment are delayed. Sudden death occurs occasionally, perhaps from sympathetic overactivity or cardiac arrhythmia.

Mental symptoms are often prominent during attacks and may include insomnia, agitation, disorientation, hallucinations, and depression. Seizures may be a neurologic manifestation of the disease or may be the result of hyponatremia. The latter results from inappropriate vasopressin secretion or from electrolyte depletion. Abdominal pain may resolve within hours and paresis within days. However, severe motor neuropathy may continue to improve over several years. Long-term risks for hypertension, impaired renal function, and hepatocellular carcinoma are increased.

Diagnosis

ALA and PBG levels are increased in plasma and urine during acute attacks [5]. Although the diagnosis of an acute attack is based on clinical findings and not the absolute level of these porphyrin precursors, the increase is expected to be substantial. PBG excretion is usually 50–200 mg/24 hr (220–880 mmol/24 hr; normal, 0–4 mg/24 hr [0–18 mmol/24 hr]), and urinary ALA excretion is 20–100 mg/24 hr (150–760 mmol/24 hr; normal, 1–7 mg/24 hr [8–53 mmol/24s hr]). Levels of these porphyrin precursors decrease after an attack but usually remain elevated, except with prolonged remissions. Decreases after hemin infusions are dramatic but usually transient (see below). A normal urinary PBG level effectively excludes AIP as a cause for current symptoms. Fecal and plasma porphyrins are normal or minimally increased in AIP, in contrast to HCP and VP. Most asymptomatic ("latent") heterozygotes with HMB-synthase deficiency, especially those who have never had symptoms, have normal urinary excretion of ALA and PBG. Therefore, measurement of HMB-synthase in erythrocytes, or better, the detection of the family's HMB-synthase mutation, is important for identification of asymptomatic family members with this enzyme deficiency.

The enzyme deficiency is detectable in erythrocytes from most AIP heterozygotes (Table 28.4). However, the activity is higher in young erythrocytes, and a concurrent condition that increases erythropoiesis may increase the enzyme into the normal range in an AIP patient. Also, because the erythroid and housekeeping forms of HMB-synthase are encoded by a single gene with two promoters [22], some mutations, usually found within exon 1, particularly in the initiation of translation codon, affect only the nonerythroid enzyme, and the erythroid enzyme is transcribed normally. Thus, patients with the rare erythroid form of AIP (erythroid, or variant, AIP) have normal enzyme levels in erythrocytes and deficient activity in nonerythroid tissues [3].

More than 240 HMB-synthase mutations have been identified in AIP, including missense, nonsense, and splicing mutations and insertions and deletions, with most mutations found

Table 28.4: Homozygous Dominant Forms of Porphyria*

Porphyria	*Deficient Enzyme*	*Clinical Onset*	*Principal Symptoms* *Neurovisceral*	*Principal Symptoms* *Cutaneous Photosensitivity*	*Other Symptoms*
Hepatic					
Homozygous dominant acute intermittent poprhyria	HMB-synthase	Infancy & childhood	+	—	Absence of acute attacks, development delay
Hepatoerythropoietic porphyria	URO-decarboxylase	Childhood	—	+	Rare anemia
Homozygous dominant coproporphyria	COPRO-oxidase	Childhood	+	+	Growth retardation
Harderoporphyria	COPRO-oxidase	Infancy & childhood	—	+	Neonatal hemolytic jaundice & anemia
Homozygous dominant variegate porphyria	PROTO-oxidase	Infancy & childhood	+	+	Absence of acute attacks, mental retardation, hand deformities
Erythropoietic					
Homozygous dominant erythropoietic protoporphyria	Ferrochelatase	Childhood	—	+	

*Modified from Elder [2].

in only one or a few families (Human Gene Mutation Database; www.hgmd.org) [18]. Identification of the gene in an index case enables detection of latent family members and prenatal diagnosis of an at-risk fetus using cultured amniotic cells or chorionic villi. However, this is seldom done because the prognosis of individuals with HMB-synthase mutations is generally favorable.

Treatment

During acute attacks, narcotic analgesics are usually required for abdominal pain, and phenothiazines are effective for nausea, vomiting, anxiety, and restlessness. Insomnia and restlessness are treated with chloral hydrate or low doses of short-acting benzodiazepines. Carbohydrate loading, usually with intravenous glucose (at least 300 g/dL), may be effective in milder acute attacks of porphyria (without paresis, hyponatremia, etc.). Because intravenous hemin is more effective and the response slower if treatment is delayed, it is no longer recommended that hemin therapy for a severe attack be started only after an unsuccessful trial of intravenous glucose for several days. Hemin should be used initially for severe attacks, and for mild attacks that do not respond to carbohydrate loading within 1–2 days. The standard regimen is 3–4 mg of heme in the form of lyophilized hematin (Ovation Pharmaceuticals), heme albumin (hematin reconstituted with human albumin), or heme arginate (Orphan Europe), infused daily for 4 days [5]. Heme arginate and heme albumin are chemically stable and are less likely than hematin to produce phlebitis or an anticoagulant effect. Recovery depends on the degree of neuronal damage and is usually rapid if therapy is started early, but patients with severe motor neuropathy may require months or years. Inciting factors are usually multiple, and removal of one or more hastens recovery and helps prevent future attacks. Frequent attacks that occur during the luteal phase of the menstrual cycle may be prevented with a gonadotropin-releasing hormone analogue, which prevents ovulation and progesterone production.

The long-term risk of hypertension and chronic renal disease is increased in AIP; a number of patients have undergone successful renal transplantation. Chronic, low-grade abnormalities in liver function tests are common, and the risk of hepatocellular carcinoma is increased. Such tumors in AIP patients have not been associated with increases in serum α-fetoprotein. Therefore, hepatic imaging is recommended at least yearly for early detection of these tumors.

An allogeneic liver transplantation was performed on a 19-year-old female AIP heterozygote who had 37 acute attacks in the 29 months before transplantation. Post transplantation, her elevated urinary ALA and PBG levels returned to normal in 24 hours, and she did not experience acute neurologic attacks for more than 18 months post transplant [1]. Liver transplantation is a high-risk procedure and should not be considered an established treatment for acute porphyrias.

Homozygous Dominant AIP

Homozygous dominant AIP is a rare form of porphyria presenting in infancy in which patients inherit HMB-synthase mutations from each of their heterozygous parents and therefore have very low (<2%) enzyme activity (Table 28.4). The disease has been described in a Dutch girl, two young British siblings, and a Spanish boy [23,24]. In these homozygous affected patients, disease manifestations included failure to thrive, developmental delay, bilateral cataracts, and/or hepatosplenomegaly. Acute attacks did not occur. Urinary ALA and PBG were markedly elevated. Interestingly, the HMB-synthase mutations (R167W, R167Q, and R172Q) in all of these patients were in exon 10 within five bases of each other. Studies of brain magnetic resonance images of children with homozygous AIP have suggested damage primarily in white matter that was myelinated postnatally, whereas tracks that myelinated prenatally were normal [24]. These findings suggest that a neurotoxic endogenous product such as ALA or PBG present in large amounts postnatally, rather than heme deficiency, caused nervous tissue damage. Prenatally, excess amounts of ALA and PBG would cross the placenta and be excreted in the mother's urine. Most children with homozygous AIP die at an early age.

Porphyria Cutanea Tarda

Porphyria cutanea tarda, the most common of the porphyrias, may be either sporadic (type 1) or familial (types 2 and 3) and may also develop after exposure to halogenated aromatic hydrocarbons. Hepatic URO-decarboxylase is deficient in all types of PCT, and for clinical symptoms to manifest, this enzyme deficiency must be substantial (~20% of normal activity or less). Generation of a URO-decarboxylase inhibitor, specifically in the liver in the presence of iron and under conditions of oxidative stress, is suspected to cause this decrease, although this inhibitor remains to be isolated and characterized [25–27].

The majority of PCT patients (~80%) have no URO-decarboxylase mutations and are said to have type 1 (sporadic) disease, or type 3 if relatives are affected. PCT patients who are heterozygous for URO-decarboxylase mutations have familial (type 2) PCT. In these patients, inheritance of a URO-decarboxylase mutation from one parent results in half-normal enzyme activity in liver and all other tissues, which is a significant predisposing factor but is insufficient by itself to cause symptomatic PCT. As discussed below, other genetic and environmental factors contribute to susceptibility to all types of PCT. For this reason, penetrance of this genetic trait is low, and many patients who present with type 2 PCT have no family history of the disease and may appear to have sporadic disease. Homozygous type 2 PCT is termed *hepatoerythropoietic porphyria* (HEP), which usually presents with clinical symptoms in childhood (see below).

Deficient hepatic URO-decarboxylase and a porphyrin pattern resembling PCT can be produced in rodents by a number of halogenated aromatic hydrocarbons, such as hexachlorobenzene and 2,3,7,8-tetrachlorodibenzo-*p*-dioxin (TCDD, dioxin). Outbreaks and isolated cases of PCT have been reported in humans exposed to these chemicals. Most notably, PCT affected thousands of children and adults in eastern Turkey during a period of food shortage, when seed wheat treated with hexachlorobenzene as a fungicide was consumed rather than planted [26].

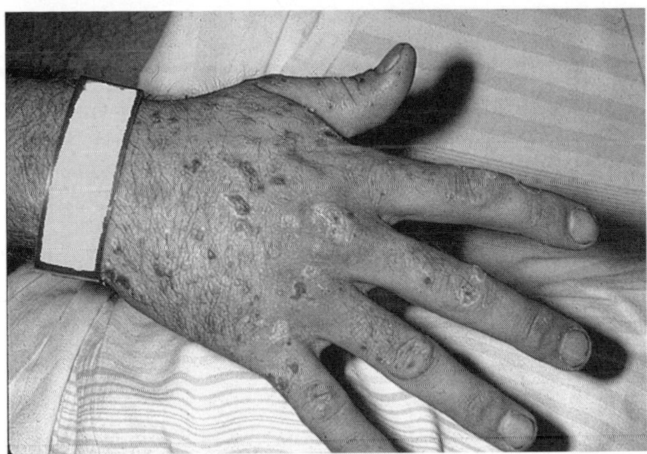

Figure 28.2. Chronic, crusted lesions resulting from blistering due to photosensitivity on the dorsum of the hand of a patient with PCT. (From Anderson et al. [3].)

Clinical Features

Blistering skin lesions that appear most commonly on the backs of the hands are the major clinical feature (Figure 28.2) [27]. These rupture and crust over, leaving areas of atrophy and scarring. Lesions may also occur on the forearms, face, legs, and feet. Skin friability and small white papules termed *milia* are common, especially on the backs of the hands and fingers. Hypertrichosis and hyperpigmentation, particularly on the face, are especially troublesome in women. Occasionally, the skin over sun-exposed areas becomes severely thickened with scarring and calcification, which resembles systemic sclerosis. Neurologic features are absent.

A number of susceptibility factors in addition to inherited URO-decarboxylase mutations in type 2 PCT can be recognized clinically and may affect management. The importance of excess hepatic iron is underscored by the increased prevalence of the common hemochromatosis-causing mutations, HFE C282Y and H63D, in patients with types 1 and 2 PCT [28–30]. PCT is strongly associated with hepatitis C in southern Europe and the United States. For example, in one series in the United States, this viral infection was found in 74% of 39 PCT patients, often in association with other risk factors [30]. Excess alcohol is a long-recognized contributor, as is estrogen use in women. Human immunodeficiency virus is probably an independent but less common risk factor, which like hepatitis C, does not occur in isolation. Multiple susceptibility factors that appear to act synergistically can be identified in the individual patient with PCT [30].

Patients with PCT characteristically have evidence of chronic liver disease, such as persistently abnormal liver function tests, even when the disease occurs in the absence of susceptibility factors that themselves cause liver damage, such as hepatitis C and excess ethanol use. Cirrhosis or hepatocellular carcinoma may develop in the long term [6].

Diagnosis

Porphyrins are increased in the liver, plasma, urine, and stool [31]. The urinary ALA level may be slightly increased, but the PBG level is normal. Urinary porphyrins consist mostly of uroporphyrin and heptacarboxylate porphyrin, which is a diagnostic pattern for PCT and HEP, with lesser amounts of coproporphyrin and hexa- and pentacarboxylate porphyrins. Plasma porphyrins are also increased, which is useful for screening. Fluorometric scanning of diluted plasma at neutral pH can rapidly distinguish VP and PCT. There is an increase in isocoproporphyrins, especially in feces, which is diagnostic for URO-decarboxylase deficiency. These tetracarboxylate porphyrins result from a normally minor pathway that is accentuated by URO-decarboxylase deficiency, whereby pentacarboxylate porphyrinogen is metabolized to isocoproporphyrinogen by COPRO-oxidase, the enzyme that follows in the pathway.

URO-decarboxylase activity in erythrocytes is generally about half-normal in type 2 PCT and normal in types 1 and 3. A genetic basis for type 3 PCT, which would clearly distinguish it from type 1, has not been established. Because most patients with familial (type 2) PCT have no family history of the disease, the finding of half-normal URO decarboxylase activity in erythrocytes is useful for identifying this predisposing genetic trait, although DNA analysis to identify a specific mutation is more reliable. More than 65 mutations have been identified in the URO-decarboxylase gene in type 2 PCT and HEP (Human Gene Mutation Database; www.hgmd.org) [18]. Of the mutations listed in the Human Gene Mutation Database, 57.4% are missense, 0.7% are nonsense, and 13.1% are splice-site mutations; most have been identified in only one or two families.

Treatment

Discontinuing risk factors, such as alcohol, estrogens, and iron supplements, is recommended but may not result in timely improvement. A complete response can almost always be achieved by the standard therapy, which at most centers is repeated phlebotomy to reduce hepatic iron [6]. A unit (450 mL) of blood can be removed approximately every 2 weeks. The aim is to gradually reduce iron until the serum ferritin reaches the lower limits of normal [26]. Hemoglobin levels or the hematocrit should be followed closely to prevent anemia. Because iron overload is not marked in most cases, the target ferritin level can often be achieved after only five or six phlebotomies; however, PCT patients with hemochromatosis may require many more phlebotomies. To document improvement in PCT, it is most convenient to follow the total plasma porphyrin concentration, which becomes normal some time after the target ferritin level is reached. After remission, continued phlebotomy may not be needed. Plasma porphyrin levels are followed at 6–12-month intervals for early detection of recurrences, which occur in a minority of patients and may be treated again by phlebotomy.

A low-dose regimen of chloroquine or hydroxychloroquine, which in some manner mobilizes excess porphyrins from the liver and promotes their excretion, is a useful alternative to phlebotomy, especially when phlebotomy is contraindicated or poorly tolerated. Small doses (e.g., 125 mg chloroquine phosphate twice weekly) should be given because standard doses may induce the rapid release of stored hepatic porphyrins; transient, marked increases in photosensitivity; and hepatocellular damage. Hepatic imaging can detect or exclude complicating hepatocellular carcinoma. Treatment of PCT in patients with end-stage renal disease is facilitated by administration of erythropoietin. Treatment of concurrent hepatitis C should be postponed until after PCT is treated and in remission.

Hepatoerythropoietic Porphyria

Hepatoerythropoietic porphyria, which is the homozygous form of familial (type 2) PCT, resembles CEP clinically (see below). Most patients have inherited different mutations from unrelated parents. In HEP, URO-decarboxylase activity is markedly deficient, with levels typically 3–10% of normal. Mutations associated with HEP are generally associated with expression of some residual enzyme activity. Excess porphyrins originate mostly from liver, with a pattern consistent with severe URO-decarboxylase deficiency (see above).

There also is a substantial increase in erythrocyte zinc protoporphyrin in HEP, as in homozygous dominant forms of the acute porphyrias, ADP, and some cases of CEP. Apparently, porphyrinogens accumulate in the marrow while hemoglobin synthesis is most active and are metabolized to protoporphyrin (and chelated with zinc by FECH) after hemoglobin synthesis is complete.

Like CEP, HEP usually presents with blistering skin lesions, hypertrichosis, scarring, and red urine in infancy or childhood. Sclerodermoid skin changes are sometimes prominent. Unusually mild cases have been described. Concurrent conditions that affect liver function may alter disease severity. For example, hepatitis A caused the disease to become manifest in a 2-year-old child and then improved with recovery from this viral infection.

Hepatoerythropoietic porphyria is readily distinguished from CEP by increases in both uroporphyrin and heptacarboxyl porphyrin in urine and in isocoproporphyrins in stool. In most cases of CEP, the excess erythrocyte porphyrins are predominantly uroporphyrin I and coproporphyrin I rather than zinc protoporphyrin. EPP is readily distinguished by its nonblistering photosensitivity and normal urine porphyrins and by demonstrating that the excess erythrocyte protoporphyrin is free and not complexed with zinc. As in CEP, avoidance of sunlight is most important in managing this disease. The outlook depends on the severity of the enzyme deficiency and may be favorable if sunlight can be avoided. Phlebotomy has shown little or no benefit.

Hereditary Coproporphyria

Hereditary coproporphyria is an autosomal dominant hepatic porphyria that results from the half-normal activity of COPRO-oxidase. The disease usually presents with acute attacks, as in AIP. However, cutaneous photosensitivity also may occur, but much less commonly than in VP [32]. In two studies of more than 100 HCP patients, over 80% had abdominal pain but only 5–29% had cutaneous symptoms [33,34]. HCP is less common than AIP or VP [34]. Homozygous dominant HCP and harderoporphyria, a biochemically distinguishable variant of HCP, present with clinical symptoms in children (see below).

Clinical Features

Hereditary coproporphyria is influenced by the same factors that cause attacks in AIP. The disease is latent before puberty, and neurovisceral symptoms, which are virtually identical to those of AIP, are more common in women. HCP is generally less severe than AIP, although severe and fatal motor neuropathy may occur. Blistering skin lesions are identical to those in PCT and VP and begin in childhood in rare homozygous cases.

Diagnosis

Coproporphyrin III is markedly increased in the urine and feces in symptomatic disease and often persists, especially in feces, when there are no symptoms [5]. Urinary ALA and PBG levels may be less increased during acute attacks and with recovery from an attack, may revert to normal more quickly than in AIP [33]. Plasma porphyrins are usually normal or only slightly increased but may be higher in cases with skin lesions. The diagnosis of HCP is readily confirmed by increased fecal porphyrins consisting almost entirely of coproporphyrin III, which distinguishes it from other porphyrias. An increase in the fecal coproporphyrin III/COPRO I ratio is useful for detecting latent cases.

Although the diagnosis can be confirmed by measuring COPRO-oxidase activity, assays for this mitochondrial enzyme are not widely available and require cells other than erythrocytes. Since the COPRO-oxidase gene was cloned, more than 35 mutations, two thirds of which are missense, have been identified in unrelated patients (Human Gene Mutation Database; www.hgmd.org) [18].

Treatment

Neurologic symptoms are treated as in AIP (see above). Phlebotomy and chloroquine are ineffective for the cutaneous manifestations.

Homozygous Dominant HCP and Harderoporphyria

Individuals with mutations in both their COPRO-oxidase alleles have been described. Several had homozygous dominant HCP and five had a variant form called harderoporphyria. One case of homozygous HCP was in a young girl, the daughter of consanguineous parents, who at the age of 4 years had symptoms of growth retardation, hypertrichosis, and skin hyperpigmentation. In her 20s, she had acute porphyric attacks. She had markedly increased fecal coproporphyrin III and 10% COPRO-oxidase activity and was homozygous for the missense mutation R331W [35].

Individuals with harderoporphyria, which is a biochemical and clinical variant form of HCP in which hemolysis and erythropoietic features are prominent, usually present in early childhood with jaundice, hemolytic anemia, hepatosplenomegaly, and skin photosensitivity [36]. However, the symptoms may be variable; one patient had only jaundice in childhood but developed mild anemia and skin lesions in adulthood, whereas two other patients had both neonatal anemia and skin photosensitivity. Acute attacks do not occur. Urinary coproporphyrin III, fecal porphyrins (66–90% harderoporphin), and erythrocyte zinc protoporphyrin are increased.

All harderoporphyria patients reported to date are either homoallelic or heteroallelic for the K404E missense mutation. Studies of the crystallized COPRO-oxidase protein and hydrophobic cluster analysis have shown that the amino acids at residues 400–404 are involved in the second step of the conversion of COPRO III to PROTO IX and mutations in any one of these amino acids may result in the release and accumulation of the reaction intermediate, harderoporphyrinogen [37,38]. Occasionally, heterozygotes for mutations in this region may develop typical HCP [37].

Variegate Porphyria

Variegate porphyria is an autosomal dominant hepatic porphyria that results from the deficient activity of PROTO-oxidase, the seventh enzyme in the heme pathway, and may present with neurologic symptoms, photosensitivity, or both. VP is particularly common in South Africa, where 3 of every 1000 whites have the disorder. Most are descendants of a couple who emigrated from Holland to South Africa in 1688 [39]. In other countries, VP is less common than AIP. Homozygous dominant VP is rare and presents early in childhood.

Clinical Features

Acute attacks identical to those in AIP and often precipitated by drugs, hormones, or diet develop in a minority of heterozygotes for PROTO-oxidase deficiency. Blistering skin manifestations are identical to those in PCT but are more difficult to treat and usually of longer duration. Attacks are generally milder than in AIP and less often fatal. In two large studies of VP patients, 59% had only skin lesions, 20% had only acute attacks, and 22% had both [38,39].

Diagnosis

Urinary excretion of ALA and PBG is increased during acute attacks but may be less increased and return to normal more quickly than in AIP. Increases in fecal protoporphyrin and coproporphyrin III and in urinary coproporphyrin III are more persistent. Plasma porphyrin levels also are increased, particularly when there are cutaneous lesions, but are increased in latent disease more commonly than fecal porphyrins. The fluorescence emission spectrum of porphyrins in plasma at neutral pH in VP is distinctive and can rapidly distinguish VP from all other porphyrias, particularly PCT, which is much more common [31,40].

Assays of PROTO-oxidase activity in cells such as lymphocytes are useful for confirming the diagnosis but not widely available, and identifying the specific PROTO-oxidase mutation is preferred once a diagnosis has been established in an index case. More than 130 mutations have been identified in the PROTO-oxidase gene from unrelated VP patients (Human Gene Mutation Database; www.hgmd.org) [18]. The missense mutation R59W is the common mutation in most South

Africans with VP of Dutch descent [41]. Five missense mutations were common among English and French VP patients [42]; however, most mutations have been found in only one or two families.

Treatment

Acute attacks are treated as in AIP, and hemin should be started early in most cases. Other than avoiding sun exposure and wearing protective clothing, there are few effective measures for treating the skin lesions. β-Carotene, phlebotomy, and chloroquine are not helpful.

Homozygous Dominant VP

Affected individuals with homozygous dominant VP have mutations affecting both PROTO-oxidase alleles, resulting in very low enzyme activity levels [43–45]. These patients generally develop cutaneous symptoms, including photosensitivity and hypertrichosis, before the age of 2 years. Scarring and deformities of the face and digits may be prominent. Most patients do not have acute attacks. Neurologic symptoms in some patients include mental retardation, convulsions, growth retardation, and nystagmus. A homozygous dominant VP patient followed for over 20 years developed mild sensory neuropathy and an unexplained immunoglobulin A nephropathy besides having severe cutaneous problems [45]. Laboratory findings include elevated erythrocyte zinc protoporphyrin levels, as in other homozygous dominant porphyrias. Missense and/or splice-site mutations have been identified in most homozygous VP patients. Expression studies have indicated that these mutations have residual activity.

THE ERYTHROPOIETIC PORPHYRIAS

In the erythropoietic porphyrias, excess porphyrins from bone marrow erythrocyte precursors are transported in plasma to the skin and lead to cutaneous photosensitivity. The most common of these, EPP, may be complicated by severe, life-threatening liver disease.

Congenital Erythropoietic Porphyria

Congenital erythropoietic porphyria is an autosomal recessive disorder, also known as Günther disease, that is the result of the markedly deficient, but not absent, activity of URO-synthase and the resultant marked accumulation of uroporphyrin I and coproporphyrin I isomers. Uroporphyrinogen I, which is derived from nonenzymatic cyclization of the substrate HMB, is metabolized by URO-decarboxylase to CORPO I, but the latter is not a substrate for CORPO-oxidase. CEP is associated with hemolytic anemia and severe cutaneous photosensitivity. Excess porphyrins are also deposited in teeth and bones.

Clinical Features

Severe cutaneous photosensitivity begins in early infancy in most cases [4]. The disease may be recognized in utero as a cause of nonimmune hydrops fetalis. The skin over light-exposed areas is friable, and bullae and vesicles are prone to rupture and infection. Skin thickening, focal hypo- and hyperpigmentation, and hypertrichosis of the face and extremities are characteristic. Secondary infection and bone resorption may lead to disfigurement of the face and hands. The teeth are reddish brown and fluoresce on exposure to long-wave ultraviolet light. Hemolysis is probably the result of the marked increase in erythrocyte porphyrins and leads to splenomegaly. A milder form of the disease in adults is often a complication of a myeloproliferative or myelodysplastic disorder.

Diagnosis

Uroporphyrin and coproporphyrin (mostly type I isomers) accumulate in the bone marrow and are also found in circulating erythrocytes, plasma, urine, and feces. The predominant porphyrin in feces is coproporphyrin I. The diagnosis can be confirmed by demonstration of markedly deficient URO-synthase activity or the identification of specific mutations in the URO-synthase gene. The disease can be detected in utero by measuring porphyrins in amniotic fluid and URO-synthase activity in cultured amniotic cells or chorionic villi or by the detection of the family's specific gene mutations. Molecular analyses of the mutant alleles from more than 50 unrelated patients have revealed the presence of 35 mutations in the URO-synthase gene, including four in the erythroid-specific promoter of the URO-synthase gene [4,46].

Treatment

Severe cases often require transfusions for anemia, which can be started in utero. Chronic transfusions sufficient to suppress erythropoiesis are effective in reducing porphyrin production but result in iron overload and other complications [47]. Splenectomy may reduce hemolysis and decrease transfusion requirements. Protection from sunlight is essential, and minor skin trauma should be avoided. Complicating bacterial infections should be treated promptly. Recently, bone marrow and cord blood transplantation have proved effective in several transfusion-dependent children [48,49], providing the rationale for stem-cell gene therapy [4,50].

Erythropoietic Protoporphyria

Erythropoietic protoporphyria is an inherited disorder resulting from the partially deficient activity of FECH, the last enzyme in the heme biosynthetic pathway. EPP is not only the most common erythropoietic porphyria but is the most common porphyria in children and the second most common in adults [51,52]. EPP patients have FECH activity as low as 15–25% in lymphocytes and cultured fibroblasts. Protoporphyrin accumulates primarily in bone marrow reticulocytes during hemoglobin synthesis, and then appears in plasma, is taken up in the liver, and is excreted in bile and feces. Protoporphyrin transported to the skin causes photosensitivity. In most patients, a disabling (i.e., causative) mutation in one FECH allele is combined with a relatively common intronic 3 (IVS3) single nucleotide alteration (IVS3–48TC) in the normal allele, which results in decreased amounts of the normal enzyme. The "C" allele results in expression of an aberrantly spliced mRNA that is degraded by a nonsense-mediated decay mechanism, thus decreasing the steady-state level of normal FECH mRNA transcribed from the "C" allele [53,54]. The low-expression allele is found in approximately 10% of the normal Caucasian population. In several studies, over 90% of symptomatic EPP patients had the "C" allele whereas no asymptomatic relatives carrying the disabling mutation did [53,55,56]. The inheritance of EPP in such families is correctly termed autosomal dominant because the IVS3–48TC alteration is a polymorphism that by itself does not cause disease, even when homozygous [7]. Another potential but clearly uncommon mechanism for decreasing FECH enzyme activity more than 50% (as predicated for a dominant mutation) is a "dominant-negative" effect – a defective subunit might interact with a normal subunit in a fashion to render the functional enzyme dimer nonfunctional so that only the 25% of dimers with two normal subunits would have enzyme activity [57,58]. In a few families, two FECH mutations and a pattern of autosomal recessive inheritance has been found. A variant form of EPP has been described in which FECH is not deficient and there are no mutations of the FECH gene; features suggesting iron-deficient erythropoiesis, but with increased ferritin, are more prominent in these patients [59]. The as yet unknown inherited defect may impair delivery of ferrous iron to the normal enzyme.

Clinical Features

Skin photosensitivity differs from that in other porphyrias, usually begins in childhood, and consists of pain, redness, and itching occurring within minutes of sunlight exposure. This occurs only in patients with substantial elevations in erythrocyte protoporphyrin and a genotype that results in FECH activity below approximately 35% of normal [7]. Vesicular lesions are uncommon. Redness, swelling, burning, and itching developing shortly after sun exposure may resemble angioedema. Symptoms may seem out of proportion to the visible skin lesions. Vesicles and bullae are sparse and occur in only about 10% of cases. Chronic skin changes may include lichenification, leathery pseudovesicles, labial grooving, and nail changes. Severe scarring is rare, as are pigment changes, friability, and hirsutism. Unless hepatic or other complications develop, protoporphyrin levels and symptoms of photosensitivity remain remarkably stable over many years in most patients. Factors that exacerbate hepatic porphyrias play little or no role in EPP.

The primary source of excess protoporphyrin is the bone marrow reticulocyte. Erythrocyte protoporphyrin is almost all free (not complexed with zinc) and is mostly bound to hemoglobin. In the variant form with normal FECH, free and zinc protoporphyrin are both increased in erythrocytes [59]. In plasma, protoporphyrin is bound to albumin. Hemolysis and anemia are usually absent or mild.

Although EPP is an erythropoietic porphyria, up to 20% of EPP patients may have minor abnormalities of liver function; in about 5% of the patients, the accumulation of protoporphyrin causes liver disease that may be chronic, but sometimes develops rapidly, and may progress to liver failure and death. Protoporphyrin is insoluble, and excess amounts form crystalline structures in liver cells and can decrease hepatic bile flow in bile fistula rats. Studies in a mouse model of EPP suggest that excess protoporphyrin alters bile composition in a manner that is toxic to bile duct epithelium, leading to ductular proliferation and fibrosis [60]. Rapidly progressive liver disease in human EPP is associated with increasing protoporphyrin levels in liver, plasma, and erythrocytes and increased photosensitivity [51]. Protoporphyric liver disease may cause severe abdominal pain, especially in the right upper quadrant, and back pain [61]. Gallstones composed at least in part of protoporphyrin may be symptomatic in EPP patients and need to be excluded as a cause of biliary obstruction in patients with hepatic decompensation.

Diagnosis

A substantial increase in erythrocyte protoporphyrin, which is predominantly free and not complexed with zinc, is the hallmark of this disease. Protoporphyrin levels are also variably increased in bone marrow, plasma, bile, and feces. Plasma and fecal porphyrins are less increased than in most other cutaneous porphyrias and are sometimes normal. Therefore, measuring erythrocyte protoporphyrin is important for diagnosis. Although erythrocyte protoporphyrin concentrations are increased in other conditions, such as lead poisoning, iron deficiency, various hemolytic disorders, and all homozygous forms of porphyria, and are sometimes somewhat increased, even in acute porphyrias, in all these conditions, in contrast to EPP, protoporphyrin is complexed with zinc. Therefore, after an increase in erythrocyte protoporphyrin is found in a suspected EPP patient, it is important to confirm the diagnosis by an assay that distinguishes free and zinc-complexed protoporphyrin. Erythrocytes in EPP exhibit red fluorescence when examined by fluorescence microscopy at 620 nm (Figure 28.3). Urinary levels of porphyrins and porphyrin precursors are normal. FECH activity in cultured lymphocytes or fibroblasts is decreased, but

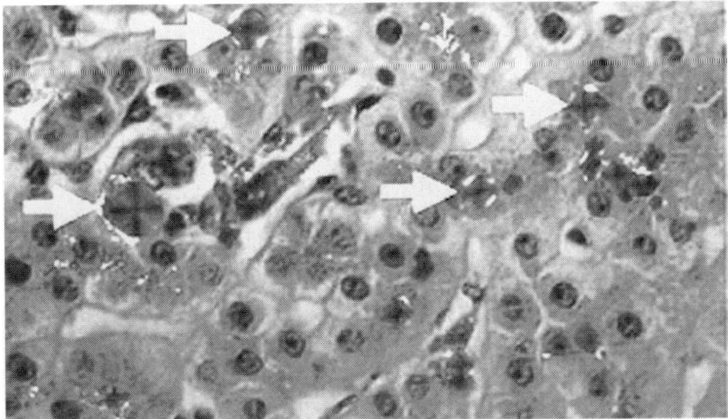

Figure 28.3. Polarization microscopy of a liver biopsy specimen from a patient with EPP shows that the pigment deposits are birefringent because of the presence of protoporphyrin crystals (*arrows*). The crystal on the left is in the form of a centrally located dark Maltese cross. (From McGuire et al. [63].)

such assays are not widely available. FECH mutation analysis is recommended to detect the causative mutation and, in most affected families, the presence of the IVS3–48TC alteration in the normal coding allele. To date, more than 90 mutations have been identified in the FECH gene, many of which result in an unstable or absent enzyme protein (null alleles; Human Gene Mutation Database; www.hgmd.org) [18]. Studies suggest that EPP patients with a null allele (and the "C" alteration at IVS3–48 in their normal allele) have a greater risk for developing severe liver complications than do those with mutations that encode some enzyme activity [62]. As noted, in a variant form of EPP, FECH mutations and decreased enzyme activity are not found, and assays for zinc and free protoporphyrin in erythrocytes show that both are increased [59].

Treatment

Avoiding sunlight exposure and wearing clothing designed to provide protection for conditions with chronic photosensitivity are essential. Oral β-carotene (120–180 mg/dL) improves tolerance to sunlight in many patients if the dose is adjusted to maintain serum carotene levels in the range of 10–15 μmol/L (600–800 μg/dL), causing mild skin discoloration due to carotenemia. The beneficial effects of β-carotene may involve quenching of singlet oxygen or free radicals.

Treatment of hepatic complications, which may be accompanied by motor neuropathy, is difficult. Cholestyramine and other porphyrin absorbents, such as activated charcoal, may interrupt the enterohepatic circulation of protoporphyrin and promote its fecal excretion, leading to some improvement. Splenectomy may be helpful if the disease is accompanied by hemolysis and significant splenomegaly. Plasmapheresis and intravenous hemin are sometimes beneficial. However, liver transplantation is sometimes necessary and is often successful in the short term (for review, see McGuire et al. [63]). Liver disease often recurs eventually in the transplanted liver because of continued bone marrow production of excess protoporphyrin. In a retrospective study of 17 liver-transplanted EPP patients, 11 (65%) had recurrent EPP liver disease [63]. Posttransplantation treatment with hemin and plasmapheresis may help prevent recurrence of this complication. Bone marrow transplantation, which has been successful in human EPP [64] and prevented liver disease in a mouse model [65], should be considered after the liver transplantation if a suitable donor can be found.

Autosomal Recessive EPP

As noted above, most individuals with EPP have one causative mutation in their FECH alleles. Rare individuals with causative mutations in both their FECH alleles have also been reported. In a study of 105 randomly selected English EPP patients, 3 patients were found to have two different missense mutations and 1 patient who had severe liver disease had one nonsense and one missense mutation [66]. These patients did not have "C" in position –48 of intron 3 in either allele. EPP patients with two mutations appear to have the same clinical symptoms as EPP patients with one mutation and the "C" variant. However, they may have an increased risk for severe liver disease. Treatment of autosomal recessive EPP is the same as that for the more common form of EPP.

DUAL PORPHYRIA

Patients with porphyria and deficiencies of two heme biosynthetic enzymes have been described, but few are documented by molecular studies. These patients are said to have dual porphyria but have diverse combinations of enzyme deficiencies and differing clinical presentations. Families with individuals having both VP and familial PCT have been described [67]. Combined deficiencies of both HMB-synthase and URO-decarboxylase may lead to symptoms of AIP, PCT, or both. An infant with severe porphyria inherited a COPRO-oxidase deficiency from one parent and URO-synthase deficiency from both [68]. Dual deficiencies of URO-synthase and URO-decarboxylase were described in a patient with features of an erythropoietic porphyria [69]. Molecular studies of a patient initially thought to have both VP and AIP revealed a PROTO-oxidase mutation but no HMB-synthase mutation [70]. A patient with both sporadic PCT and HCP due to an inherited COPRO-oxidase mutation was identified based on a urinary porphyrin pattern consistent with PCT [71]. Recently, mutations in two different heme biosynthetic pathway genes were documented in two individuals with biochemical data consistent with a dual porphyria. One patient, diagnosed after an acute porphyric attack, had a missense mutation in one COPRO-oxidase allele and a missense mutation in one ALA-dehydratase allele [72]. His urinary porphyria pattern suggested HCP except for higher-than-expected ALA levels, which suggested ADP. The second patient had a splice-site mutation in one HMB-synthase allele and a novel two-base insertion in one URO-decarboxylase allele [73]. The 25-year-old woman presented with a bullous rash in sun-exposed areas after starting on birth control pills. Her PBG was elevated, and the initial diagnosis was VP; however, studies of her urinary and plasma porphyrins did not support that diagnosis and indicated a dual porphyria. These are the first two cases of dual porphyria in which mutations in two different genes have been identified.

ANIMAL MODELS OF PORPHYRIAS

Animal models of the human porphyrias are extremely valuable in studying the pathophysiology and possible treatments of the porphyrias. Earlier models of acute hepatic porphyrias include rodents treated with chemicals such as allylisopropylacetamide and 1,4-dihydro-3,5-dicarbethoxycollidine (DDC). Rodents and hepatocytes treated with hexachlorobenzene and other halogenated polycyclic aromatic hydrocarbons have been useful models for PCT and produce URO-decarboxylase deficiency confined to the liver, as in human type 1 PCT. Mouse models produced by gene targeting technology have been generated for AIP, CEP, PCT, VP, and EPP [74–81]. In general, knockout mice that are homozygous for a null mutation have been fetal lethals with, for example, AIP [74], CEP [75], and EPP [76].

However, knockin mice, which have residual activity expressed by the targeted gene, survive and have the biochemical and/or clinical features of their human counterparts. In addition, an EPP mouse model has been generated by ethylnitrosourea-induced mutagenesis, resulting in a point mutation in the FECH gene, which is expressed as a recessive trait [82].

An AIP mouse model with HMB-synthase deficiency, produced by gene targeting, when treated with a barbiturate, has impaired motor function, ataxia, increased levels of ALA in brain and plasma, and decreased heme saturation of liver tryptophan pyrrolase. A motor neuropathy resembling that seen in AIP may develop in these mice, with normal or only slightly increased plasma or urinary ALA, suggesting a role for heme deficiency in nervous tissue [74,83,84].

Two mouse models of CEP using knockin techniques have been reported in which the mice have low URO-synthase, hepatosplenomegaly, and hemolytic anemia [77,78]; one model also had the characteristic light-induced cutaneous involvement [77].

A knockout mouse heterozygous for URO-decarboxylase, with only approximately 50% of normal activity in all tissues, did not show symptoms of PCT unless injected with iron dextran or given oral ALA [79]. These treatments decreased URO-decarboxylase activity to around 20% of normal. When the heterozygous URO-decarboxylase–null mice were bred to null *HFE*-gene mice, the combined URO-decarboxylase–null heterozygote and homozygous null *HFE* mice became uroporphyric without exogenous chemical treatment [79]. Of interest, knockin mice homozygous for the HFE C282Y mutation also developed symptoms of PCT if given 10% ethanol in their drinking water [80]. A mouse model of VP with the common South African R59W mutation in the PROTO-oxidase gene had biochemical findings similar to those of VP [81]. The heterozygous knockout mouse for EPP had skin photosensitivity but no liver disease [85], whereas the EPP mouse model generated by ethylnitrosourea-induced mutagenesis, when homozygous for the induced point mutation, has approximately 5% of normal ferrochelatase activity, skin lesions, jaundice, and severe hepatic dysfunction with massive protoporphyrin deposits [82].

ACKNOWLEDGMENTS

This work was supported in part by grants from the National Institutes of Health, including a research grant (5 R01 DK026824); the General Clinical Research Center Programs at the Mount Sinai School of Medicine (5 M01 RR00071) and the University of Texas Medical Branch (5 M01-RR0073) from the National Center for Research Resources; the U.S. Food and Drug Administration (FD-R-002604); and the American Porphyria Foundation.

REFERENCES

1. Soonawalla ZF, Orug T, Badminton MN, et al. Liver transplantation as a cure for acute intermittent porphyria. Lancet 2004;363:705–6.
2. Elder GH. Hepatic porphyrias in children. J Inherit Metab Dis 1997;20:237–46.
3. Anderson KE, Sassa S, Bishop DF, et al. Disorders of heme biosynthesis: X-linked sideroblastic anemias and the porphyrias, In: Scriver CR, Beaudet AL, Sly WS, et al., eds. The metabolic and molecular basis of inherited disease. New York: McGraw-Hill, 2001:2991–3062.
4. Desnick RJ, Astrin KH. Congenital erythropoietic porphyria: advances in pathogenesis and treatment. Br J Haematol 2002; 117:779–95.
5. Anderson KE, Bloomer JE, Bonkovsky HL, et al. Recommendations for the diagnosis and treatment of the acute porphyrias. Ann Intern Med 2005;142:439–51.
6. Desnick RJ, Anderson KE, Astrin KH. Inherited porphyrias. In: Rimoin DL, Conner JM, Pyeritz RE, et al., eds. Emery and Rimoin's principles and practice of medical genetics. Edinburgh: Churchill Livingstone, 2002;2586–623.
7. Badminton MN, Elder GH. Molecular mechanisms of dominant expression in porphyria. J Inherit Metab Dis 2005;28:277–86.
8. Kauppinen R. Porphyrias. Lancet 2005;365:241–52.
9. May BK, Dogra SC, Sadlon TJ, et al. Molecular regulation of heme biosynthesis in higher vertebrates. Prog Nucleic Acid Res Mol Biol 1995;51:1–51.
10. Kaya AH, Plewinska M, Wong DM, et al. Human δ-aminolevulinate dehydratase (ALAD) gene: structure and alternative splicing of the erythroid and housekeeping mRNAs. Genomics 1994;19:242–8.
11. Grandchamp B, De Verneuil H, Beaumont C, et al. Tissue specific expression of porphobilinogen deaminase. Two isoenzymes from a single gene. Eur J Biochem 1987;162:105–10.
12. Aizencang G, Solis C, Bishop DF, et al. Human uroporphyrinogen-III synthase: genomic organization, alternative promoters, and erythroid-specific expression. Genomics 2000; 70:223–31.
13. Sassa S. ALAD porphyria. Semin Liver Dis 1998;18:95–101.
14. Doss MO, Stauch T, Gross U, et al. The third case of Doss porphyria (delta-amino-levulinic acid dehydratase deficiency) in Germany. J Inherit Metab Dis 2004;27:529–36.
15. Akagi R, Kato N, Inoue R, et al. delta-Aminolevulinate dehydratase (ALAD) porphyria: the first case in North America with two novel ALAD mutations. Mol Genet Metab 2006;87: 329–36.
16. Maruno M, Furuyama K, Akagi R, et al. Highly heterogeneous nature of delta-aminolevulinate dehydratase (ALAD) deficiencies in ALAD porphyria. Blood 2001;97:2972–8.
17. Sassa S, Akagi R, Nishitani C, et al. Late-onset porphyrias: what are they? Cell Mol Biol (Noisy-le-grand) 2002;48:97–101.
18. Stenson PD, Ball EV, Mort M, et al. Human Gene Mutation Database (HGMD): 2003 update. Hum Mutat 2003;21:577–81.
19. Plewinska M, Thunell S, Holmberg L, et al. δ-Aminolevulinate dehydratase deficient porphyria: identification of the molecular lesions in a severely affected homozygote. Am J Hum Genet 1991;49:167–74.
20. Astrin KH, Bishop DF, Wetmur JG, et al. delta-Aminolevulinic acid dehydratase isozymes and lead toxicity. Ann N Y Acad Sci 1987;514:23–9.
21. Handschin C, Lin J, Rhee J, et al. Nutritional regulation of hepatic heme biosynthesis and porphyria through PGC-1alpha. Cell 2005;122:505–15.

22. Grandchamp B, Picat C, Mignotte V, et al. Tissue-specific splicing mutation in acute intermittent porphyria. Proc Nat Acad Sci U S A 1989;86:661–4.
23. Llewellyn DH, Smyth SJ, Elder GH, et al. Homozygous acute intermittent porphyria: compound heterozygosity for adjacent base transitions in the same codon of the porphobilinogen deaminase gene. Hum Genet 1992;89:97–8.
24. Solis C, Martinez-Bermejo A, Naidich TP, et al. Acute intermittent porphyria: studies of the severe homozygous dominant disease provides insights into the neurologic attacks in acute porphyrias. Arch Neurol 2004;61:1764–70.
25. Elder GH. Porphyria cutanea tarda. Semin Liver Dis 1998;18:67–75.
26. Thunell S, Harper P. Porphyrins, porphyrin metabolism, porphyrias. III. Diagnosis, care and monitoring in porphyria cutanea tarda – suggestions for a handling programme. Scand J Clin Lab Invest 2000;60:561–79.
27. Elder GH. Porphyria cutanea tarda and related disorders. In: Kadish KM, Smith K, Guilard R, eds. Porphyrin handbook, part II. San Diego: Academic Press, 2003:67–92.
28. Bonkovsky HL, Poh-Fitzpatrick M, Pimstone N, et al. Porphyria cutanea tarda, hepatitis C, and HFE gene mutations in North America. Hepatology 1998;27:1661–9.
29. Mehrany K, Drage LA, Brandhagen DJ, et al. Association of porphyria cutanea tarda with hereditary hemochromatosis. J Am Acad Dermatol 2004;51:205–11.
30. Egger NG, Goeger DE, Payne DA, et al. Porphyria cutanea tarda: multiplicity of risk factors including HFE mutations, hepatitis C, and inherited uroporphyrinogen decarboxylase deficiency. Dig Dis Sci 2002;47:419–26.
31. Bonkovsky HL, Barnard GF. Diagnosis of porphyric syndromes: a practical approach in the era of molecular biology. Semin Liver Dis 1998;18:57–65.
32. Anderson KE. The porphyrias. In: Goldman L, Bennett CJ, eds. Cecil textbook of medicine. Philadelphia: WB Saunders, 2000:1123–32.
33. Kuhnel A, Gross U, Doss MO. Hereditary coproporphyria in Germany: clinical-biochemical studies in 53 patients. Clin Biochem 2000;33:465–73.
34. Martasek P. Hereditary coproporphyria. Semin Liver Dis 1998; 18:25–32.
35. Martasek P, Nordmann Y, Grandchamp B. Homozygous hereditary coproporphyria caused by an arginine to tryptophane substitution in coproporphyrinogen oxidase and common intragenic polymorphisms. Hum Mol Genet 1994;3:477–80.
36. Nordmann Y, Grandchamp B, De Verneuil H, et al. Harderoporphyria: a variant hereditary coproporphyria. J Clin Invest 1983;72:1139–49.
37. Lee DS, Flachsova E, Bodnarova M, et al. Structural basis of hereditary coproporphyria. Proc Natl Acad Sci U S A 2005;102: 14232–7.
38. Schmitt C, Gouya L, Malonova E, et al. Mutations in human CPO gene predict clinical expression of either hepatic hereditary coproporphyria or erythropoietic harderoporphyria. Hum Mol Genet 2005;14:3089–98.
39. Meissner P, Hift RJ, Corrigall A. Variegate porphyria. In: Kadish KM, Smith K, Guilard R, eds. Porphyrin handbook, part II. San Diego: Academic Press, 2003:93–120.
40. Poh-Fitzpatrick MB. A plasma porphyrin fluorescence marker for variegate porphyria. Arch Dermatol 1980;116:543–7.
41. Meissner PN, Dailey TA, Hift RJ, et al. A R59W mutation in human protoporphyrinogen oxidase results in decreased enzyme activity and is prevalent in South Africans with variegate porphyria. Nat Genet 1996;13:95–7.
42. Whatley SD, Puy H, Morgan RR, et al. Variegate porphyria in Western Europe: identification of PPOX gene mutations in 104 families, extent of allelic heterogeneity, and absence of correlation between phenotype and type of mutation. Am J Hum Genet 1999;65:984–94.
43. Roberts AG, Puy H, Dailey TA, et al. Molecular characterization of homozygous variegate porphyria. Hum Mol Genet 1998;7:1921–5.
44. Palmer RA, Elder GH, Barrett DF, et al. Homozygous variegate porphyria: a compound heterozygote with novel mutations in the protoporphyrinogen oxidase gene. Br J Dermatol 2001;144:866–9.
45. Kauppinen R, Timonen K, von und zu Fraunberg M, et al. Homozygous variegate porphyria: 20 y follow-up and characterization of molecular defect. J Invest Dermatol 2001;116: 610–13.
46. Solis C, Aizencang GI, Astrin KH, et al. Uroporphyrinogen III synthase erythroid promoter mutations in adjacent GATA1 and CP2 elements cause congenital erythropoietic porphyria. J Clin Invest 2001;107:753–62.
47. Piomelli S, Poh-Fitzpatrick MB, Seaman C, et al. Complete suppression of the symptoms of congenital erythropoietic porphyria by long-term treatment with high-level transfusions. N Engl J Med 1986;314:1029–31.
48. Dupuis-Girod S, Akkari V, Ged C, et al. Successful match-unrelated donor bone marrow transplantation for congenital erythropoietic porphyria (Gunther disease). Eur J Pediatr 2005;164:104–7.
49. Shaw PH, Mancini AJ, McConnell JP, et al. Treatment of congenital erythropoietic porphyria in children by allogeneic stem cell transplantation: a case report and review of the literature. Bone Marrow Transplant 2001;27:101–5.
50. Mazurier F, Geronimi F, Lamrissi-Garcia I, et al. Correction of deficient cd34(+) cells from peripheral blood after mobilization in a patient with congenital erythropoietic porphyria. Mol Ther 2001;3:411–17.
51. Cox TM, Alexander GJ, Sarkany RP. Protoporphyria. Semin Liver Dis 1998;18:85–93.
52. Cox TM. Protoporphyria. In: Kadish KM, Smith K, Guilard R, eds. Porphyrin handbook, part II. San Diego: Academic Press, 2003:121–49.
53. Gouya L, Puy H, Robreau AM, et al. The penetrance of dominant erythropoietic protoporphyria is modulated by expression of wildtype FECH. Nat Genet 2002;30:27–8.
54. Gouya L, Martin-Schmitt C, Robreau AM, et al. Contribution of a common single-nucleotide polymorphism to the genetic predisposition for erythropoietic protoporphyria. Am J Hum Genet 2006;78:2–14.
55. Risheg H, Chen FP, Bloomer JR. Genotypic determinants of phenotype in North American patients with erythropoietic protoporphyria. Mol Genet Metab 2003;80:196–206.
56. Bloomer J, Wang Y, Singhal A, et al. Molecular studies of liver disease in erythropoietic protoporphyria. J Clin Gastroenterol 2005;39:S167–75.
57. Najahi-Missaoui W, Dailey HA. Production and characterization of erythropoietic protoporphyric heterodimeric ferrochelatases. Blood 2005;106:1098–104.

58. Ohgari Y, Sawamoto M, Yamamoto M, et al. Ferrochelatase consisting of wild-type and mutated subunits from patients with a dominant-inherited disease, erythropoietic protoporphyria, is an active but unstable dimer. Hum Mol Genet 2005;14:327–34.
59. Wilson J, Edixhoven-Bosdijk A, Koole-Lesuis R, et al. A new variant of erythropoietic protoporphyria with normal ferrochelatase activity. Physiol Res 2003;52:29S.
60. Meerman L, Koopen NR, Bloks V, et al. Biliary fibrosis associated with altered bile composition in a mouse model of erythropoietic protoporphyria. Gastroenterology 1999;117:696–705.
61. Rank JF, Carithers R, Bloomer J. Evidence for neurological dysfunction in end-stage protoporphyric liver disease. Hepatology 1993;18:1404–9.
62. Minder EI, Gouya L, Schneider-Yin X, et al. A genotype-phenotype correlation between null-allele mutations in the ferrochelatase gene and liver complication in patients with erythropoietic protoporphyria. Cell Mol Biol (Noisy-le-grand) 2002;48:91–6.
63. McGuire BM, Bonkovsky HL, Carithers RL Jr, et al. Liver transplantation for erythropoietic protoporphyria liver disease. Liver Transpl 2005;11:1590–6.
64. Poh-Fitzpatrick MB, Wang X, Anderson KE, et al. Erythropoietic protoporphyria: altered phenotype after bone marrow transplantation for myelogenous leukemia in a patient heteroallelic for ferrochelatase gene mutations. J Amer Acad Dermatol 2002;46:861–6.
65. Fontanellas A, Mazurier F, Landry M, et al. Reversion of hepatobiliary alterations by bone marrow transplantation in a murine model of erythropoietic protoporphyria. Hepatology 2000;32:73–81.
66. Whatley SD, Mason NG, Khan M, et al. Autosomal recessive erythropoietic protoporphyria in the United Kingdom: prevalence and relationship to liver disease. J Med Genet 2004;41:e105.
67. Day RS, Eales L, Meissner D. Coexistent variegate porphyria and porphyria cutanea tarda. N Engl J Med 1982;30:36–41.
68. Nordmann Y, Amram D, Deybach JC, et al. Coexistent hereditary coproporphyria and congenital erythropoietic porphyria (Günther disease). J Inherited Metab Dis 1990;13:687–91.
69. Freesemann AG, Hofweber K, Doss MO. Coexistence of deficiencies of uroporphyrinogen III synthase and decarboxylase in a patient with congenital erythropoietic porphyria and in his family. Eur J Clin Chem Clin Biochem 1997;35:35–9.
70. Weinlich G, Doss MO, Sepp N, et al. Variegate porphyria with coexistent decrease in porphobilinogen deaminase activity. Acta Derm Venereol 2001;81:356–9.
71. Doss MO, Gross U, Puy H, et al. [Coexistence of hereditary coproporphyria and porphyria cutanea tarda: a new form of dual porphyria]. Med Klin 2002;97:1–5.
72. Akagi R, Inoue R, Muranaka S, et al. Dual gene defects involving delta-aminolaevulinate dehydratase and coproporphyrinogen oxidase in a porphyria patient. Br J Haematol 2006;132:237–43.
73. Harraway JR, Florkowski CM, Sies C, et al. Dual porphyria with mutations in both the UROD and HMBS genes. Ann Clin Biochem 2006;43:80–2.
74. Lindberg RL, Porcher C, Grandchamp B, et al. Porphobilinogen deaminase deficiency in mice causes a neuropathy resembling that of human hepatic porphyria. Nat Genet 1996;12:195–9.
75. Bensidhoum M, Audine M, Fontanellas A, et al. The disruption of mouse uroporphyrinogen III synthase (uros) gene is fully lethal. Acta Haematologica 1997;98(suppl 1):100.
76. Magness ST, Brenner DA. Targeted disruption of the mouse ferrochelatase gene producing an exon 10 deletion. Biochim Biophys Acta 1999;1453:161–74.
77. Bishop DF, Johansson A, Phelps R, et al. Uroporphyrinogen III synthase knock in mice have the human congenital erythropoietic porphyria phenotype, including the characteristic light-induced cutaneous lesions. Am J Hum Genet 2006;78:645–58.
78. Ged C, Mendez M, Robert E, et al. A knock-in mouse model of congenital erythropoietic porphyria. Genomics 2006;87:84–92.
79. Phillips JD, Jackson LK, Bunting M, et al. A mouse model of familial porphyria cutanea tarda. Proc Natl Acad Sci U S A 2001;98:259–64.
80. Sinclair PR, Gorman N, Trask HW, et al. Uroporphyria caused by ethanol in Hfe(−/−) mice as a model for porphyria cutanea tarda. Hepatology 2003;37:351–8.
81. Medlock AE, Meissner PN, Davidson BP, et al. A mouse model for South African (R59W) variegate porphyria: construction and initial characterization. Cell Mol Biol (Noisy-le-grand) 2002;48:71–8.
82. Tutois S, Montagutelli X, Dasilva V, et al. Erythropoietic protoporphyria in the house mouse: a recessive inherited ferrochelatase deficiency with anemia, photosensitivity, and liver disease. J Clin Invest 1991;88:1730–6.
83. Lindberg RL, Martini R, Baumgartner M, et al. Motor neuropathy in porphobilinogen deaminase-deficient mice imitates the peripheral neuropathy of human acute porphyria. J Clin Invest 1999;103:1127–34.
84. Meyer UA, Schuurmans MM, Lindberg RLP. Acute porphyrias: pathogenesis of neurological manifestations. Semin Liver Dis 1998;18:43–52.
85. Magness ST, Maeda N, Brenner DA. An exon 10 deletion in the mouse ferrochelatase gene has a dominant negative effect and causes mild protoporphyria. Blood 2002;100:1470–7.

29

Tyrosinemia

Grant Mitchell, M.D., Pierre A. Russo, M.D., Josée Dubois, M.D., F.R.C.P., and Fernando Alvarez, M.D.

Hepatorenal tyrosinemia* is a fascinating inborn error of metabolism that can affect numerous organs, particularly the liver, kidneys, and peripheral nerves. The first report of a patient with elevated blood tyrosine was by Medes in 1932 [1]. Patients with a more typical clinical and biochemical picture of tyrosinemia were then described in the late 1950s [2–5]. Since then, more than 500 patients have been reported in the literature [6–8] or enrolled in the International NTBC [2-(2-nitro-4-trifluoromethyl benzoyl)-1,3-cyclohexanedione] Trial. Previously, almost all patients died in infancy and early childhood, and only isolated case reports described affected adults. In the 50 years since the description of tyrosinemia [3], the course of the disease has been improved successively by the introduction of diet therapy, neonatal screening, and hepatic transplantation. The advent of liver and kidney transplantation as a definitive treatment [7–11] revolutionized the outcome. Recently, the availability of NTBC, a chemical now designated as nitisinone and commercialized as Orfadin (Swedish Orphan International AB), has provided hope for a nonsurgical solution for some patients. On a fundamental level, tyrosinemia raises questions in hepatology, biochemical and population genetics, cell biology, oncology, and public health.

PATHOPHYSIOLOGY

Tyrosinemia is caused by a deficiency of fumarylacetoacetate hydrolase (FAH; enzyme [EC] 3.7.1.2), the last enzyme of tyrosine degradation (Figure 29.1A). The site of the primary metabolic block in tyrosinemia was elegantly deduced by Lindblad et al. in 1977 [12] and subsequently confirmed enzymatically by several investigators [13–15]. FAH is a 419–amino acid cytosolic homodimer present in the liver [16] and to some extent in the kidney, lymphocytes, erythrocytes, fibroblasts, and chorionic villi [17]. Human liver FAH complementary DNAs (cDNAs; GenBank accession no. NM000137) and the human *FAH* gene have been cloned and sequenced and the human gene mapped to chromosome 15q23-q25 [16]. Early studies of tyrosinemia showed that other enzymes of tyrosine degradation, particularly 4-hydroxyphenylpyruvate dioxygenase (4HPPD), are reduced in tyrosinemic liver. These changes have subsequently been shown to be secondary to the deficiency of FAH.

The mechanism of the hepatic and renal symptoms of tyrosinemia is largely conjectural, although much circumstantial evidence favors a toxic effect of the final compounds of tyrosine metabolism. Tyrosine and its early metabolites (4-hydroxyphenylpyruvate and homogentisate; Figure 29.1A) are present at high levels in other hereditary diseases that have no hepatic or renal symptoms; thus, these compounds are unlikely to cause the hepatorenal manifestations of tyrosinemia. In contrast, the compound immediately upstream from the FAH reaction, fumarylacetoacetate, and its derivatives, succinylacetoacetate and succinylacetone, have potent biologic activity. For example, fumarylacetoacetate (FAA) and its precursor, maleylacetoacetate, resemble maleic acid, a well-known toxin that can induce renal Fanconi's syndrome [18,19], and the histologic changes of maleic acid–induced Fanconi's syndrome mimic the renal changes of tyrosinemia (see Pathology). Maleylacetoacetate and FAA are reactive, unstable compounds. FAA can form glutathione adducts [12], and free glutathione concentration is somewhat reduced in tyrosinemic liver samples [20]. The significance of this observation is unknown, but free sulfhydryl groups are known to be important for protection against free radicals and other toxic compounds [21,21a].

In tyrosinemic livers, Kvittigen et al. described discrete nodules with normal FAH activity [21b] and later showed that they resulted from somatic mutations in one *FAH* gene allele that restored a normal sequence [21c]. Revertant nodules are frequent in tyrosinemic livers and may be large, presumably reflecting the highly mutagenic environment of the tyrosinemic hepatocyte and a selective growth advantage of revertant cells. Of note, fumarylacetoacetate is a mutagen [21c]. In 25 tyrosinemic livers from French Canadian patients, 20 (80%) had revertant nodules that occupied up to 36% of the surface studied;

*For simplicity, this chapter uses the generic term *tyrosinemia* to refer to hepatorenal tyrosinemia (also known as fumarylacetoacetate hydrolase deficiency, tyrosinemia type 1 or congenital tyrosinosis; assigned MIM no. 27670). Other forms of hypertyrosinemia are referred to by their specific names.

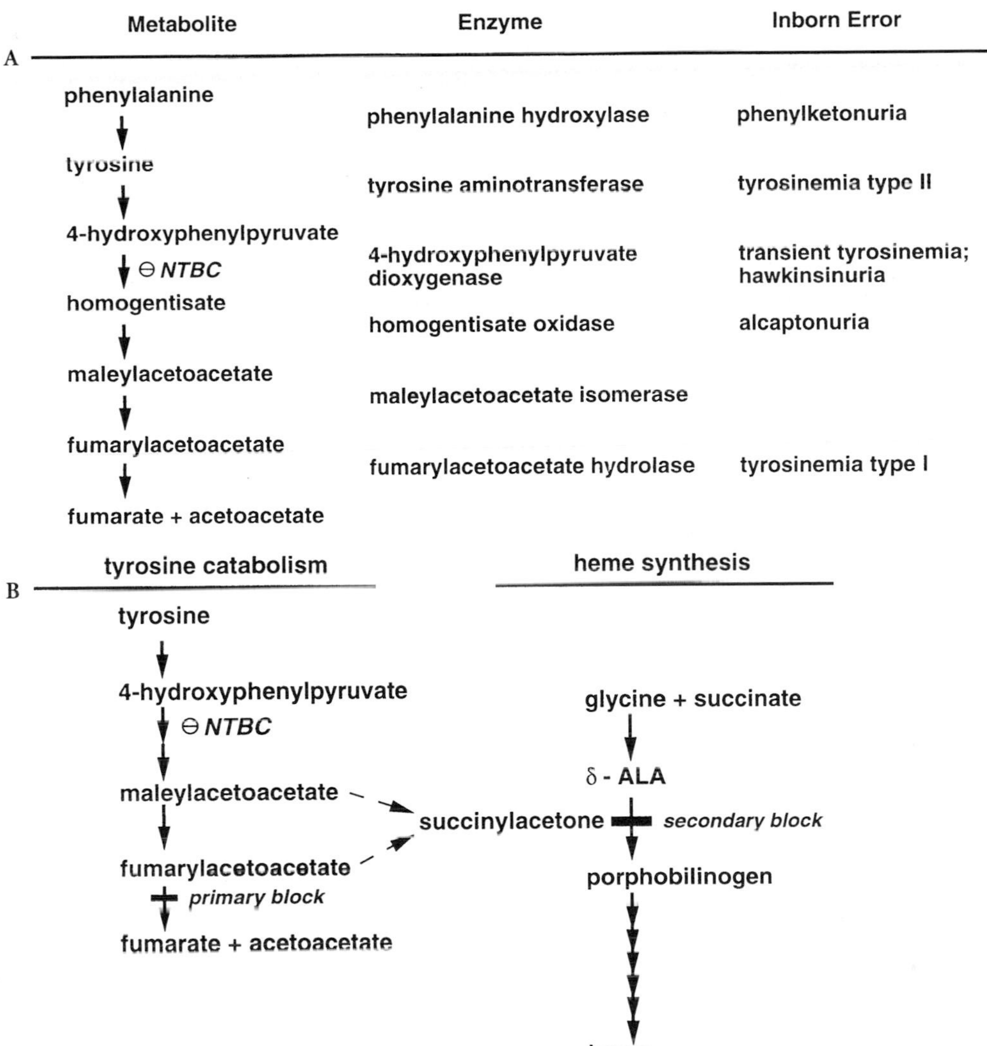

Figure 29.1. Tyrosine metabolism. (**A**) Degradation of the aromatic amino acids. The metabolic intermediates, the degradative enzymes, and the inborn errors associated with dysfunction of these enzymes are indicated. Quantitatively minor pathways of tyrosine metabolism are not shown but are of physiologic significance. These pathways include synthesis of catecholamines and the synthesis of melanin pigments and are felt to be normal in tyrosinemia. (**B**) Interrelationship of tyrosine catabolism in tyrosinemia and of heme biosynthesis. Succinylacetone is derived from the intermediates that accumulate upstream from the primary enzyme block. It inhibits the synthesis of porphobilinogen from δ-aminolevulinic acid (δ-ALA). The resulting δ-ALA accumulation is thought to cause the clinical signs of neurologic crises. Each *solid arrow* represents a single enzymatic step. The *hatched arrows* reflect the uncertainty regarding the mechanism by which succinylacetone arises from related compounds in the pathway of tyrosine degradation. In each panel, the site of action of NTBC is indicated.

interestingly, the extent of replacement by revertant nodules correlated inversely with the patients' clinical severity [21d].

Mouse models of FAH deficiency [22,23] have hepatic and renal symptoms resembling those of tyrosinemic patients but a more fulminant course, resulting in neonatal death. NTBC treatment can permit growth to adulthood, but mice rapidly develop hepatic failure if NTBC is withdrawn [24]. Also, following challenge with homogentisic acid, a tyrosine metabolite downstream from the NTBC-induced block (Figure 29.1B), hepatocytes undergo apoptosis [25,26]. FAH-deficient mice are useful for studies of the pathophysiology of tyrosinemia. However, mouse liver and nutrition have numerous differences from those of humans, such as a marked propensity to develop hepatocellular carcinoma, probably by mechanisms different from those in humans [27], and it is generally agreed that results from mouse models cannot be extrapolated directly to humans.

The most clearly established pathophysiologic mechanism in tyrosinemia is the role of succinylacetone in neurologic crises (Figure 29.1B). Succinylacetone is a potent inhibitor of the porphyrin synthetic enzyme δ-aminolevulinic acid dehydratase, and caused a marked accumulation of δ-aminolevulinic acid in children with tyrosinemia [28]. δ-Aminolevulinic acid toxicity has been shown to be associated with neurotoxicity in acute intermittent porphyria, hereditary deficiency of δ-aminolevulinic acid dehydratase, and lead poisoning [29]. Available clinical, biochemical, and pathologic evidence suggests that the neurologic crisis of tyrosinemia results from δ-aminolevulinic acid toxicity and that it represents the most severe porphyria-like condition known in humans [28–31].

GENETICS AND SCREENING

Tyrosinemia is an autosomal recessive trait [32]. It is important that couples with an affected child be aware that in each subsequent pregnancy, they have a 25% risk of having another affected child. Heterozygotes for hepatorenal tyrosinemia are asymptomatic and have normal levels of tyrosine-related metabolites.

Large numbers of cases of tyrosinemia have been reported in two regions: the province of Quebec, Canada, and northern Europe, particularly Scandinavia. In Quebec, tyrosinemia is common because of a well-documented but complex founder effect [33,34]. Tyrosinemia is particularly frequent in the Saguenay-Lac St-Jean area of northern Quebec, where the carrier rate for tyrosinemia is 1 in 20 and where 1 in 1846 live births results in an affected child [33]. Overall, the birth rate of affected children in Quebec is 1 in 16,786 [34], compared with an estimated 1 in 100,000 to 1 in 120,000 elsewhere, including Scandinavia [8]. Tyrosinemia has been reported in many ethnic groups, and lack of French Canadian or Scandinavian ancestry does not exclude the diagnosis.

Many mutations in the *FAH* gene have been described in patients with tyrosinemia [35]. The IVS12+5ga allele accounts for about 90% of mutant *FAH* alleles in the Saguenay-Lac St-Jean area of Quebec [36,37]. IVS12+5ga and IVS6–1gt are frequent in patients of diverse ethnic origins [38]. In addition, W262X is prevalent in Finns [39,40] and Q64H (192GT) in Pakistanis [41]. R341W causes pseudodeficiency [42] (see Diagnosis). In view of the protean manifestations of tyrosinemia, it will be interesting to search for genotype–phenotype correlations. However, affected subjects from the same family may have different clinical presentations [3,43]. We know of one family with three affected children, two of whom died in infancy: one from a hepatic crisis, another from a paralytic neurologic crisis. The surviving sibling is now a young adult with renal tubulopathy and modest liver disease. Clearly, environmental and genetic factors unrelated to the *FAH* gene play a major role in determining the clinical severity of tyrosinemia.

DIAGNOSIS

Tyrosinemia should be suspected in any infant or child with evidence of hepatocellular necrosis, cirrhosis, or decreased hepatic synthetic function (especially perturbed coagulation studies) for which the cause is not evident. Rarely, patients may present with coagulopathy in the absence of overt liver disease [44]. Rickets or characteristic renal or neurologic findings, especially if associated with abnormal hepatic function, also suggest this diagnosis.

Plasma tyrosine levels are initially elevated to a variable degree in almost all symptomatic patients, although older patients with a chronic course and patients treated with low-protein diets often do not show hypertyrosinemia [45]. Furthermore, hypertyrosinemia is a nonspecific finding. Blood tyrosine is elevated after meals. Therefore, hypertyrosinemia should be diagnosed only in fasting samples. Hypertyrosinemia may be associated with all forms of liver failure as well as with a diverse group of conditions involving the pathway of tyrosine catabolism (Figure 29.1). The same is true of plasma methionine levels, which may be markedly elevated in tyrosinemia, and of phenylalanine levels, which are often initially somewhat elevated at diagnosis as well. The demonstration of elevated levels of succinylacetone on dried filter paper blood samples, in plasma or in urine, is pathognomonic for tyrosinemia [46]. We have never observed a tyrosinemic patient who did not have elevated levels of succinylacetone in blood and urine. Rare case reports exist of patients with normal tyrosine levels [45] and with undetectable levels of succinylacetone [47]. We have encountered a small number of cases in which blood succinylacetone levels are very low and in which it is more convenient to demonstrate the presence of succinylacetone in urine samples.

In selected cases, it is useful to perform FAH assays as well. FAH can be assayed in lymphocytes [17] and erythrocytes [48] as well as on liver tissue. Carrier detection by these techniques is imperfect; some heterozygotes for the deficiency may have high levels of residual FAH activity. Conversely, a pseudodeficient *FAH* allele is common in certain populations [42]. This allele is not associated with clinical symptoms but has a very low activity when assayed in vitro. Enzyme assay results thus need to be interpreted in light of the patients' clinical and biochemical findings. For the above reasons, carrier detection by enzymatic means is not recommended as a screening technique.

In at-risk populations, carrier screening is possible by molecular testing for common alleles. It must be recalled that even in regions with a strong founder effect, some rare mutant alleles exist. A negative molecular screening test does not completely eliminate carrier status.

Prenatal diagnosis of tyrosinemia is possible by the measurement of succinylacetone in the amniotic fluid and by FAH assay using cultured amniocytes or chorionic villus cells [49]. Molecular diagnosis can be offered to families in which the causal mutation is known. Prenatal diagnosis should be supervised by an experienced genetician.

Neonatal screening for tyrosinemia has been under way in Quebec since 1970 [46] using blood samples dried on filter paper. Currently, succinylacetone is used as a marker for screening. Screening using blood tyrosine as a marker leads to many false-positive results in children with transient tyrosinemia (Figure 29.1A), in those with other hereditary tyrosinemias (Figure 29.1A), and occasionally in children with hepatic problems other than hepatorenal tyrosinemia. More importantly, false-negative results may be obtained in children affected with hepatorenal tyrosinemia [35], particularly in this era of low neonatal protein intake (breast-feeding, humanized formulas) and early hospital discharge, two factors that reduce the levels of blood tyrosine in predischarge samples. Succinylacetone, in contrast, is elevated in childhood (and also prenatally as a marker for diagnosis in amniotic fluid).

DIFFERENTIAL DIAGNOSIS

In practice, for tyrosinemic children presenting to the hepatologist in the first year of life, the differential diagnosis is that of diseases causing hepatic failure. In older children and young adults, the differential diagnosis includes other diseases leading to cirrhosis.

At any age, the presence of a suggestive family history or of typical neurologic crises in a patient with signs of liver dysfunction is strongly suggestive of tyrosinemia, and the demonstra tion of elevated succinylacetone in blood or urine establishes the diagnosis. Renal tubular dysfunction in patients with hepatocellular failure is suggestive of tyrosinemia but is also seen in other hereditary metabolic diseases, such as galactosemia [50], hereditary fructose intolerance [51], Wilson's disease [52], certain lactic acidoses, and glycogen storage disease type 1 [53]. Elevation of α-fetoprotein (AFP) levels is consistent with tyrosinemia, although it is not specific. In patients not treated with NTBC, the level of AFP is consistently elevated in young acutely ill patients and in most other patients but may be normal in some young adults with an indolent course of disease.

OTHER FORMS OF HYPERTYROSINEMIA

Biochemically, many patients have hypertyrosinemia secondary to hepatic failure, and the pattern of plasma amino acids is not particularly helpful in diagnosis. A practical consideration is that tyrosine can be elevated in plasma in nonfasting subjects, along with several other amino acids. Experienced interpretation and repeated plasma amino acid chromatography are necessary before initiating investigations if the clinical symptomatology does not suggest tyrosinemia.

Several inborn errors of metabolism and some acquired conditions may result in isolated hypertyrosinemia. Transient tyrosinemia of the newborn is felt to be the result of an immaturity of the enzyme 4HPPD, which causes a transient deficiency of the enzyme [54]. It is found most frequently in newborns who are premature, who receive large amounts of protein (such as are found in cow's milk), or who are deficient in vitamin C, the cofactor for 4HPPD. Transient tyrosinemia is generally felt to be a benign trait, unnoticed unless plasma amino acids are studied. It disappears spontaneously within days to weeks, although mild developmental delay has been reported. Biochemical normalization also may be hastened by the administration of vitamin C (50–100 mg/d) [54] or by dietary restriction of phenylalanine and tyrosine.

Hawkinsinuria is a rare autosomal dominant trait in which affected infants may develop acidosis and hypertyrosinemia. Clinical manifestations arise at the time of weaning from breast milk. Hawkinsinuria is hypothesized to be the result of an abnormal function of 4HPPD [55] and is diagnosed by the presence of an unusual organic compound (hawkinsin) in the urine of symptomatic patients. The prognosis seems to be excellent, and hepatic function was not markedly perturbed in the reported cases.

Tyrosinemia type III patients have primary 4HPPD deficiency. Presentations vary from asymptomatic to mental retardation and neurologic signs. It is not formally proved that this represents a true clinical phenotype and may in fact reflect an ascertainment bias (i.e., a fortuitous discovery in patients in whom amino acid chromatography was performed for mental retardation caused by unrelated factors). Conversely, because of the suspicion of neurologic risk, treatment with a phenylalanine and tyrosine–restricted diet is recommended to lower circulating tyrosine concentrations.

Tyrosinemia type II (oculocutaneous tyrosinemia) is also clinically distinct from tyrosinemia and is caused by the autosomal recessively inherited deficiency of tyrosine aminotransferase [54]. Patients affected by tyrosinemia type II develop hyperkeratosis of the palms and soles and corneal thickening, and they may have developmental delay, but hepatic and renal functions remain intact.

A preliminary communication described two siblings with severe hepatocellular dysfunction in whom succinylacetone was not detected [55]. Enzyme assay on liver from these patients revealed an isolated deficiency of maleylacetoacetate isomerase (MAI), the enzyme preceding FAH in the tyrosine catabolic pathway. This observation remains unconfirmed to date, and analysis of a large number of patients presenting with similar findings has failed to reveal cases of MAI deficiency. Furthermore, mice deficient in MAI [56] show evidence of an active glutathione-dependent shunt pathway that bypasses MAI and allows normal survival, except under extreme genetic or nutritional stress. The clinical presentation of MAI isomerase deficiency in humans is thus unknown, but we have no evidence that it resembles tyrosinemia.

Interestingly, the other inborn errors of aromatic amino acid catabolism shown in Figure 29.1 are associated neither with hypertyrosinemia nor with signs of liver disease. Phenylketonuria is usually revealed by high blood levels of phenylalanine at neonatal screening, and its major manifestation, mental retardation, can be prevented by dietary phenylalanine restriction. The signs of alcaptonuria are arthritis in middle age, a darkening of urine when exposed to air, and excessive urinary excretion of homogentisic acid.

CLINICAL FINDINGS IN NON–NTBC-TREATED PATIENTS

This section describes the natural history of tyrosinemia and the impact of diet therapy and neonatal screening. Our experience with NTBC, which radically improves the clinical course, is described later (see Treatment). Cases of tyrosinemia have traditionally been divided into acute and chronic forms based on the clinical picture. This distinction is not always clear because some children have a stormy course in the first year of life typical of the acute form but then have an indolent course compatible with the chronic form. Moreover, children over 2 years of age defined as having chronic tyrosinemia remain at risk for acute life-threatening liver and neurologic crises. The liver, kidneys, and peripheral nerves are the main organs affected by tyrosinemia.

Liver Crises

Liver crises typically present before 2 years of age and decrease in frequency and severity thereafter. In Quebec, where because of neonatal screening, diet therapy is introduced before 1 month of age, the severity of episodes of liver decompensation in infants appears to be decreased; however, these episodes may occur, and in our experience, patients treated early with diet alone all eventually develop cirrhosis. Acute episodes are often heralded by an intercurrent viral infection, with anorexia, irritability, and vomiting. Infants with liver decompensation typically emit an odor resembling that of boiled cabbage. Within a few hours to days, overt liver disease may develop, with a rapid increase in liver size, ascites, anasarca, and marked coagulopathy. Jaundice is usually a terminal event and is not a feature of most patients. Historically, over 80% of all patients with tyrosinemia died before 2 years of age from an acute liver crisis, some infants presenting with six to ten episodes in the first year of life [6].

The first laboratory indication of an impending liver crisis is disproportionate prolongation of the coagulation time [6,15,57], and a bleeding diathesis without other symptoms of liver disease may be the mode of presentation. Prothrombin and partial thromboplastin times may be alarmingly prolonged despite normal or near normal serum aminotransferase levels. These abnormalities also may be seen in clinically stable infants and are unresponsive to oral or parenteral vitamin K supplementation. Infusions of fresh frozen plasma are effective at restoring near normal coagulation in most instances. Interestingly, factor V levels, frequently used in other liver diseases as a marker of liver synthetic function, may be within or close to the normal range in tyrosinemic infants at the beginning of a crisis. In contrast, factors XI and XII, as well as vitamin K–dependent factors II, VII, IX, and X, may be exceedingly low (<15%), with normal factor VIII levels.

During a liver crisis, aminotransferase levels are initially only mildly elevated (less than twice normal values), if at all, in contrast to the pathologic coagulation profile. Serum amino acids, particularly tyrosine, methionine, and phenylalanine, are elevated and may be accompanied by generalized aminoaciduria in patients who have renal dysfunction. Serum AFP may be extremely high (up to 400,000 ng/mL), declining over several weeks to months after the crisis.

Chronic Liver Disease

A chronic course was seen in less than 40% of Quebec patients but may have been more prevalent in northern Europe [6,8]. With the systematic newborn screening program in Quebec, dietary management is instituted by 3–4 weeks of age [46]. Despite early dietary intervention, in our experience, all non–NTBC-treated children eventually develop cirrhosis, although at highly variable rates [6,7]. During the first 2 years of life, the child is particularly at risk for liver and neurologic crises. Thereafter, the dominant liver problem is the risk of hepatocarcinoma.

Clinical examination reveals hepatosplenomegaly in approximately 70% and rarely other signs of liver dysfunction, such as spider hemangiomas or clubbing. Rickets may be apparent in those with moderate or severe renal disease [58].

Forty percent of our population with a chronic course has abnormal coagulation parameters but no overt bleeding [7]. Serum AFP is elevated in virtually all patients, ranging from 100–400,000 ng/mL (normal, <10 ng/mL), with exacerbations during hepatic crises. At birth, AFP levels are extremely high and decrease to a variable extent with dietary therapy. This reduction of AFP with diet therapy alone should be recalled when evaluating results of NTBC therapy. Serum aminotransferase concentrations are usually normal or mildly elevated, with normal albumin and bilirubin in the majority. The serum γ-glutamyltransferase level is usually slightly elevated and may reflect renal involvement, although this has not been carefully evaluated.

Risk of Hepatocarcinoma

The incidence of hepatocarcinoma in tyrosinemia is difficult to estimate because systematic autopsies have not been performed in all children dying of the disease; even in autopsied patients, livers have not always been examined in detail.

At CHU Sainte-Justine, 31 tyrosinemic livers have been studied at autopsy or transplantation since 1986 (Table 29.1). In 23 of 31 livers (74%), nodules were identified by either ultrasonography or computed tomography (CT). Four livers (13%) showed one or more foci of hepatocarcinoma, and four had evidence of high-grade dysplasia [59]. The frequency of carcinoma is lower than the widely cited figure of 37% by Weinberg et al. [60], who reviewed all 42 cases of tyrosinemia published before 1976 and added their personal experience with one patient. Fourteen of their patients, from older literature, had a presumed diagnosis of tyrosinemia not always documented pathologically. The incidence of hepatocarcinoma may be less than initially reported, and this may have implications when considering the urgency of liver transplantation for children with clinically stable disease and no evidence of nodules on imaging. However, there is no question that the risk of hepatocarcinoma is high, even in infants. To our knowledge, the youngest children to develop hepatocarcinoma were 15 and 25 months old [9,61].

Table 29.1: Children with Tyrosinemia Undergoing Liver Transplantation Who Had Not Received Previous NTBC Treatment

Patient	*Age at OLT, yr*	*Nodules/HCC or Dysplasia**	*Outcome*
1	1⅔	–/Dysplasia grade 1	Death, primary nonfunction
2	8	–/–	A&W
3	9	–/–	A&W
4	3½	+/HCC and dysplasia grade 3	A&W
5	2	+/Dysplasia grade 3	A&W
6	10	+/–	A&W
7	1½	+/Dysplasia grade 1	A&W
8	12	+/–	A&W
9	1½	–/Dysplasia grade 1	A&W
10	17	–/–	Liver/kidney, A&W
11	6	+/Dysplasia grade 2	A&W
12	3	–/Dysplasia grade 2	A&W
13	2	–/Dysplasia grade 1	A&W
14	⅓	+/Dysplasia grade 2	Death, primary nonfunction
15	9½	+/Dysplasia grade 3	A&W
16	1	+/Dysplasia grade 3	A&W
17	2½	+/Dysplasia grade 1	A&W
18	2½	+/Dysplasia grade 1	A&W
19	11	+/HCC and dysplasia grade 3	A&W
20	½	+/Dysplasia grade 2	A&W
21	3	+/Dysplasia grade 1	A&W
22	11/12	+/Dysplasia grade 3	A&W
23	2	+/Dysplasia grade 2	A&W

*Dysplasia classified as in Ferrell et al. [59].
A&W, alive and well; OLT, orthotopic liver transplantation; HCC, hepatocarcinoma; –, absent; +, present.

Serial serum AFP levels do not reliably predict the presence of carcinoma. AFP levels may increase greatly following acute liver crises and do not accurately discriminate regenerating or fatty nodules from hepatocarcinoma (Figure 29.2). Hepatocarcinoma may occur in tyrosinemia in the presence of normal or low AFP levels [7]. Nevertheless, a high degree of suspicion should be maintained if there is a significant increase in AFP levels from the usual baseline in a clinically stable patient with no evidence of an acute exacerbation such as a liver crisis, because this may indicate the development of hepatocarcinoma. If a nodule is visualized radiologically or by ultrasonography, imaging characteristics cannot reliably rule out malignancy (see Imaging in Tyrosinemia).

Neurologic Crises

Neurologic crises are a hallmark of non–NTBC-treated tyrosinemia. The crises have two phases: (1) an active period of painful paresthesias, autonomic signs such as hypertension [29,62], tachycardia, and sometimes progressive paralysis and (2) a period of recuperation, seen in crises with weakness or paralysis. In our series of 48 French Canadian patients, 20 (42%) had crises [28], higher than in previous series. Crises may truly be less frequent in other populations, or perhaps crises were underreported or not identified in earlier series.

Painful crises are the most frequent. During the prodrome, which often occurs following a minor infection, the child is irritable and less active than usual. The child then develops severe pain, often in the legs. Patients frequently adopt a position of extreme hyperextension of the trunk and neck, which can be mistaken for opisthotonus or meningismus. Older patients have claimed that this alleviates the pain somewhat. This hypertonia may be mistaken for tonic convulsions, but in fact the patients are conscious. True convulsions also may be observed, often in association with severe hyponatremia.

About one third of crises in our series were associated with weakness or paralysis, and in 8 of 104 crises, mechanical ventilation was necessary because of respiratory weakness, in one case for more than 3 months. Electrophysiologically, we found evidence of axonal degeneration, with nerve conduction studies showing normal velocity but decreased wave amplitude and an increased threshold of stimulation, progressing to absence of peripheral nerve function. Recuperation from paralytic crises is possible, although patients with repeated severe crises may have chronic weakness. Patients in whom oral anesthesia develops as part of a crisis may seriously lacerate their tongue, develop severe bruxism, and dislodge teeth. Hypertension and sustained tachycardia are common during the initial phase of crises, as are electrolytic imbalances, especially in children with tubulopathy. Vomiting and ileus occur frequently and may complicate nutritional management. It is important to note that the mental development of children with tyrosinemia is normal and that during crises, their level of consciousness is not diminished. The active phase of crises usually lasts for 1–7 days.

Of note, the neurologic crises of tyrosinemia are not usually associated with deterioration of standard liver tests. Plasma transaminases, prothrombin times, and bilirubin are unchanged from periods between crises. There was no readily apparent difference between succinylacetone levels during crises when compared with values observed between crises. Urinary levels of δ-aminolevulinic acid tend to be higher during

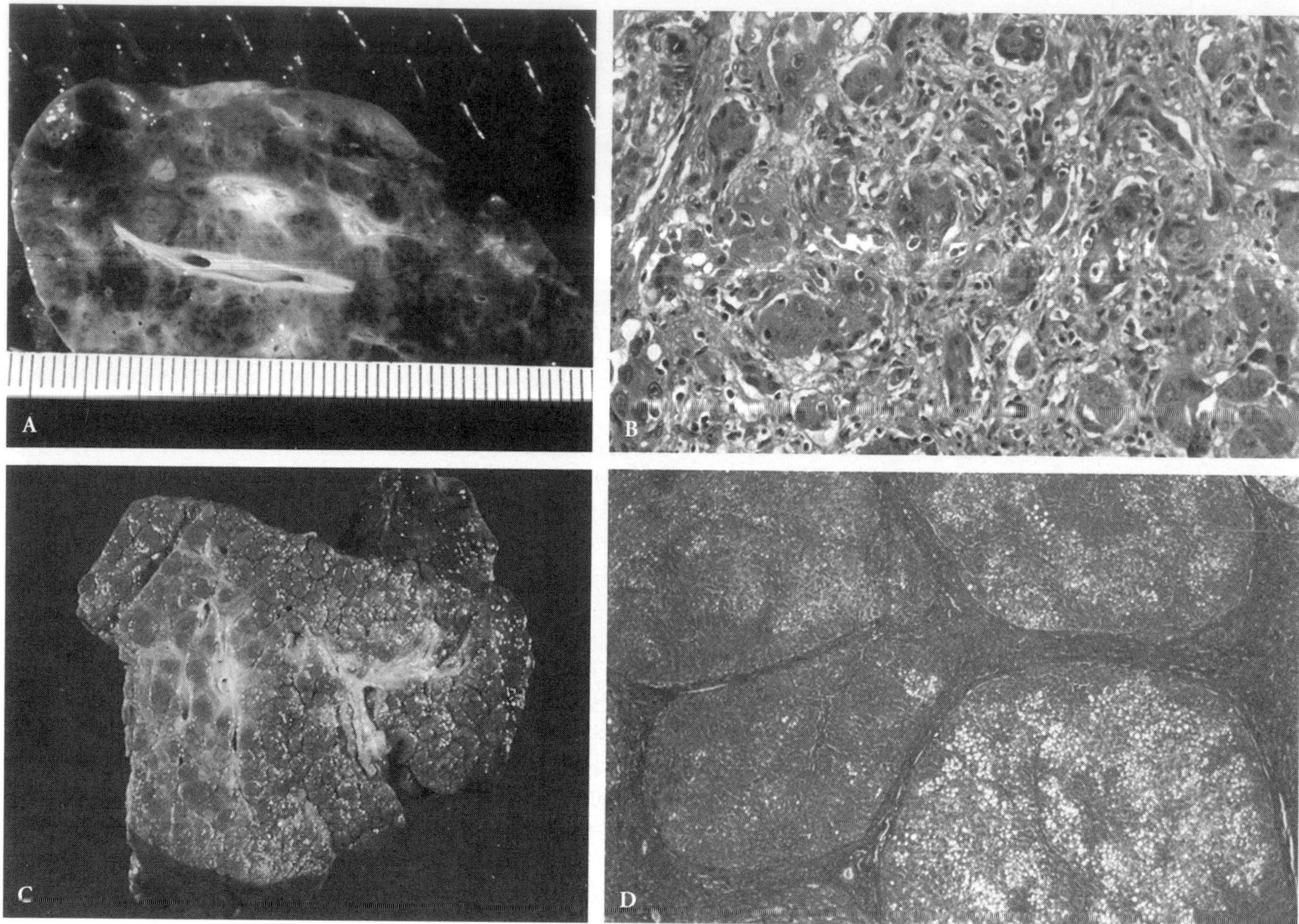

Figure 29.2. Liver pathology in tyrosinemia. Acute and chronic courses. (**A**) Microscopic appearance of liver from a 3-month-old girl with the acute form of tyrosinemia. The liver was firm, shrunken, and vaguely nodular. (**B**) Histologic examination of the liver revealed massive parenchymal collapse and fibrosis. There is cholangiolar proliferation, and surviving hepatocytes are frequently arranged in a pseudoglandular pattern. There is intracellular cholestasis and hemosiderin deposition as well as a mild, nonspecific chronic inflammatory infiltrate. (Hematoxylin-phloxine-saffron [HPS] stain, original magnification 125×.) (**C**) Enlarged, cirrhotic liver from a 2-year-old boy with a chronic form of the disease reveals a coarsely nodular external and cut surface. (**D**) Low-power histologic examination reveals a mixed macro- and micronodular cirrhosis. The nodules appear histologically heterogenous because of a variable degree of fat content in the hepatocytes. (HPS stain, original magnification 30×.) For color reproduction, see Color Plate 29.2.

crises than between crises, but in our retrospective series this had little diagnostic or predictive value for a given episode. Results of routine cerebrospinal fluid analyses are normal during neurologic crises [28,31]. In some cases, catecholamine excretion is increased [29].

Neurologic crises are a major cause of distress in non–NTBC-treated patients with tyrosinemia. There is an appreciable risk of death, particularly in paralytic crises. In our series of 20 children who had experienced at least one crisis, 11 of 14 deaths occurred during crises, and all 11 were associated with the complications of respiratory insufficiency [28]. All tyrosinemic children who are ill and who are not receiving NTBC therapy should be observed closely for the signs of neurologic decompensation, particularly respiratory insufficiency, because it may develop rapidly, thus children with signs suggestive of an impending neurologic crisis should be hospitalized.

Coma is *not* a feature of isolated neurologic crises. The development of coma in a tyrosinemic patient should not be attributed to a neurologic crisis without first ruling out other causes requiring treatment, including liver failure with encephalopathy and a false diagnosis of coma in a patient with paralysis.

The dramatic nature of painful neurologic crises is described in the following paragraph written by the mother of one of our patients, reproduced here from the first edition [62a].

> For 2 or 3 days before the crisis, P would sleep fitfully with increasing crankiness. No position seemed comfortable, and he became more unsteady on his feet. His face was drawn and pale. His appetite was poor, and he was always nauseous. His belly became bloated. He lost interest in playing and was very sensitive to the slightest touch. This was followed by periods of intense pain

for about 3 days, which decreased in frequency over the next few days. When he felt the pain coming, he would place his forearms under his chin, and would tense up and tremble. He would screw up his face and wring his hands to the point of causing bruises. He would arch his back until his head touched his heels, tear out his hair, pull out his teeth, and bite his cheeks and lips despite all the bandages we had placed to prevent him from hurting himself. He would shriek a lot but was drowsy most of the time. He would throw up a lot, and he usually had some fever. He would lose about 2–3 pounds with every crisis. It would take 2–3 weeks for him to get back to his usual state. When I asked him what the pain felt like, he would say there were two types: one was like he had large needles in his muscles and bones everywhere and the other as if he were being squeezed in a vice.

Renal Disease in Tyrosinemia

Renal involvement is almost always present in children with tyrosinemia, and it is as varied as that of the liver. Symptoms range from no evidence of renal disease to overt renal failure. Even those with no evidence of renal disease, including an intact glomerular filtration rate (GFR), may show some degree of fibrosis on biopsy (see Pathology). Both renal tubular dysfunction and glomerular involvement may occur in tyrosinemia. The severity of dysfunction is variable to some extent with the clinical state of the patient, increasing during periods of decompensation. Generalized aminoaciduria and glycosuria are sometimes seen, but rickets is the principal clinical manifestation of renal tubular dysfunction in tyrosinemia and figured prominently in its initial clinical descriptions [2]. In some patients, it is the main medical problem [63].

Some clinical evidence of proximal tubular dysfunction was present in only 10 of 37 patients evaluated at Hôpital Sainte-Justine. However, at the time of study all these patients were on a phenylalanine and tyrosine–restricted diet and some were receiving NTBC, both of which can partially reverse Fanconi's syndrome in tyrosinemia. Conversely, in an adult patient in whom chronic tubular and glomerular dysfunction is present, we have observed that tubular dysfunction may persist even after prolonged NTBC treatment, suggesting that permanent tubular abnormalities may occur [64–67]. Over 80% of the children evaluated at Hôpital Sainte-Justine have some degree of nephromegaly on ultrasonography, and 33% have evidence of mild to moderate nephrocalcinosis (Table 29.2).

Chronic renal failure may occur in adolescents and young adults [8,68]. In the Hôpital Sainte-Justine series, GFRs, as assessed by diethylenetriamine pentaacetic acid (DTPA) clearance, were generally decreased but over a wide range of severity (Table 29.2).

Other Clinical Manifestations

Some infants have episodes of hypoglycemia [69] that in our experience may be refractory to treatment. In rare patients, hypoglycemic episodes occur even during chronic NTBC treatment or after hepatic transplantation (personal observations). Although hypertrophy of the islets of Langerhans is frequent in tyrosinemia (see Pathology) and hyperinsulinism has occasionally been documented [69a], in other cases it is clearly ruled out. Therefore, hypoglycemia in a tyrosinemic patient requires a complete evaluation as for nontyrosinemic patients. One tyrosinemic child has been reported to have insulin-dependent diabetes mellitus, although the relationship of this condition to tyrosinemia is uncertain, and the pancreatic histology in this case was normal [70].

Clinically significant hypertrophic cardiomyopathy has been reported in tyrosinemia [71–72a] and has even been reported to be frequent [72b] and to respond to NTBC treatment [72a]. We have not observed this despite systematic focused evaluations, but physicians should be alert to this possibility.

IMAGING IN TYROSINEMIA

Liver

This section describes our experience before the availability of NTBC and during the first 5 years of the Quebec NTBC protocol. It is important to note that not all nodules are detectable by imaging. In cirrhotic livers examined after transplantation or at autopsy, only a minority of the nodules were detected in previous ultrasonograms or scans.
In our series of 30 patients evaluated before NTBC treatment [73], ultrasonography was more sensitive than CT in the evaluation of liver changes in tyrosinemia. However, the sensitivity is highly dependent on the experience of the ultrasonographer, and ultrasonographic examination is more difficult to standardize than are CT scans. The earliest ultrasonographic change, which may be subtle, is an inhomogeneity of the liver parenchyma without the presence of distinct nodules. Inhomogeneity is often the first sign of micronodular cirrhosis but also may be a transient finding. We speculate that transient ultrasonographic inhomogeneity may be the result of the presence of multiple small foci of fatty change, which we have observed in some biopsy samples. Subsequently, in the development of cirrhosis, hypoechogenic micronodules (<5 mm) appear and then macronodules (≥5 mm), which may be either hyper- or hypoechogenic. In our pre-NTBC series [73], the echodensity of nodules was not predictive of the presence of dysplasia or malignancy. If portal hypertension is suspected, Doppler ultrasonography should be performed.

Computed tomography scans reveal most macronodules. Of technical note, some nodules are obscured by contrast studies whereas the detection of others is enhanced. We routinely perform both examinations. Our experience with magnetic resonance imaging (MRI) is limited, but this technique merits further study in tyrosinemia, especially in children old enough to remain motionless to undergo the examination without sedation.

Table 29.2: Evaluation of Renal Disease in 37 Patients with Tyrosinemia

Patient	*Age, yr*	*Nephromegaly*	*Nephrocalcinosis*	*GFR Pretransplantation, mL/min/1.73/m²**
1	0.7	+	+	40
2	8	+	−	69
3	9	+	−	137
4	3.5	+	+	142
5	1.5	+	−	105
6	9.7	+	−	47
7	1.5	+	−	61
8	18	+	+	34
9	8	+	+	36
10	12	+	−	83
11	2.0	+	−	108
12	18	+	+	27
13	6	+	−	52
14	2.0	−	−	173
15	2.5	−	−	73
16	2.8	+	−	ND
17	3.5	+	−	ND
18	1.9	−	−	ND
19	8	+	+	ND
20	1.8	+	−	ND
21	9	+	+	117
22	0.3	+	−	82
23	4	+	+	93
24	6	+	+	65
25	2.0	+	−	86
26	0.7	+	−	182
27	0.9	+	+	155
28	2.0	−	−	147
29	2.0	+	+	125
30	0.5	−	−	141
31	2.0	+	−	107
32	9	−	−	124
33	2.0	+	+	90
34	2.5	−	−	116
35	4	+	−	128
36	1.0	−	+	120
37	3.0	−	−	128

*DTPA method
GFR, glomerular filtration rate; ND, not determined; −, absent; +, present.

Our experience with MRI of tyrosinemic nodules is limited because our patients now rarely develop cirrhotic changes. MRI can provide useful information about regenerative, dysplastic, or hepatocarcinomatous nodules. Sensitivity of detection is increased when a paramagnetic contrast agent such as mangafodipir is used. This liver-specific contrast agent is taken up by hepatocytes and excreted into bile. Nodules of functioning hepatocytes, such as in regenerative nodules, show homogeneous enhancement, whereas some hepatocellular carcinomas show reduced enhancement with this agent. This technique has been applied to one reported tyrosinemic patient who had multiple hepatic nodules and in whom the hepatic nodularity regressed and AFP levels fell when adequate NTBC treatment was instituted [73a]. The nodules enhanced normally and were felt to be benign. It should be emphasized, however, that there is not sufficient data to precisely estimate the positive predictive value of this method. Our attitude toward hepatic nodules in tyrosinemia is discussed later (see Chronic Liver Disease, under Pathology).

Kidney

In our pre-NTBC series [73], ultrasonography revealed nephromegaly in about half the patients, cortical hyperechogenicity in one third, and nephrocalcinosis in one fourth. Abdominal CT also can detect the nephromegaly. Nephrocalcinosis is best detected in scans performed without contrast. In some contrast studies, a delayed nephrogram is apparent, possibly reflecting diminished function.

Pancreas

Most patients have normal pancreatic imaging studies. Rarely, hyperechogenicity has been reported.

PATHOLOGY

Liver

Fulminant Liver Disease

In fulminant liver disease, morphologic alterations are variable, although the liver is generally slightly to moderately enlarged, frequently pale, and often nodular; in other cases, the liver may be shrunken and firm, with a brownish discoloration [74]. Histologic examination usually reveals micronodular cirrhosis and, often, marked bile duct proliferation within portal tracts and fibrotic septa (Figure 29.2). The hepatocytes are characterized by varying degrees of steatosis, and their usual regular trabecular arrangement is replaced by pseudoacinar or pseudoglandular formations around a central canaliculus often containing prominent bile plugs [74–76]. A significant accumulation of iron pigment may be seen within Kupffer cells and hepatocytes. Giant cell transformation is also occasionally observed [18]. These changes reflect the nonspecific nature of the early insult, are shared by a wide variety of infantile hepatopathies [77], and may include a neonatal hepatitis-like picture [78]. In the infant, neonatal hepatitis is a nonspecific response of the liver to a wide variety of metabolic and infectious insults and is not characteristic of any single entity.

Chronic Liver Disease

The liver is characteristically coarsely nodular and frequently enlarged as a result of usually well-established mixed micro- and macronodular cirrhosis [77]. There is steatosis, varying in extent between the various nodules or even within a single nodule. Fibrous septa vary in width and frequently contain a mild lymphoplasmacytic infiltrate. Ductular proliferation usually is minimal. Intralobular cholestasis or inflammation is usually insignificant, which correlates with the usually normal bilirubin levels of these children. Most ominous in the older child is the development of hepatic carcinoma. Sometimes, but not always, this is apparent by gross examination. In one of our cases, a single large hemorrhagic nodule was noted in the autopsy specimen. In a second case, a hepatectomy specimen was obtained at transplantation, and a large grayish white nodule of hepatoma could be easily distinguished from the surrounding nodules in the cirrhotic liver (Figure 29.3). However, numerous sections through the rest of the liver revealed multiple microscopic foci of hepatocellular carcinoma as well as multiple areas of nuclear atypia and hyperchromatism qualifying as hepatocellular dysplasia [79].

Liver cell dysplasia, either of the large cell or small cell type, has been reported in hereditary tyrosinemia in the absence of as well as in association with hepatocellular carcinoma [77]. Liver cell dysplasia, especially the small cell type, is widely accepted as a premalignant condition [79] and underlines the need for early transplantation in these patients. The occurrence of dysplasia and the high incidence of hepatocellular carcinoma in hereditary tyrosinemia, far greater than the incidence of hepatocellular carcinoma in adults with cirrhosis resulting from hepatitis, are highly suggestive of a powerful underlying carcinogenic influence, presumably related to abnormal metabolites [12,80]. Ultrastructurally, morphologic changes in the liver are quite nonspecific and characterized by the presence of fat droplets in the hepatocytes, usually without displacement of the nucleus. Mild dilatation of the endoplasmic reticulum as well as nonspecific minor changes in the mitochondria also have been noted [81,82]. In dysplastic liver cells, irregular nuclear profiles with large nucleoli and reduction of cytoplasmic organelles are characteristic ultrastructural features [79].

Kidneys

Renal tubular dysfunction, characterized by Fanconi's syndrome and hypophosphatemic rickets, may be a major clinical manifestation of tyrosinemia [6]. Renal failure, when present, has been reported in patients with longstanding disease. Although nonspecific, the characteristic morphologic change noted, especially in young patients with the fulminant form of the disease, has been nephromegaly, characterized by an increase in kidney weight with microscopically irregular dilatations of the proximal tubules and vacuolization of

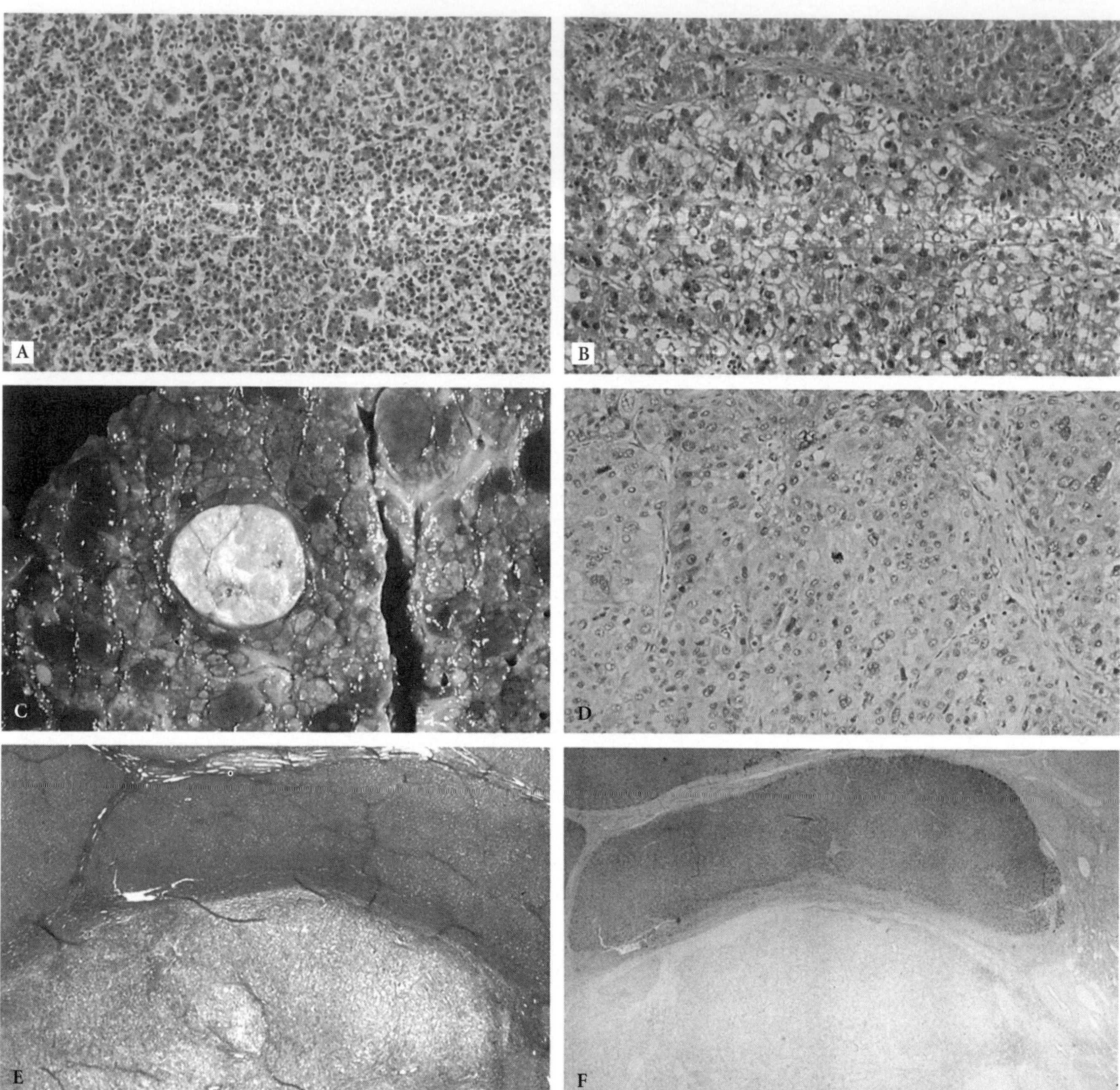

Figure 29.3. Dysplasia, carcinoma, and regenerative nodules. (**A**) Histologic examination of native liver from a 1-year-old patient undergoing a liver transplantation revealed multiple foci of dysplasia. This microphotograph shows the small cell variant, composed of fetal hepatocyte-like cells with increased nucleocytoplasmic ratio and hyperchromatic nuclei. (HPS stain, original magnification 200×.) (**B**) In the liver from the same patient, foci of large cell dysplasia are shown, characterized by irregular hyperchromatic nuclei and an increased nucleocytoplasmic ratio. Distinction from a microscopic hepatocellular carcinoma may be very difficult. (HPS stain, original magnification 200×.) (**C**) Native liver from a 4-year-old hepatic transplantation patient showing cirrhosis and one nodule that clearly stood out from the rest of the parenchyma. (**D**) Histologic examination of the nodule in the previous panel revealing hepatocellular carcinoma with extensive nuclear irregularity and many mitoses. (HPS stain, original magnification 200×.) (**E**) Native liver from an 11-year-old liver transplant recipient with extensive macronodular cirrhosis; one large focus of hepatocellular carcinoma was noted (pale staining nodule, lower portion of figure). (HPS stain, original magnification 20×.) (**F**) Immunostaining with an antibody to FAH revealed a positive reaction in many of the regenerating nodules, indicating reacquisition of the missing enzyme by the regenerating hepatocytes, suggesting reversion of the mutation. Note that the carcinomatous nodule remains negative, indicating absence of reversion. (Avidin-biotin-peroxidase technique with hematoxylin counterstaining, original magnification 20×.) For color reproduction, see Color Plate 29.3.

tubular epithelial cells [6,74]. Glycogen accumulation in collecting tubules has been reported [68]. Nephrocalcinosis, sometimes extensive and visualized by clinical imaging, is present in most samples. Ultrastructural examination reveals simplification of the epithelial cells with loss of the brush border and cytoplasmic vacuolization, especially in the periapical area. Although nonspecific, these changes are strongly reminiscent of those encountered in experimental Fanconi's syndrome induced by maleic acid [18,19].

An unusual finding was the report of hyperplasia of the juxtaglomerular apparatus in one infant [83]. This case appears to be unique: this finding has not been reported since and was absent from our series of kidney biopsies despite a careful search. The inference that this represents a secondary change is strengthened by the profound electrolytic disturbances in that case, which, as the author discussed, may have induced a change in the juxtaglomerular apparatus. Although liver transplantation may correct the metabolic derangement in many cases [7–9], some biochemical anomalies of renal tubular function may persist [84,85].

Nine of 24 cases of tyrosinemia in which renal tissue was examined at the Hôpital Sainte-Justine were characterized by a mild to moderate degree of glomerulosclerosis and interstitial fibrosis, mild glomerulosclerosis being defined as the occurrence of sclerosis in at least 10% of glomeruli accompanied by interstitial changes [18]. Significant glomerular changes have been reported infrequently in hereditary tyrosinemia [58,63]. In two cases discussed by Kvittingen et al. [63], renal failure accompanied the glomerular changes, the latter attributed to the metabolic disease rather than a consequence of pyelonephritis or an unrelated glomerulopathy. Eight of the nine patients in our series were older than 2 years, and in four of the patients, the findings were noted in renal biopsies obtained either shortly before or at the time of liver transplantation. Immunofluorescence studies usually did not reveal any significant immune deposits in the glomeruli, although the occasional presence of immunoglobulin A, a nonspecific finding related to chronic liver disease [86], was noted. No renal malignancies were observed in our series nor have any been reported to our knowledge.

Pancreas

Hyperplasia and hypertrophy of the islets of Langerhans have been reported in a large number of cases [6,76,87] and have rarely been associated with chronic hypoglycemia [83], although most patients have normal blood glucose levels. However, the variability and inconsistency of these changes are likely related both to difficulties in the accurate assessment of the relative volume of pancreatic islet cells, especially in the infant, in whom there is a relatively high proportion of islet tissue, and to probable differences in the amount of islet tissue present in different areas of the pancreas [88]. Hyalinization of the islets also has been reported in some patients [89], but whether this change may result in diabetes is purely conjectural; Lindberg et al. [70] reported a case of diabetes in association with tyrosinemia in which the islets were seen to be normal.

Heart

Myocardial hypertrophy has been associated with ultrastructural changes characterized principally by increased numbers of mitochondria in the myocytes [72]. Furthermore, this group of workers reported a significant incidence of cardiomyopathy in their tyrosinemic patients as detected by echocardiography but a low incidence of clinical heart disease. On the other hand, Edwards et al. [71] described an obstructive cardiomyopathy in two symptomatic cases. We have not observed these changes in any of our cases.

Peripheral Nerve

Three peripheral nerve specimens have been analyzed during the period of recuperation, 2–6 weeks following paralytic crises [28]. All three samples revealed axonal degeneration and secondary demyelination, similar to the changes seen in acute intermittent porphyria.

MANAGEMENT

Diet Therapy in Non–NTBC-Treated Patients

The effect of dietary restriction of phenylalanine and tyrosine on the long-term outcome of tyrosinemia has never been formally documented. Because of the highly variable clinical course and the lack of a reliable biochemical marker of optimal metabolic control, a large clinical trial would be needed to address this question; the question will remain unanswered because patients are now routinely treated with NTBC. Readers are referred to the first edition of this chapter [62a] and to other sources [90] for discussion of dietary therapy in non–NTBC-treated patients. It is logical to restrict precursor amino acids in tyrosinemic patients. Furthermore, available evidence suggests that dietary therapy improves renal tubular function in some cases and probably slows but certainly does not prevent the progression of liver disease. Cirrhosis and hepatocellular carcinoma may develop in tyrosinemic patients complying with a strict diet.

Apart from dietary intake of tyrosine and phenylalanine, the other principal variable in the control of tyrosine degradation is the metabolic state. Under catabolic stresses such as infections, fasting, surgery, or burns, muscle and other organs can liberate large amounts of amino acids. This release of endogenous phenylalanine and tyrosine can overwhelm the body's metabolic capacity. A major goal of the therapy of tyrosinemia before NTBC treatment was thus to avoid tissue catabolism by providing sufficient calories for tissue repair during catabolic states and treating the underlying acute condition.

When the diagnosis of tyrosinemia is first made in the newborn, tyrosine levels are elevated and decline gradually over days to weeks with dietary therapy [6]. Provision of high-carbohydrate, energy-rich feeds can stimulate anabolism, initially by using energy-rich nonprotein formulas. We eliminate all tyrosine and phenylalanine from the diet for 24–48 hours while providing adequate amounts of other amino acids, vitamins, and minerals by the use of special formulas. After this period, and depending on the state of the child, tyrosine and phenylalanine are gradually reintroduced in the form of humanized milk formulas or breast milk. The speed of reintroduction depends on the clinical state of the child and the levels of plasma tyrosine.

Methionine levels usually normalize with other liver functions in the days and weeks following diagnosis and therapy [6]. We do not specifically restrict methionine intake, but if prolonged hypermethioninemia is observed, dietary methionine restriction has been used by some investigators [91]. Of note, hypermethioninemia is apparently not toxic in itself, being well tolerated in other hereditary states, such as methionine adenosyltransferase deficiency [92].

After the acute phase, the intake of phenylalanine and tyrosine is titrated according to the child's growth and, to some extent, to the plasma tyrosine level. As a starting approximation, a minimum of about 90 mg/kg/d of phenylalanine plus tyrosine is sufficient for normal growth in infants, and 700–900 mg/d is sufficient for older children. Slightly more than half this amount is provided as phenylalanine. Treatment must be individualized according to the evaluation of the child's metabolic state and individual requirements for tyrosine and phenylalanine by maintaining plasma tyrosine within the normal range and ensuring adequate growth. However, in non–NTBC-treated patients, blood tyrosine and succinylacetone are imprecise indicators of the status of intracellular tyrosine metabolism in the patient's liver, and decisions about diet are based in large part on clinical evaluation of the patient.

Acute Liver Crises

In our experience, acute liver crises do not occur in NTBC-treated patients. Urgent administration of NTBC in addition to the following measures is the treatment of choice. Infections and other precipitants of liver crises should be treated aggressively. Observation in hospital; provision of sufficient energy intake, often with gavages or parenteral nutrition; and medical treatment for the accompanying complications, such as ascites, are important. A reduction or cessation of phenylalanine and tyrosine intake for 24–48 hours is usually indicated. Oral or nasogastric feeding is preferred over intravenous administration because it permits greater energy intake. In acutely ill tyrosinemic children, supplemental intravenous glucose is useful in our experience to prevent catabolism and to reduce the risk of a neurologic crisis. Most acute crises resolve within days to weeks, but fulminant liver failure may develop in non–nitisinone-treated patients, necessitating urgent liver transplantation. After the first 2 years of life, episodes of liver decompensation become less frequent. The physician should remain vigilant to this possibility at all ages.

Chronic Liver Disease and Liver Transplantation

Liver transplantation cures tyrosinemic liver disease (Table 29.1). The optimal timing for liver transplantation in the patient with chronic stable liver disease requires individual decision making. Some children with nodules found at transplantation to be hepatocarcinoma have died with recurrence of carcinoma after transplantation [9,93]. On the other hand, some children are nodule-free with normal growth. Even before NTBC therapy, we often delayed transplantation for such patients by several years. In practice, we follow patients without liver nodules who have stable renal and liver function, clinically and with serial imaging.

Some groups have advocated early liver transplantation for all patients with tyrosinemia as being both curative of the disease and preventive of the complications from neurologic crisis and liver failure [93,94]. Although small infants survive transplantation more frequently than they did previously and the reduced liver technique has allowed for greater availability of livers, children with a stable course probably would benefit from waiting until they reach at least 10 kg. This is especially true because NTBC treatment has eliminated or greatly reduced the risk of acute decompensation. Before NTBC was available, we considered a single neurologic crisis as an indication for transplantation, given the high incidence of relapse and mortality. Hepatic crises were a relative indication. We no longer accept them as indications for transplantation in NTBC-treated patients.

Patients with evidence of micronodular cirrhosis are followed closely by imaging for the development of distinct nodules. The presence of a nodule is an indication for transplantation. In some cases in which the nodule is accessible, biopsy may be an option. However, in our experience, nodules arise only in cirrhotic livers that on pathologic examination have many other nodules not detectable by CT or ultrasonography. Although the lack of dysplasia or carcinoma in a nodule examined via biopsy may reduce the urgency of transplantation, in our experience, it would not eliminate the need for transplantation.

We have not encountered the situation of an increasing AFP level in a patient without a detectable nodule. This would place the clinician in the uncomfortable position of deciding between transplantation on the basis of a (nonspecific) laboratory result and ongoing surveillance of a presumably localized, poorly differentiated population of hepatocytes. Causes unrelated to tyrosinemia, including a drug reaction, would have to be eliminated before accepting this biochemical anomaly as an indication for transplantation. More sensitive and specific tests for hepatocellular carcinomas are required for optimum medical surveillance.

Neurologic Crises

During the acute phase, we provide analgesia for the severe pain, using narcotic analgesics if necessary. A high level of carbohydrate is administered because glucose inhibits the enzyme δ-aminolevulinate synthase, reducing the production of δ-aminolevulinic acid (see Pathophysiology). Hypertension, hyponatremia, hypokalemia, and hypophosphatemia are treated symptomatically if present. Extreme hyponatremia has caused convulsions in several cases. Dental consultation and use of a protective oral prosthesis are necessary in cases with bruxism, tongue biting, and oral anesthesia. NTBC produces a striking decrease in the excretion of δ-aminolevulinic acid within 12 hours (Grant A. Mitchell, unpublished observations), suggesting that the risk of crisis is reduced almost immediately. Crises are not expected to intensify after this point, although recovery in patients with paralysis before treatment will reflect the time course of axonal regeneration. Ventilatory support and physiotherapy for muscle retraining may be necessary for several weeks during convalescence. It is important that the patient, family, and hospital personnel be aware that recuperation is possible and that an optimistic attitude be adopted during this period. In patients with tyrosinemia, we avoid the use of medications that can aggravate porphyria, such as barbiturates (see Pathophysiology), before and for at least 1 week following NTBC treatment.

Hematin, which inhibits δ-aminolevulinic acid synthetase, is an interesting therapeutic option in neurologic crises, although experience with its use is limited. Ideally, administration should begin early in the crisis. In one child receiving 3 mg/kg of hematin intravenously late in a paralytic crisis, serum δ-aminolevulinic acid decreased dramatically after administration and there was felt to be a relationship between hematin administration and motor improvement [31]. However, the course of this episode was prolonged because the child remained intubated for 2 months. In another child to whom hematin was administered during a painful crisis, the clinical course was similar to that of previous crises of the patient (J. Larochelle, personal communication). In view of the known association of coagulopathy with hematin administration, it would be especially important to monitor this parameter in tyrosinemic patients treated with hematin.

Following transplantation, none of our patients have had recurrence of neurologic symptoms [7,28]. No crises have occurred in NTBC-treated patients.

Renal Involvement

Renal tubular dysfunction in tyrosinemia usually responds to some extent to dietary therapy [64–67,95]. Rickets is the main clinical sign of tubular dysfunction in tyrosinemia. At least three mechanisms may be implicated in its pathogenesis: urinary phosphate loss, impaired hepatic hydroxylation of vitamin D, and impaired renal hydroxylation of vitamin D. Rachitic patients with tyrosinemia should be evaluated individually and treatment tailored according to the patient's needs. The need for treatment should be reassessed after several weeks of NTBC treatment. The relationship of treatment of rickets to other complications, such as nephrocalcinosis, is unclear.

Lindblad [96] has suggested that the damage in both liver and kidney is the result of decreased sulfhydryl compounds in these tissues and has advocated the use of *N*-acetylcysteine to bring about repletion of tissue glutathione content. Results of reported acute trials with oral or intravenous *N*-acetylcysteine, however, were not encouraging [15], and we have seen neurologic crises and liver progression in patients receiving this therapy orally. Whether the long-term use of *N*-acetylcysteine is of some benefit in tyrosinemia remains unproved.

Careful attention to the degree of renal involvement is required at the time of transplant evaluation (Table 29.2). This includes evaluation of tubular and glomerular functions, including phosphate reabsorption, aminoaciduria, glycosuria, and GFR by creatinine or radioisotope clearance. It would be prudent to assess the extent to which the dysfunction is reversible with NTBC treatment.

Kidney transplantation alone was performed in an adult patient with tyrosinemia and renal failure who had little clinical evidence of liver involvement, although micronodular cirrhosis was present at the time of transplantation [63]. The patient subsequently required dialysis because of chronic rejection, but liver function apparently remained normal until death 3 years after transplantation. It seems unlikely that kidney transplantation alone would significantly alter the risk of hepatocarcinoma.

Results with combined transplantation have been promising in tyrosinemia and in other hereditary diseases. Despite the fact that no cross-match (aside from ABO blood group compatibility) has been performed in our combined transplantations for tyrosinemia or other liver–kidney diseases (oxalosis type 1 and Alagille syndrome), the kidneys have not shown evidence of rejection. In fact, in combined transplantations, the liver may have fewer episodes of rejection, both in our experience and in that of others (D. Freese, personal communication).

The choice between liver alone or combined liver–kidney transplantation can be a dilemma in a patient with moderate nonreversible renal disease. Currently used immunosuppressive agents such as cyclosporine and tacrolimus are nephrotoxic and could further reduce the function of an already compromised kidney. Cyclosporine causes a significant decrease in GFR in children who undergo liver transplantation, regardless of the underlying liver disease [97]. This effect must be considered when evaluating a child with tyrosinemia for transplantation.

At our institution, 29 tyrosinemic children have undergone transplantation with livers alone, with follow-up of more than 15 years for most. In Quebec [97], decline in GFR has been of the same order in tyrosinemic patients as in children receiving transplants for other liver diseases [97a]. Some other tyrosinemic children with affected glomerular function before liver transplantation alone have improved their GFR after transplantation [98,99], but most have decreased their GFR despite low cyclosporine levels (100–120 ng/mL). Observations that the rate of decrease is similar in tyrosinemic patients and in children undergoing transplantation for other diseases suggest that liver transplantation may slow or stop the kidney disease of tyrosinemia. This is anecdotal, however, and more data are needed. Perhaps the use of three daily doses of cyclosporine may have reduced the incidence of nephrotoxicity. Alternatively, it cannot be excluded that the long-term concomitant use of calcium channel blockers [100] may have played a beneficial role. Following hepatic transplantation, there is a marked reduction but not a complete normalization of succinylacetone excretion [100a], the source of the succinylacetone presumably being the kidney itself or other extrahepatic tissues and the significance of which is unknown.

In practice, until less nephrotoxic immunosuppressive agents become available, we consider combined liver–kidney transplantation when the pretransplantation GFR is low enough (<40 mL/min/1.73 m^2) for the predicted decrease in the posttransplantation GFR to affect growth. Longer follow-up of renal function in tyrosinemic patients who have undergone hepatic transplantation may allow us to further refine our approach to the renal disease of tyrosinemia.

Gene Therapy or Hepatocyte Transplantation in Tyrosinemia

Although gene therapy and hepatocyte transplantation currently are not treatment options, they have received considerable publicity and are producing interesting results in tyrosinemic and other mice (e.g., see references [101–101c]). These approaches are intuitively appealing, and parents often spontaneously ask about them, sometimes even assuming that they are available and efficient. Gene replacement therapy is theoretically more difficult in tyrosinemia than in certain other inborn errors because the toxic intermediates in tyrosinemia are felt to be capable of inducing hepatocarcinoma and possibly kidney disease, even in the presence of normal circulating tyrosine levels. Therefore, for treatment of tyrosinemia, it would not suffice to simply produce a sufficient number of cells to normalize plasma tyrosine: all hepatocytes would have to express normal FAH to avoid the risk of progression to cancer. Biologically, cells with a functional *FAH* gene would have a selective advantage and might overgrow FAH-deficient cells, especially in mice [101–101c]. At a clinical level, it is not clear how nodules that would arise from this process could be reliably distinguished from neoplastic nodules. If major improvements occur in gene transfer technology, in vivo cell selection, and detection of hepatocellular carcinoma, they could have an important impact on the feasibility of gene therapy or hepatocyte transplantation in tyrosinemia.

NTBC (Nitisinone) Treatment for Tyrosinemia

Therapeutic trials in tyrosinemia are unusually difficult to evaluate because tyrosinemia is clinically heterogeneous and treatment is often started at different ages in patients with different degrees of clinical severity. Also, to obtain a sufficient number of patients, multicenter trials are necessary, with possible difficulties of standardization because of differences among institutions in evaluation and treatment. In Quebec, all patients are followed in a similar fashion by a small number of physicians, and nearly all are identified by neonatal screening as asymptomatic neonates. In the Quebec NTBC Study, 64 patients have been enrolled. As classified by principal clinical problem at the time of enrollment, 4 were acute hepatic, 4 acute neurologic, 5 chronic hepatic, 1 chronic neurologic, 2 chronic renal, and 48 asymptomatic, of whom 37 were under 1 month of age at the start of NTBC treatment.

Treatment Protocols

Our current protocol is discussed here, although ongoing evaluation leads to periodic changes. The protocol involves the collection of pretreatment baseline specimens of blood and urine, close observation for immediate adverse effects immediately after NTBC administration (none has been detected to date), and metabolic monitoring for 1 week in hospital and with decreasing frequency until 6 months, at which time metabolic testing is performed at 3-month intervals (with closer surveillance if clinically indicated). Metabolites (plasma tyrosine, phenylalanine, methionine, urinary δ-aminolevulinic acid dehydratase, and plasma and urine succinylacetone, every 3 months), markers of liver function (plasma levels of AFP, transaminases, and γ-glutamyltransferase, every 3 months), and coagulation tests (every 6 months) are followed. Seventy-two–hour dietary records are used to calculate phenylalanine plus tyrosine intake every 3 months. Imaging currently includes abdominal ultrasonograms every 6 months and abdominal CT once a year until age 8, annual abdominal MRI thereafter, and isotopic GFR every 3 years. Baseline ophthalmologic assessment (see Complications) is done before or soon after beginning treatment.

In the Quebec NTBC protocol, the goal for plasma tyrosine level is 250–400 μmol/L maintained by dietary phenylalanine and tyrosine restriction, which requires specialized dietary supervision and supplementation with special formulas providing the remaining nutrients for growth. Of note, whereas plasma tyrosine is a nonspecific and imprecise reflection of metabolic control in non–NTBC-treated patients, it is much more precise in those receiving NTBC because the pharmacologic block in metabolism is close to tyrosine (Figure 29.1). Plasma tyrosine therefore is a more accurate reflection of tolerance in NTBC-treated patients. NTBC is started at a dosage of 1 mg/kg/d in two divided doses and adjusted to maintain (a) an absence of detectable urinary and blood succinylacetone and (b) plasma NTBC levels greater than 50 μmol/L.

Results

In the Quebec protocol, no acute liver or neurologic crises have been seen following NTBC treatment. In follow-up of initially asymptomatic individuals for up to 9 years, none has developed detectable hepatic nodules. In contrast, four patients were unfortunately missed by neonatal screening during the transition from tyrosine to succinylacetone as a biologic marker. The unscreened patients presented at 2–8 months of age, two with hepatic failure, one with hepatomegaly, and one with hypoglycemia. Following an initial period during which hepatic imaging studies normalized, three developed cirrhosis with detectable nodules on imaging studies and underwent transplantation. It is impossible to conclude whether the development of nodules in these patients represents only the expected repair and regeneration in response to severe pretreatment liver damage or whether there was also a component of true progression of the disease during NTBC treatment. Ongoing studies with early-treated cohorts in Quebec and elsewhere will be helpful in resolving this question.

Complications

To date, in our series, the only complication attributable to NTBC has been ocular. One NTBC-treated patient developed corneal crystals, presumably representing tyrosine precipitation, which disappeared within 24 hours of initiating a strict low–phenylalanine and tyrosine diet. Similar lesions have occurred in other NTBC-treated patients [21d] and occur in rats following tyrosine loading or NTBC treatment [102]. Photophobia and ocular inflammation in an NTBC-treated patient are considered to be indications for emergency ophthalmologic examination to eliminate the presence of corneal crystals.

Regarding potential complications, the risk of hepatocellular carcinoma in early-treated patients is a major unknown factor. Hepatocarcinoma may develop in FAH-deficient mice despite NTBC treatment [24]. However, it would be inappropriate to extrapolate directly to humans, in whom (a) tyrosinemia is less severe than in mice, (b) the turnover of tyrosine and phenylalanine (milligrams/kilogram/day) is about tenfold less than in mice, (c) NTBC intake can be more reliably assured than has been the case for mice, and (d) the mechanisms of hepatocellular carcinogenesis show major differences from those in rodents [27]. However, this observation should incite physicians to perform close, well-controlled follow-ups of tyrosinemic patients treated with NTBC and to share their results in the context of multicenter trials so that nonanecdotal data can be accumulated.

It is also noteworthy that mental retardation is common in hereditary hypertyrosinemias because of deficiencies of tyrosine aminotransferase (tyrosinemia type II; Figure 29.1A) and 4HPPD, the enzyme inhibited by NTBC (tyrosinemia type III). To some extent, particularly for tyrosinemia type III, this may reflect ascertainment bias (i.e., a fortuitous discovery on amino acid chromatography performed for unrelated neurologic abnormalities). Although our cohort of NTBC-treated patients is developing and performing normally, this observation is striking enough for us to recommend continuation of the diet to maintain low levels of circulating tyrosine and ongoing surveillance of school performance and other developmental parameters.

Finally, not all complications of tyrosinemia may be reversible with NTBC therapy. In cases in which permanent damage has occurred, such as one instance in our series of an established renal tubulopathy, NTBC may not be effective although it is predicted to prevent further deterioration. We also have observed one early-treated patient who has experienced recurrent hypoglycemic episodes, in which the relation to tyrosinemia is unclear. In the Quebec series, 7 of 64 NTBC-treated patients (11%) required hepatic transplantation, all of whom had detectable liver-related symptoms of tyrosinemia when NTBC treatment was started; no screened newborns started within a month have developed detectable hepatic symptoms over a follow-up time of up to 9 years.

CONCLUSIONS

NTBC has had a major impact on the quality of life of our patients. It has eliminated the occurrence of acute liver or neurologic crises. Clinically stable patients treated chronically with NTBC are no longer hospitalized for mild infections. They are

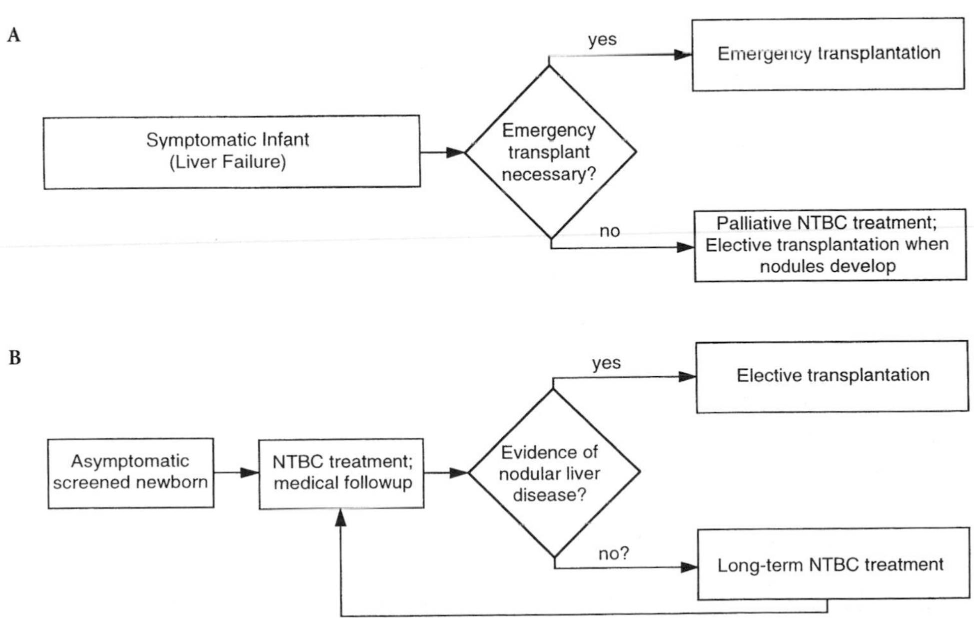

Figure 29.4. Management paradigms for hepatorenal tyrosinemia. (**A**) Without neonatal screening. (**B**) Efficient neonatal screening plus NTBC treatment. The *question mark* reflects the unknown course of tyrosinemia with long-term NTBC treatment.

vaccinated and allowed to participate fully in normal childhood activities. This contrasts starkly with the previous situation, in which families lived in daily fear of acute bouts of paralysis or liver failure. NTBC is undoubtedly the short- and mid-term treatment of choice for tyrosinemia.

It is important at this stage to guard against overconfidence. NTBC was propelled from an unlikely origin (an agricultural chemical) to the status of a therapeutic agent without passing through typical phase 2 and 3 trials. The long-term effects of NTBC administration are unknown. Vigilance, meticulous follow-up, and ongoing compilation of the world experience with NTBC treatment will be required to obtain adequate data collection.

The results may interest population geneticists and public health authorities as much as hepatologists. The efficacy of NTBC treatment has kindled debate about the optimal management paradigm for tyrosinemic patients (Figure 29.4). Should regions other than those at high risk perform neonatal screening for tyrosinemia? Most of the world's tyrosinemic patients are born outside Quebec and northern Europe, in areas where newborn screening with succinylacetone is not currently practiced. There are important technical obstacles to incorporating succinylacetone determination into expanded neonatal screening, but active research is under way to overcome these [103,104]. For the patient, there are important differences between the two alternatives of presymptomatic initiation of effective and possibly curative medical treatment and clinical detection, often when liver failure and irreversible liver damage are present.

ACKNOWLEDGMENTS

We wish to acknowledge the participation of numerous persons involved in the many facets of patient care for tyrosinemic children, including Jean Larochelle, Marie Lambert, Andrée Rasquin-Weber, Ernest Seidman, Louis Dallaire, Yolande Lefèvre, Danièlle Régimbald, Claude Roy, Sean O'Regan, C. Ronald Scott, and our other colleagues in the Quebec NTBC Study, with special thanks to Khazal Paradis. This work was supported in part by the Canadian Liver Foundation, the Garrod Association of Canada, and the U.S. Food and Drug Administration.

REFERENCES

1. Medes G. A new error of tyrosine metabolism: tyrosinosis. The intermediary metabolism of tyrosine and phenylalanine. Biochem J 1932;26:917–40.
2. Baber MD. A case of congenital cirrhosis of the liver with renal tubular defects akin to those in the Fanconi syndrome. Arch Dis Child 1956;31:335–9.
3. Sakai K, Kitagawa T. An atypical case of tyrosinosis (1-parahydroxyphenyllactic aciduria). Part 1. Clinical and laboratory findings. Jikei Med J 1957;2:1–10.
4. Sakai K, Kitagawa T. An atypical case of tyrosinosis (1-parahydroxyphenyllactic aciduria). Part 2. A research on the metabolic block. Jikei Med J 1957;2:11–15.
5. Sakai K, Kitagawa T, Yoshioka K. An atypical case of tyrosinosis (1-parahydroxyphenyllactic aciduria). Part 3. The outcome of the patient; pathological and biochemical observations of the organ tissues. Jikei Med J 1959;6:15–24.
6. Larochelle J, Privé L, Bélanger M, et al. Hereditary tyrosinemia. I. Clinical and biological study of 62 cases. Pediatrie 1973;28:5–18.
7. Paradis K, Weber A, Seidman EG, et al. Liver transplantation for hereditary tyrosinemia: the Quebec experience. Am J Hum Genet 1990;47:338–42.
8. Kvittingen EA. Hereditary tyrosinemia type I – an overview. Scand J Clin Lab Invest Suppl 1986;184:27–34.
9. Mieles LA, Esquivel CO, Van Thiel DH, et al. Liver transplantation for tyrosinemia. A review of 10 cases from the University of Pittsburgh. Dig Dis Sci 1990;35:153–7.
10. Van Thiel DH, Gartner LM, Thorp FK, et al. Resolution of the clinical features of tyrosinemia following orthotopic liver transplantation for hepatoma. J Hepatol 1986;3:42–8.
11. van Spronsen FJ, Berger R, Smit GP, et al. Tyrosinaemia type I: orthotopic liver transplantation as the only definitive answer to a metabolic as well as an oncological problem. J Inherit Metab Dis 1989;12(suppl 2):339–42.
12. Lindblad B, Lindstedt S, Steen G. On the enzymic defects in hereditary tyrosinemia. Proc Natl Acad Sci U S A 1977; 74:4641–5.
13. Kvittingen EA, Jellum E, Stokke O. Assay of fumarylacetoacetate fumarylhydrolase in human liver-deficient activity in a case of hereditary tyrosinemia. Clin Chim Acta 1981; 115:311–19.
14. Berger R, Smit GP, Stoker-de Vries SA, et al. Deficiency of fumarylacetoacetase in a patient with hereditary tyrosinemia. Clin Chim Acta 1981;114:37–44.
15. Gray RG, Patrick AD, Preston FE, et al. Acute hereditary tyrosinaemia type I: clinical, biochemical and haematological studies in twins. J Inherit Metab Dis 1981;4:37–40.
16. Phaneuf D, Labelle Y, Bérubé D, et al. Cloning and expression of the cDNA encoding human fumarylacetoacetate hydrolase, the enzyme deficient in hereditary tyrosinemia: assignment of the gene to chromosome 15. Am J Hum Genet 1991; 48:525–35.
17. Kvittingen EA, Brodtkorb E. The pre- and post-natal diagnosis of tyrosinemia type I and the detection of the carrier state by assay of fumarylacetoacetase. Scand J Clin Lab Invest Suppl 1986;184:35–40.
18. Russo P, O'Regan S. Visceral pathology of hereditary tyrosinemia type I. Am J Hum Genet 1990;47:317–24.
19. Worthen HG. Renal toxicity of maleic acid in the rat. Lab Invest 1963;12:791–801.
20. Stoner E, Starkman H, Wellner D, et al. Biochemical studies of a patient with hereditary hepatorenal tyrosinemia: evidence of glutathione deficiency. Pediatr Res 1984;18:1332–6.
21. Meister A, Larsson A. Glutathione synthetase deficiency and other disorders of the gamma-glutamyl cycle. In: Scriver CR, Beaudet AL, Sly WS, et al., eds. The metabolic basis of inherited disease. New York: McGraw-Hill, 1989:855–68.
21a. Jorquera R, Tanquay RM. The mutagenicity of the tyrosine metabolite, fumarylacetoacetate, is enhanced by glutathione depletion. Biochem Biophys Res Commun 1997;232: 42–8.

21b. Kvittingen EA, Rootwelt H, Brandtzaeg P, et al. Hereditary tyrosinemia type I: self-induced correction of the fumarylacetoacetase defect. J Clin Invest 1993;91:1816–21.
21c. Kvittingen EA, Rootwelt H, Berger R, et al. Self-induced correction of the genetic defect in tyrosinemia type I. J Clin Invest 1994;94:1657–61.
21d. Ahmad S, Teckman JH, Lueder GT. Corneal opacities associated with NTBC treatment. Am J Ophthalmol 2002;134: 266–8.
22. Niswander L, Kelsey G, Schedl A, et al. Molecular mapping of albino deletions associated with early embryonic lethality in the mouse. Genomics 1991;9:162–9.
23. Grompe M, al-Dhalimy M, Ou CN, et al. Loss of fumarylacetoacetate hydrolase is responsible for the neonatal hepatic dysfunction phenotype of lethal albino mice. Genes Dev 1993;7:2298–307.
24. Al Dhalimy M, Overturf K, Finegold M, et al. Long-term therapy with NTBC and tyrosine-restricted diet in a murine model of hereditary tyrosinemia type I. Mol Genet Metab 2002;75:38–45.
25. Endo F, Kubo S, Awata H, et al. Complete rescue of lethal albino c14CoS mice by null mutation of 4-hydroxyphenylpyruvate dioxygenase and induction of apoptosis of hepatocytes in these mice by *in vivo* retrieval of the tyrosine catabolic pathway. J Biol Chem 1997;272:24426–32.
26. Kubo S, Sun M, Miyahara M, et al. Hepatocyte injury in tyrosinemia type I is induced by fumarylacetoacetate and is inhibited by caspase inhibitors. Proc Natl Acad Sci U S A 1998;95:9552–7.
27. Grisham JW. Interspecies comparison of liver carcinogenesis: implications for cancer risk assessment. Carcinogenesis 1997;18:59–81.
28. Mitchell GA, Larochelle J, Lambert M, et al. Neurologic crises in hereditary tyrosinemia. N Engl J Med 1990;322:432–7.
29. Kappas A, Sassa S, Galbraith R. The porphyrias. In: Scriver CR, Beaudet AL, Sly WS, et al., eds. The metabolic basis of inherited disease. New York: McGraw-Hill, 1989:1305–66.
30. Strife CF, Zuroweste EL, Emmett EA, et al. Tyrosinemia with acute intermittent porphyria: aminolevulinic acid dehydratase deficiency related to elevated urinary aminolevulinic acid levels. J Pediatr 1977;90:400–4.
31. Rank JM, Pascual-Leone A, Payne W, et al. Hematin therapy for the neurologic crisis of tyrosinemia. J Pediatr 1991;118:136–9.
32. Manowski Z, Silver MM, Roberts EA, et al. Liver cell dysplasia and early liver transplantation in hereditary tyrosinemia. Mod Pathol 1990;3:694–701.
33. De Braekeleer M, Larochelle J. Genetic epidemiology of hereditary tyrosinemia in Quebec and in Saguenay-Lac-St-Jean. Am J Hum Genet 1990;47:302–7.
34. Bouchard G, Laberge C, Scriver CR. Hereditary tyrosinemia and vitamin-dependent rickets in Saguenay. A genetic and demographic approach [in French]. Union Med Can 1985;114:633–6.
35. Mitchell GA, Grompe M, Lambert M, Tanguay RM. Hypertyrosinemia. In: Scriver CR, Beaudet AL, Sly WS, Valle D, eds. The metabolic and molecular bases of inherited disease. New York: McGraw Hill, 2001: 1777–806.
36. Grompe M, St-Louis M, Demers SI, et al. A single mutation of the fumarylacetoacetate hydrolase gene in French Canadians with hereditary tyrosinemia type I. N Engl J Med 1994;331:353–7.
37. Poudrier J, St-Louis M, Lettre F, et al. Frequency of the IVS12+5G-A splice mutation of the fumarylacetoacetate hydrolase gene in carriers of hereditary tyrosinaemia in the French-Canadian population of Saguenay-Lac-St-Jean. Prenat Diagn 1996;16:59–64.
38. Ploos van Amstel JK, Bergman AJ, van Beurden EA, et al. Hereditary tyrosinemia type 1: novel missense, nonsense and splice consensus mutations in the human fumarylacetoacetate hydrolase gene; variability of the genotype-phenotype relationship. Hum Genet 1996;97:51–9.
39. St-Louis M, Leclerc B, Laine J, et al. Identification of a stop mutation in five Finnish patients suffering from hereditary tyrosinemia type I. Hum Mol Genet 1994;3:69–72.
40. Rootwelt H, Hoie K, Berger R, et al. Fumarylacetoacetate mutations in tyrosinaemia type I. Hum Mutat 1996;7:239–43.
41. Rootwelt H, Berger R, Gray G, et al. Novel splice, missense, and nonsense mutations in the fumarylacetoacetase gene causing tyrosinemia type 1. Am J Hum Genet 1994;55: 653–8.
42. Kvittingen EA, Borresen AL, Stokke O, et al. Deficiency of fumarylacetoacetase without hereditary tyrosinemia. Clin Genet 1985;27:550–4.
43. Gentz J, Johansson S, Lindblad B, et al. Excretion of delta-aminolevulinic acid in hereditary tyrosinemia. Clin Chim Acta 1969;23:257–63.
44. Croffie JM, Gupta SK, Chong SK, et al. Tyrosinemia type 1 should be suspected in infants with severe coagulopathy even in the absence of other signs of liver failure. Pediatrics 1999;103:675–8.
45. de Almeida IT, Leandro PP, Silva MF, et al. Tyrosinaemia type I with normal levels of plasma tyrosine. J Inherit Metab Dis 1990;13:305–7.
46. Grenier A, Lescault A, Laberge C, et al. Detection of succinylacetone and the use of its measurement in mass screening for hereditary tyrosinemia. Clin Chim Acta 1982;123: 93–9.
47. Haagen AAM, Duran M. Absence of increased succinylacetone in the urine of a child with hereditary tyrosinaemia type I. J Inherit Metab Dis 1987;10(suppl 2):323–5.
48. Laberge C, Grenier A, Valet JP, et al. Fumarylacetoacetase measurement as a mass-screening procedure for hereditary tyrosinemia type I. Am J Hum Genet 1990;47:325–8.
49. Jakobs C, Stellaard F, Kvittingen EA, et al. First-trimester prenatal diagnosis of tyrosinemia type 1 by amniotic fluid succinylacetone determination [letter]. Prenat Diagn 1990; 10:133–4.
50. Segal S. Disorders of galactose metabolism. In: Scriver CR, Beaudet AL, Sly WS, et al., eds. The metabolic basis of inherited disease. New York: McGraw-Hill, 1989:453–80.
51. Gitzelman R, Steinmann B, Van Der Berghe G. Disorders of fructose metabolism. In: Scriver CR, Beaudet AL, Sly WS, et al., eds. The metabolic basis of inherited disease. New York: McGraw-Hill, 1989:556–62.
52. Danks DM. Disorders of copper transport. In: Scriver CR, Beaudet AL, Sly WS, et al., eds. The metabolic basis of inherited disease. New York: McGraw-Hill, 1989:1411–32.
53. Chen YT, Coleman RA, Scheinman JI. Renal disease in type 1 glycogen storage disease. N Engl J Med 1988;318:7–11.

54. Nyhan WL. Abnormalities in amino acid metabolism in clinical medicine. Norwalk, CT: Appleton-Century-Crofts, 1984.
55. Berger R, Michals K, Galbraeth J, et al. Tyrosinemia type Ib caused by maleylacetoacetate isomerase deficiency: a new enzyme defect [abstract]. Pediatr Res 1988;23:328.
56. Fernandez-Canon JM, Baetscher MW, Finegold M, et al. Maleylacetoacetate isomerase (MAAI/GSTZ)-deficient mice reveal a glutathione-dependent nonenzymatic bypass in tyrosine catabolism. Mol Cell Biol 2002;22:4943–51.
57. Evans DI, Sardharwalla IB. Coagulation defect of congenital tyrosinaemia. Arch Dis Child 1984;59:1088–90.
58. Gentz J, Jagenburg R, Zetterström R. Tyrosinemia: an inborn error of tyrosine metabolism with cirrhosis of the liver and multiple renal tubular defects. J Pediatr 1965;66:670–96.
59. Ferrell LD, Crawford JM, Dhillon AP, et al. Proposal for standardized criteria for the diagnosis of benign, borderline, and malignant hepatocellular lesions arising in chronic advanced liver disease. Am J Surg Pathol 1993;17:1113–23.
60. Weinberg AG, Mize CE, Worthen HG. The occurrence of hepatoma in the chronic form of hereditary tyrosinemia. J Pediatr 1976;88:434–8.
61. Dionisi-Vici C, Boglino C, Marcellini M, et al. Tyrosinemia type I with early metastatic hepatocellular carcinoma: combined treatment with NTBC, chemotherapy and surgical mass removal. J Inherit Metab Dis 1997;20(suppl 1):3.
62. Cole DEC, Tithecott GA, Crocker JFS, et al. Alphaxalone/alphadolone and porphyria. Lancet 1984;1:690.
62a. Paradis K, Mitchell GA, Russo P. Tyrosinemia. In: Suchy FJ, ed. Liver disease in children. St. Louis: CV Mosby, 1994:803–18.
63. Kvittingen EA, Talseth T, Halvorsen S, et al. Renal failure in adult patients with hereditary tyrosinaemia type I. J Inherit Metab Dis 1991;14:53–62.
64. Halvorsen S. Dietary treatment of tyrosinosis. Am J Dis Child 1967;113:38–40.
65. Kogut MD, Shaw KN, Donnell GN. Tyrosinosis. Am J Dis Child 1967;113:47–53.
66. Sass-Kortsak A, Ficici S, Paunier L, et al. Observations on treatment in patients with tyrosyluria. Can Med Assoc J 1967;97:1089–95.
67. Suzuki Y, Konda M, Imai I, et al. Effect of dietary treatment on the renal tubular function in a patient with hereditary tyrosinemia. Int J Pediatr Nephrol 1987;8:171–6.
68. Bendon PW, Hug G. Glycogen accumulation in the pars recta of the proximal tubule in Fanconi syndrome. Pediatr Pathol 1986;6:411–29.
69. Parington MW, Haust MD. A patient with tyrosinemia and hypermethioninemia. Can Med Assoc J 1967;97:1059–64.
69a. Baumann U, Preece MA, Green A, et al. Hyperinsulinism in tyrosinaemia type I. J Inherit Metab Dis 2005;28:131–5.
70. Lindberg T, Nilsson KO, Jeppsson JO. Hereditary tyrosinaemia and diabetes mellitus. Acta Paediatr Scand 1979;68:619–20.
71. Edwards MA, Green A, Colli A, et al. Tyrosinaemia type I and hypertrophic obstructive cardiomyopathy [letter]. Lancet 1987;1:1437–8.
72. Lindblad B, Fällström SP, Höyer S, et al. Cardiomyopathy in fumarylacetoacetase deficiency (hereditary tyrosinaemia): a new feature of the disease. J Inherit Metab Dis 1987;10:319–22.
72a. Andre N, Roquelaure B, Jubin V, Ovaert C. Successful treatment of severe cardiomyopathy with NTBC in a child with tyrosinaemia type I. J Inherit Metab Dis 2005;28:103–6.
72b. Arora N, Stumper O, Wright J, et al. Cardiomyopathy in tyrosinaemia type I is common but usually benign. J Inherit Metab Dis 2006;29:54–7.
73. Dubois J, Garel L, Patriquin H, et al. Imaging features of type 1 hereditary tyrosinemia: a review of 30 patients. Pediatr Radiol 1996;26:845–51.
73a. Crone J, Möslinger D, Bodamer OA, et al. Reversibility of cirrhotic regenerative liver nodules upon NTBC treatment in a child with tyrosinemia type 1. Acta Pediatr 2003;92:625–8.
74. Privé L. Pathological findings in patients with tyrosinemia. Can Med Assoc J 1967;97:1054–6.
75. Carson NA, Biggart JD, Bittles AH, et al. Hereditary tyrosinaemia. Clinical, enzymatic, and pathological study of an infant with the acute form of the disease. Arch Dis Child 1976;51:106–13.
76. Halvorsen S, Pande H, Loken AC, et al. Tyrosinosis. A study of 6 cases. Arch Dis Child 1966;41:238–49.
77. Dehner LP, Snover DC, Sharp HL, et al. Hereditary tyrosinemia type I (chronic form): pathologic findings in the liver. Hum Pathol 1989;20:149–58.
78. Yu JS, Walker-Smith JA, Burnard ED. Neonatal hepatitis in premature infants simulating hereditary tyrosinosis. Arch Dis Child 1971;46:306–9.
79. Watanabe S, Okita K, Harada T. Morphologic studies of the liver cell dysplasia. Cancer 1983;51:2197–205.
80. Laberge C, Lescault A, Tanguay RM. Hereditary tyrosinemias (type I): a new vista on tyrosine toxicity and cancer. Adv Exp Med Biol 1986;206:209–21.
81. Tremblay M, Bélanger L, Larochelle J, et al. Hereditary tyrosinemia: examination of the liver by electron microscopy of hepatic biopsies: observation of 7 cases [in French]. Union Med Can 1977;106:1014–16.
82. Phillips MJ, Poucell S, Patterson J. The liver: an atlas and text of ultrastructural pathology. New York: Raven, 1987.
83. Jetvic MM, Thorp FK, Hruban Z. Hereditary tyrosinemia with hyperplasia of juxtaglomerular apparatus. Am J Clin Pathol 1974;61:423–37.
84. Tuchman M, Freese DK, Sharp HL, et al. Contribution of extrahepatic tissues to biochemical abnormalities in hereditary tyrosinemia type I: study of three patients after liver transplantation. J Pediatr 1987;110:399–403.
85. Flatmark A, Bergan A, Sodal G, et al. Does liver transplantation correct the metabolic defect in hereditary tyrosinemia? Transplant Proc 1986;18:67–8.
86. Callurel P, Feldman G, Prandi D. Immune complex type glomerulonephritis in cirrhosis of the liver. Am J Pathol 1975;80:329–36.
87. Perry TL. Tyrosinemia associated with hypermethioninemia and islet cell hyperplasia. Can Med Assoc J 1967;97:1067–75.
88. Jaffe R, Hashida Y, Yunis EJ. The endocrine pancreas of the neonate and infant. In: Rosenberg HS, Bernstein J, eds. Perspectives in pediatric pathology. Paris: Masson, 1980:137–66.
89. Hardwick DF, Dimmick JE. Metabolic cirrhoses of infancy and early childhood. In: Rosenberg HS, Bolande RP, eds. Perspectives in pediatric pathology. Chicago: Year Book, 1976:103–44.

90. Mitchell GA, Lambert M, Tanguay RM. Hypertyrosinemia. In: Scriver CR, Beaudet AL, Sly WS, et al., eds. The metabolic and molecular bases of inherited disease. New York: McGraw-Hill, 1995:1077–176.
91. Ameen VZ, Powell GK, Rassin DK. Cholestasis and hypermethioninemia during dietary management of hereditary tyrosinemia type 1. J Pediatr 1986;108:949–53.
92. Mudd SH, Levy HL, Skovby F. Disorders of transsulfuration. In: Scriver CR, Beaudet AL, Sly W, et al., eds. The metabolic basis of inherited disease. New York: McGraw-Hill, 1989:693–741.
93. Freese DK, Tuchman M, Schwarzenberg SJ, et al. Early liver transplantation is indicated for tyrosinemia type I. J Pediatr Gastroenterol Nutr 1991;13:10–15.
94. Flye MW, Riely CA, Hainline BE, et al. The effects of early treatment of hereditary tyrosinemia type I in infancy by orthotopic liver transplantation. Transplantation 1990;49:916–21.
95. Jehan P, Buchman M, Odièvre M. Dietary management of hereditary tyrosinemia. Apropos of 7 cases. Ann Pediatr (Paris) 1984;31:33–40.
96. Lindblad B. Treatment with glutathione and other sulfhydryl compounds in hereditary tyrosinemia. In: Larsson A, ed. Functions of glutathione: biochemical, physiological, toxicological, and clinical aspects. New York: Raven, 1983:337–46.
97. Herzog D, Martin S, Turpin S, Alvarez F. Normal glomerular filtration rate in long-term follow-up of children after orthotopic liver transplantation. Transplantation 2006;81:672–7.
97a. McDiarmid SV, Ettenger RB, Fine RF. Serial decrease in glomerular filtration rate in long-term pediatric liver transplantation survivors treated with cyclosporine. Transplantation 1989;47:314–18.
98. Paradis K, O'Regan S, Seidman E. Improvement in true glomerular filtration rate after cyclosporine fractionation in pediatric liver transplant recipients. Transplantation 1991;51:922–4.
99. Laine J, Salo MK, Krogerus L, et al. The nephropathy of type I tyrosinemia after liver transplantation. Pediatr Res 1995;37:640–5.
100. al Edreesi M, Caille G, Dupuis C, et al. Safety, tolerability, and pharmacokinetic actions of diltiazem in pediatric liver transplant recipients on cyclosporine. Liver Transplant Surg 1995;1:383–8.
100a. Pierik LJ, van Spronsen FJ, Bijleveld CM, van Dael CM. Renal function in tyrosinaemia type I after liver transplantation: a long-term follow-up. J Inherit Metab Dis 2005;28:871–6.
101. Overturf K, Al-Dhalimy M, Ou CN, et al. Serial transplantation reveals the stem-cell-like regenerative potential of adult mouse hepatocytes. Am J Pathol 1997;151:1273–80.
101a. Grompe M. Therapeutic liver repopulation for the treatment of metabolic liver diseases. Hum Cell 1999;12:171–80.
101b. Lee LA. Advances in hepatocyte transplantation: a myth becomes reality. J Clin Invest 2001;108:367–9.
101c. Wang X, Foster M, Al Dhalimy M, et al. The origin and liver repopulating capacity of murine oval cells. Proc Natl Acad Sci U S A 2003;100(suppl 1):11881–8.
102. Lock EA, Gaskin P, Ellis MK, et al. Tissue distribution of 2-(2-nitro-4-trifluoromethylbenzoyl)cyclohexane-1,3-dione (NTBC): effect on enzymes involved in tyrosine catabolism and relevance to ocular toxicity in the rat. Toxicol Appl Pharmacol 1996;141:439–47.
103. Magera MJ, Gunawardena ND, Hahn SH, et al. Quantitative determination of succinylacetone in dried blood spots for newborn screening of tyrosinemia type I. Mol Genet Metab 2006;88:16–21.
104. Allard P, Grenier A, Korson MS, et al. Newborn screening for hepatorenal tyrosinemia by tandem mass spectrometry: analysis of succinylacetone extracted from dried blood spots. Clin Biochem 2004;37:1010–15.

30

The Liver in Lysosomal Storage Diseases

T. Andrew Burrow, M.D., Kevin E. Bove, M.D., and Gregory A. Grabowski, M.D.

Lysosomes are membrane-bound cellular organelles that contain multiple hydrolases needed for the digestion of various macromolecules, including mucopolysaccharides, glycosphingolipids, and oligosaccharides [1]. The lysosomal storage diseases are a group of more than 40 diseases that are characterized by defective lysosomal function leading to an accumulation of specific substrates within the lysosomes and eventual impairment of cellular function. A schematic of the lysosomal system, enzyme trafficking, and substrate accumulation is shown in Figure 30.1.

These diseases are classified by the nature of the stored material that results from defects in selected lysosomal enzymes, their cofactors, and/or enzyme or substrate transport (Table 30.1). The lysosomal storage diseases are heterogeneous, progressive, multisystemic diseases that have a spectrum of ages of onset, severity, rates of progression, and organ involvement. Lysosomal storage diseases have significant morbidity and mortality in the absence of effective treatment. The majority of these diseases are autosomal recessive, and although individually each is rare, the combined birth prevalence is approximately 1 in 7000 live births [2]. The diseases are traditionally diagnosed biochemically but in many cases, may also be diagnosed molecularly by the discovery of pathogenic mutations in both copies of the particular gene.

The liver is nearly always involved in lysosomal storage diseases; this can be seen at the light or electron microscopic level. The degree of clinical involvement depends on the disorder. In many cases, mild elevations in liver studies and hepatomegaly are the only manifestations. However, significant hepatic injury may be present, resulting in considerable morbidity. For each of the diseases, the nature of the organ involvement will depend on the tissue-specific lysosomal enzyme content, substrate composition and turnover, and rate of cell turnover/replacement [3]. The resultant pathophysiologies are poorly understood but are likely the consequences of numerous proinflammatory and inflammatory events initiated by excess substrate and/or deficient products [4].

A comprehensive review of all aspects of the lysosomal storage diseases is beyond the scope of this chapter, and the reader is referred to referenced materials for such reviews. The objective of this chapter is to provide clinicians with a broad summary of the lysosomal storage diseases that significantly affect the liver.

SPHINGOLIPIDOSES

Mutations in the primary enzyme or essential cofactors – that is, sphingolipid activator proteins (saposins) – lead to defective or absent hydrolysis of specific sphingolipids and their abnormal accumulation within lysosomes. Sphingolipids are critical structural components of cell membranes that also function in protein sorting and cell signaling and recognition [5]. Among the sphingolipidoses, Gaucher's disease, Niemann–Pick disease types A and B, Farber's disease, and G_{M1} gangliosidosis are discussed here because of their specific effects on the liver.

Gaucher's Disease

Gaucher's disease, the most common lysosomal storage disease, is inherited in an autosomal recessive manner. The phenotypes result from defective cleavage of glucosylceramide by acid β-glucosidase in all nucleated cells [6]. More than 280 mutations in the gene that encodes the lysosomal enzyme acid β-glucosidase (*GBA*) have been discovered in affected patients. Gaucher's disease has a frequency of about 1 in 57,000 in the general population and around 1 in 855 in the Ashkenazi Jewish population [7].

In visceral tissues, cells of macrophage lineage are primarily involved, whereas a variety of central nervous system (CNS) neurons may be affected in some variants. These engorged macrophages, Gaucher cells, are 20–100 μm in diameter with tubular inclusions resembling wrinkled tissue paper (Figure 30.2). Gaucher cells are abundant in liver, spleen, lung, bone marrow, and lymph nodes, and can lead to hepatosplenomegaly, anemia, thrombocytopenia, pulmonary disease, lymphadenopathy, and destructive bone disease.

Three variants of Gaucher's disease have been described based on the absence or presence and severity of neuronopathic disease. *Gaucher's disease type 1*, the nonneuronopathic variant, accounts for approximately 90% of all cases of the disease

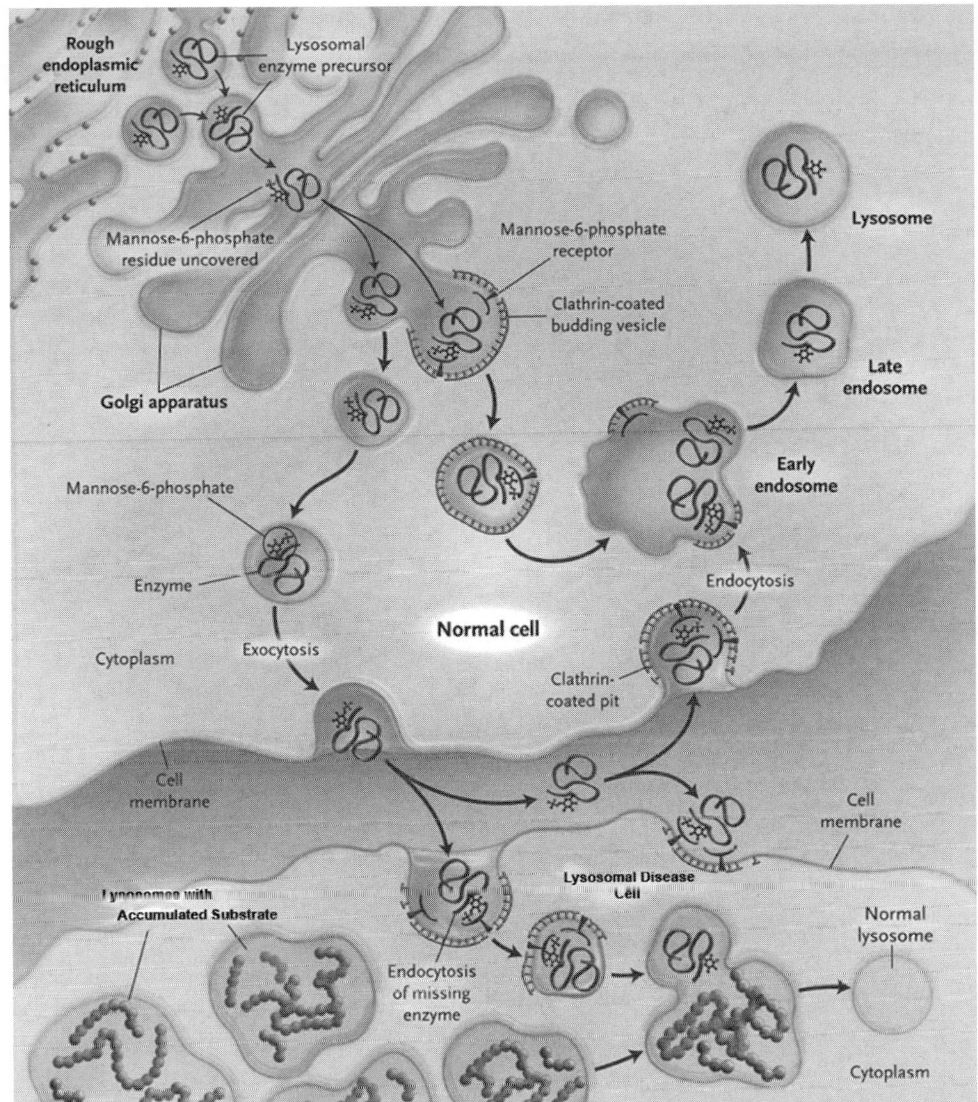

Figure 30.1. The lysosomal system in normal (*upper*) and lysosomal disease (*lower*) cells. Lysosomal enzymes are synthesized on the rough endoplasmic reticulum (RER), transported through the Golgi apparatus, and delivered to the lysosomes. In the RER, oligosaccharide chains are cotranslationally added to the nascent polypeptide. Sequential glycosidic modifications occur in the Golgi apparatus to trim terminal α-glucosidic and α-mannosidic residues, and specific glycosyltransferases add *N*-acetylglucosamine, β-galactose, and sialic acid. On selected high mannose chains, mannose-6-phosphates are exposed and used to target soluble lysosomal hydrolases to the lysosomes. Membrane-bound lysosomal proteins are targeted to lysosomes by specific peptides within the protein sequence. The glycosidic, proteolytic, and macromolecular processing of the lysosomal proteins occurs vectorially from *cis* to *trans* Golgi. The fully mature proteins and cofactors are delivered to the lysosomes after transit through the *trans* Golgi network and endosomal system. Some lysosomal enzymes are lost from the cells by exocytosis into the surrounding intercellular milieu. Such enzymes, either exogenously supplied or available by secretion, can be internalized by receptor-mediated endocytosis using the mannose-6-phosphate receptor or other receptor (e.g., macrophage mannose receptor) system. The intralysosomal deficiency of specific hydrolases or cofactors leads to an inability to cleave macromolecules (glycosaminoglycans, glycosphingolipids, oligosaccharides, etc.) and their resultant accumulation within distended lysosomes. The degree and rate of accumulation of such specific substrates will depend on the endogenous synthesis and/or exogenous delivery of substrates to particular cells and/or tissues. In the lysosomal storage diseases, the accumulated substrates elicit cellular reactions (proinflammatory, transcriptional, etc.) by mechanisms that remain undetermined. (Adapted from Muenzer J, Fisher A. Advances in the treatment of mucopolysaccharidosis type I. N Engl J Med 2004;350:1932–4.)

Table 30.1: Lysosomal Storage Disorders Involving the Liver

Disease	*Protein Defect*	*Storage Material*	*Degree of Liver Involvement*	*Established Therapy*
Sphingolipidoses				
Gaucher's disease	Acid β-glucosidase	Glucosylceramide	+→++	+
Niemann–Pick disease type A	Sphingomyelinase	Sphingomyelin	++–+++	–
Niemann–Pick disease type B	Sphingomyelinase	Sphingomyelin	++–+++	+
Farber's disease	Acid ceramidase	Ceramide	+–+++	–
G_{M1} gangliosidosis	β-Galactosidase	G_{M1} ganglioside	+–+++	–
Cholesterol transport defect				
Niemann–Pick disease type C	NPC1 or NPC2	Unesterified cholesterol/sphingolipids	+–+++	–
Glycoprotein storage diseases				
Fucosidosis	α-L-fucosidase	Fucose-rich oligosaccharides, glycolipids, and glycoproteins	+	–
α-Mannosidosis	α-Mannosidase	Mannose-rich oligosaccharides	+	–
Sialidosis	Lysosomal neuraminidase	Sialic acid–rich oligosaccharides, glycolipids, and glycoproteins	+	–
Galactosialidosis	Protective protein/cathepsin A	Gangliosides and sialic acid–rich oligosaccharides and glycoproteins	+–+++	–
Glycogen storage disease				
Pompe's disease	Acid α-glucosidase	Glycogen	+	+
Cholesteryl ester storage disorders				
Wolman's disease	Lysosomal acid lipase	Cholesteryl esters, triglycerides	+→+++	–
Cholesteryl ester storage disease	Lysosomal acid lipase	Cholesteryl esters, triglycerides	+→+++	–
Mucopolysaccharidoses				
MPS I (Hurler, Scheie, Hurler–Scheie)	α-L-iduronidase	Dermatan sulfate, heparan sulfate	+	+
MPS II (Hunter) (mild and severe)	Iduronate sulfatase	Dermatan sulfate, heparan sulfate	+	–
MPS III A (Sanfilippo A)	Heparan *N*-sulfatase	Heparan sulfate	+	–
MPS III B (Sanfilippo B)	α-*N*-acetylglucosaminidase	Heparan sulfate	+	–
MPS III C (Sanfilippo C)	Acetyl-CoA:α-glucosaminide *N*-acetyltransferase	Heparan sulfate	+	–
MPS III D (Sanfilippo D)	*N*-acetylglucosamine 6-sulfatase	Heparan sulfate	+	–
MPS IV (Morquio A)	Galactose 6-sulfatase	Keratan sulfate, chondroitin 6-sulfate	+	–
MPS IV (Morquio-B)	ß-galactosidase	Keratan sulfate	+	–
MPS VI (Maroteaux-Lamy)	Arylsulfatase B	Dermatan sulfate	+	+
MPS VII (Sly)	β-Glucuronidase	Dermatan sulfate, heparan sulfate, chondroitin 4-, 6-sulfates	+	–
MPS IX	Hyaluronidase	Hyaluronic acid	+	–
Disorder of enzyme transport				
Mucolipidosis type II (I-cell disease)	Phosphotransferase	Oligosaccharides, glycosaminoglycans, lipids	+–++	–
Mucolipidosis type III (pseudo-Hurler)	Phosphotransferase	Oligosaccharides, glycosaminoglycans, lipids	+–++	–
Miscellaneous disorder				
Multiple sulfatase deficiency	FGly-generating enzyme	Sulfated glycosaminoglycans, glycolipids, glycopeptides, and hydroxysteroids	+	–

CoA, coenzyme A; MPS, mucopolysaccharidosis; NPC, Niemann–Pick disease type C; +, ++, +++, or – refer to progressively severe involvement from absent (–) to (→) very severe (+++).

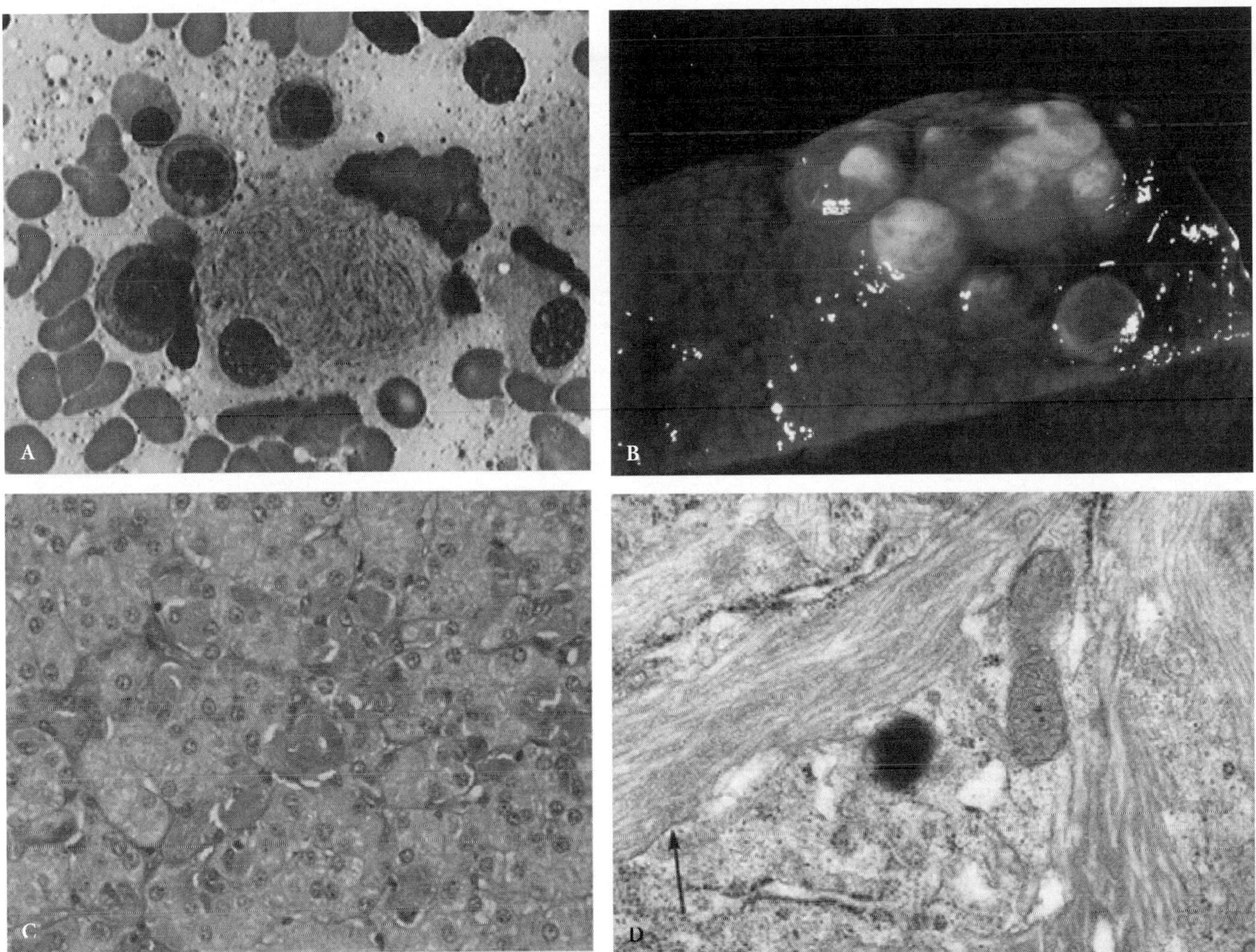

Figure 30.2. Bone marrow and liver findings in Gaucher's disease. (**A**) The bone marrow macrophage is typical of the storage cells, that is, Gaucher cells. The typical "crinkled tissue paper" cytoplasmic inclusions are evident. (**B**) Liver slice showing nodules (white/yellow) made up almost entirely of Gaucher cells. (**C**) By light microscopy, only Kupffer cells contain visible storage material, glucosylceramide, whereas the hepatocytes do not. PAS staining is negative in Kupffer cells. (**D**) Electron micrograph showing characteristic tubular storage material of Gaucher disease cellular inclusions. (Magnification 20,000×.) (Courtesy of D. Witte.) For color reproduction, see Color Plate 30.2.

in Europe and the United States. The associated phenotypes are restricted to visceral organs. The onset of disease is highly variable and occurs from childhood to adulthood. Survival is frequently reduced, but many patients live into adulthood. A significant number of patients are discovered serendipitously in the sixth to eighth decades. This variant is prevalent among those of Ashkenazi Jewish heritage.

Gaucher's disease types 2 and 3 are neuronopathic variants that are distinguished by the age of onset of neurologic signs and symptoms and their severity. Gaucher's disease type 2 may have onset in utero to 6 months of life with rapidly progressing neurologic deterioration and visceral disease. Death occurs at a mean age of 9 months. Gaucher's disease type 3 has less fulminant neuronopathic involvement. Indeed, horizontal supranuclear gaze palsy may present early without progression with concomitant variable degrees of visceral disease. Survival is usually less than 40 years [6]. The demarcation between types 2 and 3 is blurred, and these variants represent a continuum of CNS disease [8].

Hepatomegaly is the most frequent liver finding in patients with Gaucher's disease, and there is great variation in the degree of enlargement. Massive enlargement of the liver, up to tenfold normal volume, may occur, and the largest livers are in the youngest and splenectomized patients [6,8].

Typically, the liver is enlarged 1.5–2.5-fold. Clinically, some elevations of serum aminotransferase and alkaline phosphatase levels are frequent, but liver dysfunction, including hepatic failure, is unusual [6]. The most significant clinical and histologic liver disease is observed in patients who have had splenectomy [9].

Portal hypertension, with associated complications of esophageal varices, severe fibrosis and cirrhosis, and acute liver failure (ALF), has been reported [10–13] but is unusual and generally associated with concomitant viral infection.

Orthotopic liver transplantation for ALF has had varying degrees of success [10,13]. Hepatocellular carcinoma is an unusual complication of Gaucher's disease and has not been reported in children. Although this complication may be associated with secondary, known carcinogenic processes such as hepatitis B infection, one reported case had no known risk factors other than Gaucher's disease [14].

Grossly, the liver may appear yellow-brown in the presence of severe Gaucher cell replacement, grayish red with white streaks because of Gaucher cell infiltration, or dark red to purple in areas of extramedullary hematopoiesis [6]. In more severely affected patients, the liver may have micronodules or larger nodules (Figure 30.2) [10].

Examination of liver biopsies from patients with Gaucher's disease types 1, 2, and 3 (24 of 25 with hepatomegaly) showed a broad spectrum of histopathologic features [11,12]. Little difference was found in the pathologic findings among patients with any of the three disease variants. However, cirrhosis was observed only in patients with Gaucher's disease type 1 (three cases) [11,12].

Gaucher cell accumulation and fibrosis are the most common histopathologic features. The degree of involvement varied from scattered aggregates of Gaucher cells in sinusoids with few other abnormalities to more severe manifestations. Pericellular fibrosis was commonly in a diffuse pattern, but severely atrophic and diminished numbers of hepatocytes were unusual. Sixteen cases had central zonal (zone 3) distribution of Gaucher cells. The central veins were frequently compressed and obscured. Storage cell accumulation was occasionally noted in the portal zones, periportal regions, and mid-zones, but rarely to the degrees observed in the central zones. Hepatocytes close to the storage cells showed degenerative changes and atrophy. Pericellular fibrosis was observed in all sixteen cases and was characterized by thick fibrous septa surrounding the central vein with replacement of the normal hepatic parenchyma in six cases. Fibrotic linkage of adjacent central zones by fibrous bands with involvement of the portal triads was consistent with micronodular cirrhosis in three of those cases. Some regenerative activity was noted in the later six cases. Additionally, extramedullary hematopoiesis was noted in a few patients. Cholestasis was not present in these pathologic specimens [11,12].

Four patients with severe liver involvement in Gaucher's disease type 1 exhibited enlarged, nodular livers with extensive central acellular fibrosis surrounded by parenchymal nodules, frequently incorporating portal tracts. In one case, the fibrous tissue involved the portal tracts with focal ductal proliferation and surrounding small parenchymal nodules, some of which exhibited canalicular cholestasis. Gaucher cells were most often found at the fibrotic margins [10].

The diagnosis of Gaucher's disease is made by demonstration of abnormally low acid β-glucosidase activity in nucleated cells, most commonly peripheral blood leukocytes or cultured skin fibroblasts. The enzyme is not normally present in erythrocytes or plasma/serum. It may also be diagnosed by the discovery of pathogenic mutations in both copies of *GBA*. Mutational analyses are also helpful in prognostication for the risk of CNS involvement and the overall disease severity [6]. These genotype/phenotype correlations are based on associations and are not definitive. Such counseling based on risk factors is rapidly evolving and should be conducted by health care professionals with expertise in this area.

Treatment for the variants of Gaucher's disease is based on the multisystemic involvement and the need for coordinated care management plans. Although enzyme therapy (see later) has become the standard of care, treatment of patients with Gaucher's disease involves supportive management for the complications of Gaucher's disease, including appropriate orthopedic procedures and management of hematologic and CNS signs and symptoms. Bone marrow transplantation (BMT) may prove curative; however, it carries a significant risk of complications and has had limited use since the advent of enzyme therapy.

Enzyme therapy for the variants of Gaucher's disease is the standard of care for the control and reversal of visceral manifestations. Intravenous enzyme therapy has not been proven to have direct beneficial effects on the CNS involvement but plays a supportive/palliative role for type 2 and can be lifesaving in type 3 disease. Enzyme therapy is provided by regular intravenous infusions of recombinant human acid β-glucosidase that has been modified for preferential uptake into macrophages [15]. During the past decade, more than 3200 patients have received such therapy, with beneficial results. Therapeutic goals and expected outcomes have been developed and are being modified [16]. In a study of 1028 patients with Gaucher's disease type 1, a 20–30% decrease in liver volume within 1–2 years was achieved after initiating recombinant acid β-glucosidase therapy. Additional reductions to near normalcy were achieved by 5 years. In patients with massive livers, the rate of decrease was slower but overall gains were substantial. These findings were concomitant with improvements in anemia and thrombocytopenia [17]. Although enzyme therapy can stabilize existent advanced liver disease, irreversible damage may never respond [10]. Although orthotopic liver transplantation alone is not likely to be effective because of re-injury from the primary disease, orthotopic liver transplantation combined with enzyme replacement therapy has been useful in one case [10].

A secondary therapy has been approved for use in patients in whom enzyme therapy cannot be used for medical reasons. The approach inhibits the synthetic pathway for glucosylceramide, glucosylceramide synthase. The overall concept is to allow the residual mutant enzyme present in all patients with Gaucher's disease to degrade a smaller inflow of the substrate and thereby reduce storage [18,19]. Clinical trials have shown some effect on liver and splenic volumes, but the hematologic status improved only slightly. Diarrhea, the most common side effect, occurred in almost 80% of participants [20]. This approach might fill a void for patients who develop sensitivity to enzyme therapy or have additional complications that may not respond to enzyme treatment. Neither enzyme replacement therapy nor substrate reduction therapy has demonstrated effectiveness in preventing or improving neurologic dysfunction in patients with Gaucher's disease types 2 and 3 [21,22].

Acid Sphingomyelinase Deficiency (Niemann–Pick A and B)

Acid sphingomyelinase deficiencies are heterogeneous, autosomal recessive lysosomal disorders characterized by an accumulation of undegraded sphingomyelin and other lipids in the lysosomes of multiple cell types, particularly those of macrophage/monocyte lineage. The acid sphingomyelinase gene, sphingomyelin phosphodiesterase-1 (*SMPD1*), maps to chromosome 11p15.4-p15.1. More than 50 mutations have been found in the *SMPD1* gene of affected patients [23–25].

Niemann–Pick types A (NPA) and B (NPB) are phenotypes within a continuum of disease that vary by age of onset, absence or presence of neurologic disease, severity of features, and survival. Visceral features may include growth retardation; hepatomegaly, often without liver dysfunction; splenomegaly; gastrointestinal disturbances; hyperlipidemia; pulmonary disease; osteoporosis; lymphadenopathy; pancytopenia; and ocular abnormalities, particularly cherry-red maculae. NPA and NPB have a combined frequency of 1 in 248,000 in Australia [7].

Niemann–Pick type A, the more severe phenotype, displays progressive neurovisceral disease within the first several months of life. Survival depends on supportive care but usually does not extend beyond age 2–3 years. Prolonged neonatal jaundice; hepatosplenomegaly, usually without liver dysfunction; and failure to thrive are among the earliest features [26]. Affected individuals experience progressive hypotonia, muscle weakness, intellectual decline, and loss of milestones that transforms to spasticity and rigidity at the end stages of the disease [26]. NPA is particularly prevalent in the Ashkenazi Jewish population, in which about 1 in 80 persons are carriers [26].

Niemann–Pick type B is a heterogeneous, nonneuronopathic disease with visceral features as described above. The disease is frequently diagnosed in childhood to adolescence, with survival into adulthood. Hepatosplenomegaly is most prevalent during childhood but tends to become less conspicuous with age [26]. Within a subpopulation of patients with this subtype of disease, pulmonary disease is a significant source of morbidity. The disease is pan-ethnic in nature, with highest incidence in individuals of Turkish, Arabic, and North African descent and less frequency among those of Ashkenazi Jewish heritage [27].

Intermediate variants of acid sphingomyelinase deficiency are common and comprise 64% of affected individuals in central Europe. These intermediate variants are defined by a cluster of visceral features and a protracted neuronopathic course. A rapidly progressive, early fatal, visceral variant without major CNS involvement has also been described [28].

Hepatomegaly is a common finding in acid sphingomyelinase deficiency. In 29 patients with NPB, the mean liver volume was 1.91-fold increased. Mild, stable elevations of aminotransferase and bilirubin levels were common in this study [29].

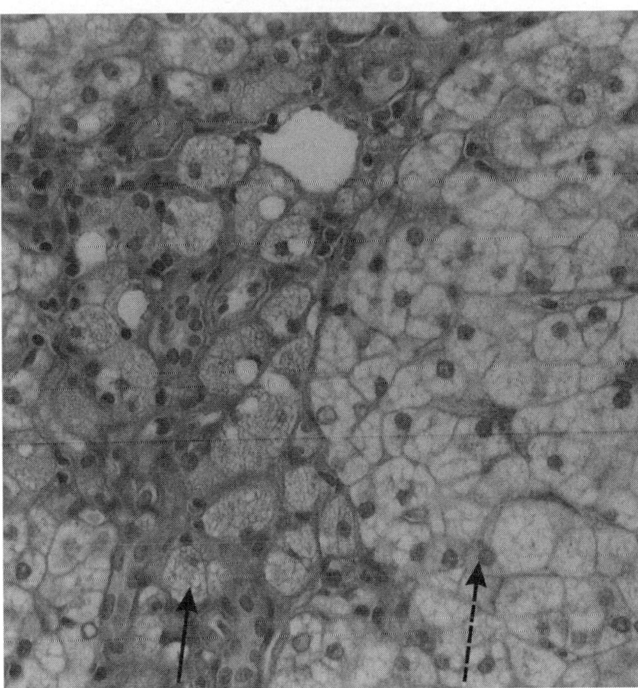

Figure 30.3. Photomicrograph of a liver section from a 6-year-old girl with NPB. Obvious "foamy" Kupffer cells are present (*hyphenated arrow*). Storage in hepatocyte is also clearly observed (*solid arrow*). The storage material is PAS diastase negative. (Magnification, 400×.) (Courtesy of M. Collins.) For color reproduction, see Color Plate 30.3.

Although not common in acid sphingomyelinase deficiency, hepatic fibrosis, cirrhosis, portal hypertension, and liver failure have been reported in adults and children, typically resulting in a poor outcome [30–33]. However, in a minority of cases, other comorbidities, such as hepatitis B, may have contributed to liver dysfunction [34]. Orthotopic liver transplantation has been successfully performed in a number of individuals with NPB due to liver dysfunction [35,36].

The liver in patients with NPB is often smooth, firm, and yellow to orange in coloration [30,32,33]. Hepatocytes and Kupffer cells contain vacuolated storage material within the cytoplasm, imparting a foamy appearance (Figure 30.3). Their distribution may initially be spotty but may become generalized in later stages of the disease. During the disease course, Niemann–Pick cells initially accumulate in the sinusoids but later extend to involvement of the portal areas [26]. These cells may accumulate to such a degree within the sinusoids that intrahepatic obstruction may result [30]. Ultrastructurally, the storage material resembles parallel membranes or concentrically laminated structures [31]. Increasing degrees of fibrosis are observed and may progress to cirrhosis in advanced cases [32,33].

The diagnosis of NPB and NPA is established by the deficiency of acid sphingomyelinase in nucleated cells. The type and severity of disease do not correlate well to the amount of residual enzyme activity. The enzyme is not present in significant amounts in erythrocytes or plasma/serum. The diseases may also be diagnosed by the discovery of pathogenic mutations in both copies of *SMPD1*. Acid sphingomyelinase deficiency leads to the accumulation of sphingomyelin, bis (monoacylglycero)phosphate, cholesterol, and other lipids in many cell types, particularly those of monocyte/macrophage lineage. These large lipid-laden cells, Niemann–Pick cells, are about 25–75 μm in size and stain negative with periodic acid–Schiff (PAS) but positive for lipid with Sudan black B and oil red O. Storage material is present in other cell types, including hepatocytes and neurons, further contributing to organ dysfunction.

Current management of NPB and NPA is symptomatic. BMT has been performed in multiple individuals with types A and B disease, and despite evidence of engraftment, the patients exhibited progression of their disease [37,38]. Enzyme replacement therapy is in development, with clinical trials begun in 2006.

Farber's Disease

Farber's disease is a very rare, progressive, autosomal recessively inherited lysosomal storage disorder resulting from mutations in the gene encoding the lysosomal enzyme acid ceramidase (*ASAH*). The diagnosis is established by detection of markedly deficient acid ceramidase activity in plasma, leukocytes, and cultured skin fibroblasts, or by molecular evaluation. The level of in vitro residual enzyme activity does not correlate with disease severity. *ASAH* is located at chromosome 8p21.3-p22. Many types of mutations result in Farber's disease; genotype/phenotype correlations are not solid because of the disease rarity [39].

Clinical diagnosis is based on a triad of features: subcutaneous nodules, particularly near the joints and pressure points; painful, progressively deformed joints; and progressive hoarseness due to laryngeal involvement [40]. Variable degrees of pulmonary, cardiac, hepatic, splenic, reticuloendothelial and nervous system involvement may also be present [40]. Several subtypes of Farber's disease are recognized, varying by phenotypic features, severity, and survival.

Classic Farber's disease, the most common subtype, is characterized by the classic triad of laryngeal, subcutaneous, and joint involvement that develops within the first months of life. Affected individuals experience failure to thrive. Swallowing dysfunction and pulmonary compromise develop as a result of granulomas in the epiglottis and larynx, requiring gastrostomy tube feedings and tracheostomies in the most severe cases [40]. These granulomatous lesions also occur in the heart, spleen, reticuloendothelial system, liver, bone, nervous system, and connective tissue, contributing to the disease process [40–42]. Hepatomegaly is observed in around 40% of affected individuals, but liver dysfunction is uncommon [40]. Death occurs in the first few years of life, often from pulmonary disease [40]. An attenuated variant displays similar, albeit milder, features of the classical disease. The age of onset is later in childhood, and survival is frequently into adulthood [40,43].

The neonatal-visceral subtype is a severe disease of neonatal or early infantile onset characterized by liver dysfunction, with death occurring in early infancy, often before the development of classic features of Farber's disease [40,44–46]. In the most severe cases, it may present as hydrops fetalis [47,48].

The progressive neurologic variant of Farber's disease is manifested by progressive, generalized, neurologic deterioration and seizures within the first few years of life, followed by death in early childhood. Although subcutaneous nodules and joint disease have been described in these patients, those features do not predominate and the visceral organs are not typically affected.

Pathologic features include an accumulation of storage material within macrophages or histiocytes as foam cells. Granulomas may be present and contain a central core of foam cells surrounded by macrophages, lymphocytes, and multinucleated cells, as well as fibrosis in older nodules [40]. Ultrastructurally, the foam cells contain distended lysosomes filled with curvilinear tubular structures, Farber bodies [40].

The liver may be firm, nodular in texture, and yellow in coloration [41,47]. The variable liver histopathology is a spectrum from microscopic normalcy to minimal fatty infiltration [41]. In more severe cases, granulomatous lesions are present [47]. The liver of neonatal-visceral Farber's disease may exhibit sinusoidal fibrosis, with weakly eosinophilic, vacuolated storage cells filling the sinusoids [44,46,47]. Mild intracellular and canalicular cholestasis may be present. Mild biliary ductal proliferation has been noted in the expanded portal zones [46].

Symptomatic management has been the therapy for the disease. Several individuals with classic Farber's disease, including neurologic dysfunction, have received BMT. A significant improvement was observed in their visceral features, but neurologic deterioration continued until death [42,49]. Recently, BMT in two patients with the attenuated phenotypes of Farber's disease and normal neurologic function led to significant reductions in the disease features, and the patients experienced improvement in their quality of life [50].

G_{M1} Gangliosidosis

G_{M1} gangliosidosis is a heterogeneous, progressive neurovisceral disorder that results from a deficiency of β-galactosidase, with resultant G_{M1} ganglioside, asialo-G_{M1} ganglioside, oligosaccharides, and keratan sulfate accumulation in a variety of tissues. The disease is autosomal recessive and caused by mutations in the β-galactosidase gene (*GLB1*). Mutations in *GLB1*, which maps to chromosome 3p21.33, are responsible for G_{M1}-gangliosidosis. The gene has been well characterized, and dozens of disease causing mutations have been identified, including missense, nonsense, duplication, insertion, and splice defect mutations [51–53].

The disorder has three variants (types 1, 2, and 3), based on age of onset, severity of neurologic involvement, presence or absence of visceral disease, and survival (Table 30.2). It has a prevalence of approximately 1 in 384,000 individuals [7]. The disease is allelic to another condition, type B Morquio's disease (a mucopolysaccharidosis lacking neurologic or hepatic features), but only G_{M1} gangliosidosis is discussed here.

Table 30.2: G_{M1} Gangliosidosis Variants

Parameter Sign	*Type 1*	*Type 2*	*Type 3*
Age at onset	0–6 mo	0.5–3 yr	Childhood/adulthood
Hepatosplenomegaly	++→++++	++→+++	+/−
CNS progression	++++	+++	+++
Cherry-red spot	+++	+/−	Rare
Dysmorphic facies	+++	+	+
Skeletal dysplasia	+++	+	+/−
Death	1–2 yr	5 yr	Adulthood

The symbols +, ++, +++, ++++ or − refer to progressively severe involvement from absent (−) to (→) very severe (++++) of different clinical manifestations.

In type 1, hepatomegaly is almost always present at or shortly after birth and is often associated with other features, such as generalized peripheral edema, ascites, or abnormalities in liver studies; however, the latter features may occur independent of hepatomegaly [54,55]. Hydrops fetalis may be observed [56]. Overt liver dysfunction is not usually present.

Adult-onset/chronic (type 3) G_{M1} gangliosidosis is a slowly progressive CNS disease. Dementia, ataxia, speech disturbances, dystonia, and parkinsonism are common neurologic features in this subtype [53,57].

In hepatocytes, neurons, glomerular cells, and myocytes, storage material accumulates, stains pink with hematoxylin–eosin, and is PAS positive [58,59]. Cells of monocyte/macrophage lineage, including Kupffer cells, also accumulate storage materials within affected organs [58,59]. Ultrastructurally, affected cells exhibit numerous pleomorphic storage material–laden lysosomes that appear empty or contain fibrillar and granular material [55,58,59]. The liver may appear normal by light microscopic examination, particularly in individuals with later-onset disease [60].

G_{M1} gangliosidosis is diagnosed by demonstrating severely decreased acid β-galactosidase activity in lymphocytes, fibroblasts, or plasma. Although the disease phenotype does not correlate well with the level of residual enzyme activity, individuals with greater degrees of residual enzyme activity have been noted to have later onset and milder disease [59]. The disease can be confirmed molecularly by the detection of *GLB1* mutations. The detection of complex carbohydrates in the urine, including keratan sulfate, adds further support to the diagnosis but is not diagnostic. The treatment for this disease is symptomatic management.

NIEMANN–PICK DISEASE TYPE C

Although originally classified with the acid sphingomyelinase deficiencies, NPA and NPB variants, Niemann–Pick disease type C (NPC) is now known to result from a lipid-trafficking defect that is unrelated to acid sphingomyelinase mutations. However, the NPC nomenclature is engrained in the literature, so it is used here.

Niemann–Pick type C is an autosomal recessive lysosomal storage disease with highly variable age of onset, pathologic features, and survival. Defective lipid trafficking, storage of lipids (unesterified cholesterol, phospholipids, sphingomyelin, and glycolipids) in lysosomes of affected cells, and secondary sphingomyelinase deficiency result in progressive neurocognitive dysfunction with visceral disease [61]. Mutations of two genes, *NPC1* and *NPC2*, are present in NPC. The *NPC1* and *NPC2* genes map to chromosomes 18q11-q12 and 14q24.3, respectively. More than 130 mutations in *NPC1* have been identified, most of which are private missense mutations, although frameshift, splice, and nonsense mutations are also described [62,63]. The *NPC1* gene product functions in the lysosomal/late-endosomal transport of cholesterol, glycolipids, and other materials [63]. The *NPC2* gene product is a lysosomal cholesterol transporter [64,65]. Abnormal function of the *NPC1* and *NPC2* proteins leads to accumulation of free cholesterol and glycolipids within the lysosomes as well as a secondary sphingomyelinase deficiency. Additionally, delayed low-density lipoprotein (LDL)-mediated regulatory responses appear to contribute to the disease process [63]. The prevalence of NPC is about 1 in 150,000, and the disease is pan-ethnic in nature [61]. Three variants are classified based on age of onset, CNS features, and survival: neonatal/early infantile, early childhood/juvenile, and adolescent/adult.

Of affected individuals, more than 90% have varying degrees of splenomegaly and/or hepatomegaly during their disease course, particularly those presenting during infancy and early childhood [66]. About 45–65% of affected children manifest liver disease/dysfunction, infantile cholestatic disease, or idiopathic neonatal hepatitis. In approximately 10% of such patients, acute liver failure develops and death occurs [67]. Those surviving show resolution by the second to fourth months of life. Hepatosplenomegaly may remain, but splenomegaly is usually predominant [66,67]. NPC was the most common metabolic/genetic cause of neonatal cholestasis at a North American center and the second most common genetic cause of liver disease in infancy in the United Kingdom, after α_1-antitrypsin deficiency [68,69].

The *neonatal/early infantile variant* accounts for around 20–30% of NPC cases [70,71]. The disease is a rapidly progressive neurovisceral disease, presenting within the first few months of life as developmental delay. Severe hepatic dysfunction can manifest prenatally as ascites or hydrops fetalis [66]. Those who recover from the liver dysfunction have progressive neurodegenerative disease with hypotonia, developmental delay, loss of acquired skills, spasticity, dystonia, dysphagia, seizures, and pyramidal signs [61,66,70].

Vertical supranuclear gaze palsy is classically observed in individuals with this disorder but is not as common in those with neonatal/infantile presentations as in those with other subtypes [61]. Generalized failure to thrive and growth retardation occur. Death often occurs from pulmonary infections by 3–5 years of age.

The *early childhood/juvenile NPC variant* accounts for about 50–70% of affected individuals [70,71]. Children with this variant may initially have normal development, but by early to late childhood, they exhibit neurocognitive deterioration, initially presenting as clumsiness, behavioral problems, and poor school performance [61,66]. Other signs of neurodegenerative disease gradually appear, including ataxia, vertical supranuclear gaze palsy, dystonia, seizures, cataplexy, dysarthria, and dysphagia [61,66,70]. Dysphagia is progressive and eventually makes oral feeding impossible [61]. Psychiatric disturbances, including psychosis, may develop around the time of puberty [61]. The individuals eventually become dependent on caregivers for all their needs. Survival into the teenage years and adulthood may occur, and death is usually the result of pulmonary infections [61]. Significant liver dysfunction is unusual. Additionally, a patient has been described with a nonneuronopathic form of the disease, primarily exhibiting splenomegaly [62,72].

The *adolescent/adult NPC* accounts for around 5–10% of cases [70,71] and presents with psychiatric and/or neurologic symptoms. The psychiatric symptoms often mimic depression or schizophrenia and may be quite debilitating [61,73]. Dementia often occurs, but at a slower rate of progression than in other subtypes of the disease. Vertical supranuclear gaze palsy may be subtle and difficult to recognize. Hepatomegaly and splenomegaly may be observed, but the latter is often more significant than in other variants. Death is usually a result of pneumonia [61].

Histopathologically, NPC exhibits accumulation of free cholesterol and sphingolipids within cells of monocyte/macrophage origin, in the visceral organs, and in neurons and glial cells of the nervous system [61]. The storage cells exhibit a foamy appearance and stain positively with PAS and filipin. Because of their microscopic appearance, storage cells of monocyte/macrophage origin are often referred to as "foam cells." Ultrastructurally, these lipid-laden cells contain numerous pleomorphic membrane–bound lipid inclusions, with structures varying from crystalline to electron-dense laminated inclusions [67,74,75].

At autopsy, the liver is enlarged and firm, with a surface that is pale yellow to green in appearance [75,76]. The neonatal liver disease may resemble idiopathic neonatal hepatitis with severe giant cell transformation of the hepatic cells and/or cholestasis, the latter suggesting biliary atresia [67,69,76,77]. Liver biopsies from 25 individuals with a history of neonatal liver disease showed cellular and canalicular cholestasis with biliary rosette formation with variable degrees of parenchymal damage and little hepatocellular necrosis but evidence of previous cell loss in the form of reticulin collapse. The latter was severe enough to produce bridging collapse and/or prominent fibrosis-induced fragmentation of the specimen core in half the cases. In addition to lobular inflammation, four patients had hematopoietic activity and multinucleated giant hepatocytes. Portal edema and ductular proliferation were also observed. In early biopsy specimens, the identification of storage cells was difficult because of the presence of activated Kupffer cells loaded with ceroid and bile pigment [67].

Liver biopsy specimens of 15 patients with a history of mild, persistent liver disease 1–8 years after resolution of fulminant signs showed that inflammation and cholestasis had vanished (12 of 15) but variable degrees of inactive postnecrotic fibrosis remained, with progression to cirrhosis in 5 cases. Storage material was noted in some hepatocytes, and storage cells were identified in the parenchyma and to a lesser extent within portal and fibrous areas [67]. In patients without a history of liver dysfunction, normal hepatic architecture was present but there was obvious storage in hepatocytes and Kupffer cells [67]. Hepatocellular carcinoma has been observed in one child with a history of infantile liver dysfunction and persisting liver disease [78].

NPC1 mutations account for approximately 95% of cases of NPC. Mutations in *NPC2* account for the remaining 5% of cases. Although mutations in both genes result in remarkably similar phenotypes, severe pulmonary disease is a unique complication in patients with *NPC2* mutations and is a cause of early demise [79].

Because of the variability in phenotypes within this disease, NPC is not always initially suspected. The diagnosis is often delayed because of the absence of hepatosplenomegaly or storage cells in the bone marrow at initial presentation. However, NPC should be considered in all cases of idiopathic neonatal hepatitis [69]. A biochemical diagnosis can be made by the demonstration of impaired cholesterol esterification and positive filipin staining in cultured fibroblasts [73]. Despite accumulation of sphingolipids in the lysosomes of affected cells, sphingomyelinase enzyme activity is normal. Molecular studies may also be employed for diagnosis; however, this method is often somewhat challenging, as many disease-causing mutations are private.

The treatment of patients with NPC relies on symptom management, particularly the neurologic and psychiatric symptoms. Cholesterol-lowering therapies [80] and BMT [81] have been studied; they had no impact on the neurologic dysfunction and ultimate disease course. Likewise, liver transplantation improved hepatic functioning, but the patient continued to exhibit progression of her disease [82].

DISORDERS OF GLYCOPROTEIN DEGRADATION

Fucosidosis, α-mannosidosis, sialidosis, and galactosialidosis are lysosomal storage diseases resulting from defects in glycoprotein degradation. Deficiencies of specific exoglycosidases result in an inability to remove terminal sugar moieties from glycoproteins and oligosaccharides and in the subsequent accumulation of excessive amounts of undigested substrates in the lysosomes of affected cells. All are inherited as autosomal recessive traits.

Fucosidosis

Fucosidosis is caused by a deficiency in the lysosomal enzyme α-L-fucosidase, which cleaves fucose moieties from the nonreducing end of a variety of oligosaccharides, glycoproteins, and glycolipids [83]. A deficiency in this enzyme results in cellular accumulation and urinary excretion of fucose-containing macromolecules, including oligosaccharides, glycoproteins, and glycolipids in the lysosomes of affected cells [83,84]. The gene for α-L-fucosidase (*FUCA1*) has been mapped to chromosome 1p34–1p36, and many types of mutations have been shown to result in fucosidosis, including point mutations, deletions, duplications, and insertions [85].

The clinical features include progressive neurologic deterioration and mental retardation, hearing loss, ocular abnormalities, coarse facial appearance, skeletal dysplasia, hepatosplenomegaly, frequent infections, growth retardation, and skin abnormalities including angiokeratoma and telangiectasia [84]. The disease is pan-ethnic, with about 100 cases being described worldwide. A relatively high number of patients have Italian and Mexican Indian (Colorado and New Mexico) backgrounds [84,85].

The two variants (types I and II) are probably more appropriately viewed as a continuum of severities [84]. In the more severe, type 1 presentations, patients experience neurologic dysfunction within the first year of life, often progressing to a vegetative, decorticate state, with death occurring before 6 years of age [83]. Conversely, individuals affected with type II disease are distinguished by a less severe and slower rate of progression of phenotypic features, usually beginning between 1 and 2 years of life, with longer survival (around three decades) [83,84]. Angiokeratoma and telangiectasia develop with age and are more common among those who survive longer. The other phenotypic features of fucosidosis are relatively consistent among individuals displaying both phenotypes.

The hepatic findings are quite mild and characterized by nonprogressive hepatomegaly and/or elevation in liver studies. Willems et al. [84] found that 40% of those affected with fucosidosis exhibited hepatomegaly and 25% of individuals had elevations in their liver enzymes independent of liver volume. Liver dysfunction does not occur and liver failure has not been described with fucosidosis.

By light microscopy, affected cells have a foamy appearance. Ultrastructurally, the storage material is quite heterogeneous in appearance (light and reticular, electron dense, or lamellar), a consequence of the many types of fucose-containing macromolecules stored in this disease [83,84,86].

Detailed and electron microscopic examination of liver biopsy tissue from a 3½-year old male with fucosidosis revealed well-preserved architecture and no signs of an inflammatory process or fibrosis. Many cell types, including Kupffer cells, hepatocytes, bile duct epithelial cells, and blood vessel endothelial cells, were packed with storage material–laden vacuoles. Foam cells were regularly seen in the portal areas. The sinusoids were frequently obscured by storage material–laden Kupffer cells, and isolated necrotic periportal cells were occasionally observed. Ultrastructurally, the storage material was heterogeneous in appearance [86].

Fucosidosis is often suspected upon recognition of the classic pattern of phenotypic features. Evidence of excessive urinary excretion of fucose-containing oligosaccharides and glycoproteins by thin-layer chromatography further supports the diagnosis. Diagnosis of fucosidosis requires the demonstration of severely diminished α-L-fucosidase activity (<5%) in cultured fibroblasts and white blood cells; however, the diagnosis must be made cautiously because 10% of the normal population carries a polymorphism that reduces the enzyme activity to 10–30% of control [84].

Treatment for this disorder relies mostly on symptomatic management. An 8-month-old boy received a BMT because of early neurologic involvement by fucosidosis. Despite evidence of mild neurodevelopmental delay, the procedure was considered a success as he consequently exhibited a less severe phenotype than did his nontransplanted sibling [87]. Similarly, an 11-month-old girl was alive 4 years after BMT despite continued neurodevelopmental delay [88]. Gene and enzyme therapies are not available for this disorder.

α-Mannosidosis

α-Mannosidosis is an autosomal recessive disorder caused by a deficiency of the lysosomal enzyme α-mannosidase, resulting in an accumulation of mannose-rich macromolecules in affected cell types. α-Mannosidase cleaves terminal mannose moieties from oligosaccharides and glycoproteins. The deficiency of α-mannosidase leads to an accumulation of α-mannosyl–terminated compounds in lysosomal cells and excretion in urine. The gene for α-mannosidase (*MANB*) has been mapped to chromosome 19p13-q12. α-Mannosidosis results from a variety of disease-causing mutations of *MANB*, including splice-site, missense, nonsense, insertion, and deletion. The missense mutation R750W has increased frequency (21%) among Europeans [89]. The variable phenotypic features include progressive mental deterioration, coarse facial appearance, deafness, ocular abnormalities, skeletal dysplasia, recurrent infections, hernias, and hepatosplenomegaly. The disease has a prevalence of approximately 1 in 500,000 [7].

Two variants (types I and II) are recognized based on age of onset and severity of disease. Individuals exhibiting type I α-mannosidosis present in infancy with severe, rapidly progressive mental deterioration and clinical features, and death often occurs within the first decade of life [83,90]. Type II α-mannosidosis has a more slowly progressive phenotype with normal early development, but mental deterioration, hearing loss, and other clinical features are apparent by childhood or adolescence [83,90,91]. Hepatomegaly is present, particularly in type I, but hepatic dysfunction does not occur.

Liver biopsies show well-preserved architecture with no signs of inflammation. Fibrosis may be present in the portal areas and around Kupffer cells. Kupffer cells, hepatocytes, bile duct epithelial cells, and blood vessel endothelial cells are engorged with storage material–laden vacuoles. Foam cells are consistently found in the portal areas. The sinusoids may be obscured by engorged Kupffer cells. The storage material is heterogeneous by election microscopy [92].

Definitive diagnosis of the disorder requires the demonstration of low levels of α-mannosidase activity in cultured fibroblasts or white blood cells or the presence of disease-causing mutations in both *MANB* alleles [83].

Symptomatic management is the mainstay of treatment. BMT in affected children (<2 years of age) has led to resolution of the sinopulmonary disease and organomegaly, improvement in the skeletal disease, and variable effects on neurocognitive function [93,94].

Sialidosis

Sialidosis is an autosomal recessive disorder caused by a deficiency of the lysosomal enzyme neuraminidase and the resultant accumulation of sialic acid–rich molecules in the lysosomes and the excretion of these molecules in the urine. Its clinical features vary according to age of onset, organ involvement, and severity of symptoms. The disease is very rare, occurring in about 1 of 4,000,000 live births [7].

The variants of sialidosis (types I and II) vary in age of onset and progression but share progressive CNS disease and macular cherry-red spots. Hepatosplenomegaly is universal in the early-onset (type II) variant. Liver dysfunction does not occur. Many infants with type II disease are stillborn [83,95,96].

The gene for lysosomal neuraminidase (*NEU1*) has been mapped to chromosome 6p21.3, and mutations in this gene are responsible for both variants of sialidosis. The enzyme exists as a multienzyme complex with β-galactosidase and protective protein/cathepsin A. The latter is critical for lysosomal transport and proper function of lysosomal neuraminidase [97,98].

Neuraminidase catalyzes the cleavage of terminal $\alpha(2,3)$- and $\alpha(2,6)$-linked sialic acid residues from numerous sialic acid–rich oligosaccharides and glycoproteins [98]. A deficiency in this enzyme results in cellular accumulation of sialic acid–containing glycopeptides and oligosaccharides in the lysosomes of affected cells, with excretion in urine.

The liver histology in type II disease shows a well-preserved architecture and membrane-bound vacuoles containing heterogeneous material in the hepatocytes, Kupffer cells, and vascular endothelial cells. The sinusoids may be widened and occluded by Kupffer cells and free foamy material. There was no evidence of necrosis, fibrosis, or inflammatory infiltration in several studies [86,99]. Hepatomegaly is not a feature of type I disease, but storage material can be observed by light microscopy [83].

Definitive diagnosis of the disorder requires the demonstration of low levels of lysosomal neuraminidase activity in cultured fibroblasts [83]. Sialidosis is often suspected when the phenotypic features described above are observed. Galactosialidosis, a similar disorder with defective β-galactosidase and neuraminidase enzyme activities, may confuse the diagnosis. The presence of large amounts of mannose-containing oligosaccharides and glycopeptides in the urine support the diagnosis. Therapy is symptomatic.

Galactosialidosis

Galactosialidosis is an autosomal recessively inherited disorder characterized by deficiencies of β-galactosidase and lysosomal neuraminidase activity. It is caused by defects in the protein protective protein/cathepsin A (PPCA), with a resultant accumulation of sialic acid–rich oligosaccharides and glycoproteins and gangliosides in affected cells and excretion of sialic acid–rich oligosaccharides in the urine [97]. Galactosialidosis has a prevalence of approximately 1 in 2.5 million in the Netherlands [2].

The disorder is classified into three variants based on age of onset, organ involvement, and severity of disease: *early infantile–*, *late infantile–*, and *juvenile/adult-onset disease* [97]. Because the disorder is partially a result of lysosomal neuraminidase deficiency, many of its phenotypic characteristics are similar to those of sialidosis. In the early infantile phenotype of disease, hepatosplenomegaly develops early and the liver can reach volumes greater than two times normal [100]. Elevations in liver studies may be observed, but overt liver dysfunction does not occur [101]. Hepatosplenomegaly of lesser degrees than that seen in the early infantile presentation may be observed in the later-onset presentations, but liver dysfunction does not occur. Hepatocytes, Kupffer cells, and epithelial cells contain numerous storage material–containing vacuoles [100]. Ultrastructurally, the storage material is quite heterogeneous in appearance [100].

The gene encoding protective protein/cathepsin A (*PPCA*) has been mapped to chromosome 20q13.1. Protective protein/cathepsin A forms a multienzyme complex with β-galactosidase and lysosomal neuraminidase and is required for proper intracellular transport and function of both enzymes [97,98]. Additionally, it has separate enzymatic functions [102–105].

A diagnosis of galactosialidosis requires the demonstration of decreased β-galactosidase, lysosomal neuraminidase, and cathepsin A enzyme activity in white blood cells or cultured skin fibroblasts [97]. Therapy relies on symptom management.

GLYCOGEN STORAGE DISEASE TYPE II (POMPE'S DISEASE)

Glycogen storage disease type II (Pompe's disease) is an autosomal recessive disorder caused by a deficiency of the lysosomal enzyme acid α-glucosidase (GAA), which results in an abnormal accumulation of glycogen in the lysosomes of cells. The gene for acid α-glucosidase (*GAA*) maps to chromosome 17q25.2-q25.3. Mutations that lead to the least amounts of residual enzyme activity are associated with infantile-onset disease and those that result in greater amounts of enzyme activity cause juvenile- and adult-onset disease [106,107].

The clinical phenotypes result primarily from glycogen accumulation in cardiac, skeletal, and smooth muscles. Many other cells contain excessive glycogen, including neurons, but this role in the disease process is not known. The three phenotypes vary by age of onset and severity and progression of symptoms: *infantile, childhood/juvenile, and adult onset.* The disease is rare, with a frequency of 1 in 14,000 to 1 in 300,000, depending on the geographic area or ethnic group [106].

The "classic" infantile phenotype of Pompe's disease is a severe, progressive disease that presents within the first few months of life with feeding problems, poor weight gain, cardiac disease, respiratory difficulties, macroglossia, and generalized myopathy [106,108,109]. Despite the presence of a severe myopathic disease, skeletal muscles are often firm and hypertrophic in appearance [106]. Cardiomegaly results from a progressive hypertrophic cardiomyopathy that affects the walls of both ventricles and the interventricular septum, with diminished volume of the ventricular chambers (Figure 30.4) [106]. Moderate hepatomegaly without liver dysfunction is noted in approximately 90% of cases [108]. Impairment of the respiratory muscles results in respiratory difficulties, and many patients require assisted ventilation. Mental development is considered grossly normal [106], but significant glycogen accumulation is present in neurons [110]. The disease is rapidly progressive, and death occurs at a median age of 9 months [106,109]. Residual tissue acid α-glucosidase levels are less than 1% of normal in affected patients [109].

A less common phenotype with early onset has been described with less severe cardiac disease. Such patients show progressive muscle weakness and hypotonia within the first few months of life and frequently require ventilatory assistance but survive for prolonged periods [111].

The childhood/juvenile-onset phenotype of Pompe's disease is primarily a myopathic variant with onset in the first decade. Cardiac disease is uncommon [106]. Typically, delayed motor milestones, progressive proximal muscle weakness, and involvement of the respiratory muscles are present [106]. Pulmonary compromise may lead to the need for ventilatory assistance, particularly during sleep. Many individuals become wheelchair bound. Moderate hepatomegaly without liver dysfunction is observed in up to 30% of affected patients [109]. The levels of residual enzyme activity in tissue are frequently less than 10% of normal [109]. Death usually results from respiratory failure [106].

The adult-onset phenotype of Pompe's disease is a slowly progressive proximal myopathy, with respiratory insufficiency in about 30% of patients with onset in the third to sixth decades [106]. However, many patients recall symptoms from childhood [112]. The lower extremities are often more significantly involved than the upper extremities, and regional variation in muscle involvement occurs [106]. Cardiac complications are

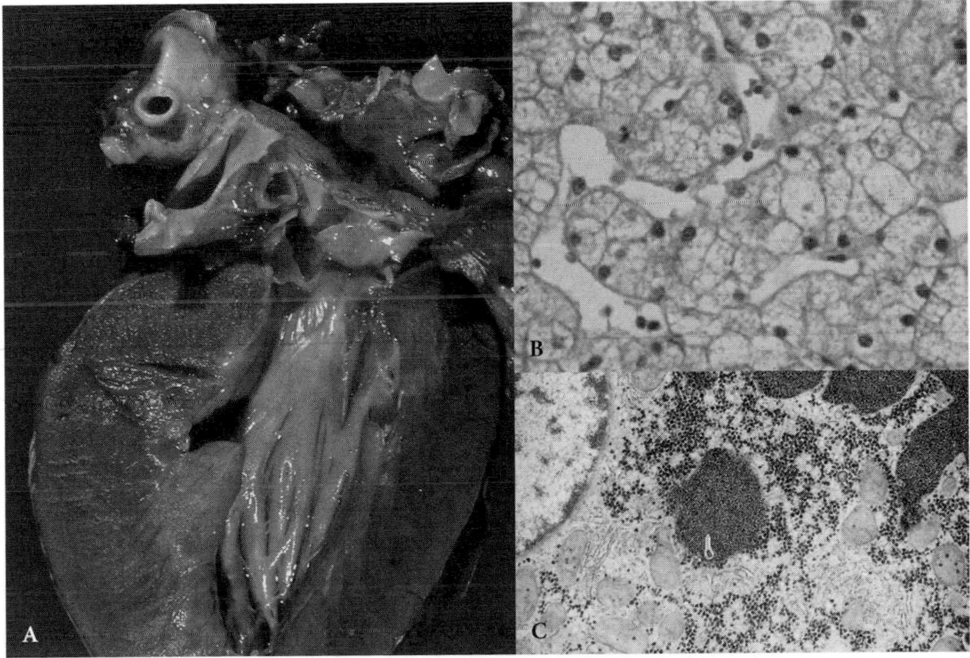

Figure 30.4. Cardiac and hepatic involvement in glycogen storage disease type II (Pompe's disease). (**A**) The massively hypertrophied myocardium of a patient younger than 1 year with infantile Pompe's disease. (**B**) Photomicrograph showing massive glycogen accumulation in hepatocytes and Kupffer cells. (Hematoxylin and eosin staining.) (**C**) Ultrastructure showing lysosomal and free cytoplasmic glycogen particles. (Magnification 20,000×.) (Courtesy of K. Bove.)

not common, and moderate hepatomegaly without liver dysfunction is observed in around 30% of patients [109]. Serum aminotransferase levels may be elevated in this population, but this may represent enzyme release from muscle tissues [113]. Individuals with adult-onset disease have higher levels of residual enzyme activity (possibly 40% of normal) than those with infantile- or childhood/juvenile-onset disease [109]. Like those with the juvenile-onset phenotype, many individuals are eventually wheelchair bound and impairment of the respiratory muscles frequently results in respiratory difficulties, often requiring ventilatory support, particularly during sleep [106,112]. Death usually occurs from respiratory failure.

Pompe's disease results from the accumulation of glycogen of normal structure within lysosomes and cytoplasm of affected cells, including liver, heart, smooth and skeletal muscle, and nervous system [106]. The storage material stains positively with PAS. Within the liver, glycogen is abundant (Figure 30.4) and is in the form of scattered cytoplasmic rosettes and smaller beta and alpha particles in the lysosomes (Figure 30.4) [106,114]. The liver architecture remains intact.

Pompe's disease is suspected in infants with massive cardiomegaly and hypotonia/muscle weakness. The diagnosis may be much more elusive in individuals with muscle weakness and lack of severe cardiac involvement. Diagnosis requires the detection of markedly diminished acid α-glucosidase activity in cultured fibroblasts and/or muscle tissue. However, the levels of residual acid α-glucosidase in adult patients can approach levels observed in unaffected carriers and the lower end values found in normal individuals, confusing the diagnosis [106]. The diagnosis can be confirmed by the discovery of disease-causing mutations in both alleles of *GAA*.

Bone marrow transplantation has been performed but has been unsuccessful [115]. Phase 3 enzyme therapy trials have been completed and indicate significant efficacy and safety [116–121]. This therapy is now FDA- and EMEA-approved. All the patients treated with recombinant enzymes survived beyond the expected survival period in nontreated individuals and showed significant improvement in cardiac structure and function. Progress in motor development was more variable; however, the results suggest that patients who begin enzyme replacement therapy at an early age experience greater improvement in motor function than do those who begin receiving enzyme replacement therapy at later ages.

Supportive therapy is an important component in the treatment of this disease and can improve the quality of life and minimize complications. However, it does not alter the disease course [109].

LYSOSOMAL ACID LIPASE DEFICIENCY (WOLMAN'S DISEASE AND CHOLESTERYL ESTER STORAGE DISEASE)

Deficiency of lysosomal acid lipase leads to the accumulation of cholesteryl esters, triglycerides, and other lipids within the lysosomes. Two major phenotypes include Wolman's disease and cholesteryl ester storage disease (CESD).

The gene for lysosomal acid lipase (*LIPA*) maps to chromosome 10q23.2-q23.3. Wolman's disease results from mutations in the *LIPA* gene that cause nearly complete deficiency of residual enzyme activity. Conversely, CESD results when residual lysosomal acid lipase enzyme activity is retained [122].

Wolman's disease presents neonatally with feeding difficulties; persistent, forceful vomiting; profuse, watery diarrhea; abdominal distention; progressive hepatomegaly; and failure to thrive due to a malabsorption syndrome. The malabsorption syndrome does not improve with medical interventions or changes in diet and may necessitate total parenteral nutrition. Generalized lymphadenopathy and splenomegaly are also present. Neurologic development is not normal, but specific signs related to CNS dysfunction are uncommon and may relate to malnutrition and severe disability [123].

Radiographic evaluation reveals enlarged adrenal glands with punctuate calcifications. Laboratory studies reveal progressive anemia, vacuolization of the lymphocytes, and elevated serum aminotransferase levels indicative of hepatic involvement. Plasma cholesterol and triglyceride levels are usually normal [124]. Death occurs within the first year of life. Wolman's disease is rare and has an incidence of about 1 in 500,000 [7].

Cholesteryl ester storage disease is a heterogeneous disorder that can present between infancy and adulthood. Hepatomegaly is the primary and sometimes sole finding in this phenotype. Hepatic involvement is often progressive, with pathologic features of steatosis and fibrosis with progression to cirrhosis. Acute or chronic liver failure may occur. Some patients affected with CESD may have a more severe course with symptoms much like those in Wolman's disease, including vomiting, watery diarrhea, failure to thrive, adrenal calcification, and liver dysfunction [125,126]. Laboratory studies often reveal hyperlipidemia, particularly type IIB hyperlipoproteinemia, and elevated aminotransferase levels.

Progressive, premature atherosclerosis occurs and may result in vascular compromise. Age of death is variable and depends on severity of hepatic and atherosclerotic disease, but survival into adulthood is common. The incidence of homozygotes for the most common mutation in CESD ($\Delta 254\text{–}277_1$) approached 1 in 300,000 in northwestern Germany [123].

Cholesteryl esters and triglycerides accumulate in the liver and other affected organs [127]. This storage material stains positively with oil red O and Sudan black, and in frozen sections, cholesterol crystals are observed under polarized light. In fixed tissues, clefts or voids can be visualized, representing lipid that was dissolved during tissue fixation. This storage material has an equally heterogeneous appearance under the electron microscope [123].

The livers in patients with Wolman's disease are markedly enlarged (often greater than two times the normal size), firm in consistency, and yellow in coloration, with a cut surface that is greasy. Hepatic architecture may be preserved early in the course but may become quite distorted [124]. Hepatocytes and Kupffer cells are engorged with lipid-laden vacuoles (Figure 30.5). Foam cells are present in the portal and periportal areas and tend to cluster between parenchymal cells. Infiltration with

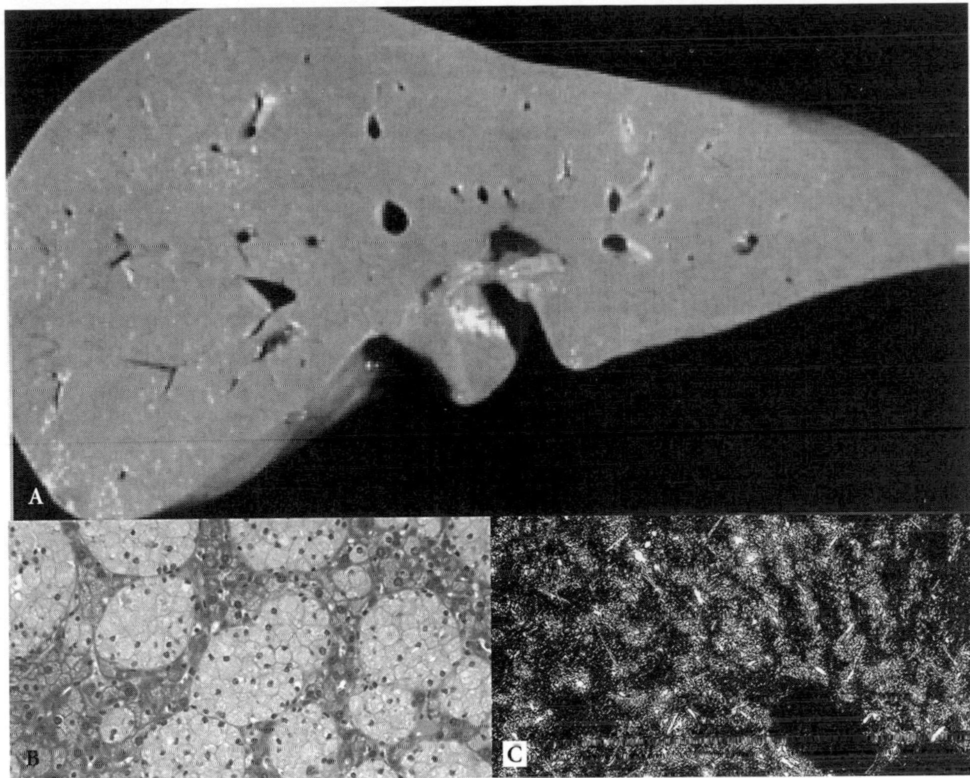

Figure 30.5. Liver from a lysosomal acid lipase–deficient human (CESD, **A**) and mouse (**B** and **C**). (**A**) Typical orange-yellow color of the liver from a patient with CESD. (**B**) Clusters of engorged Kupffer cells are evident as is the storage of neutral fats (cholesteryl esters and triglycerides) in hepatocytes. (Magnification 200×.) (**C**) Polarized light micrograph of lysosomal acid lipase–deficient mouse liver section. (Courtesy of H. Du.) Cholesterol crystals are evident as are numerous other birefringent bodies. Livers in patients with Wolman's disease and CESD are similar. For color reproduction, see Color Plate 30.5.

inflammatory cells occurs. Portal and periportal fibrosis may be observed and often progresses to micronodular cirrhosis. Ultrastructural examination reveals lipid accumulation, particularly in the lysosomes, with a heterogeneous globular to crystalline appearance [123–125,127–133].

The gross appearance of the liver in CESD is similar to that in individuals with Wolman's disease but is often more orange than yellow in coloration (Figure 30.5) [124]. Fatty infiltration of hepatocytes may be profound and may mimic nonalcoholic steatosis. Kupffer cells and foam cells are involved similarly to those in Wolman's disease. Periportal accumulation of lymphocytes and plasma cells may be quite dramatic. Fibrosis eventually develops and may progress to micronodular cirrhosis [123–126,134].

Both diseases result from defects in lysosomal acid lipase. This enzyme catalyzes the breakdown of cholesteryl esters and triglycerides that are delivered to liposomes by LDL receptor–mediated endocytosis [123]. Cleavage of these substrates leads to liberation of free cholesterol and fatty acids that are transported out of the lysosomes and into the cytoplasm. Disruption of this major pathway for neutral lipid metabolism leads to a dysregulation of the negative and positive feedback mechanisms that normally ensure intracellular cholesterol homeostasis [135,136].

Wolman's disease should be suspected in infants with a combination of gastrointestinal symptoms, hepatomegaly, and bilateral adrenal cortical calcifications [123]. Likewise, CESD should be suspected in individuals with hyperlipidemia and unexplained hepatomegaly with or without dysfunction. Diagnosis can be made by the detection of significantly diminished lysosomal acid lipase activity in leukocytes or cultured skin fibroblasts and the demonstration of disease-causing mutations in both copies of *LIPA*.

There are no specific therapies for Wolman's disease or CESD. Treatment primarily involves symptomatic management, particularly to prevent malnutrition and vitamin deficiencies. BMT has been performed in Wolman's disease, but mortality of BMT may depend on the initial status of the Wolman's disease patient. A surviving individual exhibited improvement in clinical status and normalization of lysosomal acid lipase enzyme levels in peripheral blood cells [137,138]. Orthotopic liver transplantation has been reported in two individuals with CESD, resulting in improvement in their hepatic function [122,139]. Multiple studies to determine the efficacy of 3-hydroxy-3-methylglutaryl coenzyme A (HMG-CoA) reductase inhibitors in treating reductase inhibitors in treating CESD have been performed, with mixed results; further research is necessary to determine the efficacy of this treatment for CESD [140–143]. The major benefit appears to be a decrease in serum cholesterol. The results from enzyme replacement and gene therapy studies in mice have been encouraging [144,145].

MUCOPOLYSACCHARIDOSES

The mucopolysaccharidoses (MPSs) are a group of seven lysosomal storage diseases characterized by a deficiency of various lysosomal enzymes that catalyze the degradation of glycosaminoglycans (previously called mucopolysaccharides). All are autosomal recessive in nature except for Hunter's disease (MPS II), which is X-linked. Depending on the enzyme affected, a single glycosaminoglycan or combinations of glycosaminoglycans accumulate in cells and urine.

The MPSs are quite variable with regard to age of onset, organ involvement, severity, and survival (Table 30.3). Many features are shared, including progressive course, coarse facial appearance, hearing loss, vision impairment, hepatosplenomegaly, obstructive airway disease, skeletal abnormalities, joint stiffness, and cardiac disease, with variable degrees of severity. Mental retardation and neurologic deterioration are variable between and among the types of MPSs [146]. Readers are referred to other sources [146] for a comprehensive review. The combined frequency of MPSs is approximately 1 in 22,500 in the Australian population, accounting for 35% of all lysosomal storage diseases [7].

Hepatosplenomegaly is observed in many cases of MPS, but hepatic dysfunction is not usually a feature associated with the MPSs. Liver volume assessments show about a one- to twofold increase in children and adults with late-onset variants of MPS I [147] and MPS VI [148].

Variable cytoplasmic vacuolization from deposition of incompletely degraded glycosaminoglycans is present in most organs, including the liver, although this varies according to the individual and type of MPS. Within the liver, storage material accumulates within the hepatocytes and Kupffer cells. There is an abundance of sinusoidal Kupffer cells, contributing to an obliteration of the sinusoids [149]. Ultrastructurally, these vacuoles contain heterogeneous storage material [149–151]. Significant fibrosis extending from portal to portal space and encircling the lobules, with areas of hepatocyte disintegration, may be present in patients with MPS I, II, or III [149].

The diagnosis of an MPS is suggested by the presenting phenotypic features. The observation of characteristic patterns of urine glycosaminoglycans aids in the diagnosis and helps pinpoint the enzyme deficiency. Definitive diagnosis requires the observation of deficient enzyme activity in serum, lymphocytes, or cultured fibroblasts, but residual enzyme activity is not a valid predictor of disease outcome [152]. Molecular techniques may also be employed to diagnose these disorders but requires identification of unusual mutations.

Bone marrow transplantation has been performed in several of the MPS diseases. Success in stabilizing or improving clinical features has varied with the MPS variant. The CNS dysfunction in MPS II can be ameliorated or stabilized if BMT is conducted early in the disease course (<24 months). Successful BMT outcomes for CNS function have been controversial in other MPS diseases [153–157].

Enzyme therapy has been approved for MPS I, II, and VI. Enzyme therapy for MPS I, using recombinant human α-L-iduronidase, has been approved for treating the visceral disease in all MPS I variants [147,158]. Liver volumes normalize in 70–80% of patients by 26 weeks of therapy. The recombinant enzyme does not cross the blood–brain barrier; therefore, enzyme therapy has no direct effect on neurologic function [147,158].

Enzyme replacement therapy with arylsulfatase B for MPS VI (Maroteaux–Lamy syndrome) is approved as a safe and efficacious therapy as assessed by endurance, mobility, and joint function [148]. MPS VI does not involve the CNS directly. The liver volumes normalized in four of five patients with hepatomegaly and were reduced in five of five patients [148].

MUCOLIPIDOSIS TYPES II AND III

Mucolipidosis types II and III are progressive, autosomal recessively inherited lysosomal storage diseases that result from diminished trafficking of soluble lysosomal enzymes via the mannose-6-phosphate system [159]. These phenotypes have a combined frequency of 1 in 325,000 [7].

Mucolipidosis types II and III are caused by deficient activity of uridine diphosphate–*N*-acetylglucosamine:lysosomal enzyme *N*-acetylglucosaminyl-1-phosphotransferase (phosphotransferase). Phosphotransferase contributes to the addition of a mannose-6-phosphate recognition marker on lysosomal enzymes, and it is composed of three subunits, α_2, β_2, and γ_2 [159]. Evidence suggests that the α and β subunits serve as the catalytic components of the enzyme and the γ subunit serves in substrate recognition [160]. The genes for the α and β subunits (*GNPTA*) and γ subunit (*GNPTAG*) are mapped at chromosomes 12p and 16p, respectively [160,161]. Mucolipidosis type II results from mutations in *GNPTA* (161), whereas mucolipidosis type III results from mutations in *GNPTA* and *GNPTAG* [160,162]. This recognition marker is critical for the transport of lysosomal enzymes from the Golgi apparatus to lysosomes in mesenchymal cells, and in its absence, lysosomal enzymes are secreted out of cells. The result is a deficiency of multiple lysosomal enzymes and in many, but not all, cell types, accumulations of undigested substrates within the lysosomes of affected cells [159].

In comparison, hepatocytes, Kupffer cells, and leukocytes demonstrate nearly normal levels of intracellular lysosomal enzyme activity, suggesting that alternate lysosomal enzyme transportation pathways are active within these cell types and providing a possible explanation for the diminished severity of pathologic features observed in these cells [159].

Mucolipidosis type II is often referred to as I-cell disease because of characteristic intracellular inclusions in cultured fibroblasts. The progressive phenotype presents from the

Table 30.3: The Mucopolysaccharidoses

Type	*Enzyme Defect*	*Glycosaminoglycan Stored*	*Clinical Features*
MPS I-H, severe (Hurler)	α-L-iduronidase	Dermatan sulfate, heparan sulfate	Mental retardation, corneal clouding, hepatosplenomegaly, severe dysostosis multiplex, joint stiffness, growth retardation, death in childhood
MPS I-H/S, moderate (Hurler–Scheie)	α-L-iduronidase	Dermatan sulfate, heparan sulfate	Normal intelligence, corneal clouding, hepatosplenomegaly, moderate dysostosis multiplex, joint stiffness, growth retardation, survival into adulthood
MPS I-S, attenuated (Scheie)	α-L-iduronidase	Dermatan sulfate, heparan sulfate	Normal intelligence to mild mental retardation, corneal clouding, hepatosplenomegaly, mild dysostosis multiplex, joint stiffness, normal stature, survival into adulthood
MPS II, mild (Hunter)	Iduronate-2-sulfatase	Dermatan sulfate, heparan sulfate	Normal intelligence, hepatosplenomegaly, moderate dysostosis multiplex, stiff joints, growth retardation, survival into adulthood
MPS II, severe (Hunter)	Iduronate-2-sulfatase	Dermatan sulfate, heparan sulfate	Mental retardation, retinal degeneration, hepatosplenomegaly, moderate dysostosis multiplex, stiff joints, survival into teens
MPS III A (Sanfilippo A)	Heparan *N*-sulfatase (sulfamidase)	Heparan sulfate	Neurologic deterioration, mental retardation, behavioral problems, hepatosplenomegaly, mild dysostosis multiplex, stiff joints
MPS III B (Sanfilippo B)	α-*N*-acetylglucosaminidase	Heparan sulfate	Similar to MPS III A
MPS III C (Sanfilippo C)	Acetyl CoA:α glucosaminide *N*-acetyltransferase	Heparan sulfate	Similar to MPS III A
MPS III D (Sanfilippo D)	*N*-acetylglucosamine 6-sulfatase	Heparan sulfate	Similar to MPS III A
MPS IV A (Morquio A)	Galactose 6-sulfatase (*N*-acetylgalactosamine 6-sulfatase)	Keratan sulfate, chondroitin 6-sulfate	Normal intelligence, corneal clouding, hepatosplenomegaly, severe dysostosis multiplex, survival into adulthood
MPS IV B (Morquio B)	β-Galactosidase	Keratan sulfate	Normal intelligence, corneal clouding, hepatosplenomegaly, severe dysostosis multiplex, survival into adulthood
MPS VI (Maroteaux-Lamy)	*N*-acetylgalactosamine 4-sulfatase (arylsulfatase B)	Dermatan sulfate	Mental retardation, corneal clouding, hepatosplenomegaly, severe dysostosis multiplex, variable survival
MPS VII (Sly)	β-Glucuronidase	Dermatan sulfate, heparan sulfate, chondroitin 4-, 6-sulfates	Mental retardation, no corneal opacities, hepatosplenomegaly, severe dysostosis multiplex, growth retardation, variable survival
MPS IX	Hyaluronidase	Hyaluronic acid	Short stature, periarticular soft tissue masses

neonatal period to the first year with neurologic deterioration and visceral disease, including failure to thrive, growth retardation, facial coarsening, skin thickening, corneal clouding, cardiac disease, abdominal distention, hepatosplenomegaly, skeletal dysplasia and anomalies, and joint contractures [159,163–165]. Hydrops fetalis has also been reported [166]. Death usually occurs in the first decade of life from cardiopulmonary disease [159].

Mucolipidosis type III, pseudo-Hurler polydystrophy, is a less severe and more slowly progressive phenotype of mucolipidosis that presents in childhood with variable degrees of growth retardation, coarse facial appearance, corneal clouding, cardiac valvular abnormalities, skin thickening, skeletal dysplasia, joint contractures and destruction, and carpal tunnel syndrome [159,160,162,167]. Mental retardation or learning disability occurs in approximately 50% of patients but is not as severe as in the type II phenotype [168]. Hepatosplenomegaly is not common, and the disease is not associated with liver dysfunction. Mucolipidosis type III is compatible with survival into adulthood [159,160].

In mucolipidosis II, hepatomegaly presents neonatally or shortly afterward and may be associated with elevated liver enzyme levels, but overt hepatic dysfunction is rarely observed. One infant with mucolipidosis type II presented with cholestasis and biochemical and histologic evidence of liver dysfunction. The cholestasis improved with ursodeoxycholic acid therapy [163].

The hepatic architecture remains intact, but storage material is noted in portal mononuclear cells and sinusoidal Kupffer cells, but to lesser degrees in hepatocytes [164,165,169]. Ultrastructurally, these inclusions are membrane bound and heterogeneous in appearance, appearing fibrogranular, globular, and membranous [159,169].

The diagnosis of mucolipidosis types II and III is made by finding deficient activity of multiple lysosomal enzymes in cultured fibroblasts and massive elevations of multiple lysosomal enzymes in fibroblast culture medium or serum. Additionally, phosphotransferase enzyme activity can be directly measured in white blood cells or in cultured fibroblasts. Mucolipidosis types II and III cannot be differentiated on the basis of residual enzyme activity or localization because these are similar in both disorders [159].

There are no specific treatments for either form of mucolipidosis, and therapy relies on symptom management. Physical therapy may diminish the progression of joint immobility in those with type III disease [159]. Limited experience with BMT suggests some potential benefits [163,170].

MULTIPLE SULFATASE DEFICIENCY

Multiple sulfatase deficiency is an autosomal recessive disorder characterized by impaired activity of all known cellular sulfatases caused by deficiency of an enzyme essential for posttranslational modification of an active site cysteine common to all members of the sulfatase family [171]. The phenotype is heterogeneous and combines features of the individual sulfatase deficiency disorders – metachromatic leukodystrophy, multiple mucopolysaccharidoses, X-linked ichthyosis, and chondrodysplasia punctata [171–177]. It is a very rare disease, occurring in 1 in 1.4 million people [7].

The disorder presents neonatally or during infancy with varying degrees of progressive neurologic dysfunction, developmental delays, growth retardation, facial coarsening, corneal clouding, hepatosplenomegaly, cardiac disease, ichthyosis, skeletal abnormalities, and stiff joints [172–177]. Detailed histology on liver involvement is not available, but hepatomegaly and mild elevations in liver enzyme levels occur. Microscopic studies of liver biopsy tissue in an infant with congenital multiple sulfatase deficiency and hepatomegaly exhibited normal architecture without evidence of mucopolysaccharide accumulation [173].

Sulfatases catalyze hydrolysis of sulfate ester bonds from a wide variety of substrates, including glycosaminoglycans, sulfolipids, and steroid sulfates [178]. FGly-generating enzyme, encoded by the gene *SUMF1* [179,180], activates all the known sulfatases by the oxidation of a highly conserved cysteine molecule to C_α-formylglycine [181,182]. This posttranslational modification is essential for the proper functioning of all sulfatases [180]. In individuals with multiple sulfatase deficiency, impaired activity of the sulfatases results in an accumulation of substrates within the lysosomes and cytoplasm of affected tissues [171]. Liver histology is not well documented.

Multiple sulfatase deficiency is diagnosed biochemically based on the characteristic pattern of deficient multiple sulfatase enzyme activities in leukocytes, plasma, and cultured fibroblasts. Excess mucopolysaccharides and sulfatides are usually identified in tissue samples and urine, further supporting the diagnosis. There is no known treatment for multiple sulfatase deficiency, and therapy relies on symptomatic management; however, studies into therapies for individual sulfatase deficiencies are ongoing.

NOTE

Enzyme therapy using recombinant human iduronate-2-sulfatase, idursulfase, has been approved by the FDA and EMEA for the treatment of MPS II. A randomized, double-blinded, placebo-controlled, phase II/III clinical trial spanning 53 weeks demonstrated significantly reduced hepatosplenomegaly, improved walking distance and pulmonary function, and decreased urine glycosaminoglycan excretion when the drug was infused weekly. The drug was generally well tolerated and side effects were minimal [183].

REFERENCES

1. Sabatini DD, Adesnik MB. The biogenesis of membranes and organelles. In: Scriver CR, Beaudet AL, Sly WS, et al., eds. The metabolic and molecular bases of inherited disease. New York: McGraw-Hill, 2001:433–517.
2. Poorthuis BJ, Wevers RA, Kleijer WJ, et al. The frequency of lysosomal storage diseases in The Netherlands. Hum Genet 1999;105:151–6.
3. Grabowski GA, Hopkin RJ. Enzyme therapy for lysosomal storage disease: principles, practice, and prospects. Annu Rev Genomics Hum Genet 2003;4:403–36.
4. Proia RL, Wu YP. Blood to brain to the rescue. J Clin Invest 2004;113:1108–10.
5. Degroote S, Wolthoorn J, van Meer G. The cell biology of glycosphingolipids. Semin Cell Dev Biol 2004;15:375–87.

6. Beutler E, Grabowski GA. Gaucher disease. In: Scriver CR, Beaudet AL, Sly WS, et al., eds. The metabolic and molecular bases of inherited disease. New York: McGraw Hill, 2001:3635–68.
7. Meikle PJ, Hopwood JJ, Clague AE, Carey WF. Prevalence of lysosomal storage disorders. JAMA 1999;281:249–54.
8. Grabowski GA, Kolodny EH, Weinreb NJ, et al. Gaucher disease: phenotypic and genetic variation. In: Scriver C, Beaudet A, Sly W, Valle D, eds. The metabolic and molecular bases of inherited disease. New York: McGraw-Hill, 2006: in press.
9. Malhotra A, Boxer M, Mistry PK. Hepatic response to enzyme replacement therapy (ERT) with mannose-terminated glucocerebrosidase in type 1 Gaucher disease. Hepatology 2004; 40:161.
10. Lachmann RH, Wight DG, Lomas DJ, et al. Massive hepatic fibrosis in Gaucher's disease: clinico-pathological and radiological features. Q J Med 2000;93:237–44.
11. James SP, Stromeyer FW, Chang C, Barranger JA. Liver abnormalities in patients with Gaucher's disease. Gastroenterology 1981;80:126–33.
12. James SP, Stromeyer FW, Stowens DW, Barranger JA. Gaucher disease: hepatic abnormalities in 25 patients. Prog Clin Biol Res 1982;95:131–42.
13. Perel Y, Bioulac-Sage P, Chateil JF, et al. Gaucher's disease and fatal hepatic fibrosis despite prolonged enzyme replacement therapy. Pediatrics 2002;109:1170–3.
14. Erjavec Z, Hollak CE, de Vries EG. Hepatocellular carcinoma in a patient with Gaucher disease on enzyme supplementation therapy. Ann Oncol 1999;10:243.
15. Barton NW, Brady RO, Dambrosia JM, et al. Replacement therapy for inherited enzyme deficiency – macrophage-targeted glucocerebrosidase for Gaucher's disease. N Engl J Med 1991; 324:1464–70.
16. Weinreb NJ, Aggio MC, Andersson HC, et al. Gaucher disease type 1: revised recommendations on evaluations and monitoring for adult patients. Semin Hematol 2004;41:15–22.
17. Weinreb NJ, Charrow J, Andersson HC, et al. Effectiveness of enzyme replacement therapy in 1028 patients with type 1 Gaucher disease after 2 to 5 years of treatment: a report from the Gaucher Registry. Am J Med 2002;113:112–19.
18. Radin NS. Treatment of Gaucher disease with an enzyme inhibitor. Glycoconj J 1996;13:153–7.
19. Platt FM, Jeyakumar M, Andersson U, et al. Inhibition of substrate synthesis as a strategy for glycolipid lysosomal storage disease therapy. J Inherit Metab Dis 2001;24:275–90.
20. Cox T, Lachmann R, Hollak C, et al. Novel oral treatment of Gaucher's disease with N-butyldeoxynojirimycin (OGT 918) to decrease substrate biosynthesis. Lancet 2000;355:1481–5.
21. Altarescu G, Hill S, Wiggs E, et al. The efficacy of enzyme replacement therapy in patients with chronic neuronopathic Gaucher's disease. J Pediatr 2001;138:539–47.
22. Prows CA, Sanchez N, Daugherty C, Grabowski GA. Gaucher disease: enzyme therapy in the acute neuronopathic variant. Am J Med Genet 1997;71:16–21.
23. Ricci V, Stroppiano M, Corsolini F, et al. Screening of 25 Italian patients with Niemann-Pick A reveals fourteen new mutations, one common and thirteen private, in SMPD1. Hum Mutat 2004;24:105.
24. Pittis MG, Ricci V, Guerci VI, et al. Acid sphingomyelinase: identification of nine novel mutations among Italian Niemann Pick type B patients and characterization of in vivo functional in-frame start codon. Hum Mutat 2004;24:186–7.
25. Sikora J, Pavlu-Pereira H, Elleder M, et al. Seven novel acid sphingomyelinase gene mutations in Niemann-Pick type A and B patients. Ann Hum Genet 2003;67:63–70.
26. Schuchman EH, Desnick RJ. Niemann-Pick disease types A and B: acid sphingomyelinase deficiencies. In: Scriver CR, Beaudet AL, Sly WS, et al., eds. The metabolic and molecular bases of inherited disease. New York: McGraw-Hill, 2001:3589–610.
27. Simonaro CM, Desnick RJ, McGovern MM, et al. The demographics and distribution of type B Niemann-Pick disease: novel mutations lead to new genotype/phenotype correlations. Am J Hum Genet 2002;71:1413–19.
28. Pavlu-Pereira H, Asfaw B, Poupctova H, et al. Acid sphingomyelinase deficiency. Phenotype variability with prevalence of intermediate phenotype in a series of twenty-five Czech and Slovak patients. A multi-approach study. J Inherit Metab Dis 2005;28:203–27.
29. Wasserstein MP, Desnick RJ, Schuchman EH, et al. The natural history of type B Niemann-Pick disease: results from a 10-year longitudinal study. Pediatrics 2004;114:e672–7.
30. Labrune P, Bedossa P, Huguet P, et al. Fatal liver failure in two children with Niemann-Pick disease type B. J Pediatr Gastroenterol Nutr 1991;13:104–9.
31. Sogawa H, Horino K, Nakamura F, et al. Chronic Niemann-Pick disease with sphingomyelinase deficiency in two brothers with mental retardation. Eur J Pediatr 1978;128:235–40.
32. Takahashi T, Akiyama K, Tomihara M, et al. Heterogeneity of liver disorder in type B Niemann-Pick disease. Hum Pathol 1997;28:385–8.
33. Tassoni JP Jr, Fawaz KA, Johnston DE. Cirrhosis and portal hypertension in a patient with adult Niemann-Pick disease. Gastroenterology 1991;100:567–9.
34. Wilson JA, Raufman JP. Hepatic failure in adult Niemann-Pick disease. Am J Med Sci 1986;292:168–72.
35. Kayler LK, Merion RM, Lee S, et al. Long-term survival after liver transplantation in children with metabolic disorders. Pediatr Transplant 2002;6:295–300.
36. Smanik EJ, Tavill AS, Jacobs GH, et al. Orthotopic liver transplantation in two adults with Niemann-Pick and Gaucher's diseases: implications for the treatment of inherited metabolic disease. Hepatology 1993;17:42–9.
37. Victor S, Coulter JB, Besley GT, et al. Niemann-Pick disease: sixteen-year follow-up of allogeneic bone marrow transplantation in a type B variant. J Inherit Metab Dis 2003;26:775–85.
38. Bayever E, August CS, Kamani N, et al. Allogeneic bone marrow transplantation for Niemann-Pick disease (type IA). Bone Marrow Transplant 1992;10(suppl 1):85–6.
39. Bar J, Linke T, Ferlinz K, et al. Molecular analysis of acid ceramidase deficiency in patients with Farber disease. Hum Mutat 2001;17:199–209.
40. Moser HW, Linke T, Fensom AH, et al. Acid ceramidase deficiency: Farber lipogranulomatosis. In: Scriver CR, Beaudet AL, Valle D, et al., eds. The metabolic and molecular bases of inherited disease. New York: McGraw Hill, 2001:3573–88.
41. Abul-Haj SK, Martz DG, Douglas WF, Geppert LJ. Farber's disease. Report of a case with observations on its histogenesis and notes on the nature of the stored material. J Pediatr 1962;61:221–32.
42. Zappatini-Tommasi L, Dumontel C, Guibaud P, Girod C. Farber disease: an ultrastructural study. Report of a case and review

of the literature. Virchows Arch A Pathol Anat Histopathol 1992;420:281–90.

43. Fiumara A, Nigro F, Pavone L, Moser HW. Farber disease with prolonged survival. J Inherit Metab Dis 1993;16:915–16.
44. Antonarakis SE, Valle D, Moser HW, et al. Phenotypic variability in siblings with Farber disease. J Pediatr 1984;104:406–9.
45. Cartigny B, Libert J, Fensom AH, et al. Clinical diagnosis of a new case of ceramidase deficiency (Farber's disease). J Inherit Metab Dis 1985;8:8.
46. Nowaczyk MJ, Feigenbaum A, Silver MM, et al. Bone marrow involvement and obstructive jaundice in Farber lipogranulomatosis: clinical and autopsy report of a new case. J Inherit Metab Dis 1996;19:655–60.
47. Kattner E, Schafer A, Harzer K. Hydrops fetalis: manifestation in lysosomal storage diseases including Farber disease. Eur J Pediatr 1997;156:292–5.
48. van Lijnschoten G, Groener JE, Maas SM, et al. Intrauterine fetal death due to Farber disease: case report. Pediatr Dev Pathol 2000;3:597–602.
49. Yeager AM, Uhas KA, Coles CD, et al. Bone marrow transplantation for infantile ceramidase deficiency (Farber disease). Bone Marrow Transplant 2000;26:357–63.
50. Vormoor J, Ehlert K, Groll AH, et al. Successful hematopoietic stem cell transplantation in Farber disease. J Pediatr 2004; 144:132–4.
51. Georgiou T, Drousiotou A, Campos Y, et al. Four novel mutations in patients from the Middle East with the infantile form of GM1-gangliosidosis. Hum Mutat 2004;24:352.
52. Morrone A, Bardelli T, Donati MA, et al. β-Galactosidase gene mutations affecting the lysosomal enzyme and the elastin-binding protein in GM1-gangliosidosis patients with cardiac involvement. Hum Mutat 2000;15:354–66.
53. Yoshida K, Oshima A, Sakuraba H, et al. GM1 gangliosidosis in adults: clinical and molecular analysis of 16 Japanese patients. Ann Neurol 1992;31:328–32.
54. Abu-Dalu KI, Tamary H, Livni N, et al. GM1 gangliosidosis presenting as neonatal ascites. J Pediatr 1982;100:940–3.
55. Folkerth RD, Alroy J, Bhan I, Kaye EM. Infantile G(M1) gangliosidosis: complete morphology and histochemistry of two autopsy cases, with particular reference to delayed central nervous system myelination. Pediatr Dev Pathol 2000;3:73–86.
56. Bonduelle M, Lissens W, Goossens A, et al. Lysosomal storage diseases presenting as transient or persistent hydrops fetalis. Genet Couns 1991;2:227–32.
57. Suzuki Y, Nakamura N, Fukuoka K, et al. β-Galactosidase deficiency in juvenile and adult patients. Report of six Japanese cases and review of literature. Hum Genet 1977;36:219–29.
58. Bu-Ghanim M, Sansaricq C, Gordon R, Morotti RA. Pathologic quiz case: hepatosplenomegaly in an infant with hypotonia and coarse facial features. Gangliosidosis type 1. Arch Pathol Lab Med 2004;128:1297–8.
59. Suzuki Y, Oshima A, Nanba E. β-Galactosidase deficiency (β-galactosidosis): GM1 gangliosidosis and morquio B disease. In: Scriver CR, Beaudet AL, Sly WS, et al., eds. The metabolic and molecular bases of inherited disease. New York: McGraw-Hill, 2001:3775–809.
60. Lowden JA, Callahan JW, Gravel RA, et al. Type 2 GM1 gangliosidosis with long survival and neuronal ceroid lipofuscinosis. Neurology 1981;31:719–24.
61. Patterson MC, Vanier MT, Suzuki K, et al. Niemann-Pick Disease Type C: A Lipid Trafficking Disorder. In: Scriver CR, Beaudet AL, Sly WS, et al., eds. The metabolic and molecular bases of inherited disease. New York: McGraw-Hill, 2001:3611–33.
62. Millat G, Marcais C, Tomasetto C, et al. Niemann-Pick C1 disease: correlations between NPC1 mutations, levels of NPC1 protein, and phenotypes emphasize the functional significance of the putative sterol-sensing domain and of the cysteine-rich luminal loop. Am J Hum Genet 2001;68:1373–85.
63. Vanier MT, Millat G. Niemann-Pick disease type C. Clin Genet 2003;64:269–81.
64. Naureckiene S, Sleat DE, Lackland H, et al. Identification of HE1 as the second gene of Niemann-Pick C disease. Science 2000;290:2298–301.
65. Ko DC, Binkley J, Sidow A, Scott MP. The integrity of a cholesterol-binding pocket in Niemann-Pick C2 protein is necessary to control lysosome cholesterol levels. Proc Natl Acad Sci U S A 2003;100:2518–25.
66. Vanier MT, Wenger DA, Comly ME, et al. Niemann-Pick disease group C: clinical variability and diagnosis based on defective cholesterol esterification. A collaborative study on 70 patients. Clin Genet 1988;33:331–48.
67. Kelly DA, Portmann B, Mowat AP, et al. Niemann-Pick disease type C: diagnosis and outcome in children, with particular reference to liver disease. J Pediatr 1993;123:242–7.
68. Mieli-Vergani G, Howard ER, Mowat AP. Liver disease in infancy: a 20 year perspective. Gut 1991;(suppl):S123–8.
69. Yerushalmi B, Sokol RJ, Narkewicz MR, et al. Niemann-pick disease type C in neonatal cholestasis at a North American Center. J Pediatr Gastroenterol Nutr 2002;35:44–50.
70. Fink JK, Filling-Katz MR, Sokol J, et al. Clinical spectrum of Niemann-Pick disease type C. Neurology 1989;39:1040–9.
71. Vanier MT, Pentchev P, Rodriguez-Lafrasse C, Rousson R. Niemann-Pick disease type C: an update. J Inherit Metab Dis 1991;14:580–95.
72. Fensom AH, Grant AR, Steinberg SJ, et al. An adult with a non-neuronopathic form of Niemann-Pick C disease. J Inherit Metab Dis 1999;22:84–6.
73. Imrie J, Vijayaraghaven S, Whitehouse C, et al. Niemann-Pick disease type C in adults. J Inherit Metab Dis 2002;25:491–500.
74. Dumontel C, Girod C, Dijoud F, et al. Fetal Niemann-Pick disease type C: ultrastructural and lipid findings in liver and spleen. Virchows Arch A Pathol Anat Histopathol 1993;422:253–9.
75. Gilbert EF, Callahan J, Viseskul C, Opitz JM. Niemann-Pick disease type C. Pathological, histochemical, ultrastructural and biochemical studies. Eur J Pediatr 1981;136:263–74.
76. Ashkenazi A, Yarom R, Gutman A, et al. Niemann-Pick disease and giant cell transformation of the liver. Acta Paediatr Scand 1971;60:285–94.
77. Kovesi TA, Lee J, Shuckett B, et al. Pulmonary infiltration in Niemann-Pick disease type C. J Inherit Metab Dis 1996;19: 792–3.
78. Birch NC, Radio S, Horslen S. Metastatic hepatocellular carcinoma in a patient with niemann-pick disease, type C. J Pediatr Gastroenterol Nutr 2003;37:624–6.
79. Schofer O, Mischo B, Puschel W, et al. Early-lethal pulmonary form of Niemann-Pick type C disease belonging to a second, rare genetic complementation group. Eur J Pediatr 1998;157: 45–9.
80. Patterson MC, Di Bisceglie AM, Higgins JJ, et al. The effect of cholesterol-lowering agents on hepatic and plasma cholesterol in Niemann-Pick disease type C. Neurology 1993;43:61–4.

81. Hsu YS, Hwu WL, Huang SF, et al. Niemann-Pick disease type C (a cellular cholesterol lipidosis) treated by bone marrow transplantation. Bone Marrow Transplant 1999;24:103–7.
82. Gartner JC Jr, Bergman I, Malatack JJ, et al. Progression of neurovisceral storage disease with supranuclear ophthalmoplegia following orthotopic liver transplantation. Pediatrics 1986;77:104–6.
83. Thomas GH. Disorders of glycoprotein degradation: α-mannosidosis, β-mannosidosis, fucosidosis, and sialidosis. In: Scriver CR, Beaudet AL, Valle D, et al., eds. The metabolic and molecular bases of inherited disease. New York: McGraw-Hill, 2001;3507–33.
84. Willems PJ, Gatti R, Darby JK, et al. Fucosidosis revisited: a review of 77 patients. Am J Med Genet 1991;38:111–31.
85. Willems PJ, Seo HC, Coucke P, et al. Spectrum of mutations in fucosidosis. Eur J Hum Genet 1999;7:60–7.
86. Freitag F, Blumcke S, Spranger J. Hepatic ultrastructure in mucolipidosis I (lipomucopolysaccharidosis). Virchows Arch B Cell Pathol 1971;7:189–204.
87. Vellodi A, Cragg H, Winchester B, et al. Allogeneic bone marrow transplantation for fucosidosis. Bone Marrow Transplant 1995;15:153–8.
88. Miano M, Lanino E, Gatti R, et al. Four year follow-up of a case of fucosidosis treated with unrelated donor bone marrow transplantation. Bone Marrow Transplant 2001;27:747–51.
89. Berg T, Riise HM, Hansen GM, et al. Spectrum of mutations in α-mannosidosis. Am J Hum Genet 1999;64:77–88.
90. Desnick RJ, Sharp HL, Grabowski GA, et al. Mannosidosis: clinical, morphologic, immunologic, and biochemical studies. Pediatr Res 1976;10:985–96.
91. Ara JR, Mayayo E, Marzo ME, et al. Neurological impairment in α-mannosidosis: a longitudinal clinical and MRI study of a brother and sister. Childs Nerv Syst 1999;15:369–71.
92. Monus Z, Konyar E, Szabo L. Histomorphologic and histochemical investigations in mannosidosis. A light and electron microscopic study. Virchows Arch B Cell Pathol 1977;26:159–73.
93. Wall DA, Grange DK, Goulding P, et al. Bone marrow transplantation for the treatment of α-mannosidosis. J Pediatr 1998;133:282–5.
94. Albert MH, Schuster F, Peters C, et al. T-cell-depleted peripheral blood stem cell transplantation for α-mannosidosis. Bone Marrow Transplant 2003;32:443–6.
95. Lowden JA, O'Brien JS. Sialidosis: a review of human neuraminidase deficiency. Am J Hum Genet 1979;31:1–18.
96. Young ID, Young EP, Mossman J, et al. Neuraminidase deficiency: case report and review of the phenotype. J Med Genet 1987;24:283–90.
97. d'Azzo A, Andria G, Strisciuglio P, Galjaard H. Galactosialidosis. In: Scriver CR, Beaudet AL, Valle D, eds. The metabolic and molecular bases of inherited disease. New York: McGraw Hill, 2001:3811–26.
98. van der Spoel A, Bonten E, d'Azzo A. Transport of human lysosomal neuraminidase to mature lysosomes requires protective protein/cathepsin A. EMBO J 1998;17:1588–97.
99. Aylsworth AS, Thomas GH, Hood JL, et al. A severe infantile sialidosis: clinical, biochemical, and microscopic features. J Pediatr 1980;96:662–8.
100. Nordborg C, Kyllerman M, Conradi N, Mansson JE. Early-infantile galactosialidosis with multiple brain infarctions: morphological, neuropathological and neurochemical findings. Acta Neuropathol (Berl) 1997;93:24–33.
101. Patel MS, Callahan JW, Zhang S, et al. Early-infantile galactosialidosis: prenatal presentation and postnatal follow-up. Am J Med Genet 1999;85:38–47.
102. Jackman HL, Tan FL, Tamei H, et al. A peptidase in human platelets that deamidates tachykinins. Probable identity with the lysosomal "protective protein." J Biol Chem 1990;265:11265–72.
103. Jackman HL, Morris PW, Deddish PA, et al. Inactivation of endothelin I by deamidase (lysosomal protective protein). J Biol Chem 1992;267:2872–5.
104. Kleijer WJ, Geilen GC, Janse HC, et al. Cathepsin A deficiency in galactosialidosis: studies of patients and carriers in 16 families. Pediatr Res 1996;39:1067–71.
105. Galjart NJ, Morreau H, Willemsen R, et al. Human lysosomal protective protein has cathepsin A-like activity distinct from its protective function. J Biol Chem 1991;266:14754–62.
106. Hirschhorn R, Reuser AJJ. Glycogen storage disease type II: acid α-glucosidase (acid maltase) deficiency. In: Scriver CR, Beaudet AL, Valle D, et al., eds. The metabolic and molecular bases of inherited disease. New York: McGraw-Hill, 2001;3389–420.
107. Raben N, Plotz P, Byrne BJ. Acid α-glucosidase deficiency (glycogenosis type II, Pompe disease). Curr Mol Med 2002; 2:145–66.
108. van den Hout HM, Hop W, van Diggelen OP, et al. The natural course of infantile Pompe's disease: 20 original cases compared with 133 cases from the literature. Pediatrics 2003;112:332–40.
109. Kishnani PS, Howell RR. Pompe disease in infants and children. J Pediatr 2004;144:S35–43.
110. Martin JJ, de Barsy T, van Hoof F, Palladini G. Pompe's disease: an inborn lysosomal disorder with storage of glycogen. A study of brain and striated muscle. Acta Neuropathol (Berl) 1973;23:229–44.
111. Slonim AE, Bulone L, Ritz S, et al. Identification of two subtypes of infantile acid maltase deficiency. J Pediatr 2000;137:283–5.
112. Hagemans ML, Winkel LP, Van Doorn PA, et al. Clinical manifestation and natural course of late-onset Pompe's disease in 54 Dutch patients. Brain 2005;128:671–7.
113. Di Fiore MT, Manfredi R, Marri L, et al. Elevation of transaminases as an early sign of late-onset glycogenosis type II. Eur J Pediatr 1993;152:784.
114. Bruni CB, Paluello FM. A biochemical and ultrastructural study of liver, muscle, heart and kidney in type II glycogenosis. Virchows Arch B Cell Pathol 1970;4:196–207.
115. Watson JG, Gardner-Medwin D, Goldfinch ME, Pearson AD. Bone marrow transplantation for glycogen storage disease type II (Pompe's disease). N Engl J Med 1986;314:385.
116. Klinge L, Straub V, Neudorf U, et al. Safety and efficacy of recombinant acid α-glucosidase (rhGAA) in patients with classical infantile Pompe disease: results of a phase II clinical trial. Neuromuscul Disord 2005;15:24–31.
117. Klinge L, Straub V, Neudorf U, Voit T. Enzyme replacement therapy in classical infantile Pompe disease: results of a ten-month follow-up study. Neuropediatrics 2005;36:6–11.
118. Van den Hout H, Reuser AJ, Vulto AG, et al. Recombinant human *alpha*-glucosidase from rabbit milk in Pompe patients. Lancet 2000;356:397–8.
119. Van den Hout JM, Reuser AJ, de Klerk JB, et al. Enzyme therapy for Pompe disease with recombinant human α-glucosidase from rabbit milk. J Inherit Metab Dis 2001;24:266–74.

120. Winkel LP, Van den Hout JM, Kamphoven JH, et al. Enzyme replacement therapy in late-onset Pompe's disease: a three-year follow-up. Ann Neurol 2004;55:495–502.
121. Amalfitano A, Bengur AR, Morse RP, et al. Recombinant human acid α-glucosidase enzyme therapy for infantile glycogen storage disease type II: results of a phase I/II clinical trial. Genet Med 2001;3:132–8.
122. Pagani F, Pariyarath R, Garcia R, et al. New lysosomal acid lipase gene mutants explain the phenotype of Wolman disease and cholesteryl ester storage disease. J Lipid Res 1998;39:1382–8.
123. Assmann G, Seedorf U. Acid lipase deficiency: Wolman disease and cholesteryl ester storage disease. In: Scriver CR, Beaudet AL, Valle D, et al., eds. The metabolic and molecular bases of inherited disease. New York: McGraw-Hill, 2001:3551–72.
124. Grabowski GA, Bove K, Du H. Lysosomal acid lipase deficiencies: Wolman disease and cholesteryl ester storage disease. In: Walker WA, Goulet OJ, Kleinman RE, et al., eds. Pediatric gastrointestinal disease: pathophysiology, diagnosis and management. Hamilton, Ontario: BC Decker, 2004:1429–39.
125. Boldrini R, Devito R, Biselli R, et al. Wolman disease and cholesteryl ester storage disease diagnosed by histological and ultrastructural examination of intestinal and liver biopsy. Pathol Res Pract 2004;200:231–40.
126. Drebber U, Andersen M, Kasper HU, et al. Severe chronic diarrhea and weight loss in cholesteryl ester storage disease: a case report. World J Gastroenterol 2005;11:2364–6.
127. Lough J, Fawcett J, Wiegensberg B. Wolman's disease. An electron microscopic, histochemical, and biochemical study. Arch Pathol 1970;89:103–10.
128. Bambirra EA, Tafuri WL, Borges HH, et al. Wolman's disease: a clinicopathologic, electron microscopic, and histochemical study. South Med J 1982;75:595–6.
129. Browne M, Somers G, Savoia H, Kukuruzovic R. Wolman's disease in an infant. Br J Haematol 2003;122:522.
130. Guazzi GC, Martin JJ, Philippart M, et al. Wolman's disease. Eur Neurol 1968;1:334–62.
131. Marshall WC, Ockenden BG, Fosbrooke AS, Cumings JN. Wolman's disease. A rare lipidosis with adrenal calcification. Arch Dis Child 1969;44:331–41.
132. Mitsudo S, Zucker P. Case 4. Wolman's disease. Pediatr Pathol 1989;9:193–8.
133. Wallis K, Gross M, Kohn R, Zaidman J. A case of Wolman's disease. Helv Paediatr Acta 1971;26:98–111.
134. Beaudet AL, Ferry GD, Nichols BL Jr, Rosenberg HS. Cholesterol ester storage disease: clinical, biochemical, and pathological studies. J Pediatr 1977;90:910–14.
135. Lohse P, Maas S, Sewell AC, et al. Molecular defects underlying Wolman disease appear to be more heterogeneous than those resulting in cholesteryl ester storage disease. J Lipid Res 1999;40:221–8.
136. Brown MS, Kovanen PT, Goldstein JL. Regulation of plasma cholesterol by lipoprotein receptors. Science 1981;212:628–35.
137. Krivit W, Freese D, Chan KW, Kulkarni R. Wolman's disease: a review of treatment with bone marrow transplantation and considerations for the future. Bone Marrow Transplant 1992; 10(suppl 1):97–101.
138. Krivit W, Peters C, Dusenbery K, et al. Wolman disease successfully treated by bone marrow transplantation. Bone Marrow Transplant 2000;26:567–70.
139. Arterburn JN, Lee WM, Wood RP, et al. Orthotopic liver transplantation for cholesteryl ester storage disease. J Clin Gastroenterol 1991;13:482–5.
140. Di Bisceglie AM, Ishak KG, Rabin L, Hoeg JM. Cholesteryl ester storage disease: hepatopathology and effects of therapy with lovastatin. Hepatology 1990;11:764–72.
141. Ginsberg HN, Le NA, Short MP, et al. Suppression of apolipoprotein B production during treatment of cholesteryl ester storage disease with lovastatin. Implications for regulation of apolipoprotein B synthesis. J Clin Invest 1987;80:1692–7.
142. Leone L, Ippoliti P, Antonicelli R. Use of simvastatin plus cholestyramine in the treatment of lysosomal acid lipase deficiency. J Pediatr 1991;119:1008–9.
143. Tarantino MD, McNamara DJ, Granstrom P, et al. Lovastatin therapy for cholesterol ester storage disease in two sisters. J Pediatr 1991;118:131–5.
144. Du H, Schiavi S, Levine M, et al. Enzyme therapy for lysosomal acid lipase deficiency in the mouse. Hum Mol Genet 2001;10:1639–48.
145. Du H, Heur M, Witte DP, et al. Lysosomal acid lipase deficiency: correction of lipid storage by adenovirus-mediated gene transfer in mice. Hum Gene Ther 2002;13:1361–72.
146. Neufeld EB, Muenzer J. The mucopolysaccharidoses. In: Scriver CR, Beaudet AL, Valle D, et al., eds. The metabolic and molecular bases of inherited disease. New York: McGraw-Hill, 2001:3421–51.
147. Kakkis ED, Muenzer J, Tiller GE, et al. Enzyme-replacement therapy in mucopolysaccharidosis I. N Engl J Med 2001; 344:182–8.
148. Harmatz P, Whitley CB, Waber L, et al. Enzyme replacement therapy in mucopolysaccharidosis VI (Maroteaux-Lamy syndrome). J Pediatr 2004;144:574–80.
149. Parfrey NA, Hutchins GM. Hepatic fibrosis in the mucopolysaccharidoses. Am J Med 1986;81:825–9.
150. Resnick JM, Krivit W, Snover DC, et al. Pathology of the liver in mucopolysaccharidosis: light and electron microscopic assessment before and after bone marrow transplantation. Bone Marrow Transplant 1992;10:273–80.
151. Resnick JM, Whitley CB, Leonard AS, et al. Light and electron microscopic features of the liver in mucopolysaccharidosis. Hum Pathol 1994;25:276–86.
152. Muenzer J. The mucopolysaccharidoses: a heterogeneous group of disorders with variable pediatric presentations. J Pediatr 2004;144:S27–34.
153. Herskhovitz E, Young E, Rainer J, et al. Bone marrow transplantation for Maroteaux-Lamy syndrome (MPS VI): long-term follow-up. J Inherit Metab Dis 1999;22:50–62.
154. Peters C, Balthazor M, Shapiro EG, et al. Outcome of unrelated donor bone marrow transplantation in 40 children with Hurler syndrome. Blood 1996;87:4894–902.
155. Peters C, Shapiro EG, Anderson J, et al. Hurler syndrome: II. Outcome of HLA-genotypically identical sibling and HLA-haploidentical related donor bone marrow transplantation in fifty-four children. The Storage Disease Collaborative Study Group. Blood 1998;91:2601–8.
156. Sivakumur P, Wraith JE. Bone marrow transplantation in mucopolysaccharidosis type IIIA: a comparison of an early treated patient with his untreated sibling. J Inherit Metab Dis 1999;22:849–50.
157. Yamada Y, Kato K, Sukegawa K, et al. Treatment of MPS VII (Sly disease) by allogeneic BMT in a female with homozygous

A619V mutation. Bone Marrow Transplant 1998;21:629–34.
158. Wraith JE, Clarke LA, Beck M, et al. Enzyme replacement therapy for mucopolysaccharidosis I: a randomized, double-blinded, placebo-controlled, multinational study of recombinant human α-*L*-iduronidase (laronidase). J Pediatr 2004; 144:581–8.
159. Kornfeld S, Sly WS. I-cell disease and pseudo-Hurler polydystrophy: disorders of lysosomal enzyme phosphorylation and localization. In: Scriver CR, Beaudet AL, Valle D, et al., eds. The metabolic and molecular bases of inherited disease. New York: McGraw-Hill, 2001;3469–82.
160. Raas-Rothschild A, Cormier-Daire V, Bao M, et al. Molecular basis of variant pseudo-Hurler polydystrophy (mucolipidosis IIIC). J Clin Invest 2000;105:673–81.
161. Canfield WM, Bao M, Pan J, et al. Mucolipidosis II and mucolipidosis IIIA are caused by mutations in the GlcNAc-phosphotransferace a/B gene on chromosome 12. Am J Hum Genet 1998;63:A15.
162. Tiede S, Muschol N, Reutter G, et al. Missense mutations in N-acetylglucosamine-1-phosphotransferase α/β subunit gene in a patient with mucolipidosis III and a mild clinical phenotype. Am J Med Genet A 2005;137:235–40.
163. Hochman JA, Treem WR, Dougherty F, Bentley RC. Mucolipidosis II (I-cell disease) presenting as neonatal cholestasis. J Inherit Metab Dis 2001;24:603–4.
164. Leroy JG, Spranger JW, Feingold M, et al. I-cell disease: a clinical picture. J Pediatr 1971;79:360–5.
165. Sprigz RA, Doughty RA, Spackman TJ, et al. Neonatal presentation of I-cell disease. J Pediatr 1978;93:954–8.
166. Burin MG, Scholz AP, Gus R, et al. Investigation of lysosomal storage diseases in nonimmune hydrops fetalis. Prenat Diagn 2004;24:653–7.
167. Tylki-Szymanska A, Czartoryska B, Groener JE, Lugowska A. Clinical variability in mucolipidosis III (pseudo-Hurler polydystrophy). Am J Med Genet 2002;108:214–18.
168. Kelly TE, Thomas GH, Taylor HA Jr, et al. Mucolipidosis III (pseudo-Hurler polydystrophy): Clinical and laboratory studies in a series of 12 patients. Johns Hopkins Med J 1975;137: 156–75.
169. Kenyon KR, Sensenbrenner JA, Wyllie RG. Hepatic ultrastructure and histochemistry in mucolipidosis II (I-cell disease). Pediatr Res 1973;7:560–8.
170. Grewal S, Shapiro E, Braunlin E, et al. Continued neurocognitive development and prevention of cardiopulmonary complications after successful BMT for I-cell disease: a long-term follow-up report. Bone Marrow Transplant 2003;32:957–60.
171. Hopwood JJ, Ballabio A. Multiple sulfatase deficiency and the nature of the sulfatase family. In: Scriver CR, Beaudet AL, Valle D, et al., eds. The metabolic and molecular bases of inherited disease. New York: McGraw-Hill, 2001:3725–32.
172. Blanco-Aguirre ME, Kofman-Alfaro SH, Rivera-Vega MR, et al. Unusual clinical presentation in two cases of multiple sulfatase deficiency. Pediatr Dermatol 2001;18:388–92.
173. Burch M, Fensom AH, Jackson M, et al. Multiple sulphatase deficiency presenting at birth. Clin Genet 1986;30:409–15.
174. Burk RD, Valle D, Thomas GH, et al. Early manifestations of multiple sulfatase deficiency. J Pediatr 1984;104:574–8.
175. Diaz-Font A, Santamaria R, Cozar M, et al. Clinical and mutational characterization of three patients with multiple sulfatase deficiency: report of a new splicing mutation. Mol Genet Metab 2005;86:206–11.
176. Macaulay RJ, Lowry NJ, Casey RE. Pathologic findings of multiple sulfatase deficiency reflect the pattern of enzyme deficiencies. Pediatr Neurol 1998;19:372–6.
177. Vamos E, Liebaers I, Bousard N, et al. Multiple sulphatase deficiency with early onset. J Inherit Metab Dis 1981;4:103–4.
178. Diez-Roux G, Ballabio A. Sulfatases and human disease. Annu Rev Genomics Hum Genet 2005;6:355–79.
179. Dierks T, Schmidt B, Borissenko LV, et al. Multiple sulfatase deficiency is caused by mutations in the gene encoding the human C(*alpha*)-formylglycine generating enzyme. Cell 2003;113:435–44.
180. Cosma MP, Pepe S, Annunziata I, et al. The multiple sulfatase deficiency gene encodes an essential and limiting factor for the activity of sulfatases. Cell 2003;113:445–56.
181. Schmidt B, Selmer T, Ingendoh A, von Figura K. A novel amino acid modification in sulfatases that is defective in multiple sulfatase deficiency. Cell 1995;82:271–8.
182. Dierks T, Lecca MR, Schlotterhose P, et al. Sequence determinants directing conversion of cysteine to formylglycine in eukaryotic sulfatases. EMBO J 1999;18:2084–91.
183. Muenzer J, Wraith JE, Beck M, et al. A phase II/III clinical study of enzyme replacement therapy with idursulfase in mucopolysaccharidosis II (Hunter syndrome). Genet Med 2006; 8:465–73.

31

Disorders of Bile Acid Synthesis and Metabolism: A Metabolic Basis for Liver Disease

Kenneth D. R. Setchell, Ph.D., and
Nancy C. O'Connell, M.S., C.C.R.C., C.C.R.A.

With the increased recognition of the importance of bile acid synthesis and metabolism in both normal physiology and pathophysiology, there has been a renaissance in this field in recent years. For such small and relatively simple molecules, the bile acids have amazingly diverse properties and functions. To the lipidologist, bile acid biosynthesis represents one of the major pathways for regulating cholesterol homeostasis; on the other hand, the hepatologist sees these molecules as essential for providing the major driving force for the promotion and secretion of bile and therefore as key elements in the development and maintenance of an efficient enterohepatic circulation. The gastroenterologist recognizes that bile acids play an important role in the solubilization and absorption of fats and fat-soluble vitamins in the small bowel, whereas in the large bowel, pathologists have viewed these molecules as potentially harmful in that they are cathartic, membrane damaging, and promoters of colonic disease. With regard to bile acid biosynthesis, several comprehensive reviews of the subject have been published [1–4]; therefore, this chapter provides only an overview of the pathways of bile acid synthesis and metabolism and describes specific inborn errors in bile acid synthesis that have been identified.

PATHWAYS FOR BILE ACID SYNTHESIS FROM CHOLESTEROL

Although not generally thought of as steroids, the bile acids belong to this chemical class, possessing the basic cyclopentanoperhydrophenanthrene (ABCD ring) nucleus [5,6]. They differ from steroid hormones and neutral sterols by having a five-carbon atom side chain with a terminal carboxylic acid (Figure 31.1). They are synthesized in the liver from neutral steroids by a complex series of chemical reactions catalyzed by a variety of hepatic enzymes that are located in various subcellular compartments. There is consequently a considerable amount of trafficking of the substrates and products of these enzyme reactions between subcellular compartments; although several sterol-binding proteins have been recognized [7,8], the mechanism of the transport process within this "black box" is somewhat unclear. The enzymes involved in bile acid biosynthesis have all been isolated to varying degrees of homogeneity. Complementary DNAs (cDNAs) have now been reported for most of the enzymes [9], including the rate-limiting enzyme in the bile acid biosynthetic pathway, cholesterol 7α-hydroxylase [10–13]. These have provided important tools to examine the regulation and genetics of this pathway.

Classical "Neutral" Pathway for Bile Acid Synthesis Initiated Through 7α-Hydroxylation of Cholesterol

Cholic and chenodeoxycholic acids, the two primary bile acids in man and most animal species, are synthesized from cholesterol by a sequence of reactions that leads to modifications of the ABCD ring nucleus and the side chain (Figure 31.1). Considerable substrate promiscuity for the enzymes takes place under normal conditions, and this is exaggerated during early development, when a period of physiologic cholestasis occurs [14,15], and in pathologic conditions that interfere with the integrity of the enterohepatic circulation. Overall, it is now recognized that there are two main pathways leading to primary bile acid synthesis. These have become termed the *neutral* and *acidic* pathways, the former being the classical one that is initiated by 7α-hydroxylation of cholesterol.

Cholesterol 7α-Hydroxylase, the Rate-Limiting Step for Bile Acid Synthesis

The first reaction in bile acid synthesis involves the introduction of a hydroxyl group at position C-7 of the cholesterol nucleus. This reaction is catalyzed by a microsomal cholesterol 7α-hydroxylase [16–19], a cytochrome P450 liver-specific enzyme with a molecular weight of approximately 57 kDa. The major factor influencing bile acid synthesis is negative feedback by bile acids returning via the portal vein during their enterohepatic recycling [16]. There are marked differences in the ability of different bile acids to regulate cholesterol 7α-hydroxylase [20]. For example, whereas primary bile acids down-regulate synthesis, bile acids possessing a 7β-hydroxy group, such as ursodeoxycholic acid (UDCA), do not [21]; the

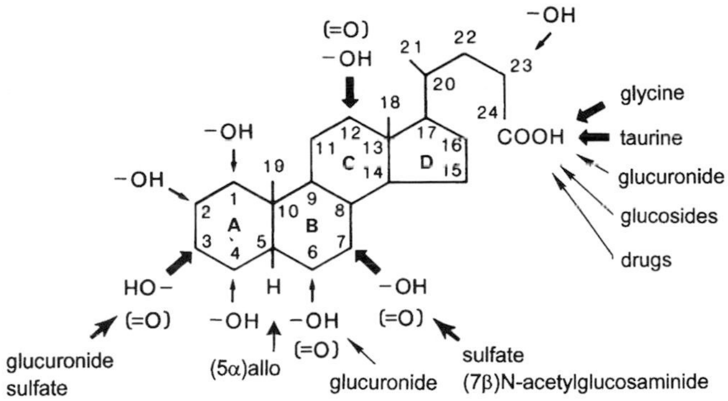

Figure 31.1. The 5β-cholanoic acid nucleus that is the basic structure of C_{24} bile acids of mammalian species. Indicated are the ABCD rings, numbering system for the carbon atoms, and positions of the principal functional groups for bile acids synthesized under normal and pathophysiologic conditions.

latter may actually increase synthesis rates [22]. This observation is relevant to the treatment of diseases involving inborn errors of bile acid synthesis [3,4]. Interruption of the enterohepatic circulation, by biliary diversion [16] or the feeding of anion exchange resins that bind bile acids in the intestinal lumen [23], results in an up-regulation of cholesterol 7α-hydroxylase activity via increased transcription [12,21,24]. In general, factors that influence cholesterol 7α-hydroxylase activity cause concomitant changes in the activity of 3-hydroxy-3-methylglutaryl–coenzyme A (HMG-CoA) reductase, the rate-limiting enzyme for cholesterol synthesis. The parallels between the control of these two enzymes lead to regulation of cholesterol synthesis and the maintenance of a constant cholesterol pool size [25]. Interestingly, cholesterol 7α-hydroxylase exhibits a diurnal rhythm that is synchronous with the activity of HMG-CoA reductase [26,27] and is reflected by diurnal changes in bile acid synthesis rates [28]. A significant nocturnal rise in bile acid synthesis takes place [22] that may be regulated by glucocorticoids because this regulation can be abolished by adrenalectomy or hypophysectomy (see Shefer et al. [18] and references therein).

Following the isolation and purification of the rat cholesterol 7α-hydroxylase enzyme [29], several groups sequenced the protein, raised antibodies, and prepared cDNAs [10,12]. Subsequently, a cDNA encoding the human cholesterol 7α-hydroxylase was prepared [11] that showed excellent homology with that of the rat enzyme. With the use of the cDNA and antibody probes, studies of the gene, mRNA, and protein demonstrated that this enzyme is exclusive to the liver [2]. This heightened awareness of the complexity in the regulation of primary bile acid synthesis [30–33]. It is now realized that there are two distinct pathways for primary bile acid synthesis: the *neutral* or classical pathway, which proceeds with initial 7α-hydroxylation of cholesterol, and the *acidic* pathway that involves initial side-chain hydroxylation by a sterol 27-hydroxylase. The relative importance of these two pathways has been long debated, but animal and clinical data now confirm that both pathways are of equal importance and that under certain conditions, they may augment each other. When activity of cholesterol 7α-hydroxylase is completely repressed by continuous infusion of squalestatin, bile acid synthesis 1 day later continues at 43% of preinfusion levels, indicating that the acidic pathway is responsible for almost half the total bile acid synthesis in the rat [34]. Furthermore, when the gene for cholesterol 7α-hydroxylase is knocked out in mice [35,36], animals die within the first few weeks of life from liver failure and the consequences of fat-soluble vitamin malabsorption. However, when fat-soluble vitamins and cholic acid are fed to these animals immediately after birth, these animals survive [37]. Despite the lack of cholesterol 7α-hydroxylase in this gene knockout model, primary bile acid synthesis occurs via the developmental expression of an oxysterol 7α-hydroxylase specific to the acidic pathway [38]. What these studies show is that primary bile acid synthesis is not exclusively dependent on cholesterol 7α-hydroxylase, and under certain conditions, alternative pathways are induced. The discovery in an infant of a genetic defect in the oxysterol 7α-hydroxylase causing fatal liver disease [39] suggests that the acidic pathway is quantitatively the most important in early human life. Overall, it appears that there are significant species differences with regard to the developmental expression of the neutral and acidic pathways.

The regulation of cholesterol 7α-hydroxylase is further complicated by the fact that a number of orphan receptors have been recognized to show specificity for bile acids and oxysterols [40–46]. A number of nuclear orphan receptors have been identified, including liver X receptor-α (LXRα), farnesoid X receptor (FXR), small heterodimer partner 1 (SHP1), pregnane X receptor (PXR), and CYP7A promoter–binding factor (CPF) [41,46–51]. These are important at two levels of regulation. These orphan receptors influence transcriptional regulation of cholesterol 7α-hydroxylase in the liver [32,52–54] and also induce transcription of the ileal bile acid–binding protein (IBABP) [55] that is involved in the ileal uptake and conservation of the bile acid pool. Chenodeoxycholic acid in particular has a high affinity for FXR [42,55–57] and is a potent regulator of cholesterol synthesis. Bile acids have been identified in the nucleus of the hepatocyte, and their concentrations are known to increase with bile acid feeding [58].

Nuclear Reactions in Bile Acid Synthesis

Following the synthesis of 7α-hydroxycholesterol, modifications to the steroid nucleus take place that result in oxidoreduction and hydroxylation, consequently preparing the sterol intermediates for direction into either the cholic acid (3α,7α,12α-trihydroxy-5β-cholan-24-oic) or chenodeoxycholic acid (3α,7α-dihydroxy-5β-cholan-24-oic) pathways. According to convention, 7α-hydroxycholesterol is converted to 7α-hydroxy-4-cholesten-3-one, a reaction catalyzed by a microsomal nicotinamide adenine dinucleotide (NAD)–dependent 3β-hydroxy-C_{27}-steroid dehydrogenase/isomerase enzyme [59], also referred to as a 3β-hydroxy-C_{27}-steroid oxidoreductase. This enzyme shows substrate specificity toward 7α-hydroxylated sterols and bile acids possessing a 3β-hydroxy-Δ^5 nucleus and is inactive on

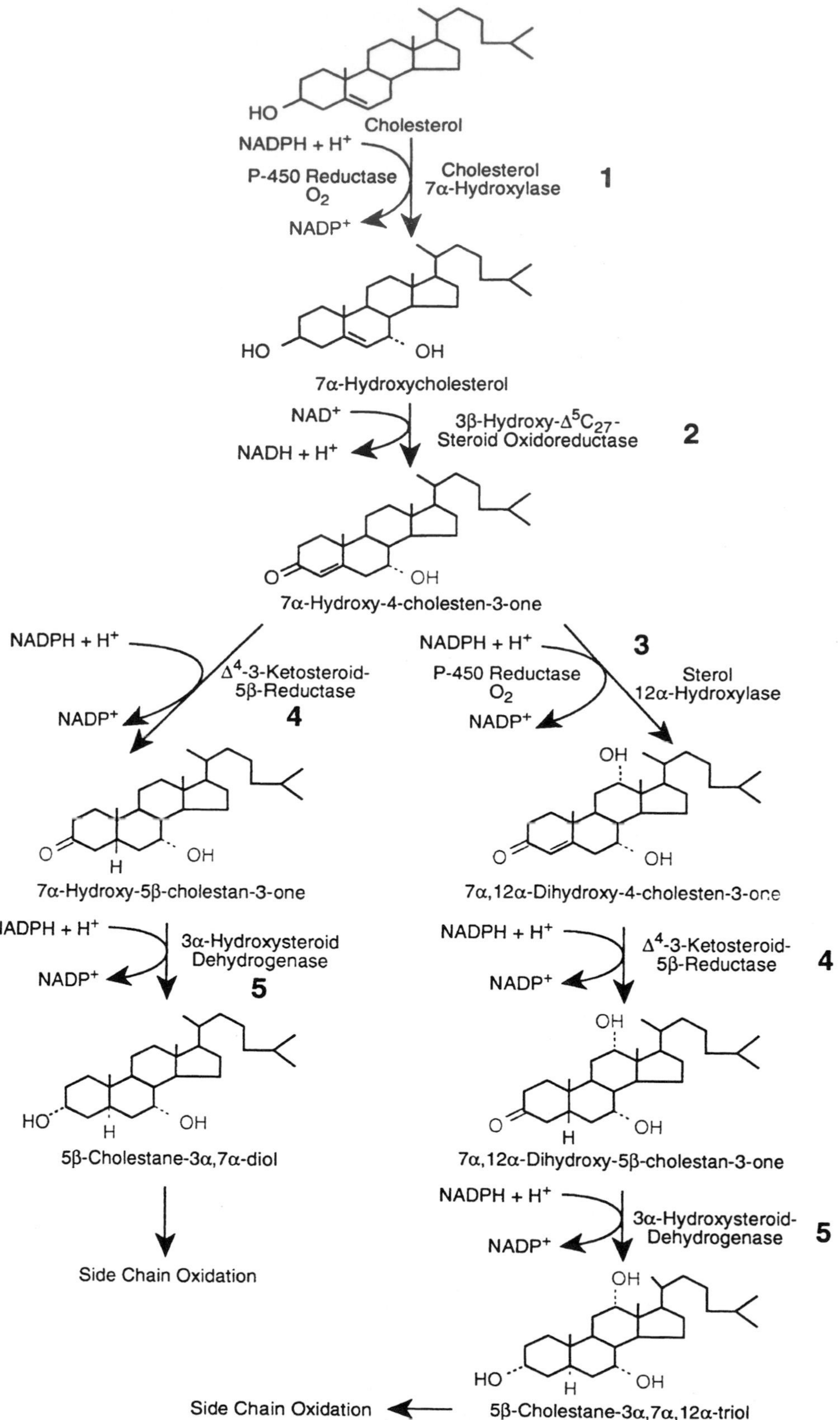

Figure 31.2. Cholesterol 7α-hydroxylase pathway for conversion of cholesterol into 5β-cholestane-3α,7α-diol and 5β-cholestane-3α,7α,12α-triol, the key intermediates in the synthesis of chenodeoxycholic and cholic acids, respectively. These steps indicate modifications to the sterol nucleus.

7β-hydroxylated analogues [60]. Comparable reactions occur in steroid hormone synthesis; however, the enzyme active on bile acid intermediates shows absolute specificity toward C_{27}-sterols [59], differing from the isozymes active on C_{19} and C_{21} neutral steroids [61–64]. 3β-Hydroxy-C_{27}-steroid dehydrogenase/isomerase is not exclusive to the liver but is also expressed in fibroblasts, which has enabled its activity to be determined in patients with defined genetic defects in this enzyme [65]. Little is known of the factors regulating this enzyme, although it is possibly influenced by the flux of bile acids in the enterohepatic circulation. Mutations in the gene encoding this enzyme have been identified and associated with progressive intrahepatic cholestasis, especially in some patients with late-onset chronic cholestasis [65,66].

12α-Hydroxylation of the product of the above reaction directs the intermediates into the cholic acid pathway. This reaction is catalyzed by a liver-specific microsomal cytochrome P450 12α-hydroxylase [67]. The primary structures of the rabbit, mouse, and human enzymes have been established by molecular cloning of their cDNAs [68,69]. It has been designated *CYP8B1* and is well expressed in rabbit and human liver, two species in which deoxycholic acid is quantitatively important. The activity of the 12α-hydroxylase enzyme determines the relative proportion and synthetic rates of cholic and chenodeoxycholic acids and appears in humans to be up-regulated by interruption of the enterohepatic circulation [70] and in animals, by starvation [71]. It is possible that in utero there may be reduced activity of this enzyme because fetal bile has a predominance of chenodeoxycholic acid [72,73]. In contrast, the ratio of cholic acid to chenodeoxycholic acid is very high in neonatal bile [74–77] compared with adult bile [78]. The neonatal period is associated with a phase of physiologic cholestasis [14,15], which may lead to an up-regulation in 12α-hydroxylase activity with a consequent increase in cholic acid synthesis.

7α-Hydroxy- and $7\alpha,12\alpha$-dihydroxy-4-cholesten-3-one both undergo reduction with formation of a 3-oxo-5β(H) structure, and this generates the basic *trans*-configuration of the A/B rings of the steroid nucleus common to the major bile acids of most mammalian species [79]. Allo(5α-H)$^-$ bile acids [80] are often major bile acid species of lower vertebrates and generally found in small proportions in humans [79]. These are formed by an analogous reaction catalyzed by a hepatic 5α-reductase. The K_m (Michaelis constant) of 5α-reductase is high, and consequently under normal conditions, 5β-reduction is favored [81]. The Δ^4-3-oxosteroid 5β-reductase has been purified, and sequence analysis of the rat and human cDNAs encoding the enzyme established its molecular weight to be 38 kDa [82]. The protein, composed of 327 amino acids [83], differs significantly in its sequence from the 5α-reductase.

Although under normal conditions this enzyme does not appear to be of regulatory importance for bile acid synthesis, its activity parallels the activity of cholesterol 7α-hydroxylase. Measurement of the plasma concentration of the product of the reaction, 7α-hydroxy-4-cholesten-3-one, strongly correlates with hepatic cholesterol 7α-hydroxylase activity [84]. The finding of elevated proportions of bile acids having a 3-oxo-Δ^4 structure in biologic fluids during severe cholestasis [85] would suggest that under pathologic conditions, it is this enzyme rather than cholesterol 7α-hydroxylase that becomes rate limiting for bile acid synthesis. A primary enzyme defect at this point in the biosynthetic pathway was first described by Setchell et al. [86]. This is manifest clinically by progressive cholestasis and biochemically by the production of large amounts of C_{24}-3-oxo-Δ^4-bile acids [86]. Mutations in the gene encoding this enzyme (*SRD5B1; AKR1D1*, OMIM 604741) have subsequently been described [87].

The enzyme catalyzing the conversion of the 3-oxo-5β(H)-sterols to the corresponding 3α-hydroxy-5β(H) intermediates is a soluble 3α-hydroxysteroid dehydrogenase that has been purified to homogeneity [88]. This enzyme catalyzes the oxidoreduction of a number of substrates, and several cDNA clones with sequence similarity to other aldo-keto reductases have been described [88–91], suggesting the existence of multiple isozymes. This is the final modification of the steroid nucleus and results in the formation of the intermediates, 5β-cholestane-3α, 7α-diol, and 5β-cholestane-$3\alpha,7\alpha,12\alpha$-triol (bile alcohols), which then undergo a sequence of reactions (Figure 31.3) leading to side-chain oxidation and consequent shortening by three carbon atoms. 3α-Hydroxysteroid dehydrogenase was also found to be the 33-kDa Y′ bile acid binder involved in the intracellular transport of bile acids [92].

Reactions Involving the Steroid Side Chain

The initial step in side-chain oxidation of the bile alcohols involves the hydroxylation of the C-27 atom, a reaction that is catalyzed by a mitochondrial cytochrome P450 27-hydroxylase [93]. This enzyme was formerly referred to as a 26-hydroxylase, but because the 25-pro-S methyl group that is attacked is now assigned the C-27 carbon [94], the enzyme is now more correctly referred to as a sterol 27-hydroxylase. cDNAs encoding the rat, rabbit, and human sterol 27-hydroxylase have been isolated [95–98]. This enzyme and its mRNA are expressed in many different tissues [95,97,99], although there are significant species differences in its regulation. When the sterol 27-hydroxylase gene was disrupted in the mouse [100], bile acid synthesis was markedly reduced; however, mutations in this gene accounting for the rare lipid storage disease cerebrotendinous xanthomatosis (CTX) have only a modest effect on bile acid synthesis [101–103]. Sterol 27-hydroxylase shows substrate specificity toward many sterols, including cholesterol and vitamin D [97,104,105]. Whether this enzyme is of regulatory importance in cholesterol synthesis, as has been suggested [106], is unclear. In addition to catalyzing the formation of a C-27 alcohol, it can perform multiple oxidation reactions at the C-27 position to yield directly the $3\alpha,7\alpha,12\alpha$-trihydroxy-5β-cholestanoic acid [107]. Sterol 27-hydroxylase appears to be the same enzyme responsible for initiating the formation of 27-hydroxycholesterol, the first step in the acidic pathway. It is expressed in many extrahepatic tissues [95,99,108–112] and appears to be important in facilitating the removal of cellular cholesterol.

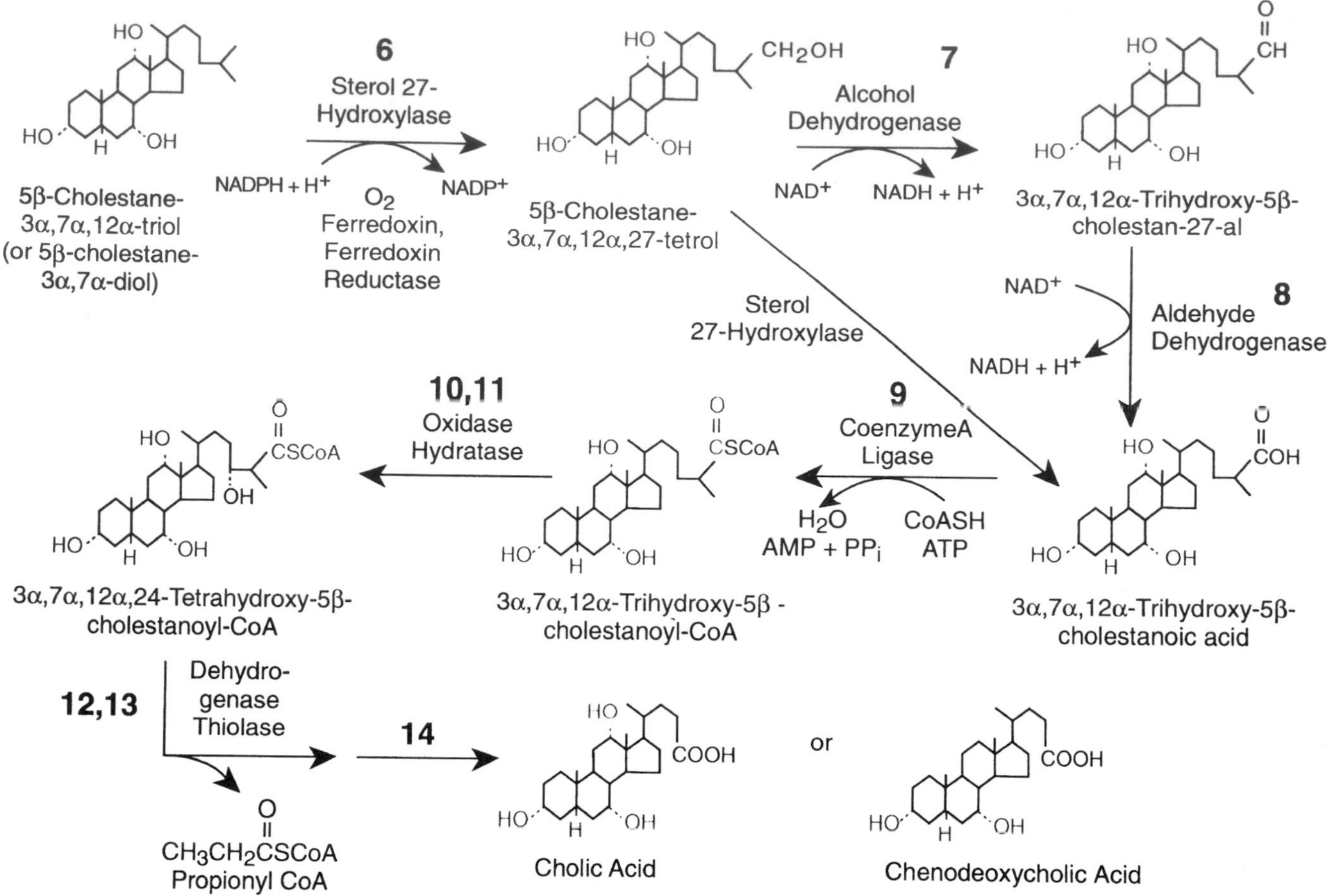

Figure 31.3. Reactions involved in the side-chain oxidation of the 5β-cholestane-$3\alpha,7\alpha,12\alpha$-triol intermediate in the pathway for primary bile acid synthesis.

The product of the sterol 27-hydroxylase catalyzed reaction, 5β-cholestane-$3\alpha,7\alpha,12\alpha,27$-tetrol, may also undergo oxidation by the combined actions of soluble or mitochondrial alcohol and aldehyde dehydrogenases [113]. The relative importance of these reactions compared with the complete 27-hydroxylase–catalyzed reaction is not known [93]. Cholestanoic acids are next converted to coenzyme A (CoA) esters by the action of a microsomal $3\alpha,7\alpha,12\alpha$-trihydroxy-5β-cholestanoic acid (THCA)-CoA ligase (synthetase), distinct from the fatty acid CoA ligases [114]. The final stage in modification of the side chain involves the β-oxidation of the cholestanoic acids, which occurs by a multiple-step reaction within peroxisomes [93]. The sequence of these reactions is analogous to the β-oxidation of fatty acids [115]. The CoA esters of the cholestanoic acid are acted on by a specific peroxisomal CoA acyl oxidase. This reaction is rate limiting, and the enzyme has been partially purified from rat liver and found to differ from the analogous CoA oxidases utilizing fatty acids as substrates [116]. The situation in humans is somewhat different in that a single peroxisomal oxidase acts on both branched-chain fatty acids and the bile acid intermediates [117]. Formation of a C-24 hydroxylated derivative occurs by the action of a bifunctional enoyl-CoA hydratase/β-hydroxyacyl-CoA dehydrogenase, a reaction that goes through a Δ^{24}-intermediate. Photoaffinity labeling experiments have demonstrated that this enzyme is the same one that is involved in the peroxisomal β-oxidation of fatty acids [118]. The dehydrogenase activity of the bifunctional enzyme yields a 24-oxo derivative that, following thiolytic cleavage, releases three carbon atoms in the form of propionic acid [119]. This results in the formation of the C_{24} bile acid CoA end product. With the exception of the CoA oxidase, defects in the other enzymes responsible for the β-oxidation of very long–chain fatty acids (VLCFAs) are also reflected by abnormalities in primary bile acid biosynthesis [2–4].

Alternative Pathways for Bile Acid Synthesis Initiated by 27-Hydroxylation of Cholesterol

Cholic and chenodeoxycholic acids can also be synthesized via different pathways (Figure 31.4), and under extreme pathologic conditions, these alternative pathways become quantitatively important [101–103,120,121]. In vitro studies of enzyme kinetics using radiolabeled intermediates first demonstrated the existence of an alternative pathway for primary bile acid synthesis

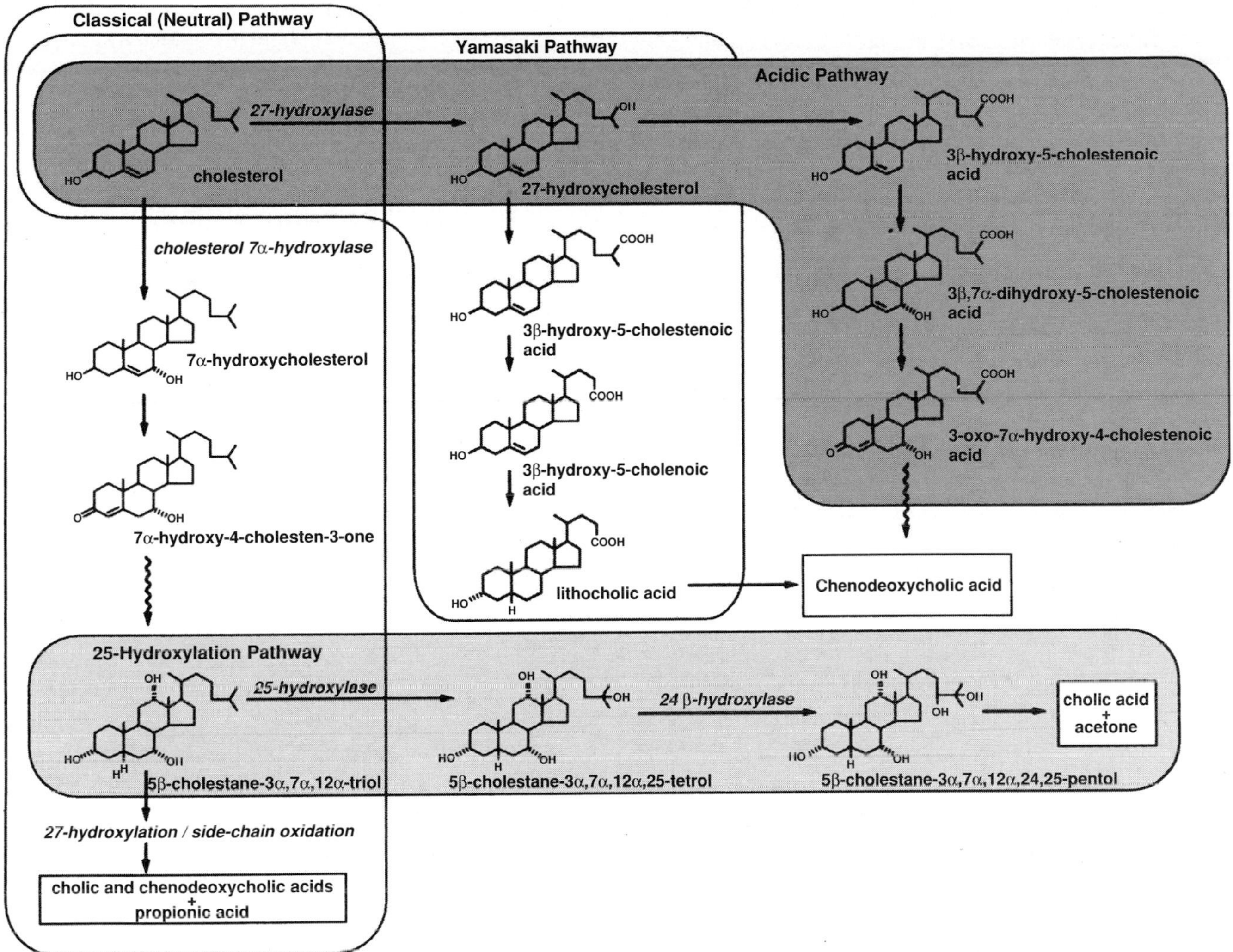

Figure 31.4. Alternative pathways for primary bile acid synthesis.

(Figure 31.4) [120,122,123]. This was confirmed in patients when it was shown that radiolabeled 27-hydroxycholesterol was more efficiently converted to chenodeoxycholic acid than 7α-hydroxycholesterol [124]. This pathway, involving initial 27-hydroxylation of cholesterol followed by 7α-hydroxylation by a specific oxysterol 7α-hydroxylase that is distinct from the rate-limiting cholesterol 7α-hydroxylase, became denoted as the acidic pathway [121]. The relative quantitative importance of this pathway is now appreciated [108,121]. 27-Hydroxylation occurs in the liver and in many other different tissues, including brain, alveolar macrophages, vascular endothelia, and fibroblasts [125–127]. The extrahepatic role of sterol 27-hydroxylase may be related to its regulation of cholesterol homeostasis by its ability to generate oxysterols that are potent repressors of cholesterol synthesis [108,111,128,129].

For some time it was evident that there were separate 7α-hydroxylases [121,130–132] and that bile acid synthesis via the acidic pathway was regulated differently and independently of the microsomal cholesterol 7α-hydroxylase [20,21,108,133]. Oxysterol 7α-hydroxylase has a high activity in human liver [131], but its regulation is not fully understood [38,134]. It has broad substrate specificity, being active on both 27- and 25-hydroxycholesterol [126,127,131,132] and 3β-hydroxy-5-cholenoic and 3β-hydroxy-5-cholestenoic acids [130], and cDNAs encoding the rat [125], mouse [38], and human [39, 134] hepatic oxysterol 7α-hydroxylase *(CYP7B1)* have been reported. The *CYP7B1* gene is localized to chromosome 8q21.3 and is in close proximity to the cholesterol 7α-hydroxylase *(CYP7A1)* gene.

It is now accepted that the acidic pathway contributes significantly to overall total bile acid synthesis and especially to chenodeoxycholic acid synthesis [108,121]. Normal levels of bile acids are synthesized by mice in which the cholesterol 7α-hydroxylase gene is knocked out, and bile acid synthesis is sustained in rats when cholesterol 7α-hydroxylase is inhibited by continuous infusion of squalestatin [34]. The oxysterol 7α-hydroxylase is developmentally induced in the rodent [35], and the failure of an infant to synthesize primary bile acids due to a mutation in oxysterol by the 7α-hydroxylase gene [39] highlights its importance in early human life. This enzyme plays an essential role in protecting the liver from hepatotoxic monohydroxy-bile acids that are otherwise formed in the acidic pathway if 7α-hydroxylation is lacking [39,135–138].

25-Hydroxylation Pathway to Cholic Acid Synthesis

In the conventional pathway described previously, side-chain oxidation takes place after C-27 hydroxylation and release of propionic acid. With the use of radiolabeled precursors, it was demonstrated that 5β-cholestane-3α,7α,12α-triol could be first 25-hydroxylated in the microsomal fraction then 24β-hydroxylated [101,120], and when oxidized to cholic acid, released acetone. This pathway is specific for cholic acid because little or no hydroxylation of 5β-cholestane-3α,7α-diol has been demonstrated. Based on studies of patients with the inborn error of CTX, it was proposed that the C-25 hydroxylation pathway may be the major pathway for cholic acid synthesis in humans [139]. The quantitative importance of this pathway was later reevaluated in vivo by measuring the production of [^{14}C]acetone after labeling the cholesterol pool with [26–^{14}C]cholesterol [103]. By this approach, it was shown that the C-25 hydroxylation pathway accounted for less than 5% of the total bile acids synthesized in healthy adults [103] and less than 2% in adult rats [102].

Yamasaki Pathway for Bile Acid Synthesis

A mitochondrial pathway involving side-chain hydroxylation of cholesterol to yield 27-hydroxycholesterol, followed by oxidation to 3β-hydroxy-5-cholenoic [140], lithocholic, and chenodeoxycholic acids [141] was first demonstrated in rats and later shown to occur in several other species [122,142–145]. In humans, it appears that this pathway, sometimes referred to as the Yamasaki pathway, is of little importance under normal conditions; however, it may account for the production of lithocholic and 3β-hydroxy-5-cholenoic acids in cholestatic liver disease and also in early life. Interestingly, lithocholic acid, which is normally formed by the action of intestinal microflora during the enterohepatic recycling of chenodeoxycholic acid, appears to become a primary bile acid under severe cholestatic conditions.

21-Hydroxylation Pathway

It is worth mentioning a proposed 21-hydroxylation pathway for the formation of bile acids from plant sterols, even though there is scant evidence to suggest that this pathway exists in humans. Plant sterols, which are normal constituents of the diet, make up a significant proportion of the neutral sterols excreted in feces because they are poorly absorbed. For this reason, the plant sterol sitosterol has been commonly employed as a nonabsorbable marker in sterol balance studies [146]. Studies by Salen et al. [147] suggested that intravenously administered [22,23–^{3}H]sitosterol could be converted to radiolabeled cholic and chenodeoxycholic acids in humans. Studies by others have confirmed that sitosterol can be converted to acidic metabolites in animals [148–150], which were not C_{24} bile acids [151] but rather C_{21} bile acids [152]. These unique bile acids were identified as C_{21} acids of pregnanetriols and pregnanetetrols, hydroxylated at positions C-3, C-11, C-15, and C-16, and were formed from radiolabeled cholesterol [153] and the plant sterol campesterol [152]. The mechanism of formation of these short-chain bile acids is presently uncertain, but it has been speculated that it may be initiated by a C-21 hydroxylation followed by oxidation to yield the 21-oic acid, and that the reactions may be facilitated by C-15 hydroxylation, a sex-specific pathway in rats. Whether the conversion of cholesterol or plant sterols to short-chain bile acids has any regulatory importance for cholesterol synthesis in animals is unknown, but studies by Bjorkhem [93] have suggested that this pathway is of no importance in humans.

27-Hydroxylation of 3-Oxo-Δ^4-Sterol Intermediates

Both 7α-hydroxy- and 7α,12α-dihydroxy-4-cholesten-3-one are good substrates for the mitochondrial sterol 27-hydroxylase (see Bjorkhem [93] and references therein). This is evident by the findings that increased concentrations of these intermediates occur in patients with CTX [154], from in vitro studies of HepG2 cells [155], and from the finding of side-chain oxidized metabolites in human plasma [121]. Side-chain oxidation of the 27-hydroxylated 3-oxo-Δ^4-sterols therefore must occur before 5β-reduction of the A ring.

Formation of Allo-bile Acids by 5α-Reduction

There are multiple pathways that can account for the presence of allo(5α-reduced)-bile acids, which under physiologic conditions account for relatively small proportions of the total bile acids of biologic fluids of humans but are major bile acid species of many lower vertebrates [79,80]. In humans, 5α-reduced bile acids are formed mainly by the action of intestinal microflora on 3-oxo-5β-bile acids during their enterohepatic circulation. Allo-bile acids consequently are excreted in significant amounts in feces. In rodents, these can be formed in the liver from 5α-cholestanol [156,157]. This pathway begins with 7α-hydroxylation of 5α-cholestanol [17], and the product is then converted to 5α-cholestane-3α,7α-diol via the intermediate 7α-hydroxy-5α-cholestan-3-one [158]. Hepatic 12α-hydroxylation of 5α-sterols is very efficient in the rat and readily leads to the formation of allo-cholic acid [158–161]. A further pathway for allo-bile acid formation involves the hepatic 5α-reduction of 7α-hydroxy- and 7α,12α-dihydroxy-3-oxo-4-cholen-24-oic acids, a reaction catalyzed by a Δ^{4-}3-oxosteroid 5α-reductase, as discussed earlier. This reaction has been demonstrated in rats, but the finding of large proportions of allo-bile acids in infants with severe cholestatic liver disease caused by a lack of Δ^{4-}3-oxosteroid 5β-reductase enzyme indicates that it is most probably of hepatic origin in humans [86].

Both 5α-reductase isozymes are expressed in the liver beginning at birth [162].

Other Cytochrome P450 Hydroxylations in the Metabolism of Bile Acids

A striking feature of bile acid synthesis and metabolism during development is the relatively large proportion of "atypical" bile acids that are not found in adult human bile. Although frequently referred to as atypical, this moniker is a misnomer because they are, in fact, very typical of the developmental phase of hepatic metabolism. Interestingly, the qualitative and quantitative bile acid composition of biologic fluids in early life closely resembles that of adults with severe cholestatic liver disease, suggesting that in the diseased liver, there is a reversion to more primitive pathways of synthesis and metabolism [72,73,163]. The most notable distinction in ontogeny is the prevalence of hydroxylation pathways that rapidly decline in importance over the first year of life. The most important hydroxylation reactions are 1β-, 4β-, and 6α-hydroxylations that are of hepatic origin. The concentrations of several of the metabolites, in particular hyocholic (3α,6α,7α-trihydroxy-5β-cholanoic) and 3α,4β,7α-trihydroxy-5β-cholanoic acids, exceed that of cholic acid in fetal bile [73]. The activities of C-1 and C-6 hydroxylases have been indirectly measured in fetal liver homogenates [164,165], whereas 4β-hydroxylation is a significant pathway in early life [166]. Relative to the enzymes involved in primary bile acid synthesis, little has been done to isolate and characterize these hydroxylases, and their activities are currently only indirectly determined from the developmental changes in the products of the reactions in bile. The role of these hydroxylation pathways is uncertain, but additional hydroxylation of the bile acid nucleus results in a significant increase in polarity, facilitating renal clearance and, at the same time, decreasing the membrane-damaging potential of their substrates. In early life and particularly in the fetus, an immaturity in canalicular and ileal bile acid transport processes leads to a sluggish enterohepatic circulation [167]. In this situation, hydroxylation presumably serves as a hepatoprotective mechanism.

Bile Acid Conjugation

Irrespective of the pathway by which cholesterol is converted to cholic and chenodeoxycholic acids, the CoA thioesters of these primary bile acids are finally conjugated to the amino acids glycine and taurine [168]. This two-step reaction is catalyzed by a rate-limiting bile acid–CoA ligase enzyme [169–172] followed by a bile acid–CoA:amino acid *N*-acyltransferase (EC 2.3.1.65) [173–176]. The genes encoding both enzymes have been cloned [177–179]. The conjugation reaction was originally believed to take place in the cytosol, but the highest activity of the conjugating enzymes was later found to be associated with peroxisomes [174,175]. A microsomal bile acid synthetase has been isolated [180] that may be involved in hydrolysis of the CoA esters and subsequent trafficking of cholic and chenodeoxycholic acids between compartments.

Genetic defects in the bile acid–CoA:amino acid *N*-acyltransferase have been associated with fat-soluble vitamin malabsorption states with variable degrees of liver disease. The bile acid–CoA:amino acid *N*-acyltransferase enzyme has been purified from human liver, has a molecular weight of 50 kDa, and utilizes glycine, taurine, and, interestingly, β-fluoroalanine, but not alanine, as substrates [173]. It also functions to conjugate VLCFAs to glycine [181]. The specificity of the enzyme has been examined in detail [176] and found to be influenced by the length of the side chain of the bile acid, bile acids having a four–carbon atom side chain. Nor(C_{23}) bile acids [182] and homo(C_{25}) bile acids are both poor substrates for amidation [183]; however, cholestanoic (C_{27}) acids found in biologic fluids of infants with peroxisomal defects are predominantly taurine conjugated [3,4]. A cDNA encoding the gene for the mouse [178] and human bile acid–CoA:amino acid *N*-acyltransferase has been isolated, characterized, and expressed in bacteria [177,179]. The human cDNA encodes a monomeric protein of 46,296 daltons, and although there is close homology with the mouse enzyme [178] and with *kan-1*, a putative rat liver *N*-acyltransferase [184], significant species differences in substrate specificity are observed. The human bile acid–CoA:amino acid *N*-acyltransferase conjugates cholic acid with both glycine and taurine, whereas the mouse enzyme showed selectivity toward only taurine. This is consistent with the mouse being an obligate taurine conjugator of bile acids, as are the rat and dog [185]. In humans, the final products of this complex multiple-step pathway are the two conjugated primary bile acids of cholic and chenodeoxycholic acids, and these are then secreted in canalicular bile and stored in gallbladder bile. In humans, glycine conjugation predominates, with a ratio of glycine to taurine conjugates of 3.1:1 for normal adults [78]. In early human life, more than 80% of the bile acids in bile are taurine conjugated [73] because of an abundance of hepatic stores of taurine [186]. Species differences in conjugation are important considerations when working with animal models.

Although the principal bile acids of humans and most mammalian species are amidated [79], other conjugates occur naturally (Figure 31.1); these include sulfates [187], glucuronide ethers and esters [188,189], glucosides [190,191], *N*-acetylglucosaminides [192], and conjugates of some drugs [193–195]. These conjugates account for a relatively large proportion of the total urinary bile acids. Conjugation significantly alters the physicochemical characteristics of the bile acid [196] and serves an important function in increasing the polarity of the molecule, thereby facilitating its renal excretion, and in minimizing the membrane-damaging potential of the more hydrophobic unconjugated species [197]. Under physiologic conditions, the various alternative conjugation pathways are quantitatively less important. However, in cholestatic liver disease, or when the liver is subjected to a bile acid load, the concentrations of these conjugates in biologic fluids increase [198,199], although the relative proportions do not appear to differ between the diseased and the healthy liver [198]. Detailed knowledge of these metabolic pathways is limited, but it is evident that there is significant localization of bile acid–conjugating enzymes in the kidneys [200,201].

Sulfation of bile acids, most commonly at the C-3 position but also at C-7 (Figure 31.1), is catalyzed by a bile acid sulfotransferase [202,203], an enzyme that in the rat, but not the human, exhibits sex-dependent differences in activity [204]. Although much has been written about the potential importance of sulfation in early life [205,206], it is evident from the finding of a relatively small proportion of bile acid sulfates in fetal bile, that hepatic sulfation is negligible in the fetus and neonate [73]. Indeed, it is most probable that urinary bile acid sulfates originate mainly by renal sulfation, which has been demonstrated both in vivo and in vitro [200,207]. Evidence in support of this contention is the fact that 60–80% of urinary bile acids are sulfated and their excretion increases in cholestasis [208]. Only traces of bile acid sulfates are found in bile [209], despite efficient canalicular transport of perfused bile acid sulfates.

A number of glucuronosyltransferases catalyze the formation of glucuronide ethers and esters [189]. The enzymes show substrate selectivity in that bile acids possessing a 6α-hydroxyl group are preferentially conjugated at the C-6 position, forming 6-O-ether glucuronides [210,211], whereas short-chain bile acids form mainly glucuronides [189]. Purification of the hyodeoxycholic acid–specific human uridine diphosphate–glucuronosyltransferase and subsequent cloning of a cDNA [212] indicate that this enzyme is highly specific toward hyodeoxycholic (3α,6α-dihydroxy-5β-cholanoic) acid; no glucuronidation of hyocholic (3α,6α,7α-trihydroxy-5β-cholanoic) acid could be detected. It is probable that there is a family of isozymes that catalyze the glucuronidation of different bile acids.

Glucosides and *N*-acetylglucosaminides of nonamidated and amidated bile acids have been identified in normal human urine [213], with quantitative excretion comparable to that of glucuronide conjugates [214]. A microsomal glucosyltransferase has been isolated and purified from human liver [190] but is also present in extrahepatic tissues [215]. The enzyme responsible for *N*-acetylglucosaminide formation exhibits remarkable substrate specificity in that it preferentially catalyzes the conjugation of bile acids having a 7β-hydroxyl group; consequently, these conjugates account for more than 20% of the urinary metabolites of patients administered UDCA [199].

The full extent to which drugs may compete for the conjugating enzymes is not known; however, bile acid conjugates of 5-fluorouracil have been identified [193,194]. The 2-fluoro-β-alanine conjugate of cholic acid was found to be a major metabolite in bile following administration of this therapeutic agent.

Formation of Secondary Bile Acids

The intestinal microflora plays an important role in bile acid synthesis and metabolism. Bacterial enzymes metabolize primary bile acids, significantly altering their physicochemical characteristics and influencing their physiologic actions during enterohepatic recycling. The result is the formation of a spectrum of secondary bile acids that are mainly excreted in feces [216]. The deconjugation of conjugated bile acids and subsequent 7α-dehydroxylation are quantitatively the most important reactions, but bacterial oxidoreduction and epimerization at various positions of the bile acid nucleus also take place along the intestinal tract [217–220]. This spatial modification is evident from bile acid profiles along the entire length of the human intestine obtained at autopsy that show relatively high proportions of secondary bile acids in the proximal jejunum and mid–small bowel [221]. The enzymes that catalyze these reactions are found in a variety of organisms, such as *Bacteroides*, *Clostridia*, *Bifidobacteria*, and *Escherichia coli*, and some of these reactions occur in the proximal small intestine [222–224]. Deconjugation precedes 7α-dehydroxylation, and the bacterial peptidases responsible for this reaction exhibit remarkable substrate specificity in that the length of the side chain is a crucial factor influencing this reaction [225,226]. The enzyme kinetics, the factors influencing the reactions, and the molecular biology of a number of the bacterial enzymes have been extensively studied by Hylemon et al. [227–229], and more detailed information can be gained from reviews by this group. 7α-Dehydroxylation of cholic and chenodeoxycholic acids, a reaction that proceeds via a 3-oxo-Δ^4-intermediate [227], results in the formation of deoxycholic and lithocholic acids, respectively, and these secondary bile acids make up the largest proportion of total fecal bile acids [216]. Lithocholic and deoxycholic acids are relatively insoluble and consequently poorly absorbed. However, both bile acids are returned to the liver and exhibit feedback inhibition of bile acid synthesis [138,230,231]. It should be noted that in rats, deoxycholic acid is very efficiently 7α-hydroxylated in the liver and converted back to cholic acid, but this reaction does not take place in humans. Serum concentrations of deoxycholic acid therefore provide a useful means of assessing the extent of impairment of the enterohepatic circulation in cholestatic liver diseases [232,233].

DEFECTS IN BILE ACID SYNTHESIS CAUSING METABOLIC LIVER DISEASE AND SYNDROMES OF FAT-SOLUBLE VITAMIN MALABSORPTION

Defects in bile acid synthesis may be expected to have profound effects on hepatic and gastrointestinal function. Working on the hypothesis that some cases of idiopathic neonatal cholestasis may be the result of genetic defects in primary bile acid synthesis, we initiated a program of screening for such defects using what then was a new innovation in mass spectrometry, fast atom bombardment ionization mass spectrometry (FAB-MS), also referred to as liquid secondary ionization mass spectrometry (LSIMS). The technique, largely considered obsolete with the introduction of electrospray mass spectrometry techniques [234], provides the basis for an international screening program for inborn errors in bile acid synthesis at the Cincinnati Children's Hospital Medical Center, Cincinnati, Ohio. The rationale

3β-Hydroxy-C_{27}-steroid-oxidoreductase

Δ^4-3-Oxosteroid 5β-reductase

Oxysterol 7α-hydroxylase

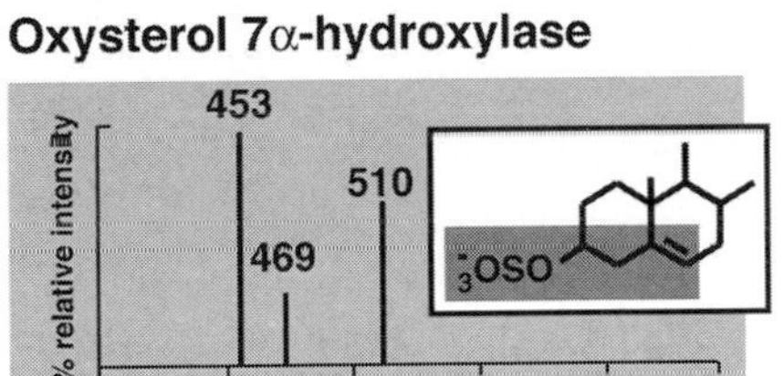

2-Methylacyl-CoA racemase

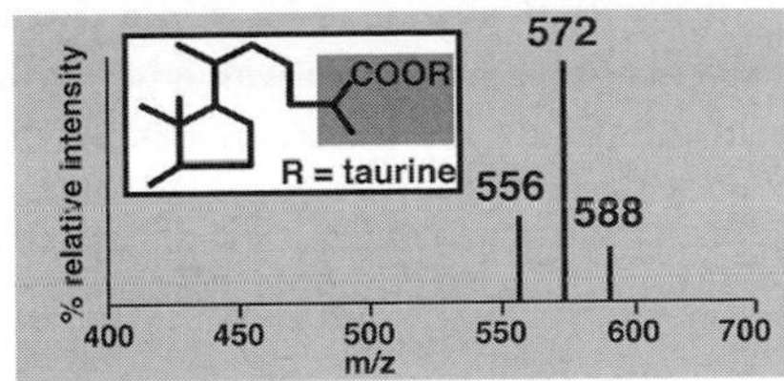

Sterol 27-hydroxylase

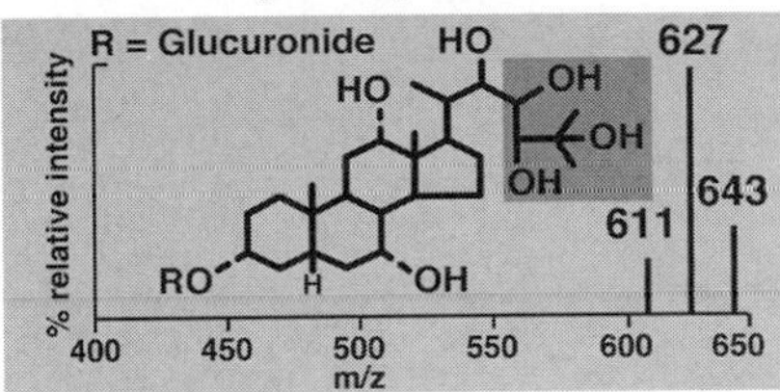

Amidation deficiency

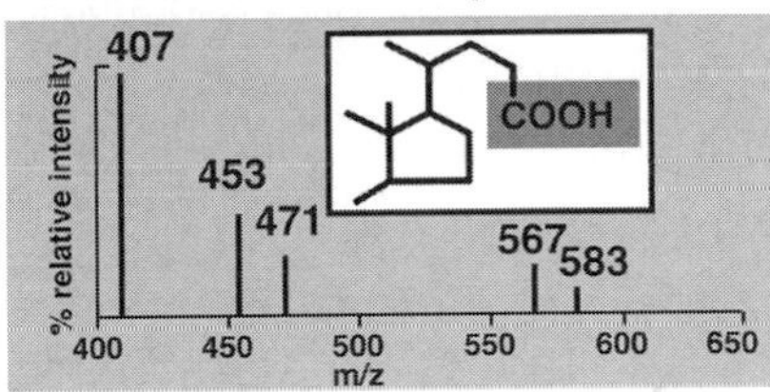

Figure 31.5. Reconstructed negative ion mass spectra generated from FAB ionization of urine extracts typically observed in patients with six different genetic defects in bile acid synthesis. Only the key diagnostic ions are shown for specific metabolites that retain the basic structure of the substrates for the deficient enzyme.

for the above hypothesis was twofold: (1) Such defects would lead to an overproduction of potentially hepatotoxic atypical bile acids synthesized from bile acid intermediates accumulating proximal to the enzyme defect, and (2) cholestasis would be exacerbated by a lack of primary bile acids that are essential for promoting bile flow. Bile acid defects were expected to manifest as progressive cholestatic conditions. Marked alterations in urinary, serum, and biliary bile acids are found in all infants and children with liver disease, but it is often difficult to ascertain whether such changes were primary or secondary to the liver dysfunction. Using FAB-MS, the direct analysis of bile acid conjugates in biologic fluids is possible. The resulting mass spectra provide characteristic profiles of specific defects in bile acid metabolism (Figure 31.5) that afford a means of "teasing out" those samples that are unique and warrant more extensive and time-consuming gas chromatography–mass spectrometry (GC-MS) analysis to elucidate potential primary defects in synthesis or metabolism. By this approach, six defects in bile acid synthesis have been defined [39,86,235–238] with a phenotypic expression of familial and progressive infantile or late-onset cholestasis or syndromes of fat-soluble vitamin malabsorption. A further defect in cholesterol 7α-hydroxylase (*CYP7A1*) has since been recognized that does not present as liver disease but rather as dyslipidemia that is unresponsive to statin [239]. Broadly, these defects may be categorized as deficiencies in the activity of enzymes responsible for catalyzing reactions in the steroid nucleus or in the side chain. It appears that disorders in bile acid synthesis account for about 2% of the screened cases of liver disease in infants and children and, in this regard, should be recognized as a distinct entity of metabolic liver disease. Further disorders are likely to be identified as screening becomes more commonplace in the work-up of patients with idiopathic liver disease.

Defects Involving Reactions to the Steroid Nucleus

Presently, three well-defined defects have been identified involving enzymes catalyzing reactions that modify the AB rings of the steroid nucleus; these are shown in Figure 31.6. A 12α-hydroxylase defect was proposed some years ago but was never definitively confirmed [240]. The clinical presentation of all these metabolic defects is variable [4], but in general, progressive cholestatic liver disease is the main manifestation in

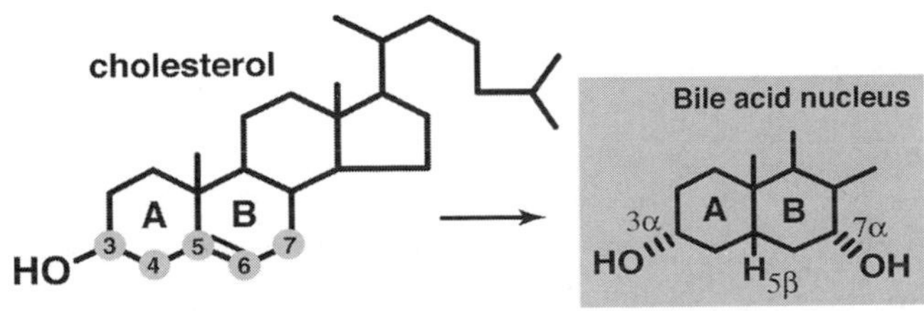

Figure 31.6. Metabolic defects involving changes to the steroid rings are clinically manifest as familial intrahepatic cholestatic syndromes.

patients with markedly impaired primary bile acid synthesis due to steroid nuclear defects. Typical biochemical abnormalities are elevations in serum liver enzymes, conjugated hyperbilirubinemia, and evidence of fat-soluble vitamin malabsorption. In the early years, subnormal levels of serum fat-soluble vitamins and, in some cases, rickets often precede any evidence of liver dysfunction [241]. These abnormalities are usually corrected with oral vitamin supplementation, but these patients eventually present later in life with hepatosplenomegaly and elevated serum liver enzymes. The 3β-hydroxy-C_{27}-steroid dehydrogenase/isomerase deficiency is the most common of the bile acid synthetic defects accounting for late-onset chronic cholestatic syndromes. A normal serum γ-glutamyl transpeptidase (γGT) level is highly associated with – although it should be stressed, not an exclusive feature of –all these bile acid synthetic defects.

3β-Hydroxy-C_{27}-Steroid Dehydrogenase/Isomerase (Oxidoreductase) Deficiency

The second step in primary bile acid synthesis involves the conversion of 7α-hydroxycholesterol into 7α-hydroxy-4-cholesten-3-one, a reaction catalyzed by a microsomal 3β-hydroxy-C_{27}-steroid dehydrogenase/isomerase [59] also referred to as the 3β-hydroxy-C_{27}-steroid oxidoreductase. A deficiency of this sterol-specific enzyme [235] leads to the accumulation of 7α-hydroxycholesterol within the hepatocyte. The remaining enzymes involved in bile acid synthesis catalyze subsequent transformations, including side-chain oxidation, with the result that in place of the normal primary bile acids, C_{24} bile acids are synthesized, retaining the 3β-hydroxy-Δ^5 structure characteristic of the substrates for the 3β-hydroxy-C_{27}-steroid dehydrogenase/isomerase.

This defect was first identified in a patient of Saudi Arabian origin who was the third infant of five to be affected by progressive idiopathic neonatal cholestasis; the two previous infants had died following a similar clinical history and were products of a consanguineous marriage [235]. Later it became appreciated that this defect explained some cases of late-onset chronic cholestasis [242,243]. All the affected infants had progressive jaundice, elevated aminotransferase levels, and conjugated hyperbilirubinemia. This general clinical presentation has been common in all the cases of 3β-hydroxy-C_{27}-steroid dehydrogenase/isomerase deficiency thus far recognized [243]. On clinical examination, patients with the 3β-hydroxy-C_{27}-steroid dehydrogenase/isomerase deficiency usually present with hepatomegaly, fat-soluble vitamin malabsorption, and mild steatorrhea. Pruritus may or may not be present. This inborn error is highly associated with elevated serum bilirubin and aminotransferase levels but a normal serum γGT concentration, and this biochemical picture is a useful clinical marker for the defect [243–245]. Furthermore, serum bile acid concentrations will be normal when measured by enzymatic or immunoassay methods and seemingly incompatible with the extent of cholestasis. Therefore, the inclusion of serum bile acid determination in the clinical evaluation may provide a further clue to this defect. As with most of the inborn errors involving the reactions responsible for nuclear modification, the 3β-hydroxy-C_{27}-steroid dehydrogenase/isomerase deficiency is familial in nature and is fatal if untreated. Age at onset and diagnosis are variable, ranging from 3 months to 14 years, indicating that cases of late-onset chronic cholestasis [243] can be explained by inborn errors in bile acid synthesis. Histologic examination of the liver of these patients shows hepatitis with the presence of giant cells and is consistent with cholestasis as evidenced by canalicular plugs, bile stasis, and inflammatory changes [235,246–249].

Definitive diagnosis of the 3β-hydroxy-C_{27}-steroid dehydrogenase/isomerase deficiency is established by FAB-MS analysis of the urine, which quantitatively indicates an elevated urinary excretion of bile acids consistent with cholestasis but qualitatively an absence of the normal glycine and taurine conjugated primary bile acids [3,4,235,243]. In place of primary bile acids, the negative ion mass spectrum (Figure 31.5) is characterized by two pairs of ions consistent with sulfate and glycosulfate conjugates of (unsaturated) dihydroxy- and trihydroxy-cholenoic acids. The structures of these bile acids were established by GC-MS analysis as 3β,7α-dihydroxy- and 3β,7α,12α-trihydroxy-5-cholenoic acids [235]. The occurrence of these atypical bile acids is explained by a deficiency in the microsomal 3β-hydroxy-C_{27}-steroid dehydrogenase/isomerase enzyme that catalyzes the conversion of 7α-hydroxycholesterol to 7α-hydroxy-4-cholesten-3-one in the normal pathway for primary bile acid synthesis. In response to a deficiency in this enzyme, C_{24} bile acids are formed that retain the 3β-hydroxy-Δ^5 structure characteristic of the substrate. Tetrahydroxy- and pentahydroxy-bile alcohols with a 3β,7α-dihydroxy-Δ^5 and 3β,7α,12α-trihydroxy-Δ^5 nucleus are also found in greatly increased amounts in the urine, plasma, and bile [250]. These bile alcohols are mainly sulfated, in contrast to the glucuronide conjugates of saturated bile alcohols observed in CTX [251]. Although primary bile acids are not detectable in the urine, the bile may contain small proportions of cholic acid resulting from intestinal bacterial metabolism of the 3β-hydroxy-Δ^5 bile acids during enterohepatic recycling. The presence of cholic acid may facilitate bile secretion and explain the longer survival of these patients.

Multiple 3β-hydroxysteroid dehydrogenase/isomerases exist that catalyze analogous reactions in steroid hormone metabolism [63,64], but the lack of overt endocrine abnormalities in these patients indicates differences in the specificity of the isozyme active on C_{27} sterols. This enzyme is expressed in fibroblasts, and further confirmation of a primary bile acid defect in the first patient to be identified with the 3β-hydroxy-C_{27}-steroid dehydrogenase/isomerase deficiency was established from assaying its enzyme activity in cultured fibroblasts using 7α-hydroxycholesterol as a substrate. In contrast to healthy controls, the patient had no detectable enzyme activity in fibroblasts whereas the parents had a low but measurable activity consistent with a heterozygous phenotype [252]. Measurement of enzyme activity to confirm the diagnosis established by mass spectrometry has now been superseded by molecular tools because DNA sequencing of the genes encoding

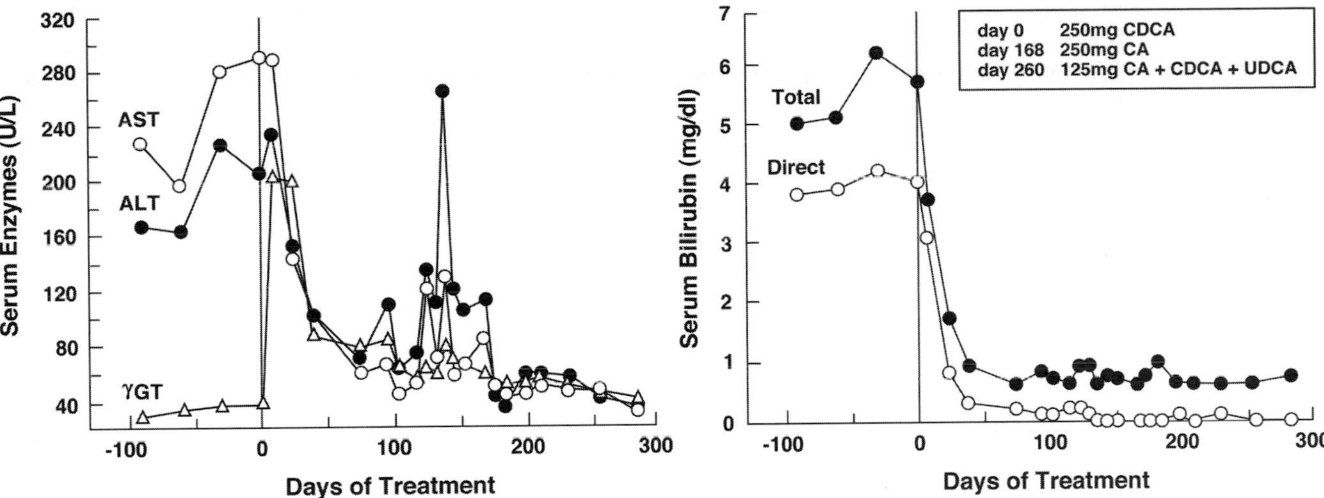

Figure 31.7. Effect of bile acid therapy on serum liver enzymes and bilirubin in a 10-year-old patient with a diagnosed 3β-hydroxy-C_{27}-steroid dehydrogenase/isomerase deficiency. ALT, alanine aminotransferase; AST, aspartate aminotransferase; CA, cholic acid; CDCA, chenodeoxycholic acid; γGT, γ-glutamyl transpeptidase; UDCA, ursodeoxycholic acid.

most of the enzymes involved in bile acid synthesis has been completed [9]. The 3β-hydroxy-C_{27}-steroid dehydrogenase/isomerase enzyme is encoded by the *HSD3B7* gene localized to chromosome 16p11.2–12, and DNA sequence analysis of 16 patients revealed 12 different mutations, including point mutations, small insertions, and deletions [66], illustrating the diverse spectrum of the genetics. In an earlier report, a 2-base pair (bp) deletion in exon 6 accounted for the inactivity of this enzyme in the index case with this bile acid defect [65]. In four cases, the mutations were compound heterozygous whereas the majority were inherited in homozygous form. When these mutations were expressed in HEK 293 cells, impaired synthesis of the protein product was demonstrated, and this lacked enzyme activity [66].

The mechanism by which liver injury occurs in this disorder is the combined result of inadequate synthesis of primary bile acids needed for the promotion of bile flow and the accumulation of atypical bile acid metabolites synthesized as a consequence of the enzyme deficiency. Interestingly, in animal models, 3β-hydroxy-5-cholenoic acid produces cholestasis [136], but this has not been found to be the case for 3β, 7α-dihydroxy-5-cholenoic acid [144] because it is rapidly metabolized to chenodeoxycholic acid in animals. This conversion does not occur in patients lacking the 3β-hydroxy-C_{27}-steroid dehydrogenase/isomerase enzyme. Studies using rat liver canalicular membrane vesicles have confirmed the cholestatic nature of the taurine conjugate of 3β,7α-dihydroxy-5-cholenoic acid [253,254]. Untreated, the progressive cholestasis characteristic of this genetic defect eventually leads to cirrhosis and liver failure.

Oral administration of primary bile acids should be the therapeutic approach. The rationale for primary bile acid therapy is that down-regulation of cholesterol 7α-hydroxylase, the rate-limiting enzyme for endogenous bile acid synthesis [19], would limit further production of hepatotoxic 3β-hydroxy-Δ^5 bile acids while additionally providing the stimulus for bile flow, thereby facilitating the hepatic clearance of endogenous bile acids and toxic substances, including bilirubin. By this approach, oral chenodeoxycholic acid (125–250 mg/d) and cholic acid (250 mg/d), the latter now the bile acid of choice (10–15 mg/kg body weight/d), has resulted in remarkable clinical and biochemical improvement, with a normalization of liver function tests and resolution of jaundice in all cases [243,245,247,249,255–257] (Figure 31.7). A number of patients with advanced liver disease who were found to have a 3β-hydroxy-C_{27}-steroid dehydrogenase/isomerase deficiency have been removed from transplantation waiting lists, and the liver disease resolved with bile acid therapy. The choice of bile acid dose is empirically derived and based on careful monitoring by FAB-MS and GC-MS of the level of endogenous bile acids in plasma and urine and by titrating dosage according to the disappearance of the unusual 3β-hydroxy-Δ^5 bile acids [243]. Although it may not be possible to completely shut down endogenous bile acid synthesis, significant down-regulation in the production of the 3β-hydroxy-Δ^5 bile acids and bile alcohols occurs and, concomitant with this response, normalization in liver function, including an improvement in liver histology, results [249].

Δ^4-3-Oxosteroid 5β-Reductase Deficiency

A deficiency of the cytosolic Δ^4-3-oxosteroid 5β-reductase enzyme responsible for the catalytic conversion of 7α-hydroxy- and 7α,12α-dihydroxy-4-cholesten-3-one into the corresponding 3-oxo-5β(H) analogues was discovered as a further cause of marked progressive and familial neonatal cholestasis [258,259]. The defect was first identified in monochorionic twin boys born with a marked and progressive cholestasis [86]. A previous sibling with neonatal hepatitis had died of liver failure following a similar clinical course. Liver function tests revealed an elevation in serum aminotransferase levels, marked hyperbilirubinemia, and coagulopathy. Unlike the 3β-hydroxy-C_{27}-steroid dehydrogenase/isomerase deficiency, serum γGT concentrations are generally elevated. Liver biopsies showed marked lobular disarray as a result of giant cell and pseudoacinar transformation of hepatocytes, hepatocellular and canalicular bile stasis, and extramedullary hematopoiesis. Electron micrographs showed small bile canaliculi that were slitlike in appearance, lacked the usual microvilli, and contained variable amounts of electron-dense material [248,249,257].

The Δ^4-3-oxosteroid 5β-reductase deficiency was identified following FAB-MS analysis, which indicated an elevated urinary bile acid excretion consistent with cholestasis and a predominance of bile acid conjugates with molecular weights consistent with (unsaturated) oxo-hydroxy- and oxo-dihydroxy-cholenoic acids (Figure 31.5). Following extraction, hydrolysis and derivatization of bile acids, GC-MS analysis confirmed two predominant metabolites, identified as 3-oxo-7α-hydroxy-4-cholenoic and 3-oxo-7α,12α-dihydroxy-4-cholenoic acids [86]. Small proportions of allo(5α-H) isomers of cholic and chenodeoxycholic acids were also present. These atypical bile acids accounted for up to 90% of the total urinary bile acids. Serum bile acids were elevated, and relatively high concentrations of allo-chenodeoxycholic, allo-cholic, and Δ^4-3-oxo-bile acids were present in serum. Only traces (<2 μmol/L) of biliary bile acids were found, confirming the findings from studies using rat canalicular membrane vesicles [253,254] that Δ^4-3-oxo-bile acids are poor substrates for the canalicular bile acid transporters, perhaps because of their poor solubility or their unique structures. The biochemical presentation of increased synthesis of Δ^4-3-oxo- and allo-bile acids in these patients is consistent with a deficiency in the activity of the nicotinamide adenine dinucleotide phosphate (NADPH)-dependent Δ^4-3-oxosteroid 5β-reductase [258,259]. The presence of high levels of allo-bile acids, normally minor metabolites, is explained by the substrates exceeding the K_m and maximum velocity (V_{max}) for the hepatic 5α-reductase in response to a lack of Δ^4-3-oxosteroid 5β-reductase activity.

Δ^4-3-Oxosteroid 5β-reductase is not expressed in fibroblasts, but further evidence for a primary enzyme defect was established by immunoblot analysis of the cytosolic fraction from the liver using a monoclonal antibody raised against the rat Δ^4-3-oxosteroid 5β-reductase. This monoclonal antibody recognized the 38-kDa protein in the liver from patients with liver disease due to other etiologies but not from the patient with the Δ^4-3-oxosteroid 5β-reductase deficiency [2]. The cDNA for the gene encoding the human Δ^4-3-oxosteroid 5β-reductase gene (*SRD5B1*) was reported [82]. Recent studies of three patients with high levels of Δ^4-3-oxo-bile acids in urine and low or absent primary bile acids revealed three different mutations in this gene, consistent with a primary enzyme defect in each case [87]. Two patients were homozygous for missense mutations (662 C>T in one patient and 385 C>T in another), and a third patient was homozygous for a single base deletion (511 delT) in exon 5 leading to a premature stop codon. The liver biopsies of all three patients were characterized by giant cell transformations, a common feature of many of the cases of inborn errors in bile acid synthesis [86,246,248,249]. In a patient from Japan who met biochemical criteria for a deficiency in this enzyme, sequence analysis of the gene revealed a single silent mutation in the coding region of the gene [82], but immunoblot analysis of the liver homogenate using a monoclonal antibody revealed expression of the normal protein [260], thus excluding a primary genetic defect. Increased production of Δ^4-3-oxo-bile acids often occurs in patients with severe liver disease [85] and also in infants during the first few weeks of life [261]. Several infants presenting with neonatal hemochromatosis have been found to have a deficiency in Δ^4-3-oxosteroid 5β-reductase [262]. Because primary bile acids are involved in the canalicular transport of iron [263], the question of whether the iron storage defect may be secondary to the bile acid inborn error, or vice versa, has been raised [262]. In the case of a suspected Δ^4-3-oxosteroid 5β-reductase deficiency, it is important to perform a repeat analysis of urine because on some occasions a resolution of the liver disease occurs and these atypical bile acids disappear [264]. This is also the case with developmental immaturity.

The liver injury in this defect is the consequence of diminished primary bile acid synthesis and the hepatotoxicity of the accumulated Δ^4-3-oxo-bile acids. A lack of canalicular secretion can be explained by the relative insolubility of these unsaturated oxo-bile acids, and the taurine conjugate of 7α-dihydroxy-3-oxo-4-cholenoic acid has been demonstrated to be cholestatic in rat canalicular plasma membrane vesicles [253,254]. The unique morphologic findings in these patients suggest that maturation of the canalicular membrane and the transport system for bile acid secretion may require a threshold concentration of primary bile acids in early development [257]. Treatment of this disorder with primary bile acid therapy (cholic acid) has, in most patients, resulted in clinical and biochemical improvement, resolution of jaundice, and normalization in liver function tests, provided that therapy is initiated before significant liver damage has occurred (Figure 31.8). The dosage of bile acid administered is based on monitoring the urine for the presence of Δ^4-3-oxo-bile acids and titrating the dose accordingly to achieve significant down-regulation in endogenous bile acid synthesis [243]. In the original infants diagnosed with this defect, bile acid therapy also led to a significant improvement in liver histology, which by electron microscopy showed a normalization of the immature-appearing bile canalicular structures with a disappearance of the electron-dense material seen in and around the canaliculi [257].

Oxysterol 7α-Hydroxylase Deficiency

The discovery of a genetic defect in oxysterol 7α-hydroxylase [39] established the acidic pathway as a quantitatively important pathway for bile acid synthesis in early life. Unlike the mouse, in which this enzyme appears to be developmentally regulated [35], or the rat, in which it is induced when there is suppression of cholesterol 7α-hydroxylase activity [34], it would appear that in the human, the oxysterol 7α-hydroxylase may be more important than cholesterol 7α-hydroxylase for

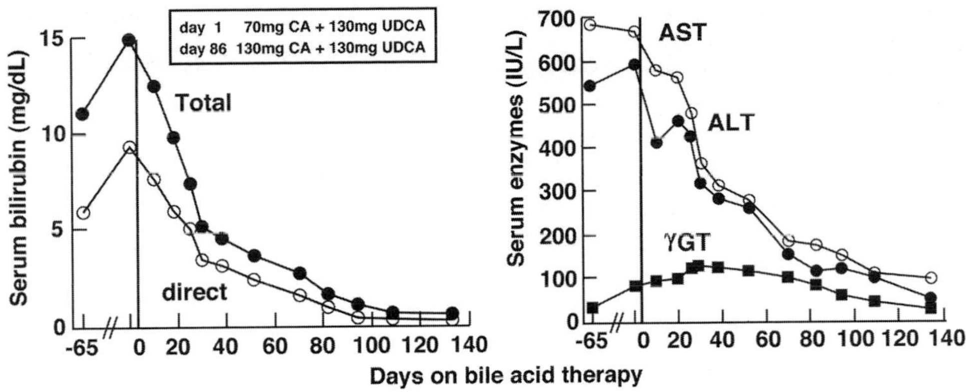

Figure 31.8. Effect of primary bile acid therapy on serum total and direct bilirubin (*left panel*) and liver enzyme (*right panel*) concentrations in a patient with a diagnosed Δ^4-3-oxosteroid 5β-reductase deficiency.

bile acid synthesis, at least in early life. In common with the 3β-hydroxy-C_{27}-steroid dehydrogenase/isomerase deficiency and the Δ^4-oxosteroid 5β-reductase deficiency, this genetic defect presents as severe progressive cholestatic liver disease. It has thus far been diagnosed in only one patient, a 10-week-old boy of parents who were first cousins [39]. This patient had severe cholestasis, cirrhosis, and liver synthetic failure from early infancy. He became progressively jaundiced by 8 weeks of age and had hepatosplenomegaly and markedly elevated serum aminotransferase levels but a normal serum γGT. The liver biopsy revealed cholestasis, bridging fibrosis, extensive giant cell transformation, and bile duct proliferation. Oral UDCA therapy interestingly led to deterioration in liver function tests, and primary bile acid therapy with cholic acid proved ineffective. The patient underwent orthotopic liver transplantation at 4.5 months of age but succumbed 3 weeks later from disseminated Epstein–Barr virus–related lymphoproliferative disease.

FAB-MS analysis of the urine revealed an absence of primary bile acids, and in their place were large concentrations of unsaturated monohydroxy-C_{24} bile acids as sulfate (mass to charge ratio [*m/z*] 453) and glycosulfate (*m/z* 510) conjugates (Figure 31.5). These were identified by GC-MS as the unsaturated monohydroxy-bile acids, 3β-hydroxy-5-cholenoic and 3β-hydroxy-5-cholestenoic acids, and accounted for 97% and 86%, respectively, of the total serum and urinary bile acids. The formation of 3β-hydroxy-5-cholenoic and 3β-hydroxy-5-cholestenoic acids occurs exclusively via the acidic pathway [265]. The biochemical features of this patient indicated a metabolic defect in the oxysterol 7α-hydroxylase enzyme. This was supported by the findings that 27-hydroxycholesterol concentrations in serum and urine were more than 4500 times normal and no 7α-hydroxylated sterols were detected. Monohydroxy-bile acids with the 3β-hydroxy-Δ^5 structure previously have been shown to be extremely cholestatic [52,137], and their hepatotoxicity in this patient would be exacerbated by the lack of primary bile acids necessary for the maintenance of bile flow.

Molecular studies of the liver tissue established the cholesterol 7α-hydroxylase gene to be normal; however, there was no measurable enzyme activity or mRNA. This may not have been surprising because cholesterol 7α-hydroxylase activity is generally low in the liver of infants [266]. It is also possible that gene expression may have been repressed by the vast amounts of oxysterol produced as a result of a deficiency in oxysterol 7α-hydroxylase. Whether these oxysterols may have acted through some of the recently described orphan receptors [41–51] is uncertain but possible. The liver tissue from the patient was found to have no oxysterol 7α-hydroxylase activity or mRNA, and analysis of the structure of the gene revealed a cytosine-to-thymidine transition mutation at position 388 in exon 5, providing unambiguous confirmation of the genetic defect in the oxysterol 7α-hydroxylase [39]. The patient was homozygous for this nonsense mutation, whereas both parents were heterozygous. When human embryonic 293 or Chinese hamster ovary cells were transfected with the cDNA having the R388* mutation, there was no detectable 7α-hydroxylase activity, and immunoblot analysis confirmed that the mutated gene encoded a truncated protein unable to catalyze 7α-hydroxylation [39]. Oxysterol 7α-hydroxylase is essential for protecting the liver from hepatotoxic and cholestatic 3β-hydroxy-Δ^5 monohydroxy-bile acids that otherwise would accumulate in the acidic pathway (Figure 31.9). The discovery

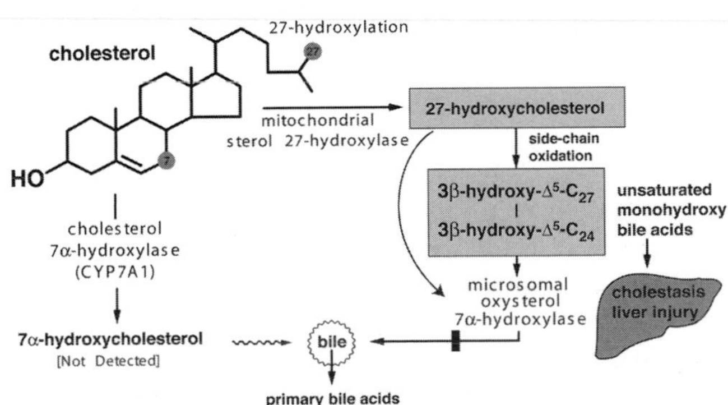

Figure 31.9. The two major pathways for primary bile acid synthesis from cholesterol depicting the biochemical presentation of a deficiency in oxysterol 7α-hydroxylase as a cause of severe neonatal cholestatic liver disease.

of this defect sheds light on the quantitative importance of the acidic pathway for bile acid synthesis in early human life. Unlike the other two previously reported nuclear defects in bile acid synthesis, the oxysterol 7α-hydroxylase deficiency seems to be particularly severe and untreatable by primary bile acid therapy. The therapeutic strategy for patients with this defect should be down-regulation in sterol 27-hydroxylase. It is possible that this cause of idiopathic liver disease may go unrecognized because of its rapid downhill course in the early months of life.

Cholesterol 7α-Hydroxylase Deficiency

Although not classified as a genetic defect responsible for cholestatic liver disease, a deficiency in cholesterol 7α-hydroxylase was reported to be responsible for hypertriglyceridemia and gallstone disease in three related adults [239]. This finding followed a screening of the *CYP7A1* gene for mutations in patients presenting with elevated low-density lipoprotein (LDL) cholesterol who were resistant to HMG-CoA reductase inhibitors. A 2-bp deletion (1302–1303 delTT) was observed in exon 6 of the gene, resulting in a frameshift mutation and causing a LeuArg substitution that when transfected into HEK 293 cells, led to an inactive protein product. All three patients were homozygous for this mutation and had serum cholesterol concentrations greater than 300 mg/dL, LDL cholesterol greater than 180 mg/dL, and elevated triglycerides [239]. The heterozygous relatives of the two patients described also had elevated cholesterol levels. There was no evidence for cholestasis, fibrosis, or inflammation, but fatty changes in the liver were reported following biopsy. Fecal bile acid analysis revealed markedly reduced total bile acid output (6% of normal) and a high (chenodeoxycholic + lithocholic)/(cholic + deoxycholic) acid ratio, consistent with preferential synthesis of chenodeoxycholic acid via the acidic pathway for bile acid synthesis.

12α-Hydroxylase Deficiency

Two separate reports have suggested the occurrence of a defect in bile acid synthesis involving 12α-hydroxylation. The first report described a 10-year-old girl with celiac disease who from the age of 3 years had steatorrhea and chronic constipation (bowel movements once every 3–6 weeks) [240]. At diagnosis, cholic acid accounted for only 17% of the biliary bile acids, and the failure to detect 12α-hydroxylase activity in a wedge biopsy of liver tissue was used in support of a hypothesis for a 12α-hydroxylation defect and the speculation that the constipation may be associated with a congenital bile acid deficiency [267]. In a later report of a premature infant with severe hypoglycemia and cholestasis diagnosed with panhypopituitarism, a low cholic/chenodeoxycholic acid ratio was found in bile, leading to speculation that the liver disease was related to an immaturity in hepatic 12α-hydroxylase [268]. In our experience, caution is required in concluding that abnormalities in bile acid metabolism are the result of enzyme defects or inborn errors, because developmental differences in bile acid synthesis and metabolism are found in early life. An immaturity in canalicular secretory function [269] and the reduced ileal uptake of bile acids [270] mean that the enterohepatic circulation of bile acids is compromised. From a practical standpoint, because of physiologic cholestasis in newborn infants, it is important to perform a follow-up analysis of urine in suspected bile acid defects diagnosed in the first few weeks of life.

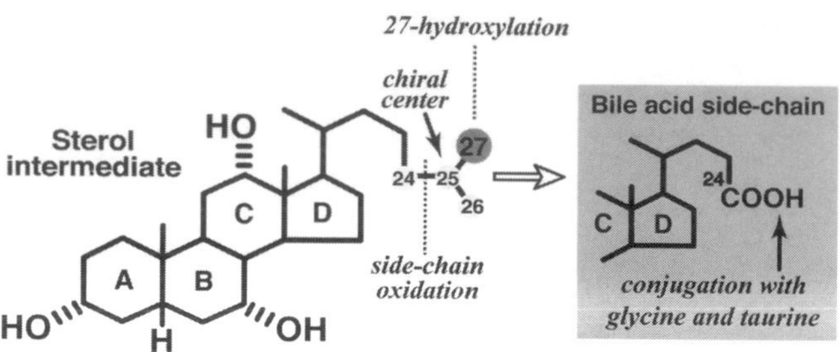

Figure 31.10. Metabolic defects involving changes to the side chain.

Defects Involving Reactions Leading to Side-Chain Modification

Defects in the reactions involved in side-chain hydroxylation and oxidation generally present as neurologic disturbances and/or syndromes of fat-soluble vitamin malabsorption. These manifestations emphasize the crucial role that bile acids play in the intestinal absorption of lipids. The structural site of these defects is indicated in Figure 31.10. Liver disease is generally mild and may not necessarily be the primary clinical presentation, because low levels of primary bile acids are often made via alternative pathways of synthesis. CTX [271] was the first defect in bile acid synthesis to be described [272] and shown conclusively to be caused by mutations in the gene for sterol 27-hydroxylase. More recently, defects in bile acid conjugation and a specific single enzyme defect in peroxisomal β-oxidation have been described. Generalized disorders in peroxisomal structure and function, distinct from single enzyme defects in the fatty acid oxidation system, ultimately lead to progressive liver disease, but this is secondary to the underlying genetic disease.

Cerebrotendinous Xanthomatosis

Cerebrotendinous xanthomatosis, a rare autosomal recessive lipid storage disease first described by Van Bogaert et al. [271], has an estimated prevalence of 1 in 70,000. The disease is usually not diagnosed until the second or third decade of life, when it becomes symptomatic, but it has been detected in a few pediatric patients [273,274]. The clinical presentation includes symptoms of progressive neurologic dysfunction, dementia, ataxia, cataracts, and the presence of xanthomas in the brain and tendons [275]. It has been suggested that the presence of bilateral juvenile cataracts and a history of chronic diarrhea, although not specific for CTX, may represent an early clinical manifestation of the disease [273,274]. More recently, it has been associated with a transient increase in serum liver enzymes in several infants, suggesting the earliest clinical picture may be that of a mild cholestasis that ultimately resolves over the first few months of life [276,277]. In one case report it was associated with fatal cholestasis in infancy [278]. The main biochemical features of this disease are (i) a significantly reduced synthesis of primary bile acids; (ii) elevated biliary, urinary, and fecal excretion of bile alcohol glucuronides; (iii) a normal or low plasma cholesterol concentration with excessive deposition of cholesterol and cholestanol in tissues; and (iv) a markedly elevated plasma cholestanol concentration.

More than two decades ago, Setoguchi et al. [272] demonstrated that the basic defect in this disorder is an impairment in side-chain oxidation and that chenodeoxycholic acid synthesis is affected to a greater extent than cholic acid synthesis [279,280]. Although there was originally controversy over the exact nature of the side-chain oxidation defect, the following lines of evidence indicated a primary enzyme defect in the sterol 27-hydroxylase enzyme: (a) A complete lack of sterol 27-hydroxylase activity was demonstrated in the mitochondrial fraction of liver biopsy tissue from a patient with CTX [281]. (b) The concentration of 5β-cholestane-3α,7α,12α-triol, the substrate for the C-27 hydroxylase, was elevated 50-fold in liver homogenates from a patient with CTX [281]. (c) The serum 27-hydroxycholesterol concentration was markedly reduced or barely detectable in CTX patients [282]. (d) Intravenous administration of radioactive precursors showed only those intermediates with a C-27 hydroxyl group were converted to cholic acid [281]. (e) Biologic fluids from patients with CTX had marked elevations in bile alcohol glucuronides having a cholestane-3α,7α,12α-triol nucleus and a hydroxyl group in positions C-22, C-23, C-24, and C-25 of the side chain [272,283,284]. (f) Cultured skin fibroblasts from patients with CTX were deficient in sterol 27-hydroxylase activity, whereas fibroblasts from healthy relatives had a markedly reduced activity consistent with the heterozygous phenotype [99]. (g) Chenodeoxycholic acid synthesis, which occurs via the acidic pathway by initial 27-hydroxylation was markedly reduced compared with cholic acid synthesis [101,120,139].

In an attempt to explain the greatly increased levels of 5β-cholestane-3α,7α,12α,25-tetrol in bile, a deficiency of the microsomal 24(S)-hydroxylase was proposed [139] because the substrate for this enzymatic reaction can be converted to cholic acid. However, under normal conditions this pathway appears to be of negligible quantitative importance for cholic acid synthesis in humans [103]; furthermore, a defect in the microsomal 24(S)-hydroxylase would not be consistent with the greatly reduced synthesis of chenodeoxycholic acid. A deficiency in 27-hydroxylation, on the other hand, adequately explains the elevation in 7α-hydroxy-4-cholesten-3-one and 5β-cholestane-3α,7α-diol, which would make these intermediates available for preferential 12α-hydroxylation and thus conversion to cholic acid via the C-25 hydroxylation pathway (Figure 31.11). This explanation is supported by the finding that hepatic 12α-hydroxylase activity is threefold higher than normal in CTX patients [285].

Conclusive evidence that the primary defect in CTX is a defect in sterol 27-hydroxylase finally came from molecular studies facilitated by the cloning of the human sterol 27-hydroxylase cDNA [98]. Using this probe, the mRNA was isolated from fibroblasts of two unrelated CTX patients and the corresponding cDNA was synthesized by reverse transcription [98]. The gene was localized to the long arm of chromosome 2, and point mutations were identified at positions 362 and 446 that convert arginine codons to cysteine codons. When these mutations were expressed in COS cells, the resulting sterol 27-hydroxylase enzyme was inactive. Recently, there have been several different types of mutations accounting for a lack of sterol 27-hydroxylase activity and mRNA in patients with CTX disease, and these have included insertion, deletion, and point mutations [98,286–304]. These studies all showed the primary defect to reside in the mitochondrial sterol 27-hydroxylase. Interestingly, the mitochondrial sterol 27-hydroxylase also catalyzes hepatic 25-hydroxylation of vitamin D [131], yet despite this, 25-hydroxyvitamin D is not usually altered in CTX patients [305].

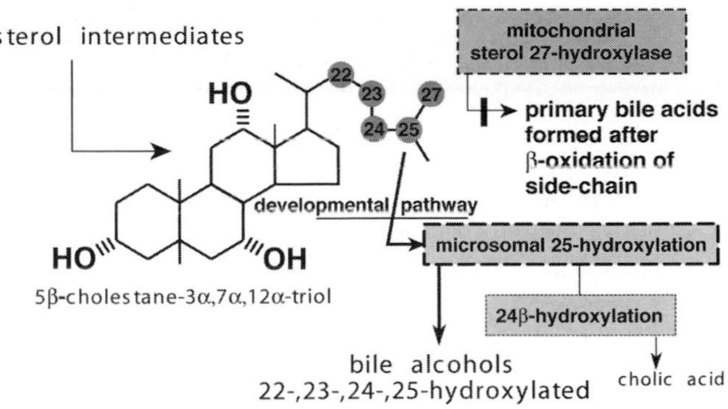

Figure 31.11. Biochemical defect in CTX leading to diminished primary bile acid synthesis and excessive production of bile alcohols.

A striking clinical feature of this disease is the accumulation of 5α-cholestan-3β-ol (cholestanol) in the nervous system and the markedly elevated concentrations of this sterol, but not cholesterol, in the plasma [306,307]. The cholestanol/cholesterol ratio in plasma may be of diagnostic value, although an elevation of this ratio and an increased urinary excretion of bile alcohol glucuronides may also occur in patients with cholestatic liver diseases [308–310]. The reason for the increased synthesis of cholestanol in CTX is discussed extensively elsewhere, and several theories have been proposed. The most plausible explanation is that cholestanol arises from sterol intermediates that accumulate because of the lack of sterol 27-hydroxylase. A pathway has been proposed involving 7α-hydroxylation of cholesterol and conversion to 7α-hydroxy-4-cholesten-3-one, followed by 7α-dehydroxylation that is hepatic rather than intestinal, and yields cholest-4,6-dien-3-one as an intermediate [311,312]. Radiolabeling studies confirm this pathway, and CTX patients have elevated plasma 7α-hydroxy-4-cholesten-3-one and cholest-4,6-dien-3-one levels. Furthermore, cholestyramine administration, which increases cholesterol 7α-hydroxylase activity, leads to increased plasma cholestanol concentrations, whereas chenodeoxycholic acid administration has the opposite effect [311,312].

Diagnosis of CTX at an early age is essential to limit neurologic and cardiovascular complications resulting from the chronic and irreversible deposition of cholesterol and cholestanol in tissues. Diagnosis is generally based on a greatly increased plasma cholestanol/cholesterol ratio [313] (although in some cases, this is not entirely reliable) and/or an elevated excretion of bile alcohols in urine. These analyses are highly specialized, time consuming, complex, and outside the scope of routine clinical laboratories. However, using mass spectrometry it is possible to rapidly and definitively diagnose CTX from an analysis of urine, which reveals the presence of increased levels of bile alcohol glucuronides [4,243,251,276]. A typical FAB-MS–negative ion spectrum from a CTX patient reveals $[M\text{-}H]^-$ ions characteristic of bile alcohol glucuronides (Figure 31.5). In health, bile acid conjugates and bile alcohol glucuronides are excreted in such low levels that these compounds are barely detectable by FAB-MS. In CTX, strong signals at *m/z* 611, *m/z* 627, and *m/z* 643, not seen in the urine of healthy people, represent the glucuronide conjugates of tetrahydroxy-, pentahydroxy-, and hexahydroxy-bile alcohols, respectively. Definitive confirmation of CTX is best achieved by complementing the mass spectrometry analysis with DNA sequencing of the sterol 27-hydroxylase gene and identification of the specific mutation.

Effective treatment of CTX has been achieved by oral bile acid administration [280,314–316]. Chenodeoxycholic acid (750 mg/d) lowers plasma cholestanol to within normal concentrations, and a concomitant decrease in urinary bile alcohol excretion occurs consistent with down-regulation in endogenous cholesterol 7α-hydroxylase, the rate-limiting enzyme in bile acid synthesis. These biochemical changes are accompanied by an improvement in clinical symptoms, particularly the neurologic disturbances [314,316,317] and are most effective when initiated before the onset of significant symptoms [318]. Cholic [315] and deoxycholic [283] acids also cause a decrease in plasma cholestanol, but UDCA is ineffective because it does not inhibit cholesterol 7α-hydroxylase [313,315]. Bile acid therapy may be more effective in CTX if combined with an HMG-CoA reductase inhibitor, which additionally inhibits endogenous cholesterol synthesis [319]. Limited studies show that the combined regimen is more effective in reducing plasma cholestanol concentrations [320].

Side-Chain Oxidation Defect in the Alternate 25-Hydroxylation Pathway

A defect in side-chain oxidation in the 25-hydroxylation pathway [101–103] was proposed by Clayton et al. [236] for a 9-week-old infant presenting with familial giant cell hepatitis and severe intrahepatic cholestasis. The diagnosis was based on the findings of reduced cholic and chenodeoxycholic acid concentrations, and elevated concentrations of bile alcohol glucuronides, specifically 5β-cholestane-3β,7α,12α,24-tetrol, 5β-cholest-24-ene-3β,7α,12α,24-tetrol, and 5β-cholestane-3β,7α,12α,25-tetrol in serum. These bile alcohols are not normally found in the plasma of infants with liver disease. Bile alcohol glucuronides were also identified as major metabolites in the urine [236]. Although the profile resembled that seen in CTX patients, it was concluded on the basis of the liver disease, which at that time was not previously described as a feature of CTX, that this represented a different side-chain defect. It was suggested to represent an oxidation defect downstream of the 25-hydroxylation step in this minor pathway for bile acid synthesis. The implications of the findings are that it could indicate that the 25-hydroxylation pathway, considered of negligible importance in adults [103], may be an important pathway for infants. The patient was treated with chenodeoxycholic and cholic acids, and this led to normalization in serum aminotransferase levels and suppression of bile alcohol production.

2-Methylacyl-CoA Racemase Deficiency

A female infant of 3 weeks of age with a mild elevation in liver enzymes and very low serum concentrations of the fat-soluble vitamins 25-hydroxyvitamin D and vitamin E was originally thought to have a single enzyme defect in THCA-CoA oxidase based on the biochemical presentation. However, continued work-up of this case has now shown this to be the result of a mutation in the gene encoding the 2-methylacyl-CoA racemase enzyme [321]. Interestingly, a deficiency in the activity of this enzyme was also ascribed to adult-onset sensory neuropathy in three patients with elevated serum phytanic and pristanic acids, but neither fat-soluble vitamin malabsorption nor liver disease was a feature in these adult cases despite the finding in two of the three patients of the mutation identical to that of this infant [322]. 2-Methylacyl-CoA racemase has been well characterized in the rat and humans [323,324]. This enzyme catalyzes the racemization of the (*25R*) diastereoisomers of THCA and 3α,7α-dihydroxy-5β-cholestanoic acid (DHCA) to the respective (*25S*) isomers [325]. This reaction is a prerequisite for the initiation of peroxisomal β-oxidation of the side chain of these C_{27} bile acid intermediates. It is also responsible for racemization of (*2R*)-pristanoyl-CoA to its (*2S*)-diastereoisomer [324] before peroxisomal β-oxidative degradation and explains why in this genetic disease, VLCFAs are normal, whereas pristanic acid, a branch-chained fatty acid, is elevated (Figure 31.12). Studies using

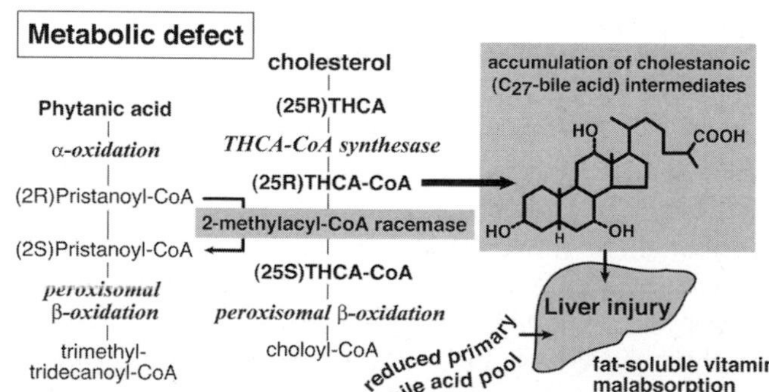

Figure 31.12. Biochemical defect in patients with a 2-methylacyl-CoA racemase deficiency.

cultured fibroblasts from the patient confirmed this pathway to be impaired [326], and molecular analysis of the gene encoding the 2-methylacyl-CoA racemase showed a missense mutation (S52P) yielding an inactive protein in this patient [321]. The urinary FAB-MS analysis gave a mass spectrum (Figure 31.5) identical to that observed in Zellweger syndrome; however, plasma VLCFAs and other peroxisomal enzyme markers were all normal. The patient responded successfully to fat-soluble vitamin supplementation and cholic acid therapy (15 mg/kg/d) and was neurologically and developmentally normal at age 3.5 years. The clinical history is remarkable for a previous sibling who was initially healthy until 5.5 months of age but died suddenly following an intracranial bleed that was found to be secondary to vitamin K deficiency. The liver of this sibling, apparently having the same bile acid synthetic defect, was transplanted, and the recipient was in good health 5 years later but receiving oral bile acid therapy. Dietary restriction of phytol should also be implemented to prevent longer-term neurologic damage caused by the accumulation of branched-chain fatty acids. A gene knockout mouse model for the 2-methylacyl-CoA deficiency was recently described, confirming the importance of phytol restriction in preventing neurologic and liver manifestations [327]. Given that the primary presentation of this infant, and her deceased sibling, was one of fat-soluble vitamin malabsorption, this discovery highlights the importance of screening for bile acid synthetic defects in patients presenting with unexplained fat-soluble vitamin malabsorption or rickets. Compromised vitamin status in the very young infant may be fatal, and early diagnosis of bile acid synthetic disorders will afford the maximum therapeutic benefit from primary bile acid therapy and fat-soluble vitamin supplementation.

Peroxisomal Disorders

The importance of the peroxisome in bile acid synthesis is apparent from the fact that disorders involving peroxisomal assembly and function have a significant impact on bile acid synthesis [328]. This is perhaps not surprising because the peroxisome packages at least 40 enzymes, including those required for the β-oxidation of fatty acids and bile acids as well as the conjugating enzymes for bile acids. Most of the disorders in bile acid synthesis in peroxisomopathies are secondary to the primary defect of organelle dysfunction. Excellent reviews of the clinical and biochemical abnormalities are published elsewhere [328–332] and in Chapter 35 of this text [333]. Consequently, this section will highlight only the features pertinent to bile acid metabolism. Early diagnosis of a peroxisomopathy is often the result of referral of the patient to a gastroenterologist for evaluation of abnormal liver biochemistries.

Many of the peroxisomal disorders show similarities and overlap in clinical and biochemical presentation. Conditions in which there is a generalized impairment in peroxisomal function exhibit abnormalities in bile acid synthesis and metabolism, and these patients often have significant liver disease. Pinpointing the exact nature of the peroxisomopathy may be challenging and requires a battery of tests to examine all steps in the β-oxidation pathway of bile acids and VLCFAs, complemented by immunoblotting techniques to identify the presence and activity of other peroxisomal enzymes and examination of the more recently recognized proteins involved in peroxisomal assembly [333]. Mass spectrometry (FAB-MS) is useful in identifying those patients in whom there are abnormalities in peroxisomal β-oxidation of bile acids, particularly when there is evidence of progressive liver disease [3,4,256,334]. Urine analysis reveals the presence the $[M\text{-}H]^-$ ions corresponding to unconjugated THCA (m/z 449), taurine conjugated THCA (m/z 556), and taurine conjugated tetrahydroxylated cholestanoic acids (m/z 572) – the spectrum being essentially identical to that observed in the 2-methylacyl-CoA racemase deficiency (Figure 31.5). Although this approach is highly definitive for the detection of abnormalities in peroxisomal β-oxidation, FAB-MS should always be complemented by detailed GC-MS analysis of plasma and urine to confirm inborn errors in peroxisomal β-oxidation, especially if there is little evidence of liver involvement. The relatives of Zellweger patients, who represent heterozygous phenotypes for this most severe form of peroxisomal defect, show normal urinary bile acid excretion with negligible or no detectable cholestanoic acids [256]. In genetic counseling of affected families, prenatal diagnosis is possible by specific detection of elevated concentrations of DHCA and THCA in amniotic fluid [335]. Elevated levels of DHCA, THCA, and a C_{29} dicarboxylic bile acid in biologic fluids are a consistent feature of patients with Zellweger syndrome, neonatal adrenoleukodystrophy, infantile Refsum's disease, and pseudo-Zellweger syndrome [235,334,336–341]. Of the single enzyme defects, X-linked adrenoleukodystrophy [342–344] and pseudoneonatal adrenoleukodystrophy [345] both show normal bile acid synthesis with no accumulation of cholestanoic acids [3,333]. DHCA concentrations are in general much lower than THCA, particularly in younger patients, and this is explained by its preferential conversion to THCA by 12α-hydroxylation. The origin of a C_{29} dicarboxylic acid found in the serum of many Zellweger patients is presumed to be the result of side-chain elongation in the endoplasmic reticulum [338]. Although bile acid synthetic rates are low in Zellweger patients, increased serum concentrations of primary bile acids are frequently found and are probably a consequence of impaired hepatic function [346,347]. Additional metabolism of THCA by microsomal hydroxylation in the side chain (to produce C-24 hydroxylated, varanic acid isomers), and in the nucleus (to produce C-1 and C-6 tetrahydroxy-cholestanoic acids) gives rise to many tetrahydroxylated cholestanoic acids that are excreted in urine and present in plasma, and these are of diagnostic value [256,334,348].

Although the diagnosis of Zellweger syndrome is often straightforward, characterizing and differentiating patients with single enzyme defects involving peroxisomal enzymes is more difficult. Two distinct acyl-CoA oxidases have been identified in humans [117], whereas the rat has three isozymes [349]. The human acyl-CoA oxidase, active on cholestanoic (C_{27}) acid intermediates, has been found in the human to be the same enzyme that catalyzes the oxidation of 2-methyl branched chain fatty acids [117]. The cDNA of the gene encoding this human enzyme has been cloned [350]. There have been several case reports of presumed THCA-CoA oxidase deficiencies, and phytanic and pristanic acids, when measured, have been elevated in these patients [344,351–354]. All presented with ataxia, and unlike the patient with a 2-methylacyl-CoA racemase deficiency who shared a similar biochemical profile, there was no evidence for any neurologic disorder [321]. With the more recent recognition of the complexity of peroxisomal biogenesis disorders, it is possible that some of these previously reported cases could have been the result of mutations in the recently described *PEX* genes [333].

Treatment of the peroxisomopathies is difficult because of the multiorgan pathophysiology of the diseases and is to a large extent restricted to managing the symptoms [355]. Dietary restriction of VLCFA and phytanic acid and administration of oleic acid have provided minimal to no benefit in the full-blown Zellweger syndrome. Clofibrate, which has been shown in rats to induce peroxisomal proliferation [356], has proved to be of no therapeutic value [357]. In general, the prognosis in most peroxisomal disorders is poor, and Zellweger syndrome patients generally succumb to respiratory failure. The progressive liver disease that commonly develops in Zellweger syndrome may in part be the result of increased synthesis and accumulation of C_{27} bile acids and reduced primary bile acid synthesis. Infusion of tauro-THCA in rats induces red cell hemolysis and produces a hepatic lesion showing mitochondrial disruption similar to that found in Zellweger patients [358]. In an attempt to limit the extent of liver injury in a Zellweger patient, primary bile acids were given orally and resulted in a marked improvement in biochemical markers of liver function and histology, most notably a decrease in the extent of bile duct proliferation and inflammation [256]. This improvement was concomitant with a decrease in the urinary and serum concentrations of cholestanoic acid. A striking and sustained increase in growth and significant improvement in neurologic symptoms were also noted. Based on this observation and following the successful treatment of patients with primary enzyme defects in bile acid synthesis, cholic acid therapy has now been used in a number of patients with peroxisomal defects and the outcomes recently summarized [243]. Thus far, eight patients with peroxisomopathies have been treated for periods ranging from 4.7–11 years. Of these, four patients had Refsum's disease whereas the remaining comprised cases of neonatal adrenoleukodystrophy or Zellweger syndrome. An additional 13 patients with peroxisomal disorders were treated with cholic acid, but 10 died or are presumed dead and 3 are lost to follow-up. The treatment failures mostly included those patients with the more severe Zellweger syndrome, in whom there was multiorgan disease. It was concluded that this group derives minimal benefit from this approach, whereas those patients with single enzyme defects in peroxisomal function causing abnormal bile acid synthesis show greater responsiveness and may benefit from oral cholic acid therapy [243].

Bile Acid–CoA Conjugation Defects

The final step in bile acid synthesis involves conjugation with the amino acids glycine and taurine [78]. Hepatic conjugation is extremely efficient, and negligible amounts of unconjugated bile acids typically appear in bile under normal and cholestatic conditions [359]. This is also the case when therapeutic dosages of the unconjugated bile acid UDCA are administered [360]. Two enzymes catalyze the reactions leading to bile acid amidation. A CoA thioester is first formed by the rate-limiting bile acid–CoA ligase enzyme [169–172], and then the amino acids glycine and taurine are coupled in a reaction catalyzed by a cytosolic bile acid–CoA:amino acid *N*-acyltransferase [173–176]. The genes encoding both enzymes involved in bile acid conjugation have been cloned [177–179], allowing the identification of gene mutations to be confirmed in patients suspected of having defects in bile acid conjugation [237,361]. For adults, glycine is the preferred substrate [78], but in the first few months of life, most of the bile acid pool will comprise taurine conjugates [73,362] because of the large store of hepatic taurine in the fetal liver [186].

A defect in bile acid amidation was first described in a 14-year-old boy presenting with fat and fat-soluble vitamin malabsorption [237]. This child was of Laotian descent and in the first 3 months of life presented with conjugated hyperbilirubinemia, elevated serum aminotransferase levels, and a normal γGT level. Two other patients, a 5-year-old Saudi Arabian boy and his 8-year-old sister, who were products of a consanguineous marriage, were soon after identified with the same bile acid defect, and remarkable was the fact that the boy had undergone a Kasai procedure for a mistakenly diagnosed biliary atresia, whereas the sister was asymptomatic at the time of diagnosis. We have since recognized this defect in several other patients with a clinical history of normal or mildly elevated liver function tests but with severe fat-soluble vitamin malabsorption and rickets. In one patient, this resulted in bone fracture. All had subnormal levels of vitamin E, vitamin K, 25-hydroxyvitamin D, and 1,25-dihydroxyvitamin D. The

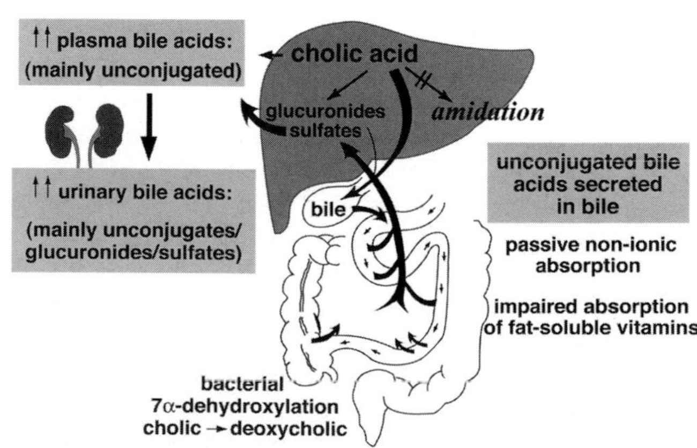

Figure 31.13. Pathophysiologic basis for a defect in bile acid conjugation causing fat-soluble vitamin malabsorption.

Table 31.1: Comparative Features of Patients with Intrahepatic Cholestasis Due to Bile Acid Synthetic Defects and PFIC1 and PFIC2

Feature	*Bile Acid Defects*	*PFIC1* and PFIC2†*
Age at presentation	Variable, late onset	<1 yr*†
Prognosis	Excellent	Fatal in first† to second* decade
Liver	Hepatosplenomegaly	Hepatosplenomegaly*†
Pruritus	Usually absent	Severe*†
Growth failure	Mild	Severe*†
Jaundice	+/−	Mild/severe*†
Serum aminotransferases	Elevated	Slight* to substantial† elevations
Serum γGT	Generally normal	Normal*†
Serum cholesterol	Normal or low	Low*†
Fat-soluble vitamins	Malabsorption	Malabsorption*†
Bile acids	No primary bile acids	Primary bile acids*†
Treatment	Bile acid therapy	Transplantation*†

*Caused by *FIC1* mutations.
†Caused by *BSEP* mutations.

phenotype of the amidation defect has been quite variable, with severe cholestasis and liver failure occurring in one recently diagnosed patient who required liver transplantation. The clinical presentation and biochemical features of defective amidation (Figure 31.13) in these patients closely parallel the predicted features hypothesized by Hofmann and Strandvik [363]. This conjugation defect has also been found in a number of patients from an Amish kindred and was associated with mutations in the *BAAT* gene encoding the bile acid–CoA:amino acid *N*-acyltransferase [361]. Additionally, mutations in the *TJP2* gene encoding tight junction protein 2 were also found in some of these patients.

Diagnosis of a bile acid conjugation defect is possible by FAB-MS analysis of the urine, serum, and bile, which reveal unique negative ion mass spectra having a major ion (m/z 407) corresponding to unconjugated cholic acid (Figure 31.5). In addition, ions characterizing sulfate and glucuronide conjugates of dihydroxy- and trihydroxy-bile acids are usually present. There is a complete lack of the usual glycine and taurine conjugated bile acids, and this may be confirmed after chromatographic separation of the individual bile acid conjugate fractions and GC-MS analysis [237]. Serum and urinary bile acids are markedly elevated in these patients and comprise predominantly cholic and deoxycholic acids.

Although inborn errors in bile acid synthesis usually present as well-defined progressive familial cholestatic liver disease, by contrast, cholestasis is not a primary manifestation of a bile acid conjugation defect, presumably because synthesis of high levels of unconjugated cholic acid is sufficient to maintain bile flow (Figure 31.13). The main feature of fat-soluble vitamin malabsorption results from reduced biliary secretion of bile acids and the inability to form mixed micelles because of rapid passive absorption of unconjugated cholic acid in the proximal small intestine [363]. Although these patients do conjugate bile acids with glucuronic and sulfuric acids, such conjugated bile acids are of little help in promoting lipid absorption [364–366]. Administration of primary conjugated bile acids should provide a therapeutic approach to correcting the fat-soluble vitamin malabsorption in this defect. The recognition that genetic defects in bile acid synthesis are associated with fat-soluble vitamin malabsorption warrants a more concerted effort to explore this patient population.

Other Disorders Affecting Bile Acid Synthesis and Metabolism

The regulation of primary bile acid synthesis is influenced by many factors [20]. In conditions that alter the integrity of the enterohepatic circulation, significant changes in bile acid synthesis and metabolism occur. Because serum bile acid concentrations reflect a balance between intestinal input and hepatic extraction, it is evident that pathophysiologic changes to the intestinal tract will be reflected by secondary changes in bile acid synthesis and metabolism. Such examples include ileal resection and bacterial overgrowth [233], whereas an inborn error in ileal bile acid transport has been shown to cause bile acid malabsorption [367,368]. Genetic defects in cholesterol synthesis, such as the Smith-Lemli-Opitz syndrome [369], will present as defects in bile acid synthesis because they impair the supply of cholesterol, the key substrate for primary bile acid synthesis.

Increased concentrations and alterations in bile acid metabolism can be found in most cases of cholestatic liver disease, but discerning whether these are primary or secondary to the liver injury may be difficult. Primary bile acid synthetic defects are a significant cause of progressive familial intrahepatic cholestasis (PFIC) and represent a distinct entity of the PFIC syndromes separate from those recognized to arise as the result of defects in the canalicular proteins responsible for organic anion transport [370–377]. It is evident that PFIC syndromes are accounted for by several defects in canalicular transporters, including BSEP (bile salt export pump) deficiency, and MDR3 (multidrug resistance protein 3) mutations [370–374]. A shared feature of PFIC type 1 and PFIC type 2 [378] with inborn errors in bile acid synthesis is a consistently low serum γGT level, but the differential diagnosis can be made based on bile acid analysis (Table 31.1). Patients with PFIC types 1 and 2 have high serum bile acid concentrations, whereas primary bile acids are absent or negligible in bile acid synthetic defects. PFIC type 3, on the other hand, is characterized by a high γGT level and defective phospholipid secretion [379]. All these defects can be recognized by a combination of molecular and analytic studies. Bile acid and phospholipid analysis of bile may facilitate differential diagnosis. For bile acid synthetic defects, except the oxysterol 7α-hydroxylase deficiency [39], the prognosis is excellent provided oral bile acid therapy is initiated before there is significant loss of quantitative liver function [243], and the need for orthotopic liver transplantation can be avoided. It is therefore important in the clinical evaluation of patients with PFIC to screen for potential defects in bile acid synthesis as early as possible.

REFERENCES

1. Bjorkhem I. Mechanism of bile acid biosynthesis in mammalian liver. In: Danielsson H, Sjovall J, eds. Sterols and bile acids. Amsterdam: BV Elsevier Science Publishers, 1985:231–77.
2. Russell DW, Setchell KDR. Bile acid biosynthesis. Biochemistry 1992;31:4737–49.
3. Setchell KDR, Street JM. Inborn errors of bile acid synthesis. Semin Liver Dis 1987;7:85–99.
4. Setchell KDR. Disorders of bile acid synthesis and metabolism. In: Walker WA, Durie PR, Hamilton JR, et al., eds. Pediatric gastrointestinal disease. Pathophysiology, diagnosis, management. Toronto/Philadelphia: BC Decker, Inc., 1996.
5. Klyne W. The chemistry of the steroids. London: Methuen and Co., Ltd., 1957.
6. Hofmann AF, Sjovall J, Kurz G, et al. A proposed nomenclature for bile acids. J Lipid Res 1992;33:599–604.
7. LeBlanc GA, Waxman DJ. Regulation and ligand-binding specificities of two sex-specific bile acid-binding proteins of rat liver cytosol. J Biol Chem 1990;265:5654–61.
8. Lin MC, Kramer W, Wilson FA. Identification of cytosolic and microsomal bile acid-binding proteins in rat ileal enterocytes. J Biol Chem 1990;265:14986–95.
9. Russell DW. The enzymes, regulation, and genetics of bile acid synthesis. Annu Rev Biochem 2003;72:137–74.
10. Noshiro M, Nishimoto M, Morohashi K, Okuda K. Molecular cloning of cDNA for cholesterol 7α-hydroxylase from rat liver microsomes. Nucleotide sequence and expression. FEBS Lett 1989;257:97–100.
11. Noshiro M, Okuda K. Molecular cloning and sequence analysis of cDNA encoding human cholesterol 7α-hydroxylase. FEBS Lett 1990;268:137–40.
12. Jelinek DF, Andersson S, Slaughter CA, Russell DW. Cloning and regulation of cholesterol 7α-hydroxylase, the rate-limiting enzyme in bile acid biosynthesis. J Biol Chem 1990;265:8190–7.
13. Li YC, Chiang JY. The expression of a catalytically active cholesterol 7α-hydroxylase cytochrome P450 in *Escherichia coli*. J Biol Chem 1991;266:19186–91.
14. Suchy FJ, Balistreri WF, Heubi JE, et al. Physiologic cholestasis: elevation of the primary serum bile acid concentrations in normal infants. Gastroenterology 1981;80:1037–41.
15. Barnes S, Berkowitz G, Hirschowitz BI, et al. Postnatal physiologic hypercholemia in both premature and full-term infants. J Clin Invest 1981;68:775–82.
16. Danielsson H, Einarsson K, Johansson G. Effect of biliary drainage on individual reactions in the conversion of cholesterol to taurochlic acid. Bile acids and steroids 180. Eur J Biochem 1967;2:44–9.
17. Shefer S, Hauser S, Mosbach EH. 7α-Hydroxylation of cholestanol by rat liver microsomes. J Lipid Res 1968;9:328–33.
18. Shefer S, Hauser S, Bekersky I, Mosbach EH. Biochemical site of regulation of bile acid biosynthesis in the rat. J Lipid Res 1970;11:404–11.
19. Myant NB, Mitropoulos KA. Cholesterol 7α-hydroxylase. J Lipid Res 1977;18:135–53.
20. Vlahcevic ZR, Heuman DM, Hylemon PB. Regulation of bile acid synthesis. Hepatology 1991;13:590–600.
21. Shefer S, Nguyen LB, Salen G, et al. Regulation of cholesterol 7α-hydroxylase by hepatic 7α-hydroxylated bile acid flux and newly synthesized cholesterol supply. J Biol Chem 1991;266:2693–6.
22. Pooler PA, Duane WC. Effects of bile acid administration on bile acid synthesis and its circadian rhythm in man. Hepatology 1988;8:1140–6.
23. Huff JW, Gilfillan JL, Hunt VM. Effect of cholestyramine, a bile-acid binding polymer on plasma cholesterol and fecal bile acid excretion in the rat. Proc Soc Exp Biol Med 1963;114:352–5.
24. Pandak WM, Li YC, Chiang JY, et al. Regulation of cholesterol 7α-hydroxylase mRNA and transcriptional activity by taurocholate and cholesterol in the chronic biliary diverted rat. J Biol Chem 1991;266:3416–21.
25. Goldstein JL, Brown MS. Regulation of the mevalonate pathway. Nature 1990;343:425–30.
26. Danielsson H. Relationship between diurnal variations in biosynthesis of cholesterol and bile acids. Steroids 1972;20:63–72.
27. Mitropoulos KA, Balasubramaniam S, Gibbons GF, Reeves BE. Diurnal variation in the activity of cholesterol 7α-hydroxylase in the livers of fed and fasted rats. FEBS Lett 1972;27:203–6.
28. Duane WC, Levitt DG, Mueller SM, Behrens JC. Regulation of bile acid synthesis in man. Presence of a diurnal rhythm. J Clin Invest 1983;72:1930–6.
29. Andersson S, Bostrom H, Danielsson H, Wikvall K. Purification from rabbit and rat liver of cytochromes P-450 involved in bile acid biosynthesis. Methods Enzymol 1985;111:364–77.

30. Pandak WM, Heuman DM, Redford K, et al. Hormonal regulation of cholesterol 7α-hydroxylase specific activity, mRNA levels, and transcriptional activity in vivo in the rat. J Lipid Res 1997;38:2483–91.
31. Goodart SA, Huynh C, Chen W, et al. Expression of the human cholesterol 7α-hydroxylase gene in transgenic mice. Biochem Biophys Res Commun 1999;266:454–9.
32. Crestani M, Sadeghpour A, Stroup D, et al. Transcriptional activation of the cholesterol 7α hydroxylase gene (*CYP7A*) by nuclear hormone receptors. J Lipid Res 1998;39:2192–200.
33. Rudling M, Parini P, Angelin B. Growth hormone and bile acid synthesis. Key role for the activity of hepatic microsomal cholesterol 7α-hydroxylase in the rat. J Clin Invest 1997;99:2239–45.
34. Vlahcevic ZR, Stravitz RT, Heuman DM, et al. Quantitative estimations of the contribution of different bile acid pathways to total bile acid synthesis in the rat [see comments]. Gastroenterology 1997;113:1949–57.
35. Schwarz M, Lund EG, Setchell KDR, et al. Disruption of cholesterol 7α-hydroxylase gene in mice. II. Bile acid deficiency is overcome by induction of oxysterol 7α-hydroxylase. J Biol Chem 1996;271:18024–31.
36. Arnon R, Yoshimura T, Reiss A, et al. Cholesterol 7-hydroxylase knockout mouse: a model for monohydroxy bile acid-related neonatal cholestasis. Gastroenterology 1998;115:1223–8.
37. Ishibashi S, Schwarz M, Frykman PK, et al. Disruption of cholesterol 7α-hydroxylase gene in mice. I. Postnatal lethality reversed by bile acid and vitamin supplementation. J Biol Chem 1996;271:18017–23.
38. Schwarz M, Lund EG, Lathe R, et al. Identification and characterization of a mouse oxysterol 7α-hydroxylase cDNA. J Biol Chem 1997;272:23995–4001.
39. Setchell KDR, Schwarz M, O'Connell NC, et al. Identification of a new inborn error in bile acid synthesis: mutation of the oxysterol 7α-hydroxylase gene causes severe neonatal liver disease. J Clin Invest 1998;102:1690–703.
40. Gustafsson JA. Seeking ligands for lonely orphan receptors [comment]. Science 1999;284:1285–6.
41. Russell DW. Nuclear orphan receptors control cholesterol catabolism. Cell 1999;97:539–42.
42. Kliewer SA, Lehmann JM, Willson TM. Orphan nuclear receptors: shifting endocrinology into reverse. Science 1999;284:757–60.
43. Willson TM, Jones SA, Moore JT, Kliewer SA. Chemical genomics: functional analysis of orphan nuclear receptors in the regulation of bile acid metabolism. Med Res Rev 2001;21:513–22.
44. Chiang JY. Bile acid regulation of gene expression: roles of nuclear hormone receptors. Endocr Rev 2002;23:443–63.
45. Goodwin B, Watson MA, Kim H, et al. Differential regulation of rat and human CYP7A1 by the nuclear oxysterol receptor liver X receptor-alpha. Mol Endocrinol 2003;17:386–94.
46. Westin S, Heyman RA, Martin R. FXR, a therapeutic target for bile acid and lipid disorders. Mini Rev Med Chem 2005;5:719–27.
47. Peet DJ, Turley SD, Ma W, et al. Cholesterol and bile acid metabolism are impaired in mice lacking the nuclear oxysterol receptor LXRα Cell 1998;93:693–704.
48. Nitta M, Ku S, Brown C, et al. CPF: an orphan nuclear receptor that regulates liver-specific expression of the human cholesterol 7α-hydroxylase gene. Proc Natl Acad Sci U S A 1999;96:6660–5.
49. Goodwin B, Jones SA, Price RR, et al. A regulatory cascade of the nuclear receptors FXR, SHP-1, and LRH-1 represses bile acid biosynthesis. Mol Cell 2000;6:517–26.
50. Rizzo G, Renga B, Mencarelli A, et al. Role of FXR in regulating bile acid homeostasis and relevance for human diseases. Curr Drug Targets Immune Endocr Metabol Disord 2005;5:289–303.
51. Handschin C, Meyer UA. Regulatory network of lipid-sensing nuclear receptors: roles for CAR, PXR, LXR, and FXR. Arch Biochem Biophys 2005;433:387–96.
52. Janowski BA, Willy PJ, Devi TR, et al. An oxysterol signalling pathway mediated by the nuclear receptor LXR alpha. Nature 1996;383:728–31.
53. Forman BM, Ruan B, Chen J, et al. The orphan nuclear receptor LXRalpha is positively and negatively regulated by distinct products of mevalonate metabolism. Proc Natl Acad Sci U S A 1997;94:10588–93.
54. Lehmann JM, McKee DD, Watson MA, et al. The human orphan nuclear receptor PXR is activated by compounds that regulate CYP3A4 gene expression and cause drug interactions. J Clin Invest 1998;102:1016–23.
55. Makishima M, Okamoto AY, Repa JJ, et al. Identification of a nuclear receptor for bile acids [see comments]. Science 1999;284:1362–5.
56. Parks DJ, Blanchard SG, Bledsoe RK, et al. Bile acids: natural ligands for an orphan nuclear receptor [see comments]. Science 1999;284:1365–8.
57. Wang H, Chen J, Hollister K, et al. Endogenous bile acids are ligands for the nuclear receptor FXR/BAR. Mol Cell 1999;3:543–53.
58. Setchell KD, Rodrigues CM, Clerici C, et al. Bile acid concentrations in human and rat liver tissue and in hepatocyte nuclei. Gastroenterology 1997;112:226–35.
59. Wikvall K. Purification and properties of a 3β-hydroxy-Δ^5-C_{27}-steroid oxidoreductase from rabbit liver microsomes. J Biol Chem 1981;256:3376–80.
60. Furster C, Zhang J, Toll A. Purification of a 3β-hydroxy-deltaΔ^5-C_{27}-steroid dehydrogenase from pig liver microsomes active in major and alternative pathways of bile acid biosynthesis. J Biol Chem 1996;271:20903–7.
61. The VL, Lachance Y, Labrie C, et al. Full length cDNA structure and deduced amino acid sequence of human 3β-hydroxy-5-ene steroid dehydrogenase. Mol Endocrinol 1989;3:1310–12.
62. Zhao HF, Simard J, Labrie C, et al. Molecular cloning, cDNA structure and predicted amino acid sequence of bovine 3β-hydroxy-5-ene steroid dehydrogenase/Δ^{5-4} isomerase. FEBS Lett 1989;259:153–7.
63. Lorence MC, Murry BA, Trant JM, Mason JI. Human 3β-hydroxysteroid dehydrogenase/Δ^{5-4} isomerase from placenta: expression in nonsteroidogenic cells of a protein that catalyzes the dehydrogenation/isomerization of C21 and C19 steroids. Endocrinology 1990;126:2493–8.
64. Zhao HF, Labrie C, Simard J, et al. Characterization of rat 3β-hydroxysteroid dehydrogenase/Δ^5-Δ^4 isomerase cDNAs and differential tissue-specific expression of the corresponding mRNAs in steroidogenic and peripheral tissues. J Biol Chem 1991;266:583–93.
65. Schwarz M, Wright AC, Davis DL, et al. The bile acid synthetic gene 3βhydroxy-Δ^5-C_{27}-steroid oxidoreductase is mutated in progressive intrahepatic cholestasis. J Clin Invest 2000;106:1175–84.

66. Cheng JB, Jacquemin E, Gerhardt M, et al. Molecular genetics of 3β-hydroxy-Δ^5-C_{27}-steroid oxidoreductase deficiency in 16 patients with loss of bile acid synthesis and liver disease. J Clin Endocrinol Metab 2003;88:1833–41.
67. Ishida H, Noshiro M, Okuda K, Coon MJ. Purification and characterization of 7α-hydroxy-4-cholesten-3-one 12α-hydroxylase. J Biol Chem 1992;267:21319–23.
68. Eggertsen G, Olin M, Andersson U, et al. Molecular cloning and expression of rabbit sterol 12α-hydroxylase. J Biol Chem 1996;271:32269–75.
69. Gafvels M, Olin M, Chowdhary BP, et al. Structure and chromosomal assignment of the sterol 12α-hydroxylase gene (CYP8B1) in human and mouse: eukaryotic cytochrome P-450 gene devoid of introns. Genomics 1999;56:184–96.
70. Einarsson K, Akerlund JE, Reihner E, Bjorkhem I. 12α-hydroxylase activity in human liver and its relation to cholesterol 7α-hydroxylase activity. J Lipid Res 1992;33:1591–5.
71. Johansson G. Effect of cholestyramine and diet on hydroxylations in the biosynthesis and metabolism of bile acids. Eur J Biochem 1970;17:292–5.
72. Colombo C, Zuliani G, Ronchi M, et al. Biliary bile acid composition of the human fetus in early gestation. Pediatr Res 1987;21:197–200.
73. Setchell KDR, Dumaswala R, Colombo C, Ronchi M. Hepatic bile acid metabolism during early development revealed from the analysis of human fetal gallbladder bile. J Biol Chem 1988;263:16637–44.
74. Encrantz JC, Sjovall J. On the bile acids in duodenal contents of infants and children. Clin Chim Acta 1959;4:793–9.
75. Poley JR, Dower JC, Owen CA, Stickler GB. Bile acids in infants and children. J Lab Clin Med 1964;63:838–46.
76. Bongiovanni AM. Bile acid content of gallbladder of infants, children and adults. J Clin Endocrinol Metab 1965;25:678–85.
77. Clayton PT, Muller DP, Lawson AM. The bile acid composition of gastric contents from neonates with high intestinal obstruction. Biochem J 1982;206:489–98.
78. Sjovall J. Dietary glycine and taurine conjugation in man. Proc Soc Exp Biol Med 1959;100:676–8.
79. Haslewood GA. Bile salt evolution. J Lipid Res 1967;8:535–50.
80. Elliott WH. Allo bile acids. In: Nair PP, Kritchevsky D, eds. The bile acids: chemistry, physiology and metabolism. New York: Plenum Press, 1971:47–93.
81. Andersson S, Bishop RW, Russell DW. Expression cloning and regulation of steroid 5α-reductase, an enzyme essential for male sexual differentiation. J Biol Chem 1989;264:16249–55.
82. Kondo KH, Kai MH, Setoguchi Y, et al. Cloning and expression of cDNA of human Δ^4-3-oxosteroid 5β-reductase and substrate specificity of the expressed enzyme. Eur J Biochem 1994;219:357–63.
83. Onishi Y, Noshiro M, Shimosato T, Okuda K. Δ^4-3-Oxosteroid 5β-reductase. Structure and function. Biol Chem Hoppe Seyler 1991;372:1039–49.
84. Axelson M, Bjorkhem I, Reihner E, Einarsson K. The plasma level of 7α-hydroxy-4-cholesten-3-one reflects the activity of hepatic cholesterol 7α-hydroxylase in man. FEBS Lett 1991;284:216–18.
85. Clayton PT, Patel E, Lawson AM, et al. 3-Oxo-Δ^4 bile acids in liver disease [letter]. Lancet 1988;1:1283–4.
86. Setchell KDR, Suchy FJ, Welsh MB, et al. Δ^4-3-oxosteroid 5β-reductase deficiency described in identical twins with neonatal hepatitis. A new inborn error in bile acid synthesis. J Clin Invest 1988;82:2148–57.
87. Lemonde HA, Custard EJ, Bouquet J, et al. Mutations in SRD5B1 (AKR1D1), the gene encoding Δ^4-3-oxosteroid 5β-reductase, in hepatitis and liver failure in infancy. Gut 2003;52:1494–9.
88. Penning TM, Abrams WR, Pawlowski JE. Affinity labeling of 3α-hydroxysteroid dehydrogenase with 3α- bromoacetoxyandrosterone and 11α-bromoacetoxyprogesterone. Isolation and sequence of active site peptides containing reactive cysteines; sequence confirmation using nucleotide sequence from a cDNA clone. J Biol Chem 1991;266:8826–34.
89. Cheng KC, White PC, Qin KN. Molecular cloning and expression of rat liver 3α-hydroxysteroid dehydrogenase. Mol Endocrinol 1991;5:823–8.
90. Pawlowski JE, Huizinga M, Penning TM. Cloning and sequencing of the cDNA for rat liver 3α-hydroxysteroid/dihydrodiol dehydrogenase. J Biol Chem 1991;266:8820–5.
91. Stolz A, Rahimi-Kiani M, Ameis D, et al. Molecular structure of rat hepatic 3α-hydroxysteroid dehydrogenase. A member of the oxidoreductase gene family. J Biol Chem 1991;266:15253–7.
92. Stolz A, Takikawa H, Sugiyama Y, et al. 3α-hydroxysteroid dehydrogenase activity of the Y' bile acid binders in rat liver cytosol. Identification, kinetics, and physiologic significance. J Clin Invest 1987;79:427–34.
93. Bjorkhem I. Mechanism of degradation of the steroid side chain in the formation of bile acids. J Lipid Res 1992;33:455–71.
94. Popjak G, Edmond J, Anet FA, Easton NR Jr. Carbon-13 NMR studies on cholesterol biosynthesized from [13C]mevalonates. J Am Chem Soc 1977;99:931–5.
95. Andersson S, Davis DL, Dahlback H, et al. Cloning, structure, and expression of the mitochondrial cytochrome P-450 sterol 26-hydroxylase, a bile acid biosynthetic enzyme. J Biol Chem 1989;264:8222–9.
96. Usui E, Noshiro M, Okuda K. Molecular cloning of cDNA for vitamin D3 25-hydroxylase from rat liver mitochondria. FEBS Lett 1990;262:135–8.
97. Su P, Rennert H, Shayiq RM, et al. A cDNA encoding a rat mitochondrial cytochrome P450 catalyzing both the 26-hydroxylation of cholesterol and 25-hydroxylation of vitamin D3: gonadotropic regulation of the cognate mRNA in ovaries. DNA Cell Biol 1990;9:657–67.
98. Cali JJ, Hsieh CL, Francke U, Russell DW. Mutations in the bile acid biosynthetic enzyme sterol 27-hydroxylase underlie cerebrotendinous xanthomatosis. J Biol Chem 1991;266:7779–83.
99. Skrede S, Bjorkhem I, Kvittingen EA, et al. Demonstration of 26-hydroxylation of C27-steroids in human skin fibroblasts, and a deficiency of this activity in cerebrotendinous xanthomatosis. J Clin Invest 1986;78:729–35.
100. Rosen H, Reshef A, Maeda N, et al. Markedly reduced bile acid synthesis but maintained levels of cholesterol and vitamin D metabolites in mice with disrupted sterol 27-hydroxylase gene. J Biol Chem 1998;273:14805–12.
101. Shefer S, Cheng FW, Dayal B, et al. A 25-hydroxylation pathway of cholic acid biosynthesis in man and rat. J Clin Invest 1976;57:897–903.
102. Duane WC, Bjorkhem I, Hamilton JN, Mueller SM. Quantitative importance of the 25-hydroxylation pathway for bile acid biosynthesis in the rat. Hepatology 1988;8:613–18.

103. Duane WC, Pooler PA, Hamilton JN. Bile acid synthesis in man. In vivo activity of the 25-hydroxylation pathway. J Clin Invest 1988;82:82–5.
104. Wikvall K. Hydroxylations in biosynthesis of bile acids. Isolation of a cytochrome P-450 from rabbit liver mitochondria catalyzing 26-hydroxylation of C27- steroids. J Biol Chem 1984;259: 3800–4.
105. Akiyoshi-Shibata M, Usui E, Sakaki T, et al. Expression of rat liver vitamin D3 25-hydroxylase cDNA in Saccharomyces cerevisiae. FEBS Lett 1991;280:367–70.
106. Javitt NB. 26-Hydroxycholesterol: synthesis, metabolism, and biologic activities. J Lipid Res 1990;31:1527–33.
107. Dahlback H, Holmberg I. Oxidation of 5β-cholestane-3α,7α, 12α-triol into 3α,7α,12α-trihydroxy-5β-cholestanoic acid by cytochrome P-450(26) from rabbit liver mitochondria. Biochem Biophys Res Commun 1990;167:391–5.
108. Javitt NB. Bile acid synthesis from cholesterol: regulatory and auxiliary pathways. FASEB J 1994;8:1308–11.
109. Bjorkhem I, Andersson O, Diczfalusy U, et al. Atherosclerosis and sterol 27-hydroxylase: evidence for a role of this enzyme in elimination of cholesterol from human macrophages. Proc Natl Acad Sci U S A 1994;91:8592–6.
110. Reiss AB, Martin KO, Javitt NB, et al. Sterol 27-hydroxylase: high levels of activity in vascular endothelium. J Lipid Res 1994; 35:1026–30.
111. Lund E, Andersson O, Zhang J, et al. Importance of a novel oxidative mechanism for elimination of intracellular cholesterol in humans. Arterioscler Thromb Vasc Biol 1996;16:208–12.
112. Babiker A, Andersson O, Lund E, et al. Elimination of cholesterol in macrophages and endothelial cells by the sterol 27-hydroxylase mechanism. Comparison with high density lipoprotein-mediated reverse cholesterol transport. J Biol Chem 1997;272:26253–61.
113. Okuda A, Okuda K. Physiological function and kinetic mechanism of human liver alcohol dehydrogenase as 5β-cholestane-3α,7α,12α,26-tetrol dehydrogenase. J Biol Chem 1983;258:2899–905.
114. Prydz K, Kase BF, Bjorkhem I, Pedersen JI. Subcellular localization of 3α,7α-dihydroxy- and 3α,7α,12α-trihydroxy-5β-cholestanoyl-coenzyme A ligase(s) in rat liver. J Lipid Res 1988;29:997–1004.
115. Lazarow PB, Fujiki Y. Biogenesis of peroxisomes. Annu Rev Cell Biol 1985;1:489–530.
116. Schepers L, Van Veldhoven PP, Casteels M, et al. Presence of three acyl-CoA oxidases in rat liver peroxisomes. An inducible fatty acyl-CoA oxidase, a noninducible fatty acyl-CoA oxidase, and a noninducible trihydroxycoprostanoyl-CoA oxidase. J Biol Chem 1990;265:5242–6.
117. Vanhove GF, Van Veldhoven PP, Fransen M, et al. The CoA esters of 2-methyl-branched chain fatty acids and of the bile acid intermediates di- and trihydroxycoprostanic acids are oxidized by one single peroxisomal branched chain acyl-CoA oxidase in human liver and kidney. J Biol Chem 1993;268:10335–44.
118. Gengenbacher T, Gerok W, Giese U, et al. Peroxisomal proteins involved in bile salt biosynthesis. In: Paumgartner G, Stiehl A, Gerok W, eds. Bile acids as therapeutic agents. Hangham, MA: Kluwer Academic Publishers, 1991:63–76.
119. Schram AW, Goldfischer S, van Roermund CW, et al. Human peroxisomal 3-oxoacyl-coenzyme A thiolase deficiency. Proc Natl Acad Sci U S A 1987;84:2494–6.
120. Swell L, Gustafsson J, Schwartz CC, et al. An in vivo evaluation of the quantitative significance of several potential pathways to cholic and chenodeoxycholic acids from cholesterol in man. J Lipid Res 1980;21:455–66.
121. Axelson M, Sjovall J. Potential bile acid precursors in plasma – possible indicators of biosynthetic pathways to cholic and chenodeoxycholic acids in man. J Steroid Biochem 1990;36:631–40.
122. Yamasaki K. Alternative biogenetic pathways of C24-bile acids with special reference to chenodeoxycholic acid. Kawasaki Med J 1978;4:227–64.
123. Vlahcevic ZR, Schwartz CC, Gustafsson J, et al. Biosynthesis of bile acids in man. Multiple pathways to cholic acid and chenodeoxycholic acid. J Biol Chem 1980;255:2925–33.
124. Anderson KE, Kok E, Javitt NB. Bile acid synthesis in man: metabolism of 7α-hydroxycholesterol-14 C and 26-hydroxycholesterol-3 H. J Clin Invest 1972;51:112–17.
125. Stapleton G, Steel M, Richardson M, et al. A novel cytochrome P450 expressed primarily in brain. J Biol Chem 1995;270:29739–45.
126. Zhang J, Akwa Y, Baulieu EE, Sjovall J. 7α-Hydroxylation of 27-hydroxycholesterol in rat brain microsomes. C R Acad Sci III 1995;318:345–9.
127. Zhang J, Larsson O, Sjovall J. 7αHydroxylation of 25-hydroxycholesterol and 27-hydroxycholesterol in human fibroblasts. Biochim Biophys Acta 1995;1256:353–9.
128. Axelson M, Larsson O, Zhang J, et al. Structural specificity in the suppression of HMG-CoA reductase in human fibroblasts by intermediates in bile acid biosynthesis. J Lipid Res 1995;36:290–8.
129. Zhang J, Dricu A, Sjovall J. Studies on the relationships between 7 alpha-hydroxylation and the ability of 25- and 27-hydroxycholesterol to suppress the activity of HMG-CoA reductase. Biochim Biophys Acta 1997;1344:241–9.
130. Toll A, Shoda J, Axelson M, et al. 7α-hydroxylation of 26-hydroxycholesterol, 3β-hydroxy-5-cholestenoic acid and 3β-hydroxy-5-cholenoic acid by cytochrome P- 450 in pig liver microsomes. FEBS Lett 1992;296:73–6.
131. Bjorkhem I, Nyberg B, Einarsson K. 7α-Hydroxylation of 27-hydroxycholesterol in human liver microsomes. Biochim Biophys Acta 1992;1128:73–6.
132. Toll A, Wikvall K, Sudjana-Sugiaman E, et al. 7α-hydroxylation of 25-hydroxycholesterol in liver microsomes. Evidence that the enzyme involved is different from cholesterol 7α-hydroxylase. Eur J Biochem 1994;224:309–16.
133. Heuman DM, Vlahcevic ZR, Bailey ML, Hylemon PB. Regulation of bile acid synthesis. II. Effect of bile acid feeding on enzymes regulating hepatic cholesterol and bile acid synthesis in the rat. Hepatology 1988;8:892–7.
134. Wu Z, Martin KO, Javitt NB, Chiang JY. Structure and functions of human oxysterol 7α-hydroxylase cDNAs and gene CYP7B1. J Lipid Res 1999;40:2195–203.
135. Emerman S, Javitt NB. Metabolism of taurolithocholic acid in the hamster. J Biol Chem 1967;242:661–4.
136. Javitt NB, Emerman S. Effect of sodium taurolithocholate on bile flow and bile acid exeretion. J Clin Invest 1968;47:1002–14.
137. Mathis U, Karlaganis G, Preisig R. Monohydroxy bile salt sulfates: tauro-3β-hydroxy-5-cholenoate-3-sulfate induces intrahepatic cholestasis in rats. Gastroenterology 1983;85:674–81.
138. Hall R, Kok E, Javitt NB. Bile acid synthesis: down-regulation by monohydroxy bile acids. FASEB J 1988;2:152–6.

139. Salen G, Shefer S, Cheng FW, et al. Cholic acid biosynthesis: the enzymatic defect in cerebrotendinous xanthomatosis. J Clin Invest 1979;63:38–44.
140. Mitropoulos KA, Avery MD, Myant NB, Gibbons GF. The formation of cholest-5-ene-3,26-diol as an intermediate in the conversion of cholesterol into bile acids by liver mitochondria. Biochem J 1972;130:363–71.
141. Mitropoulos KA, Myant NB. The formation of lithocholic acid, chenodeoxycholic acid and α- and β-muricholic acids from cholesterol incubated with rat-liver mitochondria. Biochem J 1967;103:472–9.
142. Wachtel N, Emerman S, Javitt NB. Metabolism of cholest-5-ene-3β,26-diol in the rat and hamster. J Biol Chem 1968;243:5207–12.
143. Kok E, Burstein S, Javitt NB, et al. Bile acid synthesis. Metabolism of 3β-hydroxy-5-cholenoic acid in the hamster. J Biol Chem 1981;256:6155–9.
144. Kulkarni B, Javitt NB. Chenodeoxycholic acid synthesis in the hamster: a metabolic pathway via 3β,7α-dihydroxy-5-cholen-24-oic acid. Steroids 1982;40:581–9.
145. Krisans SK, Thompson SL, Pena LA, et al. Bile acid synthesis in rat liver peroxisomes: metabolism of 26-hydroxycholesterol to 3β-hydroxy-5-cholenoic acid. J Lipid Res 1985;26:1324–32.
146. Grundy SM, Ahrens EH Jr, Salen G. Dietary β-sitosterol as an internal standard to correct for cholesterol losses in sterol balance studies. J Lipid Res 1968;9:374–87.
147. Salen G, Ahrens EH Jr, Grundy SM. Metabolism of β-sitosterol in man. J Clin Invest 1970;49:952–67.
148. Swell I, Treadwell CR. Metabolic fate of 14C-phytosterols. Proc Soc Exp Biol Med 1961;108:810–13.
149. Kritchevsky D, Davidson LM, Mosbach EH, Cohen BI. Identification of acidic steroids in feces of monkeys fed beta-sitoserol. Lipids 1981;16:77–8.
150. Skrede B, Bjorkhem I, Bergesen O, et al. The presence of 5α-sitostanol in the serum of a patient with phytosterolemia, and its biosynthesis from plant steroids in rats with bile fistula. Biochim Biophys Acta 1985;836:368–75.
151. Boberg KM, Einarsson K, Bjorkhem I. Apparent lack of conversion of sitosterol into C24-bile acids in humans. J Lipid Res 1990;31:1083–8.
152. Boberg KM, Lund E, Olund J, Bjorkhem I. Formation of C21 bile acids from plant sterols in the rat. J Biol Chem 1990;265:7967–75.
153. Lund E, Boberg KM, Bystrom S, et al. Formation of novel C21-bile acids from cholesterol in the rat. Structure identification of the major di- and trihydroxylated species. J Biol Chem 1991;266:4929–37.
154. Bjorkhem I, Oftebro H, Skrede S, Pedersen JI. Assay of intermediates in bile acid biosynthesis using isotope dilution- -mass spectrometry: hepatic levels in the normal state and in cerebrotendinous xanthomatosis. J Lipid Res 1981;22:191–200.
155. Axelson M, Mork B, Everson GT. Bile acid synthesis in cultured human hepatoblastoma cells. J Biol Chem 1991;266:17770–7.
156. Karavolas HJ, Elliott WH, Hsia SL, et al. Bile acids. XXII. Allocholic acid, a metabolite of 5α-cholestan-3β-ol in the rat. J Biol Chem 1965;240:1568–77.
157. Hofmann AF, Mosbach EH. Identification of allodeoxycholic acid as the major component of gallstones induced in the rabbit by 5α-cholestan-3β-ol. J Biol Chem 1964;239:2813–21.
158. Bjorkhem I, Gustafsson J. On the conversion of cholestanol into allocholic acid in rat liver. Eur J Biochem 1971;18:207–13.
159. Mui MM, Elliott WH. Bile acids. XXXII. Allocholic acid, a metabolite of allochenodeoxycholic acid in bile fistula rats. J Biol Chem 1971;246:302–4.
160. Blaskiewicz RJ, O'Neil GJ Jr, Elliott WH. Bile acids. XLI. Hepatic microsomal 12α-hydroxylation of allochenodeoxycholate to allocholate. Proc Soc Exp Biol Med 1974;146:92–5.
161. Ali SS, Elliott WH. Bile acids. LI. Formation of 12α-hydroxyl derivatives and companions from 5α-sterols by rabbit liver microsomes. J Lipid Res 1976;17:386–92.
162. Thigpen AE, Silver RI, Guileyardo JM, et al. Tissue distribution and ontogeny of steroid 5α-reductase isozyme expression. J Clin Invest 1993;92:903–10.
163. Shoda J, Mahara R, Osuga T, et al. Similarity of unusual bile acids in human umbilical cord blood and amniotic fluid from newborns and in sera and urine from adult patients with cholestatic liver diseases. J Lipid Res 1988;29:847–58.
164. Gustafsson J. Bile acid synthesis during development. Mitochondrial 12α-hydroxylation in human fetal liver. J Clin Invest 1985;75:604–7.
165. Gustafsson J, Anderson S, Sjovall J. Bile acid metabolism during development: metabolism of lithocholic acid in human fetal liver. Pediatr Res 1987;21:99–103.
166. Dumaswala R, Setchell KDR, Zimmer-Nechemias L, et al. Identification of 3α,4β,7α-trihydroxy-5β-cholanoic acid in human bile: reflection of a new pathway in bile acid metabolism in humans. J Lipid Res 1989;30:847–56.
167. Balistreri WF, Heubi JE, Suchy FJ. Immaturity of the enterohepatic circulation in early life: factors predisposing to "physiologic" maldigestion and cholestasis. J Pediatr Gastroenterol Nutr 1983;2:346–54.
168. Hofmann AF, Palmer KR, Yoon Y-B. The biological utility of bile acid conjugation with glycine or taurine. In: Matern S, Bock KW, Gerok W, eds. Advances in glucuronide conjugation. Lancaster U.K.: MTP Press, 1985:245–64.
169. Bremer J, Gloor V. Studies on the conjugation of cholic acid with taurine in cell subfractions. Acta Chem Scand 1955;9:689–98.
170. Killenberg PG. Measurement and subcellular distribution of choloyl-CoA synthetase and bile acid-CoA:amino acid N-acyltransferase activities in rat liver. J Lipid Res 1978;19:24–31.
171. Vessey DA, Zakim D. Characterization of microsomal choloyl-coenzyme A synthetase. Biochem J 1977;163:357–62.
172. Wheeler JB, Shaw DR, Barnes S. Purification and characterization of a rat liver bile acid coenzyme A ligase from rat liver microsomes. Arch Biochem Biophys 1997;348:15–24.
173. Johnson MR, Barnes S, Kwakye JB, Diasio RB. Purification and characterization of bile acid-CoA:amino acid N-acyltransferase from human liver. J Biol Chem 1991;266:10227–33.
174. Kase BF, Prydz K, Bjorkhem I, Pedersen JI. Conjugation of cholic acid with taurine and glycine by rat liver peroxisomes. Biochem Biophys Res Commun 1986;138:167–73.
175. Kase BF, Bjorkhem I. Peroxisomal bile acid-CoA:amino-acid N-acyltransferase in rat liver. J Biol Chem 1989;264:9220–3.
176. Shonsey EM, Sfakianos M, Johnson M, et al. Bile acid coenzyme A: amino acid N-acyltransferase in the amino acid conjugation of bile acids. Methods Enzymol 2005;400:374–94.
177. Falany CN, Johnson MR, Barnes S, Diasio RB. Glycine and taurine conjugation of bile acids by a single enzyme. Molecular cloning and expression of human liver bile acid CoA:amino acid N-acyltransferase. J Biol Chem 1994;269:19375–9.
178. Falany CN, Fortinberry H, Leiter EH, Barnes S. Cloning, expression, and chromosomal localization of mouse liver bile acid

CoA:amino acid N-acyltransferase. J Lipid Res 1997;38:1139–48.
179. Falany CN, Xie X, Wheeler JB, et al. Molecular cloning and expression of rat liver bile acid CoA ligase. J Lipid Res 2002;43:2062–72.
180. Lim WC, Jordan TW. Subcellular distribution of hepatic bile acid-conjugating enzymes. Biochem J 1981;197:611–18.
181. O'Byrne J, Hunt MC, Rai DK, et al. The human bile acid-CoA:amino acid N-acyltransferase functions in the conjugation of fatty acids to glycine. J Biol Chem 2003;278:34237–44.
182. Kirkpatrick RB, Green MD, Hagey LR, et al. Effect of side chain length on bile acid conjugation: glucuronidation, sulfation and coenzyme A formation of nor-bile acids and their natural C24 homologs by human and rat liver fractions. Hepatology 1988;8:353–7.
183. Czuba B, Vessey DA. The effect of bile acid structure on the activity of bile acid–CoA:glycine/taurine-*N*-acetyltransferase. J Biol Chem 1982;257:8761–5.
184. Furutani M, Arii S, Higashitsuji H, et al. Reduced expression of kan-1 (encoding putative bile acid-CoA-amino acid N-acyltransferase) mRNA in livers of rats after partial hepatectomy and during sepsis. Biochem J 1995;311:203–8.
185. O'Maille ER, Richards TG, Short AH. Acute taurine depletion and maximal rates of hepatic conjugation and secretion of cholic acid in the dog. J Physiol (Lond) 1965;180:67–79.
186. Sturman JA, Gaull GE. Taurine in the brain and liver of the developing human and monkey. J Neurochem 1975;25:831–5.
187. Palmer RH. The formation of bile acid sulfates: a new pathway of bile acid metabolism in humans. Proc Natl Acad Sci U S A 1967;58:1047–50.
188. Shattuck KE, Radominska-Pyrek A, Zimniak P, et al. Metabolism of 24-norlithocholic acid in the rat: formation of hydroxyl- and carboxyl-linked glucuronides and effect on bile flow. Hepatology 1986;6:869–73.
189. Radominska-Pyrek A, Zimniak P, Chari M, et al. Glucuronides of monohydroxylated bile acids: specificity of microsomal glucuronyltransferase for the glucuronidation site, C-3 configuration, and side chain length. J Lipid Res 1986;27:89–101.
190. Matern H, Matern S, Gerok W. Formation of bile acid glucosides by a sugar nucleotide-independent glucosyltransferase isolated from human liver microsomes. Proc Natl Acad Sci U S A 1984;81:7036–40.
191. Marschall HU, Egestad B, Matern H, et al. Evidence for bile acid glucosides as normal constituents in human urine. FEBS Lett 1987;213:411–14.
192. Marschall HU, Egestad B, Matern H, et al. *N*-acetylglucosaminides. A new type of bile acid conjugate in man. J Biol Chem 1989;264:12989–93.
193. Sweeny DJ, Barnes S, Heggie GD, Diasio RB. Metabolism of 5-fluorouracil to an *N*-cholyl-2-fluoro-β-alanine conjugate: previously unrecognized role for bile acids in drug conjugation. Proc Natl Acad Sci U S A 1987;84:5439–43.
194. Sweeny DJ, Barnes S, Diasio RB. Formation of conjugates of 2-fluoro-β-alanine and bile acids during the metabolism of 5-fluorouracil and 5-fluoro-2-deoxyuridine in the isolated perfused rat liver. Cancer Res 1988;48:2010–14.
195. Malet-Martino MC, Bernadou J, Martino R, Armand JP. 19F NMR spectrometry evidence for bile acid conjugates of α-fluoro-β-alanine as the main biliary metabolites of antineoplastic fluoropyrimidines in humans. Drug Metab Dispos 1988;16:78–84.
196. Hofmann AF, Roda A. Physicochemical properties of bile acids and their relationship to biological properties: an overview of the problem. J Lipid Res 1984;25:1477–89.
197. Scholmerich J, Becher MS, Schmidt K, et al. Influence of hydroxylation and conjugation of bile salts on their membrane-damaging properties – studies on isolated hepatocytes and lipid membrane vesicles. Hepatology 1984;4:661–6.
198. Setchell KDR, Balistreri WF, Lin Q, et al. Metabolism of ursodeoxycholic acid in normal subjects and in patients with cholestatic liver disease: biotransformation by conjugation and urinary excretion. In: Paumgartner G, Stiehl A, Gerok W, eds. Bile acids and the hepatobiliary system. From basic science to clinical practice. Dordrecht/Boston/London: Kluwer Academic Publishers, 1993:245–9.
199. Marschall HU, Matern H, Wietholtz H, et al. Bile acid *N*-acetylglucosaminidation. In vivo and in vitro evidence for a selective conjugation reaction of 7β-hydroxylated bile acids in humans. J Clin Invest 1992;89:1981–7.
200. Summerfield JA, Gollan JL, Billing BH. Synthesis of bile acid monosulphates by the isolated perfused rat kidney. Biochem J 1976;156:339–45.
201. Matern S, Matern H, Farthmann EH, Gerok W. Hepatic and extrahepatic glucuronidation of bile acids in man. Characterization of bile acid uridine 5′-diphosphate glucuronosyltransferase in hepatic, renal, and intestinal microsomes. J Clin Invest 1984;74:402–10.
202. Chen LJ, Bolt RJ, Admirand WH. Enzymatic sulfation of bile salts. Partial purification and characterization of an enzyme from rat liver that catalyzes the sulfation of bile salts. Biochim Biophys Acta 1977;480:219–27.
203. Loof L, Hjerten S. Partial purification of a human liver sulphotransferase active towards bile salts. Biochim Biophys Acta 1980;617:192–204.
204. Barnes S, Burhol PG, Zander R, et al. Enzymatic sulfation of glycochenodeoxycholic acid by tissue fractions from adult hamsters. J Lipid Res 1979;20:952–9.
205. Watkins JB, Goldstein E, Coryer R. Sulfation of bile acids in the fetus. In: Presig R, Bircher J, eds. The liver, quantitative aspects of structure and function. Gstaad, Switzerland: Edito Cantor Aulendorf, 1974:249–54.
206. Watkins JB. Placental transport: bile acid conjugation and sulfation in the fetus. J Pediatr Gastroenterol Nutr 1983;2:365–73.
207. Summerfield JA, Cullen J, Barnes S, Billing BH. Evidence for renal control of urinary excretion of bile acids and bile acid sulphates in the cholestatic syndrome. Clin Sci Mol Med 1977;52:51–65.
208. Back P. Urinary bile acids. In: Setchell KDR, Kritchevsky D, Nair PP, eds. The bile acids. New York: Plenum Press, 1988:405–40.
209. Nakagawa M, Colombo C, Setchell KDR. Comprehensive study of the biliary bile acid composition of patients with cystic fibrosis and associated liver disease before and after UDCA administration. Hepatology 1990;12:322–34.
210. Radominska-Pyrek A, Zimniak P, Irshaid YM, et al. Glucuronidation of 6α-hydroxy bile acids by human liver microsomes. J Clin Invest 1987;80:234–41.
211. Parquet M, Pessah M, Sacquet E, et al. Effective glucuronidation of 6α-hydroxylated bile acids by human hepatic and renal microsomes. Eur J Biochem 1988;171:329–34.
212. Fournel-Gigleux S, Sutherland L, Sabolovic N, et al. Stable expression of two human UDP-glucuronosyltransferase cDNAs in V79 cell cultures. Mol Pharmacol 1991;39:177–83.

213. Marschall HU, Green G, Egestad B, Sjovall J. Isolation of bile acid glucosides and *N*-acetylglucosaminides from human urine by ion-exchange chromatography and reversed-phase high- performance liquid chromatography. J Chromatogr 1988;452:459–68.
214. Wietholtz H, Marschall HU, Reuschenbach R, et al. Urinary excretion of bile acid glucosides and glucuronides in extrahepatic cholestasis. Hepatology 1991;13:656–62.
215. Matern H, Matern S. Formation of bile acid glucosides and dolichyl phosphoglucose by microsomal glucosyltransferases in liver, kidney and intestine of man. Biochim Biophys Acta 1987;921:1–6.
216. Setchell KDR, Street JM, Sjovall J. Fecal bile acids. In: Setchell KDR, Kritchevsky D, Nair PP, eds. The bile acids: methods and applications. New York: Plenum Press, 1988:441–570.
217. Hill MJ, Drasar BS. Degradation of bile salts by human intestinal bacteria. Gut 1968;9:22–7.
218. Hayakawa S. Microbiological transformation of bile acids. Adv Lipid Res 1973;11:143–92.
219. Macdonald IA, Bokkenheuser VD, Winter J, et al. Degradation of steroids in the human gut. J Lipid Res 1983;24:675–700.
220. Hylemon PB. Metabolism of bile acids in intestinal microflora. In: Danielsson H, Sjovall J, eds. Sterols and bile acids. Amsterdam: Elsevier Science, 1985:331–43.
221. Setchell KDR, O'Connell NC, Cummings J. Intraluminal bile acid composition along the entire length of the human intestine. FASEB J. 1993;A722.
222. Mallory A, Kern F Jr, Smith J, Savage D. Patterns of bile acids and microflora in the human small intestine. I. Bile acids. Gastroenterology 1973;64:26–33.
223. Mallory A, Savage D, Kern F Jr, Smith JG. Patterns of bile acids and microflora in the human small intestine. II. Microflora. Gastroenterology 1973;64:34–42.
224. Northfield TC, McColl I. Postprandial concentrations of free and conjugated bile acids down the length of the normal human small intestine. Gut 1973;14:513–18.
225. Huijghebaert SM, Hofmann AF. Influence of the amino acid moiety on deconjugation of bile acid amidates by cholylglycine hydrolase or human fecal cultures. J Lipid Res 1986;27:742–52.
226. Batta AK, Salen G, Shefer S. Substrate specificity of cholylglycine hydrolase for the hydrolysis of bile acid conjugates. J Biol Chem 1984;259:15035–9.
227. Bjorkhem I, Einarsson K, Melone P, Hylemon P. Mechanism of intestinal formation of deoxycholic acid from cholic acid in humans: evidence for a 3-oxo-Δ^4-steroid intermediate. J Lipid Res 1989;30:1033–9.
228. Hylemon PB. Biochemistry and genetics of intestinal bile salt metabolism. In: Paumgartner G, Gerok W, eds. Bile acids as therapeutic agents. From basic science to clinical practice. Dordrecht/Boston/London: Kluwer Academic Publishers, 1990:1–11.
229. Franklund CV, Baron SF, Hylemon PB. Characterization of the baiH gene encoding a bile acid-inducible NADH:flavin oxidoreductase from *Eubacterium* sp. strain VPI 12708. J Bacteriol 1993;175:3002–12.
230. Heuman DM, Hylemon PB, Vlahcevic ZR. Regulation of bile acid synthesis. III. Correlation between biliary bile salt hydrophobicity index and the activities of enzymes regulating cholesterol and bile acid synthesis in the rat. J Lipid Res 1989;30:1161–71.
231. Stange EF, Scheibner J, Ditschuneit H. Role of primary and secondary bile acids as feedback inhibitors of bile acid synthesis in the rat in vivo. J Clin Invest 1989;84:173–80.
232. Setchell KDR, Lawson AM, Blackstock EJ, Murphy GM. Diurnal changes in serum unconjugated bile acids in normal man. Gut 1982;23:637–42.
233. Setchell KDR, Harrison DL, Gilbert JM, Mupthy GM. Serum unconjugated bile acids: qualitative and quantitative profiles in ileal resection and bacterial overgrowth. Clin Chim Acta 1985; 152:297–306.
234. Mills KA, Mushtaq I, Johnson AW, et al. A method for the quantitation of conjugated bile acids in dried blood spots using electrospray ionization-mass spectrometry. Pediatr Res 1998;43:361–8.
235. Clayton PT, Leonard JV, Lawson AM, et al. Familial giant cell hepatitis associated with synthesis of 3β,7α-dihydroxy- and 3β,7α,12α-trihydroxy-5-cholenoic acids. J Clin Invest 1987;79:1031–8.
236. Clayton PT, Casteels M, Mieli-Vergani G, Lawson AM. Familial giant cell hepatitis with low bile acid concentrations and increased urinary excretion of specific bile alcohols: a new inborn error of bile acid synthesis? Pediatr Res 1995;37:424–31.
237. Setchell KDR, Heubi JE, O'Connell NC, et al. Identification of a unique inborn error in bile acid conjugation involving a deficiency in amidation. In: Paumgartner G, Stiehl A, Gerok W, eds. Bile acids in hepatobiliary diseases: basic research and clinical application. Dordrecht/Boston/London: Kluwer Academic Publishers, 1997:43–7.
238. Setchell KDR, O'Connell NC, Squires RH, Heubi JE. Congenital defects in bile acid synthesis cause a spectrum of diseases manifest as severe cholestasis, neurological disease, and fat-soluble vitamin malabsorption. In: Northfield TC, Ahmed H, Jazwari R, Zentler-Munro P, eds. Bile acids in hepatobiliary disease. Dordrecht: Kluwer Academic Publishers, 1999:55–63.
239. Pullinger CR, Eng C, Salen G, et al. Human cholesterol 7α-hydroxylase (CYP7A1) deficiency has a hypercholesterolemic phenotype. J Clin Invest 2002;110:109–17.
240. Iser J, Dowling R, Murphy G. Congenital bile salt deficiency associated with 28 years of intractable constipation. In: Paumgartner G, Stiehl A, eds. Bile acid metabolism in health and disease. Lancaster, U.K.: MTP Press, 1977:231–4.
241. Loomes KM, Setchell KDR, Rheingold SR, Piccoli DA. Bile acid synthetic disorder in a symptomatic patient with normal liver enzymes. J Pediatr Gastroenterol Nutr 1998;26: 579.
242. Setchell KDR, Flick R, Watkins JB, Piccoli DA. Chronic hepatitis in a 10 yr old due to an inborn error in bile acid synthesis – diagnosis and treatment with oral bile acid. Gastroenterology 1990;98:A578.
243. Setchell KDR, Heubi J. Defects in bile acid synthesis – diagnosis and treatment. J Pediatr Gastroenterol Nutr 2006;43(suppl 1): S17–22.
244. Jacquemin E, Setchell KDR, O'Connell NC, et al. A new cause of progressive intrahepatic cholestasis: 3β-hydroxy-C_{27}- steroid dehydrogenase/isomerase deficiency. J Pediatr 1994;125:379–84.
245. Setchell KDR, Balistreri WF, Piccoli DA, Clerici C. Oral bile acid therapy in the treatment of inborn errors in bile acid synthesis associated with liver disease. In: Paumgartner G, Stiehl A, Gerok W, eds. Falk symposium no. 58. Bile acids

as therapeutic agents: from basic science to clinical practice. Freiburg, Germany: Kluwer Academic Publishers, 1990:367–73.

246. Witzleben CL, Piccoli DA, Setchell KDR. A new category of causes of intrahepatic cholestasis. Pediatr Pathol 1992;12:269–74.
247. Horslen SP, Lawson AM, Malone M, Clayton PT. 3β-hydroxy-Δ^5-C_{27}-steroid dehydrogenase deficiency; Effect of chenodeoxycholic acid therapy on liver histology. J Inherit Metab Dis 1992;15:38–46.
248. Bove K, Daugherty CC, Tyson W, et al. Bile acid synthetic defects and liver disease. Pediatr Dev Pathol 2000;3:1–16.
249. Bove KE, Heubi JE, Balistreri WF, Setchell KDR. Bile acid synthetic defects and liver disease: a comprehensive review. Pediatr Dev Pathol 2004;7:315–34.
250. Ichimiya H, Egestad B, Nazer H, et al. Bile acids and bile alcohols in a child with hepatic 3β-hydroxy-Δ^5-C_{27}-steroid dehydrogenase deficiency: effects of chenodeoxycholic acid treatment. J Lipid Res 1991;32:829–41.
251. Egestad B, Pettersson P, Skrede S, Sjovall J. Fast atom bombardment mass spectrometry in the diagnosis of cerebrotendinous xanthomatosis. Scand J Clin Lab Invest 1985;45:443–6.
252. Buchmann MS, Kvittingen EA, Nazer H, et al. Lack of 3β-hydroxy-Δ^5-C_{27}-steroid dehydrogenase/isomerase in fibroblasts from a child with urinary excretion of 3β-hydroxy-Δ^5-bile acids. A new inborn error of metabolism. J Clin Invest 1990;86:2034–7.
253. Stieger B, Zhang J, O'Neill B, et al. Transport of taurine conjugates of 7α-hydroxy-3-oxo-4-cholenoic acid and 3β,7α-dihydroxy-5-cholenoic acid in rat liver plasma membrane vesicles. In: Van Berge-Henegouwen GP, Van Hock B, De Groote J, et al., eds. Cholestatic liver diseases. Dordrecht/Boston/London: Kluwer Academic Press, 1994:82–7.
254. Stieger B, Zhang J, O'Neill B, et al. Differential interaction of bile acids from patients with inborn errors of bile acid synthesis with hepatocellular bile acid transporters. Eur J Biochem 1997;244:39–44.
255. Ichimiya H, Nazer H, Gunasekaran T, et al. Treatment of chronic liver disease caused by 3β-hydroxy-Δ^5-C_{27}- steroid dehydrogenase deficiency with chenodeoxycholic acid. Arch Dis Child 1990;65:1121–4.
256. Setchell KDR, Bragetti P, Zimmer-Nechemias L, et al. Oral bile acid treatment and the patient with Zellweger syndrome. Hepatology 1992;15:198–207.
257. Daugherty CC, Setchell KDR, Heubi JE, Balistreri WF. Resolution of liver biopsy alterations in three siblings with bile acid treatment of an inborn error of bile acid metabolism (Δ^4-3- oxosteroid 5β-reductase deficiency). Hepatology 1993;18:1096–101.
258. Berseus O, Bjorkhem I. Enzymatic conversion of a Δ^4-3-ketosteroid into a 3α-hydroxy- 5β steroid: mechanism and stereochemistry of hydrogen transfer from NADPH. Bile acids and steroids 190. Eur J Biochem 1967;2:503–7.
259. Berseus O. Conversion of cholesterol to bile acids in rat: purification and properties of a Δ^4-3-ketosteroid 5β-reductase and a 3α-hydroxysteroid dehydrogenase. Eur J Biochem 1967;2:493–502.
260. Sumazaki R, Nakamura N, Shoda J, et al. Gene analysis in Δ^4-3-oxosteroid 5β-reductase deficiency [letter]. Lancet 1997; 349:329.
261. Wahlen E, Egestad B, Strandvik B, Sjoovall J. Ketonic bile acids in urine of infants during the neonatal period. J Lipid Res 1989;30:1847–57.
262. Shneider BL, Setchell KD, Whitington PF, et al. Δ^4-3-Oxosteroid 5β-reductase deficiency causing neonatal liver failure and hemochromatosis [see comments]. J Pediatr 1994;124:234–8.
263. Levy P, Dumont M, Brissot P, et al. Acute infusions of bile salts increase biliary excretion of iron in iron-loaded rats [see comments]. Gastroenterology 1991;101:1673–9.
264. Setchell KDR, O'Connell NC. Inborn errors of bile acid biosynthesis: update on biochemical aspects. In: Hofmann AF, Paumgartner G, Stiehl A, eds. Bile acids in gastroenterology. Basic and clinical advances. Dordrecht/Boston/London: Kluwer Academic Publishers, 1995:129–36.
265. Axelson M, Mork B, Sjovall J. Occurrence of 3β-hydroxy-5-cholestenoic acid, 3β,7α-dihydroxy-5-cholestenoic acid, and 7α-hydroxy-3-oxo-4-cholestenoic acid as normal constituents in human blood. J Lipid Res 1988;29:629–41.
266. Gustafsson J. Bile acid biosynthesis during development: hydroxylation of C27-sterols in human fetal liver. J Lipid Res 1986;27:801–6.
267. Dowling RH. Bile acids in constipation and diarrhoea. In: Barbara L, Dowling RH, Hofmann AF, eds. Bile acids in gastroenterology. Lancaster, U.K.: MTP Press, 1982:157–71.
268. Kimura A, Yuge K, Yukizane S, et al. Abnormal low ratio of cholic acid to chenodeoxycholic acid in a cholestatic infant with severe hypoglycemia. J Pediatr Gastroenterol Nutr 1991;12:383–7.
269. Suchy FJ. Bile formation, mechanisms and development. In: Suchy FJ, ed. Liver disease in children. Philadelphia: Mosby-Year Book, 1994.
270. Heubi JE, Balistreri WF, Suchy FJ. Bile salt metabolism in the first year of life. J Lab Clin Med 1982;100:127–36.
271. Van Bogaert L, Scherer HJ, Epstein E. Une forme cerebrale de la cholesterinose generalisee. Paris: Masson et Cie, 1937.
272. Setoguchi T, Salen G, Tint GS, Mosbach EH. A biochemical abnormality in cerebrotendinous xanthomatosis. Impairment of bile acid biosynthesis associated with incomplete degradation of the cholesterol side chain. J Clin Invest 1974;53:1393–401.
273. Cruysberg JR, Wevers RA, Tolboom JJ. Juvenile cataract associated with chronic diarrhea in pediatric cerebrotendinous xanthomatosis [letter]. Am J Ophthalmol 1991;112:606–7.
274. Wevers RA, Cruysberg JR, Van Heijst AF, et al. Paediatric cerebrotendinous xanthomatosis. J Inherit Metab Dis 1992;15:374–6.
275. Kuriyama M, Fujiyama J, Yoshidome H, et al. Cerebrotendinous xanthomatosis: clinical and biochemical evaluation of eight patients and review of the literature. J Neurol Sci 1991;102:225–32.
276. Setchell KDR. A unique case of cerebrotendinous xanthomatosis presenting in infancy with cholestatic liver disease further highlights bile acid synthetic defects as an important category of metabolic liver disease [abstract]. Den Haag, the Netherlands: Dr. Falk Pharma Gmbh, 2001:13–14.
277. Clayton PT, Verrips A, Sistermans E, et al. Mutations in the sterol 27-hydroxylase gene (CYP27A) cause hepatitis of infancy as well as cerebrotendinous xanthomatosis. J Inherit Metab Dis 2002;25:501–13.
278. von Bahr S, Bjorkhem I, Van't Hooft F, et al. Mutation in the sterol 27-hydroxylase gene associated with fatal cholestasis in infancy. J Pediatr Gastroenterol Nutr 2005;40:481–6.

279. Salen G, Grundy SM. The metabolism of cholestanol, cholesterol, and bile acids in cerebrotendinous xanthomatosis. J Clin Invest 1973;52:2822–35.
280. Salen G, Meriwether TW, Nicolau G. Chenodeoxycholic acid inhibits increased cholesterol and cholestanol synthesis in patients with cerebrotendinous xanthomatosis. Biochem Med 1975;14:57–74.
281. Oftebro H, Bjorkhem I, Skrede S, et al. Cerebrotendinous xanthomatosis: a defect in mitochondrial 26-hydroxylation required for normal biosynthesis of cholic acid. J Clin Invest 1980;65:1418–30.
282. Javitt NB, Kok E, Cohen B, Burstein S. Cerebrotendinous xanthomatosis: reduced serum 26-hydroxycholesterol. J Lipid Res 1982;23:627–30.
283. Wolthers BG, Volmer M, van der Molen J, et al. Diagnosis of cerebrotendinous xanthomatosis (CTX) and effect of chenodeoxycholic acid therapy by analysis of urine using capillary gas chromatography. Clin Chim Acta 1983;131:53–65.
284. Shimazu K, Kuwabara M, Yoshii M, et al. Bile alcohol profiles in bile, urine, and feces of a patient with cerebrotendinous xanthomatosis. J Biochem (Tokyo) 1986;99:477–83.
285. Salen G, Shefer S, Tint GS, et al. Biosynthesis of bile acids in cerebrotendinous xanthomatosis. Relationship of bile acid pool sizes and synthesis rates to hydroxylations at C-12, C-25, and C-26. J Clin Invest 1985;76:744–51.
286. Kim KS, Kubota S, Kuriyama M, et al. Identification of new mutations in sterol 27-hydroxylase gene in Japanese patients with cerebrotendinous xanthomatosis (CTX). J Lipid Res 1994;35:1031–9.
287. Leitersdorf E, Safadi R, Meiner V, et al. Cerebrotendinous xanthomatosis in the Israeli Druze: molecular genetics and phenotypic characteristics. Am J Hum Genet 1994;55:907–15.
288. Meiner V, Marais DA, Reshef A, et al. Premature termination codon at the sterol 27-hydroxylase gene causes cerebrotendinous xanthomatosis in an Afrikaner family. Hum Mol Genet 1994;3:193–4.
289. Reshef A, Meiner V, Berginer VM, Leitersdorf E. Molecular genetics of cerebrotendinous xanthomatosis in Jews of North African origin. J Lipid Res 1994;35:478–83.
290. Segev H, Reshef A, Clavey V, et al. Premature termination codon at the sterol 27-hydroxylase gene causes cerebrotendinous xanthomatosis in a French family. Hum Genet 1995;95:238–40.
291. Watts GF, Mitchell WD, Bending JJ, et al. Cerebrotendinous xanthomatosis: a family study of sterol 27-hydroxylase mutations and pharmacotherapy. Q J Med 1996;89:55–63.
292. Chen W, Kubota S, Nishimura Y, et al. Genetic analysis of a Japanese cerebrotendinous xanthomatosis family: identification of a novel mutation in the adrenodoxin binding region of the CYP27 gene. Biochim Biophys Acta 1996;1317:119–26.
293. Garuti R, Lelli N, Barozzini M, et al. Cerebrotendinous xanthomatosis caused by two new mutations of the sterol-27-hydroxylase gene that disrupt mRNA splicing. J Lipid Res 1996;37:1459–67.
294. Nagai Y, Hirano M, Mori T, et al. Japanese triplets with cerebrotendinous xanthomatosis are homozygous for a mutant gene coding for the sterol 27-hydroxylase (Arg441Trp). Neurology 1996;46:571–4.
295. Okuyama E, Tomita S, Takeuchi H, Ichikawa Y. A novel mutation in the cytochrome P450(27) (CYP27) gene caused cerebrotendinous xanthomatosis in a Japanese family. J Lipid Res 1996;37:631–9.
296. Verrips A, Steenbergen-Spanjers GC, Luyten JA, et al. Two new mutations in the sterol 27-hydroxylase gene in two families lead to cerebrotendinous xanthomatosis. Hum Genet 1996;98:735–7.
297. Verrips A, Steenbergen-Spanjers GC, Luyten JA, et al. Exon skipping in the sterol 27-hydroxylase gene leads to cerebrotendinous xanthomatosis. Hum Genet 1997;100:284–6.
298. Chen W, Kubota S, Kim KS, et al. Novel homozygous and compound heterozygous mutations of sterol 27-hydroxylase gene (CYP27) cause cerebrotendinous xanthomatosis in three Japanese patients from two unrelated families. J Lipid Res 1997;38:870–9.
299. Ahmed MS, Afsar S, Hentati A, et al. A novel mutation in the sterol 27-hydroxylase gene of a Pakistani family with autosomal recessive cerebrotendinous xanthomatosis. Neurology 1997;48:258–60.
300. Chen W, Kubota S, Seyama Y. Alternative pre-mRNA splicing of the sterol 27-hydroxylase gene (CYP27) caused by a G to A mutation at the last nucleotide of exon 6 in a patient with cerebrotendinous xanthomatosis (CTX). J Lipid Res 1998;39:509–17.
301. Chen W, Kubota S, Teramoto T, et al. Genetic analysis enables definite and rapid diagnosis of cerebrotendinous xanthomatosis. Neurology 1998;51:865–7.
302. Chen W, Kubota S, Teramoto T, et al. Silent nucleotide substitution in the sterol 27-hydroxylase gene (CYP27) leads to alternative pre-mRNA splicing by activating a cryptic 5′ splice site at the mutant codon in cerebrotendinous xanthomatosis patients. Biochemistry 1998;37:4420–8.
303. Wakamatsu N, Hayashi M, Kawai H, et al. Mutations producing premature termination of translation and an amino acid substitution in the sterol 27-hydroxylase gene cause cerebrotendinous xanthomatosis associated with parkinsonism. J Neurol Neurosurg Psychiatry 1999;67:195–8.
304. Shiga K, Fukuyama R, Kimura S, et al. Mutation of the sterol 27-hydroxylase gene (CYP27) results in truncation of mRNA expressed in leucocytes in a Japanese family with cerebrotendinous xanthomatosis. J Neurol Neurosurg Psychiatry 1999;67:675–7.
305. Berginer VM, Salen G, Shefer S. Cerebrotendinous xanthomatosis. Neurol Clin 1989;7:55–74.
306. Menkes JH, Schimschock JR, Swanson PD. Cerebrotendinous xanthomatosis. The storage of cholestanol within the nervous system. Arch Neurol 1968;19:47–53.
307. Salen G. Cholestanol deposition in cerebrotendinous xanthomatosis. A possible mechanism. Ann Intern Med 1971;75:843–51.
308. Kibe A, Nakai S, Kuramoto T, Hoshita T. Occurrence of bile alcohols in the bile of a patient with cholestasis. J Lipid Res 1980;21:594–9.
309. Hiraoka T, Kihira K, Kohda T, et al. Urinary bile alcohols in liver dysfunction. Clin Chim Acta 1987;169:127–32.
310. Weydert-Huijghebaert S, Karlaganis G, Renner EL, Preisig R. Increased urinary excretion of bile alcohol glucuronides in patients with primary biliary cirrhosis. J Lipid Res 1989;30:1673–9.
311. Skrede S, Bjorkhem I, Buchmann MS, et al. A novel pathway for biosynthesis of cholestanol with 7α-hydroxylated C_{27}-steroids as intermediates, and its importance for the accumulation of cholestanol in cerebrotendinous xanthomatosis. J Clin Invest 1985;75:448–55.

312. Skrede S, Buchmann MS, Bjorkhem I. Hepatic 7α-dehydroxylation of bile acid intermediates, and its significance for the pathogenesis of cerebrotendinous xanthomatosis. J Lipid Res 1988;29:157–64.
313. Koopman BJ, van der Molen JC, Wolthers BG, et al. Capillary gas chromatographic determination of cholestanol/cholesterol ratio in biological fluids. Its potential usefulness for the follow up of some liver diseases and its lack of specificity in diagnosing CTX (cerebrotendinous xanthomatosis). Clin Chim Acta 1984;137:305–15.
314. Berginer VM, Salen G, Shefer S. Long-term treatment of cerebrotendinous xanthomatosis with chenodeoxycholic acid. N Engl J Med 1984;311:1649–52.
315. Koopman BJ, Wolthers BG, van der Molen JC, Waterreus RJ. Bile acid therapies applied to patients suffering from cerebrotendinous xanthomatosis. Clin Chim Acta 1985;152:115–22.
316. Pedley TA, Emerson RG, Warner CL, et al. Treatment of cerebrotendinous xanthomatosis with chenodeoxycholic acid. Ann Neurol 1985;18:517–18.
317. Berginer VM, Radwan H, Korczyn AD, et al. EEG in cerebrotendinous xanthomatosis (CTX). Clin Electroencephalogr 1982;13:89–96.
318. Peynet J, Laurent A, De Liege P, et al. Cerebrotendinous xanthomatosis: treatments with simvastatin, lovastatin, and chenodeoxycholic acid in 3 siblings [see comments]. Neurology 1991;41:434–6.
319. Lewis B, Mitchell WD, Marenah CB, et al. Cerebrotendinous xanthomatosis: biochemical response to inhibition of cholesterol synthesis. Br Med J (Clin Res Ed) 1983;287:21–2.
320. Nakamura T, Matsuzawa Y, Takemura K, et al. Combined treatment with chenodeoxycholic acid and pravastatin improves plasma cholestanol levels associated with marked regression of tendon xanthomas in cerebrotendinous xanthomatosis. Metabolism 1991;40:741–6.
321. Setchell KDR, Heubi JE, Bove KE, et al. Liver disease caused by failure to racemize trihydroxycholestanoic acid: gene mutation and effect of bile acid therapy. Gastroenterology 2003;124:217–32.
322. Ferdinandusse S, Denis S, Clayton PT, et al. Mutations in the gene encoding peroxisomal 2-methyl-acyl-CoA racemase cause adult-onset sensory motor neuropathy. Nat Genet 2000;24:188–191.
323. Schmitz W, Fingerhut R, Conzelmann E. Purification and properties of an alpha-methylacyl-CoA racemase from rat liver. Eur J Biochem 1994;222:313–23.
324. Schmitz W, Albers C, Fingerhut R, Conzelmann E. Purification and characterization of an alpha-methylacyl-CoA racemase from human liver. Eur J Biochem 1995;231:815–22.
325. Cuebas DA, Phillips C, Schmitz W, et al. The role of alpha-methylacyl-CoA racemase in bile acid synthesis. Biochem J 2002;363:801–7.
326. Van Veldhoven PP, Meyhi E, Squires J, et al. Fibroblast studies documenting a case of peroxisomal 2-methylacyl-CoA racemase deficiency; possible link between racemase deficiency and malabsorption and vitamin K deficiency. Eur J Clin Invest 2001;31:714–22.
327. Savolainen K, Kotti TJ, Schmitz W, et al. A mouse model for alpha-methylacyl-CoA racemase deficiency: adjustment of bile acid synthesis and intolerance to dietary methyl-branched lipids. Hum Mol Genet 2004;13:955–65.
328. Lazarow PB, Moser HW. Disorders of peroxisome biogenesis. In: Scriver CR, Beaudet AL, Sly WS, Valle D, eds. The metabolic basis of inherited disease. New York: McGraw-Hill, 1989:1479–509.
329. Kelley RI. Review: the cerebrohepatorenal syndrome of Zellweger, morphologic and metabolic aspects. Am J Med Genet 1983;16:503–17.
330. Kaiser E, Kramar R. Clinical biochemistry of peroxisomal disorders. Clin Chim Acta 1988;173:57–80.
331. Wanders R, van Roermund C, Schutgens R, et al. The inborn errors of peroxisomal β-oxidation: A review. J Inher Metab Dis 1990;13:4–36.
332. van den Bosch H, Schutgens RB, Wanders RJ, Tager JM. Biochemistry of peroxisomes. Annu Rev Biochem 1992;61:157–97.
333. Watkins PA, Schwarz KB. Peroxisomal diseases. In: Suchy FJ, Sokol RJ, Balistreri WF, eds. Liver disease in children. 3rd ed. Philadelphia: Lippincott Williams & Wilkins, 2007:840–57.
334. Lawson AM, Madigan MJ, Shortland D, Clayton PT. Rapid diagnosis of Zellweger syndrome and infantile Refsum's disease by fast atom bombardment–mass spectrometry of urine bile salts. Clin Chim Acta 1986;161:221–31.
335. Stellaard F, Kleijer WJ, Wanders RJ, et al. Bile acids in amniotic fluid: promising metabolites for the prenatal diagnosis of peroxisomal disorders. J Inherit Metab Dis 1991;14:353–6.
336. Hanson RF, Staples AB, Williams GC. Metabolism of 5β-cholestane-3α,7α,12α,26-tetrol and 5β-cholestane-3α,7α,12α,25-tetrol into cholic acid in normal human subjects. J Lipid Res 1979;20:489–93.
337. Parmentier GG, Janssen GA, Eggermont EA, Eyssen HJ. C_{27} bile acids in infants with coprostanic acidemia and occurrence of a 3α,7α,12α-trihydroxy-5β-C_{29} dicarboxylic bile acid as a major component in their serum. Eur J Biochem 1979;102:173–83.
338. Eyssen H, Eggermont E, van Eldere J, et al. Bile acid abnormalities and the diagnosis of cerebro-hepato-renal syndrome (Zellweger syndrome). Acta Paediatr Scand 1985;74:539–44.
339. Poulos A, Whiting MJ. Identification of 3α,7α,12α-trihydroxy-5β-cholestan-26-oic acid, an intermediate in cholic acid synthesis, in the plasma of patients with infantile Refsum's disease. J Inherit Metab Dis 1985;8:13–17.
340. Clayton PT, Patel E, Lawson AM, et al. Bile acid profiles in peroxisomal 3-oxoacyl-coenzyme A thiolase deficiency. J Clin Invest 1990;85:1267–73.
341. Clayton PT. Inborn errors of bile acid metabolism. J Inherit Metab Dis 1991;14:478–96.
342. Hashmi M, Stanley W, Singh I. Lignoceroyl-CoASH ligase: enzyme defect in fatty acid beta-oxidation system in X-linked childhood adrenoleukodystrophy. FEBS Lett 1986;196:247–50.
343. Lazo O, Contreras M, Hashmi M, et al. Peroxisomal lignoceroyl-CoA ligase deficiency in childhood adrenoleukodystrophy and adrenomyeloneuropathy. Proc Natl Acad Sci U S A 1988;85:7647–51.
344. Wanders RJ, van Roermund CW, van Wijland MJ, et al. Direct demonstration that the deficient oxidation of very long chain fatty acids in X-linked adrenoleukodystrophy is due to an impaired ability of peroxisomes to activate very long chain fatty acids. Biochem Biophys Res Commun 1988;153:618–24.
345. Poll-The BT, Roels F, Ogier H, et al. A new peroxisomal disorder with enlarged peroxisomes and a specific deficiency of acyl-CoA oxidase (pseudo-neonatal adrenoleukodystrophy). Am J Hum Genet 1988;42:422–34.

346. Kase BF, Bjorkhem I, Haga P, Pedersen JI. Defective peroxisomal cleavage of the C27-steroid side chain in the cerebro-hepato-renal syndrome of Zellweger. J Clin Invest 1985;75:427–35.
347. Kase BF, Pedersen JI, Strandvik B, Bjorkhem I. In vivo and vitro studies on formation of bile acids in patients with Zellweger syndrome. Evidence that peroxisomes are of importance in the normal biosynthesis of both cholic and chenodeoxycholic acid. J Clin Invest 1985;76:2393–402.
348. Clayton PT, Lake BD, Hall NA, et al. Plasma bile acids in patients with peroxisomal dysfunction syndromes: analysis by capillary gas chromatography-mass spectrometry. Eur J Pediatr 1987;146:166–73.
349. Van Veldhoven PP, Vanhove G, Assselberghs S, et al. Substrate specificities of rat liver peroxisomal acyl-CoA oxidases: palmitoyl CoA oxidase (inducible acyl CoA oxidase), pristanoyl-CoA oxidase (non-inducible acyl-CoA oxidase), and trihydroxycoprostanoyl-CoA oxidase. J Biol Chem 1992;267:20065–74.
350. Baumgart E, Vanhooren JC, Fransen M, et al. Molecular characterization of the human peroxisomal branched-chain acyl-CoA oxidase: cDNA cloning, chromosomal assignment, tissue distribution, and evidence for the absence of the protein in Zellweger syndrome. Proc Natl Acad Sci U S A 1996;93:13748–53.
351. Christensen E, Van Eldere J, Brandt NJ, et al. A new peroxisomal disorder: di- and trihydroxycholestanaemia due to a presumed trihydroxycholestanoyl-CoA oxidase deficiency. J Inherit Metab Dis 1990;13:363–6.
352. Przyrembel H, Wanders RJ, van Roermund CW, et al. Di- and trihydroxycholestanoic acidaemia with hepatic failure. J Inherit Metab Dis 1990;13:367–70.
353. ten Brink HJ, Wanders RJ, Christensen E, et al. Heterogeneity in di/trihydroxycholestanoic acidaemia. Ann Clin Biochem 1994;31:195–7.
354. Clayton PT, Johnson AW, Mills KA, et al. Ataxia associated with increased plasma concentrations of pristanic acid, phytanic acid and C_{27} bile acids but normal fibroblast branched-chain fatty acid oxidation. J Inher Metab Dis 1996;19:761–8.
355. Kelley RI. Disorders of peroxisomal metabolism. In: Walker WA, Durie PR, Hamilton JR, eds. Pediatric gastrointestinal disease, pathophysiology, diagnosis, management. Toronto/Philadelphia: BC Decker, 1991:1032–54.
356. Lazarow PB, De Duve C. A fatty acyl-CoA oxidizing system in rat liver peroxisomes; enhancement by clofibrate, a hypolipidemic drug. Proc Natl Acad Sci U S A 1976;73:2043–6.
357. Bjorkhem I, Blomstrand S, Glaumann H, Strandvik B. Unsuccessful attempts to induce peroxisomes in two cases of Zellweger disease by treatment with clofibrate. Pediatr Res 1985;19:590–3.
358. Mathis RK, Watkins JB, Szczepanik-Van Leeuwen P, Lott IT. Liver in the cerebro-hepato-renal syndrome: defective bile acid synthesis and abnormal mitochondria. Gastroenterology 1980;79:1311–17.
359. Matoba N, Une M, Hoshita T. Identification of unconjugated bile acids in human bile. J Lipid Res 1986;27:1154–62.
360. Crosignani A, Podda M, Battezzati PM, et al. Changes in bile acid composition in patients with primary biliary cirrhosis induced by ursodeoxycholic acid administration. Hepatology 1991;14:1000–7.
361. Carlton VEH, Harris BZ, Puffenberger EG, et al. Complex inheritance of familial hypercholanemia with associated mutations in TJP2 and BAAT. Nature Genetics 2003;34:91–6.
362. Nakagawa M, Setchell KDR. Bile acid metabolism in early life: studies of amniotic fluid. J Lipid Res 1990;31:1089–98.
363. Hofmann AF, Strandvik B. Defective bile acid amidation: predicted features of a new inborn error of metabolism. Lancet 1988;2:311–13.
364. Low-Beer TS, Tyor MP, Lack L. Effects of sulfation of taurolithocholic and glycolithocholic acids on their intestinal transport. Gastroenterology 1969;56:721–6.
365. Lack L. Properties and biological significance of the ileal bile salt transport system. Environ Health Perspect 1979;33:79–90.
366. De Witt EH, Lack L. Effects of sulfation patterns on intestinal transport of bile salt sulfate esters. Am J Physiol 1980;238:G34–9.
367. Heubi JE, Balistreri WF, Partin JC, et al. Refractory infantile diarrhea due to primary bile acid malabsorption. J Pediatr 1979;94:546–51.
368. Heubi JE, Balistreri WF, Fondacaro JD, et al. Primary bile acid malabsorption: defective in vitro ileal active bile acid transport. Gastroenterology 1982;83:804–11.
369. Smith DW, Lemli L, Opitz JM. A newly recognized syndrome of multiple congenital anomalies. J Pediatr 1964;64:210–17.
370. Trauner M, Meier PJ, Boyer JL. Molecular pathogenesis of cholestasis. N Engl J Med 1998;339:1217–27.
371. Jansen PL, Sturm E. Genetic cholestasis, causes and consequences for hepatobiliary transport. Liver Int 2003;23:315–22.
372. Carlton VE, Pawlikowska L, Bull LN. Molecular basis of intrahepatic cholestasis. Ann Med 2004;36:606–17.
373. Kubitz R, Keitel V, Haussinger D. Inborn errors of biliary canalicular transport systems. Methods Enzymol 2005;400:558–69.
374. Keitel V, Burdelski M, Warskulat U, et al. Expression and localization of hepatobiliary transport proteins in progressive familial intrahepatic cholestasis. Hepatology 2005;41:1160–72.
375. Clayton RJ, Iber FL, Ruebner BH, McKusick VA. Byler disease. Fatal familial intrahepatic cholestasis in an Amish kindred. Am J Dis Child 1969;117:112–24.
376. Bull LN, Carlton VE, Stricker NL, et al. Genetic and morphological findings in progressive familial intrahepatic cholestasis (Byler disease [PFIC-1] and Byler syndrome): evidence for heterogeneity. Hepatology 1997;26:155–64.
377. Knisely AS. Progressive familial intrahepatic cholestasis: a personal perspective. Pediatr Dev Pathol 2000;3:113–25.
378. Strautnieks SS, Bull LN, Knisely AS, et al. A gene encoding a liver-specific ABC transporter is mutated in progressive familial intrahepatic cholestasis. Nat Genet 1998;20:233–8.
379. De Vree JML, Jacquemin E, Sturm E, et al. Mutations in the MDR3 gene cause progressive familial intrahepatic cholestasis. Proc Natl Acad Sci U S A 1998;95:282–7.

32

INBORN ERRORS OF MITOCHONDRIAL FATTY ACID OXIDATION

Jerry Angdisen, B.S., Majed Dasouki, M.D., and Jamal A. Ibdah, M.D., Ph.D.

Mitochondrial fatty acid β-oxidation plays a major role in energy production and homeostasis once glycogen stores are depleted because of fasting, illness, and increased muscular activity [1]. The mitochondrial β-oxidation of fatty acids provides nearly 80% of energy for cardiac and hepatic functions at all times [2]. In the liver, the β-oxidation of fatty acids generates the precursors of ketone bodies, 3-hydroxybutyrate, and acetoacetate which are used as alternate fuel by the brain and peripheral tissues, such as cardiac and skeletal muscle, when glucose supply is low [3].

Defects in the mitochondrial fatty acid oxidation pathway are inherited as autosomal recessive disorders. The first well-documented genetic defect of fatty acid oxidation (FAO), described in 1973, was carnitine palmitoyl transferase (CPT) deficiency, presenting as a skeletal muscle disorder with exercise-induced rhabdomyolysis and myoglubinuria [4]. More than 20 defects have since been discovered [2]. The growing number of FAO disorders covers a wide spectrum of phenotypes, and the disorders are characterized by a wide array of clinical presentations. FAO disorders have become an important group of inherited metabolic disorders causing morbidity and mortality. FAO disorders, if unrecognized and untreated, may cause sudden unexpected death. Previously described clinical entities such as Reye's syndrome, certain cases of sudden infant death syndrome (SIDS), cyclic vomiting syndrome, unexplained cases of liver failure, and maternal complications of pregnancy are examples of disorders associated with defects in FAO [2].

The purpose of this chapter is to review the recent advances in the field of mitochondrial FAO disorders as well as their recognition and management, with special emphasis on liver phenotypes.

REVIEW OF FATTY ACID OXIDATION

β-oxidation of fatty acids in the liver becomes an essential metabolic pathway during fasting, providing ketone bodies as alternate sources of energy that are exported to extrahepatic tissues such as cardiac and skeletal muscles when glucose supplies are low [1]. The complete oxidation of fatty acids to carbon dioxide (CO_2) is coupled to the synthesis of adenosine triphosphate (ATP). During fasting, insulin levels decline and glucagon levels rise, leading to glycogenolysis, gluconeogenesis, FAO, ketone formation in the liver, increased lipolysis, and stimulation of the release of lactate and amino acids from skeletal muscle. These adaptive mechanisms maintain plasma glucose concentrations and allow for the continued supply of glucose for brain metabolism and for peripheral organs and tissues to use as alternative fuels. Fatty acids are stored as adipose tissue in the form of triglycerides, the largest fuel reserve in the body; this is also the predominant substrate for energy production during fasting. Fatty acids provide 80% of caloric requirements after a 24-hour period of fasting in adults [5]. Infants, on the other hand, rely on FAO within 12 hours of a fast [6]. The reliance on effective ketogenesis for metabolic homeostasis during fasting renders infants and children particularly susceptible to defects in FAO.

Biochemistry of Mitochondrial Fatty Acid Metabolism

Lipid Mobilization and Cellular Uptake

Once glycogen stores are depleted, energy is acquired by alternative means. The decrease in blood glucose concentration causes a reduction in insulin levels and a rise in glucagon. Free fatty acids from adipose tissue stores are released into the plasma through the hydrolysis of triglycerides by lipoprotein lipase and hepatic lipase. Long-chain free fatty acids, such as palmitate and stearate, are the most abundant species released [7]; these are weakly soluble in plasma and readily bind to albumin. The two proposed models of long-chain fatty acid uptake are protein mediated and diffusion [8]. In the diffusion model of fatty acid uptake, fatty acids partition into membranes and become protonated and the neutral molecule is translocated into the cytosol [9]. In the protein-mediated model, fatty acid uptake occurs by sodium-dependent active transport and is dependent on carrier-mediated uptake by a family of high-affinity tissue-specific fatty acid–binding protein transporters located on liver and muscle cell membranes [9].

Table 32.1: Features of Known Fatty Acid Transport Proteins

Transporter	*Features*
FATP1	Stimulates transport and consumption of palmitate and oleate
FATP2	An isozyme of long-chain fatty acid–CoA ligase family; activates long/branched and very long–chain fatty acids ($\geq C_{22}$) to their CoA derivatives; expressed primarily in liver and kidney; present in both endoplasmic reticulum and peroxisomes but not in mitochondria; decreased in X-linked adrenoleukodystrophy
FATP4	Up-regulated in acquired obesity; a candidate gene for the insulin resistance syndrome
FATP5	Isozyme of very long–chain acyl-CoA synthetase for fatty acid elongation or complex lipid synthesis; expressed in liver and associated with endoplasmic reticulum
FATP6	Involved in heart long-chain fatty acid uptake and may play a role in pathogenesis of lipid-related cardiac disorders
FACL2	Isozymes of this family convert free long-chain fatty acids into fatty acyl-CoA esters
FACL3	Highly expressed in brain and preferentially uses myristate, arachidonate, and eicosapentaenoate as substrates
FACL4	Preferentially uses arachidonate as substrate. Heterozygous FACL4 female mice had extremely enlarged uteri and lumina filled with numerous proliferative cysts, were less fertile, and produced small litters with increased prenatal mortality. Human "hemizygous" males with FACL4 mutations had nonspecific mental retardation. Mutations in this gene may contribute to mental retardation.
FACL5	Highly expressed in uterus and spleen and expressed in trace amounts in normal brain; markedly increased levels occur in malignant gliomas
FACL6	Highly expressed in brain, fetal liver, and bone marrow

FACL, fatty acid CoA ligase; FATP, fatty acid transport protein.
Adopted with modification from Online Mendelian Inheritance in Man (OMIM), McKusick–Nathans Institute for Genetic Medicine, Johns Hopkins University (Baltimore, MD), and National Center for Biotechnology Information, National Library of Medicine (Bethesda, MD), 2000. Available at: http://www.ncbi.nlm.nih.gov/omim/.

Long-chain fatty acids are an important energy substrate used by cardiac myocytes and other cells. Using an expression cloning strategy, Schaffer and Lodish [10] identified a 63-kDa fatty acid transport protein (FATP) localized to the mouse plasma membranes of skeletal muscle, heart, and adipocytes. Hirsch et al. [11] then identified a large family of murine FATPs and their human homologues, which share a signature sequence [11]. Table 32.1 summarizes some features of this family [12].

Once the fatty acid is in the cytosol, fatty acid–binding proteins bind and transport the long-chain fatty acids intracellularly [13]; long-chain fatty acids are then esterified by *acyl coenzyme A (CoA) synthetase* to fatty acyl-CoA esters. Ubiquitously expressed acyl-CoA–binding proteins deliver the acyl-CoA esters to CPT-I [14].

Mitochondrial Uptake of Fatty Acids

Short-chain and medium-chain fatty acyl-CoA esters passively cross the mitochondrial membranes into the mitochondrial matrix, whereas long-chain fatty acyl-CoA esters are actively transported (Figure 32.1). This involves intracellular carnitine as a cofactor and is mediated by CPT-I and -II and a carnitine acylcarnitine translocase (CACT) [15]. Long chain acyl-CoA esters are first transesterified to carnitine by CPT-I, an outer mitochondrial membrane enzyme. After its transesterifcation to carnitine, long-chain acylcarnitine in the intermembrane space can cross the inner mitochondrial membrane into the mitochondrial matrix mediated by CACT in exchange for free carnitine, maintaining the mitochondrial and cytosolic carnitine pools. Acylcarnitines are re-esterified to regenerate acyl-CoA esters and free carnitine by CPT-II, located on the matrix side of the inner mitochondrial membrane.

Carnitine intake comes primarily from meat, fish, and dairy products; this accounts for 75% of total carnitine [16]. Carnitine is also synthesized endogenously from lysine and methionine, with S-adenosylmethionine required as a methyl donor [17]. It is excreted in the urine as free carnitine or as a conjugated carnitine ester. Only the liver, kidney, and brain have the enzymes necessary to synthesize carnitine, whereas other tissues depend on carnitine uptake from the circulation through a sodium-dependent carnitine transporter, the organic cation transporter (OCTN2). Carnitine is competitively inhibited by carnitine esters and is inhibited by other drugs transported by OCTN2 [18]. The OCTN2 is a high-affinity sodium-dependent active transporter found in the muscle, heart, and kidney and is encoded by the *SCL22A5* gene [19]. Elevated acyl-CoA esters are found in the urine of patients with FAO defects [20]. The formation of acylcarnitine esters buffers the depletion or accumulation of acyl-CoA during states of rapid FAO [21]. This is important as acyl-CoA esters inhibit enzymes and transporters needed for transport of ATP from the mitochondria to the cytosol [22].

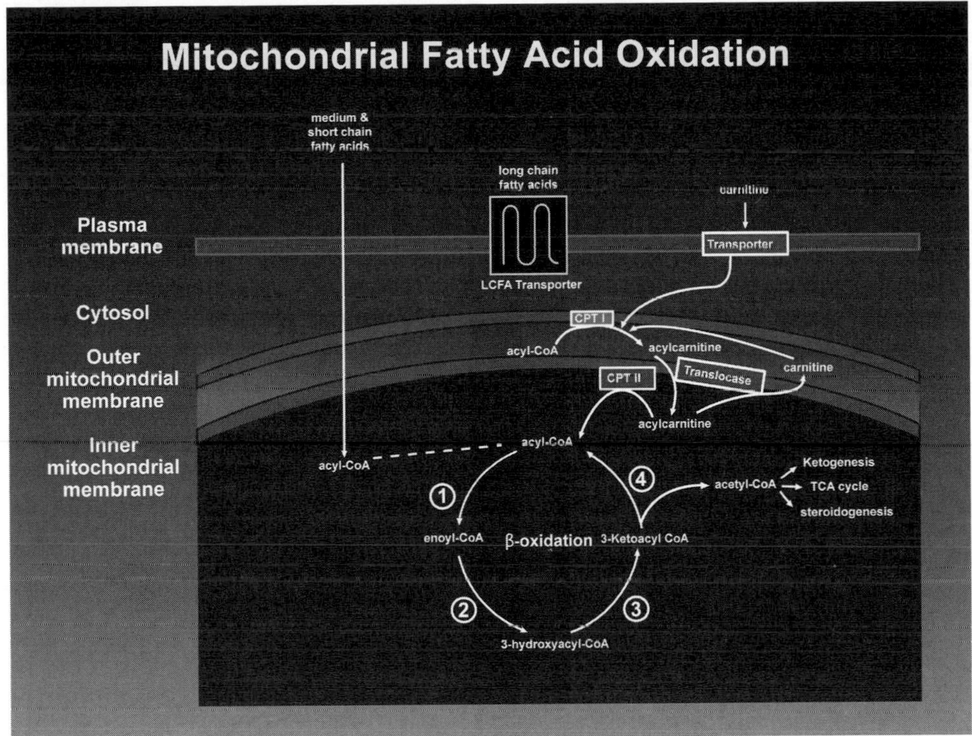

Figure 32.1. Mitochondrial fatty acid β oxidation. LCFA, long-chain fatty acid; TCA, tricarboxylic acid.

REGULATION OF INTRAMITOCHONDRIAL FATTY ACID OXIDATION

The control and regulation of fatty acid synthesis is intimately related to the regulation of FAO, glycolysis, and the tricarboxylic acid (TCA) cycle. CPT-I is a major site of regulation that determines whether fatty acids are directed toward β-oxidation or to the synthesis of triglycerides [23]. The activity, protein levels, messenger RNA (mRNA) levels, and transcription rate of CPT-I are increased in high fat feeding and starvation [24]. The peroxisome proliferator–activated receptor-α (PPARα) is a lipid-activated transcription factor that plays a role in the cellular response to fasting. In PPAR$\alpha^{+/+}$ mice, fasting induces the hepatic and cardiac expression of PPARα target genes encoding mitochondrial enzymes of the mitochondrial FAO, such as CPT-I. In PPAR$\alpha^{-/-}$ mice, fasting does not induce the same enzymes, leading to hepatic steatosis, myocardial lipid accumulation, hypoglycemia, and hypoketosis during prolonged fasting [25].

Mitochondrial Fatty Acid β-Oxidation

Once in the mitochondrial matrix, the fatty acyl-CoA esters are sequentially cleaved, two carbons shorter by the four reactions of the β-oxidation spiral producing acetyl-CoA (Figure 32.1). Each turn in the spiral also generates electrons that end up in the electron transport chain and the respiratory chain, resulting in ATP production via oxidative phosphorylation. Each step in the spiral is catalyzed by two to four distinct enzymes encoded by separate nuclear genes that exhibit different, overlapping, substrate specificities for very long–, long-, medium-, and short-chain acyl-CoA fatty acids. The enzymes with specificity for very long–chain and long-chain fatty acids are membrane associated, whereas enzymes recognizing medium-chain and short-chain fatty acids are soluble mitochondrial matrix enzymes.

ACYL-COA DEHYDROGENASES

The first reaction in the β-oxidation spiral is an acyl-CoA dehydrogenase reaction catalyzed by *very long–chain acyl-CoA dehydrogenase* (VLCAD) and its homologous enzymes, *long-chain acyl-CoA dehydrogenase* (LCAD), *medium-chain acyl-CoA dehydrogenase* (MCAD), or *short-chain acyl-CoA dehydrogenase* (SCAD) as shown in Figure 32.2. This dehydrogenation step forms a double bond at the 2–3 position of a saturated acyl CoA substrate, producing a 2,3-enoyl-CoA and generating reducing equivalents in the form of flavin adenine dinucleotide (FAD). The soluble acyl-CoA dehydrogenases show a striking homology in amino acid sequence, implying evolution from a single gene family [26]. The acyl-CoA dehydrogenases are FAD dependent.

VLCAD is a 154-kDa homodimer composed of approximate 70-kDa subunits that is loosely associated with the matrix surface of the inner mitochondrial membrane [27]. The *VLCAD* gene has been mapped to human chromosome 17p11.13-p11.2 [28]. The gene is about 5.4 kilobases (kb) long and contains 20 exons [29]. VLCAD metabolizes acyl-CoAs ranging from C_{14} to C_{20} acyl-CoAs, with palmitoyl-CoA (C_{16}) as its prime substrate. LCAD metabolizes acyl-CoAs ranging from C_{12} to C_{18} acyl-CoAs, with C_{12} as its preferred substrate. The *LCAD* gene maps to 2q34-q35 [30,31]. It is a homotetramer of four identical subunits, with each subunit containing one noncovalently

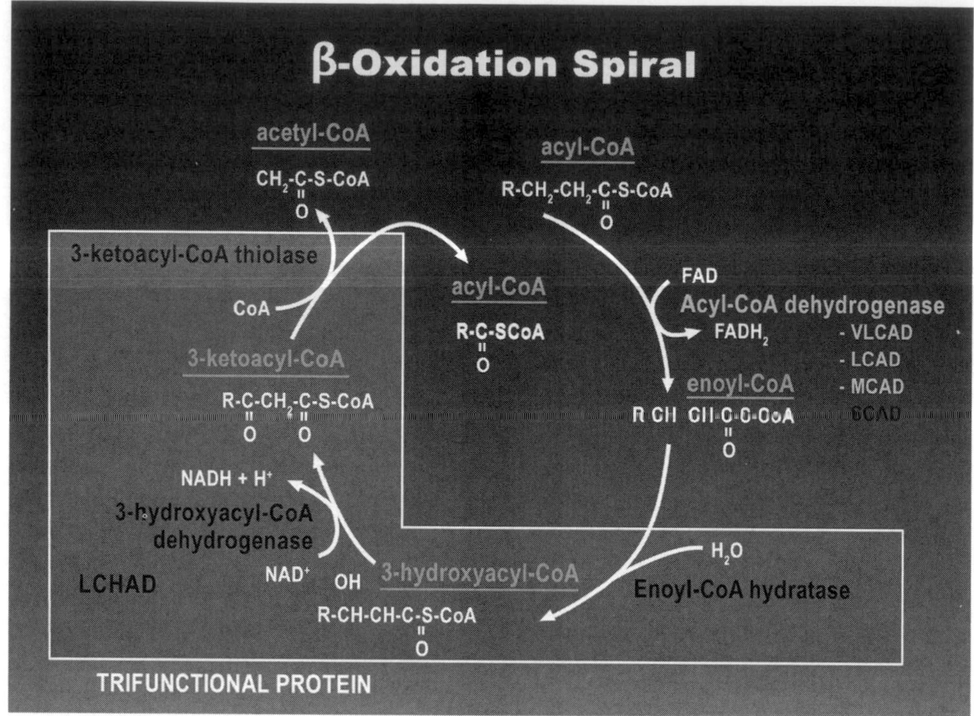

Figure 32.2. Mitochondrial β-oxidation spiral. FAD, flavin adenine dinucleotide; LCHAD, long-chain 3-hydroxyacyl-CoA dehydrogenase; NAD, nicotinamide adenine dinucleotide.

bound FAD that functions as an electron acceptor in the dehydrogenation reaction. MCAD metabolizes C_6 to C_{10} acyl-CoAs. It maps to 1p31 [32]. SCAD catalyzes C_4 to C_6 acyl-CoAs, maps to chromosome 12q, and consists of 10 exons spanning approximately 13 kb of genomic DNA [33]. Like LCAD, MCAD and SCAD are located in the mitochondrial matrix and are homotetramers [34,35].

ENOYL-COA HYDRATASES

The second step (Figure 32.2) in the pathway adds water across the double bond and is catalyzed by a long-chain 2,3-enoyl-CoA hydratase (LCEH) or a short-chain 2,3-enoyl-CoA hydratase (SCEH), which hydrates the 2,3-enoyl-CoA across the double bond. SCEH, also known as crotonase, acts on substrates with shorter chain lengths, whereas LCEH has specificities for longer–chain length substrates. LCEH is part of the mitochondrial trifunctional protein (MTP) (Figure 32.2). *SCEH*, an 11-kb gene consisting of 8 exons, was mapped to chromosome 10q26.2-q26.3 [36].

L-3-HYDROXYACYL-COA DEHYDROGENASES

The third step (Figure 32.2) is catalyzed by a long-chain 3-hydroxyacyl-CoA dehydrogenase (LCHAD) or a short-chain 3-hydroxyacyl-CoA dehydrogenase (SCHAD), which oxidizes the 3-hydroxy position, producing a 3-ketoacyl-CoA. The reaction uses oxidized nicotinamide adenine dinucleotide (NAD) as a cofactor, with a concomitant reduction of NAD to a reduced nicotinamide adenine dinucleotide (NADH). LCHAD metabolizes long-chain 3-hydroxyacyl-CoA substrates as part of MTP, whereas SCHAD reversibly metabolizes short-chain 3-hydroxyacyl-CoA substrates. SCHAD is located in the mitochondrial matrix. It consists of two identical subunits of 33 kDa, and the gene is mapped to 4q22-q26 [37].

3-KETOACYL-COA THIOLASES

The fourth and last step in the spiral is mediated by a long-chain 3-ketoacyl-CoA thiolase (LCKAT), medium-chain 3-ketoacyl-CoA thiolase (MCKAT), or short-chain 3-ketoacyl-CoA thiolase (SCKAT), which shortens the fatty acyl-CoA substrate by two carbons by cleaving off acetyl-CoA. The shortened acyl-CoA can then reenter the fatty acid β-oxidation spiral until the fatty acid is completely broken down into a two-carbon or three-carbon fatty acid species. The acetyl-CoA produced can be used for ketogenesis or steroidogenesis and as a substrate for the TCA cycle.

MCKAT catalyzes the cleavage of medium- to short-chain (C_4 to C_{12}) 3-ketoacyl-CoAs. Long-chain fatty acids are metabolized by LCKAT, part of the MTP enzyme complex.

MITOCHONDRIAL TRIFUNCTIONAL PROTEIN

In 1992, two groups of investigators independently reported that LCHAD is part of an enzyme complex, the MTP, which is associated with the inner mitochondrial membrane [38,39]. This was rapidly confirmed by other groups [40,41]. MTP, also known as trifunctional protein (TFP), is a hetero-octamer of 4α and 4β subunits (Figure 32.3). The α subunit amino-terminal domain contains the long-chain 3-enoyl-CoA hydratase enzymatic activity, whereas the LCHAD enzymatic activity resides in the carboxyl-terminal domain. The β subunit has the long-chain 3-ketoacyl-CoA thiolase enzymatic activity. The

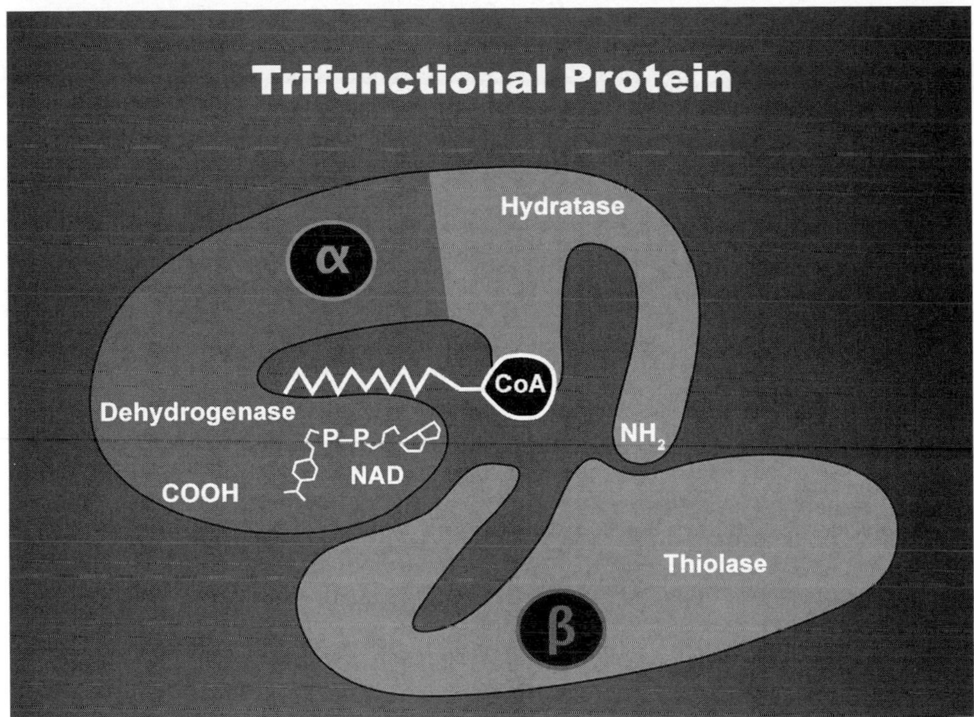

Figure 32.3. Cartoon depicting the mitochondrial trifunctional protein complex. MTP is composed of a hetero-octamer of 4α and 4β subunits. The α subunit contains the hydratase and the NAD^+-dependent dehydrogenase enzyme activities, and the β subunit contains the thiolase enzyme activities. COOH, carboxylic acid (functional group).

association of the α and β subunits to form the enzyme complex is necessary for membrane translocation and for the catalytic stability of the three enzymes [40,42]. The human complementary DNAs (cDNAs) encoding both α and β subunits have been isolated and characterized [43,44]. Both subunit genes, *HADHA* and *HADHB*, have been localized to chromosome 2p23 using *fluorescence in situ hybridization* (FISH) [45]. The α subunit gene contains 20 exons spanning more than 52 kb. In the α subunit, exons 1–2 code for the transit peptide, exons 3–7 code for the hydratase domain, exons 8–10 code for the linker region, and exons 11–20 code for the LCHAD domain. The β subunit has 16 exons, with exon 1 coding for the transit peptide and exons 2–16 coding for the thiolase enzymatic activity. Both genes have been found to be arranged in a head-to-head orientation. They both share the same 2-*cis* elements' bidirectional promoter, which is activated by the transcription factor Sp1 [46].

OXIDATION OF ODD-CHAIN FATTY ACIDS

Fatty acids with odd-numbered carbons undergo β-oxidation as do saturated fatty acids until the three-carbon "propionyl-CoA" is formed. Odd-numbered fatty acids are rare in mammals but are fairly common in plants and marine organisms. Propionyl-CoA is also generated by the metabolism of branched-chain amino acids. Three enzymes carry out the conversion of propionyl-CoA to succinyl-CoA, a TCA cycle intermediate. Propionyl-CoA is carboxylated to D-methylmalonyl-CoA by *propionyl-CoA carboxylase*, a biotin-dependent enzyme. D-Methylmalonyl-CoA is then converted to its L isomer, L-methylmalonyl CoA, by *methylmalonyl-CoA epimerase*. L-Methylmalonyl CoA is finally converted to succinyl-CoA by *methylmalonyl-CoA mutase*, a vitamin B_{12}-dependent reaction (Figure 32.4).

OXIDATION OF UNSATURATED FATTY ACIDS

Unsaturated fatty acids such as oleic ($C_{18:1}$), linoleic ($C_{18:2}$), and linolenic ($C_{18:3}$) acids undergo β-oxidation similar to saturated fatty acids until the substrate is not recognized by the enzymes of β-oxidation. Double bonds located at even and odd-numbered positions are metabolized by two additional mitochondrial enzymes, an isomerase and a reductase. A double bond between the C_3 and C_4 atoms (*cis*-3-enoyl-CoA) is metabolized by an *enoyl-CoA isomerase* that rearranges the *cis* double to a *trans* double bond that can proceed through normal β-oxidation. A double bond between the C_2 and C_3 atoms (*cis*-2-enoyl-CoA) is metabolized by *2,4-dienoyl-CoA reductase*, which produces a *trans*-3-enoyl-CoA that can then be metabolized by the enoyl-CoA isomerase, producing a *trans*-2-enoyl-CoA. The *trans*-2-enoyl-CoA can then be hydrated by the enoyl-CoA hydratase, which can proceed through normal β-oxidation (Figure 32.5).

Ketone Body Formation and Metabolism

The compounds referred to as ketone bodies are acetoacetate, 3-hydroxybutyrate (3HB), and acetone. 3HB (also known as β-hydroxybutyrate) arises from the reduction of

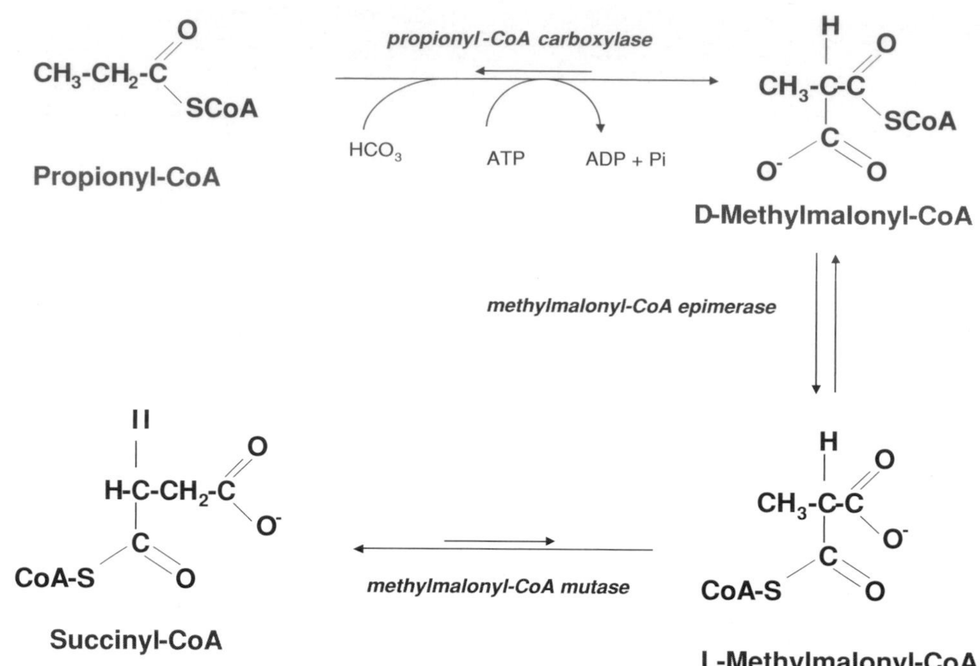

Figure 32.4. β-Oxidation of odd-carbon fatty acids. The three-carbon propionyl-CoA product of the β-oxidation of an odd-chain fatty acid is converted to succinyl-CoA by three specialized enzymes. Succinyl-CoA is a TCA cycle intermediate that can enter the TCA cycle.

acetoacetate, whereas acetone is formed from the decarboxylation of acetoacetate. Though skeletal and cardiac muscle fatty acid β-oxidation generates acetyl-CoA, only the liver can channel them into ketone formation. The liver can synthesize ketone bodies at the rate of approximately 900 g/d. The liver does not oxidize nonthiolated acetoacetate; it exports it to peripheral tissues, including brain, heart, and skeletal muscle, where acetoacetate may be oxidized to conserve glucose.

In liver mitochondria, acetyl-CoA may condense with oxaloacetate or form 3-methylglutaryl-CoA, which in turn can be

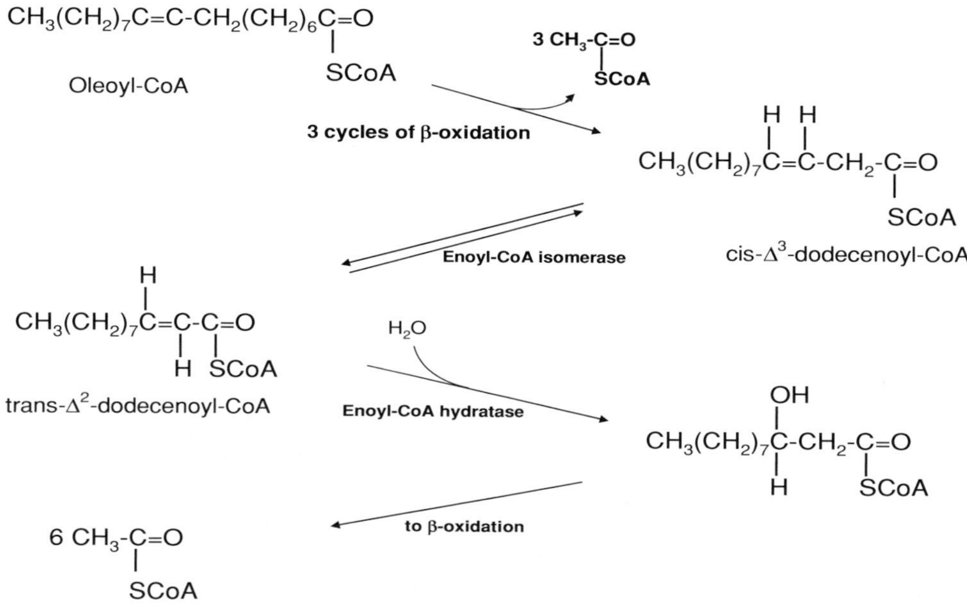

Figure 32.5. β-Oxidation of unsaturated fatty acids. The β-oxidation of unsaturated fatty acids is catabolized by two additional mitochondrial enzymes. An isomerase rearranges the *cis*-Δ^3 double bond to a *trans*-Δ^2 double bond, and the subsequent hydration by a hydratase allows the rearranged fatty acid to continue into the normal β-oxidation pathway.

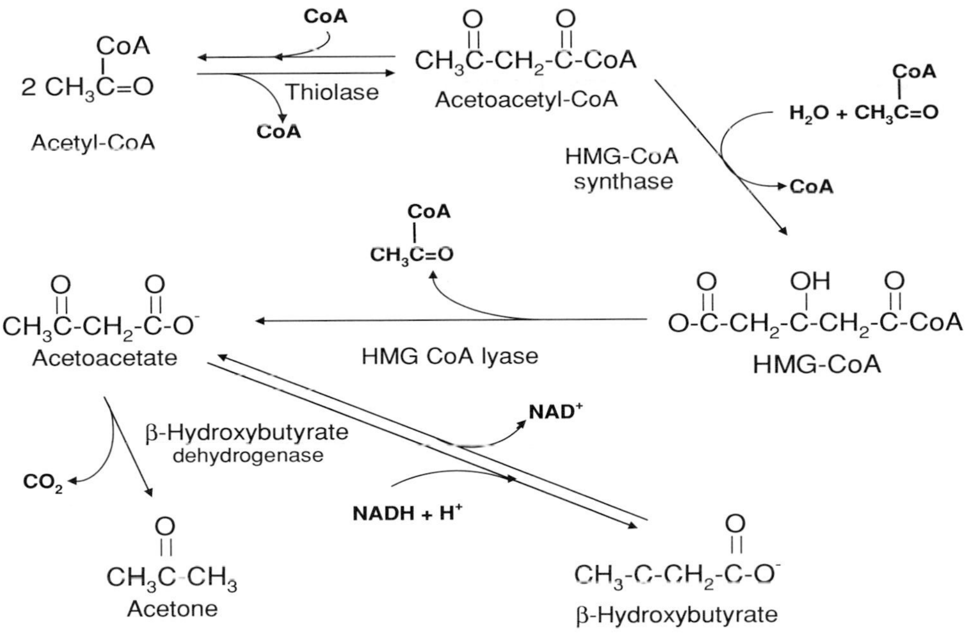

Figure 32.6. Hepatic ketogenesis.

cleaved to form ketone bodies, acetoacetate, and reduced 3HB. The concentration of oxaloacetate determines the path that acetyl-CoA takes. The acetyl-CoA formed from fatty acid β-oxidation is converted to acetoacetyl-CoA by β-ketothiolase, which is then transformed to 3-hydroxy-3-methylglutaryl (HMG)-CoA by mitochondrial *HMG-CoA synthase*. HMG-CoA is then irreversibly converted to acetoacetate by *HMG-CoA lyase*. Acetoacetate is interconverted to 3HB by *3HB dehydrogenase*, which is located in the inner mitochondrial membrane and requires phosphatidylcholine as an allosteric activator (Figure 32.6).

In nonhepatic ketolysis, occurring in the mitochondria, 3HB is converted by *3HB dehydrogenase* to acetoacetate, which is metabolized by *succinyl-CoA oxoacid transferase* (SCOT) to acetoacetate-CoA. Acetoacetate-CoA is then metabolized by *β-ketothiolase* to acetyl-CoA, which can enter the TCA cycle.

Electron Transfer to the Respiratory Chain Complex

The acyl-CoA dehydrogenases that catalyze the oxidation of the C_α–C_β bond carry noncovalent but tightly bound FAD. The dehydrogenation of the acyl-CoAs results in the generation of two electrons bound to FAD that are transferred to the electron transfer flavoprotein (ETF). The reduced ETF is reoxidized by *ETF-ubiquinone reductase*, which channels the electrons to the electron transport chain at the level of coenzyme Q.

Electron transfer flavoprotein is a mitochondrial matrix heterodimer consisting of α and β subunits [47,48]. ETF-ubiquinone reductase (ETF dehydrogenase) is a monomer associated with the inner mitochondrial membrane that contains two redox groups, an FAD cofactor and an iron–sulfur group [49].

Glycine Conjugation

A complex of enzymes exclusive to the mitochondria called acyl-CoA:amino acid *N*-acyltransferases convert acyl-CoA esters (C_4 to C_{10}) to glycine conjugates [50]. Substrates are conjugated with glycine, but glutamine and alanine may be used as the amino acid conjugate. The presence of glycine conjugates in the urine reflects the intramitochondrial accumulation of acyl-CoA esters.

Alternative Pathways for Intramitochondrial Acyl-CoA Compounds

Mitochondrial FAO is the principal pathway of fatty acid catabolism. There are other minor pathways that play important roles in the catabolism of fat in organelles such as peroxisomes and microsomes that can carry out the β-oxidation of fat as well (Figure 32.7).

PEROXISOMAL FATTY ACID OXIDATION

Very long–chain fatty acids ($>C_{20}$) are primarily metabolized in the peroxisomes. Like mitochondrial β-oxidation, peroxisomal fatty acid β-oxidation also leads to the production of acetyl-CoA (Figure 32.8). The first enzyme in the peroxisomal pathway is an FAD-dependent acyl-CoA oxidase that transfers the liberated electrons directly to oxygen instead of to the electron transport chain, forming hydrogen peroxide. It is also the rate-limiting step [51]. It metabolizes only fatty acids more than eight carbon atoms long; the short/medium-chain fatty acids produced are transported to the mitochondria for further catabolism [52]. Peroxisomal β-oxidation responds to various metabolic conditions, such as a high-fat diet and fasting, which increase the flux into the system [53,54]. Accumulation of very long–chain fatty acids is characteristic of defects in the peroxisomal system [55].

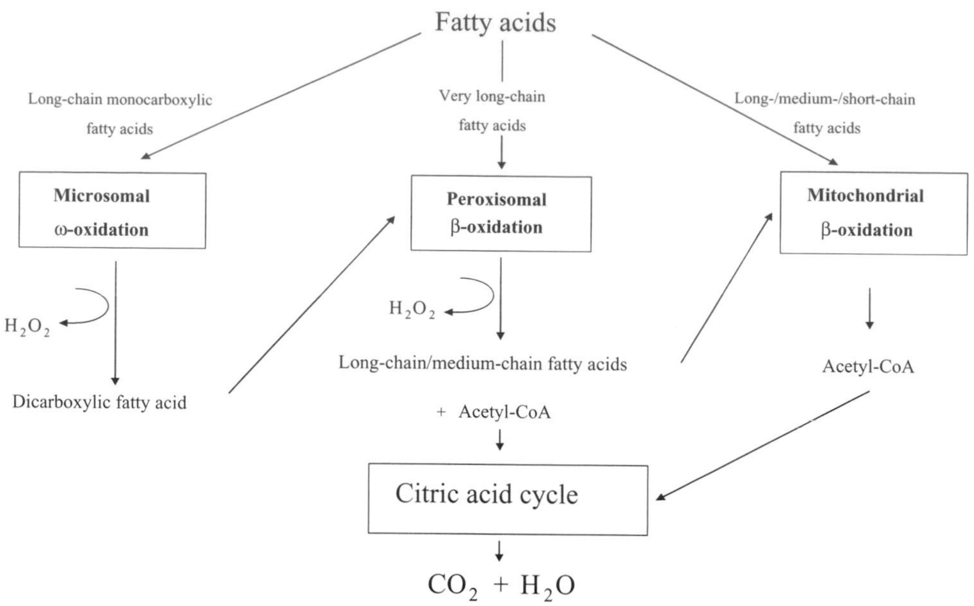

Figure 32.7. Pathways for fatty acid oxidation.

MICROSOMAL OXIDATION

The oxidation of the terminal carbon of a normal fatty acid is called omega (ω) oxidation. It occurs in liver microsomes through the actions of cytochrome P450, a monooxygenase that uses NAD phosphate (NADPH) as a coenzyme and oxygen as a substrate and places a hydroxyl group at the terminal carbon that converts the fatty acid into a dicarboxylic acid (Figure 32.9). The dicarboxylic acid can be transported to peroxisomes or to the mitochondrial matrix for β-oxidation [56]. Long-chain dicarboxylic acids can be shortened by two carbons through β-oxidation and are excreted as medium- or short-chain dicarboxylic acids in the urine. Dicarboxylic aciduria occurs as the result of a defect in β-oxidation, starvation, or ineffective mitochondrial electron transport function.

FATTY ACID OXIDATION DISORDERS

Fatty acid oxidation defects are an important group of inherited metabolic disorders characterized by a wide array of clinical

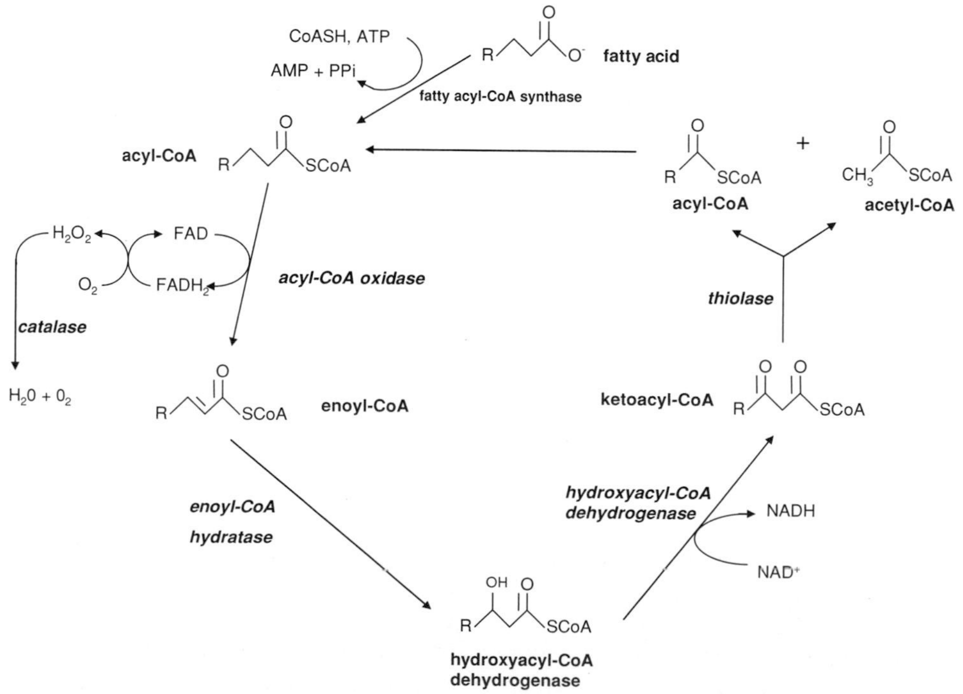

Figure 32.8. Perioxisomal β-oxidation pathway. CoASH, coenzyme A; Pii, pyrophosphate ion.

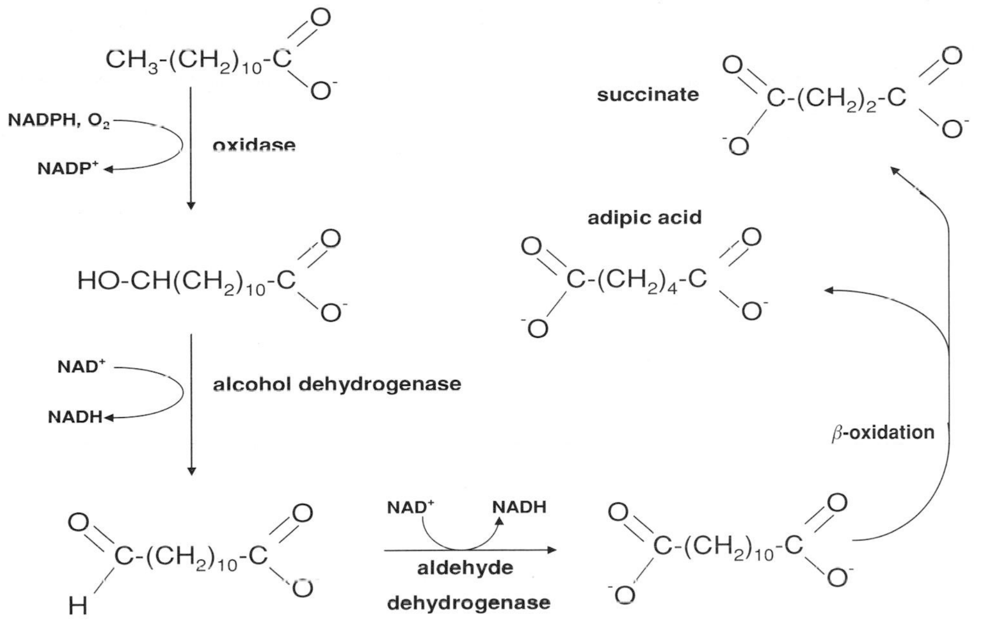

Figure 32.9. Microsomal β-oxidation. $NADP^+$, nicotinamide adenine dinocleotide phosphate.

presentations; they are considered to be important causes of pediatric morbidity and mortality. Figure 32.10 illustrates the time line for reporting various FAO defects in the literature. The first documented inherited disorder of FAO, muscle CPT-II deficiency, was described in 1973 [4]. MCAD deficiency was first reported in 1983 and is considered the most common β-oxidation defect [57]. LCHAD deficiency was first described in 1989 [58]. Overall, more than 20 different disorders that affect β-oxidation have been identified. Advances in the field of FAO disorders have been so rapid that a review article published in 1987 reported only seven documented inborn errors of FAO [59]. CPT-II, carnitine transporter, and ETF/ETF dehydrogenase (ETF-DH) deficiencies were described in the 1970s, CPT-I, SCAD, and LCHAD deficiencies in the 1980s, and FATP, CACT, VLCAD, MTP, LCKAT, SCHAD, and SCKAT deficiencies in the 1990s [60].

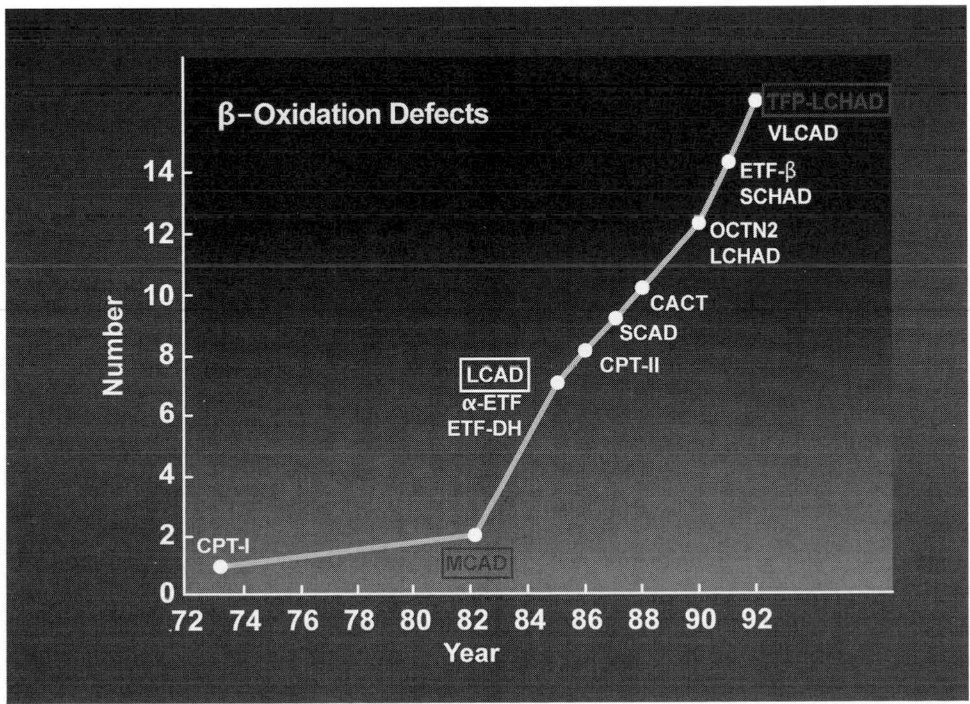

Figure 32.10. Time line of the discovery of the defects in fatty acid oxidation. ETF-DH, electron transfer flavoprotein dehydrogenase.

Rat VLCAD was first identified and purified in 1992 by Izai et al. [61]. The first human patients with VLCAD deficiency were initially described as having LCAD deficiency [62]. The discovery of VLCAD also helped explain the unusual finding of a single LCAD band in all nine LCAD-deficient fibroblast cell lines detected by using a specific anti-LCAD antibody [63]. A considerable number of patients previously diagnosed with LCAD deficiency have been reassigned as VLCAD deficient as no mutations in the *LCAD*gene were found and there was no immunoreactivity to VLCAD [64]. The failure to identify LCAD-deficient patients suggests that LCAD deficiency is either a very rare, benign metabolic disorder or a disorder with high prenatal lethality. Despite mass newborn screening for disorders of FAO using tandem mass spectrometry (MS-MS), no new cases with proven LCAD deficiency have been reported.

In clinical situations with increased energy requirements, such as prolonged fasting, illness, or prolonged exercise, an enzyme defect in an FAO pathway leads to energy depletion because of the inadequate production of acetyl-CoA, ketone bodies, and ATP in tissues with high energy demand, such as liver, heart, muscle, and brain [2,65]. The major potential clinical manifestations include fulminant liver failure, hepatic encephalopathy, cardiomyopathy, and sudden, unexpected death if unrecognized and untreated. The hallmark of FAO defects is nonhypoketotic hypoglycemia resulting from glucose depletion and the impairment of gluconeogenesis due to a lack of reducing equivalents. Nonmetabolized free fatty acids are incorporated into triglycerides and may account for the observed fat storage in liver and muscle [66]. The intracellular accumulation of acyl-CoA intermediates upstream of a block and the subsequent depletion of carnitine and CoA trigger intracellular toxicity. The toxic effects of the intermediates may be direct and/or through inhibition of other enzymes. Cardiac arrhythmias are thought to be caused by long-chain acylcarnitine accumulation [67].

Long-Chain Fatty Acid Transport/Binding Defect

The long-chain fatty acid transport/binding disorder is a defect in the transport of long-chain fatty acids across the plasma membrane. Two patients presented with recurrent episodes of acute liver failure and mild acute encephalopathy associated with nonketotic hypoglycemia and hyperammonemia often provoked by viral infections or otitis media [68]. Biochemical analysis of blood and urine showed minimal accumulation of dicarboxylic acids, acylglycines, or acylcarnitines. Biopsies showed mild, patchy necrosis of hepatocytes, hepatocellular vacuolization, mild portal inflammation, and fibrosis but no hepatic steatosis. Uptake and oxidation experiments in cultured skin fibroblasts suggested a defect in fatty acid transport. The patients received liver transplants and subsequently developed normally. The nature of the exact molecular defect is unknown as no mutations were found when genes involved in fatty acid transport were sequenced.

Carnitine Uptake/Transporter Defect

Carnitine transporter defect is an autosomal recessive disorder caused by mutations in the *SLC22A5* gene, which encodes the high-affinity carnitine transporter OCTN2 [69]. Renal reabsorption and intestinal uptake are impaired, causing systemic tissue carnitine deficiency leading to impaired long-chain fatty acid entry into mitochondria that carry out FAO. Two patients were first described in 1988 as having a defect in the active transport of carnitine in kidney, muscle, and skin fibroblasts [70]. Frameshift mutations were the first defects to be reported in the human plasma carnitine transporter gene in two patients [71]. Some patients with this defect present with acute episodes of hypoketotic hypoglycemia, lethargy, coma, and hepatic steatosis in infancy [72], whereas older children present with progressive cardiomyopathy, skeletal muscle weakness [73,74], and peripheral neuropathy [75]. Several cases of sudden and unexpected death at different ages have also been reported [72,76,77]. Microvesicular steatosis and lipid infiltration may be seen in liver and muscle biopsies. Plasma total carnitine concentrations are less than 10% of normal and are typically associated with increased urinary excretion and reduced muscle and liver carnitine concentrations. The diagnosis is confirmed either by demonstrating decreased carnitine uptake in fibroblasts or DNA mutation analysis of the *SLC22A5* gene. Multiple different mutations (microdeletions, frameshift, single base pair substitutions or insertions) resulting in premature stop codons and a truncated nonfunctional protein have been described [78–80]. Genotype–phenotype correlation has not been apparent [69]. Newborn screening using MS-MS allows presymptomatic identification [81]. Plasma free and esterified carnitines are very low. Heterozygotes for OCTN2 mutations show mildly reduced plasma carnitine levels and reduced rates of carnitine uptake [72], increased carnitine urinary loss [82], and predisposition to late-onset benign cardiac hypertrophy [83]. The absence of characteristic urinary dicarboxylic acids or glycine conjugates distinguishes patients with a defect in the carnitine cycle from patients with defects in the β-oxidation pathway. Carnitine supplementation prevents cardiomyopathy in this disorder.

Disorders of the Carnitine Cycle

Carnitine Palmitoyl Transferase I Deficiency

In CPT-I deficiency, the mitochondria cannot oxidize acyl-CoAs and remain impermeable to their entry, resulting in the cytosolic accumulation of acyl-CoAs and subsequent increase in triglyceride synthesis. CPT-I has tissue-specific, genetically distinct hepatic (CPT-IA), muscle (CPT-IB), and brain (CPT-IC) isoforms [84–86]. The "hepatic" isoform is expressed in liver, kidney, and fibroblasts and at low levels in the heart. CPT-IA is currently the only isoform for which a human deficiency disease is known; it is characterized by nonketotic hypoglycemia and liver dysfunction that may result in a fatal Reye-like syndrome. Cardiomegaly, arrhythmia, and distal renal tubular acidosis have been reported [87,88]. Pregnancy-related maternal liver disease has been reported in patients carrying

CPT-IA–deficient fetuses [89]. Urine organic acid analysis is normal and the plasma free carnitine level is elevated, whereas long-chain acylcarnitines are very low, allowing for calculation of a ratio specific for CPT-I deficiency [90]. This is in contrast to many other FAO defects, in which free carnitine is low and acylcarnitines are elevated. This is probably caused by a high renal threshold for excretion of free carnitine and a secondary increase in carnitine transport [91]. A recent study showed a distinctive organic aciduria with excretion of C_{12}-dicarboxylic acids in samples obtained from three patients a few days after presentation [92]. Although C_{12}-dicarboxylic aciduria is typically seen in severe neonatal CPT II-deficiency, it has been reported in patients with CPT-I deficiency [87,93–95]. Dodecanedioic and 3-hydroxyglutaric aciduria was also noted, suggesting that CPT-I may play a role in the uptake of long-chain dicarboxylic acids by mitochondria after their initial shortening by β-oxidation in the peroxisomes. CPT-IA deficiency can be confirmed by enzyme analysis in fibroblasts and molecular genetic analysis of the *CPTIA* gene. Most mutations are novel except for the "G710E" mutation, which is common in North American Hutterite communities [96,97].

Treatment is based on fasting avoidance and a low-fat diet supplemented with medium-chain triglycerides (MCTs). CPT-I deficiency associated with renal tubular acidosis was improved with MCT treatment [87]. A patient with CPT-I deficiency maintained on a very low–fat diet and nighttime uncooked cornstarch feeding for 5.5 years has not had a hypoglycemic episode [98]. Patients with CPT-IB and -IC deficiency have not been reported to date.

Carnitine-Acylcarnitine Translocase Deficiency

Carnitine-acylcarnitine translocase deficiency is involved in the transfer of fatty acylcarnitines into the mitochondria in exchange for free carnitine [99]. CACT deficiency was first reported by Stanley et al. in 1992 [100]. Patients typically present during the neonatal period with hypoketotic hypoglycemia, liver failure with hyperammonemia and/or hypertrophic cardiomyopathy, seizures, apnea, hypotension, ventricular arrhythmias, and cardiorespiratory arrest [101,102]. Impaired motility of the gastrointestinal tract has also been reported [103]. A low-fat diet supplemented with MCTs (which do not require CACT for crossing the mitochondrial membranes), intravenous glucose, carnitine supplementation, and preventing lipolysis are all important in the treatment of this disorder. Despite therapeutic efforts, many affected patients will die within the first year of life because of intercurrent infections and development of cardiac arrhythmias, possibly caused by the accumulation of long-chain acylcarnitines [67]. Patients without cardiac involvement have been reported to do well [104,105]. Fatty infiltration of liver, kidney, and muscle and hypertrophic cardiomyopathy are revealed after an autopsy [101,103]. Patients with residual enzyme activity have more favorable outcomes [104,106]. Patients with CACT deficiency have characteristic persistent elevation of plasma long-chain acylcarnitine concentration with prominent C_{16} and C_{18} species. Because of the similar acylcarnitine profiles observed in CACT- and CPT-II–deficient patients, enzymatic activity expressed in skin fibroblasts and/or mutational analysis of the *CACT* gene is needed to confirm the diagnosis. CACT-deficient cell lines fed with short-chain fatty acids had elevated butyrylcarnitine, which may be diagnostic [107].

Carnitine Palmitoyl Transferase II Deficiency

Carnitine palmitoyl transferase II deficiency, the first mitochondrial FAO defect to be described, was reported by DiMauro and DiMauro [4] in 1973 (Figure 32.10). CPT-II deficiency can be differentiated into several clinical presentations; a recently proposed classification is based on organ involvement, residual enzyme activity, and genotype [108]. CPT-II type I (neonatal) is the most severe form that presents in the neonatal period and affects the liver, skeletal muscle, and heart and is associated with kidney and brain abnormalities [109,110]. CPT-II type II (infantile) presents in the first years of life and affects the liver, heart, and skeletal muscle. CPT-II type III (late onset) presents in early adulthood, affects the skeletal muscle, and has a high residual enzyme activity. Acylcarnitine profiles are similar to those observed in CACT deficiency. Biochemical assays and molecular genetic tests are needed to verify the diagnosis. The most common mutation in type III is S113L, and 413delAG is common in Ashkenazi Jews [111,112]. Symptomatic heterozygotes have also been described [113]. In vitro treatment of mild-type CPT-II–deficient cells with bezafibrate (a hypolipidemic drug that acts as an agonist of PPARs) resulted in a time- and dose-dependent increase in CPT-II mRNA and residual enzyme activity and led to normalization of long-chain fatty acid cellular oxidation rates [114].

Disorders of Long-Chain Fatty Acid Metabolism

Very Long–Chain Aycl-CoA Dehydrogenase Deficiency

VLCAD deficiency can be subclassified into three forms: a severe early-onset form with high incidence of hepatopathy and cardiomyopathy, an intermediate childhood-onset form with hypoketotic hypoglycemia associated with hepatic dysfunction, and a myopathic adult-onset form with muscle weakness, myalgia, and rhabdomyolysis [115]. Hypoketotic hypoglycemia and creatinine phosphokinase elevations are characteristic during acute episodes. Plasma levels of carnitine have been low in most patients studied, with a marked increase in the fraction of esterified carnitine. The primary urinary acylcarnitine is acetylcarnitine [116]; plasma acylcarnitine analysis shows elevated levels of saturated and unsaturated C_{14} to C_{18} carnitine esters with $C_{14:1}$ as the predominant species [117]. VLCAD diagnosis can be confirmed by specific enzyme assays, in vitro probing in fibroblast cultures [118], or molecular genetic analysis of the *VLCAD* gene. Because acylcarnitine analysis can be performed in newborn screening using blood spots, early identification, intervention, and treatment of affected patients are generally possible [119,120].

Patients with VLCAD deficiency who present with hypoketotic hypoglycemia and coma have a high mortality rate. Profound hepatic steatosis is a common feature in those who survive this initial presentation; there may be residual cardiac abnormalities and muscle weakness. Another feature that occurs during an acute episode is profound hypotonia that may persist for weeks after the initial episode and eventually resolves. Profound elevation of creatine kinase is common during the acute episodes and may remain mildly elevated even when muscle strength recovers [121]. Similar to the observation of skin fibroblasts in mild CPT-II deficiency, bezafibrate was found to increase VLCAD mRNA and protein levels and decrease the production of toxic long-chain acylcarnitines in fibroblasts with VLCAD deficiency. Therefore, fibrates may be potential therapeutic agents to correct defects in FAO [122].

Mitochondrial Trifunctional Protein Defects

Human defects in the MTP complex cause either isolated LCHAD deficiency with normal or partially reduced thiolase and hydratase activity or complete MTP deficiency with markedly reduced activity of all three enzymes [123–125]. They present with cardiomyopathy, slowly progressing peripheral neuropathy, skeletal myopathy, or sudden, unexpected death [126]. In childhood, affected children present with rhabdomyolysis with muscle pain and weakness, peripheral neuropathy, or pigmentary retinopathy [127,128]. Other phenotypes reported in the literature include hypoparathyroidism [129] and hypocalcemia [130,131]. The histologic hallmark for patients with LCHAD deficiency is mixed micro- and macrovesicular steatosis (Figure 32.11). Late-onset neuromuscular disease and cholestatic disease have also been reported in MTP-deficient patients [132–134]. Higher frequencies of prematurity, intrauterine growth retardation, and intrauterine death have been reported as well [135,136]. Ophthalmic abnormalities have been seen in patients with LCHAD deficiency, with degeneration of the retinal pigment epithelium (RPE) [137–139].

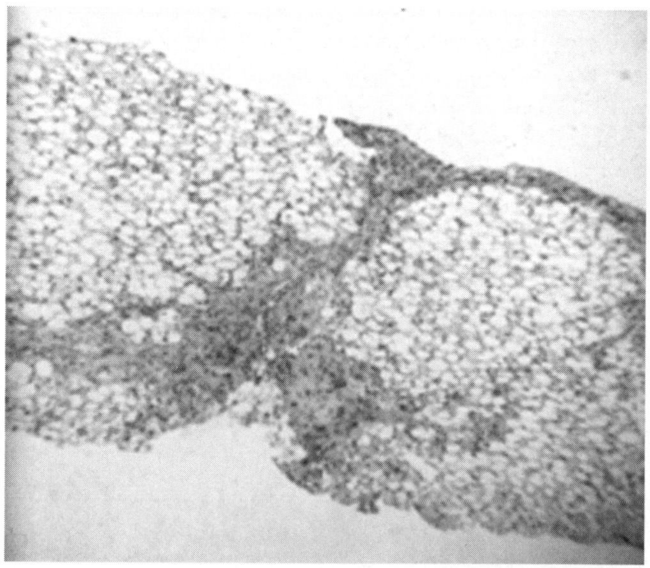

Figure 32.11. Liver histology and LCHAD deficiency. Light micrograph of a liver biopsy from a patient with LCHAD deficiency at 4 months of age showing marked steatosis.

MUTATIONS IN THE α SUBUNIT

Two teams independently delineated the G1528C mutation in exon 15 of the α subunit, which alters amino acid 474 from glutamic acid to glutamine (E474Q) and replaces the acidic and negatively charged side chain with a neutral amide-containing residue [44,125]. Ijlst et al. [125] sequenced the cDNAs encoding the MTP α and β subunits and found the G1528C mutation in 24 of the 26 Dutch patients with LCHAD deficiency [125]. Using *Saccharomyces cerevisiae* for expression studies of the wild-type and mutant protein, it was shown that the G1528C mutation was responsible for the loss of LCHAD activity [140]. Ibdah et al. [123] have reported α subunit molecular defects and phenotypes in 24 patients with documented isolated LCHAD deficiency or complete MTP deficiency. Of the 24 patients, 19 were diagnosed with isolated LCHAD deficiency and presented with a hepatic phenotype. Five were diagnosed with complete trifunctional protein deficiency, three displayed a cardiac phenotype, and the other two presented with a neuromuscular phenotype. Patients with isolated LCHAD deficiency presented predominantly with a Reye-like syndrome of liver dysfunction and carried the prevalent G1528C missense mutation on one or both alleles. Of the 19 subjects, 8 were homozygous for the common mutation E474Q whereas 11 were compound heterozygotes with one allele carrying the common mutation and the other allele having a different mutation.

The likely mechanism by which the E474Q mutation causes isolated LCHAD deficiency is that the mutation inactivates LCHAD directly within the catalytic domain, preserving the other MTP enzyme activities. The likely mechanism has been elucidated by Barycki et al. [141] based on a crystal and structural analysis of x-ray diffraction data from the human SCHAD, which is highly homologous to the LCHAD domain. E170 in SCHAD, a residue that is analogous to LCHAD E474, is located in the NAD-binding domain within the active catalytic site. E170 is also in a position to interact with another residue, H158, which serves as a base abstracting a proton from the 3-hydroxy group of the substrate. Substitution of E170 in SCHAD with glutamine disrupts the electrostatic interaction between E170 and H158, which is essential for catalysis. Similar to the E474Q in LCHAD, the E170Q mutation in SCHAD causes inactivation of the enzyme [141].

All reported patients with the complete MTP deficiency carried mutations other than the E474Q mutation [123]. Patients with MTP deficiency and cardiomyopathy had splice-site and missense mutations that caused the absence of the MTP protein complex [123]. This condition blocks the second step of the β-oxidation spiral, causing the accumulation of long-chain 3-enoyl fatty acid metabolites. Two patients with complete MTP deficiency presented with neuromyopathy. These two patients carried mutations in exon 9 that allowed stable MTP expression [124]. The exon 9 α subunit mutations resulting in a neuromuscular phenotype suggest a novel genotype–phenotype correlation [124]. Exon 9 in the MTP α subunit encodes a region described as a linker domain that may be important in subunit interaction and octamer complex formation, as suggested by crystallographic data from short-chain enoyl-CoA hydratase

[142]. The exon 9 mutations in the α subunit seem to result in defective subunit interactions and octamer formation.

MTP β SUBUNIT DEFECTS

Three clinical phenotypes are also apparent in MTP β subunit defects: hepatic, cardiac, and neuromuscular, with heterogeneity of the reported mutations [143]. The cardiac phenotype is considered lethal; patients who present with the cardiac phenotype die within days after birth as the result of severe dilated cardiomyopathy. Patients with the hepatic phenotype present with recurrent hypoketotic hypoglycemia. Patients with the mild neuromuscular phenotype present with episodic myoglobinuria. Mutational analysis revealed 16 different mutations: 12 missense mutations, 3 deletions, and 1 frameshift mutation. In compound heterozygotes with a null mutation in one allele and a missense mutation in the other allele, the milder mutation determined the clinical phenotype. Other groups have also reported β subunit mutations in a few patients involving a novel homozygous missense mutation, G976C, within a highly conserved region in the β subunit of the MTP [144]; a compound heterozygote causing a deletion; and a patient homozygous for a G1331A transition [145].

LCAD Deficiency

Human patients reported to be LCAD deficient were later reclassified as VLCAD deficient after the discovery of VLCAD in 1992 [64]. There are no confirmed human cases of LCAD deficiency, although a few suspected cases were reported. An autistic patient presented with an altered mitochondrial energy production with hypotonia and possible intermittent dicarboxylic aciduria, abnormal ammonia detoxification, and an abnormal acylcarnitine profile suggestive of LCAD deficiency [146]. This report suggests that LCAD deficiency may be one of the metabolic causes of autism. An elevated $C_{14:1}$ and $C_{14:2}$ acylcarnitine profile is noted in LCAD-deficient mice [147].

Disorders of Medium-Chain Fatty Acid Metabolism

Medium-Chain Acyl-CoA Dehydrogenase Deficiency

MCAD is responsible for the initial metabolism of acyl-CoAs with chain lengths of 4–12 carbon atoms. MCAD deficiency is the most common FAO disorder and was first described independently by three investigators [148–150]. Early reports suggested that at least 20% of undiagnosed MCAD-deficient patients die during their first metabolic crisis [151]. A prevalent missense mutation, A985G, results in an inactive enzyme [152,153]. MCAD-deficient patients present phenotypic heterogeneity. The most common symptoms are lethargy, emesis, encephalopathy, respiratory arrest, seizures, and apnea [151]. Metabolic crisis is often induced by a prolonged fast and often occurs in the midst of a viral illness with fever, vomiting, or diarrhea. Fatal outcome has been reported in a few previously asymptomatic patients with MCAD deficiency who presented later in life [154]. As with other FAO defects, histologically, MCAD deficiency is associated with microvesicular hepatic steatosis (Figure 32.12). MCAD deficiency leads to fasting-induced hypoglycemia and accumulation of medium-chain fatty acids that are metabolized to dicarboxylic acid,

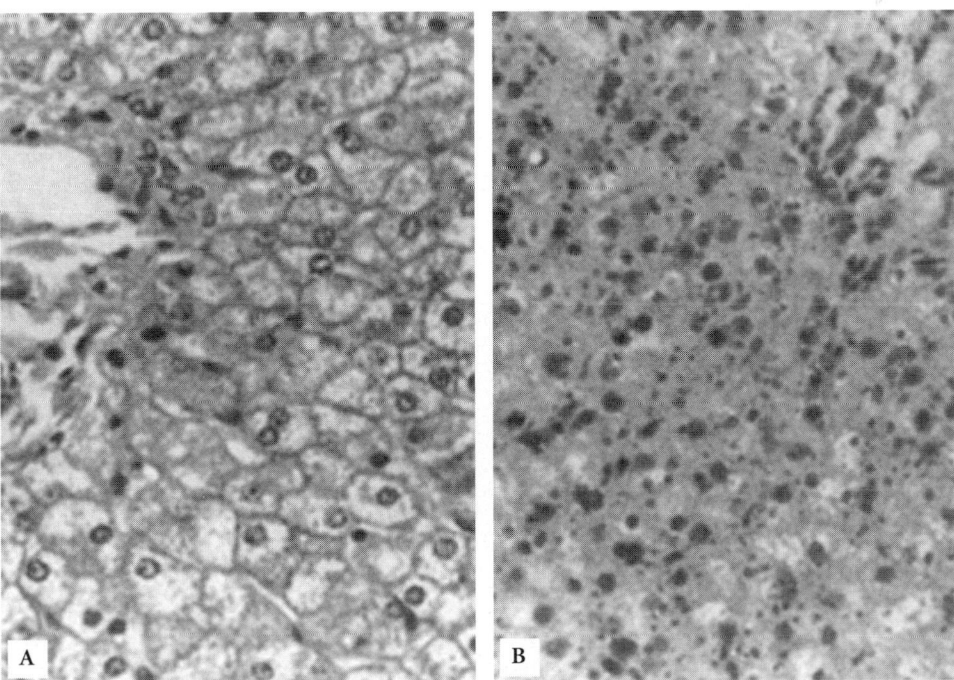

Figure 32.12. Liver histology and MCAD deficiency. Light micrograph of a liver biopsy from a patient with MCAD deficiency. (**A**) Essentially normal-appearing hepatocytes with no evident steatosis on hematoxylin and eosin (H&E) staining. (**B**) Oil red O stain on the same biopsy sample reveals abundant neutral fat in hepatocytes. (Varying-sized dark droplets; original magnification 360×.)

carnitine, and glycine esters. These metabolites can be detected by stable isotope dilution gas chromatography mass spectrometry (GC-MS), which differentiates it from other FAO defects and allows the diagnosis of asymptomatic affected individuals [155]. Analysis of plasma acylcarnitines by MS-MS reveals accumulation of C_6 to C_{10} acylcarnitine species [156]. Patients may develop secondary carnitine deficiency [157]. Diagnosis can be confirmed by fibroblast enzymatic assays and/or molecular genetic testing of the *MCAD* gene.

Medium/Short-Chain 3-Hydroxyacyl-CoA Dehydrogenase Deficiency

Medium/short-chain 3-hydroxyacyl-CoA dehydrogenase (M/SCHAD) deficiency was initially described as SCHAD deficiency, but current understanding of *SCHAD* gene function suggests that it metabolizes up to C_{10} acyl-CoAs [158]. M/SCHAD deficiency presents with different phenotypes. Cardiomyopathy with recurrent rhabdomyolysis is associated with reduction in enzymatic activity in skeletal muscle but not in liver [159]. Ketotic hypoglycemia with hepatic steatosis is associated with enzymatic reduction in the liver but not in muscle and fibroblasts [160]. Patients with hypoketotic hypoglycemia with hyperinsulinism, reduced enzyme activity in fibroblasts, and mutations in the *SCHAD* gene have been described [161,162]. Hyperinsulinism is not known to be a feature of any other known FAO defect; however, a recent study has documented that aging mice heterozygous for MTP develop hyperinsulinemia and insulin resistance [163]. A novel glucose–fatty acid cycle has been suggested [164]. Few *SCHAD* gene mutations have been found so far. SCHAD deficiency should be considered in the evaluation of an infant with persistent hyperinsulinemic hypoglycemia [162].

Medium-Chain 3-Ketoacyl-CoA Thiolase Deficiency

MCKAT deficiency has been reported in only one patient by Kamijo et al. [165]. A 2-day-old neonate presented with vomiting, dehydration, liver dysfunction, and rhabdomyolysis with myoglobinuria and died several days later. Urine organic analysis revealed lactic aciduria and significant C_6 to C_{12} dicarboxylic aciduria. Palmitate oxidation in skin fibroblast was normal, but octanoate oxidation was reduced and isolated MCKAT deficiency was demonstrated.

Disorders of Short-Chain Fatty Acid Metabolism

Short-Chain Acyl-CoA Dehydrogenase Deficiency

SCAD deficiency was first suggested by Turnbull et al. [166] in the early 1980s. Two newborns, the first reported SCAD-deficient patients, were noted to have unusually high levels of urinary ethylmalonic acid (EMA), a metabolite that accumulates when the β-oxidation of C_4 fatty acyl-CoAs cannot proceed [167]. EMA is excreted in the urine and can be measured by organic acid analysis. It also can be measured in the plasma as C_4 acylcarnitine by MS-MS. EMA in the urine and plasma is considered a biomarker for SCAD deficiency but is not exclusive to this disorder. The most common symptoms described in SCAD deficiency are developmental delay and muscle hypotonia [168]. Laboratory confirmation of SCAD deficiency is difficult because of biochemical heterogeneity complicated by gene variants. Two polymorphisms, R147W and G185S, occur in the homozygous or compound heterozygous state in 7% of the U.S. population [169]. These mutations compromise SCAD activity by affecting protein folding and thermal stability of the enzyme [170].

Ethylmalonic encephalopathy is a devastating infantile metabolic disorder characterized by widespread lesions in the brain, hyperlactic acidemia, petechiae, orthostatic acrocyanosis, and ethylmalonic aciduria. A G625A polymorphism in the *SCAD* gene was previously proposed as a cofactor in the etiology of ethylmalonic encephalopathy and other EMA syndromes. In a recent study, mutations in *ETHE1*, a gene located on chromosome 19q13, have been identified in patients affected by ethylmalonic encephalopathy [171].

Disorders of Ketogenesis

3-Hydroxy-3-Methylglutaryl-CoA Synthase Deficiency

HMG-CoA synthase deficiency is the only inborn error of metabolism that exclusively affects hepatic ketogenesis by interfering with the conversion of fatty acids to ketones [172]. A few HMG-CoA synthase–deficient patients have been described to date [172–176]. Patients presented with recurrent hypoketotic hypoglycemia leading to coma, triggered by prolonged fasting caused by gastrointestinal infections. HMG-CoA synthase is expressed in the liver, and its substrates and products are used or synthesized by other proteins that make enzymatic analysis difficult. The urinary organic profile shows elevated concentrations of various dicarboxylic acid and mitochondrial metabolites, but with the absence of ketones [172,176]. Disease-causing mutations have been discovered by mutational analysis of the human *HMGCS2* gene [172].

3-Hydroxy-3-Methylglutaryl-CoA Lyase Deficiency

HMG-CoA lyase mediates the final step of hepatic synthesis of ketones from fatty acids, and it also catalyzes the final step in leucine catabolism. Hence, its deficiency is also classified among amino acid oxidation defects. Patients present with fasting-induced metabolic acidosis, hypoketotic hypoglycemia, coma, elevated aminotransferase levels, coagulopathy, and hepatomegaly with steatosis [177–179]. Urine organic analysis shows characteristic elevation of 3-hydroxy-3-methylglutaric, 3-methylglutaconic, 3-methylglutaric, and 3-hydroxyisovaleric acids. The 3-methylglutaryl carnitine is elevated on plasma acylcarnitine analysis [180]. This disorder usually presents between 6 and 24 months of age, with 50% presenting in the first few weeks of life, and is triggered by fasting or intercurrent illness. Management of patients is based on a high-carbohydrate, low-protein or low-leucine, low-fat diet because of compromised leucine metabolism and impaired ketogenesis. A recent report on the crystal structure provides a rationale for the decrease in enzyme activity caused by pathogenic mutations that compromise the active site or enzyme stability [181].

Succinyl-CoA:3-Oxoacid CoA Transferase Deficiency

Succinyl-CoA oxoacid transferase catalyzes the first step of ketone body use in extrahepatic tissues. Patients with SCOT deficiency present with recurrent episodes of severe ketoacidosis with persistent ketonuria and hyperketonemia; onset is in the first year of life [182]. Cardiomegaly and behavioral problems have been reported [183]. No diagnostic metabolites are observed in blood and urine analysis, although acetoacetate and 3-hydroxybutyrate are elevated. Permanent or persistent ketosis is distinctively characteristic for most SCOT-deficient patients. Fukao et al. [184] reported three patients homozygous for a T435N mutation who have not had ketosis. The mutant protein had residual activity but is temperature sensitive, which may explain the ketoacidotic crises during febrile illness. Management includes limited protein intake, adequate calorie intake, and alkaline therapy to prevent aggravation of ketosis at the onset of any recurrent infection [185]. An 8-month-old child with a novel R217X mutation causing ketoacidotic crises required daily dialysis [186].

Mitochondrial β-Ketothiolase Deficiency

β-Ketothiolase is an enzyme involved in hepatic ketogenesis, nonhepatic ketolysis, and isoleucine catabolism. Most patients present with acute ketoacidosis accompanying infections and vomiting. Neurologic complications such as mental retardation and basal ganglia involvement have been described in a few patients [187,188]. Urine organic acid analysis reveals diagnostic elevation of 2-methyl-3-hydroxybutyric acid and tiglylglycine, which are products of defective isoleucine catabolism.

Other Disorders

Glutaric Acidemia Type II

Glutaric acidemia type II is also known as multiple acyl-CoA dehydrogenation (MAD) deficiency, an inborn error of fatty acid and amino acid metabolism in which the reoxidation of several mitochondrial dehydrogenases is impaired because of the inability of FAD to transfer electrons to the ETF caused by a defect in the ETF or ETF dehydrogenase. There is clinical heterogeneity, and three groups of patients have been described: those with neonatal onset with congenital abnormalities, those with neonatal onset without abnormalities, and those with a late onset with muscle weakness and carnitine deficiency [189–194]. Patients with severe neonatal onset with congenital abnormalities present with hypotonia, macrocephaly, severe hypoglycemia, metabolic acidosis, and enlarged kidneys; it is often associated with prematurity. Many of these patients die in the first week of life or early infancy. Congenital abnormalities include dysmorphic facial features, rocker-bottom feet, muscular and abdominal wall defects, and genital abnormalities [189,195,196]. Patients with the neonatal-onset form without congenital abnormalities also present with hypotonia, metabolic acidosis, hypoglycemia, tachypnea, hepatomegaly, and an acrid odor or odor of sweaty feet. Patients survive but die in a few months as the result of severe cardiomyopathy. Patients with the milder, late-onset form present with episodic vomiting, hypoglycemia, and acidosis [197]. Hepatomegaly, carnitine deficiency, and lipid storage myopathy have been described. Glutaric acidemia type II urinary organic acid profiles demonstrate an accumulation of EMA, glutaric acid, and 2-hydroxyglutaric acid. Urinary acylglycine analysis shows accumulation of isovalerylglycine and hexanoylglycine. Plasma acylcarnitine analysis reveals elevated levels of butyrylcarnitine, isovalerylcarnitine, glutarylcarnitine, and medium- and long-chain acylcarnitine species. Glutaric acidemia type II is most often caused by mutations in the genes encoding the α or β subunit of ETF or ETF-DH. Glutaric acidemia type II–deficient patients may also have mutations in the recently reported mitochondrial FAD transporter [198].

2,4-Dienoyl-CoA Reductase Deficiency

2,4-Dienoyl-CoA reductase deficiency is classified under defects in the metabolism of unsaturated fatty acids. Unsaturated fatty acids are metabolized by β-oxidation and three additional enzymes (enoyl-CoA isomerase, dienoyl-CoA isomerase, and a dienoyl-CoA reductase) that act on the double bonds. Only one patient has been reported thus far [199]. The neonate had persistent hypotonia, hyperlysinemia, hypocarnitinemia, normal organic acid profile, and an unusual acylcarnitine species "2-*trans*,4-*cis*-decadienoylcarnitine" in both urine and blood. In spite of dietary therapy, she died of respiratory acidosis at 4 months of age. Postmortem liver and muscle enzyme activities were reduced by 40% and 17%, respectively.

Maternal Liver Disease and FAO Disorders

Maternal Liver Disease

Acute fatty liver of pregnancy (AFLP) is a devastating disorder of the third trimester that carries a significant neonatal and maternal morbidity and mortality [200,201]. Its prevalence is approximately 1 in 7000–13,000 deliveries [201,202]. Women with AFLP usually present in the third trimester with initial complaints of abdominal pain, nausea, and vomiting and rapidly develop hepatic failure with coagulopathy and often encephalopathy [201,203]. Histologically, it is characterized by microvesicular hepatic steatosis and mitochondrial disruption on electron microscopy [200]. The cornerstones of management of this condition are early diagnosis and prompt delivery. There are limited reports on the risk of recurrence of AFLP in subsequent pregnancies, but several reports documented recurrence in this disorder [204–206].

HELLP (hemolysis, elevated liver enzymes, and low platelets) syndrome is also a maternal illness of the third trimester that is considered to be a complication of severe eclampsia and has a better prognosis than AFLP [201]. It is estimated to occur in 0.1–0.6% of all pregnancies and in 4–12% of women with a diagnosis of severe preeclampsia. Liver biopsy shows periportal hemorrhage and fibrin deposition [207], although both micro- and macrovesicular fatty infiltration may be present [208,209]. Similar to AFLP, prompt delivery is the treatment

Table 32.2: Genotypes and Phenotypes in 24 Families with MTP Defects

Families, No.	*Biochemical Phenotype*	*Pediatric Phenotype*	*Protein Expression*	*Pediatric Phenotype*	*Maternal Phenotype*
19	LCHAD	Homozygous (8) (E474Q)	Normal	Hepatic (7) Mixed (1)	AFLP (6) Normal (1) HELLP (1)
		Compound heterozygous (11) E474Q/splice site (3) E474Q/stop codon (7) E474Q/?*	Reduced	Hepatic (9) Mixed (1) Unknown (1)	AFLP (7) HELLP (1) Normal (3)
5	MTP	Homozygous (A-2G)	Absent	Cardiac	Normal
		Compound heterozygous (2) (G + 1A / A + 3G) (R640C/R640H)	Absent	Cardiac	Normal
		Homozygous (V246D)	Reduced	Neuromuscular	Normal
		Compound heterozygous (I269N/R255 ter)	Reduced	Neuromuscular	Normal

*Unknown mutation.

of choice. Recurrence of HELLP syndrome in subsequent pregnancies varies from 3–27% [201]. Differentiation of HELLP syndrome and AFLP may be difficult because of significant overlap in clinical and biochemical features [203,204,207,210]. For instance, thrombocytopenia is frequent in AFLP [203], and more than 20% of patients diagnosed with HELLP syndrome develop coagulopathy [211]. Both conditions are managed similarly and tend to improve after delivery. Some authors suggested that preeclampsia, HELLP syndrome, and AFLP represent different stages of the same disease and, hence, may share a common pathogenesis [203,204,208–210].

Maternal Liver Disease and LCHAD Deficiency

An interesting association between FAO disorders and severe complications during pregnancy with high maternal and fetal morbidity and mortality has been observed and well documented in women carrying LCHAD-deficient fetuses [123,212]. Schoeman et al. [205] were first to report an association between recurrent maternal AFLP with a fetal FAO disorder in two siblings who both died at 6 months of age. The authors speculated that because of the finding of similar hepatic pathology of microvesicular steatosis, AFLP and FAO defects might share a common pathogenesis.

Other case reports in the early 1990s also associated affected infants with LCHAD deficiency with the occurrence of severe preeclampsia, HELLP syndrome, or AFLP in the infants' mothers during pregnancy. Wilcken et al. [206] reported 11 pregnancies in 5 mothers in which 6 babies had LCHAD deficiency confirmed by enzymatic analysis of cultured skin fibroblasts; the mothers had either AFLP or HELLP syndrome in all 6 pregnancies with the LCHAD-deficient fetuses. Treem et al. [213] reported an LCHAD-deficient child born to a woman whose pregnancy was complicated by AFLP.

In a subsequent report published in 1995, Sims et al. [44] delineated the molecular basis of pediatric LCHAD deficiency and its association with AFLP in three families with LCHAD-deficient infants. The mothers suffered from HELLP syndrome or AFLP during pregnancies with the affected children. The analysis in two affected children revealed the G1528C mutation on both alleles, and the third child was a compound heterozygote with one allele carrying the G1528C mutation.

Another report documented an association between pediatric LCHAD deficiency and occurrence of AFLP in the mother. Isaacs et al. [214] reported a compound heterozygosity for MTP mutations in an affected child born to a woman whose pregnancy was complicated by maternal AFLP, with a novel mutation in exon 16 on one allele and the common G1528C mutation on the other allele.

Ibdah et al. [123] studied the association between MTP defects in children and liver disease in their mothers during pregnancy; 15 of the 24 women (62%) were diagnosed as having maternal liver disease, whereas 9 of the 24 women had normal pregnancies. In five of the normal pregnancies, the affected infants did not have the G1528C mutation but rather other MTP mutations. The remaining four normal pregnancies were associated with fetal LCHAD deficiency (Table 32.2). Thus 15 of 19 pregnancies associated with fetal LCHAD deficiency were complicated by maternal liver disease, and none of the pregnancies associated with complete MTP deficiency was associated with AFLP or HELLP syndrome. These results showed that when carrying a fetus that is LCHAD deficient, the mother has a 79% chance of a pregnancy complicated by AFLP or HELLP syndrome. The study also provided strong evidence that a woman whose affected fetus has the G1528C on one or both alleles of the α subunit of the mitochondrial trifunctional protein is likely to have pregnancy complications with AFLP.

In a subsequent study, Yang et al. [136] evaluated fetal genotypes and pregnancy outcomes in 83 pregnancies in 35 families with documented pediatric MTP defects; 24 pregnancies were complicated by AFLP, HELLP syndrome, or severe preeclampsia. Of the 24 pregnancies, 20 were complicated by AFLP, 2 with HELLP syndrome, and 2 with preeclampsia; in all the pregnancies, the LCHAD-deficient fetus was either homozygous or heterozygous for the G1528C mutation. Five pregnancies had fetuses with complete MTP deficiency (none of the mutations were G1528C), but there were no associated maternal complications in those pregnancies. To further assess the significance of the association between maternal AFLP and fetal LCHAD deficiency, Yang et al. [215] prospectively screened for MTP mutations in mothers who developed AFLP (n = 27) or HELLP syndrome (n = 81) and their newborn infants. The molecular screening was based solely on the maternal history. Of the 27 women who developed AFLP, 5 carried fetuses with MTP mutations, 3 were homozygous for the G1528C mutation, and 2 were compound heterozygotes for the common G1528C and another non-G1528C mutation. Only one woman diagnosed with HELLP syndrome was heterozygous for the G1528C mutation, which was not detected in her infant. None of the children born to the 81 women diagnosed with HELLP syndrome carried MTP mutations. This study documented that in approximately one out of five pregnancies complicated by AFLP, the fetus is LCHAD deficient. This strong association between AFLP and the common G1528C mutation in the fetus is significant, hence screening the offspring of women who develop AFLP at birth for this mutation may be lifesaving [215].

With the growing evidence suggesting that carrying an LCHAD-deficient fetus is associated with AFLP, we recommend that neonates born to woman with pregnancies complicated by AFLP be tested for the common G1528C mutation. Screening the newborn for the G1528C mutation in pregnancies complicated by AFLP, when done early after birth, may be lifesaving. Screening may identify LCHAD-deficient children before they manifest the disease, thus allowing early dietary intervention by instituting a diet low in fat and high in carbohydrate and by substituting long-chain fatty acids with medium-chain fatty acids. Universal newborn screening for FAO disorders by MS-MS will likely achieve the same goal.

In addition, identification of MTP mutations in the offspring of pregnancies complicated by AFLP allows appropriate genetic counseling for the mothers. Prenatal diagnosis may be performed in subsequent pregnancies to identify pregnancies at risk for development of AFLP. We performed molecular prenatal diagnosis in 11 pregnancies using chorionic villus samples and successfully identified the fetal genotype in these pregnancies as confirmed by biochemical and molecular testing of the newborn or aborted fetuses [216].

Possible Hypothesis for the Association Between Maternal Liver Disease and Fetal FAO Disorders

The precise mechanism by which an LCHAD-deficient fetus causes AFLP in a heterozygous mother is still unclear. However, several factors appear to contribute to this fetal–maternal interaction. First, the heterozygosity of the mother for an MTP defect reduces her capacity to oxidize long-chain fatty acids. Second, the stressful nature of pregnancy, with its accompanying changes in metabolism, increased lipolysis, and decreased β-oxidation, may be another contributing factor. It is possible that in the presence of the G1528C mutation, potentially hepatotoxic long-chain 3-hydroxyacyl fatty acid metabolites produced by the fetus or placenta accumulate in the maternal circulation. Accumulation of these substances occurs as a result of a block at the level of the third step, leading to the accumulation of 3-hydroxyacyl-CoA compounds. To the contrary, a block at the first step occurring in MTP deficiency will result in accumulation of enoyl-CoA metabolites, which may not be hepatotoxic.

There is evidence for FAO in a normal human placenta including LCHAD and SCHAD activity [217]. There is significant expression of fatty acid β-oxidation enzymes in human placenta as assessed by immunohistochemical and immunoblotting studies [218]. There is also high activity of FAO enzymes in human term placenta and chorionic villus samples [219]. Thus, it is highly likely that the LCHAD-deficient placenta plays a major role in the fetal–maternal interaction by producing hepatotoxic long-chain fatty acid metabolites.

Other Fatty Acid Oxidation Defects and Maternal Liver Disease

The role of other FAO defects in the development of maternal liver disease is not clear. Maternal liver disease consistent with AFLP associated with CPT-I deficiency has been reported. In a report by Innes et al. [89], a patient developed liver disease consistent with AFLP and, in a subsequent pregnancy, hyperemesis gravidarum. Both children were subsequently found to have CPT-I deficiency. Ylitalo et al. [220] described a patient who experienced complications that included a HELLP-like syndrome. She was later diagnosed to be CPT-I deficient, but her child was unaffected. Matern et al. [221] reported an SCAD-deficient infant born to a mother who developed AFLP in the course of her gestation. A pregnancy complicated by HELLP syndrome and associated with fetal MCAD deficiency has also been reported [222]. In a multicenter retrospective study by Holub et al. [223], 88 infants born to women with HELLP syndrome were screened for FAO defects; none was detected. There is also a report of three patients who developed maternal liver disease associated with fetal MTP deficiency caused by mutations other than the G1528C [224]. Bok et al. [225] reported a pregnancy complicated by HELLP syndrome associated with fetal SCAD deficiency. The infant was prematurely born and presented with unexplained cholestasis and hepatomegaly at 2 months of age. EMA and C_4 acylcarnitine levels were elevated, fibroblast SCAD activity was decreased, and DNA analysis of the *SCAD* gene showed a C1138T mutation. The mother was heterozygous for the C1138T mutation. These studies demonstrate a growing diversity of clinical presentations of FAO defects and their potential role in the development of maternal liver disease.

Sudden Infant Death Syndrome and Inherited Disorders of Fatty Acid Oxidation

Fatty acid oxidation disorders, if unrecognized and untreated, can cause sudden unexpected death. Such deaths can be certified as sudden infant death syndrome (SIDS) if FAO defects are not suspected or recognized. Postmortem studies on SIDS victims [226] and their siblings [227] attributed a small but significant number of SIDS cases to undiagnosed FAO disorders at the time of sudden infant death. The first association of FAO disorders and SIDS was made on the basis of finding hepatic fatty infiltration in 5% of 200 SIDS cases in 1976 [228]. Studies later suggested that approximately 5% of sudden infant deaths might be associated with fatty acid metabolic disorders [229–231]. A retrospective study of 418 SIDS cases using biochemical and histochemical analyses also estimated that 5% of SIDS cases may be caused by FAO disorders [227]. In a study of 189 siblings of infants who died from SIDS and 84 infants who experienced a "near-miss" episode [232,233], 28 of the 189 (15%) infants whose siblings died of SIDS had a urine metabolic profile compatible with a FAO defect, including 3 with MAD deficiency and 12 with MCAD deficiency. In the group of infants with a near-miss episode, 14 of 84 (17%) had a possible β-oxidation defect. In another study of 313 cases with SIDS, 14 had biochemical profiles seen in FAO defects, including 2 with MCAD, 4 with MAD, 4 with VLCAD/LCHAD, and 4 with carnitine transport deficiencies [227]. These studies suggest that defects in FAO account for a small but significant number of undiagnosed SIDS cases. It is strongly suggested that asymptomatic siblings and parents of those who died from SIDS be tested for defects in FAO.

DIAGNOSIS OF DEFECTS IN FATTY ACID OXIDATION

Many of the disorders of FAO present themselves with episodes of hypoketotic hypoglycemia, metabolic crisis that resembles Reye's syndrome, acute or chronic myopathy, cardiac arrhythmias, or cardiomyopathy. Most patients present very early in life [126]. The pediatric hepatologist will most likely be involved with these patients presenting early in life with hepatomegaly, elevated aminotransferase levels, hypoglycemia, hypotonia, lethargy, or coma. Many patients with defects in FAO are often symptom-free for weeks or months, whereas others present in their first hours of life. Disorders in FAO are often severe; in one study, half the patients died – 30% in the first week of life and 69% before the age of 1 year [126]. In some cases, patients suffered cardiorespiratory collapse in the first 48 hours. The acute decompensation is usually precipitated by fasting, and often children are found lethargic or comatose the morning after an overnight fast. Prolonged fasting is usually defined as more than 12 hours without food for children between 1 and 4 years old and 6–10 hours for infants less than 1 year old [234]. Liver failure with advanced hepatic fibrosis or cirrhosis is rare but has been reported in patients with LCHAD deficiency, CACT deficiency, and defects in transport of long-chain fatty acids [68,235,236]. Unique clinical findings occurring in some FAO disorders include congenital multicystic kidneys and macrocephaly in ETF-DH deficiency [126], pancreatitis in CPT-II deficiency [237], hypoparathyroidism in LCHAD deficiency [238], renal tubular acidosis in CPT-I deficiency [87], and retinitis pigmentosa and peripheral neuropathy in LCHAD deficiency [127,128]. The initial laboratory findings depend on the defect and type of presentation. Patients who present with fasting, lethargy, and coma are usually hypoglycemic with mild to moderate metabolic acidosis, mild to moderate elevations of aminotransferase levels and creatine phosphokinase, mild coagulopathy, and moderate elevations of blood urea nitrogen, uric acid, and ammonia levels.

General Approach to Diagnosis

The approach to the diagnosis of patients with disorders of FAO involves a combination of routine, specialized, and in vitro analyses, with careful consideration of the clinical condition of the patient at the time of sample collection. The concentration of key metabolites may not be significant when the patient is in an anabolic state and clinically stable. The samples collected under these conditions may not be diagnostic as the metabolic intermediates may be absent or undetectable. The most useful specimens for evaluation are those acquired during metabolic compensation, before initiation of treatment, as the metabolic profile and its interpretation rely on the clinical context at the time of sample acquisition. Although metabolite analysis may be diagnostic, cases that are highly suspicious should be followed up with molecular analysis or in vitro biochemical analysis.

Routine Laboratory Studies

Patient samples (urine and blood) should be collected at the earliest possible time during episodes of metabolic decompensation. Hypoketotic hypoglycemia is a hallmark of most disorders of FAO. Routine chemistry tests include blood gases, glucose, insulin, liver enzymes, electrolytes (with assessment of the anion gap), uric acid, triglycerides, and creatine kinase levels. Serum and urinary ketones are helpful only if obtained during the metabolic crisis. These routine studies are needed to assess the extent of organ involvement and to assess the response to therapeutic interventions. Chest radiography, electrocardiography, and echocardiography are also needed if clinical examination suggests cardiac decompensation; these are also important once a long-chain FAO disorder is diagnosed. Blood samples for plasma acylcarnitine and urine organic acid analyses should also be collected during the metabolic crisis while the patient's metabolic abnormalities are being corrected.

Providing adequate clinical information to the biochemical geneticist, including the patient's condition, medications, pregnancy history, family history, and patient's dietary history, is essential in the interpretation of the metabolic findings identified in those studies [239,240].

Specialized Metabolic Analyses

Defects associated with mitochondrial FAO result in the accumulation of metabolites proximal to the enzymatic block that can be converted into dicarboxylic or hydroxydicarboxylic acids, which in turn can be detoxified by mechanisms that produce acylglycine and acylcarnitine conjugates. Their accumulation in body fluids assists in the biochemical evaluation of these patients.

Urinary Organic Acid Analysis

Defects in FAO are often associated with abnormal and characteristic urinary organic acid profiles. Organic acids are water-soluble compounds that have at least one carboxyl group; they are best detected by GC-MS [241]. Table 32.3 shows the pattern of urine organic acids detected in various disorders of FAO. The accumulation of significant amounts of metabolites in the urine reflects the demand for energy from FAO. During metabolic stress, the presence of dicarboxylic acid in the urine signifies an impaired or defective mitochondrial FAO. Dicarboxylic acids are products of microsomal oxidation. Accumulation of urinary hexanoylglycine and suberylglycine, for example, is a characteristic signature pattern seen in MCAD deficiency. A dominant 3-hydroxy dicarboxylic aciduria of C_6 to C_{14} is seen in LCHAD deficiency. The absence of dicarboxylic aciduria does not rule out a defect in FAO as seen in patients with defects of fatty acid transport. Ketosis, a diet high in MCTs, and some peroxisomal disorders may produce dicarboxylic aciduria and therefore be confused with a mitochondrial FAO disorder. Table 32.3 lists the organic acid abnormalities most frequently observed in disorders of FAO.

Urinary Acylglycine Analysis

Other urinary metabolites are also helpful in the diagnosis of disorders of FAO. Stable-isotope dilution GC-MS allows for the quantitative determination in urine of very small quantities of metabolites, such as acylglycine, that are below the detection limit of routine urinary organic acid analysis Small quantities of acylglycine appear to be consistently excreted in children with certain FAO defects as seen in Table 32.3. MCAD deficiency can be diagnosed reliably with elevated levels of hexanoylglycine, phenylpropionylglycine, and suberylglycine, even in asymptomatic patients [155]. SCAD deficiency, MCKAT deficiency, and glutaric aciduria type II are other disorders with diagnostic acylglycine profiles [242,243].

Carnitine and Acylcarnitine Analysis

Plasma acylcarnitine analysis has become the most widely used tool for the investigation of disorders of FAO. In β-oxidation disorders, accumulated acyl-CoA compounds proximal to the metabolic block are converted to acylcarnitines, which are transported out of the cell and filtered in the kidneys [244]. The pattern of plasma acylcarnitine abnormalities is shown in Table 32.3. Low total carnitine, free carnitine, and acylcarnitine fraction are suggestive of primary carnitine deficiency. Elevated free carnitine and low acylcarnitines are seen in CPT-I deficiency. A secondary decrease in free plasma carnitine levels is seen in several FAO defects, whereas the acylcarnitines may be abnormal in a disease-specific, recognizable pattern [245]. Secondary reductions in plasma carnitine levels are generally 25–50% of normal values [91]. Very low plasma carnitine levels, approaching zero, are usually seen in patients with defects in carnitine uptake [72]. In normal fasting subjects, acetylcarnitine is the predominant carnitine ester, but in a β-oxidation disorder, the dominant acylcarnitine reflects the position of the metabolic block. Acylcarnitine profiles characteristic of MCAD, LCAD, ETF, LCHAD, CPT-II, and 2,4-dienoyl-CoA reductase deficiencies have been reported [116].

Fatty Acid Analysis

The quantitative determination of the plasma fatty acid profiles also provides useful and complementary information when assessing patients suspected of having disorders of FAO [246]. Abnormal profiles may be observed in patients with MCAD, SCHAD, LCHAD, MTP, VLCAD, and glutaric aciduria type II deficiency [247,248]. Plasma long-chain free fatty acids of C_{14} to C_{18} and 3-hydroxy fatty acids are consistently found in patients with LCHAD and MTP deficiencies. Fatty acids C_8, C_{10}, and $C_{10:1}$ predominate the profile in MCAD-deficient patients, whereas $C_{14:1}$ and $C_{14:2}$ characterize VLCAD-deficient patients.

In Vivo Loading and Stress Tests

A number of approaches have been used to test the integrity of the FAO pathway in patients suspected of having a disorder of FAO. To avoid a potentially dangerous fasting test, substrate loading has been used to provoke increased excretion of abnormal diagnostic urinary metabolites. Carnitine loading to provoke acylcarnitine excretion and phenylpropionic acid loading to provoke phenylpropionylglycine excretion have also been used [249,250]. The long-chain triglyceride loading test has been used to screen the overall hepatic FAO pathway, in which low plasma ketone body production indicates a defect somewhere in the pathway. In cases in which patients have suspected FAO defects but the data are inconclusive or cultured cells are not available, a rigidly controlled in-hospital fasting test is a useful tool; however, fasting tests on infants are not recommended. Levels of glucose, insulin, ketone bodies, β-hydroxybutyrate, free fatty acids, total and free carnitine, and urinary organic acid are important to obtain. The fast should be terminated when the child demonstrates symptoms or has a blood glucose level of 40 mg/dL or less.

Biochemical in Vitro Cell-Based Studies

Several cell-based biochemical in vitro assays are available to confirm preliminary diagnoses of disorders of FAO. Fibroblasts

Table 32.3: Metabolic Abnormalities Detected in Fatty Acid Oxidation Disorders

Fatty Acid Oxidation Disorder	*Plasma Acylcarnitine*	*Urine Organic Acids**
CUD	↓ C_0 (free carnitine) ↓ Long-chain acylcarnitines	Normal or ↑ dicarboxylic acids
CPTI	↑ C_0 ↓ Long-chain acylcarnitines	Usually normal
CPTII	↑ C_{16}, $C_{18:1}$, C_{14}, low C_2	Normal
CACT	↑ C_{16}, $C_{18:1}$, C_{14}, low C_2	Normal or ↑ dicarboxylic acids
VLCAD	↑ C_{14}, $C_{14:1}/C_{12:1}$	↑ Dicarboxylic acids
LCHAD/MTP	↑ $C_{16}OH$, $C_{18:1}OH$, $C_{14}OH$	↑ Dicarboxylic acids ↑ Hydroxydicarboxylic acids (3-hydroxyadipic acid, 3-hydroxysebacic acid)
MCKAT	Unknown	↑ Lactic, 3-hydroxybutyric, saturated and unsaturated C_6–C_{16} dicarboxylic acids
MADD/GAII	↑ C_4, C_5, C_5DC, C_6, C_8, C_{10}, C_{12}, C_{14}	↑ Glutaric acid, isobutyrylglycine, ethylmalonic acid, dicarboxylic acids, acylglycines (phenylpropionylglycine), 2-hydroxyglutaric acid
SCOT	Normal	Normal
MCAD	↑ C_8, C_{10}, $C_{10:1}$	↑ Dicarboxylic acids, acylglycines (suberylglycine, hexanoylglycine), 5-hydroxyhexanoic acid, octanedioic acid, decanedioic acid
M/SCHAD	↑ 3-OH-C_4	↑ Dicarboxylic acids, 2-hydroxyglutaric acid
SCAD	↑ C_4 (butyrylcarnitine and butyrylglycine)	↑ Ethylmalonate, methylsuccinate
ETH1	↑ C_4, C_5	↑ Lactic acid, ethylmalonate, methylsuccinate
2,4-Dienoyl reductase	Hypocarnitinemia, 2-*trans*, 4-*cis*-decadienoylcarnitine in both urine and blood	Normal
HMGCS2	Normal	Normal
HMGCL	↑ C_5OH	↑ 3-Methylglutaric acid, 3-methylglutaconic acid, 3-hydroxy-3-methylglutaric acid, 3-methylcrotonylglycine
BKT	Normal or ↓ C_0	Tiglylglycine, acetoacetic acid, 2-methylacetoacetic acid

*Normal urine organic acids usually contain small amounts of various dicarboxylic acids. In addition to disorders of fatty acid oxidation, dicarboxylic aciduria occurs in ketosis, several peroxisomal disorders, and medium-chain triglyceride supplementation.

BKT, β-ketothiolase; CACT, carnitine acylcarnitine translocase; CPTI, carnitine palmitoyl transferase I; CPTII, carnitine palmitoyl transferase II; CUD, carnitine uptake defect; ETH1, ethylmalonic encephalopathy; HMGCS2, 3-hydroxy-3-methylglutaryl-CoA synthase 2; HMGCL, 3-hydroxy-3-methylglutaryl-CoA lyase; LCHAD/MTP, long-chain 3-hydroxyacyl-CoA dehydrogenase/mitochondrial trifunctional protein; MADD/GAII, multiple acyl-CoA dehydrogenase/glutaric aciduria II; MCAD, medium-chain acyl-CoA dehydrogenase; MCKAT, medium-chain ketoacyl-CoA thiolase; M/SCHAD, medium/short-chain acyl-CoA dehydrogenase; SCAD, short-chain acyl-CoA dehydrogenase; SCOT, succinyl-CoA: oxoacid transferase; VLCAD, very long–chain acyl-CoA dehydrogenase.

cultured from skin biopsies are used to allow metabolic in vitro diagnosis of most FAO disorders in a single test [251,252].

In studies by Roe and Roe [253], cells were incubated with stable isotopes then acylcarnitine profiles were obtained from the media and cell pellets using MS-MS, high-performance liquid chromatography, or GC-MS. These in vitro studies may be helpful in differentiating certain disorders of FAO from similar defects with ambiguous plasma acylcarnitine profiles. Using specific metabolites and/or monitoring certain acylcarnitine ratios, FAO defects can be distinguished from one another

[107]. An in-depth analysis using different substrates may suggest new therapeutic strategies. As an example, LCHAD-deficient fibroblasts incubated with palmitate showed abnormal hydroxylacylcarnitine profiles, which corrected when cells were incubated with decanoate and octanoate [251].

Enzyme Activity in Cultured Skin Fibroblasts and Other Tissues

Diagnosis of specific FAO defects is also possible by directly measuring the enzyme activity. Specific enzyme assays can be performed in cultured skin fibroblasts or muscle biopsy specimens for certain enzyme deficiencies, such as CPT-I, CPT-II, SCAD, LCAD, VLCAD, LCHAD/TFP, and SCHAD. Monoclonal antibodies raised against these enzymes are also used to eliminate ambiguity and examine the overlap in substrate specificities [254].

Molecular Genetic Studies

The complete genomic sequence of all reported FAO enzymes is known as well. Confirmation of diagnosis by direct mutation analysis of DNA isolated from blood, buccal swab, skin fibroblasts, muscle, or other tissue should be sought in any patient with a diagnostic or highly suspicious biochemical profile. Molecular DNA common gene mutations have been documented for several of the deficiencies, such as the MCAD K329E and the LCHAD E474Q mutations. Genotype–phenotype correlations are emerging as well.

Prenatal Diagnosis

Amniotic fluid, amniocytes, and chorionic villus samples can be used for prenatal diagnosis [216,255,256]. Organic acid and acylcarnitine analyses may be done on amniotic fluid. Cultured amniocytes and chorionic villus samples can be analyzed for direct enzyme measurements. Direct DNA mutation analysis requires prior knowledge of the specific mutation for which the fetus is at risk and may be done on DNA isolated from cultured amniocytes and trophoblasts [216]. This is expected to help the parents prepare themselves psychologically and to allow the managing physician to provide appropriate treatment as early as possible.

Newborn Screening for Fatty Acid Oxidation Disorders

Newborn screening is a public health program whose mandate is the early identification of diseases in newborns in which timely intervention could improve the prognosis of their long-term health. Guthrie's innovative assay to detect levels of phenylalanine in dried blood spots on filter paper led to the first screening assay for phenylketonuria [257]. An increasing number of states are providing metabolic screening for disorders of FAO (U.S. National Screening Status Report, available at: http://genes-r-us.uthsca.edu). Currently, different state and commercial laboratories choose to test for certain disorders of FAO using different cut-offs and diagnostic criteria that are specific to that laboratory. MS-MS analysis allows the identification of several amino acids and organic acids as well as disorders of FAO [65]. The ability of MS-MS to screen for metabolic disorders was reported in 1990 [258]. Chace et al. [259] have applied this tool to mass newborn screening of disorders of FAO based on the profiling of acylcarnitines in blood spots.

Mass spectrometers are capable of identifying analyte-specific signatures based on their specific molecular mass to charge (*m/z*) ratio. The triple quadrupole tandem mass spectrometer is the type most commonly used in newborn screening. In this setup, two mass spectrometers (MS1 and MS3) are separated by a third one (MS2, also known as collision cell) arranged in tandem [260]. The analytic steps include analyte extraction from the blood sample followed by derivitization and then injection into the mass spectrometer (M1) for ionization, fragmentation, and then data collection. Acylcarnitines produce a common fragment (*m/z* 85) that corresponds to the carnitine backbone. Both derivitized and nonderivitized samples can be analyzed by MS-MS. The short analysis time of 1–3 minutes and capability of multianalyte detection make MS-MS a robust method suitable for mass newborn screening. A diagnostic profile of MCAD deficiency detected on newborn screening is shown in Figure 32.1. The expected metabolic abnormalities detected by MS-MS and corresponding findings on urine organic acids analysis are shown in Table 32.3. Tissue expression distribution of each enzyme determines the source most suitable for enzymatic analysis. Molecular genetic mutation analysis is available for all these genes through either clinical or research laboratories. Testing for the common MCAD (K329E) or LCHAD (E474Q) mutations is widely available in clinical laboratories using polymerase chain reaction (PCR) or direct DNA sequencing.

Results of mass newborn screening throughout the world are beginning to show the true frequency of the classic and variant forms of inborn errors of metabolism screened for in those laboratories, as shown in Table 32.4 [81,261–267]. The panel of metabolic disorders screened for is not uniform among the laboratories, neither is the analyte cut-offs used or the decision-making process. Two of the largest newborn screening studies, those reported by Naylor and Chace [261] in the United States and Schulze et al. [262] in Germany, show an overall frequency of FAO disorders of about 1 in 15,500 newborns, with MCAD deficiency being the most common disorder detected.

Cost-effectiveness studies have been published; one study suggests that screening for errors of metabolism compares favorably with other screening programs, such as those for breast and prostrate cancer, in cost per quality-adjusted life-year saved [268]. The prognosis for most patients with disorders of FAO identified presymptomatically and managed appropriately is generally favorable and suggests benefit from early diagnosis and treatment.

Postmortem Screening

The postnatal period is critical for infants with FAO defects as inadequate caloric intake and limited glycogen stores may

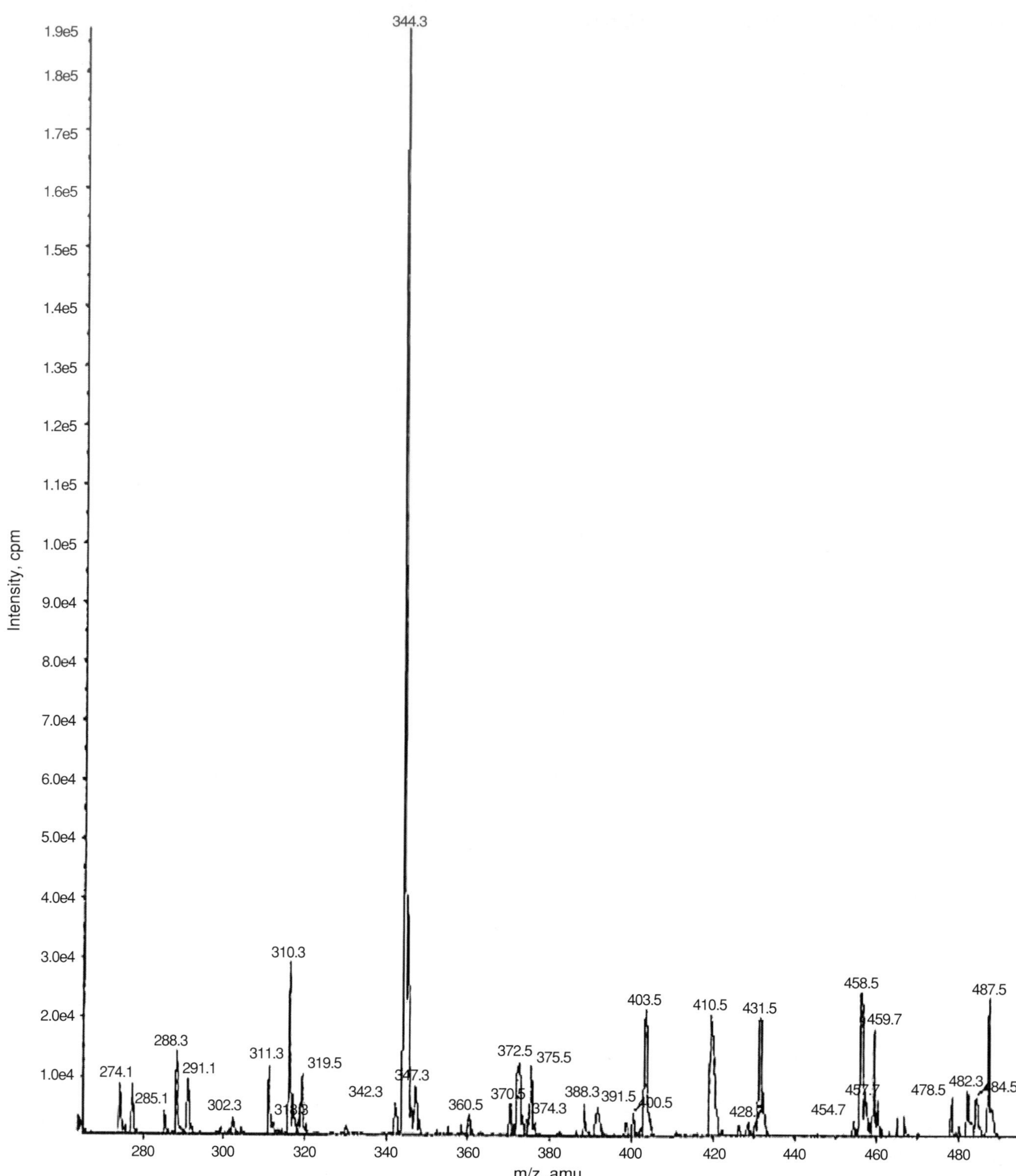

Figure 32.13. Plasma acylcarnitine profile by tandem mass spectrometry. This acylcarnitine profile was obtained using a blood sample from a newborn with MCAD deficiency. Significant elevations in C_6 (hexanoyl), C_8 (octanoyl), C_{10} (decanoyl), and $C_{10:1}$ (decenoyl) acylcarnitines are diagnostic. (Courtesy of Patrick Hopkins, Missouri Newborn Screening Laboratory.)

Table 32.4: Selected Newborn Metabolic Screening Results

Study	*Number Screened*	*Country*	*Disorders*
Wiley et al. [263]	137,120	Australia	17 PKU, 1 BH4, 3 hyperPhe, 1 MSUD, 1 Tyr I, 1 cong. lactic acid, 1 GAI, 1 BKT, 1 SCAD, 2 MCAD
Wilcken et al. [81]	149,000	Australia	4 CUD
Liebl et al. [264]	87,000	Germany	11 CAH, 9 PKU, 6 MCAD
Schulze et al. [262]	250,000	Germany	28 AA (1:8900), 12 OA (1:20,800), 16 FAO (1:15,600), total (1:2400)
Shigematsu et al. [265]	102,200	Japan	5 PA, 2 MMA, 2 MCAD, 3 ASA II, 1 PKU
Rashed et al. [266]	27,264	Saudi Arabia	20 cases (1:1381)
Naylor and Chace [261]	700,000	U.S.	86 AA, 32 OA, 45 FAO (36 MCAD)
Zytkovicz et al. [267]	>160,000	U.S.	22 AA (7 PKU, 11 hyperPhe, 1 MSUD, 1 hypermeth, 1 ASL, 1 arg), 20 FAO (10 MCAD, 5 SCAD, 2 PA, 1 CPTII, 1 MCCC, 1 VLCAD)

AA, amino acids; Arg, arginase; ASA, argininosuccinate aciduria; ASL, argininosuccinate lyase; BH4 tetrahydrobiopterin; BKT, β-ketothiolase; CAH, congenital adrenal hyperplasia; cong. lactic acid, congenital lactic acidosis; CPTII, carnitine palmitoyl transferase II; CUD, carnitine uptake defect; FAO, fatty acid oxidation; GAI, glutaric aciduria type I; hypermeth, hypermethioninemia; hyperPhe, hyperphenylalaninemia; MCAD, medium-chain acyl-CoA dehydrogenase; MCCC, 3-methylcrotonyl-CoA carboxylase; MMA, methylmalonic aciduria; MSUD, maple syrup urine disease; OA, organic acids; PA, propionic acidemia; PKU, phenylketonuria; SCAD, short-chain acyl-CoA dehydrogenase; Tyr 1, tyrosinemia type 1; VLCAD, very long–chain acyl-CoA dehydrogenase.

trigger episodes of hypoglycemia [269]. Decompensation episodes may be resolved or may be fatal, resulting in sudden and unexpected death [76,227,229,270]. Postmortem studies using histochemical and biochemical analysis of liver specimens [227], organic and fatty acid analysis of urine and plasma specimens [270], analysis of acylcarnitine profiles in bile and blood spots [259,271], and the determination of FAO rates using cultured skin fibroblasts [272] have been done to investigate sudden unexpected death in previously healthy children. Postmortem studies are important to confirm a suspected diagnosis of FAO defect for appropriate genetic counseling and future prenatal testing [273].

Differential Diagnosis

Disorders of FAO are diagnosed with increasing frequency as detection of abnormal metabolites in plasma and urine has improved using various sensitive techniques. The differential diagnosis of an infant or a young child with hypoglycemia, encephalopathy, and liver dysfunction includes fulminant hepatic failure secondary to a viral infection, toxic drug exposure, and metabolic defects of FAO. An infant or child with recurring Reye's syndrome, with a family history of Reye's syndrome or SIDS, or presenting with Reye's syndrome under the age of 2 years, should be suspected as having a disorder of FAO until proven otherwise. In Reye's syndrome, vomiting and a viral prodrome are universal, whereas they occur only in up to two thirds of FAO-deficient patients [62]. At least 85% of Reye's syndrome patients have twice the normal value of aspartate aminotransferase (AST), and most have a prolonged prothrombin time; the latter is present in less than half the patients with disorders of FAO. Patients with defects in FAO have low plasma carnitine levels (most of the carnitine is in the esterified form), whereas patients with Reye's syndrome have normal carnitine levels. Although Reye's syndrome patients excrete dicarboxylic acid in their urine, β-hydroxybutyrate levels do not decrease and ketogenesis is not inhibited. Biopsy samples from patients with disorders of FAO and Reye's syndrome look the same under light microscopy; however, ultrastructural changes in the mitochondria are not detected in biopsies obtained from patients with Reye's syndrome [62].

Some infants with FAO defects have been diagnosed with gastroesophageal reflux, and some patients with MCAD have been diagnosed with cyclic vomiting syndrome [274]. Cyclic vomiting has also been described in patients with glutaric aciduria type II and SCAD and SCHAD deficiencies. It is recommended that such infants undergo metabolic testing when they are having symptoms to maximize the chance of detecting disease-specific metabolic abnormalities.

Differentiation of disorders of FAO from other metabolic causes of hepatomegaly, hypoglycemia, and liver dysfunction can be done by specific blood or urine tests and liver biopsy if needed. Other liver metabolic diseases to be considered include α_1-antitrypsin deficiency, neonatal iron storage disease, hereditary tyrosinemia, and glycogen storage diseases. Patients with glycogen storage disease and hereditary fructose intolerance have normal ammonia levels, whereas ammonia may be elevated in patients with disorders of FAO. Patients with urea cycle defects present with Reye-like syndrome without the metabolic acidosis and hypoglycemia.

MANAGEMENT OF FATTY ACID OXIDATION DISORDERS

General Approach to Treatment of Disorders of FAO

The mainstay of treatment is fasting avoidance; a high-carbohydrate, low-fat diet; and fat substitution when applicable. Frequent feeding is recommended to avoid accumulation of toxic metabolites resulting from peripheral lipolysis and hypoglycemia [275]. Infants should be fed frequently; an every–3–4 hour schedule is sufficient. Older patients may be given uncooked starch as a source of complex carbohydrates that are slowly released in the blood to prolong feeding intervals; this allows for an overnight rest.

Management of Acute Illness

Managing acute episodes of hypoketotic hypoglycemia, coma, metabolic crisis, and acute liver dysfunction requires rapid infusion of intravenous dextrose to raise insulin levels to inhibit FAO and lipolysis from fatty acid stores. Supportive therapy including correction of coagulopathy, dehydration, metabolic acidosis, and electrolyte imbalances is important as well.

Long-Term Dietary Treatment to Reduce Fasting Stress

Fasting avoidance is the mainstay of therapy in disorders of FAO. Generally, a high-carbohydrate, low-fat diet with approximately 70% of calories from carbohydrate, 15% from protein, and 15–20% from fat is instituted. MCT substitution is recommended for patients with VLCAD, MTP/LCHAD, CPT, CACT, or carnitine transport defects as they freely diffuse into the mitochondria without the need for carnitine shuttle. However, dietary treatment of long-chain FAO defects using high carbohydrate with medium-even-chain triglycerides and reduced amounts of long-chain fats fails in some cases to prevent cardiomyopathy, rhabdomyolysis, and muscle weakness. In a study by Roe et al. [276], patients with long-chain FAO defects were fed a diet in which the fat component was switched from medium-even-chain triglycerides to medium-odd-chain triglycerides. In three patients with VLCAD deficiency, this treatment led to

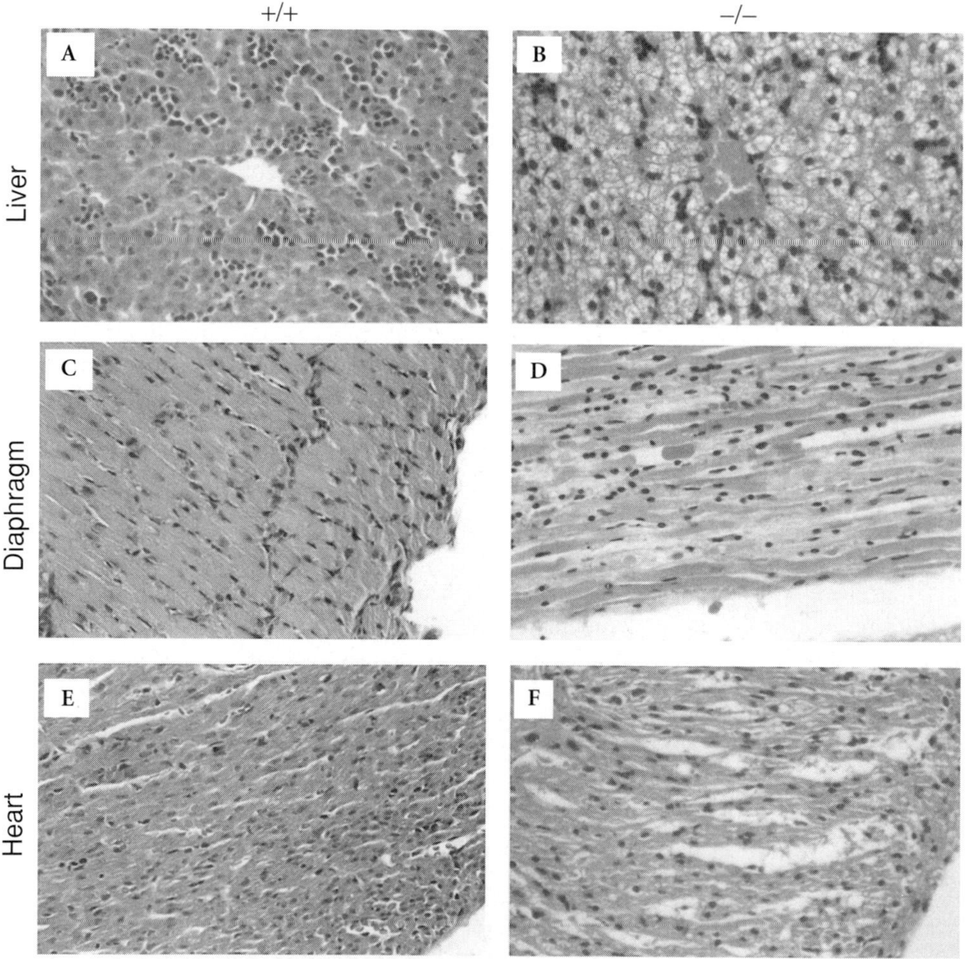

Figure 32.14. Histopathologic analysis of MTP-deficient mice. Light microscopy of sections of liver, diaphragm, and heart from 12-hour-old MTP$\alpha^{+/+}$ (**A**, **C**, and **E**) and dead MTP$\alpha^{-/-}$ (**B**, **D**, and **F**) mice at 40× magnification. Hepatic steatosis and degenerative changes in the diaphragm and heart myocytes are noted in the MTP$\alpha^{-/-}$ mice. (From Ibdah et al. [293], reproduced with permission.)

rapid clinical improvement that included the permanent disappearance of chronic cardiomyopathy, rhabdomyolysis, and muscle weakness [276]. Prior treatment with a diet containing medium-even-chain triglycerides failed to resolve these symptoms. There was no evidence of propionyl overload in these patients. The treatment has been well tolerated for up to 26 months and hence opens new avenues for the management of patients with mitochondrial FAO disorders. In another study, docosahexaenoic acid (DHA; $C_{22:6\omega\text{-}3}$) supplementation has been shown to prevent the progression of the severe chorioretinopathy that develops in children with LCHAD or MTP deficiency [277].

Although fat restriction and a high-carbohydrate intake generally have been recommended for long-term management of patients with disorders of FAO, there has been no systematic evaluation of the effect of dietary fat restriction. In patients with long-chain FAO defects, an MCT diet has been reported to be beneficial [278,279]. MCTs must not be prescribed for patients with MCAD, SCAD, ETF, or ETF-DH deficiencies. Essential fatty acid supplementation at 1–2% of total calories has been suggested when MCT supplementation is prescribed to prevent DHA deficiency, which has been hypothesized as a possible cause of the pigmentary retinopathy seen in LCHAD-deficient patients [275,280,281].

Carnitine Supplementation

The supplementation of L-carnitine has been shown to be effective only in primary carnitine deficiency, as it corrects the defect in hepatic ketogenesis and improves cardiac function and muscle strength [282]. Its use in other disorders of FAO has led to mixed results. Carnitine supplementation has the potential benefit of detoxifying accumulated acyl-CoA intermediates and replenishing the intramitochondrial carnitine pool. However, carnitine supplementation has been questioned in long-chain FAO defects because of the accumulation of long-chain fatty acylcarnitines that may cause cardiac arrhythmias [67,283]. In asymptomatic patients with MCAD deficiency, acylglycine excretion is reduced by 60% as the result of carnitine supplementation [284]. L-Carnitine supplementation in LCHAD-deficient patients resulted in improved clinical status and carnitine values [279,285]. Some patients with disorders of FAO died while being treated with carnitine [286–288], whereas others improved without carnitine supplementation [289]. Short-term L-carnitine supplementation may improve exercise tolerance in MCAD-deficient patients [290]. Recommended dosages range from 50 mg/kg/d for children to 150 mg/kg/d for adults [275].

Riboflavin Supplementation

Riboflavin supplementation with a low-fat, low-protein, and high-carbohydrate diet has been used as a therapeutic regimen in some patients with glutaric aciduria type II defects [291,292]. Its benefit is based on reducing episodes of hypoketotic hypoglycemia, vomiting, and lethargy and decreasing the excretion of urine organic acids. The recommended dosage of riboflavin is 50–150 mg/d [292].

ANIMAL MODELS FOR FATTY ACID OXIDATION DEFECTS

MTP-Deficient Mouse Model

Ibdah et al. [293] reported the generation of a mouse model that lacks the MTP. Gene targeting was used to generate an MTP α subunit null allele and produce mice that lack both the α and β subunits of the MTP. The MTP$\alpha^{-/-}$ fetuses accumulate long-chain fatty acid metabolites identical to those in humans with the deficiency. MTP$\alpha^{-/-}$ mice have low birth weight compared with heterozygous and normal littermates and suffer neonatal hypoglycemia and sudden death 6–36 hours after birth. Analysis of the histopathologic changes in the MTP$\alpha^{-/-}$ pups revealed rapid development of hepatic steatosis after birth and, later, significant necrosis and acute degeneration of the cardiac and diaphragmatic myocytes, which may be the reason for the underlying etiology of sudden death (Figure 32.14). Electron microscopy revealed swollen, hypodense mitochondria in the liver of the homozygous mice with disrupted cristae (Figure 32.15). This mouse model proves that intact mitochondrial long-chain FAO is essential for fetal development and for survival after birth. Expression studies of hepatic MTP subunits in this model revealed a significant increase in postnatal expression after birth, reaching adult expression levels within

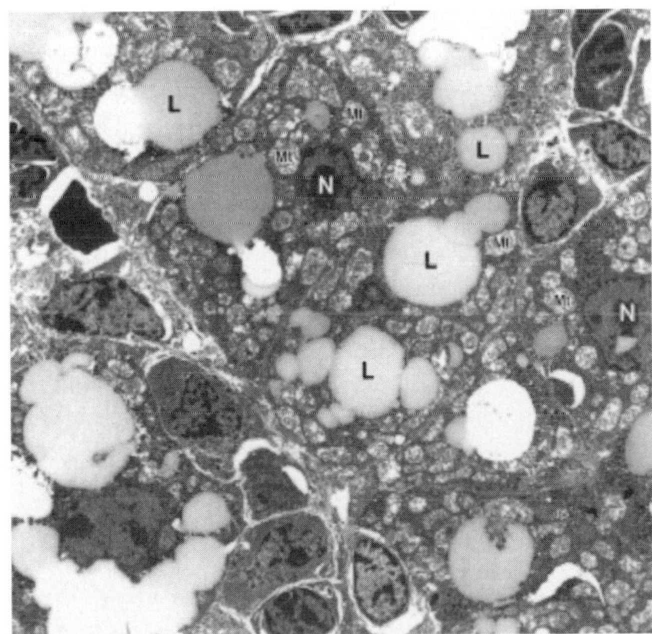

Figure 32.15. Hepatic ultrastructural changes in MTP-deficient mice. A representative electron microscopic image of a liver section from a symptomatic MTP$\alpha^{-/-}$ mouse 12 hours after birth showing extensive lipidosis, swelling, and distortion of the mitochondria. L, lipid; Mt, mitochondria; N, nucleus. (From Ibdah et al. [293], reproduced with permission.).

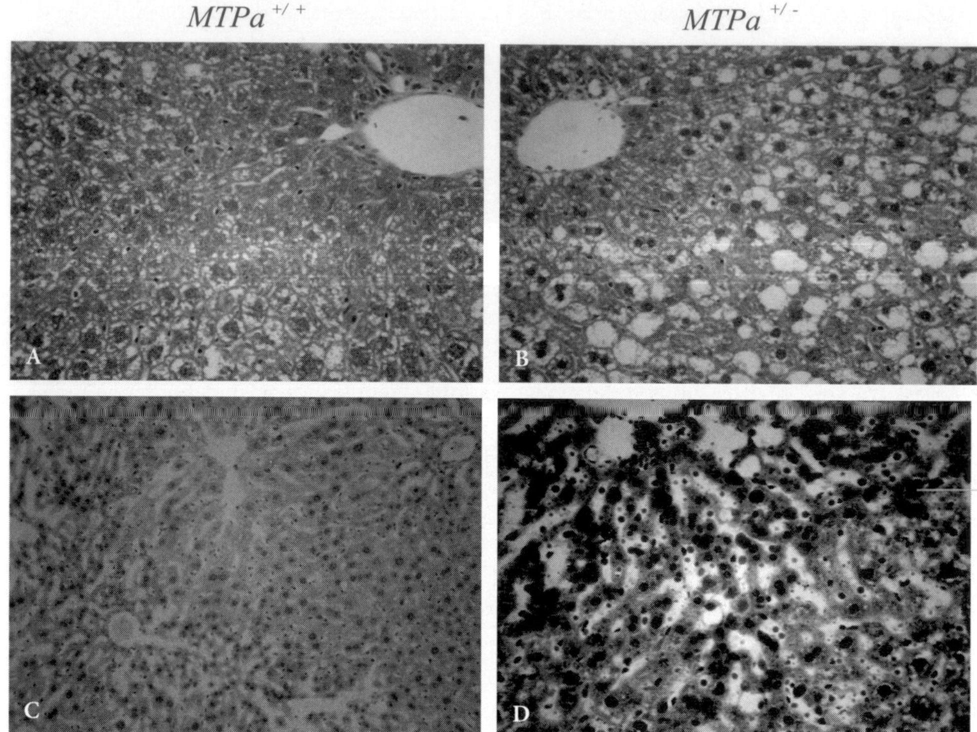

Figure 32.16. Histopathologic changes in MTP mice. Representative light microscopic images of liver sections obtained from MTP$\alpha^{+/+}$ (**A** and **C**) and MTPa$^{+/-}$ (**B** and **D**) littermates and stained with H&E (**A** and **B**) or oil red O (**C** and **D**). Micro- and macrosteatosis are noted in the liver sections from MTP$\alpha^{+/-}$ mice (dark droplets in part **D**). (From Ibdah et al. [163], reproduced with permission.)

days after birth. This suggests a reliance on FAO as a source of energy. This also coincides with the neonatal metabolic switch in nutritional fuel from glucose to maternal breast milk, which has high fat content as the nutritional source of energy. The lack of maternal phenotype in the MTP-deficient mouse model is consistent with earlier observation in families with MTP mutations causing complete MTP deficiency.

Mice heterozygous for the MTP α subunit deficiency developed hepatic steatosis and insulin resistance [163]. Aging MTP$\alpha^{+/-}$ mice, 9–10 months old, revealed hepatic macro- and microvesicular steatosis without inflammation or steatonecrosis (Figure 32.16). Electron microscopy showed swollen hepatic mitochondria with hypodense matrix and disrupted cristae. Fasting insulin levels, glucose tolerance tests, and insulin tolerance tests support the development of hyperinsulinemia and insulin resistance in aging MTP$\alpha^{+/-}$ mice. Figure 32.17 shows the histologic and ultrastructural changes in mice heterozygous for the defect compared with control wild-type littermates.

VLCAD-Deficient Mouse Model

The generation of a VLCAD-deficient mouse model was reported by Exil et al. [294]. Myocardium from VLCAD$^{-/-}$ mice showed increased fat deposition, increased collagen deposition and degenerative fibers, vacuolation, and mitochondrial proliferation compared with that from +/+ and +/− littermates. Transcription factor activator protein 2 (AP2) was moderately increased in the hearts of newborn VLCAD$^{-/-}$ mice. Adipophilin, a marker for lipid accumulation and acyl-CoA synthase 1 (ACS1), was also increased in the hearts of newborn VLCAD$^{-/-}$ mice. VLCAD deficiency in mice has a less severe phenotype compared with human VLCAD deficiency. The altered expression of genes that affect fat metabolism, ultrastructural, and physiologic changes in VLCAD-deficient mice correlates to the human disorder.

LCAD-Deficient Mouse Model

An LCAD-deficient mouse model was generated and reported in 1998 by Kurtz et al. [295]. LCAD$^{-/-}$ mice born were abnormally low in number, indicating gestational loss. LCAD$^{-/-}$ mice had reduced fasting tolerance with cardiac and hepatic lipidosis, hypoglycemia, elevated serum free fatty acids, and nonketotic dicarboxylic aciduria. Sudden death was also observed. Human patients reported to be LCAD deficient were later reclassified to be VLCAD deficient after the discovery of the *VLCAD* gene in 1992 [64]. The LCAD-deficient mouse model developed a clinical syndrome identical to human VLCAD deficiency.

MCAD-Deficient Mouse Model

The generation of an MCAD-deficient mouse model that lacked the MCAD protein was reported by Tolwani et al. [296]. Gene targeting was used to generate a truncated MCAD protein

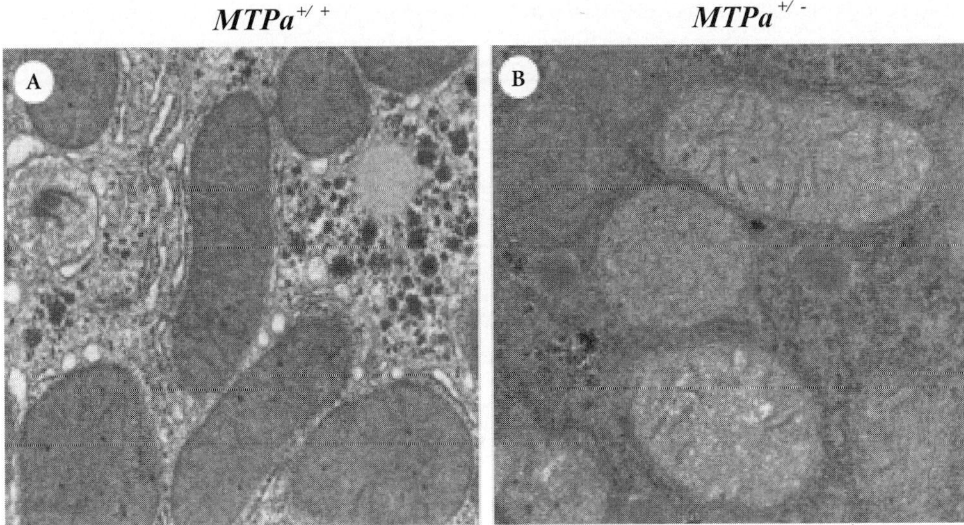

Figure 32.17. Electron micrograph of hepatocytes from MTP mice. A representative electron micrograph of hepatocytes from MTP$\alpha^{+/+}$ (**A**) and MTP$\alpha^{+/-}$ (**B**) mice at 11,700× magnification. Swollen mitochondria from MTP$\alpha^{+/-}$ can be seen, showing a hypodense matrix and disrupted cristae. (From Ibdah et al. [163], reproduced with permission.)

that was unable to tetramerize. MCAD-deficient mice developed many of the same disease characteristics seen in affected children. MCAD$^{-/-}$ pups had a high rate of neonatal loss compared with MCAD$^{+/+}$ pups. In MCAD$^{-/-}$ mice, subjection to fasting and cold stress led to lower body temperatures that resulted in death in some MCAD$^{-/-}$ mice compared with no deaths in MCAD$^{+/+}$ mice. Urine organic profiles from MCAD-deficient mice were similar to those in MCAD deficient humans. No significant differences were seen when MCAD$^{+/+}$ and MCAD$^{+/-}$ littermates were compared. Elevated $C_{10:1}$ acylcarnitine in MCAD$^{-/-}$ mice was the predominant species in contrast to C_8 acylcarnitine in humans. Histopathology revealed microvesicular and macrovesicular hepatic steatosis in MCAD$^{-/-}$ mice compared with normal histologic examination in MCAD$^{+/+}$ mice. Sporadic cardiac lesions were also observed in the MCAD$^{-/-}$ mice; these lesions have not been reported in human patients, although cardiac arrhythmias and dysfunction have been reported [297,298].

OCTN2-Deficient Mouse Model

Koizumi et al. [299] described a spontaneous mutation in a C3H-H-2(0) strain of mice that have clinical, biochemical, and histopathologic findings similar to those in Reye's syndrome. This murine model was called the juvenile visceral steatosis (JVS) mouse because of fat accumulation attributed to defective FAO caused by carnitine deficiency [300]. Nikaido et al. [301] mapped the *JVS* gene causing systemic carnitine deficiency to chromosome 11; the location was further refined by Okita et al. [302]. Subsequent work by Lu et al. [303] suggested that a missense mutation of OCTN2, a sodium-dependent carnitine cotransporter, is responsible for the phenotype in the JVS mouse. Nezu et al. [79] reported that mutations in the *SLC22A5* gene that encodes OCTN2 were responsible for loss of OCTN2 function in both the JVS mouse and in humans with primary carnitine deficiency [79].

CPT-IA–Deficient Mouse Model

A CPT-IA–deficient mouse model was generated by gene targeting producing a null allele [304]. CPT-IA deficiency in mice causes early gestational lethality, so no CPT-IA$^{-/-}$ pups, embryos, or fetuses were detected. CPT-IA$^{+/-}$ mice had decreased CPT-IA mRNA expression in the liver, heart, brain, testis, kidney, and white fat. Fasting free fatty acid concentrations were elevated and blood glucose concentrations were lower compared with CPT-IA$^{+/+}$ littermates.

SCAD-Deficient Mouse Model

The SCAD-deficient mouse was reported by Amendt et al. [305]. SCAD $^{-/-}$ mice had undetectable SCAD activity and developed severe organic aciduria and fatty liver upon fasting or dietary fat challenge. The mutant mice developed hypoglycemia after an 18-hour fast and had elevated urinary and muscle butyrylcarnitine concentrations. Ethylmalonic and methylsuccinic acids and *N*-butyrylglycine are diagnostic. Findings in the SCAD-deficient mice parallel those in the human disorder.

SUMMARY AND FUTURE DIRECTIONS

Multiple defects involving the mitochondrial oxidation of fatty acids have been recognized with significant clinical overlap and distinct biochemical signature profiles. Additional disorders of FAO are likely to be discovered. FAO disorders are associated with significant morbidity and mortality. Using MS-MS in newborn metabolic screening, it is now possible to determine the frequency of several metabolic disorders and identify affected newborns as early as possible. The availability of several mouse models for various defects of FAO will help us understand the pathophysiology of these disorders and allow testing of novel therapies, including gene therapy.

REFERENCES

1. Eaton S, Bartlett K, Pourfarzam M. Mammalian mitochondrial beta-oxidation. Biochem J 1996;320(pt 2):345–57.
2. Rinaldo P, Matern D, Bennett MJ. Fatty acid oxidation disorders. Annu Rev Physiol 2002;64:477–502.
3. Bennett MJ, Rinaldo P, Strauss AW. Inborn errors of mitochondrial fatty acid oxidation. Crit Rev Clin Lab Sci 2000;37:1–44.
4. DiMauro S, DiMauro PM. Muscle carnitine palmityltransferase deficiency and myoglobinuria. Science 1973;182:929–31.
5. McGarry JD, Foster DW. Regulation of hepatic fatty acid oxidation and ketone body production. Annu Rev Biochem 1980; 49:395–420.
6. Stanley CA, Baker L. Hyperinsulinism in infancy: diagnosis by demonstration of abnormal response to fasting hypoglycemia. Pediatrics 1976;57:702–11.
7. Eaton S. Control of mitochondrial beta-oxidation flux. Prog Lipid Res 2002;41:197–239.
8. Kalant D, Cianflone K. Regulation of fatty acid transport. Curr Opin Lipidol 2004;15:309–14.
9. Pownall HJ, Hamilton JA. Energy translocation across cell membranes and membrane models. Acta Physiol Scand 2003; 178:357–65.
10. Schaffer JE, Lodish HF. Expression cloning and characterization of a novel adipocyte long chain fatty acid transport protein. Cell 1994;79:427–36.
11. Hirsch D, Stahl A, Lodish HF. A family of fatty acid transporters conserved from mycobacterium to man. Proc Natl Acad Sci U S A 1998;95:8625–9.
12. Stahl A. A current review of fatty acid transport proteins (SLC27). Pflugers Arch 2004;447:722–7.
13. McArthur MJ, Atshaves BP, Frolov A, et al. Cellular uptake and intracellular trafficking of long chain fatty acids. J Lipid Res 1999;40:1371–83.
14. bo-Hashema KA, Cake MH, Lukas MA, Knudsen J. Evaluation of the affinity and turnover number of both hepatic mitochondrial and microsomal carnitine acyltransferases: relevance to intracellular partitioning of acyl-CoAs. Biochemistry 1999;38:15840–7.
15. McGarry JD, Brown NF. The mitochondrial carnitine palmitoyltransferase system. From concept to molecular analysis. Eur J Biochem 1997;244:1–14.
16. Steiber A, Kerner J, Hoppel CL. Carnitine: a nutritional, biosynthetic, and functional perspective. Mol Aspects Med 2004;25:455–73.
17. Bremer J. Carnitine—metabolism and functions. Physiol Rev 1983;63:1420–80.
18. Ohashi R, Tamai I, Yabuuchi H, et al. Na(+)-dependent carnitine transport by organic cation transporter (OCTN2): its pharmacological and toxicological relevance. J Pharmacol Exp Ther 1999;291:778–84.
19. Vaz FM, Wanders RJ. Carnitine biosynthesis in mammals. Biochem J 2002;361(pt 3):417–29.
20. Chalmers RA, Roe CR, Stacey TE, Hoppel CL. Urinary excretion of l-carnitine and acylcarnitines by patients with disorders of organic acid metabolism: evidence for secondary insufficiency of l-carnitine. Pediatr Res 1984;18:1325–8.
21. Corkey BE, Hale DE, Glennon MC, et al. Relationship between unusual hepatic acyl coenzyme A profiles and the pathogenesis of Reye syndrome. J Clin Invest 1988;82:782–8.
22. Latipaa PM, Peuhkurinen KJ, Hiltunen JK, Hassinen IE. Regulation of pyruvate dehydrogenase during infusion of fatty acids of varying chain lengths in the perfused rat heart. J Mol Cell Cardiol 1985;17:1161–71.
23. McGarry JD, Woeltje KF, Schroeder JG, et al. Carnitine palmitoyltransferase—structure/function/regulatory relationships. Prog Clin Biol Res 1990;321:193–208.
24. Wang L, Brady PS, Brady LJ. Hormonal regulation of carnitine palmitoyltransferase synthesis in H4IIE cells. Prog Clin Biol Res 1990;321:209–16.
25. Leone TC, Weinheimer CJ, Kelly DP. A critical role for the peroxisome proliferator-activated receptor alpha (PPARalpha) in the cellular fasting response: the PPARalpha-null mouse as a model of fatty acid oxidation disorders. Proc Natl Acad Sci U S A 1999;96:7473–8.
26. Matsubara Y, Indo Y, Naito E, et al. Molecular cloning and nucleotide sequence of cDNAs encoding the precursors of rat long chain acyl-coenzyme A, short chain acyl-coenzyme A, and isovaleryl-coenzyme A dehydrogenases. Sequence homology of four enzymes of the acyl-CoA dehydrogenase family. J Biol Chem 1989;264:16321–31.
27. Aoyama T, Souri M, Ushikubo S, et al. Purification of human very-long-chain acyl-coenzyme A dehydrogenase and characterization of its deficiency in seven patients. J Clin Invest 1995;95:2465–73.
28. Andresen BS, Bross P, Vianey-Saban C, et al. Cloning and characterization of human very-long-chain acyl-CoA dehydrogenase cDNA, chromosomal assignment of the gene and identification in four patients of nine different mutations within the VLCAD gene. Hum Mol Genet 1996;5:461–72.
29. Orii KO, Aoyama T, Souri M, et al. Genomic DNA organization of human mitochondrial very-long-chain acyl-CoA dehydrogenase and mutation analysis. Biochem Biophys Res Commun 1995;217:987–92.
30. Indo Y, Yang-Feng T, Glassberg R, Tanaka K. Molecular cloning and nucleotide sequence of cDNAs encoding human long-chain acyl-CoA dehydrogenase and assignment of the location of its gene (ACADL) to chromosome 2. Genomics 1992;12:626.
31. Indo Y, Yang-Feng T, Glassberg R, Tanaka K. Molecular cloning and nucleotide sequence of cDNAs encoding human long-chain acyl-CoA dehydrogenase and assignment of the location of its gene (ACADL) to chromosome 2. Genomics 1991;11:609–20.
32. Kidd JR, Matsubara Y, Castiglione CM, et al. The locus for the medium-chain acyl-CoA dehydrogenase gene on chromosome 1 is highly polymorphic. Genomics 1990;6:89–93.
33. Corydon MJ, Andresen BS, Bross P, et al. Structural organization of the human short-chain acyl-CoA dehydrogenase gene. Mamm Genome 1997;8:922–6.
34. Matsubara Y, Kraus JP, Yang-Feng TL, et al. Molecular cloning of cDNAs encoding rat and human medium-chain acyl-CoA dehydrogenase and assignment of the gene to human chromosome 1. Proc Natl Acad Sci U S A 1986;83:6543–7.

35. Naito E, Ozasa H, Ikeda Y, Tanaka K. Molecular cloning and nucleotide sequence of complementary DNAs encoding human short chain acyl-coenzyme A dehydrogenase and the study of the molecular basis of human short chain acyl-coenzyme A dehydrogenase deficiency. J Clin Invest 1989;83:1605–13.
36. Janssen U, Davis EM, Le Beau MM, Stoffel W. Human mitochondrial enoyl-CoA hydratase gene (ECHS1): structural organization and assignment to chromosome 10q26.2-q26.3. Genomics 1997;40:470–5.
37. Vredendaal PJ, van dB, I, Malingre HE, et al. Human short-chain L-3-hydroxyacyl-CoA dehydrogenase: cloning and characterization of the coding sequence. Biochem Biophys Res Commun 1996;223:718–23.
38. Uchida Y, Izai K, Orii T, Hashimoto T. Novel fatty acid beta-oxidation enzymes in rat liver mitochondria. II. Purification and properties of enoyl-coenzyme A (CoA) hydratase/3-hydroxyacyl-CoA dehydrogenase/3-ketoacyl-CoA thiolase trifunctional protein. J Biol Chem 1992;267:1034–41.
39. Jackson S, Kler RS, Bartlett K, et al. Combined enzyme defect of mitochondrial fatty acid oxidation. J Clin Invest 1992;90:1219–25.
40. Carpenter K, Pollitt RJ, Middleton B. Human liver long-chain 3-hydroxyacyl-coenzyme A dehydrogenase is a multifunctional membrane-bound beta-oxidation enzyme of mitochondria. Biochem Biophys Res Commun 1992;183:443–8.
41. Weinberger MJ, Rinaldo P, Strauss AW, Bennett MJ. Intact alpha-subunit is required for membrane-binding of human mitochondrial trifunctional beta-oxidation protein, but is not necessary for conferring 3-ketoacyl-CoA thiolase activity to the beta-subunit. Biochem Biophys Res Commun 1995;209:47–52.
42. Ushikubo S, Aoyama T, Kamijo T, et al. Molecular characterization of mitochondrial trifunctional protein deficiency: formation of the enzyme complex is important for stabilization of both alpha- and beta-subunits. Am J Hum Genet 1996;58: 979–88.
43. Kamijo T, Wanders RJ, Saudubray JM, et al. Mitochondrial trifunctional protein deficiency. Catalytic heterogeneity of the mutant enzyme in two patients. J Clin Invest 1994;93:1740–7.
44. Sims HF, Brackett JC, Powell CK, et al. The molecular basis of pediatric long chain 3-hydroxyacyl-CoA dehydrogenase deficiency associated with maternal acute fatty liver of pregnancy. Proc Natl Acad Sci U S A 1995;92:841–5.
45. Aoyama T, Wakui K, Orii KE, et al. Fluorescence in situ hybridization mapping of the alpha and beta subunits (HADHA and HADHB) of human mitochondrial fatty acid beta-oxidation multienzyme complex to 2p23 and their evolution. Cytogenet Cell Genet 1997;79:221–4.
46. Orii KE, Orii KO, Souri M, et al. Genes for the human mitochondrial trifunctional protein alpha- and beta-subunits are divergently transcribed from a common promoter region. J Biol Chem 1999;274:8077–84.
47. Finocchiaro G, Ito M, Ikeda Y, Tanaka K. Molecular cloning and nucleotide sequence of cDNAs encoding the alpha-subunit of human electron transfer flavoprotein. J Biol Chem 1988;263:15773–80.
48. Finocchiaro G, Colombo I, Garavaglia B, et al. cDNA cloning and mitochondrial import of the beta-subunit of the human electron-transfer flavoprotein. Eur J Biochem 1993;213: 1003–8.
49. Beard SE, Goodman SI, Bemelen K, Frerman FE. Characterization of a mutation that abolishes quinone reduction by electron transfer flavoprotein-ubiquinone oxidoreductase. Hum Mol Genet 1995;4:157–61.
50. Gregersen N. Fatty acyl-CoA dehydrogenase deficiency: enzyme measurement and studies on alternative metabolism. J Inherit Metab Dis 1984;7(suppl 1):28–32.
51. Osumi T, Hashimoto T, Ui N. Purification and properties of acyl-CoA oxidase from rat liver. J Biochem (Tokyo) 1980;87:1735–46.
52. Van Veldhoven PP, Just WW, Mannaerts GP. Permeability of the peroxisomalmembrane to cofactors of beta-oxidation. Evidence for the presence of a pore-forming protein. J Biol Chem 1987;262:4310–18.
53. Lazarow PB, De DC. A fatty acyl-CoA oxidizing system in rat liver peroxisomes; enhancement by clofibrate, a hypolipidemic drug. Proc Natl Acad Sci U S A 1976;73:2043–6.
54. Mannaerts GP, Debeer LJ, Thomas J, De Schepper PJ. Mitochondrial and peroxisomal fatty acid oxidation in liver homogenates and isolated hepatocytes from control and clofibrate-treated rats. J Biol Chem 1979;254:4585–95.
55. Wanders RJ, van Roermund CW, van Wijland MJ, et al. Peroxisomal fatty acid beta-oxidation in relation to the accumulation of very long chain fatty acids in cultured skin fibroblasts from patients with Zellweger syndrome and other peroxisomal disorders. J Clin Invest 1987;80:1778–83.
56. Gregersen N, Mortensen PB, Kolvraa S. On the biologic origin of C6-C10 dicarboxylic and C6-C10-omega-1-hydroxy monocarboxylic acids in human and rat with acyl-CoA dehydrogenation deficiencies: in vitro studies on the omega- and omega-1-oxidation of medium-chain (C6-C12) fatty acids in human and rat liver. Pediatr Res 1983;17:828–34.
57. Tanaka K, Yokota I, Coates PM, et al. Mutations in the medium chain acyl-CoA dehydrogenase (MCAD) gene. Hum Mutat 1992;1:271–9.
58. Wanders RJ, Duran M, Ijlst L et al. Sudden infant death and long-chain 3-hydroxyacyl-CoA dehydrogenase. Lancet 1989;2:52–3.
59. Vianey-Liaud C, Divry P, Gregersen N, Mathieu M. The inborn errors of mitochondrial fatty acid oxidation. J Inherit Metab Dis 1987;10(suppl 1):159–200.
60. Gregersen N, Bross P, Andresen BS. Genetic defects in fatty acid beta-oxidation and acyl-CoA dehydrogenases. Molecular pathogenesis and genotype-phenotype relationships. Eur J Biochem 2004;271:470–82.
61. Izai K, Uchida Y, Orii T, et al. Novel fatty acid beta-oxidation enzymes in rat liver mitochondria. I. Purification and properties of very-long-chain acyl-coenzyme A dehydrogenase. J Biol Chem 1992;267:1027–33.
62. Treem WR, Witzleben CA, Piccoli DA, et al. Medium-chain and long-chain acyl CoA dehydrogenase deficiency: clinical, pathologic and ultrastructural differentiation from Reye's syndrome. Hepatology 1986;6:1270–8.
63. Indo Y, Coates PM, Hale DE, Tanaka K. Immunochemical characterization of variant long-chain acyl-CoA dehydrogenase in cultured fibroblasts from nine patients with long-chain acyl-CoA dehydrogenase deficiency. Pediatr Res 1991;30:211–15.
64. Yamaguchi S, Indo Y, Coates PM, et al. Identification of very-long-chain acyl-CoA dehydrogenase deficiency in three patients previously diagnosed with long-chain acyl-CoA dehydrogenase deficiency. Pediatr Res 1993;34:111–13.
65. Rinaldo P, Matern D. Disorders of fatty acid transport and mitochondrial oxidation: challenges and dilemmas of metabolic evaluation. Genet Med 2000;2:338–44.

66. Tein I. Neonatal metabolic myopathies. Semin Perinatol 1999;23:125–51.
67. Bonnet D, Martin D, Pascale DL, et al. Arrhythmias and conduction defects as presenting symptoms of fatty acid oxidation disorders in children. Circulation 1999;100:2248–53.
68. Odaib AA, Shneider BL, Bennett MJ, et al. A defect in the transport of long-chain fatty acids associated with acute liver failure. N Engl J Med 1998;339:1752–7.
69. Wang Y, Korman SH, Ye J, et al. Phenotype and genotype variation in primary carnitine deficiency. Genet Med 2001;3:387–92.
70. Treem WR, Stanley CA, Finegold DN, et al. Primary carnitine deficiency due to a failure of carnitine transport in kidney, muscle, and fibroblasts. N Engl J Med 1988;319:1331–6.
71. Lamhonwah AM, Tein I. Carnitine uptake defect: frameshift mutations in the human plasmalemmal carnitine transporter gene. Biochem Biophys Res Commun 1998;252:396–401.
72. Stanley CA, DeLeeuw S, Coates PM, et al. Chronic cardiomyopathy and weakness or acute coma in children with a defect in carnitine uptake. Ann Neurol 1991;30:709–16.
73. Tein I, De V, Bierman F, et al. Impaired skin fibroblast carnitine uptake in primary systemic carnitine deficiency manifested by childhood carnitine-responsive cardiomyopathy. Pediatr Res 1990;28:247–55.
74. Garavaglia B, Uziel G, Dworzak F, et al. Primary carnitine deficiency: heterozygote and intrafamilial phenotypic variation. Neurology 1991;41:1691–3.
75. Makhseed N, Vallance HD, Potter M, et al. Carnitine transporter defect due to a novel mutation in the SLC22A5 gene presenting with peripheral neuropathy. J Inherit Metab Dis 2004;27:778–80.
76. Rinaldo P, Stanley CA, Hsu BY, et al. Sudden neonatal death in carnitine transporter deficiency. J Pediatr 1997;131:304–5.
77. Melegh B, Bene J, Mogyorosy G, et al. Phenotypic manifestations of the OCTN2 V295X mutation: sudden infant death and carnitine-responsive cardiomyopathy in Roma families. Am J Med Genet A 2004;131:121–6.
78. Wang Y, Ye J, Ganapathy V, Longo N. Mutations in the organic cation/carnitine transporter OCTN2 in primary carnitine deficiency. Proc Natl Acad Sci U S A 1999;96:2356–60.
79. Nezu J, Tamai I, Oku A, et al. Primary systemic carnitine deficiency is caused by mutations in a gene encoding sodium ion-dependent carnitine transporter. Nat Genet 1999;21:91–4.
80. Tang NL, Ganapathy V, Wu X, et al. Mutations of OCTN2, an organic cation/carnitine transporter, lead to deficient cellular carnitine uptake in primary carnitine deficiency. Hum Mol Genet 1999;8:655–60.
81. Wilcken B, Wiley V, Sim KG, Carpenter K. Carnitine transporter defect diagnosed by newborn screening with electrospray tandem mass spectrometry. J Pediatr 2001;138:581–4.
82. Scaglia F, Wang Y, Singh RH, et al. Defective urinary carnitine transport in heterozygotes for primary carnitine deficiency. Genet Med 1998;1:34–9.
83. Koizumi A, Nozaki J, Ohura T, et al. Genetic epidemiology of the carnitine transporter OCTN2 gene in a Japanese population and phenotypic characterization in Japanese pedigrees with primary systemic carnitine deficiency. Hum Mol Genet 1999;8:2247–54.
84. Britton CH, Schultz RA, Zhang B, et al. Human liver mitochondrial carnitine palmitoyltransferase I: characterization of its cDNA and chromosomal localization and partial analysis of the gene. Proc Natl Acad Sci U S A 1995;92:1984–8.
85. Britton CH, Mackey DW, Esser V, et al. Fine chromosome mapping of the genes for human liver and muscle carnitine palmitoyltransferase I (CPT1A and CPT1B). Genomics 1997;40:209–11.
86. Price N, van der LF, Jackson V, et al. A novel brain-expressed protein related to carnitine palmitoyltransferase I. Genomics 2002;80:433–42.
87. Falik-Borenstein ZC, Jordan SC, Saudubray JM, et al. Brief report: renal tubular acidosis in carnitine palmitoyltransferase type 1 deficiency. N Engl J Med 1992;327:24–7.
88. Olpin SE, Allen J, Bonham JR, et al. Features of carnitine palmitoyltransferase type I deficiency. J Inherit Metab Dis 2001;24:35–42.
89. Innes AM, Seargeant LE, Balachandra K, et al. Hepatic carnitine palmitoyltransferase I deficiency presenting as maternal illness in pregnancy. Pediatr Res 2000;47:43–5.
90. Fingerhut R, Roschinger W, Muntau AC, et al. Hepatic carnitine palmitoyltransferase I deficiency: acylcarnitine profiles in blood spots are highly specific. Clin Chim 2001;47:1763–8.
91. Stanley CA, Sunaryo F, Hale DE, et al. Elevated plasma carnitine in the hepatic form of carnitine palmitoyltransferase-1 deficiency. J Inherit Metab Dis 1992;15:785–9.
92. Korman SH, Waterham HR, Gutman A, et al. Novel metabolic and molecular findings in hepatic carnitine palmitoyltransferase I deficiency. Mol Genet Metab 2005;86:337–43.
93. Bergman AJ, Donckerwolcke RA, Duran M, et al. Rate-dependent distal renal tubular acidosis and carnitine palmitoyltransferase I deficiency. Pediatr Res 1994;36:582–8.
94. Bennett MJ, Boriack RL, Narayan S, et al. Novel mutations in CPT 1A define molecular heterogeneity of hepatic carnitine palmitoyltransferase I deficiency. Mol Genet Metab 2004;82:59–63.
95. Ijlst L, Mandel H, Oostheim W, et al. Molecular basis of hepatic carnitine palmitoyltransferase I deficiency. J Clin Invest 1998;102:527–31.
96. Prasad C, Johnson JP, Bonnefont JP, et al. Hepatic carnitine palmitoyl transferase 1 (CPT1 A) deficiency in North American Hutterites (Canadian and American): evidence for a founder effect and results of a pilot study on a DNA-based newborn screening program. Mol Genet Metab 2001;73:55–63.
97. Prip-Buus C, Thuillier L, Abadi N, et al. Molecular and enzymatic characterization of a unique carnitine palmitoyltransferase 1A mutation in the Hutterite community. Mol Genet Metab 2001;73:46–54.
98. Stoler JM, Sabry MA, Hanley C, et al. Successful long-term treatment of hepatic carnitine palmitoyltransferase I deficiency and a novel mutation. J Inherit Metab Dis 2004;27:679–84.
99. Pande SV, Parvin R. Carnitine-acylcarnitine translocase catalyzes an equilibrating unidirectional transport as well. J Biol Chem 1980;255:2994–3001.
100. Stanley CA, Hale DE, Berry GT, et al. Brief report: a deficiency of carnitine-acylcarnitine translocase in the inner mitochondrial membrane. N Engl J Med 1992;327:19–23.
101. Chalmers RA, Stanley CA, English N, Wigglesworth JS. Mitochondrial carnitine-acylcarnitine translocase deficiency presenting as sudden neonatal death. J Pediatr 1997;131:220–5.
102. Pande SV, Brivet M, Slama A, et al. Carnitine-acylcarnitine translocase deficiency with severe hypoglycemia and atrioventricular block. Translocase assay in permeabilized fibroblasts. J Clin Invest 1993;91:1247–52.

103. Roschinger W, Muntau AC, Duran M, et al. Carnitine-acylcarnitine translocase deficiency: metabolic consequences of an impaired mitochondrial carnitine cycle. Clin Chim Acta 2000;298:55–68.
104. Olpin SE, Bonham JR, Downing M, et al. Carnitine-acylcarnitine translocase deficiency—a mild phenotype. J Inherit Metab Dis 1997;20:714–15.
105. Morris AA, Olpin SE, Brivet M, et al. A patient with carnitine-acylcarnitine translocase deficiency with a mild phenotype. J Pediatr 1998;132(3 pt 1):514–16.
106. Pande SV. Carnitine-acylcarnitine translocase deficiency. Am J Med Sci 1999;318:22–7.
107. Roe DS, Yang BZ, Vianey-Saban C, et al. Differentiation of long-chain fatty acid oxidation disorders using alternative precursors and acylcarnitine profiling in fibroblasts. Mol Genet Metab 2006;87:40–7.
108. Thuillier L, Rostane H, Droin V, et al. Correlation between genotype, metabolic data, and clinical presentation in carnitine palmitoyltransferase 2 (CPT2) deficiency. Hum Mutat 2003;21:493–501.
109. North KN, Hoppel CL, De GU, et al. Lethal neonatal deficiency of carnitine palmitoyltransferase II associated with dysgenesis of the brain and kidneys. J Pediatr 1995;127:414–20.
110. Pierce MR, Pridjian G, Morrison S, Pickoff AS. Fatal carnitine palmitoyltransferase II deficiency in a newborn: new phenotypic features. Clin Pediatr (Phila) 1999;38:13–20.
111. Bonnefont JP, Demaugre F, Prip-Buus C, et al. Carnitine palmitoyltransferase deficiencies. Mol Genet Metab 1999;68:424–40.
112. Taggart RT, Smail D, Apolito C, Vladutiu GD. Novel mutations associated with carnitine palmitoyltransferase II deficiency. Hum Mutat 1999;13:210–20.
113. Vladutiu GD, Bennett MJ, Smail D, et al. A variable myopathy associated with heterozygosity for the R503C mutation in the carnitine palmitoyltransferase II gene. Mol Genet Metab 2000;70:134–41.
114. Djouadi F, Bonnefont JP, Thuillier L, et al. Correction of fatty acid oxidation in carnitine palmitoyl transferase 2-deficient cultured skin fibroblasts by bezafibrate. Pediatr Res 2003;54:446–51.
115. Gregersen N, Andresen BS, Corydon MJ, et al. Mutation analysis in mitochondrial fatty acid oxidation defects: exemplified by acyl-CoA dehydrogenase deficiencies, with special focus on genotype-phenotype relationship. Hum Mutat 2001;18:169–89.
116. Millington DS, Terada N, Chace DH, et al. The role of tandem mass spectrometry in the diagnosis of fatty acid oxidation disorders. Prog Clin Biol Res 1992;375:339–54.
117. Wanders RJ, Vreken P, den Boer ME, et al. Disorders of mitochondrial fatty acyl-CoA beta-oxidation. J Inherit Metab Dis 1999;22:442–87.
118. Roe DS, Vianey-Saban C, Sharma S, et al. Oxidation of unsaturated fatty acids by human fibroblasts with very-long-chain acyl-CoA dehydrogenase deficiency: aspects of substrate specificity and correlation with clinical phenotype. Clin Chim Acta 2001;312:55–67.
119. Wood JC, Magera MJ, Rinaldo P, et al. Diagnosis of very long chain acyl-dehydrogenase deficiency from an infant's newborn screening card. Pediatrics 2001;108:E19.
120. Spiekerkoetter U, Sun B, Zytkovicz T, et al. MS/MS-based newborn and family screening detects asymptomatic patients with very-long-chain acyl-CoA dehydrogenase deficiency. J Pediatr 2003;143:335–42.
121. Amendt BA, Moon A, Teel L, Rhead WJ. Long-chain acyl-coenzyme A dehydrogenase deficiency: biochemical studies in fibroblasts from three patients. Pediatr Res 1988;23:603–5.
122. Djouadi F, Aubey F, Schlemmer D, et al. Bezafibrate increases very-long-chain acyl-CoA dehydrogenase protein and mRNA expression in deficient fibroblasts and is a potential therapy for fatty acid oxidation disorders. Hum Mol Genet 2005;14:2695–703.
123. Ibdah JA, Bennett MJ, Rinaldo P, et al. A fetal fatty acid oxidation disorder as a cause of liver disease in pregnant women. N Engl J Med 1999;340:1723–31.
124. Ibdah JA, Tein I, Dionisi-Vici C, et al. Mild trifunctional protein deficiency is associated with progressive neuropathy and myopathy and suggests a novel genotype-phenotype correlation. J Clin Invest 1998;102:1193–9.
125. Ijlst L, Wanders RJ, Ushikubo S, et al. Molecular basis of long-chain 3-hydroxyacyl-CoA dehydrogenase deficiency: identification of the major disease-causing mutation in the alpha-subunit of the mitochondrial trifunctional protein. Biochim Biophys Acta 1994;1215:347–50.
126. Rinaldo P, Raymond K, al-Odaib A, Bennett MJ. Clinical and biochemical features of fatty acid oxidation disorders. Curr Opin Pediatr 1998;10:615–21.
127. Pons R, Roig M, Riudor E, et al. The clinical spectrum of long-chain 3-hydroxyacyl-CoA dehydrogenase deficiency. Pediatr Neurol 1996;14:236–43.
128. Bertini E, Dionisi-Vici C, Garavaglia B, et al. Peripheral sensory-motor polyneuropathy, pigmentary retinopathy, and fatal cardiomyopathy in long-chain 3-hydroxy-acyl-CoA dehydrogenase deficiency. Eur J Pediatr 1992;151:121–6.
129. Dionisi-Vici C, Garavaglia B, Burlina AB, et al. Hypoparathyroidism in mitochondrial trifunctional protein deficiency. J Pediatr 1996;129:159–62.
130. Ibdah JA, Dasouki MJ, Strauss AW. Long-chain 3-hydroxyacyl-CoA dehydrogenase deficiency: variable expressivity of maternal illness during pregnancy and unusual presentation with infantile cholestasis and hypocalcaemia. J Inherit Metab Dis 1999;22:811–14.
131. Amirkhan RH, Timmons CF, Brown KO, et al. Clinical, biochemical, and morphologic investigations of a case of long-chain 3-hydroxyacyl-CoA dehydrogenase deficiency. Arch Pathol Lab Med 1997;121:730–4.
132. Schaefer J, Jackson S, Dick DJ, Turnbull DM. Trifunctional enzyme deficiency: adult presentation of a usually fatal beta-oxidation defect. Ann Neurol 1996;40:597–602.
133. Tyni T, Palotie A, Viinikka L, et al. Long-chain 3-hydroxyacyl-coenzyme A dehydrogenase deficiency with the G1528C mutation: clinical presentation of thirteen patients. J Pediatr 1997;130:67–76.
134. Miyajima H, Orii KE, Shindo Y, et al. Mitochondrial trifunctional protein deficiency associated with recurrent myoglobinuria in adolescence. Neurology 1997;49:833–7.
135. Tyni T, Ekholm E, Pihko H. Pregnancy complications are frequent in long-chain 3-hydroxyacyl-coenzyme A dehydrogenase deficiency. Am J Obstet Gynecol 1998;178:603–8.
136. Yang Z, Zhao Y, Bennett MJ, et al. Fetal genotypes and pregnancy outcomes in 35 families with mitochondrial trifunctional protein mutations. Am J Obstet Gynecol 2002;187:715–20.
137. Tyni T, Kivela T, Lappi M, et al. Ophthalmologic findings in long-chain 3-hydroxyacyl-CoA dehydrogenase deficiency

caused by the G1528C mutation: a new type of hereditary metabolic chorioretinopathy. Ophthalmology 1998;105:810–24.

138. Tyni T, Pihko H, Kivela T. Ophthalmic pathology in long-chain 3-hydroxyacyl-CoA dehydrogenase deficiency caused by the G1528C mutation. Curr Eye Res 1998;17:551–9.

139. Lawlor DP, Kalina RE. Pigmentary retinopathy in long chain 3-hydroxyacyl-coenzyme A dehydrogenase deficiency. Am J Ophthalmol 1997;123:846–8.

140. Ijlst L, Ruiter JP, Hoovers JM, et al. Common missense mutation G1528C in long-chain 3-hydroxyacyl-CoA dehydrogenase deficiency. Characterization and expression of the mutant protein, mutation analysis on genomic DNA and chromosomal localization of the mitochondrial trifunctional protein alpha subunit gene. J Clin Invest 1996;98:1028–33.

141. Barycki JJ, O'Brien LK, Bratt JM, et al. Biochemical characterization and crystal structure determination of human heart short chain L-3-hydroxyacyl-CoA dehydrogenase provide insights into catalytic mechanism. Biochemistry 1999;38:5786–98.

142. Engel CK, Kiema TR, Hiltunen JK, Wierenga RK. The crystal structure of enoyl-CoA hydratase complexed with octanoyl-CoA reveals the structural adaptations required for binding of a long chain fatty acid-CoA molecule. J Mol Biol 1998;275:847–59.

143. Spiekerkoetter U, Sun B, Khuchua Z, et al. Molecular and phenotypic heterogeneity in mitochondrial trifunctional protein deficiency due to beta-subunit mutations. Hum Mutat 2003;21:598–607.

144. Schwab KO, Ensenauer R, Matern D, et al. Complete deficiency of mitochondrial trifunctional protein due to a novel mutation within the beta-subunit of the mitochondrial trifunctional protein gene leads to failure of long-chain fatty acid beta-oxidation with fatal outcome. Eur J Pediatr 2003;162:90–5.

145. Orii KE, Aoyama T, Wakui K, et al. Genomic and mutational analysis of the mitochondrial trifunctional protein beta-subunit (HADHB) gene in patients with trifunctional protein deficiency. Hum Mol Genet 1997;6:1215–24.

146. Clark-Taylor T, Clark-Taylor BE. Is autism a disorder of fatty acid metabolism? Possible dysfunction of mitochondrial beta-oxidation by long chain acyl-CoA dehydrogenase. Med Hypotheses 2004;62:970–5.

147. Cox KB, Hamm DA, Millington DS, et al. Gestational, pathologic and biochemical differences between very long-chain acyl-CoA dehydrogenase deficiency and long-chain acyl-CoA dehydrogenase deficiency in the mouse. Hum Mol Genet 2001;10:2069–77.

148. Stanley CA, Hale DE, Coates PM, et al. Medium-chain acyl-CoA dehydrogenase deficiency in children with non-ketotic hypoglycemia and low carnitine levels. Pediatr Res 1983;17:877–84.

149. Kolvraa S, Gregersen N, Christensen E, Hobolth N. In vitro fibroblast studies in a patient with C6-C10-dicarboxylic aciduria: evidence for a defect in general acyl-CoA dehydrogenase. Clin Chim Acta 1982;126:53–67.

150. Rhead WJ, Amendt BA, Fritchman KS, Felts SJ. Dicarboxylic aciduria: deficient [1–14C]octanoate oxidation and medium-chain acyl-CoA dehydrogenase in fibroblasts. Science 1983;221:73–5.

151. Iafolla AK, Thompson RJ Jr, Roe CR. Medium-chain acyl-coenzyme A dehydrogenase deficiency: clinical course in 120 affected children. J Pediatr 1994;124:409–15.

152. Kelly DP, Whelan AJ, Ogden ML, et al. Molecular characterization of inherited medium-chain acyl-CoA dehydrogenase deficiency. Proc Natl Acad Sci U S A 1990;87:9236–40.

153. Yokota I, Indo Y, Coates PM, Tanaka K. Molecular basis of medium chain acyl-coenzyme A dehydrogenase deficiency. An A to G transition at position 985 that causes a lysine-304 to glutamate substitution in the mature protein is the single prevalent mutation. J Clin Invest 1990;86:1000–3.

154. Yang BZ, Ding JH, Zhou C, et al. Identification of a novel mutation in patients with medium-chain acyl-CoA dehydrogenase deficiency. Mol Genet Metab 2000;69:259–62.

155. Rinaldo P, O'Shea JJ, Coates PM, et al. Medium-chain acyl-CoA dehydrogenase deficiency. Diagnosis by stable-isotope dilution measurement of urinary n-hexanoylglycine and 3-phenylpropionylglycine. N Engl J Med 1988;319:1308–13.

156. Van Hove JL, Zhang W, Kahler SG, et al. Medium-chain acyl-CoA dehydrogenase (MCAD) deficiency: diagnosis by acylcarnitine analysis in blood. Am J Hum Genet 1993;52:958–66.

157. Clayton PT, Doig M, Ghafari S, et al. Screening for medium chain acyl-CoA dehydrogenase deficiency using electrospray ionization tandem mass spectrometry. Arch Dis Child 1998;79:109–15.

158. Kobayashi A, Jiang LL, Hashimoto T. Two mitochondrial 3-hydroxyacyl-CoA dehydrogenases in bovine liver. J Biochem (Tokyo) 1996;119:775–82.

159. Tein I, De V, Hale DE, et al. Short-chain L-3-hydroxyacyl-CoA dehydrogenase deficiency in muscle: a new cause for recurrent myoglobinuria and encephalopathy. Ann Neurol 1991;30:415–19.

160. Bennett MJ, Weinberger MJ, Kobori JA, et al. Mitochondrial short-chain L-3-hydroxyacyl-coenzyme A dehydrogenase deficiency: a new defect of fatty acid oxidation. Pediatr Res 1996;39:185–8.

161. Clayton PT, Eaton S, Aynsley-Green A, et al. Hyperinsulinism in short-chain L-3-hydroxyacyl-CoA dehydrogenase deficiency reveals the importance of beta-oxidation in insulin secretion. J Clin Invest 2001;108:457–65.

162. Molven A, Matre GE, Duran M, et al. Familial hyperinsulinemic hypoglycemia caused by a defect in the SCHAD enzyme of mitochondrial fatty acid oxidation. Diabetes 2004;53:221–7.

163. Ibdah JA, Perlegas P, Zhao Y, et al. Mice heterozygous for a defect in mitochondrial trifunctional protein develop hepatic steatosis and insulin resistance. Gastroenterology 2005;128:1381–90.

164. Eaton S, Chatziandreou I, Krywawych S, et al. Short-chain 3-hydroxyacyl-CoA dehydrogenase deficiency associated with hyperinsulinism: a novel glucose-fatty acid cycle? Biochem Soc Trans 2003;31(pt 6):1137–9.

165. Kamijo T, Indo Y, Souri M, et al. Medium chain 3-ketoacyl-coenzyme A thiolase deficiency: a new disorder of mitochondrial fatty acid beta-oxidation. Pediatr Res 1997;42:569–76.

166. Turnbull DM, Bartlett K, Stevens DL, et al. Short-chain acyl-CoA dehydrogenase deficiency associated with a lipid-storage myopathy and secondary carnitine deficiency. N Engl J Med 1984;311:1232–6.

167. Amendt BA, Greene C, Sweetman L, et al. Short-chain acyl-coenzyme A dehydrogenase deficiency. Clinical and biochemical studies in two patients. J Clin Invest 1987;79:1303–9.

168. Corydon MJ, Vockley J, Rinaldo P, et al. Role of common gene variations in the molecular pathogenesis of short-chain acyl-CoA dehydrogenase deficiency. Pediatr Res 2001;49:18–23.

169. Nagan N, Kruckeberg KE, Tauscher AL, et al. The frequency of short-chain acyl-CoA dehydrogenase gene variants in the US population and correlation with the C(4)-acylcarnitine concentration in newborn blood spots. Mol Genet Metab 2003;78:239–46.
170. Gregersen N, Winter VS, Corydon MJ, et al. Identification of four new mutations in the short-chain acyl-CoA dehydrogenase (SCAD) gene in two patients: one of the variant alleles, 511C(r)T, is present at an unexpectedly high frequency in the general population, as was the case for 625G(→)A, together conferring susceptibility to ethylmalonic aciduria. Hum Mol Genet 1998;7:619–27.
171. Tiranti V, Briem E, Lamantea E, et al. ETHE1 mutations are specific to ethylmalonic encephalopathy. J Med Genet 2006;43:340–6.
172. Zschocke J, Penzien JM, Bielen R, et al. The diagnosis of mitochondrial HMG-CoA synthase deficiency. J Pediatr 2002;140:778–80.
173. Morris AA, Lascelles CV, Olpin SE, et al. Hepatic mitochondrial 3-hydroxy-3-methylglutaryl-coenzyme a synthase deficiency. Pediatr Res 1998;44:392–6.
174. Thompson GN, Hsu BY, Pitt JJ, et al. Fasting hypoketotic coma in a child with deficiency of mitochondrial 3-hydroxy-3-methylglutaryl-CoA synthase. N Engl J Med 1997;337:1203–7.
175. Wolf NI, Rahman S, Clayton PT, Zschocke J. Mitochondrial HMG-CoA synthase deficiency: identification of two further patients carrying two novel mutations. Eur J Pediatr 2003;162:279–80.
176. Aledo R, Zschocke J, Pie J, et al. Genetic basis of mitochondrial HMG-CoA synthase deficiency. Hum Genet 2001;109:19–23.
177. Robinson BH, Oei J, Sherwood WG, et al. Hydroxymethylglutaryl CoA lyase deficiency: features resembling Reye syndrome. Neurology 1980;30(7 pt 1):714–18.
178. Wysocki SJ, Hahnel R. 3-Hydroxy-3-methylglutaryl-coenzyme a lyase deficiency: a review. J Inherit Metab Dis 1986;9:225–33.
179. Gibson KM, Breuer J, Kaiser K , et al. 3-Hydroxy-3-methylglutaryl coenzyme A lyase deficiency: report of five new patients. J Inherit Metab Dis 1988;11:76–87.
180. Roe CR, Millington DS, Maltby DA. Identification of 3-methylglutarylcarnitine. A new diagnostic metabolite of 3-hydroxy-3-methylglutaryl-coenzyme A lyase deficiency. J Clin Invest 1986;77:1391–4.
181. Fu Z, Runquist JA, Forouhar F, et al. Crystal structure of human HMG-CoA lyase: insights into catalysis and the molecular basis for hydroxymethylglutaric aciduria. J Biol Chem 2006;281:7526–32.
182. Gregersen N, Andresen BS, Bross P. Prevalent mutations in fatty acid oxidation disorders: diagnostic considerations. Eur J Pediatr 2000;159(suppl 3):S213–18.
183. Berry GT, Fukao T, Mitchell GA, et al. Neonatal hypoglycaemia in severe succinyl-CoA: 3-oxoacid CoA-transferase deficiency. J Inherit Metab Dis 2001;24:587–95.
184. Fukao T, Shintaku H, Kusubae R, et al. Patients homozygous for the T435N mutation of succinyl-CoA:3-ketoacid CoA Transferase (SCOT) do not show permanent ketosis. Pediatr Res 2004;56:858–63.
185. Snyderman SE, Sansaricq C, Middleton B. Succinyl-CoA:3-ketoacid CoA-transferase deficiency. Pediatrics 1998;101 (4 pt 1):709–11.
186. Longo N, Fukao T, Singh R, et al. Succinyl-CoA:3-ketoacid transferase (SCOT) deficiency in a new patient homozygous for an R217X mutation. J Inherit Metab Dis 2004;27:691–2.
187. Yalcinkaya C, Apaydin H, Ozekmekci S, Gibson KM. Delayed-onset dystonia associated with 3-oxothiolase deficiency. Mov Disord 2001;16:372–5.
188. Ozand PT, Rashed M, Gascon GG, et al. 3-Ketothiolase deficiency: a review and four new patients with neurologic symptoms. Brain Dev 1994;16(suppl):38–45.
189. Bohm N, Uy J, Kiessling M, Lehnert W. Multiple acyl-CoA dehydrogenation deficiency (glutaric aciduria type II), congenital polycystic kidneys, and symmetric warty dysplasia of the cerebral cortex in two newborn brothers. II. Morphology and pathogenesis. Eur J Pediatr 1982;139:60–5.
190. Mantagos S, Genel M, Tanaka K. Ethylmalonic-adipic aciduria. In vivo and in vitro studies indicating deficiency of activities of multiple acyl-CoA dehydrogenases. J Clin Invest 1979;64:1580–9.
191. Dusheiko G, Kew MC, Joffe BI, et al. Recurrent hypoglycemia associated with glutaric aciduria type II in an adult. N Engl J Med 1979;301:1405–9.
192. Di DS, Frerman FE, Rimoldi M, et al. Systemic carnitine deficiency due to lack of electron transfer flavoprotein:ubiquinone oxidoreductase. Neurology 1986;36:957–63.
193. Loehr JP, Goodman SI, Frerman FE. Glutaric acidemia type II: heterogeneity of clinical and biochemical phenotypes. Pediatr Res 1990;27:311–15.
194. Bell RB, Brownell AK, Roe CR, et al. Electron transfer flavoprotein: ubiquinone oxidoreductase (ETF:QO) deficiency in an adult. Neurology 1990;40:1779–82.
195. Mitchell G, Saudubray JM, Gubler MC, et al. Congenital anomalies in glutaric aciduria type 2. J Pediatr 1984;104:961–2.
196. Przyrembel H, Wendel U, Becker K, et al. Glutaric aciduria type II: report on a previously undescribed metabolic disorder. Clin Chim Acta 1976;66:227–39.
197. al-Essa MA, Rashed MS, Bakheet SM, et al. Glutaric aciduria type II: observations in seven patients with neonatal- and late-onset disease. J Perinatol 2000;20:120–8.
198. Spaan AN, Ijlst L, van Roermund CW, et al. Identification of the human mitochondrial FAD transporter and its potential role in multiple acyl-CoA dehydrogenase deficiency. Mol Genet Metab 2005;86:441–7.
199. Roe CR, Millington DS, Norwood DL, et al. 2,4-Dienoyl-coenzyme A reductase deficiency: a possible new disorder of fatty acid oxidation. J Clin Invest 1990;85:1703–7.
200. Riely CA. Acute fatty liver of pregnancy. Semin Liver Dis 1987;7:47–54.
201. Knox TA, Olans LB. Liver disease in pregnancy. N Engl J Med 1996;335:569–76.
202. Castro MA, Goodwin TM, Shaw KJ, et al. Disseminated intravascular coagulation and antithrombin III depression in acute fatty liver of pregnancy. Am J Obstet Gynecol 1996;174 (1 pt 1):211–16.
203. Riely CA, Latham PS, Romero R, Duffy TP. Acute fatty liver of pregnancy. A reassessment based on observations in nine patients. Ann Intern Med 1987;106:703–6.
204. Sibai BM, Ramadan MK, Usta I, et al. Maternal morbidity and mortality in 442 pregnancies with hemolysis, elevated liver enzymes, and low platelets (HELLP syndrome). Am J Obstet Gynecol 1993;169:1000–6.

205. Schoeman MN, Batey RG, Wilcken B. Recurrent acute fatty liver of pregnancy associated with a fatty-acid oxidation defect in the offspring. Gastroenterology 1991;100:544–8.
206. Wilcken B, Leung KC, Hammond J, et al. Pregnancy and fetal long-chain 3-hydroxyacyl coenzyme A dehydrogenase deficiency. Lancet 1993;341:407–8.
207. Barton JR, Riely CA, Adamec TA, et al. Hepatic histopathologic condition does not correlate with laboratory abnormalities in HELLP syndrome (hemolysis, elevated liver enzymes, and low platelet count). Am J Obstet Gynecol 1992;167:1538–43.
208. Minakami H, Oka N, Sato T, et al. Preeclampsia: a microvesicular fat disease of the liver? Am J Obstet Gynecol 1988;159: 1043–7.
209. Dani R, Mendes GS, Medeiros JL, et al. Study of the liver changes occurring in preeclampsia and their possible pathogenetic connection with acute fatty liver of pregnancy. Am J Gastroenterol 1996;91:292–4.
210. Usta IM, Barton JR, Amon EA, et al. Acute fatty liver of pregnancy: an experience in the diagnosis and management of fourteen cases. Am J Obstet Gynecol 1994;171:1342–7.
211. Burroughs AK, Seong NH, Dojcinov DM, et al. Idiopathic acute fatty liver of pregnancy in 12 patients. Q J Med 1982;51: 481–97.
212. Ibdah JA, Yang Z, Bennett MJ. Liver disease in pregnancy and fetal fatty acid oxidation defects. Mol Genet Metab 2000;71: 182–9.
213. Treem WR, Rinaldo P, Hale DE, et al. Acute fatty liver of pregnancy and long-chain 3-hydroxyacyl-coenzyme A dehydrogenase deficiency. Hepatology 1994;19:339–45.
214. Isaacs JD Jr, Sims HF, Powell CK, et al. Maternal acute fatty liver of pregnancy associated with fetal trifunctional protein deficiency: molecular characterization of a novel maternal mutant allele. Pediatr Res 1996;40:393–8.
215. Yang Z, Yamada J, Zhao Y, et al. Prospective screening for pediatric mitochondrial trifunctional protein defects in pregnancies complicated by liver disease. JAMA 2002;288:2163–6.
216. Ibdah JA, Zhao Y, Viola J, et al. Molecular prenatal diagnosis in families with fetal mitochondrial trifunctional protein mutations. J Pediatr 2001;138:396–9.
217. Rakheja D, Bennett MJ, Foster BM, et al. Evidence for fatty acid oxidation in human placenta, and the relationship of fatty acid oxidation enzyme activities with gestational age. Placenta 2002;23:447–50.
218. Shekhawat P, Bennett MJ, Sadovsky Y, et al. Human placenta metabolizes fatty acids: implications for fetal fatty acid oxidation disorders and maternal liver diseases. Am J Physiol Endocrinol Metab 2003;284:E1098–105.
219. Oey NA, den Boer ME, Ruiter JP, et al. High activity of fatty acid oxidation enzymes in human placenta: implications for fetal-maternal disease. J Inherit Metab Dis 2003;26: 385–92.
220. Ylitalo K, Vanttinen T, Halmesmaki E, Tyni T. Serious pregnancy complications in a patient with previously undiagnosed carnitine palmitoyltransferase 1 deficiency. Am J Obstet Gynecol 2005;192:2060–2.
221. Matern D, Hart P, Murtha AP, et al. Acute fatty liver of pregnancy associated with short-chain acyl-coenzyme A dehydrogenase deficiency. J Pediatr 2001;138:585–8.
222. Nelson J, Lewis B, Walters B. The HELLP syndrome associated wiht fetal medium-chain acyl-CoA dehydrogenase deficiency. J Inherit Metab Dis 2000;23:518–19.
223. Holub M, Bodamer OA, Item C, et al. Lack of correlation between fatty acid oxidation disorders and haemolysis, elevated liver enzymes, low platelets (HELLP) syndrome? Acta Paediatr 2005;94:48–52.
224. Chakrapani A, Olpin S, Cleary M, et al. Trifunctional protein deficiency: three families with significant maternal hepatic dysfunction in pregnancy not associated with E474Q mutation. J Inherit Metab Dis 2000;23:826–34.
225. Bok LA, Vreken P, Wijburg FA, et al. Short-chain Acyl-CoA dehydrogenase deficiency: studies in a large family adding to the complexity of the disorder. Pediatrics 2003;112:1152–5.
226. Bertrand C, Largilliere C, Zabot MT, et al. Very long chain acyl-CoA dehydrogenase deficiency: identification of a new inborn error of mitochondrial fatty acid oxidation in fibroblasts. Biochim Biophys Acta 1993;1180:327–9.
227. Boles RG, Buck EA, Blitzer MG, et al. Retrospective biochemical screening of fatty acid oxidation disorders in postmortem livers of 418 cases of sudden death in the first year of life. J Pediatr 1998;132:924–33.
228. Sinclair-Smith C, Dinsdale F, Emery J. Evidence of duration and type of illness in children found unexpectedly dead. Arch Dis Child 1976;51:424–9.
229. Bennett MJ, Allison F, Pollitt RJ, Variend S. Fatty acid oxidation defects as causes of unexpected death in infancy. Prog Clin Biol Res 1990;321:349–64.
230. Pollitt RJ. Defects in mitochondrial fatty acid oxidation: clinical presentations and their role in sudden infant death. Padiatr Padol 1993;28:13–17.
231. Anonymous. Sudden infant death and inherited disorders of fat oxidation. Lancet 1986;2:1073–5.
232. Harpey JP, Charpentier C, Paturneau-Jouas M. Sudden infant death syndrome and inherited disorders of fatty acid beta-oxidation. Biol Neonate 1990;58(suppl 1):70–80.
233. Harpey JP, Charpentier C, Coude M, et al. Sudden infant death syndrome and multiple acyl-coenzyme A dehydrogenase deficiency, ethylmalonic-adipic aciduria, or systemic carnitine deficiency. J Pediatr 1987;110:881–4.
234. Chaussain JL, Georges P, Calzada L, Job JC. Glycemic response to 24-hour fast in normal children: III. Influence of age. J Pediatr 1977;91:711–14.
235. Saudubray JM, Martin D, De LP, et al. Recognition and management of fatty acid oxidation defects: a series of 107 patients. J Inherit Metab Dis 1999;22:488–502.
236. Van ML, Tuerlinckx D, Wanders RJ, et al. Long-chain 3-hydroxyacyl-CoA dehydrogenase deficiency and early-onset liver cirrhosis in two siblings. Eur J Pediatr 2000;159:108–12.
237. Tein I, Christodoulou J, Donner E, McInnes RR. Carnitine palmitoyltransferase II deficiency: a new cause of recurrent pancreatitis. J Pediatr 1994;124:938–40.
238. Tyni T, Rapola J, Palotie A, Pihko H. Hypoparathyroidism in a patient with long-chain 3-hydroxyacyl-coenzyme A dehydrogenase deficiency caused by the G1528C mutation. J Pediatr 1997;131:766–8.
239. Rinaldo P. Fatty acid transport and mitochondrial oxidation disorders. Semin Liver Dis 2001;21:489–500.
240. Sim KG, Hammond J, Wilcken B. Strategies for the diagnosis of mitochondrial fatty acid beta-oxidation disorders. Clin Chim Acta 2002;323:37–58.
241. Lehotay DC, Clarke JT. Organic acidurias and related abnormalities. Crit Rev Clin Lab Sci 1995;32:377–429.

242. Costa CG, Guerand WS, Struys EA, et al. Quantitative analysis of urinary acylglycines for the diagnosis of beta-oxidation defects using GC-NCI-MS. J Pharm Biomed Anal 2000;21:1215–24.
243. Kimura M, Yamaguchi S. Screening for fatty acid beta oxidation disorders. Acylglycine analysis by electron impact ionization gas chromatography-mass spectrometry. J Chromatogr B Biomed Sci Appl 1999;731:105–10.
244. Stanley CA, Berry GT, Bennett MJ, et al. Renal handling of carnitine in secondary carnitine deficiency disorders. Pediatr Res 1993;34:89–97.
245. Bennett MJ. The laboratory diagnosis of inborn errors of mitochondrial fatty acid oxidation. Ann Clin Biochem 1990;27 (pt 6):519–31.
246. Costa CG, Dorland L, Holwerda U, et al. Simultaneous analysis of plasma free fatty acids and their 3-hydroxy analogs in fatty acid beta-oxidation disorders. Clin Chem 1998;44:463–71.
247. Jones PM, Quinn R, Fennessey PV, et al. Improved stable isotope dilution-gas chromatography mass spectrometry method for serum or plasma free 3-hydroxy-fatty acids and its utility for the study of disorders of mitochondrial fatty acid beta-oxidation. Clin Chem 2000;46:149–55.
248. Lagerstedt SA, Hinrichs DR, Batt SM, et al. Quantitative determination of plasma c8-c26 total fatty acids for the biochemical diagnosis of nutritional and metabolic disorders. Mol Genet Metab 2001;73:38–45.
249. Roe CR, Millington DS, Maltby DA, Kinnebrew P. Recognition of medium-chain acyl-CoA dehydrogenase deficiency in asymptomatic siblings of children dying of sudden infant death or Reye-like syndromes. J Pediatr 1986;108:13–18.
250. Seakins JW, Rumsby G. The use of phenylpropionic acid as a loading test for medium-chain acyl-CoA dehydrogenase deficiency. J Inherit Metab Dis 1988;11(suppl 2):221–4.
251. Shen JJ, Matern D, Millington DS, et al. Acylcarnitines in fibroblasts of patients with long-chain 3-hydroxyacyl-CoA dehydrogenase deficiency and other fatty acid oxidation disorders. J Inherit Metab Dis 2000;23:27–44.
252. Olpin SE, Manning NJ, Pollitt RJ, et al. The use of [9,10–3H]myristate, [9,10–3H]palmitate and [9,10–3H]oleate for the detection and diagnosis of medium and long-chain fatty acid oxidation disorders in intact cultured fibroblasts. Adv Exp Med Biol 1999;466:321–5.
253. Roe CR, Roe DS. Recent developments in the investigation of inherited metabolic disorders using cultured human cells. Mol Genet Metab 1999;68:243–57.
254. Ikeda Y, Tanaka K. Immunoprecipitation and electrophoretic analysis of four human acyl-CoA dehydrogenases and electron transfer flavoprotein using antibodies raised against the corresponding rat enzymes. Biochem Med Metab Biol 1987;37:329–34.
255. Bennett MJ, Allison F, Lowther GW, et al. Prenatal diagnosis of medium-chain acyl-coenzyme A dehydrogenase deficiency. Prenat Diagn 1987;7:135–41.
256. Jakobs C, Sweetman L, Wadman SK, et al. Prenatal diagnosis of glutaric aciduria type II by direct chemical analysis of dicarboxylic acids in amniotic fluid. Eur J Pediatr 1984;141: 153–7.
257. Gutthrie R, Susi A. A simple phenylalanine method for detecting phenylketonuria in large populations of newborn infants. Pediatrics 1963;32:338–43.
258. Millington DS, Kodo N, Norwood DL, Roe CR. Tandem mass spectrometry: a new method for acylcarnitine profiling with potential for neonatal screening for inborn errors of metabolism. J Inherit Metab Dis 1990;13:321–4.
259. Chace DH, DiPerna JC, Mitchell BL, et al. Electrospray tandem mass spectrometry for analysis of acylcarnitines in dried postmortem blood specimens collected at autopsy from infants with unexplained cause of death. Clin Chem 2001;47:1166–82.
260. Garg U, Dasouki M. Expanded newborn screening of inherited metabolic disorders by tandem mass spectrometry: Clinical and laboratory aspects. Clin Biochem 2006;39:315–32.
261. Naylor EW, Chace DH. Automated tandem mass spectrometry for mass newborn screening for disorders in fatty acid, organic acid, and amino acid metabolism. J Child Neurol 1999;14(suppl 1):S4–8.
262. Schulze A, Lindner M, Kohlmuller D, et al. Expanded newborn screening for inborn errors of metabolism by electrospray ionization-tandem mass spectrometry: results, outcome, and implications. Pediatrics 2003;111(6 pt 1):1399–406.
263. Wiley V, Carpenter K, Wilcken B. Newborn screening with tandem mass spectrometry: 12 months' experience in NSW Australia. Acta Paediatr Suppl 1999;88:48–51.
264. Liebl B, Fingerhut R, Roschinger W, et al. [Model project for updating neonatal screening in Bavaria: concept and initial results]. Gesundheitswesen 2000;62:189–95.
265. Shigematsu Y, Hirano S, Hata I, et al. Newborn mass screening and selective screening using electrospray tandem mass spectrometry in Japan. J Chromatogr B Analyt Technol Biomed Life Sci 2002;776:39–48.
266. Rashed MS, Rahbeeni Z, Ozand PT. Application of electrospray tandem mass spectrometry to neonatal screening. Semin Perinatol 1999;23:183–93.
267. Zytkovicz TH, Fitzgerald EF, Marsden D, et al. Tandem mass spectrometric analysis for amino, organic, and fatty acid disorders in newborn dried blood spots: a two-year summary from the New England Newborn Screening Program. Clin Chem 2001;47:1945–55.
268. Schoen EJ, Baker JC, Colby CJ, To TT. Cost-benefit analysis of universal tandem mass spectrometry for newborn screening. Pediatrics 2002;110:781–6.
269. Seashore MR, Rinaldo P. Metabolic disease of the neonate and young infant. Semin Perinatol 1993;17:318–29.
270. Bennett MJ, Powell S. Metabolic disease and sudden, unexpected death in infancy. Hum Pathol 1994;25:742–6.
271. Rashed MS, Ozand PT, Bennett MJ, et al. Inborn errors of metabolism diagnosed in sudden death cases by acylcarnitine analysis of postmortem bile. Clin Chem 1995;41(8 pt 1):1109–14.
272. Lundemose JB, Kolvraa S, Gregersen N, et al. Fatty acid oxidation disorders as primary cause of sudden and unexpected death in infants and young children: an investigation performed on cultured fibroblasts from 79 children who died aged between 0–4 years. Mol Pathol 1997;50:212–17.
273. Gregersen N, Winter V, Jensen PK, et al. Prenatal diagnosis of medium-chain acyl-CoA dehydrogenase (MCAD) deficiency in a family with a previous fatal case of sudden unexpected death in childhood. Prenat Diagn 1995;15:82–6.
274. Rinaldo P. Mitochondrial fatty acid oxidation disorders and cyclic vomiting syndrome. Dig Dis Sci 1999;44(8 suppl):97S–102S.

275. Solis JO, Singh RH. Management of fatty acid oxidation disorders: a survey of current treatment strategies. J Am Diet Assoc 2002;102:1800–3.
276. Roe CR, Sweetman L, Roe DS, et al. Treatment of cardiomyopathy and rhabdomyolysis in long-chain fat oxidation disorders using an anaplerotic odd-chain triglyceride. J Clin Invest 2002;110:259–69.
277. Gillingham MB, Weleber RG, Neuringer M, et al. Effect of optimal dietary therapy upon visual function in children with long-chain 3-hydroxyacyl CoA dehydrogenase and trifunctional protein deficiency. Mol Genet Metab 2005;86:124–33.
278. Glasgow AM, Engel AG, Bier DM, et al. Hypoglycemia, hepatic dysfunction, muscle weakness, cardiomyopathy, free carnitine deficiency and long-chain acylcarnitine excess responsive to medium chain triglyceride diet. Pediatr Res 1983;17:319–26.
279. Duran M, Wanders RJ, de Jager JP, et al. 3-Hydroxydicarboxylic aciduria due to long-chain 3-hydroxyacyl-coenzyme A dehydrogenase deficiency associated with sudden neonatal death: protective effect of medium-chain triglyceride treatment. Eur J Pediatr 1991;150:190–5.
280. Gillingham MB, Connor WE, Matern D, et al. Optimal dietary therapy of long-chain 3-hydroxyacyl-CoA dehydrogenase deficiency. Mol Genet Metab 2003;79:114–23.
281. Harding CO, Gillingham MB, van Calcar SC, et al. Docosahexaenoic acid and retinal function in children with long-chain 3-hydroxyacyl-CoA dehydrogenase deficiency. J Inherit Metab Dis 1999;22:276–80.
282. Lamhonwah AM, Olpin SE, Pollitt RJ, et al. Novel OCTN2 mutations: no genotype-phenotype correlations: early carnitine therapy prevents cardiomyopathy. Am J Med Genet 2002;111:271–84.
283. Corr PB, Creer MH, Yamada KA, et al. Prophylaxis of early ventricular fibrillation by inhibition of acylcarnitine accumulation. J Clin Invest 1989;83:927–36.
284. Rinaldo P, Schmidt-Sommerfeld E, Posca AP, et al. Effect of treatment with glycine and L-carnitine in medium-chain acyl-coenzyme A dehydrogenase deficiency. J Pediatr 1993;122:580–4.
285. Przyrembel H, Jakobs C, Ijlst L, et al. Long-chain 3-hydroxyacyl-CoA dehydrogenase deficiency. J Inherit Metab Dis 1991;14:674–80.
286. Rocchiccioli F, Wanders RJ, Aubourg P, et al. Deficiency of long-chain 3-hydroxyacyl-CoA dehydrogenase: a cause of lethal myopathy and cardiomyopathy in early childhood. Pediatr Res 1990;28:657–62.
287. Green A, Preece MA, de Sousa SC, Pollitt RJ. Possible deleterious effect of L-carnitine supplementation in a patient with mild multiple acyl-CoA dehydrogenation deficiency (ethylmalonic-adipic aciduria). J Inherit Metab Dis 1991;14:691–7.
288. Ribes A, Riudor E, Navarro C, et al. Fatal outcome in a patient with long-chain 3-hydroxyacyl-CoA dehydrogenase deficiency. J Inherit Metab Dis 1992;15:278–9.
289. Moore R, Glasgow JF, Bingham MA, et al. Long-chain 3-hydroxyacyl-coenzyme A dehydrogenase deficiency – diagnosis, plasma carnitine fractions and management in a further patient. Eur J Pediatr 1993;152:433–6.
290. Lee PJ, Harrison EL, Jones MG, et al. L-carnitine and exercise tolerance in medium-chain acyl-coenzyme A dehydrogenase (MCAD) deficiency: a pilot study. J Inherit Metab Dis 2005;28:141–52.
291. de Visser VM, Scholte HR, Schutgens RB, et al. Riboflavin-responsive lipid-storage myopathy and glutaric aciduria type II of early adult onset. Neurology 1986;36:367–72.
292. Duran M, Cleutjens CB, Ketting D, et al. Diagnosis of medium-chain acyl-CoA dehydrogenase deficiency in lymphocytes and liver by a gas chromatographic method: the effect of oral riboflavin supplementation. Pediatr Res 1992;31:39–42.
293. Ibdah JA, Paul H, Zhao Y, et al. Lack of mitochondrial trifunctional protein in mice causes neonatal hypoglycemia and sudden death. J Clin Invest 2001;107:1403–9.
294. Exil VJ, Roberts RL, Sims H, et al. Very-long-chain acyl-coenzyme a dehydrogenase deficiency in mice. Circ Res 2003;93:448–55.
295. Kurtz DM, Rinaldo P, Rhead WJ, et al. Targeted disruption of mouse long-chain acyl-CoA dehydrogenase gene reveals crucial roles for fatty acid oxidation. Proc Natl Acad Sci U S A 1998;95:15592–7.
296. Tolwani RJ, Hamm DA, Tian L, et al. Medium-chain acyl-CoA dehydrogenase deficiency in gene-targeted mice. PLoS Genet 2005;1:e23.
297. Maclean K, Rasiah VS, Kirk EP, et al. Pulmonary haemorrhage and cardiac dysfunction in a neonate with medium-chain acyl-CoA dehydrogenase (MCAD) deficiency. Acta Paediatr 2005;94:114–16.
298. Feillet F, Steinmann G, Vianey-Saban C, et al. Adult presentation of MCAD deficiency revealed by coma and severe arrhythmias. Intensive Care Med 2003;29:1594–7.
299. Koizumi T, Nikaido H, Hayakawa J, et al. Infantile disease with microvesicular fatty infiltration of viscera spontaneously occurring in the C3H-H-2(0) strain of mouse with similarities to Reye's syndrome. Lab Anim 1988;22:83–7.
300. Kuwajima M, Kono N, Horiuchi M, et al. Animal model of systemic carnitine deficiency: analysis in C3H-H-2 degrees strain of mouse associated with juvenile visceral steatosis. Biochem Biophys Res Commun 1991;174:1090–4.
301. Nikaido H, Horiuchi M, Hashimoto N, et al. Mapping of jvs (juvenile visceral steatosis) gene, which causes systemic carnitine deficiency in mice, on chromosome 11. Mamm Genome 1995;6:369–70.
302. Okita K, Tokino T, Nishimori H, et al. Definition of the locus responsible for systemic carnitine deficiency within a 1.6-cM region of mouse chromosome 11 by detailed linkage analysis. Genomics 1996;33:289–91.
303. Lu K, Nishimori H, Nakamura Y, et al. A missense mutation of mouse OCTN2, a sodium-dependent carnitine cotransporter, in the juvenile visceral steatosis mouse. Biochem Biophys Res Commun 1998;252:590–4.
304. Nyman LR, Cox KB, Hoppel CL, et al. Homozygous carnitine palmitoyltransferase 1a (liver isoform) deficiency is lethal in the mouse. Mol Genet Metab 2005;86:179–87.
305. Amendt BA, Freneaux E, Reece C, et al. Short-chain acyl-coenzyme A dehydrogenase activity, antigen, and biosynthesis are absent in the BALB(cByJ mouse. Pediatr Res 1992;31:552–6.

33

MITOCHONDRIAL HEPATOPATHIES

Ronald J. Sokol, M.D.

Structural and functional alterations of mitochondria are now recognized as the etiology of a growing and wide variety of pathologic disorders. Genetic defects and secondary abnormalities in the synthesis of mitochondrial proteins and enzymes are the underlying cause of diseases affecting the nervous system [1], skeletal and cardiac muscle [1], the liver [2], bone marrow [3], the endocrine and exocrine pancreas [3,4], kidney, inner ear, and small and large intestines [5] (Table 33.1). Resultant perturbations in mitochondrial function yield defective oxidative phosphorylation (OXPHOS), increased generation of reactive oxygen species (ROS), accumulation of hepatocytic lipids, impairment of other mitochondrial-based metabolic processes, and activation of both apoptotic and necrotic cell death pathways. The spectrum of inherited mitochondrial hepatic and gastrointestinal disorders continues to expand. In addition, mitochondrial dysfunction may be one of the key targets and determinants for hepatocyte survival in other disorders not directly related to the mitochondrion. Thus, the concept of primary (or genetic) and secondary (or acquired) mitochondrial hepatopathies has developed. Because mitochondria possess a distinct and unique extranuclear genome, a new class of maternally inherited mitochondrial diseases has emerged as well. The tissue-specific accumulation over time of new somatic (noninherited) mutations of mitochondrial genes may also be involved in several neurodegenerative diseases [6], hepatopathies, and the process of aging itself [7]. In this chapter, recent advances are reviewed in our understanding of the genetics, the structure and the function of the mitochondrion, a classification for hepatic disorders involving mitochondrial dysfunction is proposed, and the current diagnostic armamentarium and treatment modalities for these disorders are discussed.

MITOCHONDRIAL STRUCTURE AND GENETICS

The mitochondrion is a double-membrane structure containing a soluble matrix and its own unique genome. The outer membrane serves as a "corset" to hold the highly folded inner membrane in place; as a regulator of efflux of mitochondrial enzymes, cations (including calcium), and substrates into cytosol; and a specific transport site for a variety of mitochondrial substrates that must be taken up from cytosol. The inner mitochondrial membrane contains specialized transport sites for small molecules, the electron transport chain that accepts electrons generated from the citric acid cycle, and adenosine triphosphate (ATP) synthase that carries out OXPHOS and ATP synthesis. The mitochondrial matrix is a concentrated mixture of enzymes that are active in the tricarboxylic acid (TCA) cycle, fatty acid oxidation (FAO), urea synthesis, and other metabolic pathways. Specific enzyme defects have been described for many of these matriceal enzymes, most coded for by nuclear DNA, leading to familiar, although rare, disorders of FAO, urea synthesis, gluconeogenesis, and others.

One of the most unique characteristics of mitochondria in mammalian cells is the presence of a separate genome and the enzymes necessary for the replication, transcription, translation, and expression of nucleic acids independently [1]. Virtually all mitochondrial DNA in a cell is derived from the unfertilized oocyte (sperm contribute virtually no mitochondria), and hence all characteristics encoded by the mitochondrial DNA are maternally inherited. Thus, affected men do not transmit the genetic defect. In general, deleted molecules are not transmitted from clinically affected women to their children; however, a woman with a heteroplasmic mitochondrial DNA (mtDNA) point mutation or duplications may transmit a variable amount of mutated DNA to their children [8]. The mitochondrial genome is a double-stranded, circular molecule containing 16,569 base pairs (bp) that has been fully sequenced and shown to encode 37 genes, including 2 ribosomal RNAs, 22 transfer RNAs for protein synthesis, and 13 of the subunits of complexes I, III, IV, and V of the respiratory chain (Table 33.2). Mitochondrial DNA sequences do not contain introns, as opposed to nuclear genes that include both introns and exons. Early during development of the female germline, there is a reduction of number of mtDNA molecules within each oocyte followed by an amplification to reach approximately 100,000 genomes per mature oocyte. This "genetic bottleneck" influences the variability between oocytes [9]. Mitochondrial DNA also depends on nuclear genes for its enzymes of

Table 33.1: Systemic Presentations of Mitochondrial Disorders

Cardiac	Hypertrophic cardiomyopathy
	Heart block, sudden death
	Barth syndrome (cardiomyopathy, cyclic neutropenia)
Eye	Cataracts, optic atrophy, pigmentary retinopathy
Ear	Sensorineural deafness
	Aminoglycoside deafness
Renal	Proximal tubular disorder (Fanconi's syndrome)
	Nephritis, nephrotic syndrome
Endocrine	Diabetes mellitus, short stature, and growth hormone deficiency
	Hypoparathyroidism, hypothyroidism
Hematologic	Pancytopenia, sideroblastic anemia
	Vacuolization
Gastrointestinal	Pancreatic insufficiency, pancreatitis
	Intestinal villus atrophy
	Intestinal pseudo-obstruction
Hepatic	Acute liver failure
	Cholestasis
	Hepatic steatosis
	Chronic hepatitis
	Cirrhosis and chronic liver failure
Dermatologic	Mottled pigmentation
	Hypertrichosis, dry brittle hair, alopecia
Metabolic	Lactic acidosis
	Hyperammonemia

Table 33.2: Mitochondrial Respiratory Chain Protein Complexes – Polypeptide Subunits

Complex	*Total Number of Subunits*	*Subunits Encoded by Nuclear DNA*	*Subunits Encoded by mtDNA*
I	41	34	7 – ND_1, ND_2, ND_3, ND_4, ND_{4L}, ND_5, ND_6
II	4	4	None
III	11	10	1- cyt b
IV	13	10	3-cyt oxidase I, cyt. oxidase II, cyt oxidase III
V	14	12	2 – ATPase 6, ATPase 8

replication, transcription, translation, and repair [10], and nuclear genes encode all the other proteins of the metabolic pathways located in mitochondria. It should be noted that most subunits of the respiratory chain proteins are encoded by nuclear DNA and imported into the mitochondria after assembly elsewhere in the cell (Table 33.2). Thus, abnormalities in OXPHOS can be the result of both nuclear and mitochondrial DNA mutations.

Each mitochondrion contains 2–10 copies of the genome, and because cells can contain hundreds or thousands of mitochondria, thousands of copies of this genome can be present in an individual cell [1]. Usually, all mtDNA is identical, called *homoplasmy*; however, normal and mutant mitochondrial DNA can coexist in various proportions in a single cell, a condition known as *heteroplasmy*. The phenotype of the cell is determined by the relative proportion of normal and mutated genomes. Mitochondrial DNA mutates 10–20 times as frequently as nuclear DNA, resulting in point mutations, deletions, and duplications. This DNA has neither protective histones nor an effective repair system, and it is constantly exposed to ROS generated by OXPHOS that can induce DNA damage and mutations. During cell division, mitochondria are randomly partitioned into daughter cells, resulting in nonuniform distribution of mutated mitochondrial DNA in progeny cells. The threshold of mutated mitochondrial genome needed to produce a deleterious phenotype varies among persons and organ systems and within individual tissues. The threshold for biochemical expression is about 60% mutant for mtDNA deletions and up to 95% for tRNA mutations [11]. Thus, there is variable clinical expression among patients with the same genotypic mutations, sometimes with abnormalities in OXPHOS detected only in the involved tissues. The degree of organ dysfunction will depend on a tissue's energy requirements, with brain, muscle, and liver being commonly involved tissues. During cell division, mitochondria are segregated randomly between daughter cells, shifting the proportion of mutant and wild-type mtDNA. This explains how some patients with mitochondrial disorders may actually shift from one clinical phenotype to another as they age. In addition, mutations in a new group of nuclear genes results in low synthesis of all mitochondrial genome-coded protein subunits, leading to generalized depletion of mitochondrial DNA. Cell damage in these disorders results from an inadequate supply of energy in metabolically active cells and tissues, increased generation of injurious ROS as a consequence of perturbed flow of electrons down the respiratory chain, alterations of cellular ion homeostasis, release of cytochrome c and apoptosis-inducing factor into cytoplasm, or by other undefined mechanisms.

FUNCTIONS OF MITOCHONDRIA

The essential functions of mitochondria are related to the multitude of enzyme systems located in the various compartments of this organelle. A major function of mitochondria is to synthesize ATP by the process of oxidative phosphorylation that drives energy-dependent reactions and transport processes in all cells. The transduction of energy by the transfer of electrons from substrates of the TCA cycle (via reduced nicotinamide adenine dinucleotide [NADH]) and from the FAO cycle (via NADH and reduced flavine adenine dinucleotide [$FADH_2$]) to oxygen is facilitated by the respiratory chain, a group of five large protein complexes embedded in the inner mitochondrial membrane, plus ubiquinone (coenzyme Q [CoQ]) and cytochrome c (Figure 33.1). These include complex I (NADH–CoQ reductase), complex II (succinate–CoQ reductase), complex III (reduced CoQ–cytochrome c reductase), complex IV (cytochrome c oxidase), and complex V (ATP synthase). The free energy generated from these stepwise redox reactions is converted into a transmembrane proton gradient by the extrusion of protons through the inner membrane at complexes I, III, and IV. At complex V, protons flow back into the mitochondrial matrix, and the released energy is used by ATP synthetase to synthesize ATP. When adenosine diphosphate (ADP) and inorganic phosphorus (Pi) are bound to the active site, protons are allowed to move down the concentration gradient and the free energy is enzymatically coupled to the formation of a bond between ADP and Pi. Three ATP molecules are generated for each molecule of NADH oxidized. Free NAD+ is regenerated for use in the TCA cycle and other integral mitochondrial matrix enzyme pathways. In addition to its role as the final electron receptor in the respiratory chain, 2–3% of the oxygen used by mitochondria results in the generation of superoxide by complexes I and III. This superoxide is normally converted to hydrogen peroxide by the manganese–superoxide dismutase present in the matrix or combines with nitric oxide to form peroxynitrite. The hydrogen peroxide may diffuse into cytosol or remain in the mitochondrial matrix, only to be reduced to water by glutathione peroxidases present in both the mitochondria and cell cytoplasm. If the balance of generation and scavenging of these ROS is upset, increased oxidative stress may develop within the mitochondria or cell.

Both primary and secondary defects in function of the respiratory chain have severe consequences for the metabolic homeostasis of the cell. These include a generalized deficiency of high energy molecules; a substantially increased dependence on glycolysis with increased lactate production in the cytosol; an increase in the intramitochondrial and cytoplasmic concentration of reducing equivalents; functional impairment of the TCA cycle caused by this altered redox state (an excess of NADH and lack of NAD); and an increase in the generation of oxygen free radicals with resultant oxidation of lipids in membranes, thiol-containing proteins, and mitochondrial nucleic acids, and opening of the mitochondrial permeability pore [12]. The

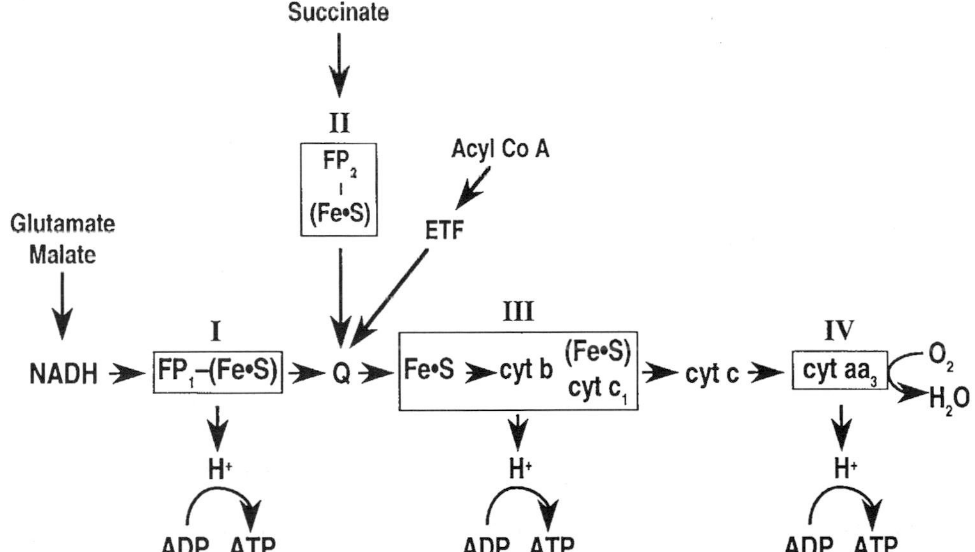

Figure 33.1. The respiratory chain protein complexes and oxidative phosphorylation of the mitochondria. During glycolysis, fatty acid oxidation (FAO), and the tricarboxylic acid (TCA) cycle, reducing equivalents are derived from the sequential metabolism of each metabolic fuel. NADH acts as a carrier of reducing equivalents from glycolysis into the mitochondria matrix, and NADH and $FADH_2$ shuttle reducing equivalents produced by FAO and the TCA cycle. Succinate carries reducing equivalents derived from the TCA cycle. To transduce this reducing power into energy, a system of electron carriers (protein complexes I–IV, coenzyme Q [Q] and cytochrome c) in the inner mitochondrial membrane convert the reducing equivalents into ATP through the efficient transport of electrons down this chain, resulting in the generation of a transmembrane proton gradient that drives the synthesis of ATP by complex V. FP, flavoprotein; Fe · S, iron sulfur cluster; cyt., cytochrome.

Table 33.3: Epidemiologic Studies of Mitochondrial Diseases

Study Population	*Mutations or Disease*	*Disease Prevalence/ 100,000 (95% CI)*	*Mutation Prevalence/ 100,000 (95% CI)*
Majamaa et al. (1998) [22] Northern Finland N = 245,201 adults	Adult point prevalence of A3243G mutation –Identified 615 patients	5.71 (4.53–6.89)	16.3 (11.3–21.4)
Chinnery et al. (2000) [20] Northern England N = 1,582,584 adults	Adult point prevalence of all mtDNA mutations –Identified 104 patients and 161 maternal relatives	6.57 (5.30–7.83)	12.48 (10.75–14.23)
Uusimaa et al. (2000) [23] Finland N = 146,482 children	All mtDNA mutations in children with respiratory chain disorders –Identified 26 children	Not able to be calculated from data	Not able to be calculated from data
Darin et al. (2001) [21] Western Sweden N = 358,616 children	Pediatric point prevalence of pediatric mitochondrial encephalomyopathies –Identified 32 children	4.76 (2.80–7.60)	Not able to be calculated from data

CI, confidence interval.
Reprinted from Gillis LA, Sokol RJ. Gastrointestinal manifestations of mitochondrial disease. Gastroenterol Clin North Am 2003;32:789–817; with permission.

mitochondrial permeability transition releases cytochrome C and apoptosis-inducing factors into cytosol, triggering the activation of caspases and the irreversible process of cellular apoptosis. In addition, the permeability transition results in loss of mitochondrial membrane potential and interruption of ATP synthesis. Thus, both metabolic failure and the induction of cellular apoptosis or necrosis could result from impairment of normal electron flow in the respiratory chain.

Another important intermediary metabolic pathway within mitochondria involves the fate of pyruvate. Glucose oxidation via glycolysis in the cytoplasmic compartment results in the formation of two moles of pyruvate from each mole of glucose. Without mitochondrial oxidation, pyruvate is anaerobically reduced to lactate; yielding only 2 of the total 38 moles of potentially available ATP if pyruvate were metabolized via the TCA cycle. Pyruvate can be translocated across the mitochondrial membrane and oxidized to acetyl coenzyme A (CoA) by the pyruvate dehydrogenase complex (PDHC), which then enters the TCA cycle by combining with oxaloacetate to form citrate. The TCA cycle enzymes are located in the mitochondrial matrix and depend on transporters imbedded in the otherwise impermeable inner mitochondrial membrane necessary for the influx of substrates and efflux of generated products.

Long-chain FAO is the predominant source of energy for cardiac and skeletal muscle at all times and becomes the major pathway for energy production during fasting in liver, cardiac, and skeletal muscle. With prolonged fasting, fatty acids are converted into ketone bodies in the liver and exported to extrahepatic tissues as an alternate fuel when the supply of glucose is limited, thus sparing glucose use for more obligate organ users such as the brain. FAO leads to the generation of electron-rich substrates for the respiratory chain, $FADH_2$, and NADH. Imbedded in the mitochondrial membrane is the enzyme that catalyzes the conversion of long-chain acyl-CoA esters to acylcarnitines, the transporters of both acyl- and free carnitine across the membrane, and the enzyme that converts acylcarnitines back to acyl-CoAs on the inner side of the inner mitochondrial membrane. In this location are the enzymes of the β-oxidation cycle, which catalyze the repetitive cleavage of two-carbon fragments from the fatty acid chain and the generation of acetyl-CoA. Acetyl-CoA either condenses with oxaloacetate to form citrate and enter the TCA cycle or becomes available for ketogenesis during fasting. Two other mitochondrial matrix enzymes catalyze the synthesis of acetoacetate and its reduction to β-hydroxybutyrate.

Other metabolic pathways partially housed in the mitochondria include the urea cycle, bile acid synthesis, methylmalonic acid and ethanol metabolism, and fatty acid synthesis. In addition, the mitochondrion plays a key role in intracellular calcium homeostasis. For purposes of this chapter, "mitochondrial diseases" that affect the respiratory chain are emphasized. These disorders are caused by primary defects or are secondary to other interrelated metabolic defects or drug interactions. In the last few years, it has become clear that a number of unexplained disorders during infancy and early childhood can be explained by disorders of electron transport and oxidative phosphorylation. In this chapter, disorders of liver, pancreatic, and intestinal dysfunction in their primary presentation either alone or as part of a more global picture of central nervous system (CNS), muscle, bone marrow, or renal disease are described, with emphasis on the clinical manifestations, diagnosis, and treatment. Other common manifestations of these disorders are diabetes, cardiomyopathy, deafness, and retinitis pigmentosa [13]. Details of the pathophysiology and molecular biology of these disorders are contained in several excellent reviews [1,11,13–16].

EPIDEMIOLOGY OF MITOCHONDRIAL DISORDERS

Pathogenic mtDNA mutations cause a wide variety of pediatric and adult mitochondrial diseases; in excess of 200 pathogenic point mutations, deletions, insertions, and rearrangements have been identified since the first mitochondrial mutations were reported in 1988 [17,18]. An estimated 90% of mitochondrial diseases are caused by mutations in nuclear genes, with only a small fraction of these nuclear mutations having been identified at this time. As a general rule, point mutations of mtDNA genes are usually maternally inherited (mtDNA genes), whereas deletions or rearrangements of mtDNA are either sporadic or inherited in an autosomal recessive manner (caused by mutations in nuclear genes).

Mitochondrial disorders are a challenge for the genetic epidemiologist. Factors that influence the prevalence of mitochondrial disorders include mutation rate, inheritance pattern, population structure, and genetic background. Accurate diagnosis is difficult, and it is not always possible to identify the underlying mitochondrial molecular genetic defect in the blood [19]. Clinical presentations vary considerably, and thus there may be significant delays in diagnosis. Moreover, transmission of a pathogenic mutation does not necessarily result in a clinical phenotype. Most epidemiologic studies determined the frequency of a specific mtDNA mutation in patients with a specific clinical presentation, failing to account for phenotypic variability. Despite these drawbacks, a number of recent studies have examined the true prevalence of mitochondrial disorders at a population level [20–23] (Table 33.3). Chinnery [24] calculated an estimated minimum prevalence of mitochondrial disease of 11.5 cases per 100,000 individuals, or 1 in 8500 members of the general population. As the spectrum of mtDNA disease continues to expand rapidly, with novel genotypes and phenotypes, epidemiologic data will accordingly require future revisions. The frequency of nuclear gene abnormalities causing mitochondrial diseases has not been accurately estimated.

NEUROMUSCULAR MITOCHONDRIAL DISORDERS

The majority of the diseases initially associated with maternal inheritance and later with mitochondrial gene mutations were neuromuscular in nature (Table 33.4). Many have been shown to be caused by large deletions or missense mutations of mitochondrial genome involving transfer RNA (tRNA) genes or subunits of the electron transport chain complexes, or mutations of nuclear genes encoding subunits of these complexes. These disorders include Leber's hereditary optic neuropathy, MELAS syndrome (mitochondrial encephalomyopathy, lactic acidosis, and strokelike episodes), MERRF syndrome (myoclonic epilepsy with ragged red fibers), Kearns–Sayre syndrome, Leigh disease, and others [1,14,16]. The A3243G mutation in tRNA is the most common single base change and has been associated with MELAS, whereas the G8344A mutation in tRNA is found in MERRF. Many of these mitochondrial encephalomyopathies have their onset in childhood and must be kept in mind by those evaluating children with neurologic and muscular disorders. The number of disorders that can be caused by mitochondrial enzyme defects, abnormal OXPHOS, or other mitochondrial DNA mutations has grown at a rapid pace and now includes several gastrointestinal diseases (discussed subsequently) as well as the mitochondrial hepatopathies. These disorders can be grouped into the primary (or congenital) and the secondary (or acquired) mitochondrial hepatopathies (Table 33.5).

Table 33.4: Mitochondrial Encephalomyopathies

Leigh syndrome: subacute necrotizing encephalomyopathy
Kearns–Sayre syndrome: ophthalmoplegia, retinal degeneration, heart block
MERRF syndrome: *m*yoclonus, *e*pilepsy, *r*agged *r*ed *f*ibers
MELAS syndrome: *m*yopathy, *e*ncephalopathy, *l*actic *a*cidosis, and *s*trokelike episodes
LHON: *L*eber's *h*ereditary *o*ptic *n*europathy
NARP: *n*europathy, *a*taxia, and *r*etinitis *p*igmentosa
MIMyCa: *m*aternally *i*nherited *my*opathy and *ca*rdiomyopathy
Myopathy and multiple deletions of mitochondrial DNA
Mitochondrial DNA depletion syndrome
MNGIE: *m*itochondrial *n*euro-*g*astro*i*ntestinal *e*ncephalomyopathy
CHERP: *c*alcification, *h*earing loss, *h*ypogonadism, *e*ncephalopathy, *r*etinitis *p*igmentosa
CPEO: *chronic* progressive *e*xternal *o*phthalmoplegia
OCRL: *o*cular *c*erebro *r*ena*l* syndrome
Alpers' disease: progressive infantile poliodystrophy
Hereditary myopathies (with or without lactic acidosis)
Fatty acid oxidation defects and other carnitine transport and deficiency states
ETF and ETF dehydrogenase deficiencies (glutaric acidemia type II)
? Parkinson's disease, Huntington's disease, Alzheimer's disease

ETF, electron-transfer flavoprotein.

CLASSIFICATION OF MITOCHONDRIAL HEPATOPATHIES

In a variety of hepatic disorders, defects in either specific biochemical pathways or more general dysfunction of mitochondria have been described. These conditions are frequently, but not universally, associated with morphologic changes of hepatic mitochondrial structure or number or with neuromuscular

Table 33.5: Classification of Mitochondrial Hepatopathies

Primary disorders

1. Electron transport (respiratory chain) defects
   - Neonatal liver failure and acute liver failure
     Complex I deficiency
     Complex IV deficiency (*SCO1* mutations)
     Complex III deficiency (*BCS1L* mutations)
     Multiple Complex deficiencies
   - Mitochondrial DNA depletion syndrome (*dGK, MPV17, POLG* mutations)
   - Delayed onset liver failure : Alpers–Huttenlocher syndrome (*POLG* mutations)
   - Pearson's marrow–pancreas syndrome (mtDNA deletion)
   - Mitochondrial neurogastrointestinal encephalomyopathy (*TP* mutations)
   - Chronic diarrhea (villus atrophy) with hepatic involvement (complex III deficiency)
   - Navajo neurohepatopathy (mtDNA depletion; *MPV17* mutations)
   - Long-chain hydroxyacyl CoA dehydrogenase deficiency
   - Acute fatty liver of pregnancy (AFLP) (LCHAD enzyme mutations)
2. Fatty acid oxidation defects
3. Carnitine palmitoyltransferase I and II deficiencies
4. Carnitine-acylcarnitine translocase deficiency
5. Urea cycle enzyme deficiencies
6. ETF and ETF-dehydrogenase deficiencies
7. Phosphoenolpyruvate carboxykinase deficiency (mitochondrial)
8. Nonketotic hyperglycinemia (glycine cleavage enzyme deficiency)

Secondary Disorders

1. Reye's syndrome
2. Hepatic copper overload
   - Wilson's disease
   - Indian childhood cirrhosis
   - Idiopathic infantile copper toxicosis
   - Cholestasis
3. Hepatic iron overload
   - Hereditary hemochromatosis, juvenile hemochromatosis
   - Neonatal iron storage disease
   - Tyrosinemia, type I
   - Zellweger syndrome
4. Drugs and toxins
   - Drugs: valproic acid, salicylic acid, nucleoside analogues (FIAU, didanosine, AZT), amiodarone, tetracycline, chloramphenicol, barbiturates
   - Chemical toxins: iron, ethanol, cyanide, antimycin A, rotenone, others.
   - Bacterial toxins: cerulide (*B. cereus* emetic toxin), Ekiri
5. Conditions causing mitochondrial lipid peroxidation:
   - Cholestasis
   - Hydrophobic bile acid toxicity (cholestasis, bile acid synthesis defects, and bile canalicular transport defects)
   - Nonalcoholic fatty liver disease and steatohepatitis – associated with obesity, insulin resistance, diabetes mellitus, drugs, parenteral nutrition, bacterial contamination of small bowel, jejuno–ileal bypass, or idiopathic
6. Cirrhosis [159]

ETF, electron-transfer flavoprotein. Adapted from Treem and Sokol [2].

involvement. We have proposed a classification scheme for mitochondrial hepatopathies. In this classification scheme (Table 33.5), the disorders are divided into *primary* disorders, in which the mitochondrial defect is the primary cause of the liver disorder, and *secondary* disorders, in which a secondary insult to mitochondria is caused by either a gene defect that affects non-mitochondrial proteins or by an acquired (exogenous) injury to mitochondria. Leonard and Schapira [11] have divided primary mitochondrial diseases into those caused by mutations affecting mtDNA genes (class 1a) and those caused by mutations in nuclear genes that encode mitochondrial respiratory chain proteins or cofactors (class 1b). Most of the nuclear gene mutations associated with oxidative phosphorylation defects that have been described result in primary neuromuscular disease. For example, a mutation in the flavoprotein of complex II causes Leigh's syndrome [11], a subunit of complex I mutation causes encephalomyopathy [25], and other mutations in complex I cause Leigh's syndrome [26]. Mutations in nuclear genes coding for non–respiratory chain mitochondrial proteins may also cause mitochondrial cytopathies. Two patients have been described with multiple deficiencies of heat shock protein 60, a chaperone protein [27]. Truncation of a mitochondrial protein homologous to a yeast mitochondrial intermembranous space protein (Tim8) has been associated with the X-linked deafness–dystonia syndrome (Mohr–Tranebjaerg syndrome) [28]. Many patients with Leigh's syndrome have now been shown to have mutations in the nuclear gene encoding Surf1, a mitochondrial protein involved in cytochrome C oxidase assembly [29]. An interesting group of mitochondrial diseases caused by nuclear genes that affect mtDNA stability has been described, including mitochondrial neurogastrointestinal encephalomyopathy (MNGIE) caused by mutations in the thymidine phosphorylase gene (*TP*), mtDNA depletion syndrome (deoxyguanosine kinase, *dGK*; thymidine kinase-2, *TK2*; DNA polymerase-γ, *POLG*; and *MPV17*), and autosomal dominant progressive external ophthalmoplegia (adenine nucleotide translocator 1, *ANT1*). These phenotypically and genotypically heterogeneous disorders appear to share a common mechanism of disturbed mitochondrial nucleoside pools. The identification and pathogenesis of many additional nuclear genes regulating mitochondrial function are the focus of exhaustive research efforts in mitochondrial medicine.

Emphasis in this chapter is placed on those mitochondrial diseases involving the electron transport proteins (respiratory chain) in the liver. These usually present either as neonatal liver failure or as a gradually progressive liver disease that may suddenly deteriorate in early childhood, frequently associated with neuromuscular symptoms. In the secondary disorders, hepatic mitochondria undergo injury, or function is impaired secondary to another pathologic process. Among these disorders are diseases of uncertain etiology but clearly involving hepatic mitochondria (e.g., Reye's syndrome); conditions caused by mitochondrial toxins, drugs, or metals; and other conditions in which mitochondrial lipid peroxidation and/or abnormal electron transport have been observed and may be involved in the pathogenesis of liver dysfunction. The remainder of this chapter focuses on prototypic and important mitochondrial hepatopathies, particularly those involving electron transport and OXPHOS. The reader is referred to other chapters for detailed discussions about the deficiencies of other specific mitochondrial enzyme systems.

Primary Mitochondrial Hepatopathies

The liver and the gastrointestinal tract are major target organs in inherited defects of mitochondrial function. Disorders of electron transport and OXPHOS affecting the liver are the first, and perhaps most severe subgroup, of the primary mitochondrial hepatopathies (Table 33.5). Reduced activity of respiratory chain complexes and OXPHOS has been associated with liver disease of varying severity and at different ages; however, neonatal and early childhood presentations predominate.

Neonatal Liver Failure

One of the more common presentations of respiratory chain defects in childhood is that dominated by severe liver failure in the first weeks to months of life. This presentation is characterized by unremitting lactic acidosis, jaundice, conjugated hyperbilirubinemia, serum alanine aminotransferase (ALT) values of 2–12 times normal, coagulopathy, ketotic hypoglycemia, and hyperammonemia [30–37]. Symptoms include lethargy and hypotonia, vomiting, a poor suck from birth, seizures, and failure to thrive. In others, after an initial normal course, a viral infection or some other undefined inciting event triggers hepatic and, sometimes, neurologic deterioration. The key biochemical features in most of these infants are the markedly elevated plasma lactate concentration, an elevated molar ratio of plasma lactate to pyruvate ($>$20 and frequently $>$30 mol/mol), and elevation of β-hydroxybutyrate and the arterial ketone body ratio of β-hydroxybutyrate to acetoacetate ($>$2.0 mol/mol). The lactic acidosis may worsen during the provision of intravenous glucose, a paradoxical finding that should increase suspicion of a respiratory chain defect.

A recent study suggests that antenatal manifestations are common in infants affected by respiratory chain disorders [38]. Low birth weight was present in 22.7% of cases, and 7% had other associated anomalies, including polyhydramnios, hypertrophic cardiomyopathy, cardiac rhythm abnormalities, hydronephrosis, ventricular septal defects, and others in excess of normal newborns. These findings suggest that metabolism is perturbed long before the infant is born.

Liver biopsy histology shows predominantly microvesicular, or a combination of microvesicular and macrovesicular, steatosis, canalicular cholestasis with bile duct thrombi and ductular proliferation, and, in some cases, hepatocellular cholestasis. Inflammation is usually absent or minimal. Periportal and centrilobular fibrosis, is characteristic, and dropout of broad bands of hepatocytes leads to a micronodular cirrhosis. Glycogen depletion is a near constant feature; and iron deposition, usually in hepatocytes, is often observed leading to confusion with neonatal iron storage disease [31]. Ultrastructural evidence of mitochondrial injury may be observed as swollen mitochondria, abnormal cristae, paracrystalline arrays, and a fluffy matrix, although normal mitochondrial morphology may be present. Increased numbers of mitochondria may also be seen in each hepatocyte, as is commonly observed in muscle biopsies from patients with mitochondrial myopathies.

These infants may progress rapidly from onset of symptoms to death from liver failure, aspiration, or sepsis in the first months of life despite available treatment [32,35,37]. It is important to note that most patients have severe neurologic involvement in infancy with a weak cry, poor suck, hypotonia, recurrent apnea, myoclonic epilepsy, or a combination of these conditions, which precludes consideration for liver transplantation [39]. However, because the degree of expression of the underlying defect in different tissues is not uniform, a number of affected infants have undergone successful liver transplantation in the absence of detectable extrahepatic manifestations [40]. Others have developed neuromuscular symptoms following liver transplantation [40]. We have successfully transplanted one such infant with cytochrome C oxidase deficiency who has shown no apparent neuromuscular, cardiac, or ocular involvement during 9 years of follow-up. The long-term outcome in these infants will not be known for some time because neuromuscular features in other mitochondrial disorders may not become apparent until adulthood [11]. Other more variable parts of the neonatal presentation include intrauterine growth retardation, hydrops fetalis, neonatal ascites, hypoalbuminemia, elevated α-fetoprotein, and renal tubular dysfunction.

The hepatic activity of either isolated or combinations of respiratory chain complexes IV, I, III, and, occasionally, II has been found to be very low in these infants. The implication is that a deficiency of these enzyme complexes, or factors regulating the activity of these enzymes, was the underlying cause of the liver failure [30–37,39–41]. Among these, cytochrome C oxidase (complex IV) deficiency is the most common. Although in most cases of cytochrome C oxidase deficiency, the disease expression includes developmental delay, progressive myopathy, or subacute necrotizing encephalomyelopathy (Leigh's syndrome), which has been observed in patients with mutations in *SURF1* and *SCO2*, other patients with cytochrome c oxidase deficiency present with predominantly hepatic failure in infancy. In one such affected family, hepatic failure, lactic acidosis, and neurodevelopmental delays were associated with mutations in the cytochrome c oxidase assembly gene *SCO1* [42]. The gene product is believed to transfer copper from a chaperone to a subunit of cytochrome c oxidase. In other cases, the use of valproic acid to treat myoclonic seizures has seemingly precipitated hepatic failure [43], even if no prior liver involvement was evident.

Mitochondrial DNA mutations or deletions have not been discovered in most patients with neonatal liver failure. Rather, many appear to have mutations in nuclear genes that are responsible for isolated respiratory chain complex deficiency or forms of mtDNA depletion syndrome (discussed later in the chapter). De Lonlay et al. [44] reported mutations in the nuclear gene *BCS1L* in infants with hepatic failure, lactic acidosis, renal tubulopathy, and variable degrees of encephalopathy who were found to have deficient activity of complex III of the respiratory chain in liver, fibroblasts, or muscle. De Meirleir et al. [45] confirmed that mutations in *BCS1L* was associated with fatal complex III deficiency, hypotonia, hypoglycemia, lactic acidosis, renal tubular dysfunction, and liver failure in two siblings. Liver histology showed microvesicular steatosis, periportal fibrosis with cholangiolar proliferation, severe cholestasis, hemosiderosis, and pseudoacinar transformation of hepatocytes. This nuclear gene encodes proteins involved in the assembly of respiratory complex III and may be responsible for a substantial portion of infants who present with neonatal liver failure and lactic acidosis. It is likely that additional novel nuclear genes encoding subunits or assembly of respiratory chain complexes will be discovered in the coming years that are responsible for other patients with this presentation.

Mitochondrial DNA Depletion Syndrome

Mitochondrial DNA depletion syndrome (MDS) is a generally fatal form of liver failure in infancy that is characterized by tissue-specific reduction in mtDNA copy number [30,31,34,46–49]. There are two clinical phenotypes of MDS: the myopathic and hepatocerebral forms. Initial reports stressed the myopathic presentation in infancy or later in childhood. However, phenotypic heterogeneity has been reported, with both myopathic and hepatocerebral presentations of MDS occurring within the same family [50]. For example, mtDNA depletion has been reported to affect the liver alone in one infant with an 88% depletion of mtDNA and the muscle alone in a second cousin whose liver mtDNA was normal [50].

Infants with the hepatocerebral form of MDS present within the first few weeks or months of life with progressive liver failure, neurologic abnormalities (including hypotonia and seizures), hypoglycemia, and unremitting lactic acidosis. Symptoms include vomiting and severe gastroesophageal reflux, failure to thrive, and developmental delay [51]. Lactic acidemia and hypoglycemia are accompanied by modestly elevated serum AST and ALT and eventually total and conjugated bilirubin. However, evidence of impaired hepatic synthetic function (prolonged prothrombin time/international normalized ratio (INR) and elevated blood ammonia) may be present even early in the course. In all reported patients, neurologic abnormalities developed before death, although the initial hypotonia may have been attributed to the lactic acidosis. Death usually occurs from liver failure, sepsis, bleeding, or aspiration by 1 year of age [52]. Histologic findings in MDS liver biopsies include microvesicular steatosis, both cytoplasmic and canalicular cholestasis, an absence of inflammation, and iron deposition in hepatocytes and sinusoidal cells (Figures 33.2–33.4). The lesion may appear quite bland for the degree of hepatic synthetic failure. Eventually loss of hepatocyte mass, cholangiolar proliferation (bile ductular reaction), and portal fibrosis develop. Ultrastructural findings [31,53] include lipid vacuoles and mitochondria having aspects of "oncocytic transformation," with pleomorphic shape, marked variation in size, dilation and other abnormalities of the cristae, and changes in matrix density (Figure 33.5). It is not uncommon to note an increased density of mitochondrial

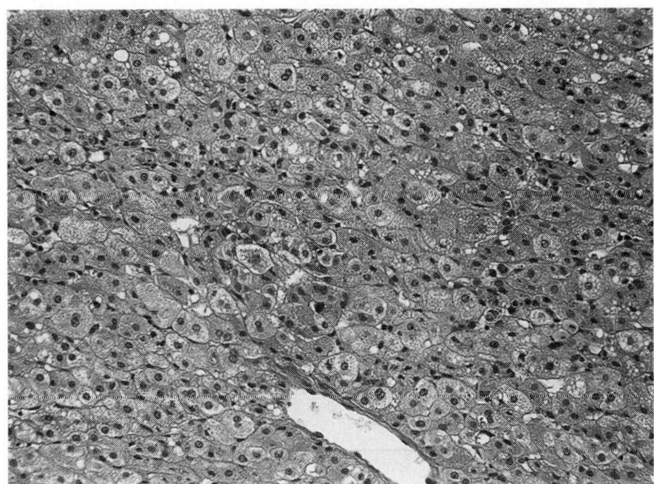

Figure 33.2. Liver histology from 11-week-old male infant with mtDNA depletion caused by *POLG* mutation. Biopsy at presentation with diarrhea, weakness, failure to thrive, and elevated AST, ALT, INR, and plasma lactate. Biopsy shows mild hepatocyte swelling with scattered microvesicular steatosis and cholestasis. Portal tracts are normal and there is no fibrosis. (Hematoxylin and eosin [H&E], ×200.) For color reproduction, see Color Plate 33.2.

number in hepatocytes. Although the individual histologic and ultrastructural findings are nonspecific, when taken together in the appropriate clinical context, they are highly suggestive of a respiratory chain disorder [54]. Diagnosis is established by the demonstration of a low ratio of amount of mtDNA to nuclear DNA in affected tissues, generally greater than 10% of normal; however, the mtDNA genome sequence is normal. In addition, there are decreased activities of the electron transport chain complexes with subunits that are coded by mtDNA (I, III, IV, and V) [30,48]. The severity of mtDNA depletion correlates with the severity of tissue involvement and biochemical defects.

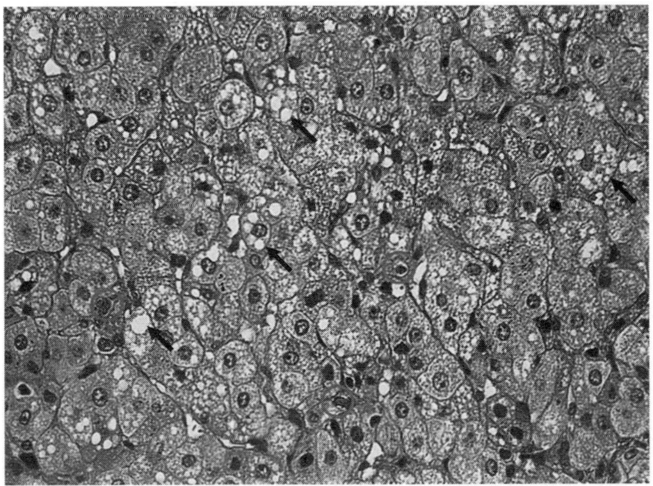

Figure 33.3. Higher power views of liver histology from patient with mtDNA depletion syndrome in Figure 33.2, showing microvesicular steatosis (*arrows*) and canalicular cholestasis (*circles*). (PAS positive diastase, ×800.) For color reproduction, see Color Plate 33.3.

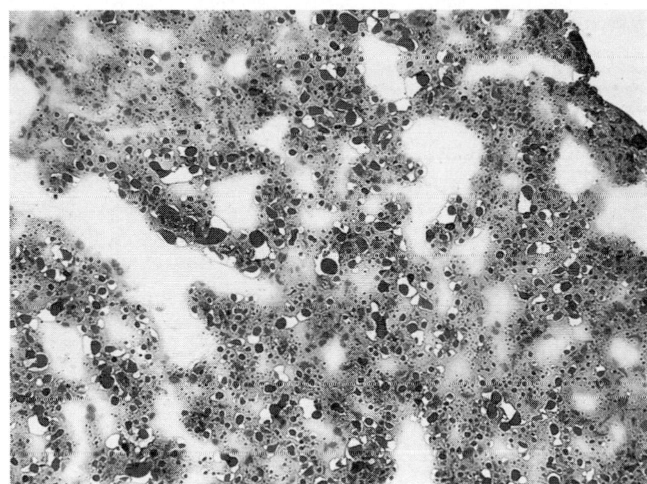

Figure 33.4. Oil-red-O stain of frozen section of liver biopsy in Figure 33.2, showing marked microvesicular steatosis in most hepatocytes, despite benign appearance of the biopsy in Figure 33.2. (Oil-red-O, ×100.) For color reproduction, see Color Plate 33.4.

Heteroplasmy of mtDNA with differential tissue involvement has suggested that MDS is a mitochondrial disease [50]; however, no convincing cases of mtDNA mutations or maternal transmission have been reported. The consanguineous origin of several of these children further suggests an autosomal recessive form of inheritance, indicating that a primary nuclear gene defect was most likely the cause of the mtDNA depletion. This hypothesis was supported by experiments in which enucleated fibroblasts from a patient with fatal neonatal hepatic failure and mtDNA depletion were fused with a human-derived rho cell line lacking mtDNA; and the hybrid cells grown in medium lacking pyruvate and uridine to select for the restoration of respiratory chain function. Growth of these cells and the demonstration by Southern blot of normal amounts of mtDNA and normal activity of respiratory chain enzymes in the F1 hybrids confirmed that mtDNA depletion was due to a defect in a nuclear gene [55,56] and led to further investigations of nuclear encoded factors that were responsible for mtDNA maintenance.

The mtDNA processing enzyme activities are dependent on several factors, including deoxyribonucleotide (dNTP) concentrations within the mitochondria, availability of ATP, and several metal cofactors. Imbalance of any of these cofactors or enzymes could affect mtDNA stability. The mitochondrial pool is maintained by either import of cytosolic dNTPs through dedicated transporters or by salvaging deoxynucleosides within the mitochondria. The mitochondrial deoxynucleoside salvage pathway is regulated by nuclear-encoded enzymes, including *dGK* and *TK2* [57,58]. Human dGK phosphorylates deoxyguanosine and deoxyadenosine, whereas TK2 phosphorylates deoxythymidine, deoxycytidine, and deoxyuridine. Imbalance of this mitochondrial dNTP pool has been proposed to be responsible for both the hepatocerebral and myopathic forms of MDS [59]. In 2001, mutations in two genes involved in this pathway were identified in patients with MDS: *dGK* in the hepatocerebral form [59] and *TK2* in the myopathic form

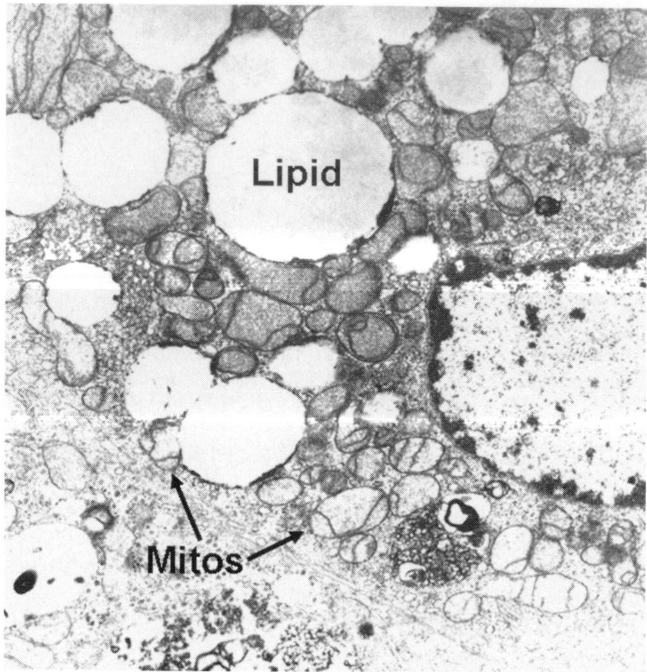

Figure 33.5. Electron microscopy (original magnification ×13,700) of liver in mtDNA depletion syndrome patient from Figure 33.2. Small droplets of neutral lipid are present in hepatocyte. Virtually all mitochondria are abnormal with enlargement and pleomorphic size and shape, unusual cristae, and flocculent matrix.

[60]. The frequency of *dGK* mutations in 21 patients with hepatocerebral MDS was only 14% in a recent study, suggesting that dGK is not the only gene responsible for mitochondrial depletion in the liver [61]. No genotype–phenotype correlation was demonstrated.

More recently two other nuclear genes have been linked to the hepatocerebral form of MDS. *POLG* is confined to mitochondria but encoded by a nuclear gene. Mutations have now been described in infants with MDS as well as older children with Alpers' disease [62–64]. Most of the cases with presentation of severe disease in infancy or with mtDNA depletion in early childhood are associated with at least one mutation in the linker region of the gene, and one in the polymerase domain. More recently, Spinazzola et al. [65] used a novel integrative genomics approach to discover mutations in *MPV17* in three families affected by the hepatocerebral form of MDS. This gene encodes an inner mitochondrial membrane protein of still uncertain function, despite prior studies suggesting this was a peroxisomal membrane protein. With the availability of clinical genotyping in commercial laboratories (see http://www.genetests.org), genetic diagnosis of mtDNA depletion syndrome is now feasible.

Later Onset Progressive Liver Failure in Early Childhood (Alpers–Huttenlocher Syndrome)

Deficiencies of respiratory chain complex I, complex IV, or combinations of respiratory chain enzymes have been associated with a later onset of recognizable liver disease in infancy and early childhood. The onset of symptoms generally occurs between 2 months and 8 years of life and is characterized by hepatomegaly and jaundice with hepatic failure evolving over time [33]. In most of these children, liver failure is preceded by the development of hypotonia, feeding difficulties, symptoms of gastroesophageal reflux or intractable vomiting, failure to thrive, and ataxia followed by the onset of relatively refractory partial motor epilepsy or multifocal myoclonus. The seizure disorder may necessitate the use of multiple anticonvulsants, including valproic acid, which may exacerbate the deficiency of respiratory chain enzyme activity. In some cases, monitoring of liver blood tests initiated solely because of the use of anticonvulsants yields the first recognition of liver function abnormality. In addition to mild to moderate elevation of aminotransferases, evidence of hepatic synthetic failure may be present (low serum albumin, prolonged prothrombin time, depressed clotting factor V or VII levels). Progressive neurologic deterioration may ensue rapidly. In other children, the neurologic features are less severe or with somewhat later onset. This clinical presentation has also been called the Alpers–Huttenlocher syndrome (Alpers' progressive infantile poliodystrophy) [66–71]. Neurologic evaluation may reveal elevated blood or cerebrospinal fluid (CSF) lactate and pyruvate levels, characteristic electroencephalogram findings (high amplitude slow activity with polyspikes [67]), asymmetric abnormal visual-evoked responses [67], and low-density areas or atrophy in the occipital or temporal lobes on computed tomography scanning of the brain [68]. A family history of an affected sibling has been reported in up to 50% of cases. In some patients, NADH oxidoreductase (complex I) deficiency has been found in liver or muscle mitochondria [33,72]. The generally accepted clinical diagnostic criteria for this syndrome are as follows: (1) refractory, mixed type seizures that often include a focal component; (2) psychomotor regression that is often episodic and triggered by intercurrent infections; and (3) hepatopathy with or without acute liver failure [73].

Striking microscopic changes in the brain include spongiosis, neuronal loss, and astrocytosis, which progress down through the cortical layers and involve the basal ganglia, cerebellum, and brainstem. Early in the course of the liver disease, liver pathology may only be notable for microvesicular steatosis, focal hepatocyte degeneration, and portal fibrosis (Figure 33.6). However, hepatic decompensation may be rapid and lead to death in 1–2 months [74]. At autopsy, the liver shows macrovesicular steatosis with accompanying micronodular cirrhosis, massive hepatocyte dropout (probably caused by apoptosis), parenchymal collapse, and bile ductular proliferation within broad bands of fibrous tissue (Figure 33.6B and 33.6C) [74,75]. On electron microscopy, there may be an increased number and density of normal appearing mitochondria in each hepatocyte or mitochondria may be swollen and pleomorphic with a less dense matrix and few cristae (Figure 33.7). Most children die by 3 years of age, but some survive into their teenage years. In those who show marked deterioration following the start of therapy for seizures, death has been attributed to hepatotoxicity caused by the valproate; however,

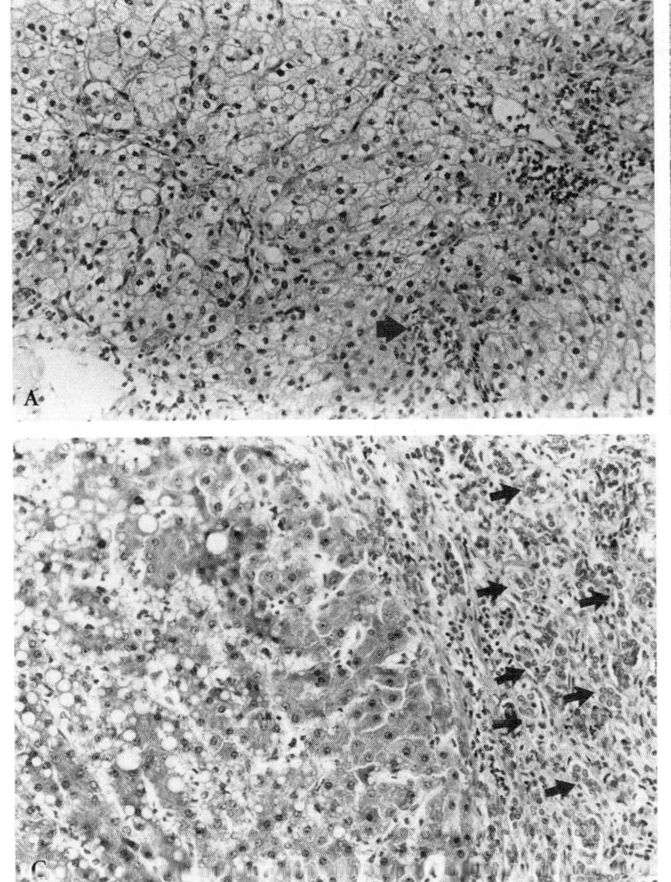

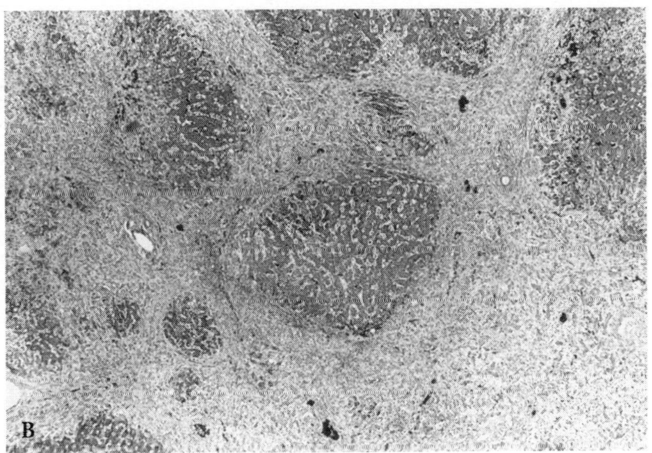

Figure 33.6. Liver histology obtained from 5-year, 7-month-old girl with Alpers' disease. (**A**) Biopsy at the time of presentation with liver involvement, showing periportal inflammation (*solid arrows*), microvesicular steatosis, and mild portal fibrosis. (**B**) Postmortem liver specimen obtained 2 months later demonstrating micronodular cirrhosis and extensive fibrosis, with prominent regenerative nodules and bile ductular proliferation. (**C**) Higher power view of edge of a regenerative nodule, demonstrating massive collapse of parenchyma with extensive portal fibrosis and bile ductular proliferation (*solid arrows*) and microvesicular steatosis in hepatocytes of regenerative nodules. (Reprinted from Narkewicz MR, Sokol RJ, Beckwith B, et al. Liver involvement in Alpers disease. J Pediatr 1991;119:260–7; with permission.)

treatment with this drug may have only accelerated the natural history of the disease [76]. Occasionally, this disorder is not recognized before liver transplantation in a child with acute liver failure; progressive neurologic deterioration may follow transplantation despite normal function of the liver allograft [39].

In recent years, it has become apparent that most children with Alpers–Huttenlocher syndrome have two mutations in the *POLG* gene that encodes the mitochondrial DNA polymerase. Naviaux and Nguyen [64] first described this association in 2004 in three children, one of whom developed acute liver failure within 3 weeks of initiation of valproic acid for refractory seizures. All three children were homozygous for a Glu873Stop mutation, which was believed to be causative, and were also heterozygous for the Ala467Thr mutation, the role of which was not known. A number of groups subsequently confirmed this association [62,63,77]. Ferrari et al. [62] found POLG mutations in 8 of 10 patients referred to their institution with Alpers–Huttenlocher syndrome and Nguyen et al. [73] in 87% of 15 sequential patients, suggesting that *POLG* mutations are responsible for the majority of cases. It should be pointed out that *POLG* mutations were first identified in families with autosomal dominant, chronic progressive external ophthalmoplegia (PEO), which is associated with accumulation

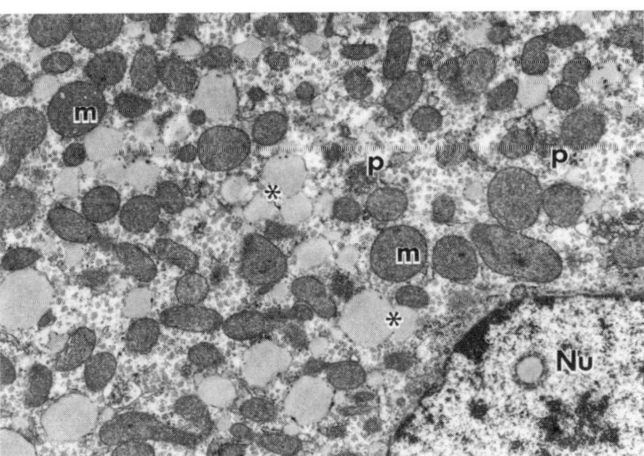

Figure 33.7. Electron microscopy (original magnification ×13,700) of liver in Alpers' disease. (**A**) Hepatocyte of same patient as in Figure 33.2, obtained at onset of liver disease. Microvesicular steatosis (*asterisk*), normal peroxisomes (*p*), and morphologically normal mitochondria (*m*) but increased in number. *Nu* denotes nucleus. (Reprinted from Narkewicz MR, Sokol RJ, Beckwith B, et al. Liver involvement in Alpers disease. J Pediatr 1991;119:260–7; with permission.)

of multiple mtDNA deletions in affected tissues [63] and then were discovered in autosomal recessive PEO. Horvath et al. [63] demonstrated that there is a wide spectrum of disease caused by mutations in this gene, with most affected children under age 7 years demonstrating significant hepatic involvement. In one series [63], all patients had either A467T or W748S mutations, so that screening for these two mutations might be an effective and sensitive means for confirming the diagnosis of Alpers–Huttenlocher syndrome. This was not confirmed in another series [63].

It has recently been suggested that children with deficiencies of one of several respiratory chain complexes may have a milder form of liver and neurologic disease [33]. Because of heteroplasmy, it is certainly conceivable that children may receive smaller "doses" of mutated mtDNA or that other modifier genes may control the oxidative stress caused by respiratory chain complex deficiencies, leading to a later onset or milder amount of liver injury. Thus, it may require accumulation of other somatic mutations of mtDNA over time, or the effect of viral illness or medications, to exceed the OXPHOS capability and free radical scavenging capacity of hepatocytes that is necessary to generate hepatic injury. Further investigation of children with these possible milder forms of respiratory chain disorders should provide guidelines for appropriate evaluation of less symptomatic children who might present with chronic hepatitis or hepatic steatosis.

Pancreatic Insufficiency, Bone Marrow Abnormalities, and Liver Involvement (Pearson's Marrow–Pancreas Syndrome)

Pearson's marrow–pancreas syndrome was described in 1979 in four children with neonatal-onset severe macrocytic anemia, variable neutropenia and thrombocytopenia, vacuolization of erythroid and myeloid precursors, and ringed-sideroblasts in the bone marrow [78]. Later in infancy or early childhood, diarrhea and fat malabsorption developed, and the patients were found to have pancreatic insufficiency caused by extensive pancreatic fibrosis and acinar atrophy. Partial villous atrophy of the small intestine was noted in a number of patients. Marked hepatomegaly, hepatic steatosis, and cirrhosis has been associated with liver failure and death in some cases before age 4 years. For years, the cause of this disorder was unknown.

It is now established that mtDNA rearrangements are present in all patients with Pearson's syndrome with large (4000–5000 bp) deletions predominating in three-quarters of reported cases [79–81]. Of the respiratory chain enzymes encoded by mtDNA, complex I is the most severely affected by this deletion; however, it also encompasses genes that encode two subunits of complex V, one subunit of complex IV, and five transfer RNA genes. Although oxidation of NADH is abnormal in lymphocytes from these patients, oxygen consumption and respiratory chain enzyme activities are normal in muscle mitochondria. Southern blotting has shown that a mixed population of normal and deleted mitochondrial genomes is present in all tissues tested (heteroplasmy), but different proportions of deleted mtDNA molecules are noted. In the clinically more severely affected tissues such as bone marrow, polymorphonuclear leukocytes, lymphocytes, pancreas, and gut, mtDNA deletions are found in 80–90% of cells but are found in only 50% of muscle cells. It appears that the phenotypic expression of Pearson's syndrome in a given tissue requires a minimum threshold number of mutated mtDNA molecules. The lack of maternal inheritance or positive family histories and the absence of mtDNA rearrangements in the lymphocytes of parents or siblings of cases suggest that many cases are caused by de novo mutations occurring during oogenesis or the early development of fertilized eggs.

Other clinical manifestations of Pearson's syndrome include renal tubular disease (Fanconi's syndrome), patchy erythematous skin lesions and photosensitivity, diabetes mellitus, hydrops fetalis, and the late development of visual impairment, tremor, ataxia, proximal muscle weakness, external ophthalmoplegia, and pigmentary retinopathy. These symptoms are similar to those found in Kearns–Sayre syndrome (KSS), a mitochondrial disease also characterized by a large 5 kilobase mtDNA deletion [82]. The occurrence of KSS in patients with Pearson's syndrome who survive to childhood is another example of the dependence of phenotypic expression on random partitioning of mutated mtDNA during cell division, changes in the proportion of rearranged mtDNA in various tissues over time, and the possible accumulation of other somatic mutations [83]. Supporting this hypothesis is the clinical observation that patients with Pearson's syndrome frequently do not require blood transfusions after age 2 years. This may be because the number of hematopoietic cells containing a high proportion of deleted mtDNA decreases with time as a result of selection of cells with normal mtDNA. When suspected, Pearson's syndrome can generally be diagnosed by analyzing for the characteristic mtDNA deletion.

Chronic Diarrhea and Intestinal Pseudo-Obstruction with Liver Involvement

Severe anorexia, vomiting, chronic diarrhea, and villus atrophy may be the initial manifestations of a rare mtDNA rearrangement syndrome appearing late in the first year or during the second year of life and associated with mild elevations of liver enzymes, hepatomegaly, and steatosis [84]. Diarrhea, vomiting, and lactic acidosis worsen in these patients with high dextrose intravenous infusions or enteral nutrition. Diarrhea improves and even resolves completely by 5 years of age in association with normalization of intestinal biopsies. However, retinitis pigmentosa, cerebellar ataxia, sensorineural deafness, and proximal muscle weakness may become evident late in the first decade of life, leading to death soon thereafter. Respiratory chain enzyme assays are normal in circulating lymphocytes but were abnormal in skeletal muscle tissue, revealing a complex III deficiency.

Mitochondrial Neurogastrointestinal Encephalomyopathy (MNGIE)

This multisystem syndrome, first described in 1983, involves skeletal muscle, peripheral and central nervous systems, the intestinal tract, and the liver [85]. In 1994, Hirano et al. [5] labeled the syndrome mitochondrial neurogastrointestinal encephalomyopathy. The syndrome is characterized by myopathy with ragged-red fibers, peripheral sensorimotor neuropathy, progressive external ophthalmoplegia, ptosis, leukoencephalopathy, and chronic intestinal pseudo-obstruction [5]. The disease onset ranges from 5 months to 43 years of age [86]. Nonspecific gastrointestinal signs and symptoms of nausea, vomiting, abdominal pain, borborygmi, diarrhea, constipation, and abdominal distention often lead to a diagnosis of intestinal dysmotility or "pseudo-obstruction" [85,87,88]. Gastrointestinal symptoms typically have onset in childhood and were the presenting complaint in 45–67% of patients [89]. Sensory neuropathy, hearing loss, or ocular symptoms were the initial manifestations in 42–49% of patients. Thin body habitus and short stature are constant findings, presumably secondary to chronic malnutrition and malabsorption. Small bowel diverticulosis, presumably secondary to markedly delayed intestinal motility, appears in early adult years in 30–67% of patients. The chronic intestinal pseudo-obstruction has been attributed to a visceral smooth muscle myopathy with atrophic fibrotic longitudinal smooth muscle in the intestinal wall but normal ganglion cells in some reported patients. In other cases, autopsy findings have suggested an autonomic neuropathy in other patients with fibrosis and vacuolization of autonomic ganglia in the myenteric plexus and decreased nerve fibers innervating intestinal smooth muscle.

Mitochondrial neurogastrointestinal encephalomyopathy is an autosomal recessive disease associated with multiple mtDNA deletions, depletion in skeletal muscle, or both. In the limited number of patients studied, skeletal muscle respiratory chain defects consisting of complex IV, complex I, or combination defects have been identified. Following the mapping of MNGIE to chromosome 22q13.32-qter region in four kindreds [90], Nishino et al. [91] reported loss-of-function mutations in the gene encoding thymidine phosphorylase (TP). More than sixteen different mutations in ethnically diverse MNGIE pedigrees have been found [92]. Thymidine phosphorylase is a multifunctional enzyme that has an important role in the nucleoside salvage pathway, catalyzing the breakdown of thymidine to be reutilized for mtDNA synthesis as dexoxythymidine triphosphate (dTTP). It also produces 2-deoxyribose, which is an endothelial cell chemoattractant in angiogenesis induction [93]. No MNGIE patients have had vascular abnormalities, suggesting that the absence of TP activity does not interfere with normal angiogenesis. Impaired thymidine metabolism has been demonstrated by biochemical analysis in 27 MNGIE patients [94], with elevated plasma levels of thymidine and depletion of the mitochondrial dTTP pool used for DNA synthesis. Recent studies have demonstrated both mtDNA depletion and deletions in smooth muscle from the small intestine of affected patients [95]. The pathogenesis of these finding in MNGIE, like mitochondrial depletion syndrome, appears to be related to an imbalance of the mitochondrial nucleoside pool.

Navajo Neurohepatopathy

Navajo neurohepatopathy (NNH) is a sensorimotor neuropathy with progressive liver disease that is confined to Navajo children. This disorder is manifested by the development of weakness, hypotonia, areflexia, loss of sensation in the extremities, acral mutilation, corneal ulceration, poor growth, short stature, and serious systemic infections [96,97]. Singleton et al. [97] reported in 1990 that there was an association of Reye's syndrome–like episodes, hepatic dysfunction, and death due to liver failure at a young age in three patients. Cerebral magnetic resonance imaging (MRI) further demonstrated the presence of progressive white matter lesions, and peripheral nerve biopsies showed severe loss of myelinated fibers. Multiple investigations of infectious, biochemical, and metabolic causes failed to yield an etiology for this multisystem disorder [98]. The inheritance appears to be autosomal recessive. The hepatic findings were recently characterized in 20 patients by Holve et al. [98]. There were three clinical presentations of NNH, including an *infantile* form, in which failure to thrive and jaundice progress to hepatic failure and death within the first 2 years of life, with or without neurologic findings; a *childhood* form presented between 1 and 5 years of age with rapid development of liver failure; and the *classical* form in which progressive neurologic findings dominate although liver dysfunction (and even cirrhosis) was present in all patients. Elevation of AST, ALT, alkaline phosphatase, and γ-glutamyl transpeptidase were present in all cases. Liver histology demonstrated portal fibrosis or micronodular cirrhosis, macrovesicular and microvesicular steatosis, pseudoacinar formation, multinucleated giant cells, cholestasis, and periportal inflammation. Nonspecific mitochondrial changes, such as swollen mitochondria and ringed cristae, were seen in several patients. Blood lactate and pyruvate levels were normal in patients tested, and skin fibroblasts had normal respiration from one patient. The liver involvement in this disorder is progressive with liver failure developing within months to years in most patients. Neurologic symptoms progressed after liver transplant in one patient. There has been no effective treatment to date for affected children.

The etiology of NNH was unknown; however, because it shares many clinical and histologic features with other mitochondrial hepatopathies, several groups pursued the possibility of NNH being a mitochondrial hepatopathy. The mtDNA genome was found to be normal in these patients. The first breakthrough came in 2001 when Vu et al. [99] demonstrated mtDNA depletion in liver biopsies from two NNH patients, consistent with the hypothesis that a nuclear gene controlling mitochondrial structure or function might be responsible for this autosomal recessive disease. A genome-wide scan, performed using 400 DNA microsatellite markers, demonstrated mapping of the disease to chromosome 2p24.2 [100]. Interestingly, *MPV17*, the gene associated in 2006 with mtDNA depletion syndrome, was located within this region. Remarkably, sequencing of *MPV17* in six NNH patients from five families demonstrated the same homozygous disease-causing R50Q mutation in exon 2 in all NNH patients [100]. Thus, it is now clear that NNH is indeed a form of mtDNA depletion with a unique clinical presentation in Navajos. This discovery now allows for the possibility of both prenatal and postnatal genetic diagnosis of NNH, even in presymptomatic patients, with the hope that an effective treatment can now be developed.

Fatty Acid Oxidation Defects and Electron Transports Deficiency

Other inborn errors of metabolism can alter the transfer of electrons and generation of ATP by the respiratory chain by generating toxic metabolites that specifically inhibit one or more of the enzyme complexes or nonspecifically damage the mitochondrial membrane and other electron transport. Long-chain 3-hydroxyacyl CoA dehydrogenase (LCHAD) deficiency is an autosomal recessively inherited defect in the third enzyme in the intramitochondrial β-oxidation pathway of FAO, which shares several features with respiratory chain disorders. For example, profound lactic acidemia occurs during episodes of metabolic crisis, in contrast to other FAO disorders. LCHAD deficiency has been associated with neonatal liver failure, progressive hepatic fibrosis, and cirrhosis, unlike other FAO defects, which usually result in micro- and macrovesicular steatosis without permanent liver damage [101]. Further, LCHAD deficiency involves the nervous system, including the inevitable development of retinitis pigmentosa in all patients who survive the neonatal and early childhood period and the appearance of a progressive peripheral neuropathy in some long-term survivors. Several groups have demonstrated that the long-chain fatty acid esters, palmityl-CoA and the 3-hydroxypalmityl-CoA, intermediates that would be expected to accumulate within mitochondria in patients with LCHAD deficiency, inhibit respiratory chain driven ATP synthesis in cultured skin fibroblasts from normal humans [102]. This inhibition of ATP synthesis appears to be localized to both the transport of succinate into mitochondria and of electrogenic ADP–ATP carrier on the inner mitochondrial membrane. Recently, a patient with complex I deficiency was described who had clinical and biochemical features of LCHAD deficiency including cardiomyopathy, liver failure, and the characteristic organic acid pattern in urine [103]. He was treated effectively with carnitine, a low-fat diet with medium chain-triglycerides (MCT) oil and essential fatty acid supplements, succinate, and ascorbate. This case underscores the need to consider respiratory chain disorders in patients who have abnormal urine organic acid patterns that suggest FAO disorders and that there is an overlap in clinical phenotype in these two types of mitochondrial hepatopathies.

Accumulating CoA esters of long-chain fatty acids found in the livers of patients with Reye's syndrome have been shown to uncouple oxidative phosphorylation and reduce intramitochondrial ATP formation. These same metabolites have been linked to liver damage in other diseases characterized histologically by intrahepatic microvesicular steatosis including acute fatty liver of pregnancy (AFLP). The recent reports of AFLP in LCHAD-deficient heterozygote mothers who are carrying an affected fetus suggest that toxic long-chain fatty acid metabolites from the fetus may enter the maternal circulation and play a role in maternal liver injury during the latter stages of pregnancy in heterozygote women [104,105]. The expression of this feto–maternal disorder requires the presence of an increased load of toxic metabolites from the fetus and a maternal liver with a limited capacity to degrade these compounds.

Other Primary Mitochondrial Hepatopathies

These disorders include nuclear gene-encoded defects in other specific enzymatic proteins or structural proteins affecting mitochondria, including FAO defects, urea cycle enzyme deficiencies, phosphoenolpyruvate carboxykinase deficiency, carnitine palmitoyl transferease (CPT)-I and II deficiency, and others (Table 33.5). The specific clinical manifestations of each disorder is dependent on the pathophysiologic consequences of the individual biochemical pathway that is disrupted and the type of toxic metabolites or precursors that accumulate. The reader is referred to other chapters of this textbook for descriptions of these conditions.

Secondary Mitochondrial Hepatopathies

Secondary mitochondrial hepatopathies are caused by an injurious metal, drug, toxin, xenobiotic, or endogenous metabolites (Table 33.5). Acquired abnormalities of mitochondrial respiration caused by these factors may be involved in the pathogenesis of these disorders. Several prototypic disorders are discussed.

Reye's Syndrome

Reye's syndrome is the classic secondary mitochondrial hepatopathy and is caused by the interaction of a viral infection (influenza, varicella, enteroviruses, other viruses) and salicylate use or some underlying undefined metabolic–genetic predisposition. In years past, many cases that were initially labeled as Reye's syndrome were undoubtedly undiagnosed metabolic diseases, such as FAO defects. However, several characteristics lead us to conclude that there are still patients who present with this clinical entity. Liver and brain electron microscopy in Reye's syndrome patients reveals striking abnormalities in mitochondrial structure (Figure 33.8) and their function is perturbed, resulting in defective ureagenesis and ketogenesis, hyperammonemia, hypoglycemia, elevated serum free fatty acids, and lactate and dicarboxylic acids [106]. Impairment of β-oxidation of fatty acids by mitochondria is also present. Salicylates have been shown to impair mitochondrial fatty acid oxidation in vitro, and recent studies indicate that this may be by reversible inhibition of LCHAD activity [106]. Cells from Reye's syndrome patients were found to be more susceptible to inhibition by low concentrations of salicylates than control subjects [106]. Glasgow et al. [106] proposed that this increased sensitivity could potentially be caused by absent or reduced activity of an uncoupling protein in mitochondria. This study provided the first biochemical evidence that might explain why only certain individuals react to aspirin in a manner that precipitates Reye's syndrome.

Most cases of Reye's syndrome traditionally occurred in the autumn and winter (influenza season), with the peak age of occurrence between ages 5 and 15 years. Symptoms developed

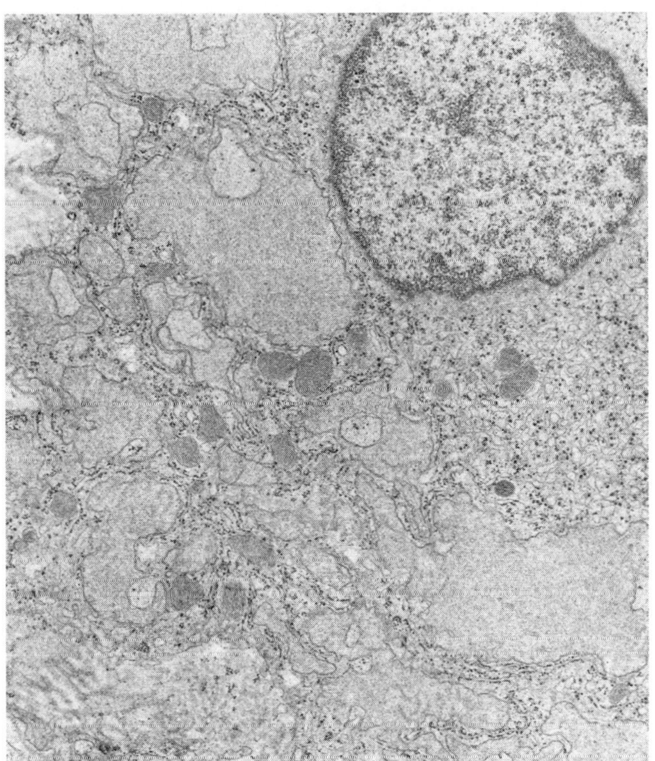

Figure 33.8. Electron micrograph (original magnification ×21,000) of hepatocyte from liver biopsy of child with Reye's syndrome. Peroxisomes are increased in number and size. There is marked reduction of cytoplasmic glycogen. Mitochondrial abnormalities include marked pleomorphism and swelling, with absent dense bodies and a flocculent matrix. (Osmium tetroxide fixation in Millonig's phosphate buffer.) (Reprinted from Partin [109], with permission.)

several days following onset of influenza A or B or varicella infection. There was a strong association of aspirin use during these illnesses and the development of Reye's syndrome [107]. Frequently, the child appeared to be recovering from a viral illness after 3–5 days when sudden, unremitting vomiting developed. After several hours of vomiting, and not uncommonly dehydration, variable degrees of encephalopathy developed [108,109]. Early mild stages of encephalopathy (grades 0–2) were associated with quietness, lethargy, and sleepiness and progressed in many affected patients to stages 3 and 4 with delirium, decorticate and decerebrate posturing, and eventually brainstem herniation, caused by cerebral edema and raised intracranial pressure. Liver dysfunction was always present when vomiting developed and was characterized by elevated AST, ALT, and blood ammonia with mild to moderate prolongation of prothrombin time, variable hypoglycemia, but normal serum bilirubin values. Metabolic support with hypertonic dextrose infusions and control of cerebral edema and intracranial pressure became the most important facets of clinical treatment, until spontaneous recovery occurred or irreversible brain injury developed. Mortality was high when patients presented in deeper stages of coma and correlated with high levels of blood ammonia at presentation [110].

Abnormal mitochondrial morphology and function characterize this disorder [108,109], with involvement of liver, brain, muscle, and kidney. Although patients present with hepatic dysfunction, hyperammonemia, and coma, the encephalopathy may be caused by direct involvement of CNS mitochondria [111] as well as the accumulating metabolic toxins. Liver biopsies are characterized by microvesicular steatosis in the absence of hepatic inflammation or necrosis and characteristic swelling and pleomorphism of mitochondria under electron microscopy [108,109] (Figure 33.8). The liver makes a full recovery in this disease, despite progressive and sometimes fatal cerebral edema. The mortality of Reye's syndrome remains high [107] primarily because most cases nowadays are diagnosed in deeper stages of coma. A detailed discussion of the pathophysiology and treatment of Reye's syndrome is found in the first edition of this textbook [109].

In more recent years, many young patients once thought to have Reye's syndrome have been found subsequently to have defects in FAO, a form of primary mitochondrial hepatopathy [112,113]. Because the incidence of Reye's syndrome has decreased dramatically in Western countries following the public warnings of salicylate use in children with viral infections [107,114], it is imperative to evaluate thoroughly all children who are diagnosed with Reye's syndrome for FAO defects, particularly those under age 5 years. Although salicylate use has not been associated with Reye's syndrome in some countries [113,114], its reduced use in the United States and England has clearly diminished the frequency of cases of Reye's syndrome [107,114]. Others believe that the increasing ability to diagnose FAO defects and other metabolic diseases over the past 2 decades also account for the decreased incidence of Reye's syndrome.

Wilson's Disease

Mitochondrial involvement in the pathogenesis of liver injury has been implicated in Wilson's disease for many years, since the early observation by Sternlieb and Feldman [115,116] of abnormal mitochondrial morphology on electron microscopy of liver biopsies that is so characteristic of this disorder of copper metabolism. Changes in mitochondrial shape, density, and size are common early in the course of Wilson's disease, including decreased matriceal density, enlarged intermembranous spaces, dilatation and vacuolization of cristae, crystalline inclusions, and vacuoles in the matrix [115,116]. Recent studies in experimental animals and naturally occurring copper toxicity in dogs and in humans have shown that the mitochondrion is a major intracellular target for copper toxicity. The accumulation of copper in the hepatic mitochondria leads to oxidant stress (increased free radical generation) with subsequent lipid peroxidation and oxidative alterations of thiol-containing proteins. In a rat model of copper overload, a 60% decrease of cytochrome c oxidase activity was demonstrated in hepatic mitochondria in conjunction with significant lipid peroxidation [117]. Similar increased lipid peroxidation has been demonstrated in hepatic mitochondria isolated from copper-overloaded dogs and from patients with Wilson's disease undergoing liver transplantation

[118]. Mansouri et al. [119] have shown that this oxidant damage in hepatic mitochondria also leads to deletions in mtDNA in young adults with Wilson's disease. These data suggest that dysfunction of hepatic mitochondrial electron transport may be an important factor in the pathogenesis of liver dysfunction and liver failure in copper overload states. The underlying defect in Wilson's disease is caused by mutations in the P type ATPase, *ATP7B*, which is present in the trans-Golgi and might be transported to hepatic mitochondria [120]. The function of ATP7b in mitochondria and how this may relate to the pathogenesis of Wilson's disease has not been determined. In addition to copper chelation therapy, treatment to reduce the oxidative stress (e.g., with antioxidants) in the liver of patients with Wilson's disease may help protect the mitochondria from injury in this disease and in other metal overload conditions.

Drugs and Toxins

Acquired abnormalities of mitochondrial respiration may be caused by a number of other drugs and toxins (Table 33.5). Valproic acid is an 8-carbon branched fatty acid that can be metabolized into a potential mitochondrial toxin, 4-envalproic acid, and it may inhibit β-oxidation by itself as well. Individual variation in mitochondrial β-oxidation may determine the sensitivity of some to a severe toxic reaction by valproic acid, causing a Reye-like syndrome or fulminant hepatic failure. Children with underlying mtDNA depletion syndrome, Alpers–Huttenlocher syndrome, and respiratory chain defects (complex I deficiency) appear to be more sensitive to valproic acid; its use has been associated with precipitating liver failure. For other drugs, the mechanism causing inhibition of mitochondrial respiration is still unclear. A number of toxins inhibit specific protein complexes of the respiratory chain (e.g., cyanide, antimycin A, rotenone) and lead to reduced ATP production and increased oxidative stress. The emetic toxin of *bacillus cereus,* cereulide, has been demonstrated to cause inhibition of respiratory chain activity and is a causative agent for fulminant liver failure [121].

In the following sections, two important toxins/drugs that cause mitochondrial injury are discussed in more detail: ethanol and nucleoside analogues.

ETHANOL TOXICITY

Acquired respiratory chain defects have been implicated in the pathogenesis of the intrahepatic microvesicular steatosis, which develops during ethanol hepatotoxicity. Ethanol consumption increases the generation of ROS by hepatic mitochondria, decreases the intrahepatic mitochondrial glutathione levels, and increases the susceptibility of hepatic mitochondria to lipid peroxidation. Because mtDNA lacks protective histones and DNA repair enzymes and lies in close proximity to the site of free radical generation, both ROS and lipid peroxidation products may damage mtDNA. Fromenty et al. [122] showed that the majority of alcoholics with microvesicular steatosis had an acquired mtDNA deletion that mimicked the large (approximately 5000 bp) deletion characteristic of Pearson's syndrome in childhood; however, it was present in a much lower percentage of cells. This mtDNA deletion was present in 6 of 10 alcoholics with microvesicular steatosis, 2 of 17 alcoholics with macrovesicular steatosis, 0 of 23 alcoholics with acute alcoholic hepatitis or cirrhosis, and 0 of 62 age-matched nonalcoholic patients with various other liver diseases or normal liver histology [122]. The pathogenesis of the microvesicular steatosis may be related to the excess of reducing equivalents (NADH) produced by ethanol in hepatic mitochondria. LCHAD is dependent on NAD as a cofactor; the accumulation of intramitochondrial NADH inhibits LCHAD activity thus decreasing β-oxidation of long-chain fatty acids. In addition, reduced reoxidation of NADH caused by an acquired complex I (mtDNA deletion) defect may also contribute to a reduction in long-chain FAO and the development of microvesicular steatosis. Strategies at improving mitochondrial respiration or reducing the generation of ROS may be of potential benefit and are under study.

NUCLEOSIDE ANALOGUES (REVERSE TRANSCRIPTASE INHIBITORS)

Several drugs directly inhibit protein complexes of the intramitochondrial respiratory chain or intramitochondrial β-oxidation enzymes or interfere with mtDNA replication (Table 33.5) and lead to hepatotoxicity and microvesicular steatosis. An example of drug-induced mitochondrial toxicity was the fatal lactic acidosis and liver failure that developed in seven adults with chronic hepatitis B who were treated with the experimental antiviral nucleoside analogue, fialuridine (FIAU) [123]. Most of these patients presented with fatigue, nausea, constipation, abdominal pain, coagulopathy, hyperammonemia, and profound lactic acidosis with only mild jaundice and minimal increases in serum aminotransferase values. Pancreatitis, peripheral neuropathy, and myopathy, reminiscent of inherited mitochondrial disorders of the respiratory chain, also developed in several patients. Liver tissue from the five patients who underwent liver transplantation showed marked microvesicular and macrovesicular steatosis, cholestasis, and swollen dysmorphic mitochondria. The mechanism of FIAU toxicity is based on its incorporation directly into mtDNA in the place of thymidine, thus interrupting transcription of mtDNA and its gene products [124]. This has a profound effect on mtDNA-encoded proteins, with impaired mitochondrial respiration and FAO that resulted in microvesicular steatosis, morphologic changes in mitochondria, and severe lactic acidosis.

Other nucleoside analogues, zidovudine, didanosine, and zalcitabine, have been shown to inhibit the DNA polymerase-γ of mitochondria and may block the elongation of mtDNA, with the potential of causing acquired mtDNA depletion over time [125]. Zidovudine has been occasionally associated with a toxic myopathy characterized by the depletion of mtDNA in myocytes and has occasionally caused lactic acidosis, hepatic steatosis, and hepatic failure in HIV-infected patients treated with the drug. Peripheral neuropathy has been reported with the use of zalcitabine, and pancreatitis occurs as a toxic consequence of didanosine in up to 50% of HIV-infected patients treated for prolonged periods. Lamivudine, another nucleoside analogue used to treat chronic hepatitis B virus infection, is not incorporated into mtDNA (as is FIAU) and shows relatively little inhibition of mtDNA synthesis at concentrations that block the synthesis of HBV DNA. Consequently, lamivudine has not been associated with myopathy or significant hepatic toxicity. Insulin resistance may also play a role in the lactic acidosis of these drugs [126]. The use of intravenous or oral L-carnitine in addition to discontinuation of the offending therapy and treatment of the acidosis are associated with survival [127].

Hydrophobic Bile Acid Toxicity

Hydrophobic bile acids [128] and metals [118] that accumulate in the liver in cholestasis appear to be toxic to hepatocytes through several mechanisms, including activation of cell death receptor and protein kinase signaling pathways, the induction of the mitochondrial membrane permeability transition, and the generation of oxidative stress. During experimental cholestasis induced by bile duct ligation in the rat, Krahenbuhl et al. [129] demonstrated reduced activity of the electron transport chain in hepatic mitochondria with an increased density of mitochondria per hepatocyte. This group further showed that hydrophobic bile acids led to inhibition of complex I and complex III activity in isolated hepatic mitochondria [130]. Pathophysiologic concentrations of hydrophobic bile acids induce the mitochondrial membrane permeability transition and hydroperoxide generation [131]. Thus, it has been proposed that, during cholestasis and in patients with bile acid synthesis and canalicular transport defects, increased concentrations of hydrophobic bile acids induce generation of reactive oxygen species from the altered electron transport chain of hepatocyte mitochondria, with the resultant opening of the permeability pore and the onset of cellular necrosis or apoptosis [132]. The antioxidant, vitamin E, has provided significant protection against bile acid toxicity in an in vivo rat model [132]. The extent of the role of mitochondrial dysfunction in human cholestatic liver disease and whether this could be targeted for new therapies has not been fully elucidated and awaits further investigation.

Nonalcoholic Steatohepatitis

Another category of secondary mitochondrial hepatopathies is the broad group of disorders now called nonalcoholic fatty liver disease (NAFLD) and nonalcoholic steatohepatitis (NASH). In these disorders micro- or macrovesicular steatosis is accompanied by varying degrees of necroinflammatory change and portal fibrosis, in the absence of intake of alcohol but generally in the presence of insulin resistance. NASH, which may be progressive and culminate in cirrhosis, is commonly associated with obesity, non–insulin dependent diabetes mellitus, jejuno–ileal bypass surgery, parenteral nutrition, bacterial overgrowth of the small intestine, and various drugs [133]. There is growing evidence that acquired mitochondrial electron transport abnormalities may underlie the oxidant stress that is generated and contribute to the intracellular accumulation of microvesicular fat [134]. Circulating lipopolysaccharide and tumor necrosis-α levels are elevated in several of the associated conditions [133] and may contribute to both the oxidant stress and mitochondrial dysfunction. The preliminary trial of vitamin E in children with obesity-related NASH that resulted in normalization of raised AST and ALT in five treated patients [135] is now being followed by a large randomized controlled trial. Further investigations into the mitochondrial pathogenesis of NASH are being conducted with a growing understanding of the role played by lipo-toxicity, inflammatory cytokines induced by obesity, and insulin resistance.

DIAGNOSIS OF RESPIRATORY CHAIN DISORDERS

General Clinical Features

Diagnosing a mitochondrial respiratory chain defect in patients with liver disease requires a high index of suspicion. Clinical events that should suggest these disorders include (1) association of neuromuscular symptoms with liver dysfunction, (2) multisystem involvement in a patient with acute or chronic liver disease, and (3) rapidly progressive course of liver disease, particularly in the presence of lactic acidosis, hepatic steatosis, or ketonemia. Although CNS and neuromuscular syndromes have been the predominant findings in many cases, a recent report of 100 patients with respiratory chain deficiencies at one European center showed that 56% of patients presented with an extra-neuromuscular problem with only 44% being referred for a neuromuscular problem [36]. A more complete list of presenting clinical symptoms at various ages has been published by Munnich et al. [36,136] (Table 33.1). Most patients with respiratory chain defects (involving any tissue) present early in life. In one large series, 36% presented before 1 month of life, 44% between 1 month and 2 years, and 20% after 2 years of age [36,136].

Screening Tests for Respiratory Chain Defects

Laboratory findings that suggest the presence of a respiratory chain defect are listed in Table 33.6 [136]. Persistent elevation of plasma lactic acid (>2.5 mmol/mL), an elevated molar ratio of plasma lactate to pyruvate (L–P >20:1), and elevation of the ketone body ratio of β-hydroxybutyrate to acetoacetate (β-OHB–AA >2:1) are highly suggestive of respiratory chain disorders. It should be stressed, however, that lactic acid and these ratios are not elevated in all patients with respiratory chain defects (e.g., Alpers–Huttenlocher syndrome). Elevated ratios are indicative of an increase in reducing equivalents (excess of NADH and lack of NAD) caused by impaired transfer of electrons from NADH to oxygen as a result of disrupted OXHPOS. The L–P ratio is a reflection of the NADH to NAD balance in the cytosol, and the β-OHB–AA ratio is a reflection of the NADH to NAD ratio within the mitochondrion. The elevated ketone body ratio is a consequence of functional impairment of the citric acid cycle, with ketone body synthesis increasing (particularly after meals) because of the channeling of acetyl CoA away from coalescence with oxalate to form citrate and into the ketogenic

Table 33.6: Screening Tests for Respiratory Chain Defects

- Plasma lactate >2.5 mmol/L (persistently elevated)
- Molar ratio of plasma lactate/pyruvate >20:1 mol/mol
- Molar ketone body ratio: Arterial 3-OH butyrate/acetoacetate >2:1 mol/mol
- Paradoxical ↑ in plasma ketone bodies or lactate after meals
- Oral glucose load (2 g/kg): repeat plasma lactate/pyruvate testing each 15 min for 90 min: elevated LP ratio
- Urine lactate, succinate, fumarate, malate, 3 methylglutaconic, 3-methylglutaric by gas chromatography–mass spectroscopy

Adapted from Treem and Sokol [2].

pathway. After feeding, the exaggerated paradoxical production of ketones is even more evident, as ketone production should normally decrease after meals because of the suppressive effect of insulin on ketogenesis. Similarly, the abnormal L–P ratio is particularly apparent in the postprandial period when more NAD is required for adequate oxidation of glycolytic substrates. In the presence of decreased NAD, pyruvate will be diverted by anaerobic metabolism to lactate. Thus, to evaluate the patient fully, some have recommended that the concentration of these substrates and their molar ratios, as well as blood glucose and free fatty acids, should be determined before and 1 hour after meals. Occasionally, it is necessary to load a fasted patient with oral glucose (2 g/kg) to provoke lactic acidemia and abnormal ratios, if the values are normal under baseline conditions. Substrates and ratios should be measured every 15 minutes for 90 minutes after the load. Lactate pyruvate molar ratios in CSF may be helpful when no elevation in plasma lactate is observed, particularly in the patient with CNS involvement. Pitfalls in interpretation of these ratios include false positives in patients with systemic hypotension or with impaired ventilation. In addition, pyruvate and acetoacetate are less stable than lactate and β-hydroxybutyrate, and artifacts of sample preparation or delayed processing may result in spuriously increased ratios. Complex II deficiency should theoretically not affect the L–P and ketone body ratios because a block at that level would not affect NADH oxidation. It should be pointed out that patients with the later presentation of liver dysfunction (e.g., Alpers–Huttenlocher syndrome) frequently do not have elevations of plasma lactate or increased L–P and arterial ketone body ratios. Patients with pyruvate dehydrogenase deficiency generally have low (<10) L–P ratios. Defects in the TCA cycle may also result in elevated L–P ratios but ketone body molar ratios should be low (<1). Renal tubular dysfunction can cause lower plasma lactate levels thus making the L–P ratio less accurate. Diabetes mellitus may impair pyruvate entry into the citric acid cycle.

Investigation of the urine is also useful. Proximal renal tubular dysfunction may lower plasma lactate and increase urinary lactate. In these cases, gas chromatography–mass spectrometry (GC-MS) can detect elevated urinary lactate, TCA cycle intermediates (succinate, fumarate, and malate), and, at times, 3-methyl-glutaconic and 3-methylglutaric acid.

It should be emphasized that these are screening tests and may not be abnormal if the respiratory chain defect is confined to one or two organs. Therefore, searching for dysfunction or abnormal histology and biochemistry of the target organs is also important.

Definitive Diagnostic Tests

Measurement of mitochondrial respiration

Analysis of oxygen consumption in mitochondrial-enriched fractions of tissues (liver, muscle, lymphocytes, and fibroblasts) can be performed by polarographic studies in the presence of a series of respiratory substrates to define the site of the respiratory impairment. Patients with complex I deficiency (NADH oxidoreductase) will show impaired respiration (oxygen consumption by mitochondria) with NADH-producing substrates, such as glutamate and malate; those with complex II (succinate oxidoreductase) with FADH-producing substrates, such as succinate; and those with complex III (ubiquinone–cytochrome c oxidoreductase) and complex IV (cytochrome c oxidase) with both types of substrates. Complex V (ATP synthetase) deficiency will produce impaired respiration with all substrates, but the addition of agents that uncouple electron transfer from phosphorylation (2,4 dinitrophenol or calcium ions) will return the respiratory rate to normal. Polarographic studies have the advantage of requiring relatively small amounts of tissue (100–200 mg of muscle; 10 mL blood for circulating lymphocytes), however, they require fresh tissue for immediate isolation and analysis of mitochondria. Therefore, biopsies must be conducted at the center performing these studies. This test is available on fresh liver biopsy specimens at very few centers around the world.

Enzymatic Activity of Respiratory Chain Complexes

Direct measurement of the enzymatic activity of the mitochondrial respiratory chain complexes is more commonly used to establish deficiency of the respiratory chain. These studies can be performed on frozen samples of small biopsies of liver, kidney, myocardium, or other tissue because they do not require the isolation of mitochondrial fractions and can be carried out on tissue homogenates, lymphocytes, or cultured skin fibroblasts. Tissue biopsy samples must be frozen immediately at the bedside or in the operating room and stored at −80°C until analyzed. Measurement of respiratory chain enzyme activities separately or in groups is performed spectrophotometrically using specific electron acceptors and donors [137]. In general, the tissues chosen for study should be those that clinically express the disease. It may also be useful to obtain skin fibroblasts and lymphocytes for testing, although a defect may be absent in these cells and confined to the involved organ. In some countries, micromethods have allowed these analyses to be performed on frozen portions of percutaneous liver and muscle biopsies specimens (10–15 mg tissue) [137]. However, in most centers, these analyses usually require open, surgical liver and muscle biopsies. Pitfalls in these measurements include the following. Normal values may have a wide range, and thus overlap may be found in affected patients. For this reason, some experts recommend expressing results as ratios of one protein complex activity to another to detect deficiencies of one enzyme that may be in the low to normal range [136]. Normal respiratory activity does not exclude a defect in mtDNA because heteroplasmy may allow for reasonably normal enzymatic activity in some areas of a given tissue. Molecular analysis of mtDNA should be performed in these instances. Certain cells (e.g., lymphocytes and cultured fibroblasts) are not good for detecting abnormalities in complex I activity. Other pitfalls in spectrophotometric analysis of tissues are further outlined in detail by Munnich et al. [136].

Histopathologic Investigations

It is possible to detect deficiencies of subunits of several of the respiratory chain complexes by histochemical examination of biopsy material. Polyclonal and monoclonal antibodies directed against cytochrome c oxidase (complex IV) subunits can be used to stain liver and muscle. Tissue specimens must be frozen immediately in liquid nitrogen-cooled isopentane for these studies. Other immunohistochemical techniques for staining NADH tetrazolium reductase and succinate dehydrogenase are also available. Histology and electron microscopy of muscle and liver may also reveal characteristic findings of respiratory chain disorders (e.g., ragged red fibers in muscle).

MtDNA and Nuclear DNA Molecular Analyses

Molecular diagnosis is becoming more useful as more nuclear genes are identified that cause specific respiratory chain and mtDNA depletion disorders. For nuclear genes, whole blood for isolation of genomic DNA will usually suffice as the "tissue" to be genotyped. For mtDNA deletions and mutations, the involved tissue may be necessary because of heteroplasmy. In addition, the DNA of biopsied tissue (including liver) can be isolated, electrophoresed, blotted, and hybridized with probes for nuclear and mitochondrial genes [136,137]. Autoradiographic signals after hybridization can be measured and the mtDNA level expressed as the ratio of the signal of the mitochondrial probe to that of the nuclear probe to determine whether mtDNA depletion is present. Mitochondrial DNA deletions and mutations can be screened by the single-strand conformational polymorphism technique. To detect mtDNA deletions, techniques using digestion of mtDNA with restriction enzymes can demonstrate two populations of mtDNA. For characterization of the nucleotide sequence at the boundaries of the mtDNA deletions, polymerase chain reaction amplification is performed followed by automated nucleotide sequencing.

Using these molecular techniques, specific mutations or deletions can be sought, and even the entire mitochondrial genome can be sequenced [138]. Genetic abnormalities in mtDNA have not been detected in most infants with neonatal liver failure caused by respiratory chain defects. However, mutations in *SCO1* and *BCS1L* may be identified in infants with neonatal hepatic failure. In patients with suspected or proven mtDNA depletion syndrome, *dGK*, *POLG*, and *MPV17* should be genotyped. In patients with the clinical presentation of MNGIE syndrome, mutations of the thymidine phosphorylase gene should be sought [91]. In patients with the later onset liver failure presentation (e.g., Alpers–Huttenlocher syndrome), *POLG* should be analyzed. Pearson's marrow–pancreas syndrome has been linked to the most common mtDNA deletion (4997 bp), as has Kearns–Sayre syndrome. In addition, multiple mtDNA duplications have been reported in Pearson's syndrome [136]. In terms of nuclear DNA abnormalities, mutations in specific genes have been associated with several neuromuscular disorders, including the flavoprotein subunit of complex II, the 18 kDa subunit of complex I, the NADH binding site of complex I, heat shock protein 60, the human homologue of *Tim8*, and *Surf1* (reviewed in [102]) [11]. Molecular DNA analysis is now becoming a useful tool in the rapid diagnosis of patients with primary respiratory chain defects and may replace the need to obtain tissue for respiratory chain enzyme activity analysis and mtDNA depletion studies, if the genetic tests become available from approved clinical laboratories (see http://www.genetests.org).

TREATMENT OF RESPIRATORY CHAIN DISORDERS

Unfortunately, there is no ideal effective therapy for most patients with respiratory chain disorders, including those with liver failure and more slowly progressive liver disease. It is not clear that any currently available medical therapy significantly alters the course of severe disease; however, some patients have experienced improvement of neuromuscular symptoms. Based on an understanding of the enzymatic and biochemical derangements, several treatment strategies have been proposed although not proved to be effective [136] (Table 33.7). Acute metabolic acidosis is treated with the slow infusion of sodium bicarbonate intravenously; anemia or thrombocytopenia are treated with transfusions; and chronic pancreatic insufficiency may require the provision of exogenous pancreatic enzymes with meals. Other strategies include supplementation with mitochondrial cofactors, scavenging of oxygen free radicals [139], symptomatic treatment, and avoidance of drugs and conditions known to have a detrimental effect on the respiratory chain. Dietary measures have also been employed. Seizure control should not include phenobarbital because it can inhibit OXPHOS. Valproic acid should likewise be used with caution in these patients because of its effects on respiration and fatty acid metabolism. Exercise is important in patients with muscle involvement. In addition to improving strength, a decrease in the proportion of mutant mtDNA in muscle can be stimulated by exercise training [140]. Even induction of muscle necrosis by drug therapy has been proposed as a means to enhance proliferation of myoblasts to attain muscle fibers with less mutated mtDNA [141].

Pharmacologic Support

A variety of antioxidant compounds have been proposed as scavengers of electrons or oxygen free radicals, as promotors of electron transport, or as stimulators of mitochondrial

Table 33.7: Proposed (but Not Proven) Pharmacologic Treatments for Respiratory Chain Disorders

Electron acceptors and cofactors		
■ Coenzyme Q_{10}	Redox bypass of complex I; Free radical scavenger (antioxidant)	Adult: 60–300 mg/d *Ped: 3–5 mg/kg/d
■ Idebenone	Redox bypass of complex I; and antioxidant	Adult: 90–270 mg/d *Ped: 5 mg/kg/d
■ Thiamine (vitamin B_1)	Cofactor of pyruvate dehydrogenase	Adult: 150–300 mg/d
■ Riboflavin (vitamin B_2)	Acts as flavin precursor for complexes I and II	Adult: 50–200 mg/d
■ Menadione (vitamin K_3)	Bypass complex III (with vitamin C)	Adult: 40–160 mg/d
Antioxidants		
■ Vitamin E	Antioxidant	Adult: 400–800 IU/d(TPGS) *Ped: 25 IU/kg/d
■ Ascorbic acid (vitamin C)	Antioxidant	Adult: 2–4 g/d
Other mechanisms of action		
■ Succinate	Donates electrons directly to complex II	Adult: 6–16 g/d
■ Carnitine	Replace secondary carnitine deficiency	*Ped: 50–100 mg/kg/d
■ Creatine monohydrate	Enhances muscle phosphocreatine	Adult: Up to 10 g/d} *Ped: 0.1–0.2 g/kg/d
■ Dichloroacetate	Reduces lactic acidosis by enhancing pyruvate dehydrogenase activity	Adult: 25 mg/kg/d *Ped: 25 mg/kg/d

TPGS, D-alpha tocopheryl polyethylene glycol-1000 succinate.
*Pediatric (Ped) doses are estimates and have not been subjected to clinical dosage trials.
Evidence for efficacy and safety of each agent is variable and not conclusive.
Adapted from Gillis LA, Sokol RJ. Gastrointestinal manifestations of mitochondrial disease. Gastroenterol Clin North Am 2003;32:789–817.

respiration [142]. Coenzyme Q_{10} (ubiquinone) has been reported to result in sustained improvement in several cases of complex III deficiency and perhaps in complex IV deficiency. CoQ is the electron acceptor from complexes I and II of the respiratory chain, receiving electrons from NADH via complex I and various feeder pathways including the TCA cycle and the β-oxidation cycle via succinate and FADH through complex II and electron-transfer flavoprotein. Using an animal model of liver injury that employed endotoxin-induced intrahepatic lipid peroxidation, exogenously administered CoQ_{10} prevented the marked reduction in hepatic levels of endogenous CoQ, α-tocopherol, and glutathione, suppressed lipid peroxidation, and increased the survival rate in endotoxemic mice [143,144]. Similar effects of CoQ_{10} were seen in a liver ischemia-reperfusion injury animal model. CoQ analogues have also been shown to promote respiration in isolated hepatic and brain mitochondria [145,146]. Hepatic mitochondrial CoQ levels have been shown to decrease after several weeks of bile duct ligation in the rat [147]; however, supplementation has not been attempted in human cases of cholestasis to our knowledge. In mitochondrial myopathies or cardiomyopathies, occasional patients have shown dramatic improvement in muscle strength and cardiac function after CoQ supplementation. There have now been numerous reports of myopathy and cerebellar ataxia patients with primary deficiencies of CoQ who respond very well to repletion with this substance [148,149]. There is little reported experience using CoQ in patients with mitochondrial hepatopathies.

Other antioxidants that have been administered to patients with respiratory chain defects include menadione (vitamin K3), ascorbic acid, and vitamin E (Table 33.6). Sustained improvement in isolated cases of complex III deficiency have been reported in patients administered menadione or CoQ. Vitamin E is incorporated into mitochondrial membranes when administered exogenously and may also be of benefit. Treatment with riboflavin has been associated with improvement in a small number of patients with complex II deficiency. Succinate has occasionally been given to patients with complex I deficiency because this substrate enters the respiratory chain via complex II. L-carnitine has been used as therapy in patients with secondary carnitine deficiency, the purpose being to scavenge potentially toxic metabolites that accumulate because of the inhibition of FAO. However, in some patients with electron transport complex abnormalities, carnitine has led to increased liver injury presumably caused by increased electron flow and increased generation of oxygen free radicals. Thus, L-carnitine supplementation in patients with mitochondrial hepatopathies should be used carefully. Dichloroacetate administration has been proposed to stimulate pyruvate dehydrogenase activity and has occasionally resulted in reduced levels of plasma lactate but not in a clear change of the natural history of respiratory chain disorders [150]. Dichloroacetate has been reported to cause a reversible peripheral neuropathy. There is a great need for the development of more effective therapeutic options for affected patients, however, it is possible that a dysfunctional respiratory chain will be incompatible with life once liver failure develops.

Drugs and compounds that can inhibit the respiratory chain either directly or through effects on the TCA cycle or the β-oxidation cycle should be avoided if there is high suspicion of a respiratory chain defect, and certainly after the diagnosis has been established. These drugs include valproate, barbiturates, salicylates, tetracycline, chloramphenicol, ibuprofen, amiodarone, and the ingestion of alcohol.

Dietary Treatment

The diet should consist of high lipid–low carbohydrate foods in patients with complex I deficiency. A high glucose diet is a metabolic challenge for patients with an impaired respiratory chain and may have precipitated hepatic failure in patients with Pearson's syndrome. Because glucose oxidation is largely aerobic in the liver, the provision of large amounts of dextrose to impaired hepatic mitochondria may result in increased lactate production and worsening acidosis and ketosis. On the basis of these considerations, the recommendation is to avoid a hypercaloric diet high in carbohydrates and parenteral infusions of solutions containing high concentrations of dextrose. Succinate (16 g/day), succinate-producing amino acids, or propionyl carnitine have occasionally been given to patients with complex I deficiency because these compounds enter the respiratory chain at complex II.

Liver Transplantation

Although the presence of neuromuscular or cardiac involvement in respiratory chain disorders should preclude the use of liver transplantation, a number of patients with defects isolated to the liver have now successfully undergone liver transplantation with excellent long-term outcomes and no extra-hepatic disease expression [39–41,151]. The prerequisite for considering liver transplantation in this setting is the exclusion of significant extrahepatic disease. This includes careful clinical and laboratory screening of potentially affected organ systems (kidneys, heart, muscle, CNS, and pancreas), MRI, or functional MRI of the brain, echocardiography, and the exclusion of depressed respiratory chain enzyme activity in muscle and skin fibroblasts. It is possible that posttransplant chimerism by which dendritic cells from the graft migrate into other tissues of the recipient could play a role in correcting the defect in extrahepatic tissues as has been proposed in patients transplanted with type IV GSD and type I Gaucher's disease [152]. However, in a few patients who have received liver transplants and had clinically unrecognized neurologic involvement before transplant, progressive neurologic symptoms occurred following transplantation [39,40]. In a series of 11 patients who underwent liver transplantation for OXPHOS deficiencies before 7 months of age, only 5 were alive and well at follow-up between 5 months and 8 years posttransplantation. Three of the six patients who died developed neurologic features only after liver transplantation. All of these patients who had liver failure and associated gastrointestinal disease died shortly after liver transplantation. Therefore, it is essential to obtain historical documentation of typical neurologic symptoms characteristic of these disorders, a complete family history, and a thorough clinical and biochemical evaluation of neuromuscular and cardiac function when evaluating young children with fulminant liver failure for liver transplantation. It must be stressed to the family that the absence of extrahepatic involvement before transplantation does not guarantee severe neurologic symptoms will not develop after transplantation.

Gene Therapy and Cell-Based Therapy

Somatic gene transfer therapy is being tested in a number of human genetic disorders, with limited success thus far. Several groups of investigators are designing novel methods to attempt to correct the underlying mtDNA defects present in some patients with mitochondrial hepatopathies. One approach has used an inhibitor of mitochondrial oxidation in cultured cells to alter the ratio of mutant to wild-type mtDNA [153]. Another uses a self-replicating copy of a normal gene sequence delivered into mitochondria in vitro [154]. A final approach is to inhibit replication of mutant mtDNA without affecting wild-type mtDNA [155]. It is hoped that these and other approaches will lead to future treatments that can alter the heteroplasmic ratios of mutant mtDNA in selected tissues and alter the course of these diseases.

Another approach is to salvage OXPHOS function in cells by importing tRNAs from cytosol into mitochondria in patients with tRNA mutations (mtDNA mutations) [156]. Finally, various in vitro approaches can be taken to prevent recurrence, such as using donor eggs. Another possibility for the future is for nuclear transfer from a maternal egg and fertilization in a donor cytoplasm using paternal sperm [156].

PRENATAL DIAGNOSIS

The ability to provide accurate prenatal diagnosis of maternally inherited mtDNA disorders is hampered by our incomplete knowledge of the actual proportion of mutant mtDNA that is necessary to produce the disease phenotype and the random distribution of mtDNA into different tissues [157]. Thus, the demonstration of the heteroplasmic presence of a known mtDNA mutation or deletion in chorionic villi or amniotic cells

Table 33.8: Comparison of Features of Primary Mitochondrial Hepatopathies

Disorder	*Onset*	*Seizures*	*Plasma Lactate*	*L–P Ratio*	*MtDNA*	*Respiratory Chain Complexes Involved*	*Genes Involved*
Neonatal liver failure	Acute	±	↑	↑	Normal	IV, III, or I	*BCS1L and SCO2*
MtDNA depletion syndrome	Acute/chronic	+	↑	↑	Depletion	I, III, IV	*MPV17, POLG, dGK*
Delayed onset liver disease (Alpers' disease)	Insidious	++	Normal	Normal	Normal	I	*POLG*
Pearson's syndrome	Insidious	–	Normal or ↑	Normal or ↑	Deletion	I, III	
Villous atrophy syndrome	Chronic	–	↑	↑	Rearrangements	III	
Navajo neurohepatopathy	Acute or chronic	–	–	±	Depletion	I, III, IV	*MPV17*

+, present sometimes; ++, present always; ±, occasionally present; –, not present; ↑, increased; L–P ratio, molar ratio of plasma lactate: pyruvate concentration.
Adapted from Sokol RJ, Treem WR. Mitochondria and childhood liver diseases. J Pediatr Gastroenterol Nutr 1999;28:4–16; used with permission.

of a progeny in an affected family does not yet have an adequate predictive value to accurately assign a disease phenotype to the fetus [36]. For the nuclear-encoded gene mutations that have been identified in a proband (e.g., *POLG, NPV17, dGK*), it is possible to assess amniocytes or chorionic villi for nuclear DNA mutations. Others have attempted to measure respiratory chain enzyme activity and ATP synthesis in digitonin-permeabilized cultured chorionic villus cells [158]. This method would be helpful only in disorders in which the defect has a mutisystemic expression in different cell types that include fibroblasts, which is not the case in all infants and young children with hepatic involvement because only 40–50% of these enzyme deficiencies are expressed in cultured fibroblasts. Therefore, prenatal diagnosis at present is not very useful in most families affected by a respiratory chain defect unless mutations are known for a nuclear-encoded causative gene.

CONCLUSIONS

Mitochondrial hepatopathies are one of the newly recognized groups of important liver disorders in childhood, particularly in infancy and in patients with liver failure. The identification of several secondary mitochondrial hepatopathies stresses the critical nature of mitochondrial function in the pathogenesis of liver injury and in the cellular processes of necrosis and apoptosis. Primary mitochondrial hepatopathies should be considered in any child with liver disease and neuromuscular involvement, multisystemic disease, lactic acidosis, or rapidly progressive disease, and when hepatic steatosis is the dominant histologic finding on liver biopsy. A comparison of salient features of six of the primary mitochondrial hepatopathies is presented in Table 33.8. Diagnosis is shifting to early genotyping of likely causative genes, as more nuclear genes responsible for these disorders are identified. Treatments are currently not satisfactory; however, liver transplantation may be successful in selected cases with isolated liver involvement.

WEB SITE INFORMATION

Additional information can be obtained from the following Internet Web sites:

Family Support Groups and Information

United Mitochondrial Disease Foundation
www.umdf.org
International Mitochondrial Disease Network
www.imdn.org

Scientific Information

Mitochondrial Interest Group
http://www.nih.gov/sigs/mito/

MitoDat – Mendelian Inheritance and the Mitochondrion
www.lecb.ncifcrf.gov/mitoDat/

Mitochondrial Research Society (MRS)
www-lecb.ncifcrf.gov/~zullo/migDB/mrs.html

Cholestatic Liver Disease Consortium
http://rarediseasesnetwork.org/clic

ACKNOWLEDGMENTS

Supported in part by NIH grants RO-DK38446, U54-DK078377, UO1-DK062453 and MO1-RR00069. The author thanks Cynthia Wyman for typing this manuscript and the Cholestatic Liver Disease Consortium for support.

REFERENCES

1. Johns DR. Seminars in medicine of the Beth Israel Hospital, Boston. Mitochondrial DNA and disease. N Engl J Med 1995;333:638–44.
2. Treem WR, Sokol RJ. Disorders of the mitochondria. Semin Liver Dis 1998;18:237–53.
3. Bernes SM, Bacino C, Prezant TR, et al. Identical mitochondrial DNA deletion in mother with progressive external ophthalmoplegia and son with Pearson marrow-pancreas syndrome. J Pediatr 1993;123:598–602.
4. Ballinger SW, Shoffner JM, Gebhart S, et al. Mitochondrial diabetes revisited. Nat Genet 1994;7:458–9.
5. Hirano M, Silvestri G, Blake DM, et al. Mitochondrial neurogastrointestinal encephalomyopathy (MNGIE): clinical, biochemical, and genetic features of an autosomal recessive mitochondrial disorder. Neurology 1994;44:721–7.
6. Beal MF, Hyman BT, Koroshetz W. Do defects in mitochondrial energy metabolism underlie the pathology of neurodegenerative diseases? Trends Neurosci 1993;16:125–31.
7. Wallace DC. Mitochondrial genetics: a paradigm for aging and degenerative diseases? Science 1992;256:628–32.
8. Lightowlers RN, Chinnery PF, Turnbull DM, Howell N. Mammalian mitochondrial genetics: heredity, heteroplasmy and disease. Trends Genet 1997;13:450–5.
9. Poulton J, Macaulay V, Marchington DR. Mitochondrial genetics '98 is the bottleneck cracked? Am J Hum Genet 1998;62:752–7.
10. Taanman JW. The mitochondrial genome: structure, transcription, translation and replication. Biochim Biophys Acta 1999;1410:103–23.
11. Leonard JV, Schapira AH. Mitochondrial respiratory chain disorders II: neurodegenerative disorders and nuclear gene defects. Lancet 2000;355:389–94.
12. Susin SA, Zamzami N, Kroemer G. Mitochondria as regulators of apoptosis: doubt no more. Biochim Biophys Acta 1998;1366:151–65.
13. Chinnery PF, Turnbull DM. Mitochondrial DNA and disease. Lancet 1999;354 Suppl 1:SI17–21.
14. Aprille JR. Mitochondrial cytopathies and mitochondrial DNA mutations. Curr Opinion Pediatr 1991;3:1045–54.
15. Munnich A. The respiratory chain. In: Fernandes J, Saudurray JM, eds. Inborn metabolic diseases: diagnosis and treatment. Berlin: Springer-Verlag, 1995:121–31.
16. Wallace DC. Mitochondrial DNA mutations in diseases of energy metabolism. J Bioenerg Biomembr 1994;26:241–50.
17. Holt IJ, Harding AE, Morgan-Hughes JA. Deletions of muscle mitochondrial DNA in patients with mitochondrial myopathies. Nature 1988;331:717–19.
18. Wallace DC, Singh G, Lott MT, et al. Mitochondrial DNA mutation associated with Leber's hereditary optic neuropathy. Science 1988;242:1427–30.
19. Chinnery PF, Howell N, Andrews RM, Turnbull DM. Mitochondrial DNA analysis: polymorphisms and pathogenicity. J Med Genet 1999;36:505–10.
20. Chinnery PF, Johnson MA, Wardell TM, et al. The epidemiology of pathogenic mitochondrial DNA mutations. Ann Neurol 2000;48:188–93.
21. Darin N, Oldfors A, Moslemi AR, et al. The incidence of mitochondrial encephalomyopathies in childhood: clinical features and morphological, biochemical, and DNA anbormalities. Ann Neurol 2001;49:377–83.
22. Majamaa K, Moilanen JS, Uimonen S, et al. Epidemiology of A3243G, the mutation for mitochondrial encephalomyopathy, lactic acidosis, and strokelike episodes: prevalence of the mutation in an adult population. Am J Hum Genet 1998;63:447–54.
23. Uusimaa J, Remes AM, Rantala H, et al. Childhood encephalopathies and myopathies: a prospective study in a defined population to assess the frequency of mitochondrial disorders. Pediatrics 2000;105:598–603.
24. Chinnery PF, Turnbull DM. Epidemiology and treatment of mitochondrial disorders. Am J Med Genet 2001;106:94–101.
25. van den Heuvel L, Ruitenbeek W, Smeets R, et al. Demonstration of a new pathogenic mutation in human complex I deficiency: a 5-bp duplication in the nuclear gene encoding the 18-kD (AQDQ) subunit. Am J Hum Genet 1998;62:262–8.
26. Schuelke M, Smeitink J, Mariman E, et al. Mutant NDUFV1 subunit of mitochondrial complex I causes leukodystrophy and myoclonic epilepsy. Nat Genet 1999;21:260–1.
27. Briones P, Vilaseca MA, Ribes A, et al. A new case of multiple mitochondrial enzyme deficiencies with decreased amount of heat shock protein 60. J Inherit Metab Dis 1997;20(4):569–577.
28. Koehler CM, Leuenberger D, Merchant S, et al. Human deafness dystonia syndrome is a mitochondrial disease. Proc Natl Acad Sci U S A 1999;96:2141–6.
29. Zhu Z, Yao J, Johns T, et al. SURF1, encoding a factor involved in the biogenesis of cytochrome c oxidase, is mutated in Leigh syndrome. Nat Genet 1998;20:337–43.
30. Bakker HD, Scholte HR, Dingemans KP, et al. Depletion of mitochondrial deoxyribonucleic acid in a family with fatal neonatal liver disease. J Pediatr 1996;128:683–7.
31. Bioulac-Sage P, Parrot-Roulaud F, Mazat JP, et al. Fatal neonatal liver failure and mitochondrial cytopathy (oxidative phosphorylation deficiency): a light and electron microscopic study of the liver. Hepatology 1993;18:839–46.
32. Cormier V, Rustin P, Bonnefont JP, et al. Hepatic failure in disorders of oxidative phosphorylation with neonatal onset. J Pediatr 1991;119:951–4.
33. Cormier-Daire V, Chretien D, Rustin P, et al. Neonatal and delayed-onset liver involvement in disorders of oxidative phosphorylation. J Pediatr 1997;130:817–22.
34. Fayon M, Lamireau T, Bioulac-Sage P, et al. Fatal neonatal liver failure and mitochondrial cytopathy: an observation with antenatal ascites. Gastroenterology 1992;103:1332–5.
35. Mazzella M, Cerone R, Bonacci W, et al. Severe complex I deficiency in a case of neonatal-onset lactic acidosis and fatal liver failure. Acta Paediatr 1997;86:326–9.
36. Munnich A, Rotig A, Chretien D, et al. Clinical presentation of mitochondrial disorders in childhood. J Inherit Metab Dis 1996;19:521–7.

37. Vilaseca MA, Briones P, Ribes A, et al. Fatal hepatic failure with lactic acidaemia, Fanconi syndrome and defective activity of succinate:cytochrome c reductase. J Inherit Metab Dis 1991;14:285–8.
38. von Kleist-Retzow JC, Cormier-Daire V, Viot G, et al. Antenatal manifestations of mitochondrial respiratory chain deficiency. J Pediatr 2003;143:208–12.
39. Thomson M, McKiernan P, Buckels J, et al. Generalised mitochondrial cytopathy is an absolute contraindication to orthotopic liver transplant in childhood. J Pediatr Gastroenterol Nutr 1998;26:478–81.
40. Sokal EM, Sokol R, Cormier V, et al. Liver transplantation in mitochondrial respiratory chain disorders. Eur J Pediatr 1999;158 Suppl 2:S81–4.
41. Goncalves I, Hermans D, Chretien D, et al. Mitochondrial respiratory chain defect: a new etiology for neonatal cholestasis and early liver insufficiency. J Hepatol 1995;23:290–4.
42. Valnot I, Osmond S, Gigarel N, et al. Mutations of the SCO1 gene in mitochondrial cytochrome c oxidase deficiency with neonatal-onset hepatic failure and encephalopathy. Am J Hum Genet 2000;67:1104–9.
43. Chabrol B, Mancini J, Chretien D, et al. Valproate-induced hepatic failure in a case of cytochrome c oxidase deficiency. Eur J Pediatr 1994;153:133–5.
44. de Lonlay P, Valnot I, Barrientos A, et al. A mutant mitochondrial respiratory chain assembly protein causes complex III deficiency in patients with tubulopathy, encephalopathy and liver failure. Nat Genet 2001;29:57–60.
45. De Meirleir L, Seneca S, Damis E, et al. Clinical and diagnostic characteristics of complex III deficiency due to mutations in the *BCS1L* gene. Am J Med Genet A 2003;121:126–31.
46. Ducluzeau PH, Lachaux A, Bouvier R, et al. Depletion of mitochondrial DNA associated with infantile cholestasis and progressive liver fibrosis. J Hepatol 1999;30:149–55.
47. Maaswinkel-Mooij PD, Van den Bogert C, Scholte HR, et al. Depletion of mitochondrial DNA in the liver of a patient with lactic acidemia and hypoketotic hypoglycemia. J Pediatr 1996;128:679–83.
48. Mazziotta MR, Ricci E, Bertini E, et al. Fatal infantile liver failure associated with mitochondrial DNA depletion. J Pediatr 1992;121:896–901.
49. Muller-Hocker J, Muntau A, Schafer S, et al. Depletion of mitochondrial DNA in the liver of an infant with neonatal giant cell hepatitis. Hum Pathol 2002;33:247–53.
50. Moraes CT, Shanske S, Tritschler HJ, et al. mtDNA depletion with variable tissue expression: a novel genetic abnormality in mitochondrial diseases. Am J Hum Genet 1991;48:492–501.
51. Tsao CY, Mendell JR, Luquette M, et al. Mitochondrial DNA depletion in children. J Child Neurol 2000;15:822–4.
52. Morris AA, Taanman JW, Blake J, et al. Liver failure associated with mitochondrial DNA depletion. J Hepatol 1998;28:556–63.
53. Mandel H, Hartman C, Berkowitz D, et al. The hepatic mitochondrial DNA depletion syndrome: ultrastructural changes in liver biopsies. Hepatology 2001;34:776–84.
54. Durand P, Debray D, Mandel R, et al. Acute liver failure in infancy: a 14-year experience of a pediatric liver transplantation center. J Pediatr 2001;139:871–6.
55. Bodnar AG, Cooper JM, Holt IJ, et al. Nuclear complementation restores mtDNA levels in cultured cells from a patient with mtDNA depletion. Am J Hum Genet 1993;53:663–9.
56. Taanman JW, Bodnar AG, Cooper JM, et al. Molecular mechanisms in mitochondrial DNA depletion syndrome. Hum Mol Genet 1997;6:935–42.
57. Jullig M, Eriksson S. Mitochondrial and submitochondrial localization of human deoxyguanosine kinase. Eur J Biochem 2000;267:5466–72.
58. Wang L, Munch-Petersen B, Herrstrom Sjoberg A, et al. Human thymidine kinase 2: molecular cloning and characterisation of the enzyme activity with antiviral and cytostatic nucleoside substrates. FEBS Lett 1999;443:170–4.
59. Mandel H, Szargel R, Labay V, et al. The deoxyguanosine kinase gene is mutated in individuals with depleted hepatocerebral mitochondrial DNA. Nat Genet 2001;29:337–41.
60. Saada A, Shaag A, Mandel H, et al. Mutant mitochondrial thymidine kinase in mitochondrial DNA depletion myopathy. Nat Genet 2001;29:342–4.
61. Salviati L, Sacconi S, Mancuso M, et al. Mitochondrial DNA depletion and dGK gene mutations. Ann Neurol 2002;52:311–17.
62. Ferrari G, Lamantea E, Donati A, et al. Infantile hepatocerebral syndromes associated with mutations in the mitochondrial DNA polymerase-gammaA. Brain 2005;128:723–31.
63. Horvath R, Hudson G, Ferrari G, et al. Phenotypic spectrum associated with mutations of the mitochondrial polymerase gamma gene. Brain 2006;129:1674–84.
64. Naviaux RK, Nguyen KV. POLG mutations associated with Alpers' syndrome and mitochondrial DNA depletion. Ann Neurol 2004;55:706–12.
65. Spinazzola A, Viscomi C, Fernandez-Vizarra E, et al. MPV17 encodes an inner mitochondrial membrane protein and is mutated in infantile hepatic mitochondrial DNA depletion. Nat Genet 2006;38:570–5.
66. Alpers BJ. Diffuse progressive degeneration of the gray matter of the cerebrum. Arch Neurol Psychiatr 1931;25:469–505.
67. Boyd SG, Harden A, Egger J, Pampiglione G. Progressive neuronal degeneration of childhood with liver disease ("Alpers' disease"): characteristic neurophysiological features. Neuropediatrics 1986;17:75–80.
68. Egger J, Harding BN, Boyd SG, et al. Progressive neuronal degeneration of childhood (PNDC) with liver disease. Clin Pediatr 1987;26:167–73.
69. Harding BN. Progressive neuronal degeneration of childhood with liver disease (Alpers–Huttenlocher syndrome): a personal review. J Child Neurol 1990;5:273–87.
70. Harding BN, Egger J, Portmann B, Erdohazi M. Progressive neuronal degeneration of childhood with liver disease. A pathological study. Brain 1986;109:181–206.
71. Hattenlocher PR, Solitare GB, Adams G. Infantile diffuse cerebral degeneration with hepatic cirrhosis. Arch Neurol 1976; 33:186–92.
72. Tulinius MH, Holme E, Kristiansson B, et al. Mitochondrial encephalomyopathies in childhood. I. Biochemical and morphologic investigations. J Pediatr 1991;119:242–50.
73. Nguyen KV, Sharief FS, Chan SS, et al. Molecular diagnosis of Alpers syndrome. J Hepatol 2006;45:108–16.
74. Narkewicz MR, Sokol RJ, Beckwith B, et al. Liver involvement in Alpers disease. J Pediatr 1991;119:260–7.
75. Wilson DC, McGibben D, Hicks EM, Allen IV. Progressive neuronal degeneration of childhood (Alpers syndrome) with hepatic cirrhosis. Eur J Pediatr 1993;152:260–2.

76. Bicknese AR, May W, Hickey WF, Dodson WE. Early childhood hepatocerebral degeneration misdiagnosed as valproate hepatotoxicity. Ann Neurol 1992;32:767–75.
77. Davidzon G, Mancuso M, Ferraris S, et al. POLG mutations and Alpers syndrome. Ann Neurol 2005;57:921–3.
78. Pearson HA, Lobel JS, Kocoshis SA, et al. A new syndrome of refractory sideroblastic anemia with vacuolization of marrow precursors and exocrine pancreatic dysfunction. J Pediatr 1979;95:976–84.
79. Morikawa Y, Matsuura N, Kakudo K, et al. Pearson's marrow/pancreas syndrome: a histological and genetic study. Virchows Arch A Pathol Anat Histopathol 1993;423:227–31.
80. Rotig A, Cormier V, Blanche S, et al. Pearson's marrow–pancreas syndrome. A multisystem mitochondrial disorder in infancy. J Clin Invest 1990;86:1601–8.
81. Sano T, Ban K, Ichiki T, et al. Molecular and genetic analyses of two patients with Pearson's marrow-pancreas syndrome. Pediatr Res 1993;34:105–10.
82. Tulinius MH, Holme E, Kristiansson B, et al. Mitochondrial encephalomyopathies in childhood. II. Clinical manifestations and syndromes. J Pediatr 1991;119:251–9.
83. McShane MA, Hammans SR, Sweeney M, et al. Pearson syndrome and mitochondrial encephalomyopathy in a patient with a deletion of mtDNA. Am J Hum Genet 1991;48:39–42.
84. Cormier-Daire V, Bonnefont JP, Rustin P, et al. Mitochondrial DNA rearrangements with onset as chronic diarrhea with villous atrophy. J Pediatr 1994;124:63–70.
85. Ionasescu V, Thompson SH, Ionasescu R, et al. Inherited ophthalmoplegia with intestinal pseudo-obstruction. J Neurol Sci 1983;59:215–28.
86. Hirano M, Vu TH. Defects of intergenomic communication: where do we stand? Brain Pathol 2000;10:451–61.
87. Cervera R, Bruix J, Bayes A, et al. Chronic intestinal pseudoobstruction and ophthalmoplegia in a patient with mitochondrial myopathy. Gut 1988;29:544–7.
88. Li V, Hostein J, Romero NB, et al. Chronic intestinal pseudoobstruction with myopathy and ophthalmoplegia. A muscular biochemical study of a mitochondrial disorder. Dig Dis Sci 1992;37:456–63.
89. Teitelbaum JE, Berde CB, Nurko S, et al. Diagnosis and management of MNGIE syndrome in children: case report and review of the literature. J Pediatr Gastroenterol Nutr 2002;35:377–83.
90. Hirano M, Garcia-de-Yebenes J, Jones AC, et al. Mitochondrial neurogastrointestinal encephalomyopathy syndrome maps to chromosome 22q13.32-qter. Am J Hum Genet 1998;63:526–33.
91. Nishino I, Spinazzola A, Hirano M. Thymidine phosphorylase gene mutations in MNGIE, a human mitochondrial disorder. Science 1999;283:689–92.
92. Nishino I, Spinazzola A, Papadimitriou A, et al. Mitochondrial neurogastrointestinal encephalomyopathy: an autosomal recessive disorder due to thymidine phosphorylase mutations. Ann Neurol 2000;47:792–800.
93. Brown NS, Bicknell R. Thymidine phosphorylase, 2-deoxy-D-ribose and angiogenesis. Biochem J 1998;334:1–8.
94. Spinazzola A, Marti R, Nishino I, et al. Altered thymidine metabolism due to defects of thymidine phosphorylase. J Biol Chem 2002;277:4128–33.
95. Giordano C, Sebastiani M, Plazzi G, et al. Mitochondrial neurogastrointestinal encephalomyopathy: evidence of mitochondrial DNA depletion in the small intestine. Gastroenterology 2006;130:893–901.
96. Appenzeller O, Kornfeld M, Snyder R. Acromutilating, paralyzing neuropathy with corneal ulceration in Navajo children. Arch Neurol 1976;33:733–8.
97. Singleton R, Helgerson SD, Snyder RD, et al. Neuropathy in Navajo children: clinical and epidemiologic features. Neurology 1990;40:363–7.
98. Holve S, Hu D, Shub M, et al. Liver disease in Navajo neuropathy. J Pediatr 1999;135:482–93.
99. Vu TH, Tanji K, Holve SA, et al. Navajo neurohepatopathy: a mitochondrial DNA depletion syndrome? Hepatology 2001;34:116–20.
100. Karadimas CL, Vu TH, Holve SA, et al. Navajo neurohepatopathy is caused by a mutation in the *MPV17* gene. Am J Hum Genet 2006;79:544–8.
101. Treem WR. Inborn defects in mitochondrial fatty acid oxidation. In: Suchy FJ, ed. Liver disease in childhood. St. Louis, MO: Mosby, 1994:852–87.
102. Ventura FV, Ruiter JP, Ijlst L, et al. Inhibitory effect of 3-hydroxyacyl-CoAs and other long-chain fatty acid beta-oxidation intermediates on mitochondrial oxidative phosphorylation. J Inherit Metab Dis 1996;19:161–4.
103. Enns GM, Bennett MJ, Hoppel CL, et al. Mitochondrial respiratory chain complex I deficiency with clinical and biochemical features of long-chain 3-hydroxyacyl-coenzyme A dehydrogenase deficiency. J Pediatr 2000;136:251–4.
104. Sims HF, Brackett JC, Powell CK, et al. The molecular basis of pediatric long chain 3-hydroxyacyl-CoA dehydrogenase deficiency associated with maternal acute fatty liver of pregnancy. Proc Natl Acad Sci U S A 1995;92:841–5.
105. Treem WR, Shoup ME, Hale DE, et al. Acute fatty liver of pregnancy, hemolysis, elevated liver enzymes, and low platelets syndrome, and long chain 3-hydroxyacyl-coenzyme A dehydrogenase deficiency. Am J Gastroenterol 1996;91:2293–300.
106. Glasgow JF, Middleton B, Moore R, et al. The mechanism of inhibition of beta-oxidation by aspirin metabolites in skin fibroblasts from Reye's syndrome patients and controls. Biochim Biophys Acta 1999;1454:115–25.
107. Belay ED, Bresee JS, Holman RC, et al. Reye's syndrome in the United States from 1981 through 1997. N Engl J Med 1999;340:1377–82.
108. De Vivo DC. Reye syndrome: a metabolic response to an acute mitochondrial insult? Neurology 1978;28:105–8.
109. Partin JC. Reye's Syndrome. In: Suchy FJ, ed. Liver disease in children. St. Louis, MO: Mosby, 1994:653–71.
110. Heubi JE, Daugherty CC, Partin JS, et al. Grade I Reye's syndrome – outcome and predictors of progression to deeper coma grades. N Engl J Med 1984;311:1539–42.
111. Partin JC, Schubert WK, Partin JS. Mitochondrial ultrastructure in Reye's syndrome (encephalopathy and fatty degeneration of the viscera). N Engl J Med 1971;285:1339–43.
112. Hou JW, Chou SP, Wang TR. Metabolic function and liver histopathology in Reye-like illnesses. Acta Paediatr 1996;85:1053–7.
113. Orlowski JP. Whatever happened to Reye's syndrome? Did it ever really exist? Crit Care Med 1999;27:1582–7.
114. Hall SM, Lynn R. Reye's syndrome. N Engl J Med 1999;341:845–6; author reply 846–7.
115. Sternlieb I. Mitochondrial and fatty changes in hepatocytes of patients with Wilson's disease. Gastroenterology 1968;55:354–67.

116. Sternlieb I, Feldmann G. Effects of anticopper therapy on hepatocellular mitochondria in patients with Wilson's disease: an ultrastructural and stereological study. Gastroenterology 1976;71:457–61.
117. Sokol RJ, Devereaux MW, O'Brien K, et al. Abnormal hepatic mitochondrial respiration and cytochrome C oxidase activity in rats with long-term copper overload. Gastroenterology 1993;105:178–87.
118. Sokol RJ, Twedt D, McKim JM Jr, et al. Oxidant injury to hepatic mitochondria in patients with Wilson's disease and Bedlington terriers with copper toxicosis. Gastroenterology 1994;107:1788–98.
119. Mansouri A, Gaou I, Fromenty B, et al. Premature oxidative aging of hepatic mitochondrial DNA in Wilson's disease. Gastroenterology 1997;113:599–605.
120. Lutsenko S, Cooper MJ. Localization of the Wilson's disease protein product to mitochondria. Proc Natl Acad Sci U S A 1998;95:6004–9.
121. Mahler H, Pasi A, Kramer JM, et al. Fulminant liver failure in association with the emetic toxin of Bacillus cereus. N Engl J Med 1997;336:1142–8.
122. Fromenty B, Grimbert S, Mansouri A, et al. Hepatic mitochondrial DNA deletion in alcoholics: association with microvesicular steatosis. Gastroenterology 1995;108:193–200.
123. McKenzie R, Fried MW, Sallie R, et al. Hepatic failure and lactic acidosis due to fialuridine (FIAU), an investigational nucleoside analogue for chronic hepatitis B. N Engl J Med 1995;333:1099–105.
124. Cui L, Yoon S, Schinazi RF, Sommadossi JP. Cellular and molecular events leading to mitochondrial toxicity of 1-(2-deoxy-2-fluoro-1-beta-D-arabinofuranosyl)-5-iodouracil in human liver cells. J Clin Invest 1995;95:555–63.
125. Swartz MN. Mitochondrial toxicity–new adverse drug effects. N Engl J Med 1995;333:1146–8.
126. Lo JC, Kazemi MR, Hsue PY, et al. The relationship between nucleoside analogue treatment duration, insulin resistance, and fasting arterialized lactate level in patients with HIV infection. Clin Infect Dis 2005;41:1335–40.
127. Claessens YE, Chiche JD, Mira JP, Cariou A. Bench-to-bedside review: severe lactic acidosis in HIV patients treated with nucleoside analogue reverse transcriptase inhibitors. Crit Care 2003;7:226–32.
128. Sokol RJ, Winklhofer-Roob BM, Devereaux MW, McKim JM, Jr. Generation of hydroperoxides in isolated rat hepatocytes and hepatic mitochondria exposed to hydrophobic bile acids. Gastroenterology 1995;109:1249–56.
129. Krahenbuhl S, Stucki J, Reichen J. Reduced activity of the electron transport chain in liver mitochondria isolated from rats with secondary biliary cirrhosis. Hepatology 1992;15:1160–6.
130. Krahenbuhl S, Talos C, Fischer S, Reichen J. Toxicity of bile acids on the electron transport chain of isolated rat liver mitochondria. Hepatology 1994;19:471–9.
131. Sokol R, Devereaux MW, Straka MS. Induction of the permeability transition in hepatic mitochondria by physiologic bile acid concentrations. Hepatology 1997;26:188A.
132. Sokol RJ, McKim JM, Jr., Goff MC, et al. Vitamin E reduces oxidant injury to mitochondria and the hepatotoxicity of taurochenodeoxycholic acid in the rat. Gastroenterology 1998;114:164–74.
133. Day CP, James OF. Hepatic steatosis: innocent bystander or guilty party? Hepatology 1998;27:1463–6.
134. Berson A, De Beco V, Letteron P, et al. Steatohepatitis-inducing drugs cause mitochondrial dysfunction and lipid peroxidation in rat hepatocytes. Gastroenterology 1998;114:764–74.
135. Lavine JE. Treatment of obesity-induced steatohepatitis with vitamin E. Gastroenterology 1998;114:A1284.
136. Munnich A, Rotig A, Chretien D, et al. Clinical presentations and laboratory investigations in respiratory chain deficiency. Eur J Pediatr 1996;155:262–74.
137. Rustin P, Chretien D, Bourgeron T, et al. Biochemical and molecular investigations in respiratory chain deficiencies. Clin Chim Acta 1994;228:35–51.
138. Verma A, Piccoli DA, Bonilla E, et al. A novel mitochondrial G8313A mutation associated with prominent initial gastrointestinal symptoms and progressive encephaloneuropathy. Pediatr Res 1997;42:448–54.
139. Pitkanen S, Robinson BH. Mitochondrial complex I deficiency leads to increased production of superoxide radicals and induction of superoxide dismutase. J Clin Invest 1996;98:345–51.
140. Taivassalo T, Fu K, Johns T, et al. Gene shifting: a novel therapy for mitochondrial myopathy. Hum Mol Genet 1999;8:1047–52.
141. Clark KM, Bindoff LA, Lightowlers RN, et al. Reversal of a mitochondrial DNA defect in human skeletal muscle. Nat Genet 1997;16:222–4.
142. Taylor RW, Chinnery PF, Clark KM, et al. Treatment of mitochondrial disease. J Bioenerg Biomembr 1997;29:195–205.
143. Frei B, Kim MC, Ames BN. Ubiquinol-10 is an effective lipid-soluble antioxidant at physiological concentrations. Proc Natl Acad Sci U S A 1990;87:4879–83.
144. Sugino K, Dohi K, Yamada K, Kawasaki T. Changes in the levels of endogenous antioxidants in the liver of mice with experimental endotoxemia and the protective effects of the antioxidants. Surgery 1989;105:200–6.
145. Imada I, Fujita T, Sugiyama Y, et al. Effects of idebenone and related compounds on respiratory activities of brain mitochondria, and on lipid peroxidation of their membranes. Arch Gerontol Geriatr 1989;8:323–41.
146. Sugiyama Y, Fujita T. Stimulation of the respiratory and phosphorylating activities in rat brain mitochondria by idebenone (CV-2619), a new agent improving cerebral metabolism. FEBS Lett 1985;184:48–51.
147. Krahenbuhl S, Talos C, Lauterburg BH, Reichen J. Reduced antioxidative capacity in liver mitochondria from bile duct ligated rats. Hepatology 1995;22:607–12.
148. Hirano M, Quinzii CM, Dimauro S. Restoring balance to ataxia with coenzyme Q10 deficiency. J Neurol Sci 2006;246:11–12.
149. Horvath R, Schneiderat P, Schoser BG, et al. Coenzyme Q10 deficiency and isolated myopathy. Neurology 2006;66:253–5.
150. Toth PP, el-Shanti H, Eivins S, et al. Transient improvement of congenital lactic acidosis in a male infant with pyruvate decarboxylase deficiency treated with dichloroacetate. J Pediatr 1993;123:427–30.
151. Rake JP, Van Spronsen FJ, Visser G. End-stage liver disease as the only consequence of a complex I and IV deficiency: liver transplantation indicated? J Inherit Metab Dis 1997;20 Suppl 1:65.
152. Starzl TE, Demetris AJ, Trucco M, et al. Chimerism after liver transplantation for type IV glycogen storage disease and type 1 Gaucher's disease. N Engl J Med 1993;328:745–9.

153. Manfredi G, Gupta N, Vazquez-Memije ME, et al. Oligomycin induces a decrease in the cellular content of a pathogenic mutation in the human mitochondrial ATPase 6 gene. J Biol Chem 1999;274:9386–91.
154. Seibel P, Trappe J, Villani G, et al. Transfection of mitochondria: strategy towards a gene therapy of mitochondrial DNA diseases. Nucleic Acids Res 1995;23:10–17.
155. Taylor RW, Chinnery PF, Turnbull DM, Lightowlers RN. Selective inhibition of mutant human mitochondrial DNA replication in vitro by peptide nucleic acids. Nat Genet 1997;15:212–15.
156. Schapira AH. Mitochondrial disease. Lancet 2006;368:70–82.
157. Ruitenbeek W, Wendel U, Hamel BC, Trijbels JM. Genetic counselling and prenatal diagnosis in disorders of the mitochondrial energy metabolism. J Inherit Metab Dis 1996;19:581–7.
158. Wanders RJ, Ruiter JP, Wijburg FA, et al. Prenatal diagnosis of systemic disorders of the respiratory chain in cultured chorionic villus fibroblasts by study of ATP-synthesis in digitonin-permeabilized cells. J Inherit Metab Dis 1996;19:133–6.
159. Muller-Hocker J, Aust D, Rohrbach H, et al. Defects of the respiratory chain in the normal human liver and in cirrhosis during aging. Hepatology 1997;26:709–19.

34

NONALCOHOLIC FATTY LIVER DISEASE

Jeffrey B. Schwimmer, M.D.

Nonalcoholic fatty liver disease (NAFLD) is a common and increasingly recognized disorder characterized by the accumulation of macrovesicular fat in hepatocytes. The condition of hepatic steatosis in association with obesity in adults was reported nearly a half century ago but received little attention compared with fatty liver associated with chronic alcohol consumption [1]. Two decades later, in 1979, Adler and Schaffner [2] reported that liver histology in a group of 29 overweight adult patients was similar to the findings of alcoholic liver disease including cases with fatty liver, fatty hepatitis, fatty fibrosis, and fatty cirrhosis. However, it was 1 year later that the field of NAFLD was truly established when a group of astute physicians at the Mayo Clinic gave the name nonalcoholic steatohepatitis (NASH) to a "hitherto unnamed disease" [3]. They too recognized that many patients had liver disease that seemed similar to alcoholic liver disease despite a clear demonstration of strict abstinence. Shortly thereafter, three cases of NASH were reported in children [4]. Over the ensuing 2 decades, much progress has been made in understanding the epidemiology, clinical features, and histology of pediatric NAFLD. Efforts at treatment are still early but deserve special attention.

TERMINOLOGY

The terminology continues to be a source of confusion and controversy. The initial term, NASH, referred to patients who had sufficiently clinically relevant disease manifestations to come to the attention of a hepatologist. The term NAFLD was developed to acknowledge that a broader spectrum of disease exists that includes steatosis alone, steatohepatitis with or without fibrosis, and cirrhosis [5]. One challenge in interpreting the literature in this young field is that the clinicopathologic definition of NASH has changed over time. Furthermore, the qualifier of "nonalcoholic" is somewhat unfortunate for use in pediatrics given that NAFLD is even seen in preschool-aged children. Another area of confusion is that of "primary" versus "secondary" NAFLD. Hepatic steatosis can be associated with multiple causes including medications, metabolic disorders, and toxin exposures. Therefore, some investigators have sought to distinguish between fatty liver that is associated with obesity and insulin resistance (primary) from that caused by other factors such as medication (secondary). The argument for this system is that the histology is similar and both are not caused by alcohol. However, using the same parent term, NAFLD, introduces noise into the understanding of the epidemiology, pathophysiology, and natural history. A final point of controversy in terminology centers around the method used to confirm the diagnosis. If a patient is believed to have NAFLD based on indirect measures only, the term used is suspected NAFLD. When a patient has a biopsy-proven diagnosis then the term applied should be NAFLD or NASH depending on the histologic findings. In interpreting the published studies, readers should be cautious to determine whether an author is discussing a patient with NAFLD that is suspected or confirmed.

EPIDEMIOLOGY

The major studies on the prevalence of pediatric NAFLD are shown in Table 34.1. Most efforts to determine the prevalence of fatty liver in children have been restricted to studies using indirect measures such as blood tests or ultrasound to predict a histologic outcome. In 1989, based on ultrasound, fatty liver prevalence was estimated to be 2.6% in school-aged children in northern Japan [6]. Most studies have been limited to children selected for the condition of obesity. Franzese et al. [7] studied 72 Italian children referred to a university obesity clinic and demonstrated elevated serum aminotransferase (ALT) activity in 25% and an abnormal liver ultrasound in 53%. Chan et al. [8] studied 84 Chinese children referred to a university obesity clinic in Hong Kong with a median age of 12 years and median body mass index (BMI) of 30.3 kg/m^2. The authors suspected fatty liver in 24% based on ALT and 77% based on liver ultrasound. Taken together, the prevalence of fatty liver in obese children in China, Italy, Japan, and the United States has been reported to be between 10 and 77% [7–10]. The wide range in estimates of prevalence is due in part to the difficulty in determining the presence or absence of fatty liver based on noninvasive tests. To address these limitations, we recently

Table 34.1: Epidemiology of Pediatric Fatty Liver

Study	*Population*	*Age*	*N*	*Prevalence of Fatty Liver*		
				ALT	*Ultrasound*	*Histology*
Tominaga et al. [6]	School-based	4–12	823	—	2.6%	—
Franzese et al. [7]	Obesity clinic	10	72	25%	53%	—
Strauss et al. [10]	NHANES 1988–1994 (obese)	15	332	10%	—	—
Chan et al. [8]	Obesity clinic	12	84	24%	77%	—
Schwimmer et al. [18]	School-based (obese)	17	127	23%	—	—
Nadeau et al. [35]	Type 2 diabetes	15	48	48%	—	—
Schwimmer et al. [11]	Community autopsy sample	2–19	954	—	—	9%

completed the Study of Child and Adolescent Liver Epidemiology (SCALE) [11]. SCALE is a 10-year study of liver histology in children aged 2–19 years who had an autopsy performed by a county medical examiner for sudden unexpected deaths that occurred outside of the in-patient hospital setting. Based on requisite histology, we estimate that fatty liver is present in 9% of children.

Clinical series of children with NAFLD uniformly demonstrate a predominance of boys versus girls [4,12–17]. Given the potential for selection bias in the subspecialty referral environment, we collaborated with the child and adolescent trial of cardiovascular health (CATCH) to conduct a geographically diverse, population-based study of obese 12th-grade students [18]. Based on the surrogate measure of ALT, suspected fatty liver was substantially more common in obese boys than obese girls even after controlling for BMI and ethnicity. In the histology-based SCALE study, it was further corroborated that after controlling for confounding factors boys are approximately 40% more likely to have fatty liver than girls [11].

In addition to gender, race and ethnicity also play a role in the development of NAFLD. Clinical series of pediatric NAFLD have included predominantly children of white or Asian race possibly reflecting the community demographics of reporting centers. Clinical series restricted to the southwestern United States raised the possibility that Mexican American children have higher rates of NAFLD than non-Hispanic children [15,19]. Although black children are known to have high rates of risk factors for NAFLD, such as obesity and insulin resistance [20–23], few children of black race are included in clinical series of NAFLD [15]. In the CATCH study of ALT in obese high school seniors, the highest rate of elevated ALT was seen in Hispanic adolescents (36%) compared with white (22%) or black adolescents (14%). Louthan et al. [24] studied a large group of obese children in a primary care setting in Kentucky. They observed elevated serum ALT activity in 21% of white children compared with only 5% of black children. Moreover, SCALE further demonstrated that fatty liver is most prevalent in children and adolescents of Hispanic ethnicity and least prevalent among children and adolescents of black race [11]. Children of Asian or white race were noted to have an intermediate prevalence of fatty liver.

DIAGNOSIS

Nonalcoholic fatty liver disease is uncommon before age 8, and the typical age at presentation is 12 years, although biopsy-proven cases have been observed in children aged 2–17 years [17]. Children with NAFLD are often asymptomatic. Therefore, clinical evaluation is typically initiated with the finding of an elevated serum ALT. This may be detected incidentally or based on clinical suspicion in relationship to obesity, acanthosis nigricans, hepatomegaly, or a combination of these. Approximately 90% of children with NAFLD are obese as defined by having a BMI that is equal to or greater than the 95th percentile for gender and age [17,25]. Therefore, some physicians perform targeted ALT or ultrasound screening of obese children based on expert committee recommendations [26,27]. However, recent data from San Francisco suggests that many pediatricians and pediatric subspecialists still have a lack of awareness of the importance of NAFLD in obese children [28]. Thus, it is incumbent on pediatric hepatologists to participate in training to improve the recognition and assessment of obesity. Acanthosis nigricans is a lesion characterized by velvety thickening and hyperpigmentation affecting localized areas of the skin on neck, axillae, and other flexural areas in persons with hyperinsulinemia [29]. Acanthosis nigricans is seen in 30–50% of children with NAFLD [14,15]. Hepatomegaly is present in 40–50% of children with NAFLD [14,15]. However, hepatomegaly may be difficult to appreciate and go undetected in obese children [30]. In addition to the physical examination findings, approximately one third of children will present with a complaint of vague abdominal pain that may be right upper quadrant in nature.

An abnormal value of serum ALT activity is the most common blood analyte used to screen for NAFLD. However, there are no data to determine the sensitivity and specificity of any given ALT cut-off point for the detection of fatty liver. Furthermore, children can have NAFLD and even NASH with a "normal" ALT value [17]. When elevated, serum ALT usually exceeds AST in a ratio of approximately 1.7:1 [31]. Children with substantially higher values of ALT and AST are believed to be much more likely to have NAFLD than those with normal serum ALT activity. However, the level of serum ALT or AST activity is not a good discriminator of histologic severity. Data suggest that serum glutamyltransferase (GGT) activity has the potential to serve as a marker of NASH with advanced fibrosis [17].

When a child is evaluated for an abnormal ALT, it is important to test for potential causes other than NAFLD. This is particularly important in the context of obesity. Although the condition of obesity makes fatty liver more common, it does not make an individual less likely to have other forms of chronic liver disease. Thus one cannot make the assumption that an abnormal ALT is entirely or even partially caused by fatty liver. One should consider the range of possibilities and test for those that are clinically reasonable. The differential diagnosis of pediatric NAFLD is shown in Table 34.2.

A number of metabolic abnormalities are common in children with NAFLD. Often patients will demonstrate dyslipidemia, particularly elevations in serum triglyceride levels. Fasting glucose is most commonly normal, whereas fasting insulin levels are typically elevated. Thus a complete evaluation for NAFLD should include an evaluation for comorbid conditions. A minimum workup would include measurements of fasting glucose, insulin, and lipids. In addition, one may consider other laboratory studies that are pertinent to obesity such as thyroid function or uric acid.

Insulin resistance results in abnormalities in both carbohydrate and fat metabolism manifested by decreased insulin-stimulated glucose transport and metabolism in adipocytes and skeletal muscle, increased lipolysis with a resultant increase in circulating free fatty acid, and increased hepatic glucose and very low-density lipoprotein output. Several studies support a role for insulin resistance in pediatric NAFLD [9,14,15]. The degree of insulin resistance seen in children with NASH exceeds that which one would expect on the basis of obesity alone [32]. Increasing evidence supports the hypothesis that fat accumulation in both the liver and skeletal muscle is a major step in the development of insulin resistance and the metabolic syndrome. Once the storage capacity of the adipocyte is exceeded, fat overflows to other tissues especially liver and skeletal muscle [33]. Thus on the basis of lipotoxicity, fatty liver may pose a risk not only for the development of steatohepatitis but may also contribute to the development of type 2 diabetes mellitus. The intracellular metabolites of triglyceride metabolism in the liver can cause acquired insulin signaling defects and insulin resistance, glucose intolerance, and type 2 diabetes mellitus [34]. Approximately 8–10% of children with NAFLD have diabetes at the time of diagnosis; however, nearly all children with biopsy-proven NAFLD are insulin resistant [15,17,32]. Furthermore, it is likely that fatty liver precedes the development of diabetes. By the time of the diagnosis of type 2 diabetes mellitus in children, approximately one half have suspected fatty liver based on elevation of alanine aminotransferase [35]. In further support of this hypothesis, in a secondary analysis of adults participating in the multicenter observational Insulin Resistance Atherosclerosis Study, a putative surrogate of fatty liver, serum aminotransferase activity, independently predicted incident type 2 diabetes mellitus [36].

Table 34.2: Differential Diagnosis of Pediatric NAFLD

Category	*Cause*
Infection	Hepatitis C virus
Immunologic disorders	Autoimmune hepatitis
	Celiac disease
	Inflammatory bowel disease
	Type 1 diabetes mellitus
Medication	Amiodarone
	Glucocorticoids
	Highly active antiretroviral therapy
	L-asparaginase
	Valproic acid
Metabolic disorders	Abetalipoproteinemia
	α-1 antitrypsin deficiency
	Alpers' syndrome
	Carnitine deficiency
	Cholesterol ester storage disease
	Cystic fibrosis
	Glycogen storage disease
	Homocystinuria
	Lipodystrophy
	Wilson's disease
Nutritional	Protein-calorie malnutrition
	Starvation
	Total parenteral nutrition
Toxins	Ethanol

Increased fat mass in obese children does not simply serve as a storage depot for excess energy. Adipose tissue participates in the regulation of homeostatic processes through the production of many biologically active molecules. These include adipokines such as adiponectin, leptin, plasminogen activator inhibitor-1, resistin, and tumor necrosis factor-alpha (TNF-α). Visceral adipose tissue in particular may produce greater amounts of TNF-α. In children with fatty liver, the amount of fat present in the liver is mildly correlated with the amount of visceral adipose tissue [37]. In animal models, TNF-α produces hepatic insulin resistance via up-regulation of suppressor of cytokines signaling (SOCS) [38]. In turn, SOCS-1 and SOCS-3, interfere with the JAK-STAT pathway, which ultimately decreases the ability of insulin to activate its signaling pathway [39]. Serum TNF-α levels are elevated in obese adults with NAFLD [40]. However, the role of TNF-α in pediatric NAFLD is unknown. Adiponectin is emerging as an integral factor linking obesity, insulin resistance, and hepatic steatosis [41–43]. In contrast to the other adipokines, the amount of adiponectin produced is decreased in the context of obesity or diabetes. Moreover, adiponectin has been implicated in NAFLD. Adiponectin enhances the action of insulin on hepatocytes, resulting in decreased hepatic glucose production and serum glucose levels. In obese, leptin-deficient ob/ob mice, circulating adiponectin levels are low [44]. When these animals were treated with adiponectin, despite no change in body weight, there is a decrease in hepatic lipid content and serum ALT levels. In adults with NAFLD, serum adiponectin is inversely correlated with the percentage of steatotic hepatocytes [45]. However, studies to date are conflicting regarding the relation between adiponectin and inflammation or fibrosis [45–47]. In children and adolescents, serum adiponectin levels are negatively correlated with percent body fat [48]. In nonobese and obese adolescents, adiponectin is inversely correlated with intramyocellular lipid content [49]. A similar relationship may be true for adiponectin and hepatic lipid content. However, in children and adolescents, the relationship between adiponectin and liver fat or NASH remains uncharacterized.

Beyond the classic associations with pediatric NAFLD, one important condition is hypothalamic and pituitary dysfunction [50–53]. These children are frequently observed to gain substantial weight, become obese, and develop NAFLD. However, the hormonal factors beyond obesity alone are likely involved. Hepatologists should have a heightened awareness because these patients have been observed to manifest the most severe cases of pediatric NASH with liver-related morbidity and mortality secondary to cirrhosis.

IMAGING

Noninvasive radiologic imaging techniques are an attractive tool for use in the diagnosis of NAFLD. Several imaging techniques have been used to examine fat within the liver. However, in children, no noninvasive method has been validated against liver histology. Furthermore, no existing imaging technology is able to discriminate between hepatic steatosis and NASH.

Liver ultrasonography is the most commonly used imaging technique to evaluate for the presence of hepatic steatosis. Advantages include low cost and wide availability. The brightness of the liver echo is compared with the kidney [54]. The sonographic features of fatty liver include increased hepatic parenchymal echotexture and vascular blurring. However, these findings are also seen in patients with other forms of chronic liver disease with fibrosis and thus are nonspecific. Also the ability to detect fatty liver by ultrasonography drops off markedly once the degree of hepatic steatosis decreases to 30% or less. Therefore, liver ultrasound can be considered a good screening test but is not diagnostic given the rate of both false positive and false negative results.

Computed tomography (CT) does provide a more specific method than ultrasonography for the detection of fatty liver. Liver attenuation values, in Hounsfield units, decrease with hepatic fat accumulation [55]. However, because of the radiation exposure, CT is rarely used clinically as a primary test for fatty liver. Fatty liver can be a common incidental finding on scans done for other reasons such as the evaluation of acute abdominal pain. Of note, the determination of fatty liver based on a contrast CT is particularly challenging and less reliable than a noncontrast CT scan [56].

Magnetic resonance (MR) methods to measure liver fat may be ideal for children because they are noninvasive, have the potential for the greatest accuracy, and do not use ionizing radiation. These include imaging (MRI) and spectroscopy (MRS). The basic MRI method is the Dixon technique, which uses sequences obtained at different values of echo time to allow a qualitative determination of fat and water content [57,58]. Images of the first sequence show the difference between fat and water (absolute value), and those of the second show their sum. A third image can be obtained to correct for inhomogeneity in the main magnetic field [59]. Fishbein et al. [60–62] developed protocols to make use of fast gradient echo techniques and four-point Dixon methods to measure hepatic fat content in children. MRS offers the opportunity for increased accuracy in tissues, such as the liver where water and fat are combined. MRS determination of fat content is strongly correlated with liver fat in adults as measured by biopsy [63,64]. A spectrum is obtained from a defined volume of tissue, the areas under the water and fat spectral peaks are measured, and corrections are applied for T_1, T2, and signal-to-weight. A direct measure of fat quantity at each spectral location is obtained. We applied MRS methodology to measure hepatic fat content in children with biopsy-proven NASH before and after treatment [32]. MRI holds the greatest promise for the future ability to assess NASH noninvasively. However, current technology is limited to the assessment of liver fat. The upper limit of normal for hepatic fat measured by MRI or MRS remains uncertain. In theory, liver fat may be best measured by a combination of Dixon imaging and MRS. Magnetic resonance imaging can be used to determine the amount of liver fat, and Dixon can be used to determine the distribution of liver fat.

LIVER BIOPSY AND HISTOLOGY

The diagnoses of NAFLD or NASH are made by an evaluation of liver pathology in conjunction with clinical information. NAFLD is characterized histologically by accumulation of macrovesicular fat in hepatocytes in a patient in whom other causes of liver disease are excluded. The issue of when to perform a liver biopsy in children with suspected NAFLD remains controversial. Biopsies are usually performed in the presence of persistently elevated serum aminotransferase values. The primary rationale for liver biopsy is that the definitive diagnosis of NAFLD and the discrimination of NASH from milder forms of fatty liver require a liver biopsy. In addition, some children with suspected NAFLD are determined to not have fatty liver, whereas in other cases, some children are proved to have an alternate diagnosis such as autoimmune hepatitis after a careful review of liver histology.

In adults with suspected NAFLD, the presence of type 2 diabetes and age older than 40 years have been proposed as clinical indications for liver biopsy [65,66]. However, neither age nor the presence of diabetes are likely to be useful determinants in children because those with advanced disease are not older than those with milder disease and may not have diabetes [17]. Retrospective models of clinical and laboratory features that predict histopathology in children have been reported [15]. Specifically, markers of insulin resistance when combined with the severity of obesity, abdominal pain, race, ALT, and AST were predictive of liver histology [15]. However, further validation and prospective analyses are needed.

The characteristic histologic features of NAFLD range from steatosis alone, to steatohepatitis with or without fibrosis, to cirrhosis. Because of the manner in which NAFLD was identified, the histologic criteria were largely derived from the understanding of the histologic features of adults with alcoholic liver disease. In adults the histologic features of NAFLD have been well described and include macrovesicular steatosis, perisinusoidal or pericellular fibrosis, ballooned hepatocytes, foci of lobular inflammation, lipid granulomas, Mallory hyaline, and megamitochondria [67]. The combination of macrovesicular steatosis with ballooning change of hepatocytes, perisinusoidal fibrosis, or both constitutes a pattern of histology considered diagnostic of NASH in an appropriate clinical context [68]. In 1999, Brunt et al. [67] proposed a system for grading and staging the histologic lesions of NASH. These "Brunt criteria" have become the most widely used scoring system for NASH. This system was derived from the review of liver biopsies from 50 adults with NASH at Saint Louis University. Recently, the National Institutes of Health NASH Clinical Research Network developed a histologic scoring system for NAFLD [69]. The pathology committee of nine hepatopathologists each reviewed liver biopsies from 32 adults and 18 children with NAFLD. An NAFLD Activity Score (NAS) was developed that includes only features that are potentially reversible in the short term. The score, ranging from 0–8, was defined as the sum of the scores for steatosis (0–3), lobular inflammation (0–3), and ballooning (0–2). Because fibrosis is less reversible and thought to be a result of disease activity, it was not included as a component of the activity score. A review of liver histology in 100 children with NAFLD demonstrated that, based on major differences in the patterns of liver injury, the Brunt criteria are not well suited for use in pediatric NASH [17]. The NAS system also relies on the feature of ballooned hepatocytes, which is uncommon in pediatric NASH.

Studies of pediatric NAFLD have described patterns of inflammation and fibrosis that differ from those reported in adults with NAFLD [4,12–14,70,71]. To develop definitions for NASH in children, we reviewed liver histology for 100 children with NAFLD [17]. Hierarchical cluster analysis was applied and demonstrated distinct histologic patterns including two forms of steatohepatitis. The definitions are shown in Table 34.3, and examples are shown in Figure 34.1. *Type 1 NASH* is consistent with NASH as described in adults and is defined as the presence of steatosis with ballooning degeneration, perisinusoidal fibrosis, or both, in the absence of portal features. *Type 2 NASH* is the predominant form of NASH observed in children and is defined as the presence of steatosis along with portal inflammation, fibrosis, or both, in the absence of ballooning degeneration and perisinusoidal fibrosis. The majority of children with advanced fibrosis were noted to manifest the type 2 NASH pattern.

Table 34.3: Histologic Definitions for NASH Types

	Type 1			*Type 2*		
Ballooning degeneration	+	+	–		–	
Perisinusoidal fibrosis	–	+	+		–	
Steatosis	+				+	
Portal inflammation		–		+	+	–
Portal fibrosis		–		–	+	+

+, feature is present; –, feature is absent.

NATURAL HISTORY

Longitudinal data in children with NAFLD are limited, although children with NAFLD may be at increased risk for both hepatic and nonhepatic morbidity and mortality [72–74]. The prognosis for a child with NAFLD is likely related to the severity of baseline liver histology. Clinical case series suggest that advanced fibrosis is present at the time of diagnosis in 5–10% of children with NAFLD. Data on the progression to cirrhosis are extremely limited. However, many investigators have reported cases of pediatric NAFLD associated with cirrhosis [14,15,17,75–77]. Moreover, there are a few reports of adolescents in the United States undergoing liver transplantation for end-stage liver disease caused by NASH [52,77]. As with any form of chronic liver disease, some children with NAFLD may develop hepatocellular carcinoma in adulthood [50,78]. Thus, pediatric NAFLD must be considered as a serious disease.

TREATMENT

Overall the approach to treatment in pediatric NAFLD is underdeveloped. Furthermore, the management leans heavily on the approach to the treatment of severe obesity, which is

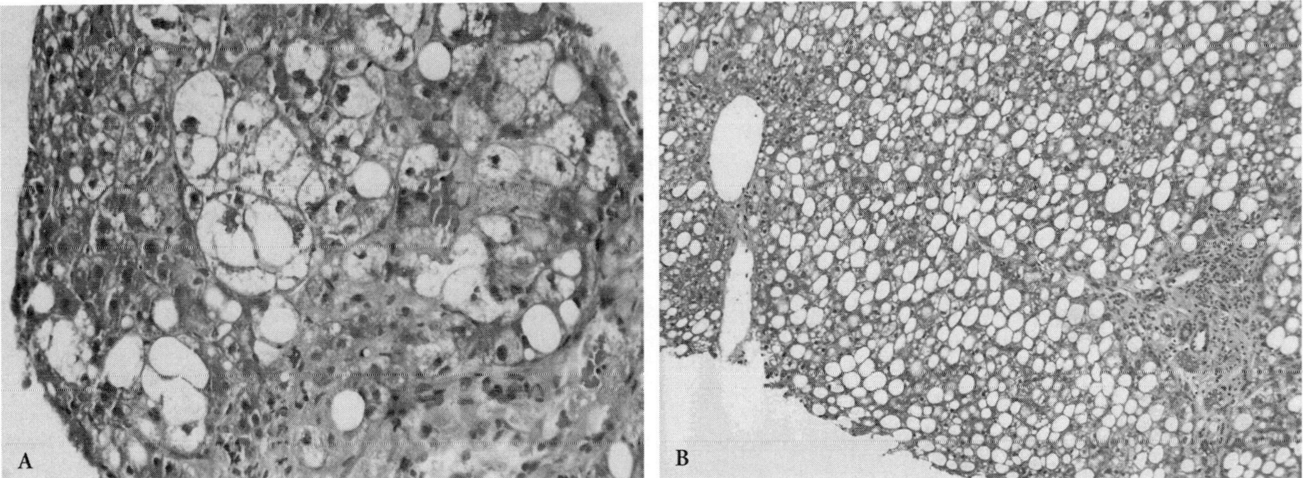

Figure 34.1. Histologic patterns of pediatric NASH. Shown are liver biopsies from two children with NASH. (**A**) A biopsy typical of type 1 NASH with ballooning degeneration of hepatocytes and perisinusoidal fibrosis. (**B**) A biopsy typical of type 2 NASH with a normal central vein, no hepatocytes ballooning but with portal inflammation and fibrosis. For color reproduction, see Color Plate 34.1.

also underdeveloped in children [25,27,79]. Determining the long-term effectiveness of therapy for NAFLD and NASH on meaningful liver-related outcomes should be a major research priority.

Lifestyle

Because the majority of children with NAFLD are obese, weight reduction via dietary change and physical activity is widely promoted. However, there are no clinical trial data available to determine the impact of such lifestyle modification on NAFLD in children. Vajro et al. [80] reported a case series of nine obese children with persistent elevation of ALT who were prescribed a balanced, individualized hypocaloric diet and physical exercise. In those patients who experienced weight loss of at least 10% of excess body weight, prolonged normalization of aminotransferase values was seen.

Experience with the effect of lifestyle therapies on histology is limited. Major questions remain about the relative efficacy of various dietary and/or physical activity strategies.

Pharmacologic

Several pilot studies of pharmacologic approaches in children have been conducted and are listed in Table 34.4. However, there is not a sufficient evidence base to make formal recommendations for the pharmacologic treatment of NAFLD. Thus, the use of a given agent in clinical practice must be balanced in terms of the evidence for efficacy and the potential for toxicity. Preliminary studies on several other agents have been conducted in adults; however, it is unclear to what extent one can extrapolate data from adults to children with NAFLD.

Obinata et al. [81] reported the first attempt at pharmacologic treatment of pediatric fatty liver. A group of 10 obese Japanese children with suspected fatty liver disease based on serum ALT and CT scan were given between 2 and 6 g of taurine powder daily for a period of 6 months or longer. Subjects were also given a "diet." Improvement in ALT and liver fat assessed by CT were seen in children regardless of changes in the severity of obesity. Many potential mechanisms for the observed effects of taurine were proposed; however, in the decade since this initial report, there has been no subsequent data on the use of taurine for the treatment of fatty liver.

One treatment strategy is to decrease oxidative stress by providing supplemental antioxidants. Lavine [82] conducted an open-label treatment trial of alpha-tocopherol in 11 obese children with elevated serum ALT and ultrasound evidence of fatty liver. Treatment consisted of escalating doses of vitamin E between 400 and 1200 IU per day for a period of 4–10 months. All subjects demonstrated normalization of serum ALT despite the absence of weight loss. In a subsequent study by Vajro et al. [83], 28 obese children with suspected NAFLD were randomized to one of two treatment groups. In 10 of the 28 children, liver biopsy was performed and confirmed the diagnosis of NAFLD. The treatment groups were diet and vitamin E versus diet and placebo. The vitamin E dose used was 400 IU per day for 2 months followed by 100 IU per day for an additional 3 months. There was no difference seen in ALT reduction between the 2 treatment groups. In one subject receiving vitamin E, there was an alarming, unexplained rise in ALT to 7 times above normal values. A post hoc analysis suggested that those children who took vitamin E and did not lose weight had a greater improvement in ALT than those children who neither lost weight nor took vitamin E.

Thus questions remain not only about the efficacy of vitamin E but also regarding patient selection, dosing, and duration of therapy.

Based on initial promise in small studies conducted in adults with NAFLD, Vajro et al. [84] conducted a pilot study using ursodeoxycholic acid in a group of 31 obese school-aged

Table 34.4: Treatment Trials for Pediatric NAFLD and NASH

Author	*Treatment*	*Treatment Group*	*Control Group*	*Diagnosis*	*Duration*	*Outcome*	*Finding*
Obinata et al. [81]	Taurine	10	n/a	Suspected NAFLD	≥6 months	ALT Steatosis (CT)	Improved Improved
Lavine [82]	Vitamin E	11	n/a	Suspected NAFLD	Variable	ALT Steatosis (US)	Normalized No change
Vajro et al. [84]	Ursodeoxycholic acid	14	17	Mixed population of Non-NAFLD, suspected NAFLD, and biopsy-proven NASH	6 months	ALT Steatosis (US)	No change No change
Vajro et al. [83]	Vitamin E	14	14	Mixed population of suspected and biopsy-proven NAFLD	5 months	ALT Steatosis (US)	No change No change
Schwimmer et al. [32]	Metformin	10	n/a	Biopsy-proven NASH	24 weeks	ALT Steatosis (MRS)	Improved Decreased

CT, computed tomography; MRS, magnetic resonance spectroscopy; US, ultrasound

children with persistent elevation of serum ALT activity. The cohort included 3 children with biopsy-proven NASH, 24 children with suspected NAFLD based on ultrasound, and 4 children with imaging evidence that did not support a diagnosis of fatty liver. Subjects who were most likely to comply with a diet and exercise program were assigned to the diet group. Those who had previously proved unable to comply with dietary and activity intervention were assigned to the medication or non-treatment group. For those in the medication group, ursodeoxycholic acid was prescribed at a dose of 10–12.5 mg/kg/d divided in 2 daily doses. Nearly 20% of the subjects assigned to diet plus medication refused to take ursodeoxycholic acid and were then reassigned to the diet only group. As expected, those children assigned to the diet group were successful in losing weight, whereas the children in the medication and nontreatment groups demonstrated further weight gain. Improvements in ALT and ultrasound appearance of the liver were seen in only those who lost weight. Treatment with ursodeoxycholic acid did not demonstrate additional improvements beyond the effect of weight loss.

We conducted the first pediatric treatment trial to only include subjects with biopsy-proven steatohepatitis [32]. Metformin was selected as the therapeutic agent because of the nearly uniform association of insulin resistance in pediatric NAFLD. Metformin reduces hepatic glucose production and increases insulin sensitivity in adolescents with type 2 diabetes mellitus [85]. Ten nondiabetic children with NASH received open-label treatment with metformin at a dose of 500 mg twice daily for a period of 24 weeks. Mean ALT and AST improved significantly from baseline to end of treatment; ALT normalized in 40% and AST normalized in 50% of subjects. Children demonstrated significant improvements in liver fat measured by MRS; insulin sensitivity measured by quantitative insulin sensitivity check index; and quality of life measured by the PedsQL 4.0. The degree to which changes in serum ALT or the amount of liver fat correlate with changes in histology remains to be established. Large multicenter randomized controlled trials are underway in the United States and England [86].

SUMMARY

In a span of only 2 decades, NAFLD has gone from a virtually unknown liver disease to a common cause of liver disease in children. Insulin resistance is an established risk factor for pediatric NASH. However, the pathogenesis is still unclear. Unfortunately, the prevalence can be expected to increase with the epidemic of pediatric obesity. An extensive understanding of the natural history is lacking, but cirrhosis can develop in childhood. Thus, pediatric NAFLD should be considered as a serious disease. In children NAFLD has both features that overlap and are distinct from NAFLD in adults. One cannot assume that data from adults with NAFLD will accurately extrapolate to children with NAFLD. No consensus exists regarding the decision and timing of liver biopsy. Moreover, the evidence base for therapeutic decision making is extremely limited. Research efforts must focus on the development of better tools for screening, diagnosis, and management. These may then form the basis of future clinical guidelines for pediatric NAFLD.

REFERENCES

1. Zelman S. The liver in obesity. Arch Intern Med. 1958;90:141–56.
2. Adler M, Schaffner F. Fatty liver hepatitis and cirrhosis in obese patients. Am J Med 1979;67:811–16.

3. Ludwig J, Viggiano TR, McGill DB, Oh BJ. Nonalcoholic steatohepatitis: Mayo Clinic experiences with a hitherto unnamed disease. Mayo Clin Proc 1980;55:434–8.
4. Moran JR, Ghishan FK, Halter SA, Greene HL. Steatohepatitis in obese children: a cause of chronic liver dysfunction. Am J Gastroenterol 1983;78:374–7.
5. Schaffner F, Thaler H. Nonalcoholic fatty liver disease. Prog Liver Dis 1986;8:283–98.
6. Tominaga K, Kurata JH, Chen YK, et al. Prevalence of fatty liver in Japanese children and relationship to obesity. An epidemiological ultrasonographic survey. Dig Dis Sci 1995;40:2002–9.
7. Franzese A, Vajro P, Argenziano A, et al. Liver involvement in obese children. Ultrasonography and liver enzyme levels at diagnosis and during follow-up in an Italian population. Dig Dis Sci 1997;42:1428–32.
8. Chan DF, Li AM, Chu WC, et al. Hepatic steatosis in obese Chinese children. Int J Obes Relat Metab Disord 2004;28:1257–63.
9. Tazawa Y, Noguchi H, Nishinomiya F, Takada G. Serum alanine aminotransferase activity in obese children. Acta Pediatr 1997;86:238–41.
10. Strauss RS, Barlow SE, Dietz WH. Prevalence of abnormal serum aminotransferase values in overweight and obese adolescents. J Pediatr 2000;136:727–33.
11. Schwimmer J, Deutsch R, Kahen T, et al. Prevalence of fatty liver in children and adolescents. Pediatrics 2006;118:1388–93.
12. Baldridge AD, Perez-Atayde AR, Graeme-Cook F, et al. Idiopathic steatohepatitis in childhood: a multicenter retrospective study. J Pediatr 1995;127:700–4.
13. Manton ND, Lipsett J, Moore DJ, et al. Non-alcoholic steatohepatitis in children and adolescents. Med J Aust 2000;173:476–9.
14. Rashid M, Roberts EA. Nonalcoholic steatohepatitis in children. J Pediatr Gastroenterol Nutr 2000;30:48–53.
15. Schwimmer JB, Deutsch R, Rauch JB, et al. Obesity, insulin resistance, and other clinicopathological correlates of pediatric nonalcoholic fatty liver disease. J Pediatr 2003;143:500–5.
16. Lavine JE, Schwimmer JB. Pediatric non-alcoholic steatohepatitis. In: Farrell G, George J, Hall P, McCollough A, eds. Nonalcoholic steatohepatitis. Oxford, England: Blackwell; 2004:229–40.
17. Schwimmer JB, Behling C, Newbury R, et al. Histopathol ogy of pediatric nonalcoholic fatty liver disease. Hepatology 2005;42:641–8.
18. Schwimmer JB, McGreal N, Deutsch R, et al. The influence of gender, race, and ethnicity on suspected fatty liver in obese adolescents. Pediatrics. 2005;115:e561–5.
19. Schwimmer JB, Burwinkle TM, Varni JW. Health-related quality of life of severely obese children and adolescents. JAMA 2003;289:1813–19.
20. Pinhas-Hamiel O, Dolan LM, Daniels SR, et al. Increased incidence of non-insulin-dependent diabetes mellitus among adolescents. J Pediatr 1996;128:608–15.
21. Gower BA. Syndrome X in children: influence of ethnicity and visceral fat. Am J Human Biol 1999;11:249–57.
22. Crawford PB, Story M, Wang MC, et al. Ethnic issues in the epidemiology of childhood obesity. Pediatr Clin North Am 2001;48:855–78.
23. Ogden CL, Flegal KM, Carroll MD, Johnson CL. Prevalence and trends in overweight among us children and adolescents, 1999–2000. JAMA 288:1728–32.
24. Louthan MV, Theriot JA, Zimmerman E, et al. Decreased prevalence of nonalcoholic fatty liver disease in black obese children. J Pediatr Gastroenterol Nutr 2005;41:426–9.
25. Committee on Prevention of Obesity in Children and Youth. Preventing childhood obesity health in the balance. Washington, D.C.: National Academies Press; 2005.
26. Barlow SE, Dietz WH. Obesity evaluation and treatment: Expert Committee recommendations. The Maternal and Child Health Bureau, Health Resources and Services Administration and the Department of Health and Human Services. Pediatrics 1998; 102:E29.
27. Speiser PW, Rudolf MC, Anhalt H, et al. Childhood obesity. J Clin Endocrinol Metab 2005;90:1871–87.
28. Riley MR, Bass NM, Rosenthal P, Merriman RB. Underdiagnosis of pediatric obesity and underscreening for fatty liver disease and metabolic syndrome by pediatricians and pediatric subspecialists. J Pediatr 2005;147:839–42.
29. Nguyen TT, Keil MF, Russell DL, et al. Relation of acanthosis nigricans to hyperinsulinemia and insulin sensitivity in overweight African American and white children. J Pediatr 2001;138:474–80.
30. Fishbein M, Mogren J, Mogren C, et al. Undetected hepatomegaly in obese children by primary care physicians: a pitfall in the diagnosis of pediatric nonalcoholic fatty liver disease. Clin Pediatr 2005;44:135–41.
31. Lavine JE, Schwimmer JB. NAFLD in the pediatric population. Clin Liver Dis 2004;8:549–58.
32. Schwimmer JB, Middleton MS, Deutsch R, Lavine JE. A phase 2 clinical trial of metformin as a treatment for non-diabetic paediatric nonalcoholic steatohepatitis. Aliment Pharmacol Ther 2005;21:871–9.
33. Bays H, Mandarino L, DeFronzo RA. Role of the adipocyte, free fatty acids, and ectopic fat in pathogenesis of type 2 diabetes mellitus: peroxisomal proliferator-activated receptor agonists provide a rational therapeutic approach. J Clin Endocrinol Metab 2004;89:463–78.
34. Shulman GI. Cellular mechanisms of insulin resistance. J Clin Invest. 2000;106:171–6.
35. Nadeau KJ, Klingensmith G, Zeitler P. Type 2 diabetes in children is frequently associated with elevated alanine aminotransferase. J Pediatr Gastroenterol Nutr 2005;41:94–8.
36. Hanley A, Williams K, Festa A, et al. Elevations in markers of liver injury and risk of type 2 diabetes: the insulin resistance atherosclerosis study. Diabetes 2004;53:2623–32.
37. Fishbein M, Mogren C, Gleason T, Stevens WR. Relationship of hepatic steatosis to adipose tissue distribution in pediatric nonalcoholic fatty liver disease. J Pediatr Gastroenterol Nutr 2006;42:83–8.
38. Ueki K, Kondo T, Tseng YH, Kahn CR. Central role of suppressors of cytokine signaling in hepatic steatosis, insulin resistance, and the metabolic syndrome in the mouse. Proc Nat Acad Sci U S A 2004;101:10422–7.
39. Ueki K, Kondo T, Kahn CR. Suppressor of cytokine signaling 1 (SOCS-1) and SOCS-3 cause insulin resistance through inhibition of tyrosine phosphorylation of insulin receptor substrate proteins by discrete mechanisms. Mol Cell Biol 2004;24: 5434–6.
40. Crespo J, Cayon A, Fernandez-Gil P, et al. Gene expression of tumor necrosis factor alpha and TNF-receptors, p55 and p75, in nonalcoholic steatohepatitis patients. Hepatology 2001;34:1158–63.

41. Tschritter O, Fritsche A, Thamer C, et al. Plasma adiponectin concentrations predict insulin sensitivity of both glucose and lipid metabolism. Diabetes 2003;52:239–43.
42. Nemet D, Wang P, Funahashi T, et al. Adipocytokines, body composition, and fitness in children. Pediatr Res 2003;53:148–52.
43. Goldfine AB, Kahn CR. Adiponectin: linking the fat cell to insulin sensitivity. Lancet 2003;362:1431–2.
44. Xu A, Wang Y, Keshaw H, et al. The fat-derived hormone adiponectin alleviates alcoholic and nonalcoholic fatty liver diseases in mice. J Clin Invest 2003;112:91–100.
45. Bugianesi E, Pagotto U, Manini R, et al. Plasma adiponectin in nonalcoholic fatty liver is related to hepatic insulin resistance and hepatic fat content, not to liver disease severity. J Clin Endocrinol Metab 2005;90:3498–504.
46. Kaser S, Moschen A, Cayon A, et al. Adiponectin and its receptors in non-alcoholic steatohepatitis. Gut 2005;54:117–21.
47. Musso G, Gambino R, Biroli G, et al. Hypoadiponectinemia predicts the severity of hepatic fibrosis and pancreatic beta-cell dysfunction in nondiabetic nonobese patients with non-alcoholic steatohepatitis. Am J Gastroenterol 2005;100:2438–46.
48. Diamond FB, Cuthbertson D, Hanna S, Eichler D. Correlates of adiponectin and the leptin/adiponectin ratio in obese and non-obese children. J Pediatr Endocrinol Metab 2004;17:1069–75.
49. Weiss R, Dufour S, Groszmann A, et al. Low adiponectin levels in adolescent obesity: a marker of increased intramyocellular lipid accumulation. J Clin Endocrinol Metab 2003;88:2014–18.
50. Adams LA, Feldstein AE, Lindor KD, Angulo P. Nonalcoholic fatty liver disease among patients with hypothalamic and pituitary dysfunction. Hepatology 2004;39:909–14.
51. Evans HM, Shaikh MG, McKiernan PJ, et al. Acute fatty liver disease after suprasellar tumor resection. J Pediatr Gastroenterol Nutr 2004;39:288–91.
52. Jonas MM, Krawczuk LE, Kim HB, et al. Rapid recurrence of nonalcoholic fatty liver disease after transplantation in a child with hypopituitarism and hepatopulmonary syndrome. Liver Transpl 2005;11:108–10.
53. Nakajima K, Hashimoto E, Kaneda H, et al. Pediatric nonalcoholic steatohepatitis associated with hypopituitarism. J Gastroenterol 2005;40:312–15.
54. Yajima Y, Ohta K, Narui T, et al. Ultrasonographical diagnosis of fatty liver: significance of the liver-kidney contrast. Tohoku J Exp Med 1983;139:43–50.
55. Bydder GM, Chapman RWG, Harry D. Computed tomography attenuation values in fatty liver. Comput Tomograph 1981;5:33–8.
56. Jacobs JE, Birnbaum BA, Shapiro MA, et al. Diagnostic criteria for fatty infiltration of the liver on contrast-enhanced helical CT. Am J Roenterol 1998;171:659–64.
57. Kim MJ, Mitchell DG, Ito K, Kim PN. Hepatic MR imaging: comparison of 2D and 3D gradient echo techniques. Abdom Imaging 2001;26:269–76.
58. Rinella ME, McCarthy R, Thakrar K, et al. Dual-echo, chemical shift gradient-echo magnetic resonance imaging to quantify hepatic steatosis: implications for living liver donation. Liver Transpl 2003;9:851–6.
59. Wang Y, Li D, Haacke EM, Brown JJ. A three-point Dixon method for water and fat separation using 2D and 3D gradient-echo techniques. J Magn Reson Imaging 1998;8:703–10.
60. Fishbein MH, Gardner KG, Potter CJ, et al. Introduction of fast MR imaging in the assessment of hepatic steatosis. Magn Reson Imaging 1997;15:287–93.
61. Fishbein M, Smith M, Li BU. A rapid MRI technique for the assessment of hepatic steatosis in a subject with medium-chain acyl-coenzyme A dehydrogenase (MCAD) deficiency. J Pediatr Gastroenterol Nutr 1998;27:224–7.
62. Fishbein MH, Miner M, Mogren C, Chalekson J. The spectrum of fatty liver in obese children and the relationship of serum aminotransferases to severity of steatosis. J Pediatr Gastroenterol Nutr 2003;36:54–61.
63. Thomsen C, Becker U, Winkler K, et al. Quantification of liver fat using magnetic resonance spectroscopy. Magn Reson Imaging 1994;12:487–95.
64. Wong WF, Northrup SR, Herrick RC, et al. Quantitation of lipid in biological tissue by chemical shift magnetic resonance imaging. Magn Reson Med 1994;32:440–6.
65. Angulo P, Keach JC, Batts KP, Lindor KD. Independent predictors of liver fibrosis in patients with nonalcoholic steatohepatitis. Hepatology 1999;30:1356–62.
66. McCullough AJ. Update on nonalcoholic fatty liver disease. J Clin Gastroenterol 2002;34:255–62.
67. Brunt EM, Janney CG, Di Bisceglie AM, et al. Nonalcoholic steatohepatitis: a proposal for grading and staging the histological lesions. Am J Gastroenterol 1999;94:2467–74.
68. Brunt EM. Nonalcoholic steatohepatitis: definition and pathology. Semin Liver Dis 2001;21:3–16.
69. Kleiner DE, Brunt EM, Van Natta M, et al. Design and validation of a histological scoring system for nonalcoholic fatty liver disease. Hepatology 2005;41:1313–21.
70. Brunt EM, Tiniakos DG. Pathology of steatohepatitis. Best Pract Res Clin Gastroenterol 2002;16:691–707
71. Schwimmer JB, Behling C, Newbury R, et al. The histological features of pediatric nonalcoholic fatty liver disease (NAFLD). Hepatology 2002;36:412A.
72. Matteoni CA, Younossi ZM, Gramlich T, et al. Nonalcoholic fatty liver disease: a spectrum of clinical and pathological severity. Gastroenterology 1999;116:1413–19.
73. Suzuki D, Hashimoto E, Kaneda K,. Liver failure caused by nonalcoholic steatohepatitis in an obese young male. J Gastroenterol Hepatol 2005;20:327–9.
74. Schwimmer JB, Deutsch R, Behling C, Lavine JE. Fatty liver as a determinant of atherosclerosis. Hepatology 2005;42:610A.
75. Kinugasa A, Tsunamoto K, Furukawa N, et al. Fatty liver and its fibrous changes found in simple obesity of children. J Pediatr Gastroenterol Nutr 1984;3:408–14.
76. Willner IR, Waters B, Patil SR, et al. Ninety patients with nonalcoholic steatohepatitis: insulin resistance, familial tendency, and severity of disease. Am J Gastroenterol 2001;96:2957–61.
77. Molleston JP, White F, Teckman J, Fitzgerald JF. Obese children with steatohepatitis can develop cirrhosis in childhood. Am J Gastroenterol 2002;97:2460–2.
78. Cuandrado A, Orive A, Garcia-Suarez C. Non-alcoholic steatohepatitis (NASH) and hepatocellular carcinoma. Obes Surg 2005;15:442–6.
79. Schwimmer JB. Managing overweight in older children and adolescents. Pediatr Ann 2004;33:39–44.
80. Vajro P, Fontanella A, Perna C, et al. Persistent hyperaminotransferasemia resolving after weight reduction in obese children. J Pediatr 1994;125:239–41.

81. Obinata K, Maruyama T, Hayashi M, et al. Effect of taurine on the fatty liver of children with simple obesity. Adv Exp Med Biol 1996;403:607–13.
82. Lavine JE. Vitamin E treatment of nonalcoholic steatohepatitis in children: a pilot study. J Pediatr 2000;136:734–8.
83. Vajro P, Mandato C, Franzese A, et al. Vitamin E treatment in pediatric obesity-related liver disease: a randomized study. J Pediatr Gastroenterol Nutr 2004;38:48–55.
84. Vajro P, Franzese A, Valerio G, et al. Lack of efficacy of ursodeoxycholic acid for the treatment of liver abnormalities in obese children. J Pediatr 2000;136:739–43.
85. Jones KL, Arslanian S, Peterokova VA, et al. Effect of metformin in pediatric patients with type 2 diabetes: a randomized controlled trial. Diabetes Care 2002;25:89–94.
86. Lavine JE, Schwimmer JB. Pediatric initiatives within the Nonalcoholic Steatohepatitis–Clinical Research Network (NASH CRN). J Pediatr Gastroenterol Nutr 2003;37:220–1.

35

Peroxisomal Diseases

Paul A. Watkins, M.D., Ph.D., and Kathleen B. Schwarz, M.D.

PEROXISOMAL STRUCTURE AND FUNCTIONS

General Aspects of Peroxisomes

Peroxisomes have the distinction of being the last true organelle discovered. They were first identified in renal proximal tubule cells by a Swedish graduate student in 1954. Initially called *microbodies*, these organelles were studied intensively by de Duve and coworkers. Because they contained enzymes that both produced (e.g., amino acid and urate oxidases) and degraded (e.g., catalase) hydrogen peroxide, de Duve and Baudhuin [1] proposed the name *peroxisomes.* Microbodies found in some lower organisms and plants were named for the specialized functions that they carry out. For example, *glyoxysomes* of fungi and plants contain the five enzymes of the glyoxylate cycle and *glycosomes* house the enzymes of glycolysis in trypanosomes [2,3]. Peroxisomes have been found in essentially all plant and animal cells with the exception of mature erythrocytes, and they range in size from about 0.1 μm (microperoxisomes of intestine and brain) up to 1.0 μm (characteristic of hepatic and renal peroxisomes; range: 0.2–1.0 μm) [4] (Figure 35.1).

A single lipid bilayer comprises the peroxisomal membrane. The organelle's matrix is finely granular, but microcrystalline cores of urate oxidase are present in the hepatic peroxisomes of some species (e.g., rats). No cores are found in human peroxisomes because humans lack urate oxidase. Unlike chloroplasts and mitochondria, peroxisomes contain no DNA, although it has been speculated that all three organelles evolved from endosymbionts. Since discovery of peroxisomes, numerous membrane proteins and matrix enzymes have been identified. Much research on peroxisomes has been fueled by the identification of patients whose cells lack either normal-appearing organelles or one or more peroxisomal metabolic functions.

Biogenesis of Peroxisomes

It was initially thought that peroxisomes, like lysosomes, originated by budding from the endoplasmic reticulum. Based primarily on two observations – that nearly all peroxisomal proteins are nonglycosylated and that both peroxisomal matrix and membrane proteins are synthesized in the cytoplasm on free polyribosomes – Lazarow et al. [5,6] hypothesized that peroxisomes arose from fission of preexisting peroxisomes. In their model, which was accepted as correct for many years, newly synthesized proteins destined for peroxisomes are posttranslationally targeted to the organelle. Following the import of both membrane and matrix proteins, peroxisomes grow in size and ultimately divide. Although considerable data in support of this model accumulated, the origin of peroxisomal membrane lipids remained unknown. This enigma, along with several experimental observations on proteins now known to be required for peroxisomal membrane protein targeting, led to a reevaluation of the contribution of the endoplasmic reticulum to peroxisome biogenesis and to a new model for peroxisome maturation [7]. Experiments following newly synthesized proteins by real-time fluorescence microscopy strongly suggest that peroxisome biogenesis begins by insertion of the peroxisomal protein Pex3p into endoplasmic reticulum membranes, and concentration of this protein into foci that then bud off and ultimately develop into mature peroxisomes [8].

Two motifs that target matrix proteins to peroxisomes have been identified. Most matrix proteins are targeted by a tripeptide sequence referred to as peroxisome targeting signal 1 (PTS1) [9]. The originally described PTS1 sequence, located at the carboxy terminus of a protein, consisted of serine-lysine-leucine, but several conserved variants have subsequently been identified. A small number of peroxisomal enzymes enter the organelle via PTS2, a nine amino acid sequence near, but not at, the amino-terminus with consensus -(R/K)-X5-(Q/H)-L-, where "X" is any amino acid [10]. Some matrix proteins contain neither PTS1 nor PTS2, and it has been suggested that they enter the organelle either via an internal PTS, or by a "piggyback" mechanism in which they bind to a PTS1-containing protein and concomitantly enter the peroxisome [11,12]. Signals for targeting peroxisomal membrane proteins (mPTS) are less well defined. Unlike PTS1 and PTS2, no consensus sequences have been identified. Rather, the signal seems to involve a group of basic amino acids adjacent to a hydrophobic domain [13].

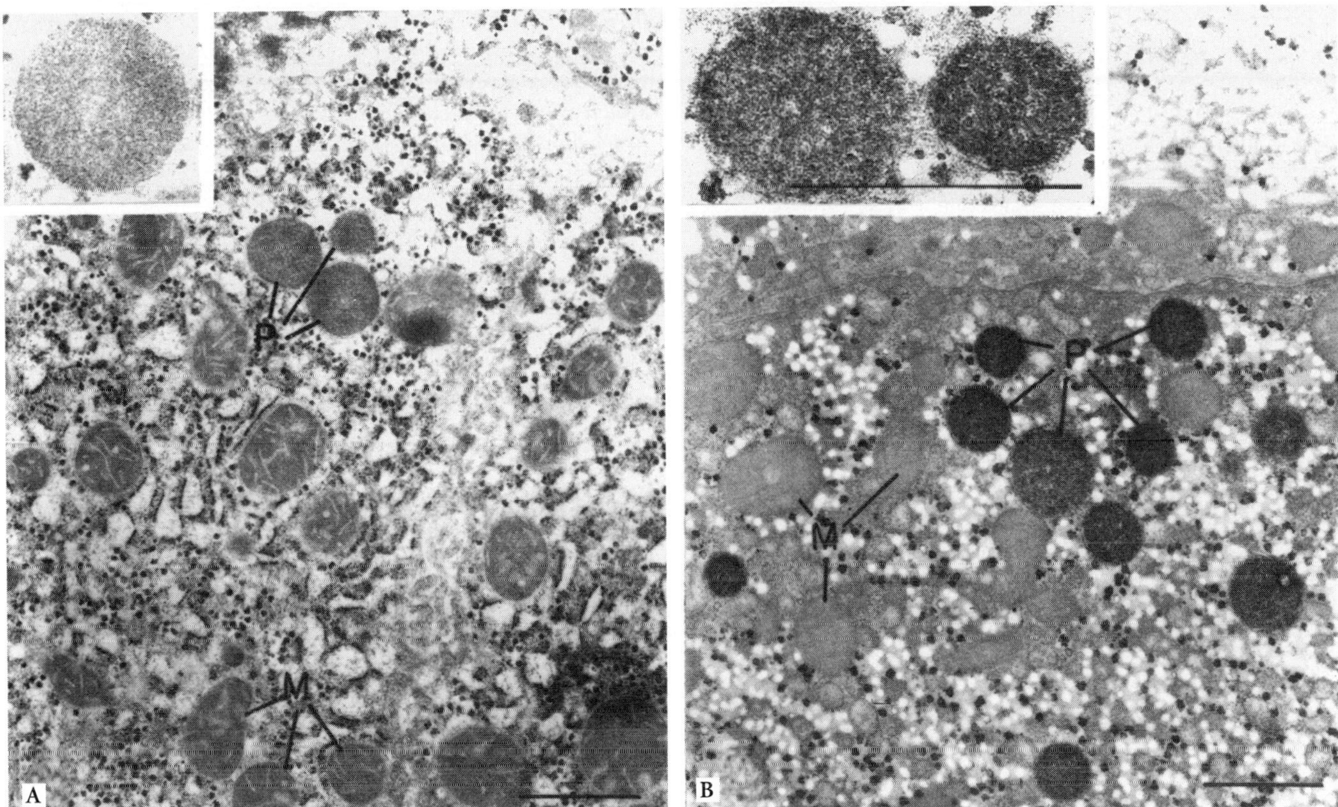

Figure 35.1. Human liver peroxisomes. Electron micrograph of normal human liver. (**A**) Peroxisomes (P) are readily distinguished from mitochondria (M) by their morphology. (**B**) Catalase cytochemistry revealing diaminobenzidine staining of peroxisomes. (Magnification ×16,000. Bar = 1 μm. Insets, magnification ×38,000.) (Lazarow PB, Black V, Shio H, et al. Zellweger syndrome: biochemical and morphological studies on two patients treated with clofibrate. Pediatr Res 1985;19:1356–64; used with permission.)

Patients whose cells lack morphologically normal peroxisomal structures have a *disorder of peroxisome biogenesis.* Skin fibroblasts from such patients may completely lack peroxisomes. More commonly, however, they have vesicular structures containing some peroxisomal membrane proteins. These cells either lack all matrix enzymes (peroxisomal "ghosts") or exhibit poor import of some matrix enzymes [14]. Complementation analysis, in which fibroblasts from two patients are chemically fused using polyethylene glycol before biochemical or morphologic analysis, revealed that multiple gene products are necessary for the normal assembly of functional peroxisomes. Currently, thirteen complementation groups of peroxisomal assembly defect patients are known [15,16]. Investigation of both human and yeast cells with defects in peroxisome biogenesis have led to the identification of at least 26 proteins required for this process [13,15]. Termed *peroxins,* these proteins are the products of *PEX* genes. Twelve of the human peroxins have been identified, and mutations in at least 10 PEX genes (complementation groups) have been described in patients [16–31]. Although some of the peroxins are found in peroxisomal membranes, others are cytosolic. Among the latter are Pex5p, Pex7p, and Pex19p, receptors for PTS1, PTS2, and peroxisome membrane proteins, respectively. Other peroxins are thought to be docking factors, to be components of import channels, or to perform other functions such as receptor recycling.

Peroxisome Proliferation

Treatment of rats or mice with clofibrate or any of a number of related hypolipidemic compounds results in hepatomegaly and a significant increase in the number of hepatic peroxisomes [32,33]. Synthesis of several hepatic peroxisomal enzymes is induced, particularly those involved in peroxisomal fatty acid β-oxidation [34]. Several other xenobiotic compounds, for example, industrial phthalate ester plasticizers, herbicides, and organic solvents, have similar effects. Chemically induced peroxisome proliferation in rodents is also associated with a significantly increased incidence of hepatic neoplasia [35,36]. Concerns that patients taking hypolipidemic drugs may have increased risk of cancer prompted intense investigation into the mechanism of action of peroxisome proliferators. The effects of these compounds are mediated by *peroxisome proliferator activated receptors* (PPARs), which are members of the steroid hormone family of nuclear receptors [37,38]. At least three isoforms of PPARs are known: PPARα, PPARδ (also called PPARβ or NUC1), and PPARγ. Although tissue expression pattern for these isoforms differ, all three are found in liver [39]. When activated by ligand binding, PPARs heterodimerize with the retinoid X receptor (RXR) and bind to *cis*-acting peroxisome proliferator response elements (PPREs) to enhance gene transcription [40–42].

The mechanism of peroxisome proliferator–induced carcinogenesis is not thought to be due to mutagenic or genotoxic properties of proliferators or their metabolites [43]. Rather, the sustained induction of peroxisomal oxidases and the resulting increased generation of intracellular hydrogen peroxide may be responsible for initiation of neoplastic transformation. Interestingly, the induction of peroxisome proliferation and enzyme induction appears to be species-specific [44]. Chronic administration of hypolipidemic agents to humans and nonhuman primates does not cause peroxisome proliferation. Furthermore, there is no evidence linking long-term treatment of patients with lipid-lowering drugs to increased incidence of hepatic tumors [45,46].

Peroxisomal Metabolic Pathways

Once considered a vestigial organelle, peroxisomes are now known to carry out a significant number of vital catabolic and anabolic processes. Many of these pathways involve lipid metabolism, but the spectrum of peroxisomal metabolic function is diverse, including amino acid, purine, and polyamine metabolism. Degradation of very long-chain fatty acids (VLCFA) and branched-chain fatty acids, synthesis of ether-linked phospholipids, bile acids, docosahexaenoic acid, and isoprenoid compounds are among the pathways of peroxisomal lipid metabolism.

Peroxisomal β-Oxidation

Degradation of dietary and stored fatty acids for energy production in humans and other higher organisms takes place in mitochondria. In lower organisms such as yeast, the oxidation of fatty acids is confined to peroxisomes. The recognition that mammalian peroxisomes also contain the enzymatic machinery for fatty acid β-oxidation came to light in 1976 [47]. Three peroxisomal enzymes catalyzing the four reactions required to chain-shorten fatty acids were subsequently found in and purified from rat liver by Hashimoto [48] (Figure 35.2).

The process by which fatty acids enter peroxisomes is not well characterized. Unlike the situation in mitochondria, carnitine is not known to be involved in this process. Peroxisomal membranes contain four members (ABCD1–4) of the ATP-binding cassette family of transmembrane proteins thought to be involved in membrane transport [49]. It has been proposed that ABCD1 functions to transport VLCFA, their CoA thioesters, or the enzyme very long-chain acyl-CoA synthetase into peroxisomes, but this remains unproved. Following an initial activation by thioesterification to coenzyme A (CoA) [50,51], saturated, unbranched fatty acids are degraded by the sequential action of three peroxisomal enzymes: acyl-CoA oxidase [52], L-bifunctional protein (LBP; also known as multifunctional enzyme 1 or MFE1) [53], and 3-ketoacyl-CoA thiolase [54], yielding acetyl-CoA and an acyl-CoA shortened by two carbons [48]. Although the enzymatic reactions are similar, there are distinct differences between the mitochondrial and peroxisomal pathways. The first mitochondrial reaction is catalyzed by a flavin adenine dinucleotide (FAD)-containing dehydrogenase that donates its electrons to the respiratory chain. In contrast, peroxisomal acyl-CoA oxidase (also an FAD enzyme) is coupled to the production of H_2O_2 from molecular oxygen. Peroxisomal LBP contains both enoyl-CoA hydratase and hydroxyacyl-CoA dehydrogenase activities. In mitochondria, these reactions are catalyzed by separate enzymes. Enoyl-CoA isomerase activity has also been attributed to LBP [55]. Distinct mitochondrial and peroxisomal enzymes catalyze the thiolytic cleavage of 3-ketoacyl-CoAs.

The relative contribution of mitochondria to the oxidation of common long-chain fatty acids (LCFA) such as palmitic and oleic acids is considerably greater than that of peroxisomes, commensurate with coupling to energy production and ketogenesis in mitochondria. However, certain fatty acids such as VLCFA, containing 22 carbons) are catabolized only in peroxisomes [56]. Dicarboxylic fatty acids, leukotrienes and other prostanoids, and certain polyunsaturated fatty acids are also degraded by this pathway.

Subsequent investigation revealed the existence of additional isoforms of peroxisomal β-oxidation enzymes and refinement of the pathways. The originally described enzymes were incapable of degrading 2-methyl-branched-chain fatty acids such as pristanic acid, the product of peroxisomal α-oxidation of phytanic acid (discussed subsequently). This led to the discovery of branched-chain acyl-CoA oxidase [57], D-bifunctional protein (DBP; also called multifunctional enzyme 2 or MFE2) [58], and the thiolase domain of sterol carrier protein X (SCPX) [59,60]. Human branched-chain acyl-CoA oxidase acts on both 2-methylacyl-CoAs and on intermediates in bile acid synthesis (discussed subsequently) [57]. Rats, on the other hand, have separate branched-chain and bile acid oxidases. The reaction is similar to that catalyzed by acyl-CoA oxidase. Like LBP, DPB contains both enoyl-CoA hydratase and hydroxyacyl-CoA dehydrogenase activities, but with different stereospecificity [61]. Interestingly, genetic deficiency of DBP in humans resulted in decreased oxidation rates of both pristanic acid and VLCFA, raising questions about the physiologic role of LBP [62,63]. SCPX is a 58-kDa protein with a carboxy-terminal 14 kDa identical to that of sterol carrier protein 2 (SCP2) and with an amino-terminal 44 kDa having thiolase activity. SCPX thiolase prefers 3-ketoacyl-CoA derivatives of branched-chain acids as substrates but will also weakly cleave the corresponding unbranched compounds [59]. In contrast, the originally described peroxisomal thiolase will not degrade branched-chain intermediates. SCP2, originally thought to be involved in cholesterol movement in cells, may function in peroxisomes as an acyl-CoA binding protein [64]. Interestingly, the carboxy terminal portion of DBP has a high degree of homology to SCP2 [65].

Additional peroxisomal enzymes required for fatty acid β-oxidation include acyl-CoA synthetases for activating LCFA and VLCFA, carnitine acetyl- and octanoyltransferases,

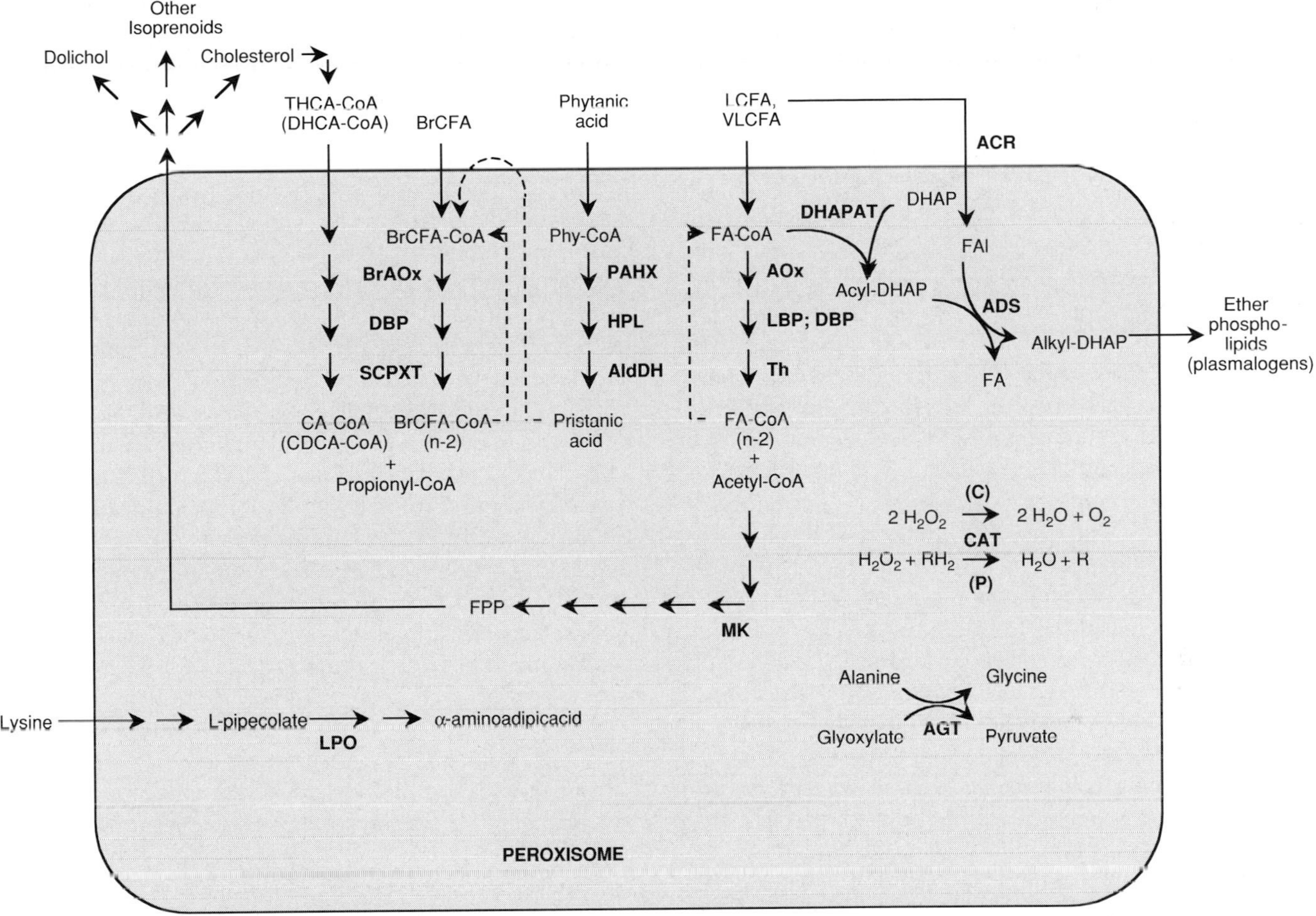

Figure 35.2. Overview of peroxisomal metabolic pathways. Peroxisomal pathways for the β-oxidation of straight-chain and branched-chain fatty acids, the α-oxidation of phytanic acid, bile acid synthesis, ether phospholipid (plasmalogen) synthesis, cholesterol synthesis, pipecolic acid metabolism, glyoxylate detoxification, and hydrogen peroxide detoxification are outlined. Enzymes necessary for β-oxidation of the CoA derivatives (FA-CoA) of long-chain fatty acids (LCFA) and very long-chain fatty acids (VLCFA) include acyl-CoA oxidase (AOx), L- or D-bifunctional protein (LBP; DBP), and 3-ketoacyl-CoA thiolase (Th). The CoA derivatives of branched-chain fatty acids (BrCFA) undergo β-oxidation by a separate but related group of enzymes that includes branched-chain acyl-CoA oxidase (BrAOx), DBP, and the thiolase domain of sterol carrier protein X (SCPXT). These enzymes also convert the CoA thioesters of the bile acid precursors tri- and dihydroxycholestanoic acids (THCA-CoA and DHCA-CoA) into the CoA derivatives of cholic acid (CA-CoA) and chenodeoxycholic acid (CDCA-CoA), respectively. The CoA derivative (Phy-CoA) of phytanic acid is converted to pristanic acid by the α-oxidation pathway, which includes the enzymes phytanoyl-CoA α-hydroxylase (PAHX), hydroxyphytanoyl-CoA lyase (HPL), and an aldehyde dehydrogenase (AldDH). Pristanic acid is further metabolized by the branched-chain β-oxidation pathway. Synthesis of ether phospholipids, including plasmalogens, requires two peroxisomal matrix enzymes: dihydroxyacetone phosphate (DHAP) acyltransferase (DHAPAT) and alkyl-DHAP synthase (ADS). The former catalyzes the acylation of DHAP and the latter the displacement of the fatty acid by a fatty alcohol (FAl). Acyl-CoA reductase (ACR) on the peroxisomal membrane is involved in FAl production. Several enzymes involved in the cholesterol biosynthetic pathway between acetyl-CoA and farnesyl-pyrophosphate (FPP) are peroxisomal, including mevalonate kinase (MK). The peroxisomal enzyme L-pipecolic acid oxidase (LPO) degrades L-pipecolic acid, an intermediate in lysine catabolism. Glyoxylate produced by peroxisomal oxidases is detoxified by the alanine:glyoxylate aminotransferase (AGT) reaction. Hydrogen peroxide generated by the numerous peroxisomal oxidases is detoxified by either the catalatic (C) or peroxidatic (P) activity of catalase (CAT). Peroxisomal enzymes for the activation (acyl-CoA synthetases) and transport of fatty acids are not shown.

α-methylacyl-CoA racemase (discussed subsequently), 2,3-dienoyl-CoA reductase, $\Delta^{3,5}$, $\Delta^{2,4}$-dienoyl-CoA isomerase, and the adrenoleukodystrophy protein (ALDP) [66].

Human diseases result from impaired peroxisomal fatty acid β-oxidation. Patients with disorders of peroxisome biogenesis have defective β-oxidation of both VLCFA and branched-chain fatty acids [56,67]. Other peroxisomal metabolic processes are affected as well. In these disorders, the absence of normal peroxisomes results in mistargeting or cytoplasmic degradation of β-oxidation enzymes. Most of these enzymes contain PTS1; however, peroxisomal thiolase is one of the few known PTS2-containing proteins [68]. Impaired β-oxidation of VLCFA is also found in patients with deficiency of either acyl-CoA oxidase [69] or DBP [70,71] and in X-linked adrenoleukodystrophy patients [72]. Branched-chain fatty acid metabolism and bile acid synthesis (discussed subsequently) are normal in acyl-CoA oxidase deficiency [73]. Patients with DBP deficiency have decreased ability to degrade 2-methyl-branched-chain fatty acids and impaired bile acid synthesis [73,74]. However, it is not clear why these patients could not break down VLCFA normally because they were initially thought to suffer from LBP deficiency [71]. Only one patient had been reported to have deficiency of the peroxisomal thiolase [75], but subsequent analysis revealed that this patient had a mutation in DBP, and not thiolase [76]. Documented deficiencies of LBP, branched-chain acyl-CoA oxidase, and SCPX thiolase have not been reported. In X-linked adrenoleukodystrophy, defects in the peroxisomal membrane protein ALDP, the product of the ABCD1 gene, result in decreased rates of VLCFA degradation by an as yet unknown mechanism [77].

Because peroxisomes lack electron transport coupled to ATP synthesis, fatty acid oxidation in this organelle must serve another purpose. In some cases, the catabolic β-oxidation pathways participate in biosynthesis processes. This is clearly the case for bile acid synthesis from cholesterol, discussed later. More recently, a requirement for peroxisomal β-oxidation in the normal synthesis of docosahexaenoic acid (DHA; C22:6ω3) has been demonstrated [78]. The precursor of DHA, eicosapentaenoic acid (EPA; C20:5ω3), undergoes two cycles of fatty acid elongation, forming C24:5ω3, followed by desaturation to yield C24:6ω3. The latter compound is then chain-shortened by one cycle of peroxisomal β-oxidation, yielding DHA. In other cases, it appears that a function of peroxisomal β-oxidation and α-oxidation (below) is degradation of compounds that are toxic when present in excess. Phytanic acid, VLCFA, and many xenobiotics fall into this category.

Peroxisomal α-Oxidation

Fatty acids with 3-methyl branches cannot be degraded by β-oxidation. Phytanic acid (3,7,11,15-tetramethylhexadecanoic acid), derived from the phytol side chain of chlorophyll, is the most significant 3-methyl-branched fatty acid in the human diet. Phytanic acid is not synthesized by humans but rather is ingested in the diet primarily in the form of ruminant meats and fats (e.g., dairy products) [79,80]. Identification of this fatty acid as the compound that accumulated in plasma and tissues of patients with Refsum disease [81], which typically presents as an adult-onset neuropathy without significant liver disease, led to the discovery of the α-oxidation pathway. After more than 3 decades of research, the details of this pathway have recently been clarified. As shown schematically in Figure 35.2, phytanic acid is activated to its CoA thioester [82] and then hydroxylated on the 2-carbon in an oxygen-requiring dioxygenase reaction catalyzed by phytanoyl-CoA α-hydroxylase [83]. Hydroxyphytanoyl-CoA lyase then catalyzes the cleavage of α-hydroxyphytanoyl-CoA to pristanal, a branched-chain fatty aldehyde, and the one-carbon metabolite formyl-CoA [84]. The latter compound rapidly degrades to formate and CoA at neutral pH. Pristanal is then oxidized to pristanic acid (2,6,10,14—tetramethylpentadecanoic acid) [85]. Pristanic acid must then be converted to its CoA derivative before subsequent metabolism, and it has been suggested that this reaction is catalyzed by peroxisomal very long-chain acyl-CoA synthetase 1 (ACSVL1) [86]. The net result of α-oxidation is the decarboxylation of phytanic acid with shift of the position of the methyl group by one carbon, allowing further degradation of pristanoyl-CoA by peroxisomal β-oxidation.

Phytanoyl-CoA α-hydroxylase, like thiolase, is a PTS2-containing protein [87]. Recently, it was found that hydroxyphytanoyl-CoA lyase contains PTS1 [88]. Because these matrix proteins are not targeted properly in disorders of peroxisome biogenesis, elevated plasma levels of phytanic acid and defective phytanic acid oxidation are observed. However, because phytanic acid is solely of dietary origin, plasma levels and total body burden in a given patient reflect both the patient's age and choice of food. In some children with defective peroxisome biogenesis, abnormal phytanic acid metabolism was the initial observation, prompting the name infantile Refsum disease (IRD) [89]. As discussed later, patients with peroxisome biogenesis disorders have multiple peroxisomal metabolic defects. The designation IRD is now used descriptively for those peroxisome biogenesis disorder patients with the longest survival.

Bile Acid Synthesis

Bile acids are synthesized in the liver from cholesterol. This process requires shortening of the acyl side-chain of the sterol and was found to take place in peroxisomes [90]. Hydroxylases and dehydrogenases located in the endoplasmic reticulum convert cholesterol into trihydroxycholestanoic acid (THCA) and dihydroxycholestanoic acid (DHCA). The side chains of THCA and DHCA resemble 2-methyl-branched-chain fatty acids and undergo a single cycle of β-oxidation to produce the primary bile acids cholic acid (CA) and chenodeoxycholic acid (CDCA), respectively. Activation of THCA and DHCA to their CoA derivatives is thought to occur mainly in the endoplasmic reticulum [91]. The mechanism for entry of these activated bile acid precursors into peroxisomes is unknown. Both THCA-CoA and DHCA-CoA are converted to the correct stereoisomers via peroxisomal methylacyl-CoA racemase (discussed later) [92] before being acted on by the D-specific branched-chain β-oxidation machinery.

As for many other peroxisomal metabolic processes, it was the observation of bile acid abnormalities in patients with peroxisome biogenesis disorders that helped elucidate the complete bile acid biosynthetic pathway. Abnormal bile acid profiles are also found in DBP deficiency [74].

α-Methylacyl-CoA Racemase

Stereoisomers of certain substrates and intermediates in the pathways of branched-chain fatty acid degradation and bile acid synthesis are found in nature. These include phytanic acid, pristanic acid, bile acid precursors, and other intermediates that contain asymmetric carbon centers. The α-oxidation of phytanic acid produces both 2*R*- and 2*S*-stereoisomers of pristanic acid; however, the branched-chain acyl-CoA oxidase can only use 2*S*-isomers as substrates [93]. These two stereoisomers of pristanic acid can be interconverted by α-methylacyl-CoA racemase, an enzyme found in both peroxisomes and mitochondria [94]. The methyl groups on carbons 6 and 10 of pristanic acid are also in the *R*-configuration and thus require α-methylacyl-CoA racemase because this fatty acid is progressively shortened via several cycles of β-oxidation.

The bile acid precursors THCA and DHCA are also normally found as both *R*- and *S*- stereoisomers. Because the carbon numbering system differs between fatty acids and sterols, it is carbon 25 in the bile acid precursors that is alpha to the carboxyl carbon in the side chain. Similar to the situation that exists with pristanic acid, only the 25*S*- stereoisomers of THCA or DHCA are substrates for branched-chain acyl-CoA oxidase and can thus be converted into mature bile acids. α-Methylacyl-CoA racemase converts 25*R*- to 25*S*, thus facilitating utilization of the *R*-isomers.

Ether Lipid Biosynthesis

Phospholipids containing an ether-linked alkyl or alkenyl chain on the first carbon of glycerol instead of an ester-linked acyl group account for about 18% of membrane phospholipids [95]. The latter (alkenyl-containing) ether lipids are also known as *plasmalogens*. Peroxisomes contain three enzymes vital to ether lipid synthesis: acyl-CoA reductase [96], dihydroxyacetone phosphate (DHAP) acyltransferase (DHAPAT) [97], and alkyl-DHAP synthase [98] (Figure 35.2). Similar to the situation for bile acid synthesis, enzymes found in the endoplasmic reticulum are also required for complete synthesis of plasmalogens. The importance of ether phospholipids is illustrated by the severity of clinical symptoms in rhizomelic chondrodysplasia punctata (RCDP). Children with RCDP have profoundly disturbed ether lipid synthesis, shortening of proximal limbs, severely disturbed endochondral bone formation and profound mental retardation [99]. RCDP is caused by defects in Pex7p, the PTS2 receptor [20–22]. Although DHAPAT is targeted to peroxisomes by PTS1 [100,101], alkyl-DHAP synthase is a PTS2-containing protein [102]. As noted earlier, phytanoyl-CoA α-hydroxylase is a PTS2 protein; thus, phytanic acid oxidation is also defective in RCDP. However, deficiency of DHAPAT alone or alkyl-DHAP synthase alone results in the RCDP clinical phenotype [101,103], indicating that ether lipids are required for normal membrane function. Because peroxisomal matrix protein import is defective in the disorders of peroxisome biogenesis, ether phospholipid synthesis is impaired in these patients.

Cholesterol and Isoprenoid Biosynthesis

One of the first indications that peroxisomes play a role in isoprenoid synthesis came from immunoelectron micrographs showing that 3-hydroxy-3-methyl glutaryl-CoA reductase was present in the organelle [104]. Subsequent studies suggested that peroxisomes are involved in cholesterol [105,106] and dolichol synthesis [107]. Several enzymes in the cholesterol biosynthetic pathway between acetyl-CoA and farnesyl pyrophosphate have now been detected in peroxisomes [108–111] (Figure 35.2). Recently, studies in human skin fibroblasts from patients with peroxisome biogenesis disorders have raised questions regarding the significance of these observations [112]. Although the overall contribution of peroxisomes to cholesterol synthesis is not known with certainty, some patients with peroxisome biogenesis disorders were found to have decreased plasma cholesterol [113]. Deficiency of the peroxisomal enzyme mevalonate kinase [110] results in mevalonic aciduria [114].

Peroxisomal Amino Acid Metabolism

Peroxisomes contain several important enzymes of amino acid metabolism, particularly alanine–gyloxylate transaminase (AGT) and L-pipecolate oxidase. AGT is found only in the liver and catalyzes the transfer of the α-amino group of alanine to glyoxylate, yielding glycine and pyruvate as products [115] (Figure 35.2). This peroxisomal enzyme is quantitatively important for degrading glyoxylate produced by two other peroxisomal enzymes – glycolate oxidase and D-amino acid oxidase [116]. These two enzymes, which convert glycolate and glycine, respectively, to glyoxylate, are typical flavin-linked peroxisomal oxidases that utilize molecular oxygen and produce H_2O_2. If not efficiently detoxified by the AGT reaction, glyoxylate is further metabolized by glycolate oxidase to oxalate. AGT is deficient in primary hyperoxaluria type I (PH1), in which accumulation of oxalate leads to the formation of calcium oxalate kidney stones and renal failure [117]. The disease is often fatal unless liver or liver–kidney transplantation is performed. AGT is targeted to peroxisomes via PTS1 [118]. Interestingly, a common polymorphism near the amino terminus of AGT unmasks a weak mitochondrial targeting signal [119]. In some patients with PH1, polymorphisms combined with additional mutations mistarget AGT to mitochondria, thus blocking the enzyme's ability to detoxify glyoxylate.

L-Pipecolic acid is synthesized in humans as an intermediate in the minor pathway of lysine catabolism [120]. The peroxisomal enzyme L-pipecolic acid oxidase is required for conversion of the imino acid pipecolic acid to Δ^1-piperideine-6-carboxylic acid [121]. The latter compound is converted to α-aminoadipic acid and ultimately to glutaric acid. Like other peroxisomal oxidases, L-pipecolic acid oxidase requires FAD and produces H_2O_2. The enzyme is targeted to peroxisomes by PTS1 [122]. Therefore, accumulation of L-pipecolic acid (hyperpipecolic acidemia; HPA) occurs in peroxisome biogenesis disorders. Most patients previously diagnosed with HPA were subsequently found to have multiple peroxisomal biochemical abnormalities. Because of this, isolated HPA was not thought to occur. Recently, however, Kerckaert et al. [123] described three children with HPA but without other peroxisomal dysfunction. No liver findings were noted in these patients. Mild elevations in plasma pipecolic acid are sometimes seen in DBP deficiency and Refsum disease (A.B. Moser, personal communication). In addition, pipecolic acid levels are elevated in the mitochondrial disorder glutaric acidemia type 2 [124]. Only about 1% of lysine is degraded via pipecolic acid in the liver [125]. A significantly greater proportion of lysine may be catabolized by this pathway in the brain, and neurotoxicity of L-pipecolate has been suggested as contributing to the neurologic problems in peroxisomal diseases [126].

Catalase

The most abundant enzyme in peroxisomes – and one of the most abundant proteins in liver – is catalase [1]. This enzyme plays a vital role in peroxisomal metabolism by decomposing H_2O_2 generated by peroxisomal oxidases. The catalase reaction proceeds via two mechanisms: a catalatic process in which H_2O_2 is degraded to water and oxygen and a peroxidatic process in which a cosubstrate is oxidized by H_2O_2 [127] (Figure 35.2). Unlike many peroxisomal enzymes, catalase remains active in the cytosol in the absence of normal peroxisomes. Assessing whether catalase is contained within organelles or free in the cytoplasm is useful for diagnosis of peroxisomal diseases [128,129]. Individuals who lack catalase (acatalasemia) are known but are either asymptomatic or have ulcerating oral lesions that are often gangrenous.

BIOCHEMICAL ABNORMALITIES IN PEROXISOMAL DISORDERS WITH LIVER INVOLVEMENT

Biochemical Assays of Peroxisomal Metabolism

Several assays have been developed to facilitate diagnosis of peroxisomal diseases. Plasma assays include quantitation of VLCFAs, phytanic acid, L-pipecolate, and bile acid intermediates by gas chromatography or gas chromatography–mass spectrometry. Urinary pipecolate and oxalate can be measured. Ether lipids (plasmalogens) in erythrocyte membranes can be quantitated. A skin biopsy and culture of fibroblasts are useful for metabolic studies. The cellular oxidation of radiolabeled phytanic acid, VLCFAs, and pristanic acid uses the α-oxidation pathway and also both β-oxidation pathways. Ether lipid synthesis can be measured in fibroblasts as well. More specialized assays such as the subcellular distribution of catalase in fibroblasts, immunofluorescence analysis for peroxisomal proteins and enzymes, and capacity to metabolize the bile acid intermediate varanyl-CoA have also facilitated diagnosis.

Wanders and Waterham [130] pointed out that the three biochemical functions that are most useful in the laboratory diagnosis of peroxisomal diseases are β-oxidation of fatty acids (e.g., VLCFA), biosynthesis of plasmalogens, and α-oxidation of phytanic acid. Initial screening tests that address the first two of these functions and that are capable of detecting a majority of patients with peroxisomal diseases include measurement of plasma VLCFA levels and erythrocyte membrane plasmalogen levels. Peduto et al. [131] also emphasized that elevations in plasma L-pipecolate levels, which are frequently measured in general metabolic screens, can raise suspicion of a peroxisomal disorder. Although the urinary bile acid profile is characteristic in both the peroxisome biogenesis disorders and DBP deficiency [132], this assay is not as widely available as other diagnostic tests.

Disorders of Peroxisome Biogenesis

Infants and children with Zellweger syndrome, neonatal-onset adrenoleukodystrophy, and infantile Refsum disease comprise the majority of patients with disorders of peroxisome biogenesis. In these disorders, hepatic peroxisomes are generally absent or at least markedly decreased in number. Also known as generalized peroxisomal disorders, these inborn errors of metabolism result from a deficiency of one of the PEX genes. Failure of peroxisomes to form normally results in a spectrum of biochemical abnormalities that reflect the various pathways present in the organelle (Table 35.1). Plasma VLCFA levels are elevated and fibroblast VLCFA oxidation is decreased [56,133]. Plasma and urine pipecolate levels are elevated [134]. Fibroblasts oxidize phytanic acid at a decreased rate and, depending on the age and diet of the patient, plasma phytanic acid levels can be elevated [135]. Erythrocyte membrane plasmalogens are decreased and fibroblast ether lipid synthesis is defective [136,137]. High plasma levels of the bile acid precursors DHCA and THCA are present [138]. Catalase is free in the cytoplasm of fibroblasts [139].

Although all of these biochemical defects are typically found in patients with PEX gene mutations, an exception is PEX7 deficiency [20–22]. This gene encodes the PTS2 receptor, and both the clinical phenotype (RCDP) and the biochemical abnormalities differ from the other disorders of peroxisome biogenesis. Impaired ether lipid synthesis and a decreased phytanic acid oxidation rate are the primary biochemical abnormalities [140].

Deficiencies of Individual Peroxisomal Enzymes

Clinically, distinction between patients with isolated deficiency of acyl-CoA oxidase or DBP and those with peroxisome biogenesis disorders is difficult. Biochemical analyses can facilitate a correct diagnosis. All of these patients have increased plasma VLCFA levels [73,141]. Patients with DBP deficiency also have impaired branched-chain fatty acid metabolism and often accumulate bile acid precursors, whereas those with acyl-CoA oxidase deficiency have normal branched-chain and bile acid metabolism [73,74,142]. Unlike in the peroxisome biogenesis diseases, plasmalogens are normal in these conditions and hepatic peroxisomes are present. However, in both acyl-CoA oxidase and DBP deficiencies, hepatic peroxisomes are both decreased in number and are larger than normal [143].

The diagnostic hallmarks of primary hyperoxaluria type I (AGT deficiency) include elevated oxalate and glycolate in urine and, occasionally, the presence of calcium oxalate crystals in liver [117]. The finding of at least a 50% decrease in AGT activity in a liver biopsy confirms the diagnosis. Interestingly, excretion of oxalate and glycolate is not usually elevated in the peroxisome biogenesis disorders.

Large amounts of mevalonic acid are excreted by patients with mevalonic aciduria (mevalonate kinase deficiency) [114]. Although decreased plasma cholesterol levels have been

Table 35.1: Biochemical Defects in Peroxisomal Disorders

	ZS/NALD/IRD	*AOx*	*DBP*	*RCDP*	*PH1*	*MK*
Plasma						
VLCFA	↑	↑	↑	N	N	N
Phytanic acid	N-↑	N	↑	↑	N	N
Pristanic acid	N-↑	N	↑	N	N	N
Bile acid precursors	↑	N	N-↑	N	N	N
Pipecolate	↑	N	N	N	N	N
Cholesterol	N-↓	N	N	N	N	N-↓
Urine						
Pipecolate	↑	N	N	N	N	N
Oxalate	N	N	N	N	↑	N
Erythrocyte membrane						
Plasmalogens	↓	N	N	↓	N	N
Fibroblast						
VLCFA β-oxidation	↓	↓	↓	N	N	N
Pristanic β-oxidation	↓	N	↓	N	N	N
Phytanic α-oxidation	↓	N	N-↓	↓	N	N
Ether lipid synthesis	↓	N	N	↓	N	N
Catalase distribution	C	P	P	P	P	P

ZS, Zellweger syndrome; NALD, neonatal adrenoleukodystrophy; IRD, infantile Refsum disease; AOx, acyl-CoA oxidase deficiency; DBP, D-bifunctional enzyme deficiency; RCDP, rhizomelic chondrodysplasia punctata; PH1, primary hyperoxaluria type 1; MK, mevalonate kinase deficiency; VLCFA, very long-chain fatty acids; N, normal; C, cytoplasmic catalase; P, peroxisomal catalase.

reported in patients with peroxisome biogenesis disorders, normal to slightly depressed levels are usually found in mevalonic aciduria [144].

Patients with elevated urine or plasma levels of pipecolic acid will generally have additional biochemical defects typical of peroxisome biogenesis disorders. However, a small number of patients with isolated hyperpipecolic acidemia have been described [123]. These patients had no overt liver disease, in contrast to the patients with biogenesis defects.

Three of the four patients with documented α-methylacyl-CoA racemase deficiency presented with increased plasma levels of both pristanic acid and the bile acid intermediates THCA and DHCA [93]. The fourth patient had increased amounts of THCA metabolites in urine but normal plasma pristanic acid levels [145]. Because phytanic acid, and thus its α-oxidation product pristanic acid, are of dietary origin, absence of the latter compound in plasma would not rule out racemase deficiency, particularly in very young children.

CLINICAL MANIFESTATIONS OF PEROXISOMAL DISORDERS

With advances in molecular biology, the family of peroxisomal disorders has grown geometrically; the estimated cumulative incidence of these peroxisomal disorders is 1:25,000 [146]. All of the abnormalities described thus far have been autosomal recessive with the exception of X-linked adrenoleukodystrophy. Parental consanguinity is common. One of the problems in attempting to classify peroxisomal disorders is that clinical syndromes have been linked to mutations in a variety of

Table 35.2: Peroxisomal Disorders

Group 1 (biogenesis defects)
Zellweger syndrome*
Neonatal adrenoleukodystrophy*
Infantile Refsum disease*
Hyperpipecolic acidemia*(?)
Rhizomelic chondrodysplasia punctata Type 1
Group 2 (single enzyme/protein deficiencies)
D-Bifunctional protein deficiency*
Acyl-CoA oxidase deficiency*
Hyperoxaluria type I (alanine glyoxylate aminotransferase deficiency)*
Mevalonate kinase deficiency*
Hyperpipecolic acidemia (?) (L-pipecolate oxidase deficiency)
X-linked adrenoleukodystrophy
Rhizomelic chondrodysplasia punctata type 2 (DHAPAT-deficiency)
Rhizomelic chondrodysplasia punctata type 3 (alkyl-DHAP synthase deficiency)
Refsum disease (classic type) (phytanoyl-CoA hydroxylase deficiency)
Glutaric aciduria type 3 (glutaryl-CoA oxidase deficiency)

*Liver abnormalities

peroxisomal genes, and there is a limited correlation between genotype and phenotype.

Two types of classifications are generally used: disorders of peroxisomal biogenesis and disorders of single enzymes (Table 35.2). Those disorders in which some sort of hepatic involvement has been reported are marked with an asterisk in Table 35.2, and the various types of liver abnormalities characteristic of those disorders are listed in Table 35.3. A brief summary of each of the peroxisomal disorders for which hepatic disease has been described are presented here, as are discussions of putative mechanisms underlying the liver disease, an approach to making a biochemical diagnosis (Table 35.1), and a suggested algorithm for the hepatologist who might encounter a child with one of these disorders.

Group 1: Disorders of Peroxisome Biogenesis

Zellweger Syndrome

Zellweger syndrome (ZS) is a generalized peroxisomal biogenesis disorder and the phenotype is caused by mutations in any of several genes involved in peroxisome biogenesis: *PEX1, PEX2, PEX5, PEX6, PEX10, PEX12, PEX13, PEX16*, and *PEX19* [147,148]. ZS, neonatal adrenoleukodystrophy, and infantile Refsum disease constitute a spectrum of overlapping features the most severe of which is ZS and the least severe infantile Refsum disease.

Zellweger syndrome is characterized by craniofacial abnormalities (wide anterior fontanelle, prominent forehead, anteverted nostrils, low nasal bridge, epicanthal folds, flattened philtrum, and narrow upper lip, together with bilateral clinodactyly and talipes equinus varus). Severe neurologic abnormalities are characteristic, including hypotonia, areflexia, absent Moro response, mental retardation, and seizures. Polycystic kidneys, cryptorchidism, and clitoromegaly have been noted. Poor sucking is usually noted in the newborn period and persists, leading to severe failure to thrive. Skeletal radiographs demonstrate stippled epiphyses, and dislocated hips are common. Cerebral ventricles may be dilated, and cerebral atrophy with an abnormal gyral pattern is characteristic, as are neonatal seizures. The average age of death is 5 months (range 1 week–18 months in one series) [149].

All children with ZS have liver disease. In normal humans, fetal liver peroxisomes are present as early as the sixth week gestation [150], but in children with ZS, hepatic peroxisomes are absent as early as midgestation. Hepatic abnormalities include hepatomegaly (which may be slight and inconsistent or marked and persistent) and conjugated hyperbilirubinemia in early infancy, possibly caused by intrahepatic biliary dysgenesis [151]. Occasionally, jaundice can be transient. Late in the first year of life, firm hepatomegaly with splenomegaly suggestive of cirrhosis and portal hypertension has been reported [149]. Hepatic histology reveals excessive hepatic iron stores and a cholangiolar lesion characterized by tiny plugs of bile in the cholangioles, particularly in the periportal area [152]. Electron microscopy of liver reveals absent peroxisomes and, occasionally, mitochondrial abnormalities. Angulated secondary lysosomes may be present in Kupffer cells and hepatocytes. Renal peroxisomes are also absent.

Mathis et al. [153] demonstrated that oxidation of the cholesterol side chain to form C-24 bile acids is impaired in ZS and that increased amounts of the C-27 bile acid intermediates (trihydroxycholestanoic acid, varanic acid, and dihydroxycholestanoic acid) are present and may contribute to ongoing liver fibrosis. Setchell et al. [154] postulated that administration of primary bile acid would be beneficial to improve liver function by down-regulation in the synthesis of these abnormal acids. Accordingly, they administered cholic acid and chenodeoxycholic acid (100 mg/d) via the oral route to a 6-month-old male infant with ZS. Biochemical indices of liver function improved, as did the hepatic histology coincident with a significant decrease in serum and urinary cholestanoic acids.

Neonatal Adrenoleukodystrophy

Neonatal adrenoleukodystrophy is also a defect of peroxisomal biogenesis. The disorder is caused by mutations in the PTS1 receptor gene or in *PEX1, PEX 5, PEX6, PEX10, PEX12*, and *PEX13* genes [23,148]. About 25% of affected children have some dysmorphic features, deafness is characteristic, psychomotor delay is progressive, and hypotonia and seizures are

Table 35.3: Hepatic Abnormalities Characteristic of Certain Peroxisomal Disorders

	Hepatic Abnormality				
Disorder	*Hepatomegaly*	*Hepatitis*	*Jaundice*	*Stones*	*Fibrosis*
Zellweger syndrome	X		X		X
Neonatal adrenoleukodystrophy	X				
Infantile Refsum disease	X		X	X	
Hyperpipecolic acidemia	X				
Acyl Co-A oxidase deficiency		X			X
D-Bifunctional enzyme deficiency	X	X			X
Primary hyperoxaluria type 1	X				
Mevalonate kinase deficiency	X		X		

common. Electroencephalograms may show hypsarrhythmia. Cortical atrophy and micropolygyria may occur. The adrenals are small with atrophic cortices. Hepatic peroxisomes are absent or greatly diminished. Survival is longer than it is in ZS, with some children surviving into the second decade [149]. A few residual peroxisomes may be seen in the liver, and hepatomegaly is characteristic. In general the liver disease is mild. An 11-year-old child with mental retardation and sensorineural deafness has been described in whom chronic liver disease was considered his major clinical problem [149].

Infantile Refsum Disease

Infantile Refsum disease, also a disorder of peroxisomal biogenesis, is caused by mutations in the *PEX1* and *PEX12* genes [17,148]. The syndrome is characterized clinically by dysmorphic features in approximately 25% of patients, including large anterior fontanelle, failure to thrive, feeding problems, and poor vision. Craniofacial abnormalities are more mild than those in ZS and may not be noted until later in the first year of life. Reported abnormalities include round facies, flat occiput, high forehead, frontal bossing, epicanthal folds, telecanthus, depressed nasal bridge, small mouth, protruding tongue, low-set ears, and short neck. Hypotonia is present occasionally although not as marked as in ZS, and peripheral reflexes are preserved. There is progressive psychomotor delay. Sensorineural deafness (100%) and rotary nystagmus have been reported along with pigmentary retinopathy (Leber congenital amaurosis). Genitourinary abnormalities reported include bilateral vesicopelvicalyceal dilation and vesicourethral reflux.

Hepatomegaly is often observed. Other hepatobiliary abnormalities include isolated neonatal cholestasis without other organ system involvement [155]. Cholelithiasis and mildly deranged liver function have been reported as early as 6 months of age [149]. Liver disease may progress and become clinically significant in children who survive the first decade. Hepatic peroxisomes are absent or deficient, and defects in bile acid metabolism are similar to those characteristic of ZS [156].

Hyperpipecolic Acidemia

The original cases described as hyperpipecolic acidemia were also probably disorders of peroxisomal biogenesis. Kelley [113] suggested that several genetic defects can lead to hyperpipecolatemia and that ZS is only one of these. Moser et al. [133] indicated that most patients with hyperpipecolatemia are part of the Zellweger–Infantile Refsum continuum. Approximately 75% of the children have dysmorphic features, most have sensorineural deafness, psychomotor delay is progressive, hypotonia occasionally occurs, and seizures are common. Most patients have hepatomegaly [157,158].

More recently, Kerckaert et al. [123] demonstrated that a deficiency of L-pipecolate oxidase leads to isolated hyperpipecolic acidemia. These authors postulated that previously reported cases of hyperpipecolic acidemia were probably unrecognized examples of ZS before the discovery of the multiple peroxisomal defects characteristic of that syndrome. The patients with the defect presented with hypotonia and enlarged fontanelles, psychomotor retardation, facial dysmorphism, and aggression. Liver disease was not mentioned in the one report of patients with the isolated enzyme deficiency.

Group 2: Isolated Peroxisomal Enzyme Deficiencies

D-Bifunctional Protein Deficiency

Patients with this disorder lack DBP (also called multifunctional enzyme 2 or MFE2) [70]. D-bifunctional protein contains both D-3-hydroxyacyl-CoA dehydratase and D-3-hydroxyacyl-CoA dehydrogenase enzyme activities. Both peroxisomal β-oxidation and oxidation of bile acid precursors are abnormal [70]. Patients are hypotonic with mild craniofacial dysmorphism, multifocal tonic–clonic seizures, and calcific stippling of certain joints. Hepatomegaly and hepatic dysfunction have been reported [159]; one patient in our institution also has liver fibrosis (G.V. Raymond, personal communication). However, the liver disease is milder than that observed in ZS [70].

Acyl-CoA Oxidase Deficiency

Patients with this disorder clinically resemble patients with neonatal adrenoleukodystrophy but differ in that their hepatic peroxisomes are not decreased in number [69]. Clinical features include profound hypotonia and dysmorphic features including hypertelorism, epicanthal folds, low nasal bridge, low-set ears, and polydactyly [160].

In a series of 6 patients with the disorder, hepatic abnormalities were not observed [73]; however, liver fibrosis and elevated serum aminotransferases have been seen in two patients in our institution (G.V. Raymond, personal communication). Neither liver failure nor portal hypertension has been reported. Transgenic knockout mice in which the fatty acyl-CoA oxidase was selectively disrupted, including the hepatic gene, have been described [161]. At 1–2 months of age, there was severe microvesicular fatty metamorphosis of hepatocytes, with few or no liver peroxisomes. By 5 months, there was hepatocyte proliferation; newly emerging hepatocytes were devoid of lipid droplets.

Primary Hyperoxaluria Type 1

Although this disorder is secondary to deficiency of the peroxisomal enzyme AGT, phenotypically the disorder is distinct from all other peroxisomal disorders. Hyperoxaluria 1 is characterized by a continuous, high urinary oxalate excretion and progressive bilateral oxalate urolithiasis and nephrocalcinosis. There are no neurologic or craniofacial abnormalities. In the pretransplant era, death from renal failure occurred in childhood or early adulthood. Extrarenal deposits of calcium oxalate have been observed in skin [162], retina [163], and myocardium [164]. We have observed massive hepatomegaly secondary to calcium oxalate deposits in liver in a 20-year-old patient with the disorder.

Pyridoxine is a cofactor in the AGT enzyme pathway and pyridoxine in doses of up to 200 mg/day has been shown to reduce and, in some cases, normalize urinary oxalate and glycolate excretion [165]. Orthophosphate supplementation may prevent the progression of calcium oxalate stones and small doses of a thiazide diuretic may be useful [166].

Because the primary enzyme defect is in the liver, renal transplantation is unsuccessful because the donor kidney is injured by continuous deposits of calcium oxalate [167]. Thus, since the late 1980s, the recommended approach for patients with end-stage renal disease secondary to hyperoxaluria 1 is to perform combined liver–kidney transplantation [168,169]. One patient suffered from livedo reticularis, peripheral gangrene, and third-degree heart block secondary to calcium oxalate sludge; all of these manifestations resolved following liver transplantation [170].

Gruessner [171] reported a successful preemptive living related liver transplant in a 22-month-old who had presented at 5 weeks of age with dehydration, uremia, and nephrocalcinosis. Kidney function stabilized after the liver transplant, without the need for dialysis or renal transplantation. Walden et al. [172] reported a 6-year follow-up in a 10-year-old boy who had undergone hepatorenal transplantation at age 4 years; radiologic bone density improved, and significant catch-up growth was noted.

Hyperoxaluria 1 is probably the only peroxisomal disorder in which percutaneous liver biopsy is needed to establish a definitive diagnosis [173] because AGT is only expressed in liver, where it is largely confined to peroxisomes. In patients with the disorder, enzyme activity in liver ranged from 11 to 47% of control values; the degree of deficiency appears to be related to clinical severity and the amount of biochemical derangement [174].

Prenatal diagnosis is possible; successful methods include enzyme assay, immunoassay, and immunoelectron microscopy of fetal liver tissues (second trimester), and linkage and mutation analysis of DNA isolated from chorionic villus samples in the first trimester [175].

Mevalonate Kinase Deficiency

Mevalonic aciduria, the first recognized defect in the biosynthesis of cholesterol and isoprenoids, is secondary to deficiency of ATP–mevalonate 5-phosphotransferase (mevalonate kinase.) Hoffmann et al. [114] described a child with severe failure to thrive, developmental delay, anemia, hepatosplenomegaly, central cataracts, and dysmorphic facies. Similar patients have been reported by others [176]. Hoffmann et al. [144] described 11 patients with the disorder; all had recurrent crises in which there was fever, lymphadenopathy, hepatosplenomegaly, arthralgia, edema, and a morbilliform rash. On occasion, patients lack significant neurologic abnormalities, and the presentation may be that of neonatal cholestasis or mimic that of congenital infections or myelodysplastic syndromes, with severe anemia, petechiae, hepatosplenomegaly, leukocytosis, and recurrent febrile episodes predominating [177].

α-Methylacyl-CoA Racemase Deficiency

Documented α-methylacyl-CoA racemase deficiency has only been reported in four patients to date. Two adults presented with adult-onset sensory motor neuropathy [93,178]. An infant with Niemann–Pick C disease was diagnosed serendipitously; no symptoms could clearly be attributed to the racemase deficiency [93]. Another infant presented with vitamin K deficiency, severe cholestasis, and giant cell neonatal hepatitis [145,179]. The infant responded well to treatment with cholic acid and fat-soluble vitamin supplementation. At age 7 years, she was reportedly in good health. This infant had an older sibling who had died of vitamin K deficiency before the infant's diagnosis of racemase deficiency. The sibling's liver had been used as a donor liver for a pediatric liver transplant procedure. The recipient had a posttransplant liver biopsy that was significant for acute rejection, bile duct proliferation, and fibrosis. It was assumed that the older sibling had succumbed to racemase deficiency. The liver recipient was then treated with ursodeoxycholic acid and is reportedly doing well 8 years posttransplant.

A mouse model for this disorder has recently been published [180]. Interestingly the knockout mice showed a 44-fold increase of C27 bile acid precursors and greater than 50% decrease in primary (C24) bile acids in bile, serum, and liver but did not develop liver disease until they were fed a diet supplemented with phytol, a source for branched-chain fatty acids. The authors thus proposed elimination of dietary phytol for patients with this disorder.

PUTATIVE MECHANISMS FOR HEPATIC ABNORMALITIES

Although mechanisms underlying the hepatic abnormalities observed in the preceding list of peroxisomal disorders have not been clarified, some generalizations can be made. Those disorders characterized by abnormalities in the metabolism of bile acids are most frequently associated with hepatomegaly, cholestasis, and hepatic fibrosis, including the Zellweger–neonatal adrenoleukodystrophy–Infantile Refsum spectrum and DBP deficiency. The experience of Setchell et al. [154] in ameliorating cholestasis and hepatic histology in a child with ZS by administration of primary bile acids suggests that in at least some patients, the liver disease results either from deficiency of primary bile acids, accumulation of toxic bile acid intermediates, or both. In one patient with ZS, the biliary profile of cysteinyl leukotrienes was markedly abnormal with increased omega oxidation metabolites of LT34 and decreased amounts of a β-oxidation metabolite of LTE3, suggesting that these abnormal metabolites might contribute to the liver disease [181]. In contrast, RCDP, in which severe bony abnormalities are characteristic, is not associated with either liver disease or abnormalities in bile acid metabolism.

The PEX5 knockout mouse model has been used to study the ontogenesis of hepatic peroxisomes and to the hepatic disease in ZS. Functional peroxisomes are not detected by the diaminobenzidine method, and catalase is mislocalized to the nucleus and cytoplasm [182]. Crystals of VLCFAs accumulate in liver, and mitochondria are abnormal both structurally and functionally, suggesting that oxidative stress may play a role in the liver injury.

As shown in Figure 35.2, both acyl-CoA oxidase and mevalonate kinase are distantly involved in the peroxisomal metabolism of bile acids through generation of THCA and DHCA from cholesterol. This relationship or the microvesicular steatosis characteristic of the acyl CoA oxidase knockout mouse (or both) described earlier may be responsible for the hepatic abnormalities noted in some patients with one of these disorders. Mouse models with targeted disruption of PPARα or peroxisomal β-oxidation enzymes have suggested a link between these deficiencies and the development of steatohepatitis [183].

APPROACH TO LABORATORY DIAGNOSIS OF PEROXISOMAL DISEASES

If a peroxisome biogenesis disorder is suspected on clinical grounds, quantitation of plasma VLCFA levels by gas chromatography is the most informative initial biochemical assay (Table 35.1). In some laboratories, phytanic and pristanic acids can be quantitated in the same analysis, although these may not be informative based on the age or diet of the patient. If elevated VLCFA levels are detected, a skin biopsy should be requested for measurement of ether phospholipid synthesis and phytanic acid oxidation. This is particularly helpful in distinguishing biogenesis disorders from DBP deficiency. Plasma and urine bile acid analysis as well as urine pipecolic acid concentration and erythrocyte membrane plasmalogen levels provide additional evidence to support a diagnosis. Although liver involvement is not generally a feature of acyl-CoA oxidase deficiency and RCDP, these analyses will distinguish these disorders from biogenesis disorders and DBP deficiency.

PRESENTATION OF PATIENTS WITH PEROXISOMAL DISEASES TO THE HEPATOLOGIST

In general, patients with peroxisomal disorders whose hepatic manifestations lead to consultation with a pediatric hepatologist would exhibit typical craniofacial and neurologic abnormalities, which should lead to analysis of plasma VLCFAs as the first step. It should be emphasized, however, that at least some patients with infantile Refsum disease have presented with neonatal cholestasis without obvious extrahepatic manifestations, so a diagnostic workup for this disorder should be considered for unexplained neonatal cholestasis that fails to resolve. Given that more than 50 peroxisomal enzymes have been described, it is likely that new peroxisomal disorders will be described in the future, and unexplained neonatal cholestasis may be a feature. Finally, the pediatric hepatologist can play a key role in establishing a definitive diagnosis of hyperoxaluria 1 by performing a percutaneous liver biopsy for enzyme analysis and by involvement regarding the appropriateness of preemptive liver transplant or hepatorenal transplant.

TREATMENT OF LIVER DISEASE IN PATIENTS WITH PEROXISOMAL DISORDERS

Although treatment options for peroxisomal diseases remain limited, Setchell et al. [154] demonstrated that the combination of cholic acid and chenodeoxycholic acid improved the liver disease of one patient with ZS. Maeda et al. [184] demonstrated that the use of chenodeoxycholic acid alone was deleterious but that the combination of this bile acid and ursodeoxycholic acid was beneficial. Using DHA, Martinez et al. [185] demonstrated dramatic clinical and biochemical improvement in patients with ZS and infantile Refsum disease and slight biochemical improvement in a child with neonatal adrenoleukodystrophy.

It is hoped that advances in our understanding of the molecular biology and genetics of peroxisomal diseases will add more to the therapeutic armamentarium for the unfortunate children with these disorders.

REFERENCES

1. de Duve C, Baudhuin P. Peroxisomes (microbodies and related particles). Physiol Rev 1966;46:323–57.
2. Breidenbach RW, Beevers H. Association of the glyoxylate cycle enzymes in a novel subcellular particle from castor bean endosperm. Biochem Biophys Res Commun 1967;27:462–9.
3. Opperdoes FR, Borst P. Localization of nine glycolytic enzymes in a microbody-like organelle in Trypanosoma brucei: the glycosome. FEBS Lett 1977;80:360–4.
4. Hruban Z, Vigil EL, Slesers Aet al. Microbodies: constituent organelles of animal cells. Lab Invest 1972;27:184–91.
5. Lazarow PB, Fujiki Y. Biogenesis of peroxisomes. Annu Rev Cell Biol 1985;1:489–530.
6. Purdue PE, Lazarow PB. Peroxisomal biogenesis: multiple pathways of protein import. J Biol Chem 1994;269:30065–8.
7. Kunau WH. Peroxisome biogenesis: end of the debate. Curr Biol 2005;15:R774–6.
8. Hoepfner D, Schildknegt D, Braakman I, et al. Contribution of the endoplasmic reticulum to peroxisome formation. Cell 2005;122:85–95.
9. Gould SJ, Keller GA, Hosken N, et al. A conserved tripeptide sorts proteins to peroxisomes. J Cell Biol 1989;108:1657–64.
10. Subramani S. Protein translocation into peroxisomes. J Biol Chem 1996;271:32483–6.
11. Klein AT, van Den Berg M, Bottger G, et al. Saccharomyces cerevisiae acyl-CoA oxidase follows a novel, non-PTS1, import pathway into peroxisomes that is dependent on Pex5p. J Biol Chem 2002;19:19.
12. Mcnew JA, Goodman JM. An oligomeric protein is imported into peroxisomes in vivo. J Cell Biol 1994;127:1245–57.
13. Michels PA, Moyersoen J, Krazy H, et al. Peroxisomes, glyoxysomes and glycosomes [review]. Mol Membr Biol 2005;22:133–45.
14. Slawecki ML, Dodt G, Steinberg S, et al. Identification of three distinct peroxisomal protein import defects in patients with peroxisome biogenesis disorders. J Cell Sci 1995;108:1817–29.
15. Weller S, Gould SJ, Valle D. Peroxisome biogenesis disorders. Annu Rev Genomics Hum Genet 2003;4:165–211.
16. Shimozawa N, Tsukamoto T, Nagase T, et al. Identification of a new complementation group of the peroxisome biogenesis disorders and PEX14 as the mutated gene. Hum Mutat 2004;23:552–8.
17. Reuber BE, Germain-Lee E, Collins CS, et al. Mutations in PEX1 are the most common cause of peroxisome biogenesis disorders. Nat Genet 1997;17:445–8.
18. Portsteffen H, Beyer A, Becker E, et al. Human PEX1 is mutated in complementation group 1 of the peroxisome biogenesis disorders. Nat Genet 1997;17:449–52.
19. Shimozawa N, Tsukamoto T, Suzuki Y, et al. A human gene responsible for Zellweger syndrome that affects peroxisome assembly. Sci 1992;255:1132–4.
20. Braverman N, Steel G, Obie C, et al. Human PEX7 encodes the peroxisomal PTS2 receptor and is responsible for rhizomelic chondrodysplasia punctata. Nat Genet 1997;15:369–76.
21. Motley AM, Hettema EH, Hogenhout EM, et al. Rhizomelic chondrodysplasia punctata is a peroxisomal protein targeting disease caused by a non-functional PTS2 receptor. Nat Genet 1997;15:377–80.
22. Purdue PE, Zhang JW, Skoneczny M, et al. Rhizomelic chondrodysplasia punctata is caused by deficiency of human PEX7, a homologue of the yeast PTS2 receptor. Nat Genet 1997;15:381–4.
23. Dodt G, Braverman N, Wong C, et al. Mutations in the PTS1 receptor gene, PXR1, define complementation group 2 of the peroxisome biogenesis disorders. Nat Genet 1995;9:115–25.
24. Wiemer EAC, Nuttley WM, Bertolaet BL, et al. Human peroxisomal targeting signal-1 receptor restores peroxisomal protein import in cells from patients with fatal peroxisomal disorders. J Cell Biol 1995;130:51–65.
25. Yahraus T, Braverman N, Dodt G, et al. The peroxisome biogenesis disorder group 4 gene, PXAAA1, encodes a cytoplasmic ATPase required for stability of the PTS1 receptor. EMBO J 1996;15:2914–23.
26. Chang CC, Lee WH, Moser H, et al. Isolation of the human PEX12 gene, mutated in group 3 of the peroxisome biogenesis disorders. Nat Genet 1997;15:385–8.
27. Okumoto K, Itoh R, Shimozawa N, et al. Mutations in PEX10 is the cause of Zellweger peroxisome deficiency syndrome of complementation group B. Hum Mol Genet 1998;7:1399–405.
28. South ST, Gould SJ. Peroxisome synthesis in the absence of preexisting peroxisomes. J Cell Biol 1999;144:255–66.
29. Matsuzono Y, Kinoshita N, Tamura S, et al. Human PEX19: cDNA cloning by functional complementation, mutation analysis in a patient with Zellweger syndrome, and potential role in peroxisomal membrane assembly. Proc Natl Acad Sci U S A 1999;96:2116–21.
30. Shimozawa N, Suzuki Y, Zhang Z, et al. Nonsense and temperature-sensitive mutations in PEX13 are the cause of complementation group H of peroxisome biogenesis disorders. Hum Mol Genet 1999;8:1077–83.
31. Honsho M, Tamura S, Shimozawa N, et al. Mutation in PEX16 is causal in the peroxisome-deficient Zellweger syndrome of complementation group D. Am J Hum Genet 1998;63:1622–30.
32. Hess R, Staubli W, Riess W. Nature of the hepatomegalic effect produced by ethyl-chlorophenoxy- isobutyrate in the rat. Nature 1965;208:856–8.
33. Subramani S. Protein import into peroxisomes and biogenesis of the organelle. Ann Rev Cell Biol 1993;9:445–78.
34. Reddy JK, Goel SK, Nemali MR, et al. Transcription regulation of peroxisomal fatty acyl-CoA oxidase and enoyl-CoA hydratase(3-hydroxyacyl-CoA dehydrogenase in rat liver by peroxisome proliferators. Proc Natl Acad Sci U S A 1986;83:1747–51.
35. Rao MS, Kokkinakis DM, Subbarao V, et al. Peroxisome proliferator-induced hepatocarcinogenesis: levels of activating and detoxifying enzymes in hepatocellular carcinomas induced by ciprofibrate. Carcinogenesis 1987;8:19–23.

36. Reddy JK, Azarnoff DL, Hignite CE. Hypolipidaemic hepatic peroxisome proliferators form a novel class of chemical carcinogens. Nature 1980;283:397–8.
37. Issemann I, Green S. Activation of a member of the steroid hormone receptor superfamily by peroxisome proliferators. Nature 1990;347:645–50.
38. Mangelsdorf DJ, Thummel C, Beato M, et al. The nuclear receptor superfamily: the second decade. Cell 1995;83:835–9.
39. Braissant O, Foufelle F, Scotto C, et al. Differential expression of peroxisome proliferator-activated receptors (PPARs): tissue distribution of PPAR-alpha, -beta, and -gamma in the adult rat. Endocrinology 1996;137:354–66.
40. Tugwood JD, Issemann I, Anderson RG, et al. The mouse peroxisome proliferator activated receptor recognizes a response element in the 5' flanking sequence of the rat acyl CoA oxidase gene. EMBO Journal 1992;11:433–9.
41. Chu RY, Lin Y, Rao MS, et al. Cooperative formation of higher order peroxisome proliferator-activated receptor and retinoid X receptor complexes on the peroxisome proliferator responsive element of the rat hydratase-dehydrogenase gene. J Biol Chem 1995;270:29636–9.
42. Kliewer SA, Umesono K, Noonan DJ, et al. Convergence of 9-Cis retinoic acid and peroxisome proliferator signalling pathways through heterodimer formation of their receptors. Nature 1992;358:771–4.
43. Rao MS, Reddy JK. Hepatocarcinogenesis of peroxisome proliferators. Ann N Y Acad Sci 1996;804:573–87.
44. Tugwood JD, Aldridge TC, Lambe KG, et al. Peroxisome proliferator-activated receptors: structures and function. Ann N Y Acad Sci 1996;804:252–65.
45. Oliver MF, Heady JA, Morris JN, et al. A cooperative trial in the primary prevention of ischemic heart disease using clofibrate. Br Heart J 1978;40:1069–118.
46. Frick MH, Elo O, Haapa K, et al. Helsinki Heart Study: primary-prevention trial with gemfibrozil in middle-aged men with dyslipidemia. Safety of treatment, changes in risk factors, and incidence of coronary heart disease. N Engl J Med 1987;317:1237–45.
47. Lazarow PB, de Duve C. A fatty acyl-CoA oxidizing system in rat liver peroxisomes; enhancement by clofibrate, a hypolipidemic drug. Proc Natl Acad Sci U S A 1976;73:2043–6.
48. Hashimoto T. Purifiation, properties and biosynthesis o fperoxisomal beta-oxidation enzymes. In: Tanaka K, Coates PW, eds. Fatty acid oxidation: clinical, biochemical and molecular aspects. New York: Alan R. Liss, 1990:138–52.
49. Almashanu S, Valle D. Peroxisomal ABC transporters. In: Holland IB, Kuchler K, Higgins CF, Cole S, eds. ABC proteins: from bacteria to man. London: Academic Press, 2003:497–513.
50. Shindo Y, Hashimoto T. Acyl-coenzyme A synthetase and fatty acid oxidation in rat liver peroxisomes. J Biochem 1978;84:1177–81.
51. Krisans SK, Mortensen RM, Lazarow PB. Acyl-CoA synthetase in rat liver peroxisomes. Computer assisted analysis of cell fractionation experiments. J Biol Chem 1980;255:9599–607.
52. Osumi T, Hashimoto T, Ui N. Purification and properties of acyl-CoA oxidase from rat liver. J Biochem (Tokyo) 1980;87:1735–46.
53. Osumi T, Hashimoto T. Peroxisomal beta-oxidation system of rat liver. Copurification of enoyl-CoA hydratase and 3-hydroxyacyl-CoA dehydrogenase. Biochem Biophys Res Commun 1979;89:580–4.
54. Miyazawa S, Osumi T, Hashimoto T. The presence of a new 3-oxoacyl-CoA thiolase in rat liver peroxisomes. Eur J Biochem 1980;103:589–96.
55. Palosaari PM, Hiltunen JK. Peroxisomal bifunctional protein from rat liver is a trifunctional enzyme possessing 2-enoyl-CoA hydratase, 3-hydroxyacyl-CoA dehydrogenase, and delta 3, delta 2-enoyl-CoA isomerase activities. J Biol Chem 1990;265:2446–9.
56. Singh I, Moser AE, Goldfischer S, et al. Lignoceric acid is oxidized in the peroxisome: implications for the Zellweger cerebro-hepato-renal syndrome and adrenoleukodystrophy. Proc Natl Acad Sci U S A 1984;81:4203–7.
57. Vanhove GF, Vanveldhoven PP, Fransen M, et al. The CoA esters of 2-methyl-branched chain fatty acids and of the bile acid intermediates dihydroxycoprostanic and trihydroxycoprostanic acids are oxidized by one single peroxisomal branched chain acyl-CoA oxidase in human liver and kidney. J Biol Chem 1993;268:10335–44.
58. Dieuaide-Noubhani M, Asselberghs S, Mannaerts GP, et al. Evidence that multifunctional protein 2, and not multifunctional protein 1, is involved in the peroxisomal beta-oxidation of pristanic acid. Biochem J 1997;325:367–73.
59. Antonenkov VD, Van Veldhoven PP, Waelkens E, et al. Substrate specificities of 3-oxoacyl-CoA thiolase A and sterol carrier protein 2/3-oxoacyl-CoA thiolase purified from normal rat liver peroxisomes. Sterol carrier protein 2/3-oxoacyl-CoA thiolase is involved in the metabolism of 2-methyl-branched fatty acids and bile acid intermediates. J Biol Chem 1997;272:26023–31.
60. Wanders RJ, Denis S, Wouters F, et al. Sterol carrier protein X (SCPx) is a peroxisomal branched-chain beta- ketothiolase specifically reacting with 3-oxo-pristanoyl-CoA: a new, unique role for SCPx in branched-chain fatty acid metabolism in peroxisomes. Biochem Biophys Res Commun 1997;236:565–9.
61. Qin YM, Poutanen MH, Helander HM, et al. Peroxisomal multifunctional enzyme of beta-oxidation metabolizing D-3- hydroxyacyl CoA esters in rat liver: molecular cloning, expression and characterization. Biochem J 1997;321:21–8.
62. Baes M, Huyghe S, Carmeliet P, et al. Inactivation of the peroxisomal multifunctional protein-2 in mice impedes the degradation of not only 2-methyl-branched fatty acids and bile acid intermediates but also of very long chain fatty acids. J Biol Chem 2000;275:16329–36.
63. Verhoeven NM, Wanders RJ, Poll-The BT, et al. The metabolism of phytanic acid and pristanic acid in man: a review. J Inherit Metab Dis 1998;21:697–728.
64. Frolov A, Cho TH, Billheimer JT, et al. Sterol carrier protein-2, a new fatty acyl coenzyme a-binding protein. J Biol Chem 1996;271:31878–84.
65. Leenders F, Tesdorpf JG, Markus M, et al. Porcine 80-kDa protein reveals intrinsic 17 beta-hydroxysteroid dehydrogenase, fatty acyl-CoA-hydratase/dehydrogenase, and sterol transfer activities. J Biol Chem 1996;271:5438–42.
66. Wanders RJ, Tager JM. Lipid metabolism in peroxisomes in relation to human disease. Mol Aspects Med 1998;19:69–154.
67. Singh H, Usher S, Johnson D, et al. A comparative study of straight chain and branched chain fatty acid oxidation in skin fibroblasts from patients with peroxisomal disorders. J Lipid Res 1990;31:217–25.
68. Swinkels BW, Gould SJ, Bodnar AG, et al. A novel, cleavable peroxisomal targeting signal at the amino-terminus of the rat 3-ketoacyl-CoA thiolase. EMBO J 1991;10:3255–62.

69. Poll-The BT, Roels F, Ogier H, et al. A new peroxisomal disorder with enlarged peroxisomes and a specific deficiency of acyl-CoA oxidase (pseudo-neonatal adrenoleukodystrophy). Am J Hum Genet 1988;42:422–34.
70. Watkins PA, Chen WW, Harris CJ, et al. Peroxisomal bifunctional enzyme deficiency. J Clin Invest 1989;83:771–7.
71. van Grunsven EG, van Berkel E, Mooijer PA, et al. Peroxisomal bifunctional protein deficiency revisited: resolution of its true enzymatic and molecular basis. Am J Hum Genet 1999;64:99–107.
72. Singh I, Moser AB, Moser HW, et al. Adrenoleukodystrophy: Impaired oxidation of very long chain fatty acids in white blood cells, cultured skin fibroblasts and amniocytes. Pediatr Res 1984;18:286–90.
73. Watkins PA, McGuinness MC, Raymond GV, et al. Distinction between peroxisomal bifunctional enzyme and Acyl-CoA oxidase deficiencies. Ann Neurol 1995;38:472–7.
74. Natowicz MR, Evans JE, Kelley RI, et al. Urinary bile acids and peroxisomal bifunctional enzyme deficiency. Am J Med Genet 1996;63:356–62.
75. Schram AW, Goldfischer S, van Roermund CWT, et al. Human peroxisomal 3-oxoacyl-coenzyme A thiolase deficiency. Proc Natl Acad Sci U S A 1987;84:2494–6.
76. Ferdinandusse S, Van Grunsven EG, Oostheim W, et al. Reinvestigation of peroxisomal 3-ketoacyl-CoA thiolase deficiency: identification of the true defect at the level of d-bifunctional protein. Am J Hum Genet 2002;70:1589–93.
77. Mosser J, Lutz Y, Stoeckel ME, et al. The gene responsible for adrenoleukodystrophy encodes a peroxisomal membrane protein. Hum Mol Genet 1994;3:265–71.
78. Moore SA, Hurt E, Yoder E, et al. Docosahexaenoic acid synthesis in human skin fibroblasts involves peroxisomal retroconversion of tetracosahexaenoic acid. J Lipid Res 1995;36:2433–43.
79. Masters-Thomas A, Bailes J, Billimoria JD, et al. Heredopathia atactica polyneuritiformis (Refsum's disease): 2. Estimation of phytanic acid in foods. J Hum Nutr 1980;34:251–4.
80. Masters-Thomas A, Bailes J, Billimoria JD, et al. Heredopathia atactica polyneuritiformis (Refsum's disease): 1. Clinical features and dietary management. J Hum Nutr 1980;34:245–50.
81. Klenk E, Kahlke W. Uber das Vorkommen der 3,7,11,15-Tetramethylhexadecansaure (Phtansaure) in den Cholesterinestern and andern Lipoidfraktionen der Organe bei einen Krankheitsfall unbekannter Genese (Verdacht auf Heredopathia atactica polyneuritiformis, Refsum's syndrome). Hoppe-Seyler's Z Physiol Chem 1963;333:133–9.
82. Watkins PA, Howard AE, Mihalik SJ. Phytanic acid must be activated to phytanoyl-CoA prior to its alpha-oxidation in rat liver peroxisomes. Biochim Biophys Acta 1994;1214:288–94.
83. Mihalik SJ, Rainville AM, Watkins PA. Phytanic acid alpha-oxidation in rat liver peroxisomes – production of alpha-hydroxyphytanoyl-CoA and formate is enhanced by dioxygenase cofactors. Eur J Biochem 1995;232:545–51.
84. Verhoeven NM, Schor DS, ten Brink HJ, et al. Resolution of the phytanic acid alpha-oxidation pathway: identification of pristanal as product of the decarboxylation of 2-hydroxyphytanoyl-CoA. Biochem Biophys Res Commun 1997;237:33–6.
85. Jansen GA, van den Brink DM, Ofman R, et al. Identification of pristanal dehydrogenase activity in peroxisomes: conclusive evidence that the complete phytanic acid alpha-oxidation pathway is localized in peroxisomes. Biochem Biophys Res Commun 2001;283:674–9.
86. Steinberg SJ, Wang SJ, Kim DG, et al. Human very-long-chain acyl-CoA synthetase: cloning, topography, and relevance to branched-chain fatty acid metabolism. Biochem Biophys Res Commun 1999;257:615–21.
87. Mihalik SJ, Morrell JC, Kim D, et al. Identification of PAHX, a Refsum disease gene. Nature Genet 1997;17:185–9.
88. Foulon V, Antonenkov VD, Croes K, et al. Purification, molecular cloning, and expression of 2-hydroxyphytanoyl- CoA lyase, a peroxisomal thiamine pyrophosphate-dependent enzyme that catalyzes the carbon-carbon bond cleavage during alpha-oxidation of 3- methyl-branched fatty acids. Proc Natl Acad Sci U S A 1999;96:10039–44.
89. Scotto JM, Hadchouel M, Odievre M, et al. Infantile phytanic acid storage disease, a possible variant of Refsum's disease: three cases, including ultrastructural studies of the liver. J Inherit Metab Dis 1982;5:83–90.
90. Kase F, Bjorkhem I, Pedersen JI. Formation of cholic acid from 3 alpha, 7 alpha, 12 alpha-trihydroxy-5 beta-cholestanoic acid by rat liver peroxisomes. J Lipid Res 1983;24:1560–7.
91. Schepers L, Casteels M, Verheyden K, et al. Subcellular distribution and characteristics of trihydroxycoprostanoyl-CoA synthetase in rat liver. Biochem J 1989;257:221–9.
92. Vanveldhoven PP, Croes K, Asselberghs S, et al. Peroxisomal beta-oxidation of 2-methyl-branched acyl-CoA esters: stereospecific recognition of the 2S-methyl compounds by trihydroxycoprostanoyl-CoA oxidase and pristanoyl-CoA oxidase. FEBS Lett 1996;388:80–4.
93. Ferdinandusse S, Overmars H, Denis S, et al. Plasma analysis of di- and trihydroxycholestanoic acid diastereoisomers in peroxisomal alpha-methylacyl-CoA racemase deficiency. J Lipid Res 2001;42:137–41.
94. Schmitz W, Conzelmann E. Stereochemistry of peroxisomal and mitochondrial beta-oxidation of alpha-methylacyl-coas. Eur J Biochem 1997;244:434–40.
95. Horrocks LA, Sharma M. Plasmalogens and O-alkyl glycerophospholipids. In: Nawthorne JN, Ansell GB, eds. Phospholipids. New comprehensive biochemistry. Amsterdam: Elsevier Biomedical Press, 1982:51–93.
96. Burdett K, Larkins LK, Das AK, et al. Peroxisomal localization of acyl-coenzyme a reductase (long chain alcohol forming) in guinea pig intestine mucosal cells. J Biol Chem 1991;266:12201–6.
97. Hajra AK, Burke CL, Jones CL. Subcellular localization of acyl coenzyme A: dihydroxyacetone phosphate acyltransferase in rat liver peroxisomes (microbodies). J Biol Chem 1979;254:10896–900.
98. Jones CL, Hajra AK. Properties of guinea pig liver peroxisomal dihydroxyacetone phosphate acyltransferase. J Biol Chem 1980;255:8289–95.
99. Lazarow PB, Moser HW. Disorders of peroxisome biogenesis. In: Scriver CR, Beaudet AL, Sly WS, Valle D, eds. The metabolic and molecular bases of inherited disease. New York: McGraw-Hill, 1995:2287–324.
100. Thai TP, Heid H, Rackwitz HR, et al. Ether lipid biosynthesis: isolation and molecular characterization of human dihydroxyacetonephosphate acyltransferase. FEBS Lett 1997;420:205–11.
101. Ofman R, Hettema EH, Hogenhout EM, et al. Acyl-CoA:dihydroxyacetonephosphate acyltransferase: cloning of the human cDNA and resolution of the molecular basis in rhizomelic chondrodysplasia punctata type 2. Hum Mol Genet 1998;7:847–53.

102. de Vet EC, van den Broek BT, van den Bosch[K8] H. Nucleotide sequence of human alkyl-dihydroxyacetonephosphate synthase cDNA reveals the presence of a peroxisomal targeting signal 2. Biochim Biophys Acta 1997;1346:25–9.
103. de Vet EC, Ijlst L, Oostheim W, et al. Alkyl-dihydroxyacetonephosphate synthase. Fate in peroxisome biogenesis disorders and identification of the point mutation underlying a single enzyme deficiency. J Biol Chem 1998;273:10296–301.
104. Keller GA, Barton MC, Shapiro DJ, et al. 3-Hydroxy-3-methylglutaryl-coenzyme A reductase is present in peroxisomes in normal rat liver cells. Proc Natl Acad Sci U S A 1985;82:770–4.
105. Appelkvist EL. In vitro labeling of peroxisomal cholesterol with radioactive precursors. Biosci Rep 1987;7:853–8.
106. Thompson SL, Burrows R, Laub RJ, et al. Cholesterol synthesis in rat liver peroxisomes. Conversion of mevalonic acid to cholesterol. J Biol Chem 1987;262:17420–5.
107. Appelkvist EL, Kalen A. Biosynthesis of dolichol by rat liver peroxisomes. Eur J Biochem 1989;185:503–9.
108. Biardi L, Krisans SK. Compartmentalization of cholesterol biosynthesis - Conversion of mevalonate to farnesyl diphosphate occurs in the peroxisomes. J Biol Chem 1996;271:1784–8.
109. Stamellos KD, Shackelford JE, Tanaka RD, et al. Mevalonate kinase is localized in rat liver peroxisomes. J Biol Chem 1992;267:5560–8.
110. Biardi L, Sreedhar A, Zokaei A, et al. Mevalonate kinase is predominantly localized in peroxisomes and is defective in patients with peroxisome deficiency disorders. J Biol Chem 1994;269:1197–205.
111. Krisans SK, Ericsson J, Edwards PA, et al. Farnesyl-diphosphate synthase is localized in peroxisomes. J Biol Chem 1994;269:14165–9.
112. Hogenboom S, Wanders RJ, Waterham HR. Cholesterol biosynthesis is not defective in peroxisome biogenesis defective fibroblasts. Mol Genet Metab 2003;80:290–5.
113. Kelley RI. Review: the cerebrohepatorenal syndrome of Zellweger, morphologic and metabolic aspects. Am J Med Genet 1983;16:503–17.
114. Hoffmann G, Gibson KM, Brandt IK, et al. Mevalonic aciduria – an inborn error of cholesterol and nonsterol isoprene biosynthesis. N Engl J Med 1986;314:1610–14.
115. Noguchi T, Takada Y. Purification and properties of peroxisomal pyruvate (glyoxylate) aminotransferase from rat liver. Biochem J 1978;175:765–8.
116. Danpure CJ, Jennings PR, Leiper JM, et al. Targeting of alanine: glyoxylate aminotransferase in normal individuals and its mistargeting in patients with primary hyperoxaluria type 1. Ann N Y Acad Sci 1996;804:477–90.
117. Danpure CJ, Purdue PE. Primary hyperoxaluria. In: Scriver CR, Beaudet AL, Sly WS, Valle D, eds. The metabolic and molecular bases of inherited disease. New York: McGraw-Hill, 1995:2385–424.
118. Motley A, Lumb MJ, Oatey PB, et al. Mammalian alanine/glyoxylate aminotransferase 1 is imported into peroxisomes via the PTS1 translocation pathway. Increased degeneracy and context specificity of the mammalian PTS1 motif and implications for the peroxisome-to-mitochondrion mistargeting of AGT in primary hyperoxaluria type 1. J Cell Biol 1995;131:95–109.
119. Danpure CJ. Variable peroxisomal and mitochondrial targeting of alanine: glyoxylate aminotransferase in mammalian evolution and disease. Bioessays 1997;19:317–26.
120. Rothstein M, Miller LL. The conversion of lysine to pipecolic acid in the rat. J Biol Chem 1954;211:851–8.
121. Mihalik SJ, Mcguinness M, Watkins PA. Purification and characterization of peroxisomal L-pipecolic acid oxidase from monkey liver. J Biol Chem 1991;266:4822–30.
122. Dodt G, Kim DG, Reimann S, et al. L-Pipecolic acid oxidase, a human enzyme essential for the degradation of L-pipecolic acid, is homologous to the monomeric sarcosine oxidases. Biochem. J. 1999;345:487–94.
123. Kerckaert I, Poll-The BT, Wanders RJA, et al. Hepatic peroxisomes in isolated hyperpipecolic acidaemia justify its classification as single peroxisomal enzyme deficiency. J Inher Metab Dis 1999;22 Suppl 1:29.
124. Frerman FE, Goodman SI. Nuclear-encoded defects of the mitochondrial respiratory chain, including glutaric acidemia type II. In: Scriver CR, Beaudet AL, Sly WS, Valle D, eds. The metabolic and molecular bases of inherited disease. New York: McGraw-Hill, 1995:1611–29.
125. Ghadimi H, Chou WS, Kesner L. Biosynthesis of saccharopine and pipecolic acid from L- and DL- 14 C- lysine by human and dog liver in vitro. Biochem Med 1971;5:56–66.
126. Chang YE. Lysine metabolism in the rat brain: the pipecolic acid-forming pathway. J Neurochem 1978;30:347–54.
127. Chance B, Oshino N. Kinetics and mechanisms of catalase in peroxisomes of the mitochondrial fraction. Biochem J 1971;122:225 33.
128. Lazarow PB, Fujiki Y, Small GM, et al. Presence of the peroxisomal 22-kDa integral membrane protein in the liver of a person lacking recognizable peroxisomes (Zellweger syndrome). Proc Natl Acad Sci U S A 1986;83:9193–6.
129. Lazarow PB, Small GM, Santos M, et al. Zellweger syndrome amniocytes: morphological appearance and a simple sedimentation method for prenatal diagnosis. Pediatr Res 1988;24:63–7.
130. Wanders RJ, Waterham HR. Peroxisomal disorders I: biochemistry and genetics of peroxisome biogenesis disorders. Clin Genet 2005;67:107–33.
131. Peduto A, Baumgartner MR, Verhoeven NM, et al. Hyperpipecolic acidaemia: a diagnostic tool for peroxisomal disorders. Mol Genet Metab 2004;82:224–30.
132. Yousef IM, Perwaiz S, Lamireau T, et al. Urinary bile acid profile in children with inborn errors of bile acid metabolism and chronic cholestasis; screening technique using Electrospray tandem mass-spectrometry (ES/MS/MS). Med Sci Monit 2003;9:MT21–31.
133. Moser AB, Singh I, Brown FRI, et al. The cerebro-hepato-renal (Zellweger) syndrome: Increased levels and impaired oxidation of very-long-chain fatty acids, and their use in prenatal diagnosis. N Engl J Med 1984;310:1141–6.
134. Danks DM, Tippett P, Adams C, et al. Cerebro-hepato-renal syndrome of Zellweger: A report of eight cases with comments upon the incidence, the liver lesion, and a fault in pipecolic acid metabolism. J Pediatr 1975;86:382–8.
135. Poulos A, Sharp P, Fellenberg AJ, et al. Cerebro-hepato-renal (Zellweger) syndrome, adrenoleukodystrophy, and Refsum's disease: plasma changes and skin fibroblast phytanic acid oxidase. Hum Genet 1985;70:172–7.

136. Heymans HS, vd Bosch H, Schutgens RB, et al. Deficiency of plasmalogens in the cerebro-hepato-renal (Zellweger) syndrome. Eur J Pediatr 1984;142:10–15.
137. Roscher A, Molzer B, Bernheimer H, et al. The cerebrohepatorenal (Zellweger) syndrome: an improved method for the biochemical diagnosis and its potential value for prenatal detection. Pediatr Res 1985;19:930–3.
138. Eyssen H, Eggermont E, van Eldere J, et al. Bile acid abnormalities and the diagnosis of cerebro-hepato-renal syndrome (Zellweger syndrome). Acta Paediatr Scand 1985;74:539–44.
139. Wanders RJ, Kos M, Roest B, et al. Activity of peroxisomal enzymes and intracellular distribution of catalase in Zellweger syndrome. Biochem Biophys Res Commun 1984;123:1054–61.
140. Hoefler G, Hoefler S, Watkins PA, et al. Biochemical abnormalities in rhizomelic chondrodysplasia punctata. J Pediatr 1988;112:726–33.
141. Mcguinness MC, Moser AB, Pollthe BT, et al. Complementation analysis of patients with intact peroxisomes and impaired peroxisomal beta-oxidation. Biochem Med Metab Biol 1993;49:228–42.
142. Tenbrink HJ, Vandenheuvel CMM, Christensen E, et al. Diagnosis of peroxisomal disorders by analysis of phytanic and pristanic acids in stored blood spots collected at neonatal screening. Clin Chem 1993;39:1904–6.
143. Roels F, Espeel M, De Craemer D. Liver pathology and immunocytochemistry in congenital peroxisomal diseases: a review. J Inherit Metab Dis 1991;14:853–75.
144. Hoffmann GF, Charpentier C, Mayatepek E, et al. Clinical and biochemical phenotype in 11 patients with mevalonic aciduria. Pediatrics 1993;91:915–21.
145. Van Veldhoven PP, Meyhi E, Squires RH, et al. Fibroblast studies documenting a case of peroxisomal 2-methylacyl-CoA racemase deficiency: possible link between racemase deficiency and malabsorption and vitamin K deficiency. Eur J Clin Invest 2001;31:714–22.
146. Roth KS. Peroxisomal disease – common ground for pediatrician, cell biologist, biochemist, pathologist, and neurologist. Clin Pediatr (Phila) 1999;38:73–5.
147. Moser AB, Rasmussen M, Naidu S, et al. Phenotype of patients with peroxisomal disorders subdivided into sixteen complementation groups. J Pediatr 1995;127:13–22.
148. Moser HW. Genotype–phenotype correlations in disorders of peroxisome biogenesis. Mol Genet Metab 1999;68:316–27.
149. Steinberg SJ, Elcioglu N, Slade CM, et al. Peroxisomal disorders: clinical and biochemical studies in 15 children and prenatal diagnosis in 7 families. Am J Med Genet 1999;85:502–10.
150. Depreter M, Espeel M, Roels F. Human peroxisomal disorders. Microsc Res Tech 2003;61:203–23.
151. Smith DW, Opitz JM, Inhorn SL. A syndrome of multiple developmental defects including polycystic kidneys and intrahepatic biliary dysgenesis in 2 siblings. J Pediatr 1965;67:617–24.
152. Bove KE, Daugherty CC, Tyson W, et al. Bile acid synthetic defects and liver disease. Pediatr Dev Pathol 2000;3:1–16.
153. Mathis RK, Watkins JB, Szczepanik-Van Leeuwen P, et al. Liver in the cerebro-hepato-renal syndrome: defective bile acid synthesis and abnormal mitochondria. Gastroenterology 1980;79:1311–17.
154. Setchell KD, Bragetti P, Zimmer-Nechemias L, et al. Oral bile acid treatment and the patient with Zellweger syndrome. Hepatology 1992;15:198–207.
155. Goez H, Meiron D, Horowitz J, et al. Infantile Refsum disease: Neonatal cholestatic jaundice presentation of a peroxisomal disorder. J Pediat Gastroenterol Nutr 1995;20:98–101.
156. Stokke O, Skrede S, Ek J, et al. Refsum's disease, adrenoleucodystrophy, and the Zellweger syndrome. Scand J Clin Lab Invest 1984;44:463–4.
157. Gatfield PD, Taller E, Hinton GG, et al. Hyperpipecolatemia: a new metabolic disorder associated with neuropathy and hepatomegaly: a case study. Can Med Assoc J 1968;99:1215–33.
158. Thomas GH, Haslam RH, Batshaw ML, et al. Hyperpipecolic acidemia associated with hepatomegaly, mental retardation, optic nerve dysplasia and progressive neurological disease. Clin Genet 1975;8:376–82.
159. Suzuki Y, Jiang LL, Souri M, et al. D-3-hydroxyacyl-CoA dehydratase(D 3 hydroxyacyl CoA dehydrogenase bifunctional protein deficiency: a newly identified peroxisomal disorder. Am J Hum Genet 1997;61:1153–62.
160. Suzuki Y, Shimozawa N, Yajima S, et al. Novel subtype of peroxisomal acyl-CoA oxidase deficiency and bifunctional enzyme deficiency with detectable enzyme protein: identification by means of complementation analysis. Am J Hum Genet 1994;54:36–43.
161. Fan CY, Pan J, Chu RY, et al. Hepatocellular and hepatic peroxisomal alterations in mice with a disrupted peroxisomal fatty acyl-coenzyme a oxidase gene. J Biol Chem 1996;271:24698–710.
162. Chesney RW, Friedman AL, Breed AL, et al. Renal failure with hypercalcemia, renal stones, multiple pathologic fractures, and growth failure. Am J Med Genet 1983;14:169–79.
163. Small KW, Letson R, Scheinman J. Ocular findings in primary hyperoxaluria. Arch Ophthalmol 1990;108:89–93.
164. Coltart DJ, Hudson RE. Primary oxalosis of the heart: a cause of heart block. Br Heart J 1971;33:315–19.
165. Yendt ER, Cohanim M. Response to a physiologic dose of pyridoxine in type I primary hyperoxaluria. N Engl J Med 1985;312:953–7.
166. Milliner DS, Eickholt JT, Bergstralh EJ, et al. Results of long-term treatment with orthophosphate and pyridoxine in patients with primary hyperoxaluria. N Engl J Med 1994;331:1553–8.
167. Klauwers J, Wolf PL, Cohn R. Failure of renal transplantation in primary oxalosis. JAMA 1969;209:551.
168. Watts RW, Calne RY, Williams R, et al. Primary hyperoxaluria (type I): attempted treatment by combined hepatic and renal transplantation. Q J Med 1985;57:697–703.
169. McDonald JC, Landreneau MD, Rohr MS, et al. Reversal by liver transplantation of the complications of primary hyperoxaluria as well as the metabolic defect. N Engl J Med 1989;321:1100–3.
170. Baethge BA, Sanusi ID, Landreneau MD, et al. Livedo reticularis and peripheral gangrene associated with primary hyperoxaluria. Arthritis Rheum 1988;31:1199–203.
171. Gruessner RW. Preemptive liver transplantation from a living related donor for primary hyperoxaluria type I. N Engl J Med 1998;338:1924.
172. Walden U, Boswald M, Dorr HG, et al. Primary hyperoxaluria 1: catch up growth and normalization of oxaluria 6 years after hepatorenal transplantation in a prepubertal boy. Eur J Pediatr 1999;158:727–9.
173. Danpure CJ, Jennings PR. Further studies on the activity and subcellular distribution of alanine:glyoxylate aminotransferase in the livers of patients with primary hyperoxaluria type 1. Clin Sci 1988;75:315–22.

174. Danpure CJ, Jennings PR, Watts RW. Enzymological diagnosis of primary hyperoxaluria type 1 by measurement of hepatic alanine: glyoxylate aminotransferase activity. Lancet 1987;1:289–91.
175. Danpure CJ, Rumsby G. Strategies for the prenatal diagnosis of primary hyperoxaluria type 1. Prenat Diagn 1996;16:587–98.
176. Mancini J, Philip N, Chabrol B, et al. Mevalonic aciduria in 3 siblings: a new recognizable metabolic encephalopathy. Pediatr Neurol 1993;9:243–6.
177. Hinson DD, Rogers ZR, Hoffmann GF, et al. Hematological abnormalities and cholestatic liver disease in two patients with mevalonate kinase deficiency. Am J Med Genet 1998;78:408–12.
178. McLean BN, Allen J, Ferdinandusse S, et al. A new defect of peroxisomal function involving pristanic acid: a case report. J Neurol Neurosurg Psychiatry 2002;72:396–9.
179. Setchell KD, Heubi JE, Bove KE, et al. Liver disease caused by failure to racemize trihydroxycholestanoic acid: gene mutation and effect of bile acid therapy. Gastroenterology 2003;124:217–32.
180. Savolainen K, Kotti TJ, Schmitz W et al. A mouse model for alpha-methylacyl-CoA racemase deficiency: adjustment of bile acid synthesis and intolerance to dietary methyl-branched lipids. Hum Mol Genet 2004.
181. Mayatepek E, Ferdinandusse S, Meissner T, et al. Analysis of cysteinyl leukotrienes and their metabolites in bile of patients with peroxisomal or mitochondrial beta-oxidation defects. Clin Chim Acta 2004;345:89–92.
182. Baumgart E, Vanhorebeek I, Grabenbauer M, et al. Mitochondrial alterations caused by defective peroxisomal biogenesis in a mouse model for Zellweger syndrome (PEX5 knockout mouse). Am J Pathol 2001;159:1477–94.
183. Reddy JK. Nonalcoholic steatosis and steatohepatitis. III. Peroxisomal beta-oxidation, PPARalpha, and steatohepatitis. Am J Physiol Gastrointest Liver Physiol 2001;281:G1333–9.
184. Maeda K, Kimura A, Yamato Y, et al. Oral bile Acid treatment in two Japanese patients with zellweger syndrome. J Pediatr Gastroenterol Nutr 2002;35:227–30.
185. Martinez M, Vazquez E, Garcia-Silva MT, et al. Therapeutic effects of docosahexaenoic acid ethyl ester in patients with generalized peroxisomal disorders. Am J Clin Nutr 2000;71:376S–85S.

36

Urea Cycle Disorders

Marshall L. Summar, M.D.

The urea cycle was first described in 1932 by Krebs and Henseleit [1] (Figure 36.1). The urea cycle disorders (UCD) result from defects in the metabolism of the extra nitrogen produced by the breakdown of protein and other nitrogen-containing molecules. The incidence of these disorders in the United States is estimated to be at least 1 in 25,000 births, but partial defects may make this number much higher. In a comprehensive Japanese study covering several years the incidence was 1 in 46,000. Severe deficiency or total absence of activity of any of the first four enzymes (CPSI, OTC, ASS, and ASL) in the urea cycle or the cofactor producer (NAGS) results in the accumulation of ammonia and other precursor metabolites during the first few days of life. In milder (or partial) urea cycle enzyme deficiencies, ammonia accumulation may be triggered by illness or stress at almost any time of life, resulting in multiple mild elevations of plasma ammonia concentration. The hyperammonemia is less severe and the symptoms more subtle. The mainstays of treatment are (1) reducing plasma ammonia concentration, (2) pharmacologic management to allow alternative pathway excretion of excess nitrogen, (3) reducing the amount of nitrogen in the diet, (4) reducing catabolism through the introduction of calories supplied by carbohydrates and fat, and (5) taking measures to reduce the risk of neurologic damage. Defects in the fifth enzyme in the pathway, arginase, result in a more subtle disease involving neurologic symptoms. Defects in the transporter proteins for ornithine (hyperammonemia–hyperornithinemia–homocitrullinemia [HHH] syndrome) and aspartate (citrullinemia II) also have presentations different from the classic disorders. In this chapter, we discuss the clinical presentation, underlying molecular pathology, treatment options, and diagnostic testing for this group of diseases. The study of this group of disorders is of particular interest in gastroenterology because many acquired or genetic diseases of the liver have an impact on this cycle and the processing of ammonia and nitrogen. Many of the treatment strategies employed in treating patients with rare urea cycle defects are exportable to the larger community of patients with hyperammonemia.

SOME BASICS OF NITROGEN METABOLISM

The bulk of the nitrogen that requires processing comes from removal of the amino group on amino acids during the process of oxidative breakdown. This occurs both during normal metabolism and at a higher rate during times of caloric insufficiency or stress as a means of energy release. The brain produces a significant amount of ammonia, which it must convert to glutamine for export through the addition of nitrogen first to -ketoglutarate to make glutamate, which is then converted to glutamine with the addition of an additional nitrogen. This is an energy expensive process for the central nervous system. Under normal conditions in 5 L of blood, there are 150 μmol of soluble ammonia and 1000 mg of urea nitrogen. The conversion to urea is therefore a very efficient and mostly one-way process. Fish on the other hand don't bother to process ammonia into urea but excrete it into the water. The urea cycle itself uses up some energy with CPSI using two adenosine triphosphate (ATP) per reaction and argininosuccinic acid synthetase (ASS) converting one ATP to adenosine monophosphate (AMP). The net expenditure, however, is only one ATP because the production of fumarate by the cycle yields one nicotinamide adenine dinucleotide (NADH) molecule, which produces three ATP. As summarized in Table 36.1, the urea, once produced, is excreted primarily in the kidneys (75%), where it is used as a concentrating agent. The remaining 25% is excreted into the gut where bacteria can convert it into ammonia or use it to make their own amino acids or proteins. This can then re-enter the body through the portal system. Ammonia levels in the portal vein normally run between 100 and 300 μM compared with 10–30 μM in the general circulation. This is an efficient way for the body to conserve nitrogen during lean times.

CLINICAL PRESENTATION OF UREA CYCLE DEFECTS

The symptoms of urea cycle defects are primarily neurologic in origin. The acute disease presentation is brought about by

Table 36.1: Disposition of Urea

Most is excreted by the kidneys and serves as a concentrating agent.

Around 25% is not excreted by the kidneys but diffuses into the gut.
  Gut bacteria convert it back to ammonia.
  Bacteria will use some to make amino acids.
  Ammonia reenters the portal system (portal levels run 100–300 μmol/mL)

cerebral edema and neurocognitive dysfunction. Elevations in ammonia are thought to have a direct effect on cerebral edema, whereas elevations in brain glutamine levels (a buffer for excess nitrogen) are thought to affect neurotransmission and perhaps the edema as well [2–6]. Depending on the age of the patient, the outward manifestations of cerebral edema can vary from increased agitation or somnolence to neurologic posturing as pressure is brought to bear on the brainstem. The closed space of the skull magnifies the effect of the swelling and unchecked progression will typically result in complete venous stasis or herniation of the brainstem. Without aggressive treatment the prognosis for a patient with hyperammonemia and cerebral edema is poor. The exception to this clinical presentation are the disorders in the transporters (HHH syndrome and citrin deficiency) and arginase deficiency, which are described separately. Although we are addressing the inborn errors of urea cycle metabolism in this chapter, the reader should remember that there a number of conditions that affect the cycle that are not primarily genetic. In patients with partial defects in the urea cycle, symptoms may not appear until a sufficiently stressful event occurs to unmask the deficit. Table 36.2 outlines a few of these conditions that should be kept in mind.

There are no consistent findings on the histopathology of liver biopsies from patients with UCDs that are distinguishing. The exception to this is patients with defects in argininosuccinic

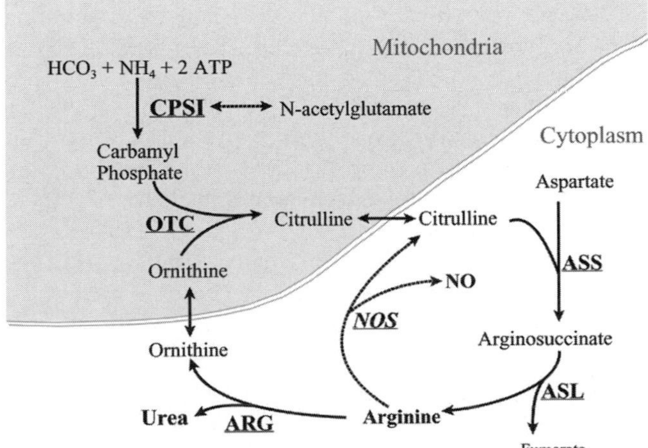

Figure 36.1. Diagram of the hepatic components of the urea cycle.

Table 36.2: Conditions That Affect or Stress Urea Cycle Function

Genetic defect in an enzyme

Damage to the liver (both chronic and acutely)
  Chemical toxins (ETOH, industrial, etc.)
  Infectious processes

Drug effects on the cycle
  Direct interference with enzymes
    Valproic acid (Depakote)
    Chemotherapy (particularly cyclophosphamide)
  Damage or general disruption of hepatic function
    Systemic antifungals
    Chemotherapy from hepatotoxic effects
    Acetaminophen

Other metabolic diseases
  Organic acidemias (such as methylmalonic, propionic, etc.)
  Pyruvate carboxylase deficiency
  Fatty acid oxidation defects
  Galactosemia
  Tyrosinemia
  Glycogen storage disease

Vascular bypass of the liver by scarring or vascular bypass

Nitrogen overload of the system
  Massive hemolysis (such as large bone fracture or trauma)
  Total parenteral nutrition
  Protein catabolism from starvation or bariatric surgery

Postpartum stress

Heart–lung transplant

Renal disease

GI bleeding

acid lyase deficiency. Many of these patients develop significant hepatomegaly (often extending to the pelvis) with progressive fibrosis of the liver. Serial biopsies of one of our patients with this disorder showed generalized cellular enlargement without a specific histologic pattern with the gradual development of fibrosis.

Neonatal Onset

This presentation typically is the result of a severe defect in urea cycle capacity. Although the stress and catabolism of the neonatal period creates an additional ammonia burden, there is clinical evidence that these patients will become hyperammonemic under even ideal conditions [7]. The difficulty with recognizing these patients is the similarity of their symptoms to other more common problems such as neonatal sepsis (Table 36.3). Infants with a UCD usually appear normal at birth but deteriorate as the ammonia, which is no longer filtered by the placenta, accumulates. This typically occurs within the first 48–72 hours of life, but may be delayed by 1–2 weeks. As they develop cerebral

Table 36.3: Symptoms of Newborns with Urea Cycle Defects

Normal appearance at birth
Somnolence progressing to lethargy then coma
Loss of thermoregulation (hypothermia)
Feeding disruption (increases catabolism)
Neurologic posturing (from cerebral edema)
Seizures
Hyperventilation and then hypoventilation

edema, they will manifest some agitation but then progress to somnolence and lethargy. They will also develop anorexia, and as their somnolence increases, their oral intake will continue to diminish. Most patients will develop some degree of dehydration from decreased intake. Although the decrease in oral intake will reduce the amount of dietary protein that can produce ammonia, the catabolism induced by poor intake and the stress of the neonatal period results in enough tissue protein breakdown to overwhelm this. As the cerebral edema and vascular stasis progresses the patient will first develop hyperventilation to adapt to the perceived blood flow changes resulting in an elevation in the blood pH from respiratory alkalosis. As the pressure increases on the brainstem and central nervous system (CNS) function fails, the patient's respiratory rate will decrease and eventually stop. A portion of patients will develop seizures of some form, although these can be difficult to detect in the context of decreasing CNS function. Unchecked, the patients will become comatose and eventually die from CNS failure often compounded by brainstem herniation.

Delayed Onset

Patients presenting in this timeframe typically have some partial function in their urea cycle [8]. The onset of their symptoms is a factor of their residual enzyme activity, diet, and environmental stressors (Table 36.4). These patients can manifest an acute hyperammonemic episode similar to the neonatal patients if they undergo a significant catabolic stress such as during an infection or after trauma. These episodes can occur anywhere from just outside the newborn period to quite late in life (sixth–seventh decade). Many of these patients will experience numerous mild hyperammonemic episodes, which can result in cumulative neurologic damage without an acute episode. It is unknown but possible that the chronic mild elevations of ammonia and glutamine affect neurologic development in these patients as well. The diagnosis of these cases is often delayed because the symptoms and signs can be quite subtle. As a probable result of mild hyperammonemia from dietary exposure, many of these patients subconsciously avoid protein in their diet, which can be an important historic clue. These patients can also have episodes triggered by drugs, which decrease urea cycle function such as valproic acid or chemotherapeutic agents [9–15]. Other reported triggers include postpartum stress, heart–lung transplant, short bowel, kidney disease, parenteral nutrition, gastrointestinal bleeding, and bariatric surgery [8].

Table 36.4: Common Clinical Features for Late Onset UCDs

Dramatic and rapid increase in nitrogen load from
Trauma
Rapid weight loss and autocatabolism
Increase in protein turnover from intravenous steroids
Patients tend to avoid protein in their diets
Patients often have history of behavioral or psychiatric illnesses
Rapid deterioration of neurolog status
Severe encephalopathy inconsistent with medical condition
Usually involve defects in first part of urea cycle
Evidence for cerebral edema by clinical exam or radiograph
Seizures in most cases
Decrease in oral intake in leading up to decompensation

HHH Syndrome (Ornithine Translocase Deficiency)

The HHH syndrome is an autosomal recessive inherited disorder in the ornithine translocase protein. The clinical symptoms are related to the hyperammonemia and resemble those of the UCD. Plasma ornithine concentrations are extremely high. The defect in ornithine translocase results in diminished ornithine transport into the mitochondria with ornithine accumulation in the cytoplasm and reduced intramitochondrial ornithine causing impaired ureagenesis and orotic aciduria. Homocitrulline is thought to originate from transcarbamylation of lysine. Most patients have intermittent hyperammonemia accompanied by vomiting, lethargy, and, in extreme cases, coma. Growth is abnormal, and intellectual development is affected. Spasticity is common, as are seizures. Adult patients are found with partial activity of the enzyme. They typically self-select low-protein diets. Diagnosis is complicated because plasma ornithine levels can normalize on a protein restricted diet. The presence of hyperammonemia and homocitrullinuria are helpful.

Citrin Deficiency (Citrullinemia II)

Citrullinemia II is an autosomal disorder that results in decreased activity in the liver of a transport molecule for aspartate. This results in limitation of activity for the enzyme argininosuccinic acid synthase, which combines aspartate and citrulline to make argininosuccinic acid (Figure 36.1). Citrin (the defective protein) is an aspartate glutamate transporter across the mitochondrial membrane. This defect can present with classic newborn hyperammonemia but is more likely to present with insidious neurologic findings in adulthood [16,17]. The majority of patients reported have been Japanese or Asian who share a common mutation. These patients can also have the dietary peculiarity of avoiding carbohydrates rather than protein. This is probably because of the overlap of this disorder

Table 36.5: Genes Directly Involved in the Urea Cycle and Urea Cycle Disorders

Gene Name	*Gene Symbol*	*Location*	*Protein Name*
Carbamylphosphate synthetase I	*CPS1*	2q35	Carbamoyl-phosphate synthase ammonia
Ornithine transcarbamylase	*OTC*	Xp21.1	Ornithine carbamoyltransferase
Argininosuccinate synthase	*ASS*	9q34	Argininosuccinate synthase
Argininosuccinate lyase	*ASL*	7cen-q11.2	Argininosuccinate lyase
Arginase	*ARG1*	6q23	Arginase 1
N-acetyl glutamate synthase	*NAGS*	17q21.3	N-acetyl glutamate synthetase
Ornithine transporter mitochondrial 1	*ORNT1*	13q14	Ornithine Transporter Mitochondrial 1
Citrin	*Citrin*	7q21.3	Proposed hepatic mitochondrial asparatate transporter

with glucose metabolism. Treatment for hyperammonemia is the same as the other UCD.

Arginase Deficiency

Arginase deficiency is not typically characterized by rapid-onset hyperammonemia. These patients often present with the development of progressive spasticity with greater severity in the lower limbs. They also develop seizures and gradually lose intellectual attainments. Growth is usually slow, and without therapy these patients usually do not reach normal adult height. Other symptoms that may present early in life include episodes of irritability, anorexia, and vomiting. Severe episodes of hyperammonemia are seen infrequently with this disorder but can be fatal. Diagnosis is made by the elevated levels of arginine in the blood and by analysis of enzymatic activity in red blood cells. Treatment is identical to other UCDs, with limitation of protein, use of essential amino acid supplements, and diversion of ammonia from the urea cycle with sodium benzoate or sodium phenylbutyrate.

MOLECULAR ASPECTS OF THE UREA CYCLE

The urea cycle is a model system for studying biochemical disease because it is the sole processing mechanism for waste nitrogen, has a manageable number of components, and is amenable to in vitro and in vivo testing of functional changes. As shown in Figure 36.1, the urea cycle is composed of five primary enzymes, one cofactor producer, and two transport molecules across the mitochondrial membrane. Inborn errors of metabolism are associated with each step in the pathway and have been well described over the years. The cycle has the interesting property of having a subset of the enzymes participate in another metabolic pathway, which produces nitric oxide (NO). The urea cycle as a nitrogen clearance system is limited primarily to the human liver and intestine with carbamyl phosphate synthetase and ornithine transcarbamylase limited exclusively to those tissues. The enzymes downstream that process citrulline into arginine are ubiquitous in their distribution. As the rate-limiting enzyme in the urea cycle, carbamyl phosphate synthetase I (CPSI) functional changes would have the greatest impact on cycle function from environmental stress. We have identified a number of polymorphisms in CPSI that appear to have functional significance, and affect disease states under environmental stress [18–22].

Other changes should also affect both the processing of ammonia and the ability to generate NO.

A brief review of the five enzymes and cofactor producer of the urea cycle is provided in Table 36.5.

Carbamyl Phosphate Synthetase I

Carbamyl phosphate synthetase I is the rate-limiting enzyme catalyzing the first committed step of the urea cycle (Figure 36.1), the primary system for removing waste nitrogen produced by protein metabolism. Expression of CPSI is limited to high levels in the liver and smaller amounts in the intestinal mucosa. It is compartmentalized within the mitochondria although it is genomically encoded. Mature CPSI is a 160-kDA protein monomer, which catalyzes the conversion of ammonia and bicarbonate to carbamyl phosphate (CP) with the expenditure of 2 ATPs. Posttranslational modification is currently unknown beyond cleavage of the first 38 residues after entry into the mitochondria [20,23–29].

Ornithine Transcarbamylase

Ornithine transcarbamylase (OTC) catalyzes the condensation of carbamyl phosphate and ornithine to citrulline. This homotrimer is encoded on the X chromosome and is the most common of the classically presenting UCDs [30–32]. Its location on the X chromosome results in a significant number of clinically affected carrier females. Unlike CPSI, human OTC can be successfully expressed in bacteria from recombinant plasmid. The crystalline structure for the gene has been determined. The X-linked nature of this disease makes the most commonly observed form of urea cycle defects.

Argininosuccinic Acid Synthase

Argininosuccinic acid synthase (ASS) catalyzes the condensation of aspartate and citrulline to form argininosuccinate. In addition to its critical role in the urea cycle, ASS is involved in the cycling of arginine and citrulline in the production of NO (Figure 36.1). Its distribution and regulation are tied into two systems, and this enzyme is found in most cells. The enzyme is found in the cytoplasm, and it requires the transport of citrulline out of the mitochondria to perform its function for the urea cycle. For NO synthesis it is located in calveolar complexes with ASL and NO synthase [33]. This enzyme also depends on the production of aspartate from either the tricarboxylic acid (TCA) cycle or protein catabolism. There exist 10 nonfunctional, widely dispersed pseudogenes for this enzyme, which suggest some method for repeated duplication within the genome [34]. Defects in this gene can present with hyperammonemia as severe as OTC and CPSI defects.

Argininocsuccinic Acid Lyase

Arginiocsuccinic acid lysase (ASL) catalyzes the cleavage of argininosuccinate into arginine and fumarate. Like ASS, it serves two masters and has a similar ubiquitous distribution and expression pattern. Of note, the enzyme resembles the Δ-crystalline gene in the eye and is a homotetramer [35]. This enzyme also demonstrates alternative splicing in a fraction of its product, which could be influenced by regional polymorphisms [36–38].

Arginase I

This enzyme is distributed throughout the body with high concentrations in the liver, kidney, and gut, as described by Cedarbaum et al. [39–44]. There is an arginase (Arg) II isozyme that has a more limited distribution and does not appear to play a significant role in ureagenesis [41]. A number of ongoing studies are looking at the role of arginase and its polymorphisms in asthma and NO metabolism [45–47]. The crystalline structure of this enzyme is known and will be helpful in elucidating the role of functional polymorphisms.

N-Acetyl Glutamate Synthetase

This enzyme and gene was recently characterized by Tuchman et al. [48–51]. Its distribution is under study but appears to match that of CPSI. This enzyme catalyzes the formation of N-acetylglutamate from glutamate and acetyl coenzyme A (CoA). This molecule is the essential allosteric cofactor for CPSI function. The production of NAG and CPSI's reliance on it may represent a key vulnerability to environmental factors in urea cycle function.

Ornithine Transporter Mitochondrial 1

This liver-expressed enzyme is responsible for the transport of ornithine across the mitochondrial membrane in the liver. It is associated with a hyperammonemia disorder known as HHH syndrome.

Citrin

Citrin or solute carrier family 25 has been reported as the causative gene for citrullinemia II almost exclusively in Asian patients [16,17,52–56]. The citrin transporter is a calcium-binding mitochondrial transporter that is thought to transport aspartate and glutamate across the mitochondrial membrane. Defects in this gene would affect the ability of ASS to produce argininosuccinate. Beyond the effects on the urea cycle, defects in this transporter also appear to cause generalized hepatic disease [17,52,53,55].

DIAGNOSIS

The first step in diagnosing UCDs is clinical suspicion. A blood ammonia level is the first laboratory test to evaluate a patient with a suspected UCD. Particular care should be taken in drawing a blood ammonia because there is significant variability depending on proper technique and handling The clinician should remember that treatment should not be delayed in efforts to reach a final diagnosis and that later stages of treatment should be tailored to the specific disorder. Laboratory data useful in the diagnosis of UCDs include plasma ammonia levels, pH, CO_2, the anion gap, plasma amino acids, and urine organic acid analyses [57,58]. Patients with true urea cycle defects typically have normal glucose and electrolyte levels. The pH and CO_2 can vary with the degree of cerebral edema and hyper- or hypoventilation. In neonates, it should be remembered that the basal ammonia level is elevated over that of adults, which typically is less than 35 μmol/L (100 μmol/L is often observed). An elevated plasma ammonia level of 150 μmol/L or higher, associated with a normal anion gap and a normal blood glucose level, is a strong indication for the presence of a urea cycle defect. Quantitative amino acid analysis can be used to evaluate these patients and arrive at a tentative diagnosis. Elevations or depressions of the intermediate amino containing molecules arginine, citrulline, and argininosuccinate (Figure 36.1) offer clues to the point of defect in the cycle. The amino acid profile in sick newborns is often quite different from those in children and adults and should be taken into account [58]. The levels of the nitrogen buffering amino acid glutamine will also be quite high and can serve as confirmation of the hyperammonemia.

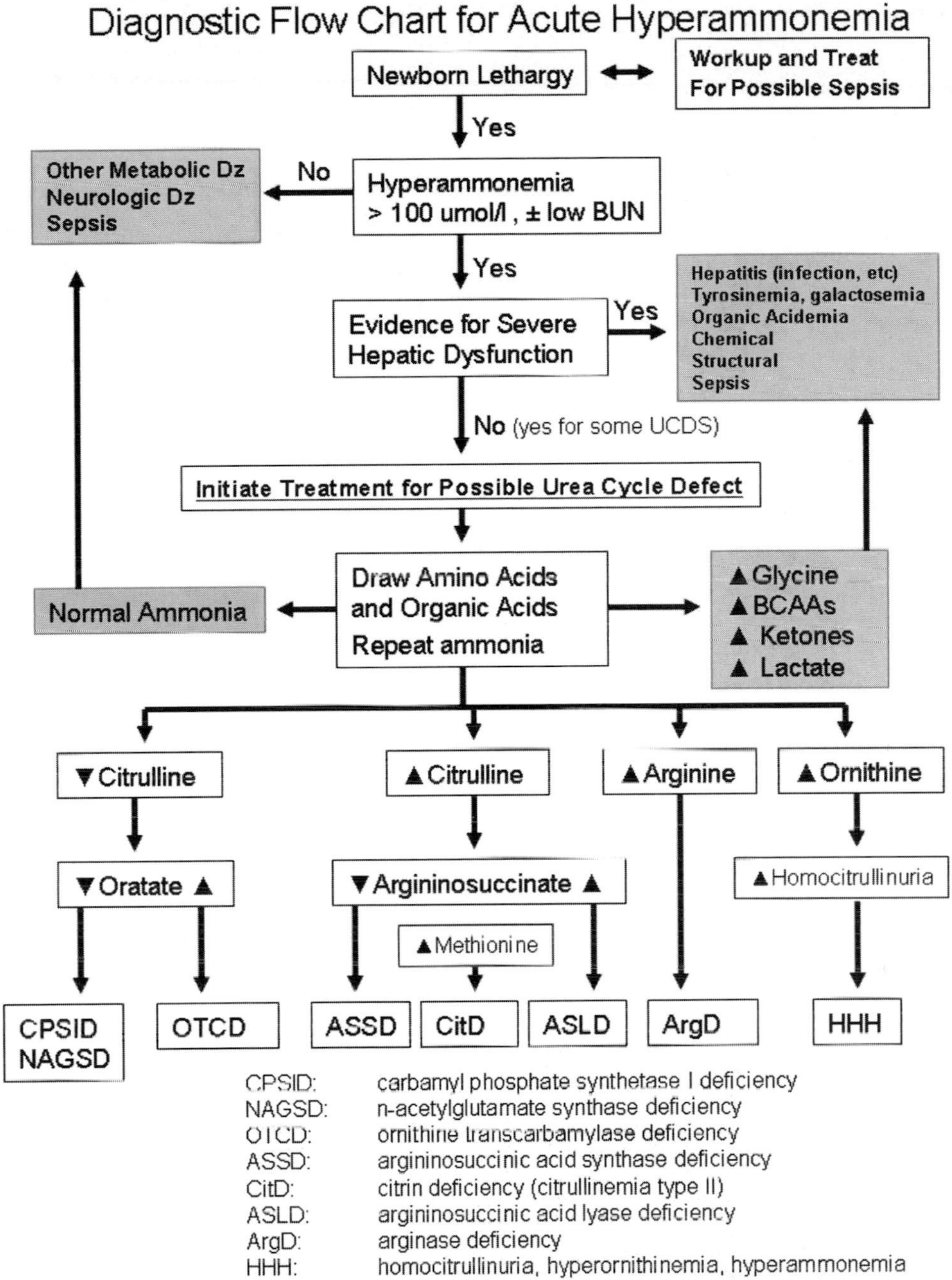

Figure 36.2. Algorithm for evaluating hyperammonemia.

If a defect in NAGS, CPSI, or OTC is suspected, the presence of the organic acid orotic acid in the urine can help distinguish the diagnosis. Orotic acid is produced when there is an overabundance of carbamyl phosphate, which spills into the pyrimidine biosynthetic system.

As shown in Figure 36.2, the process of working up a UCD can be somewhat systematized. This algorithm is useful when examining the data for these patients, but some flexibility in interpretation should always be maintained. Experience has taught that each of these patients has presentation characteristics unique to themselves.

Enzymatic and genetic diagnosis is available for all of these disorders. For CPSI, OTC, and NAGS, enzymatic diagnosis is made on a liver biopsy specimen freshly frozen in liquid nitrogen [59]. Enzymatic testing for ASS and ASL can be done on fibroblast samples, and arginase can be tested on red blood cells [57]. Clinically approved DNA sequence analysis is only available for OTC at the time of this writing, but its availability for the other disorders is anticipated soon. A frequently updated Web resource for testing information can be found at the National Institutes of Health (NIH)-sponsored site: http://www.geneclinics.org.

Table 36.6: Overall Goals of Therapy

Maximize protection of central nervous system

Physically remove large ammonia load (dialysis)

Add pharmacologic agents to remove nitrogen

Treat catabolic state

Stages of management

- Recognition
- Emergency management and stabilization
- Bulk ammonia removal and nitrogen scavenging
- Stabilization (drug/diet)

Table 36.7: Considerations in the Acute Management of Severe Hyperammonemia

Emergency management

- Fluids, dextrose, and interlipid to mitigate catabolism and typical dehydration (attempt 80 cal/kg/day)
- Antibiotics and septic workup to treat potential triggering events or primary sepsis (continue through treatment course)
- Contact and possible transport to treatment-capable institute as soon as possible
- Remove protein from intake (PO or TPN)
- Establish central venous access
- Provide physiologic support (pressors, buffering agents, etc.)
- (Renal output is critical to long-term success.)
- Stabilize airway because cerebral edema may result in sudden respiratory arrest

TREATMENT OF UREA CYCLE DISORDERS

This section provides an overview of urea cycle management (Table 36.6). The proper treatment of these patients requires a highly coordinated team of specialists trained in caring for patients with inborn errors of metabolism. An NIH-sponsored Web site with links to experts in urea cycle management and treatment protocols is available at http://www.rarediseasesnetwork.org/ucdc.

Management of patients in a urea-cycle-based hyperammonemic coma is based on three interdependent principles: first, physical removal of the ammonia by dialysis or some form of hemofiltration; second, reversal of the catabolic state through caloric supplementation and, in extreme cases, hormonal suppression (glucose/insulin drip); and third, pharmacologic scavenging of excess nitrogen.

Central venous access should be established and dialysis, if available, begun at the highest available flow rate [60]. Dialysis is effective for the removal of ammonia, and the clearance is dependent on the flow through the dialysis circuit. In severe cases of hyperammonemia, provision for hemofiltration should be made to follow the dialysis until the patient is stabilized and the catabolic state is reversed. Some patients will reaccumulate ammonia after their initial round of dialysis and may require additional periods of dialysis. Most patients will have a slight rise in ammonia after dialysis because removal by scavengers and the liver will not be as effective. This slight rise usually does not necessitate repeat dialysis.

Management of the catabolic state is often overlooked in its importance (Table 36.7). Because the catabolism of protein stores is often the triggering event for hyperammonemia, the patient will not completely stabilize until it is reversed. Fluids, dextrose, and intravenous fat emulsions (e.g., Intralipid) should be given to blunt the catabolic process. The patient should be assessed for dehydration and fluids replaced. Because these patients suffer from cerebral edema, care should be taken with overhydration. The nitrogen-scavenging drugs are usually administered in a large volume of fluid, which should be taken into consideration. A regimen of 80 cal/kg/day is a reasonable goal. Although it is not common practice at all centers, the administration of insulin and glucose are useful in profound catabolic states. At the same time, protein should be *temporarily* removed from intake (orally [PO] or total parenteral nutrition [TPN]). Supplementation of arginine serves to replace arginine not produced by the urea cycle (in addition to the partial cycle function it can stimulate) and prevents its deficiency from causing additional protein catabolism. Refeeding the patient as soon as practicable is useful because more calories can be administered this way. The use of essential amino acid formulations in feeding can reduce the amount of protein necessary to meet basic needs.

Emergency pharmacologic management (Table 36.8) with ammonia scavengers and arginine is initiated as soon as possible using the drug combination phenylacetate and benzoate (Ammonul, Ucyclyd Pharma), ideally while the dialysis is being arranged and the diagnostic workup is under way (Table 36.6). Two agents are used in combination to trap nitrogen in excretable forms. Sodium benzoate combines with glycine to make hippurate, which is excreted by the kidneys (or removed in the dialysate), and sodium phenylacetate combines with glutamine to make phenacetylglutamine, which is also excreted in the urine [61,62]. The body replaces these amino acids using excess nitrogen. It is suspected that the removal of glutamine by phenylacetate has the additional benefit of removing a compound suspected of having a major role in the neurotoxicity of these disorders [4,63–67]. Arginine is also used in the acute phase of treatment of UCDs. In addition to replenishing circulating amino acid levels, arginine can use those parts of the cycle not affected by genetic blocks and incorporate some nitrogen. Because arginine is the precursor for NO production, it is worth considering modification of the arginine dose downward if the patient develops vasodilation and hypotension. The

Table 36.8: Recommended Dosing of Urea Cycle Drugs by Diagnosis and Size

Intravenous Priming Infusion Given over 90–120 Minutes for Infants and Children

Diagnosis	*Dosing NaPA/NaBZ*	*10% Arginine*	*Dose Delivered NaPA/NaBZ (Each)*	*I 10% Arginine*
	0–20 kg			
CPSD, OTCD, NAGSD	2.5 mL/kg	2.0 mL/kg	250 mg/kg	200 mg/kg
ASSD, ASLD, unknown	2.5 mL/kg	6.0 mL/kg	250 mg/kg	600 mg/kg
ARGD	2.5 mL/kg	none	250 mg/kg	none
	>20 kg			
CPSD, OTCD, NAGSD	55 mL/m^2	2.0 mL/kg	5.5 g/m^2	200 mg/kg
ASSD, ASLD, unknown	55 mL/m^2	6.0 mL/kg	5.5 g/m^2	600 mg/kg
ARGD	55 mL/m^2	none	5.5 g/m^2	none

Intravenous Maintenance Dosing of Drugs per 24 Hours

Diagnosis	*Dosing NaPA/NaBZ*	*10% Arginine*	*Dose Delivered NaPA/NaBZ (Each)*	*I 10% Arginine*
	0–20 kg			
CPSD, OTCD, NAGSD	2.5 mL/kg	2.0 mL/kg	250 mg/kg	200 mg/kg
ASSD, ASLD, unknown	2.5 mL/kg	6.0 mL/kg	250 mg/kg	600 mg/kg
ARGD	2.5 mL/kg	none	250 mg/kg	none
	>20 kg			
CPSD, OTCD, NAGSD	55 mL/m^2	2.0 mL/kg	5.5 g/m^2	200 mg/kg
ASSD, ASLD, unknown	55 mL/m^2	6.0 mL/kg	5.5 g/m^2	600 mg/kg
ARGD	55 mL/m^2	none	5.5 g/m^2	none

NaPA/NaBZ, sodium phenylacetate, sodium benzoate (Ammonul)

dosages and administration of these drugs should only be done in consultation with an experienced specialist. A resource for finding these physicians and other treatment suggestions is the NIH-sponsored Urea Cycle Disorders Consortium found at http://www.rarediseasesnetwork.org/ucdc.

After the initial loading phase and dialysis, the patients should be converted to the maintenance doses of the ammonia scavengers listed in the manufacturers packaging insert. If the exact enzyme defect is known the amount of arginine administered can be adjusted downward. If chronic therapy is warranted, the patient can then be switched to the oral pro-drug of phenylacetate, phenylbutyrate (Buphenyl).

OTHER TREATMENT ISSUES

The use of osmotic agents such as mannitol is not considered effective in treating the cerebral edema from hyperammonemia, but this is mainly anecdotal. In canines, opening the blood–brain barrier with mannitol resulted in cerebral edema by promoting the entry of ammonia into the brain fluid compartment [5,68]. Intravenous steroids and valproic acid should be avoided. Measures to reduce cerebral metabolism to protect the brain, such as head cooling, have been proposed, but their efficacy is untested. Antibiotics and a septic workup are indicated to treat potential triggering events. Other measures include physiologic support (pressors, buffering agents to maintain pH and buffer arginine HCl, etc.) and maintenance of renal output, particularly if ammonia scavengers are being used. Finally, it is imperative to reassess continuation of care after the initial phase of treatment.

Rapid response to the hyperammonemia improves outcome. Symptomatology centers around cerebral edema and pressure on the brainstem. The resulting decrease in cerebral blood flow plus prolonged seizures, when they occur, are poor prognostic factors. In adults, because the sutures of the skull are fused, sensitivity to hyperammonemia appears considerably greater than in children. Thus, treatment should be aggressive and instituted at a lower ammonia concentration than in children.

Neurologic Evaluation

Cerebral studies should be conducted to determine the efficacy of treatment and whether continuation is warranted. Electroencephalogram should be performed because so many of these patients develop status epilepticus. If available, magnetic resonance imaging–determined cerebral blood flow can be used to establish whether venous stasis has occurred from the cerebral edema. Evaluation of brainstem function and higher cortical function are useful to assess outcome. Finally, the decision for continuation is based on baseline neurologic status, duration of the patient's coma, and potential for recovery and whether the patient is a candidate for transplantation. If the basic UCD is severe enough, then liver transplantation should be considered. Criteria for transplantation are, of course, linked back to neurologic status, duration of coma, and availability of livers.

Diagnostic samples of DNA, liver, and skin should be obtained because they can be central in family counseling and future treatment issues.

Long Term Management

Every effort should be made to avoid triggering events. In particular, intravenous steroids for asthma or valproic acid are contraindicated. Long-term diet modification with nutritional oversight is often necessary in patients with chronic episodes of hyperammonemia. Patients should also avoid dehydration, an especially common occurrence among adults in connection with alcohol intake, hiking, and airline flights. Not all adult patients who recover from a hyperammonemic episode require chronic nitrogen scavengers, but they ought to be considered because many of these patients can become more brittle as time goes on. Special precautions must be taken to avoid catabolism during subsequent illnesses or surgeries, as well as during any event resulting in significant bleeding or tissue damage.

Should psychiatric problems occur over the long term, caregivers should be alert to the possibility of hyperammonemia. In addition, many patients with citrullinemia type 2 in particular have presented with mental disturbance [16,17].

Clinical observation of patients with argininosuccinic acid lyase demonstrate a high incidence of chronic progressive cirrhosis with eventual fibrosis of the liver. This finding is not commonly seen in the other UCDs, and studies are underway to better determine the exact pathophysiology.

It is important to provide genetic counseling to assess risk to other family members.

NEW DIRECTIONS IN UREA CYCLE RESEARCH

Polymorphisms and mutations in CPSI, the rate-limiting portion of the urea cycle, are an excellent model to apply the concept of environmental–genetic interaction [21]. As shown in Figure 36.1, the urea cycle interacts with the production of NO and is the sole source for arginine, which is NO's direct precursor. The effect of these changes on intermediates and subsequent NO formation modifies a number of pathophysiologic systems [18,20–22,69]. This idea of genetic environmental interaction is not new; however, CPSI provides an excellent example of this concept. Commonly distributed functional polymorphisms in CPSI may not result in hyperammonemia but instead affect the production of downstream metabolic intermediates during key periods of need. Under duress, shortages of these precursor molecules uncouple NO synthase (NOS) from the generation of NO. Besides resulting in a paucity of NO, the enzyme can continue to donate electrons and generate additional free radicals resulting in further damage. These findings may play a role in the pathophysiology of surgically related pulmonary hypertension, bone marrow transplant toxicity, blood pressure regulation, and asthma [18,21,22,45,69,70].

There is also a long-term effort underway to study the pathophysiology and clinical outcome of these patients. The Urea Cycle Disorders Consortium and the National Urea Cycle Disorder Foundation can provide information to interested patients and families. Both of these resources can be easily located on the world wide web.

SUMMARY

The urea cycle provides an excellent model for the understanding of inborn errors of metabolism. Defects throughout the cycle affect a variety of molecular mechanisms including: catalytic enzymes, cofactor producers, and transport proteins. The timely diagnosis and treatment of these diseases directly affects the outcome of the patient, and awareness by the clinician is paramount. In addition to their clinical impact as inborn errors, mild defects in the urea cycle also affect the production of NO under physiologically stressful conditions. The availability of urea cycle intermediates, developed for the treatment of the rare diseases, in the treatment of these more common conditions may have consequences well beyond the limited number of urea cycle deficient patients.

REFERENCES

1. Krebs HA, Henseleit K. Untersuchungen uber die harnstoffbildung im tierkorper. Hoppe-Seyler's Z Physiol Chem 1932;210: 325–32.
2. Batshaw ML. Hyperammonemia. Curr Probl in Pediatr 1984;14: 1–69.
3. Brusilow SW. Urea cycle disorders: clinical paradigm of hyperammonemic encephalopathy. Prog Liver Dis 1995;13:293–309.
4. Butterworth RF. Effects of hyperammonaemia on brain function [review]. J Inherit Metab Dis 1998;21Suppl 1:6–20.
5. Fujiwara M. Role of ammonia in the pathogenesis of brain edema. Acta Medica Okayama 1986;40:313–20.
6. Takahashi H, Koehler RC, Hirata T, et al. Restoration of cerebrovascular CO_2 responsivity by glutamine synthesis inhibition in hyperammonemic rats. Circ Res 1992;71:1220–30.

7. Tuchman M, Mauer SM, Holzknecht RA, et al. Prospective versus clinical diagnosis and therapy of acute neonatal hyperammonaemia in two sisters with carbamyl phosphate synthetase deficiency. J Inherit Metab Dis 1992;15:269–77.
8. Summar ML, Barr F, Dawling S, et al. Unmasked adult-onset urea cycle disorders in the critical care setting. Crit Care Clin 2005; 21 Suppl 4:S1–8.
9. Mitchell RB, Wagner JE, Karp JE, et al. Syndrome of idiopathic hyperammonemia after high-dose chemotherapy: review of nine cases [see comments]. Am J Med 1988;85:662–7.
10. Batshaw ML, Brusilow SW. Valproate-induced hyperammonemia. Ann Neurol 1982;11:319–21.
11. Bourrier P, Varache N, Alquier P, et al. [Cerebral edema with hyperammonemia in valpromide poisoning. Manifestation in an adult, of a partial deficit in type I carbamylphosphate synthetase]. In French. Presse Med 1988;17:2063–6.
12. Castro-Gago M, Rodrigo-Saez E, Novo-Rodriguez I, et al. Hyperaminoacidemia in epileptic children treated with valproic acid. Childs Nerv Syst 1990;6:434–6.
13. Elgudin L, Hall Y, Schubert D. Ammonia induced encephalopathy from valproic acid in a bipolar patient: case report. Int J Psychiatry Med 2003;33:91–6.
14. Kugoh T, Yamamoto M, Hosokawa K. Blood ammonia level during valproic acid therapy. Jpn J Psychiatry Neurol 1986;40:663–8.
15. Vainstein G, Korzets Z, Pomeranz A, Gadot N. Deepening coma in an epileptic patient: the missing link to the urea cycle. Hyperammonaemic metabolic encephalopathy. Nephrol Dial Transplant 2002;17:1351–3.
16. Saheki T, Kobayashi K. Mitochondrial aspartate glutamate carrier (citrin) deficiency as the cause of adult-onset type II citrullinemia (CTLN2) and idiopathic neonatal hepatitis (NICCD). J Hum Genet 2002;47:333–41.
17. Saheki T, Kobayashi K, Iijima M, et al. Adult-onset type II citrullinemia and idiopathic neonatal hepatitis caused by citrin deficiency: involvement of the aspartate glutamate carrier for urea synthesis and maintenance of the urea cycle. Mol Genet Metab 2004;81 Suppl 1:S20–6.
18. Pearson DL, Dawling S, Walsh WF, et al. Neonatal pulmonary hypertension – urea-cycle intermediates, nitric oxide production, and carbamoyl-phosphate synthetase function. N Engl J Med 2001;344:1832–8.
19. Summar M. Molecular genetic research into carbamyl phosphate synthetase i: molecular defects, prenatal diagnosis, and cDNA sequence. J Inherit Metab Dis 1998;21:30–9.
20. Summar ML, Hall LD, Eeds AM, et al. Characterization of genomic structure and polymorphisms in the human carbamyl phosphate synthetase I gene. Gene 2003;311:51–7.
21. Summar ML, Hall L, Christman B, et al. Environmentally determined genetic expression: clinical correlates with molecular variants of carbamyl phosphate synthetase I. Mol Genet Metab 2004; 81 Suppl:12–19.
22. Summar ML, Gainer JV, Pretorius M, et al. Relationship between carbamoyl-phosphate synthetase genotype and systemic vascular function. Hypertension 2004;43:186–91.
23. Britton HG, Garcia-Espana A, Goya P, et al. A structure-reactivity study of the binding of acetylglutamate to carbamoyl phosphate synthetase I. Eur J Biochem 1990;188:47–53.
24. Guy HI, Evans DR. Function of the major synthetase subdomains of carbamyl-phosphate synthetase. J Biol Chem 1996;271: 13762–9.
25. Guy HI, Evans DR. Substructure of the amidotransferase domain of mammalian carbamyl phosphate synthetase. J Biol Chem 1995;270:2190–7.
26. Mareya SM, Raushel FM. Mapping the structural domains of E. coli carbamoyl phosphate synthetase using limited proteolysis. Bioorg Med Chem 1995;3:525–32.
27. Powers-Lee SG, Corina K. Domain structure of rat liver carbamoyl phosphate synthetase I. J Biol Chem 1986;261:15349–52.
28. Rubio V, Cervera J. The carbamoyl-phosphate synthase family and carbamate kinase: structure-function studies [review]. Biochem Soc Trans1995;23:879–83.
29. Rubio V. Structure-function studies in carbamoyl phosphate synthetases [review]. Biochem Soc Trans 1993;21:198–202.
30. Tuchman M, McCullough BA, Yudkoff M. The molecular basis of ornithine transcarbamylase deficiency. Eur J Pediatr 2000;159 Suppl 3:S196–8.
31. Tuchman M, Jaleel N, Morizono H, et al. Mutations and polymorphisms in the human ornithine transcarbamylase gene. Hum Mutat 2002;19:93–107.
32. Yeh SJ, Hou WL, Tsai WS, et al. Ornithine transcarbamylase deficiency. J Formos Med Assoc 1997;96:43–5.
33. Solomonson LP, Flam BR, Pendleton LC, et al. The caveolar nitric oxide synthase/arginine regeneration system for NO production in endothelial cells. J Exp Biol 2003;206:2083–7.
34. Beaudet AL, Su TS, O'Brien WE, et al. Dispersion of argininosuccinate-synthetase-like human genes to multiple autosomes and the X chromosome. Cell 1982;30:287–93.
35. Takiguchi M, Matsubasa T, Amaya Y, Mori M. Evolutionary aspects of urea cycle enzyme genes. Bioessays 1989;10:163–6.
36. Abramson RD, Barbosa P, Kalumuck K, O'Brien WE. Characterization of the human argininosuccinate lyase gene and analysis of exon skipping. Genomics 1991;10:126–32.
37. Barbosa P, Cialkowski M, O'Brien WE. Analysis of naturally occurring and site directed mutations in the argininosuccinate lyase gene. J Biol Chem 1991;266:5286–90.
38. Linnebank M, Tschiedel E, Haberle J, et al. Argininosuccinate lyase (ASL) deficiency: mutation analysis in 27 patients and a completed structure of the human ASL gene. Hum Genet 2002; 111:350–9.
39. Ash DE, Scolnick LR, Kanyo ZF, et al. Molecular basis of hyperargininemia: structure-function consequences of mutations in human liver arginase. Mol Genet Metab 1998;64:243–9.
40. Cederbaum SD, Spector EB. Arginase activity in fibroblasts. Am J Hum Genet 1978;30:91–2.
41. Cederbaum SD, Yu H, Grody WW, et al. Arginases I and II: do their functions overlap? Mol Genet Metab 2004;81Suppl 1:S38–44.
42. Dizikes GJ, Grody WW, Kern RM, Cederbaum SD. Isolation of human liver arginase cDNA and demonstration of nonhomology between the two human arginase genes. Biochem Biophys Res Commun 1986;141:53–9.
43. Dizikes GJ, Spector EB, Cederbaum SD. Cloning of rat liver arginase cDNA and elucidation of regulation of arginase gene expression in H4 rat hepatoma cells. Somat Cell Mol Genet 1986; 12:375–84.
44. Grody WW, Dizikes GJ, Cederbaum SD. Human arginase isozymes. Isozymes Curr Top Biol Med Res 1987;13:181–214.
45. Meurs H, Maarsingh H, Zaagsma J. Arginase and asthma: novel insights into nitric oxide homeostasis and airway hyperresponsiveness. Trends Pharmacol Sci 2003;24:450–5.

46. Ricciardolo FL. cNOS-iNOS paradigm and arginase in asthma. Trends Pharmacol Sci 2003;24:560–1.
47. Rudmann DG, Moore MW, Tepper JS, et al. Modulation of allergic inflammation in mice deficient in TNF receptors. Am J Physiol Lung Cell Mol Physiol 2000;279:L1047–57.
48. Caldovic L, Tuchman M. N-acetylglutamate and its changing role through evolution. Biochem J 2003;372:279–90.
49. Caldovic L, Morizono H, Gracia PM, et al. Cloning and expression of the human N-acetylglutamate synthase gene. Biochem Biophys Res Commun 2002;299:581–6.
50. Caldovic L, Morizono H, Yu X, et al. Identification, cloning and expression of the mouse N-acetylglutamate synthase gene. Biochem J 2002;364:825–31.
51. Tuchman M, Holzknecht RA. Human hepatic N-acetylglutamate content and N-acetylglutamate synthase activity. Determination by stable isotope dilution. Biochem J 1990;271:325–9.
52. Ben Shalom E, Kobayashi K, Shaag A, et al. Infantile citrullinemia caused by citrin deficiency with increased dibasic amino acids. Mol Genet Metab 2002;77:202–8.
53. Naito E, Ito M, Matsuura S, et al. Type II citrullinaemia (citrin deficiency) in a neonate with hypergalactosaemia detected by mass screening. J Inherit Metab Dis 2002;25:71–6.
54. Ohura T, Kobayashi K, Abukawa D, et al. A novel inborn error of metabolism detected by elevated methionine and/or galactose in newborn screening: neonatal intrahepatic cholestasis caused by citrin deficiency. Eur J Pediatr 2003;162:317–22.
55. Tamamori A, Okano Y, Ozaki H, et al. Neonatal intrahepatic cholestasis caused by citrin deficiency: severe hepatic dysfunction in an infant requiring liver transplantation. Eur J Pediatr 2002; 161:609–13.
56. Yamaguchi N, Kobayashi K, Yasuda T, et al. Screening of SLC25A13 mutations in early and late onset patients with citrin deficiency and in the Japanese population: identification of two novel mutations and establishment of multiple DNA diagnosis methods for nine mutations. Hum Mutat 2002;19:122–30.
57. Steiner RD, Cederbaum SD. Laboratory evaluation of urea cycle disorders. J Pediatr 2001;138 Suppl 1:S21–9.
58. Summar M. Current strategies for the management of neonatal urea cycle disorders. J Pediatr 2001;138 Suppl 1:S30–9.
59. Tuchman M, Tsai MY, Holzknecht RA, Brusilow SW. Carbamyl phosphate synthetase and ornithine transcarbamylase activities in enzyme-deficient human liver measured by radiochromatography and correlated with outcome. Pediatr Res 1989;26:77–82.
60. Summar M, Pietsch J, Deshpande J, Schulman G. Effective hemodialysis and hemofiltration driven by an extracorporeal membrane oxygenation pump in infants with hyperammonemia. J Pediatr 1996;128:379–82.
61. Batshaw ML. Sodium benzoate and arginine: alternative pathway therapy in inborn errors of urea synthesis. Prog Clin Biol Res 1983;127:69–83.
62. Batshaw ML, Brusilow SW. Evidence of lack of toxicity of sodium phenylacetate and sodium benzoate in treating urea cycle enzymopathies. J Inherit Metab Dis 1981;4:231.
63. Batshaw ML, Brusilow SW. Treatment of hyperammonemic coma caused by inborn errors of urea synthesis. J Pediatr 1980; 97:893–900.
64. Brusilow SW, Valle DL, Batshaw M. New pathways of nitrogen excretion in inborn errors of urea synthesis. Lancet 1979;2:452–4.
65. Brusilow SW. Phenylacetylglutamine may replace urea as a vehicle for waste nitrogen excretion. Pediatr Res 1991;29:147–50.
66. Connelly A, Cross JH, Gadian DG, et al. Magnetic resonance spectroscopy shows increased brain glutamine in ornithine carbamoyl transferase deficiency. Pediatr Res 1993;33:77–81.
67. Willard-Mack CL, Koehler RC, Hirata T, et al. Inhibition of glutamine synthetase reduces ammonia-induced astrocyte swelling in rat. Neuroscience 1996;71:589–99.
68. Fujiwara M, Watanabe A, Shiota T, et al. Hyperammonemia-induced cytotoxic brain edema under osmotic opening of blood-brain barrier in dogs. Res Exp Med (Berl) 1985;185:425–7.
69. Barr FE, Beverley H, VanHook K, et al. Effect of cardiopulmonary bypass on urea cycle intermediates and nitric oxide levels after congenital heart surgery. J Pediatr 2003;142:26–30.
70. Williams SM, Ritchie MD, Phillips JA III, et al. Multilocus analysis of hypertension: a hierarchical approach. Hum Hered 2004;57:28–38.

Section V: Other Conditions and Issues in Pediatric Hepatology

37

Bacterial, Parasitic, and Fungal Infections of the Liver

Donald A. Novak, M.D., Gregory Y. Lauwers, M.D., and Richard L. Kradin, M.D.

Both systemic and local infections caused by bacterial, fungal, and parasitic agents may cause significant hepatic dysfunction. This chapter attempts to delineate clinical syndromes caused by some of these organisms in the pediatric patient.

BACTERIAL INFECTIONS

Hyperbilirubinemia Associated with Sepsis

Although jaundice in association with bacterial sepsis may occur in adult patients, it appears to be significantly more common during infancy. Historically, infections of the urinary tract predominate; however, sepsis originating from other sites may contribute [1–4]. Accordingly, gram-negative bacilli, and especially *Escherichia coli*, are responsible for the majority of cases, although gram-positive organisms have been associated. Abnormal liver chemistries are found in approximately 50% of premature neonates with gram-negative bacteremia [5]. Clinical and laboratory manifestations are primarily those of the underlying disease state. Hyperbilirubinemia may be marked, with the direct fraction predominant [1]. Alkaline phosphatase levels are often elevated, and serum aminotransferase values remain normal or minimally increased [6,7]. Hepatic biopsy usually demonstrates canalicular cholestasis, with minimal evidence of hepatocyte damage or inflammatory response [6] (Figure 37.1). On occasion, the biopsy may demonstrate prominent acute cholangitis with portal bile ductular proliferation, pathologic changes often seen in large bile duct obstruction. In these cases, the possibility of large duct obstruction must be excluded by ultrasound or endoscopic retrograde cholangiopancreatography (ERCP). Jaundice resolves with appropriate treatment of the underlying infection; duration of jaundice may vary from several days to several weeks. Although the pathophysiology of sepsis-related cholestasis has not been fully elucidated, recent work suggests a role for endotoxin, known to diminish bile flow and provoke cholestasis [8,9]. Other inflammatory mediators with potential roles include tumor necrosis factor, the leukotrienes, and interleukin-1 [10]. Fatty liver has also been reported in conjunction with gram negative sepsis [11].

Pyogenic Hepatic Abscess

Pyogenic liver abscess (PLA) continues to be a significant source of morbidity, if not mortality, in the pediatric population. Although early reports (prior to 1977) quoted an incidence of 3 in 100,000 hospital admissions [12], recent studies have suggested an increasing rate of PLA, conditionally attributed to improved overall survival of immunocompromised patients [13]. Concomitantly, mortality has fallen from older estimates of 36% to approximately 15% in a recent series [12,14]; mortality rates are higher in those with multiple abscesses [15]. Patients at risk include those with impaired host defenses; chronic granulomatous disease and leukemia are commonly noted [16]. Approximately 50% of children with PLA are under age 6 years [13].

Clinical manifestations of PLA in children are nonspecific but commonly include fever, abdominal pain, right upper quadrant tenderness, and hepatomegaly [12,13,17–19]. Multiple abscesses, as well as those caused by gas-forming organisms [20], may present in a more fulminant manner. Ruptured abscesses presenting with abdominal pain and septic shock are also associated with higher mortality rates [21]. Laboratory findings may include elevation of the erythrocyte sedimentation rate, leukocytosis, anemia, and hypoalbuminemia. Serum aminotransferase and bilirubin values may be variably elevated; in series of adult patients, serum alkaline phosphatase values are more reliably increased. Diagnosis of PLA is generally made via a high index of clinical suspicion in conjunction with appropriate imaging techniques. Approximately 75% of PLAs are located in the right lobe of the liver. In a 1989 review of 109 pediatric patients with PLA, computerized tomographic (CT) scanning and angiography were noted to be the most sensitive techniques, followed by ultrasound and radioisotope scanning [13]. Magnetic resonance imaging (MRI) has been less well studied in the pediatric population but may prove useful in the detection of small lesions [22]. All techniques currently available are hampered by a lack of specificity. Because the differential diagnosis of intrahepatic cysts includes abscess due to nonpyogenic organisms, congenital cysts, tumor with central necrosis,

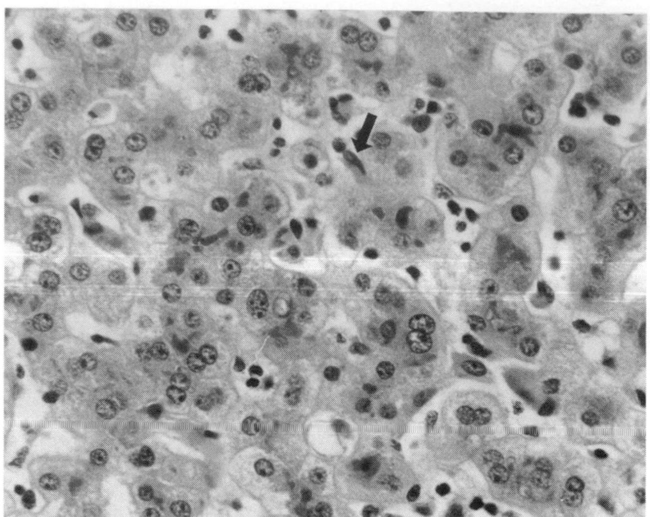

Figure 37.1. Sepsis. Perivenular hepatocytes demonstrate dilated canaliculi containing bile. The sinusoids contain a mixed inflammatory infiltrate associated with Kupffer cell hyperplasia.

hemorrhage, or a combination of these, as well as vascular malformation, specific diagnosis generally requires lesion aspiration with subsequent gram stain and culture. In appropriate clinical situations, serology for hydatid disease and *E. histolytica* should be considered before aspiration. Percutaneous drainage under CT or ultrasound guidance is often feasible, particularly in the case of large, solitary, superficial lesions (Figure 37.2) [23,24]. As opposed to adult patients, in whom gram-negative bacilli predominate, *Staphylococcus aureus* is the predominant etiologic agent in pediatric patients [12,13,17,25]. This may reflect the significant number of immunocompromised patients in pediatric series of PLA. Enteric gram-negative bacteria, predominantly *E. coli* and *Klebsiella* sp., account for approximately 31% of PLA in recent series, whereas anaerobic organisms are causative in at least 15% [26,27]. Infections may be mixed [28]. Tuberculosis is a rare cause of hepatic abscess [29,30] as is actinomycosis [31]; fungal and parasitic infections are described later in the chapter.

The etiology of PLA is variable. Adult series demonstrate a preponderance of patients with preexisting biliary tract disease, in whom PLA develops as a consequence of cholangitis [32]. Traumatic injury to the liver may result in PLA [33], as may sepsis. Extension from contiguous sites of infection may occur. Predisposition by prior infection with *Toxocara canis* has also been hypothesized [34]. In pediatric patients, altered host defenses seem to play an important role [13,35], as may portal vein bacteremia from intra-abdominal infectious processes (i.e., appendiceal abscess [32], abscess secondary to ingested foreign body [36], and inflammatory bowel disease [37]). Pyogenic liver abscess has also been associated with the use of umbilical venous catheters in the newborn population [38,39]. Approximately one half of patients in adult series had no evident etiology.

Successful therapy of PLA is contingent upon rapid and accurate diagnostic efforts. Drainage and appropriate antibiotic coverage continue to be the mainstays of therapy. Initial antibiotic coverage should be broad spectrum, including agents effective against gram-positive aerobes, gram-negative bacilli, and anaerobic organisms [28,32,40]. Subsequent therapy is dictated by culture results. Percutaneous drainage is indicated in those patients in whom lesions are accessible under CT or ultrasound guidance [23,24]. Catheters placed via these techniques are generally left in place until abscess collapse, usually 24–72 hours. Irrigation may be required. Alternatively, single or, if required, multiple discrete aspirations can be performed instead of leaving a catheter in place [41,42]. Potential contraindications to these techniques include inaccessible lesions and ascites. Complications include peritonitis, formation of additional abscess collections, fistula formation, hepatic laceration, and hemorrhage [32,43]. Patients in whom percutaneous drainage is not feasible or in whom an additional source of

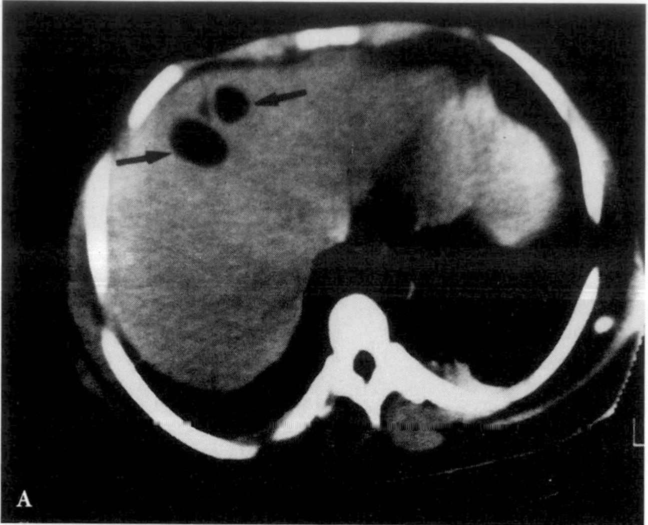

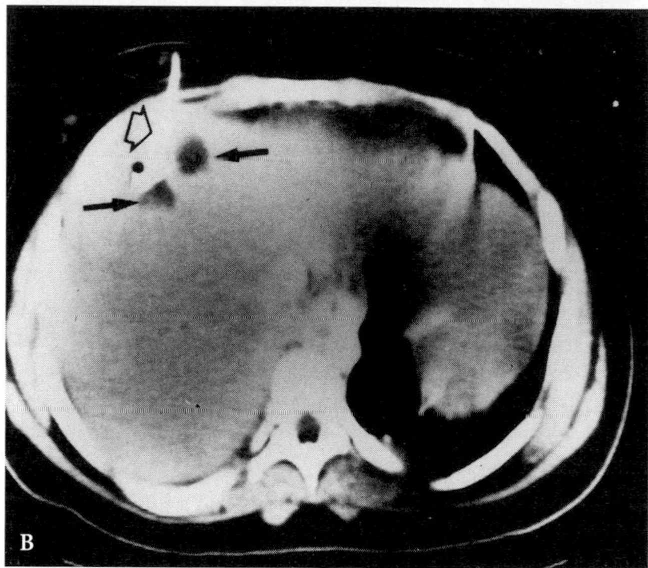

Figure 37.2. Computerized tomographic image of pyogenic liver abscess before (**A**) and after (**B**) percutaneous drainage. (**A**) *Arrows* point to abscess cavities. (**B**) *Open arrow* indicates percutaneous drainage catheter.

intra-abdominal infection (or biliary obstruction) exists, may require open drainage procedures [44]. Nonoperative management has also been reported, primarily in patients with multiple abscesses [32]. Success in this instance is more likely when abscesses are small [45]. Duration of antibiotic therapy is variable. Treatment periods of 3–6 weeks are generally accepted. Prognosis is as denoted earlier but is worse in patients with multiple abscesses.

Cholangitis

Bacterial cholangitis, or infection of the biliary system, is a relatively uncommon event in pediatrics [46]. At risk patients are those with abnormalities of the biliary tract, especially following hepatic portoenterostomy after a diagnosis of biliary atresia [47–49]. Risk of cholangitis post-Kasai procedure is approximately 40–50% [48], with highest incidence occurring in the first 3 months after surgery. Late-onset cases have also been reported [49] Other conditions that may predispose to cholangitis include choledocholithiasis, choledochal cyst, and Caroli's disease [50]. Rarely, cholangitis in the absence of other risk factors may be noted [50].

The etiology of cholangitis is multifactorial [51,52]. The normal biliary tract is sterile; the sphincter of Oddi aids in the prevention of bacterial reflux into the biliary tree from the duodenum. Destruction of this sphincter mechanism, as occurs in the Kasai procedure, may be associated with ascending bacterial colonization from the bowel. Indeed, patients in whom adequate bile drainage is attained after Kasai have a higher incidence of cholangitis than do those in whom surgery was unsuccessful [47,48]. This illustrates the importance of direct contact between the biliary system and bowel flora in the pathogenesis of cholangitis. Biliary infection may also be produced via portal bacteremia. Conversely, the presence of bacteria in the bile is probably not sufficient to produce clinically significant cholangitis. It is likely that a combination of biliary obstruction and infected bile is required. In this regard, biliary parasites may play an important role [53].

Classically, the combination of right upper quadrant abdominal pain, fever, and jaundice, denoted Charcot's triad, has been associated with the majority of adult patients with cholangitis [54]. Bowel sounds are generally present. Hypotension may be a presenting feature in approximately 5% of adult patients [52]. Presenting clinical features in a series of pediatric patients post-Kasai procedure included fever (100%), acholic stools or increase in serum bilirubin (68%), shock, and decrease in bile flow (43%) [48]. Associated laboratory findings include leukocytosis or leukopenia, elevated erythrocyte sedimentation rates, and, as noted, increased serum bilirubin. Other features often noted in series of adult patients include elevation of serum alkaline phosphatase and aminotransferase values. Further diagnostic evaluation of the patient with suspected cholangitis should include bacteriologic cultures of the blood and urine. Blood cultures may provide the etiologic organism in approximately 50% of patients [48]. Initial imaging studies should include either ultrasonography or CT scanning to evaluate for (1) abscess formation associated with cholangitis, (2) presence of calculi, (3) presence of ductal dilation, or (4) other obstructing lesions including choledochal cyst or periportal mass [52]. Magnetic resonance cholangiopancreatography (MRCP) may also be useful in selected cases [55,56]. Patients in whom culture results are negative should undergo a percutaneous hepatic biopsy, both for culture and histologic examination. Performed in the presence of normal coagulation parameters, this procedure has been shown to be relatively safe (morbidity of approximately 1%) [46], and, at least in adult series, may be safely performed in the presence of ductal dilation. Hepatic culture was positive in 32 of 69 pediatric patients with presumed cholangitis studied by Ecoffey et al. [48]. *E. coli* was the most frequently isolated pathogen (50% of first and second cholangitis episodes) in this and other studies [52]. Other commonly isolated organisms include *Klebsiella* sp., *Enterococcus*, *Bacteroides* sp., *Enterobacter* sp., and *Pseudomonas* sp. [53]. Anaerobic organisms may also be isolated; mixed cultures are not uncommon. In approximately 30% of episodes, no bacterial agent is identified. Hepatic histologic changes may be useful in these cases. Pathologic alterations include infiltration of the portal triads, bile ductules, and ductule lumens with neutrophils. Portal edema may occur, as may changes consistent with biliary obstruction (Figure 37.3) [57].

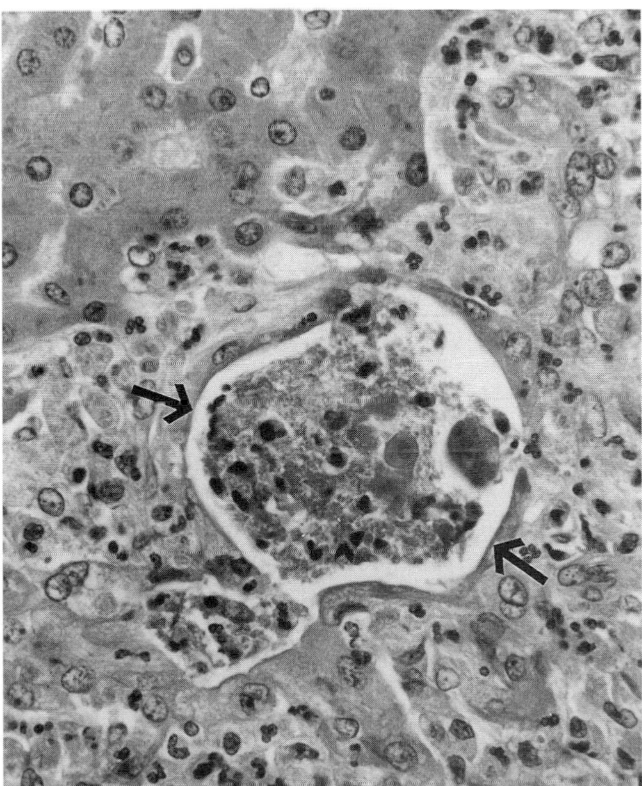

Figure 37.3. Cholangitis following hepatic portoenterostomy. The lumen of the bile duct is filled with acute inflammatory cells and necrotic debris. Neutrophils extend into the bile duct epithelium and surrounding portal tract stroma. The epithelium lining the bile duct is reactive and focally attenuated.

Therapy of acute cholangitis includes careful attention to vital signs and perfusion status, providing adequate fluid resuscitation and pressure support if needed. The patient is made nulla per os; nasogastric suction may be required in the presence of ileus [52]. Toxic patients with evidence of biliary obstruction may require emergent endoscopic, percutaneous, or, less commonly, operative intervention. In most other patients, intervention should be withheld until after several days of antibiotic therapy and defervescence of fever [55,58]. Antibiotic therapy is initially given by the parenteral route. Choice of antibiotics is governed by sensitivities of common organisms and achievable serum and biliary antibiotic levels [59]. Ampicillin, although widely used, is associated with a high percentage of treatment failures and should probably be supplanted by use of a third-generation cephalosporin (i.e., cefotaxime) in combination with an aminoglycoside [60]. Alternatively, a broad-spectrum penicillin derivative with good biliary penetration (i.e., mezlocillin) may be used. The newer penicillin derivatives have the advantage of covering *S. faecalis* as well as a variety of anaerobic organisms. Mezlocillin used alone has been prospectively compared with an ampicillin–gentamicin regimen in the treatment of cholangitis in adults and found to have a higher rate of cure in addition to a lower incidence of toxicity [60]. Ciprofloxacin has gained acceptance in the therapy of cholangitis in adults; however, use in young children continues to be debated [55]. Trimethoprim-sulfamethoxazole has also been used [48]. Particularly ill patients may require addition of specific anaerobic coverage. Duration of treatment is generally 21 days.

Biliary decompression may be required in those patients with biliary obstruction. Initial data regarding site of obstruction may be garnered through use of spiral CT or MRCP [55]. Subsequently, ERCP and placement of nasobiliary drainage tubes [52,61] after papillotomy and stone removal (if necessary) is performed. These procedures have now been safely performed in significant numbers of pediatric patients [62]. Subsequent cholangiography may delineate the site of obstruction, allowing definitive therapy to be undertaken endoscopically in select cases. Percutaneous cholangiography and decompression have also been advocated. Finally, surgical intervention may be required in some cases [54] .

The prognosis of cholangitis in pediatric patients has not been clearly delineated, but in one study of cholangitis post-Kasai, the mortality rate was approximately 1% [48]. Mortality in adult series is considerably higher, presumably because of the higher incidence of malignant lesions and debilitated patients in these groups. Repeated episodes of cholangitis can result in the cessation or diminution of bile flow in those patients who have undergone successful Kasai procedures. Therefore, aggressive diagnostic and therapeutic efforts seem justified in this population.

Cat Scratch Disease

Cat scratch disease [CSD], caused by pleomorphic gram-negative [63] bacteria identified as *Bartonella henselae* [64],

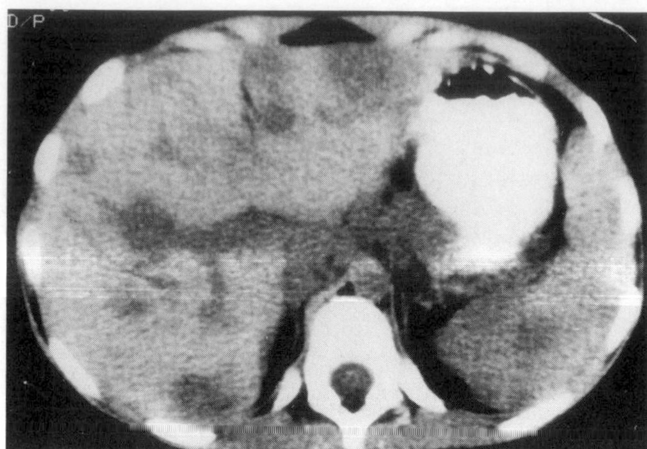

Figure 37.4. Computerized tomographic image of the liver and spleen in cat scratch disease. Multiple areas of low attenuation are visible throughout the hepatic and splenic parenchyma.

typically consists of regional lymphadenitis following inoculation of the responsible agent, usually by a cat. Clinical manifestations may also include encephalitis, pneumonitis, arthritis, osteomyelitis, and neuroretinitis [65]. Although hepatosplenomegaly and anicteric hepatitis had previously been reported in association with CSD [66,67], the association of CSD with hepatic and splenic abscesses was first noted in 1985 [68]. Affected patients often present with fever and abdominal pain [64,69]. Clinically evident adenopathy is generally but not universally present [70,71]. Elevated erythrocyte sedimentation rates are frequently observed, whereas serum aminotransferase, bilirubin, and alkaline phosphatase levels are typically normal. Abdominal imaging studies, usually performed as part of an evaluation for fever of unknown origin, reveal multiple, small, hypodense lesions in the parenchyma of the liver and spleen (Figure 37.4) [69,70]. *B. hensalae* antibody titers are characteristically elevated [72]. At surgery, firm nodules are noted. Biopsy often reveals necrotizing granulomatous hepatitis [68–70]. Organisms may be noted within the lesions (Figure 37.5). Direct confirmation of identity may be made through the demonstration of B. hensalae DNA in the hepatic tissue via polymerase chain reaction (PCR) [73]. Differential diagnosis includes other causes of hepatic granulomas, including infection with a variety of bacterial, fungal, parasitic, and viral agents. In addition, neoplasms, hypersensitivity reactions, and sarcoidosis must be considered. In the absence of widely available culture techniques for the cat scratch bacilli, precise diagnosis in the proper clinical situation, (i.e., lymphadenopathy, history of cat contact or scratch, and identification of inoculation site) necessitates elimination of other causes of granulomatous hepatitis.

Therapy remains problematic; however, some authorities recommend parenteral antibiotic treatment, often gentamicin [74], for up to 3 weeks [69]. Potentially effective oral therapy includes trimethoprim-sulfamethoxazole, rifampin,

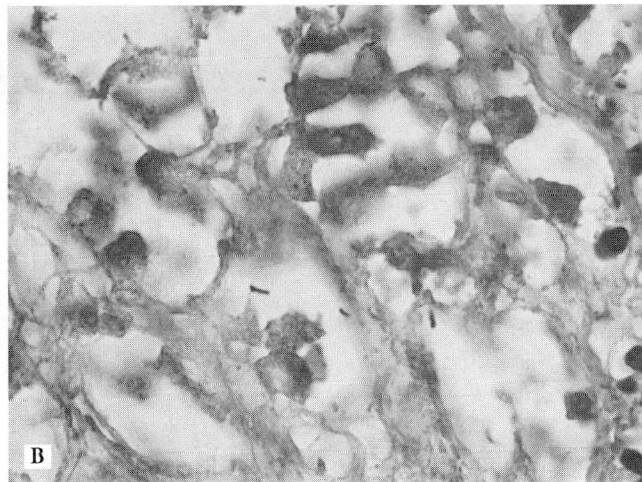

Figure 37.5. Hepatic involvement in cat scratch diease. (**A**) Portal region showing nonspecific chronic lymphocytic inflammation extending across the limiting plate of an adjacent hepatic lobule. (**B**) A Warthin-Starry silver stain shows several extracellular bacilli located within the collagenous matrix.

azithromycin dihydrate, and ciprofloxacin [74]. Corticosteroids have also been employed in cases with persistent fever [75]. Recovery appears to be complete.

Perihepatitis

First noted by Stajano in 1919, Fitz-Hugh (1934) [76] and Curtis (1930) [77] independently described the syndrome of perihepatitis associated with salpingitis that now bears their names. Generally noted in young women, symptoms include acute onset, severe right upper quadrant pain, occasionally with radiation to the shoulder and back [78]. Pain is intensified by the intake of breath or palpation of the abdomen. A friction rub may be present over the anterior liver surface. Fever may be present. The patient often has both a history of previous pelvic inflammatory disease and physical findings suggestive of same. Laboratory findings are nonspecific but often include an elevated erythrocyte sedimentation rate. Serum aminotransferase levels are normal or minimally elevated. CT scanning of the abdomen may reveal hyperemia of the anterior liver surface [79]. Laparoscopic (laparotomy) findings early in the course of perihepatitis include "violin string" adhesions between the hepatic capsule and the adjacent abdominal wall and diaphragm. Later findings consist of hemorrhagic spots and white fibrous plaques on the liver surface. The hepatic parenchyma does not appear involved. Diagnosis in the proper clinical situation is made via isolation of the causative microorganisms, *N. gonorrhoeae* or *C. trachomatis* from the cervix, urethra, or rectum [80,81]. In addition, serology for *C. trachomatis* may be sought. The pathophysiology of perihepatitis associated with salpingitis remains uncertain. Postulated mechanisms include ascending infection from the genital tract to the perihepatic region, as well as spread via the blood stream. Treatment is through eradication of the underlying infection with an appropriate antibiotic regimen.

The liver may also be involved in patients with gonococcal bacteremia; approximately 50% may have abnormalities of serum aminotransferase levels [82].

Typhoid Hepatitis

Typhoid fever, most often caused by *S. typhi* and *S. paratyphi*, is a syndrome characterized by fever, headache, and abdominal pain [83]. A relative bradycardia may be present. Subsequent findings may include pneumonia and encephalopathy. Intestinal perforation or bleeding may occur. Approximately 27% of patients have hepatomegaly [84], and 5–10% of patients will have clinical jaundice. Serum aminotransferase levels and alkaline phosphatase are mildly abnormal in 50% of cases. In one series, symptoms of hepatitis were present in 5% of patients [84]. A recent series demonstrated abnormal liver chemistries in 36% of patients with *S. enteritidis* enterocolitis [85]. Hepatic biopsy findings are relatively nonspecific and include the presence of typhoid nodules (focal areas of hepatocyte necrosis surrounded by a mononuclear cell infiltrate), sinusoidal dilation, and mononuclear cell inflammation of portal tracts. Less frequently noted were ballooning degeneration of hepatocytes, steatosis; hepatic granulomata have also been reported [86]. Typically, findings were noted in combination and could be found in biopsies from patients without hepatomegaly. Similar changes have been noted in experimental animals injected with *Salmonella* endotoxin [87], suggesting a role for endotoxin in the pathogenesis of these lesions. Diagnosis is established via culture or serology (or both). Hepatic abnormalities typically resolve with treatment of the underlying infection [85].

Brucellosis

Brucellosis, in humans generally attributable to *B. melitensis*, *B. abortus*, or *B. suis*, is an often prolonged illness characterized in children by fever, weight loss, malaise, arthralgia, back pain, and headache [88]. Complications may include abscess formation, meningoencephalitis, pneumonitis, osteomyelitis, nephritis, and endocarditis. Infection is typically acquired via contact with infected animals or ingestion of contaminated milk products.

Hepatic involvement in brucellosis is relatively common. Approximately 25% of affected children have hepatosplenomegaly on physical exam [78] (as opposed to 41% in adults) [89] and 84% have abnormal hepatic enzyme studies [89]. Clinical jaundice is relatively infrequent. Other common laboratory abnormalities in children include lymphocytosis and elevation of the erythrocyte sedimentation rate. Liver biopsy findings include portal inflammation and focal hepatocyte necrosis in 90% of patients [90], whereas noncaseating granuloma formation may be noted in up to 70% of patients primarily within the first 100 days of illness. Diagnosis is made through history of possible exposure, culture and PCR of infected tissue, as well as by specific serology [91]. Treatment is with tetracycline or doxycycline in conjunction with rifampin. Trimethoprim-sulfamethoxazole may be used in children aged under 9 years [92]. In rare cases of hepatic abscess secondary to *Brucella*, surgery made be required in addition to medical therapy [93].

Tularemia

Caused by infection with *Francisella tularensis*, tularemia may occur in typhoidal or ulceroglandular forms. Infection is typically via exposure to infected mammalian vectors (i.e., rabbits, squirrels, dogs, or cats) or through tick bites, although other more tangential methods of spread have been reported [94]. Hepatic involvement appears to be relatively infrequent; however, one series reported abnormal liver tests in 58% [95]. Hepatomegaly, clinical hepatitis, and hepatic abscess formation have all been reported [96]. Pathologic findings in tularemic hepatitis include focal coagulative necrosis with chronic inflammatory infiltrate. Diagnosis is via examination of serum *F. tularemsis* titers and culture. Treatment is with streptomycin, aminoglycoside antibiotics, or tetracycline[97].

Yersinia enterocolitica has been implicated in the development of hepatic abscesses in the setting of hemochromatosis in adults [98,99].

Toxic Shock Syndrome (TSS)

Described as a complication of tampon use, TSS is a consequence of bacterial infection generally attributable to staphylococcal and streptococcal species. Diagnostic criteria include fever, diffuse macular rash with desquamation (primarily of palms and soles 1–2 weeks after disease onset), hypotension, involvement of three or more organ systems including central nervous, hepatic, mucous membrane, renal, muscular, hematologic, or gastrointestinal systems, and negative workup for other potential causes [100]. Hepatic involvement in TSS has been described by several investigators. Cholestasis, as delineated by elevated serum bile acid and bilirubin levels, has been noted in conjunction with elevated serum aminotransferase values [101]. Pathologic changes consistent with an acute cholangitis were described by Ishak and Rogers [102]. Other observed alterations included portal inflammation and steatosis. Minimal intrahepatic cholestasis was noted. A role for staphylococcal enterotoxin (TSST-1) has been postulated [103].

Streptococcal Infection

Infections with group A β-hemolytic streptococci have long been associated with hepatic dysfunction. Jaundice has been reported as both an early and late complication of scarlet fever; the late onset component may have reflected use of serum therapy in the early 1900s [104]. Early-onset jaundice was noted in association with hepatic tenderness and hepatomegaly. Pathologic findings include focal areas of hepatocyte necrosis, as well as portal inflammatory infiltrates consisting of polymorphonuclear leukocytes and lymphocytes. Streptococci may be noted in biopsy specimens [87,104]. The etiology of observed alterations is unclear but may involve direct infection versus toxin effect. Streptococcus has also been associated with fulminant hepatic failure [105]. Hepatic abnormalities resolve with adequate anti-infective therapy, generally consisting of a β-lactamase–resistant antistaphylococcal agent in conjunction with clindamycin, which inhibits bacterial protein synthesis [106].

Pneumococcal infections, including those manifested by pneumonia, are also associated with a high incidence of hepatic enzyme abnormalities and, less frequently, jaundice [107,108]. Differential diagnosis of pneumonia associated with cholestasis must also include that caused by *Legionella* [103].

Listeriosis

Listeria monocytogenes is a gram-positive bacillus that may be acquired transplacentally, perinatally, or via genital contact [109]. Nosocomial and food-borne outbreaks have also been reported. Neonates, those with preexisting hepatic disease (including hepatic transplantation), and immunosuppressed individuals are most at risk [110–112]. The disorder is characterized by the formation of granulomas. In neonates, the liver is often diffusely involved. Hepatic involvement is noted less often in older individuals. Other clinical manifestations may include, depending on age, respiratory distress, cardiac dysfunction, meningitis, endocarditis, and osteomyelitis. Diagnosis is made through the use of cultures. Treatment is generally undertaken with ampicillin in combination with gentamycin or other aminoglycosides [113,114].

Tuberculosis

Involvement of the liver in tuberculosis is well known. In congenital tuberculosis, the liver is often the primary site of infection, perhaps because of blood flow through the ductus venosus [115]. In older patients, the liver is also frequently affected. Up to 75% of patients with extrapulmonary tuberculosis [116], as

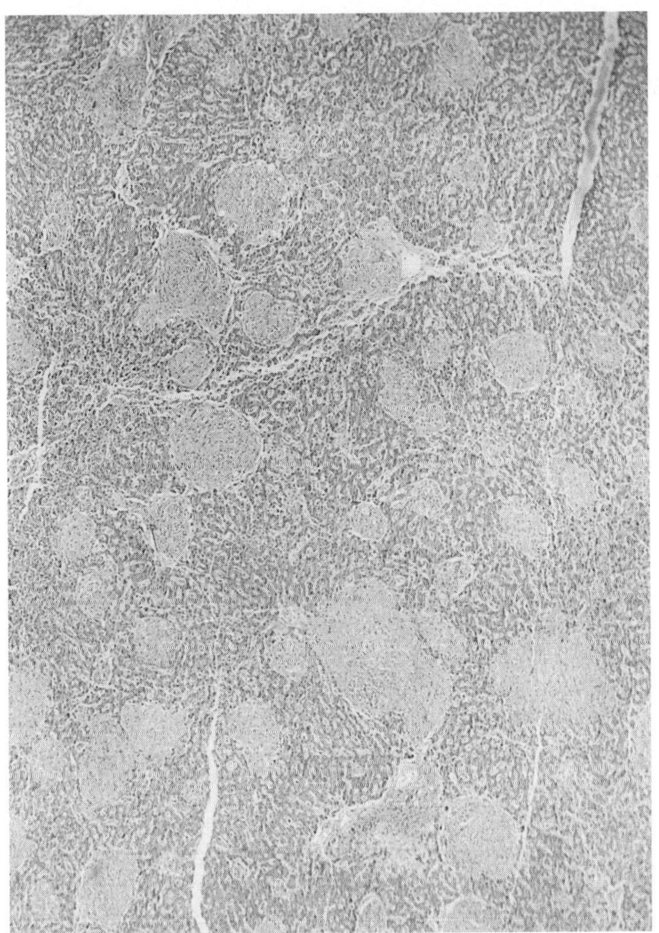

Figure 37.6. Miliary tuberculosis. Numerous oval epithelioid granulomas are scattered throughout the liver.

well as most patients with miliary tuberculosis, have hepatic involvement, as do smaller proportions of those with pulmonary involvement. Hepatic manifestations are heterogeneous; most common are small hepatic granulomas found in portal areas. Early granulomas are composed of lymphocytes and epithelioid cells; subsequently, giant cell formation and necrosis may predominate. Lesions may reach 1–2 mm in size in miliary tuberculosis [117] (Figure 37.6). Larger, 1–2 cm tuberculomata may be seen, as may tuberculous hepatic abscesses, either in conjunction with an extrahepatic foci of infection or as a primary lesion. Biliary obstruction may occur as the result of perihilar adenopathy [118]. Presenting symptoms typically depend on the location of associated disease; most hepatic disease attributed to tuberculosis is asymptomatic. Congenital tuberculosis may present in the first 1–2 weeks of life with failure to thrive; hepatosplenomegaly and jaundice may be later manifestations. In older patients, weight loss, fever, and anorexia predominate; abdominal pain is sometimes present. Hepatomegaly is common; splenomegaly is less frequently appreciated. Jaundice may occur, as may ascites. Alkaline phosphatase levels are abnormal in approximately 75% of cases, and aminotransferase levels in 35%. Plain film of the abdomen may reveal large, confluent, hepatic calcifications as well as calcifications along the course of the common bile duct [119]. CT of the liver may reveal abscess formation; ring enhancement may be present; CT may also reveal the diffuse, small, low-density lesions typical of miliary tuberculosis [120]. Duct dilation may be noted with CT or ultrasonography. Endoscopic retrograde cholangiography or percutaneous transhepatic cholangiography (or both) may be required to delineate the site of ductal obstruction [119]. Laparoscopy may be a highly specific means of diagnosing hepatic tuberculomata. Alvarez and Carpio [118] found visible lesions in 49 of 53 cases examined. Diagnosis generally requires biopsy; both histology (with appropriate stains for acid fast bacteria) and culture should be performed. Culture of other sites, including gastric aspirate, sputum, and bone marrow, may be appropriate. Polymerase chain reaction assays may also be of use [121].

Treatment is that of active tuberculosis: for susceptible strains, 2 months of isoniazid, rifampin, and pyrazinamide daily, followed by 4 months of isoniazid and rifampin [122]. Abscesses may require percutaneous catheter placement and drainage [123]; surgery is occasionally required. The prognosis of hepatic tuberculosis in children is unclear. The worst prognosis may be in neonatally acquired infection.

Mycobacterium avium complex (MAC) has also been associated with liver disease, generally in the setting of profound immunodeficiency associated with advanced human immunodeficiency virus (HIV) infection [124]. Liver disease generally occurs in the context of systemic disease. Elevated aminotransferase and alkaline phosphatase levels are frequently noted. Granulomas containing prominent foamy macrophages may be noted on liver biopsy; acid fast bacilli may be seen in some cases (Figure 37.7) [125]. Diagnosis of disseminated MAC generally is made by culture of blood, sputum, or feces. Treatment is through the use of a combination of at least two drugs with antimycobacterial activity; ethambutol and clarithromycin are most often used [126]. Prophylaxis with azithromycin or clarithromycin is recommended for HIV infected patients with profound immunosuppression [127].

Actinomycosis

Actinomycosis is caused by *Actinomyces israelli*, a ubiquitous organism found worldwide. Part of normal human oral flora, *A. israelli* may also be responsible for infections of the cervicofacial, abdominal, and thoracic regions. Hepatic infection typically occurs via direct extension or portal vein seeding from other intra-abdominal foci of infection. Hepatic infection may be primary in 15% of cases [128]. Early hepatic infection may present nonspecifically as hepatitis [129]. Subsequent infection results in hepatic abscess formation [130]. Advanced infection may also mimic hepatic neoplasia [131]. Sinus formation is common and may discourage attempts at percutaneous aspiration in suspected cases. Diagnosis is made via positive culture and demonstration of "sulfur" granules, diagnostic of actinomycosis. Therapy is undertaken with high-dose intravenous penicillin; subsequent oral therapy may include penicillin or

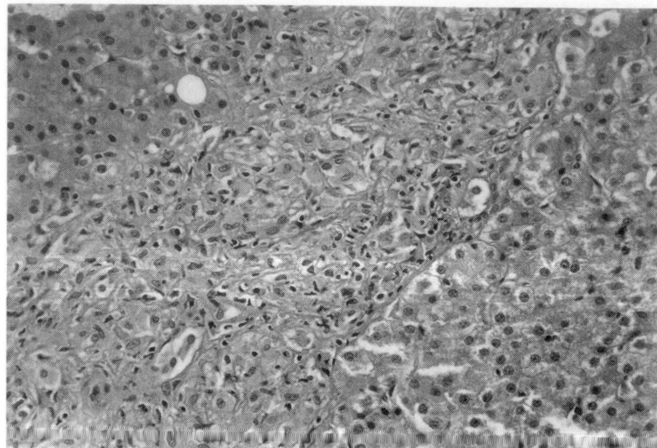

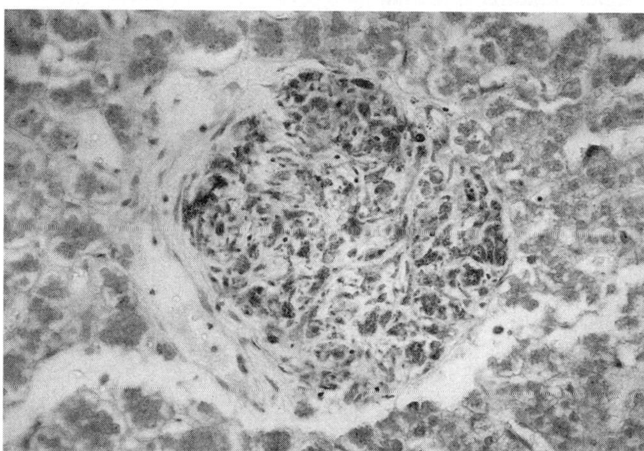

Figure 37.7 *Mycobacterium avium* complex. Non-necrotizing epithelioid granuloma formed of large foamy histiocytes (*top*). Acid-fast bacillus stain demonstrates bacilli engulfed by histiocytes (*bottom*).

tetracycline. Treatment for up to 1 year may be necessary [132]. Surgical resection of large lesions may be required [133].

Ehrlichioses

The ehrlichioses are a group of tick-borne diseases caused by bacteria of the genus ehrlichiosis [134]. These bacteria infect either human monocytes (*E. Chaffeensis,* transmitted by Lone Star ticks) or human granulocytes (human granulocyte ehrlichiosis agent, transmitted by *Ixodes scapularis* and *Ixodes pacificus*). Symptoms include fever, headache, myalgia, and malaise. Complications include prolonged fever, shock, adult respiratory distress syndrome, mental status changes, pneumonitis, and rhabdomyolysis, among others. Approximately 70–90% of affected patients demonstrate abnormal aminotransferase levels, peaking on day 6–7 of illness at approximately 10 times normal values, and then decreasing slowly as the illness resolves [135]. Liver pathology has been studied in a limited number of patients. Cholestasis, with neutrophilic infiltration of bile duct epithelium suggesting bile duct obstruction, has been noted [136,137]. Sinusoidal monocytic infiltration has been a more common finding [136–138]. Others note focal hepatic necrosis and/or ring granuloma formation [139]. Diagnosis is made through serology and the use of the PCR [140]. Treatment is generally undertaken with tetracycline derivatives [134]. Hepatic abnormalities resolve completely after therapy.

Syphilis

The liver is a common site of involvement in both congenital and secondary syphilis. Indeed, transfer of treponemes across the placenta into the fetal circulation presumably accounts for the widespread organ involvement noted in congenital syphilis [141]. Symptomatic infants are often small for gestational age, with evidence of lymphadenopathy, hemolytic anemia, and thrombocytopenia. Bony abnormalities may occur in 80–90% of affected infants, and rash occurs in 40–60%. Other associated findings include neurologic disease, dental and ocular abnormalities, and nephrosis [142–144]. Hepatic involvement is frequent, with hepatomegaly estimated to occur in 50–90% of symptomatic infants. Rarely, hepatic failure may occur [145]. Conjugated hyperbilirubinemia may also occur. Diagnosis is made through use of serology. Evaluation of the infant with findings suggestive of congenital syphilis should include serum venereal disease research laboratory (VDRL), x-ray examination of the long bones, and examination of cerebrospinal fluid. Hepatic biopsy is generally not required for diagnosis. Wright and Berry [146] reviewed liver sections from 59 children who died of congenital syphilis in the preantibiotic period; 50 of 59 sections were "histologically normal," however, 41 of 59 were "heavily infiltrated with treponemes, so much that it appeared that there were more treponemes than liver." Conversely, specimens from children treated with penicillin often show histologic changes consisting of extramedullary hematopoiesis, parenchymal and portal inflammation, and occasional focal scarring [147], leading to the hypothesis that penicillin therapy may exacerbate syphilitic hepatitis [148]. Nonetheless, penicillin remains the cornerstone of therapy for affected infants. Although syphilitic hepatitis may persist for weeks or months following treatment, the process generally resolves without sequelae.

Hepatic involvement is also a well-recognized consequence of secondary and tertiary syphilis [149,150]. Approximately 50% of patients with secondary syphilis have hepatic enzyme abnormalities, whereas jaundice is significantly less common, occurring in 1–12% of affected patients [151,152]. Alkaline phosphatase values are often disproportionately elevated. Biopsy findings are variable, but may include areas of focal necrosis encircled by lymphocytes, neutrophils, and eosinophils. Granulomatous changes may be present, as may pericholangitis. In tertiary syphilis, gumma formation is noted. Resolution is typically complete following adequate treatment of the underlying infection.

Lyme Disease

Lyme disease is caused by *Borrelia burgdorferi,* a tick-borne spirochete [153,154]. Acute signs and symptoms include erythema chronicum migrans, fever, malaise, headache, stiff neck, arthralgias, myalgias, and lymphadenopathy. Arthritis may be chronic. Hepatic involvement in humans has been described; 19–37% may have abnormal liver tests [155,156]. Symptoms consistent with hepatic dysfunction may be elicited and include nausea, vomiting, anorexia, and weight loss. Hepatomegaly and right upper quadrant pain may be noted. Liver biopsy in one case revealed infiltration of sinusoids by neutrophils and mononuclear cells. Microvesicular fat, Kupffer cell hyperplasia, ballooning hepatocytes, and increased hepatocyte mitotic activity were also noted. *Borrelia burgdorferi* organisms were present in the biopsy specimen [157,158].

Diagnosis of Lyme disease requires a high index of suspicion on the part of the investigating physician. History of travel to affected areas or of clinical signs and symptoms consistent with infection must be elicited and appropriate serologic studies (enzyme-linked immunoabsorbent assay [ELISA] or indirect fluorescent antibody) performed. PCR assays may also be of use [159]. Treatment of early disease is with doxycycline [160]; penicillin V or amoxicillin may be used in children aged under 9 years. Parenteral therapy with ceftriaxone or penicillin V may be required in those patients with severe carditis, persistent arthritis, or meningitis. Chronic hepatitis due to *Borrelia burgdorferi* has not been described.

Patients with borreliosis due to *Borrelia recurrentis* are also known to have hepatic involvement. In a series of louse-borne disease, 62% were noted to have hepatic tenderness [161]. Patients may have mild elevation of serum aminotransferase levels; jaundice may also occur. Diagnosis is via examination of blood smears for *Borrelia*. Treatment with tetracycline, chloramphenicol, erythromycin, and penicillin may be effective, particularly if the diagnosis is made early in the disease course.

Leptospirosis

Leptospirosis is caused by one of several serotypes of *L. interrogans*, a coiled, motile spirochete whose primary hosts include a variety of domestic and wild animals [162]. At-risk individuals have traditionally included those exposed to cattle, hogs, horses, and rats. Exposure to blood, other body fluids, or fluids contaminated by urine from affected animals may result in disease transmission to humans. Disease in children has been attributed to canine exposure [163]. After an incubation period of 4–20 days, one of two general disease patterns may occur. Approximately 90–95% of patients in adult series will remain anicteric and undergo an initial phase of disease lasting 4–9 days, marked by the presence of spirochetes in the peripheral circulation and characterized by fever, anorexia, abdominal pain, conjunctival erythema, lymphadenopathy, rash, and muscle tenderness. Headache and, less often, nuchal rigidity may occur. Approximately 50% of patients undergo a second period of fever, often marked by meningeal involvement, hepatitis, and, occasionally, endocarditis and myocarditis [164]. Five to ten percent of patients will undergo a more severe course marked by significant jaundice, renal failure, hemorrhage, and vascular collapse, with death occurring in up to 40%. Children with leptospirosis suffer many of the signs and symptoms noted here. Wong et al. [163] noted hepatomegaly in 5 of 9 hospitalized children with leptospirosis; acalculous cholecystitis was also noted in 5 of 9. Serum bilirubin levels greater than 1.2 was seen in 7 of 9, and elevated serum aminotransferase levels were seen in 6 of 9. More recent series have confirmed these differences in presentation between children and adults [165]. Also in contrast to data from adult series, severe disease in pediatric patients is not limited to the icterohaemmorhagiae serogroup of *L. interrogans*. Other abnormal laboratory findings may include elevated serum creatinine phosphokinase, leukocytosis, thrombocytopenia, and proteinuria. Serum prothrombin time may be elevated, but generally normalizes in response to vitamin k administration.

The pathophysiology of leptospirosis-associated hepatic disease remains uncertain. Hepatic biopsy findings include edema, disorganization of liver cell plates, and multinucleated cells reflecting hepatocyte proliferation (Figure 37.8). Erythrophagocytosis may be seen [162]. In approximately 10% of patients, small foci of hepatocellular necrosis may be present [166]. Histologic alterations do not correlate with degree of jaundice. Diagnosis of leptospirosis may be made via

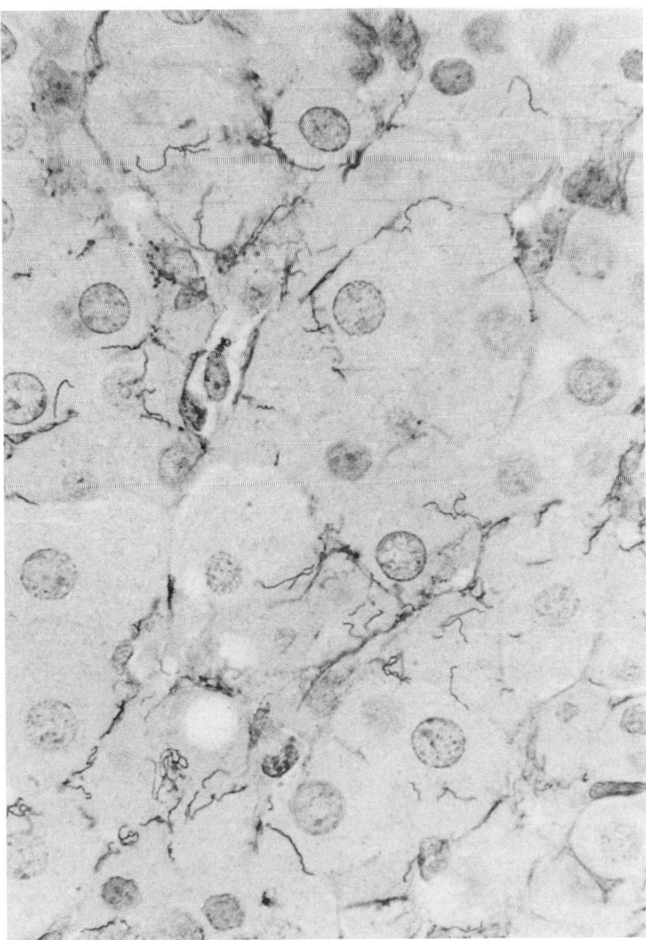

Figure 37.8. Leptospirosis. Numerous spirochetes are present. Detail of the spirochete coiling is somewhat obscured by the silver deposits in this silver impregnation–based stain (Warthin–Starry).

culture of blood or cerebrospinal fluid during early stages of illness, and from urine subsequently. Serology (ELISA, microscopic agglutination test) and PCR may also be of use. In addition, although not diagnostic, darkfield examination of the urine may provide useful information. Treatment of affected individuals with parenteral penicillin appears most efficacious if initiated within the first few days of illness [167]. Doxycycline may serve as effective prophylaxis in high-risk individuals [168].

Rickettsial Disease

Rocky Mountain Spotted Fever

Rocky Mountain spotted fever (RMSF), the clinical syndrome associated with *Rickettsia rickettsii*, is characterized by fever, petechial rash beginning peripherally, spreading to the trunk and often involving the palms and soles, and headache. Ticks serve as vectors for disease transmission [169]. Hepatic involvement may occur; clinical manifestations include hepatomegaly and, rarely, jaundice. Pathologic changes noted at autopsy have consisted of portal triaditis, portal vasculitis, and erythrophagocytosis. Rickettsial organisms may be found in portal blood vessels, sinusoidal lining cells, or both [170]. Diagnosis is via serology and high index of clinical suspicion. Treatment is with doxycycline or chloramphenicol [171].

Q Fever

Caused by *Coxiella burnetti*, Q fever is characterized by fever, headache, malaise, myalgia, and pneumonitis, although asymptomatic infection predominates in humans [172]. Transmission occurs via inhalation of the *Coxiella* organism; this mode of transmission is unique among the *rickettsiae*. Animal hosts include cattle, sheep, goats, and rodents. Transmission may also occur through ingestion of contaminated milk [173].

Symptomatic infection in humans lasts 9–16 days, although acute infection may last up to 3 months. Chronic infection may occur, primarily in the form of Q fever endocarditis. Hepatic involvement is frequent in acute Q fever. Specifically, 70–85% of patients are noted to have abnormal liver tests, and 11–65% are noted to have symptoms referable to hepatic involvement [174]. Hepatomegaly and hepatic tenderness are often present. In one center, 42% of patients with Q fever presented with hepatitis in the absence of pulmonary symptoms [174]. Five percent of cases present with jaundice. Although uncommon, hepatic failure secondary to Q fever has been documented in children [173].

Pathologic findings in the liver of patients with acute Q fever classically include fibrin ring granulomas, consisting of a central clear space surrounded by histiocytes and a fibrin ring (Figure 37.9). Early lesions may contain neutrophils, and giant cells are noted in later lesions [172]. Nonspecific changes include steatosis, mononuclear infiltration of portal areas, and Kupffer cell hyperplasia. Fibrosis may rarely occur [175]; hepatitis may rarely become chronic [176]. Diagnosis is via detection of antibodies to phase I and II antigens of *Coxiella burnetti*. Treatment is usually problematic because of the self-limited nature of most infections; however, doxycycline is efficacious [177].

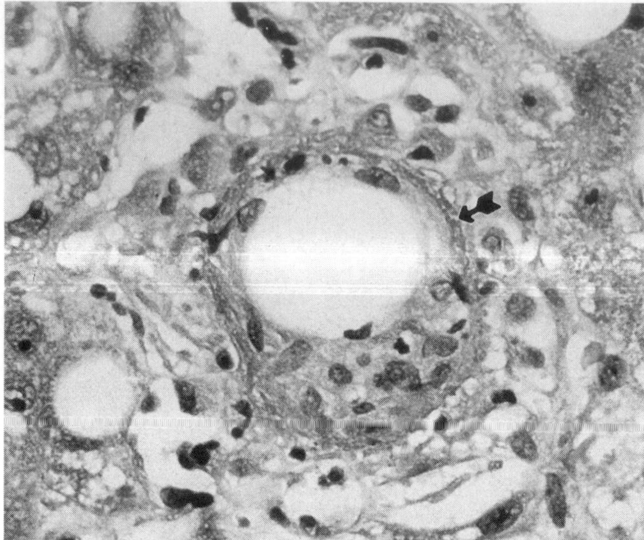

Figure 37.9. Q fever. Fibrinoid ring lesion containing a large, central lipid droplet surrounded by few inflammatory cells and encircled by a ring of fibrinoid material (*arrow*).

PARASITIC DISEASES OF THE LIVER

Entamoeba Histolytica

Entamoeba histolytica, a protozoa distributed worldwide, is estimated to occur in the United States with an incidence of approximately 3–5%. Incidence may be higher in specific groups, including residents of group homes, male homosexuals, and immigrants from endemic areas [178]. The organism is found in both trophozoite and cyst forms. Infection is via fecal–oral ingestion of cysts, thus, infected pediatric patients in the United States often live in crowded conditions marked by poor sanitation [179]. After traversing the stomach, ingested cysts dissolve during passage through the small bowel and colon where, in the presence of colonic bacteria, they mature into trophozoites. Colonic infection may be asymptomatic or may manifest as invasive disease characterized by abdominal pain, bloody diarrhea, and the presence of "pipe stem" ulcers. The cecum and ascending colon tend to be most heavily involved [180]. Hepatic disease occurs when trophozoites reach the liver, presumably via the portal vein, and are able to penetrate into the hepatic parenchyma where, through the elaboration of proteolytic enzymes, abscess formation occurs (Figure 37.10). Subsequent spread of trophozoites to other organs, including brain, lung, heart, and spleen has been described. In addition, local spread of amebic organisms may result in the presence of cutaneous ulcerations, most commonly noted in the perineal area in pediatric patients [181].

Although more common in adults, hepatic abscess formation is estimated to occur in 1–7% of pediatric patients with invasive amebiasis [180]. Children under 3 years of age seem to be most commonly affected; no male–female differential in incidence exists in this age group. Single or multiple cavities may be present; the right lobe of the liver is most commonly

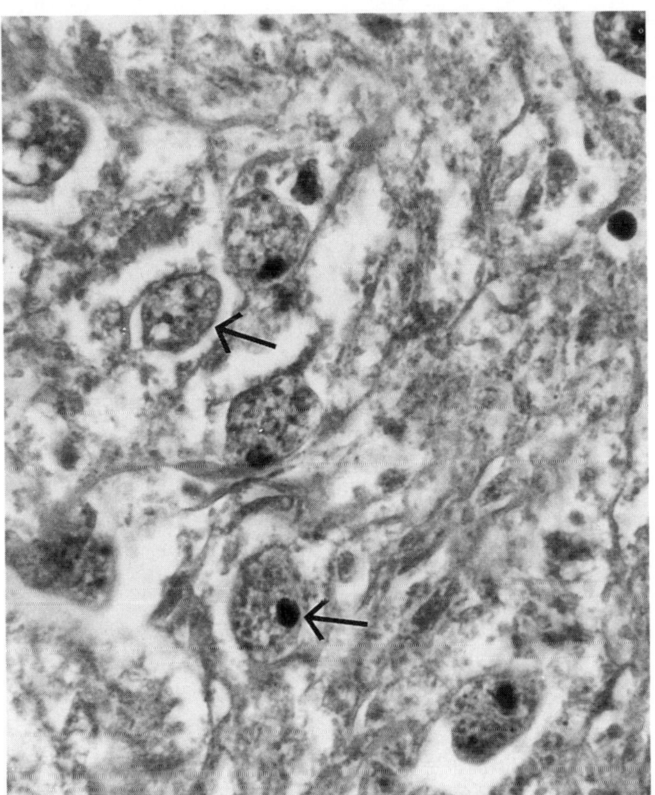

Figure 37.10. Amebic abscess. Necrotic material surrounds numerous *Entamoeba histolytica* trophozoites. The trophozoites, which are oval eosinophilic organisms, contain a single nucleus ranging in size from 10–65 μm. The cytoplasm of the trophozoites is characteristically granular and vacuolated, and often contains phagocytosed erythrocytes.

involved. The abscess cavity consists of a liquefied central area, surrounded by necrotic hepatic tissue. Ameba may be noted in the necrotic tissue or in the adjacent hepatic parenchyma [182]. Signs and symptoms of amebic abscess include fever, abdominal pain, abdominal distension, and tender hepatomegaly; however, presentation in young children may be nonspecific [179]. Patients may present with an acute abdomen secondary to intraperitoneal abscess rupture. Free perforation into the peritoneal cavity is, however, less likely than slow leakage with intra-abdominal abscess formation [183,184]. Other reported symptoms include dyspnea and productive cough, occasionally as a result of abscess rupture into the chest, with formation of a hepatobronchial fistula. Patients in whom an intrahepatic amebic abscess has ruptured into the pericardium may present in shock. Jaundice is notably uncommon. History of a preceding diarrheal episode is present in less than 50% of patients; approximately 10% have dysentery concurrent with hepatic abscess [184]. Routine laboratory examinations are of limited value in the diagnosis of hepatic amebic abscess. Serum aminotransferase levels are elevated in under 25% of affected pediatric patients, and alkaline phosphatase levels are generally normal in this age group [180]. Leukocytosis is common, as are elevated erythrocyte sedimentation rates and increased globulin fractions. Radiographs of the chest may reveal right lower lobe infiltrates, pleural effusions, or elevation of the right or left hemidiaphragms. Hepatic scintigraphy has proved useful in adult series; a filling defect is noted corresponding to abscess location. As with pyogenic liver abscess, current imaging methods of choice would seem to be CT or ultrasonography (or both). Examination of stools for trophozoites or cysts should be performed but is positive in less than 50% of patients with hepatic amebic abscess [185]. Proctosigmoidoscopy and rectal biopsy may also be of use. Serologic testing for ameba is a useful diagnostic tool, particularly in areas that have relatively low incidences of amebic disease. Approximately 95% of patients with amebic liver abscess have positive indirect hemagglutination assays (IHA) or positive complement fixation assays [180]. These studies remain positive for significant periods of time after acute infection. As a means of differentiation from pyogenic abscess, fine needle aspiration of the abscess cavity is often required. Fluid obtained in this manner is reddish-brown in color and typically sterile. Examination of this "pus" yields amebic organisms in less than one third of cases [183].

Therapy of amebic abscess consists primarily of the use of amebicidal agents, most often metronidazole, 50 mg/kg/d in divided doses for 10 days [186], followed by a luminal amebicide such as iodoquinol or paromomycin. Surgical drainage is generally not required; mortality rates appear to be significantly higher when this mode of therapy is employed [183]. Indications for surgical therapy include presentation with an acute abdomen as well as failure of other therapeutic measures. Percutaneous aspiration is more frequently used, particularly in cases that do not respond to amebecidal therapy after 4–5 days [178] or as decompressive therapy in those patients in whom rupture of the abscess cavity, into the pleural, peritoneal, or pericardial cavities, seems imminent. Repeated percutaneous aspirations in patients with amebic liver abscesses may significantly speed abscess resolution [187]. Rupture of the abscess cavity is associated with significant rates of mortality, approximately 30% when rupture into the pericardium occurs [188]. Conversely, mortality rates in adults with recognized, uncomplicated, hepatic amebic abscess are approximately 1% [183]. Current pediatric mortality rates are unclear but may be significantly higher because of delay in diagnosis.

Echinococcal Disease

Human infection with *Echinococcus granulosus* may occur after ingestion of ova excreted by infected dogs. Dogs generally acquire infection via consumption of sheep liver or intestine containing hydatid cysts. Scolices contained within the cysts then develop within the canine small intestine, maturing into adult tapeworms, 3–6 mm long. Rupture of the gravid proglottid releases 400–800 eggs, which are excreted in canine feces. Ingestion of eggs typically occurs after the handling of an infected dog or the drinking of contaminated water. The ingested embryo, after release from the egg in the duodenum, penetrates the intestinal mucosa and enters the portal circulation. Organisms may then lodge in the liver or lung of affected patients. Endemic areas include the Mediterranean basin, the Yukon territories, and parts of Africa, South America, Australia, and New Zealand, as well as sheep-rearing areas of the United States [189]. Infection is common in childhood, although symptoms may not occur for many years. Although in adult series involvement of the liver occurs 3 times more frequently, involvement of the lung is noted frequently in children. Simultaneous involvement of the liver and lung may occur. Other sites of infection in approximately 10% of children include the brain, bones, genitourinary tract, eyes, spleen, and heart. Hepatic involvement is marked by the development of "cysts" within the hepatic parenchyma, most often within the right lobe [182]. Typically, the cyst is surrounded by a fibrous capsule elaborated by the host. An acellular, hyalinized layer forms the exocyst, underlaid by a germinal layer. Extrusions of the germinal layer form brood capsules which contain protoscolices. Hydatid sand, composed of separated brood cysts and protoscolices, floats within the main cyst cavity. Septation may occur, as may formation of daughter cysts [190].

Symptoms of echinococcal cyst formation occur as a result of cyst growth and subsequent compression of surrounding tissues. Thus, right upper quadrant pain and fullness may be the only presenting features. Jaundice may occur as a result of compression of the porta hepatis; cholangitis may arise secondary to cyst rupture into the biliary tract. Compression of hepatic veins by cysts may result in Budd–Chiari syndrome. Rupture into the pericardial, peritoneal, or pleural cavities may occur. Other, atypical presentations may also occur in children [191]. Anaphylaxis may occur on release of cyst fluid. Laboratory data are typically nonspecific; elevation of serum alkaline phosphatase and aminotransferase levels may be noted. Eosinophilia may be present. Radiographs of the abdomen may show calcification of the cyst wall in adults; this change is seldom apparent in children. Ultrasonography is useful and can demonstrate the presence of hydatid sand as well as delineate septations and the presence of daughter cysts [192]. The appearance may be difficult to differentiate from simple cysts or tumors. Computed tomographic scanning and MRI demonstrate and localize lesions in a high percentage of cases [193–195]. Endoscopic retrograde cholangiography may demonstrate involvement of the biliary tree by daughter cysts following rupture of the primary hepatic cyst [192,196]. This complication appears to be less frequent in children than in adults. Definitive diagnosis rests upon demonstration of positive serology to *E. granulosus*. Commonly used studies include indirect hemagglutination and ELISA. Percutaneous aspiration for diagnostic purposes was generally not recommended secondary to risks of anaphylaxis and dissemination; however, multiple reports of cyst drainage under CT, ultrasound, or laparoscopic guidance cast some doubt on this dogma [197–199].

Historically, the primary treatment of hydatid disease has been surgical, with primary resection of peripheral and small lesions; larger lesions require cyst decompression, irrigation with scolicidal solutions, and, in some cases, omentoplasty [190,200–202]. Laproscopic approaches have also been used successfully [203]. Care is taken to avoid peritoneal dissemination at surgery; praziquantel may be used perioperatively. As alluded to earlier, however, definitive percutaneous drainage has been performed with good results and is emerging as the preferred therapy in selected cases [204,205]. Daughter cysts in the biliary tree may be removed endoscopically after sphincterotomy [206]. In addition, using ERCP, scolicidal agents have been infused into hepatic cysts that have ruptured into the biliary tract [192]. In unresectable hepatic lesions, therapy with albendazole, 15 mg/kg/day for 1–6 months, has in some cases resulted in reduction in cyst size [192]. Albendazole therapy may also be used in conjunction with percutaneous aspiration [186]. Alaskan and Canadian patients infected with *E. granulosus* may have a more benign course; thus, at present, surgery is not recommended for asymptomatic patients in this subgroup [189].

Ascariasis

Human infection with the roundworm *Ascaris lumbricoides* is extremely common in tropical and temperate regions worldwide. Infection occurs via ingestion of embryonated eggs passed in human feces and deposited in soil, where development into the infective form occurs. As a result, incidence is highest among children and in areas with poor sanitation facilities. Ingested eggs hatch in the proximal small intestine. Larvae penetrate the small bowel mucosa, are carried in the venous circulation to the lungs, and subsequently pass through the lungs and into the esophagus, once again reaching the small bowel where maturation takes place [207]. Mild hepatic abnormalities may be associated with migrating larvae; dead larvae may stimulate granuloma formation [208]. Most clinically relevant hepatic involvement, however, occurs when one or more adult worms pass thru the ampulla of Vater into the common bile duct. Worms may subsequently return to the duodenum or may reside in the gallbladder and intrahepatic bile ducts. Obstruction of the pancreatic duct may also occur [209]. Symptoms of biliary ascariasis, notably more common in children than in adults, include (in uncomplicated cases) the acute onset right upper quadrant pain (100%), vomiting (96%), history of worm infestation (64%), worm passage in stool or vomitus (50%), and fever (27%). Signs include right upper quadrant tenderness (100%), palpable gallbladder (11%), hepatomegaly (16%), and jaundice (2%). Complications of biliary ascariasis are infrequent, but may occur in a higher percentage of affected adults (53%) than children (5%) [207]. Jaundice, hepatomegaly, and fever occur in higher proportions of complicated cases. Death of ascarids within the common bile duct cause mucosal destruction and fibrosis, resulting in stricture and predisposing to stone formation. Death of worms in the intrahepatic bile ducts is associated with the release of eggs and the subsequent development of suppurative cholangitis and hepatic granuloma formation (Figure 37.11). Abscess formation may also occur [210]; rupture of abscesses into the peritoneal or pleural cavities may then follow. Other reported complications include cholecystitis, perforation of the common bile duct, and pylephlebitis of the hepatic or portal veins (or both) [87].

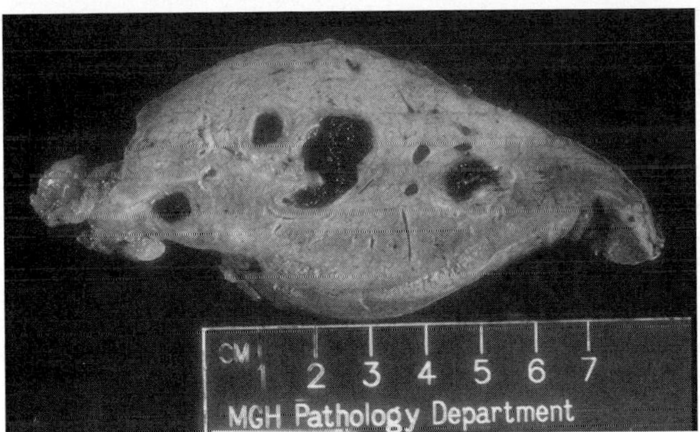

Figure 37.11. Oriental cholangitis secondary to infection by *Ascaris lumbricoides*. This section of the liver shows the characteristically cystically dilated bile ducts.

Laboratory data in uncomplicated biliary ascariasis are frequently unrevealing, with normal aminotransferase levels noted in 90% of patients [207]. Hyperamylasemia may be present in approximately 25% of patients with common duct ascarids. Ultrasonography may demonstrate the presence of ascarids in the common duct; abscess formation may be noted [211]. CT scanning is also useful [212], as is MRCP. Definitive diagnosis may be made via demonstration of adult worms or ova in stool or vomitus. Panendoscopy may demonstrate the presence of ascarids in the duodenum, whereas endoscopic retrograde cholangiography allows demonstration of adult worms throughout the biliary tree [213,214]. Therapy of biliary ascariasis in uncomplicated cases is expectant; antihelminthic therapy consists of a single dose of pyrantel pamoate, 11 mg/kg, maximum dose 1 g [186]. Alternative therapies include mebendazole and albendazole. In resistant cases, endoscopic sphincterotomy with worm extraction may be effective [211,215,216]. Nasobiliary tube placement may allow instillation of antihelminthic agents into the biliary system. Worm removal has also been performed via the percutaneous, transhepatic route [217] Surgical therapy may be required when hepatic abscess is present, as well as in the presence of common duct and gallbladder perforation.

Toxocariasis

Visceral larva migrans, caused by the nematode *T. canis*, occurs worldwide. After ingestion by a dog, embryonated ova undergo a life cycle similar to that described earlier for *A. lumbricoides*. Additionally, fetal animals may be infected in utero via transplacental spread of the organism. Human infection typically results via ingestion of soil contaminated by embryonated ova. Infection is most common in children [218]; average age is 2 years. Subsequent to ingestion, larvae penetrate the intestinal wall and migrate via lymphatics and the venous circulation, most commonly, to the liver and lung. Other affected organs include the eye, heart, and central nervous system. Symptoms include cough, wheezing, fever, pallor, and visual impairment. Hepatosplenomegaly, rales and wheezing, lymphadenopathy, and pruritic skin lesions may be present on physical exam. Marked eosinophilia and hyperglobulinemia are generally present, whereas routine biochemical indicators of hepatic injury are typically normal. Titers of isohemagglutinins to A and B blood group antigens are elevated. Serologic confirmation with an ELISA test is available. Computerized tomography may demonstrate multiple low-density lesions; MRI may also be abnormal [219]. Early pathologic findings in the liver consist of larvae surrounded by eosinophils; later findings include granulomas composed of epithelioid cells, giant cells, lymphocytes, and fibroblasts [166]. Treatment entails the administration of albendazole or mebendazole; however, the efficacy of these regimens remains uncertain [186]. Corticosteroids may be used concomitantly in children with pulmonary or ocular disease.

Capillariasis

Infection of the human liver by *Capillaria hepatica*, a nematode usually affecting rodents, cats, and dogs, is uncommon, but may be associated with a spectrum of clinical findings similar to that noted for toxocariasis. Symptoms include fever, hepatomegaly, and eosinophilia in approximately 90% of affected patients. Diagnosis is generally made through the demonstration of organisms in percutaneous hepatic biopsy specimens. Treatment options include albendazole and mebendazole [186,220,221].

Schistosomiasis

Infection with *Schistosoma haematobium*, *S. mansoni*, or *S. japonicum* occurs in 200–300 million people globally [222]. The majority of these infections occur in the pediatric population. Both *S. mansoni* and *S. japonicum* are capable of causing hepatic disease; areas of endemicity include Africa, the Middle East, South America, and sections of the Caribbean basin for *S. mansoni*, whereas *S. japonicum* is noted predominantly in Central and Southeast Asia. *S. haematobium* primarily affects the urinary tract. Schistosomal organisms infect humans via direct penetration through the skin of cercariae, previously released from a snail host. After penetration, cercariae develop into schistosomulae and eventually migrate to the liver where, in intrahepatic portal venules, they mature and mate. Single mating pairs persist within the liver for an average of 4–7 years [223]. The adult organisms then move within the portal venous system to branches of the inferior (*S. mansoni*) or superior (*S. japonicum*) mesenteric veins. Eggs subsequently produced may be excreted in feces or retained in tissue. Hepatic lesions are produced as a result of the hosts immunologic response to ova deposited in the portal venous system (Figure 37.12). Initial Th-1 and subsequently Th-2 responses to egg antigens result in the formation of granulomatous lesions composed primarily of eosinophils, epithelioid cells, lymphocytes, and plasma cells, which surround the ovum [224]. Giant cells and fibrosis become prominent after death of the ovum. Pigment may be present. Destruction of small portal radicles occurs, presumably producing the presinusoidal portal hypertension characteristic of hepatosplenic schistosomiasis [225].

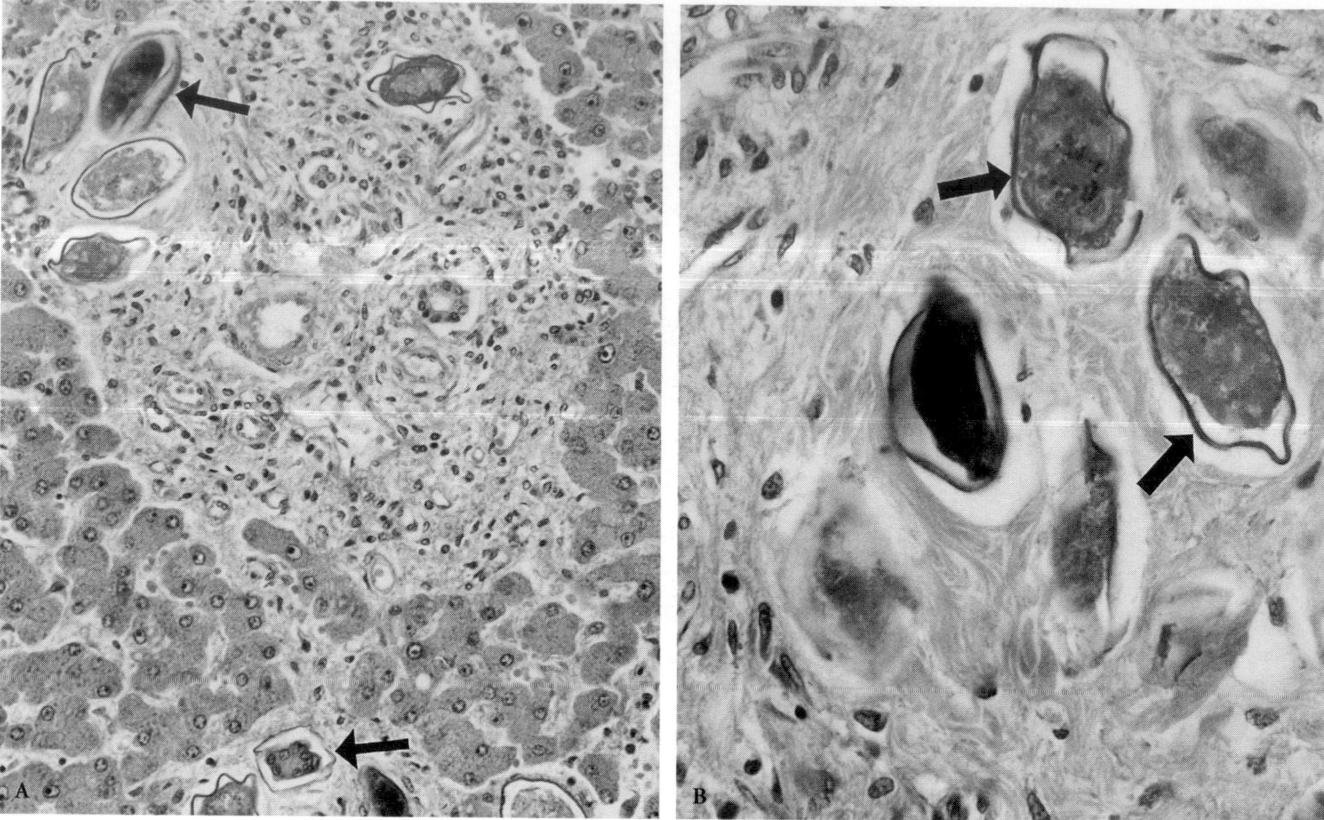

Figure 37.12. Schistosomiasis. Numerous eggs are present in the portal tracts, which are mildly expanded and fibrotic, a reaction to the presence of the eggs (*arrows*).

Fibrosis and thrombophlebitis of larger portal branches results in the "pipestem fibrosis" described by Symmers [226]. Approximately 10% of children infected with *S. mansoni* display hepatic disease with periportal fibrosis [222]. True cirrhosis is generally not seen. Clinical manifestations of schistosomiasis are protean; distinct clinical syndromes are associated with each stage of infection. Hepatic disease is marked by hepatosplenomegaly; development of hepatic disease appears to correlate with severity of infestation [225]. Symptoms of hepatic disease are few; patients may present with upper gastrointestinal bleeding from esophageal varices as the first sign of disease. Later signs may include edema and ascites. Laboratory abnormalities are also few; hypersplenism may result in anemia, thrombocytopenia, and leukopenia. Eosinophilia and hyperglobulinemia are often noted. Serum aminotransferase levels are generally not markedly elevated, but serum alkaline phosphatase levels may be increased [227]. Serologic studies (ELISA) may be useful [222]. Ultrasonography allows detection and grading of periportal fibrosis, accurate measurement of liver and spleen size, and measurement of portal vein size, as well as detection of intrabdominal varices [224,228]. CT may suggest the presence of periportal fibrosis [229]; MRI may also be of use [230]. Definitive diagnosis rests on the isolation of schistosome eggs in stool. Rectal biopsy tissue may be examined for the presence of eggs, as may hepatic biopsy [222,224]. Panendoscopy may be useful to establish the presence of varices. The pharmacologic treatment of choice is praziquantel, 40–60 mg/kg/d in divided doses. Oxamniquine may also be used in *S mansoni* infections [186]. Mild periportal fibrosis may resolve in children after effective therapy [231]. Acute variceal hemorrhage is managed in the routine manner; chronic hemorrhage may require sclerotherapy or, in some cases, shunt placement [225,232].

Liver Flukes

Infection with *Clonorchis sinensis*, a 1- to 2.5-cm trematode, is endemic throughout the Far East [233]. The life cycle of *C. sinensis*, similar to that of *Opisthorchis* species, begins when embryonated eggs are ingested by operculate snails. Development into cercariae occurs within this host; after subsequent release the cercariae penetrate freshwater fish and become encysted within their flesh. Ingestion of contaminated fish by humans allows release of metacercariae in the duodenum from whence they migrate through the ampulla and into the small bile ducts where they mature (Figure 37.13). Life span of adult flukes is 20–30 years. Perhaps as a result, most symptomatic patients are aged at least 30 years [234]. Injury to the bile ducts occurs and is manifested by adenomatous proliferation and goblet cell hyperplasia [235]. Fibrosis occurs with chronic infection. Secondary bacterial infection with *E. coli* occurs frequently and predisposes to formation of hepatic abscesses (recurrent pyogenic cholangitis [RPC]) [233,235]. Calculi are common. Repeated episodes may result in biliary stricture and periportal fibrosis.

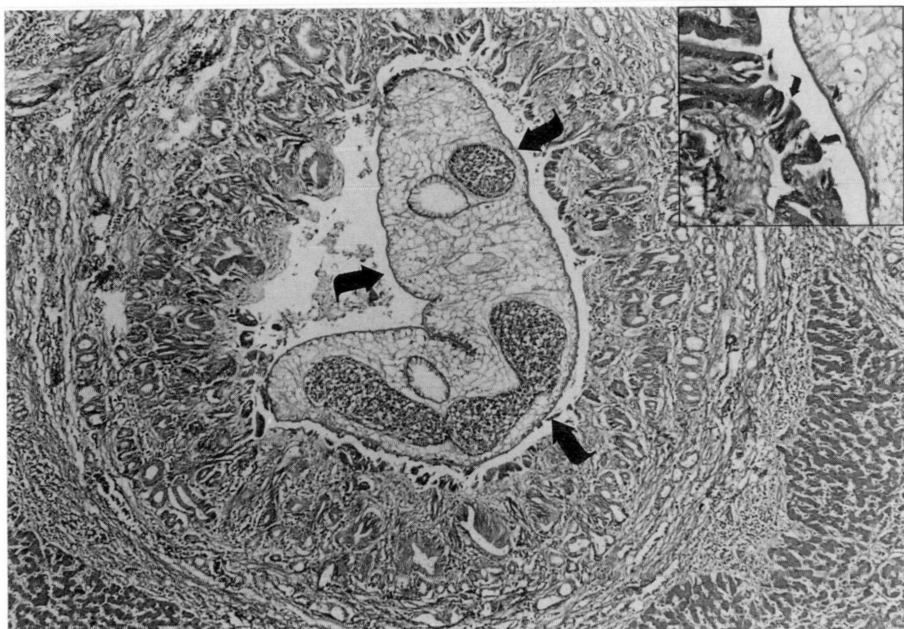

Figure 37.13. Clonorchiasis. A dilated bile duct contains an adult *Clonorchis sinensis.* Note the associated atypical hyperplasia of the lining bile duct epithelium, thought to be a premalignant epithelial process (*inset*).

Egg deposition may also be associated with the presence of giant cell reaction in the liver, as well as with portal granulomas. Development of cholangiocarcinoma may occur in those with longstanding disease [236]. Symptoms of infection vary in intensity with worm load and duration of infection. Early or mild disease may be asymptomatic; more severe cases may have fever, malaise, anorexia, jaundice, and hepatosplenomegaly. Later symptoms involve the consequences of portal hypertension and biliary obstruction [233]. Laboratory findings in late disease include elevations of serum aminotransferase, alkaline phosphatase, and bilirubin levels. Hyperglobulinemia is frequent [227]. Ultrasonography and CT may reveal duct dilation; associated cholangiocarcinomas, stones, or abscesses may also be visualized [211]. Direct visualization of the biliary system is possible with ERCP, allowing delineation of ductal morphology, identification and extraction of calculi, and detection of *Clonorchis* eggs and worms via aspiration of bile [211]. Percutaneous cholangiography may also be useful. Diagnosis may be made through stool examination, as well as through examination of bile. Therapy involves treatment with praziquantel, 75 mg/kg/d in 3 doses in 1 day [186]. Pyogenic cholangitis must be treated with appropriate antibiotics. Endoscopic papillotomy and stone extraction, as well as insertion of endoprostheses, may be required [211]. In cases of longstanding RPC, other surgical interventions may be required [237].

Fasciola Hepatica

Fasciola hepatica is a trematode found worldwide; primary hosts include sheep and cattle. The life cycle is similar to that described for *Clonorchis.* Human infection occurs after ingesting contaminated aquatic plants (i.e., watercress) [238]. In the human, metacercariae penetrate the duodenal wall, traverse the peritoneal cavity and subsequently penetrate the hepatic capsule. The organisms then migrate through the liver parenchyma until reaching the bile ducts, where they persist [239]. Symptoms and pathologic changes, therefore, reflect not only biliary tract disease as in *Clonorchis* but also parenchymal damage, manifested by the presence of necrotic microabscesses within the liver. Both sonography and CT may help to delineate these abnormalities [239,240]. Eosinophilia is common. Diagnosis rests on serology and demonstration of ova in the stool [241]. Endoscopic retrograde chalangiography may also be useful in the biliary phase of disease, both as a diagnostic (identification of eggs and intact flukes; visualization of flukes radiographically) and therapeutic (removal of flukes after sphincterotomy) measure [242]. Treatment is with triclabendazole 10 mg/kg given once. Because availability of this drug may be an issue, bithionol, 30–50 mg/kg on alternate days for 10–15 doses may also be used [186,243].

Leishmaniasis

Visceral leishmaniasis, or Kala-azar, caused by *Leishmania donovani*, is endemic throughout the Mediterranean basin, as well as parts of Africa, South America, Russia, and China [244]. Organisms are inoculated into humans via sandfly bites and are rapidly phagocytosed by dermal macrophages, where they proliferate. Rupture of infected macrophages allows organism spread to reticuloendothelial cells within the liver, spleen, bone marrow, lymph nodes, kidneys, and intestine [245]. The hepatic lesion in older children and adults is characterized by Kupffer cell hyperplasia, many of which contain parasites. Portal tract infiltration with eosinophils, lymphocytes, and plasma cells may occur, as may granuloma formation. Fibrin ring granulomas have been reported [246]. Infants may demonstrate significant hepatocellular necrosis [247]. Symptoms of infection include an incubation period of up to several months followed by fever, failure to thrive, anemia, hepatosplenomegaly, diarrhea, and bleeding diathesis. Laboratory data may reveal elevations of serum aminotransferase and alkaline phosphatase values; hypoalbuminemia and prolongation of prothrombin times may be noted with more advanced disease [227]. Bone marrow biopsy often demonstrates the presence of Leishman–Donovan bodies. Other diagnostic measures may include serology and PCR [248,249]. Nodular hepatosplenic lesions may sometimes be seen by ultrasonography or CT [250]. Prognosis of untreated Leishmaniasis is poor; Stibogluconate sodium, 20 mg/kg/day intravenously or intramuscularly (maximum dose 800 mg/day) for 20–28 days, is accepted therapy [186]. Repeated treatment may be required. Alternative therapy may be undertaken with meglumine antimonite, pentamidine, or amphotericin B.

Malaria

Malarial disease remains an important cause of morbidity and mortality throughout much of the world, occurring most frequently in tropical and subtropical climates. Deaths caused by malarial disease are most common in children 1–5 years of age [251]. Severe infection may also occur in neonates [252]. Human infection with *Plasmodium falciparum*, *P. vivax*, *P. malariae*, and *P. ovale* is initiated after passage of sporozoites into the bloodstream at the time of the bite of an infected mosquito host. Sporozoites selectively invade hepatocytes, initiating the exoerythrocytic stage of development. Parasite division then occurs until rupture of the hepatocyte releases merozoites. Erythrocytes are then invaded. Spread of disease occurs upon the development of merozoites into micro- and macrogametes, which may be ingested by feeding mosquitos and reinitiate the malarial life cycle. Other methods of spread include transfusion and shared needles. Transplacental spread appears uncommon. Symptoms of malaria include fever, gastrointestinal complaints (nausea, vomiting, and diarrhea), headache, lethargy, myalgia, and delirium. Fever in children is often continuous. Neurologic complications, noted primarily with *P. falciparum*, include seizures and coma; renal failure may occur. Tender hepatosplenomegaly is often noted, as is jaundice. Hyperbilirubinemia commonly reflects hemolysis. Although sporadic patients may become significantly jaundiced with marked elevation of serum aminotransferase levels, milder alterations of these parameters are the norm [227]. Hepatic failure, at least as characterized by coagulopathy, is uncommon, although other clinical findings including encephalopathy, may be present [253]. In jaundiced patients, pathologic findings include hepatocytes congestion, malarial pigment deposition, and inflammatory infiltrates [254]. At autopsy, the liver is noted to be congested and dark red–grey in color. Histologic findings include hypertrophied Kupffer cells containing red blood cells and malarial pigment. Sinusoids are congested with red blood cells [166]. Portal tract infiltration by lymphocytes may occur in chronic cases. If shock has occurred, centrilobular necrosis may be present [255].

Diagnosis of malarial infection may be made via detection of malarial organisms in thin and thick peripheral blood smears prepared with Giemsa stain. Treatment is initiated in most cases with chloroquine phosphate given orally, 10 mg base/kg (maximum dose 600 mg), followed by 5 mg/kg at 6 hours, 24 hours, and 48 hours [186]. Quinidine hydrochloride is the parenteral drug of choice; however, significant side effects limit its use to emergent situations when oral medications cannot be tolerated. Alternative regimens must be used in cases of chloroquine-resistant *P. falciparum* and *vivax*. Although relapse of disease may occur in individuals infected with *P. vivax* and *P. ovale*, hepatic abnormalities in treated patients typically resolve completely [256,257].

FUNGAL INFECTIONS OF THE LIVER

Candida

Hepatosplenic candidiasis occurs predominantly in neutropenic patients, primarily those receiving chemotherapy because of preexisting malignancy [16,258]. Infection of the liver and spleen may occur as a consequence of seeding during generalized fungemia [258]. Symptoms in the neutropenic patient are nonspecific; the diagnosis may be suspected in those patients in whom fever persists after the resolution of neutropenia. Fever occurs in approximately 85% of affected patients; other signs and symptoms include abdominal pain (57%), hepatomegaly (44%), and splenomegaly (43%). Serum alkaline phosphatase levels are generally elevated (60%); bilirubin and aminotransferase levels are elevated less frequently. Leukocytosis is present in approximately 30% [258]. CT may be positive in approximately 90% of cases; early lesions may be seen as areas of variably enhancing diminished attenuation; MRI is at least as sensitive [259,260]. Ultrasound appears to be less sensitive [258]; "bull's-eye" lesions are characteristic [261]. Ultrasound remains a useful technique, however, because of its portability and subsequent ease of repeated exams. All techniques may miss small lesions. Given the toxicity of antifungal therapy, tissue diagnosis is desirable. Percutaneous liver biopsy was able to confirm the diagnosis of hepatosplenic candidiasis in 70% of patients [258]. Laparoscopic and open liver biopsies are successful in higher proportions of patients; lesions are visible grossly as small yellow–white nodules throughout the liver. Early hepatic lesions are composed of pseudohyphae and yeast forms surrounded by neutrophils and an outer fibrous rim. Lesions progress to well-formed granulomas with giant cell change. Fungal organisms may be noted using periodic acid–Schiff (PAS) or silver stains. Culture of lesions is positive in 60% of untreated patients but in only 30% of those receiving prior antifungal therapy. Blood cultures may also yield candidal organisms. Polymerase chain reaction assays hold promise

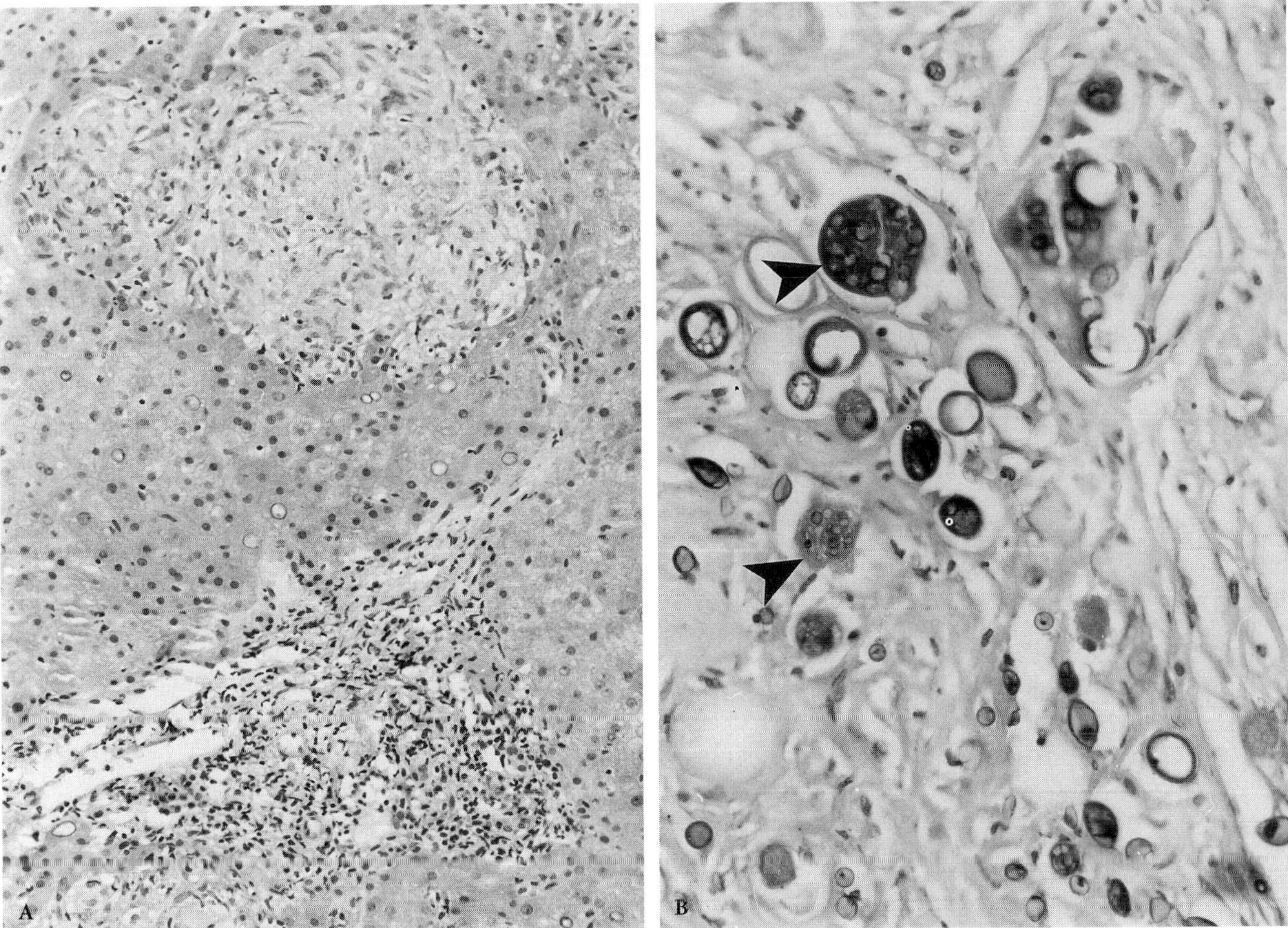

Figure 37.14. Coccidioidomycosis. (**A**) A lobular epithelioid granuloma is present containing numerous multinucleated giant cells. (**B**) Higher power examination demonstrates numerous thick walled spherules, ranging in size from 20 to 200 μm in diameter. Some of the spherules (*arrowheads*) are filled with the characteristic endospores, ranging in size from 3 to 7 μm in diameter.

for the monitoring of therapy [262]. Therapy is predicated on the use of amphotericin B, often in conjunction with 5-flourocytosine [258,263]. Newer preparations of amphotericin, primarily multi- and unilamellar liposomal suspensions, offer lower rates of drug-induced toxicity [261,264,265], although efficacy may not differ from standard preparations [266]. Fluconazole has been of use in the treatment of hepatosplenic candidiasis resistant to amphotericin B therapy [267–270] and is of particular use in prophylaxis [271]. Optimal duration of therapy is unclear; treatment regimens of several months may be required to produce radiologic resolution [266]. Prognosis in children is difficult to assess given the multiple problems of most affected patients; survival rates of approximately 60% with amphotericin therapy have been described [258].

Trichosporon Hepatitis

Trichosporon cutaneum has been rarely associated with granulomatous hepatitis in immunocompromised patients [272]. Hepatic biopsy may reveal granulomas surrounding central areas of necrosis in which fungal organisms can be visualized. Prognosis has been poor in a very limited number of patients; very long treatment periods may be required [273].

Penicillium Marneffei

Penicillium marneffei has increasingly been reported as a pathogen in immunocompromised patients, including children [274]. Multisystem involvement is the rule; however, primary hepatic disease may also occur [275]. Patterns of disease within the liver include abscesses or, in immunocompromised patients, diffuse organ infiltration with yeast. CT scan of the liver may reveal diffuse low attenuation lesions [276]. Definitive diagnosis is via culture or direct demonstration of organisms in biopsy specimens. Treatment is with a course of amphotericin B followed by itraconazole [274,277].

Coccidioidomycosis

Coccidioidomycosis, endemic in the southwestern United States as well as in parts of Mexico, Central America, and South America, is caused by the fungus *Coccidioides immitis* [278,279].

Transmission is generally via inhalation of arthrospores; accordingly, pulmonary infection is most often seen. Perinatal transmission, although uncommon, has been described [280]. Disseminated infection is most often noted in immunocompromised patients [281]. Infected infants may also have a severe disease course but, as a rule, disseminated infection is less frequent in children than in adults. Hepatic involvement is estimated to occur in 45–60% of patients with disseminated disease [282]. The lungs are infected most frequently, followed by the spleen; other involved organs include the skin, meninges, bones, and genitourinary system. Infection may begin with fever; often pulmonary symptomatology predominates. Less commonly, hepatic symptoms may predominate. Hepatomegaly may occur in conjunction with elevations in serum aminotransferase and, to a lesser degree, serum alkaline phosphatase levels. Clinically apparent jaundice is not common. Serology is often useful in patients with disseminated disease; complement fixation titers are generally high in this group of patients. Liver biopsy may be diagnostic; granuloma and giant cell formation surrounding PAS or methenamine silver-staining spherules are seen surrounded by normal-appearing hepatic parenchyma [283] (Figure 14). Hepatic abscess formation has also been reported [276]. Current treatment of disseminated disease is with amphotericin B [284].

Cryptococcosis

Cryptococcosis, associated with the fungal organism *Cryptococcus neoformans*, is responsible for human disease involving the lung, meninges, skin, and bones. The liver may be involved as part of disseminated disease; primary hepatic involvement may rarely occur [285,286]. Gross examination of the liver reveals white nodules. Histologic features are those of granuloma formation surrounding fungal organisms. Cholangitis associated with *Cryptococcus* has also been described [287,288]; ascending infection from the bowel was postulated. Therapy includes the use of amphotericin B; other useful agents include 5-fluorocytosine [289] and, presumably, fluconazole [290].

Histoplasmosis

Histoplasma capsulatum, the fungal agent responsible for histoplasmosis, is endemic in the Ohio and Mississippi River valleys in the United States. Inhalation of spores is the usual route of infection; the gastrointestinal tract may rarely act as the portal of entry [291]. Approximately 50% of patients undergo asymptomatic infection. In symptomatic, immunocompetent patients, self-limited pulmonary infection is most common. Hepatic involvement occurs in conjunction with disseminated disease, although disease limited to the liver has been reported [292]. Infants may undergo a severe, acute form characterized by fever (90%), malaise (82%), cough (42%), weight loss (42%), diarrhea (32%), nausea or vomiting (26%), and an enlarged abdomen (13%) [293]. Marked hepatosplenomegaly is noted; lymphadenopathy and pulmonary findings are less constant. Laboratory findings include anemia, thrombocytopenia, and neutropenia. Jaundice may occur, as may mild to moderate elevations of serum aminotransferase and alkaline phosphatase levels. Subacute disseminated disease occurs less frequently in children and is associated with focal involvement of the intestine, adrenal glands, meninges, oropharyngeal cavity, or heart. Hepatomegaly is also common. Chronic disease is primarily noted in adult patients. Diagnosis may be made through the use of serology and the discovery of *Histoplasma* organisms in infected secretions or tissue. Hepatic biopsy may reveal Kupffer cells loaded with fungal spores, prominent in sinusoids and periportal areas, and often associated with compression and necrosis of adjacent hepatocytes [291]. Kupffer cell infiltration of veins and arteries may be present. Granuloma formation is most commonly seen in chronic disease (Figure 37.15). Antifungal therapy is indicated in disseminated disease; untreated disseminated disease in infants is generally fatal. Amphotericin B and itraconazole have been employed as therapeutic agents [293–295].

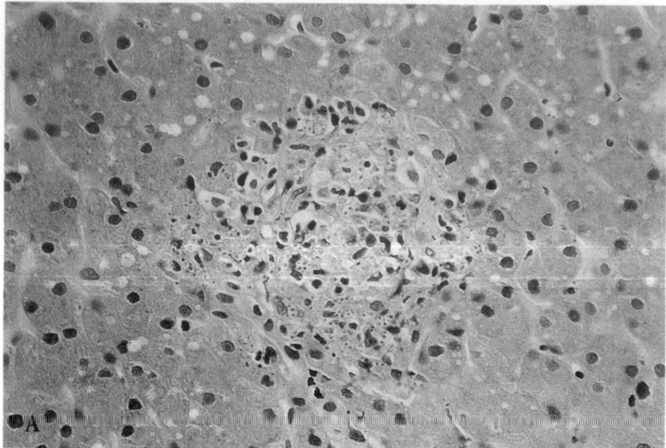

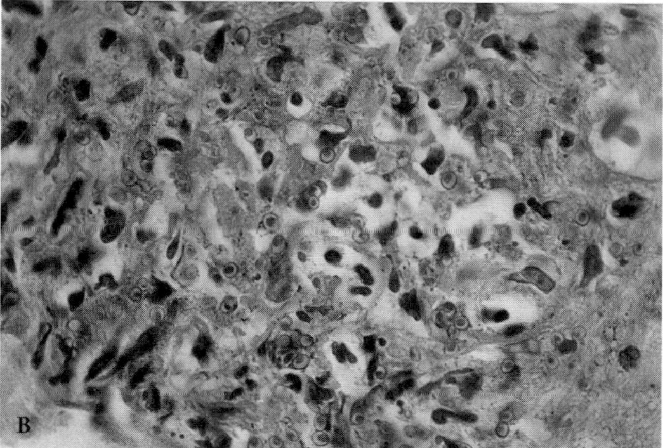

Figure 37.15. Histoplasma capsulatum. (**A**) Aggregated macrophages and Kupffer cells forming an ill-defined granuloma. (**B**) High-power magnification shows clustered fungi (periodic acid-Schiff-D stain).

Aspergillosis

A variety of *Aspergillus* species have been implicated in human disease. Pulmonary aspergillosis is the most frequent form of disease; disseminated disease most frequently occurs in immunocompromised individuals, although occurrence in infants [296], children, and immunocompetent adults has been reported [297]. Organs involved include the lungs, brain, intestines, heart, kidneys, thyroid, pancreas, esophagus, and spleen. Hepatic involvement was noted in 5 of 32 patients in an autopsy series of patients with disseminated aspergillosis; 4 of these were hepatic transplant recipients [298]. Hepatic abscess formation may be noted; aspiration with cytology and culture may be useful in diagnosis [299]. Granuloma formation has also been described. Amphotericin B and 5-flourocytosine remain the treatments of choice; liposomal amphotericin may offer advantages [300]. Itraconazole may also be of use [301]. Caspofungin acetate and voriconazole are newer agents shown efficacious in adults [302,303]; pediatric data remain limited.

Other fungal diseases of the liver associated with disseminated infections, often in immunocompromised hosts, include mucormycosis [304] and blastomycosis. Hepatic lesions in paracoccidioidomycosis occur primarily in generalized infections and include necrosis, granulomatous nodules, and portal fibrosis [305]. Obstructive jaundice due to compression of the common bile duct by infected lymph nodes has also been described [306].

REFERENCES

1. Hamilton JR, Sato N. Jaundice associated with severe bacterial infection in young infants. Pediatrics 1963;63:121–32.
2. Bernstein J, Brown AK. Sepsis and jaundice in early infancy. Pediatrics 1962;29:873–82.
3. Seeler RA, Hahn K. Jaundice in urinary tract infection in infancy. Am J Dis Child 1969;1184:553–8.
4. Rooney JC, Hill DJ, Danks DM. Jaundice associated with bacterial infection in the newborn. Am J Dis Child 1971;122:39–41.
5. Shamir R, Maayan-Metzger A, Bujanover Y, et al. Liver enzyme abnormalities in gram-negative bacteremia of premature infants. Pediatr Infect Dis J 2000;19:495–8.
6. Paton A. Sepsis and cholestasis [editorial]. Br Med J Clin Res Ed 1984;289:857.
7. Franson TR, Hierholzer WJ Jr, LaBrecque DR. Frequency and characteristics of hyperbilirubinemia associated with bacteremia. Rev Infect Dis 1985;7:1–9.
8. Utili R, Abernathy CO, Zimmerman HJ. Cholestatic effects of *Escherichia coli* endotoxin on the isolated perfused rat liver. Gastroenterology 1976;70:248–53.
9. Blaschke TF, Elin RJ, Berk PD, et al. Effects of induced fever on sulfobromophthalein kinetics in man. Ann Intern Med 1973; 78:221–6.
10. Hawker F. Liver dysfunction in critical illness. Anaesth Intensive Care 1991;19:165–81.
11. Lanza JS, Rosato EL. Regulatory factors in the development of fatty infiltration of the liver during gram-negative sepsis. Metabolism 1994;43:691–6.
12. Chusid MJ. Pyogenic hepatic abscess in infancy and childhood. Pediatrics 1978;62:554–9.
13. Pineiro CV, Andres JM. Morbidity and mortality in children with pyogenic liver abscess. Am J Dis Child 1989;14312:1424–7.
14. Hashimoto L, Hermann R, Grundfest BS. Pyogenic hepatic abscess: results of current management. Am Surg 1995;61:407–11.
15. Chou FF, Sheen CS, Chen YS, Chen MC. Single and multiple pyogenic liver abscesses: clinical course, etiology, and results of treatment. World J Surg 1997;21:384–8.
16. Chubachi A, Miura I, Ohshima A, et al. Risk factors for hepatosplenic abscesses in patients with acute leukemia receiving empiric azole treatment. Am J Med Sci 1994;308:309–12.
17. Arya LS, Ghani R, Abdali S, Singh M. Pyogenic liver abscesses in children. Clin Pediatr Phila 1982;21:89–93.
18. Kaplan SL, Feigin RD. Experience and reason – briefly recorded. Pediatrics 1976;58:14–16.
19. Dehner LP, Kissane JM. Pyogenic hepatic abscesses in infancy and childhood. J Pediatr 1969;74:763–73.
20. Chou FF, Sheen CS, Chen YS, Lee TY. The comparison of clinical course and results of treatment between gas-forming and non-gas-forming pyogenic liver abscess. Arch Surg 1995;1304: 401–5.
21. Chou FF, Sheen CS, Lee TY. Rupture of pyogenic liver abscess. Am J Gastroenterol 1995;90:767–70.
22. Mendez RJ, Schiebler ML, Outwater EK, Kressel HY. Hepatic abscesses: MR imaging findings. Radiology 1994;190:431–6.
23. Diament MJ, Stanley P, Kangarloo H, Donaldson JS. Percutaneous aspiration and catheter drainage of abscesses. J Pediatr 1986;108:204–8.
24. Wong KP. Percutaneous drainage of pyogenic liver abscesses. World J Surg 1990;14:492–7.
25. Ferreira MA, Pereira FE, Musso C, Dettogni RV. Pyogenic liver abscess in children: some observations in the Espirito Santo State, Brazil. Arq Gastroenterol 1997;34:49–54.
26. Brook I, Fraizer EH. Role of anaerobic bacteria in liver abscesses in children. Pediatr Infect Dis J 1993;12:743–7.
27. Lederman ER, Crum NF. Pyogenic liver abscess with a focus on Klebsiella pneumoniae as a primary pathogen: an emerging disease with unique clinical characteristics. Am J Gastroenterol 2005;100:322–31.
28. Brook I, Frazier EH. Microbiology of liver and spleen abscesses. J Med Microbiol 1998;47:1075–80.
29. Chakrabarti S, Varma S, Kochhar R, et al. Hepatosplenic tuberculosis: a cause of persistent fever during recovery from prolonged neutropenia. Int J Tuberc Lung Dis 1998;2:575–9.
30. Akcay MN, Polat KY, Oren D, Ozturk G. Primary tuberculous liver abscess. A case report and review of literature. Int J Clin Pract 2004;58:625–7.
31. Christodoulou N, Papadakis I, Velegrakis M. Actinomycotic liver abscess. Case report and review of the literature. Chir Ital 2004;56:141–6.
32. Zenon GJ, Cadle RM, Hamill RJ. Ampicillin-sulbactam therapy for multiple pyogenic hepatic abscesses [clinical conference]. Clin Pharm 1990;9:939–47.
33. Eng RH, Tecson TF, Corrado ML. Blunt trauma and liver abscess. Am J Gastroenterol 1981;76:252–5.
34. Rayes AA, Teixeira D, Serufo JC, et al. Human toxocariasis and pyogenic liver abscess: a possible association. Am J Gastroenterol 2001;96:563–6.
35. Muorah M, Hinds R, Verma A, et al. Liver abscesses in children: a single center experience in the developed world. J Pediatr Gastroenterol Nutr 2006;42:201–6.
36. Noel GJ, Karasic RB. Liver abscess following ingestion of a foreign body. Pediatr Infect Dis 1984;3:342–4.

37. Margalit M, Elinav H, Ilan Y, Shalit M. Liver abscess in inflammatory bowel disease: report of two cases and review of the literature. J Gastroenterol Hepatol 2004;19:1338–42.
38. Brans YW, Ceballos R, Cassady G. Umbilical catheters and hepatic abscesses. Pediatrics 1974;53:264–6.
39. Williams JW, Rittenberry A, Dillard R, Allen RG. Liver abscess in newborn. Complication of umbilical vein catheterization. Am J Dis Child 1973;125:111–13.
40. Hansen PS, Schonheyder HC. Pyogenic hepatic abscess. A 10-year population-based retrospective study. APMIS 1998;106: 396–402.
41. McFadzean AJS, Chang KPS, Wong CC. Solitary pyogenic abscess of the liver treated by closed aspiration and antibiotics. Br J Surg 1953;42:141–52.
42. Giorgio A, Tarantino L, Mariniello N, et al. Pyogenic liver abscesses: 13 years of experience in percutaneous needle aspiration with US guidance. Radiology 1995;1951:122–4.
43. Duncanson FP, Wormser GP. Nonsurgical therapy of pyogenic liver abscess. Drug Ther 1983;17–28.
44. Pitt HA. Surgical management of hepatic abscesses. World J Surg 1990;14:498–504.
45. Bamberger DM. Outcome of medical treatment of bacterial abscesses without therapeutic drainage: review of cases reported in the literature [see comments]. Clin Infect Dis 1996;23:592–603.
46. Rogers CA, Isenberg JN, Leonard AS, Sharp HL. Ascending cholangitis diagnosed by percutaneous hepatic aspiration. J Pediatr 1976;88:83–6.
47. Kobayashi A, Utsunomiya T, Obe Y, Shimizu K. Ascending cholangitis after successful surgical repair of biliary atresia. Arch Dis Child 1973;48:697–703.
48. Ecoffey C, Rothman E, Bernard O, et al. Bacterial cholangitis after surgery for biliary atresia. J Pediatr 1987;111:824–9.
49. Gottrand F, Bernard O, Hadchouel M, et al. Late cholangitis after successful surgical repair of biliary atresia. Am J Dis Child 1991;145:213–15.
50. Wyllie R, Fitzgerald JF. Bacterial cholangitis in a 10-week-old infant with fever of undetermined origin. Pediatrics 1980;65: 164–7.
51. Scott AJ. Bacteria and disease of the biliary tract. Gut 1971;12: 487–92.
52. Lipsett PA, Pitt HA. Acute cholangitis. Surg Clin North Am 1990;70:1297–312.
53. Carpenter HA. Bacterial and parasitic cholangitis. Mayo Clin Proc 1998;73:473–8.
54. Thompson JE Jr, Tompkins RK, Longmire WP Jr. Factors in management of acute cholangitis. Ann Surg 1982;195:137–45.
55. Bornman PC, van Beljon JI, Krige JE. Management of cholangitis. J Hepatobiliary Pancreat Surg 2003;10:406–14.
56. Kawamoto S, Soyer PA, Fishman EK, Bluemke DA. Nonneoplastic liver disease: evaluation with CT and MR imaging. Radiographics 1998;18:827–48.
57. Desmet DM. Cholestasis; extrahepatic obstruction and secondary biliary cirrhosis. In: Macsween RNM, Anthony PP, Scheuer PJ, editors. Pathology of the liver. Edinburgh: Churchill Livingstone, 1979:272–305.
58. Lipsett PA, Pitt HA. Acute cholangitis. Front Biosci 2003;8: s1229–39.
59. Dooley JS, Hamilton MJ, Brumfitt W, Sherlock S. Antibiotics in the treatment of biliary infection. Gut 1984;25:988–98.
60. Gerecht WB, Henry NK, Hoffman WW, et al. Prospective randomized comparison of mezlocillin therapy alone with combined ampicillin and gentamicin therapy for patients with cholangitis. Arch Intern Med 1989;149:1279–84.
61. Lee DW, Chung SC. Biliary infection. Baillieres Clin Gastroenterol 1997;11:707–24.
62. Cheng CL, Fogel EL, Sherman S, et al. Diagnostic and therapeutic endoscopic retrograde cholangiopancreatography in children: a large series report. J Pediatr Gastroenterol Nutr 2005; 41:445–53.
63. Wear DJ, Margileth AM, Hadfield TL, et al. Cat scratch disease: a bacterial infection. Science 1983;221:1403–5.
64. Dunn MW, Berkowitz FE, Miller JJ, Snitzer JA. Hepatosplenic cat-scratch disease and abdominal pain. Pediatr Infect Dis J 1997;16:269–72.
65. Carithers HA. Cat-scratch disease. An overview based on a study of 1,200 patients. Am J Dis Child 1985;139:1124–33.
66. Lambert H, Hausser E. [Anicteric hepatitis. New possible complication of cat-scratch disease]. Rev Med Suisse Romande 1965; 85:689–93.
67. Greenbaum B, Nelson P, Marchildon M, Donaldson M. Hemolytic anemia and hepatosplenomegaly associated with cat scratch fever. J Pediatr 1986;108:428–30.
68. Rocco VK, Roman RJ, Eigenbrodt EH. Cat scratch disease. Report of a case with hepatic lesions and a brief review of the literature. Gastroenterology 1985;89:1400–6.
69. Rizkallah MF, Meyer L, Ayoub EM. Hepatic and splenic abscesses in cat-scratch disease. Pediatr Infect Dis J 1988;7:191–5.
70. Lenoir AA, Storch GA, DeSchryver KK, et al. Granulomatous hepatitis associated with cat scratch disease. Lancet 1988;1: 1132–6.
71. Malatack JJ, Altman HA, Nard JA, et al. Cat-scratch disease without adenopathy. J Pediatr 1989;114:101–4.
72. Golden SE. Hepatosplenic cat-scratch disease associated with elevated anti-Rochalimaea antibody titers. Pediatr Infect Dis J 1993;12:868–71.
73. Lamps LW, Gray GF, Scott MA. The histologic spectrum of hepatic cat scratch disease. A series of six cases with confirmed Bartonella henselae infection. Am J Surg Pathol 1996;20: 1253–9.
74. American Academy of Pediatrics. Cat-scratch disease (Bartonella henselae). In: Pickering L, ed. Red Book: 2003 Report of the Committee on Infectious Diseases. Elk Grove Village, IL: American Academy of Pediatrics, 2003:232–4.
75. Bryant K, Marshall GS. Hepatosplenic cat scratch disease treated with corticosteroids. Arch Dis Child 2003;88:345–6.
76. Fitz-Hugh T. Acute gonococcic peritonitis of the right upper quadrant in women. JAMA 1934;102:2094–6.
77. Curtis AH. A cause of adhesions in the right upper quadrant. JAMA 1930;94:1221–2.
78. Bolton JP, Darougar S. Perihepatitis. Br Med Bull 1983;39:159–62.
79. Tsubuku M, Hayashi S, Terahara A, et al. Fitz-Hugh–Curtis syndrome: linear contrast enhancement of the surface of the liver on CT. J Comput Assist Tomogr 2002;26:456–8.
80. Wolner HP, Westrom L, Mardh PA. Perihepatitis and chlamydial salpingitis. Lancet 1980;1:901–3.

81. Joseph AT. Perihepatitis in women with salpingitis – an underdiagnosed clinical entity [letter]? Genitourin Med 1995;71: 331.
82. Holmes KK, Counts GW, Beaty HN. Disseminated gonococcal infection. Ann Intern Med 1971;74:979–93.
83. Cleary TG. Salmonella. In: Feigin RD, Cherry JD, Demmler GJ, Kaplan SL, eds. Textbook of pediatric infectious diseases. Philadelphia: WB Saunders, 2004:1473–87.
84. Ramachandran S, Godfrey JJ, Perera MV. Typhoid hepatitis. JAMA 1974;230:236–40.
85. Gonzalez-Quintela A, Campos J, Alende R, et al. Abnormalities in liver enzyme levels during Salmonella enteritidis enterocolitis. Rev Esp Enferm Dig 2004;96:559–62.
86. Mert A, Tabak F, Ozaras R,.Typhoid fever as a rare cause of hepatic, splenic, and bone marrow granulomas. Intern Med 2004;43:436–9.
87. Albrecht H. Bacterial and miscellaneous infections of the liver. In: Zakim D, Boyer TD, editors. Hepatology. Philadelphia: WB Saunders, 2003:1109–24.
88. Young EJ. Brucellosis. In: Feigin RD, Cherry JD, Demmler GJ, Kaplan S, eds. Textbook of pediatric infectious disease. Philadelphia: WB Saunders, 2004:1582–8.
89. Lulu AR, Araj GF, Khateeb MI, et al. Human brucellosis in Kuwait: a prospective study of 400 cases. Q J Med 1988;66:39–54.
90. Cervantes F, Bruguera M, Carbonell J, et al. Liver disease in brucellosis. A clinical and pathological study of 40 cases. Postgrad Med J 1982;58:346–50.
91. Sisteron O, Souci J, Chevallier P, et al. Hepatic abscess caused by Brucella US, CT and MRI findings: case report and review of the literature. Clin Imaging 2002;26:414–17.
92. American Academy of Pediatrics. Brucellosis. In: Pickering L, ed. Red Book: 2003 Report of the Committee on Infectious Diseases. Elk Grove Village, IL: American Academy of Pediatrics, 2003:222–4.
93. Colmenero JD, Queipo-Ortuno MI, Maria RJ, et al. Chronic hepatosplenic abscesses in Brucellosis. Clinico-therapeutic features and molecular diagnostic approach. Diagn Microbiol Infect Dis 2002;42:159–67.
94. Feigin RD, Lau CC. Tularemia. In: Feigin RD, Cherry JD, Demmler GJ, Kaplan S, eds. Textbook of pediatric infectious diseases. Philadelphia: Saunders, 2004:1628–36.
95. Evans ME, Gregory DW, Schaffner W, McGee ZA. Tularemia: a 30-year experience with 88 cases. Medicine (Baltimore) 1985; 64:251–69.
96. Ortego TJ, Hutchins LF, Rice J, Davis GR. Tularemic hepatitis presenting as obstructive jaundice. Gastroenterology 1986;91: 461–3.
97. American Academy of Pediatrics. Tularemia. In: Pickering L, ed. Red Book: 2003 Report of the Committee on Infectious Diseases. Elk Grove Village, IL: American Academy of Pediatrics, 2003:666–7.
98. Vadillo M, Corbella X, Pac V, et al. Multiple liver abscesses due to Yersinia enterocolitica discloses primary hemochromatosis: three cases reports and review [see comments]. Clin Infect Dis 1994;18:938–41.
99. Crosbie J, Varma J, Mansfield J. Yersinia enterocolitica infection in a patient with hemachromatosis masquerading as proximal colon cancer with liver metastases: report of a case. Dis Colon Rectum 2005;48:390–2.
100. Centers for Disease Control. Toxic shock syndrome. MMWR 1980;29:229–39.
101. Gourley GR, Chesney PJ, Davis JP, Odell GB. Acute cholestasis in patients with toxic-shock syndrome. Gastroenterology 1981;81:928–31.
102. Ishak KG, Rogers WA. Cryptogenic acute cholangitis – association with toxic shock syndrome. Am J Clin Pathol 1981;76:619–26.
103. Cunha BA. Systemic infections affecting the liver. Some cause jaundice, some do not. Postgrad Med 1988;84:148–3, 166.
104. Fishbein WN. Jaundice as an early manifestation of scarlet fever. Report of three cases in adults and review of the literature. Ann Intern Med 1962;57:60–72.
105. Biesel-Desthieux MN, Tissieres P, Belli DC, et al. Fulminant liver failure in a child with invasive group A streptococcal infection. Eur J Pediatr 2003;162:245–7.
106. American Academy of Pediatrics. Toxic shock syndrome. In: Pickering L, ed. Red Book: 2003 Report of the Committee on Infectious Diseases. Elk Grove Village, IL: American Academy of Pediatrics, 2003:624–30.
107. Zimmerman HJ, Thomas LJ. The liver in pneumococcal pneumonia. Observations in 94 cases on liver function and jaundice in pneumonia. J Lab Clin Med 1950;35:556–67.
108. Tugwell P, Williams AO. Jaundice associated with lobar pneumonia. A clinical, laboratory and histological study. Q J Med 1977;46:97–118.
109. Edwards MS. Listeriosis. In: McMillan JA, DeAngelis CD, Feigin RD, Warshaw JB, eds. Oski's pediatrics. Philadelphia: Lippincott Williams & Wilkins, 1999:978–80.
110. Ray CG, Wedgewood R. Neonatal listeriosis – six case reports and a review of the literature. Pediatrics 1964;34:378.
111. Vargas V, Aleman C, de TI, et al. Listeria monocytogenes-associated acute hepatitis in a liver transplant recipient. Liver 1998;18:213–15.
112. Cousens LP, Wing EJ. Innate defenses in the liver during Listeria infection. Immunol Rev 2000;174:150–9.
113. American Academy of Pediatrics. *Listeria monocytogenes* infections listeriosis. In: Pickering L, ed. Red Book: 2003 Report of the Committee on Infectious Diseases. Elk Grove Village, IL: American Academy of Pediatrics, 2003:405–7.
114. Hof H, Nichterlein T, Kretschmar M. Management of listeriosis. Clin Microbiol Rev 1997;10:345–57.
115. Starke JR, Smith KC. Tuberculosis. In: Feigin RD, Cherry JD, Demmler GJ, Kaplan S, eds. Textbook of pediatric infectious diseases. Philadelphia: W.B. Saunders, 2004:1337–79.
116. Korn RJ, Kellow WF, Heller P, et al. Hepatic involvement in extrapulmonary tuberculosis. Am J Med 1959;27:60–71.
117. Sharma S. Granulomatous diseases of the liver. In: Zakim D, Boyer TD, editors. Hepatology. Philadelphia: W.B. Saunders, 2003:1317–30.
118. Alvarez SZ, Carpio R. Hepatobiliary tuberculosis. Dig Dis Sci 1983;28:193–200.
119. Maglinte DD, Alvarez SZ, Ng AC, Lapena JL. Patterns of calcifications and cholangiographic findings in hepatobiliary tuberculosis. Gastrointest Radiol 1988;13:331–5.
120. Levine C. Primary macronodular hepatic tuberculosis: US and CT appearances. Gastrointest Radiol 1990;15:307–9.
121. Diaz ML, Herrera T, Lopez VY, et al. Polymerase chain reaction for the detection of Mycobacterium tuberculosis DNA in

tissue and assessment of its utility in the diagnosis of hepatic granulomas. J Lab Clin Med 1996;127:359–63.

122. American Academy of Pediatrics. Tuberculosis. In: Pickering L, ed. Red Book: 2003 Report of the Committee on Infectious Diseases. Elk Grove Village, IL: American Academy of Pediatrics, 2003:642–60.
123. Reed DH, Nash AF, Valabhji P. Radiological diagnosis and management of a solitary tuberculous hepatic abscess. Br J Radiol 1990;63:902–4.
124. Flegg PJ, Laing RB, Lee C, et al. Disseminated disease due to *Mycobacterium avium* complex in AIDS. QJM 1995;88:617–26.
125. Wilkins MJ, Lindley R, Dourakis SP, Goldin RD. Surgical pathology of the liver in HIV infection. Histopathology 1991;18: 459–64.
126. Wright J. Current strategies for the prevention and treatment of disseminated *Mycobacterium avium* complex infection in patients with AIDS. Pharmacotherapy 1998;18:738–47.
127. Ong EL. Prophylaxis against disseminated *Mycobacterium avium* complex in AIDS. J Infect 1999;38:6–8.
128. Jonas RB, Brasitus TA, Chowdhury L. Actinomycotic liver abscess. Case report and literature review. Dig Dis Sci 1987;32: 1435–7.
129. Meade RH. Primary hepatic actinomycosis. Gastroenterology 1980;78:355–9.
130. Sharma M, Briski LE, Khatib R. Hepatic actinomycosis: an overview of salient features and outcome of therapy. Scand J Infect Dis 2002;34:386–91.
131. Kasano Y, Tanimura H, Yamaue H, et al. Hepatic actinomycosis infiltrating the diaphragm and right lung. Am J Gastroenterol 1996;91:2418–20.
132. American Academy of Pediatrics. Actinomycosis. In: Pickering L, ed. Red Book: 2003 Report of the Committee on Infectious Diseases. Elk Grove Village, IL: American Academy of Pediatrics, 2003:189–90.
133. Felekouras E, Menenakos C, Griniatsos J, et al. Liver resection in cases of isolated hepatic actinomycosis: case report and review of the literature. Scand J Infect Dis 2004;36:535–8.
134. Dumler JS, Bakken JS. Human ehrlichioses: newly recognized infections transmitted by ticks. Annu Rev Med 1998;49:201–13.
135. Fishbein DB, Dawson JE, Robinson LE. Human ehrlichiosis in the United States, 1985 to 1990. Ann Intern Med 1994;120:736–43.
136. Moskovitz M, Fadden R, Min T. Human ehrlichiosis: a rickettsial disease associated with severe cholestasis and multisystemic disease. J Clin Gastroenterol 1991;13:86–90.
137. Sehdev AE, Dumler JS. Hepatic pathology in human monocytic ehrlichiosis. *Ehrlichia chaffeensis* infection. Am J Clin Pathol 2003;119:859–65.
138. Dumler JS, Sutker WL, Walker DH. Persistent infection with *Ehrlichia chaffeensis.* Clin Infect Dis 1993;17:903–5.
139. Dumler JS, Bakken JS. Ehrlichial diseases of humans: emerging tick-borne infections. Clin Infect Dis 1995;20:1102–10.
140. Yu X, Brouqui P, Dumler JS, Raoult D. Detection of *Ehrlichia chaffeensis* in human tissue by using a species-specific monoclonal antibody. J Clin Microbiol 1993;31:3284–8.
141. Wood A, Wilfert C, Kelsey D, Gutman L. Childhood syphilis in North Carolina. NC Med J 1980;41:443–9.
142. Tan KL. The re-emergence of early congenital syphilis. Acta Paediatr Scand 1973;62:601–7.
143. Oppenheimer EH, Hardy JB. Congenital syphilis in the newborn infant: clinical and pathological observations in recent cases. Johns Hopkins Med J 1971;129:63–82.
144. Patrick CC, McCullers JA. Syphilis. In: McMillan JA, DeAngelis CD, Feigin RD, Warshaw JB, eds. Oski's pediatrics. Philadelphia: Lippincott Williams and Wilkins, 1999:1021–5.
145. Listernick R. Liver failure in a 2-day-old infant. Pediatr Ann 2004;33:10–14.
146. Wright DJ, Berry CL. Letter: liver involvement in congenital syphilis. Br J Vener Dis 1974;50:241.
147. Brooks SE, Audretsch JJ. Hepatic ultrastructure in congenital syphilis. Arch Pathol Lab Med 1978;102:502–5.
148. Long WA, Ulshen MH, Lawson EE. Clinical manifestations of congenital syphilitic hepatitis: implications for pathogenesis. J Pediatr Gastroenterol Nutr 1984;3:551–5.
149. Ozaki T, Takemoto K, Hosono H, et al. Secondary syphilitic hepatitis in a fourteen-year-old male youth. Pediatr Infect Dis J 2002;21:439–41.
150. Ridruejo E, Mordoh A, Herrera F, et al. Severe cholestatic hepatitis as the first symptom of secondary syphilis. Dig Dis Sci 2004;49:1401–4.
151. Schlossberg D. Syphilitic hepatitis: a case report and review of the literature. Am J Gastroenterol 1987;82:552–3.
152. Comer GM, Mukherjee S, Sachdev RK, Clain DJ. Cardiolipin fluorescent (M1) antimitochondrial antibody and cholestatic hepatitis in secondary syphilis. Dig Dis Sci 1989;34:1298–302.
153. Steere AC, Grodzicki RL, Kornblatt AN, et al. The spirochetal etiology of Lyme disease. N Engl J Med 1983;308:733–40.
154. Benach JL, Bosler EM, Hanrahan JP, et al. Spirochetes isolated from the blood of two patients with Lyme disease. N Engl J Med 1983;308:740–2.
155. Steere AC, Bartenhagen NH, Craft JE, et al. The early clinical manifestations of Lyme disease. Ann Intern Med 1983;99:76–82.
156. Nadelman RB, Nowakowski J, Forseter G, et al. The clinical spectrum of early Lyme borreliosis in patients with culture-confirmed erythema migrans. Am J Med 1996;100:502–8.
157. Goellner MH, Agger WA, Burgess JH, Duray PH. Hepatitis due to recurrent Lyme disease. Ann Intern Med 1988;108:707–8.
158. Schoen RT. Relapsing or reinfectious Lyme hepatitis. Hepatology 1989;9:335–6.
159. Liveris D, Varde S, Iyer R, et al. Genetic diversity of Borrelia burgdorferi in Lyme disease patients as determined by culture versus direct PCR with clinical specimens. J Clin Microbiol 1999;373:565–9.
160. American Academy of Pediatrics. Lyme disease (Borrelia burgdorferi infection). In: Pickering L, ed. Red Book: 2003 Report of the Committee on Infectious Diseases. Elk Grove Village, IL: American Academy of Pediatrics, 2003:407–11.
161. Brown V, Larouze B, Desve G, et al. Clinical presentation of louse-borne relapsing fever among Ethiopian refugees in northern Somalia. Ann Trop Med Parasitol 1988;82:499–502.
162. Feigin RD. Leptospirosis. In: Feigin RD, Cherry JD, Demmler GJ, Kaplan S, eds. Textbook of pediatric infectious diseases. Philadelphia: W.B. Saunders, 2004:1708–22.
163. Wong ML, Kaplan S, Dunkle LM, et al. Leptospirosis: a childhood disease. J Pediatr 1977;90:532–7.
164. Jevon TR, Knudson MP, Smith PA, et al. A point-source epidemic of leptospirosis. Description of cases, cause, and prevention. Postgrad Med 1986;80:121–9.

165. Cruz ML, Andrade J, Pereira MM. Leptospirose em criancas no Rio de Janeiro [Leptospirosis in children in Rio do Janeiro]. Rev Soc Bras Med Trop 1994;27:5–9.
166. Edington GM. Other viral and infectious diseases. In: Macsween RNM, Anthony PP, Scheuer PJ, eds. Pathology of the liver. Edinburgh: Churchill Livingstone, 1979:192–220.
167. American Academy of Pediatrics. Leptospirosis. In: Pickering L, ed. Red Book: 2003 Report of the Committee on Infectious Diseases. Elk Grove Village, IL: American Academy of Pediatrics, 2003:403–5.
168. Takafuji ET, Kirkpatrick JW, Miller RN, et al. An efficacy trial of doxycycline chemoprophylaxis against leptospirosis. N Engl J Med 1984;310:497–500.
169. Feigin RD, Boom M. Rickettsial diseases. In: McMillan JA, DeAngelis CD, Feigin RD, Warshaw JB, eds. Oski's pediatrics. Philadelphia: Lippincott Williams and Wilkins, 1999:898–907.
170. Adams JS, Walker DH. The liver in Rocky Mountain spotted fever. Am J Clin Pathol 1981;75:156–61.
171. American Academy of Pediatrics. Rocky Mountain spotted fever. In: Pickering L, ed. Red Book: 2003 Report of the Committee on Infectious Diseases. Elk Grove Village, IL: American Academy of Pediatrics, 2003:532–4.
172. Westlake P, Price LM, Russell M, Kelly JK. The pathology of Q fever hepatitis. A case diagnosed by liver biopsy. J Clin Gastroenterol 1987;9:357–63.
173. Berkovitch M, Aladjem M, Beer S, Cohar K. A fatal case of Q fever hepatitis in a child. Helv Paediatr Acta 1985;40:87–91.
174. Domingo P, Orobitg J, Colomina J, et al. Liver involvement in acute Q fever [letter]. Chest 1988;94:895–6.
175. Atienza P, Ramond MJ, Degott C, et al. Chronic Q fever hepatitis complicated by extensive fibrosis. Gastroenterology 1988; 95:478–81.
176. Baquero-Artigao F, del Castillo F, Tellez A. Acute Q fever pericarditis followed by chronic hepatitis in a two-year-old girl. Pediatr Infect Dis J 2002;21:705–7.
177. American Academy of Pediatrics. Q Fever. In: Pickering L, ed. Red Book: 2003 Report of the Committee on Infectious Diseases. Elk Grove Village, IL: American Academy of Pediatrics, 2003:512–14.
178. McGowan K. How to find and treat amebiasis. Drug Ther 1984; 14:159–74.
179. Harrison HR, Crowe CP, Fulginiti VA. Amebic liver abscess in children: clinical and epidemiologic features. Pediatrics 1979; 64:923–8.
180. Hotez PJ, Strickland AD. Amebiasis. In: Feigin RD, Cherry JD, Demmler GJ, Kaplan S, eds. Textbook of pediatric infectious diseases. Philadelphia: Saunders, 2004:2660–9.
181. Rimsza ME, Berg RA. Cutaneous amebiasis. Pediatrics 1983; 71:595–8.
182. Sherlock S. Diseases of the liver and biliary system. 7th ed. Oxford: Blackwell Scientific, 1985.
183. Crane PS, Lee YT, Seel DJ. Experience in the treatment of two hundred patients with amebic abscess of the liver in Korea. Am J Surg 1972;123:332–7.
184. Chaves FJ, Cruz I, Gomes C, et al. Hepatic amebiasis-analysis of 56 cases. II. Laboratory and chest x-ray findings. Am J Gastroenterol 1977;68:273–7.
185. Barrett CE. Amebiasis, today, in the United States. Calif Med 1971;114:1–6.
186. American Academy of Pediatrics. Drugs for parasitic infections. In: Pickering L, editor. Red Book: 2003 Report of the Committee on Infectious Diseases. Elk Grove Village, IL: American Academy of Pediatrics, 2003:744–70.
187. Giorgio A, Amoroso P, Francica G, et al. Echo-guided percutaneous puncture: a safe and valuable therapeutic tool for amebic liver abscess. Gastrointest Radiol 1988;13:336–40.
188. Adams EB, MacLeod IN. Invasive amebiasis. II. Amebic liver abscess and its complications. Medicine (Baltimore) 1977;56: 325–34.
189. Turner JA. Cestodes. In: Feigin RD, Cherry JD, Demmler GJ, Kaplan S, eds. Textbook of pediatric infectious diseases. Philadelphia: W.B. Saunders, 2004:2797–816.
190. Farmer PM, Chatterley S, Spier N. Echinococcal cyst of the liver: diagnosis and surgical management. Ann Clin Lab Sci 1990; 20:385–91.
191. Gangopadhyay AN, Sahoo SP, Sharma SP, et al. Hydatid disease in children may have an atypical presentation. Pediatr Surg Int 2000;16:89–90.
192. Al Karawi MA, El Sheikh Mohamed AR, Yasawy MI. Advances in diagnosis and management of hydatid disease. Hepatogastroenterology 1990;37:327–31.
193. Agildere AM, Aytekin C, Coskun M, et al. MRI of hydatid disease of the liver: a variety of sequences. J Comput Assist Tomogr 1998;22:718–24.
194. Balci NC, Sirvanci M. MR imaging of infective liver lesions. Magn Reson Imaging Clin N Am 2002;10:121–35, vii.
195. Etlik O, Bay A, Arslan H, et al. Contrast-enhanced CT and MRI findings of atypical hepatic Echinococcus alveolaris infestation. Pediatr Radiol 2005;35:546–9.
196. Spiliadis C, Georgopoulos S, Dailianas A, et al. The use of ERCP in the study of patients with hepatic echinococcosis before and after surgical intervention. Gastrointest Endosc 1996;43:575–9.
197. Bret PM, Fond A, Bretagnolle M, et al. Percutaneous aspiration and drainage of hydatid cysts in the liver. Radiology 1988; 168:617–20.
198. Stefaniak J. Fine needle aspiration biopsy in the differential diagnosis of the liver cystic echinococcosis. Acta Trop 1997;67:107–11.
199. Bickel A, Daud G, Urbach D, et al. Laparoscopic approach to hydatid liver cysts. Is it logical? Physical, experimental, and practical aspects. Surg Endosc 1998;12:1073–7.
200. Golematis BC, Peveretos PJ. Hepatic hydatid disease: current surgical treatment. Mt Sinai J Med 1995;62:71–6.
201. Schipper HG, Kager PA. Diagnosis and treatment of hepatic echinococcosis: an overview. Scand J Gastroenterol Suppl 2004;50–5.
202. Agaoglu N, Turkyilmaz S, Arslan MK. Surgical treatment of hydatid cysts of the liver. Br J Surg 2003;90:1536–41.
203. Ertem M, Karahasanoglu T, Yavuz N, Erguney S. Laparoscopically treated liver hydatid cysts. Arch Surg 2002;137:1170–3.
204. Bosanac ZB, Lisanin L. Percutaneous drainage of hydatid cyst in the liver as a primary treatment: review of 52 consecutive cases with long-term follow-up. Clin Radiol 2000;55:839–48.
205. Ormeci N, Soykan I, Bektas A, et al. A new percutaneous approach for the treatment of hydatid cysts of the liver. Am J Gastroenterol 2001;96:2225–30.
206. Sciume C, Geraci G, Pisello F, et al. Treatment of complications of hepatic hydatid disease by ERCP: our experience. Ann Ital Chir 2004;75:531–5.
207. Louw JH. Abdominal complications of ascariasis. Surg Rounds 1981;4:54–65.

208. Sakakibara A, Baba K, Niwa S, et al. Visceral larva migrans due to Ascaris suum which presented with eosinophilic pneumonia and multiple intra-hepatic lesions with severe eosinophil infiltration — outbreak in a Japanese area other than Kyushu. Intern Med 2002;41:574–9.
209. Khuroo MS. Hepatobiliary and pancreatic ascariasis. Indian J Gastroenterol 2001;20 Suppl 1:C28–32.
210. Pinilla AE, Lopez MC, Ricaurte O, et al. Liver abscess caused by Ascaris lumbricoides: case report. Rev Inst Med Trop Sao Paulo 2001;43:343–6.
211. El Sheikh Mohamed AR, Al Karawi MA, Yasawy MI. Modern techniques in the diagnosis and treatment of gastrointestinal and biliary tree parasites. Hepatogastroenterology 1991;38: 180–8.
212. Radin DR, Vachon LA. CT findings in biliary and pancreatic ascariasis. J Comput Assist Tomogr 1986;10:508–9.
213. Bhushan B, Watal G, Mahajan R, Khuroo MS. Endoscopic retrograde cholangiopancreaticographic features of pancreaticobiliary ascariasis. Gastrointest Radiol 1988;13:327–30.
214. Reddy DN, Sriram PV, Rao GV. Endoscopic diagnosis and management of tropical parasitic infestations. Gastrointest Endosc Clin N Am 2003;13:765–73, x–xi.
215. Beckingham IJ, Cullis SN, Krige JE, et al. Management of hepatobiliary and pancreatic *Ascaris* infestation in adults after failed medical treatment. Br J Surg 1998;85:907–10.
216. Pereira-Lima JC, Jakobs R, da Silva CP, et al. Endoscopic removal of *Ascaris lumbricoides* from the biliary tract as emergency treatment for acute suppurative cholangitis. Z Gastroenterol 2001;39:793–6.
217. Ozcan N, Erdogan N, Kucuk C, Ok E. Biliary ascariasis: percutaneous transhepatic management. J Vasc Interv Radiol 2003; 14:391–3.
218. Zinkham WH. Visceral larva migrans. A review and reassessment indicating two forms of clinical expression: visceral and ocular. Am J Dis Child 1978;132:627–33.
219. Azuma K, Yashiro N, Kinoshita T, et al. Hepatic involvement of visceral larva migrans due to *Toxocara canis:* a case report – CT and MR findings. Radiat Med 2002;20:89–92.
220. Choe G, Lee HS, Seo JK, et al. Hepatic capillariasis: first case report in the Republic of Korea. Am J Trop Med Hyg 1993;48: 610–25.
221. Terrier P, Hack I, Hatz C, et al. Hepatic capillariasis in a 2-year-old boy. J Pediatr Gastroenterol Nutr 1999;28:338–40.
222. Doehring E. Schistosomiasis in childhood. Eur J Pediatr 1988; 147:2–9.
223. McKerrow JH, Sun E. Hepatic schistosomiasis. Prog Liver Dis 1994;12:121–35.
224. Bica I, Hamer DH, Stadecker MJ. Hepatic schistosomiasis. Infect Dis Clin North Am 2000;14:583–604, viii.
225. De CK. Hepatosplenic schistosomiasis: a clinical review. Gut 1986;27:734–45.
226. Symmers W. Note on a new form of liver cirrhosis due to the presence of ova of Bilharzia haematobium. J Pathol Bacteriol 1903;9:237–9.
227. DiazGranados CA, Duffus WA, Albrecht H. Parasitic diseases of the liver. In: Zakim D, Boyer TD, eds. Hepatology. Philadelphia: Saunders, 2003:1073–108.
228. Lambertucci JR, Cota GF, Pinto-Silva RA, et al. Hepatosplenic schistosomiasis in field-based studies: a combined clinical and sonographic definition. Mem Inst Oswaldo Cruz 2001;96 Suppl:147–50.
229. Palmer PE. Schistosomiasis. Semin Roentgenol 1998;33:6–25.
230. Willemsen UF, Pfluger T, Zoller WG, et al. MRI of hepatic schistosomiasis mansoni. J Comput Assist Tomogr 1995;19:811–13.
231. Doehring SE, Abdel RI, Kardorff R, et al. Ultrasonographical investigation of periportal fibrosis in children with Schistosoma mansoni infection: reversibility of morbidity twenty-three months after treatment with praziquantel. Am J Trop Med Hyg 1992;46:409–15.
232. Petroianu A, De Oliveira AE, Alberti LR. Hypersplenism in schistosomatic portal hypertension. Arch Med Res 2005;36: 496–501.
233. Lin AC, Chapman SW, Turner HR, Wofford JD. Clonorchiasis: an update. South Med J 1987;80:919–22.
234. Liu LX, Harinasuta KT. Liver and intestinal flukes. Gastroenterol Clin North Am 1996;25:627–36.
235. Sun T. Pathology and immunology of *Clonorchis sinensis* infection of the liver. Ann Clin Lab Sci 1984;14:208–15.
236. Mairiang E, Mairiang P. Clinical manifestation of opisthorchiasis and treatment. Acta Trop 2003;88:221–7.
237. Fan ST, Choi TK, Wong J. Recurrent pyogenic cholangitis: current management [see comments]. World J Surg 1991;15:248–53.
238. Jones EA, Kay JM, Milligan HP, Owens D. Massive infection with Fasciola hepatica in man. Am J Med 1977;63:836–42.
239. MacLean JD, Graeme-Cook FM. Case records of the Massachusetts General Hospital. Weekly clinicopathological exercises. Case 12-2002. A 50-year-old man with eosinophilia and fluctuating hepatic lesions. N Engl J Med 2002;346:1232–9.
240. Cosme A, Ojeda E, Poch M, et al. Sonographic findings of hepatic lesions in human fascioliasis. J Clin Ultrasound 2003;31: 358–63.
241. Hillyer GV, Soler-de GM, Rodriguez PJ, et al. Use of the Falcon assay screening test – enzyme-linked immunosorbent assay (FAST-ELISA) and the enzyme-linked immunoelectrotransfer blot (EITB) to determine the prevalence of human fascioliasis in the Bolivian Altiplano. Am J Trop Med Hyg 1992;46:603–9.
242. Sezgin O, Altintas E, Disibeyaz S, et al. Hepatobiliary fascioliasis: clinical and radiologic features and endoscopic management. J Clin Gastroenterol 2004;38:285–91.
243. Abdul HS, Contreras R, Tombazzi C, et al. Hepatic fascioliasis: case report and review. Rev Inst Med Trop Sao Paulo 1996; 38:69–73.
244. Haghighi P, Rezai HR. Leishmaniasis: a review of selected topics. Pathol Annu 1977;12 Pt 2:63–89.
245. Wittner M, Tanowitz HB. Leishmaniasis. In: Feigin RD, Cherry JD, Demmler GJ, Kaplan S, eds. Textbook of pediatric infectious diseases. Philadelphia: W.B. Saunders, 2004:2730–9.
246. Moreno A, Marazuela M, Yebra M, et al. Hepatic fibrin-ring granulomas in visceral leishmaniasis. Gastroenterology 1988; 95:1123–6.
247. Moragas A, Serrano A, Toran N. Acute form of visceral leishmaniasis in a 3-month-old infant. Pediatr Pathol 1986;6:111–17.
248. Katakura K, Kawazu S, Naya T, et al. Diagnosis of kala-azar by nested PCR based on amplification of the Leishmania mini-exon gene. J Clin Microbiol 1998;36:2173–7.
249. Noyes HA, Reyburn H, Bailey JW, Smith D. A nested-PCR-based schizodeme method for identifying Leishmania kinetoplast minicircle classes directly from clinical samples and its application to the study of the epidemiology of Leishmania tropica in Pakistan. J Clin Microbiol 1998;36:2877–81.

250. Bukte Y, Nazaroglu H, Mete A, Yilmaz F. Visceral leishmaniasis with multiple nodular lesions of the liver and spleen: CT and sonographic findings. Abdom Imaging 2004;29:82–4.
251. Barnett ED. Malaria. In: Feigin RD, Cherry JD, Demmler GJ, Kaplan S, eds. Textbook of pediatric infectious diseases. Philadelphia: Saunders, 2004:2714–40.
252. Ibhanesebhor SE. Clinical characteristics of neonatal malaria. J Trop Pediatr 1995;41:330–3.
253. Devarbhavi H, Alvares JF, Kumar KS. Severe falciparum malaria simulating fulminant hepatic failure. Mayo Clin Proc 2005;80:355–8.
254. Kochar DK, Singh P, Agarwal P, et al. Malarial hepatitis. J Assoc Physicians India 2003;51:1069–72.
255. Warrell DA. Pathophysiology of severe falciparum malaria in man. Parasitology 1987;94 Suppl:S53–76.
256. Cook GC. Malaria in the liver. Postgrad Med J 1994;70:780–4.
257. Sowunmi A. Hepatomegaly in acute falciparum malaria in children. Trans R Soc Trop Med Hyg 1996;90:540–2.
258. Thaler M, Pastakia B, Shawker TH, et al. Hepatic candidiasis in cancer patients: the evolving picture of the syndrome. Ann Intern Med 1988;108:88–100.
259. Anttila VJ, Lamminen AE, Bondestam S, et al. Magnetic resonance imaging is superior to computed tomography and ultrasonography in imaging infectious liver foci in acute leukaemia. Eur J Haematol 1996;56:82–7.
260. Semelka RC, Kelekis NL, Sallah S, et al. Hepatosplenic fungal disease: diagnostic accuracy and spectrum of appearances on MR imaging. AJR Am J Roentgenol 1997;169:1311–16.
261. Pizzo PA, Rubin M, Freifeld A, Walsh TJ. The child with cancer and infection. II. Nonbacterial infections. J Pediatr 1991;119: 845–57.
262. Einsele H, Hebart H, Roller G, et al. Detection and identification of fungal pathogens in blood by using molecular probes. J Clin Microbiol 1997;35:1353–60.
263. American Academy of Pediatrics. Candidiasis (Moniliasis, Thrush). In: Pickering L, ed. Red Book: 2003 Report of the Committee on Infectious Diseases. Elk Grove Village, IL: American Academy of Pediatrics, 2003:229–32.
264. Walsh TJ, Whitcomb P, Piscitelli S, et al. Safety, tolerance, and pharmacokinetics of amphotericin B lipid complex in children with hepatosplenic candidiasis. Antimicrob Agents Chemother 1997;41:1944–8.
265. Beovic B, Lejko ZT, Pretnar J. Sequential treatment of deep fungal infections with amphotericin B deoxycholate and amphotericin B colloidal dispersion. Eur J Clin Microbiol Infect Dis 1997;16:507–11.
266. Blot S, Vandewoude K. Management of invasive candidiasis in critically ill patients. Drugs 2004;64:2159–75.
267. Kauffman CA, Bradley SF, Ross SC, Weber DR. Hepatosplenic candidiasis: successful treatment with fluconazole. Am J Med 1991;91:137–41.
268. Anaissie E, Bodey GP, Kantarjian H, et al. Fluconazole therapy for chronic disseminated candidiasis in patients with leukemia and prior amphotericin B therapy. Am J Med 1991;91:142–50.
269. Presterl E, Graninger W. Efficacy and safety of fluconazole in the treatment of systemic fungal infections in pediatric patients. Multicentre Study Group. Eur J Clin Microbiol Infect Dis 1994; 13:347–51.
270. Driessen M, Ellis JB, Muwazi F, De VF. The treatment of systemic candidiasis in neonates with oral fluconazole. Ann Trop Paediatr 1997;17:263–71.
271. Kontoyiannis DP, Luna MA, Samuels BI, Bodey GP. Hepatosplenic candidiasis. A manifestation of chronic disseminated candidiasis. Infect Dis Clin North Am 2000;14:721–39.
272. Korinek JK, Guarda LA, Bolivar R, Stroehlein JR. Trichosporon hepatitis. Gastroenterology 1983;85:732–4.
273. Meyer MH, Letscher-Bru V, Waller J, et al. Chronic disseminated *Trichosporon asahii* infection in a leukemic child. Clin Infect Dis 2002;352:e22–5.
274. Duong TA. Infection due to Penicillium marneffei, an emerging pathogen: review of 155 reported cases [see comments]. Clin Infect Dis 1996;23:125–30.
275. Kantipong P, Panich V, Pongsurachet V, Watt G. Hepatic penicilliosis in patients without skin lesions. Clin Infect Dis 1998; 26:1215–17.
276. Viscomi SG, Mortele KJ, Cantisani V, et al. Fatal, complete splenic infarction and hepatic infection due to disseminated *Trichosporon beigelii* infection: CT findings. Abdom Imaging 2004; 29:228–30.
277. American Academy of Pediatrics. Fungal Diseases. In: Pickering L, ed. Red Book: 2003 Report of the Committee on Infectious Diseases. Elk Grove Village, IL: American Academy of Pediatrics, 2003:280–2.
278. Drutz DJ, Catanzaro A. Coccidioidomycosis. Part I. Am Rev Respir Dis 1978;117:559–85.
279. Drutz DJ, Catanzaro A. Coccidioidomycosis. Part II. Am Rev Respir Dis 1978;117:727–71.
280. Shehab ZM. Coccidiomycosis. In: Feigin RD, Cherry JD, Demmler GJ, Kaplan S, eds. Textbook of pediatric infectious diseases. Philadelphia: Saunders, 2004:2580–92.
281. Dodd LG, Nelson SD. Disseminated coccidioidomycosis detected by percutaneous liver biopsy in a liver transplant recipient. Am J Clin Pathol 1990;93:141–4.
282. Howard PF, Smith JW. Diagnosis of disseminated coccidioidomycosis by liver biopsy. Arch Intern Med 1983;143:1335–8.
283. Craig JR, Hillberg RH, Balchum OJ. Disseminated coccidioidomycosis. Diagnosis by needle biopsy of liver. West J Med 1975;122:171–4.
284. American Academy of Pediatrics. Coccidioidomycosis. In: Pickering L, ed. Red Book: 2003 Report of the Committee on Infectious Diseases. Elk Grove Village, IL: American Academy of Pediatrics, 2003:250–3.
285. Das BC, Haynes I, Weaver RM. Primary hepatic cryptococcosis. BMJ 1983;287:464.
286. Kothari AA, Kothari KA. Hepatobiliary dysfunction as initial manifestation of disseminated cryptococcosis. Indian J Gastroenterol 2004;23:145–6.
287. Lefton HB, Farmer RG, Buchwald R, Haselby R. Cryptococcal hepatitis mimicking primary sclerosing cholangitis. A case report. Gastroenterology 1974;67:511–15.
288. Bucuvalas JC, Bove KE, Kaufman RA, et al. Cholangitis associated with *Cryptococcus neoformans*. Gastroenterology 1985;88: 1055–9.
289. Lee S, Kim HJ. Cryptococcosis with cutaneous manifestations treated with 5-fluorocytosine. Dermatologica 1980;161:327–33.
290. American Academy of Pediatrics. *Cryptococcus neoformans* infections (Cryptococcosis). In: Pickering L, ed. Red Book: 2003 Report of the Committee on Infectious Diseases. Elk Grove Village, IL: American Academy of Pediatrics, 2003:254–5.
291. Goodwin-RA J, Shapiro JL, Thurman GH, et al. Disseminated histoplasmosis: clinical and pathologic correlations. Medicine (Baltimore) 1980;59:1–33.

292. Martin RC, Edwards MJ, McMasters KM. Histoplasmosis as an isolated liver lesion: review and surgical therapy. Am Surg 2001; 67:430–1.
293. Troillet N, Llor J, Kuchler H, et al. Disseminated histoplasmosis in an adopted infant from El Salvador. Eur J Pediatr 1996; 155:474–6.
294. Tobon AM, Franco L, Espinal D, et al. Disseminated histoplasmosis in children: the role of itraconazole therapy. Pediatr Infect Dis J 1996;15:1002–8.
295. American Academy of Pediatrics. Histoplasmosis. In: Pickering L, editor. Red Book: 2003 Report of the Committee on Infectious Diseases. Elk Grove Village, IL: American Academy of Pediatrics, 2003:353–6.
296. Mangurten HH, Fernandez B. Neonatal aspergillosis accompanying fulminant necrotising enterocolitis. Arch Dis Child 1979, 54:559–62.
297. Robinson SP, Remedios D, Davidson RN. Do amoebic liver abscesses start as large lesions? Case report of an evolving amoebic liver abscess. J Infect 1998;36:338–40.
298. Boon AP, O'Brien D, Adams DH. 10 year review of invasive aspergillosis detected at necropsy [see comments]. J Clin Pathol 1991;44:452–4.
299. Vairani G, Rebeschini R, Barbazza R. Hepatic and subcutaneous abscesses due to aspergillosis. Initial diagnosis of a case by intraoperative fine needle aspiration cytology. Acta Cytol 1990; 34:891–4.
300. Hospenthal DR, Byrd JC, Weiss RB. Successful treatment of invasive aspergillosis complicating prolonged treatment-related neutropenia in acute myelogenous leukemia with amphotericin B lipid complex. Med Pediatr Oncol 1995;25:119–22.
301. Lebeau B, Pelloux H, Pinel C, et al. Itraconazole in the treatment of aspergillosis: a study of 16 cases. Mycoses 1994;37:171–9.
302. Ullmann AJ. Review of the safety, tolerability, and drug interactions of the new antifungal agents caspofungin and voriconazole. Curr Med Res Opin 2003;19:263–71.
303. American Academy of Pediatrics. Aspergillosis. In: Pickering L, ed. Red Book: 2003 Report of the Committee on Infectious Diseases. Elk Grove Village, IL: American Academy of Pediatrics, 2003.200–10.
304. Camacho LL, Borges DR. Early liver dysfunction in schistosomiasis. J Hepatol 1998;29:233–240.
305. Teixeira F, Gayotto LC, De BT. Morphological patterns of the liver in South American blastomycosis. Histopathology 1978; 2:231–7.
306. Chaib E, de OC, Prado PS, Santana LL, Toloi JN, de MJ. Obstructive jaundice caused by blastomycosis of the lymph nodes around the common bile duct. Arq Gastroenterol 1988;25:198–202.

38

Systemic Disease and the Liver

Michael K. Farrell, M.D., and John C. Bucuvalas, M.D.

The liver, the largest parenchymal organ in the body, receives 25% of the resting cardiac output [1]. It is also a complex metabolic organ involved in a variety of synthetic and detoxification functions. By virtue of its size, multiple metabolic functions, and prominent position in the circulatory system, the liver is frequently involved in systemic, circulatory, and inflammatory diseases. It is often an "innocent bystander" during systemic diseases; conversely, hepatic dysfunction may be the first clue to a systemic disorder. This chapter reviews hepatic involvement in common childhood systemic diseases.

JAUNDICE IN THE CRITICALLY ILL CHILD

Hepatic dysfunction, manifest as jaundice, occurs in patients with systemic diseases associated with increased bilirubin production, ischemia, hypoxemia, or malnutrition (Table 38.1). Bilirubin production increases with hemolysis, blood transfusions, intraluminal bleeding, extracorporeal oxygenation, and resorption of blood from hematomas. The inflammatory cascade has multiple effects on hepatic function [2–9]. In the healthy patient, the liver has the capacity to conjugate and excrete bilirubin. However, with fasting, malnutrition, positive pressure ventilation, or ischemia, the liver's ability to process bilirubin is compromised and conjugated hyperbilirubinemia results [10,11] (Figure 38.1). Liver dysfunction improves with correction of the primary disorder, but inadequate or unsuccessful treatment may result in progressive hepatic dysfunction.

INFECTION

Jaundice and conjugated hyperbilirubinemia occur more frequently in infants and children with sepsis, even in the absence of shock. Patients may have mildly elevated serum alkaline phosphatase and aminotransferase levels; isolated hyperbilirubinemia is uncommon [12,13]. Serum bilirubin levels are higher in patients with preexisting hepatobiliary disease. For all age groups, jaundice may be the only sign of infection. Other signs and symptoms of liver disease are uncommon; the predominant clinical features are those of sepsis. Biochemical abnormalities are detected 2–4 days after the onset of systemic infection and resolve with appropriate therapy. These abnormalities have little prognostic significance; the prognosis is that of the underlying disease. Therapy should be directed at the primary infection. An abdominal ultrasonographic examination should be considered to exclude biliary obstruction and gallbladder disease. Any intra-abdominal infection can result in the absorption of bacteria and endotoxin into the portal venous system; septic portal thrombophlebitis and hepatic abscesses can result [14].

The liver responds to infection and injury by the initiation of a series of metabolic events, which lead to a state of negative nitrogen balance and significant loss of lean body mass. The metabolic cascade known as the acute-phase response is reflected in the clinical and biochemical findings seen with inflammation or infection, including fever, anorexia, insulin resistance, and muscle weakness. In the liver, the acute-phase response to endotoxemia is characterized by gluconeogenesis, and increased synthesis and release of coagulation factors, complement factors, and antiproteolytic enzymes. Tumor necrosis factor (TNF), interleukin-β (IL-β), and IL-6 trigger the acute-phase reaction seen with infection or injury [3,6,15–17]. The balance between proinflammatory cytokines such as TNF and the anti-inflammatory cytokines such as IL-10 and leptin may predict the clinical outcome [18,19]. In the systemic inflammatory response syndrome (SIRS), a proinflammatory state exists that is likely the cause of the end-organ dysfunction. The process is not currently completely defined, but it is apparent that it depends on the interaction among cytokines, insulin, leptin, counterregulatory hormones, insulinlike growth factors, and glucocorticoids [16,20].

The reticuloendothelial cells in the liver (Kupffer cells) serve as scavengers for endotoxin and as the major intrahepatic source of cytokines [20]. Activated Kupffer cells are protective because they produce various chemokines that attenuate the infection by recruiting inflammatory and immune cells to the liver. The released cytokines play a critical protective role. Mice with disruption of the *IL-6* gene have decreased survival following infection with *Escherichia coli* and impaired hepatic

Table 38.1: Causes of Jaundice in the Critically Ill Patient

Increased bilirubin production
- Hemolytic disease
- Hemolysis of transfused blood
- Resorption of blood from hematomas
- Intraluminal bleeding

Decreased intrahepatic processing of bilirubin
- Viral hepatitis
- Drug-induced hepatitis
- Shock/decreased perfusion
- Hypoxemia
- Fasting/malnutrition
- Preexisting liver disease

Decreased excretion of bilirubin
- Sepsis
- Extrahepatic obstruction
- Pancreatitis

regeneration following partial hepatectomy [21,22]. The release of cytokines also has adverse effects. Proinflammatory cytokines including IL-6, IL-β, and TNF contribute to the liver dysfunction common in infection or multiple organ failure [2,8, 9,23–27]. Cholestasis seen with cytokine release results from decreased expression of the Na^+,K^+ ATPase [5] and down-regulation of transport proteins that are critical to bile formation – specifically, the basolateral sodium-dependent bile salt transporter (NTCP), multidrug-resistant protein 2, a canalicular anionic conjugate transporter; and the bile salt export pump. Liver biopsies from patients with jaundice due to sepsis or endotoxinemia have intrahepatic cholestasis, Kupffer cell hyperplasia, portal mononuclear cell infiltrates, focal hepatocyte dropout and steatosis [28].

THE LIVER IN THE PRESENCE OF ALTERED SYSTEMIC CIRCULATION

Hepatic dysfunction occurs frequently in children with disorders associated with acute or chronic compromise of blood flow. Ischemic hepatopathy, which clinically may mimic toxic or infectious hepatitis, occurs in association with congestive heart failure, pericardial tamponade, shock, cardiorespiratory arrest, asphyxia, prolonged seizures, heatstroke, cardiopulmonary bypass, or severe dehydration [29–33]. The hepatic reaction may be severe enough to resemble fulminant hepatic failure [34–36]. The prognosis for children with ischemic hepatitis depends primarily on the response of the underlying disorder to therapy [37].

The liver receives approximately 25% of the cardiac output [1]. Two thirds of the hepatic blood flow arrives through the portal vein and the remainder through the hepatic artery. The hepatic artery is the sole blood supply for the major bile ducts. In the periportal zone of the hepatic acinus, the highly oxygenated blood from the hepatic artery mixes with less well-oxygenated portal blood rich in nutrients and hormones from the gastrointestinal tract. Blood flows through the hepatic sinusoids (zone 2) toward a branch of the central vein (zone 3). Blood rich in oxygen, substrates, and hormones perfuses hepatocytes in the periportal area (zone 1). The oxygen tension gradient in the hepatic lobule accounts for the increased susceptibility of pericentral hepatocytes (zone 3) to necrosis associated with decreased oxygen delivery or perfusion [38]. Regulation of hepatic blood flow occurs locally and is closely linked to adenosine clearance

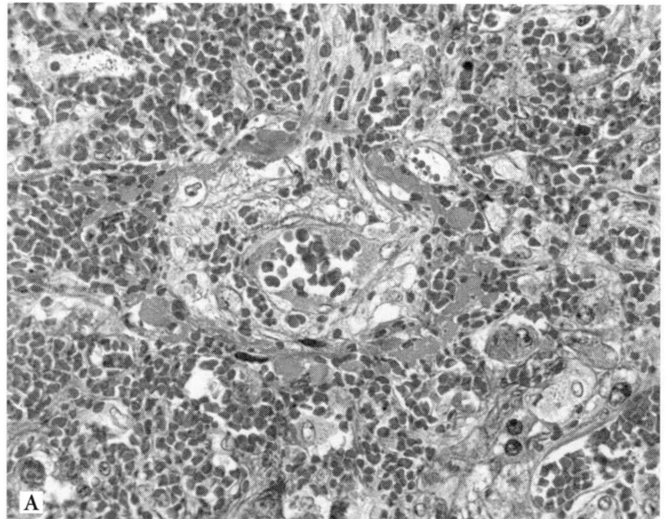

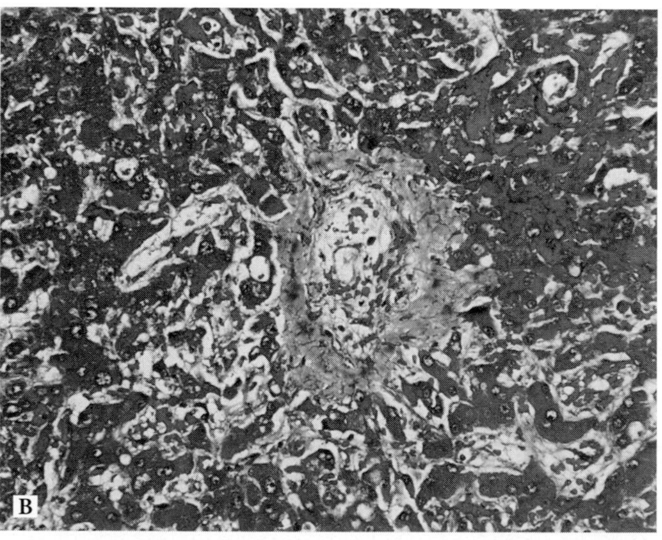

Figure 38.1. Pathology of hepatic veno-occlusion following bone marrow transplantation. (**A**) Partial occlusion of hepatic venule shows endothelial proliferation overlying cell debris. The vein wall is fibrotic. Perivenular zone is hemorrhagic because of obstruction. (**B**) Complete obstruction of a hepatic venule with sinusoidal congestion. (Hematoxylin and eosin [H&E] stain, original magnification ×350). (Courtesy of Drs. Howard Shulman and Laurie Deleve.) For color reproduction, see Color Plate 38.1.

and metabolism [1]. A change in systemic arterial pressure leads to an inverse change in hepatic arterial flow, and a change in portal blood flow leads to an inverse change in hepatic arterial flow. Adenosine, which is continuously secreted at the terminal branches of the hepatic arteriole and portal venules, acts on purinergic receptors to generate cyclic adenosine monophosphate and causes vasodilatation. As blood flow decreases, local adenosine levels increase, resulting in arterial vasodilatation; the hepatic artery delivers an increased proportion of blood flow. Reestablishment of normal hepatic blood flow increases clearance of adenosine and decreases the stimulus for arterial vasodilatation. In animal models, inhibition of nitric oxide synthase increases hepatic arterial resistance and decreases sinusoidal blood flow, suggesting that nitric oxide regulates sinusoidal perfusion by regulating vascular tone [39,40]. Nitric oxide also may serve to preserve arterial but not portal venous blood flow during and after ischemia [41–43].

Ischemic hepatopathy associated with acute compromise of blood flow is characterized by a marked and rapid elevation of serum aminotransferase levels 24–48 hours after the initial insult. Serum aminotransferase concentrations may reach 5000 to 10,000 IU/L; alkaline phosphatase levels are usually normal. Hepatomegaly, jaundice, and coagulopathy are detected in 25–50%. Elevation of serum creatine phosphokinase indicates global hypoperfusion and confirms the diagnosis [34,35]. The course is self-limited if the underlying perfusion disturbance is corrected. The half-life of aspartate aminotransferase (AST) and alanine aminotransferase (ALT) is 17–24 hours; serum concentrations return to normal in 3–11 days if perfusion and oxygenation are restored and urine output is normal [44]. This rapid decrease in aminotransferase levels in the absence of increasing hyperbilirubinemia or worsening coagulopathy distinguishes ischemic hepatopathy from viral or toxic hepatitis. Liver biopsy reveals centrilobular necrosis with preservation of the periportal zone [45–47]. Therapy should be directed toward restoring cardiac output and reversing the underlying cause of hemodynamic instability. Overly aggressive diuresis should be avoided in patients with underlying congestive heart failure.

Chronic cardiac disorders and respiratory disorders also affect the liver [48]. Typically, patients with heart failure have an insidious onset of abnormal liver chemistries. Tender hepatomegaly, distended jugular veins, and a hepatojugular reflex may be present. Complications of chronic liver disease rarely develop. However, with chronic low cardiac output, fibrous bands may form between neighboring centrilobular zones encircling normal portal areas (cardiac cirrhosis). In this situation, portal hypertension and ascites may develop [49].

Liver dysfunction occurs frequently in association with congenital heart disease. Approximately 20% of infants with severe congenital heart disease who die before 1 month of age have hepatic histologic abnormalities at autopsy [50,51]. Children who have undergone the Fontan procedure, a palliative procedure for a single functional ventricle, have an increased risk of liver dysfunction. The biochemical findings are characterized by prolongation of the prothrombin time and a low factor V level, passive congestion, and hepatic fibrosis [52,53]. Patients with right-sided heart failure are at increased risk for ischemic hepatitis, but passive congestion alone is insufficient for development of zone 3 hepatocyte necrosis [54]. Elevated aminotransferase levels are detected only in association with reduced cardiac output [29,55].

In chronic respiratory disease, elevated aminotransferase levels are detected even if the cardiac index is normal, suggesting that the liver damage occurs primarily as a result of hypoxia, not decreased blood delivery [56–58]. Severe obstructive sleep apnea has been associated with elevated serum aminotransferase levels and steatosis, independent of body weight [57].

A pattern of serum aminotransferase elevation similar to ischemic hepatopathy is seen in rhabdomyolysis or hyperpyrexia (heatstroke). The pathogenesis of these biochemical changes is multifactorial and may reflect unrecognized hypotension, alteration of local circulation, and the release of enzymes from injured muscle. If the underlying disorder is effectively treated, the biochemical abnormalities return to normal within 10–14 days [30,59]. Thus, it is important to exclude circulatory and oxygenation disorders in patients with otherwise unexplained liver abnormalities.

HEPATIC VENOUS OUTFLOW OBSTRUCTION

Budd–Chiari Syndrome

Budd–Chiari syndrome is defined as noncardiogenic hepatic venous outflow obstruction that results in ascites and liver enlargement [60]. Budd–Chiari syndrome should be suspected in patients with abdominal pain, distention, and splenic enlargement, particularly in association with thrombophilia [61]. Abdominal and chest wall vessels are prominent and distended; those below the umbilicus flow cephalad. Unlike adults, children may have only firm hepatomegaly and ascites may be absent. Mild or minimal elevation of the serum bilirubin and aminotransferase levels occur [62].

Hepatic venous outflow obstruction should be suspected in the patient with rapid onset of hepatomegaly, ascites, and abdominal pain. The goal of the evaluation of a patient with suspected Budd–Chiari syndrome is to determine the cause and level of obstruction. Diagnostic evaluation begins with pulsed Doppler sonography of the hepatic vessels. Phase forward blood flow is absent, and there is flat or reversed blood flow in the hepatic veins associated with reversed flow in the inferior vena cava [63,64]. Computed tomography (CT) or magnetic resonance imaging (MRI) scanning with contrast demonstrates no visualization of the hepatic veins and a central, fan-shaped, patchy area of increased attenuation. With acute hepatic venous flow obstruction, liver enlargement, caudate hypertrophy, and central enhancement of the liver are detected on MRI. With chronic hepatic outflow obstruction, left lobe hypertrophy, and irregular surface of the liver are also detected [65]. Hepatic venography may be necessary to determine the level of obstruction. Liver–spleen scintigraphy reveals diminished uptake in the right and left lobes and increased uptake in the caudate lobe because it

Table 38.2: Causes of Veno-Occlusive Disease

Foods
Pyrrolizidine alkaloids
Aflatoxicosis
Nitrosamines (experimental animals)
Drugs
Hypervitaminosis A
Urethane
6-Thioguanine
Vincristine
Cytosine arabinoside
6-Mercaptopurine
Dacarbazine
Indicine N-oxide
Azothioprine
Cyclophosphamide and cyclosporine
Dacarbazine
Busulfan
Cysteamine
Polysorbate
Chemoradiation for bone marrow transplantation
Miscellaneous
Alcoholic liver disease
Estrogens (cheetahs)
Familial immunodeficiency

drains directly into the interior vena cava [66,67]. A liver biopsy helps to define prognosis; cirrhosis is associated with a poor response to portosystemic decompression [68].

Hepatic venous outflow obstruction can be classified into three categories based on the level of the obstruction: intrahepatic (veno-occlusive disease [VOD]), hepatic veins, or the suprahepatic vena cava [69]. In VOD, concentric narrowing of terminal hepatic venules occurs without associated abnormalities of the hepatic veins or vena cava. VOD occurs in response to a number of insults; the most common is stem cell or bone marrow transplantation [70] (Table 38.2). VOD also occurs following chronic ingestion of herbal teas or foods containing pyrrolizidine alkaloids [71] and has been reported in a breast-fed infant whose mother drank herbal teas [72]. Outbreaks of VOD have followed the ingestion of foods contaminated with pyrrolizidine alkaloid–producing molds [73,74]. It has been reported in arsenic poisoning [75]. Infants receiving an intravenous vitamin E preparation (E-Ferol, currently unavailable) developed VOD; large doses of a polysorbate were considered the etiologic agent [76]. VOD has been associated with the use of cysteamine in the treatment of cystinosis [77]. A familial form of VOD associated with immunodeficiency has been reported [78,79]. Mutations in the gene encoding the promyelocytic leukemia nuclear protein Sp110 have recently been described in these patients [80]. Radiation-related hepatic injury is a VOD; it is potentiated by chemotherapy.

Occlusion of the hepatic veins or suprahepatic vena cava develops in a variety of conditions that predispose to thrombosis, including hyperhomocysteinemia, polycythemia vera, primary lymphoproliferative disorder, pregnancy, posttrauma, tumor invasion, inflammatory bowel disease, Behcet's disease, cirrhosis, sickle cell anemia, protein C deficiency, oral contraceptives, and collagen vascular diseases [81–91]. A clonal mutation in the Janus kinase 2 tyrosine kinase that is found in a high proportion of patients with myeloproliferative disorder was found in 59% of patients with Budd–Chiari syndrome, including 1 of 3 children with the disorder [92]. None of the patients were previously known to have a myeloproliferative disorder.

Resistance to protein C due to the factor V Leiden mutation is the most common cause of thrombophilia and accounts for 25% of cases [93,94]. Antiphospholipid syndrome predisposes patients to recurrent arterial and venous thromboses. After malignancy and myeloproliferative disorders, antiphospholipid syndrome is the most common underlying cause of the Budd–Chiari syndrome. Antiphospholipid syndrome should be strongly considered in patients with lupus erythematosus who develop hepatic venous outflow obstruction [92,95,96]. Paroxysmal nocturnal hemoglobinuria is a rare disorder of complement activation that may cause Budd–Chiari syndrome [97,98].

Congenital lesions such as hepatic venous stenosis and hypoplasia of the suprahepatic veins also may cause outflow obstruction. Constrictive pericarditis may present similarly and must be excluded [32,99,100].

Membranous obstruction of the suprahepatic vena cava is the most common cause of hepatic venous outflow obstruction worldwide and is more common in developing countries [62,101,102]. Although it has been considered a congenital defect, most patients do not develop symptoms until adulthood. The obstruction has been classified by location. In type I, there is a thin membrane at the vena cava or atrium area. In type II, there is an absent segment of the inferior vena cava of variable length. In type III, the inferior vena cava cannot be filled and only collaterals are identified [103]. The clinical presentation is different; patients frequently present with dilated veins on the trunk and abdomen rather than hepatomegaly and ascites [104]. A chest radiograph may reveal a mass that is the dilated azygous vein [105]. Histology ranges from almost normal to severe chronic congestion with fibrosis, reversed lobulation, and dilated lymphatic channels [68,103,106]. Acute congestion with massive centrilobular necrosis and fulminant hepatic failure is occasionally the presenting symptom of hepatic venous outflow obstruction [107]. A review of resected specimens suggests that the basic structure of the venous wall is maintained and that the cause is organized thrombi of various ages [103]. Affected patients are at risk for developing hepatocellular carcinoma; chronic hepatitis B infection may be a contributing factor. In one study, the incidence of hepatitis B antigenemia was 22% in affected patients compared with 9% in a control group [102].

Initial therapy is conservative, emphasizing diuresis and treatment of the predisposing factors. Medical treatment of thrombotic occlusion of the hepatic veins or suprahepatic vena cava has not been successful [60]. Percutaneous transhepatic angioplasty and venous stent placement have been successful

Table 38.3: Spectrum of Liver Disease in Sickle Cell Disease Patients

Condition	*Biopsy*	*Autopsy**
Ischemia	1	14
Viral hepatitis	1	9
Biliary obstruction	0	2
Fibrosis/cirrhosis	3	0
Cholestasis	1	0
Giant cell hepatitis	1	0
Alcoholic hepatitis	0	1
No lesion	0	5
Sarcoidosis	1	0

*Ten specimens had increased iron staining.
Modified from Omata et al. [117].

in a small number of patients [108]. Transjugular intrahepatic portosystemic shunts (TIPS) have been used to decompress portal venous pressure in adults with hepatic venous outflow obstruction, but experience in children is limited [109]. Given the risk of shunt thrombosis, TIPS is a bridge to more definitive treatment. The goal of operative decompression is excision of the obstruction or portosystemic decompression. Mesocaval, splenojugular shunt, and mesojugular shunt have been successfully used to decompress portal venous hypertension caused by hepatic venous outflow obstruction [110]. Surgery is well tolerated by patients in whom there is no evidence of cirrhosis; histologic reversal of sinusoidal congestion results [111]. Patients with evidence of progressive liver disease as defined by encephalopathy, refractory ascites, and coagulopathy are candidates for orthotopic liver transplantation. In patients with underlying thrombophilia, long-term anticoagulation is necessary to prevent recurrence [112–114].

HEMATOLOGIC DISORDERS

Hemoglobinopathies

Hepatobiliary disorders are common in children with hemoglobinopathies (Table 38.3). Virtually all children with sickle cell anemia have hepatomegaly, elevated serum aminotransferase levels, and some degree of jaundice [115–118]. Elevated unconjugated bilirubin concentrations reflect hemolysis; elevated conjugated bilirubin concentrations suggest hepatobiliary disease. Alkaline phosphatase is frequently elevated but mostly originates from bone rather than liver [119]. Elevated serum bile acid concentrations are common but do not predict the development of liver dysfunction [120]. Cholelithiasis is common and is discussed in Chapter 16.

The hepatobiliary disorders are due to several factors: an increased bilirubin load secondary to chronic hemolysis, repeated blood transfusions resulting in potential exposure to hepatotropic viruses, and iron overload. When sickling occurs, hepatocytes remove the released bilirubin. Erythrophagocytosis of the damaged red cells by the Kupffer cells leads to cell proliferation that results in sinusoidal flow obstruction. With repeated episodes of sickling, the liver is permanently injured. Chronic anemia and iron overload may lead to myocardial dysfunction and subsequent hepatic injury.

Ten percent of patients with sickle cell disease develop an acute illness characterized by severe right upper quadrant abdominal pain, leukocytosis, jaundice, and tender hepatomegaly [121,122]. In sickle cell hepatopathy or hepatic crisis, serum bilirubin and aminotransferase concentrations increase two- to tenfold, but the prothrombin time remains normal. Liver biopsy reveals sinusoidal congestion in zone 2 from erythrophagocytic Kupffer cells. Ischemic changes and steatosis are rare. Sickle cell hepatopathy is initially difficult to distinguish from viral hepatitis and cholecystitis. Imaging of the biliary tree excludes cholecystitis; in viral hepatitis, aminotransferase concentrations are more elevated and the clinical features resolve more slowly [123]. Percutaneous liver biopsy complications increase in this clinical setting [124]. Sickle cell hepatopathy is more benign than initially reported; most patients recover. Treatment is supportive, but exchange transfusion has been used in severe cases [125]. Liver transplantation has been performed in the setting of severe intrahepatic cholestasis and other comorbidities such as hepatitis C infection and sclerosing cholangitis [126,127].

Patients with sickle cell disease may be at greater risk for fulminant hepatic failure following hepatitis A infection [128]. All patients with sickle cell disease should receive the hepatitis A vaccination. Hepatitis C infection may be present in older adolescents and adults if they received transfusions prior to screening of blood products [129]. Patients with sickle cell disease have developed autoimmune liver disease [130–132]. Increasing aminotransferase concentrations or worsening jaundice mark the clinical course. Other unusual hepatic lesions noted in sickle cell anemia are hepatic vein thrombosis, focal nodular hyperplasia, and hepatic abscesses [133–136]. Bacteremia with encapsulated organisms is common because of splenic hypofunction. Impaired hepatic microcirculation may cause areas of infarction, which then act as a nidus for infection. Microinfarcts in the gastrointestinal epithelium increase intestinal permeability and allow translocation of enteric organisms; the universal splenic dysfunction impedes clearance of the bacteria [112]. Hepatic abscesses may develop, and the appropriate imaging studies confirm the diagnosis.

Multiple transfusions result in hemosiderosis. Transfusion-associated hemosiderosis occurs more frequently in patients with thalassemia than in those with other hemoglobinopathies because of the heavier transfusion requirement [137].

Coagulation Disorders

Patients with coagulation disorders are exposed to large quantities of blood products. The use of recombinant products and improved screening of the blood supply has decreased the exposure to hepatotropic viruses. Hepatitis A and B vaccinations have decreased the consequences of exposure. Prior to routine vaccination, the incidence of hepatitis B exposure in hemophiliacs was approximately 75%, with 10% having persistent antigenemia [138]. The incidence of hepatitis C exposure ranged from 60% to 90% prior to donor screening [139]. Infection with the human immunodeficiency virus (HIV) occurred frequently prior to the routine screening [140]. Coinfection with the hepatitis C virus and HIV leads to severe liver disease [140,141]. About 20% of patients with hemophilia may have persistent abnormal biochemical liver study results and histologic abnormalities ranging from chronic active hepatitis to cirrhosis [138,139]. Patients with chronic hepatitis B or C infection are at risk for the development of hepatocellular carcinoma [142]. Intravenous immune globulin prepared in 1993 and 1994 was contaminated with the hepatitis C virus; approximately 10% of patients became infected with the hepatitis C virus [143,144].

Lymphomas

Hepatomegaly, jaundice, and asymptomatic abnormalities frequently occur in patients with lymphoma, leukemia, and neuroblastoma. The processes that contribute to these hepatic abnormalities are multiple, including tumor infiltration, intrahepatic and extrahepatic obstruction, hepatotoxic chemotherapeutic agents, and protein calorie malnutrition.

Thirty percent of patients with Hodgkin's disease have hepatic involvement during the course of the disease; at autopsy, 50% have liver lesions [145]. Assessment of liver involvement is necessary to stage the disease accurately and establish the therapeutic plan. The wedge biopsy is a more sensitive method than needle biopsy, but Reed–Sternberg cells are rare, and accurate staging is often difficult to achieve [145,146]. The presence of large inflammatory cell infiltrates, acute cholangitis, portal edema, and infiltrates with atypical lymphocytes predict hepatic involvement even in the absence of Reed–Sternberg cells [145,147]. These findings suggest that an extensive search for hepatic involvement should be performed. Occasionally, idiopathic cholestasis is noted in Hodgkin's disease despite the absence of lymphomatous involvement of the liver or biliary tree [148,149]. Rarely, Hodgkin's disease may present as fulminant liver disease because of malignant infiltration of the liver parenchyma [150].

The role of the staging laparotomy is controversial; it is no longer as important as previously thought. It remains crucial if radiation therapy is being considered as the sole therapy and when the presence of intra-abdominal disease would change the therapeutic regimen [146,151]. The liver is rarely involved if the spleen is not. Hence, the staging laparotomy should include a total appendectomy, wedge and needle liver biopsy, and biopsy of the porta hepatis nodes.

In non–Hodgkin's lymphoma, liver involvement is frequently the initial presenting feature; hepatomegaly or jaundice may suggest primary liver disease [152]. Extrahepatic obstruction occurs most frequently at the hilum and the intrapancreatic duct, where the ducts are less mobile and lymph nodes are present [148,149,153]. In Burkitt's lymphoma, an abdominal mass and ascites may be the initial symptom [154]. It may present as acute Budd–Chiari syndrome [155]. Jaundice resulting from intrahepatic biliary obstruction may be due to parenchymal infiltration [156,157]. Laparotomy is usually indicated for definitive diagnosis and staging. As with Hodgkin's disease, non–Hodgkin's lymphoma can present as acute liver failure. The possibility should be considered in patients who present with acute liver failure of unknown etiology.

In the evaluation of the patient with lymphoma and liver disease, it is critical to determine whether clinical or biochemical evidence of liver disease reflects primary disease recurrence requiring tumor reduction therapy or whether it is due to causes unrelated to the tumor [152]. Non-tumor-related causes include exposure to hepatotoxic chemotherapeutic agents, radiation injury, and infection. Jaundice is uncommon in association with radiation or chemotherapy; its presence mandates further evaluation. Survivors who are at increased risk of endothelial injury from treatment with alkylating agents or and liver radiotherapy may develop focal nodular hyperplasia, a disorder that presents as a liver mass and should be differentiated from malignancy [158].

The Leukemias

Hepatic involvement is common in leukemia; 36% of patients with acute lymphoblastic leukemia have hepatosplenomegaly. Hepatic fibrosis has been noted at autopsy and is thought to be related to chemotherapy. The fibrosis is rarely of clinical significance [159,160]. In acute lymphoblastic leukemia, 6-thioguanine therapy may result in chronic liver injury including occlusive venopathy and nodular regenerative hyperplasia [161]. Hepatosplenomegaly is also common in chronic myelogenous leukemia, both the adult and juvenile type; 50% of children with acute myelogenous leukemia have hepatomegaly [162,163]. Usually liver involvement is not clinically significant, but with rapid tumor growth and extensive infiltration, liver failure or ascites may develop as a consequence of sinusoidal or venous outflow obstruction [164–172]. Chemotherapy may cause sudden tumor lysis, and the resultant hyperuricemia and hyperphosphatemia can lead to oliguric renal failure [173–175]. Marked hepatosplenomegaly in acute lymphoblastic leukemia may be an indicator of risk for early relapse [176].

STEM CELL AND ALLOGENEIC BONE MARROW TRANSPLANTATION

Hepatic injury is common in the child undergoing bone marrow transplantation [177]. Possible causes are the primary tumor, the chemotherapeutic and radiotherapy regimen, various infections, biliary sludge, parental nutrition, VOD, and graft-versus-host disease (GVHD). In regions where hepatitis B and C are endemic, risk of significant posttransplant liver disease is increased [178]. A structured approach is necessary to evaluate the stem cell–bone marrow transplant patient with hepatic injury; the goal is to seek treatable conditions. More than one pathologic process may be operative [179].

Veno-Occlusive Disease

Veno-occlusive disease occurs in about 20% of patients prepared for transplantation with total body irradiation and chemotherapy; it is more common with allogeneic than autologous transplants. The clinical course of VOD is variable. Typically, it begins with insidious weight gain within 2 weeks of transplantation followed by signs and symptoms of hepatic venous outflow obstruction. Jaundice develops after the weight gain and precedes other symptoms by 6–10 days. Fifty percent of patients develop ascites. Abdominal pain, hepatomegaly, and encephalopathy may develop [180]. Diagnosis is based on the clinical presentation and confirmed by pulsed Doppler ultrasonography [181]. It is critical to distinguish VOD from pericardial disease, which has the same mechanism of hepatic injury. If symptoms develop more than 20 days after transplantation, other etiologies such as GVHD, toxic hepatitis, or biliary disease must be considered [177,182]. The mortality from VOD ranges from 7% to 50% and is higher in those with higher total bilirubin, greater weight gain, encephalopathy, and higher peak AST levels [180,183]. More than 50% of patients with typical VOD recover within 4 weeks.

The histopathology of VOD is characterized by injury to endothelial cells in the terminal hepatic venule (Figure 38.1) [180,183]. The distribution of the lesion may be patchy. Initially, fibrin deposits are detected in the terminal venules. The subendothelial zone is widened, and subintimal edema and hemorrhage are present in small central venules. Necrosis of hepatocytes and sinusoidal congestion are prominent. After several weeks, the fibrin in the terminal hepatic venules is replaced by collagen, resulting in subtotal to complete obliteration of central venules and centrilobular sinusoidal fibrosis.

The injury to endothelial cells and hepatocytes in zone 3 provides insight into the pathogenesis of VOD. The increased risk for development of VOD after total body irradiation is well documented [183]. Injury to radiosensitive endothelial cells results in passive congestion and decreased venous outflow, thereby compromising clearance of potentially cytotoxic drugs and their metabolites. Nutritional deficiencies or exposure to drugs that alter the function of the cytochrome P450 system may further compromise the cytoprotective mechanisms of hepatocytes. Because hepatocytes in zone 3 play a central role in the metabolism of antineoplastic drugs, they are more susceptible to disorders associated with altered clearance of toxic drugs and their metabolites. Factors predictive of the development of VOD include preexisting liver disease, exposure to hepatotoxic drugs, including total body radiation during the conditioning regimen, use of matched unrelated donor transplantation, and advanced-stage malignancies [184–188]. Transfusion with platelet concentrates containing ABO-incompatible plasma also increases the risk of developing VOD. Gene polymorphisms related to drug-metabolizing enzymes may alter risk for development of VOD [189]. Busulfan and cyclophosphamide, both of which are conjugated with glutathione, have been associated with VOD [189]. The risk of VOD is increased in patients with thalassemia undergoing bone marrow transplantation who are homozygous for a glutathione S-transferase null genotype [190]. If clinicians could further stratify risk for VOD based on pharmacogenomics, mitigation of posttransplant complications might be possible.

There is no proven therapy for VOD that has been evaluated in a prospective, randomized manner. Treatment is supportive and focuses on maintaining intravascular volume while minimizing accumulation of extravascular fluid. Therapeutic paracentesis may be necessary to prevent respiratory insufficiency. Sodium restriction and diuretics may be necessary to prevent further fluid accumulation; volume depletion must be avoided to prevent compromise of hepatic and renal blood flow. Hepatic encephalopathy should be treated with lactulose and protein restriction.

There have been many therapeutic efforts to interrupt the pathologic process. Heparin can be used safely; the incidence of moderate and severe VOD is less than in historical control subjects [191]. Recombinant human tissue plasminogen activator has been used in several series. Overall it does not appear to improve survival, and it increases the risk of serious hemorrhage [192–194]. Antithrombin III has been used; improvements in organ dysfunction and reduction in mortality were noted [195]. Preliminary results indicate that prophylactic ursodeoxycholate [171] or prostaglandin E, given as a continuous intravenous infusion from day 8 to 30 after transplantation, decreased the incidence of VOD [172]. Defibrotide is a polydeoxyribonucleotide with activity in several vascular disorders that produces no systemic anticoagulant effects; an open-label, compassionate-use study suggests increased survival [173]. Glutamine and vitamin E also may improve the course of VOD [174]. Finally, N-acetyl L cysteine been used in patients who received conditioning with busulfan, for which glutathione is critical for metabolism. It appears to be safe; in a small open-label study, no cases of VOD developed [196].

Graft-Versus-Host Disease

Acute GVHD occurs when an immunocompromised host receives an allogeneic graft that contains immunocompetent T cells. The immunocompetent T cells in the graft proliferate and mount an immune response against the immunocompromised host, who is incapable of mounting an immune response against the graft [197]. Acute GVHD has been described in patients after orthotopic liver transplantation, in infants receiving intrauterine and exchange transfusions for hemolytic disease, in immunocompromised patients receiving nonirradiated blood products, and, most frequently, in recipients of allogeneic bone marrow transplants [197–201].

Acute GVHD occurs in about 70% of bone marrow transplant patients; it is more common following transplantation from unrelated donors than autologous transplantation. Myeloablative conditioning appears to increase the risk of

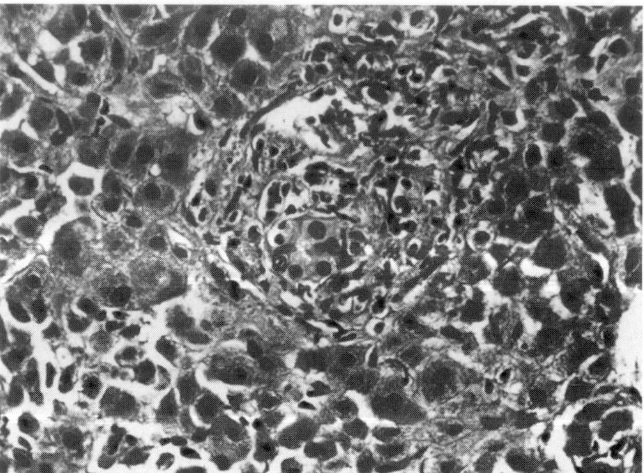

Figure 38.2. Pathology of hepatic graft-versus-host disease. Lymphocytic infiltrate in the portal area following allogeneic bone marrow engraftment. The lymphocytic infiltrate is invading the biliary epithelium causing degeneration and necrosis (*arrow*). (H&E stain, original magnification ×400.) (From Barshes et al. [220], used with permission.) For color reproduction, see Color Plate 38.2.

GVHD compared with reduced-intensity conditioning. However, this has not been confirmed in prospective controlled trials [202]. The target organs are skin, intestine, and liver, although isolated hepatic involvement may occur. Symptoms typically appear 3–6 weeks after transplantation; the predominant features are nausea, vomiting, diarrhea, and a diffuse maculopapular rash [200]. The hepatic manifestations of GVHD are jaundice and biochemical evidence of cholestasis with hepatocellular injury. Severe hepatic insufficiency rarely occurs. The characteristic histologic findings involve the small bile ducts. Segmental destruction of the bile duct epithelium and atypical bile duct epithelial cells are present [203,204] (Figure 38.2). Although GVHD typically presents with biochemical evidence of cholestasis, a hepatitic form of GVHD, characterized by higher levels of aminotransferase levels and lobular changes on biopsy, may also occur. The histologic abnormalities may be difficult to distinguish from drug-associated and viral hepatitis [205].

In the absence of VOD, sepsis, drug-related injury, or biliary obstruction, the diagnosis of acute GVHD can be made clinically or confirmed by either skin or rectal biopsy [206–208]. Endoscopic biopsies of the stomach and small bowel are also useful [209]. If skin involvement is limited or the patient has been exposed to hepatotrophic virus or hepatotoxic drugs, a definitive diagnosis may be difficult. In less typical cases, a liver biopsy may be indicated to confirm the diagnosis. Before proceeding, the clinical information to be gained from the biopsy must be weighed against the risk, because children who have undergone stem-cell transplantation are at greater risk for complications following percutaneous liver biopsy [210,211].

The prognosis is variable. Polymorphisms of cytokine genes including *TNF-α, IL-10,* interferon gamma, and *IL-6* are associated with more severe acute GVHD. Other genotypes are associated with chronic GVHD [212].

Prednisone, cyclosporine, and antithymocyte globulin have been used to treat acute GVHD. Depletion of donor T cells before transplantation decreases the incidence of acute GVHD [145,189,190] but increases the risk of graft failure and relapse. A multicenter randomized trial undertaken to determine the effects of T-cell depletion versus methotrexate and cyclosporine immunosuppression supported these single-center observations. Disease-free survival at 3 years was 27% for patients with T-cell depletion compared to 34% for patients who received treatment with methotrexate and cyclosporine. Although T-cell depletion was associated with decreased incidence of severe GVHD, there was increased higher risk disease relapse and cytomegalovirus infection [213]. Animal studies show that disruption of cytokine response and CD40 ligand ameliorates experimental models of GVHD and offers new avenues for therapy [72,191–193].

Chronic GVHD is a multisystem illness that mimics chronic hepatitis or drug-induced hepatic injury. It develops 100–400 days after transplantation and may occur in patients without a prior history of acute GVHD [214–217]. The incidence has increased with the increased use of hematopoietic stem cells collected from peripheral blood. The presenting complaints include anorexia, weight loss, and jaundice. Findings on liver biopsy include portal enlargement, fibrosis, cholestasis, Kupffer cell hyperplasia, and a decreased number of small bile ducts. Mild chronic GVHD responds to immunosuppressive therapy; prednisone and cyclosporine are the usual agents [216]. In severe long-standing chronic GVHD, a marked reduction in the number of small bile ducts is present [203,218]. Cirrhosis occasionally develops following chronic GVHD treatment with immunosuppressive therapy is usually effective [215,219]. Mortality increases with the severity of chronic GVHD [216].

Liver transplantation may be an option for patients with severe hepatic GVHD. Current 1- and 5-year survival rates are 72.4% and 62.9%, respectively [220].

COLLAGEN VASCULAR DISEASES

Hepatomegaly, splenomegaly, and biochemical abnormalities are common in the collagen vascular diseases. The hepatic involvement may be primary or secondary, particularly to drug therapy.

Juvenile Rheumatoid Arthritis

Hepatosplenomegaly is common in juvenile rheumatoid arthritis (JRA), especially the systemic form. Splenomegaly is more common than hepatomegaly. Hepatomegaly tends to decrease as the disease is treated and is often accompanied by a mild increase in serum aminotransferase levels [221]. Liver biopsy reveals nonspecific periportal collections of inflammatory cells and Kupffer cell hyperplasia [222]. Paradoxically, a flare-up of hepatic disease, regardless of etiology, often results in an improvement in rheumatic symptoms [223]. Progressive hepatomegaly is suggestive of secondary amyloidosis [224].

Therapy for JRA also may cause hepatic injury. Serum aminotransferase levels are elevated in up to 60% of children receiving long-term salicylate therapy; this is more common in young children and those with systemic-onset disease [225,226]. Aspirin causes a dose-related reversible hepatotoxic reaction that often recurs with rechallenge. Aspirin hepatotoxicity is usually asymptomatic and detected only because of mild increases in serum aminotransferase concentrations. Liver biopsy reveals a nonspecific focal hepatitis [227]. Patients with rheumatic diseases taking aspirin have a higher incidence of Reye's syndrome than the general population [228–230]. Several patients with biopsy-proven Reye's syndrome did not have the typical prodrome. Any patient with a rheumatologic disorder taking aspirin who develops vomiting or neurologic symptoms should be evaluated promptly for Reye's syndrome.

Nonsteroidal anti-inflammatory drugs (NSAIDs) have largely replaced aspirin in the treatment of JRA. Hepatotoxicity occurs less often with NSAIDs than with aspirin. In one adult study, 23 cases of NSAID-related liver injuries were detected among more than 600,000 people who received 2 million prescriptions (1.1 per 100,000 NSAID prescriptions). Patients with rheumatoid arthritis had a tenfold increase in hepatic injury compared with persons with osteoarthritis. Coinfection with hepatitis C may increase the risk [231]. Concomitant exposure to other hepatotoxic drugs also increased the risk [232–234]. Risks in children appear to be similar or less [235]. A recent review reports that only diclofenac and rofecoxib had higher rates of aminotransferase elevations than placebo and other NSAIDs; no NSAID had increased rates of liver-related serious adverse events, hospitalizations, or deaths [236].

Severe systemic reactions following medication changes in patients with JRA have been reported; it is unclear whether it is due to drug therapy or intercurrent infection [237]. Boys were more commonly affected; they developed encephalopathy, purpura, disseminated intravascular coagulopathy, renal failure, jaundice, and markedly elevated serum aminotransferase and bilirubin concentrations. Death occurred in 2 of 14 reported cases [238,239]. Liver biopsy showed diffuse macrovesicular fatty changes and marked Kupffer cell hyperplasia. A severe hepatic reaction to gold therapy also has been reported; four patients developed fulminant hepatic necrosis following the second gold injection [240]. Similar but less severe reactions have been noted after the initiation of gold or penicillamine therapy in children with systemic-onset JRA [241].

Methotrexate has become a mainstay in the treatment of refractory JRA. Initial studies in adults with psoriasis suggested that hepatic fibrosis could develop insidiously. Data from adults suggest that some patients receiving long-term methotrexate therapy develop hepatic fibrosis; comorbid factors include alcohol ingestion, obesity, and the dose and duration of therapy [242–244].

There are two forms of methotrexate toxicity: benign acute transient elevation of aminotransferase levels and hepatic fibrosis that progresses to cirrhosis. Liver biopsy is necessary to define the latter [245]. Studies have demonstrated that long-term methotrexate is safe, especially when the total cumulative dose is below 1.5 g [159,160]. However, occasional patients do develop hepatic injury. Histopathologic features include variability in nuclear size and staining, fatty changes in hepatocytes and sinusoidal lining cells, lipogranulomas, Kupffer cell hyperplasia, and periportal fibrosis [246,247].

Data from children are more reassuring: methotrexate relieves the symptoms of refractory JRA and is generally safe [248,249]. Transient increases in serum aminotransferase levels are seen in about 15% of patients receiving methotrexate, but biopsies have revealed no fibrosis or cirrhosis. A retrospective study of 25 JRA patients receiving methotrexate revealed that the frequency of biochemical abnormalities and body mass index were risk factors for increasing hepatic injury [250,251]. The American College of Rheumatology guidelines should be followed in children receiving methotrexate because fibrosis does occur [247].

Persistent hepatomegaly in a patient with long-standing JRA should point to the possibility of secondary amyloidosis, which develops in about 4% of patients. The mean onset of amyloidosis is about 8 years after the onset of JRA. Amyloidosis should be suspected if proteinuria and hepatosplenomegaly occur; the diagnosis can be confirmed by rectal biopsy [224,252,253]. Hepatic vein obstruction resulting in Budd–Chiari syndrome has been reported in JRA [68].

Felty's syndrome (long-standing rheumatoid arthritis with splenomegaly and leukopenia) is often associated with mild hepatomegaly and slightly elevated serum aminotransferase and alkaline phosphatase concentrations. The primary lesion appears to be obliteration of portal venules leading to portal hypertension, presumably due to immune complex-mediated venular injury. The liver injury may progress to nodular regeneration [82,254].

Liver involvement is common in Sjögren's syndrome, which consists of keratoconjunctivitis, xerostomia, salivary gland swelling, and autoimmune antibody positivity. Raynaud's phenomenon, achlorhydria, alopecia, splenomegaly, and leukopenia are common features. In children, primary Sjögren's syndrome is rare; it usually accompanies a connective tissue disease [255]. Forty percent of patients with Sjögren's syndrome and rheumatoid arthritis have subclinical liver disease. Antimitochondrial antibodies are common in Sjogren's syndrome Patients with antimitochondrial antibodies have a hepatic lesion that resembles primary biliary cirrhosis [256].

Liver involvement is rare in scleroderma; 25% of patients with scleroderma have positive antimitochondrial antibodies. The CREST syndrome (subcutaneous calcinosis, Raynaud's phenomena, esophageal dysfunction, sclerodactyly, and telangiectasia) has been noted in patients with primary biliary cirrhosis [257–260].

Lupus Erythematosus

Multiorgan involvement is the hallmark of systemic lupus erythematosus (SLE), but there is no consistent pattern of hepatic involvement. Hepatic disease is not a significant cause of

Table 38.4: Liver Pathology in Systemic Lupus Erythematosus

Finding	*No. of Patients (N = 52)*
Congestion	40
Fatty liver	38
Arteritis	11
Cholestasis	9
Peliosis hepatis	6
Chronic persistent hepatitis	6
Nonspecific reactive hepatitis	5
Cholangiolitis	4
Nodular regenerative hyperplasia	3
Hemangioma	3

Reprinted from Matsumoto et al. [265], with permission.

morbidity or mortality, but subclinical liver involvement is common. Hepatomegaly is detected in up to two thirds of affected children and adults. Patients usually have no hepatic symptoms; jaundice is present only in cases of hemolysis or drug reaction. Moderate splenomegaly is a feature of active disease.

A wide spectrum of hepatic disorders has been associated with SLE [261,262]. In a prospective study of 260 patients, Miller et al. [263] found serum aminotransferase elevations in 23%. Identifiable causes of liver disease included alcohol ingestion, hepatitis B infection, congestive heart failure, uncontrolled diabetes, and drug reactions. Salicylate toxicity was the most common drug reaction [263,264]. Nonsteroidal anti-inflammatory drugs may cause a cholestatic hepatitis in lupus patients [234]. In patients with unexplained aminotransferase elevations, no serious lesions were noted on biopsy. A correlation between aminotransferase elevation and lupus activity suggests that subclinical liver disease may be a manifestation of SLE. Runyon et al. [262] reviewed 238 patients; 43 had liver disease. Abnormalities included cirrhosis, chronic hepatitis, granulomatous hepatitis, and steatosis. The cirrhotic patients had an unusual form of cholestasis, and a canalicular cast of bile was noted on biopsy. Nine patients had serial biopsies: four showed progression of the liver disease, suggesting that severe and even fatal liver disease may occur in SLE. Matsumoto et al. [265] reviewed the Japanese Lupus Registry data and found that the incidence of chronic hepatitis was 2.4%, cirrhosis 1.1%, and liver fibrosis 0.8% (Table 38.4). Budd–Chiari syndrome and hepatic VOD also have been reported in SLE [96,266–268]. Massive hepatic infarction and nodular regenerative hyperplasia of the liver also have been noted [269–271].

The liver may be involved in neonatal SLE [272]. The full spectrum of neonatal lupus includes congenital heart block, transient dermatitis, and variable hematologic and systemic abnormalities. The disorder is transient and is the result of circulating maternal anti-Ro and anti-La antibodies that cross the placenta between the 12th and 16th weeks of gestation. Fetal skin, heart, and liver contain Ro and La antigens [273]. Initially liver disease was considered to be secondary to heart failure; however, recent reports have described a cholestatic syndrome that resembles biliary atresia [274]. Liver disease occurs in 10% of patients with neonatal lupus and consists of three patterns: liver failure occurring at birth or in utero, transient conjugated hyperbilirubinemia, or transient aminotransferase elevations. Cholestasis resolves by 6 months of age; the initial biopsy reveals large duct obstruction and portal fibrosis with a mixed portal inflammatory component. The mother may be asymptomatic but have circulating antibodies; hence, neonatal lupus must be considered in any cholestatic infant with cardiac arrhythmias [275].

Miscellaneous

Mixed connective tissue disease is a syndrome with overlapping features of scleroderma, polymyositis, and lupus. Hepatomegaly and splenomegaly are commonly seen. The pathologic lesion is a widespread proliferative vasculitis. Hepatic lesions have been noted. They are characterized by intimal thickening in medium-size vessels and periportal inflammatory infiltrates [255].

Dermatomyositis does not have a prominent hepatic component. Vasculitis of the gallbladder has been reported [276]. Hepatomegaly occurs in less than 5%. However, dermatomyositis may be mistaken for liver disease because of elevated serum aminotransferase concentrations secondary to rhabdomyolysis. The history of proximal muscle weakness and an elevated serum creatine phosphokinase establish the diagnosis [277]. A cholestatic picture has been described in juvenile dermatomyositis. Biopsy revealed cytoplasmic and ductal cholestasis but no abnormalities in the intrahepatic ducts. Cholestasis improved with the treatment of the dermatomyositis [278].

Hydrops of the gallbladder and hepatobiliary dysfunction have been reported in Kawasaki syndrome [279,280]. Diagnosis is made by ultrasound, and it resolves as the inflammation decreases. Hepatomegaly occurs in 14%, and abnormal biochemical studies are seen in 30% of patients. Hepatomegaly may be due to inflammation, latent heart failure, or both [281,282]. Serum gamma glutamyltransferase concentrations are often elevated [283]. Serum ALT concentrations are often elevated at diagnosis; higher levels suggest cardiac disease [284]. Serum bile acid concentrations may be elevated [285]. Autopsy findings have included portal inflammation, vasculitis, sinusoidal infiltrates, Kupffer cell hyperplasia, fatty degeneration, and severe congestive changes, presumably from cardiac disease. Intrahepatic cholangitis, bile duct epithelial necrosis, and gallbladder wall thickening have been described [286,287]. Hepatic artery aneurysms have been reported [288,289]. Salicylate hepatitis and, rarely, Reye's syndrome, may develop in patients receiving chronic salicylate therapy [290,291].

Hepatomegaly is a feature of infantile multisystem inflammatory disease, a rare disorder characterized by fever, evanescent rash and arthropathy at birth, hepatosplenomegaly, and lymphadenopathy. Hepatomegaly is present in about 50% of infants. Developmental delay, feeding difficulties, and persistent cerebrospinal fluid pleocytosis are common [292,293]. Mutations in the pyrin gene family have been described recently [294,295].

ENDOCRINE DISORDERS

Hypopituitarism

Pituitary hormones are involved in the regulation of bile secretion and flow. Experimental evidence shows that both thyroid hormone and cortisol affect bile acid–independent bile flow [296]. Cholestasis occurs in association with hypopituitarism in the neonatal period. Hypopituitarism may be familial, related to birth trauma, or part of a midline malformation syndrome [297–300]. Nonalcoholic steatohepatitis has been associated with hypopituitarism; obesity is a significant factor [301,302].

Septo-optic dysplasia is a specific syndrome involving absence of the septum pallidum and optic nerve hypoplasia, resulting in secondary hypopituitarism. Wandering eye movements are a characteristic feature of hypopituitarism secondary to septo-optic dysplasia; their presence in a cholestatic infant suggests the diagnosis [303]. Congenital hepatic fibrosis has been reported in association with septo-optic dysplasia [304].

Biochemical and histologic findings of neonatal hepatitis occur in infants with hypopituitarism. Physical examination may be normal except for micropenis. Any infant with hypoglycemia and cholestasis must be evaluated for endocrine dysfunction. If pituitary dysfunction is suspected and abnormal eye movements are present, central nervous system imaging should be performed to exclude septo-optic dysplasia. Therapy is directed at treating the endocrine insufficiency. Cholestasis resolves with the correction of the pituitary hormone insufficiency; the ultimate prognosis is that of the endocrine disorder.

Adrenal Disorders

Cholestasis has been noted in infants with primary adrenal insufficiency; Cushing's syndrome and the iatrogenic administration of corticosteroid result in steatosis and hepatomegaly [305,306]. Infants with congenital insensitivity to adrenocorticotropic hormone have cholestasis and a neonatal hepatitis–like picture [307]. Alcoholic patients may have clinical and biochemical features very similar Cushing's syndrome (alcoholic pseudo-Cushing's syndrome) [308]. A case of infantile pseudo-Cushing's syndrome has been reported from alcohol in breast milk [309].

Thyroid Disorders

Thyroid status affects bile flow and composition. In animal studies, hypothyroidism results in a decrease in bile flow, primarily because of a decrease in bile salt–independent flow. Biliary excretion of bilirubin is decreased; the fraction of bile acids conjugated with glycine increases, and there is reduction of 3-hydroxy-3-methyl-glutaryl-CoA reductase and cholesterol-7-α-hydroxylase activity [296,310]. Biochemical abnormalities are reported in 15–75% of patients with hyperthyroidism; most frequently noted are increases in serum aminotransferase and alkaline phosphatase levels [311]. There may be a slight increase in serum bilirubin levels, but overt jaundice is rare [312]. Jaundice is usually the result of cardiac failure but may occur in the absence of heart disease. Light microscopy is normal, but electron microscopy shows enlarged mitochondria, decreased glycogen, and hypertrophic smooth endoplasmic reticulum. Yao et al. [313] reported one patient with marked cholestasis without cardiac failure; liver biopsy showed centrilobular cholestasis with minimal inflammation. Thyrotoxicosis may unmask Gilbert's syndrome by reducing glucuronyl transferase activity. Severe abnormalities in liver function studies occur in thyroid storm.

Reversible abnormalities of liver function are common in hypothyroidism. Cholestasis may be the initial clinical sign of neonatal hypothyroidism. Twenty percent of infants have abnormal and prolonged jaundice; it is usually unconjugated hyperbilirubinemia. Up to one third may have cholestasis as the presenting symptom [314,315].

There is an association between Hashimoto's thyroiditis and autoimmune liver disease. Any patient with one manifestation of autoimmune disease may develop symptoms in another affected organ at any time.

Diabetes Mellitus

Evidence of liver dysfunction may be found in up to one third of patients with diabetes. The spectrum of histopathologic lesions includes increased hepatocyte glycogen, hyalin deposition, steatosis, and fibrosis leading to cirrhosis. The most common manifestation is steatosis and is discussed in detail in Chapter 34.

Myopathy Mimicking Liver Disease

Serum aminotransferase levels, AST more so than ALT, may be mildly to moderately elevated in muscle disorders, such as the congenital myopathies or dermatomyositis [316]. Early in the course of the disease, when symptoms of muscle disease are minimal, this persistent asymptomatic elevation of aminotransferase levels mimics liver disease [317]. Iorio et al. [277] studied 166 children with persistently elevated aminotransferase levels; 14 had muscular dystrophy [277]. In one series, patients with documented Duchenne's or Becker's muscular dystrophy had a ninefold increase in aminotransferase levels [318]. After acute injury, the AST declines more quickly than ALT [319]. Elevated creatine phosphokinase concentrations distinguish primary muscle disease from liver disease. The consideration of muscle disorders in children with asymptomatic ALT and AST elevations and no clinical features of liver disease prevent unnecessary diagnostic procedures.

NUTRITIONAL DISORDERS

The liver is frequently involved in nutritional disorders. Hepatic dysfunction develops in both malnutrition and obesity. Nonalcoholic fatty liver disease (NAFLD) has become a major issue in the obese child and adolescent; it is discussed elsewhere. Individual nutrient deficiencies and excesses may result in hepatic injury. Nutritional therapy is also a potential cause of hepatic injury. Many children with chronic diseases are exposed to a variety of potentially hepatotoxic drugs, herbs, and nutritional supplements [320].

The use of alternative and complementary therapies such as herbal medicines, homeopathy, and vitamin therapy is common in children, especially those with chronic disorders [320–324]. Some products are toxic in their own right; others may interfere with drug metabolism and absorption. The compounds most likely to cause direct hepatotoxicity include the pyrrolizidine alkaloids, chaparral, germander, pennyroyal, and kava [320]. VOD has been reported in a fetus as a result of maternal ingestion of pyrrolizidine alkaloids [322]. Many herbal products are contaminated with heavy metals and other substances [321].

Celiac Disease

Liver disease has been noted in celiac disease. In several series, 20–55% of patients have elevated serum aminotransferase concentrations. Alkaline phosphatase also may be elevated; it may be hepatic or osseous in origin. The prevalence in children appears to be similar. The liver disease is usually asymptomatic; hepatic biochemical abnormalities may precipitate medical evaluation. Elevated serum aminotransferase levels and hepatomegaly have been reported as the only symptoms of celiac disease. Cryptogenic cirrhosis has been reported in children with asymptomatic celiac disease. Celiac disease should be considered in the evaluation of the child with unknown liver dysfunction [325,326].

The cause of the hepatic injury remains uncertain but likely relates to the passage of antigens through the injured intestinal mucosa, because there is a prompt response to a gluten-free diet. Nutritional deficiencies also may contribute [327–332]. Pancreatic insufficiency occurs in celiac disease and may lead to diabetes mellitus and hepatic steatosis [333].

The histologic abnormalities include a nonspecific hepatitis and cryptogenic cirrhosis; cholestasis is unusual. Microvesicular and macrovesicular steatosis may develop; steatosis is more prominent when concomitant malnutrition is present. The serum and histologic abnormalities improve with a gluten-free diet. If the patient does not respond to a gluten-free diet within 1 year, other causes of liver disease should be excluded. Primary biliary cirrhosis and primary sclerosing cholangitis develop in adults with celiac disease; these do not improve with a gluten free diet.

Malnutrition

Malnutrition is associated with hepatic abnormalities; hepatic lipid increases regardless of the cause [334]. Lack of glucose availability, depletion of glycogen stores, and the eventual use of ketones as the preferred fuel source accompany starvation. Elevated serum growth hormone concentrations and increased sympathetic nervous system activity mobilize free fatty acids from adipose tissue. As free fatty acid flux increases, hepatic fat content increases [335]. In prolonged starvation, ketones are the major fuel and hepatic gluconeogenesis decreases; under these circumstances there is little fat accumulation. However, if even small amounts of carbohydrate are added to the diet, this adaptive response does not occur and steatosis develops as fatty acids are mobilized but not oxidized [336]. Any superimposed stress, such as infection or trauma, accelerates the process [337]. Protein synthesis is decreased, and decreased apoprotein concentrations may play a minor role. Lipid metabolism is altered in malnutrition, and there is disordered β-oxidation. Carnitine concentrations are decreased, and peroxisomes are virtually absent in the hepatocytes [338]. Malnutrition also leads to immunodeficiency; infection leads to further metabolic stress, creating a vicious cycle. Both the malnutrition itself and the subsequent infection affect the liver. For example, peliosis hepatis caused by the spirochete *Rochalimaea henselae* has been reported under these circumstances [339].

Kwashiorkor is a constellation of clinical features encompassing apathy, edema, skin and hair lesions, and massive hepatomegaly. The liver is characterized by massive steatosis. It usually develops after weaning and the introduction of the native diet but occasionally occurs during breast-feeding [340]. Although usually considered a condition of underdeveloped countries, kwashiorkor has occurred in nonpoverty environments [341–346]. For many years, a diet high in energy (carbohydrate) but low in protein was considered the etiologic agent [340]. Recent data challenge this simplistic notion. Kwashiorkor is the end result of multiple insults to a vulnerable child. Potential insults include poor diet, contaminated foods, infection, inflammation, and psychologic stress such as abrupt weaning [347].

The balance of oxidants and antioxidants has been proposed as the final common pathway [348,349]. Zinc is a potent antioxidant, and deficiency is common in malnourished children. Zinc deficiency also results in immunodeficiency, furthering the vicious cycle of infection and malnutrition [350]. Selenium deficiency with subsequent heart failure may develop [351]. Proinflammatory cytokines are elevated in children with kwashiorkor [352–354]. Other nutrient deficiencies also result in oxidant–antioxidant imbalance. Glutathione is a major component in antioxidant defense; its synthesis and function are affected by nutritional status, contributing to oxidant stress [355].

Aflatoxin contamination of food has been suggested as a cause of kwashiorkor. Aflatoxin is a mold product that frequently contaminates food in tropical areas; it inhibits lipid synthesis, depresses free fatty acid metabolism, and interferes with clotting factor synthesis. Aflatoxin has been found in the serum and liver of patients with kwashiorkor; it also has been found in breast milk. Aflatoxin should be considered one of (but not the only) precipitating factors in development of kwashiorkor [356,357].

Treatment of kwashiorkor consists of treating the underlying nutritional disorders [358]. Long-term hepatic damage has not been reported. Restoring antioxidant capacity with glutathione or α-lipoic acid hastens recovery and improves survival [359]. However, Cilberto et al. [360] were unable to prevent the development of kwashiorkor in susceptible Malawian infants with antioxidant supplementation.

Hepatic abnormalities have been reported in starvation conditions such as anorexia and bulimia. Mild increases in serum unconjugated bilirubin and aminotransferase levels may be noted [361–364]. A coagulopathy due to vitamin K deficiency without any evidence of liver disease occurs in bulimia [365]. Decreased caloric intake increases serum bilirubin concentrations in Gilbert's syndrome [366]. Starvation hyperbilirubinemia appears to be related to an enhanced enterohepatic circulation rather than altered hepatic transport [367].

Hepatic injury also may occur as the result of various nutritional therapies. Large doses of niacin and vitamin A can cause liver injury [368,369]. Kwashiorkor has developed in infants receiving homemade formulas or low-protein-containing drinks. [342,344,345,370]. Herbal tea remedies has been associated with liver injury [371–373]. Their use either as a remedy for the child or by a breast-feeding mother may result in a toxic hepatitis or VOD [71,72,322].

Parenteral Nutrition

The most common and best-evaluated nutrition-related hepatic disorder is total parenteral nutrition (TPN)-associated liver disease. The hepatic response depends on the age of the child and the underlying condition (Table 38.5). Cholestasis predominates in infants, and older children and adults develop steatosis and steatohepatitis. Biliary sludge and cholelithiasis occur in both age groups [374]. Cirrhosis and end-stage liver disease have replaced malnutrition and sepsis as the major causes of death in TPN-dependent infants and children. End-stage liver disease due to TPN is a common cause for liver–intestine transplantation in the infant with short bowel syndrome; chronic liver disease also develops in adults on long-term TPN [375–377]. Mortality in patients awaiting combined liver–intestine transplantation is greater than in those awaiting liver transplantation [378].

History

Soon after the introduction of parenteral nutrition, multiple reports of liver disease in infants appeared [122,379–382]. Cholestasis developed in about 25% of low birth weight infants receiving TPN; the cholestasis progressed as long as the infants received exclusive parenteral nutrition. The cholestasis persisted for a variable amount of time after discontinuation of TPN. Higher protein infusions were associated with higher bilirubin concentrations but did not affect the overall incidence of cholestasis; increased dextrose intake and increased caloric intake were also associated with cholestasis in the neonate. Lipid emulsions were suggested as a possible cause, but they could not be the sole reason because there were multiple reports of cholestasis before lipid emulsions were available in the United States [379,383]. The initial protein source in TPN was hydrolyzed protein; it was replaced with amino acids. As care improved and enteral feedings were introduced earlier, the incidence of cholestasis declined, but it still remains a significant cause of morbidity today, especially in the premature infant or those requiring prolonged therapy [384]. The infants at greatest risk currently are those with shorter bowel length, longer duration of a diverting ostomy, greater gram-positive infections, and fewer days of enteral feeding [385].

Table 38.5: Hepatobiliary Disorders Associated with Total Parenteral Nutrition

Adults
Steatosis
Steatohepatitis
Cholestasis
Fibrosis
Micronodular cirrhosis
Phospholipidosis
Biliary sludge
Cholelithiasis
Acalculous cholecystitis
Infants
Cholestasis
Fibrosis
Cirrhosis
Hepatocellular carcinoma
Biliary sludge
Abdominal pseudotumor
Cholelithiasis

Steatosis is common in older children and adults, and steatohepatitis may develop. Cholestasis also may develop [386, 387]. The histology often reflects concurrent clinical phenomena such as sepsis, preexisting liver disease, and renal failure [388]. Prolonged TPN administration may result in fibrosis and eventually cirrhosis [375,389,390].

Clinical Course

In infants, onset of cholestasis is often insidious and overlaps the period of physiologic cholestasis. Premature infants and those receiving nothing by the enteral route are at the greatest risk. The incidence is as high as 50% in low birth weight infants. The first clinical indication is mild hepatomegaly followed by biochemical evidence of cholestasis. The first biochemical abnormality is an increase in serum bile acid concentrations followed by a increase in serum conjugated bilirubin [391,392]. This begins after 2–3 weeks of parenteral nutrition. Serum alkaline phosphatase and aminotransferase levels increase days to weeks later. A portion of the increased alkaline phosphatase may be osseous in origin [393]. Early evidence of hepatic synthetic dysfunction such as hypoalbuminemia or prolonged prothrombin time should raise the suspicion of a metabolic liver disease.

Table 38.6: Evaluation of Liver Disease Associated with Total Parenteral Nutrition

Review of medical history for predisposing factors
Review of drug and transfusion exposures
Physical examination
Hepatic ultrasonography to exclude cholelithiasis and obstruction
Exclusion of common causes of neonatal cholestasis
α_1-Antitrypsin phenotype
Metabolic screen
Review of nutrient intake for excesses and deficiencies

Table 38.7: Multifactorial Causes of Parenteral Nutrition–Associated Liver Disease

Immature enterohepatic circulation
Perinatal insults
Enteral starvation
Hypoxia
Hypoperfusion
Drug toxicity (e.g., furosemide)
Gastrointestinal anomalies, diseases
Sepsis
Hepatotrophic virus exposure
Specific nutrient deficiencies
Taurine
Essential fatty acids
Carnitine
Trace metals
Vitamin E/selenium
Glutathione
Choline
Unknown
Toxicity
Amino acids
Lipid emulsions
Trace metals
Improper caloric, glucose, and protein loads
Unknown

The diagnosis of parenteral nutrition–related liver disease is one of exclusion (Table 38.6). The evaluation attempts to define potentially treatable etiologies. In most affected infants, the liver disease will resolve with time and with the institution of enteral feedings. A minority develops cirrhosis and end-stage liver disease; hepatocellular carcinoma also has occurred [394,395]. Infants receiving long-term parenteral nutrition for severe gastrointestinal dysfunction develop fibrosis and cirrhosis insidiously; the greatest risk is in those patients receiving the least enteral feedings [389]. Hyperbilirubinemia, hepatosplenomegaly, and functional hyposplenism dominate the clinical picture [396].

Older children and adolescents develop hepatomegaly and elevated serum aminotransferase concentrations. Steatosis is common; cholestasis is rarely the initial abnormality. However, if they receive long-term TPN, they do have a high incidence of liver disease, and fibrosis and cirrhosis may ultimately develop [376]. Cholestasis develops in 65% of adult patients receiving prolonged TPN; the incidence increases with duration of therapy [397].

Pathology

The pathologic changes in infants with TPN-related liver disease are nonspecific and highly variable. The major component is intralobular cholestasis either alone or in conjunction with an inflammatory portal tract lesion or bile duct proliferation suggesting possible obstruction. Canalicular and cytoplasmic bile stasis are common and tend to be more severe in the central lobular region. Giant cell transformation may occur but is relatively uncommon. Kupffer cells are often hyperplastic and contain lipofuscin pigment, a by-product of lipid peroxidation. Persistent sinusoidal erythropoiesis may be prominent but cannot be distinguished from extramedullary hematopoiesis. Portal inflammation may be accompanied by mild to moderate bile duct proliferation with occasional evidence of ductular bile plug formation, especially in infants. This may lead to portal fibrosis; some progress to cirrhosis and rarely hepatocellular carcinoma. A review of postmortem liver pathology in infants receiving TPN for more than 2 weeks revealed a progression of the lesion: bile stasis was seen after 2 weeks, followed by portal inflammation and bile duct proliferation. Portal fibrosis appeared after 8 weeks of TPN, and cirrhosis was noted after 12 weeks. The severity of the liver's histologic changes was strongly correlated with age at death, antecedent asphyxia, and neonatal gastrointestinal catastrophes [389,394,398–401]. Despite the common occurrence of hypoxia and hypoperfusion, ischemic hepatitis is rare. Results of follow-up biopsies in infants who recover are grossly normal, but electron microscopic abnormalities persist [394].

Pathophysiology

The pathogenesis of TPN-associated liver disease is unknown but is multifactorial. Infants receiving TPN have multiple comorbidities (Table 38.7). By definition, there are varying degrees of gastrointestinal dysfunction and enteral starvation [382]. Enteral starvation results in decreased gut motility, mucosal atrophy, and bacterial overgrowth. The result may be production of hepatotoxic agents such as bacterial by-products, endotoxin, and lithocholate and translocation of bacteria and bacterial products into the portal circulation [402]. Concomitant gastrointestinal injuries predispose to mucosal injury, facilitating the process. Surgical resections may facilitate bacterial translocation [403]. Hypoxic and hypotensive insults are common; these are the best predictors of TPN-associated liver disease [404]. Systemic infections that predispose to cholestasis occur frequently [405]. Patients are exposed to hepatotropic viruses through blood product transfusions and receive potentially hepatotoxic drugs. The infusate may contain potentially toxic materials or may be deficient in specific nutrients.

In infancy, the immaturity of the enterohepatic circulation is a major factor. The driving force for bile flow is bile secretion; this requires effective hepatocyte uptake, orderly intrahepatocyte processing, and canalicular excretion of bile acids. Numerous animal and human studies have demonstrated the low efficiency of this system in early life. Bile acid uptake is decreased at the sinusoidal membrane, interaction with cytosol-binding proteins is altered, and intracellular conjugation and canalicular excretion are decreased [406–409]. Ileal bile acid uptake is decreased. Several bile acid transporters are developmentally regulated. Neonatal bile flow rates are lower, and the neonatal liver has a decreased response to choleretic hormones such as secretin and glucagon. Perinatal metabolic pathways are immature both quantitatively and qualitatively, and potentially hepatotoxic compounds have been detected in meconium [399]. This physiologic immaturity results in a decreased bile pool size, elevated serum bile acid, and decreased intraluminal bile acid concentrations.

Hepatotoxic compounds then accumulate in the serum [410–417]. Among these are bile acids, particularly lithocholate. Lithocholate is the result of bacterial metabolism of primary bile acids. The inefficient enterohepatic circulation allows primary bile acids to reach the colon, where they are converted to lithocholate and absorbed. Under normal conditions, lithocholate is detoxified by the hepatocyte by sulfation or hydroxylation. This metabolic pathway is also developmentally immature; toxic compounds thereby reach the liver [418,419].

Intravenous infusions, particularly amino acids, result in decreased bile output in animal studies; a smaller decrease follows intragastric infusion. Parenteral nutrition also alters bile composition in newborn animals [420,421]. Hepatocytes preferentially take up sodium-dependent amino acids to bile acids [412]. Cholestasis develops sooner and is more severe in infants receiving higher protein loads; this effect is noted even if the protein is administered enterally [413,422]. Protein-containing parenteral nutrition solution has been shown to have an early and direct effect on the hepatocyte canalicular membrane [423]. Thus, the combination of physiologic immaturity, nutrient route, and composition favors the development of cholestasis [411].

Enteral starvation is a critical factor in the pathogenesis of TPN-associated liver disease; the most severe hepatic pathology is noted in those infants with the poorest enteral intake and, by extension, the worst intestinal function [421]. Enteral starvation results in decreased secretion of gastrointestinal hormones such as cholecystokinin, secretin, gastrin, neurotensin, and glucagon, glucagon-like peptide 2, and peptide YY [424,425]. All of these hormones have trophic effects and mediate gastrointestinal secretion and motility. Glucagon stimulates hepatic bile acid uptake; neurotensin attenuates intestinal permeability [426]. Resection or mucosal disease results in decreased secretion, especially peptide YY, which is produced in the distal small bowel and colon [427]. The premature infant has a blunted hormonal response to feeding that matures over the first several weeks of life. Additionally, the specific trophic effects of intraluminal nutrients are absent. Enteral starvation has a more pronounced effect in the premature infant [428]. The decreased enterohepatic circulation of bile acids leads to a further decrease in bile flow. Decreased vagal stimulation results in hypomotility and bacterial overgrowth; mucosal immunity is impaired, and bacterial translocation may occur [421]. All these factors contribute to an immature gastrointestinal tract that is vulnerable to a variety of insults.

Parenteral nutrition is associated with increased cecal bacterial counts in rats, increased translocation of enteric bacteria to mesenteric lymph nodes, as well as intestinal mucosal atrophy. Hepatic inflammation develops in susceptible rats and is characterized by portal tract inflammation and bile duct proliferation. Endotoxin adversely effects hepatocanalicular secretion [429]. Cholangiograms show extrahepatic ductal dilatation and ectasia; bile flow is decreased [430–435].

Anaerobic bacteria, particularly *Bacteroides* species, appear to be the responsible organisms. Treatment with metronidazole and tetracycline prevents the hepatic inflammation and decreases bile duct thickening [436]. The inflammatory lesion may be the result, not of actual bacterial infection, but of bacterial products that sensitize Kupffer cells, resulting in the release of proinflammatory cytokines [6,24,437]. Cultures of blood, liver, and peritoneal fluids are usually negative. The injection of peptidoglycan, a bacterial cell wall polymer, results in hepatic inflammation. Targeted disruption of the peptidoglycan with the enzyme mutanolysin prevents the hepatic injury [433,435]. Clinically, the bacterial overgrowth hypothesis is attractive. Most TPN patients have some degree of intestinal injury and thus are susceptible. Bacterial overgrowth results in increased conversion of primary bile acids to lithocholate, further injuring the liver. Antibiotic treatment of neonates and Crohn's disease patients with liver disease has resulted in biochemical improvement [434,438].

Sepsis is also a critical factor. Sepsis exacerbates the cholestatic state in the low birth weight infant and occurs whether the infant is receiving TPN. In a retrospective review, infants who developed severe cholestasis had more septic episodes at an earlier age than those who did not develop severe cholestasis [405]. Endotoxemia occurs in the absence of culture-proven sepsis. Endotoxins directly damage hepatocytes and induce the release of toxic free radicals and proinflammatory cytokines [439]. Antibiotics improve and prevent TPN-associated liver disease [440]. Infants and children with TPN-associated liver disease are in a proinflammatory state. There is one case report of improvement in TPN-associated liver disease in an adult following the administration of a TNF antibody [441].

Nutrient deficiencies or excesses are potential causes. Caution is necessary when interpreting these studies: the results may reflect exposure, toxicity, or an indirect effect of underlying liver disease. Taurine is an essential amino acid in infants and is required for bile acid conjugation. Taurine promotes bile flow and protects against lithocholate toxicity. Taurine supplementation has promoted bile flow in premature infants and decreased cholestasis [442–444]. Parenteral nutrition is relatively deficient in antioxidants; vitamin E and selenium levels are low, whereas copper (an oxidant) levels are high [445] Hepatic glutathione depletion occurs during TPN and renders the infantile liver susceptible to oxidant injury [446]. Intravenous methionine is hepatotoxic; elevated homocystine levels suggest an enzymatic block early in the methionine metabolic pathway [447]. Manganese has been reported to be hepatotoxic in infants; of 57 children receiving TPN, 11 had cholestasis and elevated serum manganese levels. Reduction or removal of the manganese resulted in a decline in serum bilirubin and aminotransferase concentrations [448,449]. In adults, manganese concentrations increase during TPN and reflect exposure and impaired excretion in cholestasis [450]. In one study, infants receiving higher concentrations of manganese had higher serum manganese and bilirubin levels [451]. Excessive iron in TPN solutions also may cause hepatic injury [452].

Parenteral nutrition solutions often do not contain carnitine. Low serum and tissue carnitine concentrations have been reported in infants and children receiving long-term parenteral nutrition. Premature infants appear to be particularly susceptible. Carnitine deficiency may result in steatosis and hyperbilirubinemia. Optimal dosage to prevent deficiency is not well defined; 3–10 mg/kg/d is suggested in neonates receiving TPN longer than 2 weeks. Routine carnitine supplementation has not been proven to prevent TPN-associated liver disease [453–457].

Choline deficiency has been suggested as a cause of hepatic steatosis. Patients receiving long-term parenteral nutrition have low plasma free choline levels; up to 50% may have steatosis. Oral lecithin or intravenous choline chloride increases plasma choline concentrations and results in decreased hepatic fat by MRI [458,459]. A placebo-controlled trial showed increased hepatic choline by CT, improved serum aminotransferase levels, and normal bilirubin concentrations in those receiving choline [460].

Contaminants also have been implicated as a potential etiologic factor. Sodium bisulfite degrades tryptophan and may cause cholestasis; photooxidation products of normal components may cause cholestasis [461–463]. Photoprotection of parenteral nutrition solutions has enhanced enteral feeding in premature infants [464]. Aluminium contamination of TPN solution was previously common and still occurs, particularly in small volume parenterals. Elevated serum and hepatic levels have been found and correlate with bone injury [465,466]. Cholestasis is a feature of aluminium toxicity. Polysorbates were the cause of severe liver injury associated with an intravenous vitamin E preparation [76].

Phytosterols, contaminants present in commercially available lipid emulsions, cause cholestasis in a piglet animal model, and a significant inhibition of secretory function in isolated rat hepatocytes [467]. Infants with parenteral nutrition–associated cholestasis have elevated plasma phytosterol concentrations [468]. Elevated phytosterol levels are present in other liver diseases, suggesting they are a marker of hepatic dysfunction rather than a causal agent [469].

TPN-Associated Hepatic Steatosis

Steatosis is the most frequently documented hepatic abnormality in the older patient receiving TPN [374]. It is usually asymptomatic, but mild aminotransferase and alkaline phosphatase elevations may be noted. Enzyme elevations usually occur within 2 weeks of the initiation of TPN and may spontaneously resolve. The fat is periportal in distribution; in more severe cases it may be either panlobular or centrilobular [387]. Adults on long-term TPN may develop fibrosis and cirrhosis [375].

Steatosis is the result of excess calorie infusions, usually in the form of glucose, and impaired hepatic triglyceride secretion [470,471] In the rat, infusion of carbohydrate-based TPN results in increased hepatic triglyceride content; the fatty acid content reflects endogenous synthesis. Hepatic carboxylase A–specific activity is increased. Hepatic triglyceride secretion is suppressed, and triglyceride fatty acid oxidation decreases. Excess carbohydrate, beyond the glucose oxidation capacity, is converted to triglycerides, which accumulate in the liver. A direct correlation exists between the calories administered and the hepatic triglyceride content [472]. High glucose infusions elevate serum insulin levels, promoting lipogenesis and inhibiting carnitine acyltransferase, the rate-limiting step in fatty acid oxidation [473].

Lipid emulsions have been implicated, however, it is important to remember that cholestasis was described before lipid emulsions were available in the United States [383,474,475]. Essential fatty acid deficiency causes hepatic injury. Hepatic injury occurs when large quantities of lipid are infused. Intravenous lipid emulsions promote lipid peroxidation, decrease endotoxin clearance, and affect macrophage function [475]. Lipid emulsions also increase hepatic apoptosis [476]. Cholestasis often improves when lipid infusions are decreased; this may be related to the lipid emulsion itself or the decreased calories infused. The composition of the lipid emulsion may be important. Currently available emulsions are soy-based; olive oil, fish oil, and medium chain triglyceride–based emulsions have decreased cholestasis [477–480].

Infusion of large amounts of carbohydrate calories results in an increased portal vein insulin:glucagon molar ratio [481]. The excess insulin promotes lipogenesis. Decreasing the insulin: glucagon ratio diminishes hepatic steatosis. Glucagon administration inhibits fatty acid synthesis and enhances release of fatty acids. Glutamine not only prevents intestinal atrophy in TPN-treated patients but also lessens hepatic steatosis [482]. Addition of a lipid source also decreases steatosis [470]. In general, steatosis appears to be a benign and reversible consequence of TPN and is related to the caloric and fuel mixture administered. Modification of the TPN solution can prevent steatosis.

Management

The management of TPN-associated liver disease first focuses on prevention. Aggressive recognition and management of sepsis is crucial. Every effort must be made to promote intestinal motility and prevent translocation. Oxidant stress must be minimized. Appropriate calorie amounts and a balanced solution should be administered. Protein content should be the minimum required; some data suggest that enteral administration of protein while supplying other nutrient intravenously may decrease cholestasis; however, total nutritional needs must be met [483]. Cyclic, rather than continuous, administration of TPN may decrease hepatic injury [484]. Enteral feedings must be initiated as soon as possible even if only in minimal amounts. Biochemical monitoring must be done on a routine basis, and early indications of hepatic injury should be heeded. Other causes of liver disease must be excluded. If possible, TPN should be decreased or discontinued. However, malnutrition must be avoided. Antibiotic therapy aimed at anaerobic enteral bacteria should be considered, especially when bacterial overgrowth is suspected. Cholecystokinin has been used to promote bile flow [485].

Promising new approaches are being studied. Ursodeoxycholic acid has improved bile flow in parenterally fed newborn piglets; a pilot study suggested it might be beneficial in children [486,487]. A subsequent study failed to demonstrate the value of tauroursodeoxycholic acid in either the prevention or treatment of parenteral nutrition related cholestasis [488]. Nonsteroidal anti-inflammatory drugs such as aspirin have a significant choleretic effect. Aspirin can overcome the reduction in bile flow and bile salt secretion caused by TPN, but further human studies are necessary [489,490]. In piglets given par enteral nutrition and either fish or soy oil intravenously, only those piglets receiving soy oil develop cholestasis. Basal and stimulated bile flow decreased in the soy oil–fed but not the fish oil–fed piglets. The postulated mechanism is a change in the fatty acid membrane composition [491]. It is unknown how infants with short bowel or impaired absorption would absorb enterally administered fish oil. Sincalide in preliminary studies has decreased cholestasis; it is not effective in advanced liver disease [492]. Supplementation of TPN with cysteine results in a reduction of TPN-induced hepatic lipid accumulation in the weanling rat and may protect the intestinal mucosa [493,494].

MISCELLANEOUS

Sarcoidosis

Sarcoidosis is a chronic multisystem disease of unknown etiology, which is rare in childhood. The pathologic feature is the presence of noncaseating granulomas in various tissues [495]. The pattern of symptoms in children depends on the age of presentation. Under 4 years of age, the typical presenting symptoms are rash, arthritis, and uveitis, with pulmonary involvement less common [496]. The peak age of incidence in childhood is 9 years; at this time, pulmonary symptoms predominate. Constitutional symptoms such as fatigue, weight loss, cough, bone and joint pain, and headache are common. The most common physical findings are lymphadenopathy, ocular changes, rash, and hepatosplenomegaly [496]. The liver involvement is usually asymptomatic. Sarcoidosis also may be seen in association with such systemic disorders as Crohn's disease, celiac disease, amyloidosis, lymphoma, thyroiditis, and Addison's disease [497]. Hepatomegaly is noted in up to 40% of patients. Hepatic involvement varies from minimal elevation of serum aminotransferase concentrations with no clinical symptoms to chronic liver disease and portal hypertension. Chronic intrahepatic cholestasis rarely develops. Biopsy reveals noncaseating granulomas, increased hepatic copper, and decreased interlobular bile ducts [498]. Serial biopsies occasionally reveal decreasing interlobular ducts and progression to periportal fibrosis and micronodular biliary cirrhosis. Granulomatous phlebitis of the portal and hepatic veins may be an etiologic event [499–501]. Although corticosteroids are used for treatment, the optimal dosage and duration of therapy remain uncertain. Ursodeoxycholic acid has been used [502].

Amyloidosis

Amyloidosis results when an imbalance in the production and degradation of acute-phase inflammatory protein develops and the deposition of insoluble material in various organs results [503]. The most frequently affected organs are spleen, kidney, heart, and liver. The usual hepatic presentation is hepatomegaly, elevated alkaline phosphatase, and well-preserved hepatic function. In adults, amyloidosis is associated with chronic infections or inflammatory states such as rheumatoid arthritis and tuberculosis [504–506]. In children, amyloidosis is rare. The most common causes are tuberculosis, JRA, cystic fibrosis, and familial Mediterranean fever [224,253,507]. Most pediatric cases of amyloidosis occur in patients over 15 years of age with longstanding disease. Recently, reports of amyloidosis in cystic fibrosis patients have increased; as survival increases, it is reasonable to anticipate that the incidence will continue to increase. Current incidence estimates are 6% in tuberculosis, 4–10% in JRA, and up to 33% in cystic fibrosis. Amyloidosis should be suspected in any patient with a chronic disorder who develops hepatomegaly and proteinuria; diagnosis can be confirmed by rectal or kidney biopsy.

A New Form of Systemic Disease: Congenital Disorders of Glycosylation

Congenital disorders of glycosylation (CDG) are inherited metabolic diseases caused by defective N-glycosylation of proteins [508]. Depending on the type of CDG, the carbohydrate side chains of glycoproteins are either truncated or completely absent from the protein core. The CDG syndromes can affect multiple organs and the clinical manifestations are protean and of varying severity [509]. The liver is involved in at least 11 of the 18 known subtypes (Table 38.8). Common features include dysmorphic facies, developmental delay and mental retardation, hypotonia, seizures, failure to thrive, diarrhea, protein-losing enteropathy, and recurrent infections. Coagulopathy may occur independent of the severity of liver dysfunction and is caused by the abnormal glycosylation of clotting factors. Hepatomegaly and elevated serum aminotransferase levels are often found. In several disorders with more severe liver disease, the histopathology has been defined [510]. In CDG-1b portal fibrosis and ductal plate malformation mimic the histologic findings

Table 38.8: Congenital Disorders of Glycosylation with a Liver Phenotype

Disorder	*Gene*	*Enzyme*	*Clinical Features*
CDG-1a	*PMM2*	Phosphomannomutase II	Mental retardation, hypotonia, inverted nipples, lipodystrophy, cerebellar hypoplasia, stroke-like episodes, seizures, hepatomegaly, steatosis, fibrosis
CDG-1b	*MPI*	Phosphomannose isomerase	Hepatic fibrosis, hypoglycemia, coagulopathy, protein-losing enteropathy
CDG-1c	*ALC6*	Glucosyltransferase I Dol-PGlc: Man9-GlcNAc2-P-P-Dol glucosyltransferase	Mental retardation, hypotonia, esotropia, seizures, hepatomegaly
CDG-1h	*ALG8*	dolichyl-phosphate (Dol-P)-glucose (Glc):Glc1-mannose (Man)9-N-acetylglucosamine (GlcNAc)2-PP-Dol-a-1, 3-glucosyltransferase	Hypoalbuminemia, protein-losing enteropathy (PLE), hepatomegaly, renal disease, CNS dysfunction, and coagulation factor defects.
CDG-1i	*ALG2*	Mannosyltransferase II GDPMan: Man1-GlcNAc2-P-P-Dol mannosyltransferase	Mental retardation, intractable seizures, iris colobomas, hepatomegaly, and coagulopathy
CDG –II	*ALG9*	Mannosyltransferase Dol-P-Man: Man6- and Man8-GlcNAc2-P-P-Dol mannosyltransferase	Hepatomegaly, microcephaly, hypotonia, seizures
CDG –IIb	*GLS1*	Glucosidase I	Dysmorphism, hypotonia, seizures, hepatomegaly, hepatic fibrosis, steatosis, bile ductular proliferation
CDG -11e	*COG7*	Conserved oligomeric Golgi complex subunit 7	Hepatomegaly, progressive jaundice, dysmorphism, hypotonia, intractable seizures, recurrent infections, and cardiac failure
CDG -11/COG1	*COG1*	Conserved oligomeric Golgi complex subunit 1	Hepatosplenomegaly hypotonia, growth retardation, microcephaly, and mild mental retardation
CDG-11X	*Unknown*	Unknown	Hepatic dysfunction, cirrhosis, recurrent diarrhea, failure to thrive, cerebral atrophy, and mental retardation
CDG-X	*Unknown*	Unknown	Elevated serum aminotransferases, liver fibrosis, and steatosis

of congenital hepatic fibrosis. Liver disease may be the only feature of CDG-1b for many years. Varying degrees of fibrosis and steatosis may occur in the other subtypes [511]. Cirrhosis and isolated cryptogenic liver disease has been reported in patients in whom the underlying biochemical defect has not been defined (CDG-X) [512,513].

Isoelectric focusing (IEF) of serum transferrin is the common diagnostic screening test for CDG [508,509]. Protein chip technologies and electrospray-ionization mass spectrometry are also being used to define patterns of protein glycosylation [508]. Some forms of CDG, such as CDG-IIb, cannot be detected by IEF of transferrin. Alternative methods including thin-layer chromatography of urine oligosaccharides may be required.

There are no effective treatments for most forms of CDG. Daily oral mannose supplements are being used in patients with CDG-Ib [514]. Mannose bypasses the defect in the conversion of fructose-6-phosphate to mannose-6-phosphate and reverses the altered glycosylation of proteins, coagulopathy, hypoglycemia, and protein-losing enteropathy that are associated with this disorder. The effect on liver fibrosis is uncertain.

REFERENCES

1. Lautt WW, Greenwall CV. Conceptual review of the hepatic vasculature. Hepatology 1987;7:952–63.
2. Andus T, Baier J, Gerok W. Effects of cytokines on the liver. Hepatology 1991;13:364–75.
3. Bazel S, Andrejko KM, Chen J, Deutschman CS. Hepatic gene expression and cytokine responses to sterile inflammation: comparison with cecal ligation and puncture sepsis in the rat. Shock 1999;11:347–55.

4. Geller DA, Nguyen D, Shapiro RA, et al. Cytokine induction of interferon regulatory factor-1 in hepatocytes. Surgery 1993; 114:235–42.
5. Green RM, Beier D, Gollan JL. Regulation of hepatocyte bile salt transporters by endotoxin and inflammatory cytokines in rodents. Gastroenterology 1996;111:193–8.
6. Lichtman S, Lemasters JJ. Role of cytokines and cytokine-producing cells in reperfusion injury to the liver. Sem Liver Dis 1999;19:171–87.
7. Oka Y, Murata A, Nishijima J, Ogawa M, Mori T. The mechanism of hepatic cellular injury in sepsis: an in vitro study of the implications of cytokines and neutrophils in its pathogenesis. J Surg Res 1993;55:1–8.
8. Wang P, Ayala A, Ba ZF, Zhou M, et al. Tumor necrosis factor-alpha produces hepatocellular dysfunction despite normal cardiac output and hepatic microcirculation [see comments]. Am J Physiol 1993;265:G126–32.
9. Wang P, Chaudry IH. Mechanism of hepatocellular dysfunction during hyperdynamic sepsis. Am J Physiol 1996;270:R927–38.
10. Schneider R, Laxer RM. Systemic onset juvenile rheumatoid arthritis. Baillieres Clin Rheumatol 1998;12:245–71.
11. Johnson EE, Hedley-White J. Continuous positive pressure ventilation and portal flow in dogs with pulmonary edema. J Appl Physiol 1972;22:285–9.
12. Franson TR, Hierholzer WJ, La Brecque DR. Frequency and characteristics of hyperbilrubinemia associated with bacteremia. Rev Infect Dis 1985;7:1–9.
13. Bernstein J, Brown AK. Sepsis and jaundice in early infancy. Pediatrics 1962;29:873–82.
14. Plemmons RM, Dooley DP, Longfield RN. Septic thrombophlebitis of the portal vein (pylephlebitis): diagnosis and management in the modern era. Clin Infect Dis 1995;21:1114–20.
15. Lang CH, Fan J, Cooney R, Vary TC. IL-1 receptor antagonist attenuates sepsis-induced alterations in the IGF system and protein synthesis. Am J Physiol 1996;270:E430–7.
16. Koo DJ, Chaudry IH, Wang P. Kupffer cells are responsible for producing inflammatory cytokines and hepatocellular dysfunction during early sepsis. J Surg Res 1999;83:151–7.
17. Andrejko KM, Chen J, Deutschman CS. Intrahepatic STAT-3 activation and acute phase gene expression predict outcome after CLP sepsis in the rat. Am J Physiol 1998;275:G1423–9.
18. Walley KR, Lukacs NW, Standiford TJ, et al. Balance of inflammatory cytokines related to severity and mortality of murine sepsis. Infect Immun 1996;64:4733–8.
19. Torpy DJ, Bornstein SR, Chrousos GP. Leptin and interleukin-6 in sepsis. Horm Metab Res 1998;30:726–9.
20. Szabo G, Roomics L, Frendl G. Liver in sepsis and systemic inflammatory response syndrome. Clin Liver Dis 2002;6:1045–66.
21. Cressman DE, Greenbaum LE, DeAngelis RA, et al. Liver failure and defective hepatocyte regeneration in interleukin-6-deficient mice. Science 1996;274:1379–83.
22. Dalrymple SA, Slattery R, Aud DM, et al. Interleukin-6 is required for a protective immune response to systemic *Escherichia coli* infection. Infect Immun 1996;64:3231–5.
23. Billiau A, Vandekerckhove F. Cytokines and their interaction with other inflammatory mediators in the pathogenesis of sepsis and septic shock. Eur J Clin Invest 1991;21:559–73.
24. Nolan J. Intestinal endotoxins as mediators of hepatic injury: an idea whose time has come again. Hepatology 1989;10:887–91.
25. Wang Q, Wang JJ, Boyce S, et al. Endotoxemia and IL-1 beta stimulate mucosal IL-6 production in different parts of the gastrointestinal tract. J Surg Res 1998;76:27–31.
26. Arend WP, Malyak M, Guthridge CJ, Gabay C. Interleukin-1 receptor antagonist: role in biology. Annual Review of Immunology 1998;16:27–55.
27. Buck C, Bundschu J, Gallati H, Bartmann P, Pohlandt F. Interleukin-6: a sensitive parameter for the early diagnosis of neonatal bacterial infection. Pediatrics 1994;93:54–8.
28. Moseley RH. Sepsis and cholestasis. Clin Liver Dis 2004;8:83–94.
29. Cohen JA, Kaplan MM. Left-sided heart failure presenting as hepatitis. Gastroenterology 1978;74:583–7.
30. Hassanein T, Razack A, Gavaler J, Van Thiel DH. Heatstroke: its clinical and pathologic presentation, with particular attention to the liver. Am J Gastroenterol 1992;61:1382–9.
31. Mace S, Borkat G, Liebman J. Hepatic dysfunction and cardiovascular abnormalities: occurrence in infants, children and young adults. Am J Dis Child 1985;139:60–5.
32. Strauss AW, Santa-Maria M, Goldring D. Constrictive pericarditis in children. Am J Dis Child 1975;130:822–6.
33. Sivan Y, Nutman J, Zeevi B, et al. Acute hepatic failure after open heart surgery in children. Pediatr Cardiol 1987;8:127–30.
34. Logan RG, Mowry FM, Judge RD. Cardiac failure simulating viral hepatitis: three cases with serum transaminase level above 1000. Ann Int Med 1962;56:784–8.
35. Killip T, Payne MA. High transaminase activity in heart disease. Circulation 1960;21:646–60.
36. Novel O, Henrion J, Bernuau J. Fulminant hepatic failure due to transient circulatory failure in patients with chronic heart disease. Dig Dis Sci 1980;25:49–54.
37. Garland JS, Werlin SL, Rice TB. Ischemic hepatitis in children: diagnosis and clinical course. Crit Care Med 1988;16:1209–12.
38. Jungermann K, Katz N. Functional specialization of different hepatocyte populations. Physiol Rev 1989;69:708–62.
39. Bauer C, Walcher F, Kalweit U, et al. Role of nitric oxide in the regulation of the hepatic microcirculation in vivo. J Hepatol 1997;27:1089–95.
40. Grund F, Sommerschild HT, Winecoff A, et al. Importance of nitric oxide in hepatic arterial blood flow and total hepatic blood volume regulation in pigs. Acta Physiolo Scand 1997;161: 303–9.
41. Koeppel TA, Thies JC, Schemmer P, et al. Inhibition of nitric oxide synthesis in ischemia/reperfusion of the rat liver is followed by impairment of hepatic microvascular blood flow. J Hepatol 1997;27:163–9.
42. Tanaka N, Tanaka K, Nagashima Y, et al. Nitric oxide increases hepatic arterial blood flow in rats with carbon tetrachloride-induced acute hepatic injury. Gastroenterology 1999;117:173–80.
43. Pannen BH, Bauer M, Noldge-Schomburg GF, et al. Regulation of hepatic blood flow during resuscitation from hemorrhagic shock: role of NO and endothelins. Am J Physiol 1997; 272:H2736–45.
44. Peltenburg HG, Hermens WT, Willems GM, et al. Estimation of the fractional catabolic rate constants for the elimination of cytosolic liver enzymes from plasma. Hepatology 1989;10:833–9.
45. Arcieli JM, Moore GW, Hutchins GM. Hepatic morphology in cardiac dysfunction: a clinicopathologic study of 1000 subjects at autopsy. American J of Pathology 1981;104:159–66.

46. de la Monte SM, Arcidi JM, Moore GM, Hutchins GM. Midzonal necrosis as a pattern of hepatocellular injury after shock. Gastroenterology 1984;86:627–31.
47. Kanel GC, Ucci A, Kaplan MM. A distinctive perivenular hepatic lesion associated with heart failure. Am J Clin Pathol 1980; 73:235–9.
48. Giallourakis C, Rosenberg PM, Friedman LS. The liver in heart failure. Clin Liver Dis 2002;6:947–67.
49. Katzin HM, Waller JV, Blumgart HL. "Cardiac cirrhosis" of the liver: a clinical and pathological study. Arch Int Med 1939; 64:457–70.
50. Weinberg AG, Boldande RP. The liver in congenital heart disease: effects of infantile coarctation of the aorta and the hypoplastic left heart syndrome in infancy. Am J Dis Child 1970; 119:390–4.
51. Shiraki K. Hepatic cell necrosis in the newborn: a pathologic study of 147 cases with a particular reference to congenital heart disease. Am J Dis Child 1970;119:395–400.
52. Ghaferi A, Hutchins G. Progression of liver pathology in patients undergoing the Fontan procedure: chronic passive congestion, cardiac cirrhosis, hepatic adenoma, and hepatocellular carcinoma. J Thorac Cardiovasc Surg 2005;129:1348–52.
53. Narkewicz M, Sondheimer H, Ziegler J, et al. Hepatic dysfunction following the Fontan procedure. J Pediatr Gastroenterol Nutr 2003;36:352–7.
54. Sherlock S. The liver in heart failure: relation of anatomical, functional, and circulatory changes. Br Heart J 1951;13:273–93.
55. Seeto R, Fenn B, Rockey D. Ischemic hepatitis: clinical presentation and pathogenesis. Am J Med 2000;109:109–13.
56. Henrion J, Schapira M, Luwaert R, et al. Hypoxic hepatitis: Clinical and hemodynamic study in 142 consectutive cases. Medicine 2003;82:392–406.
57. Tanne F, Gagnadoux F, Chazouilleres O, et al. Chronic liver injury during obstructive sleep apnea. Hepatology 2005;41: 1290–6.
58. Henrion J, Minette P, Colin L, et al. Hypoxic hepatitis caused by acute exacerbation of chronic respiratory failure: a case-controlled, hemodynamic study of 17 consecutive cases. Hepatology 1999;29:427–33.
59. Bianchi L, Ohnacker H, Beck K, Zimmerli-Ning M. Liver damage in heatstroke and its regression. Hum Pathol 1972;3:237–48.
60. Dilawari JB, Bambery P, Chawla Y, et al. Hepatic outflow obstruction (Budd–Chiari syndrome): experience with 177 patients and a review of the literature. Medicine 1994;73:21–56.
61. Lang H, Oldhafer KJ, Weimann A, et al. The Budd–Chiari syndrome: clinical presentation and diagnostic findings in 45 patients treated by surgery. Bildgebung 1994;61:173–81.
62. Gentil-Kocher S, Bernard O, Brunelle F, et al. Budd-Chiari syndrome in children: report of 22 cases. J Pediatr 1988;113:30–8.
63. Bolondi L, Gaiani S, LiBassi S, et al. Diagnosis of Budd–Chiari syndrome by pulsed Doppler ultrasound. Gastroenterology 1991;100:1324–31.
64. Grant GG, Schiller VL, Millener P, et al. Color Doppler imaging of the hepatic vasculature. Am J Roentgenol 1992;159:943–50.
65. Erden A, Erden I, Yurdaydin C, Karayalcin S. Hepatic outflow obstruction: enhancement patterns of the liver on MR angiography. Eur J Radiol 2003;48:203–8.
66. Meindok H, Langer B. Liver scan in Budd–syndrome. J Nucl Med 1975;17:365–86.
67. Murphy FB, Steinberg HV, Shires GT. The Budd–Chiari syndrome: a review. Am J Roentgenol 1986;147:9–15.
68. Mitchell MC, Boitnott JK, Kaufman S, et al. Budd–Chiari syndrome: etiology, diagnosis and management. Medicine 1982; 61:199–218.
69. Valla D. Obstruction of the hepatic veins. Dig Dis 1990;8:226–39.
70. McDonald GB, Sharma P, Matthews DE. Veno-occlusive disease of the liver after bone marrow transplantation: diagnosis, incidence and predisposing factors. Hepatology 1984;4:116–22.
71. Ridker PM, Ohkuma S, McDermott WV, et al. Hepatic veno-occlusive disease associated with the consumption of pyrrolizidine containing dietary supplements. Gastroenterology 1985; 88:1050–4.
72. Roulet M, Laurine R, Rivier L, Calame A. Hepatic veno-occlusive disease in the newborn infant of a woman drinking herbal tea. J Pediatr 1988;112:433–6.
73. Bach N, Thung SN, Schaffner F. Comfrey herb tea-induced hepatic veno-occlusive disease. Am J Med 1989;87:97–9.
74. Mohabbat O, Younos MS, Merzad AA, et al. A. An outbreak of hepatic veno-occlusive disease in northwestern Afghanistan. Lancet 1976;2:269–71.
75. Labadie H, Stoessel P, Callard P, Beaugrand M. Hepatic veno-occlusive disease and perisinusoidal fibrosis secondary to arsenic poisoning. Gastroenterology 1990;99:1140–3.
76. Bove KE, Kosmetatos N, Wedig K, et al. Vasculopathic hepatotoxicity assoiciated with E-Ferol syndrome in low birth weight infants. JAMA 1985;254:2422–30.
77. Avner ED, Ellis D, Jaffe R. Veno-occlusive disease of the liver associated with cysteamine treatment of nephropathic cystinosis. J Pediatr 1983;102:793–6.
78. Etzioni A, Benderly A, Rosenthal E. Defective humoral and cellular immune functions associated with veno-occlusive disease of the liver. J Pediatr 1987;112:549–54.
79. Mellis C, Bale PM. Familial hepatic veno-occlusive disease with probable immune deficiency. J Pediatr 1976;88:236–42.
80. Roscioli TR, Cliffe ST, Bloch DB, et al. Mutations in the gene encoding the PML nuclear body protein Sp110 are associated with immnodeficiency and hepatic veno-occlusive disease. Nat Genet 2006;38:620–2.
81. Li X, Wei Y, Hao H, et al. Hyperhomocysteinemia and the MTHFR C677T mutation in Budd–Chiari syndrome. Am J Hematol 2002;71:11–14.
82. Wanless IR, Godwin TA, Allen F. Nodular regenerative hyperplasia of the liver in hematologic disorders: a possible response to obliterative portal venopathy. Medicine 1980;59:367–79.
83. Sty JR. Ultrasonography: hepatic vein thrombosis in sickle cell anemia. Am J Pediatr Hematol Oncol 1982;4:213–15.
84. Khuroo Ms, Datta DV. Budd–Chiari syndrome following pregnancy: report of 16 cases, with roentgenologic, hemodynamic and histologic studies of the hepatic outflow tract. Am J Med 1980;80:113–21.
85. Goodman ZD, Ishak KG. Occlusive venous lesions in alcoholic liver disease: a study of 200 cases. Gastroenterology 1982;83: 786–96.
86. Maccini DM, Berg JC, Bell GA. Budd–Chiari syndrome and Crohn's disease. Dig Dis Sci 1989;34:1933–6.
87. Schwartz KB, Wolverson M, deMello DE, et al. Budd–Chiari syndrome in a child. J Pediatr Gastroenterol Nutr 1982;1:277–83.
88. Schraut WH, Chilcote RR. Metastatic Wilm's tumor causing acute hepatic vein occlusion (Budd–Chiari syndrome). Gastroenterology 1985;88:576–9.

89. Lewis JH, Tice Hl, Zimmerman HJ. Budd–Chiari syndrome associated with oral contraceptive steroids: review of treatment of 47 cases. Dig Dis Sci 1983;28:673–8.
90. Orloff LA, Orloff MJ. Budd–Chiari syndrome caused by Behcet's disease: treatment by side-to-side portacaval shunt. J Am Coll Surg 1999;188:396–407.
91. Broeckmans AW, Veltkamp JJ, Bertina RM. Congential protein C deficiency and venous thrombo-embolism: a study in three Dutch families. N Engl J Med 1983;309:340–3.
92. Patel RK, Lea NC, Heneghan MA, et al. Prevalence of the activating JAK2 tyrosine kinase mutation V617F in the Budd–Chiari syndrome. Gastroenterology 2006;130:2031.
93. Delarive J, Gonvers JJ. Budd–Chiari syndrome related to factor V Leiden mutation. Am J Gastroenterol 1998;93:651–2.
94. Mahmoud AE, Elias E, Beauchamp N, Wilde JT. Prevalence of the factor V Leiden mutation in hepatic and portal vein thrombosis. Gut 1997;40:798–800.
95. Tsai MS, Cheng NY, Wang CK, et al. Anticardiolipin antibody-related Budd–Chiari syndrome: report of a case. Kaohsiung J Med Sci 1998;14:48–52.
96. Pelletier S, Landi B, Piette JC, Ekert P, et al. Antiphospholipid syndrome as the second cause of non-tumorous Budd–Chiari syndrome. J Hepatol 1994;21:76–80.
97. Schattenfroh N, Bechstein WO, Blumhardt G, et al. Liver transplantation for PNH with Budd–Chiari syndrome. A case report. Transplant Int 1993;6:354–8.
98. Wyatt HA, Mowat AP, Layton M. Paroxysmal nocturnal haemoglobinuria and Budd–Chiari syndrome. Arch Dis Child 1995; 72:241–2.
99. Brockington GM, Zebede J, Pandian NG. Constrictive pericarditis. Cardiol Clin 1990;8:645–61.
100. Solano FX, Young F, Talamo TS. Constrictive pericarditis mimicking the Budd–Chiari syndrome. Am J Med 1986;80:113–16.
101. Hoffman HP, Stockland B, von der Heyden U. Membranous obstruction of the inferior vena cava with Budd Chiari syndrome: a report of nine cases. J Pediatr Gastroenterol Nutr 1987; 6:878–84.
102. Simpson IW. Membranous obstruction of the inferior vena cava and hepatocellular carcinoma in South Africa. Gastroenterology 1982;82:171–8.
103. Kage M, Arakawa M, Kojiro M. Histopathology of membranous obstruction of the inferior vena cava in the Budd–Chiari syndrome. Gastroenterology 1992;102:2081–90.
104. Okuda K, Kage M, Shrestha SM. Proposal of a new nomenclature for Budd–Chiari syndrome: hepatic vein thrombosis versus thrombosis of the inferior vena cava at its hepatic portion. Hepatology 1998;28:1191–8.
105. Cho O, Koo J, Kim Y, et al. Collateral pathways in Budd–Chiari syndrome: CT and venographic correlation. Am J of Roentgenology 1996;167:1163–7.
106. McDermott WV, Ridker PM. The Budd–Chiari syndrome and hepatic veno-occlusive disease. Arch Surg 1990;125:525–7.
107. Powell-Jackson PR, Ede RJ, Williams R. Budd–Chiari syndrome presenting as fulminant hepatic failure. Gut 1986;27:1101–5.
108. Lopez RR, Benner KG, Hall L, et al. Expandable venous stents for treatment of the Budd-Chiari syndrome. Gastroenterology 1991;100:1435–41.
109. Molmenti E, Segev D, Arepally A, et al. The utility of TIPS in the management of Budd–Chiari syndrome. Ann Surg 2005; 241:978–81.
110. Feng L, Peng Q, Li K, et al. Management of severe Budd–Chiari syndrome: report of 147 cases. Hepatobiliary Pancreat Dis Int 2004;3:522–5.
111. Hemming AW, Langer B, Greig P, et al. Treatment of Budd–Chiari syndrome with portosystemic shunt or liver transplantation. Am J Surg 1996;171:176–81.
112. Sakai Y, Wall WJ. Liver transplantation for Budd-Chiari syndrome: a retrospective study. Surg Today 1994;24:49–53.
113. Ruh J, Malago M, Busch Y, et al. Management of Budd–Chiari syndrome. Ann Surg 2005;241:978–81.
114. Murad S, Valla D, de Groen P, et al. Determinants of survival and the effect of portosystemic shunting in patients with Budd–Chiari syndrome. Hepatology 2004;39:500–8.
115. Johnson CS, Omata M, Tong MJ, et al. Liver involvement in sickle cell disease. Medicine 1985;64:349–56.
116. Bauer TW, Moore W, Hutchins GM. The liver in sickle cell disease: a clinicopathologic study of 70 patients. Am J Med 1980; 69:833–7.
117. Omata M, Johnson CS, Tong MJ, Tatter D. Pathologic spectrum of liver disease in sickle cell disease. Dig Dis Sci 1986;31:247–56.
118. Schubert TT. Hepatobiliary system in sickle cell disease. Gastroenterology 1986;86:2013–21.
119. Brody JJ, Ryan WN, Haidar MA. Serum alkaline phosphatase isoenzymes in sickle cell anemia. JAMA 1975;232:738–41.
120. Sayad AE, Farah RA, Rogers ZR, Squires RH. Correlation of serum choylglycine level with hepatic dysfunction in children with sickle cell anemia. Clin Pediatr 1999;38:293–6.
121. Ahn H, Chin-Shang L, Wang W. Sickle cell hepatopathy: clinical presentation, treatment, and outcome in pediatric and adult patients. Pediatr Blood Cancer 2005;45:184–90.
122. Buchanan GR, Glader BE. Benign course of extreme hyperbilirubinemia in sickle cell disease: analysis of six cases. J Pediatr 1977;91:21–4.
123. Barrett-Conner E. Sickle cell disease and viral hepatitis. Ann Int Med 1968;69:517–27.
124. Zakaria N, Knisely A, Portmann B, Mieli-Vergani G, Arya R, Devlin J. Acute sickle cell hepatopathy represents a potential contraindication for percutaneous liver biopsy. Blood 2003; 101:101–3.
125. Sheehy TW, Law DE, Wade BH. Exchange transfusion for sickle cell intrahepatic cholestasis. Arch Int Med 1980;140:1363–6.
126. Ross A, Graeme-Cook F, Cosimi A, Chung R. Combined liver and kidney transplantation in a patient with sickle cell disease. Transplantation 2002;73:605–8.
127. Biachi M, Arifuddin R, Mantry P, et al. Liver transplantation in sickle cell anemia: a case of acute sickle cell intrahepatic cholestasis and a case of sclerosing cholangitis. Transplantation 2005;80:1630–2.
128. Yohannan MD, Arif M, Ramia S. Aetiology of icteric hepatitis and fulminant hepatic failure in children and the possible predisposition to hepatic failure by sickle cell disease. Acta Paediatr Scand 1990;79:201–5.
129. Hassan M, Hasan D, Giday S, et al. Hepatitis C in sickle cell disease. J Nat Med Assoc 2003;95:939–42.
130. Lykavieris P, Benichou J, Benkerrou M, et al. Autoimmune liver disease in three children with sickle cell disease. J Pediatr Gastroenterol Nutr 2006;42:104–8.
131. Chuang E, Ruchelli E, Mulberg AE. Autoimmune liver disease and sickle cell anemia in children: a report of three cases. J Pediatr Hematol Oncol 1997;19:159–62.

132. el Younis C, Min A, Fiel M, et al. Autoimmune hepatitis in a patient with sickle cell disease. Am J Gastroenterol 1996;91: 1016–18.
133. Garcia-Arias M, Rodriguez-Galindo C, et al. Pyogenic hepatic abscess after percutaneous liver biopsy in a patient with sickle cell disease. J Pediatric Hematol Oncol 2005;27:103–5.
134. Shulman ST, Beem MO. An unique presentation of sickle cell disease: pyogenic hepatic abscess. Pediatrics 1971;47:1019–22.
135. Heaton ND, Pain J, Cowan NC. Focal nodular hyperplasia of the liver: a link with sickle cell disease? Arch Dis Child 1991; 66:1073–4.
136. Markowitz RI, Harcke HT, Ritchie WG, Huff DS. Focal nodular hyperplasia of the liver in a child with sickle cell anemia. Am J Roentgenol 1980;134:595–7.
137. Terzoli GS, Mauri R, Borghetti L. Cirrhosis associated with multiple transfusions in thalassemia. Arch Dis Child 1984;59:67–70.
138. Spero JA, Lewis JH, Fisher SE, et al. The high risk of chronic liver disease in multi-transfused juvenile hemophiliac patients. J Pediatr 1979;94:875–8.
139. Kanesaki T, Kinoshita S, Tsujino G, et al. Hepatitis C virus infection in children with hemophilia: characterization of antibody response to four different antigens and relationship of antibody response, viremia, and hepatic dysfunction. J Pediatr 1993; 123:381–7.
140. Goedert JJ, Eyster ME, Lederman MM, et al. End-stage liver disease in persons with hemophilia and transfusion-associated infections. Blood 2002;100:1584–9.
141. Eyster ME, Diamondstone LS, Lien J, et al. Natural history of hepatitis C infection in multitransfused hemophiliacs: effect of co-infection with human immunodeficiency virus. J Acquired Immune Defic Syndromes 1993;6:602–10.
142. El-Serag HB, Mason AC. Rising incidence of hepatocellular carcinoma in the United States. N Engl J Med 1999;340:745–50.
143. Bresee JS, Mast EE, Coleman PJ, et al. Hepatitis C virus infection associated with administration of intravenous immune globulin. JAMA 1996;276:1563–7.
144. Jonas MM, Baron MJ, Bresee JS, Schneider LC. Clinical and virologic features of hepatitis C virus infection associated with intravenous immunoglobulin. Pediatrics 1996;98:211–15.
145. Dich NH, Maj MC, Goodman ZD, Klein MA. Hepatic involvement in Hodgkin's disease. Cancer 1989;64:2121–6.
146. Urba WJ, Longo DL. Hodgkin's disease. N Engl J Med 1992; 326:678–87.
147. Abt AB, Kirschner RH, Belliveau RE. Hepatic pathology associated with Hodgkin's disease. Cancer 1974;33:1564–71.
148. Perrera DR, Greene ML, Fenster LF. Cholestasis associated with extrabiliary Hodgkin's disease. Gastroenterology 1974;67:680–85.
149. Yalcin S, Kars A, Sokmensuer C, Atahan L. Extrahepatic Hodgkin's disease with intrahepatic cholestasis: report of two cases. Oncology 1999;57:83–5.
150. Rowbotham D, Wendon J, Williams R. Acute liver failure secondary to hepatic infiltration: a single centre experience of 18 cases. Gut 1998;42:576–80.
151. Cohen IT, Higginns GR, Powars DR, Hays DM. Staging laparotomy for Hodgkin's disease in children: evaluation of the technique. Arch Surg 1977;112:948–53.
152. Birrer MJ, Young RC. Differential diagnosis of jaundice in lymphoma patients. Sem Liver Dis 1987;7:269–77.
153. Ravindra K, Stringer M, Prasad K, et al. Non–Hodgkin's lymphoma presenting with obstructive jaundice. Br J Surg 2003; 90:845–9.
154. Janus C, Edwards BK, Sartiban E, Magrath IT. Surgical resection and limited chemotherapy for abdominal undifferentiated lymphomas. Cancer Treatment Reports 1984;68:599–605.
155. Issaivanan M, Kochhar S, Poddar B, Goraya J. Burkitt's lymphoma presenting as acute Budd Chiari syndrome. Indian Pediatr 2002;39:83–7.
156. Cavalli G, Casali AM, Lambertini F, Busachi C. Changes in the small biliary passages in the hepatic localization of Hodgkin's disease. Virchow Arch 1979;384:295–306.
157. Wammanda R, Ali F, Adama S, et al. Burkitt's lymphoma presenting as obstructive jaundice. Ann Tropical Paediatr 2004; 24:103–6.
158. Bouyn C, Leclere J, Raimondo G, et al. Hepatic focal nodular hyperplasia in children previously treated for a solid tumor. Incidence, risk factors, and outcome. Cancer 2003;97:3107–15.
159. Hutter RVP, Shipsky FH, Tan CTC, et al. Hepatic fibrosis in children with acute leukemia: a complication of therapy. Cancer 1960;13:288–307.
160. Wiedrich T, Keller D, Sunita A, Gilbert E. Adverse histopathologic effects of chemotherapeutic agents in childhood leukemia and lymphoma. Pediatr Pathol 1984;2:267–83.
161. DeBruyne R, Portmann B, Samyn M, et al. Chronic liver disease related to 6-thioguanine in children with acute lymphoblastic leukemia. J Hepatol 2006;44:407–10.
162. Choi SI, Simone JV. Acute nonlymphocytic leukemia in 171 children. Med Pediatr Oncol 1976;2:119–46.
163. Castro-Malaspino H. Subacute and chronic myelomonocytic leukemia in children. Cancer 1984;54:675–86.
164. Allan RR, Wadsworth LD, Kalousek DK, Massing BG. Congenital erythroleukemia: a case report with morphological, immunophenotypic, and cytogenetic findings. Am J Hematol 1989;31:114–21.
165. Costa F, Choy CG, Seiter K, et al. Hepatic outflow obstruction and liver failure due to leukemic cell infiltration in chronic lymphocytic leukemia. Leukemia Lymphoma 1998;30:403–10.
166. Devictor D, Tahiri C, Fabre M, et al. Early pre-B acute lymphoblastic leukemia presenting as fulminant liver failure. J Pediatr Gastroenterol Nutr 1996;22:103–6.
167. McCord RG, Gilbert EF, Joo PJ. Acute leukemia presenting as jaundice with acute liver failure. Clin Pediatr 1973;12:17A.
168. Shehab TM, Kaminski MS, Lok AS. Acute liver failure due to hepatic involvement by hematologic malignancy. Dig Dis Sci 1997;42:1400–5.
169. Zafrani ES, Leclercq B, Vernant JP, et al. Massive blastic infiltration of the liver: a cause of fulminant hepatic failure. Hepatology 1983;3:428–32.
170. Kader A, Vara R, Egberongbe Y, et al. Leukaemia presenting with fulminant hepatic failure in a child. Eur J Paediatr 2004;163: 628–9.
171. Kelleher J, Monteleone P, Steele D, et al. Hepatic dysfunction as the presenting feature of acute lymphoblastic leukemia. J Pediatr Hematol Oncol 2001;23:117–21.
172. Felice M, Hammermuller E, DeDavila M, et al. Acute lymphoblastic leukemia presenting as acute hepatic failure. Leukemia Lymphoma 2000;38:633–7.
173. Saleh RA, Graham-Pole J, Cumming WA. Severe hyperphosphatemia associated with tumor lysis in a patient with T-cell leukemia. Pediatr Emerg Care 1989;5:231–3.

174. Jones DP, Mahmoud H, Chesney RW. Tumor lysis syndrome: pathogenesis and management. Pediatr Nephrol 1995;9:206–12.
175. Arrambide K, Toto RD. Tumor lysis syndrome. Sem Nephrol 1993;13:273–80.
176. Steinherz P, Gaynon P, Miller D, et al. Improved disease-free survival of children with acute lymphoblastic leukemia at high risk for early relapse with the New York regime: new intensive therapy protocol: a report from the Children's Cancer Study Group. J Clin Oncol 1986;4:744–9.
177. Wolford JL, McDonald GB. A problem oriented approach to intestinal and liver disease after marrow transplantation. J Clin Gastroenterol 1988;10:419–33.
178. El-Sayed M, El-Haddad A, Fahmy O, et al. Liver disease is a major cause of mortality following allogeneic bone-marrow transplantation. European J Gastroenterol Hepatol 2004;16: 1347–54.
179. Bertheau P, Hadengue A, Cazals-Hatem D. Chronic cholestasis in patients after allogeneic bone marrow transplantation: several diseases are often associated. Bone Marrow Transplant 1995; 16:261–5.
180. McDonald GB, Sharma P, Matthews DE. The clinical course of 53 patients with veno-occlusive disease of the liver after marrow transplantation. Transplantation 1985;39:603–8.
181. Herbetko J, Grigg AP, Buckley AR, Phillips GL. Veno-occlusive disease after bone marrow transplantation: findings at duplex sonography. Am J Roentgenol 1992;158:1001–5.
182. Farthing MJG, Clark ML, Sloane JP. Liver disease after bone marrow transplantation. Gut 1982;23:465–74.
183. Dulley FL, Kanfer EJ, Appelbaum FR, et al. Veno-occlusive disease of the liver after chemoradiotherapy and autologous bone marrow transplantation. Transplantation 1987;43:870–3.
184. Vogelsang G, Dalal J. Hepatic venoocclusive disease in blood and bone marrow transplantation in children and young adults: incidence, risk factors, and outcome in a cohort of 241 patients. J Pediatr Hematol Oncol 2002;24:746–50.
185. Baglin TP. Veno-occlusive disease of the liver complicating bone marrow transplantation. Bone Marrow Transplantation 1994;13:1–4.
186. Bearman SI. The syndrome of hepatic veno-occlusive disease after marrow transplantation. Blood 1995;85:3005–20.
187. McDonald GB, Hinds MS, Fisher LD, et al. Veno-occlusive disease of the liver and multiorgan failure after bone marrow transplantation: a cohort study of 355 patients. Ann Int Med 1993; 118:255–67.
188. Reiss U, Cowan M, McMillan A, et al. Hepatic veno-occlusive disease in blood and bone marrow transplantation in children and young adults: incidence, risk factors and outcomes in a cohort of 241 patients. J Pediatr Gastroenterol Nutr 2002;24: 706–9.
189. Lapierre V, Mahe C, Auperin A, et al. Platelet transfusion containing ABO-incompatible plasma and hepatic veno-occlusive disease after hematopoietic transplantation in children. Transplantation 2005;80:314–19.
190. Srivastava A, Poonkuzhali B, Shaji R, et al. Glutathione S-transferase M1 polymorphism: a risk factor for hepatic venoocclusive disease in bone marrow transplantation. Blood 2004; 104:1574–7.
191. Rosenthal J, Sender L, Secola R, et al. Phase II trial of heparin prophylaxis for veno-occlusive disease of the liver in children undergoing bone marrow transplantation. Bone Marrow Transplant 1996;18:185–91.
192. Bearman SI, Lee JL, Baron AE, McDonald GB. Treatment of hepatic veno-occlusive disease with recombinant human tissue plasminogen activator and heparin in 42 marrow transplant patients. Blood 1997;89:1501–6.
193. Espigado I, Rodriguez JM, Parody R, et al. Reversal of severe hepatic veno-occlusive disease by combined plasma exchange and rt-PA treatment. Bone Marrow Transplant 1995;16:313–16.
194. Heying R, Nurnberger W, Spiekerkotter U, Gobel U. Hepatic veno-occlusive disease with severe capillary leakage after peripheral stem cell transplantation: treatment with recombinant plasminogen activator and C1-estarase inhibitor concentrate. Bone Marrow Transplant 1998;21:947–9.
195. Morris JD, Harris RE, Hashmi R, et al. Antithrombin-III for the treatment of chemotherapy-induced organ dysfunction following bone marrow transplantation. Bone Marrow Transplant 1997;20:871–8.
196. Sjoo F, Aschan J, Barkholt L, et al. N-acetyl-L-cysteine does not affect the pharmacokinetics or myelosuppressive effect of busulfan during conditioning prior to allogeneic stem cell transplantation. Bone Marrow Transplant 2003;32:349–54.
197. Ferrara JLM, Deeg HG. Graft-versus-host disease. N Engl J Med 1991;324:667–74.
198. Roberts JP, Aschner NJ, Lake A, et al. Graft-versus-host disease after liver transplantation in humans: a report of four cases. Hepatology 1991;14:272–81.
199. Parkman R, Mosier D, Umansky I, et al. Graft-versus-host disease after intrauterine and exchange transfusions for hemolytic disease of the newborn. N Engl J Medic 1974;290:359–63.
200. Sullivan KM. Acute and chronic graft-versus-host disease in man. Int J Cell Cloning 1986;4:42–93.
201. Von Liedner V, Higby DJ, Kim U. Graft-versus-host reaction following blood product transfusion. American J of Medicine 1982;72:951–61.
202. Perez-Simon J, Diez-Campelo M, Martino R, et al. Influence of the intensity of the conditioning regimen on the characteristics of acute and chronic graft-versus-host disease after allogeneic transplantation. Br J Haematol 2005;130:394–403.
203. Snover DC, Weisdorf SA, Ramsay NK, et al. Hepatic graft-versus-host disease: a study of the predictive value of liver biopsy in diagnosis. Hepatology 1984;4:123–30.
204. Shulman HM, Sharma P, Amos D, et al. A coded histologic study of hepatic graft versus host disease after human bone marrow transplantation. Hepatology 1988;8:463–70.
205. Ma S, Au W, Ng I, et al. Hepatitic graft-versus-host disease after hematopoietic stem cell transplantation: clinicopathologic features and prognostic implication. Transplantation 2004;77: 1252–9.
206. Bombi JA, Nadal A, Carreras E, et al. Assessment of histopathologic changes in the colonic biopsy in acute graft-versus-host disease. Am J Clin Pathol 1995;103:690–5.
207. Epstein RJ, McDonald GB, Sale GE, et al. The diagnostic accuracy of the rectal biopsy in acute graft-versus-host disease: a prospective study of thirteen patients. Gastroenterology 1980; 78:764–71.
208. Sviland I, Pearson ADJ, Green MA. Immunopathology of early graft-versus-host disease: a prospective study of skin, rectum and peripheral blood in allogeneic and autologous bone marrow transplant recipients. Transplantation 1991;52:1029–36.
209. Ponec RJ, Hackman RC, McDonald GB. Endoscopic and histologic diagnosis of intestinal graft-versus-host disease after marrow transplantation. Gastrointest Endosc 1999;49:612–21.

210. Carreras E, Granena A, Navasa M, et al. Transjugular liver biopsy in BMT. Bone Marrow Transplant 1993;11:21–6.
211. Cohen MB, A-Kader HH, Lambers D, Heubi JE. Complications of percutaneous liver biopsy in children. Gastroenterology 1992;102:629–32.
212. Dickinson A, Middleton P, Gluckman E, et al. Genetic polymorphisms predicting the outcome of bone marrow transplants. Br J Haematol 2004;127:479–90.
213. Wagner J, Thompson J, Carter S, Kernan N. Effect of graft-versus-host disease prophylaxis on 3-year disease-free survival in recipients of unrelated donor bone marrow (T-cell Depletion Trial): a multi-centre, randomised phase II–III trial. Lancet 2005;266:743–41.
214. McDonald GD. Graft versus host disease of the intestine and liver. Immunol Allergy Clin North Am 1988;8:543–57.
215. Sullivan KM, Shulman HM, Storb R, et al. Chronic graft-versus-host disease in 52 patients: adverse natural course and successful treatment with combination immunosuppression. Blood 1981; 57:267–76.
216. Horwitz M, Sullivan K. Chronic graft-versus-host disease. Blood Rev 2006;20:15–27.
217. Bhushan V, Collins RH Jr. Chronic graft-vs-host disease. JAMA 2003;290:2599–603.
218. Shulman H, Sullivan KM, Weiden PL, et al. Chronic graft versus host syndrome in man: a long term clinicopathologic study of 20 Seattle patients. Am J Med 1980;69:204–17.
219. Couriel D, Saliba R, Escalon M, et al. Sirolimus in combination with tacrolimus and corticosteroids for the treatment of resistant chronic graft-versus-host disease. Br J Haematol 2005; 130:409–17.
220. Barshes NR, Myers GD, Lee D, et al. Liver transplantation for severe hepatic graft-versus-host disease. An analysis of aggregate survival data. Liver Transplant 2005;11:525–31.
221. Rachelefsky GS, Kar NC, Coulson A, et al. Serum enzyme abnormalities in juvenile rheumatoid arthritis. Pediatrics 1976;58: 730–6.
222. Schaller J, Beckwith B, Wedgwood RJ. Hepatic involvement in juvenile rheumatoid arthritis. J Pediatr 1970;77:203–10.
223. Korneich H, Malouf NN, Hanson V. Acute hepatic dysfunction in juvenile rheumatoid arthritis. J Pediatr 1971;79:27–35.
224. David J, Vouyiouka O, Ansell BM, et al. Amyloidosis in juvenile rheumatoid arthritis: a morbidity and mortality study. Clin Exp Rheumatol 1993;11:85–94.
225. Bernstein B, Singsen BH, King KK, Hanson V. Aspirin induced hepatotoxicity and its effect on juvenile rheumatoid arthritis. Am J Dis Child 1977;131:659–63.
226. Rich RR, Johnson JS. Salicylate hepatotoxicity in patients with juvenile rheumatoid arthritis. Arthritis Rheumatism 1973;16:1–9.
227. Athreya BH, Moser G, Cecil HS, Myers AR. Aspirin induced hepatoxicity in juvenile rheumatoid arthritis. Arthritis Rheum 1975;18:347–52.
228. Young RSK, Torretti D, Williams RH, et al. Reye syndrome associated with long term aspirin therapy. JAMA 1984;251: 754–6.
229. Remington PL, Shabino CL, McGee H, et al. Reye syndrome and juvenile rheumatoid arthritis in Michigan. Am J Dis Child 1985;139:870–2.
230. Rennebohm RM, Heubi JE, Daugherty CC, Daniels SR. Reye syndrome in children receiving salicylate therapy for connective tissue disease. J Pediatr 1985;107:877–80.
231. Riley T, Smith J. Ibuprofen-induced hepatotoxicity in patients with chronic hepatitis C. Am J Gastroenterol 1998;93:1563–5.
232. Fry SW, Seeff LB. Hepatotoxicity of analgesics and anti-inflammatory agents. Gastroenterol Clin North Am 1995;24: 875–905.
233. Garcia Rodriguez LA, Williams R, Derby LE, et al. Acute liver injury associated with nonsteroidal anti-inflammatory drugs and the role of risk factors. Arch Int Med 1994;154:311–16.
234. Teoh N, Farrell G. Hepatotoxicity associated with non-steroidal anti-inflammatory drugs. Clin Liver Dis2003;7:401–13.
235. Mortensen ME, Rennebohm RM. Clinical pharmacology and use of nonsteroidal anti-inflammatory drugs. Pediatr Clin North Am 1989;36:1113–39.
236. Rostom A, Goldkind L, Laine L. Nonsteroidal anti-inflammatory drugs and hepatic toxicity: a systematic review of randomized controlled trials in arthritis patients. Clini Gastroenterol Hepatol 2005;3:489–98.
237. Hadchouel M, Prieur A, Griscelli C. Acute hemorrhagic, hepatic and neurologic manifestations in juvenile rheumatoid arthritis: possible relationship to drugs or infection. J Pediatr 1985; 106:561–6.
238. Jacobs JC, Gorin LJ, Hanissian AS, et al. Consumptive coagulopathy after gold therapy for JRA. J Pediatr 1984;105:674–80.
239. Silverman ED, Miller JJ, Bernstein B. Consumptive coagulopathy associated with systemic juvenile rheumatoid arthritis. J Pediatr 1983;103:872–8.
240. Watkins PB, Schade R, Mills AS, Carithers RL, Van Thiel DH. Fatal hepatic necrosis associated with parenteral gold therapy. Dig Dis Sci 1988;33:1025–9.
241. Barash J, Cooper M, Tauber A. Hepatic, cutaneous, and hematologic manifestations in juvenile chronic arthritis. Clin Exp Rheumatol 1991;9:541–50.
242. Weinblatt ME, Weissman BN, Holdsworth DE, et al. Long term prospective studies of methotrexate in the treatment of rheumatoid arthritis. Arthritis Rheum 1992;35:129–37.
243. Wilkens RF, Leonard PA, Clegg DO, et al. Liver histology in patients receiving low dose pulse methotrexate for treatment of rheumatoid arthritis. Ann Rheum Dis 1990;49:591–3.
244. Kremer JM, Alarcon GS, Lightfoot RW, et al. Methotrexate for rheumatoid arthritis: suggested guidelines for monitoring liver toxicity. Arthritis Rheum 1994;37:316–28.
245. Lewis JH, Schiff E. Methotrexate-induced chronic liver injury: guidelines for detection and prevention. Am J Gastroenterol 1988;88:1337–45.
246. Kremer JM, Kaye GI, Kaye NW, et al. Light and electron microscopic analysis of sequential liver biopsy samples from rheumatoid arthritis patients receiving long-term methotrexate therapy. Arthritis Rheum 1995;38:1194–203.
247. Brick JE, Moreland LW, Al-Kawas F, et al. Prospective analysis of liver biopsies before and after methotrexate therapy in rheumatoid arthritis. Sem Arthritis Rheumatol 1989;19:31–44.
248. Giannini EH, Brewer EJ, Kuzima N, et al. Methotrexate in resistant juvenile rheumatoid arthritis: results of the U.S.A.–U.S.S.R. double-blind, placebo-controlled trial. N Engl J Med 1992;326:1043–9.
249. Wallace CA. The use of methotrexate in childhood rheumatic diseases. Arthritis Rheum 1998;41:381–91.
250. Hashkes PJ, Balistreri WF, Bove KE, et al. The relationship of hepatotoxic risk factors and liver histology in methotrexate therapy for juvenile rheumatoid arthritis. J Pediatr 1999;134:47–52.

251. Hashkes PJ, Balistreri WF, Bove KE, et al. The long-term effects of methotrexate therapy on the liver in patients with juvenile rheumatoid arthritis. Arthritis Rheum 1997;40:2226–34.
252. Smith ME, Ansell BM, Bywaters EGL. Mortality and prognosis related to the amyloidosis of Still's disease. Ann Rheum Dis 1968; 27:137–45.
253. Strauss RG, Schubert WK, McAdams AJ. Amyloidosis in childhood. J Pediatr 1969;74:272–82.
254. Thorne C, Urowitz MD, Wanless I, et al. Liver disease in Felty's syndrome. Am J Med 1982;73:35–40.
255. Cassidy JT, Petty RE. Textbook of pediatric rheumatology. Philadelphia: W.B. Saunders; 2001.
256. Whaley K, Williamson J, Dick WC, et al. Liver disease in Sjorgen's syndrome and rheumatoid arthritis. Lancet 1970;1:861–2.
257. Poirier T, Rankin G. Gastrointestinal manifestations of progressive systemic scleroderma based on a review of 364 cases. Am J Gastroenter 1972;58:30–44.
258. Powell F, Schroeter A, Dickinson E. Primary biliary cirrhosis and the CREST syndrome: a report of 22 cases. Q J Med 1987;62: 75–82.
259. D'Angelo W, Fries J, Masi A, Shulman LE. Pathologic observations in systemic sclerosis (scleroderma): a study of fifty-eight autopsy cases and fifty-eight matched controls. Am J Med 1969;46:428–40.
260. Bartholomew L, Cain J, Winkelmann R. Chronic disease of the liver with systemic scleroderma. Am J Dig Dis 1964;9:43–55.
261. Leggett BA. The liver in systemic lupus erythematosus. J Pediatr Gastroenterol Nutr 1993;8:84–8.
262. Runyon BA, LaBrecque D, Anuras S. The spectrum of liver disease in systemic lupus erythematosus: report of 33 histologically proven cases and review of the literature. Am J Med 1980;69:187–94.
263. Miller MH, Urowitz MB, Gladman DD, Blendis LM. The liver in systemic lupus erythematosus. Q J Med 1984;211:401–9.
264. Searnan WE, Ishak KG, Plotz PH. Aspirin induced hepatotoxicity in patients with systemic lupus erythematosus. Ann Int Med 1974;80:1–8.
265. Matsumoto T, Yoshimine T, Shimouchi K, et al. The liver in systemic lupus erythematosus: pathologic analysis of 52 cases and review of Japanese autopsy registry. Hum Pathol 1992;23: 1151–8.
266. Averbuch M, Levo Y. Budd–Chiari syndrome as the major thrombotic complication of systemic lupus erythematosus with the lupus anticoagulant. Ann Rheum Dis 1986;45:435–7.
267. Pappas SC, Malone DG, Rabin L, et al. Hepatic veno-occlusive disease in a patient with systemic lupus erythematosus. Arthritis Rheum 1984;27:104–8.
268. Yun YY, Yoh KA, Yang HI, et al. A case of Budd–Chiari syndrome with high antiphospholipid antibody in a patient with systemic lupus erythematosus. Korean J Int Med 1996;11:82–6.
269. Perez-Ruiz FR, Orte-Martinez FJ, Zea Mendoza AC, et al. Nodular regenerative hyperplasia of the liver in rheumatic diseases: report of seven cases and review of the literature. Sem Arthritis Rheumatol 1991;21:47–54.
270. Khoury G, Tobi M, Oren M, Traub YM. Massive hepatic infarction in systemic lupus erythematosus. Dig Dis Sci 1990;35:1557–660.
271. Colina F, Albert N, Solis JA, Martinez-Tello FJ. Diffuse nodular regenerative hyperplasia of the liver: a clinicopathologic study of 24 cases. Liver 1989;9:253–65.
272. Laxer RM, Roberts EA, Gross KR, et al. Liver disease in neonatal lupus erythematosus. J Pediatr 1984;116:238–42.
273. Watson RM, Lane AT, Barnett NK, et al. Neonatal lupus erythematosus: a clinical, serologic and immunogenetic study with review of the literature. Medicine 1984;63:362–78.
274. Rosh JR, Silverman ED, Groisman G. Intrahepatic cholestasis in neonatal lupus erythematosus. J Pediatr Gastroenterol Nutr 1993;17:310–12.
275. Lee LA, Sokol RJ, Buyon JP. Hepatobiliary disease in neonatal lupus: prevalence and clinical characteristics in cases enrolled in a national registry. Pediatrics 2002;109:e11.
276. Crowe WE, Bove KE, Levinson JE, Hilton PK. Clinical and pathogenetic implications of histopathology in childhood dermatomyositis. Arthritis Rheum 1982;25:126–32.
277. Iorio R, Sepe A, Giannattasio A, et al. Hypertransaminasemia in childhood as a marker of genetic liver disorders. J Gastroenterol 2005;40:820–6.
278. Russo R, Katsicas M, Davila M, et al. Cholestasis in juvenile dermatomyositis: report of three cases. Arthritis Rheum 2001; 44:1139–42.
279. Rowley AH, Shulman ST. Kawasaki syndrome. Pediatr Clin North Am 1999;46:313–29.
280. Burns JC, Mason WH, Glode MP, et al. Clinical and epidemiologic characteristics of patients referred for evaluation of possible Kawasaki disease. J Pediatr 1991;118:680–6.
281. Ohshio G, Furukawa F, Fujiwara H, Hamashima Y. Hepatomegaly and splenomegaly in Kawasaki disease. Pediatr Pathol 1985;4:257–64.
282. Newberger J, Takahashi M, Gerber M, et al. Diagnosis, treatment and long-term management of Kawasaki disease: a statement for health professionals from the Committee on Rheumatic Fever, Endocarditis, and Kawasaki Disease, Council on Cardiovascular Disease in the Young, American Heart Association. Pediatrics 2004;114:1708–33.
283. Ting E, Capparelli E, Billman G, et al. Elevated gamma-glutamyltransferase concentrations in patients with acute Kawasaki disease. Pediatr Infect Dis J 1998;17:431–2.
284. Uehara R, Yashiro M, Hayasaka S, et al. Serum Alanine Aminotransferase Concentrations in Patients with Kawasaki Disease. Pediatr Infect Dis J 2003;22:839–42.
285. Kimura A, Inoue O, Kato H. Serum concentrations of total bile acids in patients with acute Kawasaki syndrome. Arch Pediatr Adolesc Med 1996;150:289–92.
286. Edwards KM, Glick AD, Greene HL. Intrahepatic cholestasis associated with mucocutaneous lymph node syndrome. J Pediatr Gastroenterol Nutr 1985;4:140–2.
287. Bader-Meunier B, Hadchouel M, Fabre M, et al. Intrahepatic bile duct abnormalities in children with Kawasaki disease. J Pediatr 1992;120:750–2.
288. Landing BH, Larson EJ. Are infantile periarteritis nodosa with coronary artery involvement and fatal mucocutaneous lymph node syndrome the same: comparison of 20 patients from North America with patients from Hawaii and Japan. Pediatrics 1977;59:651–62.
289. Naoe S, Shibuya K, Takahashi K. Pathologic observations concerning the cardiovascular lesions in Kawasaki disease. Cardiol Young 1991;1:212–20.
290. Bertino JS, Willis ED, Reed MD, Speck WT. Salicylate hepatitis: a complication of the treatment of Kawasaki disease. Am J Hosp Pharm 1981;38:1171–2.

291. Lee JH, Hung HY, Huang FY. Kawasaki disease with Reye syndrome: report of one case. Zhonghua Min Xiao Er Ke Yi Xue Hui Za Zh 1992;33:67–71.
292. Hassink SG, Goldsmith DP. Neonatal onset multi-system inflammatory disease. Arthritis Rheum 1983;26:668–73.
293. Yarom A, Rennenbohm RM, Levinson JE. Infantile multisystem inflammatory disease: a specific syndrome? J Pediatr 1985; 106:390–6.
294. Feldmann J, Prieur A, Quartier P, et al. Chronic infantile neurological cutaneous and articular syndrome is caused by mutations in CIAS1, a gene highly expressed in polymorphonuclear cells and chondrocytes. Am J Hum Genet 2002;71:198–203.
295. Kilcline C, Shinkai K, Bree A, et al. Neonatal-onset multisystem inflammatory disorder: the emerging role of pyrin genes in autoinflammatory diseases. Arch Dermatol 2005;141:248–53.
296. Layden TJ, Boyer JL. Effect of thyroid hormone on bile salt independent bile flow and Na-K ATPase activity in liver plasma membrane enriched in bile canaliculi. J Clin Invest 1976;57: 1009–15.
297. Ellaway C, Silinik M, Cowell C, et al. Cholestatic jaundice and congenital hypopituitarism. J Paediatr Child Health 1995; 31:51–3.
298. Craft WH, Underwood LE, Van Wyk JJ. High incidence of perinatal insult in children with idiopathic hypopituitarism. J Pediatr 1980;96:397–402.
299. Sheehan AG, Martin SR, Stephure D, Scott RB. Neonatal cholestasis, hypoglycemia and congenital hypopituitarism. J Pediatr Gastroenterol Nutr 1992;426–30.
300. Yagi H, Nagashima K, Miyake H, et al. Familial congenital hypopituitarism with central diabetes insipidus. J Clin Endocrinol Metab 1994;78:884–9.
301. Adams L, Feldstein A, KD L, Angulo P. Nonalcoholic fatty liver disease among patients with hypothalamic and pituitary dysfunction. Hepatology 2004;39:909–14.
302. Nakajima K, Hashimoto E, Kaneda H, et al. Pediatric nonalcoholic steatohepatitis associated with hypopituitrarism. J Gastroenterol 2005;40:3312–15.
303. Willnow S, Kiess W, Butenandt O, et al. Endocrine disorders in septo-optic dysplasia (De Morsier syndrome): evaluation and follow up of 18 patients. Eur J Pediatr 1996;155:179–84.
304. Minami K, Izumi G, Yanagawa T, et al. Septo-opticdysplasia with congenital hepatic fibrosis. Paediatr Neurol 2003;29:157–9.
305. Leblanc A, Odievre M, Hadchouel M, et al. Neonatal cholestasis and hypoglycemia: possible role of cortisol deficiency. J Pediatr 1981;99:577–80.
306. Soffer LJ, Iannaccone A, Gabrilove JL. Cushing's syndrome: a study of 50 patients. Am J Med 1961;30:129–46.
307. Lacy DE, Nathavitharana KA, Tarlow MJ. Neonatal hepatitis and congenital insensitivity to adrenocorticotropin (ACTH). J Pediatr Gastroenterol Nutr 1993;17:438–40.
308. Kirkman S, Nelson D. Alcohol induced pseudo-Cushing's disease: a study of prevalence with review of the literature. Metabolism 1988;37:390–4.
309. Binkiewicz A, Robinson M, Senior B. Pseudo-Cushing syndrome caused by alcohol in breast milk. J Pediatr 1978;93: 965–7.
310. Balasubramaniam S, Mitropoulous KA, Myant NB. Hormonal control of the activities of cholesterol-7-alpha-hydroxylase and hydroxy methylglutaryl-CoA reductase in rates. In: Matern SHJ, Back P, Gerok W, eds. Advances in bile acid research. Stuttgart: Schattauer Verlag; 1975.
311. Ashkar FS, Miller R, Smoak WM, Glison AJ. Liver disease in hyperthyroidism. South Med J 1971;64:462–5.
312. Beckett GJ, Kellett HA, Gow SM. Subclinical liver damage in hyperthyroidism and in thyroxine replacement therapy. Br Med J 1985;291:427–30.
313. Yao JC, Gross JB, Ludwig J, Prunell DC. Cholestatic jaundice in hyperthyroidism. Am J Medicine 1989;86:619–20.
314. Christensen JF. Prolonged icterus neonatorum and congenital myxedema. Acta Paediatr Scand 1956;45:411–20.
315. MacGillivray MH, Crawford JD, Robey JS. Congenital hypothyroidism and prolonged neonatal hyperbilirubinemia. Pediatrics 1967;40:283–6.
316. Pearson C. Serum enzymes in muscular dystrophy and certain other muscular and neuromuscular diseases. I. Serum glutamic oxalacetic transaminase. N Engl J Med 1957;256:1069–75.
317. Zamora S, Adams C, Butzner J, et al. Elevated aminotransferase activity as an indication of muscular dystrophy: case reports and review of the literature. Can J Gastroenterol 1996;10:389–93.
318. Tay S, Ong H, Low P. Transaminitis in Duchenne's muscular dystrophy. Ann Acad Med Singapore 2000;29:719–22.
319. Nathwani R, Pais S, Reynolds T, Kaplowitz N. Serum alanine aminotransferase in skeletal muscle disease. Hepatology 2005;41:380–2.
320. Schiano T. Hepatotoxicity and complementary and alternative medicines. Clin Liver Dis 2003;7:453–73.
321. Saper R, Kales S, Paquin J, Burns M, et al. Heavy metal content of Ayurvedic herbal medicine products. JAMA 2004;292:2868–73.
322. Rasenack R, Muller C, Kleinschmidt M, et al. Veno-occlusive disease in a fetus caused by pyrrolizidine alkaloids of food origin. Fetal Diagn Ther 2003;18:223–5.
323. Lanski S, Greenwald M, Perkins A, Simon H. Herbal therapy use in a pediatric emergency department population: expect the unexpected. Pediatrics 2003;111:981–5.
324. Davis M, Darden P. Use of complementary and alternative medicine by children in the United States. Arch Pediatr Adolesc Med 2003;157:393–6.
325. Ojetti V, Fini L, Zileri Dal Verme L, et al. Acute cryptogenic liver failure in an untreated coeliac patient: a case report. Eur J Gastroenterol Hepatol 2005;17:1119–21.
326. Stevens F, McLoughlin R. Is coeliac disease a potentially treatable cause of liver failure? Eur J Gastroenterol Hepatol 2005;17: 1015–17.
327. Hay JE, Wiesner RH, Shorter RG, et al. Primary sclerosing cholangitis and coeliac disease: a novel association. Ann Int Med 1988;109:713–17.
328. Jacobsen MB, Fausa O, Elgjo K, Schrumf E. Hepatic lesions in adult coeliac disease. Scand J Gastroenterol 1990;25:656–62.
329. Logan RFA, Ferguson A, Finlayson NDC. Primary biliary cirrhosis and coeliac disease: an association? Lancet 1978;1:230–3.
330. Niveloni S, Dezi R, Pedreira S, et al. Gluten sensitivity in patients with primary biliary cirrhosis. Am J Gastroenterol 1998;93: 404–8.
331. Naschitz JE, Yeshurun D, Zuckerman E, et al. Massive hepatic steatosis complicating adult celiac disease. Am J Gastroenterol 1987;82:1186–9.
332. Cassagnou M, Boruchowicz A, Guillemore F, et al. Hepatic steatosis revealing celiac disease: a case complicated by transitory liver failure. Am J Gastroenterol 1996;91:1291–2.
333. Shamir R, Koren I, Rosenbach Y, et al. Celiac, fatty liver and pancreatic insufficiency. J Pediatr Gastroenterol Nutr 2001;32:490–2.

334. Waterlow JC. Amount and rate of disappearance of liver fat in malnourished children in Jamaica. Am J Clin Nutr 1975;28:1330–6.
335. Tenore A, Berman WF, Parks JS, Bongiovanni AM. Basal and stimulated growth hormone concentrations in inflammatory bowel disease. J Clin Endocrinol Metab 1977;44:622–8.
336. Abraira C, Virupannavar C, Nemchausky B. Protective effects of small amount of glucose on abnormal liver function tests during starvation. Metabolism 1980;29:943–8.
337. Bessey PQ, Watters JM, Aoki TT, Wilmore DW. Combined hormonal infusions simulates the metabolic response to injury. Ann Surg 1984;200:262–80.
338. Doherty JF, Golden MHN, Brooks SEH. Peroxisomes and the fatty liver of malnutrition: a hypothesis. Am J Clin Nutr 1991;54:674–7.
339. Simon DG, Krause R, Galambos JT. Peliosis hepatis in a patient with marasmus. Gastroenterology 1988;95:805–9.
340. Williams CD. Kwashiorkor: a nutritional disease associated with a maize diet. Lancet 1935;2:1151–2.
341. Eastlack JP, Grande KK, Levy ML, Nigro JF. Dermatosis in a child with kwashiorkor secondary to food aversion. Pediatr Dermatol 1999;16:95–102.
342. Sinatra FR, Merritt RJ. Iatrogenic kwashiorkor in infants. Am J Dis Child 1981;135:76–8.
343. Taitz LS, Finberg L. Kwashiorkor in the Bronx. Am J Dis Child 1966;22:76–8.
344. Liu T, Howard R, Mancini A, et al. Kwashiorkor in the United States. Fad diets, perceived and true milk allergy, and nutritional ignorance. Arch Dermatol 2006;137:630–6.
345. Katz K, Mahlberg M, Honig P, Yan A. Rice nightmare: kwashiorkor in 2 Philadelphia infants fed Rice Dream beverage. J Am Acad Dermatol 2005;52 Suppl 1:S69–72.
346. Gelfand M. Kwashiorkor in a breast-fed infant. Trans Royal Soc Trop Med 1951;45:393–6.
347. Jelliff DB, Jelliff EF. Causation of kwashiorkor: toward a multifactorial consensus. Pediatrics 1992;90:110–13.
348. Golden MH. Oedematous malnutrition. Br Med J 1998;54:433–44.
349. Golden MHN, Ramdath DD. Free radicals in the pathogenesis of kwashiorkor. Proc Nutr Soc 1987;46:53–68.
350. Prasad AS. Zinc and immunity. Mole Cell Biochem 1998;188:63–9.
351. Manar M, MacPherson G, Mcardle F, et al. Selenium status, kwashiorkor and congestive heart failure. Acta Paeditr Scand 2001;90:950–2.
352. Iputo J, Sammon A, Tindimwebwa G. Prostaglandin E2 is raised in kwashiorkor. South African Medical J 2002;92:310–12.
353. Mayatepek E, Becker K, Gana L, Hoffman G, Leichsenring M. Leukotrienes in the pathophysiology of kwashiorkor. Lancet 1993;342:958–60.
354. Dugler H, Arik M, Sekeroglu M, et al. Pro-inflammatory cytokines in Turkish children with protein-energy malnutrition. Mediators Inflamm 2002;11:363–5.
355. Wu G, Fang Y, Yang S, et al. Glutathione metabolsim and its implications for health. J Nutr 2004;134:489–92.
356. Hendrickse RG. Kwashiorkor: the hypothesis that incriminates aflatoxin. Pediatrics 1991;88:376–9.
357. Hatem N, Hassab H, Abd Al-Rahman E, et al. Prevalence of aflatoxins in blood and urine of Egyptian infants with protein-energy malnutrition. Food Nutr Bull 2005;26:49–56.
358. World Helath Organization. Management of severe malnutrition: a manual for physicians and other senior health care workers. Genva: Author, 1999.
359. Becker K, Pons-Kuhnemann J, Fechner A, et al. Effects of antioxidants on glutathione levels and clinical recovery from the malnutrition syndrome kwashiorkor – a pilot study. Redox Rep 2005;10:215–26.
360. Cilberto H, Cilberto M, Briend A, et al. Antioxidant supplementation for the prevention of kwashiorkor in Malawian children: randomised, placebo controlled trial. BMJ 2005;330:1109–13.
361. Miller KK, Grinspoon SK, Ciampa J, et al. Medical findings in outpatients with anorexia nervosa. Arch Int Med 2005;165:561–6.
362. Milner MR, McAnarney ER, Klish WJ. Metabolic abnormalities in adolescent patients with anorexia nervosa. J Adolesc Health Care 1985;6:191–5.
363. Nordgren L, von Scheele C. Hepatic and pancreatic dysfunction in anorexia nervosa. Biol Psychiatry 1977;12:681–6.
364. Barrett PVD. Hyperbilirubinemia of fasting. JAMA 1971;217:1349–53.
365. Niiya K, Kitagawa T, Fujishita M, et al. Bulimia nervosa complicated by deficiency of vitamin K-dependent coagulation factors. JAMA 1983;250:792–3.
366. Felsher BF, Rickard D, Redeker AG. The reciprocal relation between caloric intake and the degree of hyperbilirubinemia in Gilbert's syndrome. N Engl J Med 1970;283:170–4.
367. Gartner U, Goeser T, Wolkoff AW. Effect of fasting on the uptake of bilirubin and sulfobromophthalein by the isolated perfused rat liver. Gastroenterology 1997;113:1701–13.
368. Geubel AP, DeGalocsy C, Alves N, et al. Liver damage caused by therapeutic vitamin A administration: estimate of dose-related toxicity in 41 cases. Gastroenterology 1991;100:1701–09.
369. Etachason JA, Miller TD, Squires RW. Niacin-induced hepatitis: a potential side effect with low-dose-time-release niacin. Mayo Clinic Proc 1991;66:23–8.
370. Carvalho N, Kenney R, Carrington P, Dall D. Severe nutritional deficiencies in toddlers resulting from health food milk alternatives. Pediatrics 2001;107:e46–53.
371. Larrey D, Pageaux GP. Hepatotoxicity of herbal remedies and mushrooms. Sem Liver Dis 1995;15:183–7.
372. Huxtable RJ. The myth of beneficent nature: the risks of herbal preparations. Ann Int Med 1992;117:165–6.
373. Woolfe GM, Petrovic LM, Rojter SE. Acute hepatitis associated with the Chinese herbal product Jin-bu-huan. Ann Int Med 1994;121:729–35.
374. Quigley EMM, Marsh MN, Shaffer JL, Markin SS. Hepatobiliary complications of total parenteral nutrition. Gastroenterology 1993;104:286–301.
375. Bowyer BA, Fleming CR, Ludwig J, et al. Does long-term home parenteral nutrition in adult patients cause chronic liver disease? J Parenteral Enteral Nutr 1985;9:11–17.
376. Stanko RT, Nathan G, Mendelow H, Adibi SA. Development of hepatic cholestasis and fibrosis in patients with massive loss of intestine supported by prolonged parenteral nutrition. Gastroenterology 1987;92:197–202.
377. Bueno J, Ohwada S, Kocoshis S. Factors impacting the survival of children with intestinal failure referred for intestinal transplantation. J Pediatr Surg 1999;34:27–33.
378. Fryer J, Pellar S, Ormond D, et al. Mortality in candidates waiting for combined liver-intestine transplants exceeds that for

other candidates waitng for liver transplants. Liver Transplant 2003;9:748–53.
379. Benjamin SR. Hepatobiliary dysfunction in infants and children associated with long term total parenteral nutrition: a clinicopathologic study. Am J Clin Pathol 1981;76:276–83.
380. Beale EF, Nelson RM, Bucciarelli RL, et al. Intrahepatic cholestasis associated with parenteral nutrition in premature infants. Pediatrics 1979;64:342–7.
381. Peden VH, Witzleben CL, Skelton MA. Total parenteral nutrition. J Pediatr 1971;78:180–1.
382. Rager R, Finegold MJ. Cholestasis in immature newborn infants: is parenteral alimentation responsible? J Pediatr 1975;86:264–9.
383. Allardyce DB. Cholestasis caused by lipid emulsions. Surg Gynecol Obstetr 1982;154:641–7.
384. Kubota A, Yonekura T, Hoki M, et al. Total parenteral nutrition – associated intrahepatic cholestasis in infants: 25 years' experience. J Pediatr Surg 2000;35:1049–51.
385. Andorsky D, Lund D, Lillehei C, et al. Nutritional and other postoperative management of neonates with short bowel syndrome correlates with clinical outcomes. J Pediatr 2001;139:27–33.
386. Balistreri WF, Bove KE. Hepatobiliary consequences of parenteral nutrition. Prog Liver Dis 1989;9:567–600.
387. Tulikoura I, Huikun K. Morphological fatty changes and function of the liver, serum free fatty acids and triglycerides during parenteral nutrition. Scand J Gastroenterol 1982;19:177–85.
388. Wolfe BM, Walker BK, Shaul DB, et al. Effect of total parenteral nutrition on hepatic histology. Arch Surg 1988;123:1084–90.
389. Dahlstrom KA, Strandvik B, Kopple J, Ament ME. Nutritional status in patients receiving home parenteral nutrition. J Pediatr 1985;107:219–24.
390. Tu W, Kitade H, Kaibori M, Nakagawa M, et al. An enhancement of nitric oxide production regulates energy metabolism in rat hepatocytes after a partial hepatectomy. J Hepatol 1999;30:944–50.
391. Farrell MK, Balistreri WF. Parenteral nutrition and hepatobiliary dysfunction. Clin Perinatol 1986;13:197–212.
392. Demircan M, Ergun O, Avanoglu S, et al. Determination of serum bile acids routinely may prevent delay in diagnosis of parenteral nutrition-induced cholestasis. J Pediatr Surg 1999; 34:565–7.
393. Toomey F, Hoag R, Batton D, Vain N. Rickets associated with cholestasis and parenteral nutrition in premature infants. Radiology 1982;142:85–8.
394. Cohen C, Olsen MM. Pediatric total parenteral nutrition: liver histopathology. Arch Pathol Lab Med 1981;105:85–8.
395. Vileisis RA, Sorensen K, Gonzalez-Crussi F, Hunt CE. Liver malignancy after total parenteral nutrition. J Pediatr 1982;100: 88–90.
396. Kaufman SS. Prevention of parenteral nutrition-associated liver disease in children. Pediatr Transplant 2002;6:37–42.
397. Cavicchi M, Beau P, Crenn P, et al. Prevalence of liver disease and contributing factors in patients receiving home parenteral nutrition for permanent intestinal failure. Ann Int Med 2000;132:525–32.
398. Dahms BB, Halpin TC. Serial liver biopsies in parenteral nutrition associated cholestasis of early infancy. Gastroenterology 1981;81:136–44.
399. Balistreri WF. Fetal bile acid synthesis and metabolism: clinical implications. J Inherited Metab Dis 1991;14:459–77.
400. Bernstein J, Chang CH, Brough JA. Conjugated hyperbilirubinemia in infancy associated with parenteral nutrition. J Pediatr 1977;90:361–7.
401. Zambrano E, El-Hennawy M, Ehrenkranz R, et al. Total parenteral nutrition induced liver patholgy: an autopsy series of 24 newborn cases. Pediatr Dev Pathol 2004;7:425–32.
402. Steinwender G, Schimp G, Sixl B, et al. Effect of early nutritional deprivation and diet on translocation of bacteria from the gastrointestinal tract in the newborn rat. Pediatr Res 1996;39:415–20.
403. O'Brien D, Nelson L, Kemp C, et al. Intestinal permeability and bacterial translocation are uncoupled after small bowel resection. J Pediatr Surg 2002;37:390–4.
404. Dosi PC, Raut AJ, Chelliah BP, et al. Perinatal factors underlying neonatal cholestasis. J Pediatr 1985;106:471–4.
405. Sondheimer J, Asturias E, Cadnapaphornchai M. Infection and cholestasis in neonates with intestinal resection and long-term total parenteral nutrition. J Pediatr Gastroenterol Nutr 1998; 27:131–7.
406. Balasubramaniyan N, Shahid D, Suchy F, Ananthanarayanan M. Multiple mechanisms of ontogenic regulation of nuclear receptors during rat liver development. Am J Physiol Gastrointest Liver Physiol 2004 [online, DB9].
407. Hardikar W, Ananthanarayanan M, Suchy F. Differential ontogenic regulation of basolateral and canalicular bile acid transport proteins in rat liver. J Biolol Chem 1995;270:20841–6.
408. Shneider B, Dawson P, Christie D. Cloning and molecular characterization of the ontogeny of a rat ileal sodium-dependent bile acid transporter. J Clin Invest 1995;95:745–54.
409. Tomer G, Ananthanarayanan M, Weymann A, et al. Differential developmental regulation of rat liver canalicular membrane transporters Bsep and Mrp2. Pediatr Res 2003;53:288–94.
410. Back P, Walter K. Developmental pattern of bile acid metabolism as revealed by bile acid analysis of meconium. Gastroenterology 1980;78:671–6.
411. Balistreri WF, Heubi JE, Suchy FJ. Immaturity of the enterohepatic circulation in early life: factors predisposing to "physiologic" maldigestion and cholestasis. J Pediatr Gastroenterol Nutr 1983;2:346–54.
412. Bucuvalas JC, Goodrich AL, Blitzer BL, Suchy FJ. Amino acids are potent inhibitors of bile acid uptake by liver plasma membrane vesicles isolated from suckling rats. Pediatr Res 1985;19: 1298–365.
413. Senger H, Boehm G, Beyreiss A, Braun W. Evidence for amino acid induced cholestasis in very-low-birth weight infants with increasing enteral protein intake. Acta Paediatr Scand 1986; 75:724–8.
414. Suchy FJ, Courchene SM, Blitzer BL. Taurocholate transport by basolateral plasma membrane vesicles isolated from developing rat livers. Am J Physiol 1985;248:G648–54.
415. Suchy FJ, Bucuvalas JC, Novak D. Determinants of bile formation during development: ontogeny of hepatic bile acid metabolism and transport. Sem Liver Dis 1987;7:77–84.
416. Suchy FJ, Balistreri WF, Breslin JS, et al. Absence of an acinar gradient for bile acid uptake in developing rat liver. Pediatr Res 1987;21:414–21.
417. Suchy FJ, Sippel CJ, Ananthanarayanan M. Bile acid transport across the hepatocyte canalicular membrane. FASEB J 1997; 11:195–205.

418. Staudinger J, Goodwin B, Jones S, et al. The nuclear receptor PXR is a lithocholate sensor that protects against liver toxicity. Proc Nat Acad Sci U S A 2001;98:3369–74.
419. Xie W, Radominska-Pandya A, Shi Y, et al. An essential role for nuclear receptors SXR/PXR in detoxification of cholestatic bile acids. Proc Nat Acad Sci U S A 2001;98:3375–80.
420. Duerksen DR, vanAerde JE, Chan G, et al. Total parenteral nutrition impairs bile flow and alters bile composition in newborn piglets. Dig Dis Sci 1996;41:1864–70.
421. Alverdy J, Aoys E, Moss G. Total parenteral nutrition promotes bacterial translocation from the gut. Surgery 1988;104:185–90.
422. Vileisis RA, Inwood RJ, Hunt CE. Prospective controlled study of parenteral nutrition-associated cholestatic jaundice: effect of protein intake. J Pediatr 1980;96:893–7.
423. Black DD, Suttle EA, Whitington PF, et al. The effect of short term parenteral nutrition on hepatic function in the human neonate: a prospective randomized study demonstrating alteration of hepatic canalicular function. J Pediatr 1981;99:904–7.
424. Aynsley-Green A. Plasma hormone concentrations during enteral and parenteral nutrition in the human newborn. J Pediatr Gastroenterol Nutr 1983;2:S108–12.
425. Lucas A, Bloom SR, Aynsley-Green A. Gut hormones and minimal enteral feeding. Acta Paediatr Scand 1986;75:719–23.
426. Jones RS, Grossman MI. The choleretic effects of glucagon and secretin in the dog. Gastroenterology 1971;60:64–8
427. Sharman-Koendjbiharie M, Piena-Spoel M, Hopman J, et al. Gastrointestinal hormone secretion after surgery in neonates with congenital intestinal anomalies during starvation and introduction of enteral nutrition. J Pediatr Surg 2003;38:1602–6.
428. Lucas A, Bloom SR, Aynsley-Green A. Metabolic and endocrine consequences of depriving pre-term infants of enteral nutrition. Acta Paediatr Scand 1983;72:245–9.
429. Roelofsen H, Shoemaker B, Bakker C, et al. Impaired hepatocanalicular organic anion transport in endotoxemic rats. Am J Physiol 1995;269:G427–31.
430. Lichtman SN, Sartor RB, Keku J, Schwab JJ. Hepatic inflammation in rats with experimental small bowel overgrowth. Gastroenterology 1990;98:414–24.
431. Lichtman SN, Keku J, Clark RL, et al. Biliary tract disease in rats with experimental bacterial overgrowth. Hepatology 1990;13:766–72.
432. Lichtman SN, Sartor RB. Hepatobiliary injury associated with experimental small-bowel bacterial overgrowth in rats. Immunol Res 1991;10:528–31.
433. Lichtman SN, Keku J, Schwab JH, Sartor RB. Evidence for pepitoglycan absorption in rats with experimental small bowel bacterial overgrowth. Infect Immun 1991;55:555–62.
434. Lichtman SN, Keku J, Schwab JH, Sartor RB. Hepatic injury associated with small bowel bacterial overgrowth in rats is prevented by metronidazole and tetracycline. Gastroenterology 1991;100:513–19.
435. Lichtman SN, Okoruwa EE, Keku J, et al. Degradation of endogenous bacterial cell wall polymers by the muralytic enzyme mutanolysin prevents hepatobiliary injury in genetically susceptible rats with experimental intestinal bacterial overgrowth. J Clin Invest 1992;90:1313–22.
436. Kabuta A, Okada A, Imura Kea. The effect of metronidazole on TPN-associated liver dysfunction in neonates. J Pediatr Surg 1990;25:618–21.
437. Matsui J, Cameron RG, Kurian GC, Jeejeebhoy KN. Nutritional, hepatic, and metabolic effects of cachectin/tumor necrosis factor in rats receiving total parenteral nutrition. Gastroenterology 1993;104:235–43.
438. Capron JP, Ginestron JL, Herve MA, Braillon A. Metronidazole in the prevention of serum liver enzyme abnormalities during total parenteral nutrition. Lancet 1983;1:446–7.
439. Bolder U, TonNu HT, Schteingasrt CD, et al. Hepatocyte transport of bile acids and organic anions in endotoxemic rats: impaired uptake and secretion. Gastroenterology 1997;112:214–25.
440. Mosley RH. Sepsis associated cholestasis. Gastroenterology 1997;112:302–6.
441. Forrest E, Oien K, Dickson S, Galloway D, Mills P. Improvement in cholestasis associated with total parenteral nutrition after treatment with an antibody against tumor necrosis factor alpha. Liver 2002;22:317–20.
442. Belli DC, Roy CC, Fournier LA, et al. The effect of taurine on the cholestatic potential of sulfated lithocholate and its conjugates. Liver 1991;11:162–9.
443. Guertin F, Roy CC, Lepage A, et al. Effect of taurine on total parenteral nutrition associated cholestasis. J Parenteral Enteral Nutr 1991;15:294–7.
444. Rigo J, Senterre J. Is taurine essential for neonates? Biol Neonate 1977;32:221–32.
445. Korpela H, Nuutinen LS, Kumpulainen J. Low serum selenium and glutathione peroxidase activity in patients receiving short-term total parenteral nutrition. Int J Vitam Nutr Res 1989;59:80–4.
446. Sokol RJ, Taylor SF, Devereaux MW. Hepatic oxidant injury and glutathione depletion during total parenteral nutrition in weanling rats. Am J Physiol 1996;270:G691–700.
447. Moss RL, Haynes AL, Pastuszyn A, Glew RH. Methionine infusion reproduces liver injury of parenteral nutrition cholestasis. Pediatr Res 1999;45:644–8.
448. Fell JME, Reynolds AP, Meadows N. Manganese toxicity in children receiving long-term parenteral nutrition. Lancet 1996;347:1218–21.
449. Dickerson R. Manganese intoxication and parenteral nutrition. Nutrition 2001;17:689–93.
450. Wardle C, Forbers A, Roberts N, Jawhari A, Shenkin A. Hypermanganesemia in long-term intravenous nutrition and chronic liver disease. J Parenteral Enteral Nutr 1999;23:350–5.
451. Fok TF, Chui KKM, Cheung R, et al. Manganese intake and cholestatic jaundice in neonates receiving parenteral nutrition: a randomized controlled study. Acta Paediatr 2001;80:1009–15.
452. Ben-Hariz M, Goulet O, De-Potter S, et al. Iron overload in children receiving total parenteral nutrition. J Pediatr 1993;123:238–41.
453. Dahlstrom K, Ament M, Moukarzel A, et al. Low blood and plasma carnitine levels in children receiving long-term parenteral nutrition. J Pediatr Gastroenterol Nutr 1990;11:375–9.
454. Moukarzel A, Dahlstrom K, Buchman A, Ament ME. Carnitine status of children receiving long term total parenteral nutrition: a longitudinal prospective study. J Pediatr 1992;120:759–62.
455. Penn D, Schmidt-Sommerfeld E, Wolf H. Carnitine deficiency in premature infants receiving total parenteral nutrition. Early Hum Dev 1980;4:23–34.

456. Schiff D, Chan G, Secombe D, Hohn P. Plasma carnitine levels during intravenous feeding of the neonate. J Pediatr 1979; 95:1043–6.
457. Worthley L, Fishlock R, Snoswell A. Carnitine deficiency with hyperbilirubinemia, generalized muscle weakness and reactive hypoglycemia in a patient on long-term total parenteral nutrition: treatment with L-carnitine. J Parenteral Enteral Nutr 1983;7:176–80.
458. Buchman AL, Dubin M, Jenden D, et al. Lecithin increases plasma free choline and decreases hepatic steatosis in long-term parenteral nutrition patients. Gastroenterology 1992;102:1363–70.
459. Buchman AL, Dubin MD, Moukarzel AA, et al. Choline deficiency: a cause of hepatic steatosis during parenteral nutrition that can be reversed with intravenous choline supplementation. Hepatology 1995;22:1399–403.
460. Buchman A, Ament ME, Sohel M, et al. Choline deficiency causes reversible hepatic abnormalities in patients receiving parenteral nutrition: proof of a human choline requirement: a placebo-controlled trial. J Parenteral Enteral Nutr 2001;25: 260–8.
461. Bhatia J, Moslen MT, Haque AK, et al. Total parenteral nutrition-associated alterations in hepatobiliary function and histology on rats: is light exposure a clue? Pediatr Res 1993;33: 487–92.
462. Merrit RJ, Sinatra FR, Henton D, Neustein H. Cholestatic effects of intraperitoneal administration of tryptophan to suckling rat pups. Pediatr Res 1984;18:904–7.
463. Chessex P, Lavoie J, Rouleau T, et al. Photooxidation of parenteral multivitamins induces hepatic steatosis in a neonatal guinea pig model of intravenous nutrition. Pediatr Res 2002;52: 958–63.
464. Khashu M, Harrison A, Lalari V, et al. Photoprotection of parenteral nutrition enhances advancement of minimal enteral nutrition in preterm infants. Sem Perinatol 2006;30:139–45.
465. Koo WWK, Kaplan LA, Bendon R, et al. Response to aluminum in parenteral nutrition in infancy. J Pediatr 1986;5877–83.
466. Bishop NJ, Morely R, Day JP, Lucas A. Aluminum neurotoxicity in preterm infants receiving intravenous feeding solutions. N Engl J Med 1997;336:1557–61.
467. Iyer KR, Spitz L, Clayton P. New insight into mechanisms of parenteral nutrition-associated cholestasis: role of plant sterols. J Pediatric Surg 1998;33:1–6.
468. Clayton PT, Bowron A, Mills KA, et al. Phytosterolaemia in children with parenteral nutrition associated cholestatic liver disease. Gastroenterology 1993;105:1806–13.
469. Bindl L, Lutjohann D, Buderos S, et al. High plasma levels of phytosterols in patients on parenteral nutrition: a marker of liver dysfunction. J Pediatr Gastroenterol Nutr 2000;31:313–16.
470. Stein TP, Mullen JL. Hepatic fat accumulation in man with excess parenteral glucose. Nutr Res 1985;5:1347–51.
471. Buzby GP, Mullen JL, Stein TP, Rosato EF. Manipulation of TPN substrate and fatty infiltration of the liver. J Surg Res 1981; 31:46–54.
472. Hall RI, Grant JP, Ross LH, et al, Quarfordt SH. Pathogenesis of hepatic steatosis in the parenterally fed rat. J Clin Invest 1984;74:1659–67.
473. Meguid MM, Chen TY, Yang ZL. Effects of continuous graded total parenteral nutrition on feeding indexes and metabolic concomitants in rats. Am J Physiol 1991;260:E126–40.
474. Cavicchi M, Crenn P, Beau P, et al. Severe liver complications associated with long-term parenteral nutrition are dependent on lipid parenteral input. Transplant Proc 1998;30:2547.
475. Colomb V, Jobert-Giraud A, Lacaille F, et al. Role of lipid emulsions in cholestasis associated with long-term parenteral nutrition in children. J Parenteral Enteral Nutr 2000;24:345–50.
476. Tazuke Y, Drongowski R, Btaiche I, et al. Effects of lipid administration on liver apoptotic signals in a mouse model of total parenteral nutrition (TPN). Pediatr Surg Int 2004;20:224–8.
477. Mayer K, Grimm H, Grimminger F, Seeger W. Parenteral nutrition with n-3 lipids in sepsis. Br J Nutr 2002;87 Suppl 1:S69–75.
478. Mayer K, Meyer S, Reinholz-Muhly M, et al. Short-time infusion of fish oil based lipid emulsions, approved for parenteral nutrition, reduces monocyte proinflammatory cytokine generation and adhesive interaction with endothelium in humans. J Immunol 2003;171:4837–43.
479. Reimund J, Rahmi G, Escalin G, et al. Efficacy and safety of an olive-based intravenous fat emulsion in adult patients on home parenteral nutrition. Alimentary Pharmacol Ther 2005;21: 445–54.
480. Rubin M, Moser A, Vaserberg N, et al. Structured triacylglyerol emulsion, containing both medium-and long-chain fatty acids, in long-term parenteral nutrition: a double-blind randomized cross-over study. Nutrition 2000;16:95–100.
481. Li S, Nussbaum MS, Teague D, et al. Increasing dextrose concentrations in total parenteral nutrition causes alterations in hepatic morphology and plasma levels of insulin and glucagon in rats. J Surg Res 1988;44:639–48.
482. Li S, Nussbaum MS, McFadden DW, et al. Addition of L-glutamine to total parenteral nutrition and its effects on portal insulin and glucagon and the development of hepatic steatosis in rats. J Surg Res 1990;48:421–6.
483. Shamir R, Tershakovec AM, Barsky DL. Intravenous amino acids, cholestasis and kwashiorkor. J Med 1998;29:37–44.
484. Hwang T, Lue M, Chen L. Early use of cyclic TPN prevents further deterioration of liver functions for the TPN patients with impaired liver function. Hepato-Gastroenterology 2000;47: 1347–50.
485. Rintala PJ, Lindahl H, Pohjavuori M. Total parenteral nutrition-associated cholestasis in surgical neonates may be reversed by intravenous cholecystokinin: a preliminary report. J Pediatr Surg 1995;30:827–30.
486. Spagnuolo MI, Iorio R, Vegnente A, Guarino A. Ursodeoxycholic acid for treatment of cholestasis in children on long term total parenteral nutrition: a pilot study. Gastroenterology 1996;111:716–19.
487. Duerksen DR, Van Aerde JE, Granlich L, et al. Intravenous ursodeoxycholic acid reduces cholestasis in parenterally fed newborn piglets. Gastroenterology 1996;111:1111–17.
488. Heubi J, Wiechmann D, Creutzinger V, et al. Tauroursodeoxycholic acid (TUDCA) in the prevention of total parenteral nutrition-associated liver disease. J Pediatr 2002;141:237–42.
489. Demircan M, Ugural S, Mutus M, et al. The effects of acetylsalicyclic acid, interferon alpha, and vitamin E on prevention of parenteral nutrition-associated cholestasis: an experimental study. J Pediatr Gastroenterol Nutr 1999;28:291–5.
490. Nussinovitch M, Zahavi I, Marcus H, et al. The choleretic effect of nonsteroidal anti-inflammatory drugs in total parenteral nutrition-associated cholestasis. Israel J Med Sci 1996;32: 1262–4.

491. Van Aerde JE, Duerksen DR, Gramlich L, et al. Intravenous fish oil emulsion attenuates total parenteral nutrition-induced cholestasis in newborn piglets. Pediatr Res 1999;45:202–8.
492. Prescott W, Btaiche I. Sincalide in patients with parenteral nutrition-associated gallbladder disease. Annals Pharmacother 2004;38:1942–5.
493. Pollack PF, Rivera A, Rassin DK, Nishioka K. Cysteine supplementation increases glutathione, but not polyamine, concentrations of the small intestine and colon of parenterally fed rabbits. J Pediatr Gastroenterol Nutr 1996;22:364–72.
494. Narkewicz MR, Caldwell S, Jones G. Cysteine supplementation and reduction of total parenteral nutrition-induced hepatic lipid accumulation in the weanling rat. J Pediatr Gastroenterol Nutr 1995;21:18–24.
495. Newman LS, Rose CS, Maier LA. Sarcoidosis. N Engl J Med 1997;336:1224–34.
496. Fauroux B, Clement A. Paediatric sarcoidosis. Paediatr Respir Rev 2005;6:128–33.
497. Clark SK. Sarcoidosis in children. Pediatr Dermatol 1987;4:291–9.
498. Devaney K, Goodman Z, Epstein M, et al. Hepatic sarcoidosis. Am J Surg Pathol 1993;17:1271–80.
499. Ishak KG. Sarcoidosis of the liver and bile ducts. Mayo Clin Proc 1998;73:467–72.
500. Maddrey WC, Johns CJ, Boitnott JK, Iber FL. Sarcoidosis and chronic hepatic disease: a clinical and pathologic study of 20 patients. Medicine 1970;49:375–95.
501. Moreno Merlo F, Wanless IR, Shimamatsu K, et al. The role of granulomatous phlebitis and thrombosis in the pathogenesis of cirrhosis and portal hypertension in sarcoidosis. Hepatology 1997;26:554–60.
502. Becheur H, Dall'osto H, Chatellier G, et al. Effect of ursodeoxycholic acid on chronic intrahepatic cholestasis due to sarcoidosis. Dig Dis Sci 1997;42:789–91.
503. Falk RH, Comenzo RL, Skinner M. The systemic amyloidoses. N Engl J Med 1998;337:898–909.
504. Friedman S, Janowitz HD. Systemic amyloidosis and the gastrointestinal tract. Gastroenterol Clin North Am 1998;27:595–614.
505. Gertz MA, Lacy MQ, Dispenzieri A. Amyloidosis. Hematol Oncol Clin North Am 1999;13:1211–33.
506. Gillmore JD, Lovat LB, Hawkins PN. Amyloidosis and the liver. J Hepatol 1999;20 Supp 1:17–33.
507. McGlennen RC, Burke BA, Dehner LP. Systemic amyloidosis complicating cystic fibrosis. Arch Pathol Lab Med 1986;110:879–94.
508. Freeze HH. Genetic defects in the human glycome. Nat Rev Genet 2006;7:537–51.
509. Marquardt T, Denecke J. Congenital disorders of glycosylation: review of their molecular bases, clinical presentations and specific therapies. Eur J Pediatr 2003;162:359–79.
510. Damen G, de Klerk H, Huijmans J, den Hollander J, Sinaasappel M. Gastrointestinal and other clinical manifestations in 17 children with congenital disorders of glycosylation type Ia, Ib, and Ic. J Pediatr Gastroenterol Nutr 2004;38:282–7.
511. Eklund EA, Sun L, Westphal V, et al. Congenital disorder of glycosylation (CDG)-Ih patient with a severe hepato-intestinal phenotype and evolving central nervous system pathology. J Pediatr 2005;147:847–50.
512. Miura Y, Tay SK, Aw MM, et al. Clinical and biochemical characterization of a patient with congenital disorder of glycosylation (CDG) IIx. J Pediatr 2005;147:851–3.
513. Mandato C, Brive L, Miura Y, et al. Cryptogenic liver disease in four children: a novel congenital disorder of glycosylation. Pediatr Res 2006;59:293–8.
514. Harms HK, Zimmer KP, Kurnik K, et al. Oral mannose therapy persistently corrects the severe clinical symptoms and biochemical abnormalities of phosphomannose isomerase deficiency. Acta Paediatr 2002;91:1065–72.

39

Fibrocystic Liver Disease

Maureen M. Jonas, M.D., and Antonio R. Perez-Atayde, M.D.

Fibrocystic liver disease refers to a heterogeneous group of disorders that share some pathophysiologic and clinical features but have important differences. Cystic dilatation of intrahepatic bile duct structures and variable degrees of portal fibrosis are the hallmarks of fibrocystic liver disease. In most instances, there are morphologic abnormalities in the kidneys and pancreas that parallel those of the liver. For this reason, and to appreciate more thoroughly the shared pathogenesis and implications for organogenesis, fibrocystic liver disease and corresponding renal counterparts are discussed together.

It has been recognized for centuries that hepatic and renal cysts are seen in the same individuals [1], although it has not always been accepted that they are manifestations of the same diseases [2]. The older literature contains confusing descriptive classifications of fibrocystic diseases, with imprecise and overlapping definitions. Even now, attempts at describing clinical and radiographic features, prognosis, natural history, and treatment are somewhat hampered by reliance on these descriptive reports. However, much of the molecular basis for these disorders has been elucidated, and clinical diagnoses are being modified using more exact genetic criteria. The current consensus is that genetic determinants of differentiation and development of renal tubules and biliary structures result in a broad spectrum of congenital abnormalities grouped under the heading of fibrocystic liver and kidney disease [3].

Embryologic development of the liver has been discussed elsewhere (see Chapter 1) and will not be fully reviewed here. However, to understand this group of developmental disorders, it is necessary to review the stages of formation of the macroscopic and microscopic biliary tree. At about the eighth week of gestation, precursor cells that lie adjacent to the hilar portal vein vessels dramatically increase expression of cytokeratin. This sleevelike layer of cells duplicates and extends toward the periphery along small intrahepatic portal vein branches. The resultant double-layered sleeve of cytokeratin-rich cells that are separated by a slit or platelike lumen has been designated by Hammar as the ductal plate [4,5].

The ductal plate undergoes progressive remodeling from 12 weeks' gestation into the postnatal period. This process begins at the hilum and proceeds toward the periphery. As shown in Figure 39.1, short segments of the double-layered sleeve dilate to form tubules. As they form, individual bile ductules are incorporated into the periportal mesenchyme around the portal vein branches. These developing bile ductules consistently express cytokeratin 19 and begin expressing cytokeratin 7 as well as other markers of differentiated biliary epithelia by 20 weeks' gestation [6–8]. In contrast, precursor cells that are not associated with the differentiating ductal plate and bile ductules lose cytokeratin 19 expression. These cells maintain cytokeratin 8 and 18 expression and eventually give rise to hepatocytes [9].

Biliary differentiation involves a series of interactions between the mesenchyme surrounding the portal vein branches and the ductal plate epithelia [6,10,11]. As a result, the ductal plate is induced to form bile ducts, which are incorporated into the portal mesenchyme. The nontubular elements of the ductal plate involute. This remodeling of the ductal plate leads to the formation of the intrahepatic biliary tree. The largest bile ducts are formed first, followed by segmental, interlobular, and finally by the smallest ductules. Arrest or derangement in remodeling leads to the persistence of primitive bile duct configurations, or to what Jorgensen termed *ductal plate malformation* (DPM) [4]. The occurrence of DPM at different generations of the developing biliary tree gives rise to different clinicopathologic entities. Defects in ductal plate remodeling are typically accompanied by portal vein branching abnormalities [5].

Fibrocystic diseases of the liver are most often accompanied by cystic disorders of the kidney as listed in Table 39.1. Much of the work elucidating the pathogenesis of these disorders has been done using animal models, cell systems, and clinical material from affected kidneys. Thus, it is important to understand renal tubular development and how it parallels biliary development. Nephron formation begins about the eighth week of gestation, as the ureteric bud branches induce the mesenchymal cells to begin a series of stereotypical changes. The induced mesenchyme forms caplike aggregates over the advancing ureteric bud branches, which then become vesicular as they undergo a mesenchymal to epithelial transformation, polarize, and form a lumen. These vesicular structures then elongate to form S-shaped tubules. The lower portion of each tubule gives rise to the glomerular capsule and the remainder to the proximal and

Table 39.1: Renal Disorders Associated with Fibropolycystic Liver Diseases

Fibropolycystic Liver Disease	*Associated Renal Disorder*
Congenital hepatic fibrosis (CHF)	Autosomal-recessive polycystic kidney disease* Autosomal-dominant polycystic kidney disease Cystic renal dysplasia Nephronophthisis None
Caroli's syndrome (CS)	Autosomal-recessive polycystic kidney disease* Autosomal-dominant polycystic kidney disease None
Caroli's disease	Autosomal-recessive polycystic kidney disease
Von Meyenburg complexes (isolated)	?
Von Meyenburg complexes with CHF or CS	Autosomal-recessive polycystic kidney disease
Von Meyenburg complexes with polycystic liver disease	Autosomal-dominant polycystic kidney disease
Polycystic liver disease	Autosomal-dominant polycystic kidney disease* ? none

*Most common associated disorder.

distal tubules. In a reciprocal fashion, the ureteric bud continues to divide, and its terminal branches differentiate into the collecting ducts. Nephrogenesis proceeds in a centripetal pattern, from the inner cortex to the periphery, and is completed by 34 weeks' gestation [12,13].

Osathanondh and Potter [12] morphologically classified the tubular abnormalities that occur in different polycystic kidney diseases. In autosomal-recessive polycystic kidney disease (ARPKD), the cystic lesion involves 1- to 8-mm fusiform dilatations of the terminal collecting duct branches. The extent of collecting duct involvement varies inversely with age at presentation. In affected fetuses and neonates, 90% of the collecting tubules are dilated versus 10% in adolescents [14–16]. In comparison, in autosomal-dominant polycystic kidney disease (ADPKD), cysts may develop in any nephron segment or in the collecting duct, but on average they involve only 1% of the nephron population [17]. These cysts most often develop in childhood but have been detected in a fetus as early as 16 weeks' gestation [18]. They are clinically silent until the third or fourth decade of life [17].

SOLITARY NONPARASITIC CYST OF THE LIVER

Solitary nonparasitic cysts resemble the cysts seen in fibrocystic diseases in that they are developmental rather than neoplastic in origin, and lined by simple cuboidal or columnar biliary-type epithelium [19] (Figure 39.2). The surrounding hepatic parenchyma displays secondary atrophy, portal fibrosis, and bile duct proliferation [20]. However, the cysts are not associated with DPM and not seen in association with renal, pancreatic, or other cysts. Most are unilocular and do not have any clinical manifestations. When they are symptomatic, the most common presentation is that of an upper abdominal mass, although rupture, infection, or hemorrhage also may occur.

CONGENITAL HEPATIC FIBROSIS

A hereditary disorder characterized by hepatic fibrosis, portal hypertension, and renal cystic disease was described by Kerr et al. in 1961 [21] and called congenital hepatic fibrosis (CHF). Typically, CHF is associated with autosomal-recessive polycystic kidney disease (ARPKD). Some investigators considered CHF and ARPKD a single disorder with a wide spectrum of manifestations [16,22,23], whereas others argued that they are two distinct entities that share phenotypically similar biliary lesions. ARPKD is described more frequently in neonates and infants, in whom the renal lesion is clinically more severe, whereas CHF is more commonly seen in older children and adolescents, in whom the renal involvement may be minimal [24]. However, recent identification of the gene for ARPKD, *PKHD1* [25,26], has provided proof that at least most cases of ARPKD with CHF are genetically homogeneous. Using a technique for rapid screening of *PKDH1* in ARPKD pedigrees, the detection

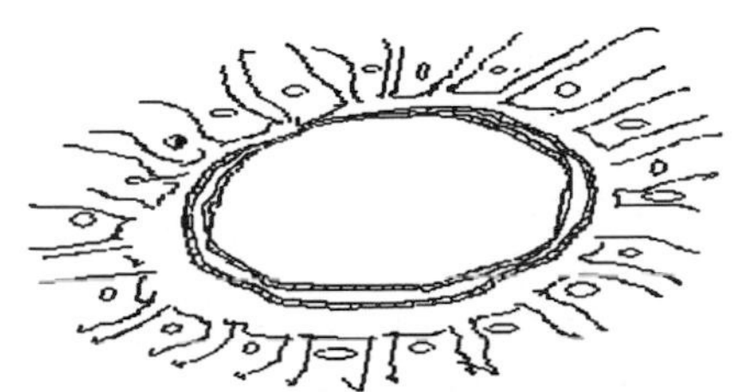
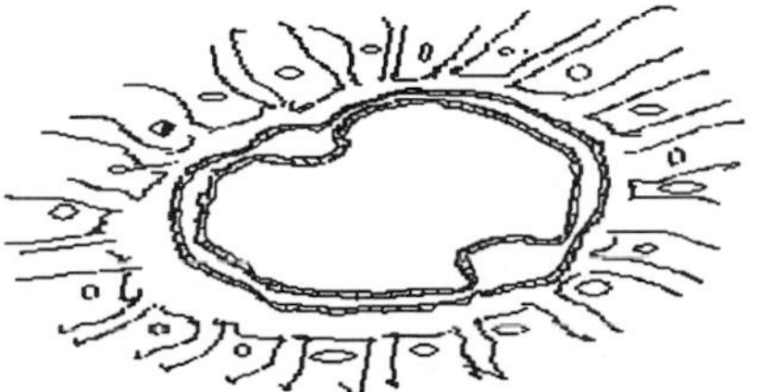
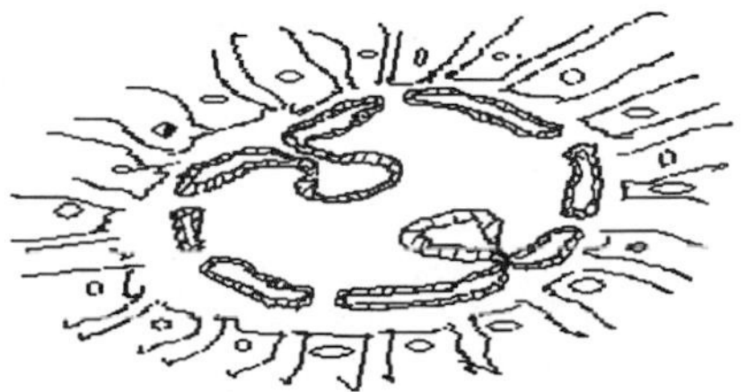

Figure 39.1. Schematic representation of the primordial ductal plate remodeling. The two layers of cells are originally separated by a slitlike lumen. Segments of the lumen dilate to form tubules, which eventually become bile ducts, incorporated into the portal tract mesenchyme. The remainder of the ductal plate involutes.

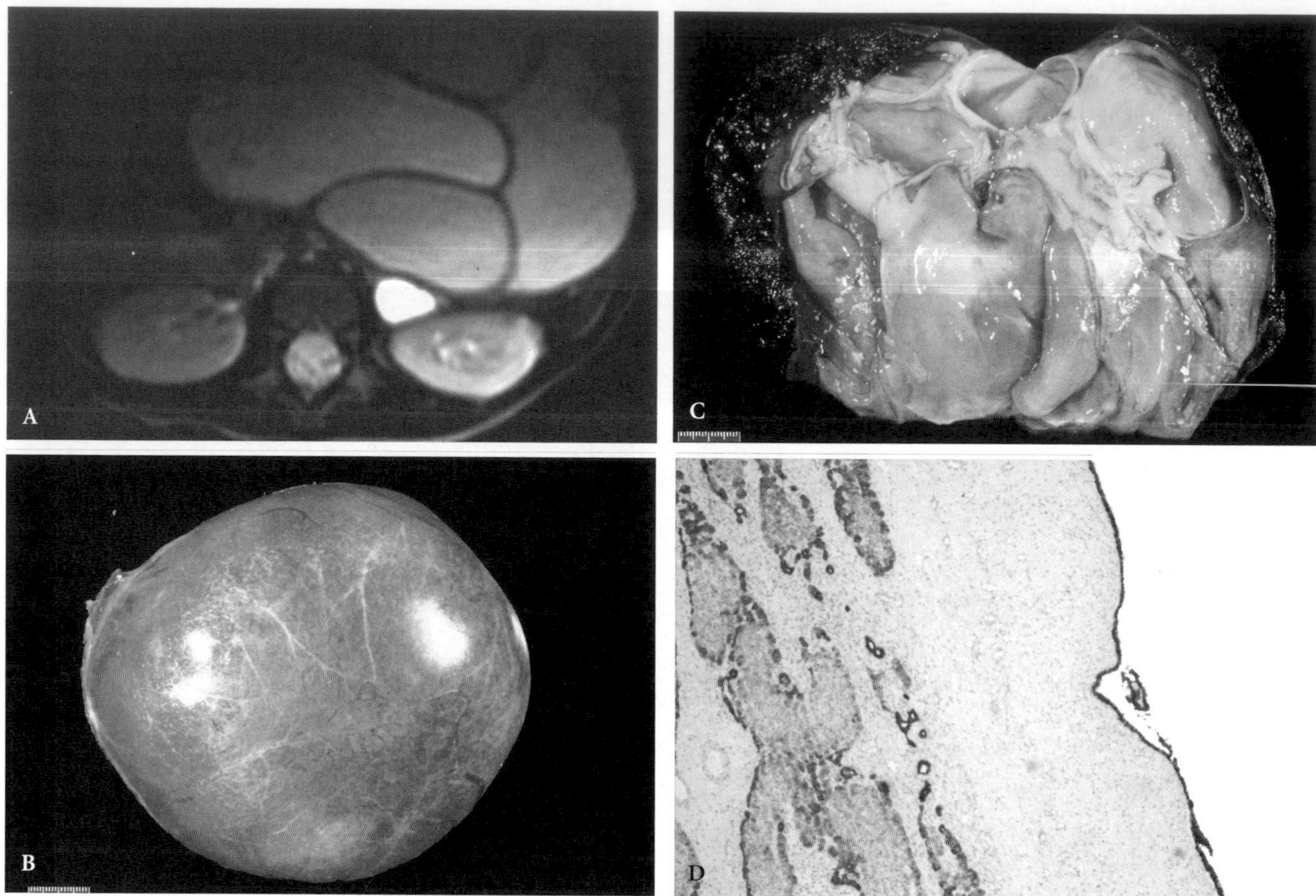

Figure 39.2 Solitary nonparasitic liver cyst. (**A**) Computed tomography scan demonstrating large multiloculated hepatic cyst. (**B**) External gross appearance of the resected cyst showing smooth, shiny surface. (**C**) Cut surface of the cyst demonstrating loculations. (**D**) Microscopically, the cyst wall is lined by AE1 cytokeratin-positive biliary epithelium. The outer part of the cyst wall contains atrophic hepatic parenchyma with portal bile duct proliferation and fibrosis.

rate of mutations was 85% in severely affected patients, 41.9% in moderate ARPKD, and 32.1% in adults with CHF or Caroli's disease [27]. For purposes of discussion, a descriptive approach is taken here; this section focuses on the biliary lesion, and the renal tubular lesion is reviewed in the discussion of ARPKD.

Although CHF is most commonly seen in association with ARPKD, it has been reported as an isolated entity [28] as well as with ADPKD [29] and nephronophthisis [30,31]. CHF also has been described in a variety of other conditions or syndromes [32–37], as listed in Table 39.2. In some of these syndromes, cystic disease of the pancreas is also observed. In most pedigrees, CHF is transmitted as an autosomal–recessive trait. Although some reports cite a higher incidence in males, this observation remains controversial. The overall incidence of CHF is unknown.

From a clinical perspective, the spectrum and severity of manifestations vary greatly. There are four clinical forms of CHF (Table 39.3): (1) portal hypertensive, which is the most common; (2) cholangitic; (3) mixed; and (4) latent. In the portal hypertensive form, clinical presentation is often esophageal variceal hemorrhage [38]. The cholangitic form is characterized by cholestasis and recurrent cholangitis [39]. The latent form is manifest late in life or is an incidental finding.

In CHF uncomplicated by either portal hypertension or cholangitis, laboratory evaluation is usually unremarkable. Serum aminotransferase and bilirubin levels are characteristically normal. Typically the liver is normal in size and quite firm in consistency. Pathologically, the liver appears grossly speckled with gray-white bands of fibrous tissue identifiable to the naked eye (Figure 39.3A and 39.3B). Microscopically, ductal plate malformation of the interlobular bile ducts is always found, and the involved ducts are in communication with the biliary system (Figure 39.3C). Prominent bands of mature fibrous tissue connect adjacent portal triads. Although the periportal fibrosis is marked, the associated inflammatory cell infiltration of the portal areas is usually mild. The intervening lobular hepatic architecture is preserved. Vascular lesions such as portal vein branch hypoplasia and hepatic arteriolar prominence have been documented [9,40,41]. Degeneration of biliary duct epithelium and mild cholestasis are occasionally seen. Although the hepatic lesions of CHF tend to become more prominent with time, the rate of progression is extremely variable.

Table 39.2: Syndromes Associated with Congenital Hepatic Fibrosis

Jeune syndrome [119]

Asphyxiating thoracic dystrophy, with cystic renal tubulary dysplasia and congenital hepatic fibrosis (15q13)

Joubert's syndrome [32]

Oculo-encephalo-hepato-renal (*AH11, HPHP1*)

COACH syndrome [37]

*C*erebellar vermis hypoplasia, *o*ligophrenia, congenital *a*taxia, ocular *coloboma,* and *h*epatic fibrosis

Meckel syndrome type 1 [33]

Cystic renal dysplasia abnormal bile duct development with fibrosis, posterior encephalocele, and polydactyly (13q13, 17q21, 8q24)

Carbohydrate-deficient glycoprotein syndrome type 1b [71]

Phosphomannose isomerase 1 deficiency (*PMI*)

Ivemark syndrome type 2 [36]

Autosomal-recessive renal-hepatic-pancreatic dysplasia

Miscellaneous syndromes

Intestinal lymphangiectasia, enterocolitis cystica [120]

Short rib (Beemer-Langer) syndrome

Osteochondrodysplasia [121]

Diagnosis of CHF is suggested by ultrasonography or computerized tomography (CT) of the abdomen. Sonographically, the liver has a patchy pattern of increased echogenicity. Sonographic evaluation should include Doppler flow studies of the portal vasculature looking for evidence of portal hypertension, such as reversal of portal flow or splenomegaly. Liver biopsy will reveal the characteristic findings described earlier.

Therapy depends on the type and manifestations of CHF. Antibiotics are provided for cholangitis. Sclerotherapy, band ligation, and portosystemic shunts have been performed effectively for variceal bleeding. The incidence of hepatic encephalopathy in CHF patients who have undergone shunting procedures is low [39]. Although transplantation is curative, it should be limited to the minority of patients with chronic cholangitis or progressive hepatic dysfunction. In most instances, CHF is a disorder characterized by well-preserved hepatic function and a good prognosis if complications such as variceal bleeding and cholangitis are controlled [42].

AUTOSOMAL-RECESSIVE POLYCYSTIC KIDNEY DISEASE

Autosomal-recessive polycystic kidney disease was once referred to as infantile polycystic disease. However, it has since been recognized in adults. ARPKD is estimated to occur in 1 in 6000 to 1 in 40,000 live births. Although ARPKD includes a spectrum of clinical and histopathologic manifestations, there are two constant features: (1) biliary tract abnormalities arising from DPM and (2) fusiform dilatation of the renal collecting ducts. In 1971, Blythe and Ockenden [24] proposed subclassification into four genetic types based on age at presentation and severity of renal disease. However, variations in disease manifestations among siblings have been noted, suggesting that these distinctions are merely descriptive and do not represent different genetic subsets [16,23]. Thus far, all cases studied have mapped to the *PKHD1* locus, at 6p21-p12 [43]. Whether isolated CHF without ARPKD also maps to this locus is as yet unknown. The *PKHD1* gene has been identified [25] and the gene product termed *fibrocystin* [26].

In affected infants, the kidneys retain their natural shape and are massively enlarged. Macroscopically, the renal surface is studded with small opalescent cysts representing the fusiform dilatation of the collecting ducts (Figure 39.4A and 39B). Microscopically, the dilated collecting ducts are arrayed at right angles to the capsule, and the corticomedullary junction is obscured (Figure 39.4C). In contrast, the glomeruli and other nephron segments appear normal. With time, progressive interstitial fibrosis develops, resulting in a progressive decline of renal function [15,16].

The hepatic lesion in ARPKD includes enlarged, irregularly fibrotic portal areas that contain tortuous and large bile ducts associated with persistence of the ductal plate. These histopathologic findings are indistinguishable from those of isolated CHF. If the process leads to macroscopic dilatation of the intrahepatic biliary tree, it will fall into the category of Caroli's syndrome (Figure 39.5).

Clinically, just as in isolated CHF, the severity of the hepatic lesion varies inversely with age. Hematemesis and melena herald the development of esophageal varices. Typically, children present with variceal bleeding at ages 5 to 13 years, but it has been reported in infants [44]. The children may have firm hepatomegaly and splenomegaly in addition to nephromegaly. Blood urea nitrogen (BUN) and serum creatinine values vary with the severity of renal involvement. Hepatic synthetic function,

Table 39.3: Manifestations of Congenital Hepatic Fibrosis

Type	*Manifestations*	*Laboratory Findings*
Portal hypertensive	Splenomegaly Varices Normal liver function Normal growth	Thrombocytopenia Neutropenia ± elevated alkaline phosphatase
Cholangitic	Cholestasis Recurrent cholangitis Hepatic dysfunction Poor growth	Elevated alkaline phosphatase ± elevated bilirubin
Mixed	Mixed	All of the above
Latent	None	None

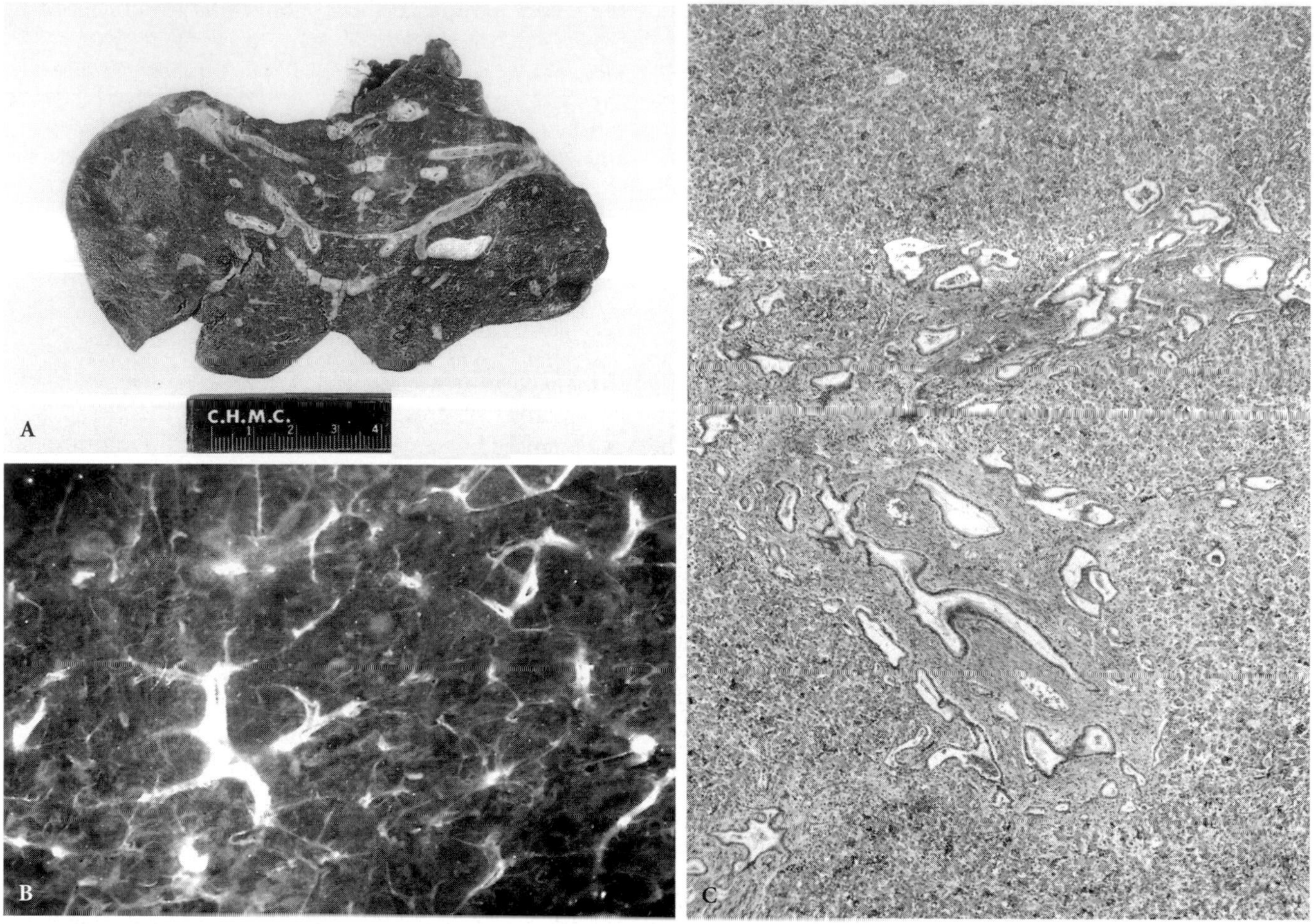

Figure 39.3. Congenital hepatic fibrosis. (**A** and **B**) Gross liver specimen demonstrating the prominent gray-white bands of fibrous tissue. (**C**) Microscopic section demonstrating dilated irregularly branching bile ducts, ductal plate malformation, and prominent portal fibrosis.

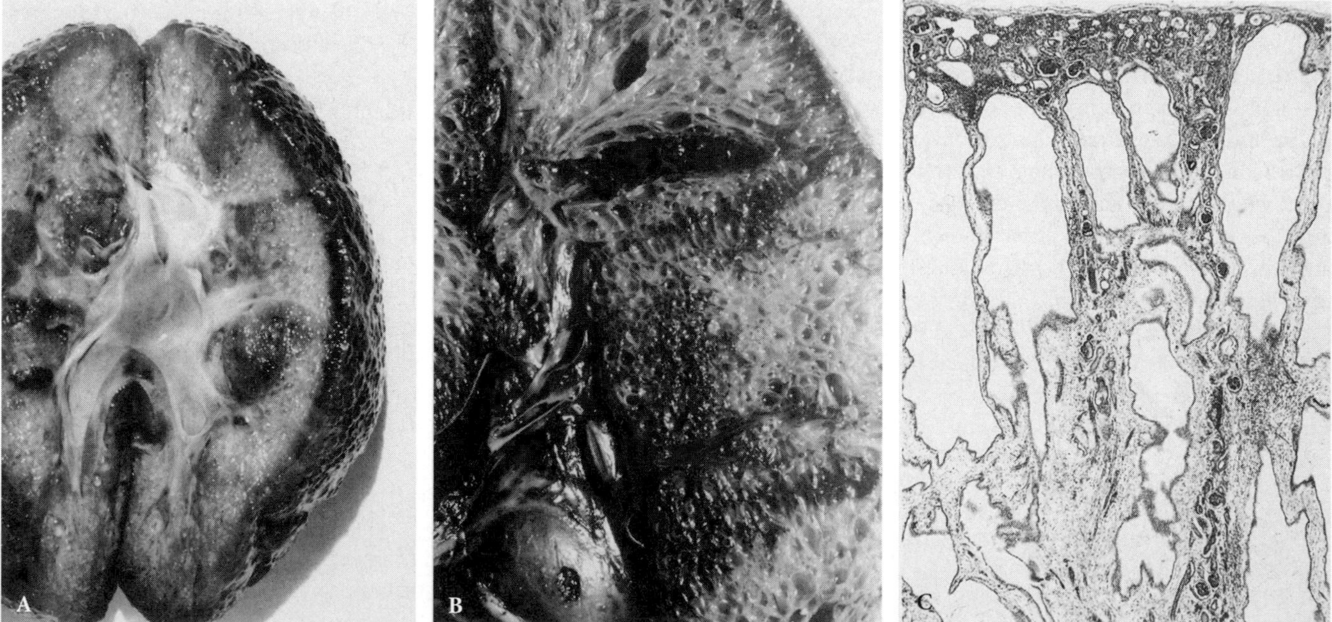

Figure 39.4. Autosomal-recessive polycystic kidney disease. (**A** and **B**) The cut surface of the kidney demonstrates innumerable small opalescent cysts of fairly uniform size. (**C**) Microscopically, the cysts represent cystically dilated collecting ducts, arranged perpendicularly to the capsule.

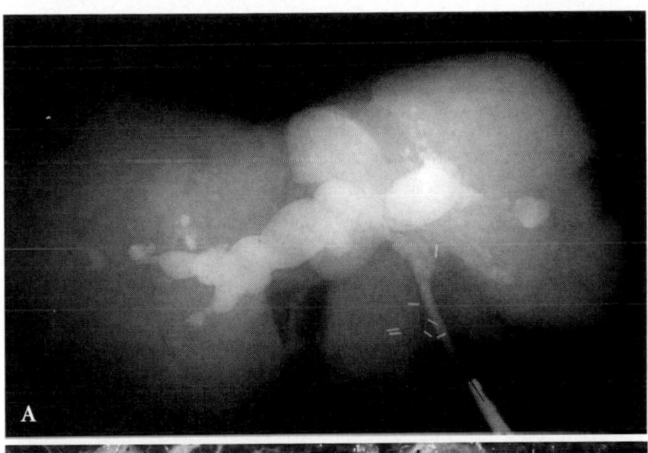

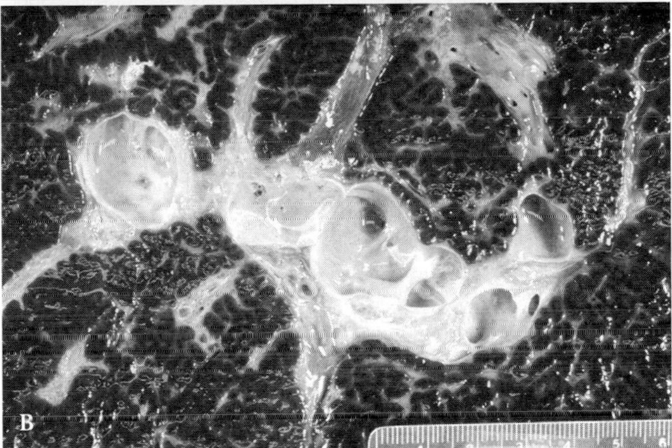

Figure 39.5. Caroli's syndrome. (**A**) Cholangiogram of a hepatic explant with marked dilatation of the intrahepatic biliary tree. (**B**) Cut surface of the same liver showing both the cystic dilatation of the biliary tree and the fibrous bands throughout the liver consistent with congenital hepatic fibrosis.

bilirubin, and aminotransferase values are generally normal. Anemia, leukopenia, and thrombocytopenia suggest associated hypersplenism. Although the disease phenotype is quite variable, many children have some degree of coexistent portal hypertension and chronic renal failure [45]. The diagnosis is suggested by the clinical presentation and radiologic studies. In the infant, ultrasonography reveals massive, hyperechoic kidneys with loss of the corticomedullary junction and a normal-sized echogenic liver. In older children, kidney size and echogenicity are more variable, and macroscopic cysts may be evident. The sonographic findings in the liver, including Doppler studies, are described in the earlier discussion on CHF. Definitive diagnosis may require renal and liver biopsies, but the diagnosis can be inferred from histology in one organ and typical sonographic findings. Treatment for the hepatic lesions in ARPKD is the same as that described above for CHF. The patients are at risk for ascending cholangitis with associated sepsis and hepatic failure; unexplained or prolonged fever warrants diagnostic liver biopsy and culture. Although portal hypertension can be managed successfully and hepatic synthetic function is generally well preserved in ARPKD, liver transplantation may be warranted in patients with chronic cholangitis. Many patients with ARPKD die in the perinatal period or during infancy from renal failure or pulmonary insufficiency. The prognosis of ARPKD in those who survive infancy, particularly those patients who undergo successful renal transplantation, has not been well defined.

CAROLI'S DISEASE AND CAROLI'S SYNDROME

Caroli described two forms of congenital dilatation of the intrahepatic biliary tree associated with renal cystic disease [46]. In the more common type, the portal tract lesion is the ductal plate malformation typical of CHF. This entity is now referred to as Caroli's syndrome. The second, much more rare type is characterized by pure ductal ectasia and is now called Caroli's disease. Both of these entities are more common in females and typically become symptomatic in adults, although they may present in childhood [47]. Both conditions are transmitted in an autosomal–recessive fashion and are associated with ARPKD [45] or, rarely, with ADPKD [48]. They also have been reported in patients with choledochal cysts, leading some researchers to classify Caroli's disease as a type of choledochal cyst [49]. However, in view of the extrahepatic biliary origin of choledochal cysts, the absence of a genetic pattern, and the lack of associated renal anomalies, this classification is probably invalid.

Caroli and Desmet have postulated that Caroli's disease results from an arrest in ductal plate remodeling at the level of the larger intrahepatic bile ducts. In contrast, Caroli's syndrome results when the full spectrum of bile duct differentiation is affected, such that the smaller interlobular ducts are involved and CHF develops [6]. Because some reports describe cases limited to the left hepatic lobe, Caroli's disease has been described in some classification schemes as either diffuse or localized [46].

Presenting signs and symptoms include intermittent abdominal pain and hepatomegaly. Steatorrhea has been described. In Caroli's syndrome, because the lesion of CHF is also present, evidence of portal hypertension is common, and usually precedes cholangitis. In both Caroli's disease and Caroli's syndrome, ductal ectasia predisposes to bile stagnation, with consequent sludge and stone formation and risk of infection. Diagnosis is confirmed by imaging studies such as abdominal CT, ultrasonography (Figure 39.6A), isotope scans, and cholangiograms (Figure 39.6B and 39.6C), which demonstrate irregular cystic dilatation of the large, proximal intrahepatic bile ducts. Cholangitis, cholelithiasis, biliary abscess, septicemia, and cholangiocarcinoma are all potential complications of these two entities. The increased risk of cholangiocarcinoma in these patients has been postulated to occur because of prolonged exposure of the ductal epithelia to high concentrations of unconjugated secondary bile acids [50].

Therapy for Caroli's syndrome is similar to that for CHF. Infection is managed with antibiotics and, in severe, localized cases, lobectomy of the affected lobe. In fact, partial hepatectomy also has been shown to be effective if the biliary lesion is predominantly confined to a discrete area [51]. In the diffuse form, liver transplantation may be necessary.

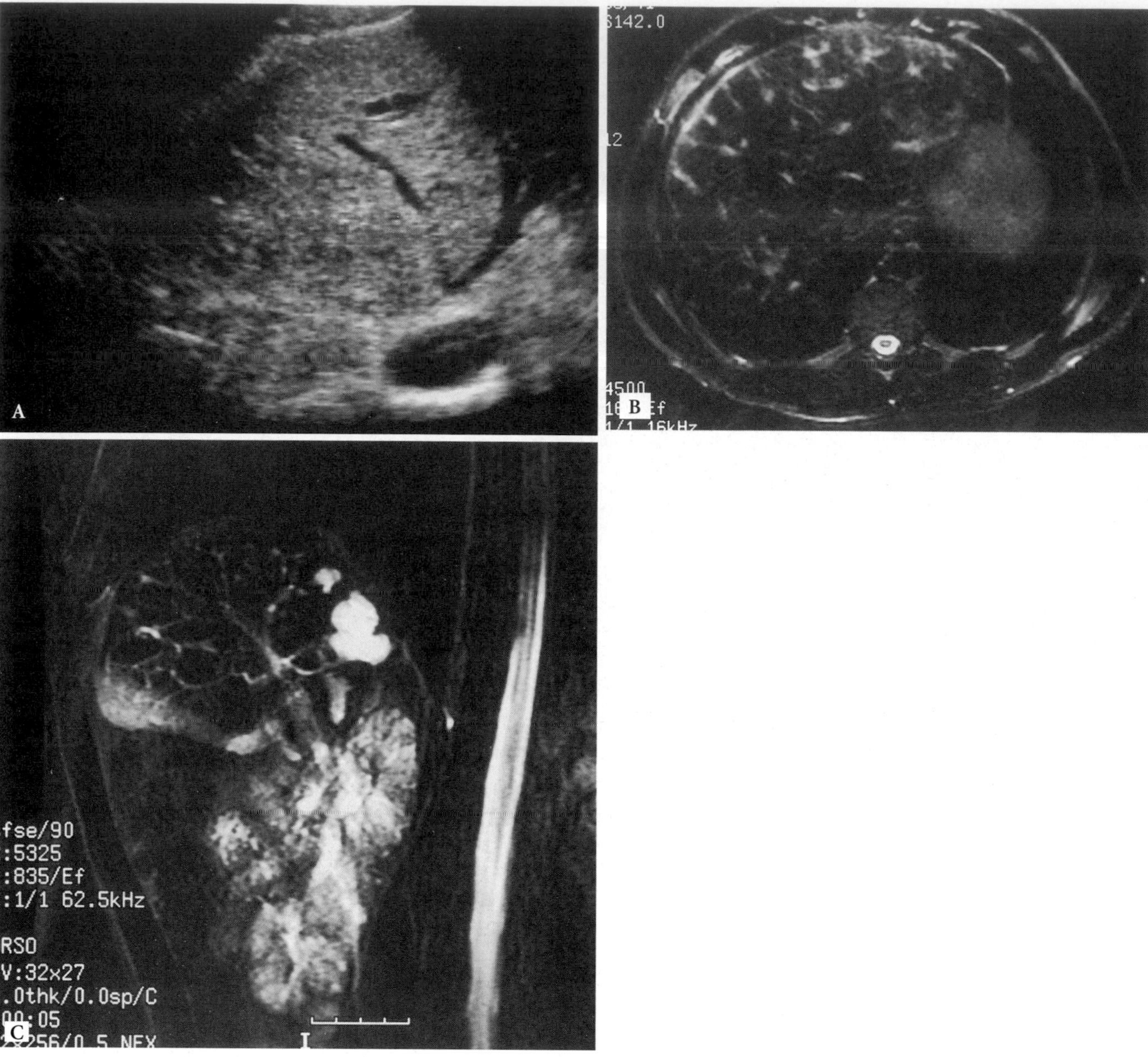

Figure 39.6. Radiographic findings in Caroli's syndrome. (**A**) Ultrasound of the liver demonstrating a large posterior cyst and a prominently dilated intrahepatic bile duct. The hepatic echotexture is coarse and heterogeneous. (**B**) Magnetic resonance cholangiogram, coronal oblique view, in the same patient, demonstrating the cysts noted on ultrasonography as well as more diffuse involvement of the intrahepatic bile ducts. (**C**) The composite transverse section provides even more detail about the extent of intrahepatic bile duct dilatation.

AUTOSOMAL DOMINANT POLYCYSTIC KIDNEY DISEASE

Bristowe [1] first described the association between hepatic and renal cysts in adults in 1856. Initially, this disorder was termed adult polycystic disease; subsequently, the nomenclature was changed to reflect the mode of genetic transmission. ADPKD occurs in 1 in 400 to 1 in 1000 individuals. It is the most common hereditary renal abnormality, affecting over 500,000 individuals in the United States; it accounts for 10% of all cases of end-stage renal disease (ESRD) [52]. Like ARPKD, ADPKD is characterized by renal and hepatic cysts, but ADPKD is often associated with other visceral anomalies as well. These include intracranial and aortic aneurysms, mitral valve prolapse and other cardiac valvular defects, pancreatic cysts, colonic diverticula, and inguinal hernias [17]. ADPKD is rarely associated with CHF [53,54] or Caroli's syndrome [48]; the more typical hepatic manifestation of ADPKD is called polycystic liver disease (PLD).

The kidneys in ADPKD contain numerous cysts of varying size in an irregular distribution, resulting in enlargement and distortion (Figure 39.7). In young children, the cysts are smaller and have a tendency to cluster; they occasionally involve the glomeruli as well as the collecting system. The kidneys of older

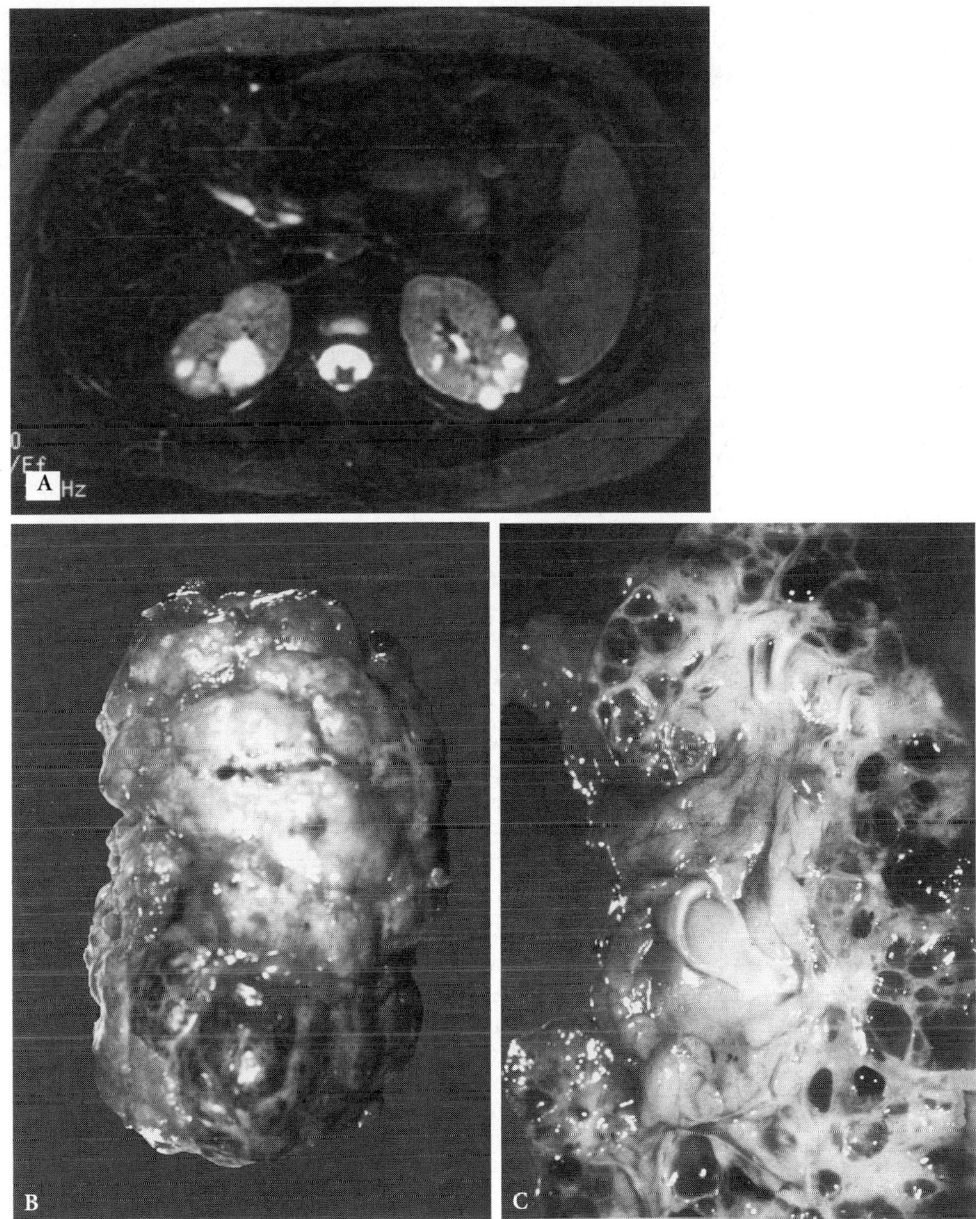

Figure 39.7. Autosomal-dominant polycystic kidney disease. (**A**) Magnetic resonance imaging demonstrates the variability in size and distribution of the renal cysts, and the normal liver and biliary tree. There is a tiny hepatic cyst in the left lobe (*tiny white dot*) that does not appear connected to the biliary tree. (**B**) Resected kidney has multiple cysts deforming the capsule and obscuring the normal contour. (**C**) The cut surface demonstrates variable size and distribution of the cysts.

children and adults have the more conventional findings of irregularly sized cysts distributed throughout the entire organ, with normal intervening renal parenchyma.

The symptomatic onset of ADPKD varies but is usually after age 40. Complications include systemic hypertension, hematuria, proteinuria, and pyelonephritis. In approximately 50% of ADPKD patients, the renal lesion progresses to ESRD [17,52]. Infection, hemorrhage, and rupture can occur in both renal and hepatic cysts.

Generally, laboratory tests are of little diagnostic value. Elevations in BUN and serum creatinine, as well as diminution of urinary concentrating ability, are related directly to the severity of renal involvement [17]. Serum alkaline phosphatase is elevated in 10–20% of patients, whereas aminotransferases and bilirubin values are usually normal. Diagnosis requires a careful family history, assessment of clinical symptoms and signs, and imaging techniques, such as ultrasonography or CT of the abdomen. Magnetic resonance imaging is a useful diagnostic modality to identify cyst infection, hemorrhage, or calcification.

In families in whom ADPKD has been identified, genetic linkage testing can be used to determine whether at-risk individuals are carrying the disease gene. In 86% of families, the

ADPKD gene defect is located on chromosome 16 (*PKD1*) [55]. A second locus (*PKD2*) has been mapped to chromosome 4 [56,57], and evidence suggests that a third, as yet unmapped, locus may exist as well [58].

VON MEYENBURG COMPLEXES (BILIARY MICROHAMARTOMAS)

Von Meyenburg complexes (VMCs) are microscopic lesions in the liver characterized by a discrete round or irregularly shaped cluster of small, often dilated bile ductules embedded in dense fibrous stroma. They also have been called biliary microhamartomas and may be found incidentally in otherwise histologically normal liver specimens. The ductular lumens within a complex are interconnecting [59]. Often VMCs are seen in livers affected with CHF, Caroli's syndrome, or PLD; in fact, they are suspected of being the cause of the latter [2]. From an embryologic perspective, these complexes appear to result from ductal plate malformation of the most peripheral interlobular bile ducts [60]. The predominantly accepted hypothesis is that the ductal structures of VMCs originally communicated with the developing biliary tree but became separated as a result of progressive dilatation, kinking, and surrounding fibrosis [59]. Although VMCs are common and generally asymptomatic, several cases of cholangiocarcinoma in association with these lesions have been reported in adults [61–63].

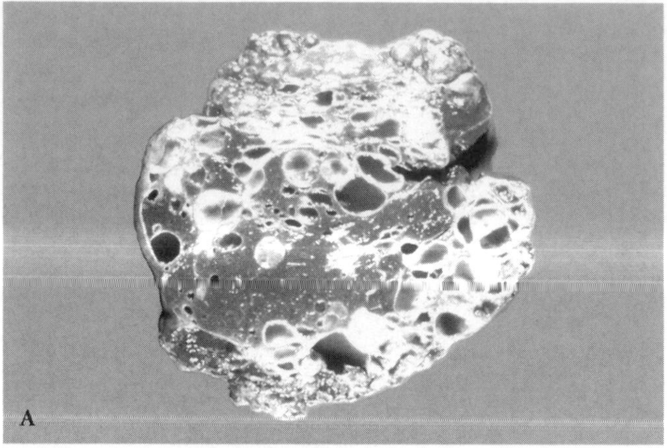

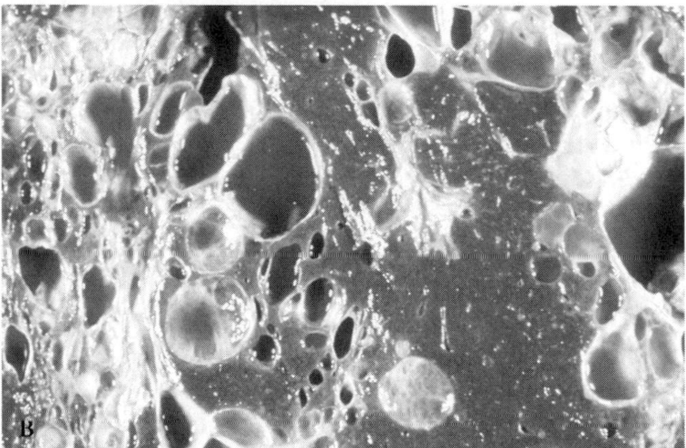

Figure 39.8. Polycystic liver disease. (**A**) The liver contains numerous cysts of varying size. The parenchyma appears compressed. (**B**) Close-up view shows thin-walled cysts, some containing mucoid clear fluid.

POLYCYSTIC LIVER DISEASE

Polycystic liver disease is the hepatic disorder most commonly associated with ADPKD. In children with ADPKD, liver cysts are rare. However, about 30% of ADPKD-affected adults have liver cysts, and the prevalence increases to 75–90% with increasing age. About 20% of affected individuals have cysts by the third decade. Development of liver cysts and associated morbidity are also influenced by female gender, pregnancy, use of oral contraceptives, and severity of renal involvement [64–66]. Typically, when PLD is present, it is associated with renal cysts, but there have been reports of isolated PLD [2,67,68].

Autosomal-dominant PLD is a distinct clinical and genetic entity in which multiple bile duct derived cysts develop and are unassociated with cystic kidney disease. Liver cysts arise from the dilatation of biliary microhamartomas and from peribiliary glands. Patients are often asymptomatic, even with large cysts. Females are more commonly affected than males, and the cysts often enlarge during pregnancy. Cysts are rarely identified in children.

The liver cysts in PLD are usually macroscopic and vary in diameter, although they are rarely larger than 10 cm. They contain clear or blood-tinged fluid. The cysts tend to be distributed in or closely associated with the portal tracts, and the lining epithelia have a biliary phenotype. These hepatic cysts arise from progressive dilatation of the ductules in VMCs, and they do not communicate with the biliary tree. Clinical manifestations of PLD may be predominant or they may be overshadowed by those of the renal disease. They include abdominal pain, abdominal mass, hepatomegaly, cyst infection with abscess formation, compression and obstruction of the biliary tree, cyst rupture, and bleeding [69]. In extreme cases, hepatic replacement with resultant hepatic insufficiency may occur (Figure 39.8). In some instances, there are no symptoms at all, and the cysts are discovered incidentally by abdominal imaging or at autopsy.

Two genes have been associated with ADPLD, *PRKCSH* and *SEC63*, which encode the β-subunit of glucosidase II (also called hepatocystin) and Sec63, respectively [70]. Hepatocystin is a protein kinase c substrate adK-H that is involved in the proper folding and maturation of glycoproteins. It is localized to the endoplasmic reticulum. SEC63 is a component of the protein translocation machinery in the ER. It is uncertain how these proteins, which are involved in regulation of glycosylation in the ER and possibly signal transduction, lead to the formation of hepatic cysts. However, a related observation is that one of the congenital disorders of glycosylation (CDG-1b) is associated with a liver pathology reminiscent of congenital hepatic fibrosis [71]. Thus, glycosylated proteins are in some way important for

Table 39.4: Genetics of Fibropolycystic Liver and Kidney Disease

Fibrocystic Disease	*Incidence*	*Onset of Symptoms*	*Genetic Loci*	*Gene Product*	*Function of Gene Product*
CHF (isolated)	Unknown	Childhood	Unknown	Unknown	Unknown
ARPKD with CHF	1/6000 to 1/40,000	Infancy	*PKHD1* 6p21-p12	Fibrocystin	Unknown
ADPKD ± PLD	1/400 to 1/1000	Adulthood	*PKD1* (chromosome 16)	Polycystin 1	Cell–cell or cell–matrix interactions
			PKD2 (chromosome 4)	Polycystin 2	?Channel protein
			Other	Unknown	? Ligand for polycystin 1 or 2
PLD (isolated)	Unknown	Adulthood	*PRKCSH*	Hepatocystin	Subunit of glucosidase II
PLD		Adulthood	*SEC63*	Sec63	Protein translocation

CHF, congenital hepatic fibrosis; ARPKD, autosomal-recessive polycystic kidney disease; ADPKD, autosomal-dominant polycystic kidney disease; PLD, polycystic liver disease.

maintaining the normal structure and function of the biliary tree.

Management of PLD is somewhat controversial and often requires a combination of medical and surgical approaches. In many instances, no treatment is necessary. Cimetidine, an H_2 receptor blocker and a secretin antagonist, has been effective in blocking secretin-induced biliary epithelial secretion, with a consequent reduction in cyst size [64]. When cysts become infected, antibiotics alone are often ineffective and should be used in conjunction with a percutaneous drainage procedure [72]. For relief of pain or biliary compression, surgical approaches have included transhepatic fenestration or a combination of fenestration and resection procedures [73]. Fenestration also may be accomplished laparoscopically and provides symptomatic relief and reduction of liver size in some patients [74–76]. For patients with extensive involvement, liver transplantation has been successful as an isolated transplant or combined with a kidney transplant [77,78].

PATHOGENESIS AND ANIMAL MODELS

Much of the work elucidating pathogenesis and genetic control of development of these organs has been done by studying humans and animals with genetic cystic renal disorders. The genetic information is summarized in Table 39.4. Three working hypotheses have been proposed to account for renal cyst development: (1) tubule obstruction, (2) defective basement membrane assembly [79], or (3) dysregulated epithelial proliferation [52,80]. The weight of the experimental evidence from human and animal model studies suggests that dysregulated epithelial proliferation is of major importance [80,81]. Experimental evidence for the role of epithelial hyperplasia in renal cyst development includes the following: increased growth potential of cyst-derived epithelial cells [82,83], detection of epidermal growth factor (EGF) in renal cyst fluid [84], and overexpression with apical mislocation of EGF receptor in cystic kidneys [85]. Animal studies have confirmed that transforming growth factor-α (TGF-α) and EGF are cystogenic in murine organ culture [86] and that mice that overexpress TGF-α develop cystic kidneys [87]. Experimental manipulation of EGF receptor activity affects cyst development in vivo [88].

Tubular fluid hypersecretion is also observed in cyst development and has been attributed to the immature pattern of Na^+,K^+ ATPase distribution, with apical rather than basolateral expression of this enzyme, in cyst epithelia from both humans and mice [89,90].

Pathogenesis and identification of genetic influences on cyst development in the kidney and liver has been elucidated with murine models. The *CPK* mouse mutant develops ARPKD and death from renal failure in the first weeks of life [91]. The heterozygote has been noted to develop hepatic cysts [92]. Abnormally elevated expression of the protooncogenes c-*myc*, c-*fos*, and c-Ki-*ras* has been demonstrated in *cpk/cpk* cystic kidneys [93]; this protooncogene expression far exceeds the extent of cell proliferation. The intrinsic proliferative capacity of *cpk* cystic cells and ADPKD cystic cells is essentially the same as that of normal controls [94]. On the basis of these observations, it has been proposed that the elevated protooncogene expression reflects a maturational arrest in renal tubuloepithelial differentiation, which in turn leads to cyst formation [80]. In other words, cystic renal epithelia are unable to differentiate terminally, and their continued proliferation, albeit at a normal rate, results in cyst formation. Several other lines of evidence support this hypothesis. As discussed, in human ADPKD and ARPKD cystic epithelia, as well as *CPK* renal cysts, there are abnormalities in the membrane localization of the Na^+,K^+ ATPase [90] and the EGF receptor [88], consistent with a less differentiated cell phenotype. Another spontaneous mutant, *BPK*, develops both massively enlarged kidneys with cysts and proliferative bile duct dilatation [95]. The observation that the biliary epithelial hyperplasia in this animal was stimulated by EGF provided additional evidence for the role of this system [96].

A novel animal model in which the responsible gene has been identified and characterized is the insertional transgenic Tg737Rpw mutant, now called *ORPK* [95]. This mouse develops renal and hepatobiliary pathology similar to that seen in ARPKD/CHF. The mutant *Tg737* gene has been mapped to the mouse chromosome 14 [81], and its human homologue to human chromosome 13 [97]. Although this location eliminates the possibility that this is the gene for human ARPKD/CHF, studies of the encoded protein have greatly added to understanding of its possible functions, as well as interactions with other implicated gene products, such as polycystin 1 [98]. Of special interest to the understanding of the hepatic lesion is the model in which the renal disease is differentially corrected by experimental expression of the cloned wild-type complementary DNA (cDNA) [99]. These animals do not have the kidney disease but continue to have functional and histologic liver abnormalities [100]. Liver epithelial cell lines from both wild-type and mutant TgN737Rpw (ORPK) mice have been isolated and studied [88]. These cells have morphologic and immunologic characteristics of oval cells, which are felt to be pluripotent hepatic stem cells of primitive bile duct origin [101]. These characteristics include an immature pattern of gene expression and rapid proliferation. In culture, the cells give rise to dysplastic ductular structures [88]. Transfection of the mutant cell line with wild-type *Tg737* cDNA decreases the proliferation rate, indicating that this gene controls proliferation and differentiation of oval cells into normal mature biliary epithelium. Further evidence for this role is the recent characterization of *Tg737* as a hepatic tumor suppressor gene [102].

The exact molecular pathogenesis of ADPKD is being elucidated [103]. There are at least three genotypes resulting in virtually indistinguishable phenotypes. A major advance in the understanding of the pathogenesis of cystic diseases has been the identification and characterization of the gene products of the best studied ADPKD genes, *PKD1* and *PKD2*.

PKD1 is the gene responsible for most cases of ADPKD. Targeted deletion of exon 34 in Pkd1, the mouse homologue of this gene, results in renal cysts and perinatal death in homozygotes [104]. *Pkd1* heterozygote mice progressively develop renal and hepatic cysts (Figure 39.9). Hepatic cysts are observed in 27% of 9- to 14-month-old mice and 87% of older mice [105]. Human *PKD1* had been localized to chromosome 16, but the specific gene was elusive until a contiguous gene deletion was recognized in a family affected by both ADPKD and tuberous sclerosis. One family member had only tuberous sclerosis, and genetic analysis revealed the site of the translocation that disconnected the two disorders, allowing exact localization of *PKD1*. The product of this gene has been called polycystin 1. Polycystin 1, with 4304 amino acids, has a large extracellular domain, a membrane-spanning region, and a short intracellular region [106]. The intracellular carboxy-terminus has been demonstrated to interact with polycystin 2 [107]. The physicochemical characteristics of polycystin 1 suggest that it is likely involved in cell–cell or cell–matrix interactions. Polycystin 1 has been localized to renal tubular epithelia, hepatic bile ductules, pancreatic ducts, and cerebral blood vessels, tissues known to be affected in ADPKD [107]. Expression of polycystin is greater in fetal than adult tissue. When the immature cyst epithelia from ADPKD patients were studied, overexpression of polycystin 1 was detected [108]. In addition, monoclonality of the epithelial cells in a cyst has been demonstrated. Because ADPKD is a germline mutation, but cyst development is sporadic and focal (in a patient or in a family), it has been postulated that a "second hit" injury to the normal allele is necessary to permit proliferation and cyst development [109]. These second hits, which are obviously frequent given the manifestations of ADPKD, occur at the somatic level, explaining the phenotypic variability.

The gene product of *PKD2* is called polycystin 2. Physicochemical characterization suggests that it is a channel protein [110], possibly a calcium channel signal. The demonstration of the interaction of polycystins 1 and 2 [109] suggests that the phenotypic expression of ADPKD results from an abnormality in either gene, causing disruption of this interaction and subsequent abnormal regulation of the epithelial development. Loss of function of either protein results in the tubular cells reverting to a less differentiated state, which is more prone to proliferation. It has been postulated that the small proportion of ADPKD families that do not have either the *PKD1* or the *PKD2* mutation have an abnormality in the ligand or an intracellular partner of polycystin 1 or 2.

The primary cilium is a specialized sensory organelle, found in many types of epithelial cells, that senses fluid flow. Recent evidence indicates that polycystin 1 and polycystin 2 mediate the sensory process in the primary cilia of renal tubular cells [111]. Support for this putative mechanism of action is provided by the finding that the homolog in the *Tg737* mouse model of PKD is also localized to the primary cilium [112].

The affected gene in ARPKD is *PKDH1*. Twenty-nine mutations and 40 mutant alleles have been identified [25,26]. Mutations are scattered throughout the gene, and most *PKHD1* mutations are unique to single families [113]. *PKDH1* is expressed during development of kidney, lung, liver, and central nervous system. Fibrocystin, the product of *PKDH1*, acts as a membrane-associated protein affiliated with the primary cilia in renal epithelial cells of mice [114,115] and humans [115]. This localization at the apical domain of polarized epithelial cells suggests that fibrocystin, like polycystin 1 and 2, may be involved in tubulogenesis or maintenance of duct-lumen architecture.

As yet, similar studies have not been conducted on human biliary tissues. However, disruption of *Pkhd1*, the rat homologue associated with the PCK rat model, results in abnormal ciliary morphology in biliary epithelium [116]. Therefore, the observations in the kidney may perhaps be extended to the ductal plate malformation model, with abnormalities in primary cilia

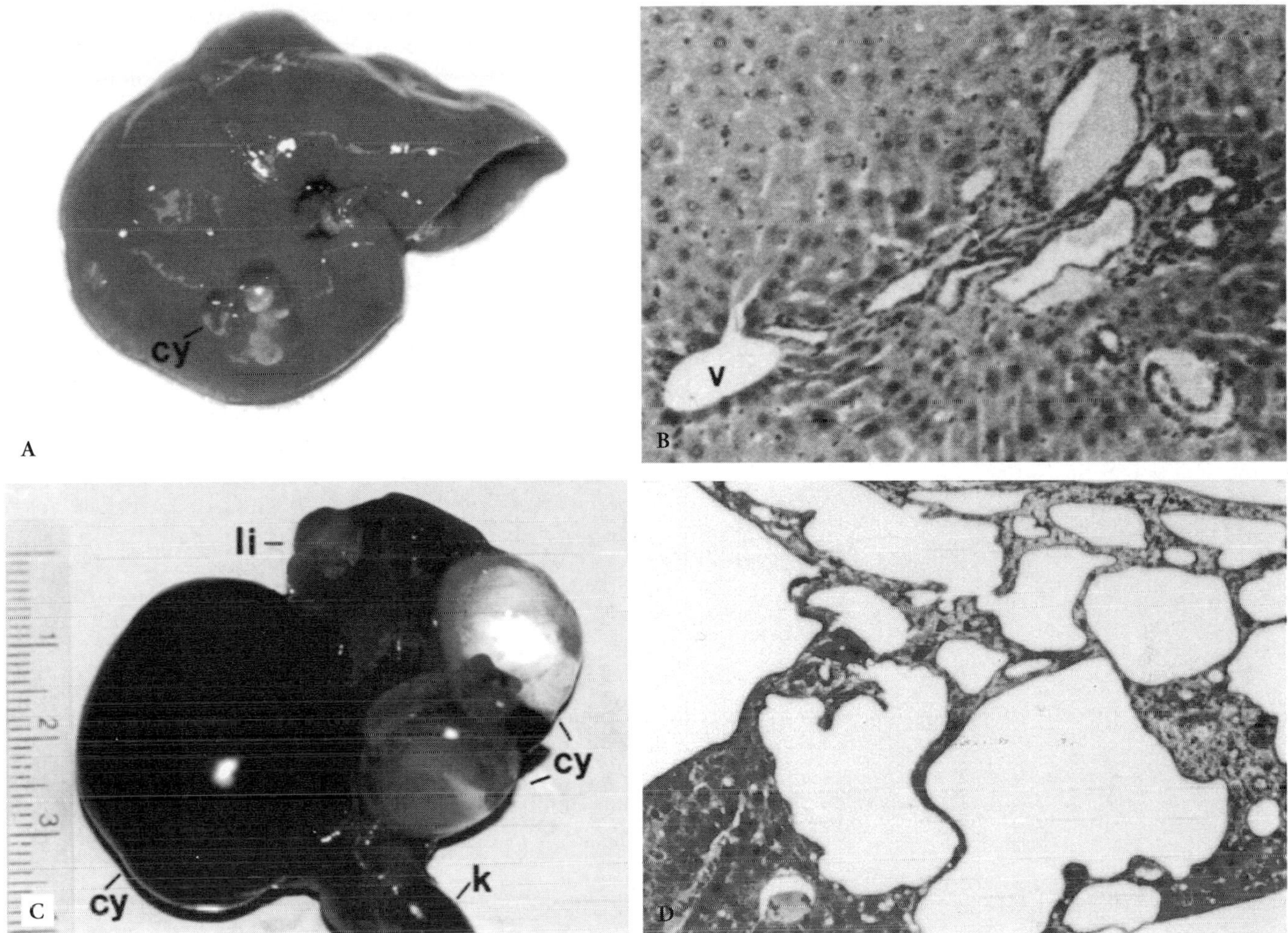

Figure 39.9. Specimens from *Pkd1* heterozygote mice. (**A**) The liver of an 11-month-old *Pkd1+/−* mouse with multilocular macroscopic cysts (cy). (**B**) Microscopic section of the liver reveals ductal plate malformation and cystic bile duct dilatation. (**C**) En bloc resection of the liver (li) and right kidney (ki). The liver contains many large cysts (cy). The kidneys are unremarkable. (**D**) Microscopic section of this liver reveals multiple back-to-back cysts.

function responsible for defective differentiation in both tissues. Jorgensen, Caroli, and Desmet have all hypothesized that ductal plate malformations arise from an arrest in the terminal differentiation of the ductal plate epithelia. This hypothesis is entirely consistent with various single gene mutations in fibrocystin causing a spectrum of disease phenotype.

Disease progression in the human polycystic kidney diseases and the CHF/Caroli's spectrum are all associated with variable degrees of necrotizing inflammation and fibrosis [5,117]. In the liver, Desmet [5] postulated that one or more fetal antigens that are expressed on the immature biliary epithelium trigger an autoimmune response. In many cases, there is no apparent inflammation in the liver, so that the stimulus to the vigorous fibrogenesis is not known. Recently, studies done in tissue homogenates from congenital hepatic fibrosis liver samples demonstrated higher levels of thrombospondin-1 and transforming growth factor-β_1 when compared with normal livers [118]. These cytokines are secreted by stellate cells, the most significant source of collagen in pathologic hepatic processes such as cirrhosis. The role of noninflammatory stellate cell activation in the pathogenesis of fibrocystic liver disease requires further study.

A proposed maturational arrest in renal and biliary tubuloepithelial differentiation could serve as a single unifying hypothesis to explain the spectrum of disease phenotypes, the development of renal cysts, and the fibrosis associated with disease progression in ARPKD, CHF, and Caroli's disease. However, although attractive, this construct is imperfect, because it does not adequately address several issues in ADPKD and PLD, that is, the less abundant fibrosis, the temporal disparity between renal and liver cyst formation, and the variable disease course in affected infants versus affected adults. Some of these discrepancies might be explained by the type of mutations identified. More precise formulation requires further work in both the human diseases and animal models to identify the genetic factors controlling renal tubular and biliary differentiation and growth. With these molecular tools, the pathogenic mechanisms operative in this spectrum of disease may be further unraveled.

REFERENCES

1. Bristowe C. Cystic disease of the liver associated with a similar disease of the kidneys. Trans Pathol Soc Lond 1856;7:229–34.
2. Karhunen PJ, Tenhu M. Adult polycystic liver and kidney diseases are separate entities. Clin Genet 1986;30:29–37.
3. D'Agata IDA, Jonas MM, Perez-Atayde AR, Guay-Woodford LM. Combined cystic disease of the liver and kidney. Semin Liv Dis 1994;14:215–28.
4. Jorgensen MJ. The ductal plate malformation. Acta Pathol Microbiol Immunol Scand Suppl A 1977;257:1–88.
5. Desmet VJ. Congenital diseases of intrahepatic bile ducts: variations on the theme "ductal plate malformation." Hepatology 1992;16:1069–83.
6. Van Eycken P, Sciot R, Callea F, et al. The development of the intrahepatic bile duct in man: a keratin-immunohistochemical study. Hepatology 1988;8:1586–95.
7. Stosiek P, Kasper M, Marsten V. Expression of cytokeratin 19 during human liver organogenesis. Liver 1990;10:59–63.
8. Desmet VJ, Van Eycken P, Scito R. Cytokeratins for probing cell lineage relation in developing liver. Hepatology 1990;12:1249–51.
9. Desmet VJ. Embryology of the liver and intrahepatic biliary tract, and an overview of malformations of the bile duct. In: McIntyre N, Benhamou J-P, Bircher J, Rizzetto M, Rodes J, eds. The Oxford textbook of clinical hepatology. Oxford, England: Oxford University Press; 1991:497–519.
10. Ruebner BH, Blankenberg TA, Burrows DA, et al. Development and transformation of the ductal plate in the developing human liver. Pediatr Pathol 1990;10:55–68.
11. Shah KD, Gerber MA. Development of intrahepatic bile ducts in humans. Arch Path Lab Med 1990;114:597–600.
12. Osathanondh V, Potter EL. Development of the human kidney as shown by microdissection. Arch Pathol 1963;76:277–302.
13. Saxen L. Organogenesis of the kidney. Cambridge, England: Cambridge University Press; 1987.
14. Black DD, Suttle EA, Whitington GL, et al. The effect of short term TPN in hepatic function in the human neonate: a prospective randomized study demonstrating alteration of hepatic canalicular function. J Pediatr 1981;99:445–9.
15. Lieberman E, Salinas-Madrigal L, Gwinn JL, et al. Infantile polycystic kidney disease of the kidney and liver: clinical, pathologic and radiologic correlations and comparison with congenital hepatic fibrosis. Medicine (Baltimore) 1971;50:277–318.
16. Zerres K, Volpel M-C, Weiss H. Cystic kidneys: genetics, pathologic anatomy, clinical picture and prenatal diagnosis. Hum Genet 1984;68:104–35.
17. Gabow PA. Autosomal dominant polycystic kidney disease. N Engl J Med 1993;329:332–42.
18. Pretorius DH, Lee ME, Manco-Johnson ML. Diagnosis of autosomal dominant polycystic kidney disease in utero and the young infant. J Ultrasound Med 1987;6:249–55.
19. Donovan MJ, Kozakewich H, Perez-Atayde A. Solitary nonparasitic cysts of the liver. Pediatr Pathol Lab Med 1995;15:419–28.
20. Pul N, Pul M. Congenital solitary nonparasitic cyst of the liver in infancy and childhood. J Pediatr Gastroenterol Nutr 1995; 21:461–2.
21. Kerr DNS, Harrison CV, Sherlock S, et al. Congenital hepatic fibrosis. Q J Med 1961;30:91–117.
22. Gang D, Herrin JT. Infantile polycystic disease of the liver and kidneys. Clin Nephrol 1986;25:28–36.
23. Kaplan BS, Fay J, Shah V, et al. Autosomal recessive polycystic kidney disease. Pediatr Nephrol 1989;3:43–9.
24. Blythe H, Ockenden BG. Polycystic disease of the kidneys and liver presenting in childhood. J Med Genet 1971;8:257–84.
25. Onuchic LF, Furu L, Nagasaka Y, et al. *PKHD1*, the polycystic kidney and hepatic disease 1 gene, encodes a novel large protein containing multiple immunogloulin-like plexin-transcription-factor domains and parallel beta-helix 1 repeats. Am J Hum Genet 2002;70:1305–17.
26. Ward CJ, Hogan MC, Rossetti S, et al. The gene mutated in autosomal recessive polycystic kidney disease encodes a large, receptor-like protein. Nat Genet 2002;30:259–69.
27. Rossetti S, Torra R, Coto E, et al. A complete mutation screen of PKHD1 in autosomal-recessive polycystic kidney disease (ARPKD) pedigrees. Kidney Int 2003;64:391–403.
28. Averback P. Congenital hepatic fibrosis: asymptomatic adults without renal anomaly. Arch Path Lab Med 1977;101:260–1.
29. Tazelaar HD, Payne JA, Patel S. Congenital hepatic fibrosis and asymptomatic familiary adult type polycystic disease in a 19 year old woman. Gastroenterology 1984;86:757–60.
30. Witzleben CL, Sharp A. Nephronophthisis-congenital hepatic fibrosis: an additional hepatorenal disorder. Hum Pathol 1982; 13:728–33.
31. Harris HW, Carpenter TO, Stanley P, et al. Progressive tubulointerstitial renal disease in infancy with associated hepatic abnormalities. Am J Med 1986;81:169–76.
32. Lewis SM, Roberts EA, Marcon MA, et al. Joubert syndrome with congenital hepatic fibrosis: an entity in the spectrum of oculo-encephalo-hepato-renal disorders. Am J Med Genet 1994;52:419–26.
33. Blankenberg TA, Ruebner BH, Ellis WG, et al. Pathology of renal and hepatic anomalies in Meckel syndrome. Am J Med Genet 1987;Suppl 3:395–410.
34. Cideciyan D, Rodriguez MM, Haun RL, et al. New findings in short rib syndrome. Am J Med Genet 1993;46:255–9.
35. Ivemark BI, Oldfelt V, Zetterstrom R. Familial dysplasia of kidneys, liver and pancreas: a probably genetically determined syndrome. Acta Paediatr 1959;48:1–11.
36. Torra R, Alos L, Ramos J, Estivill X. Renal–hepatic–pancreatic dysplasia: an autosomal recessive malformation. J Med Genet 1996;33:409–12.
37. Verloes A, Lambotte C. Further delineation of a syndrome of cerebellar vermis hypo/aplasia, oligophrenia, congenital ataxia, coloboma, and hepatic fibrosis. Am J Med Genet 1989;32:227–32.
38. Alvarez F, Bernard O, Brunelle F, et al. Congenital hepatic fibrosis in children. J Pediatr 1981;99:370–5.
39. Summerfeld JA, Nagafuchi Y, Sherlock S, et al. Hepatobiliary fibropolycystic diseases. A clinical and histologic review of 51 patients. J Hepatol 1986;2:141–56.
40. Desmet VJ. What is congenital hepatic fibrosis? Histopathology 1992;20:465–77.
41. Blankenberg TA, Lund JK, Reubner BH. Normal and abnormal development of human intrahepatic bile ducts: an immunohistochemical perspective. In: Abramowsky CR, Bernstein J, Rosenberg HS, eds. Perspectives in pediatric pathology: Transplantation pathology – hepatic morphogenesis. Basel, Switzerland: Karger; 1991:143–67.
42. Kerr DNS, Okonkwo S, Choa RG. Congenital hepatic fibrosis: the long term prognosis. Gut 1978;19:514–20.

43. Guay-Woodford LM, Bryda EC, Christine B, et al. Evidence that two phenotypically distinct mouse PKD mutations, bpk and jcpk, are allelic. Kidney Int 1996;50:1158–65.
44. Fiorillo RA, Migliorati R, Vajro P, Caldore M. Congenital hepatic fibrosis with GI bleeding in early infancy. Clin Pediatr 1982;21:183–5.
45. Bernstein J, Slovis TL. Polycystic diseases of the kidney. In: Edelmann CM Jr, ed. Pediatric jidney disease. Boston: Little, Brown; 1992:1139–53.
46. Caroli J, Couinaud C, Soupault R, et al. Une affection nouvelle, sans doute congénitale, des voies biliaires: la dilatation cystique unilobaire des canaux hépatiques. Sem Hop Paris 1958;34:136–42.
47. Kocoshis SA, Riely CA, Burrell M, Gryboski J. Cholangitis in a child due to biliary tract anomalies. Dig Dis Sci 1980;25:59–65.
48. Jordan D, Harpaz N, Thung SN. Caroli's disease and adult polycystic kidney disease: a rarely recognized association. Liver 1989;9:30–5.
49. Todani T, Watanabe Y, Narusue M, et al. Congenital bile duct cysts: classification, operative procedures and review of thirty seven cases including cancer arising from choledochal cyst. Am J Surg 1977;134:263–9.
50. Lowenfels A. Does bile promote extracolonic cancer? Lancet 1978;2:239–41.
51. Raymond M-J, Huguet C, Danan G, et al. Partial hepatectomy in the treatment of Caroli's disease. Dig Dis Sci 1984;29:367–70.
52. Welling LW, Grantham JJ. Cystic and developmental diseases of the kidney. In: Brenner BM, Rector FC Jr, eds. The kidney. Philadelphia: WB Saunders, 1991:33–6.
53. Grunfeld JP, Albouze G, Junger P. Liver changes and complications in adult polycystic kidney disease. Adv Nephrol 1985;14:1–20.
54. Lipschitz B, Berdon WE, Defelice AR, Levy J. Association of congenital hepatic fibrosis with autosomal dominant polycystic kidney disease. Pediatr Radiol 1993;23:131–3.
55. Reeders ST, Breuning MH, Davies KE, et al. A highly polymorphic DNA marker linked to adult polycystic kidney disease on chromosome 16. Nature 1985;317:542–4.
56. Kimberling WJ, Kumar S, Gabow PA, et al. Autosomal dominant polycystic kidney disease: localization of the second gene to chromosome 4q13-q23. Genomics 1993;18:467–72.
57. Peters DJM, Spruit L, Sarris JJ, et al. Chromosome 4 localization of a second gene for autosomal dominant polycystic kidney disease. Nat Genet 1993;5:359–62.
58. Ariza M, Alvarez V, Marin R, et al. A family with a milder form of adult dominant polycystic kidney disease not linked to the PKD1 (16p) or PKD2 (4q) genes. J Med Genet 1997;34:587–9.
59. Desmet VJ. Ludwig symposium on biliary disorders – part I. Pathogenesis of ductal plate abnormalities. Mayo Clin Proc 1998;73:80–9.
60. Otha W, Ushio H. Histological reconstruction of von Meyenberg's complex on the liver surface. Endoscopy 1984;16:71–4.
61. Homer LW, White HJ, Read RC. Neoplastic transformation of von Meyenburg complexes of the liver. J Pathol Bacteriol 1968;96:499–502.
62. Honda N, Cobb C, Lechago J. Bile duct carcinoma associated with multiple von Meyenburg complexes in the liver. Hum Pathol 1986;17:1287–90.
63. Burns CD, Kuhns JG, Wieman TJ. Cholangiocarcinoma in association with multiple biliary microhamartomas. Arch Path Lab Med 1990;114:1287–9.
64. Everson GT. Hepatic cysts in autosomal dominant polycystic kidney disease (editorial). Mayo Clin Proc 1990;65:1020–5.
65. Gabow PA, Johnson AM, Kaehny WD, et al. Risk factors for the development of hepatic cysts in autosomal dominant polycystic disease. Hepatology 1990;11:1033–7.
66. Ramos A, Torres VE, Holley KE, et al. The liver in autosomal dominant polycystic kidney disease. Implications for pathogenesis. Arch Path Lab Med 1990;114:180–4.
67. Pirson Y, Lannoy N, Peters D, et al. Isolated polycystic liver disease as a distinct genetic disease, unlinked to polycystic kidney disease 1 and polycystic kidney disease 2. Hepatology 1996; 23:249–52.
68. Iglesias DM, Palmitano JA, Arrizurieta E, et al. Isolated polycystic liver disease not linked to polycystic kidney disease 1 and 2. Dig Dis Sci 1999;44:385–8.
69. Qian Q, Li A, King BF, et al. Clinical profile of autosomal dominant polycystic liver disease. Hepatology 2003;37:164–71.
70. Drenth JP, Tahvanainen E, te Morsche RH, et al. Abnormal hepatocystin caused by truncating PRKCSH mutations leads to autosomal dominant polycystic liver disease. Hepatology: Official journal of the American Association for the Study of Liver Diseases 2004;39:924–31.
71. Jaeken J, Matthijs G, Saudubray J-M, et al. Phosphomannose isomerase deficiency: a carbohydrate-deficient glycoprotein syndrome with hepatic–intestinal presentation. Am J Hum Genet 1998;62:1535–9.
72. Telenti A, Torres VE, Gross JB Jr, et al. Hepatic cyst infection in autosomal dominant polycystic kidney disease. Mayo Clin Proc 1990;65:933–42.
73. Newman KD, Torres VE, Rakela J, Nagorney DN. Treatment of highly symptomatic polycystic liver disease. Ann Surg 1990; 212:30–7.
74. Kabbej M, Sauvanet A, Chauveau D, et al. Laparoscopic fenestration in polycystic liver disease. Brit J Surg 1996;83:1697–701.
75. Gigot JF, Jadoul P, Que F, et al. Adult polycystic liver disease: is fenestration the most adequate operation for long-term management? Ann Surg 1997;225:286–94.
76. Martin IJ, McKinley AJ, Currie EJ, et al. Tailoring the management of nonparasitic liver cysts. Ann Surg 1998;228:167–72.
77. Washburn WK, Johnson LB, Lewis WD, Jenkins RL. Liver transplantation for adult polycystic liver disease. Liv Transplant Surg 1996;2:17–22.
78. Swenson K, Seu P, Kinkhabwala M, et al. Liver transplantation for adult polycystic liver disease. Hepatology 1998;28:412–15.
79. Taub M, Laurie GW, Martin GR, et al. Altered basement membrane protein biosynthesis by primary cultures of *cpk/cpk* mouse kidney. Kidney Int 1990;37:1090–7.
80. Calvet JP. Polycystic kidney disease: primary extracellular matrix abnormality or defective cellular differentiation? Kidney Int 1993;43:101–8.
81. Avner ED, Studnicki FE, Young MC, et al. Congenital murine polycystic disease. Pediatr Nephrol 1987;1:587–96.
82. Wilson PD, Sherwood AC. Tubulocystic epithelium. Kidney Int 1991;39:450–63.
83. Hjelle JT, Waterds DC, Golinska BT, et al. Autosomal recessive polycystic kidney disease: characterization of human peritoneal and cystic kidney cells in vitro. Am J Kidney Dis 1990;15:123–36.
84. Wilson PD, Du J, Norman JT. Autocrine, endocrine, and paracrine regulation of growth abnormalities in autosomal dominant polycystic kidney disease. Eur J Cell Biol 1993;61:131–8.
85. Du J, Wilson PD. Abnormal polarization of EGF receptors and autocrine stimulation of cyst epithelial growth in human ADPKD. Am J Physiol 1995;269:C487–95.

86. Avner ED, Sweeney WE. Polypeptide growth factors in metanephric growth and segmental nephron differentiation. Pediatr Nephrol 1990;4:372–7.
87. Lowden Da, Lindemann gw, Merlino G, et al. Renal cysts in transgenic mice expressing transforming growth factor-alpha. J Lab Clin Med 1994;124:386–94.
88. Richards WG, Sweeney WE, Yoder BK, et al. Epidermal growth factor receptor activity mediates renal cyst formation in polycystic kidney disease. J Clin Invest 1998;101:935–9.
89. Wilson PD, Sherwood AC, Palla K, et al. Reversed polarity of Na^+K^+-ATPase: mislocation to apical plasma membranes in human polycystic kidney disease epithelia. Am J Physiol 1992; 260:F1–11.
90. Avner ED, Sweeney WE, Nelson WJ. Abnormal sodium pump distribution during renal tubulogenesis in congenital murine polycystic kidney disease. Proc Natl Acad Sci U S A 1992;89: 7447–51.
91. Gattone VH, Calvet JP, Cowley BD, et al. Autosomal recessive polycystic kidney disease in a murine model: a gross and microscopic description. Lab Invest 1988;59:231–8.
92. Crocker JFA, Blecher SR, Givner ML, et al. Polycystic kidney and liver disease and corticosterone changes in the CPK mouse. Kid Internat 1987;31:1088–91.
93. Cowley BD Jr, Chadwick LJ, Grantham JJ, et al. Elevated protooncogene expression in polycystic kidneys of the C57BL/6J (*cpk*) mouse. J Am Soc Nephrol 1991;1:1048–53.
94. Carone FA, Nakanura S, Schumacher BS, et al. Cyst-derived cells do not exhibit accelerated growth or features of transformed cells in vitro. Kidney Int 1989;35:1351–7.
95. Nauta J, Ozawa Y, Sweeney WE Jr, et al. Renal and biliary abnormalities in a new murine model of autosomal recessive polycystic kidney disease. Pediatr Nephrol 1993;7:163–72.
96. Nauta J, Sweeney WE, Rutledge JC, et al. Biliary epithelial cells from mice with congenital polycystic kidney disease are hyperresponsive to epidermal growth factor. Pediatr Res 1995;37:755–63.
97. Onuchic LF, Schrick JJ, Ma J, et al. Sequence analysis of the human hTg737gene and its polymorphic sites in patients with autosomal recessive polycystic kidney disease. Mamm Genome 1995;5:805–8.
98. Yoder BK, Wilkinson JE, Avner ED, et al. The Tg737 protein interacts with polycystin and proteins controlling epithelial polarity, EGFR stability and cellular differentiation. J Am Soc Nephrol 1997;8:386A.
99. Yoder MK, Richard WG, Sommardahl C, et al. Functional correction of renal defects in a mouse model for ARPKD through expression of the cloned wild-type *Tg737* cDNA. Kidney Int 1996;50:1240–8.
100. Yoder BK, Richards WG, Sommerdahl C, et al. Differential rescue of the renal and hepatic disease in an autosomal recessive polycystic kidney disease mouse mutant. A new model to study the liver lesion. Am J Pathol 1997;150:2231–41.
101. Tian YW, Smith PG, Yeoh GC. The oval-shaped cell as a candidate for a liver stem cell in embryonic, neonatal and precancerous liver: identification based on morphology and immunohistochemical staining for albumin and pyruvate kinase isoenzyme expression. Histochem Cell Biol 1997;107:243–50.
102. Isfort RJ, Cody DB, Doersen CJ, et al. The tetratricopeptide repeat containing Tg737 gene is a liver neoplasia tumor suppressor gene. Oncogene 1997;15:1797–803.
103. Al-Bhalal L, Akhtar M. Molecular basis of autosomal dominant polycystic kidney disease. Adv Anat Pathol 2005;12:126–33.
104. Lu W, Peissel B, Babakhanlou H, et al. Perinatal lethality with kidney and pancreas defects in mice with a targeted Pkd1 mutation. Nat Genet 1997;17:179–81.
105. Lu W, Fan X, Basora N, et al. Late onset of renal and hepatic cysts in Pkd1-targeted heterozygotes [letter]. Nat Genet 1999;21: 160–1.
106. The International Polycystic Kidney Disease Consortium. Polycystic kidney disease: the complete structure of the *PKD1* gene and its protein. Cell 1995;81:289–98.
107. Qian F, Germino FJ, Cai Y, et al. PKD1 interacts with PKD2 through a probable coiled-coil domain. Nat Genet 1997;16:179–83.
108. Geng L, Segal Y, Peissel B, et al. Identification and localization of polycystin, the PKD1 gene product. J Clin Invest 1996;98:2674–82.
109. Qian F, Watnick TJ, Onuchic LF, Germino GG. The molecular basis of focal cyst formation in human autosomal dominant polycystic kidney disease type I. Cell 1996;87:979–87.
110. Mochizuki T, Wu G, Hayashi T, et al. PKD2, a gene for polycystic kidney disease that encodes an integral membrane protein. Science 1996;272:1339–42.
111. Nauli SM, Alenghat FJ, Luo Y, et al. Polycystins 1 and 2 mediate mechanosensation in the primary cilium of kidney cells. Nat Genet 2003;33:129–37.
112. Pazour GJ, Dickert BL, Vucica Y, et al. *Chlamydomonas IFT88* and its mouse homologue, polycystic kidney disease gene *tg737*, are required for assembly of cilia and flagella. J Cell Biol 2000; 151:709–18.
113. Bergmann C, Senderek J, K1/4pper F, et al. PKHD1 mutations in autosomal recessive polycystic kidney disease ([ARPKD)]. Hum Mutat 2004;23:453–63.
114. Zhang M-Z, Mai W, Li C, et al. PKHD1 protein encoded by the gene for autosomal recessive polycystic kidney disease associates with basal bodies and primary cilia in renal epithelial cells. Proc Natl Acad Sci U S A 2004;101:2311–16.
115. Wang S, Luo Y, Wilson PD, Witman GB, Zhou J. The autosomal recessive polycystic kidney disease protein is localized to primary cilia, with concentration in the basal body area. J Am Soc Nephrol 2004;15:592–602.
116. Masyuk TV, Huang BQ, Masyuk AI, et al. Biliary dysgenesis in the PCK rat, an orthologous model of autosomal recessive polycystic kidney disease. Am J Pathol 2004;165:1719–30.
117. Hepinstall RH. Pathology of the kidney. 4th ed. Boston: Little, Brown, 1992.
118. El-Youssef M, Mu Y, Huang L, Stellmach V, Crawford SE. Increased expression of transforming growth factor-β_1 and thrombospondin-1 in congenital hepatic fibrosis: possible role of the hepatic stellate cell. J Pediatr Gastroenterol Nutr 1999;28: 386–92.
119. Whitley CB, Schwarzenberg SJ, Burke BA, et al. Direct hyperbilirubinemia and hepatic fibrosis: a new presentation of Jeune syndrome (asphyxiating thoracic dystrophy). Am J Med Genet 1987;Suppl 3:211–20.
120. Pelletier VA, Galéano N, Brochu P, et al. Secretory diarrhea with protein-losing enteropathy, enterocolitis cystica superficialis, intestinal lymphangiectasia, and congenital hepatic fibrosis: a new syndrome. J Pediatr 1985;107:61–5.
121. Nishimura G, Nakayama M, Fuke Y, Suehara N. A lethal osteochondrodysplasia with mesomelic brachymelia, round pelvis, and congenital hepatic fibrosis. Pediatr Radiol 1998;28: 43–7.

40

Tumors of the Liver

Dolores López-Terrada, M.D., Ph.D., and Milton J. Finegold, M.D.

The clinical presentation of the vast majority of liver tumors in children is an asymptomatic palpable mass. The majority of malignancies are large and may be difficult to excise without prior chemotherapy because the liver's functional capacity is rarely compromised by underlying cirrhosis. Involvement of the perihilar segments or intrahepatic dissemination may necessitate transplantation. The vascularity of the liver and ready access of cancer cells to hepatic veins make pulmonary metastasis at presentation relatively common. Therefore, knowledge of precursor conditions and screening can be lifesaving.

Approximately two thirds of all liver masses occurring in children are malignant. Twenty separate series totaling 1972 primary benign and malignant liver tumors in children from 1956 to 2001 included hepatoblastomas (HB; 37%), hepatocellular carcinomas (HCC; 21%), benign vascular tumors (15%), mesenchymal hamartomas and sarcomas (8%), adenomas and focal nodular hyperplasia (7.5%), and other tumors (4%) [1,2] (Table 40.1).

EPIDEMIOLOGY

Approximately 1.1% of all childhood tumors in the United States are malignant liver tumors according to the Surveillance, Epidemiology, and End Results (SEER) program cancer registries, with an annual incidence rate of 1.8 cases per million children younger than 15 years [3]. Of 123 children registered with malignant liver tumors in 2000, 80% had HB and they accounted for 91% of primary hepatic malignancy cases in children aged less than 5 years [4]. Primary liver tumors accounted for 6–8% of congenital tumors in Isaacs's review of 265 neoplasms discovered within 30 days of birth [5].

The mean age at diagnosis was 19 months and the median age was 16 months in the Pediatric Oncology Group (POG) series of 106 HB accrued on biologic studies, similar to findings in other studies [4,6,7]. Only 5% of cases occurred in children older than 4 years. Although rarely, HB has been reported in adults [8–10]. It is slightly more common in males with a reported male-to-female ratio of 1.4–2.0:1.0 [4].

Data from several sources have shown an increase in the number of cases of HB during the past 2 decades. In the SEER data comparing the periods 1973–1977 with 1993–1997, HB rates increased from 0.6 to 1.2 per million, and pediatric HCC rates decreased (0.45–0.29 per million) [4]. In the period 1979–1981, liver cancers represented 2% of all cancers in infants younger than 1 year, whereas a decade later, liver cancers increased to 4% of all cancers in infants [11,12].

A higher incidence of malignant liver tumors in children has been seen in Africa and Asia, where hepatitis B infection is common. It is not surprising that almost all of the tumors are HCC because this tumor has been most closely correlated with hepatitis infection. Perinatally acquired hepatitis B has also been demonstrated to have integrated into the genome in tumors from children with no clinical signs of present or past hepatitis B infection [13,14]. It is encouraging that aggressive immunization programs against hepatitis have resulted in a decrease in the number of cases [15,16].

Hepatocellular carcinoma occurs primarily after age 10 years and is the most common hepatic malignancy of adolescence. In children 15–19 years of age, HCC accounted for 87% of all malignant liver tumors, but 12.8% occurred in children under age 5 years [4]. Patients with the fibrolamellar variant of HCC are more likely to be over age 10 years [17].

ETIOLOGY

The causes of most liver tumors, similar to other types of childhood cancer, are unknown. Hepatoblastoma occurs in association with several well-described cancer genetic syndromes (Table 40.2), whereas HCC often occurs after the development of cirrhosis, which may have both genetic and environmental contributions. The strong association of HB with prematurity may account for part of the observed increase in HB overall, because survival rates continue to increase among very small premature infants [18,19]. In Japan, HB account for 58% of all malignancies occurring in surviving premature infants weighing less than 1000 g at birth [19]. The Japanese Children's Cancer

Table 40.1: Hepatic Tumors in Childhood

Primary Tumors	*Number*	*%*
Hepatoblastoma	737	37
Hepatocellular carcinoma	422	21
Adenoma	50	2.5
Focal nodular hyperplasia	94	5
Benign vascular tumors	190	15
Mesenchymal hamartoma	133	7
Sarcoma (embryonal, angio, rhabdo)	156	8
Other	90	4

Data are from Weinberg and Finegold [1] and Stocker [2].

Registry data revealed that 15 of 303 (5%) HB between 1985 and 1995 occurred in post-premature infants weighing less than 1500 g. The relative risk for infants weighing less than 1000 g at birth was 15.64 compared with 2.53 for infants weighing 1000–1499 g and 1.21 for infants weighing 2000–2499 g [20]. California's population-based cancer registry confirmed the strikingly elevated risk of HB in children who were born with very low birth weight (less than 1500 g), suggesting that the etiology may differ between children with very low birth weight and children with normal birth weight [21,22]. These data indicate the need to determine the specific factors related to prematurity that contribute to hepatic tumorigenesis, as well as the need for surveillance of the survivors of extreme prematurity. To date, no differences have been found in age of onset or histopathologic type of HB in small premature births versus term births, and even stage IV disease at presentation or recurrence did not prevent cure in a recent series of four such infants [22]. Several studies have explored relationships between perinatal and maternal factors other than congenital syndromes and low birth weight, and hepatoblastoma. A recent study documented a potential link with maternal pre-eclampsia and eclampsia [23]. Environmental factors have also been implicated in HB. An association with certain occupational exposures in fathers of children with HB has been reported [24]. These include excess exposures to metals such as in welding and soldering fumes (odds ratio 8.0), petroleum products, and paints (odds ratio 3.7). Prenatal exposure to acetaminophen in combination with petroleum products has also been noted in association with HB [25]. Parental cigarette smoking has also been reported to be associated with an increased risk of developing hepatoblastoma, doubled if both parents smoked, relative to neither parent smoking [26,27]. Cirrhosis following parenteral nutrition in infancy has been associated with the development of HCC in childhood [28,29]. Understanding the role that parenteral nutrition, which is clearly lifesaving for many premature infants, plays in the observed increase in the subsequent development of liver cancer in premature infants will await additional epidemiologic and pathophysiologic studies.

Constitutional Genetic and Metabolic Abnormalities

Associations of liver tumors in children with genetic syndromes are summarized in Table 40.2.

Beckwith–Wiedemann syndrome (BWS) is caused by genetic abnormalities in chromosomal region 11p15 and a risk of diverse intra-abdominal embryonal tumors. The National Cancer Institute's BWS support group data indicate a relative risk of HB as 2280, higher than that for other embryonal tumors, including Wilms's tumor [30]. The recognition of physical stigmata of BWS in an infant should prompt surveillance for detection for embryonal tumors by means of serial abdominal sonography and serum α-fetoprotein (AFP) measurements [31] and thus has proved beneficial to early resection. Vascular proliferations in the liver are also observed in BWS and have been misdiagnosed as HB because of serum AFP elevation (Figure 40.1).

A significantly higher risk of neoplasia was recently reported in association with certain molecular subtypes of BWS, particularly patients with uniparental disomy (UPD) and imprinting control element (IC1) defects [32]. Patients with hemihypertrophy also carry a higher risk of developing HB [31]. Hepatoblastoma has been reported in association with other over growth syndromes [33], particularly Simpson–Golabi–Behmel syndrome, an X-linked overgrowth syndrome caused by deletions in the glypican 3 (*GPC3*) gene [34–36]. The recognition of BWS as a spectrum of disorders, and the identification of molecular subtypes, has enhanced the management and surveillance of BWS children, including screening for hepatoblastoma [37].

The association of HB with familial adenomatous polyposis (FAP) was first reported in 1982 [38]. This syndrome is caused by germline mutation of the adenomatous polyposis coli (*APC*) gene [39]. Giardiello et al. [39] estimated a relative risk of 800 of HB in children in FAP families compared with the general population risk. Five of 50 children with apparently sporadic HB were found to have a constitutional mutation in *APC* [40]. In many HB cases without a family history of FAP, mutations are present in tumor [41]. The interaction of *APC* protein with β-catenin in the WNT pathway in the pathogenesis of HB is discussed later (see Acquired Genetic Changes). There are no definitive differences in age range, histologic type, or outcome in HB associated with FAP. Furthermore, FAP has been implicated in the pathogenesis of some cases of hepatocellular adenoma, HCC, and fibrolamellar carcinoma, and thus it has been suggested that mutation of the *APC* may confer a general low-level predisposition to tumorigenesis in the liver, dependent on other environmental or developmental factors [42].

Children with hereditary tyrosinemia type 1 (fumarylacetoacetate hydrolase deficiency) have a very high incidence of HCC [43,44], which has been dramatically reduced by blocking the accumulation of toxic metabolites [45,46]. Glycogen storage diseases are also associated with the development of adenomas (Figure 40.2A and 40.2B) and occasionally HCC [47–49]. HCC and cholangiocarcinomas have been observed in patients with the Alagille syndrome and other familial cholestatic syndromes (Figure 40.2C–40.2F) [50,51]. Many but not all of the latter are

Table 40.2: Constitutional Genetic Syndromes Leading to Liver Tumors

Disease	*Tumor Type*	*Chromosome Location*	*Gene*
Familial adenomatous polyposis	HB, HCC, adenoma, biliary adenoma	5q21.22	APC
Beckwith–Wiedemann syndrome	HB, vascular lesions – hemangioendothelioma	11p15.5	P57KiP2:Wnt, others
Li–Fraumeni syndrome	HB, undifferentiated sarcoma	17p13	TP53:others
Trisomy 18	HB	18	—
Glycogen storage diseases types I–IV	HB, HCC, adenoma	Several	—
Hereditary tyrosinemia, type 1	HCC	15q23–25	Fumarylacetoacetate hydrolase
Alagille syndrome	HCC	20p12	Jagged 1
Other familial cholestatic syndromes	HCC	18q21–22:2q24	FIC1:ABCB 11
Neurofibromatosis	HCC, malignant Schwannoma, angiosarcoma	17q11.2	NF-1
Ataxia telangiectasia	HCC	11q22–23	ATM
Fanconi anemia	HCC, fibrolamellar carcinoma, adenoma	1q42:3p,20q13.2–13.3:others	FAA, FAC, others (20%)
Tuberous sclerosis	Angiomyolipoma	9q34:16p13	TSC1:TSC2
Simpson–Golabi–Behmel syndrome	Hepatoblastoma and others (Wilms)	Xq26:Xp22	Glypican-3

APC, adenomatous polyposis coli; ATM, ataxia telangiectasia mutated; FAA, Fanconi anemia complementation group A; FAC, Fanconi anemia complementation group C; FIC1, familial intrahepatic cholestasis, type I; NF-1, neurofibromatosis, type 1; TSC1, tuberous sclerosis complex 1, TSC2, tuberous sclerosis complex 2.

also associated with liver dysfunction and cirrhosis of the liver. The chronic cholestasis resulting from extrahepatic biliary atresia has preceded both HCC and HB in children [52]. A case of HB in a 2-year-old child with progressive familial intrahepatic cholestasis has also been documented [53]. We have seen three HB in 2-year-old children with autosomal recessive polycystic kidney disease.

Diverse liver tumors have been reported in association with trisomy 18, neurofibromatosis, tuberous sclerosis, and ataxia–telangiectasia [54–58]. Hepatic tumors occurring in patients with Fanconi's anemia who are treated with anabolic steroids demonstrate how a genetic defect in DNA repair coupled with an exogenous agent may contribute to the development of neoplasia. In some cases, tumor regression has been observed with the withdrawal of steroids [59,60].

CLINICAL PRESENTATION

The typical age of presentation of the various hepatic tumors, both benign and malignant, is shown in Table 40.3. Yolk sac tumors, primary endocrine neoplasms, and inflammatory myofibroblastic tumors are very rare and occur in adults more often than children [61]. Most liver tumors present with an asymptomatic abdominal mass [62]. Abdominal pain, weight loss, anorexia, nausea, and vomiting may be present, particularly in advanced disease [63]. Jaundice is rare and usually a symptom of extensive disease or hilar growth of any neoplasm with compression of the major bile ducts, such as inflammatory myofibroblastic tumor at the hilum [64] or by rhabdomyosarcoma, which arises in close association with larger ducts [65]. Infants with hemangioendothelioma or hemangiomas associated with arteriovenous malformations may present with signs and symptoms of congestive heart failure [66]. In infants, diffuse hepatomegaly may occur secondary to transient myeloproliferative disorders or megakaryoblastic leukemia. In cases of severe organ dysfunction, even the former may require chemotherapy [67]. Disseminated neuroblastoma may also present as hepatic masses, as can Wilms's tumor.

Clinical symptoms of precocious puberty are due to secretion of human β-chorionic gonadotropin or testosterone [68,69]. The prognosis for seven children with HCC producing HB in Japan was very poor, with only one survivor [70]. Cushing syndrome due to corticotropin-secreting hepatic malignancies with a distinctive nested pattern has been seen in two girls aged 11 and 12 years [71,72]. Large liver hemangiomas can be associated with profound hypothyroidism [73]. Hypertension secondary to a renin-secreting mixed HB has been reported [74].

Liver enzymes and bilirubin are usually normal or only mildly elevated. A mild and normochromic, normocytic anemia is common. Thrombocytosis occurs in approximately 50–80% of patients with HB and is probably related to thrombopoietin production by the tumor [75,76]. Mild coagulation

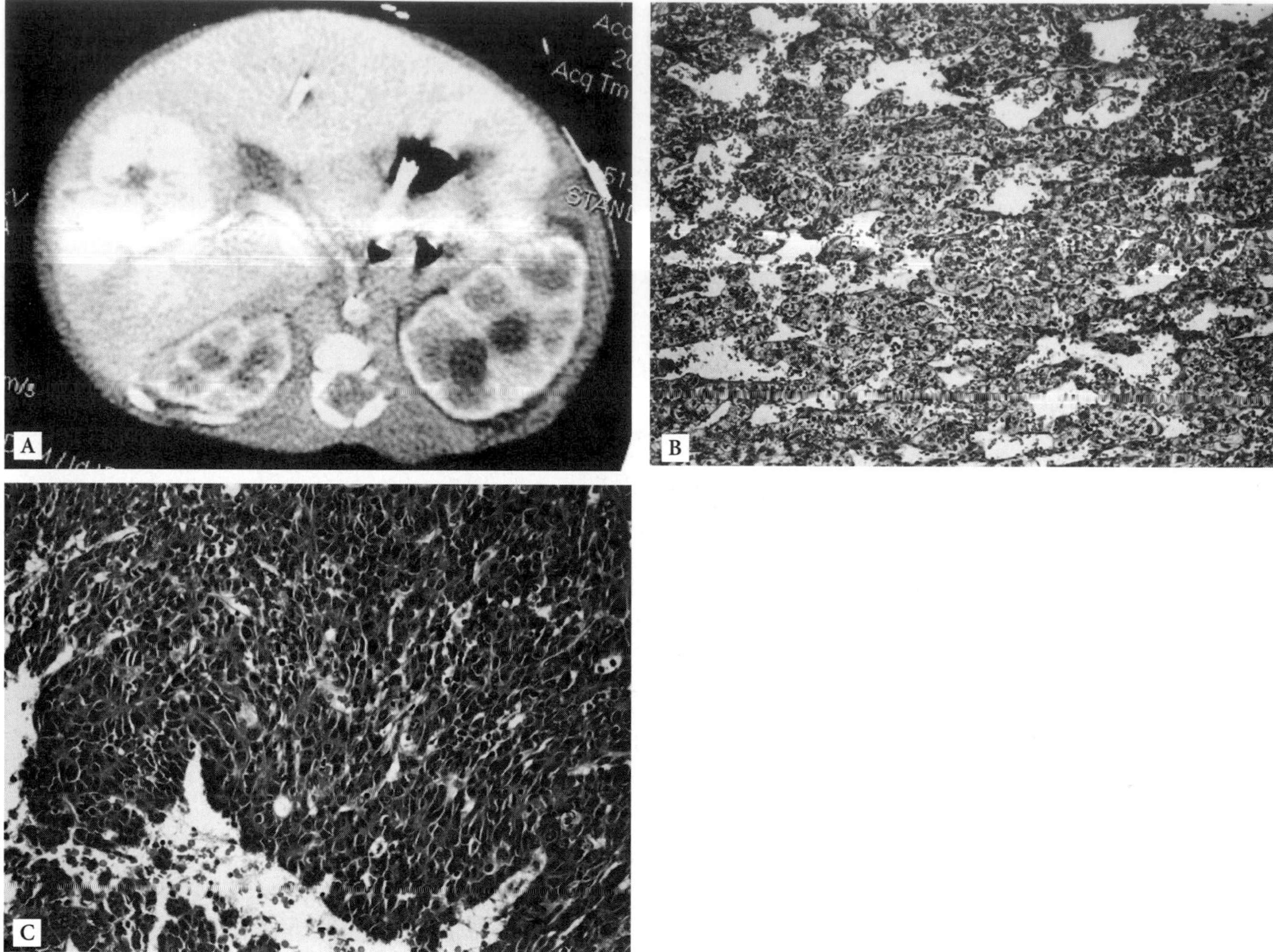

Figure 40.1. Hepatic tumors in Beckwith–Wiedemann syndrome. (**A**) CT at 1 week of age shows large enhancing mass and prominent hepatic artery. (**B**) Hemangioma with cavernous channels. No hepatocellular neoplasia. (**C**) Embryonal hepatoblastoma in an 8-month-old was detected by screening and cured by surgery and adjuvant chemotherapy.

abnormalities in children with malignant liver tumors are not unusual and a picture of a consumptive coagulopathy is sometimes associated with vascular malformations or a Kaposiform hemangioendothelioma (Kasabach–Merritt phenomenon) [77].

METHODS OF DIAGNOSIS

Assessment of a liver tumor often begins with diagnostic imaging by plain film or ultrasonography, which reveals a right upper quadrant mass. Calcifications are seen only in a minority of cases and are nonspecific and plain films are of very limited value in characterizing hepatic masses. Increased echogenicity on sonography is suggestive of malignant disease, and the diagnostic yield is increased when accompanied by Doppler flow studies to assess tumor vascularity. However, sonography is not adequate to definitively establish resectability [78]. To define the extent of disease accurately, computerized tomography (CT) scanning is used (Figure 40.3A) [79,80]. Particularly in infants, none of the imaging techniques currently available has 100% specificity. Of 26 children under age 3 months, 6 were inappropriately treated in the German cooperative liver tumor study because of imaging misinterpretations [81]. Magnetic resonance imaging (MRI) with enhancement may provide additional information and reduce exposure of young children to ionizing radiation (Figure 40.3B) [82]. For recurrent or metastatic HB, positron emission tomography scanning with F^{18}-fluorodeoxyglucose has proved to be more sensitive than MRI or CT [83]. Intrahepatic vascular dissemination of HCC is more common than in HB (Figure 40.4A), but both neoplasms have this propensity (Figure 40.4B). The most common site for metastases is the lung (Figure 40.4C), whereas metastases to the brain have been reported but are extremely rare [6,84,85]. Therefore, CT imaging of the chest, abdomen, and pelvis is essential. When bone lesions are reported, it is unclear whether these represent true metastases or areas of osteopenia, and bone marrow involvement has only very rarely been observed [86].

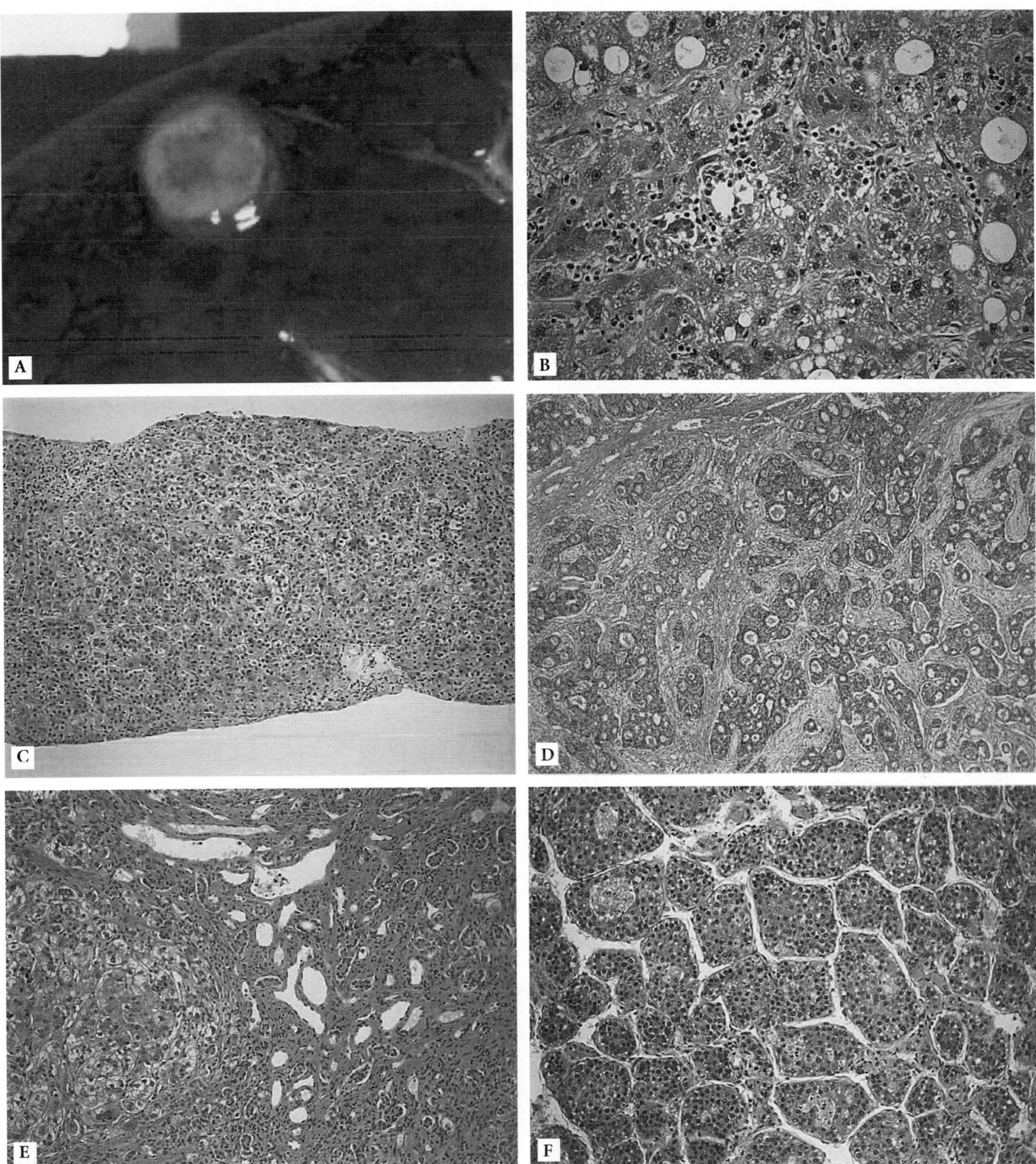

Figure 40.2. Metabolic diseases leading to neoplasia. (**A**) Adenoma in autopsy liver of a 12-year-old with glycogen storage disease (GSD), type 1A (glucose 6 phosphatase deficiency). (**B**) Adenoma in GSD 1A has "alcoholic hepatitis"–like histology with fat, Mallory bodies, and inflammation. (**C**) Alagille syndrome. Biopsy at 4 months of age shows bland cholestasis and paucity of the bile ducts. (**D**) Cholangiocarcinoma at age 8 years. (**E**) Biliary cirrhosis at age 29 months, secondary to bile salt excretory protein deficiency (progressive familial intrahepatic cholestasis type 2). (**F**) Hepatocarcinoma found in explant. For color reproduction, see Color Plate 40.2.

Table 40.3: Neoplasia of the Liver in Children According to Usual Age of Presentation

		Malignant	
Age	*Benign*	*Primary*	*Metastatic/Systemic*
Infancy (0–1 yr)	Hemangioendothelioma Mesenchymal hamartoma Teratoma	Hepatoblastoma (small cell) Rhabdoid tumor Yolk sac tumor	Langerhan's cell histiocytosis Megakaryoblastic leukemia Metastatic neuroblastoma
Early childhood (1–3 yr)	Hemangioendothelioma Mesenchymal hamartoma Inflammatory myofibroblastic tumor	Hepatoblastoma Rhabdomyosarcoma	Wilm's Pancreaticoblastoma
Later childhood (3–10 yr)	Angiomyolipoma	Hepatocellular carcinoma	Desmoplastic intra-abdominal tumor
	Adenoma	Embryonal (undifferentiated) sarcoma Angiosarcoma Nested stromal epithelial tumor	
Adolescence (10–16 yr)	Adenoma (focal nodular hyperplasia)	Hepatocellular carcinoma (fibrolamellar)	Hodgkin's lymphoma
	Biliary cystadenoma	Leiomyosarcoma Nested stromal epithelial tumor	

Serum AFP levels are markedly elevated in more than 90% of patients with HB and in two thirds of cases of HCC. α-Fetoprotein is also elevated in germ cell tumors with yolk sac components, a few cases of which arise in the liver [61,87]. The major protein produced by the fetal liver, AFP is produced in large amounts in the newborn. In the normal-term infant, the AFP level can be as high as 100,000 ng/mL or greater. The half-life of AFP is 5–7 days and levels fall throughout the first several months of life (Table 40.4). By age 1 year, the AFP level is less than 10 ng/mL [88,89]. However, it remains elevated in two genetic diseases that lead to HCC, heredity tyrosinemia type 1 and ataxia-telangiectasia. In Beckwith–Wiedemann syndrome, it serves, along with periodic abdominal ultrasonography, to detect the early onset of HB [90]. In infants younger than 1 year with HB, it may initially be difficult to distinguish the contribution to elevated AFP from reactive, normal liver versus malignant tumor. However, the AFP is a useful tumor marker to assess response to therapy as well as to monitor for disease recurrence [91,92]. After a complete resection, AFP levels should decline and approach normal ranges within several days to weeks (Table 40.5). Failure to do so indicates residual disease.

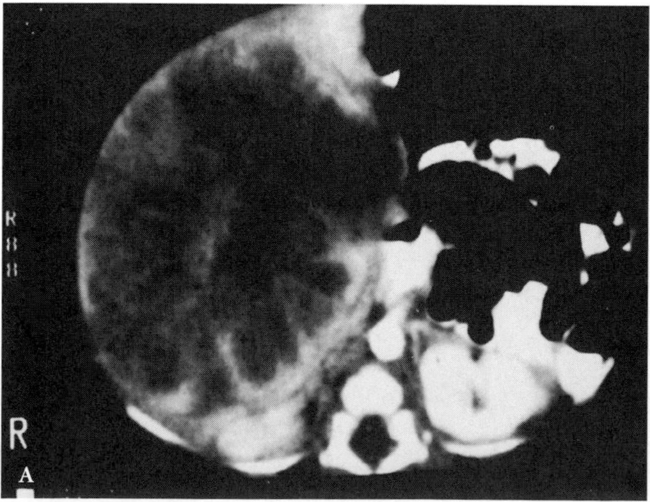

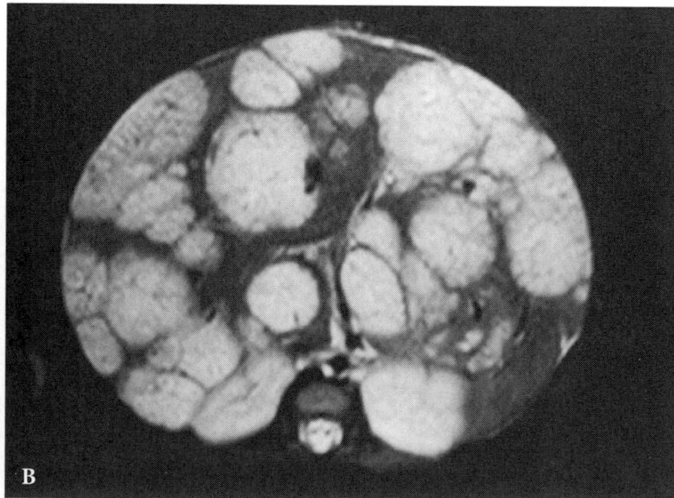

Figure 40.3. Imaging. (**A**) CT is used to demonstrate resectability of liver tumors. This patient was asymptomatic except for hepatomegaly at 5 days of age. (**B**) T1-weighted magnetic resonance image of multifocal hemangioendothelioma shows marked contrast enhancement after gadolinium (see Figure 40.14D).

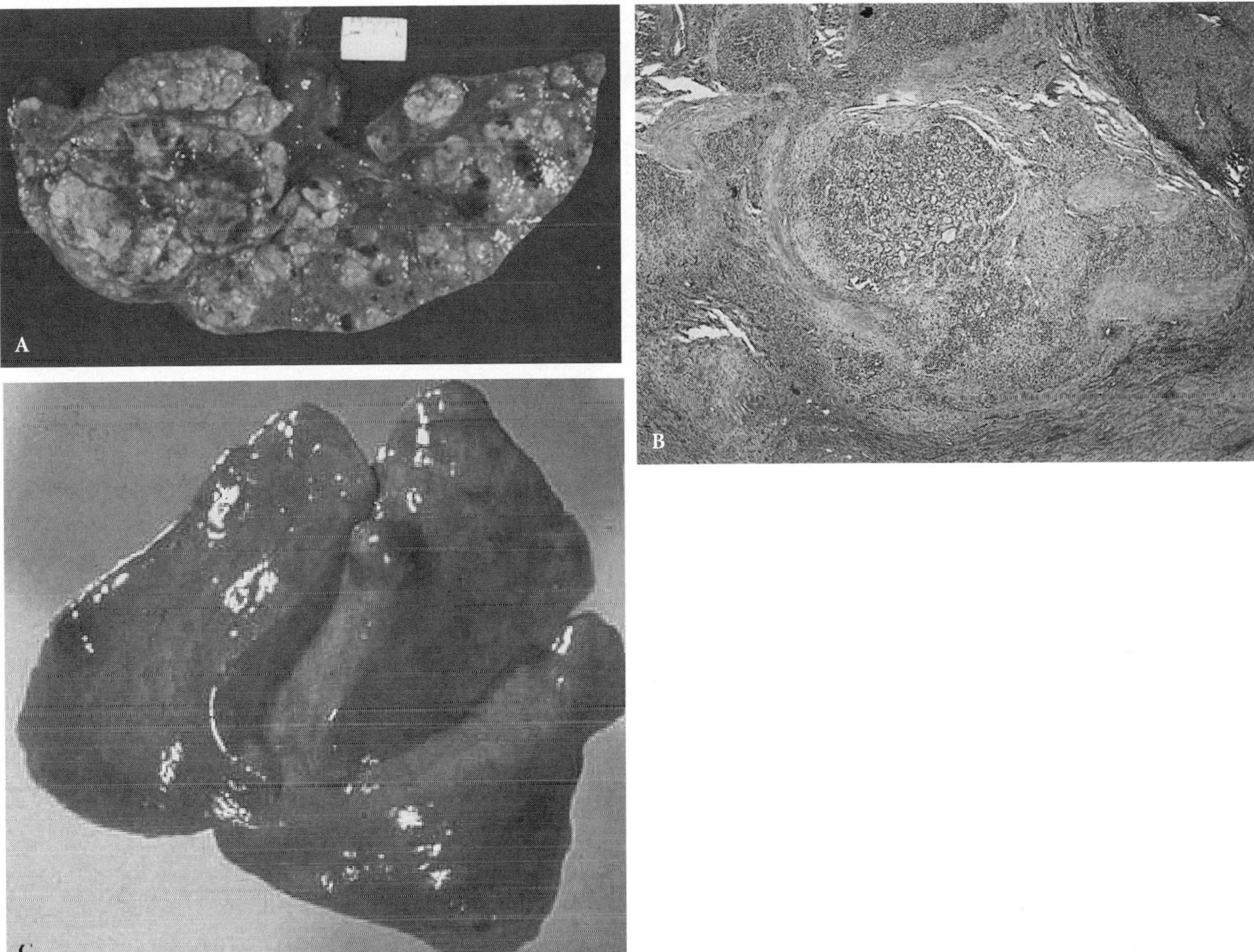

Figure 40.4. Dissemination of hepatic neoplasms. (**A**) Hepatocellular carcinoma in an 8-year-old with perinatally acquired hepatitis B. (**B**) Embryonal hepatoblastoma in hepatic vein. (**C**) Stage IV hepatoblastoma: pulmonary metastases. This is the usual reason for treatment failure, but some patients have been saved by resection.

α-Fetoprotein is usually normal with small cell undifferentiated hepatoblastoma and infantile rhabdoid tumor, the fibrolamellar variant of HCC, as well as in most benign liver tumors. However, significantly elevated AFP has been reported in cases of infantile hemangioendothelioma and mesenchymal hamartoma, which has misled clinicians into treating for HB without confirmatory diagnostic biopsy [81,93,94]. When serum AFP was combined with ultrasonography to screen high-risk adults in China, a 5-year survival rate of 62.7% was achieved in those with HCC 5 cm in diameter or less versus larger ones, which had a 37.1% rate [95]. Des-γ-carboxy prothrombin level in the serum is a marker of advanced HCC, and higher levels before transplantation indicate a poor prognosis [96].

The potential clinical use of glypican 3 oncofetal protein (GPC3) as a second diagnostic marker for HCC and HB has been reported recently [97–99]. Glypican 3, a heparan sulfate proteoglycan anchored to the membrane, is expressed at markedly elevated levels in HCC, HB, and fetal liver but is undetectable in normal hepatocytes and nonmalignant liver disease. Various studies have demonstrated that GPC3 could be used as a serologic test for the diagnosis of patients with HCC and recommended simultaneous measurement of both GPC3 and AFP for HCC screening for improved sensitivity [98].

STAGING

The conventional staging system used by the U.S. Children's Oncology Group (COG) is shown in Table 40.6 [21]. *Stage I* is defined as a tumor completely resected at diagnosis. *Stage II* refers to resection with microscopic residual disease. *Stage III* indicates gross residual disease, including involvement of local lymph nodes and inability to resect the primary tumor. *Stage IV* tumors are those with distant metastases. In the most recent COG study (P9645) from 1999 to 2001, 29% of the 153 registered cases of HB were stages I and II, and 3.4% were stage I with

Table 40.4: Physiologic α-Feto Protein Levels

Age	*Mean ± SD (ng/mL)*
Premature	134,734 ± 41,444
Newborn	48,406 ± 34,718
Newborn to 2 wk	33,113 ± 32,503
Newborn to 1 mo	9452 ± 12,610
2 mo	323 ± 278
3 mo	88 ± 87
4 mo	74 ± 56
5 mo	46.5 ± 19
6 mo	12.5 ± 9.8
7 mo	9.7 ± 7.1
8 mo	8.5 ± 5.5

"favorable" histology not requiring chemotherapy. Only 10% were stage IV, with lung disease at diagnosis, versus 20% in the 1990–94 European International Society of Pediatric Oncologie (SIOPEL-1) study [100]. In the U.S. intergroup series, HCC were amenable to primary resection only 17% of the time but seven of the eight stage I cases were 5-year survivors [101].

The staging system developed by SIOPEL is based on the number of liver segments involved [85] (Figure 40.5). This pretreatment classification scheme (PRETEXT) is intended to determine resectability by ultrasonography and CT preoperatively. This system divides the liver into four sectors – namely, an anterior and a posterior sector on the right and a medial and a lateral sector on the left. Staging groups are assigned according to tumor extension within the liver as well as the presence or absence of involvement of the hepatic vein, portal vein, regional lymph nodes, or distant metastases. When the PRETEXT stage preoperatively was compared with the pathologic examination of specimens resected *following* chemotherapy, there was only 51% agreement, with 37% of 91 specimens overstaged by imaging and four patients with positive resection margins that were missed [102]. The current COG Study of HB stratifies patients according the postsurgical staging system but will also attempt to validate the PRETEXT staging system with respect to tumor resectability and outcome.

PATHOLOGY

A primary hepatic neoplasm, whether benign or malignant, is typically an expansile solitary mass (Figure 40.6). Multiple lesions are found in some hemangiomas and hemangioendotheliomas, adenomas, and HCC, and rarely HB. Encapsulation is limited to some adenomas, although pseudocapsules secondary to compressive atrophy of the adjacent parenchyma can be deceptive with respect to an operative margin. Spontaneous focal necrosis of the rapidly growing HB is common, and many of them have large telangiectatic vessels, both of which account for highly diverse images and Doppler patterns and may lead to erroneous diagnosis, especially in infants, when the serum AFP level does not reflect the expected values [88, 102,103]. Metastatic spread of HB and HCC occurs via hepatic veins to the lungs and secondarily to the brain (Figure 40.4) [157]. Intravascular dissemination is frequent, but current chemotherapy can successfully eradicate tumor confined to the liver and even some that have metastasized [104,105].

Table 40.5: Estimated Number of Days for Elevated α-Feto Protein to Decline to Normal Levels (<10 ng/mL)

	Presumed Half-Life		
Initial AFP (ng/mL)	*5 d*	*7 d*	*10 d*
10	5	7	10
20	10	14	20
40	15	21	30
80	20	28	40
160	25	35	50
320	30	42	60
640	35	49	70
1280	40	56	80
2560	45	63	90
5120	50	70	100
10,240	55	77	110
20,480	60	84	120

Table 40.6: COG Staging of Hepatoblastoma

Stage I. Favorable histology – completely resected with pure fetal histologic pattern and low mitotic index (<2 per 10 high power fields). (Stratum 1)

Stage I. Other histology – completely resected tumors with a histologic picture other than pure fetal with low mitotic index. (Stratum 2)

Stage II. Grossly resected tumors with evidence of microscopic residual. Resected tumors with preoperative (intraoperative) rupture are stage II. (Stratum 2)

Stage III. Unresectable tumors – considered by the surgeon not to be resectable without undue risk to the patient. Lymph node involvement is considered to constitute stage III disease and may require evaluation with a second laparotomy after initial courses of chemotherapy. (Stratum 3)

Stage IV. Tumors – measurable metastatic disease to lungs or other organs. (Stratum 3)

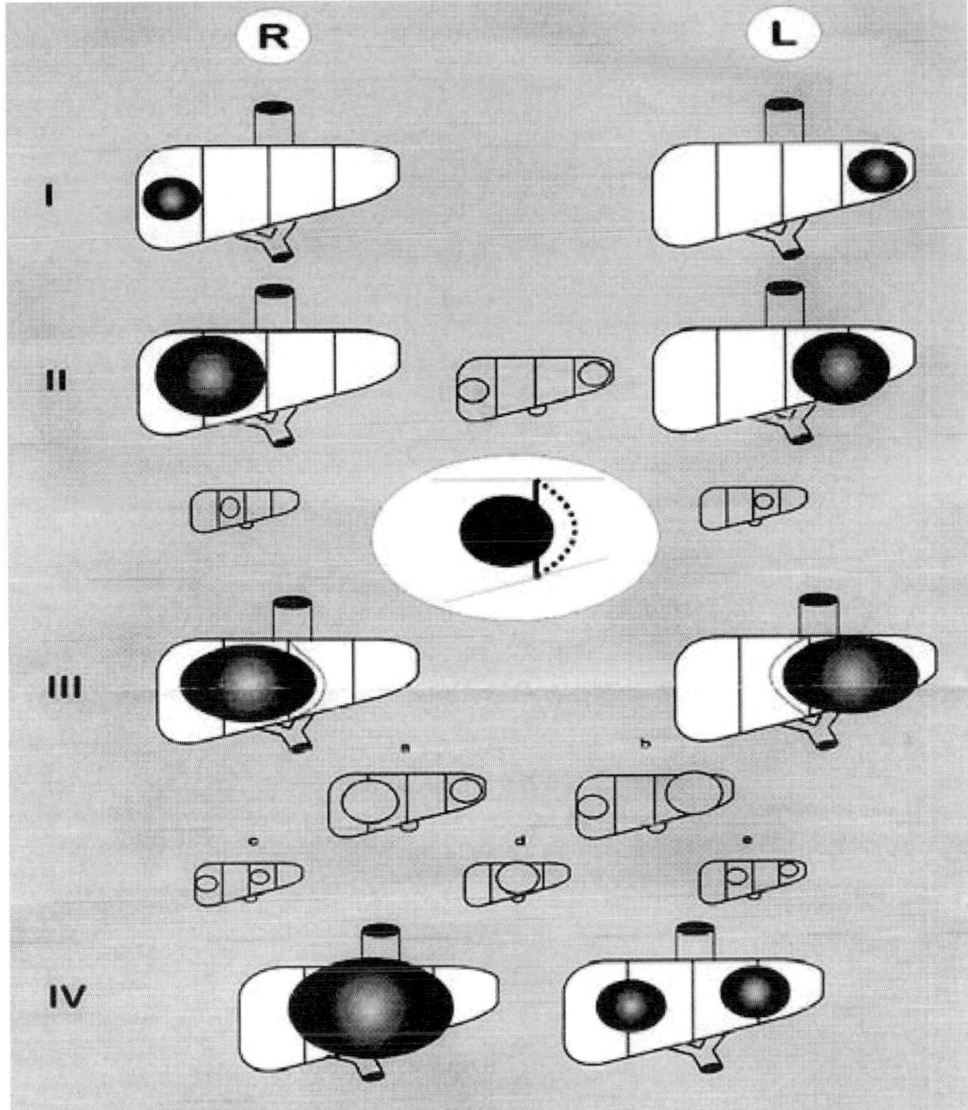

Figure 40.5. Staging. The PRETEXT scheme for preoperative evaluation of extant of tumor in the liver [85].

Hepatoblastomas arise from precursors of mature hepatocytes and most tumors display many histologic patterns reflecting diverse stages of differentiation (Table 40.7). Embryonal histology is most common and resembles the histology of the liver at 6–8 weeks of gestation (Figure 40.7A and 40.7B). Well-differentiated neoplastic fetal hepatocytes may be virtually indistinguishable in cytologic and architectural growth pattern from the normal fetal liver (Figure 40.7C) [1]. The cytoplasm is often rich in glycogen and sometimes contains neutral fats. Nuclear–cytoplasmic ratio is typically slightly higher than nonneoplastic host hepatocytes. Cholangioblastic, or ductular, differentiation (Figure 40.7D) has been reported, and this rare occurrence suggests origin from a precursor cell [106].

Hepatoblastomas may contain undifferentiated small cells that coexpress cytokeratin and vimentin reflecting neither epithelial nor stromal differentiation (Figure 40.8) [107]. Whether the small undifferentiated cell is equivalent to a "stem" cell or the "oval" cell of the rodent liver is controversial. Diverse immunohistochemical markers have led investigators to opposite conclusions [108,109]. Rarely, the entire HB is composed of only one cell type; 2.0% of the 377 cases reviewed for the POG and COG from 1986 to 2005 that could be resected without chemotherapy (stages I and II) were small cell undifferentiated, whereas 3.4% were pure well-differentiated fetal with minimal mitotic activity (Table 40.8). The remainder were mixtures of diverse epithelial cells in varying proportions and of cells intermediate among the broad categories, with either discrete nodules of a single cell type or intimate intermingling of diverse cytologies (Figure 40.8). This feature makes it difficult to predict behavior on the basis of a small biopsy of an unresectable tumor and chemotherapy affects the diverse components differently [110]. Well-differentiated fetal cells having significant mitotic activity (>2 in 10 high-power microscopic fields; Figure 40.9) very rarely occur in "pure" form except

Table 40.7: Classification of Hepatoblastoma

Classification of Hepatoblastoma
Major categories
Epithelial
Fetal, well differentiated (mitotically inactive, diploid)
Crowded fetal (mitotically active)
Embryonal
Macrotrabecular
Small cell undifferentiated
Rhabdoid
Mixed
Osteoid stroma
Undifferentiated mesenchymal-blastemal
Minor components
Ductal (cholangioblastic)
Keratinizing squamous epithelium
Intestinal glandular epithelium
Neuroid–melanocytic (teratoid)
Rhabdomyoblastic
Chondroid

in small biopsies of stages III and IV cases. They have been referred to as "crowded" fetal cells because glycogen content is usually less and the proportion of an image occupied by nuclei is consequently increased. Fifteen percent of HB are classified as "mixed" because of stromal derivatives, particularly osteoid-like protein deposits, occasional rhabdomyoblasts, and even more rarely, chondroid elements (Figure 40.10A). The osteoid-like foci become more prevalent following chemotherapy when the embryonal cells are often eradicated (Figure 40.10B) [110].

Three percent of the HB are designated "teratoid" because some cells reflecting neural or neural crest origin are present [111]. These include glial cells, neurons, and melanocytes (Figure 40.10C). True teratomas arising in the liver of infants have a full range of tissues from all embryonic germ layers, including brainlike and extra embryonal derivatives such as yolk sac and trophoblastic cells [7]. Sometimes the distinction can be difficult when histology is the only available diagnostic tool (Figure 40.10D).

Rarely, enteroendocrine derivatives containing chromogranin and diverse hormones, such as gastrin, serotonin, or

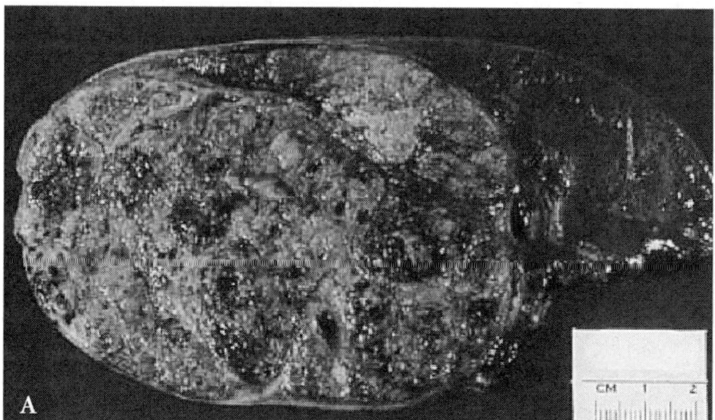

A

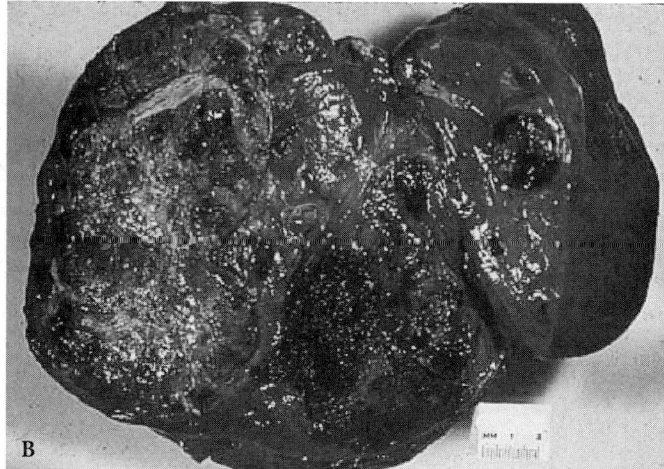

B

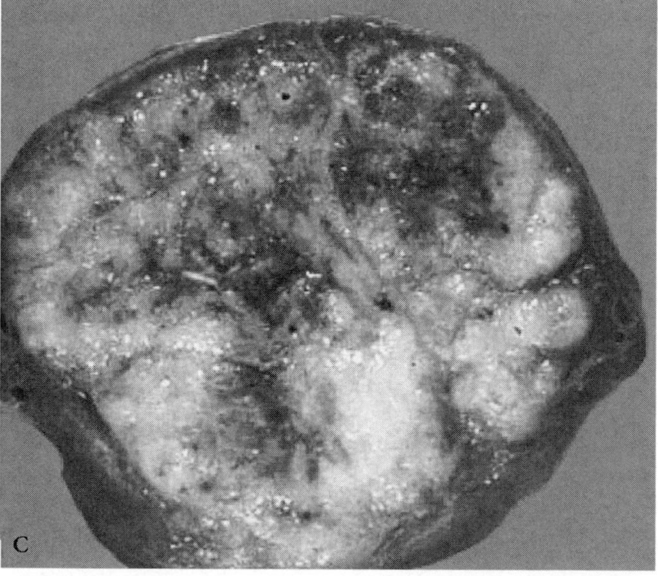

C

Figure 40.6. Gross appearance of hepatoblastoma. (**A**) Most of this tumor was composed of well-differentiated fetal hepatoblasts. (**B**) Mixed hepatoblastoma with embryonal, fetal, and mesenchymal tissues. (**C**) Small cell undifferentiated hepatoblastoma is sarcoma-like. For color reproduction, see Color Plate 40.6.

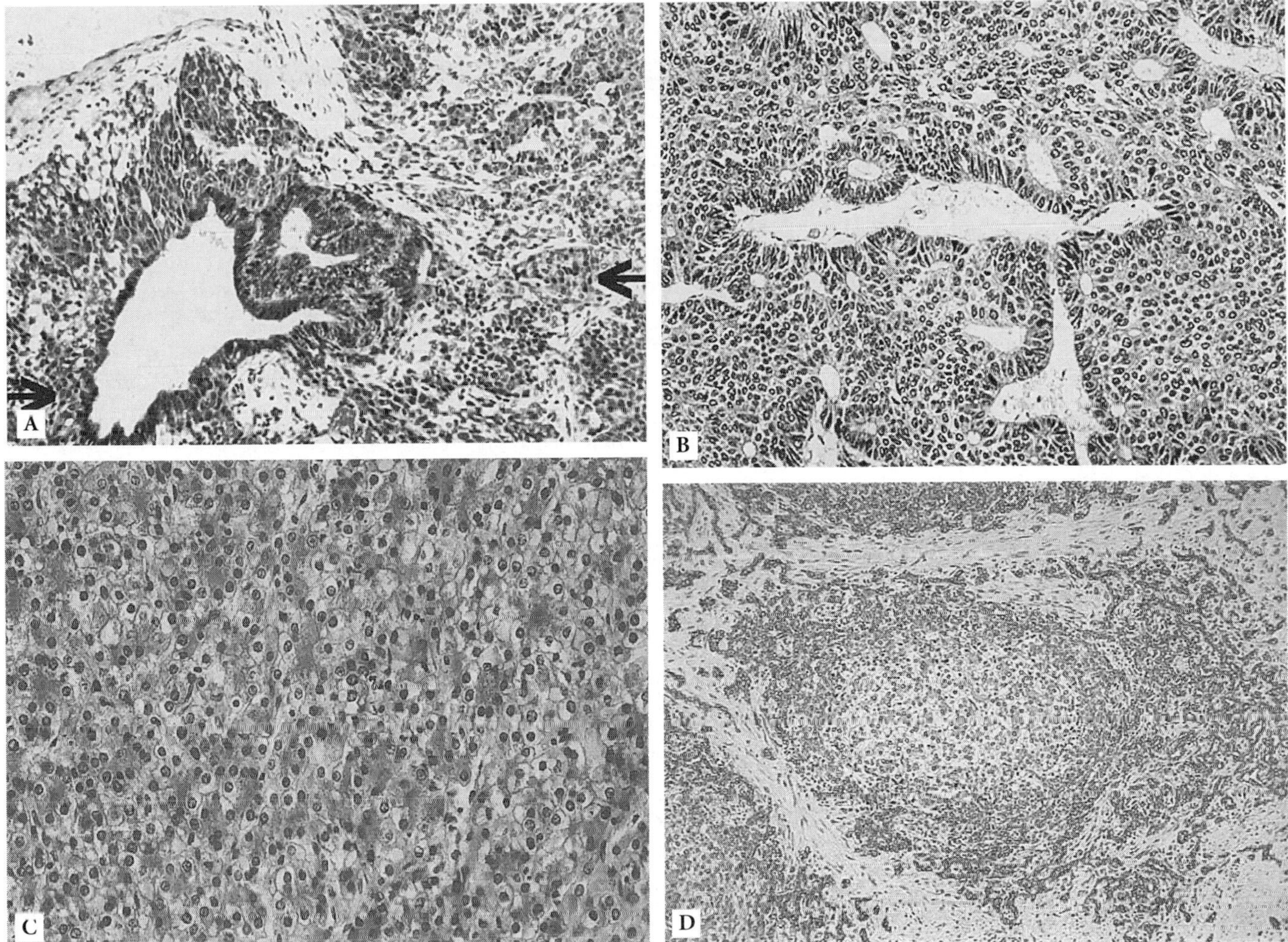

Figure 40.7. Histology of hepatoblastomas. (**A**) Histology of the embryo liver at 6–7 weeks postconception. *Arrows* call attention to differentiating hepatoblasts. (**B**) Embryonal hepatoblastoma. Mimicry of the stages of development is the basis for tumor designations. A continuum between tumor types is therefore typical of HB. (**C**) Pure fetal hepatoblastoma. The uniformity of these mature mitotically inactive cells growing in a normal cordlike manner may make them difficult to distinguish from normal hepatocytes in aspirates or small biopsies. The greater nuclear–cytoplasm is helpful. (**D**) Cholangioblastic hepatoblastoma. Cytokeratin 7 decorates the proliferative bile ductular cells, whereas hepatoblasts are unstained. For color reproduction, see Color Plate 40.7.

somatostatin, are found in mixed HB and even more rarely as pure primary hepatic tumors [112]. Small squamous pearls are frequent in mixed and teratoid tumors. Very rarely, glandular or ductal forms resembling the embryonal intestine or fetal bile ducts, are found. Primary rhabdoid tumor of the liver has yet to be included among those reported to have deletions or mutations in the *hSNF5/INI 1* tumor suppressor gene, as seen in central nervous system and renal and soft tissue primaries [113]. Expression of the *WT1* gene, normally expressed in fetal kidney and mesoderm, has been reported in rhabdoid tumors [114], suggesting the potential role of *WT1* in the process of mesodermal cells acquiring epithelial characteristics. Rhabdoid tumors share the coexpression of intermediate filaments with SCU, the onset in infancy and poor prognosis. (Figure 40.8C) [115,116]. A t(8;13) translocation has recently been documented in a malignant rhabdoid tumor of the liver [117]. Although the name rhabdoid suggests a relationship to skeletal muscle, these tumors do not contain muscle proteins. True rhabdomyoblasts may be components of HB, (Figure 40.10D) and there are full-fledged primary embryonal rhabdomyosarcomas of the liver that arise in close association to biliary epithelium, often having a polypoid growth pattern and causing obstructive jaundice [65,118].

When HB cells with either fetal or embryonal cytology grow in trabeculae of 20–100 or more cells rather than in the 2- to 4-cell-thick cords of the fetal liver, the pattern is called macrotrabecular [119]. Eighteen percent of our series contained macrotrabecular foci, and one third of them were stage IV at presentation. This aggressive behavior may reflect the fact that such histology can be indistinguishable from HCC when it occurs in pure form (Figure 40.11). Malignant tumors that have features of both HB and HCC have been observed in seven children with perinatally acquired hepatitis B infection in our consultation practice.

Table 40.8: Pediatric Liver Tumors by Stage and Histology, Pediatric and Children's Oncology Group, 1986–2005, *n* (%)

	I	*II*	*III*	*IV*	*Total*
Pure fetal	13 (3.7)		26	9	48 (14)
Fetal and Embryonal	58	10	102	48	218 (64)
Small cell undifferentiated	1		6	1	8 (2)
Mixed epithelial/ stomal	12		35	8	55 (16)
Teratoid	3	1	7	1	12 (3)
Rhabdoid			1	1	2 (0.5)
Totals	87 (25)	11 (3)	177 (52)	68 (20)	343

Hepatocarcinomas in children do not differ histologically from those in adults. The fibrolamellar variant (Figure 40.12A) occurs more commonly in adolescents and young adults [17]. The presence of a central scar with radiating fibrous bands between tumor masses suggests benign focal nodular hyperplasia (Figure 40.12B), but the histology is characteristic and the large atypical neoplastic cells are readily distinguished (Figure 40.12D). Unlike most hepatocarcinomas, fibrolamellar carcinomas arise in otherwise normal livers and for that reason are more readily resected and in many series have a higher rate of cure. However, children with fibrolamellar hepatocarcinomas do not have a more favorable prognosis and do not respond any differently to therapy from patients with typical HCC at the same stage [17]. Cholangiocarcinomas may occur in older children with antecedent cystic or cholestatic disease (Figure 40.2D) [7]. Like most adenocarcinomas, they are very resistant to treatment. Solitary benign bile duct cysts are amenable to surgical excision. Ten examples of a new variant of mixed tumor of the

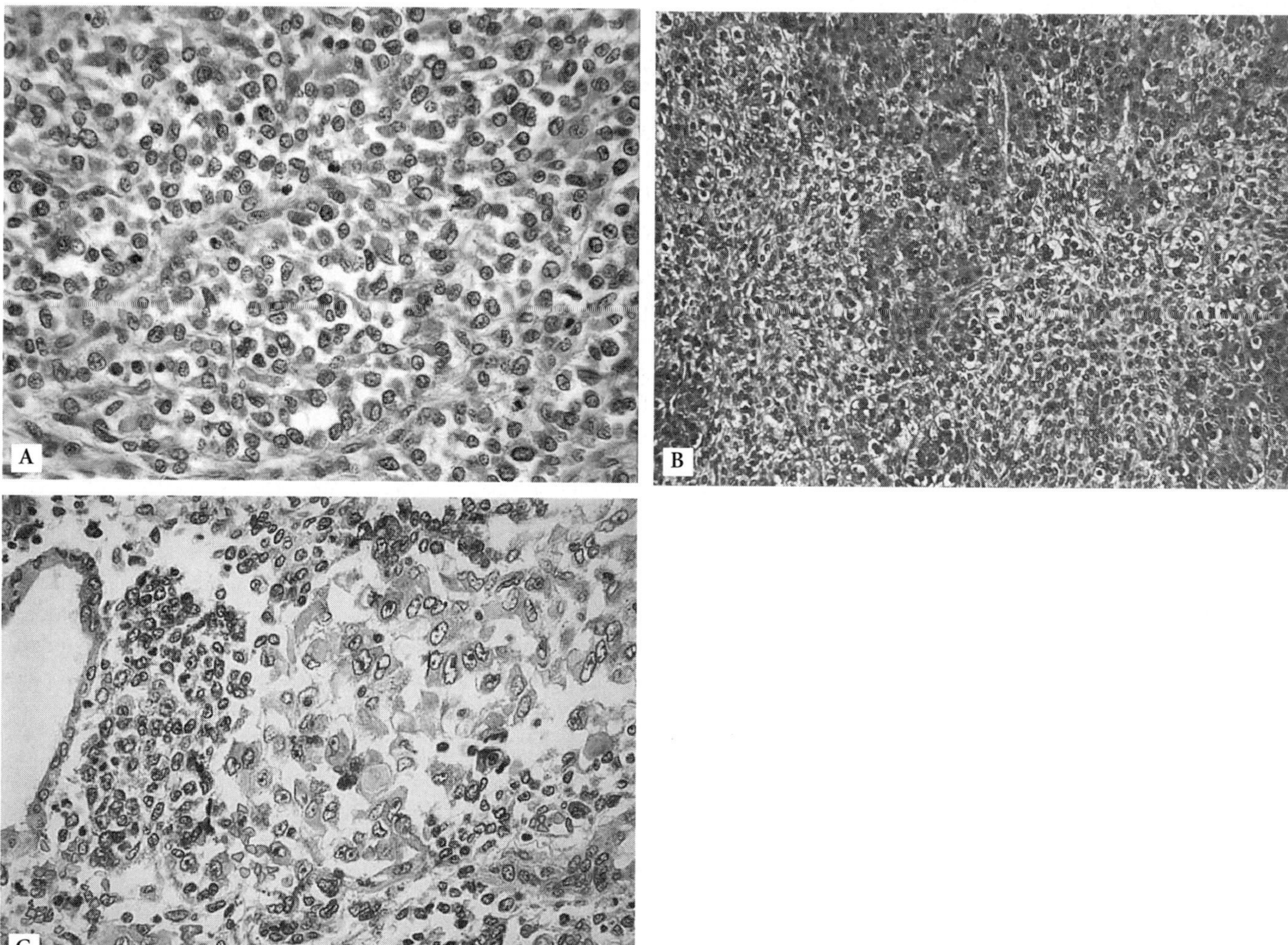

Figure 40.8. Small cell undifferentiated hepatoblastoma (SCU) and rhabdoid tumor. (**A**) When the proportion of these cells is high or are the only component, they are usually found in infants and fail to respond to standard chemotherapy [190]. (**B**) Typically, small cells and fetal or embryonal HB are haphazardly intermingled so that small biopsies may not be representative of a large neoplasm's constituents. (**C**) Intimate associate of SCU and rhabdoid tumor in an otherwise typical HB of a 7-month-old. Cells of both histotypes express cytokeratin and vimentin, intermediate filaments reflecting mesodermal–epithelial transition.

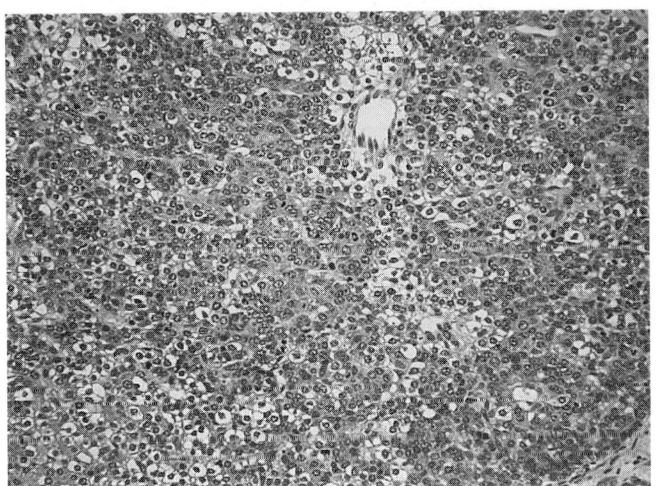

Figure 40.9. Fetal hepatoblastoma with abundant mitoses ("crowded"). Whether stage I–II tumors with this or embryonal histology could have their postexcision adjuvant chemotherapy reduced or eliminated, as can the well-differentiated fetal tumors with minimal mitoses, has not been tested.

liver have been reported in children, seven of whom were girls [71,72]. It has a distinctive pattern of epithelial nests in a spindle-cell stroma, often with calcification or ossification, and a close association with bland appearing bile ducts is observed (Figure 40.13). One patient had a recurrence and one developed a Wilms's tumor of the kidney following liver resection. Immunochemical localization of corticotropin in the epithelial nests was found in 3 patients, 2 of whom had clinical Cushing syndrome [71].

Infantile hemangiomas and hemangioendotheliomas (HE) are benign vascular tumors of the liver composed of thin vascular channels lined by a single layer of bland-appearing endothelial cells, which occur almost exclusively during the first year of life [120,121]. They are probably underreported but accounted for more than 17% of all liver tumors in children and 40% of the benign tumors in the combined series (Table 40.1). They may be single or multicentric, well demarcated, or infiltrative (Figure 40.14A and 40.14B). Single lesions are usually self-resolving or cured by surgical resection. However, some of these tumors are large, multifocal, or present with clinical complications such as congestive heart failure or coagulopathy. The latter symptoms suggest the presence of an arteriovenous malformation (Figure 40.14C). These proliferative vascular lesions can be difficult to distinguish clinically and pathologically in an infant liver. They occurred with equal frequency in a 33-year period in Cincinnati [122]. In that series, HE occurred only in female patients, and all 9 cases displayed positive expression of Glut 1, a glucose transporter, on endothelial cells (Figure 40.14D). The proliferative capillaries associated with arteriovenous malformation (AVM) were uniformly negative for Glut 1. The only patient with concurrent angiosarcoma was a 5.5-year-old with HE. Highly proliferative vasoformative endothelium can be relatively avascular and deceptive by imaging, as well as worrisome with respect to aggressiveness (Figure 40.14E).

Epithelioid hemangioendotheliomas are rare neoplasms of intermediate malignant potential observed starting from the second decade [123]. Often multinodular, they may be difficult to distinguish from metastatic adenocarcinoma because of their infiltrating growth in a fibrous stroma. Immunostains for CD34, CD31, and factor VIII serve to identify them [124] (Figure 40.14F). Angiosarcomas are rare and usually arise de novo, but a few have been reported in children as young as 4 and 5 years following biopsy or excision of benign hemangiomatous hamartomas in infancy or simultaneously in livers containing hemangiomas [125,126]. These highly infiltrative lesions disseminate widely within the liver (Figure 40.15) and metastasize to lungs and lymph nodes.

Undifferentiated, or embryonal, sarcomas present in 6- to 10-year-old children, usually de novo. However, at least seven cases have been described subsequent to or contemporaneous with a benign infantile mass lesion, the mesenchymal hamartoma [127–129]. These sarcomas generally present as large expansile masses but infiltrate the adjacent parenchyma widely, sparing bile ducts, and spread via veins through the liver and to the lungs (Figure 40.16). Many of them contain diverse elements displaying maturation of mesenchymal derivatives, including vessels, pericytes, smooth muscle, lipomatous, and fibrohistiocytic features in addition to large bizarre cells with irregular processes and multiple cytoplasmic globular inclusions containing secretory proteins such as α_1-antitrypsin (Figure 40.16C).

Mesenchymal hamartomas arise mainly in infants as typically single expansile masses composed of cystic spaces lined by either biliary epithelium or endothelial cells in a loose myxoid stroma (Figure 40.17A–40.17C). They may contain hemangiomatous foci, rarely leading to congestive failure and possibly reflecting origin from a vascular accident in utero that focally interferes with hepatocyte differentiation and growth (Figure 40.17D). Another hamartoma of the liver is the angiomyolipoma, a feature of tuberous sclerosis. There have been a few examples in children, not all of whom have had confirmed tuberous sclerosis. This is most often a tumor of adult females and can be difficult to distinguish from hepatocarcinoma on imaging and in fine needle aspirates. The antibody to homatropine methylbromide, which stains the adipocytes and myoblasts of the hamartoma but not hepatocytes, has proved useful in the examination of fine needle aspirates and biopsies. Two cases of aggressive behavior in children have been reported recently [130,131].

Hepatocellular adenoma is a benign tumor occurring in older children and adolescents that may prove problematic on imaging and in fine needle aspiration cytology. The increased incidence and hemorrhaging seen when oral contraception was first available have subsided with reduction of the estrogen content. Adenomas consist of nodular proliferation of hepatocytes in cords having no relationship to portal tracts and have a pushing border with the surrounding liver (Figure 40.2A). Adenomas may acquire fibrous capsules and some may have steatosis and even features of alcoholic hepatitis (Figure 40.2B). They may be difficult to distinguish from well-differentiated carcinoma. A few cases of carcinoma arising

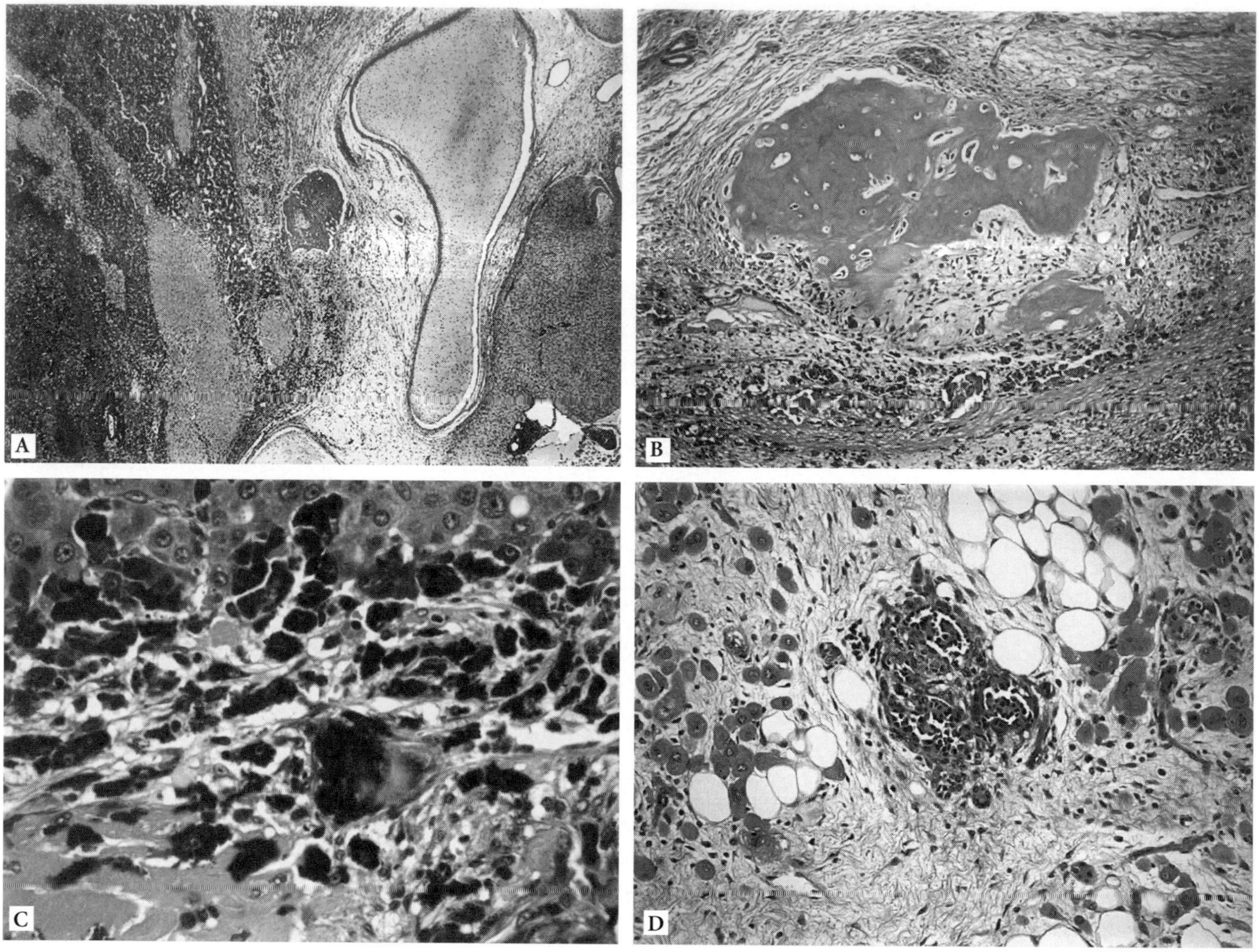

Figure 40.10. Mixed hepatoblastoma. (**A**) True bone and cartilage may be found. (**B**) Bone formation in mixed hepatoblastoma. It is especially abundant following chemotherapy. (**C**) Melanocytes along with glia and other neural derivatives that invoke the designation "teratoid." (**D**) When organoid differentiation occurs, as with this fetal kidney, the question of true teratoma arises. The primitive glomeruli and tubules are surrounded by fetal rhabdomyoblasts.

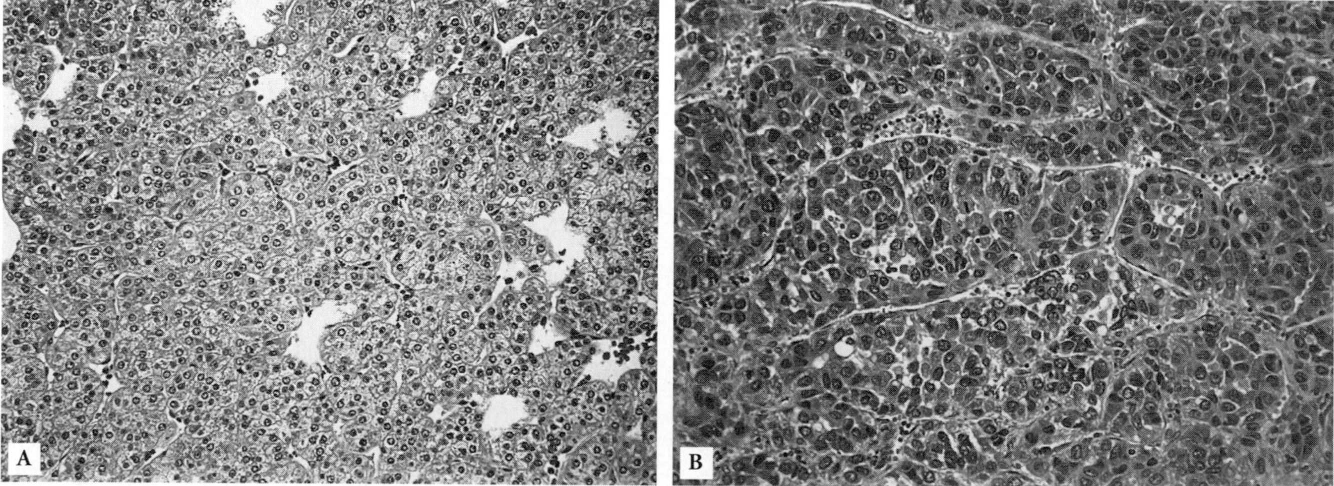

Figure 40.11. Macrotrabecular growth patterns can make HB (**A**) and HCC (**B**) difficult to distinguish, particularly in fine needle aspirates or small biopsy samples. Genetic tools, such as fluorescent in situ hybridization (FISH), are beginning to be used to resolve this difficulty.

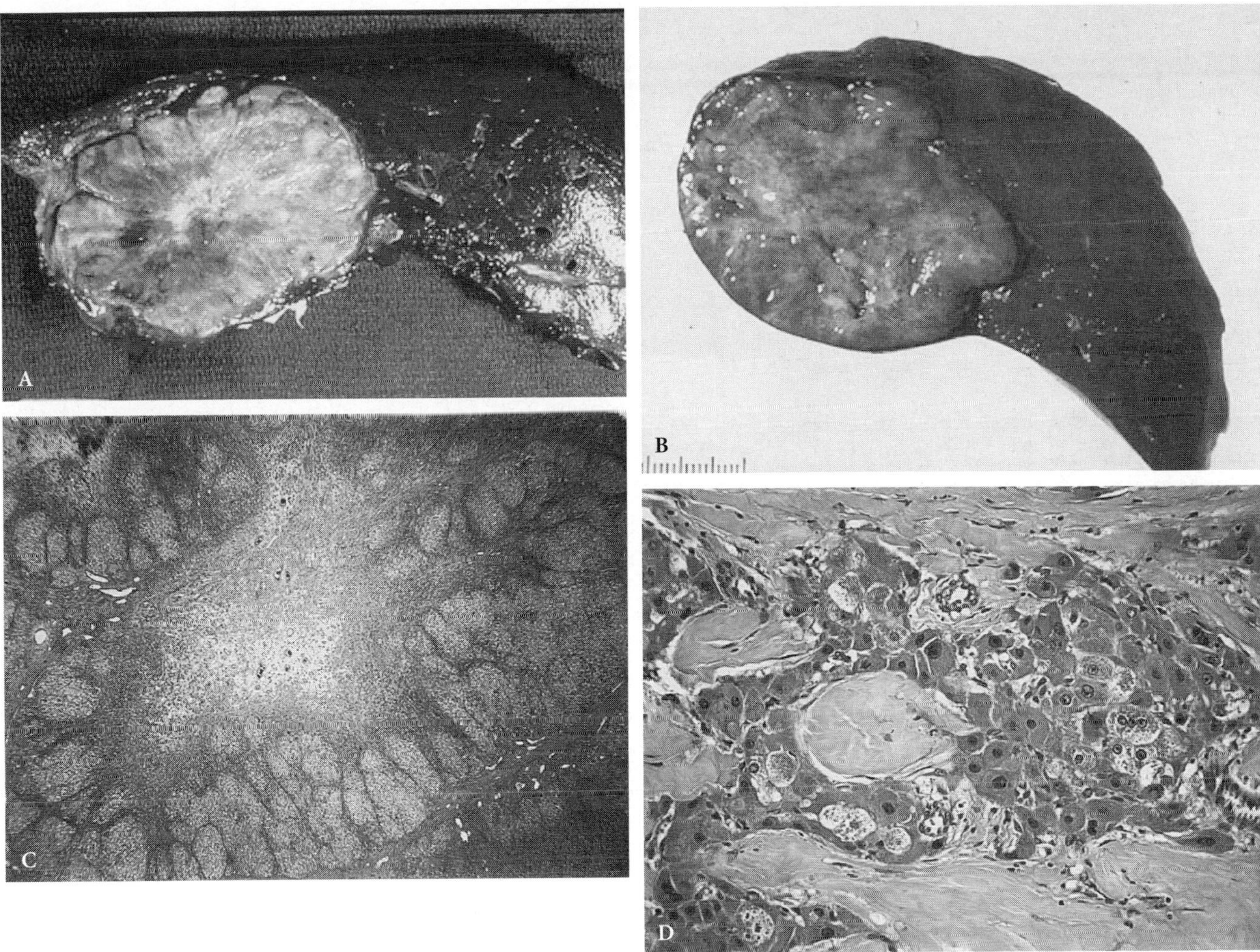

Figure 40.12. Fibrolamellar carcinoma (**A**) versus focal nodular hyperplasia (**B**). Both lesions can have a central depression due to scarring and both occur in a noncirrhotic host liver. The hepatocytes surrounding a central scar in focal nodular hyperplasia are normal in appearance (**C**). Histologically there is no difficulty in distinguishing them because large hypereosinophilic hepatocytes in the carcinoma are typically embedded in a dense fibrocollagenous stroma (**D**). For color reproduction, see Color Plate 40.12.

in young adults with glycogen storage disease have been especially confusing because even when these patients have multiple tumors, most are benign [48]. Focal nodular hyperplasia is typically a single large mass in an otherwise healthy liver characterized by central scarring that radiates between multiple nodules of regenerating parenchyma (Figure 40.12B and 40.12C). Unlike the adenoma, bile ducts are present in distorted portal tracts and these lesions are not neoplastic or preneoplastic.

The relative infrequency of liver tumors in children means that few centers care for more than one or two malignant examples each year. Therefore, it is not surprising that 10.6% of 123 biopsy cases submitted for pathology review in a U.S. Intergroup study were incorrectly interpreted. Among the errors were neuroblastoma, Wilms's tumor, and choriocarcinoma [7]. Intra-abdominal desmoplastic small cell tumors and pancreaticoblastomas metastatic to the liver have also been misinterpreted as primary hepatic malignancies.

ACQUIRED GENETIC CHANGES IN TUMORS

The COG reported cytogenetic abnormalities in approximately 50% of 111 cases of HB, with numeric abnormalities in approximately 36% of the total, particularly trisomies 2, 8, and 20, and less commonly chromosome losses. Structural changes were found in 39% of the tumors, with unbalanced translocations involving locus 1q12-21 in 18% and seven cases carrying the t(1;4) translocation [132].

Comparative genomic hybridization studies have suggested that chromosomal gains at chromosome 8 and 20 may be associated with an adverse prognosis [133,134]. Other comparative genomic hybridization studies have identified an increase in DNA copy number in the 2q24 chromosomal region, also associated with poor clinical outcome, and a high frequency of chromosome Xp and Xq gains, with little difference between epithelial and stromal components [135,136]. Occasional losses

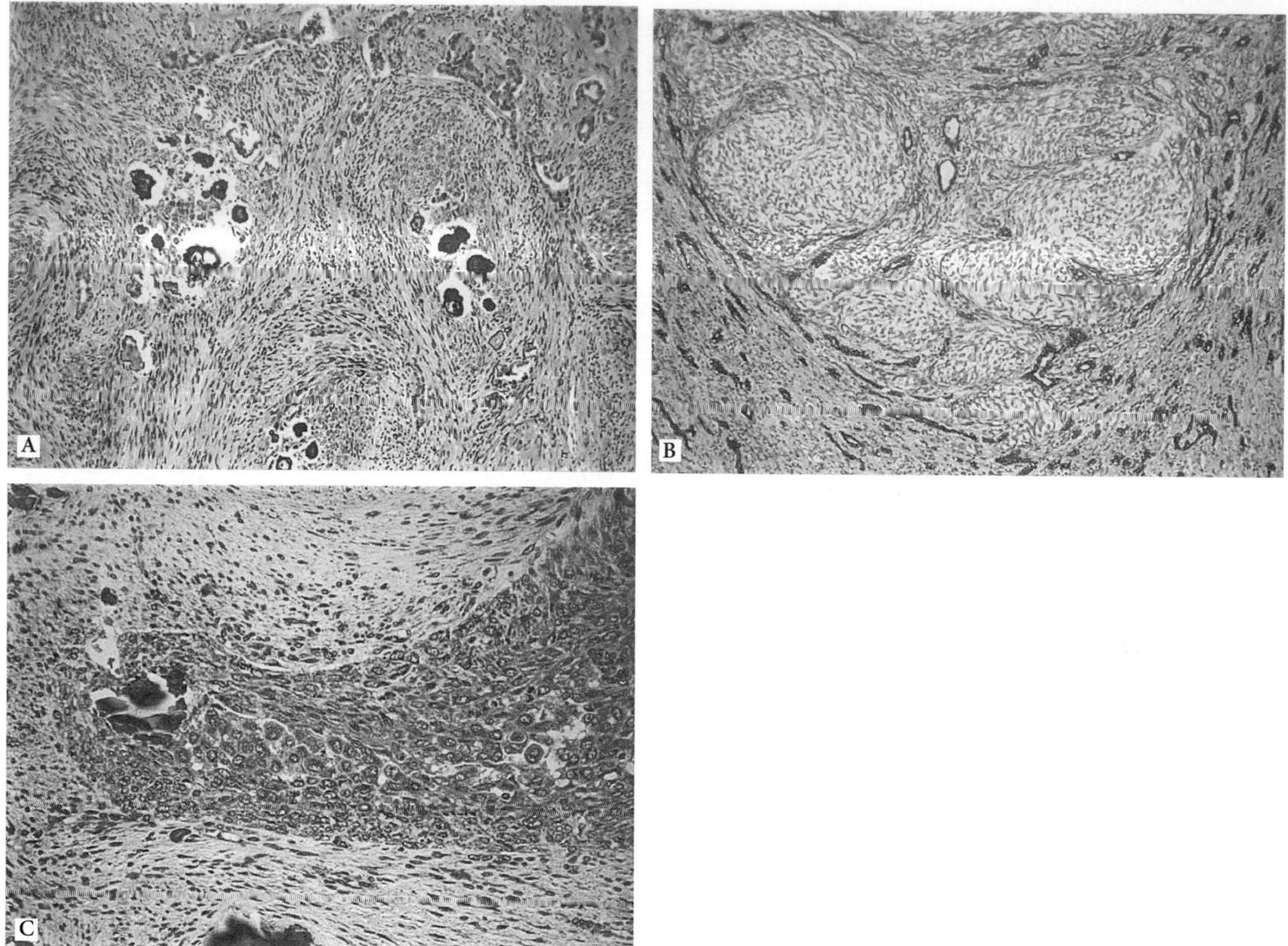

Figure 40.13. Nested stromal–epithelial tumor. (**A**) Focal calcification of the epithelial nests is typical. The behavior of these tumors is difficult to predict with only ten reported cases, but they grow very slowly, often to very large size. (**B**) Cytokeratin 19 staining reveals the intimate associate of bile ductules and the neoplastic cells. This suggests a possible origin from an endocrine precursor. (**C**) Corticotropin was demonstrable in the epithelioid nests of two patients with Cushing syndrome.

of entire chromosomes are seen and these, too, are not random. A translocation of t(1;4)(q12;q34), occurs in cases of high-stage HB [137–140]. Thus far, this abnormality has been associated with other chromosomal changes, including trisomies of 2, 8, or 20. The breakpoint has not yet been characterized. However, it is known that the region involved on chromosome 1 is heterochromatin with few structural genes. The region on chromosome 4 contains multiple genes involved in cellular growth and is also one of several genomic sites at which the hepatitis B virus is known to integrate [141]. An 8-cM interstitial deletion within 4q21-q22, overlapping with another commonly deleted region in HCC, was identified in an infant presenting with a unique congenital syndrome, manifesting with early onset HB [142]. The distal region of chromosome 4 is rearranged in 10% of HCC [143,144]. The finding of chromosome 8q amplification, and more specifically of 8q11.2-q13 associated with poor prognosis in HB, led to the investigation of the *PLAG1* oncogene at that locus. *PLAG1* transactivates transcription from the embryonic promoter P3, and overexpression may thus be responsible for the *IGF2* up-regulation [145].

Several acquired genetic changes in HB may be shared by other embryonal tumors [146,147]. An important tumor suppressor gene or growth factor gene located at 11p15.5 appears to be a factor in the development of embryonal tumors, and it is generally assumed but not proved that the critical gene lost is the same gene that is responsible for BWS. The *p57KIP2* gene at 11p15.5 is a regulator of cellular proliferation and has been shown to be mutated in some families with BWS [148]. Although not mutated, the *p57K1P2* gene may be aberrantly expressed in HB [149]. Another gene at that locus, the insulin-like growth factor *2* gene *(IGF2),* is preferentially expressed from the father in normal tissue. The parental allele specific expression is variable in tumor tissue. The *H19* gene, also at 11p15.5, shows the opposite pattern of expression of parental alleles, although the role of this nonexpressing gene in tumorigenesis is unclear [150]. When losses of genetic material

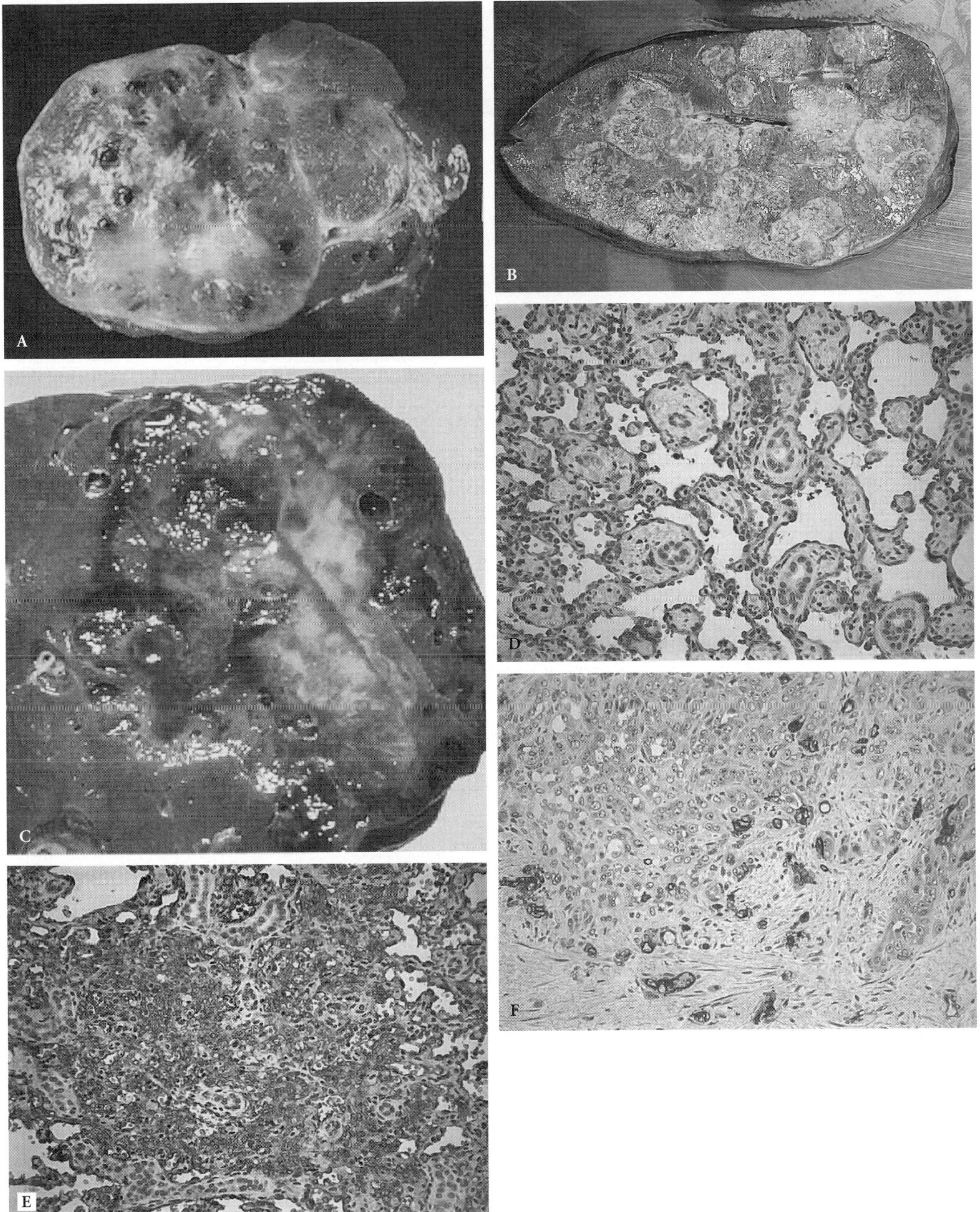

Figure 40.14. Angiomatous lesions in infancy. (**A**) Solitary hemangioendothelioma in a 5-month-old. (**B**) Multicentric hemangioendothelioma in 5-day-old (see Figure 40.3B). (**C**) Arteriovenous malformation (AVM) in a 3-week-old. (**D**) Immunohistochemical staining for glut 1 is uniformly positive in the endothelium of hemangioendothelioma and negative in the vessels of an AVM. (**E**) The active proliferation and infiltration of vasoformative positive cells as shown with CD 34 correlates with the extensive dissemination of the type 2 hemangioendothelioma. (**F**) Epithelioid hemangioendothelioma in a 15-year-old. Distinguishing this infiltrating pseudoglandular pattern from metastatic carcinoma is not difficult with immunohistochemical stains for endothelium. This is CD 34. For color reproduction, see Color Plate 40.14.

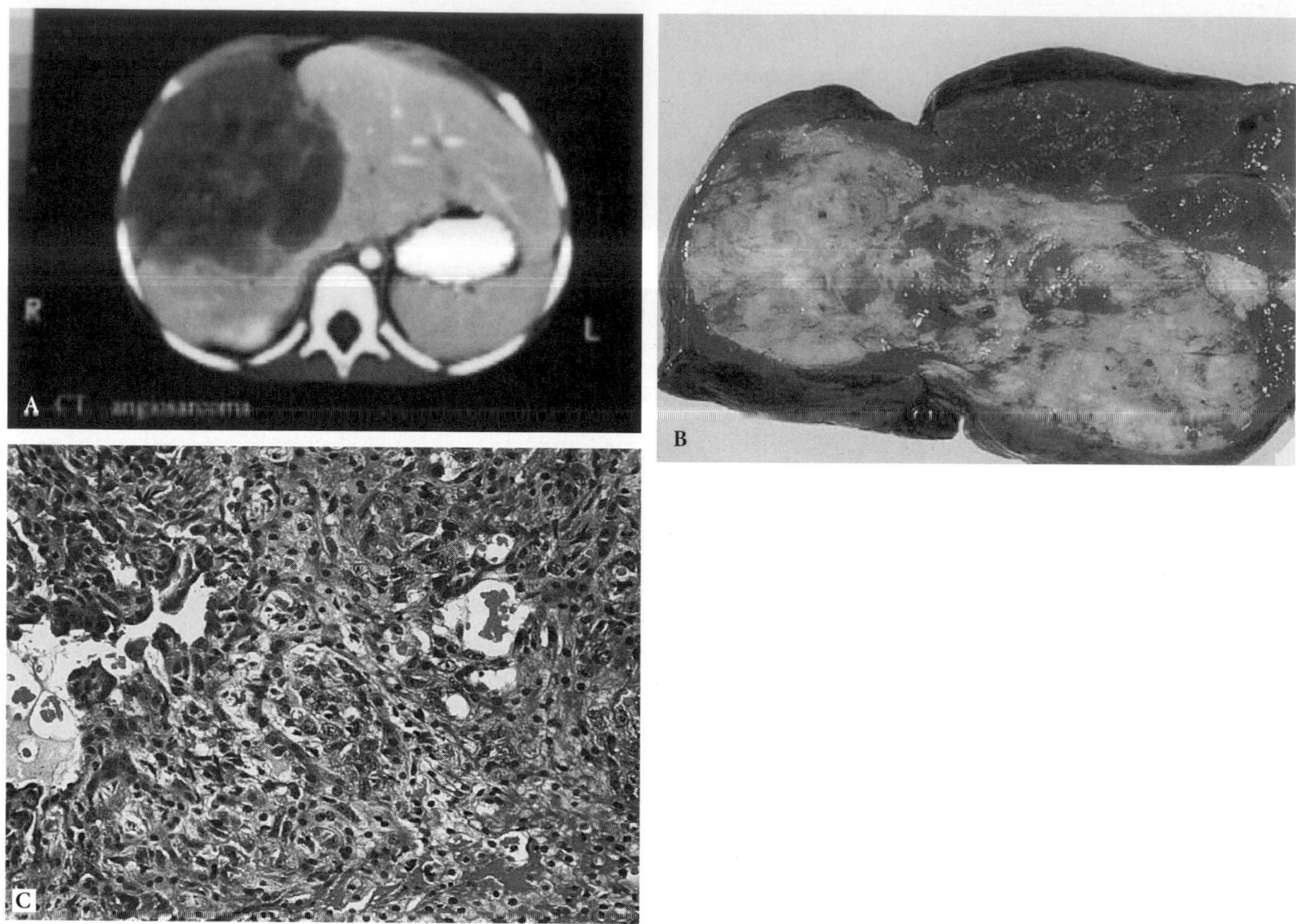

Figure 40.15. Angiosarcoma. (**A**) CT scan of a 4-year-old with an asymptomatic mass. (**B**) Resection was performed following chemotherapy. (**C**) The neoplastic cells infiltrate aggressively and only rarely form vascular channels.

at 11p15.5 occur, the losses are always of maternal origin. This suggests that the loss of imprinting of genes, or differential function depending on parental origin, may have a role in the pathogenesis of HB [151]. In HB that do not demonstrate loss of heterozygosity at 11p15.5, the differential expression of genes is lost with expression from both parental alleles [152]. Promoter-specific imprinting of the *IGF2* gene has been demonstrated in HB and fetal human liver and correlation between methylation changes in *IGF2* P3 promoter and expression has been observed in primary tumors and HB cell lines [153]. Another gene located on 11p15.5 is *BWR1A*, encoding a transmembrane transporter, highly expressed in liver, paternally imprinted, and found to be mutated in a rhabdomyosarcoma cell line, making it a possible tumor suppressor gene in HB. No mutations but allelic loss and reduced expression of *BWR1A* have been found in HB [154].

Glypican-3 (GPC3), a heparan sulfate proteoglycan possibly binding *IGF2*, is overexpressed in Wilms's tumor and HB, suggesting a growth-promoting activity for this gene product [155]. Altered gene expression of other members of the insulin-like growth factor-binding proteins indicates that the IGF axis is seriously disturbed in these tumors [156].

A few cases of HB have occurred in infants with trisomy 18, but that trisomy is not a feature of sporadic tumors. Likewise, cytogenetically detectable chromosomal aberrations of chromosome 11p15, the locus for BWS, or 5q, the locus for the *APC* gene, have not been reported in sporadic cases of HB. Acquired mutations of the *APC* gene have been reported in several cases of HB and have not been reported in other embryonal tumors [40,41]. Recent studies have focused on abnormalities of β-catenin, whose degradation is regulated by *APC*. β-catenin is more commonly altered in HB than is the *APC* gene. A German study has shown that 48% of HB have mutations of the β-catenin gene [157]. Nuclear localization of β-catenin in HB, especially in more aggressive tumors, is different from that of normal hepatocytes and well-differentiated fetal HB, which have only plasma membrane localization [158] (Figure 40.18), and it correlates with shorter survival of these patients.

López-Terrada et al. [159] investigated the status of the canonical WNT signaling pathway in a subset of hepatoblastomas and correlated the findings with histologic subtype, β-catenin immunostaining and mutation status of the *CTNNB1* gene. All tumors with embryonal–small cell histology showed either point mutations in exon 3, deletions within or confined

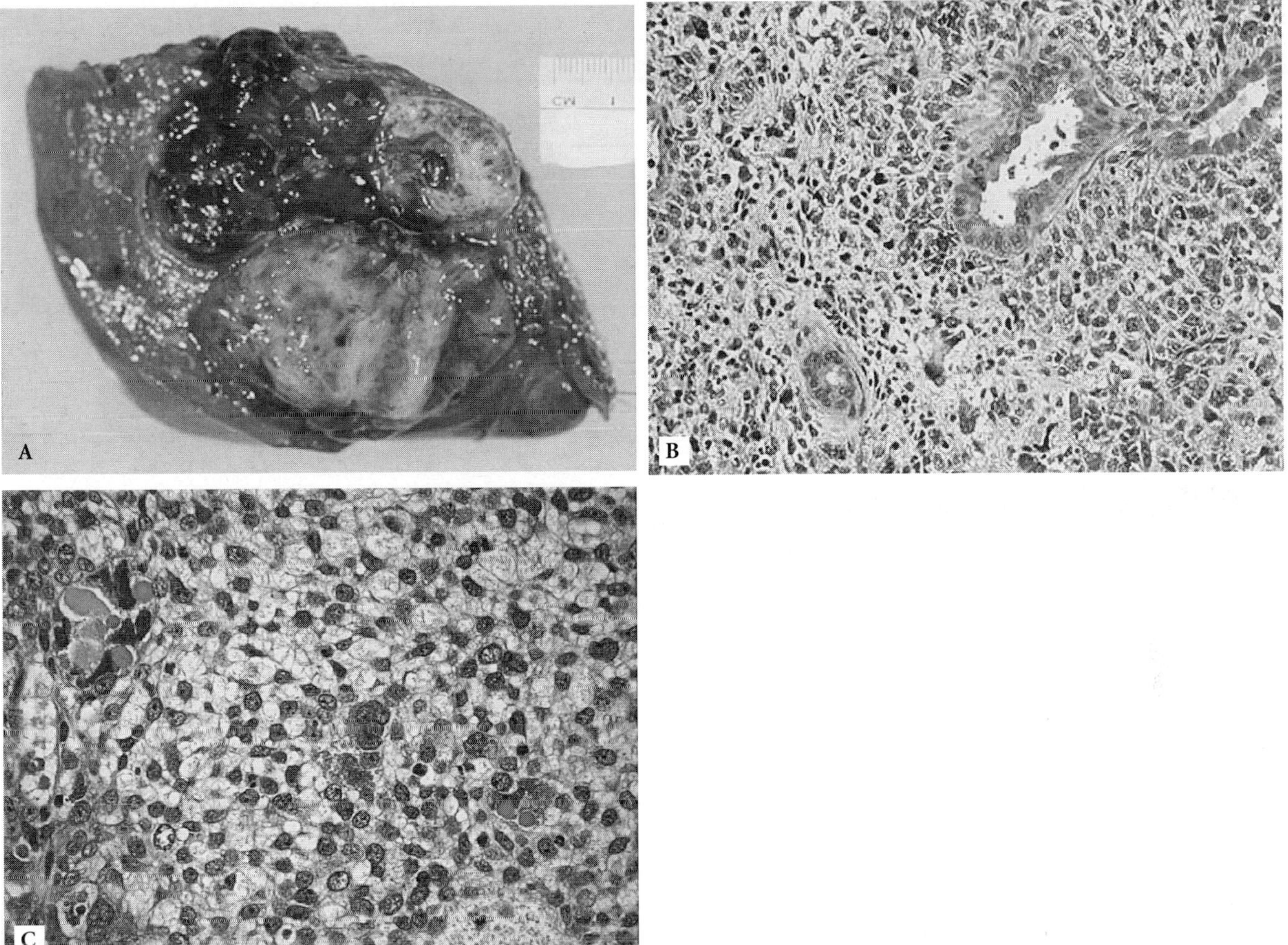

Figure 40.16. Undifferentiated or embryonal sarcoma. (**A**) Growth to a large size is typical because of the liver's enormous reserve. (**B**) Sarcomas infiltrate diffusely, sparing bile ducts. (**C**) Large eosinophilic cytoplasmic droplets of protein are common and help with the diagnosis.

to exon 3, or showed no *CTNNB1* mutations. By contrast, hepatoblastomas with pure fetal epithelial histology demonstrated predominantly large deletions of *CTNNB1* including the entire exon 3 and most of exon 4. Immunohistochemistry demonstrated a correlation between the presence of *CTNNB1* mutations confined to exon 3 and increased nuclear translocation of β-catenin, particularly in the higher-grade tumor components, whereas hepatoblastomas with large *CTNNB1* deletions showed nuclear translocation of β-catenin confined to a much smaller proportion of tumor cells or only the normal staining of cell plasma membranes. Mutations confined to exon 3 maintain the BCL9-interaction domain, essential for transcription of WNT target genes and appear to facilitate the more aggressive phenotype seen in embryonal and small cell hepatoblastoma. By contrast, large deletions including the BCL9-interactin domain, although still resulting in decreased proteosomal degradation of β-catenin, would not be as capable of facilitating canonical WNT target gene expression as wild type *CTNNB1* [159].

Wnt signal activation has also been demonstrated as a late event in BWS-associated HB involving 11p15.5 uniparental isodisomy [160]. Several studies have explored the contribution of additional Wnt pathway molecules to hepatocarcinogenesis and indicate that, in addition to the β-catenin and *APC* mutations, *AXIN1* and *AXIN2* mutations [161] and sequence variations appear to be important in 10% of HCC and HB (Figure 40.19). *Dickkopf-1*, an antagonist of wingless/WNT signaling pathway, is expressed in most HB and Wilms's tumors analyzed but is only rarely and weakly detectable in HCC and absent in normal liver and other tumor types [162]. Koch et al. [163] found elevated expression of mRNA of nine Wnt pathway antagonists in hepatoblastoma.

Investigation of potential nuclear targets associated with β-catenin/Wnt signaling and potential β-catenin binding partners, identified a correlation between deletions and mutations of the β-catenin gene, overexpression of the target genes *cyclin D1* and *fibronectin*, and poorly differentiated histology in childhood HB [164,165]. Overexpression of cyclin D1 and cdk4 proteins might play an important role in the tumorigenesis of HB, and high *cyclin D1* expression may be related with worse prognosis [166,167]. An association between a *cyclin D1* polymorphism and the age of onset of HB has been reported, similar to

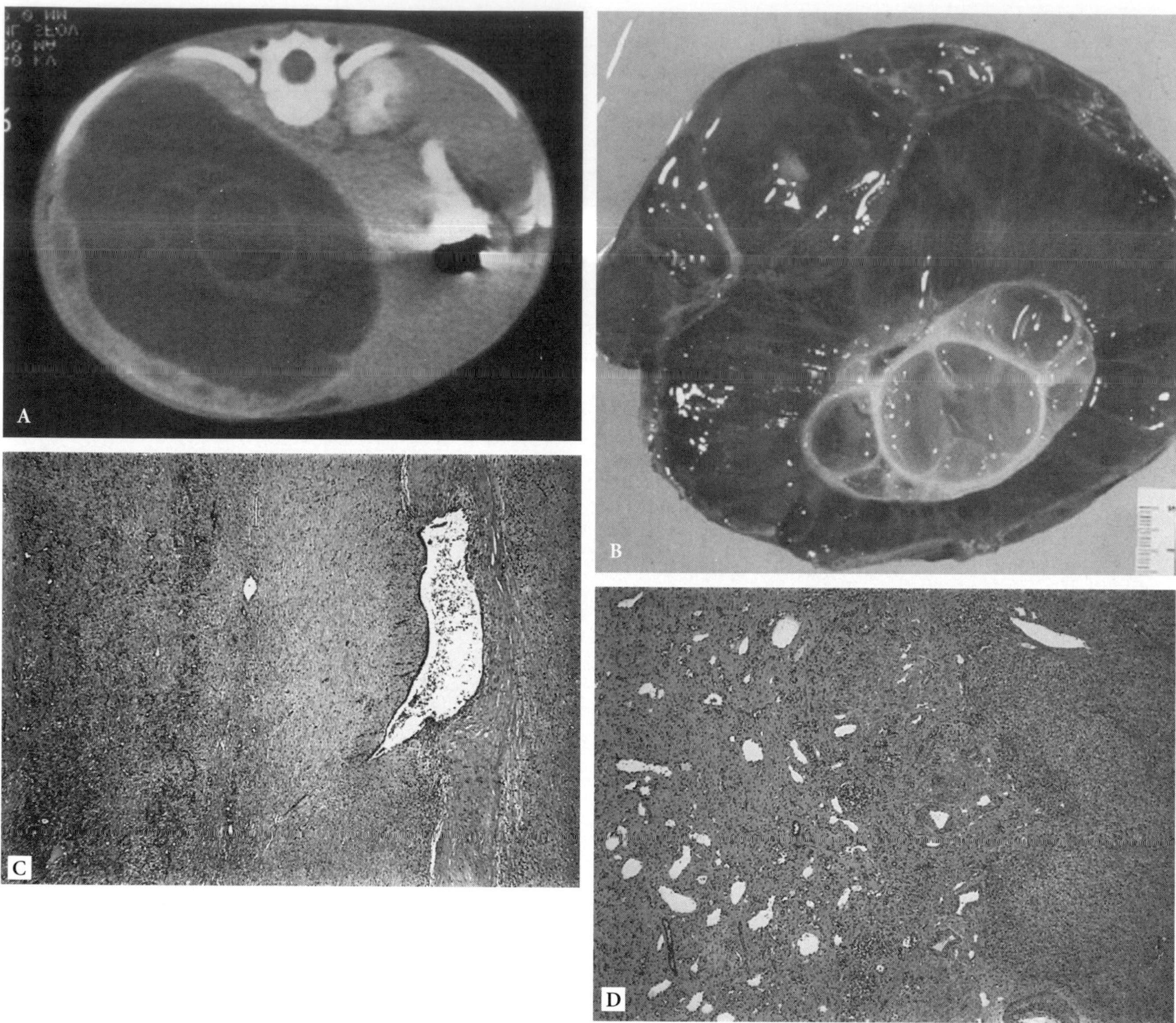

Figure 40.17. Mesenchymal hamartoma. (**A**) A multicystic mass is readily defined by CT in a 4-month-old. The apparent encapsulation is deceptive, and marsupialization is no longer suitable in view of the potential for sarcomatous growth. (**B**) A cut section of the resected specimen. (**C**) Cysts are lined by biliary epithelium or lymphatic endothelium. The stroma is myxomatous. (**D**) Vascular proliferation is frequently also present at the border with the host liver, and hypercirculation has rarely been symptomatic, simulating hemangiomas.

what was demonstrated in FAP families and colorectal cancer [167].

Other abnormalities of cell cycle genes in HB include inactivation and transcriptional repression by hypermethylation of *p16* [168] and differential p27 protein expression patterns that correlate with the degree of histologic differentiation and mitotic activity of these tumors [169]. Likewise, more expression of transforming growth factor *(TGF)-α*, a potent stimulator of cell proliferation in the liver and in liver tumors, can be detected in better differentiated HB tumor cells, suggesting that the less differentiated embryonal cells do not depend on growth stimulation provided by *TGF-α* [170].

Fas, a death receptor, and its ligand are coexpressed in HB in vivo, but some inhibitors of *Fas*-mediated apoptosis are also expressed in these tumors, suggesting that it is probably the action of inhibitory molecules of the Fas pathway that allows the tumor cells of HB to avoid apoptosis [171].

Overexpression of telomerase, a enzyme related to cellular immortality, regulated by the expression of hTERT (human telomerase reverse transcriptase), has been associated with poor outcome in patients with hepatoblastoma [172] (Table 40.8).

Many studies of HCC and its precursors have demonstrated complex and heterogeneous genetic or chromosomal abnormalities, some involving the p53 family, Rb family, and Wnt pathways [173,174]. In contrast to HB with a few characteristic chromosomal changes, HCC harbor multiple diverse chromosomal abnormalities, predominantly losses [175], with increased chromosomal instability in tumors associated with

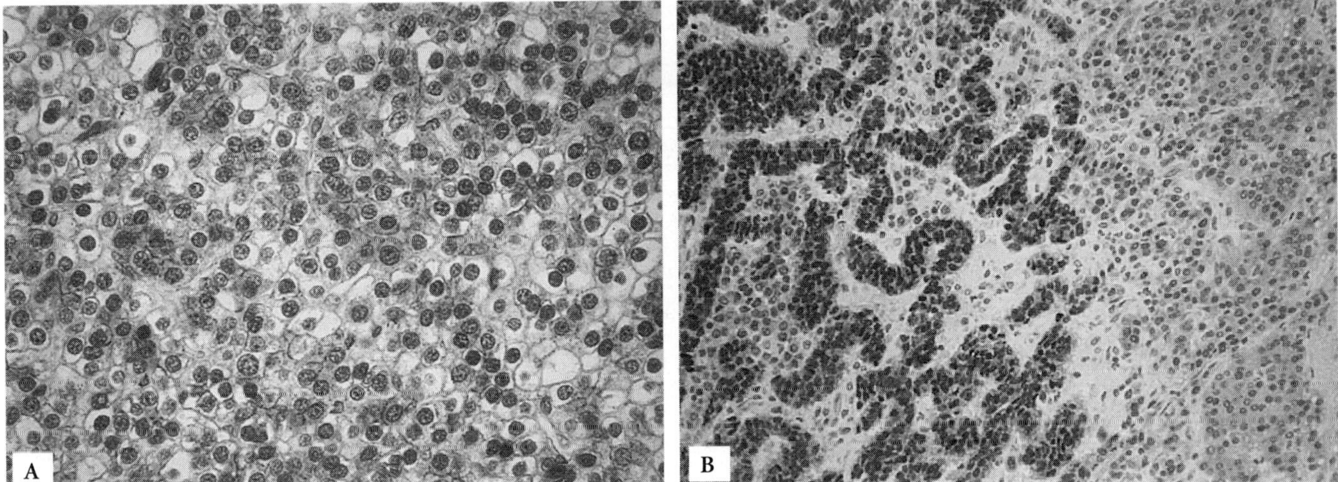

Figure 40.18. β-catenin immunostaining. (**A**) Fetal HB has staining of the plasma membranes, just as in normal hepatocytes. (**B**) In less mature cells, the protein is abundant in the cytoplasm, and in embryonal cells it is present in nuclei, where it contributes to the expression of several Wnt pathway genes. The difference can be exploited in evaluation of a stage 1 tumor for chemotherapy [158].

hepatitis B virus infection. Alterations common to HB and HCC include gain of chromosomes 1q, 8q, and 17q, and loss of 4q. Another important common feature shared by the two tumor types is the frequent activation of Wnt/β-catenin signaling by stabilizing mutations of β-catenin [176].

Karyotypic analysis demonstrated the presence of chromosomal rearrangements involving the 19q13.4 locus in primary embryonal sarcomas of the liver [177,178] as well as in a subset of mesenchymal hamartomas [127,129,178–181]. Two cases of coexistent embryonal sarcoma and mesenchymal hamartoma, one with documented chromosome 19p abnormalities [127,178] have been reported, raising the possibility of a putative pathogenic relationship and suggesting a genetic link between these two rare hepatic lesions [178,181,182].

Studies regarding the genetics of pediatric malignant vascular tumors of the liver are limited. A single case of infantile

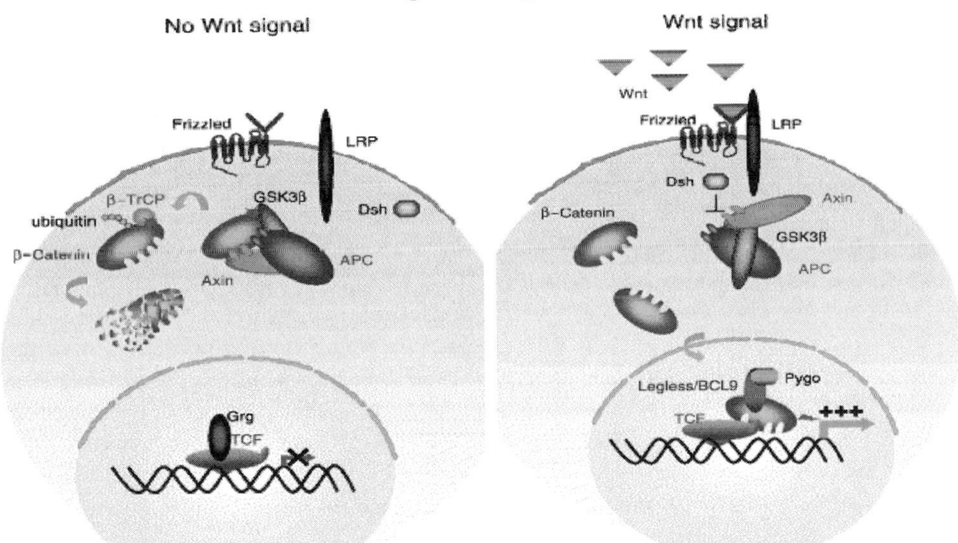

Figure 40.19. Diagram of the Wnt pathway. Oncogenes: Wnt, β-catenin, Lgs/BCL9. Tumor suppressor genes: APC, Axin, TCF1. (*Left*) In the absence of Wnt ligand β-catenin levels are regulated by a complex containing APC, Axin, and GSK3 β, and transcription of TCF targets is repressed by Grg corepressors. (*Right*) Binding a Wnt ligand destabilizes the β-catenin degradation complex, allowing transportation to the nucleus where β-catenin recruits Lgs/BCL9 and pygo and activates TCF target genes. Similar nuclear accumulation and downstream target transactivation occurs with some β-catenin mutations. (Adapted from Giles RH, van Es JH, Clevers H. Caught up in a Wnt storm: Wnt signaling in cancer. Biochimica Biophysica Acta 2003;1653:1–24.)

Table 40.9: Prognostic Factors in Hepatoblastoma

	Unfavorable Outcome	*Favorable Outcome*
Clinical		
Liver involvement	Multiple lobes	One lobe
Growth pattern	Multifocal	Unifocal
Vascular invasion	Present	Absent
Metastases	Distant metastases	Localized disease
Serum α fetoprotein	$<$ or $=$ 100 ng/mL or $>$ or $=$ 1,000,000 ng/mL	100–1,000,000 ng/mL
Serum α-fetoprotein decline	slow	rapid
Histopathology		
Differentiation	Undifferentiated small cell	Pure fetal, low mitotic activity
Genetic/Molecular		
Ploidy	aneuploidy	Diploidy
Chromosomal gains	+8q, +20	—
β-catenin expression	Nuclear	Membranous/cytoplasmic
P27/Kip1 expression	Low	High
PLK1 oncogene expression	High	Low
Cyclin D1 expression	High	Low
Telomerase expression	High	Low

hemangioendothelioma of the liver carrying an interstitial deletion of chromosome 6q was reported by Ito et al. [183]. Tannapfel et al. [184] reported inactivation of the *p16* gene, most commonly by promotor methylation, as a frequent event in angiosarcomas of the liver. *P53* gene mutations have been described as well but are an uncommon event in sporadic hepatic angiosarcomas [185].

PROGNOSTIC CONSIDERATIONS

Surgical excision is essential to cure primary liver neoplasms [186–189]. Gross venous tumor extension, distant metastatic disease, and multifocality are bad prognostic signs. Precocious puberty implies a poor outcome. The rapid decline of AFP levels in children with HB has been shown to correlate with better outcome [92]. Both exceptionally low (<100 mg/mL) and high (>1,000,000 mg/mL) values are associated with worse prognosis (Table 40.9).

Histopathologic differences in HB are important to assess prognosis and direct therapy but they cannot be fully evaluated from biopsies, which may be not representative, especially of tumors in young children. Well-differentiated, pure fetal HB with low mitotic rates can be treated with resection alone, whereas HB with a large proportion of undifferentiated small cells are associated with an unfavorable outcome [190,191]. Regrettably, only 3.4% of stage I and II cases in the POG series over 20 years fell into the "favorable histology" resectable category, but all patients were cured without chemotherapy [192]. DNA ploidy pattern analysis has demonstrated an association between aneuploidy and significantly poorer prognosis in HB [193,194]. Other genetic markers of prognostic relevance in HB include chromosomal gains on 8q and 20, associated nuclear localization of β-catenin and certain types of *CTNNB1* gene mutations with poor prognosis (discussed earlier; see Acquired Genetic Changes) [133,134,195]. Recent studies have examined the diagnostic and prognostic significance of p27/Kip1 expression in various tumors. An evaluation of 29 samples from patients with HB showed that primary well-differentiated fetal tumors without mitotic activity are strongly p27 positive, whereas the vast majority of small undifferentiated cell components are p27 negative [169], as are the fetal cells that survive chemotherapy. Whether these factors remain prognostically significant when highly active chemotherapy is administered is currently not clear.

Other molecular markers having poor prognostic significance in HB include high levels of telomerase activity, *PLK1* oncogene, and cyclin D1 overexpression [172,196,197]. None of the aforementioned molecular genetic alterations is routinely used as clinical prognostic indicators for HB at present. Ongoing molecular genetic analyses of tumor tissue, and, more specifically, of different histologic types, with careful clinical correlation may reveal prognostic markers and possible targets for therapy for this neoplasm.

TREATMENT

Surgery, either as the initial approach or after chemotherapy has rendered the tumor resectable, is the mainstay of the treatment for HB. Patients with unresectable tumors are candidates for orthotopic liver transplantation. Although only 25–30% of all HB are resectable at the time of diagnosis, cisplatin-based chemotherapy has markedly increased the number of patients who can be rendered disease-free through tumor resection after initial chemotherapy and has increased the cure rate from 25–30% (in the 1980s) to the currently achieved event-free survival of 75–80% or higher [192,198,199]. Hepatocellular carcinoma does not respond well to chemotherapy or radiotherapy; surgical resection is the only curative modality. Unfortunately, less than 30% of all HCC cases are resectable. The SIOPEL group used a pretreatment staging system (PRETEXT, Figure 40.5) and found only one patient with stage I and 14 patients with stage II among their 40 enrolled patients [100], whereas the American COG used a postsurgical staging system, which revealed eight patients with stage I (completely resected with microscopically negative margins) and 0 patients with stage II (completely resected but microscopically positive margins) among 46 enrolled children [101].

Surgery

The potential resectability of a tumor is assessed by Doppler ultrasonography, CT, or MRI, including delineation of the arterial and venous vascular supply. Resection is curative for most of the benign liver tumors, including the hepatic adenomas and mesenchymal hamartomas, where the risk for recurrences after resection alone is minimal [93,94,127,200–202]. Marsupialization of cystic mesenchymal hamartomas is no longer recommended because of the potential for the presence of sarcomatous components or transformation [201,203]. Features that prevent primary surgical resection include bilobar disease, involvement of the porta hepatitis, or tumor extension into the inferior vena cava and the right atrium [199]. With the possible exception of infants with hepatic hemangiomas/hemangioendotheliomas having characteristic imaging features (Figure 40.3B), a biopsy is necessary to establish the diagnosis in cases that cannot be primarily resected. For primary rhabdomyosarcomas or lymphomas of the liver, chemotherapy is the initial approach, but for other tumors, surgeons and oncologists in the United States believe that an attempt at primary resection should be made. The biopsy will distinguish among HB, HCC, or other, more rare, lesions including metastases. The presence of lung metastases generally dictates chemotherapy before hepatic resection but aggressive treatment, including resection of lung lesions, can be lifesaving [101,204]. There is controversy with respect to the role of preoperative chemotherapy (initial biopsy only) versus primary resection of the liver tumor [199]. In the SIOPEL 1 study, primary surgery was performed only for patients with PRETEXT group I tumors (tumor confined to left lateral sector or right posterior section). In all other cases, resection was attempted after four to six cycles of cisplatin-based chemotherapy, including the resection of any lung metastases. In that study, biopsy was found to be a safe procedure, and preoperative chemotherapy made large tumors easier to resect [199]. Our position favoring efforts at primary surgery is based on the following: (1) 3–4% of stage I HB do not require chemotherapy (well-differentiated, pure fetal histology with low mitotic rate, Table 40.8), (2) the small subgroup of tumors with a significant fraction of small undifferentiated cells does not respond to current chemotherapy, and (3) about 4% of suspected HB turn out to be benign lesions [93] or metastases [7] making up-front chemotherapy without at least an attempt at resection undesirable [205]. In two older studies performed by COG and POG, major surgical complications (hemorrhage or bile duct injuries) were significantly more common after chemotherapy than after primary resection (COG, 25% versus 8%; POG, 23% versus 0%) [105,206].

Surgical resection usually involves hepatic lobectomy or trisegmentectomy. Porta hepatis dissection and division of hepatic ligamentous attachments to examine the vessels is required to ensure that resection is possible. Extension of the tumor into the diaphragm or other adjacent organs is not considered a sign of unresectability as contiguous organs may be resected en bloc for cure. Lymph nodes at the porta hepatitis need to be sampled, and celiac and paraaortic lymph nodes should be inspected and sampled if macroscopically suspicious. Liver biopsies along the margin of resection should be subjected to frozen section examination if there is any question of tumoral infiltration. Pulmonary metastases should be removed at the time of resection if possible because this appears to improve survival rates [204,207]. Although an aggressive attitude toward total resection is encouraged, this is often complicated by the limited hepatic reserve of the patient with HCC, who may also suffer from cirrhosis or infectious hepatitis [115,208,209]. A comparison of 1000 patients (mainly adults) who underwent hepatectomy for small HCC (<5 cm in diameter) with 1366 patients with large tumors showed a higher complete resection rate (93.6% vs. 55.7%) for patients with smaller tumors [95]. More than 80% of the resections in the first group were considered curative compared with only 61% in the group with tumors larger than 5 cm. It is not surprising that this translated into improved 5-year survival rates of 63% versus 37% [95]. Hence, close follow-up and screening of children with known precursors is essential.

Chemotherapy

Combination chemotherapy has been extremely effective for most cancers in children, including HB. The most effective drug has been cisplatinum, an alkylating agent, in combination with vincristine, which disrupts microtubules, and 5-fluorouracil, an antimetabolite, or doxorubicin, which produces DNA strand breaks [188,189,210]. Irinotecan and etoposide are topoisomerase inhibitors that show promising activity but need to be studied further [101,211]. Other combinations have lately cured some angiosarcomas and embryonal sarcomas, but HCC remains resistant. The U.S. children's oncology groups compared the cisplatin, vincristine, and fluorouracil combination with cisplatinum and continuous infusion doxorubicin and did not demonstrate any statistically significant differences [192].

Patients with stage I, II, or resectable stage III did very well with a 5-year event-free survival rates of 91%, 100%, and 83%, respectively, whereas patients with unresectable or metastatic disease had only an event-free survival of 50% and 10%, respectively. Avoiding doxorubicin cardiotoxicity made the former regimen the preferred standard. In Japan, the combination of cisplatinum and Adriamycin was able to improve the 5-year survival (cure rate) of stage IV HB from 0% in 1982–90 to 57% for 1991–97 [212].

In a SIOPEL study, 37 children with HCC received preoperative chemotherapy with doxorubicin and cisplatinum. They had a disease-free survival rate of 28%, after undergoing complete resection of the tumor [100]. Event-free survival was 23% at 2 years and 17% at 5 years, but none of the patients who did not respond to preoperative chemotherapy survived. Similar results were found in the COG study in which the 46 patients were enrolled and randomized to receive either cisplatinum, vincristine, and fluorouracil or cisplatinum and continuous infusion doxorubicin [101]. Children with initially resectable tumors had a 5-year survival of 88% compared with patients who had stage III or IV disease (8% and 0%, respectively), but there was no difference between the two treatment regimens. The outcomes were no different for fibrolamellar carcinomas of comparable stage in the COG study or other studies [17]. Some promising results with intratumoral and other therapies for HCC in adults may prove useful in children as well [213].

Benign vascular tumors have a mortality of 30–80% when they cause a consumptive coagulopathy or congestive heart failure [214,215]. Large liver hemangiomas can cause severe hypothyroidism because of high levels of type 3 iodothyronine deiodinase activity in the hemangioma tissue [73]. About 30% of hemangiomas respond rapidly to corticosteroids, given orally at a dose of 2–3 mg/kg/d (rarely 4–5 mg/kg/d) for 4–6 weeks, followed by a slow taper over 9–12 months, but 40% of hemangiomas will show only a partial response and the remaining 30% do not respond [216]. Life-threatening hemangiomas that do not respond to corticosteroid therapy within 2 weeks should be considered for treatment with recombinant interferon-α (2–3 million U/m^2 body surface area) given subcutaneously every day for 9–12 months [216,217]. The most worrisome side effects are spastic diplegia, sometimes persisting even after discontinuation of interferon therapy [216,217] and rarely hypothyroidism, caused by the formation of antithyroid antibodies [218,219]. Unresectable liver hemangiomas that are unresponsive to steroids or interferon, may need to be treated with chemotherapy (vincristine, cyclophosphamide, or both) or transplantation.

Angiosarcoma of the liver is a rare but very aggressive tumor. A few cases have been cured by surgery and multidrug chemotherapy (including doxorubicin and cisplatinum) [220,221]. A positive trend is being observed in the treatment of embryonal sarcomas [222,223] and peribiliary rhabdomyosarcoma [65,224]. With typical soft tissue sarcoma protocols, including cisplatinum, doxorubicin (Adriamycin)-type drugs, actinomycin, and etoposide or ifosphamide, all children with localized and resectable rhabdomyosarcoma were cured, and 70% of the original 17 are long-term survivors.

All current chemotherapy regimens have substantial toxicities. Neutropenia occurs in about half of the patients receiving the standard regimen of vincristine, 5-FU, and cisplatinum, whereas other hematologic toxicities are uncommon [101]. Ototoxicity due to cisplatinum occurs in about 30–40% of all patients, some of them significant enough to warrant hearing aids [101,225].

Liver Transplantation

When initial chemotherapy fails to permit resection, transplantation is an effective treatment for patients with unresectable tumors confined to the liver. A recent review of the worldwide experience included 147 cases [226]. Overall survival 10 years after liver transplant was 82% for the 106 children who underwent a "primary" liver transplant and 30% for the 41 children who underwent "rescue" liver transplant after previous partial hepatectomies failed to eradicate fully the HB. Recent experience in Cincinnati supports the contention that transplantation offers a better outcome than maximal surgery in the form of trisegmentectomy: five of five patients with primary orthotopic liver transplant (OLT) and two thirds with rescue OLT were cured versus four of eight with surgery in this series [227]. In Pittsburgh, an 83% 5-year survival rate was achieved by OLT, and this was not compromised by venous invasion, lymph nodes metastases, or contiguous spread [228].

A small series of 19 children with HCC who underwent liver transplantation showed similar results with 1-, 3-, and 5-year survival rates of 79%, 68%, and 63%, respectively [228]. An analysis of 135 children with HB and 41 with HCC in the U.S. United Network for Organ Sharing database from 1987 to 2004 revealed approximately equal benefits of OLT at 1, 5, and 10 years (79%, 69%, and 66% for HB; 86%, 63%, and 58% for HCC) [229]. However, a shortage of donor livers and the fact that many patients present with metastatic disease limits the feasibility of transplantation.

Radiation Therapy

Radiation has had a limited role in the treatment of liver cancers [230]. It has occasionally been used in Europe as an adjunct treatment for unresectable HB but is unlikely to be included in any treatment protocols because liver tolerance for radiation is relatively low and the risk for intra-abdominal complications may be increased with this modality [230]. Radiation has been used with limited success in adult patients with small, nonmetastatic HCC [231–233]. Using local radiotherapy, an objective response was observed in 106 of 158 (67.1%) patients. Patients treated with greater than 50 Gy had a measurable response in 77.1%. Survivals rates at 1 and 2 years after radiotherapy were 41.8% and 19.9%, respectively, with a median survival time of 10 months [234]. Conformal radiotherapy may increase the efficacy and decrease the toxicity in the future [235].

Other Modalities

Radiotherapy has also been used in conjunction with transcatheter arterial chemoembolization (TACE) in adult patients with unresectable HCC and appears to confer additional benefits. A study of 76 patients with large unresectable HCC who were treated with TACE followed by external-beam irradiation were compared with a cohort of 89 patients with large HCC who underwent TACE alone during the same period [231]. The objective response rate in the TACE plus irradiation group was higher than that in the TACE alone group (47.4% vs. 28.1%, $P < 0.05$). The overall survival rates in TACE plus irradiation group (64.0%, 28.6%, and 19.3% at 1, 3, and 5 years, respectively) were significantly higher than those in TACE alone group (39.9%, 9.5%, and 7.2%, respectively, $P = 0.0001$) [231].

Two studies have been reported using arterial chemoembolization in children with HB with mixed results. In Japan, 6 of 8 children were free of disease for a mean of 50 months following resection [236]. In the United States, six patients with HB received hepatic arterial chemoembolization with cisplatin and doxorubicin every 2–4 weeks until their tumors became surgically resectable or they showed signs of disease progression. All patients had previously received systemic chemotherapy, and all six patients showed a partial response to the embolization treatment. However, four patients subsequently died of progressive disease, one developed a recurrence that was again treated with embolization, and another underwent OTC. The latter two patients were still alive 33 and 31 months later [237].

Interferon α has been used for the treatment of hepatitis B and C, common infections in patients with HCC. Recombinant interferon α also has an enhancing effect on the cytotoxicity of fluoropyrimidines, including the frequently used 5-fluorouracil [238,239]. Leung et al. [240] reported prolonged survival in patients who received treatment with intravenous cisplatin, doxorubicin, 5-fluorouracil, and subcutaneously administered interferon α with a median survival of 7–8 months, compared with a historical control of 2–3 months [240]. An even longer median survival of 19.5 months was achieved by using a combination of systemic continuous fluorouracil combined with subcutaneous interferon α given three times per week [241]. However, in this study only 56% of the patients had cirrhosis (vs. 83.2% in the Leung study), more patients had a negative hepatitis serology (40% vs. <10%), and the nine patients (21%) had the fibrolamellar variant of HCC [240,241]. Combining interferon α-2B with surgery was effective for epithelial hemangioendothelioma as well [242].

FUTURE PROSPECTS

Disseminated HB and unresectable HCC have an unsatisfactory prognosis. Screening of patients at increased risk for liver tumors is currently successful for children with tyrosinemia and the Beckwith–Wiedemann syndrome. It should be extended to include premature babies of very low birth weight, FAP family members, patients with glycogenoses, and chronic cholestatic syndromes, including biliary atresia and recipients of long-term parenteral nutrition.

More studies to enhance safety of efficacious treatments are needed. α-Fetoprotein is elevated in most HB and many HCC patients and has thus been explored as a potential marker in imaging studies; it may lend itself to the use as a targeted antibody-mediated therapy [243,244].

Side effects, especially ototoxicity, are common in children receiving cisplatin-based therapies. Oxaliplatin, a newer platinum agent with a more favorable toxicity profile, is being considered as a possible active agent against recurrent HB. Preclinical studies have shown oxaliplatin to be synergistic with fluorouracil and SN-38, the active metabolite of irinotecan [245]. The COG studied the role of amifostine as a chemoprotectant agent but did not see any protection against ototoxicity associated with the platinum agents [246].

The issue of multidrug resistance in patients with advanced or recurrent HB is being investigated. Increased expression of the multidrug resistance gene 1 (*MDR-1*), leading to an increase in its gene product, P-glycoprotein, results in an accelerated removal of chemotherapeutic agents from the cell's interior [247]. P-Glycoprotein inhibitors are currently undergoing phase I trials, but their role in the treatment of HB has not yet been established [248].

Both HCC and HB are highly vascular neoplasms, and thus antiangiogenic treatment approaches for this tumor are being tested. Cyclooxygenase-2 (COX-2) is overexpressed in many malignant tumors and has angiogenic activity through the increased production of vascular endothelial growth factor and prostaglandins, as well as through activation of matrix metalloproteinases, a constellation that facilitates invasion [249,250]. Future treatment protocols may include a COX-2 inhibitor, angiostatin, or even antiangiogenic gene therapy [251,252]. Thalidomide's antiangiogenic actions are being evaluated in combination with other agents, but its neurotoxicity is a serious problem. It was effective in a patient with epithelioid hemangioendothelioma [253]. The success of imatinib, a tyrosine kinase inhibitor, in treating chronic myelogenous leukemia and gastrointestinal stromal tumors prompts the hope that unraveling the complexities of signaling pathways, such as β-catenin-WNT in HB, will provide points of attack for molecular therapies specific to particular neoplasms, especially those arising from abnormalities in morphogenesis like HB.

Liver transplantation has become more acceptable, especially with the growing availability of living donor donations. The several questions that remain in regard to the appropriate selection of patients, timing, and pre- and posttransplant chemotherapy are being studied by COG and SIOPEL. The remarkable advances in treatment of rare tumors such as HB have only been possible through the multicenter collaboration of several groups (SIOP, COG, the German and Japanese liver tumor study groups). Continued cooperation regarding the development of new treatment modalities, as well as investigations of pathology and pathogenesis and of preventive and screening efforts, should further improve the medical response to these rare malignancies.

REFERENCES

1. Weinberg AG, Finegold MJ. Primary hepatic tumors of childhood. Hum Pathol 1983;14:512–37.
2. Stocker JT. Hepatic tumors in children. 2nd ed. Philadelphia: Lippincott, Williams and Wilkins, 2001.
3. See the Surveillance Epidemiology and End Results Web site, National Cancer Institute: http://seer. cancer.gov. (Accessed November 15, 2006.)
4. Darbari A, Sabin KM, Shapiro CN, Schwarz KB. Epidemiology of primary hepatic malignancies in U.S. children. Hepatology 2003;38:560–6.
5. Isaacs H Jr. Neoplasms in infants: a report of 265 cases. Pathol Annu 1983;18:165–214.
6. Tsai HL, Liu CS, Chin TW, Wei CF. Hepatoblastoma and hepatocellular carcinoma in children. J Chin Med Assoc 2004;6783–8.
7. Finegold MJ. Tumors of the liver. Semin Liver Dis 1994;14:270–81.
8. Bortolasi L, Marchiori L, Dal Dosso I, et al. Hepatoblastoma in adult age: a report of two cases. Hepatogastroenterology 1996; 43:1073–8.
9. Yamazaki M, Ryu M, Okazumi S, et al. Hepatoblastoma in an adult. A case report and clinical review of literatures. Hepatol Res 2004;30:182–8.
10. Kasper HU, Longerich T, Stippel DL, et al. Mixed hepatoblastoma in an adult. Arch Pathol Lab Med 2005;129:234–7.
11. Kenney LB, Miller BA, Ries LA, et al. Increased incidence of cancer in infants in the U.S.: 1980–1990. Cancer 1998;82:1396–400.
12. El-Serag HB, Davila JA, Petersen NJ, McGlynn KA. The continuing increase in the incidence of hepatocellular carcinoma in the United States: an update. Ann Intern Med 2003;139:817–23.
13. Pontisso P, Morsica G, Ruvoletto MG, et al. Latent hepatitis B virus infection in childhood hepatocellular carcinoma. Analysis by polymerase chain reaction. Cancer 1992;69:2731–5.
14. Cheah PL, Looi LM, Lin HP, Yap SF. A case of childhood hepatitis B virus infection related primary hepatocellular carcinoma with short malignant transformation time. Pathology 1991; 23:66–8.
15. Chang MH. Decreasing incidence of hepatocellular carcinoma among children following universal hepatitis B immunization. Liver Int 2003;23:309–14.
16. Montesano R. Hepatitis B immunization and hepatocellular carcinoma: The Gambia Hepatitis Intervention Study. J Med Virol 2002;67:444–6.
17. Katzenstein HM, Krailo MD, Malogolowkin MH, et al. Fibrolamellar hepatocellular carcinoma in children and adolescents. Cancer 2003;97:2006–12.
18. Oue T, Kubota A, Okuyama H, et al. Hepatoblastoma in children of extremely low birth weight: a report from a single perinatal center. J Pediatr Surg 2003;38:134–7; discussion 134–7.
19. Ikeda H, Hachitanda Y, Tanimura M, et al. Development of unfavorable hepatoblastoma in children of very low birth weight: results of a surgical and pathologic review. Cancer 1998; 82:1789–96.
20. Tanimura M, Matsui I, Abe J, et al. Increased risk of hepatoblastoma among immature children with a lower birth weight. Cancer Res 1998;58:3032–5.
21. Reynolds M. Current status of liver tumors in children. Semin Pediatr Surg 2001;10:140–5.
22. Kapfer SA, Petruzzi MJ, Caty MG. Hepatoblastoma in low birth weight infants: an institutional review. Pediatr Surg Int 2004;20:753–6.
23. Ansell P, Mitchell CD, Roman E, et al. Relationships between perinatal and maternal characteristics and hepatoblastoma: a report from the UKCCS. Eur J Cancer 2004;41:741–8.
24. Buckley JD, Sather H, Ruccione K, et al. A case–control study of risk factors for hepatoblastoma. A report from the Childrens Cancer Study Group. Cancer 1989;64:1169–76.
25. Satge D, Sasco AJ, Little J. Antenatal therapeutic drug exposure and fetal/neonatal tumours: review of 89 cases. Paediatr Perinat Epidemiol 1998;12:84–117.
26. Sorahan T, Lancashire RJ. Parental cigarette smoking and childhood risks of hepatoblastoma: OSCC data. Br J Cancer 2004; 90:1016–18.
27. Pang D, McNally R, Birch JM. Parental smoking and childhood cancer: results from the United Kingdom Childhood Cancer Study. Br J Cancer 2003;88:373–81.
28. Vileisis RA, Sorensen K, Gonzalez-Crussi F, Hunt CE. Liver malignancy after parenteral nutrition. J Pediatr 1982;100:88–90.
29. Patterson K, Kapur SP, Chandra RS. Hepatocellular carcinoma in a noncirrhotic infant after prolonged parenteral nutrition. J Pediatr 1985;106:797–800.
30. DeBaun MR, Tucker MA. Risk of cancer during the first four years of life in children from The Beckwith–Wiedemann Syndrome Registry. J Pediatr 1998;132:398–400.
31. Clericuzio CL, Chen E, McNeil DE, et al. Serum alphafetoprotein screening for hepatoblastoma in children with Beckwith–Wiedemann syndrome or isolated hemihyperplasia. J Pediatr 2003;143:270–2.
32. Cooper WN, Luharia A, Evans GA, et al. Molecular subtypes and phenotypic expression of Beckwith–Wiedemann syndrome. Eur J Hum Genet 2005;13:1025–32.
33. Gracia Bouthelier R, Lapunzina P. Follow-up and risk of tumors in overgrowth syndromes. J Pediatr Endocrinol Metab 2005;18 Suppl 1:1227–35.
34. Li M, Shuman C, Fei YL, et al. GPC3 mutation analysis in a spectrum of patients with overgrowth expands the phenotype of Simpson–Golabi–Behmel syndrome. Am J Med Genet 2001; 102:161–8.
35. Buonuomo, P.S, Ruggiero A, Vasta I, Attina G, Riccardi R, Zampino G. Second case of hepatoblastoma in a young patient with Simpson-Golabi-Behmel syndrome. Pediatr Hematol Oncol 2005;22:623–8.
36. Rodriguez-Criado, G, Magano, L, Segovia, M, et al. Clinical and molecular studies on two further families with Simpson–Golabi–Behmel syndrome. Am J Med Genet A 2005;138:272–7.
37. Cohen MM Jr. Beckwith–Wiedemann syndrome: historical, clinicopathological, and etiopathogenetic perspectives. Pediatr Dev Pathol 2005;8:287–304.
38. Kingston JE, Draper GJ, Mann JR. Hepatoblastoma and polyposis coli. Lancet 1982;1:457.
39. Giardiello FM, Petersen GM, Brensinger JD, et al. Hepatoblastoma and APC gene mutation in familial adenomatous polyposis. Gut 1996;39:867–9.
40. Aretz S, Koch A, Uhlhaas S, et al. Should children at risk for familial adenomatous polyposis be screened for hepatoblastoma and children with apparently sporadic hepatoblastoma be screened for APC germline mutations? Pediatr Blood Cancer 2006;47:811–18.

41. Oda H, Imai Y, Nakatsuru Y, et al. Somatic mutations of the APC gene in sporadic hepatoblastomas. Cancer Res 1996;56: 3320–3.
42. Thomas D, Pritchard J, Davidson R, et al. Familial hepatoblastoma and APC gene mutations: renewed call for molecular research. Eur J Cancer 2003;39:2200–4.
43. Weinberg AG, Mize CE, Worthen HG. The occurrence of hepatoma in the chronic form of hereditary tyrosinemia. J Pediatr 1976;88:434–8.
44. Demers SI, Russo P, Lettre F, Tanguay RM. Frequent mutation reversion inversely correlates with clinical severity in a genetic liver disease, hereditary tyrosinemia. Hum Pathol 2003; 34:1313–20.
45. Lindstedt S, Holme E, Lock EA, et al. Treatment of hereditary tyrosinaemia type I by inhibition of 4-hydroxyphenylpyruvate dioxygenase. Lancet 1992;340:813–17.
46. Holme E, Lindstedt S. Nontransplant treatment of tyrosinemia. Clin Liver Dis 2000;4:805–14.
47. Bianchi L. Glycogen storage disease I and hepatocellular tumours. Eur J Pediatr 1993;152 Suppl 1:S63–70.
48. Coire CI, Qizilbash AH, Castelli MF. Hepatic adenomata in type Ia glycogen storage disease. Arch Pathol Lab Med 1987;111: 166–9.
49. Siciliano M, De Candia E, Ballari, S, et al. Hepatocellular carcinoma complicating liver cirrhosis in type IIIa glycogen storage disease. J Clin Gastroenterol 2000;31:80–2.
50. Kaufman SS, Wood RP, Shaw BW Jr, et al. Hepatocarcinoma in a child with the Alagille syndrome. Am J Dis Child 1987;141:698–700.
51. Rabinovitz M, Imperial JC, Schade RR, Van Thiel DH. Hepatocellular carcinoma in Alagille's syndrome: a family study. J Pediatr Gastroenterol Nutr 1989;8:26–30.
52. Taat F, Bosman DK, Aronson DC. Hepatoblastoma in a girl with biliary atresia: coincidence or co-incidence. Pediatr Blood Cancer 2004;43:603–5.
53. Richter A, Grabhorn E, Schulz A, et al. Hepatoblastoma in a child with progressive familial intrahepatic cholestasis. Pediatr Transplant 2005;9:805–8.
54. Lederman SM, Martin EC, Laffey KT, Lefkowitch JH. Hepatic neurofibromatosis, malignant schwannoma, and angiosarcoma in von Recklinghausen's disease. Gastroenterology 1987; 92:234–9.
55. Geoffroy-Perez B, Janin N, Ossian K, et al. Cancer risk in heterozygotes for ataxia-telangiectasia. Int J Cancer 2001;93:288–93.
56. Tsui WM, Colombari R, Portmann BC, et al. Hepatic angiomyolipoma: a clinicopathologic study of 30 cases and delineation of unusual morphologic variants. Am J Surg Pathol 1999;23:34–48.
57. Fricke BL, Donnelly LF, Casper KA, Bissler JJ. Frequency and imaging appearance of hepatic angiomyolipomas in pediatric and adult patients with tuberous sclerosis. AJR Am J Roentgenol 2004;182:1027–30.
58. Ucar C, Caliskan U, Toy H, Gunel E. Hepatoblastoma in a child with neurofibromatosis type I. Pediatr Blood Cancer 2005, Nov. 10; Epub ahead of print.
59. Abbondanzo SL, Manz HJ, Klappenbach RS, Gootenberg JE. Hepatocellular carcinoma in an 11-year-old girl with Fanconi's anemia. Report of a case and review of the literature. Am J Pediatr Hematol Oncol 1986;8:334–7.
60. Touraine RL, Bertrand Y, Foray P, et al. Hepatic tumours during androgen therapy in Fanconi anaemia. Eur J Pediatr 1993;152:691–3.
61. Ishak KG, Goodman ZD, Stocker JT. Tumor of the liver and intrahepatic bile ducts. Washington, D.C.: Armed Forces Institute of Pathology, 2001.
62. Stringer MD. Liver tumors. Semin Pediatr Surg 2001;9:196–208.
63. Jung SE, Kim KH, Kim MY, et al. Clinical characteristics and prognosis of patients with hepatoblastoma. World J Surg 2001; 25:126–30.
64. Dasgupta D, Guthrie A, McClean P, et al. Liver transplantation for a hilar inflammatory myofibroblastic tumor. Pediatr Transplant 2005;8:517–21.
65. Horowitz ME, Etcubanas E, Webber BL, et al. Hepatic undifferentiated (embryonal) sarcoma and rhabdomyosarcoma in children. Results of therapy. Cancer 1987;59:396–402.
66. Mueller BU, Mulliken JB. The infant with a vascular tumor. Semin Perinatol 1999;23:332–40.
67. Shiozawa Y, Fujita H, Fujimura J, et al. A fetal case of transient abnormal myelopoiesis with severe liver failure in Down syndrome: prognostic value of serum markers. Pediatr Hematol Oncol 2004;21:273–8.
68. Arshad RR, Woo SY, Abbassi V, et al. Virilizing hepatoblastoma: precocious sexual development and partial response of pulmonary metastases to cis-platinum. CA Cancer J Clin 1982; 32:293–300.
69. Galifer RB, Sultan C, Margueritte G, Barneon G. Testosterone-producing hepatoblastoma in a 3-year-old boy with precocious puberty. J Pediatr Surg 1985;20:713–14.
70. Watanabe I, Yamaguchi M, Kasai M. Histologic characteristics of gonadotropin-producing hepatoblastoma: a survey of seven cases from Japan. J Pediatr Surg 1987;22:406–11.
71. Heerema-McKenney A, Leuschner I, Smith N, et al. Nested stromal epithelial tumor of the liver: six cases of a distinctive pediatric neoplasm with frequent calcifications and association with cushing syndrome. Am J Surg Pathol 2005;29:10–20.
72. Hill DA, Swanson PE, Anderson K, et al. Desmoplastic nested spindle cell tumor of liver: report of four cases of a proposed new entity. Am J Surg Pathol 2005;29:1–9.
73. Huang K, Lin S. Nationwide vaccination: a success story in Taiwan. Vaccine 2000;18 Suppl 1:S35–8.
74. Moritake H, Taketomi A, Kamimura S, et al. Renin-producing hepatoblastoma. J Pediatr Hematol Oncol 2000;22:78–80.
75. Nickerson HJ, Silberman TL, McDonald TP. Hepatoblastoma, thrombocytosis, and increased thrombopoietin. Cancer 1980; 45:315–17.
76. Shafford EA, Pritchard J. Extreme thrombocytosis as a diagnostic clue to hepatoblastoma. Arch Dis Child 1993;69:171.
77. Enjolras O, Wassef M, Mazoyer E, et al. Infants with Kasabach–Merritt syndrome do not have "true" hemangiomas. J Pediatr 1997;130:631–40.
78. Ravindra KV, Guthrie JA, Woodley H, et al. Preoperative vascular imaging in pediatric liver transplantation. J Pediatr Surg 40:643–7.
79. Foulner D, Cremin B. Childhood hepatocellular carcinoma and hepatoblastoma: integrated sonography and dynamic CT. Australas Radiol 1991;35:346–9.
80. King SJ, Babyn PS, Greenberg ML, et al. Value of CT in determining the resectability of hepatoblastoma before and after chemotherapy. Am J Roentgenol 1993;160:793–8.

81. von Schweinitz D, Gluer S, Mildenberger H. Liver tumors in neonates and very young infants: diagnostic pitfalls and therapeutic problems. Eur J Pediatr Surg 1995;5:72–6.
82. Hoffer FA. Magnetic resonance imaging of abdominal masses in the pediatric patient. Semin Ultrasound CT MR 2005;26:212–23.
83. Philip I, Shun A, McCowage G, Howman-Giles R. Positron emission tomography in recurrent hepatoblastoma. Pediatr Surg Int 21:341–5.
84. Begemann M, Trippett TM, Lis E, Antunes NL. Brain metastases in hepatoblastoma. Pediatr Neurol 2004;30:295–7.
85. Perilongo G, Brown J, Shafford E, et al. Hepatoblastoma presenting with lung metastases: treatment results of the first cooperative, prospective study of the International Society of Paediatric Oncology on childhood liver tumors. Cancer 2000;89:1845–53.
86. Archer D, Babyn P, Gilday D, Greenberg MA. Potentially misleading bone scan findings in patients with hepatoblastoma. Clin Nucl Med 1993;18:1026–31.
87. Abramson LP, Pillai S, Acton R, et al. Successful orthotopic liver transplantation for treatment of a hepatic yolk sac tumor. J Pediatr Surg 2005;40:1185–7.
88. Blohm ME, Vesterling-Horner D, Calaminus G, Gobel U. Alpha 1-fetoprotein (AFP) reference values in infants up to 2 years of age. Pediatr Hematol Oncol 1998;15:135–42.
89. Schneider DT, Calaminus G, Gobel U. Diagnostic value of alpha 1-fetoprotein and beta-human chorionic gonadotropin in infancy and childhood. Pediatr Hematol Oncol 2001;18:11–26.
90. Vaughan WG, Sanders DW, Grosfeld JL, et al. Favorable outcome in children with Beckwith–Wiedemann syndrome and intraabdominal malignant tumors. J Pediatr Surg 1995;30:1042–4; discussion 1044–5.
91. Pompili M, Rapaccini GL, Covino M, et al. Prognostic factors for survival in patients with compensated cirrhosis and small hepatocellular carcinoma after percutaneous ethanol injection therapy. Cancer 2001;92:126–35.
92. Van Tornout JM, Buckley JD, Quinn JJ, et al. Timing and magnitude of decline in alpha-fetoprotein levels in treated children with unresectable or metastatic hepatoblastoma are predictors of outcome: a report from the Children's Cancer Group. J Clin Oncol 1997;15:1190–7.
93. Boman F, Bossard C, Fabre M, et al. Mesenchymal hamartomas of the liver may be associated with increased serum alpha foetoprotein concentrations and mimic hepatoblastomas. Eur J Pediatr Surg 2004;14:63–6.
94. Stocker JT, Ishak KG. Mesenchymal hamartoma of the liver: report of 30 cases and review of the literature. Pediatr Pathol 1983;1:245–67.
95. Zhou XD, Tang ZY, Yang BH, et al. Experience of 1000 patients who underwent hepatectomy for small hepatocellular carcinoma. Cancer 2001;91:1479–86.
96. Shimada M, Yonemura Y, Ijichi H, et al. Living donor liver transplantation for hepatocellular carcinoma: a special reference to a preoperative des-gamma-carboxy prothrombin value. Transplant Proc 2005;37:1177–9.
97. Capurro M, Wanless IR, Sherman M, et al. Glypican-3: a novel serum and histochemical marker for hepatocellular carcinoma. Gastroenterology 2003;125:89–97.
98. Filmus J, Capurro M. Glypican-3 and alphafetoprotein as diagnostic tests for hepatocellular carcinoma. Mol Diagn 2004;8:207–12.
99. Yamauchi N, Watanabe A, Hishinuma M, et al. The glypican 3 oncofetal protein is a promising diagnostic marker for hepatocellular carcinoma. Mod Pathol 2005;18:1591–8.
100. Czauderna P, Mackinlay G, Perilongo G, et al. Hepatocellular carcinoma in children: results of the first prospective study of the International Society of Pediatric Oncology group. J Clin Oncol 2002;20:2798–804.
101. Katzenstein HM, London WB, Douglass EC, et al. Treatment of unresectable and metastatic hepatoblastoma: a pediatric oncology group phase II study. J Clin Oncol 2002;20:3438–44.
102. Aronson DC, Schnater JM, Staalman CR, et al. Predictive value of the pretreatment extent of disease system in hepatoblastoma: results from the International Society of Pediatric Oncology Liver Tumor Study Group SIOPEL-1 study. J Clin Oncol 2005;23:1245–52.
103. Wu JT, Book L, Sudar K. Serum alpha fetoprotein (AFP) levels in normal infants. Pediatr Res 1981;15:50–2.
104. Reynolds M. Conversion of unresectable to resectable hepatoblastoma and long-term follow-up study. World J Surg 1995;19:814–16.
105. Ortega JA, Krailo MD, Haas JE, et al. Effective treatment of unresectable or metastatic hepatoblastoma with cisplatin and continuous infusion doxorubicin chemotherapy: a report from the Childrens Cancer Study Group. J Clin Oncol 1991;9:2167–76.
106. Zimmermann A. Hepatoblastoma with cholangioblastic features ("cholangioblastic hepatoblastoma") and other liver tumors with bimodal differentiation in young patients. Med Pediatr Oncol 39:487–91.
107. Ruck P, Xiao JC, Kaiserling E. Small epithelial cells and the histogenesis of hepatoblastoma. Electron microscopic, immunoelectron microscopic, and immunohistochemical findings. Am J Pathol 1996;148:321–9.
108. Badve S, Logdberg L, Lal A, et al. Small cells in hepatoblastoma lack "oval" cell phenotype. Mod Pathol 2003;16:930–6.
109. Fiegel HC, Gluer S, Roth B, et al. Stem-like cells in human hepatoblastoma. J Histochem Cytochem 2004;52:1495–501.
110. Heifetz SA, French M, Correa M, Grosfeld JL. Hepatoblastoma: the Indiana experience with preoperative chemotherapy for inoperable tumors; clinicopathological considerations. Pediatr Pathol Lab Med 1997;17:857–74.
111. Manivel C, Wick MR, Abenoza P, Dehner LP. Teratoid hepatoblastoma. The nosologic dilemma of solid embryonic neoplasms of childhood. Cancer 1986;57:2168–74.
112. Ruck P, Harms D, Kaiserling E. Neuroendocrine differentiation in hepatoblastoma. An immunohistochemical investigation. Am J Surg Pathol 1990;14:847–55.
113. Biegel JA, Tan L, Zhang F, et al. Alterations of the hSNF5/INI1 gene in central nervous system atypical teratoid/rhabdoid tumors and renal and extrarenal rhabdoid tumors. Clin Cancer Res 2002;8:3461–7.
114. Thorner P, Squire J, Plavsic N, et al. Expression of WT1 in pediatric small cell tumors: report of two cases with a possible mesothelial origin. Pediatr Dev Pathol 1999;2:33–41.
115. Katzenstein HM, Kletzel M, Reynolds M, et al. Metastatic malignant rhabdoid tumor of the liver treated with tandem high-dose therapy and autologous peripheral blood stem cell rescue. Med Pediatr Oncol 2003;40:199–201.
116. Scheimberg I, Cullinane C, Kelsey A, Malone M. Primary hepatic malignant tumor with rhabdoid features. A histological, immunocytochemical, and electron microscopic study of four

cases and a review of the literature. Am J Surg Pathol 1996; 20:1394–400.

117. Donner LR, Rao A, Truss LM, Dobin SM. Translocation (8;13)(q24.2;q33) in a malignant rhabdoid tumor of the liver. Cancer Genet Cytogenet 2000;116:153–7.
118. Mann JR, Kasthuri N, Raafat F, et al. Malignant hepatic tumours in children: incidence, clinical features and aetiology. Paediatr Perinat Epidemiol 1990;4:276–89.
119. Gonzalez-Crussi F, Upton MP, Maurer HS. Hepatoblastoma. Attempt at characterization of histologic subtypes. Am J Surg Pathol 1982;6:599–612.
120. Daller JA, Bueno J, Gutierrez J, et al. Hepatic hemangioendothelioma: clinical experience and management strategy. J Pediatr Surg 34:98–105; discussion 105–6.
121. Selby DM, Stocker JT, Waclawiw MA, et al. Infantile hemangioendothelioma of the liver. Hepatology 1994;20:39–45.
122. Mo JQ, Dimashkieh HH, Bove KE. GLUT1 endothelial reactivity distinguishes hepatic infantile hemangioma from congenital hepatic vascular malformation with associated capillary proliferation. Hum Pathol 2004;35:200–9.
123. Adler B, Naheedy J, Yeager N, et al. Multifocal epithelioid hemangioendothelioma in a 16-year-old boy. Pediatr Radiol 35:1014–18.
124. Radin DR, Craig JR, Colletti PM, et al. Hepatic epithelioid hemangioendothelioma. Radiology 1988;169:145–8.
125. Selby DM, Stocker JT, Ishak KG. Angiosarcoma of the liver in childhood: a clinicopathologic and follow-up study of 10 cases. Pediatr Pathol 1992;12:485–98.
126. Awan S, Davenport M, Portmann B, Howard ER. Angiosarcoma of the liver in children. J Pediatr Surg 1996;31:1729–32.
127. de Chadarevian JP, Pawel BR, Faerber EN, Weintraub WH. Undifferentiated (embryonal) sarcoma arising in conjunction with mesenchymal hamartoma of the liver. Mod Pathol 1994; 7:490–3.
128. Walker NI, Horn MJ, Strong RW, et al. Undifferentiated (embryonal) sarcoma of the liver. Pathologic findings and long-term survival after complete surgical resection. Cancer 1992;69: 52–9.
129. Lauwers GY, Grant LD, Donnelly WH, et al. Hepatic undifferentiated (embryonal) sarcoma arising in a mesenchymal hamartoma. Am J Surg Pathol 1997;21:1248–54.
130. Dalle I, Sciot R, de Vos R, et al. Malignant angiomyolipoma of the liver: a hitherto unreported variant. Histopathology 2000; 36:443–50.
131. McKinney CA, Geiger JD, Castle VP, et al. Aggressive hepatic angiomyolipoma in a child. Pediatr Hematol Oncol 2005;22:17–24.
132. Tomlinson GE, Douglass EC, Pollock BH, et al. Cytogenetic evaluation of a large series of hepatoblastomas: numerical abnormalities with recurring aberrations involving 1q12-q21. Genes Chromosomes Cancer 2005;44:177–84.
133. Weber RG, Pietsch T, von Schweinitz D, Lichter P. Characterization of genomic alterations in hepatoblastomas. A role for gains on chromosomes 8q and 20 as predictors of poor outcome. Am J Pathol 2000;157:571–8.
134. Mullarkey M, Breen CJ, McDermott M, et al. Genetic abnormalities in a pre and post-chemotherapy hepatoblastoma. Cytogenet Cell Genet 2001;95:9–11.
135. Kumon K, Kobayashi H, Namiki T, et al. Frequent increase of DNA copy number in the 2q24 chromosomal region and its association with a poor clinical outcome in hepatoblastoma: cytogenetic and comparative genomic hybridization analysis. Jpn J Cancer Res 2001;92:854–62.
136. Terracciano LM, Bernasconi B, Ruck P, et al. Comparative genomic hybridization analysis of hepatoblastoma reveals high frequency of X-chromosome gains and similarities between epithelial and stromal components. Hum Pathol 2003;34:864–71.
137. Sainati L, Leszl A, Stella M, et al. Cytogenetic analysis of hepatoblastoma: hypothesis of cytogenetic evolution in such tumors and results of a multicentric study. Cancer Genet Cytogenet 104: 39–44.
138. Ma SK, Cheung AN, Choy C, et al. Cytogenetic characterization of childhood hepatoblastoma. Cancer Genet Cytogenet 2000;119:32–6.
139. Schneider NR, Cooley LD, Finegold MJ, et al. The first recurring chromosome translocation in hepatoblastoma: der(4)t (1;4)(q12;q34). Genes Chromosomes Cancer 1997;19:291–4.
140. Parada LA, Limon J, Iliszko M, et al. Cytogenetics of hepatoblastoma: further characterization of 1q rearrangements by fluorescence in situ hybridization: an international collaborative study. Med Pediatr Oncol 2000;34:165–70.
141. Blanquet V, Garreau F, Chenivesse X, et al. Regional mapping to 4q32.1 by in situ hybridization of a DNA domain rearranged in human liver cancer. Hum Genet 1988;80:274–6.
142. Terada Y, Imoto I, Nagai H, et al. An 8-cM interstitial deletion on 4q21-q22 in DNA from an infant with hepatoblastoma overlaps with a commonly deleted region in adult liver cancers. Am J Med Genet 2001;103:176–80.
143. Pasquinelli C, Garreau F, Bougueleret L, et al. Rearrangement of a common cellular DNA domain on chromosome 4 in human primary liver tumors. J Virol 1988;62:629–32.
144. Chou YH, Chung KC, Jeng LB, et al. Frequent allelic loss on chromosomes 4q and 16q associated with human hepatocellular carcinoma in Taiwan. Cancer Lett 1998;123:1–6.
145. Zatkova A, Rouillard JM, Hartmann W, et al. Amplification and overexpression of the IGF2 regulator PLAG1 in hepatoblastoma. Genes Chromosomes Cancer 2004;39:126–37.
146. Fletcher JA, Kozakewich HP, Pavelka K, et al. Consistent cytogenetic aberrations in hepatoblastoma: a common pathway of genetic alterations in embryonal liver and skeletal muscle malignancies? Genes Chromosomes Cancer 1991;3:37–43.
147. Steenman M, Westerveld A, Mannens M. Genetics of Beckwith–Wiedemann syndrome-associated tumors: common genetic pathways. Genes Chromosomes Cancer 2000;28:1–13.
148. Hatada I, Ohashi H, Fukushima Y, et al. An imprinted gene p57KIP2 is mutated in Beckwith-Wiedemann syndrome. Nat Genet 1996;14:171–3.
149. Hartmann W, Waha A, Koch A, et al. p57(KIP2) is not mutated in hepatoblastoma but shows increased transcriptional activity in a comparative analysis of the three imprinted genes p57(KIP2), IGF2:and H19. Am J Pathol 2000;157:1393–403.
150. Ross JA, Radloff GA, Davies SM. H19 and IGF-2 allele-specific expression in hepatoblastoma. Br J Cancer 2000;82:753–6.
151. Albrecht S, von Schweinitz D, Waha A, et al. Loss of maternal alleles on chromosome arm 11p in hepatoblastoma. Cancer Res 1994;54:5041–4.
152. Rainier S, Dobry CJ, Feinberg AP. Loss of imprinting in hepatoblastoma. Cancer Res 1995;55:1836–8.
153. Eriksson T, Frisk T, Gray SG, et al. Methylation changes in the human IGF2 p3 promoter parallel IGF2 expression in the primary tumor, established cell line, and xenograft of a human hepatoblastoma. Exp Cell Res 2001;270:88–95.

154. Albrecht S, Hartmann W, Houshdaran F, et al. Allelic loss but absence of mutations in the polyspecific transporter gene BWR1A on 11p15.5 in hepatoblastoma. Int J Cancer 2004;111: 627–32.
155. Toretsky JA, Zitomersky NL, Eskenazi AE, et al. Glypican-3 expression in Wilms tumor and hepatoblastoma. J Pediatr Hematol Oncol 2001;23:496–9.
156. von Horn H, Tally M, Hall K, et al. Expression levels of insulin-like growth factor binding proteins and insulin receptor isoforms in hepatoblastomas. Cancer Lett 2001;162:253–60.
157. Koch A, Denkhaus D, Albrecht S, et al. Childhood hepatoblastomas frequently carry a mutated degradation targeting box of the beta-catenin gene. Cancer Res 1999;59:269–73.
158. Wei Y, Fabre M, Branchereau S, et al. Activation of beta-catenin in epithelial and mesenchymal hepatoblastomas. Oncogene 2000;19:498–504.
159. López-Terrada DG, Pulliam JF, Adesina A, et al. Analysis of beta-catenin status and Wnt pathway in different histologic subtypes of hepatoblastoma. Mod Pathol 2005;302.
160. Fukuzawa R, Hata J, Hayashi Y, et al. Beckwith–Wiedemann syndrome-associated hepatoblastoma: wnt signal activation occurs later in tumorigenesis in patients with 11p15.5 uniparental disomy. Pediatr Dev Pathol 2003;6:299–306.
161. Taniguchi K, Robert, LR, Aderca IN, et al. Mutational spectrum of beta-catenin, AXIN1:and AXIN2 in hepatocellular carcinomas and hepatoblastomas. Oncogene 2002;21:4863–71.
162. Wirths O, Waha A, Weggen S, et al. Overexpression of human Dickkopf-1:an antagonist of wingless/WNT signaling, in human hepatoblastomas and Wilms' tumors. Lab Invest 2003; 83:429–34.
163. Koch A, Waha A, Hartmann W, et al. Elevated expression of Wnt antagonists is a common event in hepatoblastomas. Clin Cancer Res 11:4295–304.
164. Takayasu H, Horie H, Hiyama E, et al. Frequent deletions and mutations of the beta-catenin gene are associated with overexpression of cyclin D1 and fibronectin and poorly differentiated histology in childhood hepatoblastoma. Clin Cancer Res 2001;7:901–8.
165. Anna CH, Iida M, Sills RC, Devereux TR. Expression of potential beta-catenin targets, cyclin D1:c-Jun, c-Myc, E-cadherin, and EGFR in chemically induced hepatocellular neoplasms from B6C3F1 mice. Toxicol Appl Pharmacol, 2003;190:135–45.
166. Kim H, Ham EK, Kim YI, et al. Overexpression of cyclin D1 and cdk4 in tumorigenesis of sporadic hepatoblastomas. Cancer Lett 1998;131:177–83.
167. Pakakasama S, Chen TT, Frawley W, et al. CCND1 polymorphism and age of onset of hepatoblastoma. Oncogene 2004;23: 4789–92.
168. Shim YH, Park HJ, Choi MS, et al. Hypermethylation of the p16 gene and lack of p16 expression in hepatoblastoma. Mod Pathol 2003;16:430–6.
169. Brotto M, Finegold MJ. Distinct patterns of p27/KIP 1 gene expression in hepatoblastoma and prognostic implications with correlation before and after chemotherapy. Hum Pathol 2002; 33:198–205.
170. Kiss A, Szepesi A, Lotz G, et al. Expression of transforming growth factor-alpha in hepatoblastoma. Cancer 1998;83:690–7.
171. Lee SH, Shin MS, Lee JY, et al. In vivo expression of soluble Fas and FAP-1: possible mechanisms of Fas resistance in human hepatoblastomas. J Pathol 1999;188:207–12.
172. Hiyama E, Yamaoka H, Matsunaga T, et al. High expression of telomerase is an independent prognostic indicator of poor outcome in hepatoblastoma. Br J Cancer 2004;91:972–9.
173. Buendia MA. Genetics of hepatocellular carcinoma. Semin Cancer Biol 2000;10:185–200.
174. Suriawinata A, Xu R. An update on the molecular genetics of hepatocellular carcinoma. Semin Liver Dis 2004;24:77–88.
175. Wong N, Lai P, Pang E, et al. A comprehensive karyotypic study on human hepatocellular carcinoma by spectral karyotyping. Hepatology 2000;32:1060–8.
176. Buendia MA. Genetic alterations in hepatoblastoma and hepatocellular carcinoma: common and distinctive aspects. Med Pediatr Oncol 2002;39:530–5.
177. Iliszko M, Czauderna P, Babinska M, et al. Cytogenetic findings in an embryonal sarcoma of the liver. Cancer Genet Cytogenet 1998;102:142–4.
178. O'Sullivan MJ, Swanson PE, Knoll J, et al. Undifferentiated embryonal sarcoma with unusual features arising within mesenchymal hamartoma of the liver: report of a case and review of the literature. Pediatr Dev Pathol 2001;4:482–9.
179. Speleman F, De Telder V, De Potter KR, et al. Cytogenetic analysis of a mesenchymal hamartoma of the liver. Cancer Genet Cytogenet 1989;40:29–32.
180. Mascarello JT, Krous HF. Second report of a translocation involving 19q13.4 in a mesenchymal hamartoma of the liver. Cancer Genet Cytogenet 1992;58:141–2.
181. Rakheja D, Margraf LR, Tomlinson GE, Schneider NR. Hepatic mesenchymal hamartoma with translocation involving chromosome band 19q13.4: a recurrent abnormality. Cancer Genet Cytogenet 2004;153:60–3.
182. Bove KE, Blough RI, Soukup S. Third report of t(19q)(13.4) in mesenchymal hamartoma of liver with comments on link to embryonal sarcoma. Pediatr Dev Pathol 1998;1:438–42.
183. Ito H, Yamasaki T, Okamoto O, Tahara E. Infantile hemangioendothelioma of the liver in patient with interstitial deletion of chromosome 6q: report of an autopsy case. Am J Med Genet 1989;34:325–9.
184. Tannapfel A, Weihrauch M, Benicke M, et al. p16INK4A-alterations in primary angiosarcoma of the liver. J Hepatol 2001; 35:62–7.
185. Soini Y, Welsh JA, Ishak KG, Bennett WP. p53 mutations in primary hepatic angiosarcomas not associated with vinyl chloride exposure. Carcinogenesis 1995;16:2879–81.
186. Fuchs J, Rydzynski J, Von Schweinitz D, et al. Pretreatment prognostic factors and treatment results in children with hepatoblastoma: a report from the German Cooperative Pediatric Liver Tumor Study HB 94. Cancer 2002;95:172–82.
187. von Schweinitz D, Hecker H, Schmidt-von-Arndt G, Harms D. Prognostic factors and staging systems in childhood hepatoblastoma. Int J Cancer 1997;74:593–9.
188. Brown J, Perilongo G, Shafford E, et al. Pretreatment prognostic factors for children with hepatoblastoma – results from the International Society of Paediatric Oncology (SIOP) study SIOPEL 1. Eur J Cancer 2000;36:1418–25.
189. von Schweinitz D, Byrd DJ, Hecker H, et al. Efficiency and toxicity of ifosfamide, cisplatin and doxorubicin in the treatment of childhood hepatoblastoma. Study Committee of the Cooperative Paediatric Liver Tumour Study HB89 of the German Society for Paediatric Oncology and Haematology. Eur J Cancer 1997;33:1243–9.

190. Haas JE, Feusner JH, Finegold MJ. Small cell undifferentiated histology in hepatoblastoma may be unfavorable. Cancer 2001; 92:3130–4.
191. Haas JE, Muczynski KA, Krailo M, et al. Histopathology and prognosis in childhood hepatoblastoma and hepatocarcinoma. Cancer 1989;64:1082–95.
192. Ortega JA, Douglass EC, Feusner JH, et al. Randomized comparison of cisplatin/vincristine/fluorouracil and cisplatin/continuous infusion doxorubicin for treatment of pediatric hepatoblastoma: a report from the Children's Cancer Group and the Pediatric Oncology Group. J Clin Oncol 2000;18:2665–75.
193. Hata Y, Ishizu H, Ohmori K, et al. Flow cytometric analysis of the nuclear DNA content of hepatoblastoma. Cancer 1991;68:2566–70.
194. Zerbini MC, Sredni ST, Grier H, et al. Primary malignant epithelial tumors of the liver in children: a study of DNA content and oncogene expression. Pediatr Dev Pathol 1998;1:270–80.
195. Park WS, Oh RR, Park JY, et al. Nuclear localization of beta-catenin is an important prognostic factor in hepatoblastoma. J Pathol 2001;193:483–90.
196. Yamaoka H, Ohtsu K, Sueda T, et al. Diagnostic and prognostic impact of beta-catenin alterations in pediatric liver tumors. Oncol Rep 2006;15:551–6.
197. Yamada S, Ohira M, Horie H, et al. Expression profiling and differential screening between hepatoblastomas and the corresponding normal livers: identification of high expression of the PLK1 oncogene as a poor-prognostic indicator of hepatoblastomas. Oncogene 2004;23:5901–11.
198. King DR, Ortega J, Campbell J, et al. The surgical management of children with incompletely resected hepatic cancer is facilitated by intensive chemotherapy. J Pediatr Surg 1991;26:1074–80; discussion 1080–1.
199. Schnater JM, Aronson DC, Plaschkes J, et al. Surgical view of the treatment of patients with hepatoblastoma: results from the first prospective trial of the International Society of Pediatric Oncology Liver Tumor Study Group. Cancer 2002;94:1111–20.
200. Luks FI, Yazbeck S, Brandt ML, et al. Benign liver tumors in children: a 25-year experience. J Pediatr Surg 1991;26:1326–30.
201. Ramanujam TM, Ramesh JC, Goh DW, et al. Malignant transformation of mesenchymal hamartoma of the liver: case report and review of the literature. J Pediatr Surg 1999;34:1684–6.
202. Gangopadhyay AN, Sharma SP, Gopal SC, et al. Mesenchymal hamartoma of liver. Indian Pediatr 1995;32:1109–11.
203. Rosenberg AS, Kirk J, Morgan MB. Rhabdomyomatous mesenchymal hamartoma: an unusual dermal entity with a report of two cases and a review of the literature. J Cutan Pathol 2002; 29:238–43.
204. Black CT, Cangir A, Choroszy M, Andrassy RJ. Marked response to preoperative high-dose cis-platinum in children with unresectable hepatoblastoma. J Pediatr Surg 1991;26:1070–3.
205. Finegold MJ. Chemotherapy for suspected hepatoblastoma without efforts at surgical resection is a bad practice. Med Pediatr Oncol 2002;39:484–6.
206. Reynolds M, Douglass EC, Finegold M, et al. Chemotherapy can convert unresectable hepatoblastoma. J Pediatr Surg 1992;27: 1080–3; discussion 1083–4.
207. Passmore SJ, Noblett HR, Wisheart JD, Mott MG. Prolonged survival following multiple thoracotomies for metastatic hepatoblastoma. Med Pediatr Oncol 1995;24:58–60.
208. Vivarelli M, Guglielmi A, Ruzzenente A, et al. Surgical resection versus percutaneous radiofrequency ablation in the treatment of hepatocellular carcinoma on cirrhotic liver. Ann Surg 240: 102–7.
209. Kubo S, Taukamoto T, Hirohashi K, et al. Appropriate surgical management of small hepatocellular carcinomas in patients infected with hepatitis C virus. World J Surg 2003;27:437–42.
210. Suita S, Tajiri T, Takamatsu H, et al. Improved survival outcome for hepatoblastoma based on an optimal chemotherapeutic regimen–a report from the study group for pediatric solid malignant tumors in the Kyushu area. J Pediatr Surg 2004;39: 195–8; discussion 195–8.
211. Casanova M, Massimino M, Ferrari A, et al. Etoposide, cisplatin, epirubicin chemotherapy in the treatment of pediatric liver tumors. Pediatr Hematol Oncol 2005;22:189–98.
212. Matsunaga T, Sasaki F, Ohira M, et al. Analysis of treatment outcome for children with recurrent or metastatic hepatoblastoma. Pediatr Surg Int 2003;19:142–6.
213. Katzenstein HM, Krailo MD, Malogolowkin MH, et al. Hepatocellular carcinoma in children and adolescents: results from the Pediatric Oncology Group and the Children's Cancer Group intergroup study. J Clin Oncol 2002;20:2789–97.
214. Enjolras O, Riche MC, Merland JJ, Escande JP. Management of alarming hemangiomas in infancy: a review of 25 cases. Pediatrics 1990;85:491–8.
215. Iyer CP, Stanley P, Mahoure GH. Hepatic hemangiomas in infants and children: a review of 30 cases. Am Surg 1996;62:356–60.
216. Mulliken JB, Boon LM, Takahashi K, et al. Pharmacologic therapy for endangering hemangiomas. Curr Opin Dermatol 1995; 2:109–13.
217. Barlow CF, Priebe CJ, Mulliken JB, et al. Spastic diplegia as a complication of interferon alfa-2a treatment of hemangiomas of infancy. J Pediatr 1998;132:527–30.
218. Koh LK, Greenspan FS, Yeo PP. Interferon-alpha induced thyroid dysfunction: three clinical presentations and a review of the literature. Thyroid 1997;7:891–6.
219. Jones TH, Wadler S, Hupart KH. Endocrine-mediated mechanisms of fatigue during treatment with interferon-alpha. Semin Oncol 1998;25:54–63.
220. Gunawardena SW, Trautwein LM, Finegold MJ, Ogden AK. Hepatic angiosarcoma in a child: successful therapy with surgery and adjuvant chemotherapy. Med Pediatr Oncol 1997;28:139–43.
221. Prokurat A, Chrupek M, Kosciesza A, et al. Hemangioma of the liver in children – conservative versus operative treatment. Surg Childh Intern 2000;3:202–7.
222. Bisogno G, Pilz T, Perilongo G, et al. Undifferentiated sarcoma of the liver in childhood: a curable disease. Cancer 2002;94: 252–7.
223. Kim DY, Kim KH, Jung SE, et al. Undifferentiated (embryonal) sarcoma of the liver: combination treatment by surgery and chemotherapy. J Pediatr Surg 2002;37:1419–23.
224. Spunt SL, Lobe TE, Pappo AS, et al. Aggressive surgery is unwarranted for biliary tract rhabdomyosarcoma. J Pediatr Surg 2000;35:309–16.
225. Pritchard J, Brown J, Shafford E, et al. Cisplatin, doxorubicin, and delayed surgery for childhood hepatoblastoma: a successful approach – results of the first prospective study of the International Society of Pediatric Oncology. J Clin Oncol 2000;18:3819–28.

226. Otte JB, Pritchard J, Aronson DC, et al. Liver transplantation for hepatoblastoma: results from the International Society of Pediatric Oncology [SIOP] study SIOPEL-1 and review of the world experience. Pediatr Blood Cancer 2004;42:74–83.
227. Tiao GM, Bobey N, Allen S, et al. The current management of hepatoblastoma: a combination of chemotherapy, conventional resection, and liver transplantation. J Pediatr 146:204–11.
228. Reyes JD, Carr B, Dvorchik I, et al. Liver transplantation and chemotherapy for hepatoblastoma and hepatocellular cancer in childhood and adolescence. J Pediatr 2000;136:795–804.
229. Austin MT, Leys CM, Feurer ID, et al. Liver transplantation for childhood hepatic malignancy: a review of the United Network for Organ Sharing (UNOS) database. J Pediatr Surg 2006; 41:182–6.
230. Habrand JL, Pritchard J. Role of radiotherapy in hepatoblastoma and hepatocellular carcinoma in children and adolescents: results of a survey conducted by the SIOP Liver Tumour Study Group. Med Pediatr Oncol 1991;19:208.
231. Guo WJ, Yu EX, Liu LM, et al. Comparison between chemoembolization combined with radiotherapy and chemoembolization alone for large hepatocellular carcinoma. World J Gastroenterol 2003;9:1697–701.
232. Cheng JC,, Wu JKHuang CM, et al. Radiation-induced liver disease after three-dimensional conformal radiotherapy for patients with hepatocellular carcinoma: dosimetric analysis and implication. Int J Radiat Oncol Biol Phys 2002;54:156–62.
233. Habrand JL, Nehme D, Kalifa C, et al. Is there a place for radiation therapy in the management of hepatoblastomas and hepatocellular carcinomas in children? Int J Radiat Oncol Biol Phys 1992;23:525–31.
234. Park HC, Seong J, Han KH, et al. Dose-response relationship in local radiotherapy for hepatocellular carcinoma. Int J Radiat Oncol Biol Phys 2002;54:150–5.
235. Dawson LA, McGinn CJ, Lawrence TS. Conformal chemoradiation for primary and metastatic liver malignancies. Semin Surg Oncol 2003;21:249–55.
236. Oue T, Fukuzawa M, Kusafuka T, et al. Transcatheter arterial chemoembolization in the treatment of hepatoblastoma. J Pediatr Surg 1998;33:1771–5.
237. Malogolowkin MH, Stanley P, Steele DA, Ortega JA. Feasibility and toxicity of chemoembolization for children with liver tumors. J Clin Oncol 2000;18:1279–84.
238. Braybrooke JP, Propper DJ, O'Byrne KJ, et al. Induction of thymidine phosphorylase as a pharmacodynamic end-point in patients with advanced carcinoma treated with 5-fluorouracil, folinic acid and interferon alpha. Br J Cancer 2000;83:219–24.
239. Marchetti S, Chazal M, Dubreuil A, et al. Impact of thymidine phosphorylase surexpression on fluoropyrimidine activity and on tumour angiogenesis. Br J Cancer 2001;85:439–45.
240. Leung TW, Tang AM, Zee B, et al. Factors predicting response and survival in 149 patients with unresectable hepatocellular carcinoma treated by combination cisplatin, interferon-alpha, doxorubicin and 5-fluorouracil chemotherapy. Cancer 2002; 94:421–7.
241. Patt YZ, Hassan MM, Lozano RD, et al. Phase II trial of systemic continuous fluorouracil and subcutaneous recombinant interferon Alfa-2b for treatment of hepatocellular carcinoma. J Clin Oncol 2003;21:421–7.
242. Galvao FH, Bakonyi-Neto A, Machado MA, et al. Interferon alpha-2B and liver resection to treat multifocal hepatic epithelioid hemangioendothelioma: a relevant approach to avoid liver transplantation. Transplant Proc 2005;37:4354–8.
243. Mizejewski GJ. Biological role of alpha-fetoprotein in cancer: prospects for anticancer therapy. Expert Rev Anticancer Ther 2002;2:709–35.
244. Kairemo KJ, Lindahl H, Merenmies J, et al. Anti-alpha-fetoprotein imaging is useful for staging hepatoblastoma. Transplantation 2002;73:1151–4.
245. Raymond E, Faivre S, Chaney S, et al. Cellular and molecular pharmacology of oxaliplatin. Mol Cancer Ther 2002;1:227–35.
246. Katzenstein H, Chang KC, Krailo M, et al.Presented at the American Society of Clinical Oncology, New Orleans, Louisiana, 2004.
247. Warmann S, Hunger M, Teichmann B, et al. The role of the MDR1 gene in the development of multidrug resistance in human hepatoblastoma: clinical course and in vivo model. Cancer 2002;95:1795–801.
248. Schnater JM, Kohler SE, Lamers WH, et al. Where do we stand with hepatoblastoma? A review. Cancer 2003;98:668–78.
249. Murono S, Yoshizaki T, Sato H, et al. Aspirin inhibits tumor cell invasiveness induced by Epstein-Barr virus latent membrane protein 1 through suppression of matrix metalloproteinase-9 expression. Cancer Res 2000;60:2555–61.
250. Cianchi F, Cortesini C, Bechi P, et al. Up-regulation of cyclooxygenase 2 gene expression correlates with tumor angiogenesis in human colorectal cancer. Gastroenterology 2001;121:1339–47.
251. Ishikawa H, Nakao K, Matsumoto K, et al. Antiangiogenic gene therapy for hepatocellular carcinoma using angiostatin gene. Hepatology 2003;37:696–704.
252. Koga H. Hepatocellular carcinoma: is there a potential for chemoprevention using cyclooxygenase-2 inhibitors? Cancer 2003;98:661–7.
253. Mascarenhas RC, Sanghvi AN, Friedlander L, et al. Thalidomide inhibits the growth and progression of hepatic epithelioid hemangioendothelioma. Oncology 2004;67:471–5.

41

Liver Transplantation in Children

Greg Tiao, M.D., Maria H. Alonso, M.D., and Frederick C. Ryckman, M.D.

Pediatric hepatologists and transplant surgeons have transformed the outcome of severe end-stage liver disease in children from hopelessness to success. Liver and combined multivisceral transplantation procedures have become the state-of-the-art treatment for these complex clinical problems, with anticipated success. The progressive improvement appreciated has been advanced through the use of innovative operative procedures using unique technical solutions in response to donor shortages. Although preoperative care advancements have significantly improved pretransplant morbidity, the full potential of improved transplant success has been limited by longer waiting lists and limited donor availability. Expanding indications for transplantation to children and adults with previously fatal diseases have increased this discrepancy. Parallel advances in critical care, immunosuppression, and postoperative management have also played a pivotal role in improved survival. However, the success of the past has bred unique problems that must be met in the future. If we are to succeed in meeting the needs of the increasing number of candidates, improved donor awareness and availability must occur. A delicate balance between the risks assumed by living donors and the needs of their children must be struck. The increasing numbers of surviving patients present unique challenges and complications related to lifelong immunosuppression. The future success of pediatric liver transplantation will require appreciation of the increasingly complex care needs of this population and a national focus on donor organ shortages.

THE SELECTION PROCESS

The primary aim of the evaluation process is to identify appropriate candidates for liver transplantation (LTx) and establish an effective pretransplant management plan. With the ever-increasing scarcity of suitable donor organs and prolonged pretransplant waiting times, referral for transplantation must occur before the development of progressive deterioration and life-threatening complications. Our collective experience suggests that the progression of liver failure is not linear, but exponential. This suggests that early warning signs of hepatic compromise, such as deteriorating synthetic function and refractory nutritional failure, should lead to prompt evaluation and clarity of future needs. The primary pretransplant evaluation identifies areas for intervention to optimize success, such as nutritional improvement, immunizations, and preventive dental care. In children with fulminant hepatic failure (FHF) or rapidly progressive deterioration, aggressive critical care intervention is essential to maintain and support all other physiologic systems until a suitable donor organ can be found.

INDICATIONS

The most common clinical presentations prompting transplant evaluation in children can be classified as follows: (1) progressive primary liver disease, with anticipated hepatic failure; (2) stable liver disease with a remarkable morbidity or mortality; (3) hepatic-based metabolic disease; (4) FHF; (5) unresectable primary liver tumors confined to the liver; and (6) complex hepatic-based vascular malformations leading to progressive heart failure. Table 41.1 reviews the primary diagnoses leading to pediatric liver transplantation.

PRIMARY LIVER DISEASES LEADING TO LIVER TRANSPLANTATION

Neonatal Cholestatic Syndromes: Biliary Atresia

Children with biliary atresia (BA) constitute at least 50% of the pediatric liver transplant population. The Kasai portoenterostomy should be the primary surgical intervention for all infants with BA unless the initial presentation is late in infancy (>120 days of age), the liver biopsy shows advanced cirrhosis, or the clinical course is unfavorable. In these exceptional patients, primary LTx is indicated [1,2].

Progressive liver decompensation following the Kasai procedure can be manifest by various combinations of complications such as recurrent bacterial cholangitis, ascites, progressive portal hypertension, malnutrition, progressive hepatic synthetic failure, or a combination of these. Approximately

Table 41.1: Indications for Liver Transplantation, Primary Liver Transplants ($N = 317$)

	N	%
Cholestatic liver disease	157	50
Biliary atresia	136	
Alagille syndrome	8	
Familial cholestasis	1	
Primary sclerosing cholangitis	8	
Ideopathic	4	
Metabolic disease	55	17
α-1 antitrypsin deficiency	27	
Tyrosinemia	7	
Urea cycle defect	9	
Glycogen storage disease	5	
Wilson's disease	2	
Primary hyperoxaluria	4	
Cystic fibrosis		1
Fulminant liver failure	47	15
Cirrhosis/hepatitis	28	9
Cryptogenic cirrhosis	15	
Autoimmune	7	
Neonatal nepatitis	4	
Hepatitis C	1	
Congenital hepatic fibrosis	1	
Tumor	12	4
Hepatoblastoma	10	
Hepatocellular carcinoma	1	
Sarcoma	1	
Other	18	6
Hemangioendothelioma	2	
Hemachromatosis	2	
Budd–Chiari	1	
Total parenteral nutrition–related	5	
Megacystis/microcolon	1	
Portal vein atresia/hepatopulmonary	1	
Intestinal pseudo-obstruction (L/SI/P)	1	
Short gut syndrome (L/SI/P)	4	
Necrotizing enterocolitis (L/SI/P)	1	

L/SI/P, liver/small intestine/pancreas

half of all BA infants develop these warning signs within the first 6 months following surgery. Most require LTx within the first 2 years of life. Children with the successful establishment of biliary drainage with normal postoperative serum bilirubin levels may still develop progressive cirrhosis with eventual hepatic decompensation. Although these complications eventually lead to LTx, many do not access LTx until they are older than 2–5 years of age. The development of hepatopulmonary syndrome is increasingly recognized in these longer-term survivors and can occur with stable liver function. These children have undergone liver transplantation to avoid progressive hypoxia or later fixed pulmonary hypertension. Despite the high failure rate following the Kasai procedure, approximately 15–20% of

Table 41.2: Transplantation for Metabolic Disease in Children

Wilson's disease	Hemophilia A
α-1-antitrypsin deficiency	Protoporphyria
Crigler–Najjar syndrome (type I)	Homozygous hypercholesterolemia
Tyrosinemia	Urea cycle enzyme deficiencies
Cystic fibrosis	Primary hyperoxaluria
Glycogen storage disease IV	Neonatal iron storage disease

all BA patients may not require LTx [3,4]. The sequential use of the Kasai procedure and LTx optimizes overall survival and organ utilization [2,5].

On occasion, other cholestatic conditions, such as Alagille syndrome, may cause cirrhosis and require LTx [6–8].

Hepatic-Based Metabolic Disease

A leading indication for hepatic transplantation in children is hepatic-based metabolic disease (Table 41.2). In these patients, LTx is not only lifesaving, it also accomplishes phenotypic and functional cure of the disease. Hepatic replacement to correct the metabolic defect should be considered before other organ systems are affected, or the consequences of the defect result in irreversible quality-of-life compromises or complications that would prove to be contraindications for transplantation. For example, patients with urea cycle defects (UCD) who have repetitive hyperammonemic crisis sustain significant neurologic injury with resulting mental retardation. Early transplantation allows the potential for neurologic protection and recovery with preserved neurologic function and quality of life [9,10]. The use of living donors or carriers of UCD has been successful and allows planned early transplantation [11]. Patients with tyrosinemia historically had a high risk of developing hepatocellular carcinoma (HCC), requiring LTx before extrahepatic spread of the tumor occurred. Experience using 2-(2-nitro-4-trifluoromethylbenzoyl)-1, 3-cyclohexanedione (NTBC) has been successful in preventing dysplasia and avoiding the need for LTx. Successful prevention of HCC also seems to occur with NTBC therapy. Neonatal hemochromatosis presents a challenge in diagnosis and management. Most affected infants present at birth or within weeks with FHF. The use of antioxidant cocktails as described later has not improved patients with severe disease [12,13]. Liver transplantation is lifesaving, but success rates of approximately 50% are reported [12]. It is hoped that the use of novel gene therapy and further innovative strategies will limit the need for whole organ replacement for many of these cellular-based diseases [14,15].

Fulminant Hepatic Failure

Patients who develop FHF without recognized antecedent liver disease present diagnostic and prognostic difficulties. Rapid clinical deterioration frequently makes establishment of a primary diagnosis impossible before the need for urgent transplantation. The most common cause of FHF is viral hepatitis of undefined type, followed by drug toxicity, toxin exposure, and previously unrecognized metabolic disease. In infants, causes of FHF such as neonatal hemochromatosis are due to chronic in utero liver disease and present with decompensated cirrhosis but lesser elevation of transaminases. Timely administration of antioxidant cocktails containing desferrioxamine, M-acetylcysteine, selenium, vitamin E, and prostaglandin E-1, even while awaiting confirmatory diagnosis, appear to improve the clinical course in selected infants, although scientific support for their use is lacking. Failure to respond within 48–72 hours mandates transplantation [16]. Mitochondrial respiratory chain abnormalities representing disorders in the electron transport proteins present both as FHF or progressive liver disease with sudden decompensation [17,18]. They are especially important to recognize during the evaluation process because they represent multiorgan progressive diseases; transplantation is neither curative nor indicated.

We have recently treated several children with congenital or acquired hemophagocytic lymphohistiocytosis (HLH) induced FHF. These can be congenital, acquired, or triggered by infection in an immunocompromised host. In children who have HLH, inappropriate activation of macrophages and natural killer cells causes severe hepatocyte injury [19]. The role of liver transplantation in the treatment of patients with HLH has not been clearly established because recurrence in the graft has been shown to occur. The primary treatment is hematologic rather then organ replacement.

Selection of FHF candidates for transplantation is difficult because the natural history of each disease is not clearly established. The King's College Institute of Liver Studies has developed a scoring system for children with FHF, stratifying their risk [20]. Factors predictive of poor outcome included international normalized ratio (INR) bilirubin greater than 235 μmol/L, age under 2 years, and white blood cell count (WBC) greater than 9000/mm^3. Sensitivity and predictive ability increase when multiple factors are present. Similarly, predictive risk factors in other independent studies include the onset of encephalopathy greater than 7 days, prothrombin time greater than 55 seconds, and alanine aminotransferase (ALT) less than 2384 IU/L on admission, grade IV encephalopathy, infants less than 1 year of age, or the need for dialysis [21,22]. Although these criteria are helpful, careful observation for progression and clinical change is most rewarding. The role of liver biopsy is in evolution in our center. In all cases in which autoimmune hepatitis is considered, biopsy is undertaken as medical treatment may salvage individual patients [23].

The prognosis for patients with FHF is difficult to predict, and neurologic outcome is potentially suboptimal. Failure to maintain a cerebral perfusion pressure (mean blood pressure minus intracranial pressure [ICP]) of greater than 50 mm Hg and an ICP less than 20 mm Hg has been associated with very poor neurologic recovery [24]. For short-term stabilization, we have used repetitive courses of plasmapheresis to ameliorate the clinical manifestations of FHF. Daily exchanges of volume equal to the extracellular volume (20% of body weight) are undertaken. Replacement fluids include fresh frozen plasma, platelets, and cryoprecipitate as needed. Coagulation correction is excellent, and fluid overload before transplantation is also avoided. Neurologic improvement is common but not sustained, and no suggestion of enhanced native liver recovery has occurred. Daily repetitive courses are helpful, but ultimately, transplantation is the only effective treatment modality [25,26]. The initial degree of encephalopathy is not predictive of the need for transplantation; however, progressive and increasing encephalopathy is associated with poor outcome (grade I–II, 44%; grade III–IV, 78%) without transplantation [20]. When candidates undergo transplantation before the development of irreversible neurologic abnormalities, the results can be dramatic [24]. Isolated hepatocyte transplantation has been used in an attempt to provide neurologic protection while awaiting organ acquisition or spontaneous recovery [27,28]. The use of auxiliary partial orthotopic transplantation (APOLT), which can allow later recovery of the native liver, may substantially change the long-term prognosis in these complex patients [29,30]. Although technically feasible, success with APOLT is far from assured. Biliary complications, the need for retransplantation, and acute cellular rejection were all increased in the APOLT group, and survival was decreased compared with conventional transplantation. In the Hospital Paul Brousse experience, only 17% of patients had full success (i.e., patient survival, liver regeneration, and immunosuppression withdrawal leading to graft removal) [31]. Further experience with this procedure will define its role in the treatment of FHF. In cases of FHF, recovery of the native liver allows for termination of immunosuppression and allograft atrophy [29,30,32,33].

Malignancy

Hepatoblastoma and HCC are the two most common primary hepatic malignancies found in children. Outcomes for children who underwent liver transplantation for these lesions was poor in initial studies. More recent experience has documented the efficacy of liver transplantation in a subset of patients who have a hepatoblastoma and established transplantation as an integral part of the treatment strategy for these children [34–39].

In children who present with a hepatoblastoma, complete surgical resection of the primary liver lesion remains the most crucial intervention required to achieve long-term survival. Adjuvant chemotherapy and conventional resection should be employed when feasible; however, some children have lesions that remain unresectable. In these children, complete hepatectomy and transplantation serves as the only option to achieve complete resection. In these children, transplantation is best undertaken before completing chemotherapy, so that the final 1–2 cycles of chemotherapy can be given after successful LTx. Results using this and similar protocols are shown in Table 41.3.

Unlike the adult population, the frequency of HCC in the pediatric population is low; therefore, the experience in the application of liver transplantation in the pediatric population

Table 41.3: Liver Transplantation for Hepatoblastoma

Study	*No. of Patients*	*Preoperative Chemotherapy*	*Prior Resection (%)*	*Recurrence (%)*	*Transplant Mortality (%)*	*Overall Survival (%)*
Penn [38], 1991	18	No	N/A	50	N/A	50
Koneru et al. [44], 1991	12	No	33	25	25	50
Al-Qabandi et al. [43], 1999	8	Yes	25	25	12	63
Reyes et al. [40], 2000	12	Yes	8	17	0	83
Srinivasan et al. [35], 2002	13	Yes	8	8	7	93
Molmenti et al. [36], 2001	9	Yes	33	13	33	63
Pimpalwar et al. [34], 2002	12	Yes	0	17	8	83
Tiao et al. [37], 2003	8	Yes	38	0	12	88

for HCC is limited [35,40–44] (Table 41.4). In patients whose disease is confined to the liver or who have no underlying metabolic liver disease, the use of liver transplantation is indicated. Because chemotherapy is not beneficial at present in this group, results in patients with more extensive disease are poor. Although no specific criteria for transplant candidacy are established for children, adults criteria include patients with TMN classified T1 and T2 lesions by the revised Milan Criteria [45] (Table 41.5). Reason would suggest that these criteria should be applied to children as well.

Cystic Fibrosis

Prolonged survival of many children with cystic fibrosis has increased consideration of selected individuals for liver transplantation. Liver disease occurs in approximately one quarter of all children, and significant portal hypertension in approximately 10% [46]. Direct management of portal hypertensive variceal bleeding by variceal banding and portosystemic shunting allows prolonged survival [47–49]. Patients with hepatic decompensation can successfully undergo LTx. Postoperative long-term survival is compromised by the increased risk of polymicrobial or fungal sepsis, although short-term recovery is similar to other pediatric recipients [50,51].

CONTRAINDICATIONS

Contraindications to transplantation include the following: (1) HIV positive serology, (2) primary extrahepatic unresectable malignancy, (3) progressive terminal nonhepatic disease, (4) uncontrolled systemic sepsis, and (5) irreversible neurologic injury. Conditions that may present as relative contraindications to transplantation but that need to be individually evaluated include (1) advanced or partially treated systemic infection, (2) advanced hepatic encephalopathy – grade IV, (3) severe psychosocial abnormalities, (4) portal venous thrombosis extending throughout the mesenteric venous system, (5) malignancy metastatic to the liver, and (6) metastatic liver tumors unresponsive to chemotherapy.

PREOPERATIVE PREPARATION

Efforts to correct abnormalities noted during candidate evaluation will decrease both the operative risk and postoperative complications. Particular attention to the nutritional status of the recipient will improve postoperative recovery; placement of nasogastric feeding tubes and calorie-enhanced formula is often necessary to achieve this goal in small children. Assessment of prior viral exposure and meticulous attention to the delivery of all normal, well-child immunizations, particularly the live-virus vaccines, is imperative if time allows before LTx. Additionally, patients receive a one-time inoculation with pneumococcal vaccine, as well as hepatitis B vaccine.

PRIORITIZATION

Candidate evaluation and selection is undertaken by a multidisciplinary team, candidate acceptability and medical urgency are established, and preoperative intervention and education are initiated.

In the early 1980s, the Organ Procurement and Transplantation Network (OPTN) was established by the U.S. government to develop a system to distribute organs in an equitable fashion. Time accrued waiting on the pretransplant list and severity of illness, as expressed by patient location (home, hospital, intensive care unit), were the primary factors used to stratify patients. It was shown that waiting time had no relationship to death, except for urgent status 1 patients, leading to dissatisfaction with the existing system [52]. A reevaluation of this system by the Health Resources and Services Administration in 1998 established the "Final Rule," requiring allocation policies

Table 41.4: Liver Transplantation for Hepatocellular Carcinoma in Children

Study	*No. of Patients*	*Preoperative Chemotherapy*	*Prexisting Liver Diseases (%)*	*Recurrence (%)*	*Transplant Mortality (%)*	*Overall 5-Year Survival (%)*
Tagge et al. [39], 1992	9	Selected	N/A	45	11	44
Superina and Bilik [41], 1996	3	Yes	66	0	0	100
Achilleos et al. [42], 1996	2	Yes	100	50	50	0
Reyes et al. [40], 2000	19	Selected	79	32	10	68

to be based on sound medical judgment using defined criteria to achieve the best use of donated organs and avoid wasting of organs [53]. Using knowledge gained from the Mayo End-Stage Liver Disease (MELD) model, the MELD was established for adults, based on three biochemical values: serum creatinine, serum bilirubin, and INR. Based on similar information derived from the Studies of Pediatric Liver Transplantation (SPLIT), a pediatric specific score (PELD) was established using bilirubin, INR, serum albumin, age less than 1 year, and growth failure. Initial evaluation of this scoring system to predict death on the waiting list at 3 months showed a c statistic of 0.92 [54]. The effect of this matching system has been to (1) slightly increase the percentage of children and adults who receive a deceased donor organ and (2) decrease death or removal from the waiting list. The preferential policy to direct pediatric organs (< 18 year old donor) to pediatric recipients was maintained, and status 1 priority was maintained for children with chronic or acute liver disease. Candidates for combined liver–intestinal transplantation were noted to have 3.6 times the death rate awaiting transplantation as children awaiting isolated liver transplantation. This equated to 12 PELD points for the average patient, and the PELD score was modified to include these additional points for these candidates. Additional PELD points are also awarded for specific risk factors not identified in the PELD equation, such as hepatopulmonary syndrome, urea cycle abnormalities, hepatic neoplasms, gastrointestinal bleeding. Although the PELD system improved numerical quantification of candidates and removed waiting time from the scoring equation, the PELD score has not proven to be a successful predictor of 30-day or long-term outcome following transplantation [55,56]. A rapid increase in the PELD score while awaiting donor availability may identify patients with accelerated deterioration and increased postoperative risk. Concerns that identification and transplantation of "sicker patients first" would lead to decreased survival have not proved correct [56]. In a review of the first year of PELD, graft and patient survival remained unchanged from the prior allocation system [54]. Of greater concern is the perceived failure of the PELD system to quantitate candidate risk appropriately. The majority of infants and children allocated organs have achieved a PELD score sufficient for transplantation through special exception points, or status 1 (emergency transplantation) [57,58]. Further modeling and analysis will allow this system to be modified to reflect identified predictive factors and continually improve access and equity to all potential recipients.

DONOR ORGAN OPTIONS AND SELECTION

The limited availability of pediatric donor organs and an increasing waiting list population has stimulated the development of innovative surgical procedures to increase donor options. *Whole organ transplantation*, replacing the recipient's liver with a size matched liver, remains the primary goal for most children and teenagers. The limited supply and increased early complications associated with whole organ transplantation using infant donors led to the development of *reduced-size transplantation* (RSLTx), transplanting only the left lobe, or left lateral segment from a deceased donor liver. Although operative reduction of a larger sized donor liver expanded the number of donor organs available to small recipients and allowed the use of donors with improved stability, it merely shifted donor resources rather than increasing donor availability. The rapid expansion in the waiting-list population called into question the wisdom of shifting these donors into pediatric recipients as other older patients suffered increased mortality while awaiting transplantation. However, the success of the operative techniques perfected doing reduced-size transplantation has allowed the development of both *split-liver transplantation* (SLTx), where a single liver is used to transplant two recipients, and *living-donor transplantation* (LD) (Figure 41.1).

Several factors must be considered when donor options are evaluated for specific patients.

Hepatocellular Mass

The selection of a donor organ or segment with an appropriate parenchymal mass for adequate function is critical to success. Unfortunately, the minimal hepatic mass necessary for recovery is not clearly established. Any calculation must take into account the temporary loss of function caused by the donor's primary injury or illness and comorbidity, as well as the possibility of preservation damage, early acute rejection, or technical problems. Because preservation injury is greater in deceased donors, the hepatic mass needed using a whole, reduced-size, or split-liver graft should be greater than the calculated mass necessary using a living donor liver segment. The

Table 41.5: Milan Criteria for Hepatocellular Carcinoma

Classification	*Definition*	*Liver Transplant Candidate*
T1	1 nodule <2 cm	Yes
T2	1 nodule 2–5 cm, 2–3 nodules all <3 cm	Yes
T3	1 nodule >5 cm, 2–3 nodules, 1 >3 cm	No
T4	>4 nodules, any size	No

Any patients with node involvement or metastatic disease as well as gross intrahepatic portal or hepatic vein involvement detected by computerized tomography scan, magnetic resonance imaging, or ultrasound are excluded from transplantation. Adapted from Hertl and Cosimi [45].

normal liver volume in a child can be calculated using the following formula: Estimated Liver Volume $= 706.2 \times \text{BSA}(\text{m}^2) + 2.4$ [59]. A donor weight range of 15–20% above or below that of the recipient is usually appropriate for whole organ donors, taking into consideration body habitus and factors that would increase recipient abdominal size such as ascites, hepatosplenomegaly, and others. When selecting donor segments, transplantation of at least 40–50% of this ideal calculated estimated liver volume is recommended [60–62]. Estimates of donor graft to recipient body weight ratio (GRWR) may prove to be the most accurate predictor of adequate graft volume. A minimum graft fraction of 1% recipient body mass meets this need [54]. A GRWR of 1–3% is optimum. In cases in which the GRWR is less than 0.7%, overall allograft and patient survival suffered. In extreme cases where small for size grafts are used, excessive portal flow can lead to hemorrhagic necrosis of the graft. Large for size allografts (GRWR >5.0%) have a better relative outcome compared to small allografts but still show compromised survival [61,63,64].

Donor Stability

The initial success of liver transplantation is closely related to the stability and quality of the donor. Assessment of donor organ suitability is primarily undertaken by evaluating clinical information and static biochemical tests. Clinical factors of concern include donors who are at the limits of age, have had prolonged intensive care hospitalization with potential sepsis, and have vasomotor instability requiring excessive vasoconstricting inotropic agents. Static biochemical tests (liver function, coagulation) identify preexisting functional abnormalities or the consequences of organ trauma but do not serve as good

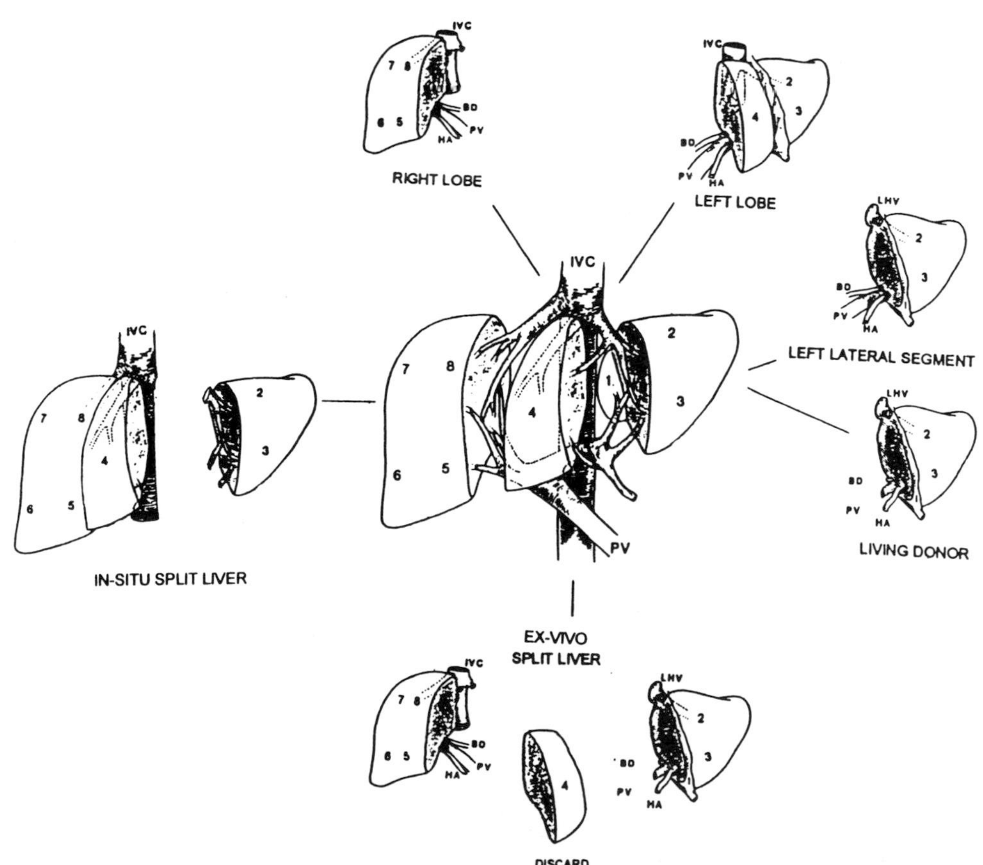

Figure 41.1. Schematic diagram of reduced-sized allografts, living donor, and split-liver transplants. Anatomic subdivisions as described by Couinard.

Table 41.6: Suggested Criteria for Identifying "Split-Liver" Deceased Donors

Donor Characteristic	*Ideal Donor for Split Liver*
Age	10–50 yr
Serum sodium	<150 meq/L
Hemodynamics	≤1 vasopressor, cardiac arrest <30 min (prefer no arrest)
Hospital stay	<5 days
Aspartate aminotransferase/alanine aminotransferase	<5× normal range (<250 mg/dL)

benchmarks of functional capability to differentiate acceptable and poor donor allografts. Severe electrolyte disturbances and deteriorating trends identify increased risk. Although marginal donor organs can be used as whole allografts, especially when ischemic time is limited, they have proved to be very high risk when used as donors for reduced-size or split-liver allografts. Suggested criteria for identifying these critical "ideal" split-liver donors are shown in Table 41.6. Children can serve as excellent split-liver donors, with results comparable to those achieved using adults [56]. Special concern for allocation of adequate hepatic mass and biliary and vascular structures for both split-liver recipients is critical for recipient recovery and should be part of the initial donor evaluation and decision to split. Any decrement in donor organ function adversely affects this hepatic mass calculation and must be considered in the final allocation of segments. Donor liver biopsy at the time of organ harvest, or during evaluation in liver donors, is helpful in questionable cases to identify preexisting liver disease or donor liver steatosis. The transplant team must undertake the difficult process of balancing the stability and quality of the donor organ versus the risk and health status of the potential recipient(s).

Age of Donor

Donor age can affect the long-term results of pediatric liver transplantation; however, the spectrum of influence is not completely clear. When the UNOS database was used with the UNOS Liver Allocation Model, Kaplan–Meier graft survivals showed that pediatric patients receiving livers from pediatric aged donors had a 3-year graft survival rate of 81% compared with 63% if children received livers from donors aged 18 years or older. In contrast, adult recipients had similar 3-year graft survivals irrespective of donor age. In the multivariate analysis, the odds of graft failure were reduced to 0.66 if pediatric recipients received livers from pediatric aged donors. The odds of graft failure were not affected at any time point for adults whether they received an adult or pediatric-aged donor [65]. The primary use of pediatric donors for pediatric recipients is further supported by evaluating adult experience with pediatric donor organs. In the Mount Sinai Hospital adult series, adult (>18 years age) recipients of pediatric donor organs had an increased risk of hepatic artery thrombosis (HAT) and poor function compared with recipients of adult donors, an effect that increased with increasing donor-to-recipient size discrepancy [66]. This was confirmed in the Mayo Clinic series, in which the 1-year graft survival rate in adult transplant recipients receiving grafts from donors less than 12 years of age was 64.3% compared with 87.5% when the donor was 12–18 years of age ($P = .015$) [67]. The main cause of graft loss was again vascular complications. This data strongly support the use of pediatric donors when possible in pediatric recipients when deceased donors are used. Because the outcome of small pediatric donor livers in adult recipients is poor and small pediatric donors are the only source of lifesaving organs for the infant recipient, the use of small pediatric donor livers in adults should be avoided. The upper limit of donor age acceptable is balanced by the needs of each individual recipient; we limit donor age at 45 years unless urgency demands exception.

Living Donor Selection

A similar critical element of living donor transplantation is the proper evaluation and selection of a donor, usually a parent or first-degree relative. This procedure is performed on the assumption that donor safety can be reasonably assured and that the donor liver function is normal. Donors should be 18–55 years of age, have an ABO compatible blood type, and have no acute or chronic medical condition. Significant efforts are made to identify potential donors who have thrombophilic events or risk factors because pulmonary emboli have accompanied fatal complications in several donors. A history of thrombosis, significant varicosities, body mass index greater than 30, or homozygous protein-S, protein-C, or factor V Leiden mutation all should exclude living donation [68]. Following a satisfactory medical and psychologic examination by a physician not directly involved with the transplant program, vascular imaging (magnetic resonance angiography, computed tomographic angiogram, or angiography) is undertaken to assess the hepatic arterial anatomy, excluding potential donors with multiple or intrahepatic arteries to segments 2 and 3. Experience has shown that when donors are deemed unacceptable, 90% were rejected on the basis of history, physical exam, laboratory screening, and ABO type. Only 10% were excluded following angiography. Donor safety has been excellent in all living donor series [69–72].

Ethical Issues

The ethical issues that arise when using this large variety of surgically reduced allografts are complex [73]. Although whole, RSLTx, SLTx, and LD all have similar survival and complication profiles in experienced centers, a significant "learning curve" exists in the complex donor and recipients operations. Maximizing the number of available donor organs cannot justify compromising patient safety or survival. The ethical obligation to maximize available organs must be balanced by clear and concise discussions at the time of evaluation with patients and families regarding risks, center experience, and success with these technically difficult grafts. Parents and patients must maintain the right to refuse offered organs without risk of decreased access. Surgeons and hepatologists must be responsible for the moral stewardship of precious donor organs.

DONOR LIVER HARVEST AND LIVER TRANSPLANTATION

Whole organ harvest is now a well-described procedure and is nearly always part of the harvest of multiple organs. The principles of minimum mobilization to define vascular structures, in situ perfusion with 4°C preservation solution and sequential en-block harvest of organs yield good allograft preservation. When reduction hepatectomy is needed for reduced-size grafts, this is accomplished following en-block harvest. The operative techniques for this reduction are well described [74,75]. Modifications of these procedures with in situ division of liver parenchyma form the basis for living donor and split-liver transplant procedures.

Split-liver grafting involves the preparation of two allografts from a single donor [76,77]. In most cases, the extended right lobe allograft (segments 4–8) is used in an adult or large child, and the left lateral segment allograft (segments 2 and 3) is transplanted into a small recipient. Generally, the celiac trunk remains with the left lateral segment graft (LLS) and the main portal vein and the common hepatic duct remain with the extended right lobe allograft [78,79]. Conventional techniques for implanting the respective allografts preserving the native inferior vena cava (IVC) are used. The use of in situ division of the left lateral segment (LLS), as during living donor liver procurement, is our preferred method for split-liver donor preparation at the present time, although comparable results using ex vivo division have also been achieved [76].

Creative use of these techniques has allowed additional transplant options in individual cases. Resection of the left lobe of the native liver followed by *auxiliary partial orthotopic transplantation* of a left lateral segment allograft (APOLT) has been successfully undertaken for patients with metabolic disease (urea cycle abnormalities, Crigler–Najjar syndrome), FHF, and as a "bridge" with small for size syndrome [80,81]. This provides for normal hepatic synthesis and function while leaving the right lobe of the native liver in situ [82]. The possible competition for adequate portal venous flow between the allograft and primary liver has led some centers to undertake preemptive portal vein diversion to the graft; others have not found this necessary. Overall technical success is good; however, the role and success of the procedure is most related to the primary indication, with patients having FHF showing the least predictable success and patients with metabolic disease seem enjoying better outcomes [83].

The technical details of these pediatric liver transplant procedures are well described [84,85]. However, the following concepts deserve emphasis:

1. The most underestimated portion of this complex operative procedure entails the removal of the native liver. Multiple prior operations or revisions for BA, or multiple episodes of spontaneous bacterial peritonitis lead to extensive vascularized adhesions and scarring. These increase the risk of intestinal perforation and bleeding at transplantation.
2. Optimal arterial inflow is essential for donor liver recovery. When the native hepatic artery is less than 4–5 mm in diameter, we prefer to implant the celiac axis of the donor liver directly into the infrarenal aorta. When adequate length is lacking, a donor iliac arterial vascular interposition graft is used to accomplish this anastomosis. Access to the infrarenal aorta is provided by mobilizing the right colon and duodenum. A large experience with microvascular reconstruction techniques for the hepatic artery, using both operating microscope and high-power 6× loupes, have both been shown to be very successful techniques [86,87].
3. Allograft outflow must be unimpeded. This is especially important in "piggyback" implantation to the native IVC in small children, where a confluence of all three hepatic venous orifices is our preference to achieve wide and effective outflow. Addition of a longitudinal incision in the anterior wall of the IVC augments the size of the outflow and provides stability to the graft in the right upper abdomen [88]. Impaired outflow leads to allograft swelling, increased vascular resistance, and subsequent inflow thrombosis.
4. Immediate postoperative and daily Doppler ultrasound will assist in recognizing correctable blood flow abnormalities before graft compromise.
5. Bile duct reconstruction as an end-to-side choledochojejunostomy into an isoperistaltic Roux-en-Y jejunal limb is our preference in young recipients. Older children without primary biliary pathology can undergo direct stent-free choledochal reconstruction.
6. When closing the abdomen, increased intra-abdominal pressure should be avoided. In many cases, avoidance of fascial closure and the use of mobilized skin flaps and running monofilament skin closure is advisable. Musculofascial abdominal wall closure can be completed approximately 1 week postoperatively. Most allografts assume a suitable position within the abdomen at the time of closure. Left lateral segment and living donor allografts are at great risk for hepatic venous obstruction if the left hepatic vein experiences any torsion.

Immunosuppressive Management

Over the last 15 years, some of the most significant developments in the care of children who require liver transplantation have occurred in the management of immunosuppression. New medications have been developed giving transplant teams more alternatives in the care of their patients. Immunosuppressive protocols following transplantation typically use a combination of the following medications.

Tacrolimus and Cyclosporine

The calcineurin inhibitors (CNIs) tacrolimus or cyclosporine remain the backbone of most protocols. The CNIs selectively target T cells binding to form a complex with the intracellular proteins tacrolimus binding protein (FKBP) for tacrolimus and cyclophilin for cyclosporine. Once bound, the complex inhibits the ability of the enzyme calcineurin to dephosphorylate nuclear regulatory elements, which are required for T-cell activation and proliferation. The introduction of cyclosporine and tacrolimus into the immunosuppression pharmaceutical armamentarium markedly improved the success of solid organ transplantation; however, CNIs have significant side effects and require therapeutic drug level monitoring.

In the pediatric population, studies comparing tacrolimus with the microemulsion form of cyclosporine have shown that tacrolimus is more effective in the control of acute rejection following transplantation [89,90]. Overall graft and patient survival was similar in patients treated with either medication but because of these results tacrolimus has become the most commonly used CNI.

Corticosteroids

Although the precise mechanism by which corticosteroids inhibit the immune system has not been established, corticosteroids bind to glucocorticoid receptors found within the cytoplasm that translocate to the nucleus and inhibit gene transcription. Corticosteroids have been used in virtually all immunosuppressive regimens since the advent of solid organ transplantation; however, corticosteroids negatively impact childhood growth and development. In addition, the cushingoid appearance of patients on long-term steroids affects the recipients self-image reducing adherence to therapy. As a result, steroid withdrawal within a few months after transplantation has become common [91,92]. Recently, steroid-free immunosuppressive protocols have been tested and their efficacy established [93].

Mycophenolate Mofetil (MMF) and Azathioprine (Aza)

The antimetabolites MMF and Aza are inhibitors of DNA synthesis. MMF selectively inhibits the purine synthesis pathway in lymphocytes reducing T-cell proliferation, and Aza, a purine analogue, is incorporated into cellular DNA where it inhibits DNA synthesis and RNA metabolism. Because Aza is nonspecific, affecting all rapidly proliferating cells, it has been supplanted by MMF in most immunosuppressive regimens; MMF is administered orally and can cause gastrointestinal discomfort.

In the pediatric liver transplant population, no prospective randomized trials have been performed that demonstrated efficacy of MMF; however, in adult liver transplant recipients, MMF has been shown to effectively reduce the incidence of rejection [94]. As a result, MMF has been incorporated into many immunosuppression protocols. In addition, MMF can be used in patients in whom recurrent acute rejection has occurred and more maintenance immunosuppression is required [95].

Immunomodulatory Agents (Monoclonal and Polyclonal Antibodies)

OKT-3, a monoclonal antibody directed against the CD3 marker found on all T cells, and Thymoglobulin (anti-thymocyte globulin), a rabbit polyclonal antibody directed against human lymphocytes, are potent modulators of the immune response. Induction therapy, the use of immunomodulatory agents at the time of transplant, suppresses the host immune system and allows the administration of a CNI to begin several days after the transplant procedure has been completed. In so doing, the side effects of a CNI, which may be exacerbated by the hemodynamic changes that occur around the transplant procedure, are minimized. Refractory rejection can also be treated with antilymphocyte antibodies.

Basiliximab and daclizumab, humanized monoclonal antibodies against the interleukin 2 receptor, specifically target the proliferative T-cell response of the immune system. Alemtuzumab, which targets the CD 52 surface protein, is the most recently developed monoclonal antibody shown to be effective in the treatment of adult liver transplant patients [96]. Induction therapy using basiliximab has decreased the rate of acute rejection following liver transplantation in children; however, the rate of steroid refractory rejection episodes and chronic rejection remained unchanged [97,98].

Rapamycin

Rapamycin (Sirolimus) is the most recently developed immunosuppressive medication. Rapamycin binds to the intracellular protein TOR and inhibits T-cell recruitment. Although it has been shown to be efficacious in patients undergoing renal transplantation, it has been associated with poor wound healing and increased hepatic artery thrombosis in patients who have undergone liver transplantation therefore is not recommended for use early after liver transplantation [99]. Rapamycin is often considered in patients in whom CNI toxicity (i.e., renal insufficiency) precludes long-term use [100].

At our program, the immunosuppression protocol that is employed following liver transplantation consists of the combination of tacrolimus and corticosteroids. Corticosteroids are tapered over a 3-month period after transplantation. In patients with renal dysfunction, induction therapy with Thymoglobulin and corticosteroids is followed by the administration of low-dose tacrolimus beginning on postoperative day 4. At 1 month posttransplant, patients are converted from tacrolimus to rapamycin. Using these regimens, we have experienced an acceptable incidence of acute rejection with overall good graft and patient survival.

Yet although survival rates after transplantation have improved markedly, as a result, the consequences of long-term immunosuppression have become apparent. Side effects of chronic calcineurin inhibitor use include renal insufficiency,

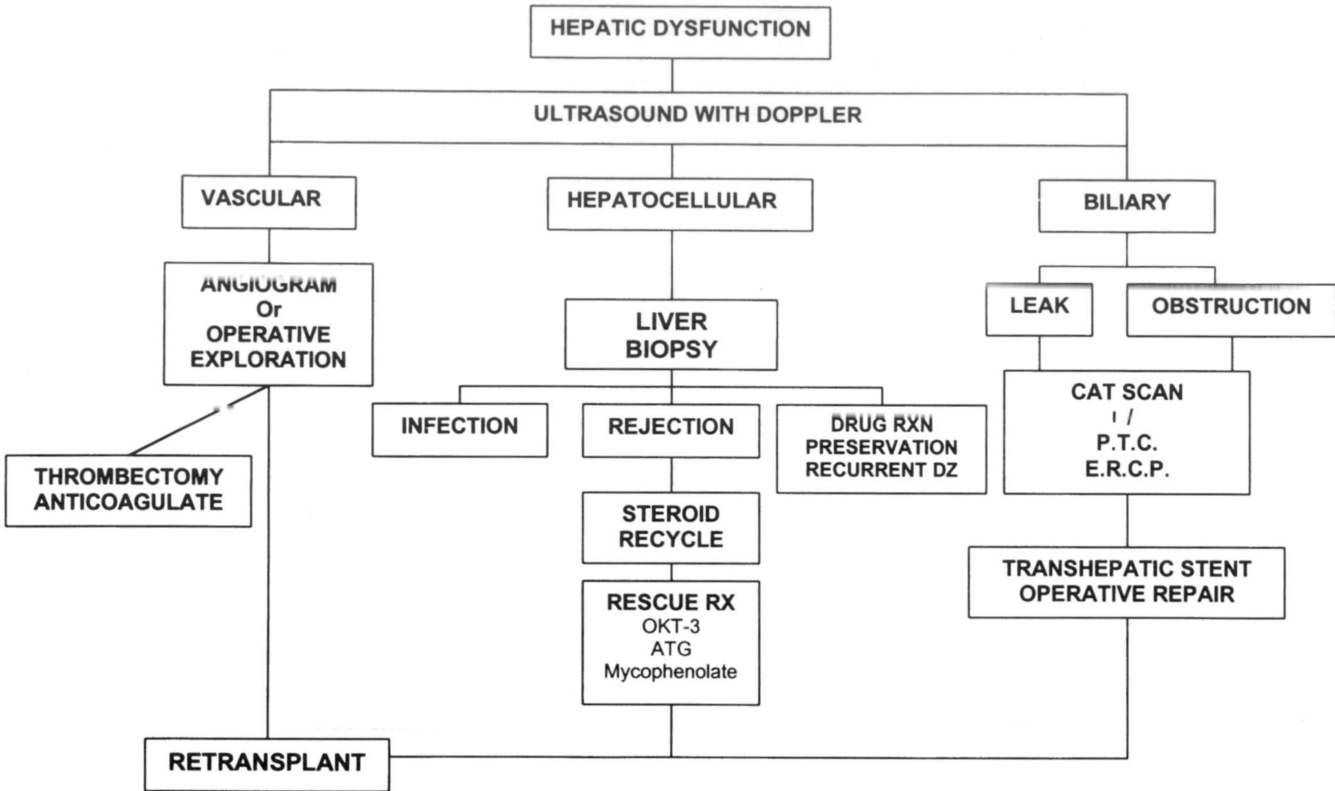

Figure 41.2. Schematic flow diagram for the management of postoperative hepatic allograft dysfunction.

diabetes mellitus, hypertension, and atherosclerosis and coronary artery disease. Strategies are being developed that eliminate the long-term use of calcineurin inhibitors [68,91]. Ultimately, immunologic tolerance, eliminating the need for long-term immunosuppression is the goal in solid organ transplantation [101].

Postoperative Complications

Most postoperative complications present with some combination of cholestasis, rising hepatocellular enzyme levels, and variable fever, lethargy, and anorexia. This nonspecific symptom complex requires specific diagnostic evaluation before beginning treatment (Figure 41.2). Therapy directed at the specific causes of allograft dysfunction is essential; empiric therapy of presumed complications is fraught with misdiagnosis, morbidity, and mortality.

Vascular Thrombosis

Vascular thrombosis is the most common cause of early postoperative allograft loss. Hepatic artery thrombosis occurs in children 3–4 times more frequently then in adult transplant series, occurring most often within the first 30 days following transplantation. The overall incidence of vascular thrombosis is similar in whole, SLTx, and LD transplants in experienced centers [76,77]. A variable clinical picture may be seen, including (1) fulminant allograft failure, (2) biliary disruption or obstruction, or (3) systemic sepsis. When identified early, successful thrombectomy and allograft salvage is possible when reconstruction is undertaken before allograft necrosis [102]. Acute HAT with allograft failure requires immediate transplantation. Biliary complications are particularly common following HAT. Percutaneous drainage and biliary stenting may control bile leakage and infection until retransplantation is undertaken.

Late postoperative thrombosis can be asymptomatic or present with slowly progressive bile duct stenosis. Rarely, allograft necrosis occurs. Arterial collaterals from the Roux-en-Y limb can provide a source of revascularization of the thrombosed allograft through hilar collaterals. These collateral channels develop during the first postoperative months, making late thrombosis an often silent clinical event. Conversely, disruption of this collateral supply during operative reconstruction of the central bile ducts in patients with HAT can precipitate hepatic ischemia and parenchymal necrosis. When HAT is asymptomatic, careful follow-up alone is indicated.

Portal vein thrombosis occurs in 5–10% of recipients. It is uncommon in whole organ allografts unless prior portosystemic shunting has altered the flow within the splanchnic vascular bed or severe portal vein stenosis in the recipient has impaired inflow into the allograft. In infant recipients with BA, preexisting portal vein hypoplasia often requires replacement of the entire portal vein to the superior mesenteric vein/splenic vein confluence with donor portal vein to avoid low flow related thrombosis. In LD allografts, size mismatch between donor and recipient and short venous pedicles may require grafting with donor gonadal or inferior mesenteric vein segments [103]. Preexisting portal vein thrombosis in the recipient can be overcome by thrombectomy or portal vein replacement or extra-anatomic venous bypass using donor portal–iliac vein. Early thrombosis following transplantation, detected by Doppler screening, requires immediate anastomotic revision and thrombectomy. Later thrombosis is detected by decreased platelet counts and increasing spleen size or gastrointestinal bleeding. Interventional radiographic stent placement or balloon dilation has been successful in patients with portal anastomotic stenosis, but is less successful when occlusion has occurred [103]. Portal venous shunting may be needed in selected patients with progressive portal hypertensive complications.

PRIMARY NONFUNCTION

Primary nonfunction (PNF) of the hepatic allograft implies the absence of metabolic and synthetic activity following transplantation. Complete nonfunction requires immediate retransplantation. Lesser degrees of allograft dysfunction occur more frequently but are usually reversible. The status of the donor liver contributes significantly to the potential for PNF. Ischemic injury secondary to anemia, hypotension, hypoxia, or direct tissue injury is often difficult to ascertain in the history of multiple trauma victims. Donor liver macrovesicular steatosis has also been recognized as a factor contributing to severe dysfunction or nonfunction in the donor liver. Livers with severe fatty infiltration (>40–50%) should be discarded, and donors with moderate involvement are used with some concern [104,105]. Microvascular steatosis is not related to PNF [106].

Biliary Complications

Biliary complications have been referred to as the Achilles heel of liver transplantation, occurring in approximately 10% of pediatric liver transplant recipients. Their spectrum and treatment is determined by the status of the hepatic artery and the type of allograft used. Although whole and surgically reduced allografts (RSLTx, SLTx, and LD) as a group have an equivalent risk of biliary complications, the spectrum of complications differs [77,107,108]. Late complications following any type of primary duct-to-duct biliary reconstruction include anastomotic stricture, biliary sludge formation, and recurrent cholangitis. Endoscopic dilation and internal stenting of anastomotic strictures or minimal biliary leaks has been successful in early postoperative cases. With recurrent stenosis or persistent postoperative leak, Roux-en-Y choledochojejunostomy is the preferred treatment. This is also the reconstruction of choice in small children and in all patients with BA. Recurrent cholangitis, a theoretical risk, suggests anastomotic or intrahepatic biliary stricture formation, or small bowel obstruction at or distal to the Roux-en-Y anastomosis.

The complexity of the biliary reconstruction is increased in both SLTx and LD allograft, which often require the anastomosis of two individual segmental bile ducts. The presence of multiple bile ducts in surgically reduced allografts has a documented increased risk for biliary leak following reimplantation. Parenchymal bile leaks and anastomotic leaks were slightly more common in SLTx, whereas anastomotic strictures are more common in LD [77]. These complications seem most related to graft type rather then patient illness (UNOS Status). This increased complexity and risk of complications is the known trade-off for increased organ availability. Dissection remote from the vasobiliary sheath in the donor liver has significantly decreased the incidence of these complications of surgical reduction by decreasing microvascular disruption.

Acute Cellular Rejection

Allograft biopsy is essential to establish the diagnosis of acute rejection before treatment. Acute rejection is characterized by the histologic triad of endothelialitis, portal triad lymphocyte infiltration with bile duct injury, and hepatic parenchymal cell damage [109]. The rapidity of the rejection process and its response to therapy dictates the intensity and duration of antirejection treatment.

Acute rejection occurs in approximately two thirds of patients following LTx using tacrolimus- or cyclosporine-based immunotherapy [110]. The primary treatment of rejection is a short course of high-dose steroids. Bolus doses administered over a several-day period with a rapid taper to baseline therapy is successful in 75–80% of cases [111]. When refractory or recurrent rejection occurs, antilymphocyte therapy using the monoclonal antibody, OKT-3, is successful in 90% of cases [112].

Retransplantation for refractory rejection is necessary in fulminant cases in which vascular thrombosis occurs and in cases unresponsive to treatment. In refractory cases, retransplantation should be undertaken before the use of multiple courses of corticosteroids or antilymphocyte agents to avoid the overwhelming risks of infection or lymphoproliferative disease. Fortunately, modern immunosuppressive treatment makes this an uncommon event.

Chronic Rejection

Chronic rejection occurs in 5–10% of transplanted patients and with equal frequency in children and adults. The primary clinical manifestation is a progressive rise in biliary ductal enzymes (alkaline phosphatase, γ-glutamyl transpeptidase) and progressive cholestasis. This course can be initially asymptomatic or follow an unsuccessful and often protracted treatment course for acute rejection. The syndrome can occur within weeks of transplantation or later in the clinical course.

Chronic rejection can follow one of the two clinical forms [113]. In the first, the injury is primarily to the biliary epithelium; the clinical course is characterized as "acute vanishing bile duct syndrome" in which severe ductopenia is seen in at least 20 portal tracts [114]. The eventual spontaneous resolution of nearly half of affected patients when they were administered tacrolimus therapy has led to the development of enhanced immunosuppression protocols for this patient subgroup. Retransplantation is occasionally necessary but rarely emergent. The second subtype is characterized by the early development of progressive ischemic injury to both bile ducts and hepatocytes leading to ductopenia and ischemic necrosis with fibrosis. The clinical course is relentlessly progressive and nearly always requires retransplantation. Recurrence of chronic rejection in the retransplanted allograft is a common event with both subtypes [113].

Infection

Infectious complications now represent the most common source of morbidity and mortality following transplantation. Bacterial infections occur in the immediate posttransplant period and are most often caused by gram-negative enteric organisms, *Enterococcus*, or *Staphylococcus* species. Sepsis originating at sites of invasive monitoring lines can be minimized by replacing or removing all intraoperative lines soon after transplantation. Antibacterial prophylactic antibiotics are discontinued as soon as possible to prevent the development of resistant organisms.

Fungal sepsis represents a significant potential problem in the early posttransplant period. Aggressive protocols for pretransplant prophylaxis are based on the concept that fungal infections originate from organisms colonizing the gastrointestinal tract of the recipient. Selective preoperative bowel decontamination was successful in eliminating pathogenic gram-negative bacteria from the gastrointestinal tract in 87% of adult patients; in all cases, *Candida* was eliminated [115]. However, these protocols have not been practical in pediatric patients because there is a long waiting time for pediatric organs, and the taste of the antibiotics used is poorly accepted. Fungal infection most often occurs in patients requiring multiple operative procedures and those who have had multiple antibiotic courses. All patients undergoing LTx receive antifungal prophylaxis with fluconazole at our center.

The majority of early and severe viral infections are caused by viruses of the Herpes family, including Epstein–Barr virus (EBV), cytomegalovirus (CMV), and herpes simplex virus (HSV) [116]. The likelihood of developing either CMV or EBV infection is influenced by the preoperative serologic status of the transplant donor and recipient [117,118]. Seronegative recipients receiving seropositive donor organs are at greatest risk. Use of various immune-based prophylactic protocols including intravenous immunoglobulin G (IgG) or hyperimmune anti-CMV IgG, coupled with acyclovir or ganciclovir, have all achieved success in decreasing the incidence of symptomatic CMV and EBV infection, although seroconversion in naïve recipients inevitably occurs [117,119].

The clinical diagnosis of CMV infection is suggested by the development of fever, leukopenia, maculopapular rash and hepatocellular abnormalities, respiratory insufficiency, or gastrointestinal hemorrhage. Hepatic biopsy or endoscopic biopsy of colonic or gastroduodenal sites allows early diagnosis with immunohistochemical recognition. Early treatment with hyperimmune anti-CMV IgG and ganciclovir is now successful in most cases.

Herpes simplex virus syndromes, similar to those seen in nontransplant patients, require treatment with acyclovir when diagnosed.

Epstein–Barr virus infection occurring in the perioperative period represents a significant risk to the pediatric transplant recipient. It can occur as a primary infection or following reactivation of a past primary infection. It has a variable presentation including a mononucleosis-like syndrome, hepatitis-simulating rejection, extranodal lymphoproliferative infiltration with bowel perforation, peritonsillar or lymph node enlargement, or encephalopathy. When serologic evidence of active infection exists, an acute reduction in immunosuppression is indicated. Surveillance screening of EBV blood viral load by quantitative polymerase chain reaction (PCR) appears to be the best predictor at present of risk. We recommend monthly EBV-DNA PCR counts to monitor increased genomic expression. Increasing viral load levels warrant more frequent monitoring every 1–2 weeks. In the EBV seronegative pretransplant patients, greater than 40 genomes/10^5 peripheral blood leukocytes (PBL), and greater than 200 genomes/10^5 PBL identify patients for reduction in primary immunosuppression by 25–100%. Institution of antiviral therapy with ganciclovir and CMV-IgG is also used in most cases, although only nonrandomized observational studies support their use. Treatment should be continued until symptoms such as lymphadenopathy have resolved and viral EBV-DNA PCR has returned to baseline [120,121]. It should, however, be cautioned that posttransplant lymphoproliferative disease (PTLD) can develop and progress without increases in EBV-PCR viral load [122]. The balance between viral load measured by quantitative PCR and specific cellular immune response, perhaps mediated by CD8 T cells specific to EBV, may explain this lack of specificity to viral load alone [123–125].

A potentially fatal abnormal proliferation of B lymphocytes, PTLD can occur in any situation in which immunosuppression is undertaken. The importance of PTLD in pediatric liver transplantation is a result of the intensity of the immunosuppression required, its lifetime duration, and the absence of prior exposure to EBV infection in 60–80% of pediatric recipients. PTLD is the most common tumor in children following transplantation, representing 52% of all tumors compared with 15% in adults. About 80% occur within the first 2 years following transplantation [123]. Multiple studies analyzing immunosuppressive therapy and the development of PTLD have shown a progressive increase in the incidence of PTLD with (1) an increase in total immunosuppression load, (2) EBV-naïve recipients, and (3) the intensity of active viral load [126,127]. No single immunosuppressive agent has been directly related to PTLD. The second pathogenic feature encouraging PTLD appears to be EBV infection. Treatment of PTLD is stratified according to the immunologic cell typing and clinical presentation [128]. Documented PTLD requires an immediate decrease or discontinuation of immunosuppression and institution of anti-EBV therapy. Patients with polyclonal B-cell proliferation frequently show regression with this treatment [120,121]. If tumor cells express B-cell marker CD 20 at histology, the anti-CD 20 monoclonal antibody rituximab has been used with increasing success. When given alone, its response rate was 46%, and it has a 54% relapse–progression rate. The combination of cyclophosphamide and prednisone yielded a response rate exceeding 80%, but 2-year event-free survival was only 58%. Recently, chemoimmunotherapy using cyclophosphamide, prednisone, and rituximab has shown response rate of 100%, with minimal toxicity. Further use of this combination will clarify its future role [129,130]. Patients with aggressive monoclonal malignancies have poor survival even with immunosuppressive reduction, acyclovir, and conventional chemotherapy or radiation therapy.

Other viruses leading to significant posttransplant infectious complications include adenovirus hepatitis, varicella, and enterovirus-induced gastroenteritis. Recurrent viral hepatitis is an uncommon problem in pediatric transplantation. Pneumocystis infection has been nearly eliminated by the prophylactic administration of sulfisoxazole: trimethoprim or aerosolized pentamidine.

REOPERATION

Early reoperation has become a common occurrence with the use of surgically reduced allografts of all types. Infants and small children with initial skin closure only require secondary laparotomy in 5–7 days for musculofascial closure. Long-term intravenous access can be established at this time for future blood access for immunosuppression monitoring and biochemistry surveillance. Complications related to biliary leak, hemorrhage, bowel injury secondary to multiple intraabdominal adhesions, and sepsis can be diagnosed and initially treated during this operative procedure. Clear discussion of these needs with the family before transplantation decreases the anxiety associated with reoperation and facilitates postoperative decision making.

Retransplantation

The majority of retransplantation (58%, SPLIT Registry) in pediatrics occurs because of acute allograft demise caused by HAT or primary nonfunction; chronic rejection and biliary complications are more uncommon causes. When retransplantation is promptly undertaken for acute organ failure, patient survival in our experience is 84%. However, when retransplantation was undertaken following prolonged immunosuppression for chronic allograft failure, often complicated by multiple organ system insufficiency, the survival was only 50%. The overall incidence of retransplantation is 14% in our series, and ranges from 8% to 29%. Although the technical complexity of pediatric LTx increases with surgically reduced allografts, the incidence of retransplantation is similar when primary whole organ allografts are compared with primary reduced-size allografts.

OUTCOME FOLLOWING TRANSPLANTATION

Although the potential complications following liver transplantation are frequent and occasionally severe, the overall results are rewarding. Overall patient and allograft survival reported to the SPLIT Transplant Registry, representing 1611 patients, is shown in Figure 41.3 [131]. Similar data for our center for 185 patients followed for over 4 years is also shown. Overall 1-year patient and graft survival has reached 88% and 82%, respectively, in the SPLIT registry and 92% and 84% in our own center. The highest risk of mortality occurs in all groups during the first year, with the majority of this risk within the first 3-month following transplantation. Long-term survival beyond 1 year is excellent (83% and 74% in SPLIT, 4 years) and is similar in all ages and for all diagnostic groups. Specific factors influencing early survival include age, diagnosis, severity of illness, and possibly allograft type.

Age

Survival has improved dramatically in infants and small children over recent years. Infants less than 1 year of age or less than 10 Kg have a reported survival of 65–88% overall, an improvement over previously reported rates of 50–60% [132]. Experienced programs and the SPLIT registry presently record patient survival (Pt) of 88% and graft survival (Gt) of 83% at 3 months. Although this is 5% below the best recipient group (1–5 years of age, 92%/88% [Pt/Gt]), it demonstrates the technical success currently achieved in this difficult subgroup. In our experience, 70% of all mortalities occurred within the first posttransplant year. One year survival in this under 1-year-old group at our center was 88%/81% (Pt/Gt), with the SPLIT registry being 85%/79% (Pt/Gt) [133]. Improved survival in these small recipients is consistent throughout all levels of medical urgency and results from both technical innovations in graft preparation and avoidance of life- and graft-threatening complications such as HAT and PNF. These young recipients are particularly at risk for EBV disease and consequences of over immunosuppression, making PTLD and sepsis contributors to poor survival.

Infants less than 3 months of age represent a particularly challenging and unique group. All present in accelerated or fulminant liver failure, requiring urgent access to transplantation. Because of the limitations in infant cadaveric donors, nearly all require surgically reduced or living-donor allografts. Long-term appropriate neurodevelopmental outcomes depend on rapid and successful transplantation. Although their challenges are substantial, our experience with seven patients in the past decade demonstrates an 86% lifetime survival, justifying efforts to continue to offer LTx in appropriate circumstances.

Diagnosis

Posttransplant survival is similar in patients with cholestatic and metabolic liver disease; patients with FHF have poorer

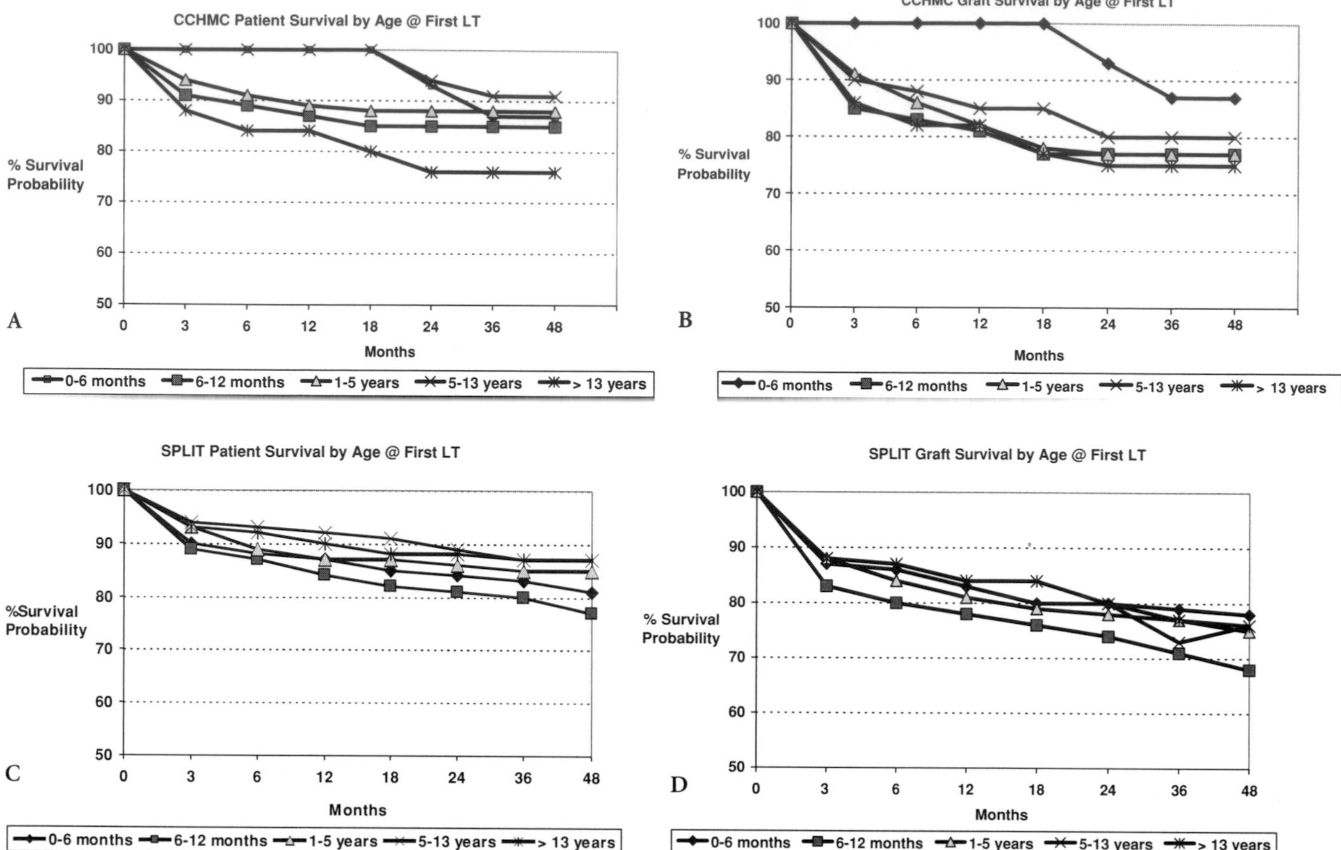

Figure 41.3. Liver transplant patient survival, SPLIT Registry and Cincinnati Children's Hospital Medical Center experience.

initial survival for the first 6 months but similar long-term survival to other recipients. Associated multiorgan failure and a limited donor acquisition time frame influence this result. Similar decreased survival trends are seen in patients with a PELD score greater than 20 and status 1 recipients or in those with significant deterioration in their PELD score before transplant [56].

Graft Type

Donor factors decreasing patient and graft survival include donor age less than 6 months or greater than 50 years. The influence of graft type – whole, reduced, split, or living donor – is less clear. In the U.S. Scientific Registry of Transplant Recipients database review (N = 6467), for patients aged younger

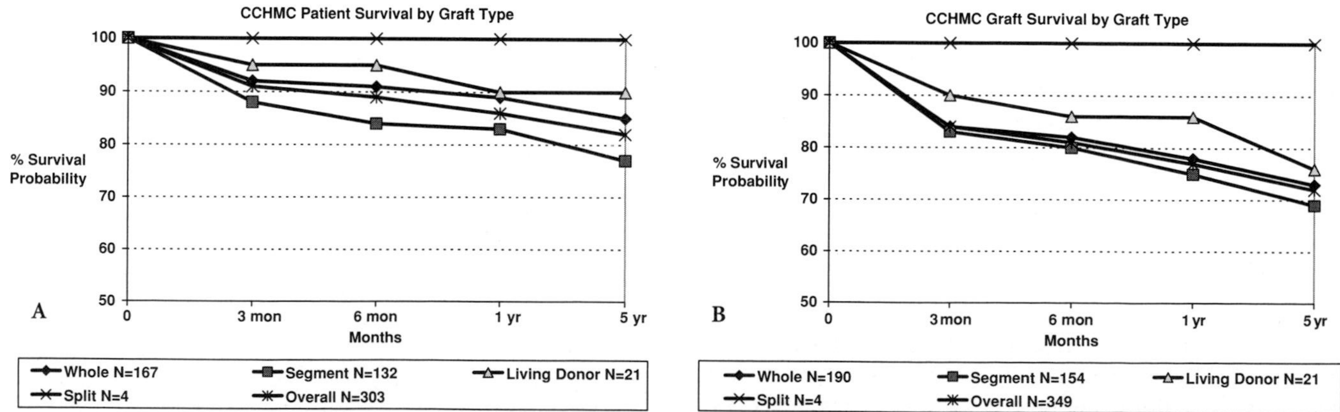

Figure 41.4. Liver transplant patient and graft survival subdivided by the anatomic subtype of the allograft, Cincinnati Children's Hospital experience, 1986–2005.

than 2 years, LD transplant allografts had a significantly lower risk of graft failure compared with whole and split (including reduced) allografts. This advantage was lost with the recipient age older than 2 years, whereas older recipients showed a higher risk of graft loss and subsequent mortality with LD transplantation [134]. In the combined SPLIT registry, whole organ recipients had better patient and graft survival than any surgically reduced liver, split liver, or LD recipients [135]. These results may be influenced by the diverse nature of the experience accumulated in these registries. When whole organ, living donor, and split-liver recipients were directly compared in experienced centers, there was no difference in patient or graft survival or biliary or vascular complications [77,136–138]. Transplantation of extremely small recipients (<5 Kg) with monosegments has been successful in 27 reported cases, with 85% survival at a mean of 21 months [139]. Further experience is needed with this newest extension of surgical reduction. These combined results suggest that best results will be achieved at centers with extensive experience with all age groups and allograft types, allowing transplantation to be tailored to the needs of the recipient and family, rather then identifying specific graft types for patient subgroups (Figure 41.4). When using any surgically reduced graft option, provision for transfer of adequate hepatic mass must be accounted for relative to the quality of the donor.

The most important factor determining survival is the severity of the patient's illness at the time of transplantation [140]. The good survival enjoyed by most LD transplant patients is positively influenced by the ability to plan transplantation before the development of life-threatening complications or severe nutritional depletion [141]. Patients presenting with FHF, PELD greater than 20, and growth failure greater than 2 SDs have overall survival significantly lower than other diagnostic groups. Prior surgical procedures, especially in multiply reoperated patients, influence the incidence of complications, especially bowel perforation, but do not adversely affect overall patient or graft survival. Reoperation for technical and bleeding complications or for delayed closure of the abdomen, is more common in infants and recipients of all complex technical grafts (split, reduced size, LD) and is essential to maintain optimal outcomes. Long-term survival is most influenced by the unintended consequences of immunosuppression – infection and PTLD [142]. The effect of secondary consequences of calcineurin inhibitors, such as renal insufficiency, hypertension, diabetes mellitus, and coronary artery disease have not been fully appreciated in this growing population but will be a challenge for future management.

SUMMARY

Liver transplantation has evolved from an experimental procedure used in disparate conditions to the state-of-the-art therapy for most patients with end-stage liver disease. The wide variety of surgical options developed to increase donor availability in pediatric transplantation have both improved survival and decreased waiting-list mortality. However, the ideal implementation of the higher potential risk options such as split-liver and living donor transplantation require their use in candidates with satisfactory stability. Early referral of the potential recipient allows timely evaluation of potential living donors or suitable time for acquisition of a cadaveric donor organ. Meticulous operative management and improved postoperative care have combined to offer excellent long-term survival and quality of life in pediatric recipients. The continued development of future options such as hepatocellular transplantation, gene therapy for hereditary diseases affecting the liver, and improved immunosuppressive management, should yield greater success for the future.

REFERENCES

1. Kasai M, Mochizuki I, Ohkohchi N, et al. Surgical limitation for biliary atresia: indication for liver transplantation. J Pediatr Surg 1989;24:851–4.
2. Ryckman F, Fisher R, Pedersen S, et al. Improved survival in biliary atresia patients in the present era of liver transplantation. J Pediatr Surg 1993;28:382–5; discussion 386.
3. Nio M, Ohi R, Hayashi Y, et al. Current status of 21 patients who have survived more than 20 years since undergoing surgery for biliary atresia. J Pediatr Surg 1996;31:381–4.
4. Altman RP, Lilly JR, Greenfeld J, et al. A multivariable risk factor analysis of the portoenterostomy (Kasai) procedure for biliary atresia: twenty-five years of experience from two centers. Ann Surg 1997;226:348–53; discussion 353–5.
5. Otte JB, de Ville de Goyet J, Reding R, et al. Sequential treatment of biliary atresia with Kasai portoenterostomy and liver transplantation: a review. Hepatology 1994;20:41S–8S.
6. Cardona J, Houssin D, Gauthier F, et al. Liver transplantation in children with Alagille syndrome — a study of twelve cases. Transplantation 1995;60:339–42.
7. Hoffenberg EJ, Narkewicz MR, Sondheimer JM, et al. Outcome of syndromic paucity of interlobular bile ducts (Alagille syndrome) with onset of cholestasis in infancy. J Pediatr 1995;127:220–4.
8. Tzakis AG, Reyes J, Tepetes K, et al. Liver transplantation for Alagille's syndrome. Arch Surg 1993;128:337–9.
9. Ryckman FC, Alonso MH. Transplantation for hepatic malignancy in children. In: Busuttil RW, Klintmalm G, eds. Transplantation of the Liver. Philadelphia: W.B. Sanders, 1996:216–26.
10. McBride KL, Miller G, Carter S, et al. Developmental outcomes with early orthotopic liver transplantation for infants with neonatal-onset urea cycle defects and a female patient with late-onset ornithine transcarbamylase deficiency. Pediatrics 2004;114:e523–6.
11. Morioka D, Kasahara M, Takada Y, et al. Current role of liver transplantation for the treatment of urea cycle disorders: a review of the worldwide English literature and 13 cases at Kyoto University. Liver Transpl 2005;11:1332–42.
12. Rodrigues F, Kallas M, Nash R, et al. Neonatal hemochromatosis – medical treatment vs. transplantation: the king's experience. Liver Transpl 2005;11:1417–24.
13. Leonis MA, Balistreri WF. Neonatal hemochromatosis: it's OK to say "NO" to antioxidant-chelator therapy. Liver Transpl 2005;11:1323–5.

14. Mito M, Kusano M, Kawaura Y. Hepatocyte transplantation in man. Transplant Proc 1992;24:3052–3.
15. Jan D, Poggi F, Laurent J, et al. Liver transplantation: new indications in metabolic disorders? Transplant Proc 1994;26:189–90.
16. Flynn DM, Mohan N, McKiernan P, et al. Progress in treatment and outcome for children with neonatal haemochromatosis. Arch Dis Child Fetal Neonatal Ed 2003;88:F124–7.
17. McClean P, Davison SM. Neonatal liver failure. Semin Neonatol 2003;8:393–401.
18. Sokol RJ, Treem WR. Mitochondria and childhood liver diseases. J Pediatr Gastroenterol Nutr 1999;28:4–16.
19. Filipovich AH. Life-threatening hemophagocytic syndromes: Current outcomes with hematopoietic stem cell transplantation. Pediatr Transplant 2005;9 Suppl 7:87–91.
20. Dhawan A, Cheeseman P, Mieli-Vergani G. Approaches to acute liver failure in children. Pediatr Transplant 2004;8:584–8.
21. Lee WS, McKiernan P, Kelly DA. Etiology, outcome and prognostic indicators of childhood fulminant hepatic failure in the United Kingdom. J Pediatr Gastroenterol Nutr 2005;40:575–81.
22. Baliga P, Alvarez S, Lindblad A, Zeng L. Posttransplant survival in pediatric fulminant hepatic failure: the SPLIT experience. Liver Transpl 2004;10:1364–71.
23. Santos RG, Alissa F, Reyes J, et al. Fulminant hepatic failure: Wilson's disease or autoimmune hepatitis? Implications for transplantation. Pediatr Transplant 2005;9:112–16.
24. Rivera-Penera T, Moreno J, Skaff C, et al. Delayed encephalopathy in fulminant hepatic failure in the pediatric population and the role of liver transplantation. J Pediatr Gastroenterol Nutr 1997;24:128–34.
25. Kondrup J, Almdal T, Vilstrup H, Tygstrup N. High volume plasma exchange in fulminant hepatic failure. Int J Artif Organs 1992;15:669–76.
26. Singer AL, Olthoff KM, Kim H, et al. Role of plasmapheresis in the management of acute hepatic failure in children. Ann Surg 2001;234:418–24.
27. Strom S, Fisher R. Hepatocyte transplantation: new possibilities for therapy. Gastroenterology 2003;124:568–71.
28. Lee SW, Wang X, Chowdhury NR, Roy-Chowdhury J. Hepatocyte transplantation: state of the art and strategies for overcoming existing hurdles. Ann Hepatol 2004;3:48–53.
29. van Hoek B, de Boer J, Boudjema K, et al. Auxiliary versus orthotopic liver transplantation for acute liver failure. EURALT Study Group. European Auxiliary Liver Transplant Registry. J Hepatol 1999;30:699–705.
30. Boudjema K, Bachellier P, Wolf P, et al. Auxiliary liver transplantation and bioartificial bridging procedures in treatment of acute liver failure. World J Surg 2002;26:264–74.
31. Azoulay D, Samuel D, Ichai P, et al. Auxiliary partial orthotopic versus standard orthotopic whole liver transplantation for acute liver failure: a reappraisal from a single center by a case-control study. Ann Surg 2001;234:723–31.
32. Girlanda R, Rela M, Williams R, et al. Long-term outcome of immunosuppression withdrawal after liver transplantation. Transplant Proc 2005;37:1708–9.
33. Girlanda R, Vilca-Melendez H, Srinivasan P, et al. Immunosuppression withdrawal after auxiliary liver transplantation for acute liver failure. Transplant Proc 2005;37:1720–1.
34. Pimpalwar AP, Sharif K, Ramani P, et al. Strategy for hepatoblastoma management: Transplant versus nontransplant surgery. J Pediatr Surg 2002;37:240–5.
35. Srinivasan P, McCall J, Pritchard J, et al. Orthotopic liver transplantation for unresectable hepatoblastoma. Transplantation 2002;74:652–5.
36. Molmenti EP, Nagata D, Roden J, et al. Liver transplantation for hepatoblastoma in the pediatric population. Transplant Proc 2001;33:1749.
37. Tiao GM, Bobey N, Allen S, et al. The current management of hepatoblastoma: a combination of chemotherapy, conventional resection, and liver transplantation. J Pediatr 2005;146:204–11.
38. Penn I. Hepatic transplantation for primary and metastatic cancers of the liver. Surgery 1991;110:726–34; discussion 734–5.
39. Tagge EP, Tagge DU, Reyes J, et al. Resection, including transplantation, for hepatoblastoma and hepatocellular carcinoma: impact on survival. J Pediatr Surg 1992;27:292–6; discussion 297.
40. Reyes JD, Carr B, Dvorchik I, et al. Liver transplantation and chemotherapy for hepatoblastoma and hepatocellular cancer in childhood and adolescence. J Pediatr 2000;136:795–804.
41. Superina R, Bilik R. Results of liver transplantation in children with unresectable liver tumors. J Pediatr Surg 1996;31:835–9.
42. Achilleos OA, Buist LJ, Kelly DA, et al. Unresectable hepatic tumors in childhood and the role of liver transplantation. J Pediatr Surg 1996;31:1563–7.
43. Al-Qabandi W, Jenkinson HC, Buckels JA, et al. Orthotopic liver transplantation for unresectable hepatoblastoma: a single center's experience. J Pediatr Surg 1999;34:1261–4.
44. Koneru B, Flye MW, Busuttil RW, et al. Liver transplantation for hepatoblastoma. the American experience. Ann Surg 1991;213:118–21.
45. Hertl M, Cosimi AB. Liver transplantation for malignancy. Oncologist 2005;10:269–81.
46. Genyk YS, Quiros JA, Jabbour N, et al. Liver transplantation in cystic fibrosis. Curr Opin Pulm Med 2001;7:441–7.
47. Debray D, Lykavieris P, Gauthier F, et al. Outcome of cystic fibrosis-associated liver cirrhosis: management of portal hypertension. J Hepatol 1999;31:77–83.
48. Gooding I, Dondos V, Gyi KM, et al. Variceal hemorrhage and cystic fibrosis: Outcomes and implications for liver transplantation. Liver Transpl 2005;11:1522–6.
49. Diwakar V, Pearson L, Beath S. Liver disease in children with cystic fibrosis. Paediatr Respir Rev 2001;2:340–9.
50. Fridell JA, Bond GJ, Mazariegos GV, et al. Liver transplantation in children with cystic fibrosis: a long-term longitudinal review of a single center's experience. J Pediatr Surg 2003;38:1152–6.
51. Molmenti EP, Squires RH, Nagata D, et al. Liver transplantation for cholestasis associated with cystic fibrosis in the pediatric population. Pediatr Transplant 2003;7:93–7.
52. Freeman RB, Jr., Edwards EB. Liver transplant waiting time does not correlate with waiting list mortality: implications for liver allocation policy. Liver Transpl 2000;6:543–52.
53. Organ Procurement and Transplantation Network – HRSA. Final rule with comment period. Fed Regist 1998;63:16296–338.
54. Freeman RB, Jr., Wiesner RH, Roberts JP, et al. Improving liver allocation: MELD and PELD. Am J Transplant 2004;4 Suppl 9:114–31.
55. McDiarmid SV, Merion RM, Dykstra DM, Harper AM. Selection of pediatric candidates under the PELD system. Liver Transpl 2004;10Suppl 2:S23–30.
56. Bourdeaux C, Tri TT, Gras J, et al. PELD score and posttransplant outcome in pediatric liver transplantation: a retrospective study of 100 recipients. Transplantation 2005;79:1273–6.

57. Shneider BL, Suchy FJ, Emre S. National and regional analysis of exceptions to the pediatric end-stage liver disease scoring system (2003–2004). Liver Transpl 2006;12:40–5.
58. Shneider BL, Neimark E, Frankenberg T, et al. Critical analysis of the pediatric end-stage liver disease scoring system: a single center experience. Liver Transpl 2005;11:788–95.
59. Urata K, Kawasaki S, Matsunami H, et al. Calculation of child and adult standard liver volume for liver transplantation. Hepatology 1995;21:1317–21.
60. Ozawa K. Living related donor liver transplantation. Basel: Karger, 1994:58–60.
61. Higashiyama H, Yamaguchi T, Mori K, et al. Graft size assessment by preoperative computed tomography in living related partial liver transplantation. Br J Surg 1993;80:489–92.
62. Dahm F, Georgiev P, Clavien PA. Small-for-size syndrome after partial liver transplantation: definition, mechanisms of disease and clinical implications. Am J Transplant 2005;5:2605–10.
63. Morimoto T, Ichimiya M, Tanaka A, et al. Guidelines for donor selection and an overview of the donor operation in living related liver transplantation. Transpl Int 1996;9:208–13.
64. Corno V, Torri E, Bertani A, et al. Early portal vein thrombosis after pediatric split liver transplantation with left lateral segment graft. Transplant Proc 2005;37:1141–2.
65. McDiarmid SV, Davies DB, Edwards EB. Improved graft survival of pediatric liver recipients transplanted with pediatric-aged liver donors. Transplantation 2000;70:1283–91.
66. Emre S, Soejima Y, Altaca G, et al. Safety and risk of using pediatric donor livers in adult liver transplantation. Liver Transpl 2001;7:41–7.
67. Yasutomi M, Harmsmen S, Innocenti F, et al. Outcome of the use of pediatric donor livers in adult recipients. Liver Transpl 2001;7:38–40.
68. Burdelski MM, Rogiers X. What lessons have we learned in pediatric liver transplantation? J Hepatol 2005;42:28–33.
69. Dazzi A, Lauro A, Di Benedetto F, et al. Living donor liver transplantation in adult patients: our experience. Transplant Proc 2005;37:2595–6.
70. Shackleton CR, Vierling JM, Nissen N, et al. Morbidity in live liver donors: standards-based adverse event reporting further refined. Arch Surg 2005;140:888–95; discussion 895–6.
71. Olthoff KM, Merion RM, Ghobrial RM, et al. Outcomes of 385 adult-to-adult living donor liver transplant recipients: a report from the A2ALL Consortium. Ann Surg 2005;242:314–23, discussion 323–5.
72. Wiederkehr JC, Pereira JC, Ekermann M, et al. Results of 132 hepatectomies for living donor liver transplantation: report of one death. Transplant Proc 2005;37:1079–80.
73. Vulchev A, Roberts JP, Stock PG. Ethical issues in split versus whole liver transplantation. Am J Transplant 2004;4:1737–40.
74. Broelsch CE, Emond JC, Whitington PF, et al. Application of reduced-size liver transplants as split grafts, auxiliary orthotopic grafts, and living related segmental transplants. Ann Surg 1990;212:368–75; discussion 375–7.
75. Ryckman FC, Flake AW, Fisher RA, et al. Segmental orthotopic hepatic transplantation as a means to improve patient survival and diminish waiting-list mortality. J Pediatr Surg 1991;26:422–7; discussion 427–8.
76. Renz JF, Yersiz H, Reichert PR, et al. Split-liver transplantation: a review. Am J Transplant 2003;3:1323–35.
77. Yersiz H, Renz JF, Farmer DG, et al. One hundred in situ split-liver transplantations: a single-center experience. Ann Surg 2003;238:496–505; discussion 506–7.
78. Lee TC, Barshes NR, Washburn WK, et al. Split-liver transplantation using the left lateral segment: a collaborative sharing experience between two distant centers. Am J Transplant 2005;5:1646–51.
79. Yan JQ, Becker T, Neipp M, et al. Surgical experience in splitting donor liver into left lateral and right extended lobes. World J Gastroenterol 2005;11:4220–4.
80. Gubernatis G, Pichlmayr R, Kemnitz J, Gratz K. Auxiliary partial orthotopic liver transplantation (APOLT) for fulminant hepatic failure: first successful case report. World J Surg 1991;15:660–5;discussion 665–6.
81. Uemoto S, Yabe S, Inomata Y, et al. Coexistence of a graft with the preserved native liver in auxiliary partial orthotopic liver transplantation from a living donor for ornithine transcarbamylase deficiency. Transplantation 1997;63:1026–8.
82. Terpstra OT, Metselaar HJ, Hesselink EJ, et al. Auxiliary partial liver transplantation for acute and chronic liver disease. Transplant Proc 1990;22:1564.
83. Kasahara M, Takada Y, Egawa H, et al. Auxiliary partial orthotopic living donor liver transplantation: Kyoto University experience. Am J Transplant 2005;5:558–65.
84. Ryckman FC, Fisher RA, Pedersen SH, Balistreri WF. Liver transplantation in children. Semin Pediatr Surg 1992;1:162–72.
85. Otte JB, de Ville de Goyet J, Sokal E, et al. Size reduction of the donor liver is a safe way to alleviate the shortage of size-matched organs in pediatric liver transplantation. Ann Surg 1990;211: 146–57.
86. Inomoto T, Nishizawa F, Sasaki H, et al. Experiences of 120 microsurgical reconstructions of hepatic artery in living related liver transplantation. Surgery 1996;119:20–6.
87. Guarrera JV, Sinha P, Lobritto SJ, et al. Microvascular hepatic artery anastomosis in pediatric segmental liver transplantation: microscope vs loupe. Transpl Int 2004;17:585–8.
88. Tannuri U, Mello ES, Carnevale FC, et al. Hepatic venous reconstruction in pediatric living-related donor liver transplantation – experience of a single center. Pediatr Transplant 2005;9: 293–8.
89. Cacciarelli TV, Reyes J, Jaffe R, et al. Primary tacrolimus (FK506) therapy and the long term risk of post-transplant lymphoproliferative disease in pediatric liver transplant recipients. Pediatr Transplant 2001;5:359–64.
90. Kelly D, Jara P, Rodeck B, et al. Tacrolimus and steroids versus ciclosporin microemulsion, steroids, and azathioprine in children undergoing liver transplantation: randomised European multicentre trial. Lancet 2004;364:1054–61.
91. Reding R, Webber SA, Fine R. Getting rid of steroids in pediatric solid-organ transplantation? Pediatr Transplant 2004;8:526–30.
92. Diem HV, Sokal EM, Janssen M, et al. Steroid withdrawal after pediatric liver transplantation: a long-term follow-up study in 109 recipients. Transplantation 2003;75:1664–70.
93. Boillot O, Mayer DA, Boudjema K, et al. Corticosteroid-free immunosuppression with tacrolimus following induction with daclizumab: a large randomized clinical study. Liver Transpl 2005;11:61–7.
94. Wiesner RH, Shorr JS, Steffen BJ, et al. Mycophenolate mofetil combination therapy improves long-term outcomes after liver

transplantation in patients with and without hepatitis C. Liver Transpl 2005;11:750–9.

95. Chardot C, Nicoluzzi JE, Janssen M, et al. Use of mycophenolate mofetil as rescue therapy after pediatric liver transplantation. Transplantation 2001;71:224–9.
96. Tryphonopoulos P, Madariaga JR, Kato T, et al. The impact of Campath 1H induction in adult liver allotransplantation. Transplant Proc 2005;37:1203–4.
97. Ganschow R, Lyons M, Grabhorn E, et al. Experience with basiliximab in pediatric liver graft recipients. Transplant Proc 2001;33:3606–7.
98. Ganschow R, Grabhorn E, Schulz A, et al. Long-term results of basiliximab induction immunosuppression in pediatric liver transplant recipients. Pediatr Transplant 2005;9:741–5.
99. Trotter JF. Sirolimus in liver transplantation. Transplant Proc 2003;35 Suppl 3:193S–200S.
100. Sindhi R, Seward J, Mazariegos G, et al. Replacing calcineurin inhibitors with mTOR inhibitors in children. Pediatr Transplant 2005;9:391–7.
101. Starzl TE, Murase N, Abu-Elmagd K, et al. Tolerogenic immunosuppression for organ transplantation. Lancet 2003;361:1502–10.
102. Langnas AN, Marujo W, Stratta RJ, et al. Hepatic allograft rescue following arterial thrombosis. Role of urgent revascularization. Transplantation 1991;51:86–90.
103. Ueda M, Egawa H, Ogawa K, et al. Portal vein complications in the long-term course after pediatric living donor liver transplantation. Transplant Proc 2005;37:1138–40.
104. Todo S, Demetris AJ, Makowka L, et al. Primary nonfunction of hepatic allografts with preexisting fatty infiltration. Transplantation 1989;47:903–5.
105. D'Alessandro AM, Kalayoglu M, Sollinger HW, et al. The predictive value of donor liver biopsies on the development of primary nonfunction after orthotopic liver transplantation. Transplant Proc 1991;23:1536–7.
106. Fishbein TM, Fiel MI, Emre S, et al. Use of livers with microvesicular fat safely expands the donor pool. Transplantation 1997; 64:248–51.
107. Heffron TG, Emond JC, Whitington PF, et al. Biliary complications in pediatric liver transplantation. A comparison of reduced-size and whole grafts. Transplantation 1992;53:391–5.
108. Peclet MH, Ryckman FC, Pedersen SH, et al. The spectrum of bile duct complications in pediatric liver transplantation. J Pediatr Surg 1994;29:214–19; discussion 219–20.
109. Snover DC, Sibley RK, Freese DK, et al. Orthotopic liver transplantation: a pathological study of 63 serial liver biopsies from 17 patients with special reference to the diagnostic features and natural history of rejection. Hepatology 1984;4:1212–22.
110. Mor E, Solomon H, Gibbs JF, et al. Acute cellular rejection following liver transplantation: clinical pathologic features and effect on outcome. Semin Liver Dis 1992;12:28–40.
111. Adams DH, Neuberger JM. Treatment of acute rejection. Semin Liver Dis 1992;12:80–8.
112. Ryckman FC, Schroeder T, Pedersen S. Use of monoclonal antibody immunosuppressive therapy in pediatric renal and liver transplantation. Clin Transplant 1991;5:186–90.
113. Freese DK, Snover DC, Sharp HL, et al. Chronic rejection after liver transplantation: a study of clinical, histopathological and immunological features. Hepatology 1991;13:882–91.
114. Ludwig J, Wiesner RH, Batts KP, et al. The acute vanishing bile duct syndrome (acute irreversible rejection) after orthotopic liver transplantation. Hepatology 1987;7:476–83.
115. Wiesner RH, Hermans PE, Rakela J, et al. Selective bowel decontamination to decrease gram-negative aerobic bacterial and Candida colonization and prevent infection after orthotopic liver transplantation. Transplantation 1988;45:570–4.
116. Singh N, Carrigan DR, Gayowski T, Marino IR. Human herpesvirus-6 infection in liver transplant recipients: documentation of pathogenicity. Transplantation 1997;64:674–8.
117. Patel R, Snydman DR, Rubin RH, et al. Cytomegalovirus prophylaxis in solid organ transplant recipients. Transplantation 1996;61:1279–89
118. Fox AS, Tolpin MD, Baker AL, et al. Seropositivity in liver transplant recipients as a predictor of cytomegalovirus disease. J Infect Dis 1988;157:383–5.
119. Darenkov IA, Marcarelli MA, Basadonna GP, et al. Reduced incidence of Epstein-Barr virus-associated posttransplant lymphoproliferative disorder using preemptive antiviral therapy. Transplantation 1997;64:848–52.
120. Holmes RD, Orban-Eller K, Karrer FR, et al. Response of elevated Epstein–Barr virus DNA levels to therapeutic changes in pediatric liver transplant patients: 56-month follow up and outcome. Transplantation 2002;74:367–72.
121. Holmes RD, Sokol RJ. Epstein-Barr virus and post-transplant lymphoproliferative disease. Pediatr Transplant 2002;6:456–64.
122. Axelrod DA, Holmes R, Thomas SE, Magee JC. Limitations of EBV-PCR monitoring to detect EBV associated post-transplant lymphoproliferative disorder. Pediatr Transplant 2003;7:223–7.
123. Smets F, Sokal EM. Lymphoproliferation in children after liver transplantation. J Pediatr Gastroenterol Nutr 2002;34:499–505.
124. Smets F, Sokal EM. Epstein-Barr virus-related lymphoproliferation in children after liver transplant: role of immunity, diagnosis, and management. Pediatr Transplant 2002;6:280–7.
125. Sokal EM, Antunes H, Beguin C, et al. Early signs and risk factors for the increased incidence of Epstein–Barr virus-related posttransplant lymphoproliferative diseases in pediatric liver transplant recipients treated with tacrolimus. Transplantation 1997;64:1438–42.
126. Guthery SL, Heubi JE, Bucuvalas JC, et al. Determination of risk factors for Epstein-Barr virus-associated posttransplant lymphoproliferative disorder in pediatric liver transplant recipients using objective case ascertainment. Transplantation 2003;75:987–93.
127. Penn I. Post-transplant malignancy: the role of immunosuppression. Drug Saf 2000;23:101–13.
128. Hanto DW, Frizzera G, Gajl-Peczalska KJ, Simmons RL. Epstein–Barr virus, immunodeficiency, and B cell lymphoproliferation. Transplantation 1985;39:461–72.
129. Orjuela M, Gross TG, Cheung YK, et al. A pilot study of chemoimmunotherapy (cyclophosphamide, prednisone, and rituximab) in patients with post-transplant lymphoproliferative disorder following solid organ transplantation. Clin Cancer Res 2003;9:3945S–3952S.
130. Gross TG. Low-dose chemotherapy for children with post-transplant lymphoproliferative disease. Recent Results Cancer Res 2002;159:96–103.
131. Studies of Pediatric Liver Transplantation (SPLIT): Annual Report. 2004:6.1–6.27.
132. Sokal EM, Veyckemans F, de Ville de Goyet J, et al. Liver transplantation in children less than 1 year of age. J Pediatr 1990; 117:205–10.
133. Tiao GM, Alonso M, Bezerra J, et al. Liver transplantation in children younger than 1 year – the Cincinnati experience. J Pediatr Surg 2005;40:268–73; discussion 273.

134. Roberts JP, Hulbert-Shearon TE, Merion RM, et al. Influence of graft type on outcomes after pediatric liver transplantation. Am J Transplant 2004;4:373–7.
135. Lozanov J, Millis JM, Anand R, Group TSR. Surgical Outcomes in Primary Pediatric Liver Transplantation: SPLIT Database Report. Abstract 1453. Annual meeting of American Society of Transplantation, Seattle, Washington, 2005.
136. Deshpande RR, Bowles MJ, Vilca-Melendez H, et al. Results of split liver transplantation in children. Ann Surg 2002;236:248–53.
137. Kim JS, Broering DC, Tustas RY, et al. Split liver transplantation: past, present and future. Pediatr Transplant 2004;8:644–8.
138. Busuttil RW, Farmer DG, Yersiz H, et al. Analysis of long-term outcomes of 3200 Liver transplantations over two decades: a single-center experience. Ann Surg 2005;241:905–18.
139. Enne M, Pacheco-Moreira L, Balbi E, et al. Liver transplantation with monosegments. Technical aspects and outcome: A meta-analysis. Liver Transpl 2005;11:564–9.
140. Bilik R, Greig P, Langer B, Superina RA. Survival after reduced-size liver transplantation is dependent on pretransplant status. J Pediatr Surg 1993;28:1307–11.
141. Austin MT, Feurer ID, Chari RS, et al. Survival after pediatric liver transplantation: why does living donation offer an advantage? Arch Surg 2005;140:465–70; discussion 470–1.
142. Ryckman FC, Alonso MH, Bucuvalas JC, Balistreri WF. Long-term survival after liver transplantation. J Pediatr Surg 1999;34:845–9;discussion 849–50.

INDEX

Page numbers followed by "*f*" indicate figures, and those followed by "*t*" indicate tables.